U0358846

《活体形态学（*VIVOMORPHOLOGY*）》的姐妹篇

当代医学影像误诊学

CONTEMPORARY MEDICAL IMAGING MISDIAGNOSIS

第四卷

VOLUME Ⅳ

总主编　巫北海

天津出版传媒集团

天津科学技术出版社

编者名单

总 主 编 巫北海 主任医师、教授、博士生导师（原第三军医大学第一附属医院，现陆军军医大学第一附属医院）

副总主编 刘 筠 主任医师、教授、博士生导师（天津南开大学人民医院）

刘昌华 副主任医师（厦门大学成功医院）

颜志平 主任医师、教授、硕士生导师（厦门弘爱医院）

吕维富 主任医师、教授、博士生导师（中国科学技术大学附属第一医院 / 安徽省立医院）

黄学全 主任医师、教授、博士生导师（陆军军医大学第一附属医院）

陈 伟 副主任医师、副教授、博士生导师（陆军军医大学第一附属医院）

韩 丹 主任医师、教授、博士生导师（昆明医科大学第一附属医院）

秦 伟 主任医师、教授、硕士生导师（重庆北部宽仁医院）

秦将均 主任医师、教授、硕士生导师（海南三亚中心医院 / 海南省第三人民医院）

邝 菲 副主任医师、副教授（厦门大学第一医院）

第一卷（颅脑与脊髓卷）主编 巫北海 颜志平 张伟国 黎海涛 陆 明 张晓宏

第二卷（面颈及多系统多部位疾病卷）主编 巫北海 刘 筠 韩 丹 秦 伟 唐 震

第三卷（胸心卷）主编 巫北海 吕维富 俞安乐 牟 玮 邱明国

第四卷（腹盆上卷）主编 巫北海 刘昌华 黄学全 秦将均 王 毅

第五卷（腹盆下卷）主编 巫北海 蔡 萍 邝 菲 周代全 薛跃辉 傅 绢

第六卷（肌骨及脊柱卷）主编 巫北海 陈 伟 汪庆华 刘士辰 胡荣惠

编写人员（按姓氏笔画为序）

马 奎 王 毅 邓 学 刘 筠 刘士辰 刘昌华 邝 菲 冯 浩 吕维富
牟 玮 伍宝忠 张伟国 张晓宏 陈 伟 陈丙丁 陈思敏 陈春梅 陈海燕
汪庆华 陆 明 杨利根 巫北海 巫登锦 肖贵玉 邱明国 周代全 林怀雄
林建坤 俞安乐 郑妙琼 秦 伟 秦将均 胡 雄 胡荣惠 韩 丹 唐 震
谢 斌 曾英琅 常 诚 黄学全 蔡 萍 郭春生 康绍磊 颜志平 傅 绢
黎海涛 薛跃辉

序

在62年的医疗实践中，个人深深体会到一个问题，作为临床影像诊断的医务工作者，日常工作中，为成千上万的患者诊断正确是理所应当的，没有人在意这些工作，但是如果出现误诊或漏诊，则将引起不小的震动，小则上级领导批评，大则引发医疗纠纷、医疗事故，甚至导致不良的社会影响，对于患者、医务工作者个人、医疗单位等都可能造成不必要的损失。

1996年，拙著《影像诊断中的误诊》问世后，许多读者来信称该书对于临床工作帮助甚大，但唯一的缺点是该书主要是文字，没有图像可供阅读，希望再版时增加内容和配以图像，以对临床工作更有益处。

误诊学是医学诊断学的一部分，它是一门专门研究诊断错误的学科，其内容涵盖甚广，既包括医学，又包括医学以外的许多学科。

作为《活体形态学（Vitomorphology）》的姐妹篇，《当代医学影像误诊学（Contemporary Medical Image Misdiagnosis）》也分为六卷：颅脑与脊髓卷、面颈与多系统多部位疾病卷、胸心卷、腹盆上卷、腹盆下卷、肌骨与脊柱卷。

《当代医学影像误诊学》是医学诊断学中专门研究影像诊断错误的专著，它既包括医学影像诊断学，又包括医学影像诊断学以外的许多学科；它主要讨论医学影像诊断中的误诊和漏诊，既有影像诊断学的丰富内容，又有许多相应临床各科的资料。

众所周知，作为影像诊断医生的我们，在多年临床工作中，诊断正确者成千上万，一点都记不住，可是，对误诊的病人却会牢牢记住一辈子，因为误诊给人的印象太深了，甚至于可以这样说，误诊给人的打击太重了。

误诊和漏诊在临床上的重要性是我们编写《当代医学影像误诊学》的动力，几十年来，我们一边工作，一边学习，一边收集资料，一边整理总结，一边深入研究、分析和编写，现在终于完成了这项艰巨的任务，呈送给同仁和读者们，由于我们才疏学浅，手边资料十分有限，难免存在许多错误和瑕疵，敬请同仁和读者们不吝批评和指正。

我们深知，医学影像的误诊学确实是一门很深奥的学问，涉及面十分广泛，而且相当有深度，从编写过程中我们学习到许多以往从未接触到的知识，真是长见识不少，这对提高我们的工作水平和质量十分有益。

本书编写时间跨度较大，长达三十余年，收集文献较多，由于出版规定参考文献篇幅有限，在此只能将5年内的外文文献和8年内的中华系列杂志文献列出,参考的绝大多数文献都无法一一列出,敬请各位作者鉴谅,在此谨致谢意。

由于作者们才疏学浅,对医学影像学的学习和研究甚感力不从心,对诊断思维的深入研究更是欠缺,加之收集资料范围有限,今冒昧将点滴学习和研究的经验和体会整理成册,与同仁们进行学术交流,因此,本书多有不当之处,衷心希望各地同仁和读者不吝批评指正。

致谢:本书编写历时甚长,编写过程中得到了全国各地多位老师的大力支持和热情关怀,学生有幸登门拜见多位老师,老师们不厌其烦地介绍他们亲身经历的误诊病例,并对误诊的教训和经验进行归纳和总结,昔日谆谆教诲,至今仍历历在目,在此,请允许学生向众多老师致谢:荣独山、汪绍训、朱大成、邹仲、左立梁、孔庆德、郭庆林、江海寿、杨竞飞、王其源、刘国相、周成刚、陈官玺、刘承志、魏大藻、刘玉清、吴恩惠、王云钊、曹来宾、兰宝森、蔡锡类、贾雨辰、郭俊渊、陈种、和毓天。

在本书的编写过程中,得到了厦门大学成功医院领导及医学影像科同仁们的大力支持,在此一并致谢。

巫北海

谨识于厦门

2020年9月

Preface

In the past 62 years of medical practice, I, as a medical professional dealing with radiological diagnostics, recognize that making correct diagnoses for thousands of patients in our routine work has been taken for granted. Nobody cares about our daily activities. However, if we make a misdiagnosis or overlook a diagnosis, an unneglectable shock triggered by our mistake would be initiated around our working environment. If the consequence of misdiagnosis is not serious, we may just incur fierce criticism from our administration and related parties. If serious, we will be involved in disputes of malpractice and law sues and the mistakes we made even may directly lead to medical accidents. Furthermore, the impacts given rise from our mistakes on our society would be negative, causing unnecessary losses to the patients, medical personnel and hospitals.

After my book Misdiagnosis in Imaging Diagnostics was published in 1996, I successively received positive feedbacks from the readers. They stated that the book was helpful for their clinical work. However, one obvious drawback in that book was that it only had character descriptions but had no medical images as illustrations. The readers hope more character contents and medical images could be added in the upcoming edition. It is expected that supplemented contents and medical images will be more beneficial to their clinical practice.

Misdiagnosis is a part of medical diagnostics. It is a discipline that specializes in studying diagnostic mistakes, covering a wide range of topics in medicine as well as in many other non-medical fields.

As a sibling of serial works Vitomorphology, Contemporary Medical Image Misdiagnosis also composes of six volumes: Cranial and Spinal Cord, Face, Neck and Diseases in Multi-systems and Multi-locations, Heart and Thorax, Abdomen and Pelvis I, Abdomen and Pelvis II, and Musculoskeletal and Spine.

Contemporary Medical Image Misdiagnosis is a series of works that specialize in studying mistakes of imaging diagnosis in medical diagnostics. This series of books cover but are not limited to medical-imaging diagnostics, instead, the books also cover extensive information in other specialties of clinical medicine. This series of books discussed misdiagnosis and overlook of diagnosis in imaging diagnosis, containing affluent contents in diagnostic radiology as well as in a variety of other relevant clinical specialties.

It is known that we, radiologists, can't remember correct diagnoses we had made for thousands of cases in the past years. However, if we make mistakes in diagnosis, we will keep the misdiagnosed cases in mind for life because misdiagnosis gives us impression too deeply to be forgotten. In another word, we will be severely injured by the misdiagnosis.

That misdiagnosis and overlook are clinically important motivates us to work on this series of books Contemporary Medical Image Misdiagnosis. During the past decades, while we were working and studying, we collected clinical data, and organized and summarized those raw materials. In the meantime, we did researches and analyses on the data we accumulated and then started writing. After continuously hard working for decades, we eventually completed this mission which seemed to be impossible at the very beginning and we are pleasant to present the works to our fellow colleagues and readers today. Since we can't be experts in all fields the works involved in, and the data and references in our hands can't cover everywhere in details, our works, more or less, are unable to be free of drawbacks and mistakes. Additionally, our ability in studying medical imaging may not always help reach our goals and furthermore，we might be short of further study on diagnostic logics. Regardless of those excuses，we still daringly accomplished this series of books with our experiences accumulated in our long term of studies and researches in attempt to deal with academic exchanges with our fellow colleagues and readers. Therefore，we sincerely welcome that our fellow colleagues and readers feel free to express their critics and advices on this series of books.

We deeply recognize that misdiagnosis in the field of radiological diagnostics is indeed a discipline of sciences. It involves a lot of fields and its contents are extensive in scope and depth. Meanwhile，we were also filled of knowledge which was unknown to us before. We really learnt a lot during working on the books，which is beneficial to improve the quality of our daily clinical work.

The timeframe we spent on this series of books spanned more than 30 years. During the period，huge amount of references were searched and collected. Due to the limited space of reference listing，only abroad literature published five years ago and the Chinese national journals of medicine published eight years ago were listed in this series of books. We would specifically pay our apology to the authors whose publications had been referenced but had no chances to be listed in this series of books，meanwhile，we would like to express our sincere respect and gratitude to them.

Acknowledgement：It spanned long time for us to edit this series of books，during which we have been blessed to receive the generous supports and warmhearted cares from many well-known senior academic experts in radiology nationwide. I was honored to have chances to meet some of them. They had done a lot of work in abstracting and summarizing the lessons they learnt from their past clinical practice and always patiently shared their own experiencing misdiagnoses with me. With their mentoring opinions and advices being so deeply impressed in my mind，I feel that our conversations，which have past years and even decades，just took place minutes ago. On behalf of my fellow authors in this series of books，I would like to cordially express our gratitude to them whose names are listed as follows：Rong Dushan(荣独山)，Wang Shaoxun(汪绍训)，Zhu Dacheng(朱大成)，Zou Zhong(邹仲)，Zuo Liliang(左立梁)，Kong Qingde(孔庆德)，Guo Qinglin(郭庆林)，Jiang Haishou(江海寿)，Yang Jingfei(杨竞飞)，Wang Qiyuan(王其源)，Liu Guoxiang(刘国相)，Zhou Chenggang(周成刚)，Chen Guanxi(陈官玺)，Liu Chengzhi(刘承志)，Wei Dazao(魏大藻)，Liu Yuqing(刘玉清)，Wu Enhui(吴恩惠)，Wang Yunzhao(王云钊)，Cao Laibin(曹来宾)，Lan Baosen(兰宝森)，Cai Xinei(蔡锡类)，Jia Yuchen(贾雨辰)，Guo Junyuan(郭俊渊)，Chen Zhong(陈种)，and Ho Yutian(和毓天).

In the process of writing this book, I am grateful for the strong support of the leaders of Xiamen University Hospital and colleagues in the medical imaging department.

Beihai Wu，Professor
At Xiamen，Fujian，China
In September 2020

前　言

影像诊断学误诊对临床学科的影响

我们不敢奢谈医学的误诊问题，因身处医学影像诊断学，只是临床医学的一部分，在此谨讨论分析影像诊断中的误诊和漏诊问题，至于涉及影像诊断的临床科室和临床病理学的有关误诊的问题，我们也进行了一些研究，在本书有关章节向读者逐一介绍，也许对有关科室的临床工作有所帮助。

影像诊断与临床

关于影像诊断学与临床医学的关系问题讨论甚多。我们认为，说影像诊断引导临床诊断不合适，将医学影像科室说成是辅助科室，不仅不符合实际情况，而且早已过时。影像诊断学对于临床医学不是指导，也不是领导、辅助、辅导，是侦察、是检查、是寻找、是探索症状与体征的根源，是分辨体内正常与异常，区别生理情况与病理表现，辨别病灶的部位、大小、范围及性质等。

我们大力提倡影像诊断学工作者与临床各科及病理学工作者合作进行科学研究，一起筹划、申报、完成同一课题，一起分析研究、撰写文章，使影像诊断与临床及病理结合更为紧密，更好地减少和避免出现误诊和漏诊。

关于临床医师的职责

临床医师申请影像诊断时，申请单上寥寥数语，未能提供病人主要的症状及体征。这种简单、潦草一是对病人不负责，二是浪费影像诊断的资源。影像诊断医师毫无重点地读片，浪费观察、分析、研究图像的时间，不但导致诊断质量明显降低，以致造成误诊和漏诊，还会耽误诊断的时间，这在临床上屡见不鲜。

我们认为，临床各科的医师应正确认识自己应尽的职责，应认真研究病人的症状和体征，倾听病人的主诉，重点扼要地填写影像诊断申请单，让不在门诊坐诊和病房查房的影像诊断医师基本了解病人的情况，重点地观察、分析、研究可能产生症状和体征的部位，这对减少和避免误诊和漏诊十分重要。

诊断的个性化

临床和中医诊断的个性化，与病人直接接触，深入了解病情、病史、症状和体征，再做出诊断，进行个性化的治疗，可能会比我们不接触病人即做出诊断的误诊少许多！如何在影像诊断中应用这类个性化原则?真值得研究!在此,我们不得不联想到临床科室医生的职责,如果临床医生能够真正做到尽职尽责,尽量多给予病人的信息资料,对于减少和避免影像诊断误诊将起到十分重要的作用。

不断更新知识,防止误诊与漏诊

努力学习新的知识是避免和减少误诊的最重要、最行之有效的方法和途径。不断更新知识,扩大知识面,广开思路,对防止误诊与漏诊十分有用!本书在有关章节对近期出现的影像组学、精准医学、人工智能等,以及近年影像诊断的新理论、新技术、新仪器等作了简要介绍,力图帮助读者更新有关方面的认识和了解。

新式仪器或新技术与活体形态学研究

对新式仪器或新技术钻研不够,过于迷信、盲从,导致误诊。例如 PET 等影像技术手段,对于“异常”的发现过于敏感或敏感性过高,常造成过度诊断。

由于新的影像诊断技术问世不久,人们积累的临床经验相对不足,或对正常与异常间差别掌握较差,对正常标准研究少,了解肤浅,认识不清,直接影响诊断的能力和诊断的水平。如何区分正常与异常?这就要求活体形态学进一步深入研究,这也是我们当年编写《活体形态学》的初衷。

影像诊断各项诊断技术的通力协作是减少误诊的基础

目前,在一所普通的综合医院,医学影像科一个科室的固定资产占全院固定资产总额的30%左右,是高科技,也是高成本。各项影像诊断手段虽然都是独自工作,各项影像诊断手段和技术理应通力协作,尊重兄弟科室,扬长避短,发挥各自优势,合力最大,经常讨论、协商、会诊,形成比较一致的诊断意见,对提高影像诊断水平十分重要,这对院内院外都是这样。然而,纵观近三十年临床影像诊断工作,一些医院的临床经验证明,影像诊断各项手段之间不协作是导致影像诊断误诊的一大原因。

影像诊断与病理

目前,免疫组织化学检测是病理学诊断金标准,它有无误诊的可能?标本的采集,观测的准确性,选择检测的项目是否合适,如何结合临床,如何结合影像等问题都值得我们深入学习和分析研究。

为了确保影像诊断的正确性,本书中所介绍的病例都是经过手术病理证实的,如无病理证实者都属于淘汰之列。我们认为,对于影像诊断的研究,应该有病理的证实,千万不要用影像证实影像,对于部分杂志上发表的一些文章中的病例要辨证地看,有的是经过病理证实的,有的却不一定经过病理证实,只是滥竽充数而已。

关于肿瘤分类的一些思考

四肢短骨的软骨瘤,根据组织学检查可能有恶性征象,但临床上此种肿瘤很少有恶性发展者;反之,扁骨或长骨的软骨瘤,从显微镜下的组织表现为良性,而发展为恶性者却甚多。

还有长骨的骨软骨瘤或软骨瘤,临床表现确已恶性变,且有转移,而显微镜下的组织学改变仍不明显。因此,对骨软骨瘤或软骨瘤恶变而来的骨软骨肉瘤或软骨肉瘤的病理诊断,必须密切结合临床和影像学表现。

子宫肌瘤一直划归良性肿瘤,可是有的子宫肌瘤却可沿着血管转移到其他部位,这种生物学行为是恶性?还是良性?

这里提出一个问题,就是如何处理病理组织学观察与病变的生物学行为之间的关系,因此,单纯按照组织细胞学表现称良性、恶性似有不妥之处。

关于“四结合”的临床诊断模式的建议

实践是检验真理的唯一标准,在与疾病的斗争中,诊断治疗是否正确?检验的唯一标准是疗效,诊断错误者疗效绝对不可能满意,疗效满意就是检验临床影像学诊断是否正确的唯一标准。

临床诊断金标准的讨论一直在进行。普遍认为,临床诊断的金标准以前是病理诊断,长期临床实践告诉我们,临床诊断的金标准,应为临床、影像、病理和疗效追踪随访四个方面的资料适当结合起来分析研究的结果(简称“四结合”),才更为正确,更符合病人的实际情况。

建议国内一些杂志放开对“个案报告”的字数的限制

国外一些杂志的“个案报告”深受读者的欢迎,因为那些个案报告不只是简单地报告一个病例,而是通过一个病例具体情况报告一类新发现的疾病;或是通过一个病例深入分析研究某种疾病的误诊和漏诊;或是通过一个病例深入浅出地讨论临床和影像诊断对某种疾病的诊断和治疗的新的动向;或是通过一个病例全面系统地综述全球对该类疾病的研究进展和趋势……。此类个案报告,无字数的限制,让作者畅所欲言,讨论十分深入细致,让读者受益匪浅。反观国内一些杂志对“个案报告”的字数的限制十分严格,我们建议应放开限制,让作者畅所欲言,深入讨论。

怎样阅读本书

我们建议读者阅读本书的方法是:在临床上有需要分析和研究的病例时,按照病人影像表现的异常征象所在的器官和组织,查阅有关章节;然后再按拟诊的可能性,及可能性的大与小,分别查阅该章节内该疾病的有关部分,这样就可以事半功倍地取得效果。自然,如果你有时间愿意将本书通读,然后再用上述方法查阅,那效果更好。

在学习和研究误诊学期间,我们发现一些疾病可以出现在多个系统,多个器官和某个器官的多个部位,导致误诊和诊断困难。我们特地将多系统多器官疾病尽可能集中在一起,安排于本书面颈与多系统多部位疾病卷进行介绍和讨论,作为该卷的第二部分内容,以供读者参考。但对每一种病常见部位、常见器官,则在该常见部位、常见器官另写一章或一节,更为具体、详细,这样全书合成一体,互相呼应,更有利于读者在临床实践中查阅。

病理学与影像诊断关系十分密切,病理学基本知识的了解,对于影像诊断十分必要,非常重要,尤其是免疫组织化学检测对疾病的最后诊断所起的决定性作用,更应让现代的影像诊断医生有所初步了解,我们专门在本书面颈与多系统多部位疾病卷作一简介,作为该卷的第三部分。

随着现代科技的飞跃发展,现代医学进展也非常迅速,作为影像诊断医生,知识更新是每天的必修课,近期出现的影像组学、精准医学、人工智能等,我们安排在本书面颈与多系统多部位疾病卷第四部分进行简要的介绍,只能起到扫盲的作用。该部分还介绍了一些规范及专家共识。

《当代医学影像误诊学》讨论内容非常广泛,前言与总论的内容十分庞杂,但限于前言与总论篇幅有限,只能扼要地提纲挈领地进行简要的介绍,有关前言与总论内容的更详细的介绍和讨论,集中安排在本书面颈与多系统多部位疾病卷,作为该卷的第五部分内容,欢迎同仁和读者们参阅并提出宝贵意见。

有关活体形态学的资料,请查阅科学出版社 2006 年出版,巫北海总主编《活体形态学》第一版各卷,在此不再赘述。

Forward

Misdiagnosis in radiology and its Impacts on disciplines of clinical medicine.

It might be beyond the scope of this series of books to discuss the diagnostic errors in medical sciences since diagnostic radiology is just a discipline of clinical medicine. However, we are focusing on discussing and analyzing the misdiagnosis and overlook of diagnosis in imaging diagnosis. We also analyzed and discussed misdiagnosis caused by other clinical disciplines including pathology, which is closely relevant to imaging diagnosis, hoping benefit our colleagues in other clinical departments.

Radiological diagnostics and clinical medicine

There have been a myriad of discussions regarding the relationship between radiology and clinical medicine. From our standpoint of view, diagnostic imaging should not be improperly treated as guiding discipline over other clinical disciplines in diagnosis, nor is it just an auxiliary branch of clinical medicine, a misperception, which had existed for a while and was outdated now. Diagnostic radiology does not function as a guideline for clinical medicine, nor does it bear features of leadership, auxiliary and consultancy. Instead, it is an approach to explore sources of symptoms and signs, identify normality and abnormality in human anatomy, differentiate physiological and pathological manifestations in the body, disclose location, size, scope and nature of a lesion and so forth.

We strongly encourage radiologists to work with physicians in other clinical departments and pathologists to practice clinical medicine and scientific research in a collaborative manner, including drafting proposals and applying for research funding on the same subjects and sharing data analyses and research results, a way of cooperation, which is able to establish a closer link between radiology and other clinical disciplines as well as pathology to reduce and avoid misdiagnosis and overlook of any lesions.

Responsibilities of clinical physicians in imaging diagnosis

It is not a good practice for clinical physicians to request diagnostic imaging assessment with no basically required information regarding signs and symptoms from the patients. Simplicity of imaging request forms which have no detailed main description regarding the symptoms and signs is irresponsible for the patients and wastes sources of imaging study. Radiologists have no focus in reading, which is time-consuming in observing, analyzing and studying the images, resulting in poor quality of imaging diagnosis, even bringing about misdiagnosis and overlook. As a result, processing of clinical diagnosis could be delayed. Unfortunately, it is not individual case in the clinical practice.

We do believe that clinical physicians should bear full awareness of their responsibilities when requesting imaging examinations. They should tell radiologists main findings they collect from their patients as much as possible. By this way, radiologists, who don't meet the patients in person, still are knowledgeable of cases, being able to focus on potential locations of lesions which are possibly implicated by the symptoms and signs. It is very important for reducing and avoiding misdiagnosis and overlook.

Individualization of diagnosis

Doctors of the traditional Chinese medicine make diagnosis by directly contacting patients via a cascade of process which consists of 4 steps, i.e. wang-wen-wen-qie (Literally they are observation, auscultation and olfaction, inquiry as well as pulse feeling and palpation, respectively). They exhaustively collect medical history, symptoms and signs from their patients and make individualized treatment plans. Their misdiagnosis ratio could be prospectively lower than ours, probably because radiologists don't directly obtain information from the patients. It is remarkably worthy of studying how to apply the principle of individualization in imaging diagnosis. Thus, it reiterates responsibilities from the clinicians. Should the clinicians provide us the information of the patients as in detail as they can when requesting imaging examinations, it would be much more helpful for us to reduce and avoid radiological misdiagnosis.

Prevention of misdiagnosis and overlook via knowledge update

The most significant and efficient method and approach to reduce and avoid misdiagnosis and overlook are to diligently update our knowledge. In order to reach this goal, we need to continuously learn new technologies, broaden our scope of view on other clinical specialties and establish closer communications with other clinical departments. In the relevant chapters of this series of books, we briefly introduce recently developed edging-cut technologies such as radiomics, precision medicine, and artificial intelligence, as well as new imaging theories, new techniques, and the-state-of-art equipment in imaging diagnosis in an effort to help readers refresh their understanding and knowledge.

Innovative equipment, new technologies and research on vitomorphology

If we lack fully understanding of unique features each of innovative equipment or new techniques possesses or if we are over confident to depend upon those latest developed technologies, misdiagnosis still may occur. For instance, overdiagnoses are coming out from time to time when detected "abnormalities" result from oversensitivity produced by imaging approaches such as PET, etc.

Along with advent of innovative imaging approaches, continuous education of radiologists may not be timely in pace of development of new imaging technologies. With less experience, or poor recognition between normality and abnormality, or insufficiency of study on standards of normality, or lack of deep understanding, or incapacity of judgement, our capability in imaging diagnosis could be impacted. How to tell normality vs. abnormality? An opportunity for further study has been brought to the vitomorphology.

Basics of reducing and avoiding misdiagnosis upon comprehensive collaboration of various diagnostic imaging techniques

At present, in a general hospital, the fixed assets for a department of radiology usually account for about 30 percent of the total fixed assets of the hospital. Diagnostic imaging is an advanced technology but expensive in cost. Various imaging techniques are working independently but they should be collaboratively and fully used in order to take the advantages and avoid disadvantages each of them possesses. In clinical work, we should pay respect to our colleagues in other clinical departments and make full use of each other's advantages to maximize efficiency in diagnosis and treatment. We, radiologists and clinicians in correspondent departments, should take an active engagement by academic conferences, discussions and consultations. Eventually we are able to reach consents upon diagnoses. It would magnificently help improve quality of radiological diagnosis, a model of cooperation, which not only should be used in internal consultations in a hospital but also in any other consultations among hospitals. However, throughout the past 30 years of clinical practice in imaging diagnosis, our lessons are that lack of effective collaboration among imaging diagnostic techniques in some hospitals is a major cause of imaging misdiagnosis.

Radiological diagnosis and pathology

At present, immunohistochemistry testing is the golden standard for pathological diagnosis. Is it possible for a misdiagnosis made by this technique? Is every procedure, including the collection of specimens, the accuracy of observation, and the suitability of the applied techniques, appropriate? How to combine the pathological observation with clinical data and imaging data? To answer those questions, we need to do further broad investigations and studies.

In order to ensure the accuracy of the image diagnosis, the diagnoses of cases illustrated in this series of books all had been confirmed by pathological testing. Those with no pathological results were all excluded. We believe that the imaging diagnosis must be supported by the pathological testing. It is extremely inappropriate to confirm an imaging diagnosis with another imaging techniques. When we go over literature, we need to read with a dialectical view because cases in some of articles had been confirmed with pathological evidences, whereas some of others might not but just made up numbers in amount.

Thoughts on Tumor Classifications

The chondroma in the short bones of the four limbs may have malignant signs on histological examination, but clinically those tumors rarely witness malignant development. On the contrast, the chondroma in the flat or long bones appears benign under the microscope but many of cases evolve to malignant stages.

Furthermore, osteochondroma or chondroma located in long bones clinically may manifest as malignancy because metastases in remote organs already occur, but histologically, malignant signs under microscope are still not obvious. Therefore, pathologically diagnosing osteochondrosarcoma or chondrosarcoma cancerated from osteochondroma or chondroma should reference clinical manifestations and imaging findings.

Hysteromyoma has been classified as benign tumor, but in some cases, the tumors can be transferred along the blood vessels to other sites. Biologically, is this kind of behavior malignant or still benign?

Therefore a question is raised on how to deal with the relationship between pathological-histological observations and the biological behaviors of lesions. As the result of fact, it appears to be inappropriate to judge benign or malignancy only simply based on histological cytology.

Suggestions on the four-in-one model of clinical diagnosis

Practice is the sole criterion for judging true or false. Are a diagnosis and a treatment plan correct in the battle against illness? Treatment effectiveness is the sole criterion for judging the accuracy of diagnosis and intervention. Incorrect diagnosis absolutely is unable to produce satisfying treatment effectiveness. Satisfying therapeutic effectiveness is the only criterion for judging the accuracy of clinical diagnosis, in which, diagnostic radiology plays a role.

Discussions on the golden standard of clinical diagnoses continuously are ongoing. In the past, it was generally believed that the golden standard for clinical diagnoses was pathological testing. Nevertheless, long term of clinical practice indicates that the golden standard of clinical diagnoses could be regarded as a combination of results obtained from analyses and studies via clinical examination, imaging diagnosis, pathological testing as well as therapeutic follow-up (Briefly called Four-in-One model). The description of the golden standard based on acknowledgement of Four-in-One model appears to be more accurate and therefor, more realistic in clinical medicine.

Suggestion for restriction of word count on "Case Report" by domestic journals

"Case Report" in some oversea journals is very popularly welcome by readers, because "Case Report" not only simply reports cases, but by analyzing and studying a typical individual case, it may lead to find new entities of diseases, or it may investigate misdiagnosis and overlook on a certain category of diseases, or it may explore the new trend of diagnosis and treatment made by clinical methods and radiology on a type of diseases, or it may systematically illustrate the development status and trend of global researches on the same species of diseases and so on.

"Case Report" in abroad journals has no restriction on number of words. The authors are able to fully express their opinions. Discussions in "Case Report" cover broad scope of topics, which much better benefits the readers.

On the other hand, some domestic journals have strict limitation on word count. We suggest the limitation on word count should be lifted and the authors are allowed for making full discussions on reported cases in scope and depth.

How to read this series of books

We would recommend some tips on how to read this series of books: Whenever clinically needed in analyzing and studying cases, the readers are able to search for correspondent chapters based on tissues and organs where abnormal imaging findings are located at, and then read relevant sessions of the diseases in that specific chapter based on impression of potential diagnoses and priority of possibilities. Thus, the readers may double efficiently obtain information they are searching for. Absolutely, it is recommended for readers to go over all the chapters of this series of books and then employ the tips suggested above.

While doing analyses and studies on misdiagnosis, we found that some diseases could occur in multiple systems, multiple organs and multiple sites within a certain of organ, leading to difficulty in making diagnosis and even resulting in misdiagnosis. We specifically tried our best to collect those diseases which involve in multi-systems and multi-organs in one book, Volume of the Face and the Neck, particularly arranging them as the second part of the volume for readers' references. However, for common locations and organs of the diseases, more detailed description and discussion in specific chapter or section can be found in volumes which cover the locations and organs the diseases are commonly located at. By doing so, all the volumes of this series of books are consistently integrated and reciprocally cited each other, which is more productive for the readers to search for literature in clinical practice.

The relationship between pathology and radiological diagnostics is very close. Understanding the basics of pathology in imaging diagnosis is necessary and important. Specifically, the decisive role immunohistochemical testing plays in finalizing diagnoses of diseases requires radiologists be knowledgeable in this field. We particularly brief the immunohistochemical technology which has been arranged in the third part of the Volume of the Face and Neck.

With the rapid development of modern sciences and technologies, the progress of modern medicine is also very speedy. As radiologists, updating our knowledge should be our daily requirement. Regarding the recent advent of radiomics, precision medicine and artificial intelligence, we arranged the topics in the fourth part of the Volume of the Face and Neck. Since our introductory contents are very concise, it is just elementary for our readers' awareness of those new imaging technologies.

The spectrum of discussion on misdiagnosis is very extensive. The information contained in the Preface and the Executive Summary is giant in amount and complex in structure. However, due to the limitation of space for the Preface and the Executive Summary, we are only able to synopsize hot spots of misdiagnosis. More detailed description and discussion about the contents mentioned here have been arranged as the fifth part of the Volume of Face and Neck. We sincerely welcome the feedbacks and comments from our readers.

With regard to detailed information on vitomorphology, please refer to the first edition of Vitomorphology edited by Professor Beihai Wu and published by Science Publishing House, China in 2006.

总论一　医学影像误诊研究

与前人比较，我们这一代是相当幸运的，赶上了前所未有的好时代，科技发展突飞猛进，知识大爆炸，信息交流活动日新月异，信息种类之多，信息量之大，传送速度之快，真让人喘不过气来，影像诊断技术的飞跃，更让人力不从心，我们的先辈、同辈、晚辈都忙于学习、研究影像诊断的新技术、新设备在临床的应用和科研教学，成了影像诊断各方面的专家，在影像诊断的进步和诊断水平的提升做出了傲人的成绩。

随着影像诊断的新技术、新设备的引进和广泛应用，临床上一些问题逐渐暴露出来：检查技术的规范化，各个疾病诊断标准的建立，正常与异常的鉴别，健康与疾病的划界，亚健康情况的出现，过度诊断和过度治疗的发现，误诊和漏诊的情况都是我们必须面对的问题。

误诊、漏诊研究相当复杂

我们在工作中发现，日常临床工作中所遇到的疾病大约有 80% 是教科书上写的典型表现，工作一段时间后，不少医生都可胜任诊断，其诊断的准确性也较高；另外 20% 左右的疾病没有教科书上描写的那么典型和简单，准确地对其诊断存在着一定的难度，常常导致误诊，这就是误诊学研究的主要内容；在典型疾病中有时出现漏诊，其原因有时颇耐人寻味；在常见疾病中偶尔见到十分少见的表现，也给诊断带来相当困难；在少见疾病中时不时表现为教科书上的典型表现，引起诊断混淆；在临床工作中，经常暗藏着诊断陷阱，导致误诊与漏诊。凡此等等，都是误诊学应该研究的对象。

由于误诊和漏诊的研究是一类相当复杂的问题，涉及的内容的深度远比以往想象的深刻，误诊和漏诊的原因是多方面的，多层次的，且涉及面十分广泛，因此《当代医学影像误诊学》研究和讨论的内容甚为丰富多彩：既有误诊原因的分析，又有鉴别诊断的内容；既有误诊、漏诊的经验教训介绍，又有防止误诊、漏诊的理论性研究；既有诊断思维的研究，又有知识更新的信息；既有活体形态学的研究，又有发育变异的表现；既有影像检查技术的进展，又有影像诊断研究的学术总结；既有临床常见症状、体征的观察分析，又有病理学、免疫组织化学的研究简介；既有少见疾病影像学表现，又有常见疾病的不典型征象；既有按照断面影像分卷、分章讨论，又有各个生理解剖系统疾病的分析；既有各个系统特有疾病的研究，又有多系统多部位疾病的介绍。本书不是一般的诊断学教科书，而是适用于临床工作的参考书，本着有话则长，无话则短的原则进行撰写和编纂。

国内、外对误诊的研究

造成误诊的原因有很多,国内、外学者研究不少,但专著不多,而且都是从单一的角度进行研究和分析,例如:有的从发育变异入手,专门研究导致误诊的发育变异,尤其是骨骼系统的发育变异,国内也有译本;有的从检查手段入手,专门研究影像检查中因机器设备和检查技术不当引起的各类伪影,专业期刊中不断有文章发表;有的从影像诊断的思维分析方法研究入手,还在专业期刊上辟专栏进行讨论;有的地方专业学会学术活动每次都讨论误诊病例,但报告的多,讨论分析的少,多只是以吸收错误的教训而告终;不少作者对误诊都感兴趣,许多专业期刊的个案报告都是此类内容,只不过一些作者诚实地承认对该病例发生了误诊,一些作者却碍于情面,放不下架子,不提误诊这两个字,只提经验教训一笔带过。

在研究误诊学时,我们发现,在临床工作中,对待误诊的态度真是千奇百怪:有的老实承认错误,仔细分析研究导致错误的原因,认真总结经验教训,写出研究误诊的文章,诊断水平不断提高;有的医生避重就轻,称“太忙,我只看了一眼”不负责任的推脱;有的主任在科室内是“权威”,当有人告诉他出现误诊时,他只是一笑置之,立刻转移话题,从不总结经验,故步自封,当有人追究责任时,则推给下级医生,自己永远都是“正确”的。

活体形态学研究

现代影像学的发展给我们研究活体形态学提供了前所未有的条件,研究活体形态学是时代给我们的要求,临床影像诊断医生应加大研究活体形态学的力度,这是临床影像诊断医生工作的主要研究范围之一,活体的功能、形态学研究应该是将来工作的重点。

我们一直认为,临床诊断标准的建立——金标准是活体研究而非尸体研究。每个人青壮年时期健康的活体形态学表现,可作为该个体的正常活体形态学最佳标准,可用它来检查和发现该个体患病早期出现的轻微异常,这是早期发现疾病较好的方法。因此,可以这样说,个人青壮年时期健康的活体形态学资料是检查和发现该个体患病的早期表现的最佳标准。

本书讨论活体形态学的具体内容有:关于发育变异;活体研究与非活体研究;对发育变异与先天异常的认识;变异的观点——先天发育与后天发育;关于影像诊断的个性化;正常与异常;动态生理与影像诊断的误诊;医学生物学的发展;活体的动态观察;从目前情况看,活体形态学的研究任重而道远。

诊断方法研究

对于诊断方法的研究,本书着重指出,影像诊断报告务必要留有余地。关于循证放射学和循证医学的出现和进展,我们进行了深入介绍。在影像诊断中,一定要注意保证正确诊断必需的时间。我们对于避免误诊的思维方法研究、误诊与鉴别诊断、影像诊断中的讨论、综合影像检查和诊断试验研究等也作了讨论。

影像诊断报告务必要留有余地，我们告诉读者关于四点注意事项：影像诊断应有自知之明；关于文责自负；现代问题，人人都是专家，见仁见智；放射科医生应该如何在现代环境下进行工作。希望在临床工作中，尽量减少和避免误诊和漏诊的出现。

本书还着重讨论放射科医生的视野问题，内容包括：放射科医生的视野必须超越影像；影像征象的定义；影像征象的特点；影像征象的分类；基本功训练点滴；知识更新与诊断标准。

常见共性征象的研究与分析

常见的有共性的 CT 或 / 和 MRI 征象的研究与分析，包括：颅脑及脊髓占位、脑病、脑白质疾病、癫痫、痴呆、面颈部病变、颅颈连接区病变、颈胸连接区病变、肺门包块、肺门与纵隔区域的淋巴结肿大、孤立性肺结节、肺磨玻璃密度影、肺肿块、弥漫性肺疾病、慢性阻塞性肺病与通气障碍、乳腺癌、冠状动脉疾病、胸腹连接区病变、肝占位、黄疸、胆胰管十二指肠连接区疾病、门静脉疾病、上腹包块、血尿、腹腔积液、腹膜外间隙疾病、妊娠与胎儿病变、软组织疾病、骨肿瘤及肿瘤样病变、脊柱占位性病变、骨质疏松、骨髓疾病的分析与鉴别诊断。

影像学技术

影像学技术不当造成的误诊有：不同影像手段选择应用程序的研究，投照因素不正确，投照角度不准确，伪影出现的识别和造成伪影的原因的认识，扫描序列选择和组合的应用不恰当，CT 三维重建技术不当，对不同技术（如 CT 与 MR）的诊断标准及诊断能力的评价与其评价的年代关系甚为密切，因为近年技术进步相当快速，如不注意此点，难免出现一些完全可能避免的误诊和分析意见。

相关学科与医学影像学

在相关学科与医学影像学通力合作方面，本书详细介绍了相关学科与医学影像学；手术学科对医学影像学的依赖性越来越高；医学影像学科自身的发展；医学影像学信息系统的发展；携手兄弟科室共同发展；影像诊断与临床；观察者的差异；CT 肺动脉成像之肺动脉栓塞的影像诊断读片者间的一致性研究；影像诊断各项诊断技术的通力协作是减少误诊的基础。

规范及与误诊学相关的部分资料

本书详细介绍了目前我们可以收集到的有关规范、专家共识及诊断标准，并对新的设备与检查技术的进展作了讨论，关于新近出现的影像组学、精准医学和人工智能有关资料，本书不仅介绍，而且还建议读者更深入地学习和研究。

关于病理学检查的认识

我们认为应当重视临床病理的工作和科学研究，欢迎临床病理医生到影像科室指导工作，还讨论了：病理误导与误诊；关于临床诊断金标准的认识；关于病理证实的问题；关于病理报告与误诊；临床生物学行为和组织病理表现。

影像学诊断质量评价和管理

在影像诊断学中十分重要的一个问题是影像学诊断质量评价和管理,本书对此作了比较详尽的介绍,首先简介关于影像学诊断质量评价和管理问题的重要性,并对医学生物学的发展;我国医学影像学的发展;开展影像诊断的质量保证诸多事项进行必要的讨论。

此外,本书在有关章节内,还对下述问题分别进行了详尽的研究和讨论。

影像变化与临床症状:颈椎序列及颈椎椎间盘的研究,活体的功能变化与机械的观察的矛盾,有的椎间盘膨出明显,可见突出,却一点症状都没有;有的症状明显,却未见膨出和突出;可见临床症状与膨出和突出的关系值得研究,也说明具体有无临床症状,其中还有其他许多因素在起作用。

对于误诊与病变的发现问题:我们着重强调指出,只有熟悉正常才能发现异常,并对阴影的意义,对疾病的早期发现、早期诊断,及关于读片的程序进行了深入讨论。

动态观察:在讨论动态观察与影像诊断的误诊时,除了简单扼要地分析研究身体各部位的动态观察与影像诊断的误诊以外,本书着重强调指出,一定要注意检查时间与观察的时间的差异。

影像诊断学近来的发展:本书介绍了不少疾病影像诊断研究的进展,一些检查技术及扫描序列的研究,新近发现的疾病或综合征的影像诊断学表现。

本书不是一般的诊断学教科书,而是适用于临床工作的参考书,适用于临床影像诊断医务工作者、临床各科医生、医学院校学生阅读,有利于扩大知识面,增加信息量,是有关临床影像诊断继续教育和自学较好的参考资料。

Pandect Ⅰ Study on Misdiagnosis (Medical Imaging)

Executive Summary

We are much more blessed than our last generation because we catch up an unprecedented era, during which, science and technology are developing speedily. Intellectuality and knowledge are explosively increasing. The activities of information exchange keep changing at daily base. We are experiencing shortness of breath when we have to deal with the information which is numerous in categories, giant in amount as well as fast in velocity of transmission. Facing speedy development of new technologies and the-state-of-art equipment, we are worry about that our capability in imaging diagnosis may not be able to confront the challenges. Our pioneers, peers and younger generation all are busy in learning and studying those new imaging technologies and equipment which are successively employed in clinical practice, research and teaching. They grew up to become professional experts in imaging diagnostics. We are proud of their accomplishment in improving accuracy and quality of imaging diagnosis.

Along with applications of innovative techniques and equipment in radiological diagnostics, some clinical problems gradually are surfacing, including standardization of examination procedures, establishment of diagnostic criterion for individual disease, differentiation between normality and abnormality, discrimination between healthy status and morbidity, appearance of sub-healthy status, discoveries of overdiagnosis and overtreatment as well as misdiagnosis and overlook of diagnosis, all of them need to be resolved.

Complexity in studying misdiagnosis and overlook of diagnosis

We found that 80% of diseases clinically manifest as typically described in the textbooks and are able to be diagnosed by most of physicians who already have had some clinical experiences. The ratio of diagnostic accuracy on those diseases is relatively high. Nevertheless, the manifestations of remaining percentage of diseases are not so straightforward and typical as appeared in the textbooks, bringing about difficulty in diagnosis and even leading to misdiagnosis. As a result of fact, it gives rise to a research subject for misdiagnosis. Clinically, some of typical diseases sometimes are overlooked. We need to explore the reasons why we miss the diagnoses. Sometimes, unusual manifestations may occur in typical diseases, bringing about difficulty for diagnosis, too. Meanwhile, classic manifestations described in the textbooks could be seen in non-typical diseases, causing confusion in diagnosis. The traps of diagnosis are hidden in clinical practice from time to time, leading to misdiagnosis and overlook. All of these phenomena constitute subjects the misdiagnosis is studied on.

Since misdiagnosis and overlook are complicated, the meaning of the involved contents in scope and depth is beyond what we imagined before. Misdiagnosis and overlook may result from varying causes and may occur at multi-levels of diagnostic processing. With touching each of aspects in diagnostic radiology, the topics discussed and studied in Contemporary Medical Image Misdiagnosis are diverse and plentiful, which involve in analyses on causes of misdiagnosis as well as differential diagnosis, demonstration of lessons and experiences from misdiagnosis and overlook as well as theoretical research how to prevent them, study on diagnostic logics as well as information of knowledge update, research on vitomorphology as well as findings of developmental anomaly, the latest progress of imaging technologies as well as academic summarization of researches on imaging diagnostics, observation and analysis on clinically typical symptoms and signs as well as introduction on the progress of immunohistochemical technique, discussion about sectional imaging by separate chapters and volumes as well as analysis on the diseases by their physiological and pathological systems, study on special diseases by systems as well as introduction on diseases which appear in multi-systems and multi-sites in one system, etc. This series of books are not general textbooks in diagnosis but reference books which are citable in clinical work. The books are edited based on the principles that describe topics as fully as possible if needed and just brief them if no details are required.

Domestic and abroad studies on misdiagnosis

Misdiagnosis could be brought about by varying causes. A number of domestic and abroad scholars had done researches on it, but a few of specific works on the topic had been published, almost all of them conducted studies and analyses from a single of viewpoint. Some abroad researchers, for instance, started with developmental anomaly, focusing on developmental anomaly which gives rise to misdiagnosis, specifically on developmental anomaly in skeletal system. Their research reports in Chinese version were published in domestic publications. Some started with procedures of examinations, specializing in a variety of artificial imaging resulting from inappropriate use of facilities and procedures during the imaging examinations. Their publications continuously appear in journals. Some began with the methods of logic analysis in imaging diagnosis, opening forums on the topics in special columns of academic journals. Discussions on misdiagnosed cases almost exclusively appear in academic seminars and conferences, but most of them were just case reports with little exploration and analysis in depth, ending up with a conclusion that lessons should be learnt from the mistakes.

A lot of authors expressed interest in misdiagnosis and case reports published in academic journals almost were about the topic related. However, only some of authors honestly confessed that they mistakenly diagnosed the cases, whereas some of others embarrassedly never mentioned “misdiagnosis” but just concluded that the lessons must be learnt from the reported cases.

When studying misdiagnosis, we found that the people's attitudes toward misdiagnosis were strangely diverse in clinical practice. Some of them honestly accepted the facts that they made mistakes. They carefully studied possible causes which resulted in the misdiagnosis and seriously thought of lessons they experienced. And they published research reports of the cases and had quality of their diagnosis improved. Some didn't willingly touch key factors in misdiagnosis and irresponsibly gave their excuses, for instance, “too busy to carefully deal with the case”. Some ones who were in leadership positions in the departments were absolutely “authoritative” in making diagnosis. When being aware of mistakes they made, they dismissed with smile and skipped the topic. They never recalled lessons they experienced. They stopped at what they learnt, which might be outdated years ago and were self-constrained. When being blamed of responsibility, they exclusively attributed the charges to others whom they supervised and kept themselves “correct” forever.

Study on vitomorphology

Development of modern imaging provides us with unprecedented conditions to study vitomorphology. We are given of an accountability for studying vitomorphology by the era we are currently in. Radiologists should pay much more efforts to the research of vitomorphology, which will be one of our major research subjects. Study on functions and morphologies of live bodies will be emphasized in our future work.

We always believe that the establishment of clinical diagnostic criterion, golden standard, should be dependent upon study on live bodies rather than on cadavers. Everyone's healthy vitomorphological findings in 30s of adulthood could be regarded as optimal reference standard of normal vitomorphology for the individual body, which could be employed to examine and find any subtle early stage of abnormality in the individual body in future. It is a better solution to find early stage of diseases. Therefore, it is reasonably to state that information of healthy vitomorphology in the adulthood is the best standard for examining and detecting early stage of morbidity which occurs in the individual body.

The following contents in this series of books which will be discussed in detail include developmental anomaly, study on live bodes and cadavers, recognition on developmental anomaly and congenital anomaly, standpoint of view on anomaly – congenital development and acquired development, individualization of diagnostic imaging, normality and abnormality, dynamic physiology and misdiagnosis in imaging diagnostics, the progress of medical biology, dynamic observation on live bodies, etc. All in all, we have a lot of work to do and a long way to go in vitomorphology.

Study on diagnostic approaches

Regarding study on diagnostic approaches, we highlighted that the diagnostic reports of imaging should be necessarily conservative for conclusions. We also introduced the latest progress of evidence-based radiology and evidence-based medicine in depth. In order to make correct imaging diagnosis, enough time should be guaranteed. We also discussed study on logic thinking how to avoid misdiagnosis, misdiagnosis vs. differential diagnosis, forums in imaging diagnosis, combined examinations of imaging approaches as well as study on diagnostic experiment.

We are trying to tell our readers that conclusions of imaging diagnosis should necessarily be conservative and attention should be paid to the following four aspects: It is out of question that diagnostic imaging is important in clinical diagnoses, but radiologists also should clearly recognize its own limitations; We are responsible for what are recorded in the imaging reports; With regard to existed problems in the modern society, everyone is professionally able to make their own annotation from their standpoints of view and how radiologists should implement their work under modern environment. We hope that we always try our best to decrease and avoid misdiagnosis and overlook in our clinical work.

In this series of books, we specially emphasized radiologists' scope of view, which always should be beyond the imaging. We also discussed definitions, features and categories the imaging signs possess, tips of basic training and knowledge update as well as diagnostic criteria.

Study and analysis on common generality of imaging signs

Study and analysis on common generality of signs displayed on CT and/or MRI cover the following diseases: Occupying lesions in brain and spinal cord, encephalopathy, white matter diseases, epilepsy, dementia, lesions in face and cervix, Lesions in junction of cranium and cervix, Lesions in junction of cervix and thorax, masses in hilus pulmonis, enlargement of lymph nodes in hilar and mediastinal areas, solitary pulmonary nodules, ground-glass like density shadow in lungs, masses in lungs, diffuse pulmonary diseases, chronic obstructive pulmonary diseases and dysfunction of ventilation, breast cancer, coronary artery disease, Lesions in junction of thorax and abdomen, occupying lesions in liver, jaundice, lesions in junction of biliary-pancreatic duct and duodenum, lesions in portal vein, masses in upper abdomen, hematuria, ascites, lesions in extraperitoneal space, Lesions in pregnancy and fetus, lesions in soft tissues, tumors and tumor-like lesions in bones, occupying lesions in spine, osteoporosis, analysis and differential diagnosis on lesions in bone marrow.

Imaging techniques

Misdiagnosis due to inappropriate application of imaging techniques includes incorrectly selected procedures of imaging approaches, incorrect projection and inaccurate angles of projection, identification of artificial shadows and unawareness of causes for the shadows, improperly selected scanning sequences, inappropriate 3D-reconstruction of CT. Evaluation on diagnostic criteria and ability of different imaging approaches such as CT, MRI, etc. is closely in correlation with time when the evaluation had been completed. Since the progress of techniques is very fast in the recent years, if neglect the facts, it is hard for us to avoid misdiagnosis and incorrect analytic opinions which originally are avoidable.

Relevant disciplines and medical imaging

With regard to collaboration among clinical specialties, this series of books introduced relevant disciplines and medical imaging, increased dependency of surgical specialties upon medical imaging, development of medical imaging as well as development of information system on the imaging's own, collaborative development with other specialties, imaging diagnostics and clinical medicine, differences among observers, study on consensus among readers with regard to imaging diagnosis of pulmonary artery thrombosis on CT imaging of pulmonary artery. Full collaboration among a variety of imaging approaches is basic in decreasing misdiagnosis.

Standard and information relevant to misdiagnosis

This series of books described in details about standard, experts' consensus and diagnostic criteria and discussed the progressive status of innovative equipment and techniques. In term of latest developed radiomics, precision medicine and artificial intelligence, we not only had description but also suggested readers to do further investigation and research.

Recognition on pathological testing

We are emphasizing the importance of clinical pathology and its scientific research, and always welcome pathologists to come to departments of diagnostic radiology for consultations and guidance. We also discussed pathology and misdiagnosis, pathological misleading and misdiagnosis, recognition on golden standard of clinical diagnosis, pathological evidences and clinically biological behaviors vs. histologically pathological manifestations.

Quality assurance and management of imaging diagnostics

An important issue in radiology is the quality assurance and management of imaging diagnostics, which had been fully detailed in this series of books. First of all, we emphasized why they were important, and then necessarily discussed the development of medical biology, domestic development of medical imaging and how to implement quality assurance of imaging diagnostics, etc.

Additionally, the following topics also had been fully discussed and studied in correspondent chapters of the books.

Radiological manifestations vs. clinical symptoms: We studied the sequence of cervical spine and cervical intervertebral discs, discrepancy between functional changes of live bodies and mechanical observation. We found that in some cases, herniation of intervertebral disc was obvious and protrusion was clearly displayed, but the patients had no symptoms at all. Whereas some demonstrated very obvious symptoms, but no herniation of intervertebral disc was seen. Obviously, it deserves further study on the relationship between clinical symptoms and extrusion or herniation. Meanwhile, it indicates that existence of clinical symptoms lies on many other factors.

Misdiagnosis vs. discovery of morbidity: We reiterate that only normality has been well recognized, can abnormality be detected. We also discussed in depth significance of shadows, early detection and diagnosis of diseases as well as procedures of image reading.

Dynamic observation: When discussing dynamic observation vs. imaging misdiagnosis, we briefly analyzed and studied dynamic observation on organs and systems. In addition, we specifically emphasized lapse between time of examination and time of observation.

The latest development of diagnostic radiology: In this series of books, we introduced the latest research progress of imaging diagnostics on a number of diseases, exploration on techniques of examination and scanning sequences along with the radiological manifestations of newly discovered diseases and syndromes.

This series of books are not general textbooks in diagnosis but reference books which are citable in clinical work. So the objects our books are edited for are radiologists, physicians in clinical departments and medical students. They are beneficiary in broadening scope of knowledge and obtaining additional information. Therefore, this series of books are good tutorials in continuous education and self-learning.

总论二　客观评价人工智能在医学影像学中的作用

在过去几十年间，计算机科学有了快速的发展，给人工智能（AI）的开发带来了前所未有的机遇。随着卷积神经网络（CNN）在2012年的引入，使得深度学习（DL）升级到更高台阶，其结果就是人工智能在医学影像领域日益地活跃起来。

深度学习算法不需要事先预设的资料，它可以通过训练数据集学习，而训练数据集可以是来自研究机构或医院多年积累起来的样本，或是来自已经构建起来的对公众开放的数据库。在训练期间，深度学习算法从样本提取特征和参数，然后构建模型。模型要经过验证数据集的评估，如有必要，其参数会得到修订。训练和验证的连续迭代，可以使算法得到最佳化，从而避免过度拟合。训练完成后，测试数据集会用于确认模型的分类，准确及泛化能力。除了两端的输入和输出，居于中间的层次及处理过程都是看不见的，被称作为隐藏层，或黑匣子。

人工智能在处理医学影像中的优势

接受训练后，借助强大的计算能力，人工智能能够在短时间内处理数据繁杂的图像，并能从正常人体解剖中辨识出异常。于是，人工智能有可能把医学影像医生从繁重的工作中解脱出来。这些医学影像医生每天花费大量时间在海量的医学影像中试图寻找异常。这样他们可以专注于病灶的分析与判断。大量研究报告显示，人工智能在检测病灶及做出鉴别诊断方面的能力能够达到高年资放射科医生的水平。于是人工智能有助于帮助低年资医学影像医生改善他们的诊断质量。对于肺癌的早期检测，卷积神经网络积分也能达到现有积分模型的水平，如像Brock模型等。但在假阴性判断方面，卷积神经网络积分系统优于Brock模型。卷积神经网络还能增强现有的影像诊断辅助设施的执行能力，如像计算机辅助检测（CADe）、计算机辅助诊断（CADx）及计算机辅助容积测量（CADv）等。卷积神经网络还能使影像组学（Radiomics）技术得以升级换代。

人工智能的局限性与减少和避免误诊

在医学影像中，人工智能对于良、恶性病灶的鉴别诊断及预测的高准确率已经有了广泛的报道，但同时它的一些局限性也引起了人们的注意。

首先，为了训练的目的，卷积神经网络需要大量的数据来学习，从中提取各种不同的影像特征。如果数据集来自一家研究机构及它的协作单位，所包含的病种总是有限的。对公众开放的数据库也难以解决这个问题，因为在设计之初，这些不同来源的数据集的组合彼此之间难以保持高度一致。有了组合数据集，病种是增加了，但基于这些组合数据集的模型难以避免地带有偏差。

其次，人工智能在胸部放射学有着令人鼓舞的应用，其成就主要聚焦在肺部结节。然而，如果结节过大（直径 >5cm），或者邻近胸膜，或者晚期肿瘤已经侵犯到了相邻结构，人工智能检测病灶的能力显著下降，于是导致误诊。

再其次，人工智能在检测病灶的假阳性率也是不能忽略的。文献中有报道指出，人工智能的假阳性率可以高达 41%，其构成包括肺异常膨出症（dystelectases）、肺内血管、肺门钙化淋巴结、肋骨、呼吸伪影等。

在知悉人工智能的优势及局限性后，我们认识到人工智能在医学影像的临床应用方面的确有着光明的前景，但目前仍然在继续开发中。人工智能所接受的训练过程其实也就是医学影像医生经历过的。这就解释了人工智能的诊断能力只是与高年资放射科医生的水平相当，还未实现超越。虽然人工智能有其独特的能力测量医学影像上密度及信号的细微差别，而这些细微差别有时是人的肉眼所不能感知的，它甚至可以直接去利用在扫描时获取的原始数据，但这些技术所提供的帮助仍然是有限的。因此，当我们在临床和研究工作中应用人工智能的时候，时刻警惕它的局限性，在某种特定情况下，例如假阳性、晚期肿瘤等，随时准备人为的干预。

Pandect Ⅱ Objectively Evaluate the Role of artificial intelligence in Medical Imaging

In the past decades, the computer science has been experiencing a speedy progress. It brings about an unprecedented chance to the development of artificial intelligence (AI). With convolutional neural network (CNN) introduced in 2012, deep learning (DL) has been escalated to a higher level. As a fact of result, exploration and study of AI in medical imaging are increasingly active.

Deep learning algorithms do not require an intermediate feature extraction or preprocessed data. It is able to learn from training data set assigned from examples and/or from existing tremendous amount of data accumulated in the institutes and hospitals in the past years or from publicly available databases. During training, the DL algorithms abstract features and parameters, and then establishes the models. The models will be evaluated by validation data set and parameters for the models get tuned if needed. Successive iterations of training and validation may be performed to optimize the algorithms and avoid overfitting. After the training is completed, testing data set is used to confirm the models' performance of classifications, accuracy and generalizability. The whole processing experiences input of imaging, convolutional layer, pooling layer, flatten, fully connected layer and output of classification. Except input and output, all those layers and processes are invisible. So those invisible structures also are called hidden layers or black box.

Advantages of AI in Processing Medical Images

After training, with powerful computation, AI is able to deal with huge amount of images in short time and discriminate abnormalities from normal human anatomy. So it is possible for AI to free medical image doctor from spending a lot of time on a sea of images at daily work in searching for abnormalities and let them pay special attentions to analyze and judge the lesions. A lot of studies have showed that capability of AI in detecting lesions and making differential diagnosis could reach the level of senior medical image doctor. Thus, AI is useful to help junior medical image doctor improve their quality of diagnosis. With respect to early detection of lung cancer, CNN score are at the lever of existing models like Brock model, etc. but CNN score is superior to Brock model in false negative. CNN is able to improve performance for existing auxiliary utilities of imaging diagnosis, such as, computer-aided detection (CADe), computer-aided diagnosis (CADx), computer-aided detection of volume (CADv), etc. and escalate Radiomics technology.

Limitations of AI Versus Misdiagnosis

While the high accuracy of AI in differentiating and predicting benign and malignant lesions are widely reported, some limitations also have been noticed. First of all, CNN needs to learn from a large amount of data for the purpose of training and then is able to abstract a variety of imaging features from the training. If dataset comes from one institute and its collaboration institutes, the categories of diseases are always limited after all. Publicly available databases can't resolve this issue either because if combination of datasets from diverse resources is unable to be consistent each other in designs, the models based on the combined datasets could be inevitably biased.

Secondly, while AI encouragingly displays its application in chest radiology, its achievements are mainly focusing on pulmonary nodules. However, if nodules are too large in size (>5cm) or their locations contact pleura or the advanced tumors invades structures adjacent to the lung, the capability of AI in detecting lesions could be remarkably decreased. Thus misdiagnosis would take place.

Thirdly, the false-positive rate of AI in detecting lesions also is not negligible. In the literature, it was reported that false-positive of AI could be as high as 41%, among which are dystelectases, intrapulmonary vessels, hilar calcified lymph nodes, detection of ribs, and a breathing artifact.

Being aware of advantages and limitations of AI, we realize that AI indeed displays promising future in the clinical application of medical imaging but currently is still under development. The training processing AI received actually is what medical image doctor experienced. It may explain that diagnostic capability of AI has not been beyond but is just equivalent to senior medical image doctor. Though AI has its unique ability to measure the minute differences of densities and signals which may not be discerned by human's eyes, and it even is able to directly use raw data acquired from scanning, the assistance provided by these technologies is still limited. Therefore, while we make use of AI in study and clinical work, we should be alert to its limitations and be prepare to manual intervention anytime under certain circumstances, such as false-positive, advanced tumore, etc.

全书总目录

第一卷(颅脑与脊髓卷)

第一篇　颅脑疾病概论 / 1
第二篇　颅脑肿块一般情况 / 41
第三篇　脑 胶 质 瘤 / 61
第四篇　脑 膜 肿 瘤 / 127
第五篇　脑 膜 疾 病 / 171
第六篇　其他颅脑肿块 / 199
第七篇　脑　　病 / 263
第八篇　颅脑囊性病变 / 329
第九篇　颅脑与脊髓血管性疾病 / 351
第十篇　脑白质疾病 / 463
第十一篇　颅 脑 神 经 / 505
第十二篇　脊髓与椎管 / 535
第十三篇　鞍区及其毗邻疾病 / 603
第十四篇　颅 底 疾 病 / 645
第十五篇　颅骨及头皮疾病 / 669
第十六篇　脑 室 疾 病 / 705
第十七篇　小 脑 疾 病 / 745
第十八篇　颅脑发育及先天异常 / 785
第十九篇　颅 脑 炎 症 / 805
第二十篇　颅脑与脊髓损伤 / 837
第二十一篇　小儿脑及脊髓 / 863
第二十二篇　关于痴呆 / 929
第二十三篇　关 于 癫 痫 / 951
第二十四篇　颅脑功能成像 / 961
第二十五篇　精神功能异常与影像学检查 / 975
第二十六篇　基底节区海马杏仁核及丘脑 / 983
第二十七篇　桥小脑角区、脑干及其他 / 1003
第二十八篇　颅与颅外沟通性疾病 / 1035
第二十九篇　颅脑内金属沉积 / 1053
第三十篇　头痛与颅脑手术后 / 1075
参考文献 / 1085
本卷有关医学影像词汇 / 1091

第二卷(面颈及多系统多部位疾病卷)

第一部分　面颈疾病 / 1
第一篇　眼及眼眶 / 3
第二篇　鼻咽、鼻窦与鼻 / 55
第三篇　口咽与喉咽 / 111
第四篇　口腔与涎腺 / 127
第五篇　喉与周围 / 177
第六篇　甲状腺与甲状旁腺 / 189
第七篇　耳与颞骨 / 229
第八篇　颅底区及颅内外沟通性疾病 / 273
第九篇　颅颈连接区 / 295
第十篇　颈胸连接区 / 323
第十一篇　面颈部血管 / 339
第十二篇　面颈部淋巴 / 365
第十三篇　面颈部骨与关节 / 393
第十四篇　小儿面颈部疾病 / 421
第十五篇　面颈部创伤 / 443
第十六篇　面颈部其他疾病 / 449
第二部分　多系统多部位疾病 / 483
第一篇　神经源性疾病 / 485
第二篇　纤维组织源性肿瘤 / 497
第三篇　血管源性疾病 / 513
第四篇　与淋巴有关的疾病 / 533
第五篇　与血液有关的疾病 / 571
第六篇　与免疫功能抑制有关的疾病 / 587
第七篇　免疫缺陷性疾病 / 603
第八篇　小儿多系统多部位疾病 / 613
第九篇　其他多系统多部位肿块 / 639
第十篇　其他多系统多部位疾病 / 681
第三部分　与误诊学有关的基础临床病理学概要 / 725
第一篇　临床病理学 / 727
第二篇　免疫组织化学 / 741
第三篇　分子病理学 / 759
第四部分　规范及与误诊学相关的部分资料 / 769
第一篇　有关规范及诊断标准 / 771
第二篇　设备与检查技术 / 783
第三篇　关于基因组 / 857
第五部分　总论有关问题深入讨论 / 863

第一篇 人工智能与医学影像的发展 / 865
第二篇 误诊学是一门学科 / 891
第三篇 诊断方法研究 / 927
第四篇 误诊与影像学研究 / 963
参考文献 / 1013
本卷有关医学影像词汇 / 1021

第三卷(胸心卷)

第一篇 胸部疾病 / 1
第二篇 孤立性肺结节 / 47
第三篇 肺结节 / 65
第四篇 肺癌 / 121
第五篇 胸部其他肿块 / 177
第六篇 肺结核病 / 249
第七篇 慢性阻塞性肺病和通气障碍 / 271
第八篇 肺部感染 / 289
第九篇 肺弥漫性疾病 / 325
第十篇 全身疾病的胸部表现 / 349
第十一篇 气管及支气管疾病 / 367
第十二篇 心脏大血管疾病 / 401
第十三篇 冠状动脉疾病 / 457
第十四篇 心肌疾病 / 537
第十五篇 肺血管 / 571
第十六篇 纵隔 / 627
第十七篇 食管疾病 / 699
第十八篇 胸腹连接区 / 729
第十九篇 胸膜与胸壁 / 767
第二十篇 乳腺疾病 / 823
第二十一篇 胸部淋巴 / 913
第二十二篇 胸部先天异常和发育变异 / 945
第二十三篇 小儿胸部疾病 / 955
第二十四篇 胸部创伤和胸部手术 / 985
参考文献 / 994
本卷有关医学影像词汇 / 1006

第四卷(腹盆上卷)

第一篇 肝局灶性病变 / 1
第二篇 肝转移瘤 / 75
第三篇 肝细胞性肝癌 / 91
第四篇 肝细胞性肝癌以外的肝恶性肿瘤 / 181
第五篇 肝的其他局灶性疾病 / 211
第六篇 肝结节性病变 / 279
第七篇 肝囊性病变 / 287
第八篇 儿童肝占位性病变 / 297
第九篇 肝脏弥漫性病变 / 311
第十篇 肝血管性疾病 / 363
第十一篇 肝的先天异常和发育变异 / 395
第十二篇 肝与肝外 / 409
第十三篇 肝创伤和肝手术后 / 427
第十四篇 关于肝移植 / 433
第十五篇 胆系疾病 / 445
第十六篇 胆管疾病 / 471
第十七篇 胆囊疾病 / 553
第十八篇 胆囊管疾病 / 601
第十九篇 胆胰管十二指肠连接区疾病 / 631
第二十篇 胰腺疾病 / 701
第二十一篇 脾脏疾病 / 849
第二十二篇 腹盆部多器官多系统疾病 / 901
第二十三篇 胃的疾病 / 943
第二十四篇 十二指肠 / 1009
第二十五篇 空、回肠疾病 / 1041
第二十六篇 大肠疾病 / 1091
第二十七篇 阑尾疾病 / 1151
第二十八篇 门静脉疾病 / 1169
第二十九篇 急腹症与腹盆创伤 / 1207
第三十篇 小儿腹盆部疾病(上) / 1217
第三十一篇 腹盆部影像学检查技术 / 1241
参考文献 / 1257
本卷有关医学影像词汇 / 1267

第五卷(腹盆下卷)

第一篇 腹膜与腹膜腔 / 1
第二篇 腹膜外间隙疾病 / 79
第三篇 肾上腺疾病 / 157
第四篇 肾及肾周疾病 / 207
第五篇 尿系疾病 / 303
第六篇 前列腺疾病 / 369
第七篇 男性生殖系统 / 401
第八篇 卵巢疾病 / 429
第九篇 女性生殖系统 / 473
第十篇 妊娠与胎儿 / 519
第十一篇 腹盆腔其他包块和恶性肿瘤 / 553
第十二篇 腹盆部结核 / 571
第十三篇 腹盆部其他疾病之一 / 581
第十四篇 腹盆部血管疾病 / 599
第十五篇 腹盆部创伤 / 627

第十六篇　小儿腹盆部疾病（下）/ 637
第十七篇　腹盆部淋巴 / 679
第十八篇　腹盆部其他疾病之二 / 707
参考文献 / 742
本卷有关医学影像词汇 / 751

第六卷（肌骨及脊柱卷）

第一篇　软组织疾病 / 1
第二篇　骨与骨肿瘤一般情况 / 91
第三篇　骨肿瘤及肿瘤样病变 / 113
第四篇　关节疾病 / 211
第五篇　脊柱占位性病变 / 239
第六篇　脊柱关节病和脊柱炎症 / 257
第七篇　关于椎间盘 / 279
第八篇　脊柱各段疾病 / 291
第九篇　软骨疾病 / 361
第十篇　骨与软骨损伤 / 381
第十一篇　关于骨髓 / 411
第十二篇　四肢疾病 / 429
第十三篇　上肢及肩带 / 459
第十四篇　下肢与骨盆 / 543
第十五篇　膝部疾病 / 689
第十六篇　小儿肌骨与脊柱 / 749
第十七篇　肌骨遗传代谢性疾病和先天异常 / 803
第十八篇　骨关节炎症 / 819
第十九篇　骨质疏松症 / 829
第二十篇　肌骨系统其他疾病 / 841
参考文献 / 851
本卷有关医学影像词汇 / 857

第四卷(腹盆上卷)目录

第一篇　肝局灶性病变

第一章　肝脏疾病研究 / 3
第一节　肝肿瘤样病变的简要鉴别诊断 / 3
第二节　机器学习在肝脏疾病影像诊断中的研究 / 4
第三节　代谢组学在肝脏疾病的应用 / 7
第二章　肝局灶性病变定位研究 / 8
第三章　具有脂肪特征的肝脏疾病 / 12
第一节　肝脏内含脂肪与脂质的病变 / 12
第二节　肝内含肉眼可见脂肪的病变 / 13
第三节　含脂肪成分的肝脏病变 / 14
第四节　肝脂肪浸润 / 15
第五节　关于脂肪肝背景 / 15
第六节　肝的脂肪浸润与诊断陷阱 / 16
第七节　肝的脂肪浸润与超声的跳跃区 / 17
第八节　局灶性脂肪变和局灶性肝岛 / 17
第九节　肝脏多灶性结节状脂肪浸润 / 18
第四章　肝脏富血管性病变 / 20
第一节　肝脏富血管(供)性疾病 / 20
第二节　肝脏富血供良性病变 / 21
第三节　十六种肝富血管病变 / 24
第五章　伴有其他影像学特征的肝脏疾病 / 29
第一节　伴包膜回缩的肝脏疾病 / 29
第二节　伴钙化的肝脏疾病 / 30
第三节　并发出血的肝脏疾病 / 31
第四节　伴中央瘢痕的肝脏疾病 / 33
第五节　延迟或延长强化的肝脏病变 / 34
第六节　密度 / 信号局限性异常与肿瘤 / 35
第六章　有关肝肿瘤的几个问题 / 38
第一节　肝肿瘤成像的几个问题 / 38
第二节　代谢组学在肝脏疾病的应用 / 39
第三节　肝肿瘤性病变的诊断与鉴别 / 41
第四节　肝脏少见肿瘤及肿瘤样病变简介 / 42
第五节　人工智能及影像组学在肝脏肿瘤中的应用 / 44
第七章　部分肿瘤的不典型表现 / 46
第一节　肝脏部分肿瘤的不典型 CT 表现 / 46
第二节　CT 增强扫描:肝脏单发不典型强化病灶 / 48
第八章　关于良、恶性肝肿瘤 / 50
第一节　DWI 与肝良、恶性肿瘤 / 50
第二节　良、恶性肝脏疾病的鉴别 / 51
第三节　肝局灶性结节增生病例 / 51
第四节　MR 和 CT 发现穿过肝脏肿瘤的血管 / 52
第五节　肝细胞性肝癌与 DWI 及 Gd-DTPA 动态增强 / 52
第六节　周边廓清:局灶性肝脏病变钆增强 MRI 的一种恶性征象 / 53
第九章　肝局灶性病变与超声 / 54
第一节　超声低回声晕环鉴别肝良、恶性肿瘤 / 54
第二节　左肝叶伪似肝内包块或胰腺包块 / 54
第三节　超声检查时肝的假性病变 / 54
第四节　肝脏超声的伪影与误诊 / 55
第十章　肝局灶性病变与 CT / 56
第一节　CT 平扫呈低密度的肝脏局灶性病变 / 56
第二节　肝脏第Ⅰ、Ⅳ段的假性病变 / 57
第三节　动脉门静脉造影 CT 出现的迷走胃右静脉引流所致肝Ⅱ及Ⅲ节段假性病灶 / 60
第四节　肝右叶局灶性结节增生病例 / 60
第五节　CT 增强扫描后显示的肝脏低密度病变 / 61
第六节　肝 CT 检查中的假性病变 / 62
第七节　肝左右叶多发性巨大外生性海绵状血管瘤病例 / 62
第八节　肝脏假肿瘤性病变 / 63
第九节　关于经动脉门静脉 CT 成像(CTAP)的误诊 / 64
第十节　关于肝 CT 扫描中的伪影 / 66
第十一章　肝局灶性病变与 MRI / 67
第一节　肝脏局灶性病变的 MRI 表现 / 67
第二节　MRI 镰状韧带旁伪影及肝功对比研究 / 69
第三节　多层面动态 MRI 中肝左叶内段早期增强的假病灶 / 69
第四节　肝脏成像中常见的 MRI 伪影 / 70
第五节　MRI 动态增强误诊 / 70
第十二章　一些诊断陷阱 / 71
第一节　肝的假性占位性病变 / 71
第二节　肝的假良性肿瘤 / 71

第三节　肝肿瘤的误诊 / 72
第四节　关于肝左叶占位病变血管造影诊断 / 72
第五节　肝外肿块与肝肿块 / 72
第六节　肝脏第Ⅰ、Ⅳ段的假性病变 / 73
第七节　肝核素显像时的假阳性 / 73

第二篇　肝转移瘤

第一章　肝转移瘤 / 77
第一节　关于肝脏转移性肿瘤影像学研究 / 77
第二节　恶性胃肠道间质瘤肝脏转移病例 / 78
第二章　不典型的肝转移瘤 / 80
第一节　源自消化系统黏液癌钙化性转移瘤 / 80
第二节　孤立性多血性肝转移瘤 / 80
第三节　肝脏囊性转移瘤 / 81
第四节　肝转移瘤坏死 / 82
第五节　误诊病例简介:原发性肝内胆管细胞癌与肝转移性肿瘤及胰腺癌 / 83
第六节　肝脏转移性平滑肌肉瘤 / 83
第七节　肝淋巴道转移癌 / 84
第八节　恶性黑色素瘤肝转移 / 85
第九节　影像诊断中的假性肝转移瘤 / 85
第十节　误诊病例简介:肝腺癌与肝结核瘤 / 86
第三章　肝转移瘤与 CT 及 MRI / 87
第一节　肝脏转移瘤不典型 CT 表现 / 87
第二节　肝内胆管细胞癌与转移性肝癌的鉴别 / 87
第四章　肝转移瘤与血管造影 / 89

第三篇　肝细胞性肝癌

第一章　诊疗规范和专家共识 / 93
第二章　肝癌一般情况 / 97
第一节　原发性肝癌包膜形成 / 97
第二节　血管周上皮样细胞肿瘤(简称 PEComa)/ 98
第三节　含脂肪肝癌 / 99
第四节　增强扫描时不同密度的肝癌 / 100
第五节　含脂肝细胞肝癌 / 100
第六节　代谢组学在肝脏疾病的应用 / 101
第七节　原发性肝细胞性肝癌的少见征象 / 101
第八节　关于原发性肝癌的分期 / 102
第九节　假肝癌 / 104
第十节　关于浸润型肝癌 / 104
第十一节　误诊病例简介:原发性肝细胞性肝癌与转移性肝癌 / 106
第三章　小肝癌 / 108
第一节　肝纤维化、肝癌前期病变及早癌的影像学研究 / 108
第二节　早期肝细胞癌与小肝癌 / 109
第三节　早期肝细胞性肝癌病例 / 110
第四节　早期肝癌与高分化肝细胞癌 / 111
第五节　小肝癌不典型的影像表现 / 111
第六节　关于小肝癌的漏诊 / 113
第七节　小肝癌的不典型增强表现 / 113
第八节　误诊病例简介:小肝癌与良性病灶 / 114
第四章　肝癌基础研究点滴 / 116
第五章　透明细胞型肝癌 / 119
第一节　原发性透明细胞型肝癌 / 119
第二节　原发性肝细胞性肝癌(透明细胞型)/ 120
第三节　肝脏原发性透明细胞癌 / 121
第六章　纤维板层型肝细胞癌 / 122
第七章　外生型肝癌 / 124
第一节　外生型肝癌 / 124
第二节　误诊病例简介:外生性肝癌,低分化肝细胞性肝癌淋巴转移 / 127
第八章　硬化型肝癌 / 128
第九章　肉瘤样肝细胞癌 / 130
第十章　混合型肝癌 / 132
第一节　混合型肝细胞癌 - 胆管细胞癌 / 132
第二节　肝内混合型肝癌(胆管细胞癌 + 肝细胞癌)病例 / 133
第十一章　肝细胞癌的扩散和转移 / 135
第一节　肝细胞性肝癌伴有胆管癌栓 / 135
第二节　肝脏肿瘤侵犯胆管的 MRI 楔形征 / 136
第三节　肝细胞癌侵犯胆管 / 137
第四节　关于浸润型肝癌 / 140
第十二章　肝癌与门静脉 / 141
第十三章　肝癌与 CT / 143
第一节　肝的 CT 扫描技巧点滴 / 143
第二节　肝癌内 CT 所见钙化 / 143
第三节　左肝内段低分化肝细胞性肝癌伴坏死 / 144
第四节　MSCT 双动脉期与门脉期增强扫描对原发性肝癌检出比较 / 144
第十四章　肝癌与 MRI / 146
第一节　关于原发性肝癌的动态增强 MRI / 146
第二节　MRI 动态增强误诊 / 146
第三节　误诊病例简介:高分化肝细胞性肝癌与血管平滑肌脂肪瘤 / 147
第十五章　肝癌与超声 / 149

第十六章　肝癌与 DSA / 152
第十七章　肝癌破裂出血 / 155
第十八章　关于肝占位性病变的鉴别诊断 / 158
第十九章　关于肝癌的误诊 / 160
第一节　螺旋 CT 三期增强扫描误诊或漏诊肝细胞性肝癌 / 160
第二节　乏血供型肝细胞癌 / 162
第三节　CT 平扫为等密度的肝癌 / 163
第四节　慢进快出型肝细胞肝癌 / 165
第五节　肝占位性病变 CT 误诊为原发性肝癌 / 166
第六节　误诊病例简介：高分化肝细胞性肝癌与肝结核 / 168
第七节　误诊病例简介：不典型肝癌误诊为囊腺瘤 / 170
第八节　肝癌误诊与漏诊 / 171
第九节　肝细胞性肝癌强化表现 / 171
第十节　假肝癌 / 172
第十一节　肝细胞癌误为脾肿瘤 / 172
第十二节　肝癌的不典型表现和少见 CT 表现 / 172
第十三节　肝癌影像诊断误诊研究点滴体会（基层医院讲课提纲）/ 173
第十四节　MRI 误诊为肝细胞癌的肝巨淋巴结增生症 / 175
第二十章　关于肝癌的治疗与复发 / 176
第一节　肝癌的复发 / 176
第二节　原发性肝癌术后复发的肝动脉造影表现 / 177
第三节　肝癌治疗中的 CT 观察 / 178
第四节　肝癌射频消融术后特殊征象 / 179
第五节　误诊病例简介：布加综合征合并原发性肝癌 / 180

第四篇　肝细胞性肝癌以外的肝恶性肿瘤

第一章　胆管细胞型肝癌 / 183
第一节　误诊病例简介：肝内胆管细胞癌与肝结核瘤 / 183
第二节　误诊病例简介：肝内胆管细胞癌与肝脓肿 / 184
第三节　不典型的肝内胆管细胞癌 / 184
第四节　不同生长方式肝内胆管细胞癌 / 186
第五节　肝内胆管细胞癌淋巴结转移 / 187
第六节　无胆管扩张的肝内胆管细胞癌 / 188
第七节　肝内胆管细胞癌与转移性肝癌的鉴别 / 189
第二章　肝脏恶性纤维组织细胞瘤 / 190
第三章　肝血管源性恶性肿瘤 / 191
第一节　肝脏原发性血管肉瘤 / 191
第二节　肝脏上皮样血管内皮瘤 / 192
第四章　成人肝未分化肉瘤 / 194
第五章　癌肉瘤 / 196
第一节　肝脏原发性癌肉瘤 / 196
第二节　误诊病例简介：肝肉瘤样癌（梭形细胞癌）与腹膜后占位 / 196
第三节　肝肉瘤样癌肝门淋巴转移 / 198
第六章　其他肝肉瘤 / 199
第一节　误诊病例简介：膈下腹膜间皮肉瘤与血管瘤 / 199
第二节　误诊病例简介：左肝外叶平滑肌肉瘤与肝血管平滑肌脂肪瘤 / 199
第三节　误诊病例简介：肝平滑肌肉瘤与肝血管平滑肌脂肪瘤 / 200
第七章　肝淋巴瘤 / 201
第一节　肝淋巴瘤 / 201
第二节　肝脏弥漫大 B 细胞淋巴瘤病例 / 202
第八章　肝恶性肿瘤的一些检查方法和影像学表现 / 203
第九章　原发性肝脏神经内分泌肿瘤 / 205
第一节　原发性肝脏神经内分泌癌 / 205
第二节　原发性肝胆神经内分泌肿瘤 / 206
第十章　肝其他恶性肿瘤 / 207
第一节　误诊病例简介：肝左外叶导管内乳头状腺癌 / 207
第二节　肝上皮样血管内皮瘤 / 207
第三节　误诊病例简介：原发性肝间质瘤并多发性转移与多发性巨大血管瘤 / 208
第四节　肝门部肿瘤 MRI 误诊分析 / 209

第五篇　肝的其他局灶性疾病

第一章　关于肝局灶性病变 / 213
第二章　肝血管瘤 / 216
第一节　不典型血管瘤 / 216
第二节　误诊病例简介：肝外生性海绵状血管瘤与胃肠间质瘤 / 218
第三节　肝脏血管瘤不常见 CT 和 MRI 表现 / 219
第四节　肝不典型海绵状血管瘤 / 221
第五节　不典型和不常见的血管瘤 / 221
第六节　肝左右叶多发性巨大外生型海绵状血管瘤 / 222
第三章　肝脏局灶性结节增生 / 224

第一节 误诊病例简介:右肝炎性肌纤维细胞瘤被误诊为局灶结节性增生 / 224
第二节 误诊病例简介:局灶性结节性增生与肝癌 / 225
第三节 肝左外段局灶性结节性增生 / 226
第四节 肝局灶性结节性增生 / 227
第五节 左肝局灶性结节增生 / 227
第六节 局灶性结节增生合并局灶性海绵状淋巴管瘤 / 228
第七节 肝局灶结节性增生 / 229
第八节 局灶性结节增生之不典型表现 / 230
第九节 右肝局灶性结节性增生 / 233
第十节 肝脏局灶结节增生不典型 CT 表现 / 233
第十一节 肝局灶结节性增生 / 234
第十二节 关于肝脏局灶性结节增生的鉴别诊断 / 235
第十三节 肝脏多发性局灶性结节增生 / 236
第十四节 几个问题的讨论 / 237

第四章 肝肉芽肿性疾病 / 239

第五章 肝细胞腺瘤 / 240

第一节 误诊病例简介:老年男性肝细胞腺瘤与肝癌 / 240
第二节 多发性肝细胞腺瘤与先天性Ⅰ型糖原累积症 / 240
第三节 肝细胞腺瘤 / 241
第四节 肝腺瘤 / 242

第六章 肝脏间叶性肿瘤 / 244

第一节 移动性肝副叶上皮样血管平滑肌脂肪瘤 / 244
第二节 肝血管平滑肌脂肪瘤不典型 CT 表现 / 244
第三节 肝脏炎性肌纤维母细胞瘤 / 245
第四节 误诊病例简介:肝脏上皮样血管内皮细胞瘤与血管瘤及转移瘤 / 246
第五节 误诊病例简介:肝脏上皮样血管内皮瘤与多发肝囊肿 / 247
第六节 肝血管周上皮样细胞肿瘤 / 248
第七节 肝脏血管平滑肌脂肪瘤不同表现 / 249

第七章 肝脏炎性疾病 / 250

第一节 误诊病例简介:肝炎性肌成纤维细胞瘤与局灶性结节增生 / 250
第二节 肝脏炎性假瘤 / 250
第三节 误诊病例简介:肝脏孤立性坏死性结节被误诊为炎性假瘤 / 251
第四节 中度慢性肝炎(肝脏假性占位) / 252
第五节 肝脓肿 / 252
第六节 容易误诊的含气肝脓肿破裂 / 253
第七节 左肝外段肝脓肿 / 254
第八节 误诊病例简介:嗜酸性肝脓肿与肝的恶性肿瘤 / 254
第九节 细菌性肝脓肿的误诊与置管引流 / 255
第十节 误诊病例简介:肝脏 IgG4 相关性炎性假瘤 / 256

第八章 肝寄生虫病 / 257

第一节 肝泡性包虫病与肝癌的鉴别 / 257
第二节 不典型的肝血吸虫病表现 / 257
第三节 误诊病例简介:肝肺吸虫病误诊为肝癌并腹腔多发转移 / 258

第九章 肝脏孤立性坏死结节 / 260

第一节 误诊病例简介:肝孤立性坏死结节与肝炎性假瘤 / 260
第二节 误诊病例简介:肝脏孤立性坏死性结节与肝脓肿 / 260
第三节 误诊病例简介:肝脏孤立性坏死结节与炎性假瘤 / 261
第四节 肝脏孤立性坏死性结节与海绵状血管瘤同存 / 262

第十章 肝神经源性肿瘤 / 263

第一节 误诊病例简介:神经纤维瘤病侵犯肝脏与肝脏多发占位病变 / 263
第二节 误诊病例简介:肝脏副神经节瘤 / 263

第十一章 肝脏淋巴动力学异常 / 265

第十二章 朗格汉斯细胞组织细胞增生症 / 266

第十三章 肝脏真菌感染 / 268

第一节 免疫抑制状态下并发肝脏真菌感染 / 268
第二节 原发性肝脏隐球菌病 / 269

第十四章 肝紫癜 / 271

第十五章 肝平滑肌瘤 / 273

第一节 肝脏良性转移性平滑肌瘤 / 273
第二节 原发性肝脏平滑肌瘤 / 273

第十六章 肝横纹肌样瘤和肝门区横纹肌母细胞瘤 / 274

第一节 误诊病例简介:肝横纹肌样瘤 / 274
第二节 肝门区横纹肌母细胞瘤 / 274

第十七章 其他肝局灶疾病 / 275

第一节 类似肝脏肿瘤的肝内异位脾组织植入 / 275
第二节 猫抓伤病 / 275
第三节 肝包膜下血肿误诊 / 275
第四节 镰状韧带脂肪瘤 / 276
第五节 肝脏多灶性结节状脂肪浸润 / 276

第六节 肝的不规则局灶性脂肪浸润 / 276
第七节 肝裂中的脂肪 / 277
第八节 局灶性肝脂肪浸润 / 277
第九节 肝脏假性淋巴瘤 / 277
第十节 局灶性脂肪变和局灶性肝岛 / 278

第六篇 肝结节性病变

第一章 肝结节性病变 / 281
第二章 肝再生性结节 / 284
第三章 肝硬化结节 / 286

第七篇 肝囊性病变

第一章 肝脏囊性病变 / 289
第一节 肝囊肿 CT 诊断的陷阱 / 289
第二节 误诊病例简介:肝囊肿与肝胆管囊腺瘤 / 290
第二章 肝脏肿瘤性囊性病变 / 291
第一节 肝脏肿瘤性囊性病变 CT 诊断 / 291
第二节 横纹肌母细胞瘤 / 293
第三章 其他肝囊性病变 / 294

第八篇 儿童肝占位性病变

第一章 肝恶性肿瘤 / 299
第一节 儿童肝母细胞瘤 / 299
第二节 非分化性(胚胎性)肉瘤 / 300
第三节 丛状纤维组织细胞瘤侵犯肝脏 / 301
第二章 肝良性肿瘤 / 302
第一节 婴儿血管内皮瘤 / 302
第二节 误诊病例简介:肝脏间叶错构瘤与多房性肝囊肿 / 303
第三章 先天性囊性疾病 / 305
第一节 先天性囊肿 / 305
第二节 间叶性错构瘤 / 305
第三节 先天性肝内胆管囊肿 / 305
第四节 肝外胆管囊肿 / 305
第四章 后天性囊性疾病 / 306
第一节 包囊虫病 / 306
第二节 感染性疾病 / 306
第五章 肉芽肿性病变 / 307
第一节 慢性肉芽肿性疾病 / 307
第二节 霉菌和肉芽肿性病变 / 307
第六章 儿童肝占位的误诊 / 308
第一节 化疗后继发肝、脾、肾霉菌感染 / 308
第二节 可能误诊为肝肿块的病变 / 309
第三节 新生儿特发性肝内巨大血肿的误诊 / 309

第九篇 肝脏弥漫性病变

第一章 肝脏弥漫性病变简介 / 313
第二章 肝弥漫均匀型病变——密度升高 / 315
第一节 弥漫均匀型病变 / 315
第二节 不典型原发性血色素沉着症 / 315
第三节 肝豆状核变性 / 316
第四节 CT 平扫呈弥漫性高密度的肝脏疾病 / 316
第三章 肝弥漫性病变——密度降低 / 317
第一节 脂肪肝背景导致的漏诊 / 317
第二节 脂肪肝背景 / 319
第三节 弥漫性脂肪肝与占位病变同时存在 / 319
第四节 肝弥漫性病变——密度降低 / 319
第四章 密度下降——肝弥漫性节段型病变 / 320
第一节 局灶性脂肪变和局灶性肝岛 / 320
第二节 脂肪肝迅速地出现和消失 / 320
第三节 局灶性脂肪肝与更重要的占位病变的区别 / 320
第四节 诊断陷阱:肝的局灶性脂肪浸润 / 320
第五节 肝的脂肪浸润与超声:脂肪变性中的局灶性跳跃区 / 320
第六节 弥漫性脂肪肝的局部未受累区域 / 321
第七节 肝弥漫性节段型病变 / 321
第五章 布 - 加综合征 / 322
第六章 肝结节状再生性增生 / 323
第七章 肝脏淋巴动力学异常 / 324
第一节 肝脏淋巴异常动力学改变的 CT 研究 / 324
第二节 门静脉周围晕:肝病的一个 CT 征象 / 326
第八章 自身免疫性肝病和 IgG4 相关性疾病(IgG4-RD) / 327
第一节 自身免疫性肝炎、原发性胆汁性肝硬化、原发性硬化性胆管炎重叠综合征 / 327
第二节 免疫球蛋白 G4 相关肝胆疾病的诊断和鉴别诊断 / 327
第九章 肝炎 / 330
第一节 肝炎 / 330
第二节 急性戊型肝炎致肝内淋巴淤滞 / 330
第三节 病毒感染后的肝硬化 / 331
第十章 肝脏体积和形态变化 / 332
第一节 肝脏肿大 / 332
第二节 淀粉样变性 / 333
第三节 Niemann-Pick 病和 Gaucher 病 / 334

第四节 肝肾淀粉样变性 / 334
第十一章 肝纤维化形态学研究 / 336
第一节 肝纤维化程度的诊断 / 336
第二节 融合性肝纤维化 / 336
第十二章 肝纤维化功能代谢研究 / 337
第十三章 肝弥漫性病变中的血管疾病 / 339
第一节 肝窦阻塞综合征 / 339
第二节 肝淤血 / 339
第三节 日本血吸虫病 / 339
第十四章 肝弥漫性病变中胆管疾病 / 340
第一节 胆管微小错构瘤 / 340
第二节 继发性肝内胆汁淤滞 / 340
第三节 肝弥漫性病变的胆管造影表现 / 340
第四节 先天性肝内胆管囊性扩张症(Caroli 病) / 340
第十五章 肝脏弥漫性病变与 MR 扩散加权成像 / 341
第十六章 肝弥漫性病变与灌注成像 / 344
第十七章 肝硬化相关结节 / 345
第一节 早期肝癌(不典型增生伴恶性灶) / 345
第二节 肝硬化结节 / 345
第三节 弥漫性结节性肝硬化,伴局灶结节性增生 / 346
第四节 肝硬化与癌前病变 / 347
第十八章 肝硬化与脑 / 348
第十九章 肝硬化与骨 / 349
第二十章 肝铁过载 / 351
第一节 肝铁质沉积病 / 351
第二节 MR 磁敏感加权成像检出肝硬化铁沉积结节 / 352
第二十一章 药物性和放射性肝损伤 / 354
第一节 药物性肝病 / 354
第二节 放射性肝损伤 / 355
第二十二章 部分肝弥漫性肿瘤 / 356
第一节 弥漫型肝脏上皮样血管内皮细胞瘤 / 356
第二节 恶性组织细胞病 / 356
第三节 弥漫型的肝细胞癌与胆管癌合并存在 / 357
第二十三章 关于肝富血管性疾病 / 358
第一节 肝富血管性疾病 / 358
第二节 局灶性结节增生与肝腺瘤的鉴别 / 358
第三节 肝血管瘤与肝富血管肿瘤鉴别 / 359
第四节 肝硬化中的肝脏富血管病变 / 359
第五节 不常见的肝脏富血管病变的诊断与鉴别诊断 / 359
第二十四章 肝弥漫性病变的其他情况 / 361
第一节 肝衰竭 CT 表现 / 361
第二节 结节病侵犯肝脏 / 362
第三节 弥漫性病变中的部分局灶性病变 / 362

第十篇 肝血管性疾病

第一章 布 - 加综合征 / 365
第一节 误诊病例简介:布 - 加综合征合并原发性肝癌 / 365
第二节 布 - 加综合征与结节性再生性增生 / 365
第三节 肝窦阻塞综合征 / 365
第四节 诊断陷阱:脾肺固定术后 / 367
第五节 关于布 - 加综合征的误诊 / 367
第六节 布 - 加综合征误诊为肝癌 / 368
第二章 肝动脉 / 369
第一节 肝动脉变异影像学研究 / 369
第二节 关于肝动脉的发育变异 / 371
第三节 肝总动脉变异 / 372
第四节 肝动脉的假性动脉瘤 / 373
第五节 肝动脉成像中的误诊 / 373
第三章 一过性肝实质强化 / 375
第一节 一过性肝实质强化 / 375
第二节 一过性(暂时性)肝实质强化 / 378
第三节 肝外胆管细胞癌所致肝实质一过性密度差异 / 379
第四章 肝脏血流灌注异常 / 380
第一节 多层面动态 MRI 中肝左叶内段早期增强的假病灶 / 380
第二节 肝脏的高灌注异常 / 380
第三节 肝脏的第三供血血管与"假性病变" / 381
第五章 肝血管性疾病 / 384
第一节 肝动脉瘤 / 384
第二节 肝动脉的假性动脉瘤 / 385
第三节 肝脏遗传性出血性毛细血管扩张症 / 385
第六章 肝动静脉分流 / 387
第一节 肝脏动静脉短路的病因和分类 / 387
第二节 少见的肝动脉 - 门静脉瘘 / 387
第七章 肝静脉 / 389
第一节 肝静脉发育变异 / 389
第二节 肝窦阻塞综合征 / 389
第三节 副肝静脉 / 389
第四节 肝静脉发育变异与诊断陷阱 / 392
第八章 肝血管其他疾病 / 393

第十一篇 肝的先天异常和发育变异

第一章 肝的先天性异常 / 397

第一节 糖原蓄积病 / 397

第二节 囊性纤维化 / 398

第三节 肝发育不全和发育不良 / 398

第二章 肝的发育与活体形态学简介 / 399

第一节 腹腔动脉与肠系膜上动脉的发育变异 / 399

第二节 腹腔动脉发育变异 / 399

第三节 肝动脉的发育变异 / 400

第四节 误诊与诊断陷阱 / 400

第三章 肝发育变异与诊断陷阱 / 403

第一节 肝脏形态发育变异 / 403

第二节 肝动脉诸分支起源变异、形态变化 / 404

第三节 镰状韧带及镰状韧带周围的假性病灶 / 405

第四节 病人的体位和肝脏的位置 / 406

第五节 肝核素显像与肝脏实质的柔软性 / 406

第六节 肝胃韧带及肝的毗邻关系 / 407

第七节 动态扫描 / 407

第八节 肝脏大小的变异 / 407

第九节 肝右叶发育不良 / 407

第十二篇 肝与肝外

第一章 肝外疾病侵犯肝脏和诊断陷阱 / 411

第一节 肺癌直接侵犯肝脏 / 411

第二节 误诊病例简介：神经纤维瘤病侵犯肝脏 / 411

第三节 腹膜后、肝尾叶炎性假瘤与肝尾叶肝癌 / 412

第四节 白血病肝浸润 / 413

第五节 丛状纤维组织细胞瘤侵犯肝脏 / 413

第六节 急性胰腺炎对肝脏损害的 CT 观察 / 413

第七节 膈肌附着点与假性病变 / 414

第八节 肝外的假性病变 / 414

第二章 其他疾病影响肝脏 / 415

第一节 肝脏多发脾种植 / 415

第二节 上腔静脉阻塞综合征肝内异常强化灶 / 416

第三节 误诊病例简介：CT 诊断不典型药物性肝损害与肝内多发肿瘤 / 417

第三章 肝周 / 419

第一节 HELLP 综合征相关肝脏并发症 / 419

第二节 误诊病例简介：肝包膜下血肿误诊为囊实性占位病变 / 420

第三节 肝裂或隐窝内局限性积液可误为肝内病变 / 420

第四节 肝周超声检查的一些情况 / 420

第五节 关于腹水 / 421

第四章 肝脏疾病与肝外 / 422

第一节 肝肾综合征（HRS）/ 422

第二节 获得性肝脑变性：一种少见的肝病相关神经系统病变 / 423

第十三篇 肝创伤和肝手术后

第一章 肝创伤 / 429

第一节 肝创伤 / 429

第二节 肝、脾动脉破裂出血 / 429

第三节 肝内胆汁肿与亚急性血肿 MRI 鉴别诊断 / 429

第四节 肝损伤的其他情况 / 430

第二章 肝的放射性损伤 / 431

第三章 肝手术后 / 432

第一节 部分肝切除术后 / 432

第二节 活检通道 / 432

第三节 肝叶切除术后的误诊 / 432

第十四篇 关于肝移植

第一章 肝移植 / 435

第一节 CTA 与肝移植 / 435

第二节 活体供肝者肝血管与胆管发育变异之间的关系 / 435

第二章 肝移植术后 / 436

第一节 肝移植术后并发症 / 436

第二节 肝移植术后排斥反应 / 438

第三章 肝移植后的胆系并发症 / 440

第十五篇 胆系疾病

第一章 胆系结石类疾病 / 447

第一节 误诊病例简介：非肝移植胆管铸型综合征 / 447

第二节 黏稠胆汁和胆泥 / 447

第三节 误诊病例简介：黏胆症与黏液性乳头状癌 / 447

第四节 肺内胆石 / 448

第五节 黏胆症 / 448

第二章 胆系积气、胆系损伤和胆系出血 / 450

第一节 胆系积气 / 450

第二节 假性胆系积气 / 450

第三节 有关胆系积气的诊断陷阱 / 450

第四节 十二指肠 - 胆系逆流的少见原因之一 / 451

第五节 胆囊腺鳞癌伴坏死，胆囊穿孔，腹膜炎 / 451

第三章 胆系肿块 / 453

第一节 肝门部肿瘤 MRI 误诊分析 / 453
第二节 误诊病例简介:胆系横纹肌肉瘤与胆总管囊肿合并感染 / 453
第四章 胆系炎症 / 454
第五章 胆系其他疾病 / 455
第一节 活体供肝者肝血管与胆管发育变异之间的关系 / 455
第二节 胆肠 Roux-Y 吻合术后空肠桥袢结石 / 455
第三节 门静脉性胆病 / 456
第六章 磁共振胆胰管成像(MRCP) / 457
第一节 磁共振胆胰管成像误诊 / 457
第二节 胆汁流动伪影的 MRCP / 459
第三节 磁共振胆胰管成像的误诊 / 460
第七章 胆系 MRI / 462
第一节 肝胆成像中常见的 MRI 伪影 / 462
第二节 MRI 动态增强误诊 / 462
第八章 胆系其他影像学检查技术 / 463
第一节 MRCP 与 ERCP 的比较 / 463
第二节 术中胆系造影 / 464
第九章 胆系手术后 / 466
第一节 手术损伤性胆管狭窄 / 466
第二节 腹腔镜胆囊切除术后并发症 / 466
第三节 胆管空肠吻合术后吻合口狭窄 / 467
第四节 术后引流管造影 / 468
第五节 黏胆症 / 469

第十六篇 胆管疾病

第一章 胆管梗阻一般情况 / 473
第一节 误诊病例简介:非肝移植胆管铸型综合征 / 473
第二节 Mirizzi 综合征 / 474
第二章 梗阻性黄疸 / 475
第一节 恶性胆管梗阻 / 475
第二节 左肝外段低分化肝内胆管细胞癌 / 476
第三节 胆汁淤滞 / 476
第四节 梗阻性黄疸和门静脉钙化 / 482
第五节 假性肝外胆管梗阻 / 482
第六节 肝细胞性肝癌合并胆管癌栓 / 482
第七节 误诊病例简介:胆管黏液性乳头状腺癌 / 484
第八节 继发性肝内胆汁淤滞 / 484
第九节 黏胆症 / 484
第三章 良、恶性胆管梗阻的鉴别 / 485
第一节 MRI、超声、CT 对胆系良、恶性梗阻鉴别诊断的对比研究 / 485
第二节 胆管扩张的研究 / 486
第四章 胆管囊肿 / 488
第一节 肝外胆管憩室(Ⅱ型肝外胆管囊肿)/ 488
第二节 总胆管壁内囊肿 / 488
第三节 先天性肝内胆管囊肿 / 489
第四节 胆总管囊肿破裂 / 489
第五章 胆管肿块 / 490
第一节 假胆管癌征 / 490
第二节 原发性肝癌侵犯胆管 / 490
第三节 肝细胞性肝癌伴有胆管癌栓 / 490
第六章 肝内胆管细胞癌 / 491
第一节 误诊病例简介:肝内胆管细胞癌与肝脓肿 / 491
第二节 肝内胆管细胞癌,累及大网膜组织 / 492
第三节 肝细胞癌和肝内胆管细胞癌共存 / 492
第四节 肝内混合型癌(肝细胞癌 - 胆管细胞癌)/ 493
第五节 不同生长方式肝内胆管细胞癌的 CT 表现 / 494
第六节 原发性肝内胆管细胞癌与肝转移性肿瘤及胰腺癌 / 494
第七节 肝左内叶中分化肝内胆管细胞癌 / 494
第八节 左肝高分化肝内胆管细胞癌 / 495
第九节 囊性肝内胆管细胞癌与肝脓肿 / 496
第十节 右肝内胆管癌(乳头状腺癌)/ 497
第十一节 肝内胆管细胞癌淋巴结转移 / 498
第十二节 左肝外段胆管细胞癌 / 498
第十三节 左肝外叶肝内胆管腺癌,高分化,侵犯广泛 / 500
第十四节 肿块型胆管细胞癌 / 500
第十五节 肝内胆管细胞癌与转移性肝癌的鉴别 / 502
第十六节 左肝中分化胆管细胞癌 / 502
第七章 肝内胆管囊腺瘤和囊腺癌 / 504
第一节 肝内胆管囊腺癌 / 504
第二节 肝胆管囊腺瘤 / 506
第八章 肝内胆管乳头状肿瘤 / 507
第九章 先天性肝内胆管囊肿 / 509
第一节 先天性肝内胆管扩张(Caroli 病)/ 509
第二节 先天性肝内胆管囊性扩张症 / 510
第十章 肝内胆管其他疾病 / 511
第一节 胆管性错构瘤 / 511
第二节 左肝内胆管腺癌,高分化 / 512
第三节 肝内胆管成像中的误诊和诊断陷阱 / 514
第十一章 肝门胆管癌 / 515
第一节 肝门部浸润型胆管癌的早期诊断 / 515
第二节 肝门部胆管癌 MR 3D-VIBE 序列和 MRCP / 516

第三节　肝门部胆管癌与肝门肿大淋巴结 / 518
第四节　肝门胆管中分化腺癌 / 518
第五节　肝门胆管癌 MSCT 误诊 / 519
第十二章　肝门区其他疾病 / 521
第一节　肝门部肿瘤 MRI 误诊分析 / 521
第二节　PTC 检查时肝管汇合处的假性肿瘤 / 522
第三节　假胆管癌征 / 522
第十三章　肝外胆管肿块 / 523
第一节　肝外胆管细胞癌所致肝实质一过性密度差异 / 523
第二节　误诊病例简介：肝外胆管囊腺瘤与胆总管囊肿 / 524
第十四章　胆管结石 / 526
第一节　肝外胆管结石 MRCP 的表现 / 526
第二节　MRCP 结合 T_2WI 与 MSCT 诊断肝外胆管结石 / 527
第三节　胆管内的假结石 / 529
第四节　MSCT 胆系三维成像与胆管系统结石 / 529
第五节　胆管内未怀疑的结石 / 530
第六节　胆管结石的诊断陷阱和误诊 / 531
第七节　肝内胆管变异与胆管结石 / 531
第八节　黏胆症 / 533
第十五章　肝外胆管其他情况 / 534
第一节　胆总管十二指肠瘘 / 534
第二节　总胆管 - 十二指肠瘘并十二指肠溃疡 / 534
第三节　肝外胆管的正确识别 / 534
第四节　肝外胆管测量 / 535
第五节　肝外胆管胰上段 / 536
第六节　肝外胆管胰腺段 / 537
第七节　肝外胆管成像中的误诊 / 538
第八节　胆钙乳的动态观察 / 540
第十六章　胆管狭窄 / 541
第一节　慢性胰腺炎引起的胆管狭窄 / 541
第二节　手术损伤性胆管狭窄 / 542
第三节　胆管狭窄与异位血管压迫 / 543
第四节　胆管狭窄的误诊 / 544
第十七章　胆管先天异常和发育变异 / 545
第一节　胆管先天性异常 / 545
第二节　肝间管 / 545
第三节　先天性双胆管 / 546
第四节　MRCP 与发育变异 / 546
第五节　诊断陷阱 / 546
第十八章　原发性硬化性胆管炎 / 547
第十九章　胆系寄生虫病 / 551
第一节　胆系蛔虫病 / 551
第二节　肝吸虫胆管炎 / 552

第十七篇　胆囊疾病

第一章　胆囊癌 / 555
第一节　早期胆囊癌 / 555
第二节　误诊病例简介：直径 0.8cm 胆囊低分化腺癌，侵及浆膜层与胆囊结石 / 557
第三节　误诊病例简介：胆囊高分化胆管型腺癌 / 557
第四节　厚壁型胆囊癌与慢性胆囊炎鉴别 / 558
第五节　误诊病例简介：高密度胆囊癌与胆囊炎及胆囊结石 / 559
第六节　误诊病例简介：胆囊癌误诊为肝脓肿 / 560
第七节　误诊病例简介：胆囊癌与肝门胆管癌 / 560
第二章　胆囊神经内分泌癌 / 562
第三章　淋巴瘤与淋巴管瘤 / 564
第一节　胆囊黏膜相关淋巴组织型淋巴瘤 / 564
第二节　胆囊淋巴管瘤 / 564
第四章　肉芽肿性胆囊炎 / 566
第一节　黄色肉芽肿性胆囊炎误诊为胆囊癌 / 566
第二节　肉芽肿性胆囊炎（软斑病）/ 566
第三节　黄色肉芽肿性胆囊炎和厚壁型胆囊癌及误诊分析 / 567
第五章　胆囊腺肌增生症 / 569
第一节　胆囊腺肌增生症及误诊分析 / 569
第二节　胆囊腺肌增生症病例之一 / 573
第三节　胆囊腺肌增生症病例之二 / 573
第四节　慢性胆囊炎伴腺肌病及结石形成 / 574
第六章　胆囊其他肿块 / 575
第一节　胆囊胆甾醇沉积病 / 575
第二节　胆囊腺瘤 / 575
第三节　迷走胰腺 / 576
第四节　胆囊的假肿瘤 / 576
第五节　胆囊息肉 / 576
第六节　肝细胞癌侵犯胆囊 / 577
第七节　发生于胆囊的胃肠道外间质瘤 / 577
第七章　胆囊结石 / 578
第一节　单能量成像及能谱曲线与胆囊等密度胆固醇结石 / 578
第二节　漂浮结石 / 579
第三节　肺内胆石 / 579
第四节　同一胆囊内各种类型结石 / 579

第五节 CT 对胆石化学性质预测 / 580
第六节 胆肠瘘伴结石性肠梗阻 / 581
第七节 胆囊结石化学类型 / 581
第八节 X 线检查胆囊结石进入胃壁和胃腔 / 582
第九节 胆石性肠梗阻 / 582
第十节 假性胆囊结石 / 583
第十一节 Mirizzi 综合征 / 584
第八章 胆囊炎症 / 585
第一节 误诊病例简介:胆囊结石并胆囊结核与胆囊癌 / 585
第二节 肝局灶性结节增生,慢性胆囊炎伴多发胆固醇息肉 / 585
第三节 胆囊结核 / 586
第四节 慢性坏疽性胆囊炎伴结石形成 / 587
第五节 钙胆汁(乳状胆汁)/ 588
第九章 胆囊壁的其他情况 / 589
第一节 胆囊的连接皱襞 / 589
第二节 超声和 CT 所见胆囊壁的厚度 / 589
第三节 慢性乙型肝炎患者胆囊壁水肿 / 589
第四节 误诊病例简介:胆囊穿孔、腹腔包裹性积液误诊肝包虫 / 590
第十章 胆囊发育变异和先天异常 / 591
第一节 胆囊形态变异和异常 / 591
第二节 胆囊结构变异和异常 / 592
第三节 胆囊数目的变异和异常 / 593
第四节 假的双胆囊 / 594
第五节 胆囊位置的变异和异常 / 594
第六节 胆囊大小的异常 / 596
第十一章 胆囊创伤与胆囊术后 / 597
第一节 腹腔镜胆囊切除术的并发症 / 597
第二节 诊断陷阱:胆囊切除术后银夹 / 597
第三节 误诊病例简介:胆囊切除术后,肝内胆管细胞癌与炎症性纤维增生 / 597
第十二章 胆囊其他疾病和诊断陷阱 / 599
第一节 胆囊的假肿瘤 / 599
第二节 胆囊核素显像的假阴性 / 599
第三节 超声扫描中的假胆囊 / 599
第四节 胆囊内众多小的回声区 / 599
第五节 胆囊的影像学检查及诊断陷阱 / 599

第十八篇 胆囊管疾病

第一章 胆囊管疾病 / 603
第一节 胆囊管发育变异及病变 / 603
第二节 胆囊管疾病 / 604
第三节 胆囊管疾病影像学检查 / 606
第四节 胆囊管 MRCP / 609
第五节 误诊病例简介:胆囊管与胆钙乳 / 610
第二章 胆囊管的发育变异和先天性异常 / 612
第一节 胆囊管的发育变异和先天性异常 / 612
第二节 胆囊管的活体形态学 / 616
第三节 胆囊管先天异常 / 617
第四节 先天性胆囊及胆囊管缺如 / 618
第五节 胆囊管发育变异 / 618
第六节 胆囊管低位汇入综合征 / 620
第三章 Mirizzi 综合征 / 624
第一节 Mirizzi 综合征之一 / 624
第二节 Mirizzi 综合征之二 / 628
第四章 关于胆囊管残端 / 629
第一节 胆囊管残端 - 十二指肠瘘 / 629
第二节 再显性胆囊 / 629
第三节 胆囊管残端与胆囊管低位汇入 / 630

第十九篇 胆胰管十二指肠连接区疾病

第一章 胆管低位梗阻 / 633
第一节 低位梗阻性黄疸的分型 / 633
第二节 胆管低位梗阻 CT 诊断标准 / 634
第三节 低位梗阻性黄疸病因病理 / 634
第四节 胆胰管连接区梗阻 / 635
第五节 十二指肠壁内胆胰共同管内异位胰腺致梗阻性黄疸 / 636
第六节 胆管下端高分化胆管型腺癌 / 637
第七节 MRCP 双管征的讨论 / 638
第八节 胆胰管括约肌段狭窄 / 640
第九节 胆胰管十二指肠连接区梗阻鉴别诊断 / 640
第十节 假胆管癌征 / 642
第二章 胆胰管十二指肠连接区癌 / 643
第一节 胆胰管十二指肠连接区癌 / 643
第二节 胆胰共同管周围癌 / 645
第三节 “壶腹”周围癌 / 647
第四节 胆胰管十二指肠连接区高中分化腺癌 / 648
第五节 胆胰管十二指肠连接区癌 / 649
第六节 共同管癌 / 655
第七节 胆管下端小的高分化胆管型腺癌 / 656
第八节 误诊和漏诊病例简介:胆胰共同管周围高中分化腺癌 / 657

第三章 胆胰管十二指肠连接区其他肿瘤 / 658
第一节 胆胰共同管的腺瘤及有关问题 / 658
第二节 十二指肠乳头肿瘤样表现的鉴别诊断 / 659
第三节 括约肌区域病变分类 / 660
第四节 胆胰共同管肿瘤分类 / 660
第五节 胆胰共同管错构瘤 / 661
第四章 十二指肠乳头及乳头区憩室 / 662
第一节 MRCP 诊断乳头区憩室综合征 / 662
第二节 乳头区憩室和憩室内乳头 / 663
第五章 胆胰管十二指肠连接区结石 / 670
第一节 胆胰管十二指肠连接区结石 / 670
第二节 结石的影像学研究 / 671
第三节 胰头区的高密度影 / 673
第六章 胆胰管下端括约肌闭锁不全 / 674
第一节 新生儿胆胰管下端括约肌闭锁不全 / 674
第二节 成人胆胰管下端括约肌闭锁不全 / 674
第三节 十二指肠 - 胆系逆流的少见原因 / 674
第四节 胆胰管下端括约肌闭锁不全鉴别诊断 / 675
第七章 胆胰管下端括约肌段狭窄 / 676
第一节 胆胰管括约肌段狭窄 / 676
第二节 括约肌段狭窄的影像诊断 / 678
第三节 括约肌段的良性狭窄 / 678
第四节 胆胰共同管假性肿瘤 / 678
第八章 胆胰共同管及其周围疾病 / 679
第一节 胆胰共同管周围病变 / 679
第二节 胆胰共同管假性肿瘤 / 684
第三节 PTCD 术中对比剂胰管逆流与共同管的关系探讨 / 684
第四节 共同管的暂时性水肿或痉挛 / 686
第五节 共同管区的误诊 / 686
第六节 十二指肠壁内胆胰共同管内异位胰腺致梗阻性黄疸 / 686
第九章 连接区的检查技术 / 687
第一节 MRCP 与低位梗阻定位、定性 / 687
第二节 脂餐和胰泌素刺激后的 MRCP / 688
第十章 胆胰管异常连接 / 689
第一节 胆胰管异常连接与 MRCP / 689
第二节 关于胆胰管异常连接的形成 / 691
第三节 胆胰管异常连接 / 691
第四节 胆胰管异常连接合并胆管扩张 / 695
第五节 胆胰管异常连接与胆囊管最低位汇入总肝管 / 696
第六节 十二指肠乳头异位与胆胰管异常连接 / 698
第七节 PTCD 术中对比剂胰管逆流与共同管的关系探讨 / 699
第八节 胆胰管异常连接合并胰腺融合畸形 / 699
第九节 胆胰管异常连接合并胰管环状重复畸形 / 699
第十节 胆胰管汇合情况与急性胰腺炎发病关系的研究 / 700

第二十篇 胰腺疾病

第一章 关于胰腺肿瘤 / 703
第一节 诊断陷阱:酷似原发性胰腺肿瘤的胰腺及胰周疾病 / 703
第二节 浸润性胰腺导管腺癌,高分化 / 704
第三节 胰腺肿瘤的分类 / 705
第四节 易与原发性胰腺肿瘤混淆的胰和胰周疾病 / 705
第五节 胰腺实性假乳头状肿瘤(SPN)/ 709
第二章 早期胰癌与小胰癌 / 710
第一节 关于早期胰癌与小胰癌 / 710
第二节 早期胰腺癌 / 710
第三节 关于小胰癌 / 713
第四节 有关钩突的病变 / 714
第三章 胰腺癌的术前分期与手术切除性评价 / 715
第一节 不可切除的主要原因 / 715
第二节 胰头癌周围淋巴结转移 / 716
第三节 远处转移灶 / 717
第四节 术前分期 / 717
第五节 胰腺低分化癌伴坏死,侵犯脾脏 / 717
第四章 胰腺癌 / 719
第一节 误诊病例简介:胰腺中低分化囊性腺癌与间质瘤 / 719
第二节 胰腺导管腺癌,Ⅱ级 / 720
第三节 中低分化胰腺导管腺癌,侵及十二指肠黏膜下层 / 721
第四节 胰腺间变细胞癌 / 722
第五节 表现为囊性肿块的胰腺癌 / 723
第六节 胰颈中高分化腺癌伴大量坏死 / 723
第七节 胰头腺癌 / 724
第五章 胰腺的部分影像学检查 / 725
第一节 逆行胰管造影术中的充盈缺损原因 / 725
第二节 胰腺疾病中不熟悉的 X 线征象 / 726
第三节 胰腺超声检查的误诊 / 726
第六章 MRI、CT 与胰腺癌 / 727

第一节 3.0 T MR 不同扩散加权成像与胰腺癌 / 727
第二节 误诊病例简介:胰腺癌与实性假乳头状瘤 / 728
第三节 误诊病例简介:胰腺中低分化囊性腺癌,侵及十二指肠黏膜下层 / 729
第七章 CT、MRI 以外的其他影像学检查 / 731
第八章 胰腺癌的综合诊断 / 732
第一节 胰腺癌的综合诊断 / 732
第二节 MR 多种成像技术综合诊断 / 733
第九章 胰腺癌的鉴别诊断 / 735
第一节 假肿瘤性慢性胰腺炎 / 735
第二节 误诊病例简介 / 736
第三节 慢性胰腺炎误诊为胰腺癌 / 736
第四节 误诊病例简介:胃与十二指肠交界处慢性炎性增生团块与胰头癌 / 738
第五节 胰腺癌和炎性胰腺肿块鉴别 / 739
第六节 胰腺癌与慢性胰腺炎鉴别诊断 / 740
第七节 胰头部肿块型慢性胰腺炎 / 741
第八节 胰十二指肠沟区病变的鉴别诊断 / 742
第十章 胰腺囊性病变 / 747
第一节 胰腺囊性肿瘤 CT 诊断与处理对策 / 747
第二节 胰腺囊性病变钙化 / 747
第三节 关于胰腺囊性病变 / 748
第四节 误诊病例简介:胰腺癌被误诊为胰腺囊腺癌 / 748
第十一章 胰腺囊腺瘤与囊腺癌 / 750
第一节 CT 能谱成像鉴别胰腺寡囊型浆液性囊腺瘤与黏液性囊性肿瘤 / 750
第二节 浆液性囊腺瘤 / 751
第三节 胰体浆液性囊腺瘤 / 751
第四节 小囊性囊腺瘤,大囊性囊腺瘤或腺癌 / 752
第五节 胰体尾浆液性微囊性腺瘤 / 752
第六节 胰腺先天性囊肿 / 753
第七节 胰管黏液囊性瘤的导管淤积变型 / 753
第八节 胰腺浆液性囊腺瘤病例 / 753
第九节 浆液性囊腺瘤与黏液性囊性肿瘤的鉴别 / 753
第十节 胰腺浆液性囊腺瘤 / 754
第十一节 胰腺黏液性囊腺瘤 / 755
第十二节 误诊病例简介:胰腺浆液性囊腺瘤与扩张的主胰管 / 757
第十二章 胰腺假性囊肿 / 758
第一节 位于纵隔的胰腺假性囊肿 / 758
第二节 胰腺假性囊肿表现类似肾囊肿或肾周囊肿及脓肿 / 758
第三节 胰腺假性囊肿对肾脏的犯及 / 758
第四节 胰腺假性囊肿的自发性内引流 / 759
第五节 胰腺假性囊肿 / 759
第六节 其他少见部位的胰腺假性囊肿 / 760
第七节 胰腺假性囊肿的并发症 / 760
第八节 胰腺假性囊肿与左肾 / 761
第九节 胰腺假性囊肿蛋壳状钙化 / 761
第十节 不典型部位胰腺假性囊肿与 CT / 761
第十一节 误诊为胰腺假性囊肿的一些情况 / 762
第十二节 胰腺假性囊肿 / 763
第十三节 胰腺假性囊肿的动态变化 / 763
第十三章 胰腺导管内乳头状黏液性肿瘤 / 764
第一节 MSCT 及 MRI 对胰腺导管内乳头状黏液性肿瘤的诊断 / 764
第二节 胰腺导管内良、恶性黏蛋白性肿瘤的 MRCP 鉴别诊断 / 765
第十四章 胰腺实性假乳头状瘤和胰腺实性假乳头状癌 / 767
第一节 胰腺实性假乳头状瘤肝转移 / 767
第二节 胰腺实性假乳头状瘤 / 768
第三节 误诊病例简介:胰腺乳头状囊性肿瘤 / 768
第四节 胰腺实性假乳头状肿瘤 / 769
第五节 胰腺实性假乳头状瘤误诊分析 / 769
第六节 误诊病例简介:胰头实性假乳头状肿瘤与胰腺假性囊肿 / 771
第七节 胰腺实性假乳头状瘤与恶性胰腺实性假乳头状瘤 / 772
第八节 胰腺囊实性乳头状瘤误诊分析 / 773
第九节 胰腺实性假乳头状肿瘤(SPN)/ 773
第十节 胰腺实性假乳头状瘤典型与不典型表现 / 774
第十一节 胰腺实性假乳头状瘤误诊讨论 / 775
第十五章 胰腺内分泌肿瘤 / 777
第一节 胰岛素瘤 MRI 漏诊 / 777
第二节 胰腺小功能性腺瘤的检出:MR 成像序列选择 / 778
第十六章 胰腺神经内分泌肿瘤 / 780
第一节 胰腺神经内分泌肿瘤的良、恶性 / 780
第二节 胰腺神经内分泌肿瘤,肝脏转移性胰腺神经内分泌肿瘤 / 782
第三节 胰腺类癌 / 782
第四节 胰腺神经内分泌肿瘤转移至肝脏和周围淋巴结 / 784
第十七章 胰腺其他恶性肿瘤 / 786

第一节 胰腺单发转移瘤与胰腺癌的 CT 鉴别诊断 / 786
第二节 误诊病例简介:肾癌胰腺转移瘤 / 787
第三节 胰腺巨大非霍奇金 B 细胞淋巴瘤,倾向 Burkitt 淋巴瘤 / 787
第四节 胰腺转移瘤 / 788
第五节 误诊病例简介:起源于胰腺的孤立性纤维瘤 / 789

第十八章 胰腺其他包块 / 790
第一节 误诊病例简介:胰腺结核与胰腺癌 / 790
第二节 假肿瘤性慢性胰腺炎 / 791
第三节 误诊病例简介:胰头神经鞘瘤与胰头癌 / 792
第四节 误诊病例简介:胰腺内异位副脾 / 793
第五节 胰腺的假性肿瘤 / 794
第六节 误诊病例简介:脾脏破裂伴出血,胰体尾部及胃后壁之间侵袭性纤维瘤病 / 795

第十九章 胰腺先天异常和发育变异 / 796
第一节 胰腺分裂与诊断陷阱 / 796
第二节 成人完全性环状胰腺并急性胰腺炎 / 796
第三节 环状胰腺和半环状胰腺 / 797
第四节 误诊病例简介:异位胰腺与胃肠间质瘤 / 797
第五节 误诊病例简介:胃异位胰腺囊腺癌 / 797
第六节 误诊病例简介:胃体小弯异位胰腺与固有肌层间质瘤 / 798
第七节 背侧胰腺发育不全和假性发育不全 / 799
第八节 消化道异位胰腺 / 799
第九节 迷走胰腺或副胰及误诊漏诊分析 / 800
第十节 异位胰腺肿瘤 / 802
第十一节 背胰发育变异 / 804
第十二节 误诊病例简介:小肠脂肪瘤伴异位胰腺致小肠套叠 / 804

第二十章 胰腺其他囊性疾病 / 805
第一节 胰腺囊实性乳头状瘤误诊分析 / 805
第二节 误诊病例简介:胰腺乳头状囊性肿瘤 / 806
第三节 胰腺囊性畸胎瘤 / 806
第四节 其他胰腺恶性或潜在恶性囊性肿瘤 / 806
第五节 胰腺囊性病变钙化 / 807
第六节 胰管黏液囊性瘤的导管淤积变型 / 807
第七节 胰腺先天性囊性病变 / 808
第八节 胰腺囊性和囊实性病例误诊分析 / 808

第二十一章 重症急性胰腺炎 / 810
第一节 重症急性胰腺炎的影像分类 / 810
第二节 胰管中断综合征 / 811

第二十二章 急性胰腺炎 / 813
第一节 胆胰管汇合与急性胰腺炎 / 813
第二节 急性胰腺炎对肝脏损害的 CT 观察 / 814

第二十三章 自身免疫性胰腺炎 / 815
第一节 IgG4 相关自身免疫性胰腺炎误诊为胰腺癌 / 815
第二节 IgG4 相关疾病的影像学表现 / 816

第二十四章 胆源性胰腺炎 / 819

第二十五章 胰腺结石和胰腺钙化 / 821
第一节 胰腺结石 / 821
第二节 胰腺结石与胰腺癌 / 823
第三节 胰腺结石并发胰癌 / 824
第四节 胰腺钙化的区别诊断 / 824
第五节 胰腺囊性病变钙化 / 825

第二十六章 胰腺结核 / 826
第一节 误诊病例简介:胰腺结核与胰腺癌 / 826
第二节 极易误诊的胰腺结核 / 826
第三节 胰腺结核的诊断思维 / 827
第四节 胰腺结核 / 828

第二十七章 慢性胰腺炎 / 829
第一节 三种慢性胰腺炎 / 829
第二节 有关慢性胰腺炎的诊断标准 / 829
第三节 CT 检查中胰管扩张的意义 / 829
第四节 假肿瘤性慢性胰腺炎 / 830
第五节 误诊病例简介:慢性胰腺炎所致的良性病变与恶性肿瘤 / 830
第六节 自身免疫性胰腺炎 / 831
第七节 误诊病例简介:胰体尾部慢性胰腺炎与胰体尾部肿瘤 / 831

第二十八章 关于糖尿病 / 832
第一节 糖尿病胰腺的密度、轮廓和厚度 / 832
第二节 脂肪萎缩性糖尿病 / 832

第二十九章 关于胰腺周围血管 / 834

第三十章 MRCP 与胆胰疾病 / 837

第三十一章 胰腺创伤及手术后 / 840
第一节 胰腺断裂 / 840
第二节 假性胰腺折断 / 840
第三节 胰十二指肠切除术后改变 / 840

第三十二章 与胰腺有关的周围组织疾病及全身性疾病 / 841
第一节 周围病变累及胰头与胰头 - 连接区癌累及周围结构的 CT 鉴别诊断 / 841
第二节 位于纵隔的胰腺假性囊肿 / 842
第三节 坏死性脂膜炎 / 842

第四节 胰十二指肠沟区疾病及其鉴别诊断 / 842
第三十三章 胰腺疾病的一些诊断陷阱 / 843
第一节 胰腺脂肪浸润 / 843
第二节 胰腺脂肪裂和胰腺假性破裂 / 843
第三节 胰腺超声检查的误诊 / 844
第四节 CT 部分诊断陷阱 / 844
第五节 假性胰腺折断 / 844
第六节 假胰管 / 844
第七节 易与原发胰腺肿瘤混淆的胰和胰周疾病 / 845
第八节 诊断陷阱:酷似原发性胰腺肿瘤一些影像学表现 / 845
第九节 胰腺移植可能造成的诊断陷阱 / 846
第三十四章 胰腺活体形态学研究 / 847
第一节 胰腺大小和形状 / 847
第二节 老年人的胰腺 / 847

第二十一篇 脾脏疾病

第一章 脾脏占位性病变与脾脏肿瘤 / 851
第一节 脾脏肿瘤及误诊病例 / 851
第二节 误诊病例简介:脾脏上皮样血管内皮瘤合并肝和肾上腺囊肿 / 852
第三节 误诊病例简介:脾脏纤维瘤病 / 852
第二章 脾脏错构瘤 / 854
第一节 脾脏错构瘤 / 854
第二节 误诊病例简介:脾脏错构瘤与血管瘤 / 855
第三章 脾脏炎性假瘤 / 856
第一节 脾脏炎性假瘤 / 856
第二节 脾原发性炎性肌成纤维细胞瘤 / 857
第四章 脾恶性肿瘤 / 858
第一节 脾淋巴瘤 / 858
第二节 脾血管肉瘤 / 859
第三节 脾非霍奇金 B 细胞淋巴瘤 / 860
第四节 脾脏恶性纤维组织细胞瘤 / 860
第五节 恶性组织细胞病 / 861
第六节 脾转移瘤 / 861
第七节 脾脏 B 细胞淋巴瘤,累及胰腺和肾上腺 / 862
第五章 脾脏淋巴管瘤 / 864
第一节 不常见 CT 增强表现的脾脏海绵状淋巴管瘤 / 864
第二节 脾脏海绵状淋巴管瘤的不典型影像学表现 / 864
第三节 误诊病例分析:脾血管淋巴管瘤与淋巴瘤或转移性肿瘤 / 866
第六章 关于脾脏病变 / 867
第一节 脾脏病变 / 867
第二节 脾多灶性病变及误诊分析 / 868
第七章 脾窦岸细胞血管瘤 / 870
第一节 脾窦岸细胞血管瘤 / 870
第二节 脾硬化性血管瘤样结节性转化 / 871
第八章 脾硬化性血管瘤样结节性转化 / 872
第一节 误诊病例介绍:脾脏硬化性血管瘤样结节性转化 / 872
第二节 误诊病例介绍:脾脏硬化性血管瘤样结节性转化与血管肉瘤、淋巴瘤 / 873
第九章 其他脾血管性疾病 / 875
第一节 脾动脉瘤与胃出血 / 875
第二节 Klippel-Trenaunay 综合征伴脾血管瘤 / 875
第三节 治疗性脾动脉栓塞与腹腔内游离气体 / 875
第十章 脾囊性病变 / 876
第一节 脾脏表皮样囊肿 / 876
第二节 多发脾假性囊肿伴钙化 / 876
第三节 脾脏内的胰腺假性囊肿 / 877
第四节 先天性脾囊肿 / 877
第五节 出血性脾假性囊肿 / 877
第十一章 脾脏创伤 / 878
第一节 CT 图像上的假性脾破裂 / 878
第二节 误诊病例简介:脾脏破裂伴出血,胰体尾部及胃后壁之间侵袭性纤维瘤病 / 878
第三节 外伤性膈疝和脾的疝入 / 879
第四节 自发性脾破裂 / 879
第五节 脾外伤诊断的一次教训 / 879
第十二章 脾的发育变异和先天异常 / 880
第一节 副脾与诊断陷阱 / 880
第二节 脾活体位置与体型关系 / 880
第三节 病理误诊病例简介:副脾伴大量钙化与淋巴瘤 / 881
第四节 胰腺内副脾 / 881
第五节 副脾有关误诊分析 / 882
第六节 倒置的脾 / 883
第七节 CT 图像上的假性脾破裂 / 883
第八节 脾组织的分叶和切迹 / 883
第九节 活体脾的大小和重量的变异 / 884
第十节 脾形状发育变异引起的混淆 / 884
第十一节 脾脏位置变异 / 885
第十三章 游走脾及其疾病 / 886
第一节 游走脾与腹部包块 / 886

第二节 游走脾合并脾扭转 / 886
第三节 游走脾与脾梗死 / 887
第四节 游走脾影像学检查 / 887
第十四章 脾脏感染性疾病 / 888
第一节 脾脏结核 / 888
第二节 胃内金属异物穿破胃刺入脾引发脾脓肿 / 889
第三节 胰腺炎的脾实质并发症 / 889
第四节 肝脾结核 / 890
第十五章 脾脏增大(脾肿大) / 891
第一节 脾肿大与急性胰腺炎 / 891
第二节 脾结节病 / 891
第三节 饮水以后脾体积的变化 / 892
第四节 脾肿大指数 / 892
第五节 脾肿大的其他重要原因 / 892
第十六章 脾种植 / 893
第一节 腹部脾组织植入 / 893
第二节 误诊病例简介:胸壁异位种植脾 / 894
第三节 大网膜内部分脾自体移植术后观察 / 894
第十七章 脾脏其他疾病 / 896
第一节 胸内脾功能亢进 / 896
第二节 脾假性囊肿与脾的钙化 / 896
第三节 脾妊娠 / 896
第十八章 脾影像诊断的一些陷阱 / 897
第一节 不均匀强化 / 897
第二节 正常的脾门脂肪伪似脾内病变 / 897
第三节 脾切除术后真、假性包块的超声诊断 / 897
第四节 CT 扫描及一些诊断陷阱 / 898
第五节 经动脉门静脉血管造影 CT(CTAP)的脾灌注缺损 / 898
第六节 脾的假性病变 / 898
第七节 诊断陷阱:脾肺固定术后 / 899
第八节 MRI 的一些诊断陷阱 / 899

第二十二篇 腹盆部多器官多系统疾

第一章 免疫缺陷疾病 / 903
第二章 自身免疫性疾病 / 908
第三章 腹部淋巴瘤 / 909
第一节 原发性胃肠道淋巴瘤及误诊分析 / 909
第二节 胃肠道假性淋巴瘤 / 910
第三节 黏膜相关性淋巴样组织淋巴瘤 / 910
第四节 弥漫性大 B 细胞淋巴瘤侵犯肠道、肾上腺、腹膜及腹膜后 / 910
第四章 胃肠道间叶组织肿瘤 / 912
第一节 胃肠道间质瘤的误诊和漏诊 / 912
第二节 胃肠道间质瘤误诊及漏诊病例简介 / 913
第三节 空肠胃肠道间质瘤 / 914
第四节 十二指肠球部远端胃肠道间质瘤(极低危险度) / 915
第五章 腹部其他恶性肿瘤 / 916
第六章 腹盆部其他肿瘤 / 917
第一节 上皮内瘤样病变 / 917
第二节 表现较为特殊的腹内侵袭性纤维瘤病 / 918
第三节 腹部不典型神经鞘瘤 / 919
第七章 胃肠道疾病 / 921
第一节 误诊病例简介:血友病患者之胃肠壁内病变与胃窦癌及胃壁血肿 / 921
第二节 胃肠道的假性病变 / 921
第三节 钡剂被覆不良或胃肠扩张不佳 / 921
第四节 胃弥漫浸润型低分化腺癌 / 922
第五节 胃肠道假性淋巴瘤 / 922
第六节 胃肠淋巴增生呈现少见的脐样息肉病变 / 922
第七节 诊断陷阱: CT 图像上一些情况类似胃肠病变 / 923
第八节 吻壁现象 / 923
第九节 不同检查方法的误诊教训 / 924
第八章 胃肠道炎症 / 925
第一节 嗜酸细胞性胃肠炎 / 925
第二节 胃肠道结核 / 926
第三节 嗜酸性粒细胞性胃肠炎 / 927
第九章 克罗恩病 / 929
第十章 胃肠道息肉 / 932
第一节 胃肠道息肉病综合征 / 932
第二节 胃肠道假性息肉 / 932
第十一章 腹部手术后改变 / 934
第一节 Billroth Ⅰ式术后改变 / 934
第二节 Billroth Ⅱ式术后改变 / 934
第三节 贲门胃底切除术后改变 / 934
第四节 全胃切除术后改变 / 934
第五节 胰十二指肠切除术后改变 / 934
第六节 术后缺损或术后假肿瘤 / 935
第七节 近期造口、吻合术等造成的误诊 / 935
第十二章 腹部淋巴结及肿瘤转移 / 936
第一节 淋巴结转移是胃癌转移的主要方式 / 936
第二节 淋巴结和淋巴滤泡的发育变异 / 936
第十三章 腹盆部其他疾病 / 937
第一节 消化道出血的常见病因及其 DSA 诊断 / 937

第二节 胃肠出血的部分原因 / 938
第三节 胃肠和肠系膜的创伤 / 938
第四节 胃肠道内异物 / 939
第五节 误诊病例简介:肠系膜、网膜及淋巴结结核与小肠间质瘤 / 940
第六节 胃肠道充盈缺损较难见到的原因 / 940
第七节 胃肠淋巴增生呈现少见的脐样息肉病变 / 941

第二十三篇 胃的疾病

第一章 胃癌术前分期 / 945
第一节 MSCT 对胃癌分期误诊病例分析简介(过度分期与分期不足)/ 945
第二节 国际抗癌联盟及美国癌症联合会胃癌 TNM 分期系统(第 8 版)影像相关更新解读 / 945
第二章 胃癌分型 / 948
第三章 关于进展期胃癌 / 949
第一节 进展期胃癌手术可根治性的 CT 评估 / 949
第二节 进展期胃癌与胃淋巴瘤鉴别 / 950
第三节 胃弥漫浸润型低分化腺癌 / 951
第四章 早期胃癌和肿瘤血管生成 / 953
第一节 早期胃癌影像学诊断 / 953
第二节 误诊病例简介:胃小弯印戒细胞癌与胃窦壁稍增厚 / 955
第五章 胃癌的转移 / 956
第一节 胃癌的淋巴结转移 / 956
第二节 淋巴结转移是胃癌的主要转移途径 / 956
第三节 误诊病例简介:以阻塞淋巴管、深静脉为首发症状的右肩转移性胃癌 / 958
第六章 胃癌部分检查技术 / 959
第一节 漏诊病例简介:临床要求与全面观察 / 959
第二节 MSCT 在胃癌诊断中的临床应用 / 959
第七章 胃癌的少见表现 / 962
第一节 钙化性胃癌 / 962
第二节 胃癌合并胃脂肪瘤 / 963
第三节 胃癌与十二指肠溃疡同存 / 963
第八章 胃淋巴瘤 / 964
第一节 胃的孤立性霍奇金病 / 964
第二节 进展期胃癌与胃淋巴瘤鉴别 / 964
第三节 误诊病例简介:胃非霍奇金 B 细胞淋巴瘤与胃溃疡 / 964
第九章 胃间质瘤 / 966
第一节 胃肠道间质瘤的 CT / 966
第二节 胃肠道间质瘤(低危险度)/ 967
第三节 胃底胃肠道间质瘤(低危险度)/ 967
第四节 胃间质瘤良、恶性区别研究 / 968
第五节 胃底胃肠道间质瘤(低危险度)/ 969
第六节 转移性胃间质瘤 / 969
第七节 胃底小的胃肠道间质瘤 / 970
第十章 其他胃恶性肿瘤 / 972
第一节 胃类癌 / 972
第二节 胃低度恶性肌成纤维细胞肉瘤 / 972
第三节 胃粒状细胞肌胚细胞瘤 / 973
第四节 误诊病例简介:胃神经内分泌瘤与间质瘤 / 974
第五节 原发性胃恶性黑色素瘤 / 974
第六节 误诊病例简介:胃体部神经内分泌肿瘤(类癌)与平滑肌瘤伴大溃疡 / 975
第七节 胃原发外周原始神经外胚叶肿瘤 / 975
第十一章 胃其他肿瘤和囊肿 / 977
第一节 胃脂肪瘤与 CT / 977
第二节 胃粒状细胞肌胚细胞瘤 / 977
第三节 误诊病例简介:胃底梭形细胞肿瘤与胃息肉 / 977
第四节 胃癌合并胃脂肪瘤 / 978
第五节 胃血管瘤 / 978
第六节 误诊病例简介:胃体神经鞘瘤与胃窦黏膜腺癌 / 979
第七节 误诊病例简介:胃窦部神经鞘瘤与间质瘤 / 979
第八节 胃底平滑肌瘤 / 980
第九节 胃少见的原发性肿瘤及误诊分析 / 980
第十节 胃窦囊肿 / 982
第十一节 胃窦后壁巨大息肉脱垂入空肠 / 983
第十二节 胃底胃肠道间质瘤 / 983
第十二章 关于胃黏膜 / 985
第一节 胃黏膜的乳头样形状变异 / 985
第二节 胃底平滑肌瘤病例 / 985
第三节 胃窦的黏膜隔 / 985
第四节 误诊病例简介:胃体小弯异位胰腺与间质瘤 / 985
第五节 一些诊断陷阱 / 986
第十三章 胃的炎症 / 987
第一节 息肉型胃炎与胃癌 / 987
第二节 诊断困难的放射治疗后的胃炎 / 987
第十四章 消化道出血与胃 / 988
第一节 肿块状胃壁静脉曲张 / 988
第二节 胃间质瘤伴出血 / 989
第三节 Dieulafoy 病 / 990

第十五章 胃的假性病变 / 991
第一节 误诊病例简介:青少年胃反应性结节性纤维性假瘤误诊为胃恶性肿瘤 / 991
第二节 胃的假瘤 / 992
第三节 CT 诊断陷阱之一:胃底和胃憩室及充盈液体的脏器 / 992
第四节 幽门管与贲门星 / 992
第五节 关于瀑布胃的诊断陷阱 / 992
第六节 胃反应性结节状纤维性假瘤 / 993
第七节 胃的假性溃疡 / 994
第十六章 关于胃的血管 / 995
第一节 CTA 显示胃周动脉及其变异 / 995
第二节 胃的动脉性压迹 / 995
第三节 肿块状胃壁静脉曲张 / 996
第四节 胃静脉曲张的诊断陷阱 / 996
第十七章 胃的其他疾病 / 997
第一节 误诊病例简介:胃结核 / 997
第二节 胃支气管瘘 / 997
第三节 胃异位胰腺 / 997
第四节 胃肠道间质瘤,伴黏液样变性 / 998
第五节 植物性胃石与肠梗阻 / 998
第六节 牙刷穿透胃壁致右髂窝脓肿 / 1000
第七节 胃窦局限性血管炎 / 1000
第八节 关于胃壁增厚 / 1001
第九节 误诊病例简介:胃黏膜下巨大陈旧性血肿与左上腹囊液性肿块性质待定 / 1002
第十节 误诊病例简介:异物导致慢性胃穿孔与胃窦占位 / 1002
第十一节 诊断陷阱:胃底憩室与左侧肾上腺区疾病 / 1003
第十二节 一些诊断陷阱 / 1003
第十八章 胃手术后 / 1005
第一节 Biliroth Ⅰ式术后改变 / 1005
第二节 Billroth Ⅱ式术后改变 / 1005
第三节 贲门胃底切除术后改变 / 1006
第四节 全胃切除术后改变 / 1006
第五节 胃术后缝合处的肉芽肿 / 1006
第六节 胃大部切除术后假性肿瘤变形 / 1007

第二十四篇 十二指肠

第一章 十二指肠恶性肿瘤 / 1011
第一节 十二指肠恶性淋巴瘤 / 1011
第二节 误诊病例简介:十二指肠空肠低分化癌或肉瘤样癌与肠壁血肿 / 1011
第三节 原发性十二指肠癌及误诊分析 / 1013
第四节 十二指肠平滑肌肉瘤 / 1015
第五节 十二指肠弥漫性大 B 细胞淋巴瘤 / 1015
第二章 十二指肠间质瘤 / 1017
第一节 十二指肠间质瘤 MSCT / 1017
第二节 十二指肠球部胃肠道间质瘤 / 1018
第三节 十二指肠胃肠道间质瘤 / 1019
第三章 十二指肠肿块 / 1020
第一节 非乳头区十二指肠肿瘤 / 1020
第二节 关于十二指肠肿瘤 CT 检查注意事项 / 1021
第三节 十二指肠上部肿瘤及肿瘤样病变 / 1021
第四节 十二指肠血管瘤 / 1023
第五节 十二指肠的假性息肉 / 1023
第六节 十二指肠袢伪似脓肿 / 1023
第七节 邻近的肠袢 / 1023
第四章 十二指肠乳头 / 1024
第一节 十二指肠乳头癌 / 1024
第二节 十二指肠乳头异位与胆胰管合流异常的相关性分析 / 1025
第五章 关于十二指肠溃疡 / 1026
第一节 胃癌与十二指肠溃疡同存 / 1026
第二节 十二指肠慢性溃疡合并梗阻性黄疸 / 1026
第六章 十二指肠乳头区憩室 / 1027
第一节 十二指肠乳头旁憩室 / 1027
第二节 误诊病例简介:十二指肠腔内憩室 / 1028
第三节 诊断陷阱:十二指肠乳头旁憩室与胆胰管下端恶性占位性病变 / 1029
第四节 乳头区憩室和憩室内乳头 / 1029
第七章 十二指肠梗阻和狭窄 / 1030
第一节 十二指肠结石性梗阻 / 1030
第二节 十二指肠外压性狭窄 / 1030
第三节 弯曲引起的狭窄 / 1031
第四节 十二指肠结核 / 1031
第五节 十二指肠淤积症 / 1031
第六节 十二指肠的占位性病变 / 1032
第八章 十二指肠先天异常与发育变异 / 1033
第一节 先天性巨十二指肠 / 1033
第二节 巨大十二指肠重复畸形 / 1033
第三节 成人完全性环状胰腺并急性胰腺炎 / 1034
第四节 十二指肠一些发育变异 / 1034
第九章 十二指肠创伤 / 1035
第一节 十二指肠肠壁内血肿 / 1035

第二节 十二指肠壁内血肿 / 1036
第十章 十二指肠瘘 / 1037
第十一章 十二指肠其他疾病 / 1038
第一节 右侧十二指肠旁疝 / 1038
第二节 十二指肠结石 / 1038
第三节 十二指肠邻近病变 / 1039
第四节 十二指肠弯曲部假性病变 / 1039
第五节 胆囊病变引起胃流出道梗阻 / 1039
第六节 一些诊断陷阱 / 1039
第十二章 十二指肠疾病的影像学检查 / 1040
第一节 CT 显示十二指肠病变 / 1040
第二节 十二指肠在 X 线腹部正位片上的诊断陷阱 / 1040

第二十五篇 空、回肠疾病

第一章 淋巴瘤 / 1043
第一节 小肠动脉瘤性淋巴瘤 / 1043
第二节 误诊病例简介:回肠 T 细胞相关性(巨大)淋巴瘤伴破裂与肠壁型间质瘤 / 1043
第三节 小肠与阑尾弥漫性大 B 细胞淋巴瘤 / 1044
第二章 小肠间质瘤 / 1046
第一节 不典型小肠恶性间质瘤的 MSCT 表现(误诊讨论)/ 1046
第二节 胃肠道间质瘤 / 1048
第三节 不同侵袭危险度的小肠间质瘤 / 1049
第四节 小肠胃肠道间质瘤(中等危险度或潜在恶性)/ 1050
第五节 小肠系膜恶性间质瘤 / 1050
第六节 小肠胃肠道间质瘤 / 1051
第七节 关于小肠间质瘤及小肠肿物的影像诊断思维 / 1052
第三章 空回肠其他恶性肿瘤 / 1054
第一节 空回肠类癌 / 1054
第二节 麦克尔憩室类癌 / 1055
第三节 回肠原发性黑色素瘤 / 1055
第四章 小肠包块 / 1056
第一节 病理误诊病例简介:小肠炎性肌纤维母细胞瘤与间质瘤 / 1056
第二节 误诊病例简介:大部分钙化的空肠炎性肌纤维母细胞瘤与畸胎类肿瘤 / 1057
第三节 小肠梭形细胞肿瘤 / 1058
第四节 误诊病例简介:回肠系膜淋巴管肌瘤病并累及肠系膜淋巴结 50/55 枚 / 1059
第五章 炎症性肠病 / 1060
第一节 炎症性肠病 / 1060
第二节 炎症性肠病 / 1063
第六章 空、回肠克罗恩病 / 1064
第一节 空回肠克罗恩病与 MRI / 1064
第二节 MSCT 小肠造影与克罗恩病 / 1065
第三节 有关鉴别诊断 / 1066
第七章 小肠梗阻 / 1068
第一节 误诊病例简介:小肠脂肪瘤伴异位胰腺致小肠套叠 / 1068
第二节 腺瘤、息肉和脂肪瘤同时并存引起成人肠套叠 / 1068
第三节 柿石性小肠梗阻 / 1069
第四节 MSCT 诊断肿瘤性肠梗阻 / 1070
第五节 “假肾征”在诊断肠套叠中的价值 / 1071
第六节 肠梗阻的少见病因 / 1071
第七节 小肠假性梗阻 / 1071
第八节 腹内疝 / 1072
第九节 腹膜腔内疝及其误诊与漏诊的分析 / 1073
第八章 小肠淋巴管扩张症 / 1074
第九章 小肠创伤 / 1076
第一节 延迟性小肠破裂 / 1076
第二节 腹腔游离气体与胸腔积气 / 1077
第十章 肠壁积气和成人小肠中气体 / 1078
第一节 肠壁积气 / 1078
第二节 成人小肠内的气体 / 1078
第三节 “透光”伪影 / 1078
第四节 分成小腔的气腹酷似肠壁内气体 / 1079
第十一章 肠道缺血 / 1080
第一节 肠缺血 / 1080
第二节 关于小肠“狭窄” / 1081
第三节 小肠梗死肠壁内积气的难见表现 / 1081
第十二章 空肠和回肠的其他疾病 / 1083
第一节 导致肠壁增厚的良性疾病 / 1083
第二节 回盲瓣逆行脱垂 / 1083
第三节 回盲瓣的脂肪瘤样肥大抑或是肿瘤 / 1083
第四节 小肠出血性梗死 / 1084
第五节 小肠发育变异和诊断陷阱 / 1084
第六节 一些诊断陷阱 / 1085
第七节 空肠与回肠的少见病 / 1085
第十三章 小肠疾病影像检查技术 / 1087
第一节 小肠磁共振水成像 / 1087
第二节 腹腔多发占位性病变 - 胃肠道间质瘤病例 /

1088
第三节 肠壁 CT 增强后的密度改变 / 1089

第二十六篇 大肠疾病

第一章 大肠癌 / 1093
第一节 大肠癌的少见表现 / 1093
第二节 异物所致炎性肉芽肿误诊为肿瘤 / 1093
第三节 升结肠黏液腺癌病例 / 1093
第四节 多个误诊病例简介:非大肠病变与大肠癌 / 1094
第五节 炎性病变类似于大肠癌 / 1095
第六节 结肠恶性肿瘤少见 CT 表现 / 1096
第七节 回盲部隆起型中分化腺癌伴套迭病例 / 1098
第八节 人工智能及影像组学在结直肠肿瘤中的应用简介 / 1099
第二章 大肠淋巴瘤 / 1101
第一节 大肠淋巴瘤 / 1101
第二节 弥漫性大 B 细胞淋巴瘤病例 / 1102
第三节 结肠外周 T 细胞淋巴瘤与结肠炎性病变 / 1103
第四节 降结肠 T 细胞淋巴瘤病例 / 1104
第三章 大肠其他肿块 / 1106
第一节 肠管恶性黑色素瘤 / 1106
第二节 大肠类癌 / 1107
第三节 升结肠胃肠道型神经鞘瘤病例 / 1107
第四节 结肠绒毛状肿瘤 / 1108
第五节 右半结肠黏膜下脂肪瘤,肠外膜局部区呈化脓性炎伴脓肿形成 / 1109
第六节 Gardner 综合征 / 1110
第七节 胃肠道间质瘤(高危险度)/ 1111
第四章 大肠炎症 / 1113
第一节 原发性肠脂垂炎:急腹症的鉴别诊断 / 1113
第二节 炎症性肠病 / 1114
第三节 慢性溃疡性结肠炎的不常见的并发症 / 1114
第四节 克罗恩病病例之一 / 1115
第五节 转移性癌误诊为结肠炎 / 1116
第六节 肉芽肿性结肠炎之少见的结肠中毒性扩张 / 1116
第七节 克罗恩病 / 1116
第八节 慢性缓泻性结肠炎 / 1116
第九节 炎性病变类似于大肠癌 / 1117
第十节 异物所致炎性肉芽肿误诊为肿瘤 / 1117
第十一节 克罗恩病病例之二 / 1117
第五章 回盲部疾病 / 1118
第一节 回盲瓣逆行脱垂,回盲瓣的脂肪瘤样肥大抑或是肿瘤 / 1118
第二节 回盲部少见病 / 1118
第三节 诊断的混淆 / 1118
第四节 误诊病例简介:回盲部腺癌与类癌、恶性间质瘤 / 1118
第六章 盲肠疾病 / 1119
第一节 误诊病例简介:盲肠炎与肿瘤 / 1119
第二节 盲肠腺癌需与慢性炎症性病变鉴别 / 1119
第三节 误诊病例简介:盲肠腺瘤 / 1119
第四节 盲肠发育变异 / 1120
第五节 盲肠悬吊 / 1120
第七章 横结肠与升结肠疾病 / 1121
第一节 横结肠系膜病变的 CT 研究 / 1121
第二节 横结肠脂肪瘤并肠套叠 / 1122
第三节 横结肠韧带样型纤维瘤病 / 1123
第四节 升结肠黏膜下黏液纤维肉瘤 / 1124
第五节 病理误诊漏诊病例简介:横结肠癌、胃神经鞘瘤与胃间质瘤、胃窦黏膜腺癌 / 1124
第八章 乙状结肠疾病 / 1126
第一节 巨大的乙状结肠憩室 / 1126
第二节 误诊病例简介:乙状结肠副神经节瘤与腺癌 / 1126
第三节 乙状结肠暂时性腔外的充盈缺损 / 1127
第四节 卵巢癌复发浸润乙状结肠误为粪石 / 1127
第五节 乙状结肠粪结误为肿瘤 / 1127
第六节 诊断陷阱:尿滞留引起乙状结肠 - 直肠的假性狭窄 / 1127
第七节 异物所致炎性肉芽肿误诊为肿瘤 / 1128
第九章 直肠癌 / 1129
第一节 前列腺癌及直肠癌对盆腔筋膜侵犯 / 1129
第二节 直肠癌浸润周围筋膜的 MRI 表现 / 1130
第十章 结直肠癌 / 1131
第一节 直肠结肠癌诊断与 MSCT / 1131
第二节 双对比检查中结肠直肠癌的误诊和漏诊 / 1132
第十一章 直肠与肛的其他疾病 / 1133
第一节 盆底直肠周围恶性血管外皮瘤 / 1133
第二节 直肠后间隙的动态表现 / 1133
第三节 MSCT 与肛缘定位 / 1134
第十二章 关于排粪 / 1136
第十三章 下胃肠道出血和大肠憩室 / 1137
第一节 大肠的憩室病 / 1137
第二节 肠道血管畸形伴血管瘤形成 / 1138

第十四章 大肠的影像学检查技术 / 1139
第一节 大肠双对比技术检查中的诊断陷阱 / 1139
第二节 对大肠影像认识与解释不当导致误诊 / 1139
第三节 胆石性肠梗阻的不常见的诊断手段 / 1140
第十五章 大肠的发育变异和诊断陷阱 / 1141
第一节 大肠一般情况的改变与误诊 / 1141
第二节 关于结肠息肉 / 1142
第三节 消化道钡剂检查中的一些诊断陷阱 / 1142
第四节 关于回盲部 / 1143
第五节 乙状结肠、直肠与肛 / 1144
第六节 大肠的位置异常 / 1145
第七节 肠道的肝膈间位 / 1145
第八节 结肠壁的厚度 / 1146
第九节 结肠与肾脏关系 / 1146
第十六章 大肠的其他疾病 / 1147
第一节 结肠袋被侵 / 1147
第二节 大肠破裂 / 1148
第三节 关于结肠"狭窄" / 1148
第四节 结肠黏膜下脂肪沉积 / 1148
第五节 结肠缺血 / 1148
第六节 结肠水肿 / 1149
第七节 结肠孤立性良性溃疡 / 1149
第八节 关于大肠的内容物 / 1149
第九节 大肠的淋巴滤泡 / 1149
第十节 卡拉兹综合征(Chilaiditi's syndrome) / 1150

第二十七篇 阑尾疾病

第一章 炎症 / 1153
第一节 阑尾周围脓肿误诊为右侧髂窝恶性肿瘤 / 1153
第二节 急性化脓性阑尾炎病例 / 1153
第三节 急性阑尾炎 CT 检查的限度与诊断的问题 / 1154
第四节 急性阑尾炎 CT 诊断中的几个问题 / 1154
第五节 急性阑尾炎诊断假阴性的分析 / 1155
第六节 有液体充盈的远端回肠酷似急性阑尾炎 / 1155
第七节 急性化脓性阑尾炎病例 / 1156
第八节 老人非急性阑尾炎 / 1156
第九节 急性化脓性阑尾炎,局部坏疽,周围脓肿 / 1158
第十节 急性阑尾炎与阑尾的位置 / 1158
第二章 阑尾结石 / 1160
第三章 阑尾囊性病变 / 1161
第一节 阑尾黏液囊肿 / 1161
第二节 阑尾黏液囊肿与回盲部黏膜下黏液囊肿病例 / 1162
第三节 阑尾黏液性囊腺瘤病例 / 1162
第四章 阑尾肿瘤 / 1164
第一节 原发性阑尾肿瘤 / 1164
第二节 阑尾黏液性囊腺瘤病例 / 1165
第三节 误诊病例简介:阑尾周围脓肿与盆腔高代谢肿块 / 1165
第四节 阑尾类癌 / 1166
第五章 阑尾的活体形态学 / 1167

第二十八篇 门静脉疾病

第一章 肝硬化门静脉高压 / 1171
第一节 肝硬化合并不同病变对门静脉成像延迟时间的影响 / 1171
第二节 门脉高压时的钡餐检查 / 1172
第三节 肝脏门静脉成像延迟时间选择 / 1172
第二章 非肝硬化性门静脉高压 / 1173
第三章 门静脉高压时的侧支循环 / 1175
第一节 门脉 - 系统侧支引流血管与超声检查 / 1175
第二节 自发性肝内型门静脉 - 下腔静脉分流 / 1176
第四章 门静脉海绵样变与门静脉胆病 / 1177
第一节 门静脉海绵样变性 / 1177
第二节 门静脉性胆病 / 1178
第五章 关于门静脉血流 / 1180
第一节 门脉血流量的研究 / 1180
第二节 门静脉循环与体循环 / 1180
第六章 肝动脉 - 门静脉分流 / 1181
第一节 肝内肉眼可见的肝 - 门静脉分流的 MR / 1181
第二节 诊断陷阱:肝硬化中非肿瘤性肝动脉门静脉分流之 MSCT / 1181
第三节 少见的肝动脉 - 门静脉瘘 / 1183
第七章 门静脉系血栓形成 / 1184
第一节 门静脉血栓形成 / 1184
第二节 急性门静脉和肠系膜上静脉血栓形成 / 1184
第八章 门脉癌栓 / 1186
第一节 原发性肝癌门脉癌栓 / 1186
第二节 门脉癌栓与血栓的超声检查 / 1187
第九章 门脉先天异常和发育变异 / 1188
第一节 门静脉先天畸形 / 1188
第二节 先天性门 - 腔静脉分流畸形 / 1188
第三节 先天性肝内门静脉 - 肝静脉瘘 / 1189
第四节 先天性门静脉缺如 / 1190
第五节 门静脉 - 系统静脉的腹膜后侧支通路 / 1190

第六节 门静脉-腔静脉之间可能出现的侧支循环 / 1191
第七节 门静脉发育变异 / 1191
第八节 少见的副门脉形成 / 1192
第九节 门静脉先天性异常 / 1192
第十章 关于门腔静脉间隙 / 1194
第一节 门腔静脉间隙 / 1194
第二节 门腔静脉间隙淋巴结 / 1195
第三节 门腔间隙 / 1195
第四节 门腔间隙病变 / 1197
第十一章 门静脉瘤 / 1198
第一节 门静脉瘤 / 1198
第二节 肝外型门静脉瘤 / 1198
第十二章 关于门静脉周围 / 1200
第一节 门静脉周围的晕圈 / 1200
第二节 门静脉周围脂肪 / 1200
第三节 门静脉周围窦性扩张和肝紫癜 / 1200
第四节 门静脉周围晕:肝病的一个 CT 征象 / 1201
第五节 肝的门静脉周围的透光区或水肿 / 1201
第十三章 关于门静脉的影像检查技术 / 1203
第一节 肝脏门静脉成像延迟时间选择 / 1203
第二节 肝硬化合并不同病变对门静脉成像延迟时间的影响 / 1204
第十四章 门静脉其他疾病及活体形态学 / 1205
第一节 门静脉积气 / 1205
第二节 门静脉受侵 / 1205
第三节 门静脉异常 / 1205
第四节 门静脉造影的一些问题 / 1206

第二十九篇 急腹症与腹盆创伤

第一章 急腹症 / 1209
第一节 小肠梗阻 / 1209
第二节 腹部空腔脏器穿孔 MSCT / 1209
第三节 原发性肠脂垂炎:急腹症的鉴别诊断 / 1210
第四节 坏死性小肠结肠炎 / 1210
第五节 儿童急性阑尾炎 / 1210
第六节 胆石性肠梗阻 / 1210
第七节 成人肠套叠的 CT 表现 / 1211
第二章 腹盆创伤 / 1213
第三章 消化道出血 / 1215
第一节 消化道出血的常见病因及其 DSA 诊断 / 1215
第二节 胃肠出血的少见原因 / 1216
第三节 消化道出血与胃 / 1216

第三十篇 小儿腹盆部疾病(上)

第一章 胃十二指肠疾病 / 1219
第一节 十二指肠壁内血肿及误诊病例简介 / 1219
第二节 一些诊断陷阱 / 1220
第二章 胃肠道疾病 / 1221
第一节 新生儿胃肠穿孔 X 线征 / 1221
第二节 新生儿上消化道出血 / 1222
第三节 小儿胃肠道特点 / 1222
第三章 肠道疾病 / 1223
第一节 儿童一过性小肠套叠 / 1223
第二节 儿童慢性特发性小肠假性梗阻综合征 / 1223
第三节 儿童急性阑尾炎 / 1223
第四章 肝脏疾病 / 1226
第一节 儿童肝占位性病变 / 1226
第二节 小儿肝钝伤 / 1226
第五章 小儿黄疸 / 1228
第六章 小儿胆系疾病 / 1229
第一节 先天性胆总管囊肿自发穿孔 / 1229
第二节 先天性气管胆管瘘 / 1230
第三节 误诊病例简介:小儿胆总管管状乳头状腺瘤与胆总管囊肿 / 1230
第四节 新生儿胆胰管下端括约肌闭锁不全 / 1231
第七章 小儿胰腺疾病 / 1232
第一节 MR 诊断小儿环状胰腺 / 1232
第二节 胰母细胞瘤 / 1232
第三节 胰腺胚胎细胞瘤 / 1233
第四节 胰腺损伤 / 1233
第八章 小儿脾脏疾病 / 1235
第一节 脾硬化性血管瘤样结节性转化 / 1235
第二节 多脾综合征伴腹腔脏器转位 / 1235
第三节 脾尖部的重叠引起 CT 误诊 / 1235
第四节 婴儿急性脾扭转 / 1235
第九章 小儿门静脉疾病 / 1237
第十章 小儿其他疾病 / 1239

第三十一篇 腹盆部影像学检查技术

第一章 腹盆部影像学检查 / 1243
第二章 CT 与腹盆部疾病 / 1245
第一节 CT 检查意外发现胃肠疾病 / 1245
第二节 CT 灌注有利于肿瘤的分期 / 1245
第三章 其他影像学检查技术 / 1246
第一节 胃肠疾病的核素检查 / 1246

第二节 胃肠疾患与超声检查 / 1246
第三节 肝脏术中超声 / 1247
第四章 关于伪影 / 1248
第一节 腹部和盆腔血管多普勒超声伪影 / 1248
第二节 MRI 运动伪影的形成与处理 / 1251
第四节 流动相关伪影 / 1253
第五节 MRI 与伪影 / 1254

参考文献 / 1257
本卷有关医学影像词汇 / 1267

第一篇　肝局灶性病变

第一章　肝脏疾病研究

第一节　肝肿瘤样病变的简要鉴别诊断

表 1-1-1　肝硬化中肝细胞结节新旧名词对照

新名词	旧名词
再生结节（regenerative nodule，RN）	再生结节（regenerative nodule）
发育不良性结节（dysplastic nodules，DNs）	巨再生结节，Ⅰ型
	普通腺瘤样增生（adenomatous hyperplasia，AH，低级）
发育不良性结节（DNs），高级	巨再生结节，Ⅱ型
	腺瘤样增生，非典型（adenomatoid hyperplasia with atypia，AAH）
发育不良性结节伴癌亚灶（dysplastic nodules with subfocus of HCC）	早癌（early HCC），腺瘤样增生伴镜检 HCC
小癌（small HCC）<2 cm	腺瘤样增生伴可视癌灶（adenomatoid hyperplasia with macroscopic HCC）

注：HCC 系肝细胞性肝癌。

1. 肝硬化癌前病变　再生结节（RN）：肝硬化的再生结节是由再生的肝细胞为纤维间隔包绕所形成，结节的直径多在 3 mm 以下，但可融合成为较大的结节，进一步发展为发育不良结节（DN）。CT 表现：在 CT 平扫不易发现，偶尔显示为稍高密度病灶。少数大的 RN 平扫呈等密度；增强 CT 的动脉期、门静脉期和平衡期均显示为低密度病灶。此外，在肝硬化的肝脏中，还可见到坏死结节，不易与小肝癌鉴别。

2. 肝脏发育不良性结节（DN）　DN 属于癌前病变，在肝硬化中占 15%~25%。DN 的直径常为 1 mm~10 mm，但有达 20 mm 者。DN 在 CT 上检出率不高，平扫上可呈高或低密度，在增强扫描上呈等或高密度。96% 的 DN 主要由门静脉供血，而 94% 的肝细胞性肝癌由主要肝动脉供血，当肝硬化患者的肝脏有多结节时，其中较大的结节可考虑为 DN。DN 的 MR 表现：在 MR 上，典型 DN 在 T_1- 为略高信号，T_2- 低信号。增强扫描动脉期无强化或轻度强化，门静脉期轻度强化，延迟期呈等信号；肿块都呈均质性，边缘清楚，无包膜。

3. 融合性肝脏纤维化　融合性肝脏纤维化常见于肝硬化的后期，有 14%。多为楔形，自肝门向外放射，常伴有肝包膜的内陷和肝段实质的收缩，有时纤维化病灶位于肝脏的外围不伸向肝门。增强 CT 扫描融合纤维化区的密度可有等、低、高三种密度差别。

4. 肝脏暂时性高密度　肝脏暂时性高密度，亦称暂时性肝脏密度差（THAD），是在肝硬化基础上，肝内出现自发性动 - 门静脉交通（瘘）的表现。在双期螺旋 CT 扫描上，动脉期表现为明显的高密度，在门静脉期呈稍高或等密度。暂时性肝脏密度差常位于肝包膜下，在动脉期显示为楔状，边缘平直的密度增高区，有时少数暂时性肝脏密度差呈假结节形，不易与肝细胞性肝癌鉴别，但结节形暂时性肝脏密度差常位于包膜下，在门静脉期呈等密度，而肝细胞性肝癌多呈低密度。

5. 布 - 加综合征　近年来由于 CT、MRI 等先进技术的发展，能发现布 - 加综合征的多发性结节表现，由于肝静脉的血流量的减少或闭塞，引致多灶性肝动脉扩张，久之则形成结节状肝细胞增生，被称为“大再生结节”（larger regenerative nodule），这种结节需与癌前病变的“发育不良结节”相鉴别。大再生结节多见于慢性布-加综合征，数目较多，常在10个以上，大小在数毫米至4厘米。CT平扫呈高密度，增强扫描密度更高或呈外低中高的结节。极少数大再生结节向肝外生长，易误诊为肝外肿瘤。

6. 局灶性肝脂肪浸润 CT表现：局灶性肝脂肪浸润主要见于肝裂周围，表现为孤立的或多发的球形、扇弧形或大片状不规则形低密度病灶，CT值约为0~30 HU，对其周围血管无推移，无占位效应。增强扫描如动态CT扫描，病灶不强化或轻微强化，其动态增强曲线与正常肝组织相似。肝脂肪浸润MRI表现：在常规SE序列T_1WI及T_2WI像上局灶性肝脂肪浸润呈略高信号，脂肪抑制序列扫描，该病灶表现为低信号。

7. 正常肝岛 弥散型脂肪肝中有时可见无脂肪化的正常肝岛，多见于左内叶后部Ⅳ段和胆囊窝周围，有时不易与肝肿瘤区别。

8. 肝脏炎性假瘤 炎性假瘤以往名称繁多，目前病理学家认为炎性肌成纤维细胞瘤的名称更为贴切。CT表现：由于肝脏炎性假瘤包含多种成分，因而肝脏炎性假瘤的CT表现多种多样，诸如：病灶始终无强化，病灶一般边缘清晰，呈圆形或类圆形，少数病灶呈特殊的哑铃形、香蕉形、多结节融合形、不规则形等；周边环状强化，可见轻至中度环状强化；周边呈突起状或钟乳石状部分强化，纤维间隔可有强化，病灶中心结节状强化。

9. 肝梗死 肝脏梗死或梗死是肝脏局部组织因动脉血流阻断而引起的坏死。CT表现：根据梗死区所累及肝脏位置不同，可将肝梗死大致分为如下三型：①中央实质梗死型，最为常见，病灶平扫呈指向肝门楔形低密度影，边缘较为清晰锐利，并延伸至肝包膜，部分低密度病灶内可有更低气体低密度影，增强后低密度区无强化；②包膜下梗死型，多出现于肝脏移植后，病变比较局限，表现为内缘不规则，外缘为光滑的肝包膜低密度影；③胆管周围梗死型，梗死灶表现为与受累胆管一致的不规则分支状低密度区，胆管可扩张积气，周围不规则低密度区边缘较为清晰。

第二节 机器学习在肝脏疾病影像诊断中的研究

由于呼吸运动影响、组织天然对比较差及肝脏影像分割难度较大等原因，机器学习在肝脏疾病影像诊断方面的研究相对较少，但随着算法的改进和硬件设备的升级，此方面的研究正在逐步增多。慢性肝病筛查及严重程度评估：慢性肝病(CLD)主要包括乙型肝炎病毒和丙型肝炎病毒感染、酒精性肝病、非酒精性脂肪肝病以及相关的肝硬化和肝癌。目前，支持向量机已经用于慢性肝病的诊断。Gatos等(2017)将基于硬度评估和机器学习算法的计算机辅助诊断系统应用于超声剪切波弹性成像(SWE)，进而对慢性肝病进行评估。通过分析126例受试者(56名健康对照，70例慢性肝病)的临床资料，提取了超声剪切波弹性成像影像中存在的35个物理特征的(每个集群7个)，采用逐步回归分析的特征简化方法推导出一个简化的特征子集，将其输入到支持向量机分类算法中，从而把慢性肝病分类出来。

支持向量机模型对慢性肝病受试者的健康分类最高准确度为87.3%，敏感度和特异度分别为93.5%和81.2%，受试者操作特征(ROC)曲线下面积(AUC)为0.87(95%CI：0.77~0.92)。该研究还介绍了一种基于超声剪切波弹性成像影像的硬度值对颜色信息进行量化的机器学习算法，并从健康的样本中识别慢性肝病。

目前研究提供的慢性肝病诊断的新客观参数和标准可以被认为是基于颜色解释的重要一步，并且可以在检查后立即使用个人计算机安装的软件进行分析，从而协助放射科医生的诊断工作。除了传统的支持向量机，也有研究者进一步开发新的模型，并将神经网络应用于疾病风险程度分级。Kuppili等(2017)提出了一种可靠的、快速的极端学习机器(extreme learning machine，ELM)组织特征系统，用于肝脏超声成像的脂肪肝风险程度分级。极端学习机器用于训练单层前馈神经网络。该研究中使用美国肝脏数据库的63例样本(27例正常，36例异常)训练，结果表明极端学习机器性能优于支持向量机，使用肝S8段数据集的K10交叉验证协议，极端学习机器和支持向量机的准确度分别为96.75%和89.01%，ROC AUC分别为0.97和0.91。进一步的研究显示极端学习机器分类器的平均可靠性为

99%，并且使用极端学习机器的平均速度比使用支持向量机提高 40%。该研究结果表明，基于超声成像的机器学习方法，特别是极端学习机器可以较好地用于脂肪肝风险程度分级，有助于临床决策。

肝纤维化早期的临床干预可以减缓肝硬化的发展，降低肝癌的发病风险。肝脏活检是肝纤维化诊断的金标准，但具有有创性和较高的抽样误差等缺点。而超声实时组织弹性成像（real-time tissue elastography，RTE）可以对肝纤维化进行准确评估且具无创性，可能成为很有前景的成像技术。但从临床的实时组织弹性成像影像中确定肝纤维化的程度是很困难的。Chen 等（2017）的多中心合作研究中，采用实时组织弹性成像 影像和多元回归分析预测诊断分级，并采用了 4 种经典分类器（支持向量机、朴素贝叶斯算法、随机森林、k-NN）建立一个决策支持系统，来提高肝纤维化诊断效能。他们对 513 例接受肝脏活检的受试者的影像进行分析，共获得 11 个实时组织弹性成像 影像特征，研究中所采用的分类器明显优于传统的肝纤维化指数方法，而随机森林分类器在 4 种机器算法中具有最高的平均精度。这一结果表明，复杂的机器学习方法可以成为评估肝纤维化分级的有力工具，并显示出较好的临床应用前景。

近期，Yasaka 等（2018）探讨了卷积神经网络深度学习模型在肝纤维化分期中的应用价值，其采用钆塞酸二钠增强肝胆期 MRI 影像作为输入数据，其中训练集包括 534 例病人，测试集为 100 例病人。训练集中（纤维化分期为 F0、F1、F2、F3 和 F4 的病人分别为 54、53、81、113 和 233 例），MRI 原始图像上增加了 90 倍因素扩增（旋转、平行移位、亮度改变和对比度变化，共得到 144 180 张图像）。在测试集中评估卷积神经网络模型的效能（纤维化分期为 F0、F1、F2、F3 和 F4 的病人分别为 0、10、15、20 和 45 例）。结果深度学习对肝纤维化的评分与纤维化分期显著相关（Spearman 等级相关系数为 0.63；$P<0.001$）。纤维化分期为 F4、F3 和 F2 的 ROC AUC 分别为 0.84、0.84 和 0.85，结果表明卷积神经网络模型在肝纤维化分期中表现出较高的诊断效能。

Wang 等（2018）也探讨了基于卷积神经网络深度学习的弹性成像影像组学模型评估肝纤维化分期的价值，采用二维超声剪切波弹性成像 影像作为输入数据，共收集 398 例病人（1 990 幅影像），266 例病人作为训练集，132 例病人作为测试集，分别计算肝硬化（F4）、晚期纤维化（≥ F3）和显著纤维化（≥ F2）的 ROC AUC。结果显示，卷积神经网络深度学习弹性成像影像组学模型预测肝纤维化为 F4 期、≥ F3 期和≥ F2 期的 AUC 分别为 0.97（95%CI：0.94~0.99）、0.98（95%CI：0.96~1.00）和 0.85（95%CI：0.81~0.89）。该研究结果提示，与二维超声剪切波弹性成像和生物标志物相比，深度学习的弹性成像影像组学模型显示出更好的肝纤维化预测效能，对乙型肝炎病毒感染病人肝纤维化分期的无创性诊断具有重要的实用价值。除此之外，卷积神经网络深度学习模型近期还被用于正常肝脏和肝硬化的筛查。Liu 等（2017）首先提出一种超声影像提取肝包膜的方法，然后根据提取的肝包膜，对一个深层卷积神经网络模型进行微调，从肝包膜周围的影像块中提取特征。最后，应用训练支持向量机分类器将样本分为正常或异常。该方法能有效提取肝脏包膜，并准确地对超声影像进行分类，识别正常肝脏和异常肝脏。

肝脏局灶性病变的影像鉴别诊断一直是临床的重点和难点，近期基于机器学习的方法不断应用于肝脏局灶性病变的鉴别诊断并取得了较好的结果，神经网络有望辅助临床进行鉴别诊断。Hwang 等（2015）利用 99 例肝脏病灶（包括 29 例肝囊肿、37 例血管瘤、33 例恶性肿瘤）超声成像，提取了共 42 个混合结构纹理特征，主成分分析选取 29 个关键特征，作为前馈神经网络的一组输入。结果显示，超声成像在肝局灶性病变之间（囊肿与血管瘤、囊肿与恶性肿瘤、血管瘤与恶性肿瘤）的诊断准确度高达 96% 以上。在最优特征集内，当回声被包括在内时，准确度略有提高。该研究表明所提出的方法在临床上是可行的，有望帮助临床进行疾病鉴别诊断。

近期最突出的应用是将卷积神经网络深度学习模型应用于肝脏 CT 影像局灶性病变的鉴别诊断。Yasaka 等（2018）利用有肝脏肿块的 3 个时相（平扫、动脉期、延迟期）CT 影像，共 55 536 个影像进行了卷积神经网络 模型监督训练，从 460 例病人中获得 1 068 个原始图像，并在原始图像上增加了 52 倍的因素扩增（旋转、平行移动、增强放大、噪声添加），随后用 100 个肝脏肿块影像进行卷积神经网络模型测试（男 74 例、女 26 例；A、B、C、D、E 类的影像分别有 21、9、35、20、15 例）。训练和测试各进行了 5 次，使用分别构建的平扫、动脉期、延迟期、动脉-延迟期联合、三期联合卷积神经网络 模型对肝脏肿块进行分类,并计算出不同类别 A-B 和 C-E 分类的 AUC。肝脏肿块的鉴别诊断准确度为 0.84。不同类别 A-B 和 C-E 分类的 AUC 的中位数为 0.92。结果表明,基于卷积神经网络 的深度学习在动态增强 CT 鉴别肝脏肿块方面具有较高的诊断效能,并且深度学习可以不需要专家自主提取特征,更加接近真实数据,减少了人为的影响。

Diamant 等(2017)提出了一种新的 Bag of Visual-Words(BoVW)模型的自动医学影像分类的方法。这种方法通过使用基于互信息的标准学习每个任务的最相关的视觉词的任务驱动字典来改进 BoVW 模型。其将肝脏病灶 CT 影像分为 4 类(32 例血管瘤、35 例转移瘤、29 例肝癌、22 例肝囊肿),对 118 例肝脏门静脉期 CT 影像进行验证。新的 BoVW 模型与以往 BoVW 模型对比,在肝脏病变分类方面,敏感度提高了 6%,特异度提高 2%($P<0.001$)。结果表明,基于信息选择词汇的分类结果有显著的改善。

新的 BoVW 方法在临床上显示了很好的结果,它可以发现当前任务的相关影像部分,而不需要对训练数据进行明确的标注,从而能为影像分析任务的医学专家提供计算机辅助支持。Depeursinge 等(2014)描述了一个框架,用于 CT 影像中对肝脏病变的视觉语义进行建模,以预测放射科医生在描述这些病变时所报告的视觉语义术语(visual semantic terms, VST)。利用高阶可控 Riesz 小波和支持向量机的线性组合,从图像数据中学习计算 VST 模型。在第 1 步中,这些模型用于预测描述肝脏病变的每一个语义术语的存在;在第 2 步中,计算所有 VST 模型之间的距离,建立一个包含术语间同义和互补性的非分层计算性 VST 本体;最后使用来自 RadLex 本体的 18 个 VST 注释的 74 个肝脏病变对所提出的框架进行了初步评估。病人交叉验证 ROC 曲线下平均面积为 0.853。该研究中提出的框架预计能够促进影像学中影像解释的人机协同作用,同时使用 VST 的旋转-协变计算模型来量化它们的局部可能性,并明确地将它们与基于像素的影像内容联系起来。以上研究表明,机器学习有望辅助医生进行肝脏局灶性病变的鉴别诊断,具有广阔的研究前景。

肝病影像分割算法的改进及影像质量的自动评估:肝脏病变的影像分割一直是限制机器学习 在肝脏疾病应用的重要原因,也有一些研究者进行尝试和改进算法,包括尝试使用神经网络方法。Le 等(2016)提出了一种新的计算机化的 MRI 影像肝肿瘤分割方法。该方法包括 4 个主要阶段。首先利用种子点提取包含 T_1WI 序列中肝肿瘤区域的兴趣区(ROI)影像,降低 ROI 影像中的噪声,增强边界;应用 3D 快速推进算法生成被认为是教师区域的初始标记区域;采用非迭代算法训练的单隐层前馈神经网络对未标记体素进行分类;最后,后处理阶段被用来提取和细化肝肿瘤边界。该方法对 16 例病人的 25 个肿瘤进行了 2 个数据集的评估,提出的方法获得的肿瘤体积重叠误差为 27.43%,平均百分比容量误差为 15.73%。平均表面距离、均方根表面距离和最大表面距离的平均值分别为 0.58 mm、1.20 mm、6.29 mm。此方法有望改进肝癌 MR 影像的分割,进一步增进机器学习的肝癌的应用研究。

Esses 等(2018)开发和测试了一种新的卷积神经网络 深度学习方法,用于对 T_2WI 肝脏影像的非诊断影像进行自动筛选,并将该方法与 2 名放射科医师的评估相比较。研究纳入了 522 例来自 1.5 T 和 3.0 T 的肝脏 MRI 影像,351 例 T_2WI 影像用于训练卷积神经网络模型,每个病例都有一个诊断或非诊断的标记。另外 171 例由 2 名放射科医师对其 T_2WI 影像进行独立评估,并被标注为诊断或非诊断。将该算法的影像质量输出与 2 位放射科医师的结果进行比较。卷积神经网络 算法在识别非诊断性影像质量的敏感度和特异度分别为 67% 和 81%(观察者 1)、47% 和 80%(观察者 2)。卷积神经网络 算法识别非诊断性影像质量的阴性预测值为 94%(观察者 1)、86%(观察者 2)。采用这种卷积神经网络 算法对肝脏的非诊断性 T_2WI 影像筛查具有很高的预测价值,这表明计算机可以应用于影像质量的筛查,有助于减轻临床工作量。

小结与展望:我国医疗数据资源丰富,但在医疗数据机器学习应用方面与欧美国家相比还有一定的差距,与我国医疗数据缺乏规范化、没有统一的标准、缺乏多中心的协同共享以及统一监管等有关。2017 年 7 月 20 日,国务院发布《新一代人工智能发展规划》,标志着人工智能正式纳入国家战略规划,我国机器学习的研究今后也将更上一个台阶。目前,基于医学影像数据分析的机器学习 在肝病诊断中的应用已逐渐成为研究热点,也是研究难点。在算法应用方面,深度学习,特别是卷积神经网络算法将成为肝病影像诊断机器学习研究的主要工具。在临床应用方面，肝脏局限性病变的鉴别诊断是临床关注的问题，未来可以进一步开展更深入的研究。

第三节　代谢组学在肝脏疾病的应用

详见本书 本卷 本篇 第六章 第二节 代谢组学在肝脏疾病的应用。

第二章　肝局灶性病变定位研究

肝段的非活体解剖学及活体形态学划分

现代外科学的发展已经能够开展肝段、亚肝段甚至楔形切除,这就要求术前对肝脏病变的解剖部位与切除平面进行更加精确的定位。随着活体的医学影像学的发展, PTC、ERCP 以及螺旋 CT 血管成像及 MR 血管成像等技术能从不同方向确定病变的部位及其与周围管道的关系。目前有多种肝段的划分法,并且关于划分肝段的解剖标志及肝段间真正边界的确定一直存在争议,造成外科实践中肝段划分及肝段概念的使用无法统一。

(一)肝脏分叶、分段的发展历史

传统上,以肝脏表面解剖标志为界限,将肝简单地分为右、左叶。右叶大,左叶小,方叶和尾叶均归为右叶。但这种分法与肝内管道分布情况不符,不能满足外科肝段切除的要求。

Glisson(1654)首次描述了肝内解剖结构。Rex(1888)通过观察哺乳动物肝脏标本,发现肝门静脉左、右干的分布构成肝脏真正的两叶。Cantile(1898)提出肝脏功能解剖的概念,根据肝左、右动脉在肝内的分布将肝脏分为左、右两叶,并依据门静脉的流向,认为由胆囊窝至下腔静脉窝的平面为左右半肝的真正分界,后来此平面被称为: Rex-Cantlie 线。

20 世纪四五十年代,很多学者应用腐蚀法、色素明胶注射法、肝内血管及胆管造影以及肝脏血管灌注等方法对肝脏进行了深入研究,提出肝动脉、门静脉及肝胆管可分为 2 个左、右独立的系统,分别供应肝左、右叶;供应肝左、右叶的 2 个系统间无肝内交通。

随后又出现多种肝段划分法。Hjortsjo(1951)基于用腐蚀标本和尸体胆管造影,确定了肝动脉的分布区域、肝静脉的引流范围以及胆管树的分布,认为肝管以肝段的形式分支和引流,从而提出肝段的概念,使得对肝脏分叶、分段及肝内解剖的研究取得较大进展。

在肝脏的分叶方法中将其一致地分为左外叶、左内叶、右前叶、右后叶和尾状叶,但对于肝段的进一步划分意见不一。Healey 和 Schroy(1953)依据肝动脉及伴随肝管的分支作为肝内区段的分界线,将肝脏分成 2 叶、10 区。

Couinaud(1954)经过大量的尸肝解剖研究,提出肝脏的功能分段应以门静脉鞘系供血在肝内的分布作为依据,各段均有 Glisson 系统的一个分支供血并引流胆汁,以引流相邻肝段回心血液的肝静脉为分段界限来描述肝段解剖,将肝分为左、右半肝, 4 部及 8 段,每一肝段均可视为肝的功能解剖单位。

Couinaud(库氏)肝段法是以 3 个肝静脉作垂直平面形成纵行主裂(正中裂、左叶间裂及右叶间裂),并以左右门静脉主干进行分段。正中裂有肝中静脉经过,将肝分为左右两半;左叶间裂有肝左静脉经过,将左半肝分为左内区和左外区;右叶间裂有肝右静脉经过,将右半肝分为右内区和右外区。每一个区又被一个通过左右门脉支的假想平面分为上下段,共分为血流动力学上独立的 8 个肝段。这些段在正面观,从尾状叶(S_1 段)开始顺时针依次为 S_1、S_2、S_3、S_4、S_5、S_6、S_7、S_8 段。Couinaud 分段法建立在门静脉分支和肝静脉走行基础上,各段之间分界明确,命名简单实用,因而很长一段时间被国际上广泛采用。但其结论是以离体肝铸型标本为依据,因其失去了韧带等支持固定结构,血管等结构发生移位,因而 Couinaud 分段法的肝段方位与在体肝不尽相符。

Goldsmith 和 Woodburne(1957)根据肝静脉分布提出肝段命名法,将肝分为 2 叶、5 段和 8 个亚段,即肝中静脉分肝为左、右叶,右叶被肝右静脉分为右前、右后段,左叶被肝左静脉分为左内、左外段,每一个段又分为上、下两亚段,尾状叶为一独立段。有研究依据 Glisson 系统和肝静脉走行将肝分为两半肝、5 叶、6 段,即尾状叶(左、右段)、左外叶(上、下段)、左内叶、右前叶以及右后叶(上、下段)。另有研究依 Glisson 系统和肝静脉将肝分为 5 叶、

10段。

1982年，有研究者在Couinaud肝段法的基础上，结合Goldsmith和Woodburne肝段命名法，用亚段代替段进行命名，即尾状叶（Ⅰ段）；左外侧上亚段（Ⅱ段）、左外侧下亚段（Ⅲ段）；左内侧亚段（Ⅳ段，左内侧上、下两亚段均用Ⅳ）；右前下亚段（Ⅴ段）、右前上亚段（Ⅷ段）；右后下亚段（Ⅵ段）以及右后上亚段（Ⅶ段）。为避免左内侧上、下两亚段的混淆，Sugarbaker提出修改方案分别以$Ⅳ_a$、$Ⅳ_b$亚段指代其上、下亚段。

近年，有学者认为，既然$Ⅳ_a$、$Ⅳ_b$亚段是独立的实体结构，在临床上可单独切除，就应该与其他亚段同等的进行排序，建议以1代替$Ⅳ_a$亚段，以9代替原Ⅰ亚段（尾状叶），用阿拉伯数字来表达1~9段分别代表肝脏的9个亚段。

（二）肝脏分段的解剖基础

Glisson系统和肝静脉：肝脏是人体内唯一具有4套管道系统的器官，这些管道的走行分布构成了不同肝段划分方法的解剖基础。

1. 格里申（Glisson）系统　Glisson系统为互相伴行的肝门静脉、肝动脉、肝管在肝内的各级分支被结缔组织纤维鞘包绕而形成的三联管道系统，似树枝状分布于肝段内。其中，门静脉管径最粗，易于显示和观察，且分支相对恒定，较肝动脉和肝管变异少，因此，以它为中心代表肝动脉和肝管作为划分肝段的解剖基础和标志。肝门静脉主干多分为左、右2支：①门静脉左支细而长，分为横部、角部、矢状部及囊部4部分，沿途发出分支供应尾状叶左侧及肝左叶各亚段；②门静脉右支粗而短，发出分支供应尾状叶右侧及肝右叶各亚段。肝段是以肝门静脉分支为基础进行划分，但门静脉也存在多种变异，给临床工作肝段的划分带来困难。

2. 肝静脉系统　肝静脉系统包括肝左、中、右静脉以及它们的属支，肝左、中、右静脉分别走行于左段间裂、正中裂及右叶间裂内，引流相邻肝段的静脉血，三者于第二肝门汇入下腔静脉；此外还有一些肝短静脉，为收集右后叶脏面和尾状叶的一些小静脉的总称，有3~10支，口径细，于第三肝门位置汇入下腔静脉。

3. 肝脏的大体解剖学分段　根据修改后的肝段划分法，门静脉是确定肝段的关键标志，以肝静脉确定肝段范围，用肝的自然沟、裂、窝及韧带作为确定肝段的重要辅助标志。

肝裂：正中裂：即主门裂或Cantlie线，内有肝中静脉走行。表面标志为肝膈面前下方胆囊窝中份至后上方下腔静脉的左壁的连线，该裂与水平面形成一开口向左的75°夹角。

右叶间裂：即右门裂，内有肝右静脉走行。表面标志为肝膈面后上方下腔静脉右壁至前下方肝下缘胆囊窝中份与肝右角距离中外1/3交点的连线。

右段间裂：即横裂，内有门静脉右支走行，主要依门静脉右支确定此裂。表面标志为肝脏面起于肝门横沟右端，向右经肝右缘中点达膈面，再水平向左与右叶间裂汇合。

左叶间裂：即脐裂，相当于左纵沟位置，内有左叶间静脉和门静脉左支矢状部走行。表面标志为肝膈面肝镰状韧带左侧1 cm处与下腔静脉左壁的连线，于脏面则为肝圆韧带。

左段间裂：即左门裂，内有肝左静脉走行，表面标志为肝膈面起于肝左静脉汇入下腔静脉处，向左达肝左缘中、后1/3交界处，转到脏面，多止于脐静脉窝上1/3处。

背裂：将尾状叶（Ⅰ段）同左内叶和右前叶，表面标志为上起三大肝静脉出肝处，下至第一肝门。

肝段：根据上述肝裂位置，肝脏被正中裂分为左、右半肝，左、右半肝又被左、右叶间裂及背裂分为5叶，即左内叶、左外叶、右前叶、右后叶、尾状叶。以门静脉左、右支所在水平充当横裂，将左内叶、左外叶、右前叶、右后叶又分别分为上、下两亚段，共8亚段，即尾叶（Ⅰ段）、左外侧上亚段（Ⅱ段）、左外侧下亚段（Ⅲ段）、左内侧上亚段（$Ⅳ_a$亚段）、左内侧下亚段（$Ⅳ_b$亚段）、右前下亚段（Ⅴ段）、右前上亚段（Ⅷ段）、右后下亚段（Ⅵ段）以及右后上亚段（Ⅶ段）。

肝亚段解剖：现在普遍采用的肝亚段解剖是由Couinard（1975）首先描述，后来由Bismuth修改的肝亚段分段法。这一分段方法中，依据门静脉和肝静脉的分布将肝分为若干个肝段。尾状叶是第1肝段，肝脏另有8个肝段和肝亚段（2、3、4a、4b、5、6、7、8），这些肝段由三个垂直平面和一个水平平面划分而成。第一个垂直平面包含有肝中静脉，并将肝脏分成左、右肝叶，第二个垂直平面包含有肝右静脉，并将肝右叶分成前、后肝段。第三个垂直平面包含有肝左静脉，并将肝左叶分为内侧段和外侧段。然后，肝段被一个经由门静脉左、右主干的横向平面分成肝亚段。标准轴面CT判定肝亚段时有困难。但是应用计算机进行肝亚段解剖的研究已取得进展，已成为研究三维肝亚段解剖的有效方法，如何将其应用到标准轴面CT切面上尚有待研究。

(三)肝脏的影像学分段

在横断面上，肝动脉和肝管细小，难以识别，故肝静脉的走行和门静脉的分支是划分肝段的主要依据，同时也参照肝的自然沟、裂、窝及韧带。

1. 肝段在横断面上的划分　以目前的影像学水平所能显示的肝内结构来看，从第二肝门平面至第一肝门平面是观察肝段的主要断面。在较高层面，可以肝静脉作为肝段间分界标志；在较低层面上，因看不到各主肝静脉，必须借助于其他结构进行定位。以含有不等量脂肪及胆囊的正中裂划分左、右叶，以左段间裂、左门静脉段间部及镰状韧带、肝圆韧带划分左内、外叶；最低层以肝圆韧带作为段的界限；右门静脉及其进入右前、后段的分支作为段间标志，以左右门静脉水平作为左内侧段、左外侧段、右前段以及右后段划分上、下亚段的标志。

CT检查可在下述4个层面上明确识别主肝静脉和门静脉左、右支，据此可在CT影像上区分各肝段，其他扫描层面则可参照与这4个层面的关系进行定位：①最头端的层面，为3支主肝静脉汇入下腔静脉的层面；②肝门静脉左支层面；③肝门静脉右支层面；④最尾端的层面，为肝门静脉主干和胆囊水平的层面。

横断面影像上各肝裂的位置确定如下：

正中裂——上部，为肝中静脉长轴到下腔静脉左前壁的连线；下部，在第一肝门上、下平面水平，肝中静脉主干会被其左、右根所取代，而缺乏识别正中裂的标志结构，故以下平面以胆囊窝中点至下腔静脉左前壁的连线作为正中裂的标志。

左叶间裂——上部(门静脉左支矢状部以上)为镰状韧带在肝的附着点左缘向下腔静脉中点连线；如果左叶间静脉出现，就为左叶间裂上份的天然标志，即左叶间静脉长轴或中点至下腔静脉左前壁的连线；中部为门静脉左支矢状部的长轴；下部为肝圆韧带裂。

左段间裂——依肝左静脉长轴或其段间支确定此裂。

右叶间裂——为肝右静脉长轴或中点至下腔静脉左前壁的连线。

右段间裂——主要依门静脉右支确定此裂，当门静脉呈三叉形分支方式，可以此分叉处确定此裂。

背裂——其上部为肝左、中静脉汇入下腔静脉左前壁至静脉韧带裂右端的弧形线，下部为下腔静脉右壁至肝门或门静脉的连线。

2. 矢状面划分肝段　矢状面影像上，单独在一个断面很难划分肝段，必须对肝内管道进行连续的追踪观察，因此选择一个最佳开始断面对于正确划分肝段是十分必要的。

矢状面上划分肝段，左叶间裂常作为最佳开始平面，原因有以下几点：①6个肝裂，仅左叶间裂近于矢状位，识别标志是肝门静脉左支矢状部；②肝门静脉左支矢状部极短或缺如者少见，常与下腔静脉同层或出现于其右侧的第一个断面上，易于寻找，也易于追踪左、右肝静脉走行；③门脉左支矢状部出现的断面常是门静脉分左、右支的起始点，这一断面向右侧的断面，出现肝门静脉右支，这一断面向左侧的断面，出现肝门静脉左支。

矢状面影像上肝裂的位置确定如下：

左叶间裂——应首先确定最佳开始断面，即左叶间裂所在的断面，肝门静脉左支是确定此裂的明显标志。此平面上30%可见显示肝左静脉的属支左叶间静脉的全程，这条静脉也有助于寻找左叶间裂。

左段间裂——其识别标志为肝左静脉，肝左静脉口径较大，位于左外叶中间部位。

背裂——肝中静脉根部至肝门静脉左支横部或右支主干的连线即为背裂，Ⅰ段左份位于静脉韧带裂与膈之间，右份则位于背裂与下腔静脉之间。

正中裂——肝中静脉至胆囊窝连线即为正中裂，此裂呈左后上至右前下斜位，因此，于矢状断面上不会出现肝中静脉全长。

右叶间裂——在矢状断面上，肝右静脉至肝门静脉右支或胆囊后端的连线可作为右叶间裂；在肝右静脉细小或胆囊以右的断面上，只能以前、后两组肝门静脉分支之间的“无血管带”作为标志。

右段间裂——肝门静脉左、右支大致位于肝上下径中份，以此来确定此裂。

3. 冠状面划分肝段　左叶间裂：其前部为肝圆韧带或门静脉左支矢状部至镰状韧带附着缘左侧1cm处的连线，后部为天然标志——静脉韧带裂。如果镰状韧带显示不清，则以肝左静脉根部(走行于左叶间裂上份内)或肝左静脉的属支左叶间静脉与肝门静脉左支矢状部的连线作为确定此裂的标志。左段间裂：其标志线为肝左静脉至肝左缘中点的连线。正中裂：其前部为肝中静脉至胆囊窝中点的连线，后部为肝中静脉至门静脉或肝门的连线。右叶间裂：右叶间裂近乎冠状位且稍偏向前下方，在冠状断面上，肝右静脉常显示其全长，并且常与下腔静脉同层。右段间裂：在右前叶，主要依门静脉右支或右前支来区分；在右后叶，此区无恒定结构来作为分段的标志，可用分别供应两段的门静脉支之间的无血管区作为分段标志。背裂：背裂的前部为肝左、中静脉注入下腔静脉处至门静脉主干中点的连线，其后部为下腔静脉右缘。

4. 易致错分肝段的肝脏血管因素　以上所述为正常大多数的肝内管道结构对肝段划分的标志性意义，但是肝脏血管变异情况复杂多变，使肝段形态、大小变化较大，因此划分肝段不能简单地依赖肝外结构，必须认真辨识和追踪肝内血管走行，据此来划分的肝段才是可靠的。但是，对某些血管应引起注意，它们易致错分肝段。

肝右后上缘静脉：肝右后上缘静脉在胎肝管道铸型中出现率为 48.8%。有时较粗大，易被误认为肝右静脉，导致误识右叶间裂。两者的区别是肝右后上缘静脉位置较表浅，在横断面仅见于头端的 1~2 个层面，不会伸入右叶间裂内。

肝右后下静脉：肝右后下静脉的出现率为 84%，口径在 0.40~0.89cm 之间，其中一半以上的口径大于 0.5cm。该静脉不位于右叶间裂，引流肝右后叶脏面的静脉血，于第三肝门位置汇入下腔静脉，不能作为分段的标志。

在肝段划分中，易将粗大的肝右后下静脉误认为肝右静脉，导致误识右叶间裂，两者的区别是：①横断面上，肝右静脉常出现在门静脉右后支的头侧，而肝右后下静脉常出现在门静脉右后支的尾侧；②肝右静脉在近头端的横断面上较粗大，截面呈椭圆形，而肝右后下静脉多在肝门上下高度的横断层面出现，常表现为一注入下腔静脉的长而直的管道；③在矢状断面上，肝右静脉呈椭圆形，出第二肝门，肝右后下静脉呈圆形，出第三肝门；④肝右静脉位置较深，而肝右后下静脉位置表浅，多位于肾压迹处。此外，肝右后静脉有时可与门静脉右后支平行而呈平行管征，此时应注意与扩张的胆管相鉴别。

肝左叶间裂静脉：肝左叶间裂静脉在胎肝管道铸型中存在率为 85.4%，约有 22% 的左叶间裂静脉同肝左静脉一样粗大，汇入肝中静脉或直接注入下腔静脉（双肝左静脉）。两者的区别是：①矢状断面上，肝左静脉与肝门静脉左外叶上、下段支同层，而左叶间裂静脉常与下腔静脉和（或）肝门静脉左支矢状部同层；②肝左静脉位于左段间裂内，而左叶间静脉位于左叶间裂内。

肝左后上缘静脉：肝左后上缘静脉口径较小，位于左外叶后上缘，在近下腔静脉入口处常位于肝外，出现率为 63.4%；而肝左静脉口径较大，多居于左外叶中间。在左外叶左份，左后上缘静脉易被误认为肝左静脉本干。

尽管对于肝段划分的研究已经非常深入，但由于各地区使用的肝段划分方法和名称不统一、肝静脉显影不理想、影像学上标志不明确以及血管变异现象普遍等问题的存在，使临床上划分肝段仍存在困难。Strunk 等（2003）和 Fasel 等（1998）在相关研究中发现，CT 横断面像上显示的肝区，有 17.3% ± 6.5% 被归于错误的肝段；在中心区域错误率高达 51.6% ± 19.9%；影像学方法确定肝段的亚段边界与实际测量的解剖结构确定的真实亚段边界的最大偏差值高达 40 mm。有不同研究者在各自的研究中均发现肝脏亚段的定位与亚段的实际范围分别为 31% 或 22% 不相符。此外，从下腔静脉沿着肝右静脉、肝中静脉及肝左静脉所画的 3 条线并不完全符合对应的肝门静脉段和亚段之间的真正边界，肝段间的边界并不是简单的平面，而是呈波浪状的裂隙。虽然 Couinaud 肝段法已经得到认可，但亚段边界的形状和位置仍有很大变异，这无疑增大了临床工作中肝段精确定位的难度。由此可见，肝段的影像学划分与解剖学划分的真实情况相差甚远，临床工作中尚有许多问题亟待解决，也需要一种影像学上确定肝段和亚段解剖的更准确的方法，将肝段的解剖学、影像学、外科手术中的划分方法及肝段名称统一起来，以满足临床工作的需要。

第三章 具有脂肪特征的肝脏疾病

第一节 肝脏内含脂肪与脂质的病变

表 1-3-1 含脂肪(肉眼、镜下)的肝脏病变

含脂肪(肉眼)的肝脏病变	含细胞内脂质(镜下)的肝脏病变
	局灶性肝脂肪变性
	再生性结节:罕见
肝细胞癌	肝细胞癌
肝腺瘤/腺瘤病	肝腺瘤
肝转移	肝转移:罕见
局灶性结节样增生:罕见	局灶性结节样增生:罕见
血管平滑肌脂肪瘤	
脂肪瘤	
脂肪肉瘤	
包虫囊肿	
脂肪性肝紫癜症	
肝肾上腺剩余肿瘤	
腔静脉周围脂肪	
假脂肪瘤	
肝畸胎瘤	
髓外血细胞生成	
髓质脂肪瘤	
嗜伊红细胞性肉芽肿	

有些肝脏病变内可含有肉眼可见的脂肪,而有些病变的细胞内可含有镜下脂质(表 1-3-1),肝细胞癌、肝腺瘤、肝转移和局灶性结节样增生既可含有脂肪亦可含有(细胞内)脂质。

最常见的含有脂肪和/或脂质的肿瘤是肝细胞癌和肝腺瘤,肝转移和局灶结节增生较罕见。腺瘤病中脂肪变较单个腺瘤更多见;局灶结节增生中,肉眼脂肪与镜下脂质均罕见。在 CT、MRI 和超声横断面影像上显示病变内含有脂肪或类脂质有助于肝局灶性病变的定性或缩小鉴别诊断范围。

肝内脂肪浸润的 CT 与 MRI 表现:CT 上表现为肝脏密度低于脾(正常时脾 CT 值为 36~42HU,低于肝脏);脂肪出现和消失快;肝内血管结构显示"相对密度增高";脂肪沉积可呈局灶性、叶性、节段性或补丁样分布;脂肪较少沉积区域:尾叶、方叶、被膜下、胆囊窝。MRI 上表现为 T_1WI 和 T_2WI 上无明显信号改变;在反相位像、自旋回波、脂肪抑制技术和短 T_1 反转恢复序列(ST1R)上,脂肪呈低信号强度。因此,肝脏病变内所含肉眼脂肪容易在 CT(低密度、负 CT 值)和 MRI(T_1WI 和 T_2WI 上呈高信号,在脂肪抑制影像上信号丢失)上分别被定性。在包虫囊肿内则可见脂肪小滴。

而肝脏病变细胞内所含的镜下脂质只能被 MRI 化学位移、正相和反相(T_1WI, In- 和 out-of-phase)梯度回波序列表现为信号丢失以及在动态钆剂增强上加以确定。

肝细胞内含镜下脂质的肝脏病变:局灶性脂肪变性,肝局灶性脂肪变性因过多的甘油三酯沉积引起,它可以呈均匀的、片样或点样。局灶性脂肪变性在超声上可显示呈高回波的肿块性病变,如血管瘤、血管脂肪瘤或转移性肿瘤。CT 上诊断弥漫性肝脂肪变性需在平扫时 CT 值较脾低 8~10HU。局灶性肝脂肪变性常表现为肝左叶内段、邻近镰状韧带、Ⅳ段的顶部和沿胆囊部位的局部病变,可呈多灶性。有时肝脏内可发生不同程度的肝脂肪变性,CT 上在肝脏弥漫性脂肪变性的基础上,可显示有局部更低密度(含更多脂肪)区。MRI 对评估局灶性脂肪变性有一定价值。反相 T_1W 梯度回波成像对鉴别局

灶性脂肪变性与肿瘤性肿块具有较高正确性。局灶性脂肪变性在正相影像上呈等或高信号，同时在反相影像上呈均匀性信号丧失。其形态大多能与肿瘤内脂肪区别，如肝细胞癌、腺瘤、血管平滑肌脂肪瘤或脂肪瘤。局灶性脂肪变性在 MR T_1WI 钆增强影像上表现为有角的、楔形边缘，境界常相对清楚、与肝脏等信号。对肝血管或胆管均无占位效应，且常可见血管影横（越）过脂肪变性区，这也可与肿瘤性病变鉴别。

肝细胞癌：在组织学上，肿瘤的分化程度、纤维组织的数量、出现瘤内坏死或出血，以及细胞内糖原、脂肪或金属离子等都严重地影响肝细胞癌的影像学表现，特别是对 MRI 的影响，在 T_1WI 上，可从低信号到等或高信号，以及在 T_2WI 上从低信号至高信号中的不同信号表现。有时肝细胞癌可含有脂肪。有脂肪变态的肝细胞癌约占 17%。有些研究已提示脂肪变态是一些肝细胞癌在 T_1WI 上呈高信号的原因，认为这一表现有助于确诊。然而，在常规自旋回波 T_1WI 上呈现高信号的其他原因包括糖原的含量、亚急性出血、透明细胞形成和过多的铜积聚等。Semelka 等（2002）认为应用化学位移成像在硬化的肝脏中发现脂瘤性结节可对肝细胞癌中脂肪成分定性。然而，肝内良性再生结节也可能含有脂肪。

局灶结节增生：局灶结节增生是一个有明确境界的肿块，并无真正的包膜，但有特征性的中心瘢痕。其典型的 MRI 表现为在 T_1WI 和 T_2WI 上呈等信号或接近等信号。中央瘢痕在 T_1WI 上呈低信号，而在 T_2WI 上呈高信号。在 MRI 钆剂动态增强动脉期，病变显示高度强化，而中央瘢痕不强化。在门静脉期病变内对比剂快速洗脱，成为与肝脏等信号。而中央瘢痕可显示延迟强化。Stanley 等（2003）报道由于病变内大量脂肪，使局灶结节增生成为明显不均质。

肝细胞腺瘤 / 腺瘤病：肝细胞腺瘤是一种不常见的原发性良性肿瘤。口服避孕药和雄激素治疗已可明确其病因。在大多数病例中，腺瘤表现为单发、境界清楚的肿瘤。组织学上腺瘤由糖原和脂肪增多的肝细胞索组成。糖原和脂肪是 T_1WI 上形成腺瘤高信号的主要因素。然而病变内亚急性出血区也可在 T_1WI 上呈明显高信号。依据化学位移在反相影像上所显示的肿瘤信号降低可确认存在脂肪成分，而不是由出血所引起。在 MRI 动态增强动脉期病变显示早期强化并快速洗脱，表明其典型的富血供特性。

第二节　肝内含肉眼可见脂肪的病变

血管平滑肌脂肪瘤：发生于肝脏的血管平滑肌脂肪瘤较少见。可呈一个孤立的肿块性病变，亦可伴同结节性硬化发生。组织学上是由成熟脂肪、平滑肌和血管混合组成的良性间质性肿瘤。瘤体因其组成比例［脂肪、血管和平滑肌三者相等；脂肪成分明显为多（达 90%）；脂肪成分较少（仅 10%）］不同致其影像学表现多变。Hooper 等（1994）报道在 12 例血管平滑肌脂肪瘤中有 11 例在未增强 CT 上表现为低密度病变，而在增强动脉期有 8 例中心血管明显强化。门静脉期 8 例中有 6 例中心血管保持强化。认为在病变内出现中心血管是肝血管平滑肌脂肪瘤的特征性表现。尽管富供应血管也可见于其他富血供病变，如肝细胞癌和局灶结节增生，但它们常位于病变的外围。MRI 脂肪抑制和多相动态增强扫描时，病变也因其组成比例不同，可有不同的信号强度，在 T_2WI 上可有从弱到强的高信号强度。MRI 的动态增强也能在病变内见中心血管强化。影像学上，脂肪成分占优的血管平滑肌脂肪瘤常不能与髓质脂肪瘤或脂肪瘤区别。而脂肪成分较少者又常与肝细胞癌伴有脂肪变者难以区别。两者都可以表现为富血供、伴有脂肪区的肿块。但仍有一些特性有助于两者鉴别（表 1-3-2）。

表 1-3-2　肝血管平滑肌脂肪瘤与肝细胞癌的特性比较

疾病	脂肪成分	早期强化	持续强化	包膜	供应血管
血管平滑肌脂肪瘤	大量	+（峰值较晚）	+	-	中心部
肝细胞癌	少量	+	-	+	周边部

肝转移瘤：肝脏转移瘤中有脂肪者较少见。转移瘤常反映原发肿瘤的组织特性，含脂肪的原发肿瘤，如畸胎瘤、脂肪肉瘤、肾母细胞瘤、肾细胞癌以及转移性卵巢皮样囊肿等可转移至肝脏。在 MR T_1WI

上呈高信号强度。

脂肪瘤和脂肪肉瘤:肝脂肪瘤较血管平滑肌脂肪瘤更少见。呈局限性、均质性病变,脂肪瘤也能多发。CT 上呈脂肪密度,增强后不强化。MRI 上与脂肪类肿瘤一样,在 T_1WI 上呈高信号, T_2WI 脂肪抑制序列上呈低信号。脂肪肉瘤是罕见的间质性恶性肿瘤,常起源于后腹膜和四肢。原发性肝脂肪肉瘤极罕见,首例报道于 1987 年。肝脂肪肉瘤超声上显示为境界不清、分叶的、浸润性回声肿瘤,伴有因继发出血和坏死而呈现的不均质阴影区。CT 上则可由脂肪密度的低 CT 值肿块加以佐证。

脂肪性肝紫癜:肝紫癜症是以肝窦状隙扩大、充满血液为特征。然而,脂肪性肝紫癜症被认为是另一截然不同的紫癜样病变,其发生于被移植的、因小叶中央肝细胞损害和坏死后脂肪变的肝脏,是一种不常见的肝脏疾病。肝窦状隙被脂肪液滴充满。虽然脂肪性肝紫癜是指发生在移植肝脏的肝细胞脂肪坏死,但任何受缺血性损害的肝脏脂肪都可引起相似病变。

包虫病:肝脏是最常被包虫囊肿感染的器官。Mendez Montero 等(1996)报道在包虫囊肿内可显示有脂 - 液平面或脂肪小滴。并确认囊壁上有大穿孔,与主要肝胆管交通,认为包虫囊肿内脂肪滴是由胆汁中脂质成分所衍生。

邻近肝内下腔静脉的局限脂肪:在 CT 上可于邻近下腔静脉见局限脂肪,这一改变可看作正常的发育变异,但更常见于慢性肝病病人。也可被误认为含脂肪肝病。

其他:肝肾上腺剩余肿瘤、格利森包膜假性脂肪瘤及肝畸胎瘤也可含有脂肪。有研究报道,肝内局灶性髓外血细胞生成也含有脂肪。

第三节　含脂肪成分的肝脏病变

肝脏多种病变,不管是良性还是恶性,都有可能含有脂肪,病变内脂肪的检出对判断病变特征及帮助鉴别诊断有较高的价值。

肝脏病变内脂肪成分的病理学基础:病变内脂肪可分为巨观脂肪和细胞内脂肪。巨观脂肪 MSCT 上表现为负值密度,CT 值 -10 HU 以下;细胞内脂肪肉眼不可见,CT 值为正值。该组病例主要讨论含巨观脂肪肝脏病变在 CT 上的表现。肿瘤成分中形成脂肪的原因主要包括:①成熟脂肪细胞,包括脂肪瘤、脂肪肉瘤、肝血管平滑肌脂肪瘤、畸胎瘤等;②网膜成分,包括肝脏包膜假脂瘤、肝胆术后网膜充填;③先天变异,如腔静脉旁脂肪;④肝细胞脂肪变性,包括肝腺瘤、肝细胞性肝癌、肝局灶结节增生;⑤与起源组织或原发灶成分类似的病变,包括肝脏肾上腺迷离瘤、转移性脂肪肉瘤、转移性肾癌、转移性胃肠道肿瘤等。

含脂肪成分肝脏病变的 CT 鉴别诊断: CT 扫描对巨观脂肪极为敏感,以下几个方面对鉴别诊断有重要价值。

临床特征:肝细胞性肝癌患者多有乙型肝炎、肝硬化病史,甲胎蛋白阳性。肝血管平滑肌脂肪瘤 6% 与结节性硬化相关。该组病例中未发现含巨观脂肪的肝腺瘤、畸胎瘤。肝腺瘤患者一般为口服避孕药和 I 型糖原贮积病的年轻女性。肝脏畸胎瘤好发于 3 岁以下的女性婴幼儿,可有肝功能损害和甲胎蛋白增高,肝脏原发罕见,多为腹膜内或腹膜后畸胎瘤侵犯肝脏所致。肝胆术后网膜填充物均有肝区手术病史,该组病例为原发性肝细胞性肝癌术后。脂肪肉瘤多数有后腹膜及肢体脂肪肉瘤病史,原发于肝脏者仅占 10%。

发生部位:肝包膜假脂瘤为位于肝脏表面、膈肌与肝上表面之间的脂性结节,该组 2 例表现典型,位于肝右后叶包膜下,并紧贴包膜。术后网膜脂肪填充位于术区肝裂附近。肝脏肾上腺迷离瘤好发于肝右后叶包膜下,部分与肾上腺分界不清。

病灶大小:肝细胞性肝癌早期即可发生脂肪变性,但一般在进展期才会出现巨观脂肪,所以含巨观脂肪的肝细胞性肝癌均较大。Balci 等(2009)的一组 11 例含脂肪成分的肝细胞性肝癌中,仅 1 例含巨观脂肪(CT 值为 ~11 HU),直径为 12 cm。该组 3 例肝细胞性肝癌中 2 例直径 >10cm。

形态、密度:肝细胞性肝癌有包膜,密度不均匀,中央可见坏死、囊变、脂肪变性;肝血管平滑肌脂肪瘤为实性肿块,边界清晰,但无包膜,密度不均匀,坏死、囊变少见;肝腺瘤易出血,表现为肿瘤内不均匀高密度;肝局灶性结节性增生有时可见低密度车辐状中央瘢痕；肝脏囊性畸胎瘤有包膜，密度不均匀，为局灶复杂囊性肿块，伴肉眼脂肪、钙化或骨化和软组织成分。

脂肪体积所占比例：肝细胞性肝癌脂肪含量较少，夹杂于坏死、囊变组织内，脂肪含量一般少于10%，该组病例脂肪含量为0.6%~1.5%。肝血管平滑肌脂肪瘤含血管、平滑肌、脂肪三种成分，脂肪含量10%~90%不等，该组肝血管平滑肌脂肪瘤脂肪含量为43%~91%，远高于肝细胞性肝癌，提示有一定鉴别诊断意义。肝脂肪瘤含均匀脂肪密度，增强后无强化，该组4例与之相符，另1例含纤细纤维分隔。肝脂肪肉瘤与脂肪瘤表现相仿，即使在病理上也难以区分。

脂肪分布：肝细胞性肝癌脂肪分布比较散在，呈镶嵌状，这与其病理基础相符合，肿瘤中央发生坏死伴脂肪变性，故发生在病灶坏死区域内并呈散在分布；肝血管平滑肌脂肪瘤脂肪成分及脂肪内血管影和围绕平滑肌构成洋葱皮样或类似旋涡状强化具有一定特征；肝腺瘤细胞内富含糖原和脂肪，但仅7%CT可显示巨观脂肪，表现为均匀片状分布的脂肪沉积；肝局灶性结节性增生内脂肪通常呈斑片状分布。

增强表现：尽管脂肪的存在对肝细胞性肝癌动脉期强化有所影响，大多数肝细胞性肝癌仍表现为动脉期富血供。此外，门静脉期廓清可与肝血管平滑肌脂肪瘤相区别。肝血管平滑肌脂肪瘤动脉期强化但强化高峰迟于肝细胞性肝癌。有学者研究发现：肝血管平滑肌脂肪瘤脂肪区域血供丰富，早期有强化；肝细胞性肝癌脂变区域相对乏血供而无强化。肝血管平滑肌脂肪瘤动脉期病灶中央血管的显示是其特征，肝细胞性肝癌、肝局灶性结节性增生也可见供血血管，但一般位于病灶周围。该组4例肝血管平滑肌脂肪瘤均见中央血管，1例肝细胞性肝癌周围见肝动脉血供。

总之，病灶内脂质成分的检出以及脂质存在形式的准确监测对于病变的定性诊断具有非常重要的意义。仔细分析病变的形态特征，尤其是脂肪的分布、含量及增强后表现，并且结合临床可以缩小鉴别诊断范围，甚至明确诊断。

第四节　肝脂肪浸润

肝脂肪浸润，又称为脂肪肝、肝的脂肪沉积、脂肪增生、地图状的或弥漫性脂肪浸润，多伴存于下述不同疾病中。

常见的有：①酒精性肝病；②糖尿病；③肥胖；④蛋白质-热能营养不良；⑤慢性疾病，如结核病、感染性肠病、充血性心力衰竭；⑥重症肝炎；⑦内生的和外生的皮质类固醇；⑧肠外营养；⑨因为肥胖而作肠道旁路；⑩毒肝素，如四氯化碳、磷、化学治疗。

不常见的有：①囊性纤维化；②创伤；③Reye综合征*；④妊娠时的急性脂肪肝；⑤糖原蓄积症；⑥大量的四环素药物治疗；⑦酶的缺乏，如糖原合成酶。①

虽然上述各种肝脏疾病有种种不同，但它们都有肝肿大，肝细胞功能紊乱，还可能有瘢痕形成与门脉高压。

第五节　关于脂肪肝背景

脂肪肝的病理基础及诱发因素：脂肪肝是肝脏的一种常见病，主要由于肝细胞内甘油三酯过多沉积所致，诱发因素有：肥胖、饮酒、糖尿病、药物性损伤（激素、化疗药物等）、病毒性肝炎、高血脂、肝代谢异常及先天性代谢异常等。有作者报告一组弥漫型脂肪肝中，大部分为肿瘤患者接受化疗后CT随访发现，尤其多见于乳癌术后使用三苯氧胺辅助化疗者，推测系化疗药物对肝细胞的毒性作用所致。1

① *Reye综合征：为童年时罕见的急性的，有时为致死性的疾病，常发生于水痘或病毒性上呼吸道感染之后。其特点为反复发作的呕吐及血清转氨酶升高，伴有肝脏及其他内脏的特殊性改变；可继以急性脑肿胀性脑病、意识障碍及抽搐发作。

例肝糖原沉积病伴脂肪肝,为糖代谢异常继发脂肪代谢异常所致。

脂肪肝背景对肝内局灶性病变CT检出的影响:正常情况下,肝脏实质密度均匀,其内局灶性病变常表现为低密度。脂肪肝背景下,CT对肝内局灶性病变检测的敏感性及特异性均有下降。轻度脂肪肝时,大部分肝内局灶性病变CT平扫仍表现为低或稍低密度影;当脂肪肝达到一定程度时,肝内局灶性病变呈等密度或相对高密度,多界限不清,鉴别诊断困难,易造成漏诊或误诊。此外,中重度脂肪肝内残存的正常肝岛组织也易误诊为肝内占位性病变。该组病例显示,当肝实质脂肪变性CT值低于或等于肝内局灶性病变时,常规低密度病灶则显示为高或等密度影,而CT增强扫描发现这些病变仍具有原来各自的特征表现。由此可见,CT增强检查对脂肪肝背景下肝内局灶性病变的诊断和鉴别具有重要意义。

弥漫型脂肪肝中各种常见局灶性病变CT表现:该组病例中,肝转移瘤最多,共18例,其中17例为多发病灶。CT平扫呈低、等或高密度,界限不清,这与脂肪肝背景造成的病灶与肝组织间密度差异减小有关,其相对密度的高低取决于脂肪肝的严重程度。增强扫描大部分病灶呈周边环形强化,界限较平扫清,这是因为富血供转移灶门静脉血供主要位于肿瘤边缘。增强CT结合原发肿瘤病史,脂肪肝背景下转移性病变的诊断并不难。该组2例多发肝细胞肝癌中,1例病灶在平扫、增强动脉期及门静脉期均呈高密度,但动脉期强化明显,强化表现为肝细胞肝癌所特有的"快进快出"方式。该组8例血管瘤中,3例(包括1例多发病灶)病灶平扫呈等或稍高密度,增强后7例呈典型的血管瘤强化方式,即动态增强早期边缘结节样强化,后逐渐由边缘向中央充填。由此可见,脂肪肝背景会改变病灶的相对密度,但强化方式一般不改变,故双期动态增强对鉴别诊断不可缺少。

肝腺瘤常见于口服避孕药的育龄期女性,多为单发,多发较少。该病常与糖原沉积病有关。CT平扫为界限清楚的低密度灶,动脉期呈均匀或不均匀强化的高密度,门静脉期为等密度或略高密度,病灶几乎均有包膜。该组1例经活检证实的肝多发腺瘤继发于糖原沉积病,其增强表现典型,且增强后期有典型包膜,但因有脂肪肝背景,平扫部分病灶呈稍高密度、部分呈等密度而不能显示。肝囊肿一般具有典型表现,诊断不难。在重度脂肪肝背景下,囊肿可呈相对高密度,增强后有时还可见环形薄壁样强化。在有恶性肿瘤病史且肝内病灶多发时,易误诊为转移,随访对照、CT值的测定及增强后无强化等有助于诊断。

脂肪肝内残存肝岛的诊断与鉴别:肝岛为弥漫型脂肪肝中的局灶性未受累区,为残存的正常肝组织,表现为整个肝脏低密度背景下的局灶性高密度影,有时易误诊为肿瘤。

肝岛多见于肝包膜下、胆囊床周围、镰状韧带旁以及肝门前缘区,其形成主要与肝内门静脉血供异常有关。CT平扫呈稍高或高密度,增强方式与正常肝组织一致,即门静脉期以均匀强化为主。该组5例肝岛表现典型,其中2例经穿刺证实者经保肝治疗后随访,脂肪肝消失,肝组织密度均匀,3例经1年以上多次随访无变化。对于已知恶性肿瘤患者,弥漫型脂肪肝内的局灶性高密度影,肝岛的诊断应该慎重,若要除外转移性病变,随访或穿刺活检是必要的。总之,弥漫型脂肪肝内局灶性病变,其CT表现与正常背景下有所不同,由于相对密度的差异变化容易导致误诊、漏诊。增强检查尤其是动态增强对病变的诊断与鉴别具有重要意义,随访复查也有助于正确诊断。

第六节　肝的脂肪浸润与诊断陷阱

肝内局灶性脂肪浸润可类似肝之低密度包块,仔细分析图像,可发现它缺少血管影像的移位,这与真正包块不一样。此类肝脏与脾脏比较,肝则呈现普遍性密度减低,可见较大的脂肪蓄积的局限性区域,或是局灶性脂肪浸润的线状、地图状表现。

Lewis等(1983)报告1例酒精性肝硬化病人,肝脂肪浸润产生大片均匀的密度减低区,尾叶既肿大又分叶类似一肝包块,增强扫描时密度增强的肝血管类似该包块的边缘。另有学者指出,肝内脂肪浸润偶尔也可表现为高密度病变而被误为肝转移性病变。在CT扫描图像上,肝裂内的脂肪可误认为扩张之肝内胆管。

Yates 和 Streight（1986）报告 2 例肝的多发性边界清楚的病变，超声与 CT 皆发现，考虑为恶性转移性病变，然而从核素显像与活检（其中 1 例手术）看，正确诊断仍是脂肪浸润。该作者指出，在见到多发性散在的肝的病变时，应考虑此类局灶性脂肪浸润的可能性，特别在有脂肪蓄积倾向的病人更应如此考虑。核素显像与活检可用来确诊 CT 的发现。

Kawashima 等（1986）指出肝的局灶性脂肪浸润伴似肿瘤，他们在一无症状的女性病人超声发现肝的局灶性脂肪浸润的不常见表现，CT 图像示一锐利边界的球形团块病变，平扫为软组织密度，CT 值 30HU，增强扫描为 50HU。用超声与 CT 对该病例追踪随访，见其完全消逝殆尽。该作者强调，此类病例务必追踪随访以除外原发性或转移性肿瘤。

Rampal 等（1986）在讨论不规则的肝脂肪变性时指出，不规则的肝脂肪变性常与肝的转移性病变混淆，他们报告 6 例，均为肝活检证实诊断，而临床和生物学检查皆系非特异性的发现。3 例肝超声示回声增强；另 3 例病变（脂肪变性）范围较大者，超声把非病变的正常肝组织误为回声减弱区，而将脂肪变性区视作“正常”。在 CT 检查时，不规则的肝脂肪变性通常表现较为特殊：非球状的形态；肿块占位效应的缺乏；其密度值接近于水（3 例）。当脂肪变性较局限（3 例）时，CT 图像上特点较少，肝活检可证实诊断。当已作脂肪肝治疗以后，再行 CT 扫描可观察病变部分或全部消散。

肝脏脂肪浸润与肥胖、饮酒、糖尿病、使用类固醇、营养过剩或营养不良有关。在螺旋 CT 增强的早期，因为肝脏没有完全强化而表现为低密度。在这种情况下，很难对比肝 / 脾的密度差别，因此有必要将肌肉作为参考标准。CT 图像上脂肪肝表现为均匀或不均匀的低密度。由于低密度病变与脂肪肝密度的对比度降低，CT 在脂肪肝基础上检出肝内病变常有困难。由于灌注差异，肝脏脂肪浸润偶尔呈区域或局灶性改变，不应误认为是肝脏肿块或梗死。如果有脂肪浸润，在脂肪浸润区域内可见到正常血管影像，而无占位效应。然而，当局灶性脂肪肝表现为一小团块时，可与肝脏肿块或转移瘤混淆。局灶性脂肪肝常发生在镰状韧带邻近区域，即肝动脉供血的分水岭区域。

局限性脂肪浸润所致的非均匀性脂肪肝偶可误诊为肝脏占位病变，这种改变在门静脉周围区域最为常见。为鉴别局灶性脂肪浸润抑或肝脏肿块，进一步的影像学检查是必要的，其中超声与 MRI 检查有助于区别二者。偶尔需要经皮活检。

第七节　肝的脂肪浸润与超声的跳跃区

Kissin 等（1986）报告 4 例肝的弥漫性脂肪浸润中出现局灶性的缺乏，超声、CT 与核素显像均清楚显示出此类表现，该作者强调超声检查时，如未觉察到肝脏大部分回声的增强，就有可能把正常肝实质的正常回声区误解为局灶性的病理性低回声病变。Marchal 等（1986）就超声与血管造影检查讨论了肝脂肪变性中的跳跃区，他们建议将脂肪变性中的局灶性跳跃区描写为新的亚节段型，它不同于局灶性脂肪变性的更典型的叶型或节段型的范围和形态。在亚节段型，脂肪均匀浸润整个肝脏，除少数称作跳跃区的不受影响的小的肝实质区以外。这些跳跃区主要位于包膜下区，或沿着叶间裂或胆囊床。活体的超声检查和死后的血管造影，都提示此跳跃区的范围，局部解剖学能够用血管解剖学的局灶性区别来做解释。

第八节　局灶性脂肪变和局灶性肝岛

肝脂肪浸润既可为均匀的，又可为不均匀的；既可呈局灶性，又可弥漫分布于全肝，其边界清楚或模糊。偶尔，肝内脂肪灶可类似于病变，通过比较同相位与异相位 T_1WI 可鉴别脂肪灶与病变。利用化学位移选择抑制技术（脂肪饱和技术）诊断脂肪浸润并不可靠。当一个体素内脂肪和水含量大致相等如肝脂肪浸润时，异相位成像显示最大的信号丢失。

当脂肪成分接近 100% 时，脂肪饱和抑制成像则显示最大的信号丢失,后者常出现于局灶性脂肪病变,包括脂肪瘤和血管肌脂肪瘤。肝脏假性病变常发生于镰状韧带周围,应与脂肪浸润相鉴别。肝弥漫性脂肪浸润时可伴有正常不含脂肪的肝组织,即肝岛。肝岛常见于胆囊窝、镰状韧带周围及第4肝段。异相位成像可鉴别残留的局灶性正常肝实质与局灶性肿块。

第九节 肝脏多灶性结节状脂肪浸润

肝脏多灶性结节状脂肪浸润(HMNFI)是一种良性非肿瘤性病变,临床少见,因其具有“类肿瘤”样的影像学表现,而易导致误诊。

肝脏脂肪浸润,又称肝脏脂肪变性或脂肪肝,是指由于肥胖、糖尿病、酗酒、营养不良、组织缺血缺氧以及肝毒性物质等因素导致肝脏脂肪代谢功能发生障碍,造成过多脂肪(甘油三酯和脂肪酸)在肝细胞质内蓄积而导致的肝细胞脂肪变性,其发病机制目前尚无确切定论。肝细胞脂肪变性也是慢性丙型肝炎的主要组织学表现之一,有文献报道约50%的成人慢性丙型肝炎患者伴有肝脂肪变性。脂肪肝患者一般没有临床症状及体征,多数通过影像学体检发现。一组5例患者中1例有丙肝病史,1例患有糖尿病,1例感皮肤及口唇干燥,2例没有特殊临床症状。

根据脂肪浸润的范围和程度不同,脂肪肝可分为弥漫型和局灶型两大类。其中弥漫型临床常见,CT平扫表现为肝实质密度普遍减低,低于脾,有时可在弥漫脂肪变性的肝实质内残存少量相对高密度的正常肝组织,称为肝岛。

局灶型脂肪肝可有多种表现形式,脂肪浸润可以累及肝的一段、一叶,或两个以上的段或叶,也可呈单发或多发的小灶状分布。

Tang-Barton等(1985)将肝脏局灶型脂肪变性分为五种类型:①均匀分布于叶或段内的病变;②段或叶内的结节状病变;③肝门附近的病变;④弥漫分布的斑片状病变;⑤散在多发的结节状病变。以前三型较多见,诊断也较容易,后两者相对少见,特别是呈多发结节状改变的局灶脂肪变性(即HMNFI)更加罕见,加之其“类肿瘤”样的影像学表现,容易被误诊为肝脏多发性肿瘤,如肝转移瘤、多灶型小肝癌、肝海绵状血管瘤等,因此需要引起重视。

肝脏多灶性结节状脂肪浸润的CT平扫表现为肝实质内散在多发的结节状密度减低区,各叶分布无规律,大小不一,密度欠均匀,动态增强扫描其强化方式与正常肝实质一致,肝脏的形态及大小正常,表面光滑。

一些作者认为肝脏多灶性结节状脂肪浸润的CT影像特征除上述共性之外,还可细分为以下三种类型:①结节边界稍模糊,可相互融合呈串珠状,多期增强扫描病灶强化程度始终低于正常肝实质,无动脉期高强化及门静脉/平衡期廓清或延迟强化等表现;②结节边界较为清晰,边缘可见环形极低密度影包绕,动态增强扫描病灶中央在动脉期几乎无强化或者轻度强化,门静脉期及平衡期呈中等~明显强化,而边缘极低密度环几乎无强化,病灶酷似“牛眼”,而可能误诊为肝脏转移瘤,分析此极低密度环可能与该处肝细胞脂肪变性更加彻底有关;③平扫结节边界较模糊,动脉期无确切强化,门静脉期及平衡期强化明显,与肝实质呈等强化,而致病变形态轮廓变得模糊甚至消失。

无论上述哪一种类型的结节,结合多平面重建观察病灶均没有明显的占位效应,肝内的血管及胆管无变形移位,也没有扩张及狭窄;有时可以观察到强化的血管穿行于病灶内,但走行自然柔和,没有受压、扭曲等表现。

肝脏多灶性结节状脂肪浸润的MRI常规T_1WI及T_2WI平扫表现为肝实质内散在分布的多个结节状等或稍高信号区,边界较模糊,信号欠均匀,有时病灶与正常肝实质信号没有显著差异,容易造成漏诊。分析其原因可能是对于含脂病变来说,其内脂肪含量越多,在常规T_1WI及T_2WI平扫上信号越高,但是对于肝脏多灶性结节状脂肪浸润来说,病灶内脂肪变性的肝细胞数量不足以使其产生明显的或可检测到的显著信号强度改变,所以常规的T_1WI及T_2WI图像对于肝脏多灶性结节状脂肪浸润诊断的敏感性和特异性不高。

随着化学位移成像技术的发展,MRI诊断肝脏多灶性结节状脂肪浸润不再是难题。目前,临床多采用扰相梯度回波T_1WI序列,利用水和脂肪中氢质子的共振频率不同，通过选择不同的 TE 时间，运用双回波技术，一次扫描同时获得反相位（OP）及同相位（IP）T_1WI 图像，具有很强的对比性，易于发现局灶型脂肪浸润并进行定性诊断。

反相位图像的效果是水和脂肪中氢质子信号之差，反相位图像的效果是二者之和，故两者对比时，若反相位图像上信号强度有所下降（变黑），则说明病灶内含有脂肪成分，这种方法对于病灶内少量脂肪的检出也很敏感。

此外，反相位图像具有独特的勾边效应，可以在病变结节边缘脂肪变性较彻底（富含脂肪成分）的区域与邻近肝实质交界处呈现出环形低信号黑边，使病灶边界勾勒更加清晰。所以肝脏多灶性结节状脂肪浸润在反相位 T_1WI 上的影像学表现具有特征性，表现为肝实质内散在分布的多个大小不一的结节状低或稍低信号区，边界清楚，部分病灶边缘可以见到极低信号环，与 CT 图像所见的极低密度环相对应。

而肝脏多灶性结节状脂肪浸润在反相位 T_1WI 上的表现与常规 T_1WI 图像相似，呈等信号。该组研究中，运用动态增强成像的扰相梯度回波腹部屏气三维 T_1WI 序列以及脂肪饱和法进行脂肪抑制，因该组序列的 TE 时间接近反相位的 TE 时间，故病灶也能表现出类似在反相位图像所见的特征，病灶的强化情况与 CT 增强扫描类似。

根据上述 CT、MRI 反相位、反相位及动态增强影像学特征，再结合患者肿瘤标志物等实验室检查资料，肝脏多灶性结节状脂肪浸润的诊断不难，但因该病临床较少见，加之放射科及临床医师对肿瘤性病变的警惕性较高，在遇到这样“类肿瘤”样病变的时候，容易先入为主而造成误诊。

第四章 肝脏富血管性病变

第一节 肝脏富血管(供)性疾病

原发与继发:肝脏富血管性病变分为原发于肝脏的富血管性疾病和继发的肝脏转移性富血管肿瘤。肾细胞癌、乳腺癌、甲状腺癌、黑色素瘤、类癌、胰岛细胞癌和肉瘤等是最常见的富血管性肝转移的来源。而最常见的原发于肝脏的单个较大的富血管性肿块是局灶性结节增生、肝腺瘤和肝细胞性肝癌,较小的肝血管瘤在早期增强影像上有时亦可表现为一小富血管病变。

肝脏的富血管病变主要包括:肝细胞癌、纤维板层肝细胞癌、富血管性肝转移、肝硬化发育不良结节(西方罕见)、肝硬化再生结节(西方罕见)、布加综合征中再生结节(和其他血管性疾病中的再生结节)、(上皮样)血管内皮细胞瘤、血管肉瘤、肝内胆管癌(罕见)、血管瘤(小)、肝腺瘤、血管平滑肌脂肪瘤、局灶性结节增生、肝紫癜症、动静脉畸形(先天性或介入手术后)、肝动脉动脉瘤(创伤性或炎症性)。

大多数肝细胞癌可依据其侵袭特性和临床背景做出鉴别。但伴有中央瘢痕的局灶结节增生难以与纤维板层肝细胞癌鉴别,肝腺瘤也常难与低度恶性肝细胞癌鉴别。

局灶结节增生与肝腺瘤的鉴别:两者都可发生于中青年女性,肝腺瘤可有服用避孕药的病史。影像学检查有助于两者鉴别(表 1-4-1)。应用特殊 MRI 对比剂会对鉴别更有帮助。与常规钆剂不同,3%~5% 钆贝葡胺莫迪司(Gd-BOPTA)是通过肝胆管路径排出,由于肝腺瘤内无胆管结构,Gd-BOPTA 增强时,延迟(1~3h)影像上呈低信号。而局灶结节增生含有畸形的胆小管,故在延迟影像上几乎都呈高信号或与肝脏呈等信号。此外,因局灶结节增生和肝腺瘤对超顺磁性氧化铁颗粒(SPIO)摄取类似,故对局灶结节增生的定性诊断,Gd-BOPTA 优于 SPIO。

表 1-4-1 局灶结节增生与肝腺瘤的影像学鉴别要点

病变类型	中央瘢痕	不均质*	强化不均匀	被膜下供血动脉	动脉期强化程度	门脉期瘤体强化程度	出血	T_1WI 高信号	Gd-BOPTA** 延迟摄取
FNH	+	-	-	-	>	+	-	+/-	+
腺瘤	-	+	+	+	<	++	+/-	+/-	-

注:动脉期局灶结节增生强化程度远高于腺瘤;局灶结节增生强化率 >1.6(动脉期衰减值与平扫时衰减值比);腺瘤强化率 <1.6。在门静脉期局灶结节增生常为等密度,而腺瘤则为高密度;*:含 CT 密度与 MRI 信号强度;**:中译名为钆贝葡胺莫迪司

肝血管瘤与肝富血管肿瘤鉴别:依据血管瘤的球形、周围性、进行性强化特点,很容易与其他病变进行鉴别。然而,小血管瘤可以在动脉期或门静脉期呈均匀性强化,难以与其他富血管性病变进行鉴别。有些方法可协助区别。强化程度:血管瘤的强化程度在动脉期与主动脉相当;而在门静脉期则与血管湖相当;而其他富血管性病变则强化程度稍低;强化延长:在延迟影像上,血管瘤持续存在着相当于血管湖的衰减值,而其他病变则已被洗脱,成为相对于肝脏的低密度;MRI T_2WI:在重 T_2WI 上,血管瘤较其他富血管性病变有更高的高信号;病灶周围强化:在动脉期,血管瘤有时可在病变周围显示有一过性强化差异。但这一现象也见于肝细胞癌。

不常见的肝脏富血管病变的诊断与鉴别诊断:布-加综合征中的再生结节:这类再生结节常较小,多发且富血管。可能是由于肝血供不足区发生萎缩,而有适当血供的区域发生代偿性结节增生的结

果。这类结节也在造成肝血供损害（减少）的其他全身性疾病中被报道，如自身免疫性疾病、淋巴 - 骨髓增生性疾病和类固醇与抗肿瘤药物治疗后。相似的结节也见于自身免疫性肝炎中。这些再生结节是来自结节性再生性增生（NRH）。结节之间没有纤维变性。如结节直径 >1cm，则可见中央瘢痕。有时结节在 MR T1WI 上呈高信号，通常在 T_2WI 呈等信号到低信号。同局灶结节增生一样，它们也可延迟摄取 Gd-BOPTA。结节的多样性特征有助于它们与其他的肝脏富血管病变鉴别。发生于布 - 加综合征的再生结节，在这些方面不同于继发于肝硬化中的再生结节。布 - 加综合征中的再生结节的鉴别特征：MR T_1WI 呈高信号；动脉期常强化；直径 >1cm 的病变常有中央瘢痕。

肝血管肉瘤：肝血管肉瘤的强化并不同于血管瘤。肝血管肉瘤可表现为不规则形、中心或环形局部强化，强化程度低于主动脉。通常延迟期还呈进行性强化，这有助于血管肉瘤与肝细胞癌鉴别。此外，在肝血管肉瘤中，有脾转移时可与肝细胞癌鉴别。

肝紫癜症：肝紫癜症的特征是肝内多发性、不同大小的充有血液的囊肿。它常由恶性病变、慢性感染、获得性免疫缺陷综合征（AIDS）和各种药物 [如口服避孕药和蛋白同化甾体（anabolic steroids）药物] 引起。其增强模式有从周围向中央扩展（模拟血管瘤），以及从中央向周围扩展（更常见）。典型的表现：病变缺乏占位效应，这有助于与其他肝脏病变进行鉴别；病变在延迟期强化延长，这有助于与其他富血管性肝脏病变进行鉴别。

肝内胆管（腺）癌：富血管性肝内胆管癌极罕见。它们在延迟期强化延长，可与肝细胞癌进行鉴别。

第二节　肝脏富血供良性病变

一、血管瘤

CT 平扫表现：血管瘤平扫多为低密度，边界清楚，少数因脂肪肝的存在可表现为等密度或高密度。如为等密度，血管瘤较小时，其内密度较均匀一致；病灶较大时，病灶中央可见更低密度区，多为偏心性，呈不规则形、裂隙状或星形，这种低密度改变可以是中心瘢痕或为出血和血栓形成。中心瘢痕形成与病灶大小相关，6~7cm 以上的病灶多数可见到瘢痕，3~4cm 以内的甚少见。血管瘤钙化极为少见。

CT 增强表现：肝血管瘤增强后的 CT 表现与诸多因素有关，一方面是血管瘤本身的组织结构和大小，另一方面与对比剂注射的方式和速度、扫描方式等因素密切相关。应用高压注射器注射足够量的对比剂（总量按 1.5ml/kg 体重计算），采用动脉期、门脉期和延迟期扫描，对 95% 的血管瘤病灶的诊断可以满足要求。延迟扫描的时间应根据病灶大小确定，一般为 3~5 分钟。血管瘤的典型表现为增强动脉期边缘强化，呈结节状、片状或环状，其强化密度极高，接近腹主动脉的密度。门脉期强化区逐渐向病灶中央扩展，延迟后病灶呈等密度或略高密度。血管瘤填充的时间与病灶大小有关，小的病灶约 1~4 分钟，大的病灶长达十多分钟或更长。也有少数血管瘤仅在门脉期或 / 和延迟期出现点状强化，称为“点状征”，这也是血管瘤的典型表现。有作者认为，如出现“点状征”，也可明确血管瘤的诊断，不必加做进一步的延迟扫描。平扫中央有低密度区的血管瘤，增强后该部分无充填表现。此表现多见于较大的血管瘤。

较小的血管瘤（<3cm），其增强表现多样化，主要有以下几种表现：

（1）管壁较薄，管腔较大的小血管瘤，早期整个病灶均匀强化呈高密度，和肝细胞癌的表现相似，但两者不同的是血管瘤的强化密度更高，有作者统计，血管瘤强化后的 CT 值比肝细胞癌高 50HU 左右。另外血管瘤强化持续的时间较长，可从动脉期持续到门脉期和 / 或延迟期。故螺旋 CT 多期动态扫描是必要的，可充分显示血管瘤的强化特征，其时间 - 密度曲线为“快进慢出”，和肝细胞癌的“快进快出”完全不同，因此对增强早期均匀强化的血管瘤的诊断是容易的。

（2）病灶一部分明显强化，呈点状、球状或片状，随时间延长，强化区逐步扩大，直至完全充填，即小的血管瘤也象大的血管瘤一样具有典型表现。

（3）增强早期病灶无强化，呈低密度表现，但门脉期和延迟期病灶可出现强化。常为边缘或中心点状强化,如强化程度高,和血管的密度接近,则易于做出诊断,否则容易误诊。

(4)增强动脉期病灶均匀强化,门脉期和/或延迟期呈等密度。此种表现的血管瘤和肝细胞癌及局灶性结节样增生易于混淆,属真正意义上的不典型血管瘤。动脉期病灶强化的程度对鉴别有一定的帮助,但还需结合其他检查。

(5)病灶始终未出现强化表现。这类血管瘤管壁厚,管腔小,对比剂进入慢,有些病灶在增强后5分钟才可出现强化表现,但目前多数单位均使用螺旋CT,扫描速度很快,在一般的检查过程中极少会长时间的等待,因此对这部分血管瘤的诊断有一些困难。

另外,罕见的是纤维性血管瘤,病灶内有大量的纤维组织增生使对比剂也难以进入。

上述五种表现以第1、2种最多见,第3、4、5种表现均少见。从定性来说,第4、5种强化方式的血管瘤定性较难。

在血管瘤CT检查中,因目前所采用的对比剂注射速率均较快(3ml/s以上),因此动脉期扫描有时能见到高灌注异常的表现。一种表现为病灶周围的环状略高密度,一种为病灶邻近的肝实质呈片状或楔形的高密度区。后者往往提示有动静脉瘘的形成。有时在片状高灌注异常区内,还可见到早显的静脉。以往的观点认为,动静脉瘘的形成为肝细胞癌的特征性表现,但也有少数作者认为也见于血管瘤。

在脂肪肝存在的情况下,血管瘤的CT表现应重新认识,特别是中度和重度脂肪肝。由于肝脏实质密度的降低,在平扫时血管瘤表现为等密度,或呈高密度病灶,给显示病灶和诊断带来一定困难。但增强后的表现多与一般血管瘤一致,对比剂由周边向中央扩展,最后将病灶充填,而延迟扫描血管瘤表现为高密度。或增强早期明显强化呈高密度,持续至门脉期和延迟期。此时血管瘤的密度不应与存在脂肪肝的肝实质密度相比较,可以密度相对恒定的脾脏作为参考。但在少数情况下,血管瘤表现不典型,则易于误诊。MRI是非常有价值的补充手段。

MRI表现:T_2WI多回波技术对血管瘤的诊断最为重要。随TE时间的延长,血管瘤的信号逐渐增高,在重T_2WI上,病灶的信号极高,称之为"亮灯征",为血管瘤的典型表现。但值得注意的是富血供肿瘤的肝内转移灶以及血窦扩张型的血管平滑肌脂肪瘤,在T_2WI上也可出现"亮灯征"。在T_1WI上血管瘤多表现为圆形或卵圆形的低信号,边界清楚、锐利。纤维瘢痕在T_1WI和T_2WI均为低信号,如纤维瘢痕组织内有出血或血栓,T_2WI上可为高信号。文献报道MR对血管瘤的诊断准确率达95%以上,一般不需增强即可明确诊断。Gd-DTPA动态增强可进一步观察血管瘤的强化方式,有助于鉴别诊断。在增强扫描中血管瘤的强化方式和CT增强扫描一致。

二、肝细胞腺瘤

CT表现:CT平扫时由于肿瘤的密度与正常肝实质相近,因此不仔细观察容易漏诊,通常表现为等密度或略低密度。伴有脂肪肝时,可呈高密度。平扫极少显示包膜,新鲜出血可表现为病灶内高密度,陈旧性出血则为低密度。腺瘤的囊变区域为低密度。肿瘤血供丰富,增强后,特别是双期扫描动脉期可见肿瘤强化呈高密度,囊变、出血区无强化。门脉期和延迟期病灶呈等密度或略低密度。病灶内的出血则无强化,包膜可延迟强化呈环形高密度带。

MR表现:在T_1WI上从略低信号到略高信号,T_2WI上为略高信号,病灶内可含有脂肪、坏死、出血或钙化,因此信号往往不均匀。T_1WI还可显示病灶的包膜,完整或不完整的低信号带,厚薄不一,和肝细胞癌的包膜相似。因腺瘤细胞和正常肝细胞一样,因此也可以在所有序列上和正常肝实质的信号一致而不能被发现。Gd-DTPA动态增强可进一步观察病灶的血供。腺瘤为富血供的肿瘤,增强动脉期有明显强化,但往往不均匀。门脉期和延迟期可为等低信号或等高信号。其强化方式和局灶性结节样增生相似,但腺瘤多有包膜,而局灶性结节样增生常出现中心瘢痕。此外,MR特异性对比剂的应用有一定帮助。

三、血管平滑肌脂肪瘤(AML)

病理上血管平滑肌脂肪瘤可分为四型,混合型最为常见,占70%左右,各种成分均存在。脂肪瘤型以脂肪细胞为主,肌瘤型以平滑肌细胞为主。血管瘤型又可分为二种,以厚壁血管为主或以扩张血窦为主。有作者报道肝脏血管平滑肌脂肪瘤和肾脏血管平滑肌脂肪瘤可同时存在并伴有结节硬化。大多数患者无明显症状和体征,多由体检发现,因此掌握其影像学表现是非常重要的,可酌情避免不必要的手术，因其无恶变倾向。

CT 和 MRI 表现：因组成成分的比例各不相同，其 CT 表现也多种多样。含脂肪成分多的血管平滑肌脂肪瘤其 CT 表现和单纯型脂肪瘤相似，而含血管及平滑肌成分多的肿瘤，多为富血供的肿瘤。脂肪成分的存在是特征之一，但病灶内脂肪组织的含量有很大差异，由 5%~90%。含量少的 CT 和 MRI 不易显示，而有些根本不含脂肪。含有脂肪成分者也会误诊为肝癌伴脂肪变性。病理上病灶中的脂肪为成熟的脂肪细胞，可伴有空泡变性，而肝癌中的脂肪为肝细胞的脂肪变性，两者在病理上易于鉴别，但在 CT 上两者的鉴别有一定难度。

MR 显示脂肪成分比 CT 更敏感，其中的脂肪成分表现为 T_1WI 上高信号，加用脂肪抑制后，病灶的信号下降。采用 FSE T_2WI 加脂肪抑制后病灶内脂肪信号强度也有下降。

血管平滑肌脂肪瘤可伴有出血，平扫可呈高密度。增强扫描动脉期，绝大多数病灶明显强化，多为不均匀强化。中心血管影的显示高度提示血管平滑肌脂肪瘤的诊断。有作者报道的一组 12 个病例中，9 个病灶可显示中心血管影，呈粗大或扭曲细小的血管影，特别是脂肪成分中见到血管影更具诊断意义。增强晚期病灶的表现也多种多样，和其病理分型有关。混合型、肌瘤型和血窦扩张型的可有持续强化，呈略高密度或略低密度，也可显示血管影。以厚壁血管为主的则表现为低密度，因血管内的对比剂已排泄。此型的强化方式和肝细胞肝癌一致，中心血管影的显示对两者的鉴别有帮助。

四、局灶性结节增生

CT 表现：CT 平扫显示肿块密度均匀，呈等密度或略低密度，部分病灶可显示中心的低密度瘢痕，其形态多种多样，星芒状、点状、条状或不规则形。局灶性结节样增生很少有钙化出现。局灶性结节样增生增强动脉期明显强化呈高密度。其强化特征为除瘢痕以外的区域强化均匀一致。有些病灶还可显示供血动脉，位于病灶中心或周边，粗大而扭曲。中心瘢痕无早期增强而呈低密度。门脉期和延迟期病灶强化程度下降，为等密度或略低密度，此时病灶边界往往不清楚。中心瘢痕延迟强化为其特征。

Mortele 等指出不典型的局灶性结节样增生有以下几点：①年龄：80%~95% 的局灶性结节样增生发生于 30~40 岁的妇女，而在儿童期（0~16 岁），其发病率仅占肝脏肿瘤的 2%。②肿瘤大小：85% 的局灶性结节样增生直径 <5cm，12% 在 5~10cm 之间，而 3% 的局灶性结节样增生病灶的直径 >10cm。大的病灶可引起症状，如腹部疼痛，可扪及肿块。③病灶多发。④病灶内出血、坏死和脂肪堆积。是极为少见的表现，因多数局灶性结节样增生呈密度均匀的实质性肿块。⑤无中心瘢痕。有些病例其中心瘢痕特别小，在 CT 上无法显示，约占 16%~40%。这类病例有时和肝实质的密度一致甚至不能发现，仅表现为肝脏轮廓的改变和邻近血管的受压。⑥假包膜样强化。以往认为局灶性结节样增生无包膜，而且这是和肝细胞癌鉴别的一个重要特征。但也有文献报道，局灶性结节样增生可以有假包膜，不过概率很低。包膜的出现表明病灶的生长缓慢，使周围正常肝实质受压。包膜由增厚的、透明的纤维组织构成。须注意勿将正常受压的血管或增粗的、病灶周围的滋养血管误认为包膜。⑦部分中心瘢痕无强化。此类瘢痕为胶原性的，和腺瘤、纤维板层样肝细胞癌等的瘢痕一样缺乏血管，因此增强扫描后无强化表现。

以上列举的几点局灶性结节样增生不典型表现，从局部看虽为不典型，但从整体分析也许仍较典型，不影响诊断。如病灶的大小，年龄并非关键因素。中心瘢痕显示高度提示诊断，延迟强化则更为可靠。

MR 表现：局灶性结节样增生在 T_1WI 上多为等信号或略低信号，中心瘢痕为更低信号，边界多不清楚，有时病灶中心或周边可见到流空的血管影，代表有血管畸形存在。T_2WI 上多为略高信号或等信号，中心瘢痕为更高信号，反映了局灶性结节样增生由正常肝细胞构成，因此和正常肝实质之间信号差异不大。中心瘢痕在 T_2WI 上为高信号颇具特征性，主要是内含慢血流的血管所致。MR 显示瘢痕的敏感性较高，达 49%~100%，但显示细薄的纤维分隔有一定困难。小的局灶性结节样增生中心瘢痕不明显，信号较均匀。

局灶性结节样增生含有枯否细胞，因此可以反映枯否细胞活动的影像学技术均可用于局灶性结节样增生的诊断。80% 的局灶性结节样增生可吸收 ^{99m}Tc，但腺瘤和肝细胞癌也可吸收 ^{99m}Tc，但吸收量不如局灶性结节样增生多，因此 ^{99m}Tc 的浓聚可提示局灶性结节样增生的诊断，但并非病理诊断。肝细胞特异性对比剂如 Gd-EOB-DTPA 或 Mn-DPDP 等也可用于诊断,局灶性结节样增生含正常肝细胞因而可以吸收 Gd-EOB-DTPA 或 Mn-DPDP 而明显强化,表明病灶为肝细胞性,其强化的程度高,峰值持续的时间长,和肝细胞癌有别,但和高分化的肝细胞癌相似。而且中心瘢痕的显示率提高。网状内皮细胞特异性对比剂如 SPIO 也可被局灶性结节样增生中的枯否细胞吞噬,病灶的信号在 T_2WI 上受到抑制。该项检查同样可与肝细胞癌、转移灶等区分,但高分化肝细胞癌也可枯否细胞,须结合其他资料综合分析。

第三节　十六种肝富血管病变

1. 原发性肝细胞性肝癌(HCC)　原发性肝细胞性肝癌是肝脏最常见的恶性肿瘤之一, 90% 合并肝硬化,原发性肝细胞癌的大体病理分型:结节型、巨块型、弥漫型。结节型:肿瘤呈结节状,与周围组织境界清楚,可有假被膜。一般早期无或极少向被膜外浸润或形成门脉内瘤栓。可进一步分为单结节型,多结节型。单结节型:与周围组织境界清楚单发结节。多结节型:可见两个以上基本相同的癌结节。巨块型:癌组织向周围呈浸润性生长,与周围组织分界不清,不规则,形成巨大肿块。其内常有坏死,周围可有小结节。常形成门脉内肿瘤栓塞。弥漫型:肿瘤呈 5~10mm 直径大小之无数散在性小癌结节,不相互融合,分布于全肝,结节大小比较一致。常于门脉、肝静脉内形成瘤栓。

与影像诊断有关的病理组织学特征:肿瘤由肝动脉供血,癌结节内分布于动脉性肿瘤血管。肿瘤细胞间之血窦形成及动静脉瘘均很明显。门静脉、肝静脉内肿瘤栓塞发生率高。肿瘤与周围组织交界部部分可见富于血管集簇之结缔组织被膜形成。

CT 表现:平扫:肿瘤一般呈低密度,少数呈等密度。动脉期:肝癌血供丰富,动脉期肿瘤明显强化,小肝癌常为均一增强浓染,大肝癌由于内部形成分隔,有不同的血管结构,而呈不均匀强化,其差别较大。门脉期:呈低密度或等密度。延时扫描为低密度。

2. 纤维板层型肝癌　临床表现:该型肝癌有如下特征:青年人多见,女多于男(1.07:1);血清乙型肝炎病毒标志物多阴性;血清甲胎蛋白阴性;不伴肝硬化;肿瘤常为单个,多位于肝左叶,瘤体内可有钙化灶或中心瘢痕;肿瘤发现时体积常超过 10cm。分化程度好,生长缓慢;切除后生存期长,平均 32~68 个月。该型肝癌在我国少见,在肝癌低发的某些西方国家多见。病理学:肿瘤大多为单个实性结节,以癌细胞巢间出现大量平行排列的板层状纤维组织及强嗜 酸性颗粒状的癌细胞浆为其主要病理特点。癌细胞索被平行的板层状排列的胶质纤维隔开,因而称为纤维板层型肝细胞癌。CT 表现:CT 表现呈巨块型,边缘可有分叶,CT 平扫呈等或低密度灶,分界清楚,可有包膜,中央有星状更低密度纤维瘢痕向周围放射。动脉期肿块明显强化,门静脉期肿块强化消退,中央瘢痕在动脉期及门脉期无明显强化,可见斑点状钙化。极少伴门静脉瘤栓形成。局灶性结节增生中央瘢痕有延迟强化,而纤维板层型肝癌的瘢痕无强化。

3. 肝血管瘤　肝血管瘤在组织学上分为海绵状血管瘤、硬化性血管瘤、血管内皮细胞瘤和毛细血管瘤。肝血管瘤是肝脏最常见的良性肿瘤。肝脏的血管瘤多数为海绵状血管瘤。多无临床症状。病理表现:单发或多发,可位于肝包膜下,向外突出于肝表面,也可比较深在。肿瘤被覆结缔组织被膜,与周围肝组织分界清楚,由充满血液的血管囊腔构成,囊腔间有纤维性分隔。肿瘤可发生纤维化,钙化及血栓形成。CT 表现:病灶多为圆形或类圆形,边界清楚但无假包膜。平扫呈均匀低密度,增强扫描病灶边缘呈明显的不连续的结节状强化,强化区域进行性向中心扩展。延迟扫描病灶呈高密度充填。较大的病灶中心可见始终不充填。血管瘤与其他富血供肿瘤的鉴别:血管瘤的强化与血管相当;血管瘤在延迟影像上呈持续强化;血管瘤有周围结节样强化,其环内缘呈波浪状,而肝转移瘤其强化环内缘凹凸不平;血管瘤增强后呈进行性持续性、向心性强化,无“周围洗脱”现象。

4. 肝腺瘤　肝腺瘤,包括肝细胞腺瘤和肝胆管腺瘤,通常所指的腺瘤为肝细胞腺瘤,而肝胆管腺瘤因其常含有囊性成分,又称为肝囊腺瘤。肝腺瘤多见于长期口服避孕药的育龄期妇女,偶见于儿童和男性。病理表现:肿块常较大(有时直径达 8~10cm)。单发,圆球形,边界清晰,有包膜。位于肝脏外表面。易并发出血及囊变。CT 表现：平扫呈边界清楚的低密度灶。增强扫描动脉期明显均匀强化。门脉期高密度或者等密度，延时期为低密度。少部分病例始终不强化，一直表现为低密度灶。

5. 局灶性结节增生　临床表现：多见于 30~60 岁女性。与肝腺瘤的区别，在于肝腺瘤无胆管存在，巨噬细胞少见。局灶性结节增生无出血倾向。常无症状。病理学：良性占位，常为单发，20% 为多发。它是由结构紊乱的正常肝细胞、肝巨噬细胞、血管和胆管等构成。边界清晰，无包膜。主要是由中央纤维瘢痕和周围增生的肝细胞结节与胆小管组成。缺乏正常的中央静脉和脉管结构，但穿行于纤维瘢痕内的血管丰富。CT 表现：平扫：呈均质的等密度或轻度低密度肿块影，少数呈等密度。动脉期：明显均匀强化，呈高密度。14%~44% 的肿瘤中心可见星状未强化的低密度纤维瘢痕组织。门脉期：动态扫描有时可见离心性增强。中央瘢痕门脉期均匀强化，呈高密度或低密度（中央瘢痕强化延迟），延迟期呈高密度（因所含的黏液瘤样间质内对比剂洗脱延迟）。

局灶性结节增生与肝腺瘤的鉴别：动脉期强化较肝腺瘤强；门静脉期较肝腺瘤更趋于等密度；较肝腺瘤更具均质性；局灶性结节增生出血少见，而肝腺瘤出血常见；肝腺瘤可出现脂肪变，而在局灶性结节增生中罕见。

局灶性结节增生与纤维板层肝细胞癌的鉴别：中央瘢痕在 T_2WI 上，局灶性结节增生呈高信号，而纤维板层肝细胞癌呈低信号；局灶性结节增生的中央瘢痕可有延迟强化，而纤维板层肝细胞癌中不出现；局灶性结节增生的中央瘢痕较小。纤维板层肝细胞癌的中央瘢痕较大，更具分叶，更具不均质；纤维板层肝细胞癌可见钙化，而局灶性结节增生罕见。

6. 胆管癌（末梢型）　胆管癌以 50 岁以上男性多见，可分为肝内型（即肝内胆管细胞癌）和肝外型（包括肝门部胆管癌及肝外远侧段胆管癌）。肝内胆管细胞癌富于纤维间质。根据其发生部位又可分为末梢型胆管细胞癌及肝门部胆管细胞癌。末梢型胆管细胞癌大体病理与腺癌形态大致相同，与腺癌之肝转移癌很类似，不易鉴别。肿瘤边缘部存活癌细胞多而稍隆起，与肝组织之界线呈波状。肿瘤中心富于纤维组织而坚硬。临床症状主要为上腹痛及进行性梗阻性黄疸。末梢型胆管细胞癌早期多无症状，晚期可有上腹部不适，肝大等。CT 表现：平扫表现为边缘不规则的低密度占位性病变，密度比较均匀。动脉期：肿瘤边缘呈轻度环状强化。门静脉期：于肿瘤边缘显示为低密度环，而中心表现为高密度灶。并可见肿瘤末梢侧肝内胆管扩张的征象。延迟期：延迟后强化逐渐明显，呈持续性。胆管细胞癌利于诊断的几点：病史（胆系多发结石、CA199 增高）；血供表现（周边强化、延迟强化）；病变密度较低（CT 值 20~30HU）；肝左叶呈轻度萎缩表现，边缘局部内陷。

7. 转移瘤　肝脏是恶性肿瘤易发生转移的器官，为转移癌的好发部位之一。肝转移的来源途径包括：血行性转移，经门脉及肝动脉转移；邻近脏器直接浸润；经腹膜种植。病理学：转移瘤的病理标本呈白色，与周围肝组织境界清楚，肿瘤中心多发生坏死，退变，而于表面形成中心性凹陷。CT 表现：肝转移癌的 CT 表现因原发癌及病理组织类型不同而异。平扫时：显示为多发性大小不等的低密度肿瘤结节，也可为单发结节。多在低密度内存在更低密度区域，从而显示为同心圆状或等高线状双重轮廓为其特征。增强扫描：肿瘤境界清楚，边缘部分可增强而密度增高。1cm 大小转移癌可出现类似环状增强的表现。平滑肌肉瘤、软骨肉瘤、类癌、肾癌、胰岛素瘤、甲状腺癌等的肝转移癌血供丰富，动脉期及门脉期可见明显肿瘤增强征象。有时候与肝细胞癌难以鉴别，但其总体以环状强化为主要特征，再结合临床诊断很重要。

8. 肝母细胞瘤　肝母细胞瘤是原发于肝的一种高度恶性胚胎源性上皮组织的肿瘤，好发于 3 岁以下的婴儿和儿童，以 1 岁以下更多见。与乙型肝炎及肝硬化无关。特点是甲胎蛋白明显升高。患儿可有腹部肿块，贫血、腹水等症状，并可出现黄疸。病理学：单个或多个瘤块结构，边界清晰，可有包膜。大体病理分为：块状型、多结节型、弥漫型。CT 表现：肿块单发或多发，多为圆形或类圆形，平扫呈低密度灶，边界清晰。钙化多见。增强扫描呈轻度到明显强化，密度可高于周围肝组织，亦可低于正常肝组织。延迟扫描呈等密度或低密度。

9. 血管肉瘤　血管肉瘤，又称恶性血管内皮细胞瘤，是一种肝血窦壁细胞异常增生所形成的原发性恶 性肿瘤，肉眼观肿瘤为灰棕色结节性肿块，可多放，肿瘤易发生出血。发病年龄 50~60 岁，男性多见。本病可为先天性血管内皮恶变，也可为后天发生。有报告发现肿瘤与酒精性肝硬化及接触放射性物质有关。肝血管肉瘤预后差,早期常发生肺、骨转移。CT 表现:平扫时呈低密度肿块灶,境界多较清楚。增强扫描早期病变示边缘强化,随着时间的延伸,强化逐渐向中心扩张,仍为低密度。表现与海绵状血管瘤相似,但与之相比,肿瘤染色、增强更为显著,内部结构形态更为复杂,并可为多发性病变,弥漫性侵及全肝。且有恶性征象。

10. 上皮样血管内皮瘤(EHE) 上皮样血管内皮瘤发生于肝脏,较少见,典型的发病年龄为 10~20 岁,也见于成人,好发于女性。病理学:表现为潜在恶性,病灶以多灶性,多中心性为主,且不会自行消亡。肿瘤由上皮样和树突细胞组成,中心有明显的纤维间质。病灶周边强化外围可见有低密度的晕环征。CT 表现:肝外围、靶样强化、包膜回缩。肿瘤多位于肝脏的周边区域,肝脏包膜无膨隆。CT 平扫为低密度影,病灶中心更低密度,约 20% 病灶可有钙化,增强后动脉期主要表现为周边强化为主,延迟后肿瘤实质内对比剂进入,而中央低密度区无强化。

上皮样血管内皮瘤与肝母细胞瘤的鉴别:肝母细胞瘤为儿童最常见的肝脏恶性肿瘤,发病年龄 1~5 岁,罕见于新生儿;肝母细胞瘤血清甲胎蛋白明显增高;肝母细胞瘤 CT 平扫呈低密度,增强动脉期多呈不均匀的高强化,门静脉期洗脱低密度,与上皮样血管内皮瘤的向心性强化、延迟期持续强化或强化减弱而呈等密度者不同。

11. 肝血管平滑肌脂肪瘤 肝血管平滑肌脂肪瘤,又称为肝错构瘤,它是一种极罕见的先天性肝脏肿瘤样畸形。根据组成的组织多少,分为起源于内胚层和起源于中胚层两类;起源于内胚层者又分为实质性错构瘤(以肝细胞增生为主体)和胆管错构瘤(以胆管和纤维胶原基质的增生为主体);起源于中胚层者又分为间质性错构瘤(以间质性组织的增生为主体)和血管性错构瘤(以血管和纤维组织的增生为主体)。病理学:肿瘤常发生于肝包膜下,多为单发,偶为多发性。肿瘤质地坚硬似橡皮,表面凹凸不平呈结节状,切面呈棕灰色。显微镜下可见大量结缔组织呈中心性星状排列,肝细胞排列不规则,不形成肝小叶,胆管上皮及血管多数已纤维化。肿瘤与正常肝细胞间的界线较清楚,一般无真正的包膜,但可形成假膜。肿瘤内多有囊肿存在。CT 表现:为囊实性包块,邻近结构受压移位。动脉期增强扫描实性部分呈不均匀强化,囊性部分不强化,门脉期及延时期逐渐呈等密度。肿瘤内有脂肪密度影为其特点。本病多见于幼儿,男女之比为 3∶1,早期无任何症状,随肿瘤增大,上腹部可扪及坚硬的肿块,可随呼吸上下移动,通常无压痛。肿瘤压迫邻近脏器,可引起恶心、呕吐、便秘、腹胀等症状。本病的最佳治疗方案是手术切除,预后良好。

鉴别诊断:肝癌瘤灶内有脂肪变性时,分布弥散,界限不具体,常伴液化坏死和血管侵犯,而血管平滑肌脂肪瘤为成熟脂肪,常位于周边。肝癌 80% 合并肝硬化及甲胎蛋白阳性。局灶性结节增生(FNH)强化方式与血管平滑肌脂肪瘤相似,但血管平滑肌脂肪瘤中心 CT 强化常可见到供应血管,磁共振呈流空低信号影,而局灶性结节增生中心为纤维瘢痕,随延迟可逐渐强化或不强化。肝脂肪瘤完全由成熟的脂肪组织构成,病理切面为均匀黄色脂肪,成分单一,见不到血管影。肝血管瘤的 CT、MRI 表现更加典型,表现为由周边到中心的“充填式”、“快进慢出”样强化,MRI 在 T_2WI 相上呈现“灯泡征”。

12. 肝硬化再生结节 肝硬化结节的病理:肝细胞大量坏死,肝细胞肥大再生而形成肝硬化结节,同时伴有肝内广泛纤维化致肝小叶结构紊乱,从而导致肝脏收缩、体积缩小及肝脏表面高低不平。纤维化,结节再生,变性坏死和脂肪变性等病理改变致肝脏密度的高低不均。病理上分为 3 型,直径大于 3cm 的为大结节型,最大可达 12cm,直径位于 1~3cm 为小结节型,二者混存为混合型;有研究表明,肝硬化再生结节以门脉供血为主,缺乏动脉供血。

小结节的再生性结节:在螺旋 CT 的平扫及动态增强扫描中常不能发现,因为肝实质的密度都较均匀。少数大结节的再生性结节在增强扫描中可见,表现为平衡期呈略低密度,而少数的较大的再生性结节在增强扫描的三期中均呈略低密度,类似于少血供的原发性肝细胞性肝癌。肝硬化再生结节平扫一般为高密度或等密度;注射对比剂后动脉期不同程度强化或强化不明显,在门脉期及延迟期肝硬化再生结节与肝实质密度趋向一致,这是诊断肝硬化结节的主要征象;肝硬化结节是发生在肝硬化基础上的良性增生结节,肝硬化,脾大,腹水,门静脉迂曲也是诊断肝硬化再生结节的一个征象。肝脏的密度由平扫时的不均匀变为增强后的均匀,这都是诊断肝硬化结节的重要征象。

需与肝癌鉴别，肝癌平扫绝大多数呈低密度，少数呈等密度或高密度，肝癌瘤灶内的密度更低区有其多数性，多形性及多层面显示的特征；肿瘤边缘的“晕圈征”和CT平扫边缘不清而常规增强后缘变清楚且肿瘤随之变小及周围的“卫星”结节直径3~5cm时，其动脉期强化一般是不均匀的，极少数是均匀的；增强过程癌结节对比剂的充盈呈“快进快出”的表现。值得注意的是肝癌与肝硬化结节共存时，容易漏诊。

13. 肝紫癜症　肝紫癜（peliosis hepatis，HP）是一种较少见的肝脏良性病变，表现为肝脏多发的大小不等的充满血液的囊腔。本病可见于任何年龄，但成人多见。病理表现：囊样扩大的肝窦状隙和与之相交通且充有血液的腔隙，伴有支持肝细胞和肝窦的网状纤维破裂为特征。腔隙大小不等，小者1mm，大者可达3cm。肝紫癜症的病因不明，可能与恶性疾病，慢性感染。药物等有关。CT表现：病灶多发，大小自1mm至数厘米不等。平扫呈低密度，增强扫描：强化模式多样，自周围向中央扩展或中央强化后离心扩展，持续至延迟期。 诊断特征：无肿块效应，病灶多样性，自中央或周围扩展进行性强化模式及强化延长。

肝紫癜症与局灶性结节增生鉴别要点：局灶性结节增生的典型CT和MRI非持续强化模式：动脉期为均匀性强化，门脉期和延迟期病灶常为等密度。与肝紫癜症鉴别常无困难；局灶性结节增生的病灶中常有中央瘢痕，其强化模式为增强动脉期呈相对低密度，门脉期密度或信号仍偏低，延迟期瘢痕则可出现强化表现，肝紫癜症则无中央瘢痕；动态增强时，肝紫癜症病灶内有时可因存在血栓而不强化；局灶性结节增生如无典型的强化模式和中央瘢痕时，则鉴别困难。

肝紫癜症与血管瘤鉴别要点：肝紫癜症缺乏肿瘤效应；肝紫癜症有周围性强化，且呈持续性强化，实质期和静脉期强化更慢；血管瘤呈向心性强化的病灶常较大，有明显占位效 应；血管瘤增强早期常呈周边结节样强化，且为非持续性。

肝紫癜症与富血供的转移瘤鉴别要点：肝转移性肿瘤一般为非持续性强化，动脉期强化，门静脉期和延迟期强化消退；含纤维成分较多的富血管肝转移性肿瘤，亦可见门静脉期和延迟期仍强化；结合临床病史和临床症状易做出鉴别。

14. 肝炎性假瘤　病因：肝脏炎性假瘤少见，发病情况不详，肿瘤是纤维结缔组织增生伴大量炎性细胞浸润形成的结节状病变。目前认为与自身免疫性疾病、硬化性胆管炎、溃疡性结肠炎等有关。基本病理特征是：炎性增生肿块主要由纤维基质和浆细胞为主的各种慢性炎性细胞浸 润所构成的局灶性病变，多呈圆形或椭圆形直径1~25cm。CT平扫均为低密度占位，增强后动脉像基本不出现强化，中晚期边缘和中间部出现局灶性充填，这点和肝癌有明显区别，因为肝癌血供来自肝动脉。而肝胆管细胞癌其强化后改变基本和肝炎性假瘤相同，均在门静脉期出现边缘强化和瘤体中间局灶性强化。

15. 肝脏结核　肝结核主要是由全身粟粒性结核循肝动脉血流入肝和消化道结核杆菌经门静脉入肝造 成感染。只有当机体免疫力极度低下，大量结核杆菌侵入肝脏时才致病。近年来，HIV感染者肝结核发病率明显增加，提示细胞免疫与肝结核关系密切。肝结核的基本病理变化为肉芽肿，在不同的病变阶段可表现为不同的形式，包括干酪样坏死、液化坏死、纤维组织增生及钙化等。同时并存的肉芽肿可以融合形成较大的形状不规则的纤维囊性包裹的干酪样脓肿。

需与肝结核鉴别的疾病有：肝脓肿，单发或多发圆形或不规则形低密度区，单房或多房，部分病灶内见气体影，增强扫描呈单环或多环状强化，具有特征性。肝转移瘤，肝实质内见多发圆形类圆形低密度区，有时病灶呈囊性或病灶内出现钙化，增强扫描，病灶边缘不规则强化，门静脉期病灶均匀或不均匀强化，但低于正常肝实质。胆管细胞癌，CT平扫为低密度灶，部分病灶内有不规则的高密度钙化灶，其特点是钙化位于病灶内，数目多而小，密度高形态不规则；增强后病灶不均匀强化，但增强程度低于 正常肝实质。纤维板层样肝细胞癌，CT平扫为边缘清晰的低密度区，可显示内部条索状结构和坏死区，病灶内出现钙化为其特点，钙化呈点状或小圆形，密度较高且位于病灶内，病灶周围可出现小的卫星灶，形成一个多结节的病灶。

16. 肝脓肿　肝脓肿可由溶组织阿米巴原虫或细菌感染所引起。阿米巴肝脓肿的发病与阿米巴结肠 炎有密切关系，且脓肿大多数为单发；细菌性肝脓肿的细菌侵入途径除败血症外，可由腹腔内感染直接蔓延所引起，亦可因脐部感染经脐血管，门静脉而入肝脏，胆道蛔虫亦可为引起细菌性肝脓肿的诱因。常见的细菌有金黄色葡萄球菌、链球菌等。此外,在开放性肝损伤时,细菌可随致伤异物或从创口直接侵入引起肝脓肿。肝脓肿的病理改变为肝组织局部充血、水肿、蜂窝织炎,继而坏死、液化形成脓腔。脓肿壁由炎症充血带或纤维肉芽组织形成。临床主要表现为发烧和肝区疼痛。实验室检查一般可伴有白细胞增高。肝脓肿的典型 CT 表现为:肝内低密度占位,边缘多模糊,内可见分隔及气体;增强后低密度病灶周边可见环形强化,可以是单环、双环和三环。单环为脓肿壁,双环代表脓肿壁(内环)和周围水肿带(外环),三环则表示除外环水肿带外,脓肿壁有内外两层构成,外层(中环)一般为纤维肉芽组织,强化最明显,内层(内环)由炎症组织构成。增强后脓肿内分隔强化,呈“簇状征”,即肝内呈蜂窝状的小低密度脓肿。“肝段强化”征是指动态增强扫描动脉期脓肿旁的一过性强化。胆源性肝脓肿的特征性改变为脓肿与扩张的胆管相通或紧邻、胆系积气、胆系结石。

肝脓肿的鉴别诊断:原发性肝癌及肝转移瘤:肝脓肿与原发性肝癌平扫同为低密度的病灶,增强扫描有助于鉴别诊断。原发性肝癌在动脉期出现明显强化,但是持续时间短,呈现“快进快出”的特点,一般不会出现持续强化及病灶缩小。少数肝转移瘤可表现全部或部分囊变,增强后呈环形强化,与肝脓肿相似,但肝转移瘤出现一过性肝实质强化的概率明显低于肝脓肿,具有“簇状征”“病灶缩小征”。肝血管瘤:肝血管瘤在增强早期有边缘不规则强化,周围肝组织正常,不会出现明显强化,增强区域逐渐向中心延伸,最后完全充填均匀,强化过程呈“快进慢出”特点。而无网格状及蜂窝状持续强化的特点。胆管细胞癌:纤维肉芽肿性肝脓肿和胆管细胞癌的 CT 表现有所重叠,胆管细胞癌的强化主要表现为轻度不规则强化,以边缘为主,而且常伴有邻近肝内胆管的扩张;纤维肉芽肿性肝脓肿,表现为逐渐明显的延迟强化和内部细小的无强化区,再结合临床表现两者多能鉴别。

第五章　伴有其他影像学特征的肝脏疾病

第一节　伴包膜回缩的肝脏疾病

肝包膜回缩常与邻近的肝肿瘤伴同发生，但也见于非肝肿瘤的病变中（表 1-5-1），是一个非特异性征象。如果伴有肿瘤发生，它可能是继发于肿瘤坏死和促结缔组织增生性反应。

表 1-5-1　伴有肝包膜回缩征的肝肿瘤和非肝肿瘤疾病（肝内、外病变）

肝肿瘤	非肝肿瘤病变
肝转移：可发生于治疗前或治疗后，以及病变增大或缩小时	肝硬化：融合性肝纤维化
肝内胆管癌	胆管阻塞
上皮样血管内皮细胞瘤	原发性硬化性胆管炎
血管瘤：常见于直径 >4cm 的病变	外伤
肝细胞癌	复发性化脓性胆管炎
纤维板层肝细胞癌	胆管坏死
局灶性结节增生	

从表 1-5-1 可以看出肝包膜回缩多见于肝脏恶性肿瘤，影像学检查有助于对它们进行鉴别。

肝上皮样血管内皮细胞瘤：典型的包膜回缩征象出现于较罕见的肝脏肿瘤——肝上皮样血管内皮细胞瘤。它是一种低度恶性的血管性肝肿瘤，其临床病程是介于海绵样血管瘤与血管肉瘤之间的中间型，发生于成人，平均年龄 45 岁，女性略占优势。

肿瘤由上皮样细胞在纤维黏液样基质上组成。除肿瘤的纤维基质成分和在包膜下的位置常造成肿瘤的包膜回缩外，其他影像学表现有多发性、周围性结节样肿块及其聚集、相互融合成的肝包膜下大肿瘤。由于肿瘤中心的相对少血管和肿瘤周围的相对富血管的特性，在增强后可形成特征性的“靶”样表现，中心低密度，四周有强化的边缘和围绕高密度“缘”的低密度“晕影”，构成低 - 高 - 低三层结构。

伴发肝包膜回缩的肝细胞癌：McLarney 等（1999）认为纤维板层肝细胞癌含有大量纤维组织和瘢痕，常发生肝包膜回缩改变（发生率约占 10%），如瘤块过大（已替代了肝脏全段）则回缩征可能不被发现。在纤维化不显著或未经治疗的肝细胞癌中极少见到肝包膜回缩，但经化疗或消融治疗后的肝细胞癌，病变缩小和纤维化增加，更易引起包膜回缩。罕见的硬化型肝癌或胆管 - 肝细胞混合癌有引起包膜回缩倾向。纤维板层肝细胞癌具有常发生于年轻人，肿块常较大（直径 >10cm）、呈均质性、境界清楚和分叶状，病灶中心可见钙化和大量纤维瘢痕和间隔，60% 以上病人可有淋巴结肿大等特征。此外，由肝细胞癌引起肝包膜回缩者，可有慢性肝病的临床病史，血液中肿瘤标记物升高，以及有关影像学表现和门静脉或肝静脉受侵犯等表现有助于鉴别。

胆管癌：胆管癌内有明显的纤维基质，易引起肝内胆管阻塞；而慢性周围性胆管阻塞常是节段性肝实质萎缩和包膜回缩的原因，故胆管癌亦常会造成肝包膜回缩。临床诊断胆管癌的依据有原发性硬化性胆管炎，或其他慢性胆系炎症的病史。最常伴有肝包膜回缩的周围型胆管癌，在 CT 平扫影像上常显示为一个低密度的球形肿块。注射对比剂 10 min 后，可显示含大量纤维组织肿瘤强化的特征性表现，即延长的中等度强化。

肝转移瘤：肝转移瘤也是极常见的局灶性肝包膜回缩的原因。其形成机制包括：肿瘤内存在纤维基质、邻近肝实质的局部萎缩、肿瘤治疗后发生体积缩小和纤维化。包膜回缩常发生于邻近包膜下的转移性肿瘤化疗、放疗或射频消融治疗后。未经治疗的转移灶也可引起包膜回缩,尤其是含有或能产生纤维组织的原发瘤,如肺癌、乳腺癌、结肠癌和类癌。确定转移性肝包膜回缩的病因,需依据临床(原发肿瘤病史)和影像学资料。肝转移在CT上常表现为多发、球形病变,大多是乏血供,在CT平扫和增强扫描时,均表现为低密度(CT值低于正常肝脏);如原发瘤为富血供者(来自胰岛细胞、甲状腺和类癌等内分泌性肿瘤),则可在CT增强动脉期时出现一过(暂时)性高于肝脏密度。重度的包膜回缩形成的假性肝硬化表现是经化疗的乳腺转移癌的特征。

肝纤维化:在非肿瘤病变中,包膜回缩征则多见于晚期肝硬化的融合性肝纤维化,呈楔形,常发生在肝前段和内段。肝脏其他良性病变(如肝血管瘤、胆管阻塞或肝创伤等)能引起肝实质纤维化、瘢痕形成和萎缩者都可能并发邻近肝包膜回缩现象。CT检查能提供这些病变的特征,大多数情况下,能找出“肝包膜回缩征”的原始病因。

肝恶性肿瘤:Soyer(1994)回顾性研究了8例已证实为肝恶性肿瘤CT图像示有肝包膜凹陷者,4例转移癌,余4例为肝内原发性胆管癌、胆囊癌、类肉瘤和分化良好的肝细胞癌各1例。包膜凹陷可分为两种类型:包膜凹陷边缘规则;中心病灶累及肝包膜不规则凹陷。该作者以此为标准前瞻性观察分析253例患有良恶性肝肿瘤的CT表现,其中恶性肿瘤178例,良性肿瘤75例。CT扫描包括平扫和增强扫描。在回顾性研究8例中,肿瘤均位于肝右叶,直径为15~70mm;中心坏死3例,胆管癌1例见小片状钙化。7例肝包膜凹陷边缘规则,其中1例凹陷包膜附近有局限性腹腔积液;另1例胆囊癌,肿瘤中心溃烂,累及肝表面边缘不规则。在前瞻性研究的253例中, 4例(2%)肿瘤附近肝包膜凹陷,均为恶性肿瘤: 1例纤维板层肝细胞癌,2例类肉瘤,1例直肠癌转移; 3例肿瘤位于肝右叶, 1例纤维板层肝细胞癌位于左叶; 4例肝包膜凹陷均为规则型。肝包膜凹陷发生于各种肝恶性肿瘤附近的肝表面,以往描述仅见于肝上皮性血管内皮细胞瘤。然而,此种表现也可见于其他肝恶性肿瘤。在此项研究中未发现伴存于良性肝肿瘤者。

第二节 伴钙化的肝脏疾病

肝内病变伴有钙化并不具特异性,它能在大多数感染性疾病以及原发和转移性肿块中出现。某些情况下,钙化的出现可缩小鉴别诊断范围。例如:一个伴有中央瘢痕的肝脏病变,若出现钙化,应考虑诊断纤维板层肝细胞癌,而不是局灶性结节增生。

伴有钙化的肝脏疾病分类:①寄生虫病,包括肝血吸虫病、包囊虫病等;②炎症,包括慢性化脓性或阿米巴脓肿、肝结核、肝胆管炎及布氏杆菌肉芽肿、梅毒树胶肿等;③血管病变,包括肝动脉动脉瘤、门静脉血栓、血肿(陈旧性);④肝转移,包括黏液腺瘤(来源于结肠直肠、乳腺、胃、胰腺、卵巢和甲状腺)、眼黑色素瘤、神经母细胞瘤、间皮瘤、直肠癌、骨肉瘤、软骨肉瘤;⑤原发肝脏疾病,包括纤维板层肝细胞癌、肝内胆管癌、血管瘤(海绵样)、肝细胞癌、肝细胞腺瘤、局灶结节增生(罕见)、胆管囊腺瘤/胆管囊腺癌、血管内皮细胞瘤、肝上皮样血管内皮瘤、婴儿血管内皮瘤、肝母细胞瘤、间叶性错构瘤。

肝脏肿瘤钙化的特点:纤维板层肝细胞癌钙化发生率高达68%,常是小钙化,位于纤维瘢痕中央。血管瘤的钙化可表现为多“斑点”状(静脉石样)或较大的、中心区钙化。胆管癌钙化继发于黏液分泌后,较未经治疗的肝细胞癌更常见。肝细胞癌钙化常呈离心性(偏心),常见于出血、坏死后囊变区。局灶性结节增生钙化极罕见,出现率仅1.4%。肝母细胞瘤是发生于5岁以下儿童最常见的、有症状的肝肿瘤,男孩好发,常见有钙化,浓密、粗糙的钙化常提示为肝母细胞瘤,而不是婴儿血管内皮瘤。婴儿血管内皮瘤常发生在6个月内婴儿,女孩好发,钙化常见(组织病理检查者中50%可见),与肝母细胞瘤相比,钙化常较为细小且呈颗粒样。

肝血吸虫病的肝钙化发生率极高,达90%以上,可谓居各种原因钙化发病率之首,但是,此类钙化在X线腹部平片一般难以发现,是慢性肝血吸虫病有诊断价值的CT征象。肝内钙化的分布,以右叶为最多,次为方叶和左叶,尾叶最少。钙化的程度,以右叶重于其他叶,肝外围重于中心区,而且愈接近肝表面,钙化愈明显,钙化带也愈宽。肝血吸虫病肝内钙化的形态颇具特征性。约65.2%为地图状，表现为线条状钙化相互交错，将肝脏分隔成大小不等形态不一的小区，形如地图；条状钙化约占17.4%；蟹状钙化约占13%，其中心钙化聚集成团，周围有条状影似蟹腿伸出。有作者推测，小叶间纤细钙化在CT图像上表现为条状；汇管区局部集结的死卵钙化呈蟹状；在大面积内小叶间与汇管区钙化相互连结，则呈典型的地图状。因而，三型钙化的本质相同，只是程度和范围的差异而已。

第三节　并发出血的肝脏疾病

在没有创伤或抗凝治疗下，肝脏自发性破裂、出血相对较少见。非创伤性肝出血主要由潜在的肝内疾病所致，也可由肝外病变引起。最常发生的肝内病变是肝细胞癌和肝细胞腺瘤（表1-5-2）。

表1-5-2　致肝脏自发性破裂出血的疾病分类

分类	疾病
肝脏疾病	
较常发生的	肝细胞癌、肝细胞腺瘤、肝血管瘤
较少发生的	局灶性结节增生、肝转移瘤、肝血管内瘤、肝淀粉样变、肝紫癜、结节性再生性增生、肝血管平滑肌脂肪瘤
血管瘤：常见于直径>4cm的病变	外伤
其他疾病	HELLP综合征*、结节性多动脉炎、系统性红斑狼疮、伤寒热、疟疾

注：*HELLP综合征（溶血、肝酶增高和低血小板综合征）

影像学对其诊断和处理有特殊作用。在临床资料基础上，当超声检查见一个高回声肿块或一个肿块伴有低回声区时，或是在CT上发现一个高CT值肿块时，抑或在MR T_1WI上显示肿块伴有高信号区都应怀疑肝脏出血病变。

（一）出血性肝细胞癌

发病机制：肝细胞癌自发破裂机制有多种假说：①认为是由于寄生动脉或静脉［如膈下血管、供应或引流血管］破裂；②来自体外或体内的轻微损伤造成肿瘤浅表撕裂；③因癌肿阻塞或完全阻塞肝静脉或其分支，使瘤内急速充血、压力增高后发生破裂。形成肝包膜下血肿或/和腹腔积血。临床表现为突然上腹部或右季肋骨下剧烈疼痛、低血压、休克（59%~90%）、腹膜炎（60%~100%）、血性腹水、肝脏急速增大和腹部肿大。腹腔穿刺86%积血阳性。发生率：在亚洲和非洲，肝细胞癌破裂达6.9%~14%，发生率与肿瘤发现和诊断时的大小有关，是男性最常见的非创伤性腹腔积血原因。有些病人可能有极轻微的腹部钝性损伤史。影像学研究：超声：可见肝脏不规则增大、硬化肝脏内显示有高回声肿块或一个肿块内有高回声区。CT：可提示潜在病变：位于肝脏周边部位、突入腹腔内、较大的、不规则状高密度肿块，并且周围缺乏正常肝实质组织；可以确定血肿的期龄和范围：急性期（24~72h内）呈高密度，随后（10~30d）CT值逐步降低，且有假包膜形成；CT上包膜下血肿或腹腔积血显示为围绕肝脏和脾的高密度液体影，有时可见分层的血凝集现象。MRI：T_1WI上肿块内有高信号区，提示为出血性肝细胞癌。血液的信号强度改变依出血期龄而异。除出血外，肝细胞癌脂肪性变、细胞内糖原或铜贮积等也可引起。

（二）肝细胞腺瘤

病理学：肝细胞腺瘤是不确定原因的良性肿瘤之一。自1960年口服避孕药开始使用后，其发生率迅速增加。在每10万个长期服用口服避孕药者中约有4人发病。组织学上，肝细胞腺瘤是以分化良好的肝细胞束为特征，而没有能分泌胆汁的胆小管存在。肿瘤框架内也缺乏门静脉管道和终末肝静脉，有别于正常肝组织或腺瘤性增生。但肝腺瘤有恶变危险，亦可以发生破裂、出血，导致右上腹痛，而被拟诊为急性胆囊炎。偶见严重出血致休克。

出血性肝腺瘤的影像学研究：超声，出血性肝腺瘤可表现为低回声肿块，内有高回声区，或一个高回声肿块伴包膜下区或腹腔内由液体形成的中间回声。彩色多普勒可在肿瘤周围显示有大血管。CT平扫：女性服口服避孕药者，肝肿瘤内发现有高CT值影、伴有邻近包膜下血肿或腹腔积血，则应做出疑似本病的诊断。MRI：肝细胞腺瘤出血表现无特异性。T_1WI和T_2WI上均为高信号，大多呈不均质。但出血在T_1WI上的高信号与脂肪存在相当，增强扫描有助于鉴别;在动态增强 MRI 上可见早期动脉强化。但其强化模式又与局灶性结节增生相似,然而局灶性结节增生可有中央“星状”瘢痕,可资区别;有时超声、CT 或 MRI 影像显示为继发于小腺瘤的包膜下血肿,而其原发病变并不被发现。

(三)肝血管瘤

病理学:肝血管瘤是最常见的肝脏良性肿瘤,尸检发现率约为 20%。女性好发(女:男为 5:1)。雌激素可以导致肝血管瘤生长。肝血管瘤大多较小(直径 <3cm),无症状。直径 >4cm 者,被称为巨大(海绵样)血管瘤,易自发性破裂出血,并出现严重腹痛等症状。组织学上表现为互相连接的衬有内皮的血管被包围在疏散的成纤维基质内。切面上可见有纤维化、出血、钙化,尤其是在较大的血管瘤中。影像学研究:在已知血管瘤病人中,如病变较大,超声上显示有增高的回波发生;在 CT 上有密度增高区;或在 MR T_1WI 上有高信号区时,应诊断出血性血管瘤。出血量较多者,还可伴有包膜下血肿或腹腔积血发生。

(四)肝转移瘤

病理学和临床:原发于肺、胰腺、胃、肾、乳腺、前列腺、睾丸、胆囊、皮肤(黑色素瘤)和鼻咽部肿瘤的肝转移,以及来自绒毛膜癌和肝淋巴瘤的肝转移,可引起自发性破裂后出现腹腔积血。其中肺癌、肾癌和黑色素瘤的肝转移是最常见的出血性肝转移。临床表现多变,可表现为不明原因的、不同程度的失血、休克或类似急腹症征象。出血性肝转移在临床上很少能在术前做出诊断。当出现急腹症表现时,常被误诊为胃或十二指肠溃疡穿孔。影像学研究:在已知有肝转移或已知有原发肿瘤存在的影像上,如在一个或多个肝脏病变内能确定有血液存在时,则应怀疑出血性肝转移。如果出血严重,可见到包膜下血肿或腹腔积血。然而腹腔积血更常见于原发性肝脏肿瘤,因为它们较转移性病变有更丰富的血供。转移瘤则倾向于更多纤维化与较少血供。对转移性腹腔积血的唯一措施是控制出血,但预后极差,多数病人生存期不足 6 个月,有的仅 6 周。

(五)局灶性结节增生

病理学:局灶性结节增生是继血管瘤后第 2 位常见肝脏良性肿瘤,发生率约为 3%。发病年龄可从 3 周 ~74 岁,但最常出现在 30~40 岁间,女性好发(男女比例约为 1:2)。口服避孕药可促使其生长。病变大多为偶然发现。仅 20% 病人可有继发于肝脏肿块的症状和体征。局灶性结节增生并不具侵袭性或恶性病程。局灶性结节增生极少出血。但曾有腹腔出血伴有局灶性结节增生者的文献报道。局灶性结节增生大多呈实质性、结节性肿块,常位于肝脏表面,清楚界限,无包膜。中央见“星形”含多血管的瘢痕是其特征。有较大的动脉和静脉出现在病灶周围以及中央瘢痕部位。腹内出血可由这些血管糜烂而引起。

影像学研究:虽然局灶性结节增生破裂、出血远比肝细胞腺瘤少见,但仍可以发生。如服用避孕药的年轻妇女突然出现激烈腹痛时,这一情况还是应当加以考虑或排除。CT 平扫对局灶性结节增生并发出血诊断有价值,可显示为病灶密度不均匀、孤立的包膜下或腹腔内积血。CT:平扫时局灶性结节增生常表现为等密度、等或轻度低密度肿块,30% 病例伴有更低密度的中央瘢痕。由于局灶性结节增生的供应血管主要来自动脉,故在 CT 动态增强动脉早期(20~30s)病变明显强化;而在门静脉期(注射 70~90s 后)局灶性结节增生与正常肝组织呈等密度,并伴有低密度的中央瘢痕。但中央瘢痕对对比剂的洗脱较缓,故在延迟期可显示有延迟强化。局灶性结节增生的典型“轮辐征”并不常见,一旦出现有助于诊断。MRI:在非增强 MR T_1WI 上病变与正常肝组织呈等或略低信号,而在 T_2WI 上呈等或稍高信号。中央瘢痕在 T_1WI 上则呈低信号,T_2WI 呈高信号。局灶性结节增生含有较多的枯否细胞,静脉注射超顺磁性氧化铁颗粒(SPIO)被病灶内枯否细胞吞噬,由于 T_2 缩短,使局灶性结节增生在 T_2WI 上信号强度明显降低,这有助于病变定性以及与肝转移肿瘤、肝细胞腺瘤等鉴别。

(六)肝淀粉样变

淀粉样变被定义为细胞外淀粉样纤维蛋白沉积,它可发生在躯体的一个或多个部位,尤其在肝脏、肾脏、脾和心脏较明显。肝脏常受淀粉样变侵犯,淀粉样蛋白无固定形态,沉积于肝窦间隙内,然后进行性侵犯邻近肝实质细胞及肝窦。出现大面积的肝组织被替代,质地似橡胶样、肝体积增大,肝细胞破裂少见。也有自发性肝破裂伴有淀粉样变的报道。肝淀粉样变中自发性肝破裂被认为是由于淀粉样侵犯造成肝实质变硬以及受累血管变脆所致。腹腔积血或包膜下血肿可由超声或 CT 做出诊断。淀粉样肝破裂的病例少见,大多数已报道病例均在几小时到几天内死亡。

肝结节性再生性增生：肝结节性再生性增生是由类似于正常肝细胞组成的弥漫性增生结节为特征。在结节周围没有纤维变性。肝结节性再生性增生的病因不确定。它能伴同于骨髓增生性或淋巴增生性疾病。男女发病比例相等，但年龄范围较大。病人可无症状或出现于非肝硬化门静脉高压。肝CT和MRI可显示正常，也可显示有多发性结节，而误认为肝转移性病变。但也可罕见有肝硬化表现者。在结节病灶间无纤维变性的特征，使肝结节性再生性增生可与出现于布-加综合征中的再生结节区别。再生结节的结节间有纤维变性发生。肝结节性再生性增生可有出血，但较少见。

（七）肝血管肉瘤

在肝脏血管肉瘤中强化通常并不表示是血管性病变。在肝脏血管肉瘤中的局灶性强化区，其CT值要稍低于主动脉且形态不规则，可位于中央或呈“环状”。在延迟期进行性强化，这有助于与肝细胞癌鉴别。此外，在肝脏血管肉瘤中最常见的脾转移对与肝细胞癌的鉴别亦有帮助。

（八）HELLP 综合征

病理学：Weinstein（1982）描述了溶血、肝酶升高和低血小板综合征（HELLP 综合征）。其在子痫或先兆子痫妇女分娩前或婴儿出生后瞬间发生，很快即出现严重并发症，即弥漫性血管内凝血、肝坏死和出血性梗死。组织学上，肝门区被纤维蛋白沉积、出血和肝细胞坏死所包围。纤维蛋白沉积在窦状隙、门静脉管道和肝动脉，可继发于弥漫性血管内凝血。但也有假说是节段性血管痉挛促使血管内皮细胞损害，使纤维蛋白沉淀。继发于休克的低灌注也促使肝坏死和梗死。然而肝梗死较门静脉周围坏死或出血更为少见，可能是缘于肝脏的双重血供关系。虽然肝梗死是严重的肝脏受侵，但肝实质内出血可发展成包膜下积血，甚至破裂入腹腔，是更为严重的危及生命的并发症。影像学研究：HELLP 综合征在临床早期常因病人出现右上腹痛而应用超声来排除胆囊病变，超声能发现肝包膜下和肝内血肿。CT可显示包膜下血肿和肝破裂伴有腹腔内出血；肝梗死也可在CT上显示为肝周边区低CT值的楔形区，并无肿块效应。

第四节　伴中央瘢痕的肝脏疾病

肝脏中最常见的伴中央瘢痕的病变是局灶性结节增生、血管瘤（大、海绵样）和纤维板层肝细胞癌（FLC），其次有胆管细胞癌、肝细胞腺瘤、肝细胞癌、富血管性肝转移和布-加综合征（或其他血管病变）中的再生结节。其中以肝细胞癌和局灶性结节增生的中央瘢痕更具特征，通常在超声上呈高回声的线状或星芒状。血管瘤常因有特征性的强化模式而得以鉴别，但局灶性结节增生与纤维板层肝细胞癌同为好发于年轻病人且伴中央瘢痕的富血管性肿瘤性病变，鉴别困难。一些影像学特征可有助于两者的鉴别（表 1-5-3）。

表 1-5-3　局灶性结节增生与纤维板层肝细胞癌的病理与影像学鉴别要点

疾病	性别	结节大小	分叶状表面	不均质	钙化	被膜回缩	瘢痕大小	T_2WI上所见的瘢痕信号	瘢痕延迟强化	被膜[1]	假被膜[2]	细胞内脂质	恶性特征[3]
FNH	女性	<5cm	-	-	-	-	<2cm	高信号	-	-	+/-	-	-
FLC	无偏向	>5cm	+	+	+/-	罕见	>2cm	低信号	-	+/-	+/-	-	+/-

注：1. 肝细胞癌可有一个真正的被膜，它在 T_1WI 和 T_2WI 上呈低信号，且显示延迟或延长强化；

2. 局灶性结节增生的假被膜可由周围血管或肝实质受压继发，在 T_2WI 上呈高信号，且有延迟强化；肝细胞癌也可有假被膜，与真被膜连同一起，在 T_2WI 上表现为低信号环被高信号所围；

3. 指肝血管和胆管受侵犯，淋巴结增大，肝外病变。

布-加综合征可以表现为多发性富血管病变并伴有中央瘢痕。良性再生性肝结节在布-加综合征中显示为多发、小和富血管病灶。可能是因肝脏血供不足出现萎缩，而在有适当血供部位出现代偿性结节增生的结果。这类结节也见于其他损害肝血流的系统性疾病，如自身免疫性疾病、淋巴增生性和骨髓增生性疾病，以及用类固醇和抗肿瘤药物治疗后。

相似的结节也见于自身免疫性肝炎。这些再生性结节与结节性再生性增生（NRH）不同，后者结节与结节之间并无纤维化，而再生性结节（尤其是直径 >1 cm 者）中央可有瘢痕。在 MR T_1WI 上，结节有时呈高信号，在 T_2WI 常呈等或低信号。这类结节的多样性有助于与其他富血管性肝脏病变区别。布 - 加综合征中的再生结节与继发于肝硬化的再生结节存在以下不同：T_1WI 上更常呈高信号；在动脉期影像上常强化；>1 cm 病灶常见有中央瘢痕。

第五节　延迟或延长强化的肝脏病变

具有延长 / 延迟强化的肝脏病变：延迟强化是指主要和显著的强化于动脉期后才发生者。肝脏病变中延迟强化常与纤维组织相对应。有些病变，如海绵状血管瘤可有延长强化，即病变从早期强化一直持续至延迟期。肝脏内兼具延迟与延长强化特性的病变包括：海绵状血管瘤、胆管癌（肝内）、局灶性结节增生（中央瘢痕）、肝细胞癌［常为（假）包膜增强］、肝转移、融合性肝纤维化、淋巴瘤、脓肿、上皮样血管内皮细胞瘤、肝紫癜病、炎性假瘤、肝腺瘤病（紫癜型和混合型）。

具有延长 / 延迟强化肝脏病变的特征：肝细胞癌：肝细胞癌病灶主要接受肝动脉供血，其强化程度与动脉血管内对比剂浓度相当，在 CT 增强动脉期呈明显高密度。门静脉期时主动脉内对比剂明显减少，肝细胞癌病灶密度也随之下降，而正常肝组织因接受门静脉供血密度增高，病灶相对于高密度的肝实质背景更表现为低密度。极大多数肝细胞癌典型的动态强化模式为动脉期强化，门静脉期对比剂洗脱。而 Gabata 等（1998）获得一组 30 例肝细胞癌 MRI 钆剂延迟（6min）强化与超延迟强化（1.4h）影像，13 例在 MR 延迟影像上、22 例在 MR 超延迟影像上显示有肿瘤中心延迟强化。对照病理确认病灶内延迟强化部位与病变内高纤维基质区相符。研究认为在硬癌性肝细胞癌中含有丰富的纤维基质，在 MRI（对比分辨率较 CT 为高）上可见延迟和延长强化。

此外，肝细胞癌（假）包膜的动态强化也与癌瘤体者不同，有其特征性。在动脉期表现为低密度环；在门静脉或平衡期强化；延迟期仍可见延长强化。Itoh 等（1987）认为肝细胞癌（假）包膜如显示这一特性，常提示该瘤肿组织分化较好，生长缓慢，预后相对较好。

融合性肝纤维化：各型肝硬化都可发生融合性肝纤维化。约 32% 晚期肝硬化中能见到融合性肝纤维化，因肝硬化行肝移植者也常并发融合性肝纤维化。常侵犯肝右叶前段和左叶内段，少数可呈弥漫性肝纤维化。CT 上显示为从肝门向外放射的楔形病变。平扫时呈低密度，增强门静脉期，病变可表现为等密度或仍为低密度。但由于对比剂在纤维间质内潴留，在延迟的增强影像上，部分融合性纤维斑块可表现为高密度，并伴有肝实质节段性萎缩和“包膜回缩征”。

炎性假瘤：炎性假瘤是极罕见的良性肿瘤样病变。病理特征为增生性纤维血管组织与炎性细胞相混合。肝脏居肺之后，是第二位最常发生炎性假瘤的部位。其真正病因不知。目前认为炎性假瘤可能与炎症性肠病、原发性硬化性胆管炎有关。炎性假瘤病灶常较大（>3.0cm）。CT 平扫病变呈低密度或与肝实质等密度。动态增强时常显示动脉早期强化，门静脉期呈等密度或呈轻度强化，延迟期病变内显示较正常肝实质有更多对比剂留存。能在病变周围见“缘样”或间隔的延迟强化。MRI 上，在增强前 T_1WI 和 T_2WI 都呈现自低到高的不同信号。但大多数在 T_2WI 上见到的是高信号。MRI 的对比剂强化与 CT 所见相似。

肝紫癜症：肝紫癜症的特征是肝内多发、不同大小、充满血液的囊肿。它常伴存有恶性病变、慢性感染、获得性免疫缺陷综合征和各种药物，如口服避孕药与蛋白同化甾类。其强化模式有周围强化向中央进展（模拟血管瘤模式）以及中央强化后向外离心地进展。但不管何种强化模式，肝紫癜症在动态增强成像中于病灶外围（环状）、中央（靶样）或全部呈现为高或等密度，具有延长强化效应。通常无肿块效应，有助于与其他肝脏病变进行鉴别。

肝腺瘤病：肝腺瘤病是常分布于肝两叶的多个肝腺瘤（≥ 4 个），常发生于年轻女性，有 3 种病理类型：脂肪变型、紫癜型和混合型。多灶性腺瘤病变在 MR T_1WI 上呈等至高信号；在 T_2WI 呈高信号。紫癜型在脂肪抑制影像上没有信号丢失，且动脉增强后可持续至延迟期。而脂肪变型在脂肪抑制影像上有信号丢失，且动脉增强后病灶无延迟期强化。影像学上，肝细胞腺瘤病易与其他的增生性肝细胞疾病相混淆，如结节性再生性增生、肝硬化的巨再生结节或腺瘤性增生结节鉴别。

第六节 密度/信号局限性异常与肿瘤

CT/MR 平扫或增强扫描出现的密度/信号的局限性异常减低或增高，并非一定反映了肿瘤自身或肿瘤的实际范围。在肿瘤病例中，异常密度区或异常信号区可能包括肿瘤以外的区域，或只是肿瘤的一部分，这种情况在增强扫描时尤为多见。此处从增强扫描的角度来讨论 CT 和 MR 上不代表肿瘤或肿瘤实际范围的异常区域，并介绍相关的平扫表现。

增强研究：CT 和 MR 成像设备的发展使全肝动态扫描（动脉期和门脉期）成为可能，肝脏的增强扫描对于发现肝脏肿块并予以定性有很大的意义。因为肝脏是有着双重血供系统的特殊器官，而且除了分化良好的肝细胞癌及某些肿瘤的周边部分之外，肝脏肿瘤多由动脉单独供血，所以动脉期扫描是观察富血供肿瘤的最有效方法。但动态扫描，尤其是动脉期扫描和血管造影 CT 常出现假阳性的强化区域。

分析门脉血流只能借助 CTAP（经动脉门脉造影 CT）来进行。经动脉门脉造影 CT 用于发现肝脏小肿瘤，这种方法为创伤性，假阳性高，再加上肝脏专用的 MR 对比剂的冲击，目前在欧美已很少应用，而在日本这种方法一直在使用，甚至有进一步推广的趋势，原因是门脉血流及动脉血流的综合评估对研究肝细胞癌的多步发生有非常重要的意义。若将经动脉门脉造影 CT 和 CTHA（动脉造影 CT）结合起来，可借助影像更好地评估肝脏的血流状况。

肝实质在动脉期呈显著强化的区域分以下五种情况来讨论：①血管变异；②血管畸形；③增生性结节以及与弥漫性肝病有关的状况；④瘤周表现；⑤其他情况。

血管变异：肝脏接受来自门静脉和肝固有动脉的血流，但肝脏的某些区域也接收来自非门静脉主干的静脉血，其来源可以是非门脉的内脏静脉之一，例如，不经过门静脉主干，直接进入肝脏的来自胆囊、胰头、胃窦等消化器官的静脉。这类静脉不像门静脉那样含有自空肠吸收的丰富营养物质，所以称之为“非门脉血管”或“来自于体静脉的血管”。

因为静脉回流早，“非门脉”静脉供血区早于正常肝实质强化，在动脉造影 CT 更明显。这种强化区可根据以下 3 方面直接诊断：①好发部位，多在肝门旁及胆囊窝；②形状，与肝被膜宽基底相贴，不像一个局限的病灶；③动态扫描中出现的时期，动脉晚期之后，如果发生于脂肪肝，这类区域表现为局部不受累的区域，在 CT 平扫上呈现局部密度增高。强化区如果在平扫时即为高密度，则强烈提示为非肿瘤性；但如果没有平扫图像，原来已有的高密度会使局部强化更加明显，从而导致误诊为富血供肿瘤。

肝的体静脉供血常见于上腔静脉综合征的病人，显著强化的区域可见于 S4 和 S3 的前中部（经由副脐下静脉），和/或见于 S4/2 的头侧部（经由副脐上静脉）。由于肝脏存在门-体静脉侧支通道（由体静脉和肝内门静脉之间的生理性静脉连接构成），这种情况还可出现于肝裸区。根据上腔静脉综合征的血流动力学可知，自腋静脉注入的对比剂在动脉前期就可通过体静脉丛的侧支通道进入肝实质。

即使在生理状况下也有 S4 前中部的小部分区域由体静脉供血的情况。即增强或平扫上均为局部低密度，经动脉门脉造影 CT 上表现为灌注缺失。Ohashi 等用经内乳动脉增强 CT 扫描观察到局部强化的现象，但在非上腔静脉综合征病人经静脉动态增强 CT 很少观察到这种现象。人们猜测经动脉门脉造影 CT 上呈现灌注缺损的病例是因为对比剂在静脉动态扫描的动脉前期就到达了肝实质，或直接通过与腋静脉相连的静脉丛和来自内乳动脉的静脉，在体循环中缓慢地释放。

血管畸形：很多疾病都可引起局部血流减少或衰竭。血管畸形是动脉期出现显著强化区的重要成因。首先，门静脉和肝动脉间的病理性沟通形成动脉门脉瘘；因为肝动脉与门静脉之间的压力差，受累区域表现为仅由肝动脉供血。而且,在远段肝动脉与门静脉之间存在生理性沟通,即胆旁丛和经肝窦的沟通。如果门静脉阻塞或门静脉血流功能性中断(如肝静脉栓塞),就会由肝动脉单独供血,而且只要动脉系统完好,供血量还会有所增加。

过去,动脉 - 门脉分流被定义为血管造影中门静脉远段分支或近段分支提前显影,而在动态 CT/MR 成像的时代,动脉 - 门脉分流有更广泛的定义:CT/MR 图像上可见的经门静脉的早期一过性或过多的动脉血供应。这样,伴有或不伴有可见门静脉的肝实质提前强化都可以归入广义的动脉 - 门脉分流,如:伴有或不伴有肝肿瘤的门静脉或肝静脉阻塞(即"肿瘤性"或"非肿瘤性"分流)、瘤栓或瘤周强化(见瘤周情况)。

除了瘤周强化,很多原因可引起动脉 - 门脉分流表现为弓形朝向肝被膜的楔形影,所以,除了靠近膈顶的肝实质,其他部位的动脉 - 门脉分流易于诊断。但有些门静脉或肝静脉并未到达肝被膜,而是在距肝被膜较远的肝实质内。如果这些静脉阻塞,会形成非典型的动脉 - 门脉分流,不到达肝被膜,那么增强扫描上表现为肝内类圆形的不与肝被膜相接的强化区。动脉 - 门脉分流也可出现于肝被膜旁。此类病灶与真正的富血管肿瘤在动态 CT/MR 扫描上的强化过程和表现是不同的,可资鉴别。

另一种有用的鉴别方法是超顺磁性氧化铁(SPIO)MR 成像,这是一种 20 世纪 90 年代兴起的用于发现肝局灶性病变的方法,超顺磁性氧化铁是一种组织特异性对比剂,有缩短 T_2 的效应,静脉注射后主要积聚于网状内皮系统的枯否细胞。富血供的恶性肿瘤没有枯否细胞,超顺磁性氧化铁摄取少,且肿瘤性动脉 - 门脉分流会使组织病理学表现正常的肝实质摄取超顺磁性氧化铁的能力减低,所以上述区域表现为 T_2WI 上较周围肝实质高的信号。非肿瘤性动脉门脉分流区域超顺磁性氧化铁摄取多,表现为 T_2WI 上较周围肝实质低的信号。

但应注意以下特殊情况的存在:①有些富血管肝细胞癌超顺磁性氧化铁摄取多,呈现低信号;②完全没有门静脉血供的区域(如肿瘤或门静脉血栓以远的缺乏门静脉血供的区域)网状内皮系统破坏,无法摄取超顺磁性氧化铁,因而呈现高信号。

典型的非肿瘤性动脉 - 门脉分流,因血管未受侵蚀,故而血管容量恒定,门静脉分流量受动脉及门静脉压力和流量的影响。Tochio 等用彩色多普勒观察到非肿瘤性动脉门脉分流区餐后门静脉血流增加,动脉 - 门静脉分流消失,这说明此类区域网状内皮系统仍保持功能。

肝血管的局部扩张在对比剂到达后呈现显著强化。伴有或不伴有门脉 - 肝静脉分流的门脉血管瘤在门脉期呈现明显、均一、持续强化,而动脉瘤及一些特殊的动脉 - 门脉分流在增强扫描的动脉早期即可出现类似的强化。影像所见的肝紫癜(肝实质内出现可导致充血或坏死的微血池)是一种少见的现象,供血血管为单独的肝动脉、门静脉或两者都有。

增生性结节:局灶性增生结节是发生于非硬化肝脏的富血供非肿瘤结节,既往研究认为门静脉血流的减少或缺如可导致局灶性增生性结节的形成。门静脉系统缺如属罕见病,表现为肝内门静脉缺失(周边门静脉走行区可见未充分发育的门静脉),门静脉血流通过门静脉 - 下腔静脉通路回流。越来越多的报道称某些特殊的弥漫性肝病可导致富血供结节的形成。布 - 加综合征可合并肝细胞癌,也可合并很多富血供结节。酒精性肝病病人肝细胞癌罹患率极高,同时也易形成小的富血供结节,组织病理学上为过度增生性结节。有少量文献报道,约半数酒精性肝病病例可见超顺磁性氧化铁高摄取现象。应与富血供肝细胞癌鉴别的血供丰富的良性肿瘤及肿瘤样病变有很多,但其不在此讨论范围内。这里只简单列出其中几种病变的名称:局灶性增生结节、肝腺瘤、血管平滑肌脂肪瘤(尤其在脂肪成分过少时)及胆管腺瘤。

瘤周情况:借助对比剂可清楚显示肿瘤,但对比增强也可能使肿瘤确切范围的划定及周边是否有卫星病灶的判定变得困难。因为肿瘤的范围对判断肿瘤的可切除性及病人的预后情况至关重要。Irie 等通过研究暴露于肝被膜的转移瘤发现,强化环只在肿瘤突向肝被膜处中断,指出动脉造影 CT(应用灌注技术作单时相研究)时,转移瘤的强化环并不反映肿瘤边缘,而代表肿瘤之外的肝实质。有作者根据强化环与下腔静脉或肝静脉相贴的转移瘤可以完全切除而无需切除这些静脉,得出与 Irie 相同的结论。

肿瘤边缘强化在判断病人预后方面有一定的意义。在分析肿瘤边缘增强方面,严格的动态扫描较有优势。Ueda 应用同一层面动态动脉造影 CT(自团注对比剂后 10 秒开始,每秒扫描 1 幅图像,持续 40 秒)观察结节及富血供肝细胞癌,指出注入肿瘤的对比剂几乎都是经由门静脉流入到肿瘤周围的肝实质；研究者将日冕式强化归于肿瘤血管引流所致的肿瘤边缘强化。应用同一层面动态经动脉门脉造影CT和动脉造影CT技术研究后，研究者认为，因为明显的日冕式强化没有时相的相关性，所以这种明显的周边强化应解释为肿瘤周围的卫星病灶所致。有些研究者应用经静脉同一层面动态CT已有20多年历史，他们观察发现，有一小部分少血供的转移瘤在动脉期呈现一过性瘤周强化。Ueda应用同一层面动态动脉造影CT研究转移瘤，也观察到有些少血供转移瘤在动脉早期呈现明显的瘤周强化。有些结肠癌转移瘤在静注动态增强CT上呈现瘤周强化，这类肿瘤的预后明显差于无此征象者。少血供肿瘤的这种早期强化的机制尚未阐明，但现在可应用全肝动态双动脉期或三动脉期的CT、MR扫描技术来研究这种强化方式。

在动态CT/MR成像上可清楚显示动脉-门脉分流，这一征象曾被认为是肝细胞癌的特征影像学表现，但现在的研究发现，海绵状血管瘤也常有肿瘤边缘强化及静脉显现；在肝脓肿形成过程中常有楔形强化（脓肿灶在强化区内，此楔形区域将随脓肿的成熟而消失或在强化程度上减低）。肝细胞癌常形成门静脉瘤栓。当瘤栓栓塞了近侧门脉，则在动脉期会有楔形强化，动脉造影CT上强化程度类似富血管肿瘤。

其他情况：放射性肝炎及暴发型肝炎或严重肝损害后的肝脏改变表现为受累区域动脉期强化。动脉晚期，大多数对比剂进入间质间隙内，瘢痕及纤维部分可见强化。同理，转移瘤的中心部分也在动脉晚期强化（与分布于周边的活跃的肿瘤细胞不同，中心部分为液化坏死区）。如前所述，经动脉门脉造影CT和动脉造影CT结合应用或经静脉注射对比剂行动脉期动态扫描对分析对比增强的机制有重要意义。比较兴趣区域与余部肝实质（正常或弥漫性肝病如肝硬化、肝炎及脂肪肝）所含门静脉及动脉血流的相对数量，可以说没有在门静脉期和肝动脉期都增强的区域。一般除囊肿及少血供肿瘤外，如果门静脉血流减少或衰竭，则动脉血流常增加。

当经动脉门脉造影CT上清楚显示灌注缺损或减少，而动脉期动脉血流无任何改变，则应考虑"非门脉"供血或体静脉供血和肋骨压迫肝实质的可能。门静脉血流增多较少见，但某些异常增生结节或早期肝细胞癌可呈经动脉门脉造影CT上强化及动脉造影CT上动脉血流显著减少的征象。有些再生结节经动脉门脉造影CT呈等密度强化，动脉造影CT不强化。

平扫研究：脂肪肝的脂肪浸润可发生于整个肝脏，可呈解剖分布，也可呈非解剖分布。非解剖分布者可分为规则性、局灶、多发结节和周边带状等亚型。局灶亚型多见于镰状韧带周围，其他部位有S4前中部、S4肝门侧、S3前侧部、除S4以外的肝门区。镰状韧带旁脂肪变的病因为由体静脉代替门静脉所致的肝实质损害。另一常见的部位是S4的肝门侧，被认为是来源于胰头的富含激素（尤其是来源于胰腺的胰岛素）的非门静脉内脏静脉供血所致。脂肪的存在是通过脂肪抑制MR扫描与常规MR扫描对比来证实。局部脂肪变也出现于常见部位之外，且病因不明。若发现自肝外而来的表现正常的血管，则可排除脂肪性肿瘤。

弥漫性脂肪肝的局部未受累区域：弥漫性脂肪肝病例中常可见局部未受累区域，应与脂肪肝合并肿瘤相鉴别，其常见部位为肝门部及胆囊窝周围的肝实质。病因学方面的解释为非门脉性内脏静脉供血所致，更普遍的观点认为，病因为富含甘油三酯和脂肪酸等营养物质的门静脉血供缺失，因而在增强扫描章节里讨论的缺乏门静脉供血的区域会形成脂肪肝中的未受累区。另外发现肿瘤周围的肝实质在脂肪肝时可不发生脂肪变，而脂肪肝的成因正是营养过剩。局部未受累区域偶尔可发生于肝被膜下的肝实质，但诊断较发生于常见部位者困难。

其他情况：任何原因引起的门静脉血流衰竭都可导致肝实质损伤，T_2WI呈高信号，偶尔在CT平扫上呈低密度。脓肿形成或其他炎症过程中的充血在T_2WI上也呈高信号。肝硬化引起的纤维化和暴发型肝炎所致的肝损伤，在CT平扫上呈低密度，T_2WI上呈高信号，需与肝脏肿瘤鉴别。肝损伤病例可见呈解剖分布或非解剖分布的局灶性的铁沉积，尤其常见于肝硬化再生结节，在梯度回波MRI表现较明显。梗阻性黄疸病人可见沿解剖分布的异常密度，但与肝肿瘤易于鉴别。另外，一些肝囊肿难与囊性肿瘤（复合型囊肿）或液性肿瘤（肝纤毛前肠囊肿）鉴别。

第六章　有关肝肿瘤的几个问题

第一节　肝肿瘤成像的几个问题

多年来，肝肿瘤成像一直作为衡量腹部影像学发展的标准。现代的原发性和继发性肝肿瘤成像采用运动抑制、组织特异性对比剂、多维成像、血流成像等技术。放射诊断技术的不断改进提高了诊断水平。

一般原则：首先，影像诊断要确定以下问题：①肝内是否存在病灶？ ②有多少病灶？ ③病灶的特征是什么？ ④是否适合切除？ 其次，比较成像方法时应考虑其损伤性。通常检测肝肿瘤最敏感的手段对机体的损伤最大，而受检者很多为正常人，必须尽可能不损伤身体。

最后，“外科”肝转移和“内科”肝转移的概念涉及以下情况：像结肠腺癌和内脏肉瘤等原发性肿瘤转移至肝的病灶通常数目少，散在分布于周边部，适合局部切除或其他根治术；而像乳腺和胰腺肿瘤转移至肝的病灶通常弥散于全肝，一般只适合内科治疗。这样的病例只要求影像诊断为实施治疗做出“阳性”或“阴性”的回答。

直径小于10mm的结节：到目前为止，普通CT可满意显示10mm直径的病灶，但仍有30%~50%的孤立病灶漏诊。高性能的MR技术常可显示直径小于10mm的良性或恶性结节。尽管很多文献报道其敏感性高，但普通MR不能描述此类病灶的形态学特征。由于部分容积效应，普通CT在10mm水平难以准确鉴别肝囊肿和转移瘤。这样的小病灶难以活检只有进一步检查和随访影像学检查切实可行。

肝实质的表现：影像学所见肝肿瘤常伴有相应肝实质局限或弥散，增生或代谢，与新生物相关或不相关的改变。肝恶性肿瘤常有散在或局限性脂肪浸润，给诊断带来困难，需要多种技术综合处理。所有这些病例在超声检查和硫胶显像核素闪烁图上可以帮助诊断。

不少文献把局限性脂肪浸润灶描述为边缘锐利的圆形低密度灶，几乎与转移灶难以区分，它常呈多灶性，可增大或浸润，多见于镰状韧带附近。MR常规序列对弥散性脂肪浸润不敏感，但在局限性病灶呈典型短T1强信号。必要时可以采用化学位移技术帮助诊断。

疾病分期：解剖：影像学检查分期意在确定①肝内病灶的部位和范围；②是否累及关键部位（如：肝门、下腔静脉、大胆管）；③是否存在肝外病灶。目前影像诊断多以法国应用解剖学家Couinaund和Bismuth的肝分段标准进行描述，即以三条大的肝静脉（即：左、中、右）和门静脉将肝分为8段。以这种分段进行多叶段切除允许清除肝实质的量可达80%。位于中央部位，累及门静脉或下腔静脉的肿瘤，切除治疗就不大可能了。

成像技术：在评估肝肿瘤时，CT或/和MRI多用于筛选，而CT动脉性门脉造影（CTAP）和术中超声检查（IOUS）则用于临床分期。CTAP发现小的肝病灶极其精确，Matsui等在18例直径小于15mm的结肠癌肝转移中发现10例都是经CT、超声和血管造影未检出的病例。Heiken等的研究表明CTAP对转移灶的检出率为81%，而CT只检出38%，CTAP对直径大于10mm的病灶检出率为100%。Nelson等的研究结果与此接近。

可能由于动脉变异、静脉性梗阻以及导管因素的影响，CTAP显示层流灌注缺损的假阳性率高达30%~40%。不过，此类灌注缺损通常呈典型的楔形，位于周边部，而转移瘤则呈圆形。Fernandez和Bernardino研究表明灌注缺损常出现于肝左叶内段

（占 14%），这可能与沿胆囊窝包膜下组织的供养血管变异有关。CTAP 的假阳性所见很容易通过 4~6 小时延迟扫描发现，假阳性病灶显示等密度灌注，而转移灶则持续存在。术中超声检查是对近中央部位且术中无法触及的病灶进行判定的备选方法。Sugarbaker 认为，如果术前已获得高质量的成像，术中超声就不很重要了，但可做为肝切除性手术的备择手段。

CT 与 MR 的比较：CT 对 MR 肝肿瘤成像的相对优势是前者在以往多年中已有大量的科学研究和论证。不少综述总结了当前的看法，大多认为 MR 探查病灶的能力和 CT 相似，而描述病灶特征的能力可能优于 CT。暂且不说 CT 造影技术，就 MR 场强、脉冲序列、运动抑制技术等的应用就有非常之多的组合，这样，各家的意见难以苟同。

关于海绵状血管瘤：CT 评价海绵状血管瘤存在下列问题：①与转移瘤鉴别的标准仅在 55% 的病例中是典型的；②很多情况下，给予对比剂后需延迟扫描达 30 分钟以证实典型的周边向心灌注表现；③由于灌注表现短暂，很难在不同 CT 层面对多发性病灶进行评估，还需采用重复 CT 扫描、核素血池期扫描、经皮活检、MR 扫描等。当采用不进床单层面动态 CT 评估单个病灶的灌注类型时，这种局限性尤为明显。

这种新的单层面方法采用快速扫描和对比剂团注技术显示出酷似 X 线动脉造影灌注形式的末稍球形增强。而 MR 在多层面显示多中心病灶不需延迟扫描或其他成像。在 2.0 T 以内不同场强下鉴别转移瘤和血管瘤的准确度超过 85%，100ms 以上的 TE 序列 T_2WI 自旋回波成像能有效地显示典型慢血流表现的长 T_2 超强度亮信号。海绵状血管瘤可显示“灯泡”征形态学表现，而且高的对比 - 噪声比率和信号 - 噪声比率可以准确鉴别血管瘤和转移瘤。

MR 肝对比剂：超顺磁铁氧化物（SPIO）颗粒已引起大多数学者关注。颗粒大小为 20~200nm，外裹以葡聚糖或糖原，能够被肝和脾的网状内皮系统封存，而肿瘤组织却不能。与 SPIO 颗粒相关的大磁矩产生局部不均匀磁场，正常肝实质 T_2 信号变短，变暗。信号噪声比和对比噪声比的提高增加了检出病灶的能力，可以发现直径 2~3mm 的病灶。第二代不超过 10nm 的超微 SPIO 颗粒已应用于肝细胞成像，这种对比剂外包以阿拉伯半乳糖，可特异地被肝细胞乏唾液酸基糖蛋白识别系统捕获。用量比大的 SPIO 颗粒少，评价肝功能的能力强，还可能用来区别良、恶性肿瘤。特异性肝顺磁对比剂锰 DPDP 是一种维生素 B_6 衍化物，诱发正常肝实质选择性地 T_1 信号变短，却不能影响转移瘤。具有相对较长的成像窗位，毒性可以忽略。象肝细胞癌，腺癌等原发性肿瘤对锰 DPDP 亲合力较强，使组织特异性鉴别诊断成为可能。

MR 快速成像：很多种快速屏气梯度回声序列已经引入临床使用，包括快速获得自旋回波，梯度回波小角度快速拍照，预磁化快速获得梯度回波 MR。大多数快速成像技术需应用像钆等顺磁对比剂来缩短肝实质 T_1 弛豫，增强信号噪声比和病灶 - 正常肝的对比噪声比。动态给予对比剂可以显示血管瘤的慢血流灌注形式，类似增强 CT 所见。

第二节　代谢组学在肝脏疾病的应用

肝脏作为全身最重要的代谢器官，糖类、脂类及氨基酸 3 大营养物质的代谢过程均在肝脏完成，一旦肝功能受损，机体多个重要脏器功能亦可能出现障碍。由于其在代谢方面的重要性，从代谢的角度对肝脏及其疾病进行系统研究就显得尤为重要。

肝细胞性肝癌（HCC）早期诊断、早期治疗对改善肝细胞癌预后、提高生存率至关重要。目前，甲胎蛋白（AFP）作为肝细胞癌的客观诊断指标。但甲胎蛋白在重型肝炎肝细胞坏死后再生时也可升高，非肝癌所特有。因此，Yin 等（2009）利用快速液相色谱联合 4 级杆高分辨飞行时间质谱对肝硬化组和肝细胞癌组的血清进行研究。该研究在样本分离阶段结合使用了高效液相色谱和亲水相互作用色谱（HILIC）分离技术，进行多元分析，发现甘胆酸、鹅脱氧甘胆酸、牛黄胆酸和牛黄鹅脱氧胆酸为与肝硬化相关的潜在生物标志物，而二氢鞘胺醇和植物鞘胺醇则为肝细胞癌的潜在生物标志物。

Chen 等（2008）利用超高效液相色谱 - 质谱联用技术（UPLC-MS）对原发性肝癌患者及健康志愿者的尿液进行了代谢组学研究。该研究中利用亲水相互作用色谱和反相液相色谱进行代谢物分离,结合模式识别技术,发现21种代谢组可作为潜在标志物。同时表明亲水相互作用色谱比反相液相色谱更好地将肝癌患者与健康志愿者分开,而且更适合对尿液进行代谢组学分析。Wang等(2012)应用超高效液相色谱-质谱联用技术为基础的代谢组学方法,对肝细胞癌患者、肝硬化患者和健康志愿者的血清进行研究,通过多元统计方法和受试者工作特征曲线进行数据分析,表明代谢物轮廓可以将肝细胞癌与肝硬化和健康者区分开,敏感度和特异性为100%。鉴定出肝细胞癌中13种物质和几种有意义的主要代谢通路。发现刀豆氨酸琥珀酸在肝硬化中降低,在肝细胞癌中增高。另外,鹅脱氧胆酰甘氨酸被认为是肝细胞癌诊断及预后的重要物质。UPLC-MS单独或联合甲胎蛋白可作为诊断肝细胞癌和高危人群筛选的有效和便利工具。

肝衰竭早期预测和及时治疗,可明显改善患者的预后。Yang等(2006)采用高效液相色谱-质谱联用的方法对37名慢性乙型肝炎急性发作患者与50名健康对照人群的血清进行分析,发现溶血性磷脂酰胆碱及甘氨鹅去氧胆酸等成分在两组间存在显著性差异,这些产物可用于疾病恶化的早期预测。Amathieu等(2011)应用质子磁共振波谱技术(^{1}H-MRS)对肝硬化患者的血清进行代谢组学分析。建立的正交投影模型具有较高的检测变异和预测变异。显示多种代谢物在肝衰竭严重程度不同时出现显著差异:高密度脂蛋白和磷酸胆碱共振态在轻度慢性肝衰竭患者血清中明显高于重度慢性肝衰竭患者;而乳酸、丙酮酸、氨基酸和肌酐在重度慢性肝衰竭患者血清中的水平明显高于轻度患者。该研究表明^{1}H-MRS为肝硬化患者肝功能损伤严重程度有关的代谢过程提供了新的见解。

药物和毒物等非病毒性因素引起的肝脏损伤病死率高,很难察觉,已成为一大健康威胁。Heijne等(2005)对溴苯诱导的急性肝坏死小鼠进行代谢组学研究,发现处理组小鼠血清及尿中某些代谢产物如乳酸盐、酪氨酸等与正常对照组小鼠不同。并且证明转录组学及代谢组学的整合能更敏感地检测到肝毒性有关的改变并发现相关的生物标志物。同时对溴苯诱导急性肝坏死的多种生物学通路的作用有了更深的见解。Lin等(2009)建立了由四氯化碳引起肝损伤的小鼠模型,应用液相色谱质谱联用的代谢组学方法对小鼠尿液进行分析,最终发现23种内源性代谢物可作为四氯化碳引起的肝损伤的潜在生物学标志物。

非酒精性脂肪性肝病(NAFLD)发病机制至今尚未明确,目前大多数学者认为它与肥胖、脂代谢紊乱、胰岛素抵抗等有关,是代谢综合征在肝脏的表现。Barr等(2010)利用超高效液相色谱-质谱联用方法对非酒精性脂肪性肝病患者的血浆进行代谢组学研究,发现多种代谢物在疾病组与对照组之间存在显著差异,这些物质可能与肝功能障碍及肝细胞炎症有关。且同样的差异也存在于非酒精性脂肪性肝病模型鼠与野生型鼠之间。Li等(2011)利用蛋氨酸及胆碱缺乏饮食喂养的雄性C57BL/6小鼠代表非酒精性脂肪性肝病的不同阶段,应用^{1}H-MRS波谱为基础的代谢组学方法,发现4种标志物:葡萄糖、乳酸、牛磺酸及谷氨酸。并检测了这4种物质在非酒精性脂肪性肝病的不同阶段血浆中的浓度。确定这4种物质可作为诊断非酒精性脂肪性肝病不同阶段的潜在标志物。

代谢组学的发展是“整合化”的发展,“整合化”的代谢组学是代谢组学发展的必然趋势。目前“整合化”的代谢组学不仅在不同原因、不同阶段肝病的研究中取得了巨大的成就,在其他疾病的早期诊断、新药的研发、植物、微生物等领域也获得了可喜的成果及广阔的发展前景。代谢组学的整合虽可解决一些问题,但在前进过程中仍会遇到严峻的挑战,只有代谢组学更好的发展,才能实现更全面、更准确寻找能够作为生物标志物的关键化合物,探索这些标志物在机体的代谢作用的目标。因代谢组学最根本的是技术问题,所以需要不断探索并改善方法,创造新的技术,实现组学研究的技术创新,最终实现系统生物学的全面整合。

第三节 肝肿瘤性病变的诊断与鉴别

表 1-6-1 肝脏原发性良、恶性肿瘤的分类

良性肿瘤	恶性肿瘤
上皮性	**上皮性**
肝细胞性：再生结节	肝细胞性：肝母细胞瘤（儿童发病）
腺瘤性增生结节（异形增生结节）	肝细胞癌
肝腺瘤	
胆管细胞性：胆管腺瘤	胆管细胞性：胆管腺癌
胆管囊腺瘤	胆管囊腺癌
间质性	**间质性**
脂肪性：脂肪瘤、肌脂瘤、血管平滑肌脂肪瘤	肌肿瘤：平滑肌肉瘤
肌肿瘤：平滑肌瘤	横纹肌肉瘤
脉管肿瘤：血管瘤	脉管肿瘤：血管肉瘤
婴儿血管内皮细胞瘤	上皮样血管内皮细胞瘤
肝紫癜病	卡波西肉瘤
其他：间皮瘤	其他：胚胎性未分化肉瘤、纤维肉瘤
混合组织性	**其他**
间叶性（充质）错构瘤	癌肉瘤、鳞状癌
良性畸胎瘤	畸胎瘤、卵黄囊瘤
其他	类癌
肾上腺剩余肿瘤、胰腺剩余肿瘤	淋巴瘤

肝脏原发肿瘤分类：肝脏原发性良、恶性肿瘤均可起源于上皮组织、间质（脉管、肌肉、脂肪）以及其他胚胎性组织等（表 1-6-1），且大多具有相对应的良恶性病变，然而两者在临床处理及其预后截然不同。为此，影像学诊断极为必要。

肝脏肿块（肿瘤）性病变的鉴别：在评估肝脏肿块性病变时除高质量的影像学资料外，临床病史也极为重要，两者结合有利于明确诊断或缩小鉴别诊断范围。

临床表现：在诊断中必须重视的 3 个重要因素是：病人的年龄、性别以及是否（或已经）存在肝外的恶性病变。

年龄因素：①成人，小于 40 岁可见的肝肿瘤包括肝转移、纤维板层型肝癌、局灶性结节增生和肝细胞腺瘤；而大于 50 岁者最常见的肝肿瘤有肝转移、典型的肝细胞肝癌、肝内胆管腺癌、血管肉瘤和血管瘤。②儿童，血管性（婴儿血管内皮细胞瘤和血管瘤）肿瘤可见于 6 个月以内婴儿；而肝母细胞瘤常出现于 3 岁儿童（虽然也见有出生时发病者，但高峰年龄是 18 个月）；良性间叶性错构瘤的发病也与肝母细胞瘤相似。③较年长儿童和青春期。则可发生肝细胞肝癌和胚胎性未分化肉瘤。在年龄因素中，值得注意的是，无论是在儿童或成人中，肝转移性肿瘤的发病都较原发性肝肿瘤更为常见。

性别因素：男性以肝脏原发性恶性肿瘤更常见；女性则以肝脏原发性良性肿瘤更常见。

药物史：有长期使用类固醇类药物和口服避孕药史，与使用类固醇有关的肝肿瘤主要是肝细胞腺瘤，其次有局灶性结节增生、结节状再生性增生、血管瘤和肝细胞肝癌。

影像学研究：应用多种影像学检查有利于对肝肿瘤的评估。动态增强 CT、MRI 和超声能提供重要的诊断线索以获得最终诊断。当分析肝脏影像时，应考虑的参数有是单个抑或是多个肿块，大小和密度（均匀、不均匀），分布（局限、弥漫），肿块轮廓（锐利、模糊），病变质地（实质性、囊性、囊实性），钙化的有和无，对比剂强化（有、无、持续性），血管开放或闭塞与血供（富或乏）以及有无向肝外扩展等。在全面客观地获得上述各种影像学的参数后，尚需进行综合分析，如病灶大小常需结合病变的数目，甚至需与其分布、质地等一并加以分析。

目前横断面影像学技术已能发现更多、更小的肝内病变，但也带来了许多新问题，被发现的较小（直径 <15mm）病变其临床意义更不确定（可无临床意义，但也可能是极为严重病变的早期）。如前所述，依据影像学表现做出"肝脏小囊肿"诊断时，并不能完全否定（即使概率很小）这是一个正在发展中的"肝转移病灶"。

Rappeport 等（2007）应用 CT 技术研究一组拟诊肝肿瘤者。发现单个、小（直径 <1.5cm）病变中，良性病例占 65%；多个（2~4 个）微小病变中，良性病例也占 59%。当病变数目增加或另有较大病变出现时（结合病变数与病变大小不均匀分析），则恶性可能性增加。

同样，即使有肝外恶性病变存在，这类小病变中仍有 51% 是良性者。这一发现提示，肝内多发性、小病变并非都是肝转移性病变。对将行肝手术切除的肝转移病人，应考虑其他病变仍有可能是良性的。事实上，肝内多发占位病变不只是肝转移。尚有许多其他病变，如脓肿、囊肿、髓外造血、肝内胆管腺癌、多灶性或弥漫性肝细胞肝癌、血管肉瘤、结节状再生性增生或 / 和血管瘤等都有可能是多发的。影像学的诊断与鉴别诊断必须按照循证放射学的要求，参阅文献中的前瞻性研究和可靠的资料荟萃成果，正确认识和运用敏感性、特异性和正确性较高的影像学征象，进行全面和科学的分析。

手术与非手术：分析影像学表现并做出诊断后，医师应决定该肝脏肿块是能手术，还是非（不应）手术或不能手术（晚期）的病变。成人中主要的非手术原发肿瘤是血管瘤和局灶性结节增生，影像学医师应先加以确定或排除。在儿童中，婴儿血管内皮细胞瘤也是不需要手术者，通常经保守、支持或经栓塞治疗肿瘤能自发回缩。

而对成人肝转移、肝细胞肝癌、纤维板层型肝癌、肝内胆管腺癌、血管肉瘤和肝细胞腺癌，儿童的肝母细胞瘤、未分化性胚胎性肉瘤、肝细胞肝癌和间叶性错构瘤，理论上都是需经外科手术治疗的病变。此时，影像学医师应根据影像学表现（病变的大小，周围扩展，有否重要器官受侵，肝外有无浸润、转移等）为病变做出手术能否切除或取得疗效提供依据，协助临床做出判断。

非手术病变的诊断：①肝血管瘤在超声、CT、MRI 和核素显像上都有特征性表现。然而最理想的影像学技术应是 MRI 钆剂动态增强和 CT 增强。②局灶性结节增生在超声、CT 和非增强 MRI 上的表现都非特异性，除非出现中央瘢痕，或者重叠发生有纤维板层型肝癌和肝细胞腺瘤。然而钆剂增强 MRI 或 MR T_2WI SPIO 增强影像可显示缩小鉴别诊断范围的局灶性结节增生特征。典型的局灶性结节增生显示动态信号缺失，信号缺失的程度要大于肝细胞腺瘤和肝转移等其他病变，是局灶性结节增生有价值的诊断特征。

组织活检：无可否认的事实是，有时所获得的影像学表现不典型或不能得出结论时，应考虑作经皮穿刺活检。通常，在 CT 或超声引导下，进行肝活检并无危险性。如穿刺活检取材不能做出诊断时，应作剖腹活检。因此，经多种不同的影像学检查获得的资料和临床表现能明确诊断或显著地缩小肝肿瘤性病变的鉴别诊断范围。如缺乏特征性的影像学表现时，经皮穿刺活检可用于对肿瘤定性。

第四节　肝脏少见肿瘤及肿瘤样病变简介

多种肿瘤及肿瘤样病变可发生于肝脏。常见的恶性肿瘤主要为原发性肝细胞肝癌、胆管细胞癌及各种继发性肝转移瘤。常见的良性肿瘤及肿瘤样病变包括囊肿、血管瘤、肝脓肿及肝硬化结节等。其他病变在肝脏相对少见，部分仅有个例报告。

一、恶性肿瘤

包括胆管囊腺癌、神经内分泌癌、肉瘤样肝细胞癌及未分化肉瘤等。

（一）胆管囊腺癌

胆管囊腺癌为少见的胆管来源囊性恶性肿瘤。胆管囊腺瘤为其良性病变，但有恶变倾向，临床也需手术切除，常一同描述。胆管囊腺类肿瘤85%发生于肝内，约占全部胆管来源肝内囊性肿瘤的5%，好发于中年女性，平均发病年龄38岁。这类肿瘤虽然少见，但特征明显，影像表现典型者术前可做出正确诊断。

肝脏的胆管囊腺类肿瘤的影像学表现与卵巢和胰腺的囊腺类肿瘤相似。肿瘤常境界清楚，有包膜，瘤周可见胆管扩张。切面呈多房性，囊腔内有浓淡不等的浆液或黏液，可发生囊内出血，后者多见于恶性。囊内表面光滑，伴有乳头及壁结节，以恶性多见。CT扫描可以反映病变的大体病理特征，囊腺瘤表现为多房性囊性病变，囊壁及囊内分隔厚薄均匀、光整，可有钙化，各房腔之间的CT值可因囊液成分有较大差异。囊腺癌病变一般较大，可为单房，囊壁及分隔厚薄不均，常可见瘤结节，增强扫描囊壁、间隔及瘤结节可见明显强化，钙化则粗大、不规则。

（二）神经内分泌癌

神经内分泌癌，也称为类癌。肝脏是神经内分泌癌最常转移的部位，而原发于肝脏者非常少见，故诊断时应首先排除转移性肿瘤。肝脏神经内分泌癌的来源说法不一。一般认为起源于肝内毛细胆管的神经内分泌细胞（Kulchitsky细胞），或起源于肝内异位的胰腺或肾上腺组织。原发肝脏神经内分泌癌多见于成人，预后较肝细胞肝癌好。肿瘤一般为无功能性，类癌综合征等肿瘤分泌症状主要见于转移。肝脏原发神经内分泌癌多为单发，右叶多见。平扫呈低密度，增强扫描动脉期肿瘤明显强化，呈高密度，静脉期及延迟扫描多呈略高或等密度，可与肝癌鉴别。肿瘤内常可见多发小囊状无强化区，病理提示为含陈旧血液成分的小血管腔，这种表现有一定特征性，也可出现于转移性神经内分泌癌。

（三）肉瘤样肝细胞癌

肉瘤样肝细胞癌，是指肿瘤的大部分或全部被肉瘤样梭形细胞替代，约占肝癌尸检的3.9%~9.4%，占肝癌外科手术切除的1.8%。肿瘤好发于50~60岁，男性明显高于女性（约5∶1）。46%可见甲胎蛋白升高，但多数不超过400μg/ml。病变生长快，恶性度高，边缘不规则，无明确的包膜，易侵犯周围组织、发生肝内播散、肝外转移和腹膜种植等。关于肉瘤样肝细胞癌影像表现的描述非常少见，且缺乏图像资料。一般认为肿瘤低血供，影像表现缺乏特异性，与转移瘤不易鉴别。有作者总结肿瘤CT呈囊性低密度，中心可见不规则分隔，边缘部可见乳头状或结节状软组织密度影，但描述更类似下述的未分化肉瘤。一组两例肉瘤样肝细胞癌表现相似：动脉期及静脉期均为相对低密度，边缘不清，可累及肝被膜及周围组织。肿瘤内可见大片低密度坏死区。

（四）未分化肉瘤

未分化肉瘤，也称恶性间叶细胞瘤、胚胎性肉瘤等。好发年龄3~37岁，在小儿肝脏肿瘤中居第3位。肿瘤体积较大，直径10~25 cm，多单发，分界清，部分可见假包膜形成。病变大体虽多为实性肿物（83%），但由于肿瘤内含大量黏液基质成分，而在CT上主要呈囊性表现，多数有出血、坏死，少数可有钙化。病情进展快，转移发生早，多数死于肝功能衰竭。肿瘤在影像上有一定特征，多表现为肝内巨大单发、边界清楚的病灶，分两种类型：一种以囊性为主，较为多见，可单房或多房，内含乳头状或不规则的软组织影，可合并出血，钙化较为少见，多表现为病灶边缘针尖样钙化；另一种以实性为主，病灶内可见若干小囊，较为少见，可能为病变的早期表现。囊性病变需与肝包虫鉴别，后者多见于流行区，囊内囊及囊壁环形或弧形钙化是其特征表现。

二、肝脏少见良性肿瘤及肿瘤样病变

主要包括肝细胞腺瘤、局灶性结节增生、血管平滑肌脂肪瘤和孤立性坏死结节。

（一）肝细胞腺瘤

肝细胞腺瘤，即肝腺瘤，为少见的肝细胞起源的良性肿瘤。多见于育龄的妇女，与口服避孕药有一定关系，在停药后肿瘤可缩小或消失。由于肝腺瘤有出现急症及恶变的可能，治疗上一般主张手术切除。肝腺瘤常发生于没有肝硬化背景的正常肝，70%~80%为单发，67%位于肝右叶，约2/3的病例肿瘤直径大于5cm，多发者常见于糖原贮积症或肝腺瘤病患者，可同时发生10余个肿瘤，但大小常小于单发病变。肿瘤边缘清楚，无分叶，30%有包膜，病变较大或多发时，常伴有出血及坏死。肿瘤细胞较正常肝细胞大，内含大量糖原和脂质，并可有脂肪变性。CT平扫肿瘤表现为等密度或低密度，可见出血（25%）和脂肪（7%~10%），增强扫描动脉期肿瘤可见均匀或不均匀强化，静脉期和延迟期主要表现为等密度。肿瘤脂肪变明显时，在CT扫描各期均表现为低密度。部分病变静脉期表现为相对低密度,容易误诊为肝癌,但患者没有肝硬化背景,甲胎蛋白不增高,可帮助鉴别。

(二)肝局灶性结节增生

肝局灶性结节增生,并非真性肿瘤,但常作为良性肿瘤进行统计及研究,近几年发病率明显增高,在全部肝脏原发肿瘤中约占8%,在欧美是仅次于肝血管瘤的肝脏第二常见的良性肿瘤。约86%~95%的肿瘤见于30~40岁的妇女,约20%为多发。口服避孕药可促进局灶性结节增生的生长但并非其发生的真正原因。局灶性结节增生不会恶变,可不行手术治疗。约1/2的病灶在随访中可见肿瘤缩小,个别可以完全消失。

目前认为,局灶性结节增生是肝细胞对先天性血管发育异常的一种增生性反应,是正常肝细胞异常排列形成,内可有小胆管,但不与大胆管相通,有枯否细胞,但常没有功能。与肝腺瘤相比,其病灶通常较小,约84%直径<5 cm,并较少出现坏死、出血。病变中央的"星形"瘢痕并非真性瘢痕,而是血管与胆管的聚积。有30%的局灶性结节增生不出现中心瘢痕。典型局灶性结节增生可见分叶,平扫呈低或等密度,增强扫描动脉期肿瘤实质部分明显均匀强化,瘢痕呈相对低密度,门静脉期及延迟扫描多数病灶的实质部分呈略高或低密度,中心瘢痕可呈相对强化。小的局灶性结节增生在延迟期的表现有时不典型,且常常无明显的中央瘢痕,甚至呈相对低密度,很难与小血管瘤或肝癌相鉴别。

(三)血管平滑肌脂肪瘤

血管平滑肌脂肪瘤,为间叶来源的良性肿瘤,多见于肾脏,与结节性硬化有一定关系。发生于肝脏者仅占5%~10%,以单发常见,与结节性硬化的关系不及肾脏血管平滑肌脂肪瘤明显。肝脏血管平滑肌脂肪瘤常见于中青年女性,肿瘤直径0.3~36.0cm,肿瘤较大时容易出血。血管平滑肌脂肪瘤为成熟脂肪组织,平滑肌细胞和纡曲厚壁血管3种成分按不同比例混杂,其中脂肪成分可从10%至90%。Tsui等(1999)按血管、平滑肌和脂肪在肿瘤中所占比例及分布,将血管平滑肌脂肪瘤分为4型:Ⅰ型,混合型,最常见;Ⅱ型,脂肪瘤型,脂肪含量大于70%;Ⅲ型,肌瘤型,脂肪含量小于10%;Ⅳ型,血管瘤型,由许多粗大厚壁血管组成,细胞成分少。肿物无包膜,但一般边缘较清楚,CT表现取决于病灶内各种组织成分的比例,诊断主要依靠脂肪的检出,如于脂肪成分中见到血管影更具诊断意义。增强扫描肿瘤于动脉期、门静脉期明显强化,脂肪含量少时,可能被周围强化掩盖,平扫及薄层扫描有助于脂肪的检出。

部分血管平滑肌脂肪瘤内可出现假性动脉瘤,光镜下为明显扩张的厚壁畸形血管,CT表现瘤内"团块"样强化。与肾脏血管平滑肌脂肪瘤不同,50%的肝脏血管平滑肌脂肪瘤不能检出脂肪成分,且部分病例在增强扫描也表现为"快进快出",而与肝细胞肝癌鉴别困难。

(四)孤立性坏死结节

孤立性坏死结节,是一种罕见的肝脏良性病变。发病年龄在50~70岁,男性多于女性,临床一般无症状。病灶多位于肝右叶表面,可单发或多发,直径一般小于3cm。病理特点为纤维层包裹的结节状凝固坏死灶,较大病灶内可含有小片液化坏死裂隙。病因不清,可能为血管病变、感染或免疫反应等原因造成肝组织凝固性坏死,继而出现纤维包裹所致。坏死结节可为类圆形、哑铃形及不规则形等。病变边缘较清楚,位于肝被膜下时,可略突出肝脏轮廓。平扫呈低密度,在大于2cm的病灶中,部分病灶内可见更低密度的点状或小片状液化坏死。增强扫描可见病灶于动脉期及门静脉期均无强化,部分病例于延迟扫描显示边缘部有轻度强化,呈细环状。坏死结节在MRI的T_2WI序列表现相对特异,较易获得明确诊断。CT表现可不典型,有时需与转移瘤相鉴别。

肝脏少见病变虽然诊断困难,但部分病变仍具有特异性相对较高的影像表现特点,熟悉这些病变的典型表现有利于早期获得正确诊断,辅助制定治疗计划。对于表现典型的病例应明确诊断,而对于表现不典型者应结合临床、发病率及多种影像表现进行综合分析,并给出合理的鉴别诊断及定性评价。

第五节 人工智能及影像组学在肝脏肿瘤中的应用

随着信息技术的迅速发展和计算机算法的不断革新,人工智能(AI)已广泛涉及临床诊疗的诸多环节。其中，人工智能与影像学的结合具有巨大的发展潜力，并已初步应用于临床。

影像组学是人工智能在肿瘤影像方面的应用热点，它通过高通量地提取影像特征，结合机器学习等人工智能算法，为肝脏肿瘤的精确诊断、个体化治疗提供更多信息。

1. 人工智能技术　在肿瘤表型判断上，临床上主要依靠病理活检，存在有创、取材局限等问题。影像学具有无创、全面、可反复等优势，在人工智能的帮助下有望术前预测肿瘤表型。一组学者基于肝癌患者的超声灰阶图像，先后使用最大相关最小冗余和稀疏表示法筛选了 8 个特征组成最优子集，进一步构建支持向量机预测肝癌细胞 Ki-67 表达，留一验证的 AUC 为 0.75。Yao 等（2018）综合 3 种超声图像组建多模态模型，分别构建支持向量机预测肝癌细胞的 PD-1、Ki-67 表达及微血管侵犯情况，留一验证的结果表明 3 个模型的 AUC 分别为 0.97、0.94、0.98，为人工智能预测肿瘤表型提供了可行性依据。

以上两项研究均将 Ki-67 以特定阈值转换为分类数据进行预测，未来能否对 Ki-67 进行更精确的定量评价，有待进一步探索。

在人工智能辅助肿瘤诊断方面，有学者利用超声组学特征构建支持向量机以鉴别肝脏良恶性病变，AUC 为 0.94。Li 等（2017）基于 T2WI 发现了 35 个有助于鉴别肝血管瘤、肝癌和肝转移瘤的 MRI 特征，并分别构建 K 最近邻分类、神经网络和支持向量机对上述肿瘤进行鉴别，结果显示神经网络的准确性最优。Yasaka 等（2018）在 CT 图像的基础上使用卷积神经网络鉴别 5 类肝脏肿瘤，经过 5 次训练和验证，平均准确率和 AUC 分别为 0.84、0.92。有研究者使用卷积神经网络在 DWI 图像上对原发性、转移性肝癌进行鉴别，并比较了三维和二维卷积神经网络的分类性能，发现前者的准确性优于后者。

2. 影像组学　预后评价对肿瘤个体化治疗至关重要，影像组学从肿瘤异质性、微环境等角度出发，有望更精确地预测预后。Brenet Defour 等（2019）对肝细胞癌患者的增强 CT 进行特征提取，发现门静脉期的偏度与总生存期显著相关。Zheng 等（2018）回顾性收集了 319 例肝癌患者的术前 CT 图像，发现由 6 个组学特征构建的组学分数是预后的独立预测因素，并且组学模型的预测性能优于 TNM 分期。同时，Cozzi 等（2017）提出影像组学模型可以评估接受容积调强放疗的肝癌患者的总生存期。一些学者分别基于增强 CT 动脉期和门静脉期构建影像组学模型，发现两个模型均可预测肝癌患者经肝动脉化疗栓塞术后的 3 年生存期。

在肝癌病理学分级方面，Zhou 等（2017）发现，增强 MRI 的动脉期均值和灰阶步长不均匀性等特征在高、低级别肝癌间具有区分能力。Wu 等（2019）在 125 例患者的 T_1WI 和 T_2WI 上进行组学分析并构建模型，联合组学标签和临床资料的预测模型在验证集中的 AUC 为 0.8。

肝衰竭是肝癌术后的严重并发症，Cai 等（2019）发现，与现有肝病评分系统相比，整合了影像组学的预测模型在预测术后肝衰竭上区分度更优，该研究还进一步进行前瞻性验证，AUC 为 0.833。

挑战与展望：尽管人工智能及影像组学等相关研究方兴未艾，但应该认识到，人工智能与影像的融合仍处于起步阶段。首先，目前应用于临床的商业化人工智能影像产品多集中于单纯的图像识别、病变检出和良恶性判断等，人工智能仅作为影像医师的辅助工具以减少重复性工作，避免漏诊，提高阅片效率。而对于肿瘤影像而言，人工智能及影像组学在预测肿瘤的表型、预后、疗效评估等方面的探索尚未成功转化应用于临床。

其次，腹部和肝脏的肿瘤种类较多、胃肠道形态位置不固定等因素导致肿瘤在自动分割上具有挑战性，目前大多数研究仍依赖人工分割，这个过程需要耗费大量的时间和精力，难以友好地融入影像医师的日常诊断流程中。此外，在临床上应用人工智能技术同样带来一些伦理、社会层面的问题，诸如医疗责任的划分、数据处理流程中患者隐私的保护等，未来有待更深入的讨论及立法规范。综上所述，当下医学影像已经步入大数据时代，作为人工智能和影像大数据共同促进的时代产物，人工智能影像的发展具有巨大的价值和广阔的前景。相信在不远的将来，人工智能及影像组学会克服现有不足，进一步帮助影像医师实现更高效、准确的诊断，并对临床实践产生深远的影响。

第七章　部分肿瘤的不典型表现

第一节　肝脏部分肿瘤的不典型CT表现

1. 肝癌的不典型表现　肝细胞肝癌（HCC）主要由肝动脉供血，动脉期CT值迅速上升达到峰值，由于肝脏实质主要由门静脉供血，动脉期增强不明显，平扫时为低密度的病灶此时明显高于正常肝实质，出现早期高密度强化征象；病灶增强峰值停留时间很短，迅速下降，与浓密显影的主动脉下降速度几乎一致。门静脉期肝脏实质明显强化，而肝细胞癌密度降低，表现为明显低密度影，即表现为“快进快出”的特点。采用螺旋CT机，其出现率可高达90%，意味着大部分肝癌血供是比较丰富的。

（1）动脉期和门静脉期均强化，密度高于肝脏：Loyer等报告一组肝癌病例，27%表现为动脉期和门静脉期均强化，密度高于肝脏。可能与病人的血液循环较慢，门静脉期时肝动脉内碘浓度较高有关。发生于肝脏顶部的肝癌出现这种表现可能与门静脉期扫描先扫查肝脏顶部有关。脂肪肝背景下的肝癌可有此种表现。此时必须加扫延迟期，这些病灶在延迟期为低密度，即可诊断为肝癌。应注意与肝脏血管瘤和局灶性结节增生鉴别。

（2）动脉期和门静脉期均为低密度：这类肝癌血供较少，动脉期和门静脉期不强化或轻度强化，均表现为低密度。可能与病灶脂肪变性或纤维组织较多有关。应注意与肝脏转移瘤、炎性病变及淋巴瘤等鉴别。

（3）动脉期或门静脉期或动、门静脉双期呈等密度：肝癌病灶的密度从低到高再到低早于肝脏实质密度的变化，但两者有密度相等的交汇点，如果扫描时间恰好碰上此交汇点，病灶表现为等密度。也与患者血液循环的个体差异有关。重要的是病灶在延迟期若表现为低密度，即可诊断为肝癌。可见延迟扫描在肝癌定性诊断中的重要性。疑难病例应结合临床资料，大部分肝癌病例甲胎蛋白增高或明显增高以及乙肝表面抗原（HbsAg）阳性，30%左右甲胎蛋白正常。有研究认为，甲胎蛋白>200μg/L，可诊断为肝癌。

2. 胆管细胞肝癌　胆管细胞肝癌占肝脏原发恶性肿瘤的3%~5%，预后较差。男性明显多于女性，2∶1~6∶1。临床表现更像肝细胞癌。病理分为：混合型和合并型。一种认为是肝细胞肝癌的变体，另一种认为是由肝脏多能干细胞发展而来。影像学具有肝细胞癌和胆管细胞癌的特征。混合型是肝细胞癌成分和胆管细胞癌成分混合存在，合并型是肝细胞癌成分和胆管细胞癌成分各占一部分。肿块一般较大，CT平扫呈均匀或不均匀低密度。增强扫描动脉期密度不均匀，肝细胞癌部分强化，胆管细胞癌部分为低密度。门静脉期肝细胞癌部分降为低密度，胆管细胞癌部分仍为低密度。延迟扫描肝细胞癌部分仍为低密度，胆管细胞癌部分纤维成分较多延迟强化为高密度。诊断要点是延迟扫描时部分低密度区变为高密度，并以此与坏死鉴别。

3. 肝脏转移瘤　肝脏转移瘤是肝脏最常见的恶性肿瘤。肝脏转移瘤CT平扫时多呈低密度，有出血或钙化时呈较高密度，有钙化的肝转移瘤多见于结肠、直肠癌，也可见于其他器官（胃、乳腺、卵巢等）的黏液腺癌。转移瘤发生钙化的机制可以是肿瘤本身所产生，也常由营养不良或出血后所致。增强扫描示大多数转移瘤为乏血供，其密度较正常肝实质低，但由于周边有生长活跃的肿瘤组织，血供较丰富，在肝动脉期及门静脉期均或呈环形强化，为其典型表现，另一典型表现是增强扫描无强化而呈低密度。

转移瘤多保留原发肿瘤的病理组织学特征，囊性转移灶较少见，其原发肿瘤常为卵巢、胰腺等的囊腺癌或产生大量黏液的肿瘤，子宫恶性间叶瘤、间质肉瘤的肝转移瘤内常可因坏死而可见液平面。高血供的原发肿瘤有肾细胞癌、类癌、恶性胰岛细胞瘤、甲状腺癌、恶性嗜铬细胞瘤等。脂肪肝内转移瘤的影像表现比较复杂，平扫时转移瘤的表现与脂肪浸润程度密切相关。在重度脂肪肝时转移瘤密度往往高于肝背景而呈相对高密度影，与一般转移瘤密度低于肝实质不同，小的转移瘤有时不易与血管影鉴别。中度脂肪肝内转移瘤往往呈等密度，有时其周围有一极薄的低密度环，稍一疏忽即易漏诊。增强扫描对检出和诊断脂肪肝内转移瘤至关重要，但应注意与血管瘤、脂肪肝内残留正常肝岛等鉴别。

大多数血管瘤的强化与同层血管相仿，边缘常可呈结节状，而转移瘤的强化一般低于同层的血管，常呈环形强化。应注意此时不可只根据目测密度差进行诊断，细致测量有关部位的 CT 值十分重要。残余肝岛好发于肝的周边部位，包括贴邻肝裂、胆囊窝边缘等处，而转移瘤常发生在肝边缘。一般而言，转移瘤与肝缘的交界多为锐角，而肝岛的交界多为钝角，边缘模糊。诊断疑难时可行 MRI 扫描。

4. 肝脏血管瘤　肝海绵状血管瘤是最常见的肝脏良性肿瘤。CT 平扫常呈均匀低密度，与邻近血管密度相仿。在脂肪肝背景下可呈相对高密度。在增强扫描时，一般早期（动脉期）呈周边结节状或弧形强化，其密度与同层面的血管密度相仿，随着时间延迟向中央渐进性充填，注药后 5~7 分钟，逐渐扩大至全瘤强化，强化密度逐渐降至稍高于或等于正常肝脏。大的血管瘤往往中央有星形、大的低密度区，可以为纤维化或囊性变所致，纤维化成分可在延迟 20 分钟时完全充填，呈等密度，但囊变区则不会强化。

不典型 CT 表现常见于≤ 3cm 的小血管瘤。小的血管瘤可以在动脉期即呈全部致密的均匀强化，不呈典型的周边结节状强化表现，但其密度往往较高，与主动脉相仿，在延迟期呈高或等密度。其他不典型的 CT 表现有：增强扫描强化不明显，呈点状较轻程度的强化，充填慢，可能与供血动脉较细和较大的血管间隙有关；以及中央先强化等。

5. 肝脏局灶结节增生　肝脏局灶结节增生在西方国家发病率较高，我国近几年发病率也明显增高，目前局灶性结节样增生在肝脏良性肿瘤中的发病率仅次于血管瘤居第二位。中青年女性多见。早期文献认为局灶性结节样增生的发生与使用避孕药有关，目前的研究认为雌激素与局灶性结节样增生的发病机制无关。

目前认为局灶性结节样增生是肝脏细胞对血管发育异常或损伤的一种增生性反应，由正常形态的肝细胞围绕富于胆管和血管的纤维结缔组织间隔生长，间隔中有枯否细胞等。

大体病理特点为无包膜、轮廓光整的良性肝脏肿物。中央为“星状瘢痕”，瘢痕内有一条或数条较大的动脉，也可以有门静脉，但动脉与静脉的关系与正常门脉汇管区者不同。瘢痕内有增生的胆管，其管径较动脉小，还有结缔组织及炎性细胞。

局灶性结节样增生多为单发实性肿物，约 7%~20% 为多灶，好发于肝脏的游离缘。局灶性结节样增生无特征性的临床症状、体征及实验室检查异常，常由影像检查偶然发现。

CT 平扫局灶性结节样增生表现为等密度或略低密度影。局灶性结节样增生血供丰富，并由肝动脉供血，增强扫描动脉期表现为均匀的明显强化影。门静脉期密度下降表现为高密度或略高密度，延迟后平衡期扫描表现为高密度、略高密度或等密度，可能与局灶性结节样增生的结构异常、对比剂的排泄及廓清较慢有关，与肝癌的“快进快出”不同，表现为“快进慢出”。19%~78% 的病灶内有纤维分隔或瘢痕，动脉期和门静脉期为低密度，延迟扫描纤维分隔或瘢痕可表现为高密度或仍为低密度。文献报道 1.4% 的局灶性结节样增生含有钙化。

局灶性结节样增生的不典型影像表现并不少见，可能与其细胞增生及不典型增生等有关。局灶性结节样增生不典型表现有：CT 平扫呈不均匀的低密度，增强扫描呈低血供，有假包膜及钙化等，无中心瘢痕和纤维分隔等。

不典型的局灶性结节样增生也需与肝腺瘤、肝细胞癌鉴别，用 ^{99m}Tc 硫胶做核素显像，由于局灶性结节样增生内有枯否细胞，可浓聚核素，而肝细胞癌及肝腺瘤无浓聚。

6. 肝血管平滑肌脂肪瘤　肝血管平滑肌脂肪瘤（AML）多见于肾脏，发生在肝脏者仅占 5%~10%，为罕见的肝良性肿瘤。组织学特点为含有血管、平滑肌及成熟脂肪成分。Tsui 把血管平滑肌脂肪瘤病理分为 4 型：混合型、脂肪型（脂肪≥ 70%）、平滑肌型（脂肪≤ 10%）和血管型，其中混合型最常见。

血管平滑肌脂肪瘤病理组成不同决定其影像学表现存在多样性，加之扫描技术使用是否合理和肿块大小等因素的影响,使血管平滑肌脂肪瘤的影像诊断有一定困难。

CT检查中发现脂肪成分是提示血管平滑肌脂肪瘤的关键,脂肪成分的CT值呈负值(-20HU以下)。平滑肌型和血管型脂肪成分较少或不含脂肪成分影像诊断困难,肿瘤在CT表现为混杂密度,平滑肌成分动脉期一般中度或明显强化,血管主要由扭曲的动脉、静脉构成,强化程度与同层主动脉相仿,两者对比剂廓清慢,在门静脉期仍为高密度。巨大的血管平滑肌脂肪瘤,由于其内含有较大的不成熟血管可形成"假性动脉瘤"。

肝癌、肝转移瘤、肝腺瘤和局灶性结节样增生等也可有脂肪成分,含有较少的脂肪成分而有较丰富血供的血管平滑肌脂肪瘤与上述肿瘤鉴别有困难时,超声引导下的穿刺活检有助于明确诊断。

第二节 CT增强扫描:肝脏单发不典型强化病灶

肝脏病变CT征象分析:肝脏病变种类繁多,影像表现多样。既往对肝癌、胆管细胞癌、炎性假瘤、不典型增生结节、肝腺瘤、非霍奇金淋巴瘤等典型表现均有报道,此节仅对一些不典型病灶的增强CT表现加以分析,以提高对不典型病例的诊断水平,降低误诊率。

快进快出征象:快进快出是肝癌的典型影像表现,但是,在一组病例中,不典型增生结节和炎性假瘤、肝腺瘤亦出现了类似征象。其中,不典型增生结节属于癌前病变,但组织学尚无恶性肿瘤证据,在既往研究中主要表现为无明显强化或轻度强化,但该组病例均表现为动脉期明显强化,病理提示除肝细胞不典型增生外都伴有不同程度组织血管化,与高分化肝癌具有一定相似表现,因此属于不典型增生结节晚期,需要随诊观察或按照肝癌进行处理。不过,虽然动脉期都有明显强化,但门脉期病灶2/3例仍呈等密度,与典型肝癌仍有区别,可能与其血管化程度仍低于肝癌有关。

该组5例肝癌表现亦不典型,延迟期均呈等密度,这主要是由于基础性肝病如脂肪肝或肝硬化导致肝癌病灶平扫时即对比不明显或呈等密度,此时更应注意分析动静脉期的密度变化,结合对照平扫表现,不要被延迟期呈等密度的征象蒙蔽。

另外,该组病例中1/5例炎性假瘤表现出明显的快进快出征象,既往尚无类似报道,病理提示为大量分化成熟的淋巴细胞伴多量成熟浆细胞,未见肿瘤细胞,复习其影像特点,无肝硬化、伴有病灶周围强化征、境界光整有助于与肝癌鉴别。此外,该组1/2例肝腺瘤由于血供丰富亦表现为快进快出,不过延迟期趋于等密度是其鉴别特点。

除了以上不典型病例外,有时局灶性结节增生、多血性转移瘤(如类癌或乳腺癌等)及不典型血管瘤亦需要加以鉴别。不典型局灶性结节增生可以表现为快进快出,延迟呈等或低密度,但是多数境界清楚且不具有包膜,常见中央瘢痕伴延迟强化,多见于年轻人,无肝硬化基础,由于局灶性结节增生一般不会恶变和出血,故大多不需治疗,因此术前诊断很重要。

伴有肝动脉门静脉瘘的血管瘤可以表现为动脉期病灶快速均匀强化、类似肝癌,临床诊断中亦需要特别注意,其鉴别点在于病灶周边由于动静脉瘘常导致灌注不均匀、病灶周边出现不规则轻度密度增高表现,另外磁共振成像T_2WI呈明显高信号仍为其特征性表现。

周围强化征象:此征为炎性假瘤或肉芽肿的重要征象,在该组(5/5)炎性假瘤中均有表现,主要反映了病灶周围组织的炎细胞浸润和炎性充血。有作者将炎性假瘤强化方式分为无明显强化型、分隔状强化型、环状边缘强化型、中心结节状延迟强化型,其中部分病例特别是强化明显的病灶常伴有周围强化征。

胆管细胞癌有时也可以表现出周围强化征象,该组3例中有1例出现病灶周围薄雾样轻度强化,可能与其周围伴有炎性改变有关。胆管细胞癌常可以伴有胆结石或远段胆管扩张,因此也可能伴有继发炎性改变,另外,胆管细胞癌大多境界欠清,无明显包膜,可能伴有向周围组织的浸润,继而也能导致周围强化反应。

(假)包膜征象:是指病灶边缘形成的包膜或类似包膜的结构在CT形成的征象,它既可以是真正的包膜结构,也可以是由于肿块压迫周围组织形成的假包膜结构,病理上均表现为纤维组织,真包膜相对非薄和光整些，CT 显示包膜征在门脉期或延迟期更为明显。

肝癌（特别是肿块较大时）比较容易形成假包膜结构，这也成为其在 CT 上经常出现的征象。而炎性假瘤由于慢性炎性增生反应亦容易形成包膜结构，但其往往还伴有周围强化征，可以与肝癌加以鉴别。肝腺瘤和局灶性结节增生有时也可以出现包膜，前者发生概率约为 25%，后者相对更少一些。该组中有 1 例巨大肝腺瘤表现出明显包膜征象。

渐进性强化：临床最多见于血管瘤，其特点为边缘结节样明显强化并向病灶中心逐渐强化，典型者容易诊断。胆管细胞癌亦常见此征象，不过典型的胆管细胞癌主要为周边强化（强化程度较血管瘤低），渐进性强化后（约 15 min 达到高峰，强化过程一般较血管瘤缓慢）强化病灶可能呈等或略高密度，但病灶中心一般仍呈略低密度（坏死区），肿块较大时低密度范围也会相应增大。炎性假瘤或肉芽肿由于含有血管纤维组织也可以表现为逐渐强化征象，其强化程度与所含组织成分相关。此外，该组病例中有 1 例少见的原发性非霍奇金淋巴瘤，亦表现为渐进性强化过程，与 Beaty 等（2008）报道个案有一定相似性。

延迟呈等密度征象：该征象常与渐进性强化具有一致性，由于该征象最常见于血管瘤，容易形成良性征象的分析定势，但是事实上，该组病例中的各种疾病均具有延迟呈等密度的可能性，因此在定性诊断中应注意其局限性。此外，在分析此征象时，务必还要结合其他征象表现，例如平扫呈等密度则需要考虑等密度肝癌或不典型增生结节的可能，如果合并出现以上提到的其他征象，亦需分别加以鉴别分析。

该组病例的局限性：该组均为不典型病例，病例数相对较少，不过，该项研究的目的并非统计某一征象在某种疾病中的出现率，而主要是通过一些不典型表现揭示各种征象的局限性，减少诊断定势的误导。另外，需要说明的是有一类病例（转移瘤）没有包括，而既往研究表明，转移瘤可以表现为多种强化方式，除了典型的环形强化表现外，转移瘤还可以具有整体病灶快进快出，延迟性强化并呈等密度（类似血管瘤）等表现，因此，在临床诊断工作中针对不典型病例还需要排除转移瘤的可能。总之，肝脏不典型强化病变诊断较为困难，需要在临床工作中不断总结经验，提高影像征象的分析能力。另外，借助综合影像诊断的优势也非常重要。

第八章 关于良、恶性肝肿瘤

第一节 DWI与肝良、恶性肿瘤

DWI原理是在常规自旋回波(SE)T_2加权扫描序列180º脉冲前后加入两个大小相等、方向相反对称性的扩散敏感梯度场，两个扩散敏感梯度场分别造成质子的去相位和相位重聚，水分子沿梯度磁场方向的布朗运动导致自旋质子的失相位从而引起MRI信号衰减，扩散受限区域则信号保留，从而形成DWI信号改变。

根据不同b值条件下(b为0、1000)的扩散信号S10、S11，由公式ADC=ln($S10/S11$)/($b1-b0$)可以得到ADC值。通过测量病灶实质性部分ADC值、信号强度，对病灶进行定性。

选用高b值或较大b值差进行计算时ADC值更稳定，更能反映病变水分子扩散真实情况，但信号强度、信噪比及图像质量随着b值增力或b值差增大明显下降，组织T_2值可以影响ADC值及DWI图像信号。小b值更多反映组织灌注水平的信息。因此一些作者选择b值为1000 s/mm²时分别对肝细胞癌、胆管细胞癌、血管瘤、肝囊肿、局灶性结节增生及正常肝组织进行ADC值测量。

该项研究结果表明，单纯囊肿、血管瘤ADC值明显高于肝脏恶性肿瘤，有显著性统计学意义。肝脏囊肿ADC值最高，与胆囊信号相仿，依次为血管瘤。肝细胞癌、胆管细胞癌及转移瘤ADC值较低，且相互之间差异无统计学意义，这与文献报道相符合。该项研究结果进一步证实了DWI对良、恶性肿瘤之间的鉴别具有稳定性。正常肝组织和局灶性结节增生ADC值位于上述良恶性肿瘤之间。该组作者分析局灶性结节增生并非真正意义上肝脏肿瘤，病理改变为肝细胞异常增生、排列紊乱并被星形纤维瘢痕分隔成结节状。因此可以解释局灶性结节增生与正常肝组织ADC值较相近，两者均与恶性肿瘤ADC值差异有统计学意义。

大量动物实验及临床实验表明，组织成分及水分子扩散程度决定ADC值。肝囊肿含有大量自由水，水分子扩散无受限制，ADC值最高，因囊肿为无血供病变，ADC值随着b值改变相差不大。

血管瘤主要由纤维间隔及血窦形成，水分子在血窦内扩散相对自由，运动较快，ADC值主要受病灶内纤维成分多少及血流灌注影响，因此含纤维成分较多血管瘤水分子扩散运动受限较为明显，ADC值相对较低，血管瘤血流丰富，低b值时ADC值较高，随着b值增加，ADC值下降明显，DWI信号衰减较快。

肝细胞癌、胆管细胞癌及转移瘤肿瘤细胞核较大，排列紧密，细胞外隙很小，自由水相对较少，故水分子扩散受限较为明显，ADC值较低，且肿瘤血供丰富，高b值时DWI肿瘤组织实性部分呈明显高信号，可以提高病变检出率。肿瘤内坏死区水分子扩散受限程度减轻，ADC值较高。

ADC值在肝脏良、恶性肿瘤间存在显著性差异，在文献上已得到广泛的公认，并在临床应用上起到重要的作用。但两者间存在较多重叠区域，目前仍然未能采用统一的ADC值来区分肝脏良、恶性肿瘤。

Erturk等(2008)将ADC值$1.63\times10^{-3}mm^2/s$(b=1000)作为肝脏肿瘤鉴别阈值时，良、恶性肿瘤诊断的敏感度95.2%，特异度91.0%。

由于肝脏恶性肿瘤性病变ADC值无显著性差异，特别在不典型肝癌、胆管细胞癌及转移瘤的诊断及鉴别诊断上有很大困难。Sun等(2005)对肝癌和转移瘤进行瘤-肝ADC比值分析，发现肝癌的瘤肝比为0.91，转移瘤的瘤肝比为1.21，两者有显著统计学意义，认为与肝硬化患者常伴有不同程度肝纤维化等病理改变有关。

该项研究的价值在于进一步证实了 DWI 鉴别肝脏良、恶性肿瘤的价值。各种局灶性实质性病变 ADC 值具有差异，同时分析了局灶性结节增生 ADC 值的特点，关于局灶性结节增生 ADC 值在文献报道较少，说明该项研究在 DWI 研究肝脏局灶性病变有了一定的深入。

该项研究局限性：研究仅局限于肝单纯囊肿、血管瘤、肝细胞癌、胆管细胞癌、转移瘤及局灶性结节增生的研究，缺乏对肝脏再生结节、腺瘤等病变的研究，有待积累较多的病例进行观察。虽然平面回波序列在腹部尤其肝脏已有较深入研究。但图像信噪比较低，伪影较大，易受心脏搏动、相邻肺组织及肠管气体磁敏感伪影影响，严重影响病灶检出及 ADC 值测量，在成像技术上需改进。

综上所述，DWI 为一种新的 MRI 功能成像技术，在分子水平反映病变组织的功能状况，能敏感地发现肝脏早期病变。ADC 值能对病变水分子扩散程度进行定量分析，在肝脏局灶性占位性病变诊断及鉴别诊断方面，提供了可靠的定量指标。

第二节　良、恶性肝脏疾病的鉴别

无论是原发性肝癌还是肝转移瘤均由肝动脉供血，所以恶性肝肿瘤的肝动脉灌注指数增高，一般 >0.25 $ml \cdot min^{-1} \cdot ml^{-1}$，良性肿瘤多不由肝动脉供血，其肝动脉灌注量多正常，肝动脉灌注量增加对诊断肝脏恶性肿瘤的敏感性为 82%，特异性为 62%。

在此值得一提的是，肝硬化的肝动脉灌注量也增加，但多伴有脾脏灌注增加，而肝脏恶性肿瘤多不伴有脾脏灌注的增加。

肝脏恶性肿瘤门静脉期多正常或轻度增加，少数也可下降，因此无定性价值，但门静脉期下降可能代表疾病的进展。

Leggett 等（1997）对 8 例结肠癌患者进行肝脏 CTP 的研究，发现 4 例门静脉期下降，经随访观察发现其中 3 例肝内出现明显转移灶，1 例虽无肝脏病变，但结肠局部肿瘤广泛复发，他认为这是由于肿瘤本身释放一些血管活性物质，使血管收缩，这些物质可以是原发瘤释放也可以由转移瘤释放，随病变进展，血管活性物质增多，使得门静脉期下降。

在一段时间中，对动脉造影 CT 和动脉性门静脉造影 CT 研究较多。动脉造影 CT 是将导管置入肝动脉内造影，同时行肝区动态扫描，主要显示肝动脉供血丰富的肿瘤。动脉性门静脉造影 CT 是将导管置入肠系膜上动脉或脾动脉内，注射对比剂后 20~25 s 开始扫描，不论肝脏肿瘤供血丰富与否，均表现为低密度灶。在一段时间中认为此 2 种方法联合运用，对小肝癌，特别是 1 cm 以下小肝癌最为敏感。

Kikkawa 和 Ichilcawa（1998）曾对 58 例病人共 144 个肝细胞癌，用常规 CT 增强扫描、延迟扫描、动脉造影 CT、动脉性门静脉造影 CT 或动脉造影 CT 与动脉性门静脉造影 CT 联合检查，结果检出率为动脉造影 CT 95.8%，动脉性门静脉造影 CT 90.3%，动脉性门静脉造影 CT 和动脉造影 CT 合用为 98.6%。联合运用动脉性门静脉造影 CT 和动脉造影 CT 技术，能很好提高肝癌结节的检出率。

第三节　肝局灶性结节增生病例

见图 1-8-1。

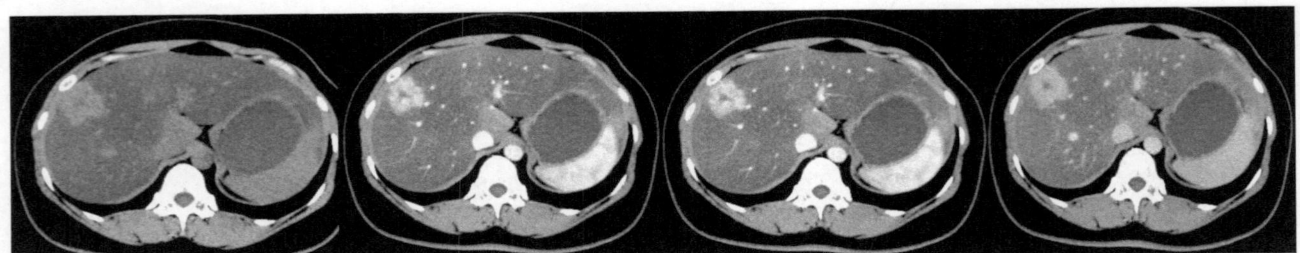

图 1-8-1 患者,女,27 岁。手术病理证实肝局灶性结节增生。影像学表现瘢痕明显,多结节显示清楚。脂肪肝

第四节 MR 和 CT 发现穿过肝脏肿瘤的血管

一般认为,在肝脏 CT 和 MRI 图像上显示的异常密度或信号区内有正常走行的血管穿过是良性局灶性脂肪浸润的指征。但是,Apicella(1994)报道 5 例恶性肝肿瘤病人也有类似情况出现。5 例病人进行肝脏 CT 增强扫描(n=4)或肝脏 MRI(n=5)或两者均进行。5 例肝脏病灶内均有门静脉或肝静脉穿过。肝脏病变对血管无明显的占位效应,没有阻塞或血管移位的证据。在影像学检查之后,对 4 例病人肝脏病灶进行针刺活检,1 例行楔形切除,病理检查结果皆是恶性肿瘤,包括肝淋巴瘤 2 例,转移性黑色素瘤 1 例,转移性腺癌 2 例。

尽管发现血管穿过病灶常常考虑为局灶性脂肪浸润,但上述所见提示,相对较大的血管也可穿越肝肿瘤而无血管结构受压或移位的现象,因此,观察到血管穿过病灶不应作为排除恶性肿瘤可能性的严格标准,应仔细检查恶性肿瘤的其他征象,包括信号强度的特征和对比剂增强的类型等。

第五节 肝细胞性肝癌与 DWI 及 Gd-DTPA 动态增强

国内外进行了多种 MR 技术的研究以寻求一种最适合肝脏病变的检测和定性的成像方法。然而,单用一种 MR 成像技术很难对小病变进行良、恶性鉴别诊断。虽然各种 T_1 和 T_2 增强对比剂的应用提高了小病灶诊断的敏感性及特异性,但还是不能从影像角度充分评价肝硬化患者中肝脏结节的性质,如肝脏再生结节、发育不良结节及微小肝癌等。直径小于 10mm 的结节也可能含有肝癌细胞,但是明确的诊断确是很困难的。

研究表明,多数(95.1%)肝细胞性肝癌于 DWI 图像上表现为高信号。DWI 不受新生血管密度及血流循环速度的影响,它反映的是肿瘤的超微结构变化。肝细胞性肝癌在 DWI 图像的信号增加主要由于扩散对比,肝细胞性肝癌细胞增殖导致细胞密度增加,细胞板层增厚,肝脏血窦毛细血管化,组织细胞间隙缩小,以及细胞内大分子物质和细胞器的增加均会使水分子运动受限制,而致使肿瘤信号增强。

而且 DWI 有很好的背景抑制效果,血管、胆管及腹腔脂肪等都呈明显低信号,肝脏实质也因为扩散运动快而呈较低信号,所以 DWI 有很高的信噪比及对比噪声比,使病变显示明显,更方便读片者发现病变,减少漏诊。6 个肝细胞性肝癌在 DWI 图像上表现为等信号,这 6 个肝细胞性肝癌都有严重的肝硬化背景。Ichikawa 等(1998)发现肝硬化肝脏比正常肝脏 ADC 值下降,肝硬化肝脏实质 DWI 图像信号会增高,肝硬化实质和肿瘤本身的因素可能使肝细胞性肝癌与周围肝的对比降低,而呈等信号,这可能会影响 DWI 检测能力,肝硬化程度越严重,则影响可能越大,关于此情况还需要进一步研究。101 个(82.8%)的肝细胞性肝癌在动脉期强化明显,其中 99 个门静脉及平衡期表现为低信号,符合典型的肝细胞性肝癌增强表现,主要是因为肝细胞性肝癌主要为动脉供血,而无门静脉血供或很少。但 20 个(16.4%)肝细胞性肝癌在动脉期表现为等强化,在 DWI 均表现为高信号,其中有 18 个直径 <20mm,

这为肝细胞性肝癌的明确诊断带来一定困难。

因为动态增强扫描主要通过检测肿瘤动脉血供增加情况发现肿瘤，以往研究表明，小细胞性肝癌的强化程度与肿瘤内的新生血管相关，不同分化程度的肝细胞性肝癌，瘤体内部的异常小动脉密度有明显差异，与血管造影结果明显相关。微小肝细胞性肝癌中，一些高分化的肿瘤，可能新生血管增加不明显，或因为部分容积效应等因素使其与周围肝脏实质对比下降而不能被检测。

而且不同患者血流循环速度不同，经验性扫描延迟时间长短及扫描速度将影响肝细胞性肝癌的强化程度及检出率，增强前进行循环血流测试可能会增加检出率。这 20 个肝细胞性肝癌中有 6 个靠近心底及血管，可能是因为靠近血管及心底的小病灶即使有强化，有时也很难与强化的血管横断面鉴别，或者受心脏及大血管搏动影响，这也可能也是造成动态增强检查对微小肝细胞性肝癌检出率不高的原因之一。

14 个良性病变中，有 1 个病变病理证实为再生结节，此结节在 T_1WI 平扫表现为稍高信号，DWI 均为高信号，增强后动脉期明显强化，门静脉期及平衡期呈等信号，术后病理示结节内纤维间隔有明显的炎性细胞浸润。动脉期强化的异型增生结节在以往的研究中曾有报道，但强化如此明显的再生结节尚未见相关报道，炎性细胞浸润导致组织充血水肿可能是其强化的原因，炎性水肿导致 T_2 透过效应可能是造成 DWI 高信号的原因。

7 个动态增强均无强化病变，在 DWI 上表现为高信号，因为 DWI 表现为高信号，与肝细胞性肝癌不能完全鉴别，1 个术后为再生结节，另外 6 个随访无变化。所以在 DWI 上表现为高信号的结节，要考虑到再生结节的可能。另外 6 个动态增强动脉期表现强化的病变，在 DWI 上表现为等信号。以往的研究表明，异型增生结节、动静脉瘘或肝脏纤维化可致动脉期强化。总之，Gd-DTPA 动态增强与 DWI 结合可能会提高肝细胞性肝癌诊断的敏感性。部分良性病变，如再生结节在 DWI 也可以表现为高信号，需要结合 Gd-DTPA 动态增强或其他检查以明确诊断。

第六节　周边廓清：局灶性肝脏病变钆增强 MRI 的一种恶性征象

Mahfouz（1994）指出，肝肿块性病变周边廓清征定义应为：在延迟增强 MRI 时，病灶周边出现相对于病灶中心的低信号强度环；此征可用以评价和鉴别良、恶性肝脏局灶性病变。

该作者用 1.5 T MR 机对 102 例肝脏肿块病变（含恶性 49 例，良性 53 例）进行研究，发现周边廓清征在良、恶性病变的差异于统计学上具有显著性意义（$P<0.001$），该征象诊断恶性病变的敏感性为 24.5%，特异性为 100%，周边廓清征象仅见于恶性肿瘤的现象可以用病灶周边和中心部位血管状态不同来解释，恶性肿瘤的生长前缘具有丰富的血管似乎在钆增强 MRI 周边廓清效应方面具有重要的作用，尽管此征的敏感性仅为 24.5%，但特异性为 100%，在某些病例，这种外周廓清现象可能是增强 MRI 时唯一的恶性征象。

第九章　肝局灶性病变与超声

第一节　超声低回声晕环鉴别肝良、恶性肿瘤

肝脏的强回声和等回声病灶较难区别，因为肝血管瘤和转移瘤这两种肝脏最常见的良、恶性肿瘤均可呈这两种声象改变。

与血管瘤不同的是等回声和强回声转移瘤边缘常绕以低回声晕环。在超声组织学对照研究中，Wernecke（1992）发现该征象主要与肿瘤内的肿瘤细胞增生环相一致。该作者采用双盲法分析100例肝脏病变，良、恶性各50例。低回声晕环在恶性肿瘤中显示44例，良性病灶仅7例。对良、恶性肿瘤的鉴别，该征象的敏感性为88%，特异性为86%，阳性和阴性预示价值分别为86%和88%。7例原发性恶性肿瘤5例显示低回声晕环，转移瘤43例中有39例显示低回声环；良性肿瘤中，血管瘤29例仅2例显示低回声晕环；4例脓肿中1例有该征象；所有9例肝脂肪浸润、2例肝脓肿和1例再生结节均未见此环。值得注意的是所有3例局限性结节状增生和2例肝腺瘤中的1例出现此环。在等回声或强回声转移瘤与血管瘤鉴别中，晕环征的敏感性为88%，特异性为93%，预计阳性和阴性价值分别为95%和87%。

在鉴别强回声和等回声肝良、恶性肿瘤方面，晕环征是一较客观的诊断标准。此研究中29例血管瘤仅2例出现低回声晕环，与其他作者报道一致。1例血管瘤组织学检查显示该晕环是由一层菲薄的纤维性假包膜引起。低回声晕环是等回声或强回声肝转移瘤最常见最重要的征象，在鉴别肝转移瘤和血管瘤方面很有价值。

第二节　左肝叶伪似肝内包块或胰腺包块

在超声检查时，肝左叶外段的后份常常出现回声减弱，有时还出现分叶，伪似肝内或胰腺包块。但此部肝脏围绕正常的门静脉可减少此类混淆。该部肝脏与其前方的肝脏之间回声的差异是造成此种假象的原因。

第三节　超声检查时肝的假性病变

Mitchell等（1982）介绍低回声的尾叶为超声扫描的一种肝假性病变。由于门静脉左干与静脉韧带位于该尾叶的前方，围绕这些结构的纤维组织吸收声波而产生低回声区。类似的表现还可见于肝静脉梗阻的布-加综合征病人。在超声检查过程中，操作技巧不良和发育变异常造成肝的假性病变，这包括镰状韧带、肝周围脂肪，与血管和胆管有关的声影，胆管树内的空气，心脏房室，超声穿透不适及肋下缺损等。Prando等（1979）曾对此类问题详细讨论，在此不拟赘述。

另外，肾周围脂肪也可伪似肝内的病变，此时肾周围脂肪多挤压肝的右叶，只横断扫描可能误诊，再

辅以纵断扫描，多可减少此类混淆。

第四节　肝脏超声的伪影与误诊

声影伪影：肝圆韧带声影或仅其本身的强回声特性可酷似钙化团块。静脉韧带对声束的衰减作用常导致其后方肝尾叶内出现类似低回声的病变。多切面扫查常可排除病变的存在。

镜像伪影：当肝脏病变邻近膈肌，特别是强回声病变，可以产生镜像伪影。这种伪影是由于声束在两个相邻的曲面即病变表面与膈肌间的反射所致。在一些病例的扫描中，镜像伪影与真正的病变不同，因此，镜像伪影与真正的病变不可能见于同一声像图中。在这种情况下，投射在肺组织中伪影的位置有助于判定病变的实际情况。

高回声伪影：肝脏内高回声区包括肝上部表面嵌入的膈肌和自后方凹入肝脏的肝周脂肪。柔软的肝实质使这些酷似肝部病变的结构穿入肝实质内。其形态、膈肌复合体在声像图上的分层表现，肝被膜嵌入的脂肪及其在动态扫查中相对于肝脏的独立运动，均有助于将其与真正的肝脏病变区分开来。并且，通过纵切和横切面上仔细观察，将有助于正确的诊断。肝脏内另一强回声伪影可能是声加强效应，可使肝静脉后方的肝组织回声增强。

肝叶扩展伪影：在左侧膈下，偶尔在左半膈肌与脾上部之间的肝左叶延伸部位可在脾上部产生一个新月形的低回声团块样结构（正常肝）或高回声团块样结构（脂肪肝），可能被误诊为脾被膜下血肿。但肝脏中的门静脉分支和脾脏之间的独立运动有助于确定这种正常肝脏变异的存在。增大的肝左叶外段也可因位于胃与脾之间而类似肿块表现。

肝右叶也可变异拉长（里德尔叶），向下可延伸至右髂嵴而酷似盆腔内包块或被误认为肝肿大。这种正常变异可通过观察肝实质回声情况及其与肝脏的连续性而与盆腔内肿块区别。

双管征（平行管征）：肝脏内的双管征通常提示存在胆管扩张。偶尔门静脉和伴行的肝动脉也可形成双管征。这种情况多见于肝硬化病人，此时门静脉血流减少，而肝动脉由于代偿而扩张。多普勒超声检查可明确诊断。

折射伪影：在超声扫描时，常见门静脉边缘的回声影，偶尔出现折射伪影而佯似肝内结石或胆囊颈结石声影。另有作者报道，肝内的数枚折射伪影可类似转移病灶的声影，表现为数个小的团絮影，它们可能来源于换能器使用不当。

第十章　肝局灶性病变与CT

第一节　CT平扫呈低密度的肝脏局灶性病变

正常肝实质的密度均匀，但较肝血管内血液为高，故CT平扫时，肝内血管常显示为低密度的分支状影。CT检查时，肝内病变只有与正常肝实质背景密度存在密度差（衰减）时才得以呈现。肝脏病变低于正常肝实质密度而得以显示者，统称为低密度病变；高于肝实质密度而显示者则统称为高密度病变。其高或低的密度差可用CT值量化（表1-10-1）。

表1-10-1　CT平扫呈局灶性低密度的肝脏病变及其表现

肝脏病变	CT平扫表现
恶性肿瘤	
肝细胞癌：少血管性病变及富血管性伴有血色素沉着病者可呈低密度	病灶多灶性、多样性，边界不清、浸润性、坏死、钙化、侵犯门静脉
肝转移瘤：以结肠黏液癌、乳腺癌和肺癌为主	可表现似囊样低密度，可伴有点状钙化
间充质肉瘤：以血管肉瘤为主	以及其他少见间充质肉瘤都可表现为低密度病变
肝内胆管癌：低密度病变以肿块形成型为主	病灶中央常见扩张的胆管，有可能延迟强化
良性肿瘤	
血管瘤：海绵状血管瘤；>5cm为巨大血管瘤	低CT值病变，可发生钙化。增强后呈周围结节状强化，向中央进展，灌注增强，逐渐被对比剂充满，延迟期持续强化
腺瘤：大者可出血	低密度肿块、富血管性、有包膜、动脉早期强化，但较快减弱
局灶性增生结节：<20%为多发	外周分布、富血管性，可见中央瘢痕，中央瘢痕动脉早期强化，较快减弱
囊性	
囊肿：良性、单纯性	多发，大小均有，水样密度，增强后不强化。但边缘可清晰，可见极细微的囊壁
包虫病：以细粒棘球蚴多见，泡状棘球蚴少见	厚壁或薄壁的单房或多房囊性肿块，于母囊边缘部可见更低密度的子囊结构
成人型多囊性肝脏疾病：胆管上皮源性囊肿	肝内囊肿：肝外围多发、多而大的水样密度区；增强后，囊腔与囊壁均不强化
	胆管周围囊肿：管状和串珠型都沿门静脉或胆管分布；散在型难与肝内囊肿区别
脓肿	
化脓性：囊性病变，也可呈"簇"状	少数可含有气体、呈气液平面周围强化，伴病变四周水肿的邻近肝实质强化
阿米巴性（溶组织内阿米巴）	常发生于肝右叶，圆形或椭圆形的低密度灶，增强后可见3~5mm厚强化脓肿壁
真菌性：念珠菌、隐球菌属	多发、低密度、微小脓肿

续表

肝脏病变	CT 平扫表现
局部脂肪浸润：胆囊窝、肝门及韧带周围	地图样低密度，无肿块效应，增强后密度无变化，但脂肪浸润区显示更清楚
血管性	
血肿：创伤后，位于肝实质内或包膜下	血肿和撕裂呈低密度，新出血为高密度，增强后无改变，但病灶显示更为显著
梗死：肝脏有双重供血，故不常见	多位于肝外周，呈楔形灌注缺损造成低密度区，伸至肝包膜下，无占位效应
胆系扩张	
胆汁瘤	创伤或介入手术后
肝内胆管囊肿、胆管囊肿	非阻塞性胆管囊性扩张性疾病，扩张的胆管为水样密度

第二节　肝脏第Ⅰ、Ⅳ段的假性病变

体循环的某些静脉可以向肝脏第Ⅰ、Ⅳ段供血，形成独特的血流动力学，并因此在该区形成假性病变，增强 CT 检查时表现为异常灌注区，以及在异常灌注区的基础上所形成的易与肝脏肿瘤性病变相混淆的局灶性脂肪肝和弥漫性脂肪肝中的正常“肝岛”。

人们对肝脏的双重血供已熟知，却很少注意到部分肝组织还有一些其他的供血血管，Yoshimitsu 等（2001）称之为肝脏的第 3 供血血管，它常由体循环的一些正常或迷走的静脉不经门静脉系统直接进入肝脏而形成。由于这些血管常对肝脏的第Ⅰ、Ⅳ段供血，故在该区易形成这种独特的血流动力学状况，并由此导致该区门静脉血供的减少或缺失，在动脉性门静脉造影 CT（CTAP）上形成灌注缺损区。

所谓“假性病变”，是指能够在 CTAP 图像上形成的灌注缺损区，而其本身并不是一种有临床意义的真性病变。多种因素均可导致假性病变形成，如因肝硬化或明显的肝内血管受压而致的侧支循环开放，各种原因所致的肝内肝动脉 - 门静脉瘘等，均可在 CTAP 图像上形成灌注缺损区而形成假性病变。

此处所描述的肝脏第Ⅰ、Ⅳ段假性病变仅限于上述独特的血流动力学所致者，其在 CT 平扫和经静脉动态增强 CT 扫描中可有两种类型的表现：第 1 种类型为 CT 平扫上无异常发现，而在动态增强 CT 图像上，Ⅰ、Ⅳ段肝实质可出现一过性的异常灌注区。第 2 种类型为在 CT 平扫上，该区出现相对的低或高密度灶，在动态增强 CT 图像上亦有明显的异常灌注表现。两者的区别在于 CT 平扫上假性病变是否出现密度的异常。若这种独特的血流动力学状况已持续很久，那么就有可能造成局部肝实质的代谢发生变化，形成局灶性脂肪肝，或在肝实质代谢改变而出现脂肪浸润时，该区则形成弥漫性脂肪肝中所谓的正常‘肝岛’，此两者在 CT 平扫上均有密度的异常，即为第 2 种类型的假性病变表现。

一、胆囊静脉

胆囊静脉可以分成两组，第 1 组为一些细小的分支，直接进入肝脏第Ⅳ、Ⅴ段，这些分支向胆囊体和底部周围的肝实质供血，其在肝内与门静脉的周围分支相交通，从而稀释了该区的门静脉血流，为假性病变的形成提供了基础。

这种血供特点可在胆囊旁区形成动态增强扫描中的一过性异常灌注表现（即第 1 种类型的假性病变），也可形成弥漫性脂肪肝中的正常‘肝岛’，而目前尚未见到该区可形成局灶性脂肪浸润的报道（Paulson 等，1993；Ito 等，1997），其原因可能是胆囊静脉血成分中各种营养物质、激素及其他因子对局部肝组织的作用，使之不会产生脂肪浸润（Kawamori 等，1996）。

CT 平扫表现：第 1 种类型假性病变无密度异常，而‘肝岛’则表现为在周围相对密度较低的肝组织衬托下，围绕胆囊周围的薄层相对高密度区，其他典型表现还包括非结节样的外形、不清楚的边界和无定形的形态。动态增强CT扫描：由于解剖关系的邻近，流经该组静脉的血液快速进入肝脏，故在动脉期有可能出现胆囊旁区的肝实质提早强化的表现，类似于肿瘤的早期强化。尤其在急性胆囊炎以及胆囊癌时，胆囊的血供异常增加，这种早期强化的假性病变可能更加明显，因而在胆囊癌中不应将这种提早强化区与胆囊癌的局部肝实质侵犯相混淆（Yoshimitsu等，1997）。在门静脉期，第1种假性病变基本呈等密度，即仅在动脉期出现一过性高灌注表现。而'肝岛'并不是想当然的表现为等密度或相对低密度区，其原因有以下两方面：①假性病变区只是门静脉血供被稀释，并不是完全被替代，故该区在门脉期仍有一定程度的强化。②周围受脂肪浸润的肝组织，其强化程度较正常时略低，故多数病例中，假性病变区在门静脉期仍表现为相对高密度。由于这组胆囊静脉较短小，故它们在静脉性增强CT扫描中大多不显示。

CT血管成像（CTA）和CTAP表现：在经导管选择性胆囊动脉造影的CTA图像上，这两种类型的假性病变均表现为浓密的高密度区，而在CTAP图像上则表现为局部的灌注缺损区。结合CTA和CTAP的灌注表现，常能将假性病变与肿瘤鉴别开。第2组胆囊静脉穿过胆囊三角汇入肝门区的胆管旁静脉丛，并构成该静脉丛的前上部分，再引流入肝脏的第Ⅰ、Ⅳ段，亦可形成假性病变，见下述胆管旁静脉系统节。

二、胆管旁静脉系统

该静脉丛走行于肝十二指肠韧带中，主要由3组静脉汇成，即包括上述第2组胆囊静脉，收集胰头区静脉血的胰十二指肠静脉和收集胃远端小网膜囊侧静脉血的胃右静脉（或称幽门静脉），并分别构成该静脉丛的前上、下外侧和内侧部分（Yamagami等，1999）。多数情况下，这些静脉引流入门静脉主干或门静脉系统的较大分支。但偶尔它们在肝门附近汇合形成静脉网并附着于胆管壁上，沿着胆管直接进入肝脏，该静脉系统由此得名。入肝后，该静脉系统或与门静脉系统的小分支汇合，或继续分支形成一支向某个肝段单独灌注的血管（Couinaud，1988）。胆管旁静脉丛进入肝内可以与除Ⅷ段外的所有肝段内的门静脉分支相交通，其中交通频率最大的是第Ⅰ、Ⅳ段内的门静脉分支。而且，由胆管旁静脉丛向肝段的供血中，不经与门静脉小分支的广泛交通，而直接以较大分支形式向肝段供血的情况仅发生在第Ⅰ、Ⅳ段。

其向第Ⅳ段的供血包括以下两种形式：一种是一个较大的胆管旁静脉分支独立于门静脉左支，直接进入Ⅳ段；另一种形式是与门静脉左支的分支相汇合后向Ⅳ段供血（Matsui等，1994）。以上述方式向肝脏Ⅳ段供血的血管多来自于胃右静脉，且在Ⅳ段背侧假性病变的研究中，有关迷走胃右静脉的报道也最多（Matsui等，1995）。但各家报道的迷走胃右静脉的影像学检出率不尽相同，Takayasu等（1990）统计的血管造影检出率为1.5%，Fernandez和Bernardino（1991）在其50例研究中，检出率为14%，而Matsui等（1994）在其300例研究中，检出率为6%。由于胆管旁静脉丛的血管分支间有着丰富的交通，故在三组中，何组静脉在形成假性病变中成为主要因素，是由这些交通血管中的血流方向和血流量来决定，也有可能假性病变是由多根静脉共同形成。

至于形成的假性病变是局灶性脂肪肝，还是弥漫性脂肪肝中的正常'肝岛'，有作者提出可能与迷走血管中的血液成分有关，由胰十二指肠静脉灌注Ⅳ段形成的假性病变多为局灶性脂肪肝，其原因可能与该血管中富含胰岛素有关，而由第2组胆囊静脉和迷走的胃右静脉灌注形成的假性病变中，两者均可发生，但以弥漫性脂肪肝中的正常'肝岛'为多，出现这种同样部位、同样的血供变异为什么在某些病例中形成局灶性脂肪肝，而在另一些病例中却形成弥漫性脂肪肝中的正常'肝岛'，其具体机制目前尚不明确。

CT平扫表现：第1种类型的假性病变无异常密度，局灶性脂肪肝表现为局限性低密度，而'肝岛'则为局限性相对高密度区。动态增强CT表现：第1种类型的假性病变并不一定都显示出异常灌注的特点，因为胆管旁静脉丛常在Ⅰ、Ⅳ段肝内与门静脉的分支相交通，故含对比剂的血液经门静脉血液的稀释后对肝实质的强化作用已明显下降；只有在胆管旁静脉丛的分支向Ⅰ、Ⅳ段单独供血的情况下，假性病变区才有可能出现一过性高灌注表现。

局灶性脂肪肝和'肝岛'在CT动态增强扫描的动脉晚期均有强化表现，因为含对比剂的血液经胆管旁静脉丛流入Ⅳ段假性病变区的时间要短于经肠系膜上静脉回流至肝脏的血流（Kawamori等，

1996）。

故在门静脉期肝实质增强之前，假性病变区先发生强化。但局灶性脂肪肝仍表现为相对低密度区，只是与周围肝实质的密度差有所缩小；而弥漫性脂肪肝中的正常‘肝岛’仍为相对高密度区，但与周围肝实质的密度差进一步加大。门静脉期由于周围肝实质明显强化，故两种假性病变与周围肝实质的密度差分别增大和缩小，但仍为相对低和高密度区。

由胆管旁静脉丛供血引起的假性病变中，Ⅳ段背侧的典型部位非常关键，对诊断的确立有很大的价值。另外，假性病变的边界可以不清晰，也可较清晰，这取决于胆管旁静脉丛在肝内是否与门脉分支有丰富的交通，若有，则假性病变区有这两种静脉共同供血，其间无明确分界，故常显示边界不清晰；反之，则边界清晰。由通过胆囊三角的胆囊静脉和迷走的胰十二指肠静脉向Ⅳ段供血形成的假性病变中，在静脉性对比增强的 CT 扫描中一般很难发现这些静脉，因为胆囊静脉较短小，而胰十二指肠静脉也因为太小，且走行与肝动脉较靠近而不易区分；而在高质量的动态增强 CT 扫描上，有时可以显示迷走的胃右静脉，表现为动脉晚期一条由肝门区向Ⅳ段背侧引流的细小血管影，同时可见该区肝实质的强化。

CTA 和 CTAP 表现：在选择性胆囊动脉、胰十二指肠动脉和胃右动脉成像的 CTA 上，无论是局灶性脂肪肝还是弥漫性脂肪肝中的正常‘肝岛’，假性病变区都会出现浓密的强化，证实有迷走静脉的灌注；在 CTAP 图像上，假性病变区均显示为对比剂的灌注缺损区，表明局部门静脉血流的减少或缺失。

三、腹壁 - 附脐静脉系统

该静脉系统由镰状韧带旁的小静脉组成，引流腹壁前部的静脉血直接进入肝脏，稀释局部的门静脉血液，形成假性病变。该系统由 3 组静脉构成：Sappey 上、下静脉（即附脐静脉）和 Burow 静脉。

Sappey 上静脉引流镰状韧带上部和膈肌内侧的静脉血进入肝左叶，并与门静脉的周围分支相汇合，它也与腹壁上静脉或胸廓内静脉的分支相交通。Sappey 下静脉引流镰状韧带下部的静脉血进入肝左叶的门静脉分支，它沿着圆韧带下行与脐周的腹壁下静脉的分支相交通。Burow 静脉是由两条腹壁下静脉和一条发自膀胱的静脉汇合而成，它终止于闭锁的脐静脉的中部，并不直接进入门静脉。它引流腹壁前部和部分膀胱的静脉血。Burow 静脉与 Sappey 下静脉之间也有一些小的交通支，称为插入静脉（intercalary veins）。

所有这些静脉在出现腔静脉梗阻时，向肝内的血流量则加大（Kakihara 等，2000）。而在门静脉高压时，这些血管内的血液会反向流动，成为离肝的血流。由该静脉系统形成的假性病变可以为局灶性脂肪肝和弥漫性脂肪肝中的正常‘肝岛’。

CT 平扫表现：多在Ⅳ段前缘的镰状韧带及肝圆韧带旁出现相对的低和高密度区，边界常不清晰，分别代表局灶性脂肪肝和‘肝岛’。而第 1 种类型的假性病变则无异常密度。CT 动态增强扫描：局灶性脂肪肝和‘肝岛’的表现与胆管旁静脉丛形成的假性病变的表现一致，而第 1 种假性病变在动脉期常无强化表现，这可能是由于血液从腹壁回流到假性病变区的解剖距离较远所致（Ohashi，1995）。

然而，在腔静脉梗阻的情况下，则其 CT 增强表现要根据梗阻的血管是上或下腔静脉以及注药部位而有所不同。若上腔静脉阻塞，而从上肢注药扫描时，早期对比剂经胸廓内静脉、腹壁上静脉和 Sappey 上静脉进入肝脏，可在Ⅳ段前缘出现浓密的增强表现，而门静脉期转为低密度区；若从下肢静脉注药，由于对比剂到达肝脏的时间要晚，故不能表现出早期的增强。在下腔静脉梗阻的病例中会出现上述现象的镜像表现，即从下肢注药后扫描，对比剂早期即经腹壁下静脉、Sappey 下静脉以及 Burow 静脉进入肝脏形成明显的强化区，若从上肢注药则无早期强化表现。在这些情况下，沿着胸、腹壁走行的相关侧支血管的显影也有助于假性病变的诊断。

CTA 和 CTAP 表现：很少行选择性胸廓内动脉或腹壁上、下动脉插管的 CTA 及 CTAP，若行肠系膜上动脉插管的 CTAP，则假性病变区形成灌注缺损。

总之，肝脏第Ⅰ、Ⅳ段独特的血流动力学是形成假性病变的重要因素。肝脏第Ⅰ、Ⅳ段易于发生这些血管变异主要是胚胎发育所造成。肝动脉、胆管、胆管旁静脉系统及肝脏的第Ⅰ、Ⅳ段发育较晚（约在妊娠第 32~34 天，而大部分的肝组织和门静脉系统发育较早（约在妊娠第 26~28 天），故第Ⅰ、Ⅳ段形成时，这两段可由胆管旁静脉系统等血管供血（Couinaud，1988）。了解这些供血血管的有关情况，有助于理解假性病变形成的基础及相关的 CT 表现，以减少其对诊断的干扰。

第三节 动脉门静脉造影CT出现的迷走胃右静脉引流所致肝Ⅱ及Ⅲ节段假性病灶

Yoon等(1999)报道3例在动脉门静脉造影CT(CTAP)上出现的由迷走胃右静脉引流(AGVD)所致的肝Ⅱ/Ⅲ节段假性病灶。

例1为59岁男性,系肝细胞癌复发伴有与C型肝炎有关的肝硬化,1年前曾用碘油及明胶海绵颗粒作过经导管化学栓塞。CTAP上,肝左叶后缘(Ⅱ节段)显示直径2cm的楔形灌注缺损区,而在常规CT、超声或MRI上,该区域未见确切异常。肝总动脉造影的静脉期见到一支迷走的胃静脉。CT上当对比剂灌注到肝总动脉时,看到一支迷走胃右静脉从其下后方进入Ⅱ节段,并在肝内分支,认为迷走胃右静脉灌注区与CTAP上显示的灌注缺损区一致。影像检查随访1年以上,该区未见异常病灶。

例2系56岁男性,因胰腺囊性肿块入院,增强CT见胰尾有2.5cm大小、边界清楚的单房厚壁囊性肿块,考虑为胰腺囊性肿瘤,为了解肝转移的可能性,作了CTAP及肝动脉造影。CTAP显示Ⅲ节段后缘有楔形灌注缺损区,在次选择性胃右动脉造影的静脉期,见迷走胃右静脉引流从胃进入肝脏Ⅲ节段,并见到它在肝内的分支。CT扫描在注入的对比剂进入胃右动脉时,见迷走胃右静脉进入Ⅲ节段后缘。该区与CTAP上的低密度区一致。1周后,患者作胰腺远端切除,诊断为胰腺黏蛋白囊性癌,术中肝区未见确切肿瘤。

例3为患慢性B型及C型肝炎的76岁女性,作螺旋CT发现肝脏前上段有一0.7cm强化结节。CTAP上见前上段小的灌注缺损及肝外侧段(Ⅲ段)前缘有一个1.5cm楔形灌注缺损区。肝固有动脉造影的静脉期显示从肝左叶处外侧段引流的迷走胃右静脉,它的分支在肝内。然而,该区在常规CT、超声或MRI上未见确切异常病灶。

Yoon等(1999)认为,CTAP是显示肝肿瘤及门静脉阻塞最敏感的方法,而采用这种技术容易出现假性病灶。假性病灶的起因之一是供应肝脏的系统静脉,病灶呈楔形或少见的圆形灌注缺损。它们独特的位置,如在内段后缘、中段和前下段胆囊周围、邻近镰状韧带的内侧段腹侧正中部分,可疑为它的起因。另有报道肝脏Ⅱ/Ⅲ节段是假性病灶发生部位之一。Yoon等(1999)指出,当CTAP上见到Ⅱ和Ⅲ节段后缘或前缘楔形灌注缺损区时,应疑为迷走胃右静脉引流引起的假性病灶。

第四节 肝右叶局灶性结节增生病例

见图1-10-1。

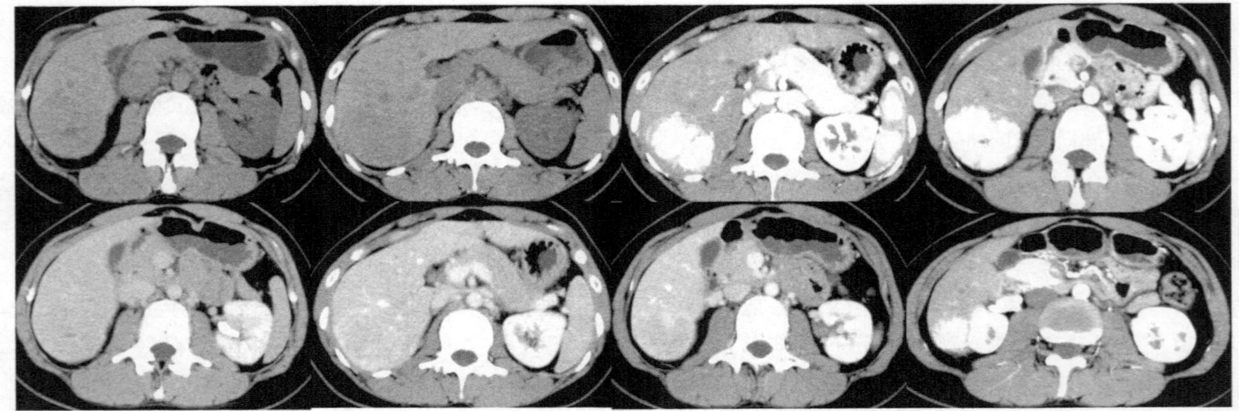

图1-10-1 患者,女,25岁。CT:动脉期明显强化,门脉期强化轻微,3分钟延迟期扫描只见肿瘤中心裂隙,其余均已消逝。术后病理免疫组化诊断:肝局灶性结节增生

第五节　CT增强扫描后显示的肝脏低密度病变

注射对比剂增强后，有些病变，或在有些情况下，并未如预期可见的病灶强化、肝脏实质密度升高以及病灶内出现密度对比差。而是病变仍呈现为相对偏低密度，或在肝实质内出现补丁样低密度区（表1-10-2）。

表1-10-2　CT增强扫描不同特征对应的肝脏病变

CT特征	对应病变
增强后呈低密度的肝脏病变	肝转移：以肺、乳腺、结肠癌等为主
	巨大血管瘤：直径≥5.0cm者
	囊性肿瘤：胆管囊腺瘤（癌）、肝内胆管囊肿、淋巴管瘤
	原发性肿瘤：延迟强化的胆管癌
	再生结节：增强前为高密度的结节、肝脏硬化
	囊肿：多发性囊肿增强后，病变发现可增加
	局灶性脂肪浸润：分布于肝周韧带、胆囊窝以及肝门周围
	脓肿：增强可显示多层脓肿壁，肝右叶好发
	血肿（外伤后、潜在病变：肝腺瘤）
增强后呈相对低密度的补丁样区	常见：布加综合征、肝硬化、心力衰竭、肝炎、门静脉血栓形成
	不常见：淋巴瘤浸润、结节病、血吸虫病、甲状腺毒症、三尖瓣闭锁

增强后呈现为相对偏低密度病变的原因：原病变（如囊肿、脓肿和血肿）内的液性部分不被强化，低密度性质不变；但对比剂增强对其仍有作用，有利于发现额外的病变；对病变大小、形态、周边情况，特别是脓肿或囊肿壁的显示更清晰。原病变（如良、恶性肿瘤）所并发的病灶中心坏死、液化或出血所形成的低密度区增强后不强化。瘤块越大、生长速度越快者出现概率越高。

增强后肝实质内出现“补丁”样低密度区的病变：大多见于血管性病变中，如布卡综合征、心力衰竭、三尖瓣闭锁、门静脉血栓形成以及肝硬化等，造成肝淤血、灌注低下、异常分流等血流动力学改变。

心源性肝硬化：肝脏被动性充血是充血性心力衰竭和缩窄性心包炎最常见的并发症。由肝静脉回流受阻引起的肝实质内血液淤滞，中心静脉压升高，压力由右心房传递到肝静脉，肝窦状隙充盈和充血膨（扩）大。如为慢性右心衰竭则将导致心源性肝硬化。

CT增强时，团注对比剂自衰竭的右心房直接进入、充盈和扩张下腔静脉和肝静脉；肝内受损静脉的外流可导致肝脏血流动力学和肝实质影像改变，显示为密度不均匀的、斑片状和网格样表现；线状和弧线状不强化区可因小～中等肝静脉的延迟强化所致；而在肝脏外围的较大或片状（补丁样）不强化或延迟强化区可能是由于肝静脉高压造成的血流停滞。其他表现尚有心脏增大、肝肿大、淋巴水肿导致的肝内门静脉周围透亮度增加、胸腔积液、腹水和心包积液。MR早期增强影像上肝脏可呈马赛克样强化伴有低信号的条纹构成的网格。肝脏的信号强度趋向同一性。肝静脉和下腔静脉肝上段扩张。如CT所见一样，臂静脉注射对比剂也可反流到肝静脉和肝上段下腔静脉，使它们在门静脉期前显示。在梯度回波MRI上，下腔静脉内见到缓慢甚至缺乏顺行性血流可以确诊。

布加综合征：CT平扫表现为肝脏正常或增大，伴肝实质充血所致弥漫性肝密度减低与下腔静脉和肝静脉腔内见高密度血栓以及腹水。动态增强动脉期和门静脉期，可因肝内不同部位（中央、周边）的不同血流灌注（正常、低下）呈现不同密度（高、低）的“补丁样”区（参阅本书 本卷 第十篇 第一章　布加综合征）。

门静脉血栓形成：门静脉血栓形成后，CT动态增强门静脉期除显示门静脉分支无对比剂充盈外，还可显示与门静脉血栓形成有关肝段血供改变的间接征象：节段门静脉阻塞部分的肝萎缩和由营养性缺血继发的脂肪浸润，造成CT平扫时呈低密度；血栓形成远端肝实质，因门静脉灌注低下造成增强门静脉期的低密度区；肝动脉-门静脉分流是门静脉阻塞的另一个间接征象，于动态增强动脉早期受累的门静脉分支可强化；因门静脉灌注低下，肝动脉代偿性供血增加，于CT增强动脉期时动脉血流增加，显示呈相对高密度区。

第六节　肝CT检查中的假性病变

Jolles和Coulam（1980）在讨论腹水的CT鉴别诊断时提到环形伪影可佯似腹水。他们发现沿着肝的外侧缘有一低密度带状影，类似腹水表现，究其原因方了解到此低密度带实为一环形伪影，乃由于CT扫描器中的X线探测器口径不当所致。Kollins（1978）发现有时在腹部CT横断图像上可见到肝右叶后段的外侧表面的分叶，不应将其误认为一包块或断裂，它乃属正常发育变异。CT扫描在诊断肝的疾病上作用确实不小，但需注意，因为它只是横断图像，对肝的大体解剖的改变，在缺乏其他参考资料（诸如：超声、血管造影、CT矢状面重建等）时，实难分析。

左半膈的反向，源于大量胸腔积液的报告早见于文献（Swingle等，1969；Malvey，1965），然而，由于右上腹有肝脏存在，右半膈反向出现极少。Katzen等（1978）报告1例肝脏明显下移，伴右膈反向，乃源于右侧胸腔积液，CT图像呈现为肝的假肿瘤。Hertzanuy和Solomon（1986）报告1例大量胸腔积液导致右膈反向，指出这是胸腹连接区CT检查的一个陷阱。他们认为，如观察CT图像疑及右膈反向导致出现肝的假性肿瘤时，可辅以矢状重建，或另行超声或MR扫描，常可澄清此类混淆。Kressel等（1977）指出，腹部CT平扫图像上，部分肝脏与门静脉结构可显示为一低密度的病变区，且类似扩张的胆管，经手术证实并非真正病变。Miraldi（1983）与Young等（1983）相继报告光束硬化（beam hardening）和邻近肋骨的运动可造成肝的假性的明显低密度的病变，这些伪影恰位于肋下。

另外，CT图像上有的肝裂内脂肪可类似于扩张的肝内胆管，造成误诊。

第七节　肝左右叶多发性巨大外生性海绵状血管瘤病例

见图1-10-2。

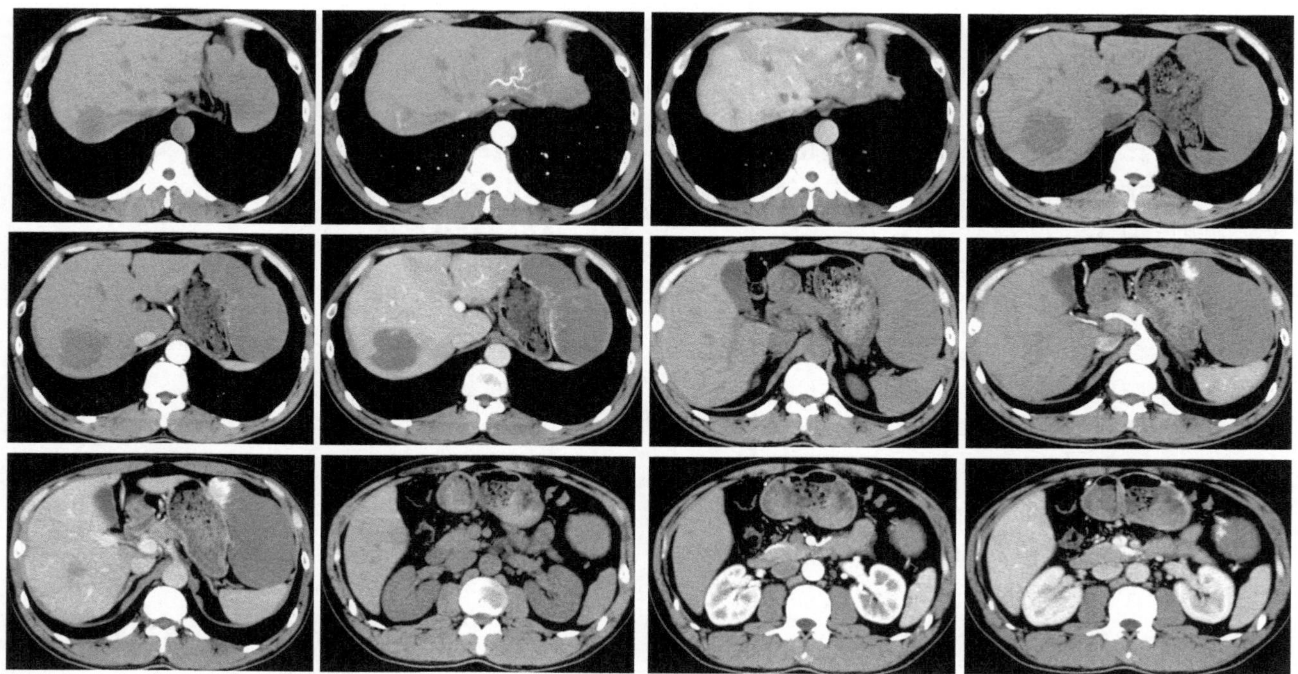

图 1-10-2　患者，男，36 岁。术后病理诊断：左侧及右侧肝肿物切除标本：多发性海绵状血管瘤

第八节　肝脏假肿瘤性病变

所谓肝脏假肿瘤性病变其本身并不是一种有临床意义的真性病变，而是肝局部血流动力学异常所导致的异常灌注区或局灶性肝脂肪浸润。最初见于 CT 肝门静脉造影（CTAP）图像上，随着 MSCT 动态增强的临床应用日益普及，更加深了肝假肿瘤性病变表现的认识。

肝内假肿瘤性病灶最初是在 CTAP 图像上发现的异常灌注区，随着 MSCT 动态增强技术的成熟，这种假性病变的特殊表现引起了临床的关注，其发生并不少见。一组 25 例研究发现其发生率约为 12.52%。究其形成基础与肝脏的胚胎发育密切相关。

肝脏动脉、胆管、胆管旁静脉系统及肝脏Ⅰ、Ⅳ段发育晚于门静脉系统和大部分肝组织，故肝脏Ⅰ、Ⅳ段可由胆管旁静脉系统等血管供血。肝脏第Ⅰ、Ⅳ段这种独特的血流动力学如不造成肝脏局部代谢改变，CT 平扫不显示，仅在增强扫描显示。如造成代谢改变则形成局灶性脂肪沉积或弥漫性脂肪肝中的肝岛，平扫也能显示为低密度或高密度。

按 MSCT 表现可分为高密度和低密度的假性病变，高密度假性病灶包括肝岛和增强扫描动脉期的高灌注，低密度的假性病变主要为局部脂肪浸润和增强扫描门静脉期的低灌注。

动脉期高灌注假肿瘤灶平扫表现为等密度，增强扫描动脉早期或晚期呈一过性高密度强化，边界清楚，可呈楔形、片状、条带状或结节状，门静脉期为略高或等密度，平衡期呈等密度，多位于肝包膜下和胆囊窝周围。该组 9 例为此表现。此种假肿瘤灶形成机制为：胆囊周围肝实质及Ⅰ、Ⅳ段背侧由胆囊静脉和迷走胃右静脉供血，其回流早于门静脉，故在动脉后期表现为相应区域一过性高灌注；来自于体循环的肝包膜血管供血肝包膜下肝组织，表现为增强动脉早期肝包膜下片状或楔形强化；肝硬化时门静脉结构重建，导致小的肝动脉和门静脉分支交通，硬化肝脏在肝动脉期可见高密度灶在门静脉期呈等密度是小的动 - 门静脉分支沟通的表现，其分布无明显特点，可为结节或片状。

门静脉期低灌注假肿瘤灶主要表现为门静脉期呈低密度，平扫可为等密度或低密度，这类病灶多位于镰状韧带旁。此类病灶动脉期和平衡期呈等密度，门静脉期呈低密度，提示该区域门静脉血供减少或缺失，其血供可能来源于附脐静脉，附脐静脉回收前腹壁肌肉的静脉血而后入肝，供血镰旁区域肝组织,其回流略晚于门静脉,因而造成局部附脐静脉供血区门静脉期强化低于周围肝实质,从而出现镰旁区域低密度假病灶;进入平衡期或延迟期后,动脉和静脉中的对比剂含量达到平衡,这种强化差别即消失,即低密度假病灶又转为等密度而不能分辨,此种表现该组占 41.4%(12/29)。

平扫即呈低密度的镰旁肝假病灶可能代表局部脂肪浸润,肝圆韧带和肝镰状韧带中,有细小的静脉供应肝镰状韧带周围肝组织,当这些细小静脉因韧带牵拉发生闭塞,肝镰状韧带周围肝脏缺血时引起肝组织脂肪变性。除 CT 平扫呈低密度外,在螺旋 CT 肝动脉期和门静脉期仍呈相对低密度。该组有 4 例门静脉期密度较平扫和肝动脉期有所增高,这是因肝局部虽有脂肪浸润,但仍能正常强化, 1 例内见门静脉分支, 1 例脂肪肝基础上假肿瘤灶呈更低密度。

肝岛是弥漫性脂肪肝中正常的肝组织,肝脏局部来自其他静脉供血如胆囊静脉、胆管周围静脉、上腹脐周静脉等均可导致局部肝组织代谢改变,在弥漫性脂肪肝基础上形成相对正常的肝岛,平扫为相对高密度,在动态 CT 增强图像上肝岛与周围脂肪浸润的肝组织强化同步,只是动脉期强化肝岛与周围脂肪肝背景的密度差进一步加大,门静脉期由于周围肝实质明显强化,肝岛与周围肝实质的密度差缩小,但仍为相对高密度区,平衡期呈等或相对高密度。该组平扫高密度灶 3 个。

肝脏假肿瘤性病灶发生部位特殊,正确认识其在平扫及多期增强扫描中的特征性表现与密度变化过程,则不难与真正的病灶,特别是恶性病灶如肝细胞癌和肝转移瘤相鉴别。

肝细胞癌多见于有肝硬化基础的患者,可发生在肝任何部位,以结节形为主,增强扫描强化曲线呈速升速降型;而肝脏假肿瘤病灶绝大多数见于无肝硬化基础的患者,该组 23 例病变为楔形和不规则形比例明显高于肝癌。

肝转移瘤可发生于肝任何部位,常为多发,且可有原发恶性肿瘤史。肝假肿瘤病灶发生部位特殊,常为单发,偶为两个呈对称性分布于肝左叶内、外侧段前缘镰状韧带旁。若鉴别困难,可行 MRI 进一步检查(平扫任何序列均呈等信号)或密切随访。

第九节　关于经动脉门静脉 CT 成像(CTAP)的误诊

经动脉门静脉 CT 成像技术:经动脉门静脉 CT 成像的 X 线输出和扫描床的移动是无间隔连续进行的,一次屏气 20s 即可获得整个肝脏的容积数据,消除了运动伪影和错位登录。经动脉门静脉 CT 成像是通过脾动脉或肠系膜上动脉注入对比剂,使对比剂选择性地进入肝内门静脉系统。为获得肝实质非强化病变与强化正常组织间最大的 CT 衰减值差别,应在对比剂进入体循环前完成全肝扫描。病变与正常组织间衰减值的差异是由于正常肝实质的血供 75% 来自门静脉,而转移瘤和原发性肝脏肿瘤与之相反,均主要由肝动脉供血,没有明显的门静脉期增强。为显示肝动脉和确定正常发育变异(即异位肝动脉),应行常规腹腔动脉和肠系膜上动脉血管造影检查,通过造影可观察到肠系膜上动脉、脾动脉、脾静脉、肠系膜上静脉及门静脉的开放情况。为避免通过动脉灌注引起肿瘤增强和避免随后经动脉门静脉 CT 成像肝实质与病灶之间 CT 衰减值差异的缩小,应减少血管造影时对比剂的用量。

有作者提出将导管置于脾动脉内而非肠系膜上动脉内,可使肝实质的强化更显著,更均匀,并使少数几种非肿瘤性病变发生灌注缺损。但该方法不适合于脾切除术后或脾静脉血栓形成的病人。约 25% 的病人出现异位肝右动脉,它是造成经动脉门静脉 CT 成像误诊的原因之一。异位的肝右动脉起源于肠系膜上动脉近端而非腹腔动脉干,直接供应肝右叶的一部分。这种变异将可导致经动脉门静脉 CT 成像上的误诊。进入肠系膜上动脉的对比剂使异位的肝右动脉显著优先增强,随后,由肝右动脉供血的肝右叶肝段内的局灶性病变消失。由于此时可用于经动脉门静脉 CT 成像的对比剂减少、稀释,导致不甚理想的门静脉造影效果。

完成常规血管造影检查后,将导管留置于肠系膜上动脉的近端,并将导管的另一端与肝素 - 盐水输液器连接在一起,固定并保护好导管,将病人转送至 CT 室。

正常表现:经动脉门静脉 CT 成像中,正常肝实质呈均匀一致性密度升高, CT 值达 150~175HU。由于对比剂在血管外间隙的积蓄,当从膈顶向肝下界扫描时，较低层面肝实质 CT 值呈轻微的进行性升高。非门静脉供血的结构，包括胆囊、胆管分支、肝动脉、肝裂、肝包膜、膈肌和其他肝周结构不发生强化。门静脉和肝静脉呈均匀一致的密度升高，CT 值达 250~300HU。下腔静脉可不显示，呈混杂密度或高密度。经动脉门静脉 CT 成像时主动脉可显示某种程度的增强，可能是由于某种原因对比剂在体循环再循环的结果，或由于最初的介入血管造影所致。经肠系膜上动脉注射对比剂时，胰腺或肠壁显著强化；而经脾动脉注射对比剂时，脾脏则明显强化。

经动脉门静脉 CT 成像的误诊：经动脉门静脉 CT 成像是诊断肝脏恶性肿瘤最敏感的术前成像方法。然而，与其他诊断技术如静脉增强 CT、经腹超声或 MRI 比较，经动脉门静脉 CT 成像的假阴性率为 9%~19%，对直径小于 1.0cm 的肿块更是如此。

经动脉门静脉 CT 成像的假阴性也出现于局灶性脂肪肝、伴在门静脉高压的弥漫性肝细胞病变、包膜及包膜下转移、腹膜癌以及进展期的肝转移瘤。病变位于肝脏的中心部位可引起门静脉的压迫或闭塞。此外，对于严重肝硬化的病人，经动脉门静脉 CT 成像很难鉴别再生结节，发育不良性结节抑或肝细胞癌。经动脉门静脉 CT 成像的假阳性是造成误诊的另一个重要原因，常见于肝局灶性良性病变、肝外胆管癌以及未强化的正常肝内、外结构，也见于门静脉系统的血管变异、中心部位肿瘤压迫或闭塞门静脉后出现的肝实质灌注缺损区和罕见的及病因不明的所谓圆形中心性灌注缺损区。经动脉门静脉 CT 成像灌注缺损可分为肿瘤性和非肿瘤性灌注缺损，由于二者治疗原则不同，临床上必须鉴别。

肿瘤性灌注缺损：肿瘤性灌注缺损可为转移瘤、肝细胞癌或良性肿瘤所致。转移瘤由肝动脉供血，经动脉门静脉 CT 成像表现为边界清楚局限性圆形低密度病灶，与邻近强化的正常肝组织形成鲜明对比。转移瘤与其他肝实质局灶性病变的鉴别可能是困难的。

肝细胞癌也可见类似的表现，这种灌注缺损可由门静脉内的瘤栓所致，呈肝段或肝叶分布。经动脉门静脉 CT 成像诊断肝细胞癌的敏感性为 72%，低于转移瘤，可能与下列情况有关：肝细胞癌呈多中心起源，约 25% 的病例有多个小于 2.0cm 卫星癌灶；肝细胞癌通常由肝动脉供血，大约 6% 的病例由于肿瘤外周动静脉瘘的形成，而伴有门静脉血供；如果有一个大的肝细胞癌位于肝中心区，由于门静脉内瘤栓或门静脉分支受压导致外周部灌注缺损，可使多个外周部病变漏诊。

不恰当的经动脉门静脉 CT 成像检查技术通常可导致假阴性结果，如在肝实质强化减弱区或高密度区以及非肿瘤性的弥漫性斑点状病灶区。假阳性结果见于肝细胞病变，如伴有发育不良结节的肝硬化和融合纤维化病灶，但多数发育不良结节主要由门静脉系统供血，常出现某种程度的强化。

经动脉门静脉 CT 成像中局灶性灌注缺损也见于肝良性肿瘤和其他良性局灶性病变，包括肝血管瘤、局灶性结节增生、肝细胞腺瘤、局灶性脂肪变、局灶性纤维化、经消融技术治疗后肿瘤细胞消失的转移瘤、包膜下及实质内血肿、脓肿和囊肿。良性局灶性病变一般不会出现因血管闭塞而引起灌注缺损的情况。

非肿瘤性灌注缺损：经动脉门静脉 CT 成像中由非正常解剖结构或良恶性肿瘤引起的单发或多发港湾缺损并非少见。这些灌注缺损分为：假性病变（小的三角形或方形、外周或中心灌注缺损）；大的圆形中心性灌注缺损；流动灌注缺损（较大的亚段、段或肝叶灌注缺损）。

假性病变最常见于肝左叶内侧段。15% 的经动脉门静脉 CT 成像可出现假性病变，形态为圆形、卵圆形或方形，肝周静脉异常被认为是其形成的原因。人群中大约 6%~14% 的胃右静脉直接回流到第 4 肝段，而不注入门静脉干。发生于肝脏中心部位邻近镰状裂隙的假性病变，一般认为是胆囊周围静脉系统迷走血管所造成。此外，肝外周包膜下假性病灶被认为是由外周包膜下肝实质的微血管系统向门静脉回流时的发育变异所引起。

大的圆形中心性灌注缺损类似于肿瘤，然而，这些罕见的灌注缺损既不是由肝局灶性实质性病变引起，也不具有假性病变或流动灌注缺损的特征，其因不明，但最可能的原因是门静脉系统的异常静脉血管或变异所致。流动灌注缺损继发于阻塞性或非阻塞性病变，范围常较假性病变更大。在阻塞性流动灌注缺损中，可见位于肝中心部位的转移瘤或肝细胞癌及其压迫、侵犯邻近的门静脉分支或在其内形成血栓的影像。较大的流动灌注缺损呈段或叶分布，边界清楚，周围为正常强化的肝实质，这一征象称为“直线征”。

非阻塞性流动灌注缺损是由于门静脉血流分布

不均所致的肝实质不均匀强化。

补偿技术与成像:为增加经动脉门静脉CT成像的准确性和敏感性,可同时进行肝动脉造影CT。该技术可提供转移瘤和肝细胞癌的动脉供血特征,对于诊断多血供的肿瘤更准确。但该方法需在肝动脉内置入另一个导管,操作时间长而且复杂。对于有异位肝右动脉的病人此项检查所获得的信息更有限。

有作者提出注射对比剂后4~5h进行延迟经动脉门静脉CT成像,可进一步提供肿瘤与非肿瘤的灌注缺损特征。延迟经动脉门静脉CT成像中,非肿瘤灌注缺损显示一定程度的类似于正常肝实质的强化。而且,延迟经动脉门静脉CT成像可见到早期经动脉门静脉CT成像所不能显示的灌注缺损区。最早在注射对比剂10min后就可得到延迟经动脉门静脉CT成像。

经动脉门静脉CT成像的另一不足是缺乏诊断特异性,因而多数病人为明确诊断需要进一步超声或CT导引下经皮活检。偶尔,延迟经动脉门静脉CT成像可提高其特异性。

由于经动脉门静脉CT成像的误诊和侵袭性以及目前螺旋CT和MR的发展,经动脉门静脉CT成像逐渐受到冷落。近来CT和MRI的发展极大提高了对肝脏肿瘤的诊断水平。螺旋CT多期扫描可在一次屏气时使肝脏获得满意的强化。MRI利用肝脏特异性对比剂来增加肿瘤与肝脏间对比,已用于肝脏肿瘤的诊断。对于诊断肝脏病变,多期螺旋CT和MRI与经动脉门静脉CT成像检出肝脏病灶具有同样的价值,但前二者具有更高的诊断特异性。有作者提出诊断肝脏病变,特别是转移瘤,应使用氧化铁(ferumoxide)增强MRI,而不是经动脉门静脉CT成像。氧化铁增强MRI与经动脉门静脉CT成像一样敏感,但无侵袭性,且更有效,特异性更高。经动脉门静脉CT成像被认为是检出肝局灶性病变如肝细胞癌和转移瘤的最敏感的影像方法,不足之处是存在许多误诊。多数的误诊来自于正常或变异的血供,常见于肝脏恒定的部位。充分了解经动脉门静脉CT成像的误诊和正常变异是进行正确诊断的前提。

第十节　关于肝CT扫描中的伪影

部分容积效应:因为每一CT像素值代表相应体素的平均密度,当两个相邻组织具有明显的密度差别时均可发生部分容积效应,因此,部分容积效应可以在体内任何一部分发生。如果一个像素包含着具有不同衰减系数的组织,那么组合成的像素就有一个中间的衰减值,使不同组织的界限模糊。在普通CT图像上,可以通过减小层厚来降低或防止发生部分容积效应,尽管螺旋CT的部分容积效应比普通CT更明显,但它可用重叠重建来减小。研究表明,利用螺旋CT检出肝脏局灶性病变,可以通过减小层间距提高检出率。螺旋CT可对兴趣区进行额外地后处理,而不需要再行扫描,这种后处理避免了病人的额外再次照射,并可基本消除部分容积效应的影响。部分容积效应还导致将肝外结构误诊为肝内病变,常遇见的问题是增大的右肾上腺、肾脏肿块或门静脉周围淋巴结与原发肝肿瘤的鉴别。这一问题在儿童或腹部脂肪少的消瘦成年人中尤其多见。缩小扫描层厚和进行三维重建有助于疑难病例的鉴别。

线束状伪影:当X线束穿透骨质和坚硬物体时,可能发生线束状伪影。这种伪影可见于肋骨附近的肝组织内,导致邻近右侧下位肋骨的肝组织内出现边缘不清的低密度伪影;这种伪影也可见于高密度导管或手术银夹的周围。不应将线束状伪影误认为肝内肿块或肝破裂。在特定病例中,采用高电流进行延迟或重复CT扫描有助于克服这种潜在的误诊。

条纹状伪影:Moon 和 Federle(1983)指出,在肝CT横断扫描图像上有时出现条纹状伪影,可遮蔽低密度的肝的撕裂,导致误诊。空气与对比剂界面的条纹状伪影也可遮蔽肝左叶内段或/和外段的低密度的微小脓肿,有作者介绍弥漫性念珠菌病人肝内多发性脓肿CT扫描时发现此类情况,在无条纹状伪影的区域清楚可见小脓肿。

手术夹和金属缝线伪影:在CT检查和超声扫描时,肝区及附近的手术夹和/或金属缝线皆可干扰而出现伪影,此类伪影可遮蔽低密度的肝内脓肿,Lewandowski 等(1985)专门著文讨论此类问题。

第十一章　肝局灶性病变与MRI

第一节　肝脏局灶性病变的MRI表现

由于T_1、T_2、质子密度、磁化率等组织参数不同，MRI对肝脏正常和病变组织结构显示是不同的。MRI扫描的基本序列包括T_1WI、T_2WI平扫及增强后T1WI扫描，分析这些序列的不同表现，有利于多数肝脏疾病进行检测及定性诊断（表1-11-1）。

表1-11-1　肝脏病变在不同MRI序列中的表现

肝脏病变	T_1WI信号强度	T_2WI信号强度	钆剂增强后信号强度
肝细胞癌	低、等、高	高	高
肝转移（除黑色素瘤外）	低	高	*
黑色素瘤肝转移	高	低	*
肝血管瘤	低	极高	高
肝腺瘤	高	低	不强化
FNH：中央瘢痕	低	更高	高
边缘部	等	高	*
再生结节（RN）	低、等	低、高	不强化
血色素沉着病/铁沉积	低	极低	不强化

注：*为动脉期与肝实质呈等信号，而于门静脉期呈低信号。

T_1WI序列可反映病灶的病理特性。囊肿、血管瘤以及含较多液体的病灶常表现为明显的低信号；含有较多纤维组织的病灶，亦表现为T_1WI低信号，如经治疗后的脓肿、化疗后的转移灶都有纤维化；而出血性病灶（包括出血性转移，含蛋白、含较多脂肪组织的病灶）则表现为高信号，如肝细胞癌、肝腺瘤及富含黑色素的黑色素瘤。

T_2WI结合T_1WI表现分析有助于病变的定性。T_2WI上脂肪呈显著高信号，为消除脂肪伪影，可加用脂肪抑制技术。液体成分较多的病灶在T_2WI上呈高信号，含铁的病灶则表现为低信号。在重T_2WI时，含有大量液体以及含缓慢血流的肝内局灶性病变均表现为极高信号。而含有中量液体的肝实质病变（如肝细胞癌等）T_2较短，则表现一般强度的高信号。因而，基于T_2WI序列表现可以鉴别肝囊肿、血管瘤与转移性肿瘤或肝细胞癌。

MRI动态增强T_1WI是肝脏占位病变诊断中的重要序列。肝脏由肝动脉和门静脉双重血供，故动态增强成像的动脉期对显示肝动脉供血为主的病变（如肝细胞癌等）十分重要。

肝脏肿瘤的MRI：Hermine（1992）分析179例肝脏肿瘤的MRI征象。106例恶性肿瘤中44例为转移，62例为原发。73例良性肿瘤中血管瘤46例，13例为腺瘤，14例为结节状增生。超导，0.5T，层厚10mm。

转移性肝癌MRI诊断优于CT检查，对于小的病灶敏感，可清晰地显示20 mm以下病灶较强的梯度信号，T_2WI对于胃肠道肿瘤的肝内转移特别敏感，可以发现直径小于5mm的转移灶，甚至粟粒样病灶。MRI对原发性肝癌与CT检查结果相仿。

肝脏原发性恶性肿瘤和腺瘤在大多数病例中表现相似不易区别。在某个程序肝肿瘤可较好显示，或将两个程序结合使用更好。肿瘤界限清晰，在T_1WI有低信号的环。

高信号的存在和延长T_2WI可判断肿瘤内有无坏死囊变，在缺血性坏死灶不含液体时T_2WI低信号，T_1WI高信号可见于经化疗栓塞后肝癌肿块中的自发性缺血性坏死。肿瘤内出血在T_2WI为高信号。由于肿瘤内脂肪变，肝细胞性肝癌T_1WI常为高信号。海绵状血管瘤在T_2WI延长150ms为高信号，43% 为不均匀的，在第一回波有低信号区，另有高信号的间隔，T_2WI 短时间内病变结构变化是海绵状血管瘤的特征，有利于血管瘤的诊断。在 MRI 图像上局限性结节状增生病变中央有血管蒂，在 T_1WI 病灶中央为星状的低信号区，在 T_2WI 为高信号，形态多变的中央血管蒂是局限性结节状增生的特点，应注意不要与肝癌中央星状纤维化相混淆。T_1WI、T_2WI 图像病变中央有星状高信号区是肝癌纤维化的特点。

MR T_1WI 呈高信号强度的肝脏病变：肝脏病变内如伴发宏观肉眼可见脂肪或出血，在 MR T_1WI 上可呈高信号，但有些呈高信号的肝脏病变并无出血或肉眼可见的脂肪，则可能是病变细胞内含有继发的镜下脂质、铜、蛋白质、黏蛋白或黑色素等成分。MR T_1WI 呈高信号的肝脏病变见下表(表 1-11-2)。

表 1-11-2 MR T_1WI 上呈高信号强度的肝脏病变及其形成机制和表现

肝脏病变	形成机制和表现
脂肪变性	伴有宏观肉眼脂肪的病变，如局灶性肝脂肪变性
肝内出血	伴有出血的病变
肝细胞腺瘤(HCA)	由瘤内出血或含脂肪组织所致，T_1WI 低信号区提示肿瘤内有坏死区。少数肿瘤周围纤维包膜可呈现为病灶周边环状影，T_1WI、T_2WI 均表现为低信号；应注意与肝细胞癌的假包膜相鉴别。偶见中央瘢痕表现。肝腺瘤常是高血供型肿瘤， 增强后常强化
局灶性结节性增生(FNH)	为富血供实质性肿块，其内部结构均匀，出血和坏死少见。呈球形，无包膜。切面为实性，中央可见星状瘢痕，呈放射状向四周分布。FNH 在 T_1WI 上表现为等信号或略低信号灶肝细胞癌(HCC)依据 HCC 细胞内脂肪变程度、含有纤维成分多少及肿瘤的组织学类型，在 T_1WI 可表现为低、等信号或高信号；分化良好的 HCC，细胞内有脂肪组织沉积，在 T_1WI 上表现为高信号(有特征性)，因大多数肝内恶性肿瘤 T_1WI 表现为低信号。瘤内出血也可呈高信号
肝转移	转移灶内含有黏蛋白、脂肪、亚急性出血或黑色素，可在 T1WI 上表现为高信号，出血的转移灶如类癌，黑色素瘤，结肠、卵巢、胰腺黏液囊性和骨髓瘤等转移常在 T1WI 上呈高信号
肝硬化中异形增生结节(DN，发育不良性)	硬化肝脏的肝细胞内可有铁质沉着，沉着于细胞质内者为铁蛋白，沉着于溶酶体内者为含铁血红素，以沉着于 RN 和 DN 内为多。沉着于肝内的铁质是超顺磁性的，在 T_2WI 和 T_2WI 上显示为低信号。非铁质沉着 DN 在 T_1WI 上呈等信号，但硬化的背景肝脏其纤维化在 T_1W1 上呈低信号，从而使非铁质沉着 DN 在 T_1WI 上呈相对高信号；部分含有脂质的 DN，在 T_1WI 上可呈高信号
肝硬化中再生结节(RN)	RN 可分为铁质沉着 RN 和非铁质沉着 RN。前者比较多见，在 T_1WI 上呈低信号，非铁质沉着 RN 在 T_1WI 上大多数为等信号，即与其背景信号相仿，少数为 T_1WI 高信号，其原因与脂质和血供无关，可能与含有其他顺磁性物质(如铜等)有关
布加综合征中的再生结节(RN)	布加综合征慢性期出现再生结节。在 T_1WI 平扫上常呈高信号，可能与含铜有关。结节与结节间有纤维组织包绕。大于 1cm 者有时可见低密度的中心瘢痕。增强后 30s 常不能显示，120s 时显示消退的低信号结节中心可有一强化的高信号中心瘢痕
胆管囊腺瘤 / 囊腺癌	常较大；囊内有间隔样改变与见附壁结节者常提示为囊腺癌。囊腺瘤和囊腺癌常为黏液性(含黏蛋白)和出血。在 T_1WI 上高信号常代表血性液体成分

MR T_2WI 呈低信号强度的肝脏病变：肝脏病变内如继发有出血、钙化，以及纤维化、促结缔组织增生的基质、细胞坏死、黏蛋白或铁沉积时，在 MR T_2WI 上可表现为病变内含有低信号区。呈弥漫性低信号表现者有铁沉着再生结节；呈不均质的低信号区者可伴有出血；呈中央低信号者可见于胆管癌的中央纤维性瘢痕(表 1-11-3)。

表 1-11-3 MR T_2WI 上不同强度的低信号所对应的肝脏病变

信号强度	肝脏病变
T_2WI 呈低信号	①出血性病变；②伴发钙化的病变；③肝硬化中的再生结节；④布加综合征再生结节；⑤发育不良性(异形增生)结节；⑥肝细胞癌(坏死)：罕见(肝细胞癌在 T_2WI 上常呈高信号)；⑦黑色素瘤转移；⑧结核(纤维化期)；⑨泡状棘球蚴病(浸润)；⑩肝豆状核变性等
病变中心在 T_2WI 呈低信号	①肿瘤内的纤维化 / 瘢痕如纤维板层肝细胞癌、胆管癌、血管肉瘤等；②肝转移，如结直肠癌

第二节　MRI 镰状韧带旁伪影及肝功对比研究

关于 MR 扫描中肝脏的伪影相关文献的报道已经很多，识别这些伪影有助于我们的诊断，其中一种被认为是由于镰状韧带压迫所引起的，伪影位于肝脏左内段镰状韧带旁，其产生的原因可能为镰状韧带压迫肝实质导致局限性、暂时性的门脉血流受阻，而不影响动脉的血供。动物实验表明随着腹膜腔内压力的增高，门脉的压力同时增加，而腹主动脉的压力不变，从而推断门脉的血流比动脉更易受压力的影响。有作者收集 120 例 MR 检查的病例就快速动态增强中伪影出现率与肝功能的联系做出初步的研究。

镰状韧带位于肝脏膈面呈矢状位，前方与肝圆韧带融合构成划分肝脏左内段与左外段的标志。附脐静脉起源于脐周静脉网的数条小静脉，主要收集前腹壁与脐周的血液，沿着肝圆韧带向下注入肝内门脉的左侧分支。通过脐周皮下组织内的脐周围静脉网使肝门静脉系的附脐静脉与上腔静脉系的腹壁上静脉和胸腹壁静脉间相吻合；或者与下腔静脉系的腹壁下静脉和腹壁浅静脉间吻合。

以往关于镰状韧带所致肝脏伪影的研究都是以 CT 的三期扫描为检查方法的，而关于 MR 动态扫描的相关文献少见报道，这可能是早期 MR 扫描速度较慢无法在相应的时间内完成三期扫描。随着 MR 硬件及软件的发展，现在已经可以在短时间内完成高质量 3D 扫描，使图像的质量与扫描时间都达到了要求，如在该研究中所采用的 3D-SPGR 序列，其单期扫描的时间为 15 s，必要时调整参数可以达到 11 s，并且所得图像质量能够达到诊断的要求。

Ohashi 等（1995）研究发现在 CT 的三期扫描中，门脉期肝左内段出现相对低密度影，而在动脉期及平衡期无此现象。所发现伪影的发生率为 24.7%，这与该研究中总的发生率是相符合的。Peterson 等（1992）在早期也对此类伪影做过研究，据其报道伪影的发生率为 17.3%，与该研究对比略低，可能与早期螺旋 CT 的扫描速度慢及对比剂注射量有关，其对伪影的解释为局限性的缺氧、低氧造成局限性肝脏脂肪浸润。Bluemke 等（1995）对此的解释为由于镰状韧带的压迫导致在门脉期相对短暂的供血不足，从而导致该区域 CT 图像表现为相对低密度影。该研究中以肝功能的 Child-Paugh 分级为标准，所有伪影均发现在组 1 病人（即正常肝功与肝功异常较轻者 A 类）中。开始该作者对此的解释为由于肝硬化病人的肝叶萎缩，肝裂增宽导致冠状韧带与左内段的间隙加大，故不易产生伪影。但在研究组 1 的病例中，发现肝裂增宽时也可发生伪影，因此推测伪影的产生与肝实质的弹性与硬度有关。肝硬化的演变过程中，随着肝实质纤维化肝功能随着受损，同时肝脏质地变硬，当镰状韧带局限性压迫的肝实质柔软有弹性时，其压力局限程度明显，相对应的门脉血供因此也受到影响而产生伪影，相反当镰状韧带局限性压迫的肝实质坚硬时，其所致受压程度分散，所引起的血供变化不明显故不产生伪影。

（以肝功能的 Child-Paugh 分级为标准，主要参考 5 个因素：肝性脑病、腹水、总胆红素水平、总蛋白水平及凝血时间。每个因素权重 1~3 分不等。肝功异常分为 3 类：A，5~6 分；B，7~9 分；C，10~15 分）

第三节　多层面动态 MRI 中肝左叶内段早期增强的假病灶

Ito（1993）采用多层面动态 MRI 诊断肝脏肿瘤或肝硬化时，在动脉期影像上偶尔发现一个早期增强的假病灶，他为探讨引起这种现象的机制及其临床意义，特意回顾分析了 185 例怀疑肝脏疾患的多层面动态 MRI 图像，包括 93 例肝细胞癌，肝硬化 35 例，肝海绵状血管瘤 26 例，转移瘤 14 例，囊肿 9 例，脂肪肝 4 例，胆管癌和恶性淋巴瘤各 2 例。

使用 1.5T 超导机，首先应用常规自旋回波 T_1WI（500/15）和 T_2WI（2000/90）横断扫描，然后进行梯度回波的屏气多层面动态 MRI 扫描（150/6），偏转角 60°，屏一口气采集 10 幅图像，平扫后静脉注射 Gd-DTPA，在 20~46 秒时扫描获得动脉期图像，3 分钟时行延迟扫描。6 例疑假病灶的患者在行 MRI 的前和后两周都作了超声和 CT 检查，4 例作了血管造影,此6例均进行了6个月的超声和CT随访。

结果见到,185例患者中,6例在动脉期时可见肝左叶内段早期增强的假病灶,4例肝硬化,1例肝细胞癌,1例脂肪肝,病灶都位于肝左叶内段靠近肝门处的包膜下,病灶直径为10~25mm,5例为卵圆形,1例为三角形。在T_1WI和T_2WI,除1例脂肪肝患者外,其余5例在早期增强假病灶的相应位置处未见异常,在增强前及延迟的多层面动态扫描MRI图像上假病灶与周围肝脏组织呈等信号;超声、CT及血管造影上均未见相应的病灶。1例脂肪肝患者,CT平扫假病灶呈高密度,MRI T_1WI像呈低信号,增强前快速小角度激发成像呈稍高信号区。该作者推测,引起早期增强假病灶的原因可能是由于肝左叶内段近肝门处包膜下区接受胆囊动脉和肝动脉的供血,使该区较周围肝实质有较丰富的血液供应;胆囊的引流静脉系统亦与门静脉周围小支有交通,通过此门-体交通,胆囊静脉血供较门脉系统血液更快地进入肝窦,在动脉期造成假病灶出现。

在延迟期,门脉血进入肝窦使得病灶与周围肝脏实质呈等信号。在多层面动态MRI图像上,富血管肿瘤在动脉期显示增强,肝左叶内段早期增强的假病灶可误认为肿瘤,所以在多层面动态MR成像上出现典型部位的早期增强病灶应考虑到假病灶的可能。

第四节　肝脏成像中常见的MRI伪影

一般而言,MRI伪影不是来自于被检病人身体真正的解剖结构。

在肝脏的成像过程中,不仅显示了基本的解剖结构,同时还会显示某个部位实际上并不存在的假性信号。根据不同的来源伪影可分为三类:

(1)来自于扫描过程中病人有关的运动,包括血液的流动和由呼吸或胃肠蠕动引起的肝脏运动所产生的伪影;

(2)与扫描时间无关,而与特殊的扫描技术或特殊的扫描参数有关的伪影,包括化学位移伪影,相消伪影、磁敏感性伪影、折叠伪影及截断伪影;

(3)与系统相关的伪影,指在数据采集过程中由于一个或多个扫描仪部件出现故障或错误校准所引起的伪影,包括磁场的紊乱、系统不稳定性或错误校准、尖峰信号和噪声。

总之,伪影与正常肝脏易于或不易于分辨,主要取决于伪影能否再现。讨论伪影的目的是认识肝脏MRI中常见的伪影,以采取措施减少或消除对最终图像的负面影响。

第五节　MRI动态增强误诊

MRI动态增强扫描是诊断肝脏疾病的重要检查方法,但可能出现以下几种误诊:肝叶、段、亚段及包膜下过度灌注异常;早期强化的假性病变,尤其易发生在肝左叶内侧段;全肝的不均匀过度灌注异常;由血管伪影、不增强的肝血管、部分容积伪影、磁敏感性伪影和肝硬化再生结节等所致的低信号假病变。

在动态MRI增强动脉期,这些异常表现有时类似于真正的病变或类似于肿瘤向周围肝实质的侵犯。然而,多数情况下,在其他序列或延迟期MRI增强时没有相应的异常改变,而且,过度灌注异常的特定部位有助于同真正的肿瘤鉴别。

第十二章　一些诊断陷阱

第一节　肝的假性占位性病变

在肝脏影像诊断中，产生肝脏假性占位性病变的原因甚多，除肝内局灶性脂肪浸润、胸腔积液与膈的反向、医源性的肝显像缺损及邻近器官疾病对肝脏的挤压外，还有：

关于晕征：所谓晕征（halo）一般在肝血管造影时被认为是肝内肿瘤的一种可靠征象，然而有时一个腹膜后肿瘤也可产生此种表现。Chuang 和 Lorman（1977）即报告 2 例此类肝假性肿瘤。Rossi 等（1967，1970）讨论肝内外包块区别诊断的血管造影标准，Shanser 等（1974）指出这些标准在区别无血管性或少血管性包块的病例时不总是那么可靠，近年来一些作者著文赞成后者的看法。当此类矛盾的晕征出现时，有几个因素支持诊断为肝外包块：①肝动脉或门静脉仅轻度伸展、移位；②环绕包块的肝动脉缺乏皱折；③可见邻近器官或组织的异常血管或包块。

在一无血管或少血管的肝内包块，肝血管造影时可呈现透光的缺损区，且伴肝实质期的一致密边缘，即称晕征。致密边缘环绕一无血管包块，此表现或为肝实质受挤压，或是环绕一囊状结构的反应性充血，或是炎症性病变。无血管性包块动脉期肝动脉常呈现皱折，或弓状围绕包块的边缘。肝由于具有巨大的柔韧性，易为邻近器官挤压或压凹，腹膜后包块直接从后方挤压肝脏，此类肝外包块从周围推挤肝实质，也可形成晕征而伪似一肝内包块，此即为矛盾的晕征。

鉴别二者甚为重要。如细心研究连续照片，假肿瘤之肝动脉和门静脉的伸直或移位常常十分轻微，与包块大小颇不相称；肝动脉分支似乎皆自由延伸越过包块；围绕包块的动脉缺乏皱折或变形，提示血管与包块之间缺乏密切的关系，这些都是肝假性肿瘤的矛盾的晕征的特点。另外，在肝血管造影时使用斜位投照以便在切线位观察肝外包块，对邻近器官进行选择性血管造影，都有助于诊断肝外包块。

左肝叶伪似肝内包块或胰腺包块：在超声检查时，肝左叶外段的后份常常出现回声减弱，有时还出现分叶，伪似肝内或胰腺包块。但此部肝脏围绕正常的门静脉可减少此类混淆。该部肝脏与其前方的肝脏之间回声的差异是造成此种假象的原因。

第二节　肝的假良性肿瘤

肥大的膈肌肌束伪似血管瘤：横膈腱膜部分中的肥大肌束在超声检查中少有见到，肌束的迂曲最有可能反映病理学上描写的所谓肝叶征象。Oyen 等（1984）指出，孤立的肥大的膈肌肌束极为类似于血管瘤，可导致误诊。此类肌束的鉴别甚为困难，有时可在横断扫描时使此迂曲肌束显示更清楚，从而有助于区别。

血管类似肝囊肿：超声检查肝静脉，只见其短的轴面象时，极为类似于肝囊肿的表现；如改变扫描断面 90°，使其沿着肝静脉的长轴进行观察，即可减少此类误诊。

第三节　肝肿瘤的误诊

Longmaid 等（1986）指出，在 CT 检查时，肝细胞性肝癌可表现为原发性肝外包块，他们报告 7 例肝癌均如此误诊，全部病例皆经皮穿刺活检、手术切除或尸检证实。这些病例在临床资料与 X 线检查发现的基础上事前无一怀疑为肝癌，其中 3 例起初疑及肝癌，但因其病史、甲胎蛋白阴性、CT 扫描示包块位于肝外而考虑为其他疾病。该作者强调，尽管此类情况并不多见，但在怀疑肝癌的诊断时应想到它的可能性。Laing 等（1984）指出，肝硬化病人的肝的再生结节在 CT 扫描时可表现为等密度分叶性肝包块，这也是值得注意的问题。

第四节　关于肝左叶占位病变血管造影诊断

少血性原发性肝细胞癌于动脉期表现为肿瘤血管呈弧形移位，牵张拉直，动脉侵蚀，较少或无明显新生血管，其动脉侵蚀程度不一，呈内壁不光整，偏心性狭窄，环形狭窄甚至完全中断，多在肝左动脉或肝总动脉主干，亦见于其分支；少数于肿瘤周边部出现少量新生血管，部分有门脉分支提前显影。肝实质期显示肿瘤不染色或周边部少量染色。

多血性原发性肝细胞癌表现为大量新生血管，肿瘤染色，血管弧形移位，血管湖，门脉早显。胆管细胞癌主要显示为肿瘤染色及血管侵蚀，较少新生血管，其染色亦位于肿瘤周边部，缺乏特征性表现。转移瘤中来自胃癌直接浸润及直肠癌血行转移者，多为少血性表现，即显示肿瘤周围血管推压移位等占位征象，而未见新生血管和肿瘤染色。

肝左叶较右叶薄，与脊柱重叠，加上胃、脾和胰腺血管的干扰，故病变显示常欠清晰，导致诊断出现困难。但是，肝左叶病变手术切除率高，尤其是肝左叶外段病变，手术切除效果更佳。肝左叶占位病变的误诊率和漏诊率较右叶为高。一些作者报告 27 例原发性肝细胞癌，误诊原因主要是少血性原发性肝细胞癌缺乏特异性表现，它缺少恶性肿瘤的新生血管、肿瘤静脉、动 - 静脉分流和肿瘤染色等特征。

为提高肝左叶占位病变的正确诊断率，须注意以下问题：使用 IA-DSA，可消除脊柱，胃肠气体及其他组织结构的干扰，提高成像质量；密切结合病史及临床其他检查，是提高正确诊断率的关键；原发性肝细胞癌常有甲胎蛋白、γ-GT 和铁蛋白的增高，且检验甲胎蛋白变异体更具特异性，可与非原发性肝细胞癌病变鉴别；转移瘤常能查到原发病灶；放射性核素血池扫描对血管瘤的特异性高，可提高不典型血管瘤的正确诊断率；在排除其他病变之后，对少血性的占位病变，应想到胆管细胞癌的可能。此外，结合 CT、MRI 和超声检查等影像学手段，亦能为鉴别诊断提供有力证据。一些作者提出，在肝左叶占位病变中，其肝左动脉直径大于或等于 4mm，肝左动脉直径 / 肝固有动脉直径比值大于或等于 0.65 提示原发性肝细胞癌的可能性大。

第五节　肝外肿块与肝肿块

不少作者指出，在 CT 平扫图像上，邻近肝脏的其他脏器或组织的肿块，偶尔可表现伪似肝内原发性肿块，此刻，应用 CT 增强扫描及其他多方位性的影像诊断技术（如超声、磁共振成像等）常有助于正确地鉴别诊断。

第六节　肝脏第Ⅰ、Ⅳ段的假性病变

详见本书 本卷 本篇 第十章 第六节　肝脏第　Ⅰ、Ⅳ段的假性病变。

第七节　肝核素显像时的假阳性

局限性肝叶变薄：Bolich 和 Tyson（1973）报告 1 例核素检查时肝左叶中心部位出现计数减少的局部区域，疑为病变，手术见该区肝叶极为菲薄，故强调肝的网状内皮组织的厚度对核素检查十分重要。一些作者还提示肝结构的变形，如肝硬化或脂肪浸润，均可减少局部的计数，产生此类假阳性的肝扫描。

肝方叶和门静脉分支异常：Suzuki 等（1977）报告 1 例早期肝硬化核素检查时发现接近肝门处沿着肝的下内缘有一稀疏的扫描缺损，考虑为病变，很小的肝左叶为低度活跃，肿大的脾活跃明显增加，脊柱为中度活跃。腹腔镜检查发现一小的肝左叶，方叶下表面内有一舌样组织突到胆囊窝的左缘。经肝穿刺门脉造影发现门静脉异常分支和右侧门静脉分支中度扩张。腹腔动脉造影未发现异常，无方叶区肿块的征象，但却看到正常的血管供应上述肝的副叶，因此，该作者认为此系核素检查的假阳性。

乳腺的衰减：在 ^{99m}Tc 核素显像时，一个下垂的乳腺或一人工文胸可造成局灶性缺损，而误为肝脏的病变。这通常出现于前方观察时，偶尔也见于右前斜位观察时。由于此缺损密度一致，边缘光滑而容易认识，加之它常伴存一活动相当增加的窄条影。此窄条影考虑由肝与乳腺组织和 / 或空气的界面发出的小角度散射的光子所造成。如怀疑此类伪影，应将下垂乳腺上提或去除人造文胸后再行核素显像，即可澄清。

第二篇　肝转移瘤

第一章　肝转移瘤

第一节　关于肝脏转移性肿瘤影像学研究

流行病学研究发现，肝转移瘤是肝内最多见的恶性肿瘤。

影像学研究：超声，肝转移性肿瘤，多为回声明显增强的团块影。有作者认为，结肠癌转移到肝，多呈现反射增强的团块影；但由淋巴瘤所致的肝转移，则呈多发性无回声区；肝转移肿瘤经化疗和放疗后，产生坏死、液化，可出现无回声反射区。

CT：肝脏转移瘤 CT 平扫时多呈低密度，有出血或钙化时呈较高密度。囊性肝转移灶，有钙化的肝转移瘤，转移瘤坏死，淋巴道转移癌，恶性黑色素瘤肝转移均较少见，且有其特殊性。增强扫描示大多数转移瘤为乏血供，其密度较正常肝实质低，但由于周边有生长活跃的肿瘤组织，血供较丰富，在肝动脉期及门静脉期均或呈环形强化，为其典型表现，另一典型表现是增强扫描无强化而呈低密度。少数肝转移癌与原发性肝癌在形态学上难以鉴别，动态增强 MRI 对两者的鉴别诊断有一定的帮助。由于多数肝转移瘤是少血管的，动态扫描的血管期和组织期均表现为低密度。

在不知道有原发癌存在的情况下，血管期表现低密度提示有转移瘤的可能（一般认为单发肝转移癌与原发性肝癌 CT 图像鉴别甚难，对少血管肿瘤，从机会上转移瘤的可能性要大些，但与个别原发性肝癌也不好鉴别）。动态增强检查，肝转移癌常表现为少血管性肿瘤的增强形式，增强早期（注药后 1 分钟之内）一般不出现强化。

在增强晚期和延迟期，对比剂由血管内向肝细胞外间隙和瘤组织细胞间隙扩散，使转移癌表现为中等程度强化，但其信号升高程度始终低于正常肝组织，病灶和肝脏之间的对比差异较增强前明显增大。有时，肝转移癌可出现周边强化和不均匀的混杂强化信号。

血管丰富的肝转移癌在增强检查早期可出现强化高峰，随后信号下降并呈不均匀表现，一般在增强晚期和延迟期不出现均匀一致的强化形式。

MRI：MR 增强早期图像上，肝转移瘤周围的短暂周边强化与组织学上肿瘤边缘厚度的增加及肝实质的改变有关。化疗药物能降低肿瘤的生长速度、炎症反应和血管生成，从而使病变周边强化减弱，据此可以通过肿瘤周边强化的厚度和程度推测肿瘤对治疗的反应。

一般认为，转移性肝癌 MRI 诊断优于 CT 检查，对于小的病灶敏感，可清晰地显示 20mm 以下病灶较强的梯度信号，T_2WI 对于胃肠道肿瘤的肝内转移特别敏感，可以发现直径小于 5mm 的转移灶，甚至粟粒样病灶。

脂肪肝内的转移瘤：脂肪肝内转移瘤的影像表现比较复杂，平扫时转移瘤的表现与脂肪浸润程度密切相关。在重度脂肪肝时转移瘤密度往往高于肝背景而呈相对高密度影，与一般转移瘤密度低于肝实质不同，小的转移瘤有时不易与血管影鉴别。中度脂肪肝内转移瘤往往呈等密度，有时其周围有一极薄的低密度环，稍疏忽即易漏诊。增强扫描对检出和诊断脂肪肝内转移瘤至关重要，但应注意与血管瘤、脂肪肝内残留正常肝岛等鉴别。大多数血管瘤的强化与同层血管相仿，边缘常可呈结节状，而转移瘤的强化一般低于同层的血管，常呈环形强化。应注意此时不可只根据目测密度差进行诊断，细致测量有关部位的 CT 值十分重要。残余肝岛好发于肝的周边部位，包括贴邻肝裂、胆囊窝边缘等处，而转移瘤常发生在肝边缘。一般而言，转移瘤与肝缘的交界多为锐角，而肝岛的交界多为钝角，边缘模糊。诊断疑难时可行 MRI 扫描。

发现微小转移瘤:所谓微小转移灶是指病变非常小,仅可导致血流动力学改变,而无肝内形态学改变。由于肝癌术后复发率可达 60%,是影响患者长期生存的关键问题,多数研究表明这是由于术前影像学未发现的微小转移灶所导致。

还有一种可能是癌旁灶中存在微转移灶,而这种微转移灶由于太小而不能在常规 CT 上显示。肝癌组、癌旁肝和正常肝脏之间灌注参数存在明显差别,不同病理级别的肝动脉灌注量明显不同,说明了 CT 灌注成像可以较好地反映肿瘤的血管生成活性,不但提供肿瘤的解剖信息,而且提供了肿瘤血管生成情况,并进一步推断肿瘤的生物学特性,从影像学方面无创性地给临床治疗和预后以指导。此外,结肠癌患者 10%~30% 在手术时已有肝隐匿性转移,从而导致进一步治疗的失败。Miles 等(1993)实验证明转移灶内肝动脉灌注量为 0.620 ml·min^{-1}·ml^{-1},邻近肝组织内的肝动脉灌注量为 0.51 ml·min^{-1}·ml^{-1},均有明显升高,病灶内肝动脉灌注量升高与局部微血管密集有关,组织学可见动脉形成;邻近肝组织肝动脉灌注量升高意味着新生血管化可能是恶性的。

第二节　恶性胃肠道间质瘤肝脏转移病例

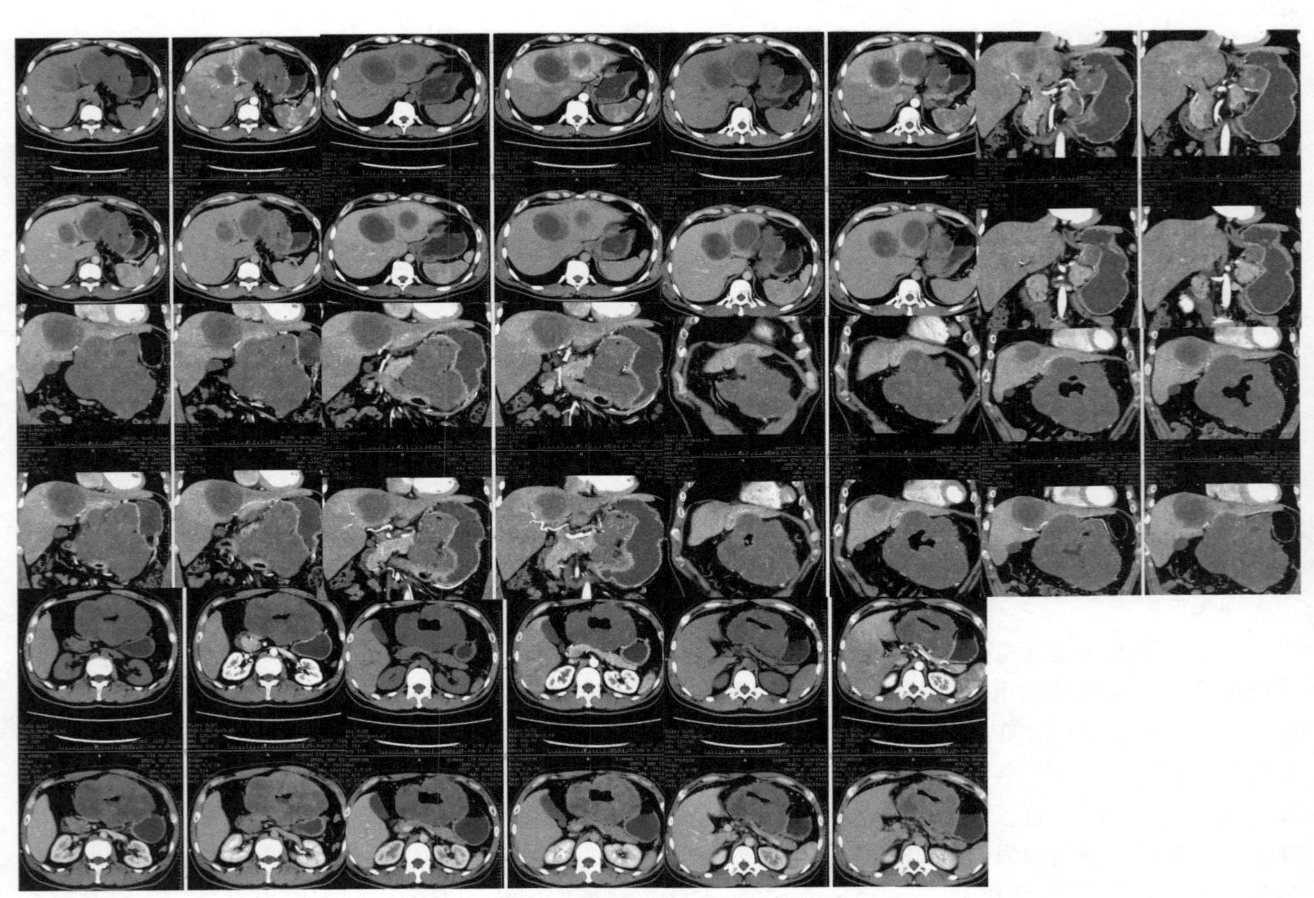

图 2-1-1　恶性胃肠道间质瘤肝脏转移

患者,男, 42 岁。间歇性酒后黑便 1 年,腹痛、腹胀 1 月余入院。

胃黏膜活检及腹腔肿块穿刺活检后行手术切除肿瘤,手术所见:腹腔巨大肿瘤,位于胃体中部前壁及小弯侧,约 14cm × 15cm × 8cm,表面可见粗大供血的血管,包块质中,边界清楚,与周围组织无明显粘连,胃周围淋巴结未及明显肿大。左肝可扪及多发肿物,最大者位于左肝内叶,并突出肝表面,肿物质中,与左肝粘连明显,与周围其余组织轻度粘连，切开后见左肝内叶肿物推挤肝中静脉。右肝未及明显肿物。胆、脾、胰、十二指肠、空回肠、结直肠、盆腹壁未及明显肿物。盆腹腔无明显积液。

病理检查：A 胃肿瘤切除标本：结节状肿物一块，大小 18cm×15 cm×11 cm，重 1600 克。表面一侧附胃组织一块，大小 8 cm×7 cm×0.7 cm，胃黏膜光滑，肿物位于胃组织外侧壁，肿物切面灰白灰褐，质中偏软。另见网膜组织一块，大小 20 cm×20 cm×4 cm。B 左肝切除标本：肝组织一块，大小 18 cm×7.5 cm×4.5 cm，表现可见 2 枚结节状肿物，直径分别为 1.7cm、7cm。切面灰白，质中，与周围肝组织界限较清。其余肝组织切面黄褐，质中。常规病理诊断：胃肿瘤切除标本：胃壁胃肠道间质瘤，伴黏液样变性（与穿刺活检图像相似），大小 18cm×15 cm×11 cm，重 1600 克，符合高危性或恶性。局部侵及黏膜层，大网膜未见肿瘤累及。左肝切除标本：肝脏梭形细胞肿瘤，2 个，直径分别为 1.7cm 和 7cm，考虑为间质瘤转移，待做免疫组化检测进一步证实。合并轻度慢性肝炎，门静脉切缘阴性。免疫组化检测：阳性：CD117，CD34，DOG1（弱+），CK18，Nestin，Ki-67（+，约 20%）；阴性：Actin，Desmin，SMA，Calponin，S-100，CK8，HBsAg，HBcAg。免疫组化诊断：左肝切除标本：胃肠道间质瘤肝脏转移，合并轻度慢性肝炎，HBsAg，HBcAg 均阴性。其他情况参见常规组织学报告（图 2-1-1）。

第二章 不典型的肝转移瘤

第一节 源自消化系统黏液癌钙化性转移瘤

脑内及肝脏内转移瘤多为低密度灶,可单发或多发,大多为多发,单发少见,转移瘤内可发生坏死、囊变和出血,偶可出现钙化。

钙化性转移:钙化性转移少见,是全身性钙、磷代谢障碍致血钙和/或血磷升高,使钙盐在未受损的组织上沉积所致。好发生钙化性转移的疾病有:结肠黏液癌、胃黏液腺癌、卵巢癌、乳腺癌,其他尚有胰岛细胞瘤、平滑肌肉瘤、黑色素瘤和骨肉瘤。转移瘤密度的高低取决于原发病变的性质以及转移瘤内是否有出血,CT值的测定无疑是确定是否钙化的比较简单的方法。瘤内出现钙化灶,并不是特异性表现,钙化的有无及钙化的分布和形态对鉴别诊断无重要意义,但是转移瘤内出现钙化往往可以提示原发肿瘤的范围,有助于缩短原发肿瘤的检出时间,减少患者的经济负担。发生钙化性转移瘤首先应该排除消化系统黏液癌。

颅内转移瘤:颅内转移瘤灶周常伴有与瘤体本身大小不相称的显著性水肿,灶周明显水肿是转移瘤的一个显著特征,当转移灶单发,灶周水肿不明显,瘤内有钙化时则确诊困难。该组误诊4/9例。CT、MRI是当前颅脑转移瘤检查的主要方法,但MRI对于钙化的显示仍不及CT。

肝脏转移瘤:肝脏内转移瘤平扫多为低密度,如合并脂肪肝,转移灶的密度可高于或等于肝实质。肝脏内出现钙化性转移瘤较少见,转移瘤可表现为中心低密度坏死区,边缘呈同心圆状高密度钙化,即“向日葵”征,也可以表现为较为均一的高密度,或者低密度的转移瘤内出现不规则的高密度钙化灶,转移瘤内钙化灶的多少可能与转移瘤出现的时间长短有关。原发病及转移灶的治疗方法不同,单发性转移瘤可采用手术切除,原发灶与转移瘤都切除的患者预后较好,多发性转移瘤不宜手术,及时确诊病因对原发病的治疗以及避免不必要的手术具有重要的临床意义。转移瘤的表现多种多样,钙化性转移是其中的一种少见的转移方式,消化系统黏液癌易发生钙化性转移瘤,必要的影像学检查、原发病灶的检出是诊断的关键,CT扫描对诊断钙化性转移瘤有重要价值。

第二节 孤立性多血性肝转移瘤

孤立性肝转移瘤(含多血性与少血性)约占肝转移瘤的15%~19%,而孤立性多血性肝转移瘤约占肝转移瘤的10%左右。多血性肝转移瘤的原发病灶,常见为绒毛膜上皮癌、肾上腺癌、肾癌、平滑肌肉瘤和类癌等,来自于消化道的癌肿较为少见。来自于胃和食管癌者,多累及肝右叶,这与门静脉血液在肝脏两叶的引流和分布存在明显差异有关。

孤立性多血性肝转移瘤在影像诊断时,容易与肝细胞癌、肝血管瘤和肝脓肿等混淆。有作者指出,下列四种影像学表现有助于孤立性多血性肝转移瘤与肝细胞癌鉴别:①孤立性多血性肝转移瘤,在CT增强扫描显中央液化的低密度肿块的周边强化,尤其是厚环状强化和“牛眼征”;②在MRI的T_1WI呈周边高信号,中央低信号强度(即面包圈征),和T_2WI示周边低信号,中央高信号强度(靶征);③DSA示轮胎状肿瘤染色;④肿瘤供血动脉不增粗。

孤立性多血性肝转移瘤出现上述影像学表现，与其巨块瘤灶的迅速生长和血供不成比例，肿瘤细胞生长旺盛的边缘血供较中心丰富，以及肿瘤中央易出现坏死或囊性变的病理基础有关。肝转移瘤病例的甲胎蛋白多呈阴性，但源自胃癌或胰腺癌的肝转移瘤，甲胎蛋白值可以升高（约占 1%），临床需谨慎识别。癌胚抗原（CEA）值升高可提示胃肠道癌肿或其转移灶的存在，瘤灶完全切除后 1~2 月，其值可恢复正常。孤立性肝转移瘤的瘤灶如能完全手术切除，可延长其生存期。不能手术切除的肝转移瘤，现多采用介入放射学治疗。

第三节　肝脏囊性转移瘤

肝脏囊性转移瘤原发肿瘤的性质及病理基础：肝脏囊性转移瘤在肝脏转移性肿瘤中并不常见，文献报道肝转移性肿瘤囊变发生率为 3.3%。囊性转移灶较少见，其原发肿瘤常为卵巢、胰腺等的囊腺癌或产生大量黏液的肿瘤，子宫恶性间叶瘤、间质肉瘤的肝转移瘤内常可因坏死而可见液平面。

最常见的原发肿瘤：肝脏囊性转移瘤最常见的原发肿瘤有：鼻咽癌、消化道平滑肌肉瘤、大肠癌、胃癌、肺癌、胰腺癌、贲门癌等。有关原发肿瘤中各种类型肿瘤最常见发病率的报道并不一致，有作者报道鼻咽癌为最常见的原发肿瘤；另有作者报道消化道平滑肌肉瘤和大肠癌为最常见的原发肿瘤；一项 11 例的研究发现鼻咽癌肝脏囊性转移瘤发病率较高，在鼻咽癌中，4 例为分化差的鳞状细胞癌。

囊性变的原因：肝脏转移瘤囊性变的原因，主要有三：一是肿瘤自身分泌囊液；二是肿瘤内部广泛出血；三是肿瘤自发液化坏死或栓塞化疗后液化坏死。对于上皮来源的肿瘤如囊腺癌和鼻咽癌等，肿瘤组织能自身分泌是转移瘤囊变的主要原因；对于血供丰富、生长快的原发性肿瘤肝转移，转移瘤内部出现出血、液化、坏死以致囊腔形成，如肉瘤、肾癌等。

影像学研究：肝脏囊性转移瘤具有一般转移瘤的 CT 影像特点，即病灶多为多发，呈类圆形。该组仅 1/11 例为单发，其余均为多发。

其主要的 CT 表现可分为三种形式，包括单囊型、单囊附壁结节型及分隔型，最常见的是单囊附壁结节型。囊壁可薄可厚，大多不均匀。该组病例单囊型 3 例，单囊附壁结节型 5 例，分隔型 1 例。增强扫描后大部分囊壁、壁结节及分隔有强化，而囊腔不出现强化。

该组病例均见不同程度的囊壁、壁结节及分隔增强，其中贲门癌、胃癌及结肠癌肝内转移以动脉期增强明显，而鼻咽癌及胰腺囊腺癌以静脉期增强为明显，囊腔不增强。该组病例转移灶可以位于左叶，也可以位于右叶，可以在肝包膜下，也可以在肝中心，各部位的发病率没有显著差异。肝脏囊性转移瘤一般发生于肿瘤患者的晚期，可以同时伴发其他部位的转移，该组资料显示在发生肝脏囊性转移瘤时，45.5% 的患者已有其他部位的转移，对于肝脏囊性转移瘤的诊断很有帮助。

鉴别诊断：单发或多发性肝脓肿：肝脓肿 CT 平扫没有明显的特异性，增强扫描却具有一定的特异性，表现为除脓肿壁及房隔有明显的强化外，尤其是动态 CT 脓肿壁表现为典型内低、中高、外低 3 层不同密度特征，另外肝脓肿周围肝实质可出现片状或楔形一过性增强征。肝囊肿：肝囊肿 CT 平扫一般均表现病灶边缘清晰，囊肿壁厚薄均匀、光整。增强扫描囊壁及囊腔均无增强征象，一般也不会出现囊壁结节。当囊肿发生恶变时，与囊性转移瘤的鉴别就变得有些困难，结合原发肿瘤病史，囊性转移瘤诊断不难。

肝脏囊腺瘤或囊腺癌：肝囊腺瘤或囊腺癌是来源于胆管上皮细胞的少见肿瘤，因而又称为胆管性囊腺瘤或囊腺癌。本病多见于中年女性，恶性程度低，病史较长，以多房囊性病变为其特点，可有壁结节，壁上可有钙化及有卫星灶、胆管扩张等特征。囊腺瘤或囊腺癌的房隔较多而纤细，并且从病理基础上说，两种有明显的区别，肝囊腺瘤或癌的分隔为纤维组织，而囊腺转移瘤的分隔由残存的肿瘤组织构成。

第四节 肝转移瘤坏死

肝转移瘤可以坏死,CT 扫描是显示肿瘤坏死改变的重要方法。一些作者报道 16 例肝转移瘤,其原发肿瘤为:胃肠道平滑肌肉瘤 5 例,胃癌 4 例,大肠腺癌 4 例,左前壁腺泡状肉瘤、鼻咽癌、膀胱癌各 1 例。该组肝转移瘤在 CT 图像上表现为肝内散在分布的、多发的、大小不等的圆形或椭圆形低密度区,边缘大致清楚,较大的瘤灶边缘轻度分叶,增强扫描后病灶轻度强化,边缘更加清楚。除上述表现外,还出现以下几种反映肿瘤坏死的较特异的表现。

中心性密度更低区:CT 平扫时,在肝转移瘤的部分低密度瘤灶内,中心部清楚可见或隐约可见比周围瘤灶密度更低的区域, CT 值为 -2~16HU,其边界模糊或清楚。增强扫描后此密度更低区无强化,且边界清楚,但周围的低密度瘤灶则有强化。手术病理研究证实,密度更低区的病理基础是肿瘤坏死或 / 和坏死后液化组织。这些密度更低区,不论其形态是圆形还是不规则形,也不论密度更低区所在的瘤灶大小如何,其密度更低区都位于该瘤灶的中心部分,形成了中心性坏死的特征。这些中心性坏死区又以圆形表现为多。

比较原发性肝癌的 CT 表现,中心性圆形密度更低区实为转移性肝肿瘤的特异性征象。尤其是当肿瘤较小(直径在 10mm 左右)就出现中心性圆形密度更低区(即瞳孔征)时,更是肝转移瘤的特征,因为原发性肝癌属多血供肿瘤,肿瘤较小时一般不出现中心性坏死。这些密度更低区按其形态、大小及与周围组织的关系,可出现三种 CT 表现:①厚环征:增强扫描时,瘤灶中心的密度更低区呈圆形,且直径较大,边界清楚,当包绕它的瘤组织(即周围环绕的低密度带)较少时,这些瘤组织即形成类似环形的厚壁,此环壁厚薄一致或略为不匀。有作者称这种改变为厚环征。②瞳孔征:增强扫描时,瘤灶中心的密度更低区呈边界清楚的小圆形,且其范围明显小于由瘤组织形成的周围低密度区时,即形成类似瞳孔的形态,称瞳孔征。③不规则的密度更低区:增强扫描时,瘤灶中心的密度更低区形态不规则,边界清楚或不清楚。上述中心性圆形密度更低区须与肝脓肿进行鉴别。肝脓肿在 CT 增强扫描时可出现特征性双靶征,即肝脓肿的内壁(或内环)有密度增高的环形增强,环形增强的周围又出现厚薄不等的低密度带包绕。

双靶征与肝转移瘤中心圆形坏死的主要区别是:增强扫描时,前者的内环有环形增强,而后者的内环从不出现环形增强。此外,在肝脓肿的脓腔内可包含气体,这也是肝脓肿不同于肝转移瘤的又一征象。至于那些既无双靶征,脓腔内又不含气体的肝脓肿,单凭 CT 表现,则难以和有中心性圆形坏死的肝转移瘤鉴别,此刻,就必须结合临床病史体征和临床检验才能进行鉴别。一些作者报告 44 例平滑肌肉瘤的肝转移, 29 例(65.9%)出现中心性坏死的 CT 表现,其中 19 例肝转移瘤的原发灶来源于胃肠道平滑肌肉瘤。可见,坏死性肝转移瘤的原发瘤灶,多数来自胃肠道的平滑肌肉瘤或大肠癌。

壁结节征:厚的环壁内缘上有与环壁密度相同的小的结节状突起,Mcleod 等(1984)称之为壁结节征,为瘤组织突起所致。

液 - 液平征:密度更低区内可出现水平状分界,在平扫时,其下方密度不仅高于上方密度,而且略高于密度更低区周围瘤组织的密度。由于水平状分界的上下方都是坏死液化组织,故称液 - 液平征。此征的病理基础可能是肿瘤中心性坏死液化时,同时有出血,血液沉积在下方并形成水平状分界,故平扫时分界下方密度略有增高。增强扫描时,出血不强化而周围瘤组织强化,故使分界下方密度与周围瘤组织一致。

第五节　误诊病例简介：原发性肝内胆管细胞癌与肝转移性肿瘤及胰腺癌

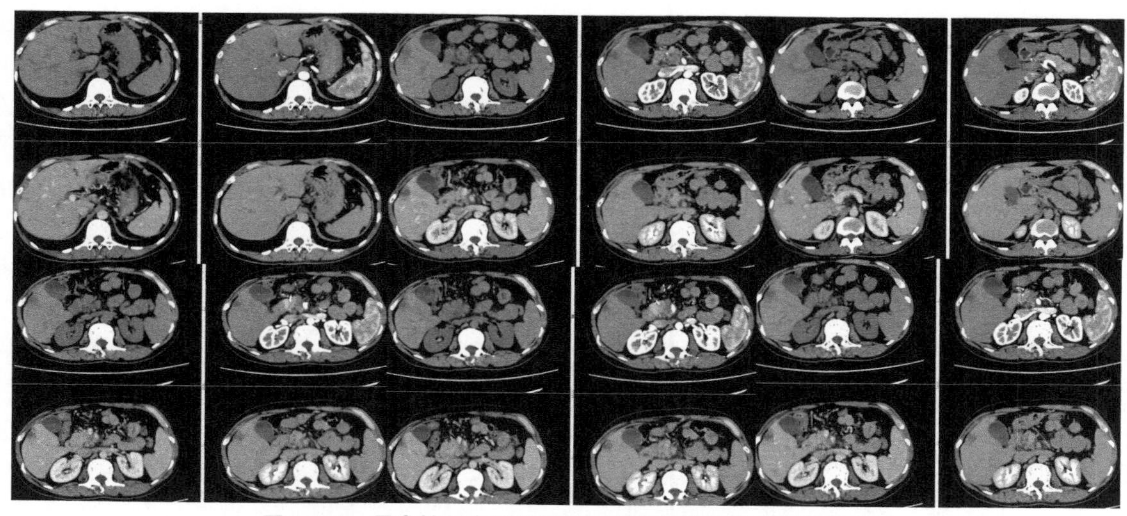

图 2-2-1　原发性肝内胆管细胞癌与肝转移性肿瘤及胰腺癌

患者，男，38 岁。反复上腹痛 1 余年入院。缘于 1 年前无明显诱因出现上腹部疼痛，以剑突下及右上腹明显，无放射至其他部位，无畏寒、发热、腹胀、腹泻、咳嗽、咳痰等不适，遂就诊于外院，查肝胆彩超示“胰头部实质性占位伴主胰管扩张，腹膜后淋巴结肿大”，行上腹部 MR 提示“胰腺囊肿，胰头占位”；未行治疗；10 月前在上海长征医院行胰腺增强 CT 示“胰腺钩突占位，肿瘤可能性大，胰尾部假性囊肿”，未行治疗；于同月就诊他院，诊断“胰腺癌、胰尾部假性囊肿”，行“选择性胰腺肿瘤供血动脉灌注化疗、栓塞术”2 次；术后仍反复出现上腹部疼痛。

手术记录：行肝转移瘤切除 + 腹腔肿瘤特殊治疗（胰头肿物无水酒精注射术 + 肝转移瘤电刀烧灼 + 腹腔氟尿嘧啶植入剂联合吉西他滨腹腔植入）。游离肝圆韧带、肝镰状韧带，显露肝脏，于肝左叶边缘切除一大小约 1cm × 1cm 转移瘤送术中冰冻病理检查，余肝脏表面转移瘤用电刀逐个烧灼。

病理检查：冰冻病理和常规病理：肝脏转移瘤切除标本：肝组织两块，大小分别为 1.8cm × 1.6cm × 1cm 和 1.4cm × 1cm × 0.7cm。切面红褐色，质中。局灶灰白色。

冰冻病理诊断：肝脏转移瘤切除标本：肝内腺癌，来源待定，不排除原发性可能。常规病理诊断：肝脏转移瘤切除标本：左肝内腺癌，待免疫组化进一步确诊。免疫组化诊断：肝脏转移瘤切除标本：左肝内腺癌，考虑为原发性肝内胆管细胞癌。注：腺癌免疫表型与肝内胆管一致，且 CA19-9（-），故考虑为肝内原发性胆管细胞癌。可排除胃肠道癌转移。胰腺癌的免疫表型与胆管细胞癌有重叠，且常高表达 CA19-9，但本例 CA19-9 阴性。请结合临床考虑（图 2-2-1）。

第六节　肝脏转移性平滑肌肉瘤

肝脏转移性平滑肌肉瘤在肝脏肿瘤中较为少见，自 Longmire（1966）首次手术切除肝脏转移性平滑肌肉瘤后，文献上偶有报道。

一、发病情况

肝脏转移性平滑肌肉瘤发病率低，上海医科大学肝癌研究所手术及病理证实的肝恶性肿瘤 1430 例中，有肝转移性恶性肿瘤 89 例，其中肝脏转移性平滑肌肉瘤 15 例，占肝恶性肿瘤 1.04%，占肝转移性恶性肿瘤 16.9%。肝脏转移性平滑肌肉瘤可来源于多个器官与组织，以来源于消化道的平滑肌肉瘤较为多见，也可来源于肠系膜及泌尿、生殖系统等。

该组3例来源于肠系膜，2例来源于消化道。消化道平滑肌肉瘤起源于消化道平滑肌，包括黏膜层、黏膜下层及浆膜层的平滑肌纤维束，也可来源于血管壁的肌层。消化道各段均可发生。转移途径以血行转移为主，以肝脏受累最多见。

McGrath等(1987)报告肝转移率高达65%。Dougherty等(1991)报道55例胃肠道平滑肌肉瘤，19例发生远处转移，其中肝转移15例，占79%。一些作者报道胃肠道平滑肌肉瘤116例，其中24例发生肝转移。也可有腹腔种植和淋巴转移，但少见。另有作者报告28例胃肠道平滑肌肉瘤，其中手术中和手术后发现肝转移伴腹腔种植8例。

该组5例肝脏转移性平滑肌肉瘤中，下腔静脉癌栓2例，腹膜后淋巴结转移2例，肺及肾上腺转移1例，小肠、阑尾及大网膜转移1例，盆腔转移1例。

二、CT表现

体积较大的肝脏转移性平滑肌肉瘤，因血供不足往往引起肿瘤出血、坏死、囊变，CT扫描肿块可表现为囊性、实性、囊实性，坏死、液化、囊变区无强化，周边实质部分可呈明显的富血管特征，强化明显。肿瘤表现为富血供的不均一强化。体积较小的肝脏转移性平滑肌肉瘤亦可出现中央囊变、坏死区。

虽然绝大多数巨块型病灶有液化、坏死、囊变，但部分巨块型病灶反而非常均匀一致，明显强化的包膜清晰可见，肿瘤呈膨胀性生长，向外挤压周边组织。该组未发现门脉受侵迹象，而是明显受挤压推移。一些作者报告44例平滑肌肉瘤的肝转移，29例(65.9%)出现中心性坏死的CT表现，其中19例肝转移瘤的原发灶来源于胃肠道平滑肌肉瘤。可见，坏死性肝转移瘤的原发瘤灶，多数来自胃肠道的平滑肌肉瘤或大肠癌。有报道指出肝脏转移性平滑肌肉瘤在CT表现上可与原发灶表现不同，可能与肝脏血供有关，尚不明了，但腹腔、盆腔内广泛转移灶的CT表现与原发灶是一致的。

三、鉴别诊断

肝细胞肝癌：肝细胞肝癌患者往往有乙肝病史和肝硬化背景，甲胎蛋白可呈阳性；小肝癌强化明显，呈“快进快出”表现；较小的肝癌中央发生液化坏死的概率远较肝脏转移性平滑肌肉瘤低；巨块型肝癌虽然中央可发生坏死，但囊性变很少，且门脉受侵和癌栓的发生率较高，与肝脏转移性平滑肌肉瘤不难鉴别。

消化道腺癌肝转移：肝脏转移性平滑肌肉瘤以周边强化明显，也有环形强化特点，但与消化道腺癌肝转移仍有不同，腺癌肝转移也表现为环形强化，但中央很少有肝脏转移性平滑肌肉瘤那样的极低密度。

肝脏囊腺癌：肝脏囊腺癌的表现与平滑肌肉瘤较相似，囊腺癌边界清晰，但囊腺癌边缘经常可以发现典型的壁结节向腔内突出生长。该组1例术前误诊为肝囊腺癌，主要是因过于关注该例病灶平扫时呈囊性的影像征象，而忽略了病灶增强时的强化特点，应引起重视。

肝脓肿：肝脓肿往往壁厚且不规则，液化坏死形成的脓腔以多房性多见，且多有发热、血常规改变等病史。

原发性肝平滑肌肉瘤：原发性肝平滑肌肉瘤极为罕见，其CT表现与肝脏转移性平滑肌肉瘤相似。

由于肝脏转移性平滑肌肉瘤的血供丰富，增强扫描强化明显，该组1例早期曾误诊为肝血管瘤及局灶性结节增生，后CT复查发现病灶明显增大，追问病史发现患者有胃平滑肌肉瘤手术史。因此，胃肠道平滑肌肉瘤的原发病史、肝内典型的囊性、囊实性占位及其强化特征仍是肝脏转移性平滑肌肉瘤鉴别诊断的主要依据。综上所述，较小的肝脏转移性平滑肌肉瘤血供丰富，中央有液化坏死，较大的转移可以表现为实性、囊实性，周边实质部分强化，中央坏死囊变无强化。影像检查未发现门脉癌栓，临床有原发病史，无阳性肿瘤标志物，无肝炎病史，在肝的富血供占位病变的鉴别诊断中，应该考虑到肝脏转移性平滑肌肉瘤的可能。

第七节　肝淋巴道转移癌

有作者对4例肝淋巴道转移癌的影像学和病理学表现进行了分析，男女各2例，年龄62~81岁，原发于胆囊 2 例，胃和胰腺各 1 例，均为腺癌。超声和 CT 图像示门脉束扩大，边缘模糊，肝内胆管扩张，肝静脉边缘清楚，肝实质内无肿块；X 线胆管造影示肝内胆管多发不同程度狭窄和扩张；1 例 X 线血管造影示肝动脉和门静脉分支扭曲、移位及闭塞。

大体病理检查见肿瘤沿门脉行径，由肝门至外周呈线样放射，并有小结节。立体显微镜下，这些病变由受肿瘤侵犯而扩大的门脉束组成，组织学检查示病变由充满大量癌栓而扩张的淋巴管周围门静脉、胆管和肝动脉组成，并压迫这些管道。淋巴管内癌细胞浸润周围结缔组织并继发纤维化导致门脉束扩大。超声和 CT 识别门脉束的扩大对肝淋巴道转移癌的诊断很重要。

第八节　恶性黑色素瘤肝转移

恶性黑色素瘤原发于表皮和真皮交界处，转移到肝者十分少见。约 10%~20% 的病例找不到原发灶。肿瘤有包膜，易出血、坏死、囊变，瘤细胞富含色素颗粒。

临床表现：可有乏力、纳差、肝区疼痛、胸背疼痛等。查体可见肝肿大、质硬、表现不光滑或光滑，有或无压痛及扣击痛。

影像学研究：超声成像，可见多发性低回声病变，示内部有坏死。CT 扫描：平扫示肝肿大，内有多个结节影，CT 值 30~70HU 左右，部分病灶有低密度包膜，部分瘤体可轻度至中度强化。

肝脏恶性黑色素瘤影像学表现较为复杂，下述几点可能对诊断有所帮助：①肝内多发占位性病变，呈膨胀性生长，可有包膜，易出血、坏死、囊变，实体部分可轻度强化，肝外可有类似病灶；②各个瘤体的 CT 表现可互不相同，但单一病灶表现较为单纯，偶可有钙斑；③MRI 可见瘤体表现形式多样，活组织在 T_2WI 呈稍高信号，可被 Gd-DTPA 强化，富含含铁血黄素的陈旧性出血在各加权象上均为低信号强度，是其最特征性的影像学表现。

第九节　影像诊断中的假性肝转移瘤

肝圆韧带类似肝转移瘤：一些作者指出，在肝圆韧带处常可见到局灶性回声增高区域，而伪似肝的转移瘤。此类影像可能是围绕肝圆韧带的纤维组织或脂肪组织造成的，该处的纵断扫描可展现左肝叶的段间裂，此裂分肝左叶为外侧段和内侧段。

食管胃连接区伪似肝周病变：超声检查时，在膈下食管胃连接区可见一肠道特有的靶征，这不应混淆于肝的靶形病变，后者可见于肝的转移性病变时。

超声检查操作技巧不当：在肝超声检查时，操作技巧不当可产生低回声区，而伪似囊性或转移性肝癌，这尤其常见于肝右叶后部。虽然这常常容易确定为伪影，但有时也颇难与一真性回声减弱区鉴别。

肝的假性转移：肝静脉血流梗阻引起的临床表现称为布加综合征，梗阻的部位是肝静脉本身或下腔静脉。临床表现与肝穿刺活检通常可提示本病，而只有影像诊断方法才能建立诊断，并显示梗阻部位。

有作者报告 1 例血管造影及核素显像误诊为肝转移癌的布加综合征。此病人为女性 28 岁，口服含雌激素的避孕药已 3 年，现肝肿大，有触痛，无黄疸，脾不肿大。^{99m}Tc 显像示肝肿大，其内有数个充盈缺损，提示为多发性转移。腹腔动脉造影示肝动脉狭窄、伸展及变直。先后 3 次肝活检皆示肝硬化，静脉阻塞而无新生物的证据，观察 3 年病人健存且照常工作，该作者考虑此例为口服避孕药引起的肝脏小静脉血栓形成，导致表现为肝静脉血流梗阻。

第十节 误诊病例简介:肝腺癌与肝结核瘤

患者,女,57 岁。体检发现肝占位 1 月余入院。胸部 CT:扫描范围内见肝实质密度不均匀减低,CT 值 35~43HU,肝左内叶见一 5.4cm×5.1cm 稍低密度影,CT 值 33HU,边界尚清。CT 诊断:肝左内叶稍低密度影性质?炎性假瘤?请结合 MRI 检查。

MRI:肝左内叶见一分叶状异常信号影,大小约 4.1cm×5.2cm,T_1WI 低信号,T_2WI 压脂高低信号,扩散成像呈不均匀高信号,边界清楚,周围可见轻度水肿带;增强扫描动脉期病灶边缘呈环状强化,中间无强化,静脉期及延迟期病灶内部逐渐强化呈条片状高信号,散在无强化区,边缘变环形低信号,外周片状强化呈高信号,范围较平扫扩大,肝内外胆管无明显扩张,肝门部可见多个肿大淋巴结影,大小约 2.6cm×1.8cm,边界清楚,胆囊未见异常。MRI 诊断:肝左内叶占位伴肝门部淋巴结肿大,考虑结核瘤,肿瘤待排?

病理检查:冰冻病理与常规病理:右肝肿物切除标本,红褐色碎组织一堆,总体积 1.8 cm×1.5 cm×1.5 cm,其中一切面见一结节,直径 0.6 cm,结节切面灰白质中;第 8 组淋巴结,结节一个,大小 2.8 cm×1.8 cm×1.8 cm,切面灰红灰白,质中;第 12 组淋巴结,灰红色组织三块,大小 2.8 cm×1.6 cm×0.8 cm,切面灰红,质中。冰冻病理诊断:右肝肿物切除标本:腺癌;第 8 组淋巴结:转移性腺癌;第 12 组淋巴结:未见癌转移。常规病理诊断:右肝肿物切除标本:腺癌;第 8 组淋巴结:转移性腺癌;第 12L 淋巴结:转移性腺癌。建议免疫组化标记探讨其来源。

免疫组化检测:第 8 组淋巴结:阳性:CK7(+++)、CK19(+++)、CA19-9(+++)、Villin(+++)、Vimentin(+)、CD10(+);阴性:CK20、CA125、TTF-1、Tg、ER、PR、CDX2。免疫组化诊断:第 8 组淋巴结,转移性腺癌,可能来自肝内外胆管系统或胰腺。建议临床进一步检查胆管、胰腺,并注意肾脏、子宫内膜情况,明确原发病灶。

同日第二次病理检查:左肝内叶及胆囊切除标本,肝组织一块,大小 6.5cm×6cm×5.5cm,切面见一不规则结节,大小 6.5cm×5cm,呈灰白、综绿色,质中,与周围界限不清;肝组织一侧附胆囊组织,胆囊大小 5.5cm×2cm×1.5cm,黏膜呈粗网状,囊壁厚 0.2cm;门静脉旁淋巴结清扫标本,结节样组织一块,大小 2.5cm×1.5cm×1cm,切面灰白,质中。常规病理诊断:左肝内叶及胆囊切除标本,镜下可见腺癌样癌组织侵犯周围正常肝组织,待做免疫组化检测进一步明确癌肿类型,胆囊组织呈慢性炎,未受癌组织累及;门静脉旁淋巴结清扫标本,检出淋巴结 1 枚,可见癌转移。免疫组化检测:阳性:CK19、CK8、CK18、CK7、Villin、CA19-9、Vimentin(灶+)、CEA(散在+)、CD10(散在+);阴性:Hepatocyte、HBsAg、HBcAg、AFP、CK20、CD34。免疫组化诊断:左肝内叶切除标本:结合临床病史、影像学检查、免疫组化检测结果及组织学图像,诊断为中低分化腺癌,癌组织侵犯周围正常肝组织,并可见脉管内癌栓,考虑来源于肝内外胆管系统(胆管细胞癌)。

第三章　肝转移瘤与 CT 及 MRI

第一节　肝脏转移瘤不典型 CT 表现

肝脏转移瘤是肝脏最常见的恶性肿瘤。

肝脏转移瘤 CT 平扫时多呈低密度，有出血或钙化时呈较高密度，有钙化的肝转移瘤多见于结肠、直肠癌，也可见于其他器官（胃、乳腺、卵巢等）的黏液腺癌。转移瘤发生钙化的机制可以是肿瘤本身所产生，也常由营养不良或出血后所致。

增强扫描示大多数转移瘤为乏血供，其密度较正常肝实质低，但由于周边有生长活跃的肿瘤组织，血供较丰富，在肝动脉期及门静脉期均或呈环形强化，为其典型表现，另一典型表现是增强扫描无强化而呈低密度。

转移瘤多保留原发肿瘤的病理组织学特征，囊性转移灶较少见，其原发肿瘤常为卵巢、胰腺等的囊腺癌或产生大量黏液的肿瘤，子宫恶性间叶瘤、间质肉瘤的肝转移瘤内常可因坏死而可见液平面。高血供的原发肿瘤有肾细胞癌、类癌、恶性胰岛细胞瘤、甲状腺癌、恶性嗜铬细胞瘤等。

脂肪肝内转移瘤的影像表现比较复杂，平扫时转移瘤的表现与脂肪浸润程度密切相关。在重度脂肪肝时转移瘤密度往往高于肝背景而呈相对高密度影，与一般转移瘤密度低于肝实质不同，小的转移瘤有时不易与血管影鉴别。

中度脂肪肝内转移瘤往往呈等密度，有时其周围有一极薄的低密度环，稍一疏忽即易漏诊。增强扫描对检出和诊断脂肪肝内转移瘤至关重要，但应注意与血管瘤、脂肪肝内残留正常肝岛等鉴别。

大多数血管瘤的强化与同层血管相仿，边缘常可呈结节状，而转移瘤的强化一般低于同层的血管，常呈环形强化。应注意此时不可只根据目测密度差进行诊断，细致测量有关部位的 CT 值十分重要。残余肝岛好发于肝的周边部位，包括贴邻肝裂、胆囊窝边缘等处，而转移瘤常发生在肝边缘。一般而言，转移瘤与肝缘的交界多为锐角，而肝岛的交界多为钝角，边缘模糊。诊断疑难时可行 MRI 扫描。

第二节　肝内胆管细胞癌与转移性肝癌的鉴别

在甲胎蛋白阴性的肝脏恶性肿瘤中，发病率最高的是转移性肝癌和肝内胆管细胞癌，两者的发病率约为 10 : 1，其 MRI 表现特征有交叉和相似的部分，故两者的鉴别诊断有时相当困难。转移性肝癌的治疗方式主要为化疗，肝内胆管细胞癌的治疗方式主要为早期手术切除，因此，两者的早期鉴别诊断至关重要。

发病率：肝内胆管细胞癌约占肝脏原发性肿瘤的 15%~20%，在原发性肝脏恶性肿瘤中居第 2 位，仅次于肝细胞性肝癌，与胆系的相关疾病有关。转移性肝癌为肝脏最常见的恶性肿瘤之一，居所有肝脏恶性肿瘤首位，其发病率与原发性肝癌相近。转移性肝癌可来源于全身各个部位的转移。原发灶主要为恶性消化道肿瘤、肺癌、乳腺癌等。

影像学研究：肝内胆管细胞癌与转移性肝癌的 MRI 影像特征有多方面的不同，具有一定的特征性。肝内胆管细胞癌的 MRI 平扫主要表现为不规则状及结节状，边界多不清楚，肿瘤在 T_1WI 上表现为均匀的低信号，极少数可表现为斑点状、片状极低信号，可能与肿瘤内出血及含有胆汁、黏液成分有关,在 T_2WI 上表现为稍高信号,部分中心为星芒状、条状或者片状低信号。胆管扩张是肝内胆管细胞癌诊断的又一特征,当肿瘤侵犯肝总管分叉部时,会有广泛的胆总管扩张,一项研究中 22 例肝内胆管细胞癌中 12 例伴有胆管扩张,占 54.5 %。

肝脏包膜凹陷在 22 例肝内胆管细胞癌中有 8 例,占 36.4%,肝脏包膜凹陷征象的病理基础是由于病灶内有大量纤维成分致局部肝包膜受牵拉所致,既往认为肝包膜凹陷征对肝内胆管细胞癌鉴别诊断有重要的价值,但该征象也可见于多种恶性肿瘤,如肠道、胰腺来源的肝转移瘤,融合性肝纤维化转移性肝癌,也可见于良性病变,如肝硬化性血管瘤,因为这些肿瘤也会引起纤维间质反应。该研究中 24 例转移性肝癌中 2 例有包膜牵拉凹陷。由此可见,肝脏包膜凹陷征并不是肝内胆管细胞癌的特异性征象。

转移性肝癌的 MRI 表现与原发灶有关, T_1WI 上均为低信号,有时病灶中央会有更低信号区。T_2WI 信号变化较多,该项研究 146 个病灶中 T_2WI 均匀稍高信号占 71.1%(69/96),中间高信号占 22.7%(22/96),不均匀高信号占 4.1%(4/96),边缘高信号占 1%(1/96)。

观察发现,直径在 <3 mm 的转移性肝癌病灶中, T_2WI 多表现为均匀高信号;直径 >3 mm 病灶多表现中间高信号。T_2WI 上中央高信号即为文献所报道的“牛眼征”和“靶征”,此为转移性肝癌的特征性表现。中间高信号区代表含水量的增加或者坏死。

转移性肝癌多为多发病灶,与肝内胆管细胞癌所见多发病灶不同,转移性肝癌的多发病灶多为类圆形,边缘清晰,大小较一致,并且影像表现也大都相似,多弥漫分布。其为一个较大病灶,其他为卫星病灶,大小不一致,病灶多局限分布。此征象在文献中有相似报道。

MRI 动态增强: MRI 动态增强对两者鉴别诊断有重要价值,肝内胆管细胞癌的典型表现为“快进慢出”型,即动脉期周边出现环状、花边状强化,程度不一,不同于血管瘤的点片状或结节状明显强化特性;门静脉期强化范围向中心扩展,延迟期中心呈渐进性填充式强化,而此时周边强化程度无明显减弱。该组 46 个病灶中 14 个为这种强化方式,占 29.8%。研究报道,肿块型肝内胆管细胞癌 CT 上这种征象出现率为 71%,可能与病例数较少及研究对象不同有关。肝内胆管细胞癌的另一个特征性表现为动脉期病灶内出现网格状、索条状、羽毛状强化,是肝内胆管细胞癌呈浸润性生长、瘤灶内肿瘤血管被肿瘤组织浸润或包埋、对比剂进入所致,或因肿瘤内部形成动静脉瘘,导致动静脉早显引起。

转移性肝癌的强化方式多为动脉期环形强化,门静脉期强化程度与动脉期相似,延迟期强化程度下降,该研究中这种强化方式占 79.1%(76/96),显然要比肝内胆管细胞癌 17.3%(8/46)多。在动脉期,肝内胆管细胞癌表现为环形强化的比例占 85.1%(40/46),整体高信号占 2.1%(1/46),部分高信号占 8.5%(4/46),转移性肝癌所占比例分别为 60.8%(59/96)、32%(31/96)、4.1%(4/96),文献报道肝内胆管细胞癌环形强化的比例为 84%~89%,转移性肝癌环形强化占 72%~80%。动脉期环形强化为两者的共同特征。

病理证实,肝内胆管细胞癌在病灶外周有大量的肿瘤细胞,中央区主要有纤维组织构成,肿瘤细胞在其中分布稀疏。成活的肿瘤细胞是产生肿瘤早期强化的基础,而纤维组织是肿瘤延迟强化的基础。转移性肝癌中乳腺癌肝脏转移病理证实,病灶中央由间质和纤维成分的细胞反应组成,周围有高血供的肿瘤细胞。因此两者的动脉期环形强化具有相似的病理基础,在动脉期两者鉴别相当困难。Al Ansari 等(2014)研究也表明,动脉期环形强化虽然在两者之间有差异,但没有明确鉴别诊断价值。因此,需要结合动态增强及其他序列征象进行鉴别。

综上所述,肝内胆管细胞癌与转移性肝癌影像特征表现各异,其中病灶的形状、边缘、T_2WI 表现、强化方式具有重要鉴别诊断价值,结合伴随症状中包膜凹陷、肝叶萎缩、胆管扩张($P<0.01$),可提高鉴别诊断能力。病灶的个数、长径,动态增强各期的表现对两者的鉴别诊断有一定作用($P<0.05$)。填充进展的强化模式、胆管扩张、包膜凹陷、肝叶萎缩等提示为肝内胆管细胞癌。动脉期环形强化、门静脉期强化与动脉期相似,延迟期强化稍减退、病灶大小一致、T_2WI 中央相对高信号等有助于转移性肝癌的诊断。

第四章　肝转移瘤与血管造影

肝动脉造影与腹腔动脉造影对肿瘤的血供差异的反映

与正常肝脏有双重血供不同，肝肿瘤主要由肝动脉供血，少数作者指出肝肿瘤血供中门静脉也起一定作用，但从血管造影研究角度分析，纵然门静脉对血供有作用，然而对血流动力学意义却不大。这种血供的差别，为诊断肿瘤提供了简单而有效的鉴别方法。肝动脉造影初期，正常肝实质与肿瘤均显影，随后肝实质中的对比剂立即被大量不显影的门脉血流稀释、冲刷和冲走，但肿瘤由于缺乏门脉血流冲洗而成为多血管的团块，此即所谓门静脉冲洗阴性。

然而，在腹腔动脉造影，对比剂平分到肝、脾动脉。因为仅一半对比剂通过肝总动脉到达肝脏，所以造影初期，肝实质和肿瘤都不完全显影。当另一半对比剂通过门静脉到达肝脏时，仅正常肝组织显影，密度继续增加。动脉相的肿瘤血管和染色很淡的肝肿瘤，与正常染色增加的肝实质相比，成为相对少血管区，此即为假性门静脉冲洗阳性效应，它可解释为什么在肝肿瘤诊断中腹腔动脉造影敏感性差，可靠性低，它同样解释了为何在早期研究报告中部分转移性肿瘤被认为是“等血管区”或“少血管区”。

由于肿瘤血管的多或少是与周围肝实质相比而言，少血管或中等血管的肿瘤，如大部分转移性肝肿瘤，在腹腔动脉造影时表现为“少血管”，而在肝动脉造影中却表现为显著“多血管”。多血管肿瘤，如大部分原发性肝癌，在腹腔动脉造影和肝动脉造影均为“多血管”。由于人的眼睛对于鉴别密度增加较亮度更为敏感，小部分少血管肿瘤的诊断只能靠灌注法肝动脉造影，因为阴性门静脉冲洗效应仅能增强微弱的肿瘤染色。因为所有存活的肝肿瘤均由肝动脉分支供养，而且在肝动脉造影中皆现肿瘤染色，所以肿瘤染色可作为评价肿瘤治疗效果的一个重要标志。治疗后肿瘤从显著“多血管”变为“少血管”或“无血管”，即认为治疗有效。

第三篇　肝细胞性肝癌

第一章　诊疗规范和专家共识

肝细胞性肝癌国际诊断指南与国内诊疗规范的比较与解读

肝细胞性肝癌（hepatocellular carcinoma，HCC）是原发性肝癌的最常见病理类型，占85%~90%。目前，全球各国和地区均积极制定适合自身国情的肝细胞性肝癌临床实践指南，主要包括美国国立综合癌症网络（National Comprehensive Cancer Network，NCCN）指南、美国肝病研究学会（American Association for the Study of Liver Diseases，AASLD）指南、欧洲肝病研究学会（European Association for the Study of the Liver，EASL）指南、亚太肝病研究学会（Asian Pacific Association for the Study of the Liver，APASL）指南、日本肝病学会（Japan Society of Hepatology，JSH）指南、韩国肝癌研究组（Korean Liver Cancer Study Group，KLCSG）和国家癌症中心（National Cancer Center，NCC）指南等。

2011年，中国卫生和计划生育委员会（原卫生部）颁布了原发性肝癌诊疗规范（以下简称规范），并于2017年修订更新。这些指南和规范均由多学科专家团队结合最新循证医学证据经充分讨论而建立，并定期更新，对规范和指导肝细胞性肝癌的临床实践起到了积极推动作用。影像检查是高危人群中肝细胞性肝癌筛查及诊断的主要方法。全球不同地区肝细胞性肝癌发病率不一，基础肝病背景也显著不同，导致筛查方案、检查技术及诊断流程均有很大差异。一组作者通过深入解读我国2017年版规范相关内容，并与国际诊断指南进行对比，旨在提高对肝细胞性肝癌的诊断水平。

（一）2017年版诊疗规范解读

1. 筛查监测　2017年版规范中明确提出，我国肝细胞性肝癌的高危人群主要包括：乙型肝炎病毒（hepatitis B virus，HBV）和/或丙型肝炎病毒（hepatitis C virus，HCV）感染、长期酗酒、非酒精脂肪性肝炎、食用被黄曲霉毒素污染的食物、各种原因引起的肝硬化以及有肝癌家族史等患者。超声（ultrasonography，US）联合甲胎蛋白（alpha-fetoprotein，AFP）是筛查监测肝细胞性肝癌的主要手段。对US检查阴性但AFP持续升高者需进一步行动态增强影像扫描；仍为阴性者，在排除妊娠、活动性肝病、生殖胚胎源性肿瘤以及消化道癌的前提下，需要密切随访AFP水平以及每隔2~3个月进行一次影像复查。

2. 诊断工具　对于超声筛查检出的结节，2017年版规范推荐了4种诊断工具，包括超声增强造影（contrast-enhanced ultrasonography，CEUS）、动态增强CT、Gd-DTPA动态增强MRI、钆塞酸二钠（gadoxetate disodium，Gd-EOB-DTPA）增强MRI（EOB-MRI），对CEUS对比剂的类型未做明确规定。PET/CT和单光子发射计算机体层成像（single photon emlssion computed tomography，SPECT）/CT主要用于明确肝外转移情况进行分期，DSA基本被取代。

2017年版规范更推崇肝细胞性肝癌的无创性诊断理念，对穿刺活检的实施有了更严格、精确的规定，明确了在高危人群中，对于直径>2 cm的结节，如果上述4种影像检查均无典型的肝细胞性肝癌特征，则需进行肝穿刺活检；直径≤2 cm结节，若上述4种影像检查中≤1项有典型的肝细胞性肝癌特征，可进行肝穿刺活检或每2~3个月间隔进行影像随访。

3. 诊断路径　与2011年版规范比较，2017年版规范将AFP在诊断流程中删除，主要依赖影像方法进行肝细胞性肝癌诊断，这与国际上的理念更为统一。在动态增强影像上，肝细胞性肝癌的典型表现为动脉期显著强化伴门静脉期和/或延迟期对比剂廓清（“快进快出”）。

在高危人群中，对于直径>2 cm的结节，4项检查中≥1项显示有肝细胞性肝癌典型特征，可做出肝细胞性肝癌的临床诊断；对于直径≤2 cm结节，4项检查中≥2项显示有肝细胞性肝癌典型特征，可做出临床诊断。

旧版规范中，对于≤1 cm的结节仅推荐随访监测，不做诊断要求，但新版规范中则推荐积极诊断，这主要得益于以DWI为代表的MRI功能影像技术和肝胆特异性对比剂的临床应用提高了微小病灶的检出率及定性诊断准确性。

需要强调的是，上述肝细胞性肝癌诊断路径针对的是慢性病毒性肝炎、肝硬化等高危人群，并非普通人群；而且即使对于这类高危人群，也应谨慎地除外其他常见的良性实性肿块，如海绵状血管瘤、肝脏局灶性结节增生（focal nodular hyperplasia，FNH）等，避免不必要的有创性检查。

4. 肝胆特异性对比剂　与2011年版比较，2017年版规范新增了EOB-MRI作为一线诊断工具。Gd-EOB-DTPA是一种双功能对比剂，既可以静脉团注得到血供信息，还可以通过肝细胞膜上的有机阴离子转运多肽（orgamcamon transporting polypeptides，OATP）吸收进入肝细胞（摄取率约50%），进行肝胆特异期成像（延迟20 min）。大多数良性肝硬化结节可摄取Gd-EOB-DTPA，在肝胆特异期呈等或高信号；但约90%的肝细胞性肝癌不能摄取Gd-EOB-DTPA，在肝胆特异期呈低信号。

钆贝葡胺（gadobenate dimeglumine，Gd-BOPTA）也是一种肝胆特异性对比剂，诊断原理与Gd-EOB-DTPA类似，肝细胞摄取率约5%，也可用于多期动态增强扫描和肝胆特异期成像（延迟40~120 min，平均90 min）。Gd-EOB-DTPA与Gd-BOPTA对肝细胞性肝癌的诊断效能无明显差异，在临床实践中可结合医院实际、综合时间成本及患者个体化问题灵活选择应用。

肝胆特异性对比剂对检出乏血供肝细胞性肝癌和直径1 cm以下的微小肝细胞性肝癌极具优势，有助于肝细胞性肝癌与肝腺瘤及FNH的鉴别。肝腺瘤在肝胆特异期多为稍低信号（部分炎症型和β-catenin突变型可呈稍高信号），FNH则多为高信号（尤其是环形高信号更具特异性）。但价格较为昂贵，技术操作相对复杂，病灶显示受肝功能影响，因缺少传统意义上的延迟期而影响包膜显示，严格的肝细胞性肝癌诊断标准尚未完全统一，图像判读经验还有待进一步积累。

（二）欧美地区肝细胞性肝癌诊断指南

1.NCCN指南　高危人群包括肝硬化和HBV携带者，推荐间隔6~12个月监测US联合AFP。对于AFP持续升高但US未检出结节者，应进一步行增强CT或MRI检查。推荐诊断工具包括增强CT和动态MRI。对于直径≤1 cm结节，不做诊断要求，但需采用增强CT、MRI或CEUS进行严密监测随访（3~6个月间隔，持续2年）。对于直径>1 cm结节，需进行增强CT或MRI检查，2种检查结果均阳性可确诊为肝细胞性肝癌；1种检查结果阳性需要行另一种增强影像检查；如检查结果为阴性，直径>2 cm者行穿刺活检，直径为1~2 cm者可穿刺活检或间隔3个月行增强影像监测。

2.AASLD指南　仅将肝硬化列为高危人群，推荐US 6个月间隔筛查监测，联合或不联合AFP。推荐诊断工具包括增强CT和动态MRI。对于直径≤1 cm结节，采用US随访（间隔3个月）。对于直径>1 cm结节，经≥1种影像检查结果显示为“快进快出”强化者即可诊断为肝细胞性肝癌；如二者检查结果均为阴性，需行穿刺活检。

3.EASL指南　内容与AASLD指南类似，只是对于直径≤1 cm结节的随访间隔为4个月，均未将CEUS作为诊断工具，这是由于肝内胆管细胞癌在CEUS可表现出与肝细胞性肝癌类似的强化特征，导致假阳性。直径≥2 cm结节推荐行增强CT或MRI，≥1种检查结果最示为“快进快出”强化者即可诊断肝细胞性肝癌，如二者均阴性需进行穿刺活检。对于直径1~2 cm的结节，要求必须同时行CT和MRI检查（减少假阴性），≥1种检查结果为阳性即可诊断，如二者均为阴性，需进行穿刺活检。

（三）亚太地区肝细胞性肝癌诊断指南

1.APASL指南　2017版APASL指南中的高危人群包括肝硬化和HBV患者，推荐间隔6个月行US联合AFP检查监测。推荐诊断工具包括增强CT、动态MRI和EOB-MRI，CEUS仅列为二线诊断工具，且对比剂仅限定为Sonazoid。在增强CT和动态MRI上表现为“快进快出”强化者，不管结节大小，即可诊断为肝细胞性肝癌；不表现为“快进快出”强化者，直径≥1 cm结节，动脉期无强化或动脉期强化但无对比剂廓清者，推荐行穿刺活检；直径<1cm结节推荐间隔3~6个月行增强CT、动态MRI检查随访。

在EOB-MRI上，APASL指南强调需在门静脉期图像上判定病灶对比剂“廓清”，因为在移行期（3 min）肝实质已出现强化，可表现为病灶假性廓清，导致假阳性。

诊断分为以下4种情况：①动脉期强化伴对比剂廓清，可确诊为肝细胞性肝癌；②动脉期强化、无对比剂廓清，肝胆特异期低信号，可确诊为肝细胞性肝癌；③动脉期无强化，肝胆特异期出现等或高信号，推荐间隔6个月行US随访；④动脉期无强化，肝胆特异期低信号，推荐行CEUS检查；CEUS仍无法明确者，直径≥1 cm结节推荐行穿刺活检，直径<1 cm结节推荐行EOB-MRI或间隔3~6个月行增强CT随访。

2.JSH指南 于2007年首次推出，最新版于2014年修订，比其他指南更为严格。高危人群包括肝硬化、HBV和HCV患者，又将HBV和HCV后肝硬化定义为极高危人群。对高危人群，JSH指南中推荐间隔6个月行US联合多种血清学标志物监测，血清学标志物包括AFP、甲胎蛋白异质体AFP-L3、维生素K缺乏诱导凝血酶原Ⅱ等。对极高危人群，随访间隔缩短为3~4个月，同时建议每6~12个月行动态增强CT或MRI检查。对于有条件的肝癌专科医疗中心，推荐将EOB-MRI作为一线筛查及诊断工具，可以替代增强CT。另外还推荐了补充影像检查方法，包括超顺磁性氧化铁增强MRI、CEUS和CT血管成像。

2014版JSH指南中细化了EOB-MRI的诊断流程，具体内容包括：①动脉期强化，伴对比剂廓清，可确诊为肝细胞性肝癌；②动脉期强化，无对比剂廓清，肝胆特异期呈低信号，结合其他序列或影像方法除外高流量血管瘤，可确诊为肝细胞性肝癌；③动脉期强化，无对比剂廓清，肝胆特异期呈等或高信号，需行穿刺活检；④动脉期无强化，肝胆特异期低信号，推荐CEUS。CEUS显示动脉期强化和Kupffer期缺损可确诊为肝细胞性肝癌；不能确诊的直径≥1.0~1.5 cm结节行穿刺活检，<1.0~1.5 cm结节间隔3~6个月行EOB-MRI随访；⑤动脉期无强化，在肝胆期呈等或高信号者，再次进入常规随访流程。

3.KLCSG-NCC指南 于2003年提出，并于2014年更新。高危人群包括肝硬化、HBV和HCV患者。推荐的诊断工具包括增强CT、MRI和EOB-MRI，未包括CEUS。与AASLD指南不同，KLCSG-NCC允许在门静脉期和移行期评价EOB-MRI上病灶内对比剂廓清情况。对于直径≥1 cm结节，≥1种影像检查显示为“快进快出”可诊断为肝细胞性肝癌，否则需进行穿刺活检；对于直径<1 cm结节，必须同时满足≥2种影像检查显示肝细胞性肝癌特征，且伴有AFP持续升高（肝炎活动已控制）才能诊断肝细胞性肝癌，否则需进行穿刺活检。

（四）国际指南与国内规范的比较

前国际指南与国内规范均提倡采用以影像检查为主导的无创性诊断理念，基于显示血供特征的动态增强影像技术已经成为肝细胞性肝癌的主要诊断方法，但国际指南与国内规范中对肝细胞性肝癌的筛查监测和诊断流程仍存在较大差异（表3-1-1，3-1-2）。

表3-1-1 肝细胞性肝癌国际诊断指南与国内原发性肝癌诊疗规范的筛查监测方案比较

指南、规范名称	高危人群	血清学检查	影像方法	时间间隔
NCCN	肝硬化、HBV	AFP	US	6~12个月
ASSLD	肝硬化、部分特定的HBV	无	US	6个月
EASL	肝硬化、HCV伴进展期纤维化（F3期）	无	US	4个月
APASL	肝硬化、HBV	AFP	US	6个月
JSH	肝硬化、HBV、HCV，HBV和HCV后肝硬化为极高危	AFP、AFP-13、PIVKA-Ⅱ	US；增强CT或EOB-MRI（极高危人群）	6个月；极高危人群为3~4个月，同时每6~12个月行增强CT或EOB-MRI检查
KLCSG-NCC	肝硬化、HBV和HCV	AFP	US	6个月
原发性肝癌诊疗规范	肝硬化、各类慢性肝病患者	AFP	US	6个月

注：HCC：肝细胞性肝癌；NCCN：美国国立综合癌症网络；AASLD：美国肝病学会；EASL：欧洲肝脏学会欧洲肝脏研究联合会；APASL：亚太肝脏学会；JSH：日本肝病学会；KLCSG-NCC：韩国肝癌研究组.韩国国立癌症中心；HBV：乙型肝炎病毒；HCV：丙型肝炎病毒；AFP：甲胎蛋白；AFP-L3：甲胎蛋白异质体；PIVKA-Ⅱ：维生素K缺乏诱导凝血酶原Ⅱ；US：超声；EOB-MRI：钆塞酸二钠增强MRI；原发性肝癌诊疗规范为2017年版

表 3-1-2　肝细胞性肝癌国际诊断指南与国内原发性肝癌诊疗规范的诊断流程比较

指南、规范名称	AFP	影像检查方法	直径< 1 cm 结节	影像检查次数
NCCN	无	CEUS;增强 CT;动态 MRI	不做诊断;间隔 3~6 个月行增强 CT、MRI 或 CEUS 随访,持续 2 年	直径≥ 1 cm:1 次
AASLD	未强制要求	增强 CT;动态 MRI	不做诊断;间隔 3 个月 US 随访	直径≥ 1 cm:1 次
EASL	无	增强 CT;动态 MRI	不做诊断;间隔 4 个月 US 随访	直径≥ 2 cm:1 次;1 cm <直径< 2 cm:2 次
APASL	无	CEUS;增强 CT;动态 MRI;EOB-MRI	影像诊断	乏血供结节:2 次
JSH	无	CEUS;增强 CT;EOB-MRI;必要时可选用 SPIO-MRI、CEUS 或 CT 血管成像	影像诊断	EOB-MRI 无动脉期强化、肝胆特异期低信号结节:2 次
KLCSG-NCC	适用于直径< 1 cm 结节	增强 CT;动态 MRI;EOB-MRI	AFP+ 影像诊断	直径≥ 1 cm:1 次;直径< 1 cm:2 次
原发性肝癌诊疗规范	无	CEUS;增强 CT;动态 MRI;EOB-MRI	影像诊断	直径≥ 2 cm:1 次;直径< 2 cm:2 次

注: HCC:肝细胞性肝癌; NCCN:美国国立综合癌症网络; AASLD:美国肝病学会; EASL:欧洲肝脏学会欧洲肝脏研究联合会; APASL:亚太肝脏学会; JSH:日本肝病学会; KLCSG-NCC:韩国肝癌研究组一韩国国立癌症中心; AFP:甲胎蛋白; CEUS:超声增强造影; EOB-MRI:钆塞酸二钠增强 MRI; SPIO:超顺磁性氧化铁;原发性肝癌诊疗规范为 2017 年版

与欧美地区指南相比,亚太地区指南和国内规范中的肝细胞性肝癌监测方案更为严格,均联合了 US 和血清学指标,并将 EOB-MRI 作为一线诊断工具,积极提倡对直径 <1 cm 结节进行定性诊断。这是由于在东方人群中,约 80% 的肝细胞性肝癌经历了由再生结节到异型增生结节再癌变为肝细胞性肝癌的过程。肝硬化结节多步癌变过程中,除了血供改变,还存在细胞密度、铁含量等变化,这构成了 MRI 多模态成像的病理基础,是对动态增强影像技术的重要补充。肝细胞膜表面 OATP 表达的减低要先于门静脉血流减少和完全性动脉血流增加,使得 EOB-MRI 对不表现为典型"快进快出"强化的肝细胞性肝癌具有诊断优势。肝硬化背景下肝细胞性肝癌的诊断,保持尽可能高的敏感性与合理的高特异性,更有助于实现肝细胞性肝癌的根治性治疗(射频消融术、手术切除等),使患者获益。

需要强调的是,2017 版诊疗规范所推荐的是基本规范,鉴于国内各地区医疗水平不均衡,诊断流程未做进一步细致的规定,在临床实践中应结合医院实际灵活掌握应用。

另外,2017 版规范仍然基于专家共识层面,循证医学证据的强度还有待提高,尤其是缺少高质量的基于中国人群的临床研究数据支持,在后续推广使用中还需要更进一步的科学验证。

第二章　肝癌一般情况

第一节　原发性肝癌包膜形成

原发性肝癌是肝脏最常见的原发恶性肿瘤，我国是世界肝癌的高发区之一，早期发现和早期诊断已成为提高肝癌手术切除率及生存率的重要因素之一。近几年随着MR成像技术的飞速发展，使它日益成为肝癌的诊断与鉴别诊断中重要的诊断方法。

纤维包膜或"假包膜"是肝癌的特征性影像学表现之一。肝癌包膜也是经导管肝动脉化疗栓塞术治疗中晚期原发性肝癌的有利预后因素。原发性肝癌包膜不仅可以阻碍肿瘤的肝内或远隔转移，同时可以阻隔动脉化疗栓塞术时化疗药物、超液化碘油乳液等物质进入周围正常肝组织，在一定程度上可以减轻对正常肝组织的损害，对患者肝功能起到保护作用。因此无论是肝癌的鉴别诊断还是临床治疗、预后，包膜都有重要意义。其他影像学检查对肝癌包膜显示欠佳，而MRI多个序列对包膜都有良好的显示。一项研究通过回顾性分析233例肝癌的MRI图像，对应用高场强MRI各序列对肝癌包膜的显示情况进行评价。

肝癌MRI主要特异性表现：肝癌MRI主要特异性表现包括：脂肪变性、包膜征、门静脉癌栓、镶嵌征等。肝内的局灶性病变，除腺瘤外，其他的病变（局灶性结节增生、转移瘤、血管瘤等）很少有包膜形成。肝腺瘤相对少见，多见于青年女性并常有避孕药口服史。我国肝癌则多发生在慢性乙型肝炎及肝硬化的基础上。

包膜形成机制：包膜形成机制是：当肿瘤血管生成较多、营养供应丰富，瘤细胞生长活跃并呈膨胀性生长压迫周围的正常肝组织，从而使肿瘤边界清楚；另外部分生长较慢的癌细胞对邻近肝组织的压迫可导致纤维结缔组织增生；同时，由于肿瘤细胞及其间质细胞产生大量促进血管生成的细胞因子，使纤维结缔组织内血管生成活跃也促进形成肿瘤包膜。

肝癌包膜信号特点：包膜在T_1WI上都呈低信号；在T_2WI上大部分亦呈低信号，只有包膜较厚时（4.6 mm ± 1.0 mm）可呈双层环状改变（内层呈低信号，外层高信号），与包膜外层富含小血管和新生胆管有关。Gd-DTPA增强早期，包膜不强化，门静脉期及延迟期时因包膜内的微血管密度较高，细胞外间隙较大，病灶周边被挤压的肝实质内的血窦受压，对比剂扩散和滞留的时间长，而病灶内的对比剂已开始排出，故包膜呈欠规则的环形高信号带。一组病例包膜信号特点与报道一致。据病理证实肝癌的包膜主要是由纤维组织构成，纤维组织水分含量少，缺乏可运动质子，因而在T_1WI及T_2WI上均呈低信号。

T_1WI、T_2WI和LAVA增强对肝癌包膜显示的比较：该项研究显示，T_1WI对肝癌包膜的显示优于T_2WI，一些作者认为T_1WI发现包膜比T_2WI敏感的观点一致。这是由于T_1WI的解剖分辨率最好，善于显示病灶外形及毗邻关系，故T_1WI显示肿瘤包膜为低信号带；另外，包膜内含胶原蛋白并将肿瘤与正常组织分开，在T_1WI上观察更为清楚，但T_2WI因信噪比降低而难以显示包膜。LAVA增强在显示完整肝癌包膜方面优于T_1WI、T_2WI。文献报道包膜厚度为0.2~6 mm，当包膜厚度<0.4 mm时，不能被MRI显示。因此肝癌包膜厚度是其是否能在MRI显示的重要因素。

因常规T_1WI、T_2WI序列均存在扫描速度较慢、层厚及层间距较大等缺点，对原发性肝癌细节显示存在明显不足。而LAVA多期动态增强，扫描层厚更薄，能清楚地显示病灶的边缘与细节；尤其是LAVA增强门脉期和延时期，病灶内的对比剂已开始排出,而包膜呈环形高信号带,使得瘤灶与包膜形成了良好对比,有利于对肝癌包膜的显示。另外,包膜清楚、完整病灶经导管动脉内化疗栓塞治疗后可获得较好的疗效,因此包膜的完整与否还可作为判断肿瘤治疗预后的一个因素。如出现不完整环状强化征象时,可提示肝癌分化程度低,预后较差。因此LAVA增强在显示完整肝癌包膜方面、判断预后具有重要意义。

T_1WI及T_2WI对直径较小的肝癌包膜的显示较差,尤其是小肝癌,随着直径的增大,这2种序列对肝癌包膜的显示率逐渐提高,对巨块型肝癌的包膜显示最好。因肝癌包膜厚度随肿瘤大小的增加而增厚,病灶越大,包膜越厚;同时小肝癌包膜的出现、完整与否与癌结节大小也呈正相关,因此癌结节大小对包膜显示的贡献最大。该组小肝癌包膜厚度明显小于巨块型肝癌,因此随着肿瘤直径的增大、包膜的增厚,T_1WI及T_2WI的优势愈加明显。

该项研究显示MRI LAVA增强序列对结节型肝癌包膜显示率最高。一些研究报道直径2~5 cm肝癌包膜形成率最高,而<2 cm肝癌包膜形成少见,并认为纤维包膜是随着肝癌发生、发展而逐渐形成的。有作者报道小肝癌62.2%病灶可见包膜,小肝癌>1 cm的病灶多可见包膜,发生率随着肿瘤体积增大而增高,2 cm以上的肿瘤更为常见。该组小肝癌包膜显示为38. 9%,低于一些报道,该组认为可能与病例中小肝癌大小比例有关。该组肝癌包膜显示率为58.16%(139/239),高于一项研究报道的50%。可能的原因为:该项研究为回顾性研究,可能存在选择性偏倚;扫描层厚为4.4 mm的LAVA序列增强扫描有利于包膜显示。

有包膜与无包膜肝癌门静脉癌栓的形成比较:该项研究显示,无包膜肝癌较有包膜肝癌易形成门静脉癌栓,与一些研究一致。门静脉瘤栓的形成与肿瘤本身有无包膜关系密切,一般认为有包膜者是癌细胞分化程度较高的一种类型,而无包膜肿瘤因分化程度较差,癌灶侵入门静脉形成瘤栓的倾向性更大。研究表明肝癌包膜完整与否对其预后有很大影响,它可以阻碍肿瘤向肝内或远隔转移;同时包膜完整的病灶的手术切除率高、复发率低,生存期延长。

总之,高场强MRI平扫及LAVA增强序列可以较好显示肝癌包膜,LAVA增强(门脉期+延时期)显示肝癌包膜优于T_1WI、T_2WI。肝癌直径的增加,更加有利于T_1WI及T_2WI显示。高场强MRI平扫及LAVA增强序列对肝癌包膜的显示,不仅促进肝癌的诊断及鉴别诊断,也可为肝癌术前方案的确定及术后评估预后提供更多信息。

第二节 血管周上皮样细胞肿瘤(简称PEComa)

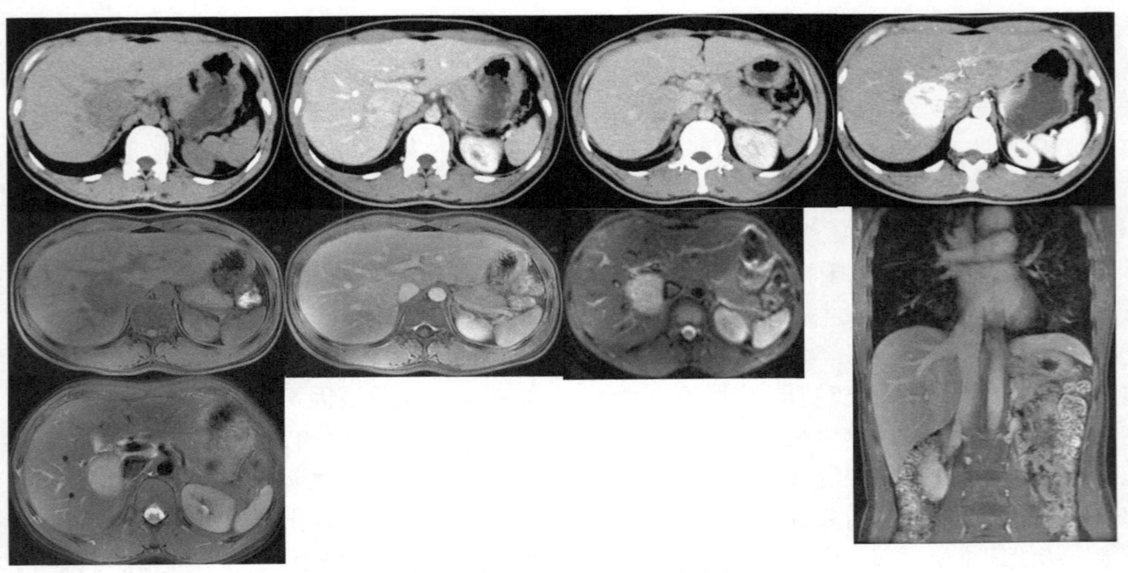

图3-2-1 血管周上皮样细胞肿瘤

患者,女,42 岁。查体发现肝占位性病变,实验室检验各项阴性(图 3-2-1)。

术后病理诊断:肝细胞癌;免疫组化诊断为血管周上皮样细胞肿瘤(简称 PEComa)。

第三节　含脂肪肝癌

一组 11 例含脂肪肝癌,影像学术前 5 例确诊,4 例误诊为肝血管平滑肌脂肪瘤,1 例误诊为恶性脂肪瘤,另 1 例无明确诊断,仅描述性诊断为含脂肪性肿瘤。

原发性肝细胞肝癌是一种常见的肝脏恶性肿瘤,临床上多有慢性肝病史,甲胎蛋白常明显升高,在影像学上常表现为有包膜的结节或团块状改变,有时呈弥漫性病变,增强扫描动脉期不均匀强化,实质期强化明显减退,延迟扫描多恢复为低密度或低信号状态,呈"快进快出"改变,门静脉内常可见癌栓形成。典型的肝细胞癌比较容易诊断。

含脂肪肝癌是原发性肝细胞癌的一种比较罕见的特殊类型,常易误诊。国外报道约占肝细胞癌的 0%~2%,但也有作者认为采用 MRI 化学位移梯度回波序列可提高含脂肪肝癌在肝癌中的百分率。Martin 等(1995)用 MR 化学位移梯度回波序列对 63 例肝癌患者的 69 个病灶进行成像,含脂肪肝癌的比例达 14%。

组织病理学发现肝细胞癌可有不同程度的脂肪变性,早期的肝细胞癌的脂肪变性多均匀分布于病变,不易被检测到,但可导致肝细胞癌病灶的密度降低,此时,CT 和常规 MRI 序列检查常检测不到脂肪成分,磁共振化学位移梯度回波序列可检测到肝细胞癌中包含的少量脂肪,在反相位像上呈信号明显减低,是目前检出肝内病灶脂肪成分较敏感的影像学方法。

而在晚期可在肝细胞癌中形成脂肪瘤样改变。此时,在 CT 上可表现为 CT 值在 -10~-40 HU 的低密度灶,在 MRI 上表现为 T_1WI 及 T_2WI 均呈高信号,脂肪抑制序列低信号的典型脂肪组织的表现。该组有 2 例做了 MRI 检查,仅在脂肪抑制序列上表现为信号减低,没有显示出 MRI 检查的优点,可能与病例数少和病变较大有关,也与检查技术的应用有关。加做同反相位图像对显示肿瘤的脂肪成分是必要的。含脂肪肝癌的实质部分的影像学表现与普通肝细胞癌相似。在 CT 图像上呈不均质低密度灶,在 MRI 图像上呈长 T_1 长 T_2 信号,信号不均匀,增强扫描多呈较典型的快进快出改变,少数病例强化可不典型多有包膜。

其与普通肝细胞癌最大的区别是在肿瘤组织中含有脂肪成分,当肝细胞癌较小时,可因脂肪变性而致病灶密度降低,强化程度减轻。Cem Balci 等(2009)认为是脂肪均匀分布所致。此时 CT 往往不容易检出,而磁共振化学位移梯度回波序列检查时在反相位像上则呈特征性的信号明显减低。当肝细胞癌较大所含脂肪成分可呈脂肪瘤样改变,在 CT 上表现为 CT 值在 -10~-40 HU 左右的均匀或不均匀低密度影,在 MRI 上表现为 T_1WI 高信号,T_2WI 低信号,脂肪抑制序列呈低信号的特征性改变。Eguchi 等(1992)认为肝结节内脂肪成分的检出是腺瘤样退变结节转变为肝细胞癌的重要指征。

鉴别诊断:含脂肪肝癌主要需与其他的肝脏含脂肪成分的肿块相鉴别,其中,最常误诊的是肝脏的血管平滑肌脂肪瘤。该组中术前误诊为肝血管平滑肌脂肪瘤共 4 例,占了近半数。血管平滑肌脂肪瘤好发于肾脏,在肝脏中少见,肝血管平滑肌脂肪瘤由成熟的脂肪细胞、血管和平滑肌组织构成。多见于女性,与肾脏的血管平滑肌脂肪瘤不同,肝脏的血管平滑肌脂肪瘤脂肪成分常很少,CT 多不易检出。Hogemann 等(2001)报告的 7 例中只有 4 例检出脂肪,但是,肿瘤内常可见较粗大的血管影,即所谓"中心血管影"。

一些作者曾搜集肝血管平滑肌脂肪瘤 9 例,其中 8 例 CT 检查的病例中只有 1 例内见大片脂肪密度,其余 7 例均未检测出典型的脂肪密度,其中 3 例呈均匀低密度,4 例呈不均匀低密度,1 例行 MRI 检查的肝血管平滑肌脂肪瘤在常规序列上均未显示明确脂肪信号,在反相位图像上信号有较明显的降低。与其他部位的血管平滑肌脂肪瘤有较大的不同。但 9 例中有 7 例出现较典型的中心血管影。

而在该组含脂肪肝癌病例中,均未见明显中心血管影,且脂肪成分的显示率也明显比肝血管平滑肌脂肪瘤高,可能有助于两者之间的影像学鉴别。肝脏血管平滑肌脂肪瘤多无慢性肝炎和肝硬化病史,甲胎蛋白多阴性,均有利于与含脂肪肝癌相鉴别。此外,含脂肪肝癌还需要与肝细胞腺瘤、肝脏脂肪瘤、畸胎瘤等相鉴别。

该组病例中误诊病例都发生在早期,与当时医生对本病的认识不足有关。在近几年发现的病例均没有发生误诊。可见,提高对本病的认识是正确诊断本病的关键。总之,含脂肪肝癌比较少见,常易误诊,慢性肝病史、甲胎蛋白阳性、包膜显示及增强扫描实质部分的"快进快出"强化是诊断要点,需与肝脏其他含脂肪肿瘤尤其是血管平滑肌脂肪瘤相鉴别。

第四节 增强扫描时不同密度的肝癌

高密度肝癌:血供丰富的肝癌在肝动脉期增强,显示为相对较正常肝组织浓密的高密度影,而在门静脉增强期,同一病变显示为相对较正常肝组织淡的低密度影像。对于直径为30~50mm的肝内低密度病灶,单层动态扫描有较大的诊断意义。典型肝癌在注药后前30秒CT图像常是高密度,而在随后的门脉期迅速变为低密度,5分钟以上的延时扫描也不变为等密度。肝癌时间-密度曲线峰值高,且早于正常肝组织峰值10~15秒出现,与肝血管瘤截然不同。这种表现是与大部分肝癌血供丰富的特点相一致的。

等密度肝癌:动态增强的门脉期CT值在正常肝组织可以提高45HU以上,而肝内病变一般增强程度较小。因此,增强扫描可以增加病变对正常肝组织的密度差异达20HU。此点对诊断肝内等密度肝癌极富诊断意义。有作者报告10例平扫为等密度病变者,由于平扫较难确定病变部位,无法用单层动态扫描,而只能用移动式动态增强扫描,扫描基本在门脉期内完成。其CT表现为:①病变区和周围正常肝组织的密度差异增大,达10~20HU;②病变边界较平扫时清楚,这是由于注药后可出现代表肝癌包膜的环形密度增高影像,此种增强环与肝血管瘤比较窄得多,既不规则也不完整;③沿增强环出现花边状肿瘤分隔;④肿瘤与周围正常肝组织之间出现比较明显的低密度晕环;⑤增强后,肿瘤内部不均匀现象较平扫时显著,从而有助于对病变的识别。

低密度肝癌:如果原发性肝癌是少血管型的,动态增强扫描血管期表现为低密度。

第五节 含脂肝细胞肝癌

原发性肝细胞性肝癌为富血供肿瘤,瘤内脂肪少见,比较容易诊断。而含脂肝细胞肝癌是原发性肝细胞性肝癌的一种比较少见的特殊类型,由癌细胞脂肪代谢紊乱导致,其与普通肝细胞性肝癌最大的区别是在肿瘤组织中含有脂肪成分,一组14例中,13例病灶的脂肪变性细胞以小斑块状散在分布于肿瘤中,并且分布于周边区域为主,脂肪变性区域大小不等;仅有1例病灶呈弥漫性脂肪变性表现,脂肪变性区域>90%。

影像学研究:早期的肝细胞性肝癌脂肪变性程度较轻或范围较小,脂肪变性细胞夹杂在没有脂肪变性的肿瘤细胞中,此时在病理切片中能检出脂肪成分,但CT和MRI序列常检测不到,这是由于此时的脂肪变性程度和范围尚不足以在CT上表现出密度降低或者明显影响MRI的弛豫时间;当肝细胞性肝癌脂肪变性进展到一定程度,在磁共振氢谱(^{1}H-MRS)或梯度回波序列等MRI序列中才能检测到脂肪成分,但是由于脂肪变性程度不一致,在MRI上表现为数个散在含脂小斑块,然而在病理切片上大多表现为连续性的脂肪变性区域(只是脂肪变性程度稍有差异);晚期可在肝细胞性肝癌中形成局部脂肪沉积样改变,从而在CT上可表现为小斑块状明显低密度灶,MRI上表现为T_1WI、T_2WI高信号、脂肪抑制序列低信号的典型表现,以致容易误诊。

但其仍有一些特征性影像学表现:①含脂肝细胞肝癌多位于肝脏边缘,该组14例中13例位于肝脏包膜下,1例邻近肝脏包膜,即病灶以位于肝脏外周区域为主,这与文献报道基本一致;②脂肪变性细胞主要以斑片状形式散在分布于病灶周围区域,中心区域相对少见，利用MRI正、反相位扫描，对脂肪的检出更具有敏感性；③该组含脂肝细胞肝癌具有普通肝细胞性肝癌的典型影像表现形式，即“快进快出型”强化，动脉期可见扭曲强化血管影及不规则的强化分隔，延迟期分隔强化减退程度不明显，病灶边缘包膜逐渐强化。

有学者利用MRI梯度回波序列在69个肝癌病灶中检出10个病灶含有脂肪成分，含脂肝细胞肝癌比例达14%。MRI梯度回波序列被认为是目前检出肝脏病灶中脂肪成分较为敏感的影像学方法。但该序列对轻度脂肪变性检测较难，加之MRI信号受组织 T_1、T_2 弛豫时间及其他因素（如脂肪变合并出血、含铁血黄素沉着、纤维化）等影响，准确性和敏感性还有待提高。而 ^{1}H-MRS对组织脂肪含量的定性和定量分析更具有优越性，但扫描时间相对较长。

鉴别诊断：由于含脂肝细胞肝癌内的脂肪成分，需与以下几种肝内含脂病变进行鉴别。

（1）肝脏血管平滑肌脂肪瘤：肝脏血管平滑肌脂肪瘤内脂肪含量5%~90%不等，其中乏脂型肝脏血管平滑肌脂肪瘤内脂肪含量<10%。脂肪成分以团块状表现为主，管状大血管以大静脉湖为主，所以动态增强强化血管影多在门静脉期达到强化峰值，病灶以延迟强化为主而脂肪组织无强化。

（2）肝腺瘤：肝腺瘤约占肝脏良性肿瘤的1.6%，具有恶性潜能，脂肪变性区域CT的显示率不到10%，有文献报道用MRI梯度双回波序列显示肝腺瘤肿瘤脂肪变性发生率高达90%。而病理组织学切片显示肝腺瘤均有不同程度局灶性或弥漫性脂肪变性（100%）。肿瘤好发于年轻女性，与正常肝组织分界清晰，周围常见低密度“透明环”，瘤内易伴发出血或坏死以及脂肪变性使MRI信号复杂多变、混杂；动态增强动脉期可见肿瘤供血动脉与明显强化的病灶相连，肿瘤实性部分显著较均匀强化。

（3）肝硬化结节脂肪沉积：在肝退变结节（DN）和小肝细胞性肝癌中均可出现脂肪沉积，一些作者对25个肝细胞性肝癌结节进行组织学病理检查，其中23个结节出现脂肪沉积（95%）。其与原发性含脂肝细胞肝癌主要区别是肝硬化背景下的小结节（直径<3cm），对肝硬化结节脂肪沉积的随访动态观察是区别原发含脂肝细胞性肝癌的有效手段之一。

（4）透明细胞性肝癌：透明细胞性肝癌发病率不足肝细胞性肝癌的10%，是肝细胞性肝癌的一种少见的临床病理类型。由于癌细胞胞质内因富含糖原而呈透明状，当癌细胞中透明细胞比例超过50%时，应诊断为透明细胞性肝癌。其影像学表现形式无明显特异性，依靠影像学检查难以与含脂肝细胞肝癌鉴别，其确诊和鉴别需依赖病理和免疫组织化学检查。

（5）假结节样脂肪浸润：假结节样脂肪浸润多见于局灶性脂肪肝或弥漫性脂肪肝背景下，表现为肝内低密度结节影，无占位效应，增强扫描均匀强化，病灶内有正常血管穿行，其强化形式与正常肝脏组织一致。

（6）其他罕见的肝脏含脂肿瘤：良性如肝脏肾上腺残余瘤、错构瘤；恶性如脂肪肉瘤等。

总之，含脂肝细胞肝癌在CT和MRI图像上有一定特异性表现，其仍然具有肝细胞肝癌典型的强化方式和临床表现，与肝脏其他含脂性病变可资鉴别，在影像学检查难以鉴别时，可采取术前穿刺病理等手段确诊。

第六节　代谢组学在肝脏疾病的应用

请详见本书 本卷 第一篇 第六章 第二节　代谢组学在肝脏疾病的应用。

第七节　原发性肝细胞性肝癌的少见征象

1. 外生型肝癌　外生型肝癌是肝癌中一种较少见类型，可分有蒂型和突出型两种。有蒂型极为罕见，而突出型则相对多见。

2. 肝癌侵犯血管和右心房　原发性肝癌易侵犯门静脉，形成动静脉短路和门静脉癌栓，而发生于肝静脉、下腔静脉和右心房的癌栓较为少见。

3. 肝癌侵犯胆管　肝癌侵犯胆管可引起黄疸，故又称为黄疸型肝癌。MRCP/ERCP：可表现为充盈缺损、肝总管单纯性闭塞性狭窄、肝总管截断和混合性表现。CT：可呈肝门部胆管内圆形低密度影，密度较肝脏实质低，但较扩张的胆管密度高，可有轻度强化或无明显强化，肝内胆管有较显著的扩张。

4. 肝癌内髓脂肪瘤　髓脂肪瘤的病因不清，可能与组织坏死脂肪变性有关。肝癌内髓脂肪瘤大体观为位于肝癌组织中央的边界清楚的结节，直径约1.0cm。平扫CT表现为低密度肿块，中央可见脂肪密度结节。增强扫描，肝癌强化，中央区域直至延迟期也无明显强化。

5. 囊性肝癌　囊性肝癌多见于转移性肝癌，而原发性肿瘤甚少见，可能是肿瘤的异常生长或为肿瘤缺血坏死所致。CT发现左右肝多个边缘清楚的囊腔，并有液平可见。

6. 肝细胞性肝癌自发性完全坏死或消退　肝癌自发性坏死并不少见，但完全坏死肿瘤消退，则甚为罕见。其原因一是缺血坏死；其次是免疫机制。2003年报道肝细胞性肝癌自发性坏死者英文文献为25例，但完全坏死者仅4例。肝细胞性肝癌经导管动脉栓塞治疗后肿瘤坏死合并气体生成：在CT上表现为肿瘤内大量碘油沉积，其间夹杂以极低密度气体，周边可见包膜存在。

7. 肝癌自发性破裂　肝细胞性肝癌破裂可分自发性破裂和经导管动脉栓塞治疗后癌破裂。肝细胞性肝癌发生自发性破裂的概率可高达10%，占肝细胞性肝癌死亡率的10%~15%。其原因可能是：肿瘤缺血坏死；肿瘤出血，瘤内压力升高而破裂出血。

8. 原发性肝癌种植转移　①腹腔内种植：腹腔内种植多为表浅部位肝细胞性肝癌的破裂所造成，少数为腹腔手术或介入治疗的种植。发生率在2%~16%之间。肝细胞性肝癌的种植转移远较有些肝内原发性肿瘤为低，如肝母细胞瘤(33.3%)、胆管细胞(46.3%)、胆管肝细胞混合癌(66.6%)。种植转移灶常位于胃肠道、内脏的浆膜面，或散在于腹膜腔网膜上。CT表现：为多发性结节，腹膜、网膜增厚和腹水；增强扫描可见结节状强化。种植性转移多见于外生性肝癌，肝内原发灶可能较小，而转移灶相对较大。②肝细胞性肝癌的腹壁种植转移。经皮酒精注射穿刺部位种植转移瘤出现的时间，大约3年。CT平扫可见腹壁内圆形或椭圆形肿块，边界清晰，密度均匀；增强后肿块不均匀强化。血管造影显示右下前胸壁之肿块血管丰富，由内乳动脉供血。

9. 混合细胞型肝癌　混合细胞型肝癌是由肝细胞癌和胆管细胞癌混合而成，其发生率在2.4%~5%之间。就其混合的形式，分为3种类型：Ⅰ型，肝细胞性肝癌和胆管细胞癌两个分开的肿块；Ⅱ型，两瘤靠近，但各自独立的肿块；Ⅲ型，一个肿块混有两种组织成分。CT：平扫病灶可呈低密度或等密度；增强扫描可表现为周围环形低密度，而瘤体呈等密度的圆形病灶。肝动脉造影：多数显示为少血性肿块，少数病例显示为肿块外围少血而中心浓染的"靶征。

10. 肝癌与血管瘤并发　肝癌和血管瘤二者都是肝脏常见的肿瘤，因此合并存在的概率也比较高，多为分别存在，少数紧密相连两个病灶，诊断比较困难。在CT上必须强调三期增强扫描，延迟期十分重要，因二者的强化特点明显不同，肝细胞性肝癌为速升速降，而血管瘤在门静脉期和延迟期仍有强化。

第八节　关于原发性肝癌的分期

原发性肝癌是指发生于肝细胞或肝内胆管细胞的癌，是我国常见的恶性肿瘤之一。

肝细胞性肝癌的大体分类可分四型。块状型：病灶直径≥ 5cm，>10cm称巨块型。结节型：3cm<病灶直径<5cm。弥漫型：多发小结节弥漫性均匀分布。小癌型：单个癌结节最大直径≤ 3cm，多个癌结节数目不超过两个，最大直径总和≤ 3cm。

原发性肝癌的组织学类型：原发性肝癌主要有3个组织学类型，即肝细胞性肝癌(HCC)，肝内胆管细胞癌、混合性癌。我国90%以上为肝细胞性肝癌。还有一种特殊类型的肝癌，即纤维板层性肝癌，这种肝癌以癌细胞巢内出现大量平行排列的板层状纤维组织为主要特点，国内少见。

早期肝癌诊断：以甲胎蛋白(AFP)升高为主要表现，在排除妊娠和生殖腺胚胎瘤的基础上，甲胎蛋白>500μg/L持续4周；或甲胎蛋白低浓度逐渐升高不降；或甲胎蛋白大于200μg/L以上持续8周，应高度怀疑肝细胞性肝癌。

中晚期肝细胞性肝癌临床表现：①肝区疼痛，多为持续性钝痛或胀痛；②肝脏肿大，肝脏进行性增大，质地硬；③黄疸，一般在晚期出现；④肝硬化门脉高压，脾脏增大，腹水等；⑤全身及消化道症状，低热、纳差、消瘦等。

典型肝细胞性肝癌的 CT 表现：CT 平扫病灶为低密度，增强动脉期明显强化，高于正常肝实质，门脉期呈轻度强化，密度低于正常肝实质，延迟期强化进一步减低，呈"快进快出"征象。

肝细胞性肝癌的鉴别诊断：

肝海绵状血管瘤：病灶平扫呈低密度，增强动脉期瘤灶周边结节状强化，动态扫描逐渐向中心强化，延迟扫描呈等或稍高密度填充，呈"快进慢出"征象。

肝细胞腺瘤：肝细胞腺瘤好发于女性，与长期服用避孕药有关。CT 平扫病灶呈低密度，增强动脉期多呈均匀明显强化，门脉期呈等或稍高密度，延迟期呈等或稍低密度。

肝脏局灶性结节增生：平扫稍低密度或等密度，增强动脉期病灶除中央瘢痕组织低密度外，全瘤均匀强化，门脉期等于或稍高于正常肝组织，病灶中心呈星状或车辐状低密度。

原发性肝癌 TNM 分期（UICC/AJCC，2010）：T-原发病灶：Tx：原发肿瘤不能确定；T0：无原发肿瘤的证据；T1：孤立肿瘤，没有血管受侵；T2：孤立肿瘤，有血管受侵或多发肿瘤直径≤ 5cm；T3a：多发肿瘤直径 >5cm；T3b：孤立肿瘤或多发肿瘤侵及门静脉或肝静脉主要分支；T4：肿瘤直接侵及周围组织，或至胆囊或脏器穿孔。

N- 区域淋巴结：Nx：区域内淋巴结不能测定；N0：无淋巴结转移；N1：区域淋巴结转移。

M- 远处转移：Mx：远侧转移不能测定；M0：无远处转移；M1：有远处转移。

肝癌分期：Ⅰ期：T1N0M0；Ⅱ期：T2N0M0；Ⅲ A 期：T3aN0M0；Ⅲ B 期：T3bN0M0；Ⅲ C 期：T4，N0M0；Ⅳ A 期：任何 T，N1M0；Ⅳ B 期：任何 T，任何 N，M1。

我国对肝癌的临床分期以往采用 1977 年全国肝癌防治协作会议的方案：Ⅰ期：无明显肝癌症状和体征；Ⅱ期：超过Ⅰ期的标准而无Ⅲ期的证据；Ⅲ期：有明确恶病质、黄疸、腹水或肝外转移之一。

表 3-1-3　肝功能 Child-Pugh 分级

指标	A 级	B 级	C 级
血清总胆红素（mg/L）	<2	2~3	>3
白蛋白（g/L）	>35	28~35	<28
腹水	无	轻度，可控制	顽固性腹水
肝性脑病	无	轻度	重度
凝血酶原时间延长（秒）	<4	4~6	>6
	（<1.7）*	（1.7~2.2）*	（>2.2）*

* 国际标准化比值（INR）

我国肝癌分期（2001 年全国肝癌会议制定）

Ⅰ a 期：单个肿瘤最长径小于 3cm，无癌栓，无腹腔淋巴结及远处转移；肝功能分级为 Child A。

Ⅰ b 期：单个或两个肿瘤最长径之和小于 5cm，位于半肝，无癌栓，无腹腔淋巴结转移及远处转移；肝功能分级为 Child A。

Ⅱ a 期：单个或两个肿瘤最长径之和不超过 10cm，位于半肝，或两个肿瘤最长径之和不超过 5cm，在左右两半肝，无癌栓，无腹腔淋巴结及远处转移；肝功能分级为 Child A。

Ⅱ b 期：单个或两个肿瘤最长径之和大于 10cm，在半肝，或两个肿瘤最长径之和大于 5cm，在左右两半肝，或多个肿瘤，无癌栓、无腹腔淋巴结及远处转移；肝功能分级为 Child A。肿瘤情况不论，有门静脉分支、肝静脉或胆管癌栓和 / 或肝功能分级为 Child B。

Ⅲ a 期：肿瘤情况不论，有门静脉主干或下腔静脉癌栓、腹腔淋巴结或远处转移之一；肝功能分级为 Child A 或 Child B。

Ⅲ b 期：肿瘤情况不论，癌栓、转移情况不论；肝功能分级为 Child C。

第九节　假肝癌

肝再生中的动静脉瘘类似肝癌：肝癌常表现为多血管性病变，而无血管性肝癌的继发征象(诸如动静脉瘘、染色区域与不规则的血管等)有助于诊断。Farrell 等(1972)报道一例经剖腹探查肝楔形切除证实的活动性肝硬化的再生结节，被误诊为无血管性肝癌。此病例在硬化的肝脏中有一显著的动静脉瘘，核素扫描时在肝右叶外侧缘上可见明显充盈缺损，而导致诊断为无血管的肝癌。

血管瘤伪似肝癌：在肝超声检查时，常可见到小的回声增强的局灶区，当单发的小灶回声增强区出现于无症状的病人时，几乎总是血管瘤。但当它们邻近横膈时，扫描可在膈上发现它的镜面像，而伪似肝癌。这类病变可用超声或其他影像检查技术(如 CT)追踪观察和确定性质。

肝硬化病人的假肝癌血管造影表现：肝硬化的血管造影表现常与其病变的阶段有关，在进展期，血管造影的征象有时类似于肝癌，或是原发性或是继发性肝癌。Passariello 等(1978)指出这些异常血管造影表现包括：动脉 - 门静脉瘘；肝门的狭窄或实质内血管分支的狭窄；富血管区的增加或减少；实质内动脉分支走行的变化。这些异常表现出现于 154 例肝硬化中的 12 例病人，其中 8 例类似原发性肝癌，4 例为弥漫性而颇似肝转移癌。

超声技术不当与假肝癌：不适当的超声检查技巧可使肝的某部出现回声增强区而类似于肝癌，但此类人工伪影的本质可借助于下述因素加以确定：极难见到肝癌不引起肝的动、静脉和门脉走行变化，而此类病例血管走行分布均属正常；此回声增强区常常延伸超越肝的周界，更说明系伪影；此类回声增强区可能与换能器固有的局灶带(focal zone)有关。

第十节　关于浸润型肝癌

尽管约有 13%~26% 的病例报道有肝内胆管扩张，但这并不是浸润型肝癌的特征性表现。10%~22% 的病例，肝外转移累及上腹部淋巴结。13%~23% 的病例远处转移出现在肺、骨骼及肾上腺。类似浸润型肝癌的疾病：多种肝脏疾病，包括局灶融合性纤维化、脂肪沉积、微脓肿、胆管癌和弥漫转移性疾病，都可以有类似于浸润性肝癌的影像表现(见表 3-1-4)。

局灶融合性纤维化：凭 CT 及 MR 影像表现较难鉴别局灶融合性纤维化与肝脏恶性病变，原因在于无论瘢痕或是肿瘤取代正常肝细胞，都可以改变的肝脏的结构及强化方式。融合性纤维化通常累及肝的前段及内侧段，从肝门向外周成辐射，呈典型的楔形表现。不像浸润型肝癌，融合性纤维化会导致包膜叠加回缩和血管丛集。与正常肝实质相比，融合性纤维化 CT 平扫表现为典型的低密度区域；纤维化区域在 MR T_1WI 图像上呈低信号，T_2WI 图像中呈轻度高信号。恶性病变的磁共振 T1WI 图像与 T_2WI 图像有相似的表现，因此，增强特性的分析显得尤其关键。与肝细胞性肝癌不同，肝局灶融合纤维化在增强扫描早期表现为乏血供、继而延迟强化。有作者报道 8 例局灶融合纤维化患者中，7 例出现延迟强化，而 19 例浸润型肝癌均未见此征像。用肝胆特异性对比剂行肝脏 MRI 时，由于肿瘤和纤维化都对其摄取缺乏，所以仅凭肝胆期表现不足以鉴别。

该组作者的同一研究显示 18/19 例浸润型肝癌和 5/7 例局灶融合纤维化病灶由于对肝特异对比剂缺乏摄取而在肝胆期成像上表现为呈低信号。并且发现浸润型肝癌的表观扩散系数较融合性纤维化(±标准差)更低(分别为 $0.97cm^2/s \pm 0.19$ 和 $1.35cm^2/s \pm 0.39$；p=0.001)，门静脉栓子和肝内卫星灶的出现率更高。一例患者，男，60 岁。浸润型肝癌及门静脉、肝静脉瘤栓形成，血色素沉着病史，甲胎蛋白明显升高(14.546ng/mL)，在轴位动脉期 CT 示肝右叶轻度不均匀强化及门脉右支富血供恶性瘤栓；轴位门脉期 CT 示肝右叶病变与累及门静脉右支的瘤栓均显示对比剂不均匀廓清；肝固有动脉造影(局部介入化疗栓塞术)显示门静脉瘤栓及肝静脉瘤栓的肿瘤新生血管。

表 3-1-4　浸润型肝细胞癌与类似疾病的鉴别

类似病变	影像学特点	不同于浸润型肝细胞癌的表现
肝局灶融合纤维化	CT 为地图样分布的相对低密度区；T_1WI 相对低信号，T_2WI 轻度高信号	常累及前部及内侧肝段，楔形、尖端指向肝门；包膜回缩，延迟强化
肝脂肪沉积	地图样或结节样分布的异常密度 / 信号区；MRI 肝胆期累及区域呈低信号	常见部位（胆囊窝旁或镰状韧带旁）容易鉴别；双回波同反相位梯度回波 T_1WI 可见信号减低
肝脏微脓肿	CT 示多发低密度灶；T_2WI 高信号伴轻度扩散受限及周边 / 分隔强化	临床病史
肝内胆管细胞癌	边界不清的肿块，T_1WI 低信号，T_2WI 高信号	不规则周边强化，渐进性中心强化；包膜回缩；瘤栓表现不典型
肝弥漫转移瘤（假性纤维化）	弥漫转移病变和肝脏形态的改变类似肝硬化	恶性原发肿瘤临床病史（如乳腺癌）

肝脏脂肪沉积：肝脏脂肪沉积表现多样，局灶性脂肪及局灶性脂肪缺失的常见部位，如胆囊窝或镰状韧带旁，勿需额外评估。但地图样及多灶性脂肪变性表现与浸润型肝癌相似，受累区域在注射肝细胞特异性钆螯合物（钆贝葡胺和钆塞酸等）行增强 MR（脂肪抑制）扫描时，肝胆期为低信号。双回波 T_1WI 同反相位成像表现均一低信号，常提示脂肪沉积。

一例患者，女，63 岁。局灶融合纤维化，溃疡性结肠炎继发胆汁性肝硬化病史，血清甲胎蛋白及 CA19-9 正常，CT 发现肝Ⅴ段肿块而进一步检查。轴位增强 T_1WI 的动脉期和门脉期均显示肝Ⅴ段大片异常信号，动脉期周边强化、内部延迟强化。轴位 T_2WI 为轻度高信号。轴位 T_1WI 肝胆期（钆塞酸注射后 20 分钟成像）为低信号。注意邻近的肝包膜回缩。超声介导穿刺活检提示肝硬化、未见恶性征象。另例患者，女，65 岁。地图样脂肪变性，原发性胆汁性肝硬化病史；轴位门脉期 CT 显示肝Ⅳ段地图样低密度；轴位同相位和反相位见相应区域信号减低，诊断地图样脂肪沉积。

肝内多发微脓肿：肝内多发微脓肿是在 CT 成像上表现为多发低密度病变的又一原因，坏死及脓性碎屑在 MR T_2WI 呈高信号。脓细胞碎屑可致轻度扩散受限，与浸润型肝癌表现类似。此外，脓肿还可成簇出现、互相融合，导致强化不均匀，与肝细胞性肝癌不同，脓肿在增强 CT 和 MRI 典型征象为周边和分隔强化。其周边可见水肿所致 T_2WI 高信号。

临床病史常有助于肝恶性肿瘤与感染性病变的鉴别，肝脓肿可发生于免疫抑制基础上或免疫功能正常的败血症患者及肠道术后患者，且肝脏感染性病变只有形态学改变，不似肝细胞性肝癌常伴有肝硬化。一例患者，男，49 岁。肝内微脓肿，乙型肝炎后肝硬化和结直肠癌病史。轴位动脉期增强 T_1WI 和轴位 T_2WI 平扫显示肝硬化的形态学改变和肝内无数边缘模糊的小结节，前者表现明显强化，后者为高信号。延迟期未见对比剂廓清。同时可见脾大和腹水，符合门静脉高压改变，门静脉通畅，血清甲胎蛋白正常。病灶部位细针穿刺抽吸活检示嗜中性粒细胞浸润，与微脓肿诊断相符。未分离出微生物。

肝内胆管细胞癌：胆管细胞癌，包括一系列亚型，根据肿瘤的形态和从胆管系统浸润至邻近肝实质的程度，肿瘤的生长方式分为：外生型或肿块型、导管周围型或浸润型、导管内型或息肉样型，或者是混合型。典型的肿块型肝内胆管细胞癌表现为边界不清的肿块，并伴纤维性假包膜和继发性肝包膜回缩。在 CT 和 MR 平扫（T_1WI 呈低信号，T2WI 呈高信号）上表现与肝细胞性肝癌相似。增强扫描与浸润型肝细胞性肝癌不同，胆管细胞癌表现为不规则周边强化并渐进性中心强化。

肝内胆管细胞癌在 T_2WI 表现为高信号的部分可能是黏蛋白或坏死成分，这不是浸润型肝细胞性肝癌的非典型征象。浸润性胆管癌可一个肝叶或节段性沿管周生长，这种生长方式导致肝内胆管壁不规则增厚，长段胆管狭窄，周围胆管扩张，而肝细胞性肝癌可导致肿瘤内胆管扩张。虽然典型的胆管细胞癌边界清楚，但其浸润的属性使得其与浸润型肝细胞性肝癌鉴别困难。胆管细胞癌可使血管受压、移位，但是一般不会伴有瘤栓形成。

肝细胞性及胆管细胞性混合型肝癌少见。混合型肝癌常为肿块型，包含不同比例的肝细胞及胆管上皮成分，导致不均质的影像学特性。增强的方式和伴随表现与胆管细胞癌相似。然而，卫星灶和血管侵犯常与浸润型肝细胞性肝癌相混淆。虽然结合影像表现和肿瘤标志物（CA19-9，甲胎蛋白）的升高可以提示混合型肝癌，但是确诊也取决于组织学检查。

一例患者，男，43 岁。肝内胆管细胞癌，原发性硬化性胆管炎病史，黄疸、瘙痒，实验室检查结果异常。血清癌胚抗原和癌抗原 19-9 均显著增高，血清甲胎蛋白正常。轴位增强 MR T_1WI 动脉期和静脉期）肝Ⅴ、Ⅷ段见巨大肿块，动脉期边缘不规则强化，延迟渐进性中心强化。DWI 示相应区域高信号。行超声引导下活检，结果符合低到中等分化肝内胆管细胞癌。胆管扩张或包膜回缩未看到。

弥漫性转移瘤（假性肝硬化）：典型的浸润型肝细胞性肝癌常发生在肝硬化基础上，任何发生过程中扭曲肝脏结构的疾病均应具有影像上的相似性。乳腺癌肝转移瘤治疗后相关的假性肝硬化就是一例，治疗后肝脏改变包括肝萎缩、纤维化、增生，并导致肝形态改变和门脉高压征象，这些表现与肝硬化相似。原发肿瘤临床病史（如乳腺癌）对正确诊断十分重要。

一例患者，女，65 岁。乳腺癌转移瘤（假性肝硬化）浸润性乳腺导管癌转移病史。横断位静脉期增强 CT 示肝硬化形态特点伴肝内弥漫性结节。DWI 显示肝内弥漫性高信号结节。门静脉通畅。

浸润型肝细胞性肝癌患者的治疗和预后：浸润型肝细胞性肝癌患者预后差，生存率低，这与发现时肿瘤呈进展期表现并常侵犯血管有关。手术切除后生存率反而降低，因此浸润型肝癌是手术切除及肝移植的禁忌证。经动脉介入治疗，如经动脉栓塞术对浸润型肝细胞性肝癌患者生存率的作用还不明确。Lopez 等研究表明经动脉栓塞术对于弥漫型肝细胞性肝癌无益，术后发病率和死亡率增高，远期生存率反而降低。Kneuertz 等大宗病例研究发现：与仅使用支持治疗时中期生存率为 3 个月相比，经动脉治疗可提高浸润型肝细胞性肝癌患者的耐受性和收益，中期生存率可延长至 12 个月。在他们的病例中，大部分经动脉治疗的患者 Child-Pugh 评分为 A 和 B，胆红素 <2mg/dl、甲胎蛋白 <400ng/ml 的患者中经动脉栓塞术效果更好。

同样，在近期研究中，Jang 等认为选择合适的浸润型肝细胞性肝癌患者并注意保护肝功能，经动脉栓塞治疗是安全的，并且可以提高生存期（>2 年）。总之，全身化疗对浸润型肝细胞性肝癌无效。近日研究表明索菲拉尼（多酪氨酸激酶分子抑制剂）对晚期肝细胞性肝癌包括浸润型肝细胞性肝癌有一定作用。随着肝细胞性肝癌发病率越来越高，掌握不同类型肿瘤的知识对疾病正确的诊断和治疗十分重要。浸润型肝细胞性肝癌与肝硬化不易鉴别，确诊时常常已经是晚期，预后较差。影像科医生掌握其独特的影像特点以及将浸润型肝细胞性肝癌从其他一系列类似表现的疾病中区分出来，可以使患者得到及时治疗。

第十一节　误诊病例简介：原发性肝细胞性肝癌与转移性肝癌

病例，女，60 岁。体检发现肝占位性病变 4 天入院。2 年前曾因乙状结肠溃疡型中分化腺癌在本院手术切除，术后病理发现肿瘤浸润至肠系膜外纤维脂肪层。4 天前体检彩色超声发现肝内实性包块，2.6cm × 1.3cm。CT：肝左外叶类圆形低密度灶，大小约 2.2 cm × 1.8 cm，边界尚清，CT 值 39HU，肝内外胆管无扩张，肝门结构清楚。CT 诊断：肝左外叶占位，性质待定，转移瘤？建议增强扫描。MRI：肝左外叶可见结节状异常信号影，T_1WI 稍低信号，T_2WI 压脂稍高信号，DWI 呈明显高信号，大小约 2.2 cm × 1.9 cm，边界清；增强扫描明显强化呈高信号，静脉期及延迟期强化程度有所减低，肝门结构清楚，门脉不增宽。MRI 诊断：肝左外叶占位，结合病史考虑转移瘤，请结合临床。

手术所见：腹腔无腹水，肝脏表面无硬化结节，腹腔内可见广泛粘连，肿瘤位于左外叶，大小约 3.0 cm × 2.0 cm，质中，边界清楚，包膜完整，局部突出肝脏表面。余肝未扪及明显肿物。肠管、脾脏、胰腺、盆腔未见肿瘤转移。

病理检查：肝左外叶肿瘤切除标本：部分肝组织一块，大小 9 cm × 6 cm × 2 cm，切面见一灰白结节，直径 2 cm，其余切面淡黄，质中。常规病理诊断：肝左外叶肿瘤切除标本：初步诊断肝细胞癌，待做免疫组化检测进一步明确诊断。

免疫组化检测：阳性有 CK8、CK18、Villin、AFP、Hepatocyte、CD34（肝窦 +）、Ki-67（+，约 20%）；阴性有 CK7、CK20、CK19、CEA、CD10、CDX2、CA19-9、Mucin-2、CgA、Syn、HMB45、S-100。免疫组化诊断：肝左外叶肿瘤切除标本：肝细胞性肝癌。

误诊病例分析：该病例的肿瘤病史误导为原因之一；其次，没有仔细分析所见影像，尤其是 MRI，

CT 只做了平扫，MRI 不仅平扫，还做了增强，却未能认真仔细地分析强化的表现，导致误诊；三是年老病人多病，可以多个肿瘤同存；另外，在有肿瘤病史的病人，切不可一见他处（特别是肝与肺）有肿块时，立即想到是转移性肿瘤，还应多增添一个考虑，想到存在该器官原发性肿瘤的可能性，这也是此类误诊病例给我们的教训。

第三章 小肝癌

第一节 肝纤维化、肝癌前期病变及早癌的影像学研究

肝细胞癌是我国居第三位的恶性肿瘤，每年患者数高达 11 万之多，其预后甚差。而小肝细胞癌的手术切除率高，5 年生存率达 60% 以上。因此，小肝细胞癌的早期发现和诊断给影像诊断学提出了挑战。肝癌的发生往往与慢性肝病有关。手术切除标本上除主要的肝癌外，有时可见无明确癌特征的小结节性病变。用于这些小结节性病变的适当术语一直有争论，称它们为：腺瘤性增生，腺瘤样增生，巨大再生性结节，结节性增生，腺瘤增生性结节，非典型性腺瘤性增生，以及腺瘤性增生伴恶性灶。

这些病变中有些表现有严重的异型性，目前认为是癌前病变和癌早期。这些病变组织学上表现不同，可以是明显良性的大的再生性结节，或可疑恶性结节，或含明显恶性灶的结节。区分良、恶性结节在临床上是重要的，因为对小恶性结节的最有效的治疗措施是手术切除，而手术对良性结节则是不必要的。

一般认为，小肝癌是指直径小于 30mm 的进展型肝癌，外周有纤维包膜，其内见镶嵌征，镜下见为中度或低度分化，相当于 Edmondson 2 或 3 级。有作者指出，小肝细胞癌指直径小于 30mm，内有镶嵌征象，外有纤维包膜的中等或低分化古典肝细胞癌，相当于 Edmondson 2 级或以上。

肝癌在非洲、东南亚以及中国尤其沿海地区是发生率和致死率较高的恶性肿瘤。人群中高的乙型肝炎感染率、水、食品及环境污染是很重要的因素。肝癌的诊断手段主要有血清学检测，超声、CT、MRI 检查以及活检。经多年努力，小肝癌和微小肝癌的影像学检测和诊断已取得了重大突破，分别达到 86% 和 95% 以上的检出率。

但以往的研究均以肿瘤的形态学改变为主。今后研究的主要方向为肝脏的弥漫性病变以及肝癌的前期病变，前者包括多种原因引起的肝纤维化和肝硬化，后者包括在肝硬化基础上形成的良性结节，如增生结节（RN）、退变结节（DN）以及上述结节逐步向癌演变的过程。

上述病变的及时诊断有极其重要的临床意义，如能在肝纤维化阶段发现病变，加以临床治疗和干预，也许可以终止病情的发展，减少肝癌的发生；如能在肝癌演变的早期及时发现病变，其治疗效果和预后将大为改观，一些癌前期病变可以密切随访，一旦有癌变可能，再加以治疗，其预后也完全不一样。

到目前为止，临床上尚无有效的手段诊断肝纤维化和癌前期病变，必须依赖肝穿刺活检。肝穿刺活检为有创性的，不能作为常规方法。因此探讨肝纤维化和癌前期病变的影像学诊断无疑极富挑战性，也是热门课题。下面综合讨论一下这方面的研究。

肝纤维化和肝硬化：在病理学，肝纤维化按程度分成 Ⅰ～Ⅳ 级，伴肝细胞功能不同程度的损害，此外，肝脏的枯否细胞在数量和功能上也有不同程度的减少和损害，随着肝纤维化程度的加重直至肝硬化，肝内门静脉阻力不断升高，门脉血流量也逐步减少。

超声、CT 和 MRI 对典型肝硬化病例也许不难诊断，但对肝纤维化，尤其早期肝纤维化，常规影像学方法难以判断，因其形态学改变尚不明显。而功能影像学可以反映伴随肝纤维化而发生的肝功能改变，以往和目前的研究包括以下几个方面：

肝细胞性 MR 特异性对比剂如 Mn-DPDP 进行的大鼠四氯化碳诱发的肝纤维化模型研究结果表明，其增强曲线在 Ⅰ～Ⅳ级肝纤维化中是不同的；在

同样的肝纤维化模型中，采用 SPIO 对比剂行动态增强研究，结果表明，其增强曲线在不同级别的肝纤维化中是不同的，两组研究均表明，随肝纤维化程度的加重，肝细胞功能和枯否细胞功能（量和质）均呈下降趋势，低级别和高级别肝纤维化之间存在显著差异，但两两之间差异不明显；MR 扩散成像（DWI）在肝脏方面的应用报道较多的是肝实质性肿瘤与囊性肿瘤、血管瘤的鉴别。该技术反映微观的水分子运动情况，肝纤维化时，间质的水分子运动受到一定限制，近来动脉模型研究表明，肝硬化与非肝硬化的 ADC（表观扩散系数）有显著差异；肝纤维化患者，随门脉阻力升高，门脉血流量减少，肝脏灌注成像表明，肝硬化患者其肝的门脉灌注量以及全肝总灌注量下降。

上述研究说明，肝脏的 MR、CT 功能成像确实可以反映肝纤维化导致的肝功能改变，正常肝脏或早中期肝纤维化与晚期肝纤维化（肝硬化）之间，多数参数存在显著差异，但正常组与早期肝纤维化之间不存在显著差异，所以影像学确定早期肝纤维化以及相互分级是有困难的，但可确定中晚期肝纤维化诊断，通过随访了解病变演变也是有价值的。

肝癌和癌前期病变：超声、CT 和 MRI 动态增强对小肝癌和微小肝癌结节的诊断是行之有效的，并被列为检查常规，这些技术的综合应用可使小肝细胞癌和中等大小的肝细胞癌的检出率达到 85% 和 92% 左右，但在许多增生结节中，识别小病灶，尤其是癌前期结节鉴别仍然是困难的。MRI 对某些癌前期病变的诊断也是有益的，但有很大限度。如欲取得突破，宏观与微观，即形态、功能与代谢方面的研究都应值得重视，或双管齐下。

从癌前期结节到癌结节的演变过程中，从病理到分子代谢水平均发生一系列变化，病理改变包括：①肝窦毛细血管化；②肿瘤新生血管形成；③门脉血流减少，肝动脉血流量增加；④细胞间变到癌细胞形成（见表）；⑤代谢方面包括葡萄糖、脂肪糖原和胆碱等一系列代谢改变。

表 3-3-1　5 种结节的结构：从细胞间变到癌细胞形成

	增生结节	低度退变结节	高度退变结节	早期肝细胞癌	小肝细胞癌
病理形态	肝细胞增生结节	含少量间变细胞	含多量间变细胞	含肝细胞癌	
观察重点	完全由肝细胞组成				
门脉血管	完全	↓	↓↓	↓↓↓	进一步减少
动脉血管	无	少量	增多	增多	进一步增多

影像学检查：①动态增强从宏观上反映结节的血流（供）变化，有助于病变的检测和定性；②CTHA 和 CTAP 的结合可以更客观，更准确地反映结节的动脉、门脉血供情况，从而有助于结节性质的判断，但属有创性；③结节的 PWI 扫描，可以从微观水平反映结节的微循环，了解结节的动脉、门脉血供状况，如能克服技术上的问题，对结节性质的判断很有发展前景；④结节的 DWI 扫描，探讨其 ADC 值，也许有一定帮助。一组研究表明 DWI 对小癌结节的显示较 T_2 敏感；⑤采用 MRS 测定结节的代谢产物，如胆碱和脂肪酸。肝脏的 MRS 目前存在技术困难；⑥^{18}F-FDG PET 和 ^{11}C acetate PET 检测结节的葡萄糖和碳水化合物代谢，研究认为，低分化的肝细胞癌常表现为 ^{18}F-FDG 的高摄取，而高分化的肝细胞癌表现为等或低摄取，对 ^{11}C acetate，高分化的肝细胞癌则为高摄取，两者结合可提高结节的鉴别能力以及对肝细胞癌分化程度的了解。

上述几个方面为我们对肝结节的研究提供了重要手段，但都处于实验阶段，也很不成熟，随着技术的改进，研究的深入，也许会取得一定的预期结果。

第二节　早期肝细胞癌与小肝癌

为确定 CT 在诊断早期肝细胞癌的敏感性及其 CT 表现，Takayasu 等（1995）回顾性研究了 31 例共 39 个病理证实的早期肝细胞癌（平均直径 17mm），除 2 个病灶外，其余均是术前确诊。诊断方法有超声检查、CT、DSA 和 MRI。另有病理证实的 18 个小肝癌（平均直径 23mm）为对照组。

病理学:早期肝细胞癌的病理学特点为分化良好,无纤维包膜;而小肝癌则为中度分化及分化不良并有纤维包膜。其中 9 例组织病理示以往有慢性肝炎, 22 例有肝硬化。

影像学研究:39 个癌灶由 CT 检出 32 个,在 CT 增强早期检出 12 个,其中 10 个为低密度, 2 个为高密度;增强晚期检出 20 个,均为低密度;另平扫检出 9 个,均为低密度。肿块越大,CT 敏感性越高。

平扫、增强早期、增强晚期表现:早期肝癌最常见类型在平扫、增强早期、增强晚期均为等密度,这一类型在 37 个早期肝细胞癌灶中有 17 个;其次常见类型为 CT 平扫、增强早期为等密度,增强晚期为低密度,有 8 个病灶;再其次为 CT 平扫、增强早期、增强晚期均为低密度,有 7 个病灶;另有 5 个病灶为混杂型, CT 平扫、增强早期、增强晚期分别表现为等 - 高 - 等(2 个),等 - 低 - 低(1 个),低 - 等 - 低(1 个),低 - 等 - 等(1 个),未做 - 低 - 低(2 个)。

早期肝细胞癌中既无 CT 平扫的低密度环,也无增强晚期的高密度环,而这些表现在有包膜的小肝癌中较常见。病理也证实早期肝细胞癌中无纤维包膜组织, CT 平扫低密度表示轻度或中度脂肪变,而等密度表示无或极少脂肪变。该作者指出,虽然 CT 诊断早期肝细胞癌的敏感度为 56%,然而,当增强早期与晚期病变表现为等 - 低密度或低 - 低密度型时,应考虑早期肝细胞癌的诊断,尤其是在有慢性肝病的病人。

CT 动脉造影、动脉性门静脉造影 CT 及动态 CT 扫描:应用 CT 动脉造影、动脉性门静脉造影 CT 、及动态 CT 扫描技术, Takayasu(1995)报道早期肝癌的 CT 表现。CT 动脉造影检查的 20 例早期肝癌,11 例呈低密度,6 例为高密度,3 例为等密度;动脉性门静脉造影 CT 检查 35 例早期肝癌,23 例为低密度,12 例为等密度。

肿瘤密度与大小之间的关系为:较大早期肝癌在动脉性门静脉造影 CT 检查时呈低密度的频率增高,而在 CT 动脉造影呈高密度的频率减低;较小的早期肝癌动脉性门静脉造影 CT 呈等密度的频率增高。结合 CT 动脉造影和动脉性门静脉造影 CT 的表现,有利于区别小肝细胞癌和早期肝癌,二者最显著的差异是增强模式的不同。

在动态 CT 扫描时,早期肝癌在平扫、早期和后期增强时,37 个病灶,8 个呈等 - 等 - 低密度模式,7 个呈低 - 低 - 低密度模式,呈此两种模式者可考虑早期肝癌。

第三节　早期肝细胞性肝癌病例

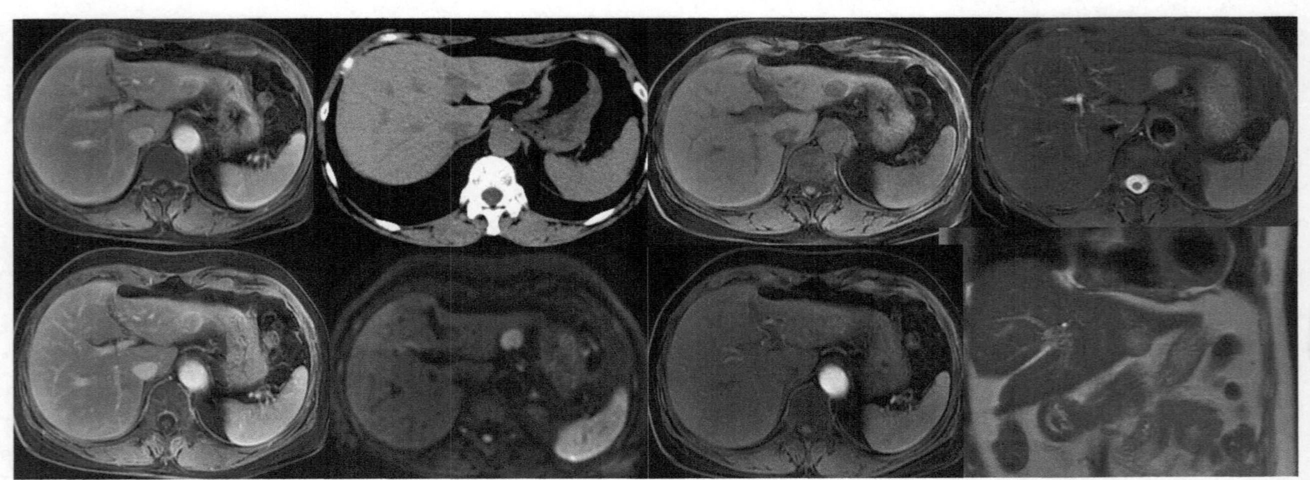

图 2-3-1　早期肝细胞性肝癌

患者,女, 60 岁。缘于上周体检彩超发现肝内实性包块(26 mm × 13mm),行 CT 检查示肝左外叶占位,转移瘤? 原发性肝癌? 甲胎蛋白 122.54ng/ml。

病理检查:部分肝组织一块,大小 9cm × 6cm × 2cm,切面见一灰白色结节,直径 2cm,其余切面淡黄,质中。常规病理诊断:肝左外叶肿瘤切除标本:初步诊断肝细胞癌,待免疫组化进一步明确诊断。

免疫组化检测：阳性：CK8，CK18，Villin，AFP，Hepatocyte，CD34（肝窦＋），Ki-67（＋，约 20%）；阴性：CK7，CK20，CK19，CEA，CD10，CDX2，CA19-9，Mucin-2，CgA，Syn，HMB45，S-100。免疫组化诊断：肝左外叶肿瘤切除标本：肝细胞性肝癌（图 3-3-1）。

第四节　早期肝癌与高分化肝细胞癌

早期肝癌，是一种结节性病变，它的存在不破坏肝脏基本结构，在细小的小梁和腺泡结构中包含几个肝癌细胞。镜下癌细胞分化良好，类似于 Edmondson 1 级。“早期”一词仅提示病变相当于肝癌发生的早期阶段，而不能预示治疗后临床预后一定很好。早期肝癌极微小，肉眼观呈黄色。癌细胞系局部替代性生长，肝小叶或假小叶结构无破坏。肿瘤可涉及多个假小叶，但仍保存原有的小叶间微细结构。无周围组织因膨胀性生长的受压表现。这些病变可能代表原位肝癌或微小侵袭性肝癌，其表现有别于前述四型小肝细胞癌。

显微镜下，早期肝癌是高分化的，并表现结构上的异型性，如薄的小梁形式或腺泡形成与伴轻度核异型的细胞结构增加；它与明显的肝癌不同在于它没有假包膜和没有肝结构的根本性破坏。

另一方面，含早期成分的明显的肝癌（进展性早期肝癌）是早期肝癌的进一步发展，瘤内肝癌结节大，足以能在大体检查中被发现，且通常表现富血管性，多数是高分化的。

Matsui 等（1991）发现，肝癌的动脉和门脉血供比例，与病变的恶性程度有关，即随病变恶性程度增加，门脉血供趋于减少直至消失，而代之以动脉血供为主或单独动脉供血，几乎所有明显肝癌都为肝动脉单独供血，早期肝癌可能也遵循这规律。而其他作者，如 Takayasu 等（1990）发现早期肝癌的血供并不完全符合这种门脉血和肝动脉血互补规律，他们认为，肝癌病变的这种血供互补机制的建立，可能发生在从早期到明显病变的过渡过程中。

高分化肝细胞癌：高分化肝细胞癌相当于 Edmondson 1 级，日本国立癌中心的病理学者称其为早期肝癌。

脂肪变性：早期肝癌和小肝细胞癌均可发生脂肪变性。Takayasu 等（1995）在对一组 39 个早期肝癌的研究中，发现其中 26 个肿瘤（67%）有程度不等的脂肪变性，而 Yoshikawa 等（1988）报道 600 例进展型肝癌中仅见 10 例（1.7%）肿瘤内有脂肪变性。Kadoya 等（1992）的报道与 Yoshikawa 等（1988）类似，在 67 例进展型肝癌中仅见 6 例肿瘤细胞有脂肪变性。有作者认为，脂肪能在肝癌细胞中产生，提示肝癌细胞分化良好，早期肝癌脂肪变性发生率高可能与其分化良好有关。

第五节　小肝癌不典型的影像表现

肝细胞癌在我国的发病率较高，多数患者具有慢性肝病背景，特别是肝硬化的出现使影像检查对小肝癌的检出受到影响。

关于诊断标准：近年美国肝脏病研究协会（AASLD）实践指南修改了前期有关肝细胞癌的诊断标准，将过去 >10 mm 的肝细胞癌诊断应根据 MSCT 和 MR 2 种增强检查出现典型的影像表现（即动脉期的高血供和静脉期或延迟期的流出），修改为上述 1 种影像检查出现典型表现即可，对 <10 mm 的肝脏内结节样病变应采取间隔 3 个月复查超声的动态观察。

指南给影像诊断提出了更高的要求，但临床上小肝细胞癌常出现不典型的影像表现，这就需要影像科医生不断提高发现更小肝细胞癌的能力，让患者得到有效和及时的治疗。

典型与不典型：肝细胞癌是肝硬化患者死亡的重要原因，早期诊断是长期生存的关键因素。肝细胞癌的典型影像表现为动脉期强化，静脉期和延迟期因对比剂的快速流出表现为低密度。肿瘤的动脉血供特征和门静脉血供缺乏导致了肿瘤的流出效应，出现动脉期高密度，静脉期和延迟期的低密度表现，有时这种效应仅表现在延迟期。目前 MSCT 和

MR 检查是临床诊断肝细胞癌的主要方法，癌变结节的血流动力学改变是影像检查发现肝细胞癌的病理基础，但发生在肝硬化患者的肝细胞癌诊断具有一定的困难。

国内有关 <20 mm 肝细胞癌的影像表现报道不多，一项研究使用 MSCT 对 39 例 <20 mm 肝细胞癌的影像表现进行初步总结，其中肝细胞癌典型的影像表现 20 例，占 51.3%(20/39)；不典型表现 19 例，占 48.7%(19/39)。

不典型影像表现：不典型影像表现以静脉期等密度和延迟期低密度最多见，占不典型表现的 31.6%(6/19)。该组 19 例不典型表现中有 6 例动脉期未出现强化，占 31.6%(6/19)；延迟期表现为低密度者多达 18 例，占 94.7%(18/19)；仅 1 例在静脉期和延迟期等密度。

双期增强 CT，即增强后行动脉期和门静脉期扫描是诊断肝癌的主要手段。动脉期强化是肝癌影像表现的最常见和最重要特征，但门静脉期敏感性稍差，这是因为部分肿瘤与周围肝实质等密度，降低了肿瘤的显示率。

文献报道肝细胞癌在延迟期较门静脉期有更好的显示度，即增强 3 期扫描优于双期扫描。该组病例中延迟期为低密度而静脉期为高和等密度表现者分别为 4 例和 6 例，共占 25.6%(10/39)，如果不结合延迟期图像而只进行双期增强扫描，可能与血管瘤或异型增生结节混淆。

肿瘤的血管密度和肝脏的不同血供决定了肿瘤的显示度，高血供肿瘤强化明显易于识别，低血供肿瘤的动脉血供差，在动脉期表现为等密度时可能被忽略。

肿瘤的血供与恶性度相关，低度恶性以门静脉血供为主，随着恶性度的增加，肿瘤会出现新生血管和动脉血供的增加。门静脉期高分化和中 - 低分化肿瘤的密度差异不大，许多情况下肿瘤密度与肝实质同步性增加，这是因为含有对比剂的动脉血的连续供应，动脉期时肿瘤内对比剂的残留，肿瘤的双血供等。

不论肿瘤分化情况如何，绝大多数在延迟期表现为低密度，其原因包括肿瘤的对比剂流出、门脉高压导致肝实质的延迟强化、肿瘤细胞较周围肝组织致密等。该组 39 例患者除 1 例延迟期等密度外，皆表现为低密度；另该组中 - 低分化和高分化肝细胞癌分别有 48.1% 和 50% 出现不典型表现。

不典型影像表现的形成机制：小肝细胞癌不典型影像表现的形成机制多样，该组内有 3 例低血供病灶(即增强后动脉期未出现强化)的组织学检查为原发性肝癌高分化透明细胞癌，肿瘤组织内血窦不丰富，肿瘤细胞大泡性脂变，肿瘤排列实体型。

文献报道这种低血供表现是因为肿瘤动脉新生血管不足、门静脉血供降低、肿瘤内坏死、脂肪变和透明细胞变，这也是低血供病变只在延迟期出现低密度的原因。

肿瘤在门静脉期出现持续强化的原因为肿瘤存在双重血供，动脉血供增加的同时门静脉血供未减少。该组中这种以静脉期持续强化的不典型影像表现最多见，说明肿瘤血管处于向动脉化过渡的过程中。

肿瘤包膜强化为门静脉期或延迟期出现在肿瘤周围的强化环，表示对比剂在肿瘤边缘的纤维或血管结构内的滞留，包膜很少见于 10 mm 以下肿瘤，可能此时纤维包膜还未形成。该组病例可见 2 例包膜强化，均见于典型表现中，未见 10 mm 以下肿瘤出现包膜强化。该组中 1 例增强后动脉期病灶边缘呈环形强化，静脉期强化持续，这种表现可能与大量纤维组织的存在使对比剂在灶周滞留时间长有关。

另 1 例静脉期肿瘤周围出现低密度环的原因是瘤周为肝血窦结构较少的纤维组织，文献中少有报道"结中结"表现是一种少见但具有特征性的肝细胞癌影像表现，通常指肝细胞癌位于增生结节或再生结节内。影像表现为动脉期肿瘤强化，周围的结节部分不强化，MR 表现更特异。该例"结中结"的组织学检查可见肿瘤内血窦丰富、瘤周大量脂肪浸润和周围肝组织受压推移，后者是静脉期包膜强化的主要原因。

重视甲胎蛋白阴性：长期以来，尽管甲胎蛋白作为肝细胞癌的诊断和监测指标，但还缺乏足够的敏感性和特异性，因为部分胆管细胞癌和肝转移癌也会升高，因此美国肝脏病研究协会指南推荐肝细胞癌的诊断应该依靠放射学和组织学表现。该组病例均行甲胎蛋白检查，其中 21 例升高，占 53.8%(21/39)；18 例正常，占 46.2%(18/39)，表明实际工作中应重视甲胎蛋白阴性患者小肝细胞癌发生的可能性。

鉴别诊断：小肝细胞癌的鉴别诊断包括再生结节，异型增生结节和小血管瘤等。结合小肝细胞癌的典型表现鉴别不困难，对于不典型表现应结合患者的病史和临床资料，必要时还应考虑其他影像检查，如 MR 或 DSA。该项研究的结果也提示对于小肝细胞癌除了动脉期的强化，其他期相的表现也同样重要，特别是延迟期的表现，对于目前以 MSCT 为肝脏病变主要检查手段的临床机构非常重要。

第六节　关于小肝癌的漏诊

有作者报告一例肝细胞癌患者，CT 和超声检查均未见异常，而因其甲胎蛋白高达 11 340μg/L 而作血管造影，发现肝左叶有一低密度病灶，术中见该病灶为 7mm × 16mm × 16mm 大小。一项研究报告 14 例直径在 30mm 以下的小肝癌，其中有 4 例常规 CT 扫描未见异常：1 例因外院 CT 机分辨力较差，另 1 例可能系病灶太小（仅 10 × 10mm），也可能因病人每次扫描时屏气状态不一致而遗漏，此二例均因甲胎蛋白值升高后为血管造影和 / 或 CTAP 所检出和确诊；1 例因平扫时病灶呈等密度，且病灶较小（直径为 26mm）和较深在，肝局部轮廓无异常，增强扫描自上而下进行，仍呈等密度表现，因超声检查疑肝细胞癌故及时做双期 CT 发现异常，后经血管造影和 CTA 确诊；1 例漏诊的原因是增强扫描技术不当，尽管 CT 平扫已发现低密度病灶，注射对比剂后未首先对病灶层实施扫描，而是按自上而下的顺序扫描，在首层扫描后 73 秒才扫描病灶区，早已错过了显示肝细胞癌特点的血管期。

由此看来，在这些病例防止漏检的措施，主要应改进扫描技术：如平扫时已发现病变，增强时要在血管期（即 40 秒内）对病灶层实施扫描；如临床疑有肝细胞癌（甲胎蛋白值升高，或超声检查疑有肝细胞癌等）而常规 CT 扫描又无异常时，应不失时机地实施双期 CT 扫描、X 线血管造影、CTA 以及 CTAP 等检查。

该组作者还报告 1 例甲胎蛋白正常，作了常规 CT、X 线血管造影和 CTA 等检查，虽发现其自内向外顺序染色征象有别于典型的血管瘤表现，但未引起足够注意，再次就诊时，肿瘤直径已从 2cm 增至 8cm，正是由于此例误诊教训，才使他们特别重视由内向外顺序染色这一有价值的征象。

病变检出遗漏原因分析和防止漏检的措施：一组作者报告 14 例直径在 30mm 以下的小肝癌中，有 9 例行 X 线血管造影，8 例富血管病灶均呈自内向外顺序染色，其中 3 例的这一征象为 CTA 的单层动态扫描所证实。除 1 例（首例 CTA）因缺乏经验误诊外，此后所见的 7 例（含 1 例甲胎蛋白正常和 2 例甲胎蛋白轻度升高而 CT 诊断为性质待查者）的定性诊断均正确，因此，该组作者认为自内向外顺序染色这一征象对小肝癌的诊断价值应予肯定。

肝细胞癌血供研究观察发现，大多数的肝细胞癌或小肝癌结节有肝动脉分支直接伸入到癌结节中心，由肝动脉灌注乳胶或硅酮的癌结节呈血管球样表现，可能是癌灶自内向外顺序染色征象的病理基础。识别自内向外顺序染色征象，一定要从一系列图像作动态分析，否则容易误判。Honda 等（1992）指出，在早期和晚期呈边缘性强化的病灶分别有 62.8%（22/35）和 70%（7/10），可能是血管瘤。有的病理证实的血管瘤，从常规 CT 增强图像看，显然属全部强化者，但从血管造影系列图像动态分析，则无疑属从边缘向中心顺序染色者。所以，识别自内向外顺序染色征象，一定要动态分析一系列图像。大约有 1/4 的局灶性结节状增生亦呈自内向外顺序染色征象，它与肝细胞癌的鉴别可借助核素扫描，摄取核素正常或高于正常者，以前者可能性较大；摄取核素偏低或不摄取核素而呈充盈缺损时，则应首先考虑肝细胞癌。

第七节　小肝癌的不典型增强表现

小肝癌（SHCC）为单发直径≤ 3 cm 的肝癌或 2 个癌结节直径之和≤ 3 cm。小肝癌 CT 平扫多数表现为低密度，脂肪肝背景基础上可为等密度或高密度。一组研究 CT 平扫小肝癌的检出率为 76.19%。CT 平扫因不能反映癌灶内的血供情况，对小肝癌的定性诊断意义不大，但对小肝癌的检出及增强后的对比有一定的价值，为增强扫描提供必要的技术参数。增强后病灶的强化不仅应与周围肝实质相比，也需与病灶本身相比才能肯定。因此，一般认为平扫仍然是增强扫描所不可缺少的。

CT 增强检查可反映正常肝脏及小肝癌灶的血供情况，正常肝脏 75% 由门静脉供血，在发生癌变的肝结节中，动脉新生血管增多，正常的肝血窦遭到破坏，门静脉供血减少，因此在 CT 增强动脉期肝癌结节呈明显强化，而在门静脉期由于缺少门静脉供血癌结节不强化，低于或等于周围正常肝实质密度，延迟期密度仍低于正常肝实质。这也是小肝癌 CT 增强的典型表现。在一组研究中，符合小肝癌典型影像表现的癌灶共 29 个（29/42，69.04%），其中 23 个病灶表现为动脉期高密度，门静脉期低密度，延迟期低密度，3 种组合模式均可做出定性诊断；另 6 个癌灶动脉期表现为高密度但门静脉期表现为等密度，此种表现动脉期 + 门静脉期组合不能对其做出定性诊断而易漏诊。

对表现较为典型的小肝癌，多期 CT 增强诊断并不困难，正确诊断率可达 90% 以上。但在该组研究中，还有部分病灶并不符合小肝癌的典型影像学特征，不典型增强表现可分为以下 3 种：①动脉期与门静脉期均为高密度，延迟期低密度，该组有 7 个，占 16.67%。这可能与小肝癌灶中动脉新生血管增多而肝血窦尚未完全破坏，导致癌结节既由新生的肝动脉供血同时还存在残留的门静脉供血，动脉期与门静脉期均有强化，此类结节在动脉期加门静脉期组合中不能做出明确诊断易漏诊，而在动脉期加延迟期组合及 3 期联合诊断中可做出定性诊断。②动脉期为等密度，门静脉期、延迟期为低密度，该组有 4 个，占 9.52%。此种表现除扫描时间延迟的因素外，可能的原因是这些病灶肝动脉血供有轻度增加，还不足以使病灶在动脉期扫描呈高密度，而在延迟期由于门脉血供的减少呈略低密度。还有学者认为此种不典型表现的原因是这类小肝癌瘤体内存在肝动脉和门静脉瘘，导致动脉期时不含碘的门静脉血流入瘤体，稀释了瘤体内含碘的肝动脉血的浓度，因此肝动脉期呈等密度；此种增强表现 3 种组合模式均可做出定性诊断。③动脉期、门静脉期与延迟期均为低密度，该组有 2 个，占 4.76%。此类小肝癌动脉与门静脉供血均少于正常肝实质，属少血供小肝癌，有学者认为癌灶内坏死、脂肪变是小肝癌动脉期不强化或无明显强化的主要因素。还有学者认为癌细胞透明样变也是原因之一。此种增强表现 3 种组合均未能做出定性诊断。

在此值得一提的是，并非所有螺旋 CT 动脉期不强化的病灶都是少血供的，这和扫描持续时间的选择密切相关。虽然螺旋 CT 1 次屏气可完成全肝扫描，并且可以在肝脏增强的不同时期进行扫描，但螺旋 CT 扫描是逐层进行的，每个层面的采集时间都不同。动脉期采用头尾方向扫描时，膈顶层面和肝脏下极层面的扫描时间差较大，开始动脉期扫描时，膈顶的癌灶也许尚未开始强化，而肝脏下极层面的病灶，则可能强化的峰值已过，因而均未能见到强化表现。肝癌的早期诊断和治疗是提高生存率的重要途径，也是临床不断探索的课题。双期或多期螺旋 CT 扫描是小肝癌首选检查方法之一。经长期探索，在双期或多期扫描中，小肝癌的表现较为典型，诊断并不困难。但双期（动脉期 + 门静脉期）扫描会遗漏不典型小肝癌的诊断，不利于小肝癌的早期发现，对肝癌病灶的定性，延迟期扫描很有必要。该组研究表明，在小肝癌的检出和定性方面动脉期价值最大，与以往报道结果一致。在小肝癌增强扫描不同组合模式中，动脉期 + 延迟期扫描组合模式对小肝癌的定性诊断率为 95.24%，优于动脉期 + 门脉期组合（64.28%，P=0.001）。由于动脉期 + 延迟期扫描可减少 1 次辐射剂量，在减少患者辐射剂量方面，优于 3 期联合扫描。因此，一些作者认为动脉期 + 延迟期扫描可满足小肝癌的早期定性诊断，可作为小肝癌 CT 增强常规扫描方式。

但是，门脉期小肝癌的表现说明它的门脉期血液供应差，正是它的特征性表现，因此，不少作者认为，门脉期对于小肝癌的定性十分重要，不宜放弃。

第八节　误诊病例简介：小肝癌与良性病灶

患者，女，68 岁。发现肝占位病变一月余入院。在一月内定期复查甲胎蛋白逐渐升高。CT：左肝外叶见一约 1.0cm × 1.2cm 类圆形稍低密度影，边界尚清，平扫 CT 值 33HU，增强后动脉早期轻度强化，

CT 值 49HU，静脉期明显强化，CT 值 102HU，延迟期强化稍减低，CT 值 90HU。CT 诊断：左肝外叶稍低密度影性质？考虑良性病变可能，建议随访复查。

手术所见：见肝左外叶一大小约 3.0 cm × 2.5 cm 肿块突出肝表面，形态欠规则，边界欠清，腹腔内无积液。病理检查，肝左外叶肿物切除标本：肝组织一块，大小 4.5 cm × 2.8 cm × 1.5 cm，切面见两个灰白色结节，直径 0.6~1.0cm，与周围界限尚清，其余切面土黄，质中。常规病理诊断：肝左外叶肿物切除标本：初步诊断原发性肝细胞性肝癌，待做免疫组化检测进一步证实。免疫组化检测，阳性：CK18、CK8、AFP（灶 +）、CD34（肝窦内皮 +）、Hepatocyte（灶 +）、Villin（灶 +）、CD（P）、HBsAg、Ki-67（+，约 30%）；阴性：EMA、CEA、CD10、Vimentin、CK19、CK7、CK20、HBcAg。免疫组化诊断（肝左外叶肿物切除标本）：原发性肝细胞性肝癌（透明细胞型）。

误诊病例回顾分析：该病例在发现病灶后一个月内定期复查甲胎蛋白逐渐升高的情况，被影像诊断医师完全忽略，这是一条沉痛教训。在小肝癌的三期增强扫描中影像学表现，常常出现不典型的情况，给定性分析造成一定困难，此例即如此，此时，密切结合临床尤其显得重要，这也是应该经常交流的经验之一。

第四章　肝癌基础研究点滴

肝癌相关基因

肝细胞癌的生物学行为,可通过CT来反映,从而作出较明确的判定。随着现代分子生物学技术的发展,对肝细胞癌的认识已深入到基因水平,这有助于解释肝细胞癌影像学表现的多样性和复杂性。目前,影像学(大体形态学)和相关肿瘤基因(微观)的系统研究已成为影像学研究的热点。肝细胞性肝癌(简称肝癌)的生物学行为,如生长、转移方式和血供特点等,目前已公认CT可做出较明确的判定,螺旋CT快速成像技术的应用能更多地反映肝细胞性肝癌的特性。随着现代分子生物学技术的发展,对肝癌的认识已深入到基因水平,故而可以从蛋白质和mRNA水平解释肝癌的发生、发展、侵袭性、转移及预后,并有助于解释肝细胞性肝癌影像学表现的多样性和复杂性。

肝癌CT表现与病理学特性的相关性:20世纪80年代中期日本学者Okuda等(1984)将肝细胞性肝癌分为5种病理学类型,即:①膨胀型:癌肿边界清,有纤维包膜形成(假包膜),常伴肝硬化,且分化较好。②浸润型:癌肿边界不清,多不伴有肝硬化。③混合型。④弥漫型。⑤特殊型。这种分类能较准确地反映肝癌的生物学行为。

CT能较为可靠地反映肝癌的病理学特性,即肿块的数目、大小、卫星结节、肿块的生长方式(膨胀式和浸润式)、癌栓形成和远处转移,以及肿块的血液供应情况,而且对伴随的肝脏弥漫性病变,如肝硬化、脂肪肝等也可全面了解,肝癌CT表现与病理学特性有密切关系。癌肿浸润、癌栓形成以及卫星结节和转移与肿瘤大小成正比,肝癌分化程度与肝癌大小也成正比关系。小肝癌分化良好,其中Edmondson分级Ⅰ级占75%,Ⅱ级占25%;随着肿瘤的增大,分化较差,Ⅱ~Ⅳ占优势,而晚期大多为Ⅳ级。门脉系统受侵犯及癌栓形成与病灶大小或病程密切相关,也与病理类型和肿瘤生长方式密切相关。

p53基因:p53基因是一种肿瘤抑制基因,基因表达产物为p53蛋白,它与特定的DNA序列结合,诱导WAFl(wild type p53 activated fragment 1)基因表达产物p21蛋白的生成,而p21蛋白则与肿瘤增殖细胞核抗原(PCNA)结合,阻抑DNA多聚酶delta的功能,从而抑制DNA复制;p21蛋白也抑制细胞周期素/细胞周期素依赖性激酶(CDK)的底物磷酸化,阻止细胞周期从G1到S期。突变型p53蛋白不具备这一功能。

人类各种癌症中,60%左右存在p53基因突变,其中约85.6%为错义突变,野生型p53基因功能由此丧失,突变型p53基因具有癌基因的作用,促进细胞恶性转化。免疫组化和PCR-SSCP(聚合酶式反应-单链构象多态性)已被广泛应用于p53基因突变的检测。

但有研究表明,p53表达并不能很好地 反映p53基因突变(Batsakis等,1995)。以前的研究认为野生型p53蛋白的半衰期短(6~20秒)、降解快,而突变型p53蛋白半衰期长(4~12小时)、降解慢,故免疫组化只能检出突变型p53蛋白,而野生型p53蛋白却难以检出。

Battifora(1994)的研究表明,有一种p53结合蛋白,如mdm-2或病毒癌蛋白可能抑制野生型p53蛋白降解,导致非突变型p53蛋白过度表达。Kirk等(2000)对1组肝细胞性肝癌病例的血浆DNA检测发现,p53基因249位点突变是p53基因突变的“热点”。Heize等(1999)研究发现,p53突变是人类恶性肿瘤中常见的现象。肝细胞性肝癌中,p53表达高者1年和2年生存率低于p53表达低者。Hsu等(1993)揭示,外侵型肝细胞性肝癌其p53表达水平高于非外侵型。p53基因突变及其编码蛋白的异常表达是肝细胞性肝癌的不良预后因子。

众多的研究表明,p53基因异常对肝癌的发生有重要作用,p53基因异常和突变型p53蛋白过度表达导致肝癌侵袭性的增加。肝癌体积较小,癌细胞分化较高,则基因突变率较低,蛋白过度表达也较低且强度偏弱;肝癌肿块大,癌细胞分化低,有侵袭性转移者，则 p53 基因突变率高，p53 蛋白过度表达也较高。因此，可以认为 p53 基因异常和突变型 p53 蛋白过度表达与肝细胞性肝癌肝内播散和门脉癌栓的形成、突破包膜生长，以及肝细胞性肝癌分化程度密切相关。

基于肝癌 CT 表现和肝癌病理特性的密切关系，通过肝癌的 CT 图像来间接反映肝癌的分子病理学特性是可能的。

nm23-H1 基因：nm23 基因是一种转移抑制基因。在人类基因组中，存在 nm23-H1 和 H2 基因，它们编码 17kD 蛋白质。nm23-H1 和 H2 基因产物与人体二磷酸核苷激酶是同一种物质（Stahl 等，1991），它在肝细胞性肝癌细胞浆内和核内均有表达。Boix 等（1994）认为 nm23-H1 的表达与肝细胞性肝癌肝内转移、门静脉癌栓形成、侵袭性生长和肝硬化程度呈负相关；对单发小肝癌，nm23-H1 过度表达，则其术后复发率低，预后好。

Lin 等（1998）对 1 组肝细胞性肝癌的 nm23-H1 mRNA 表达的研究表明，nm23-H1 高表达与肝细胞性肝癌的发展有关。肝细胞性肝癌病灶周围的微环境对肝细胞性肝癌肝内转移有很重要的作用，nm23-H1 mRNA 的减少使 nm23-H1 阴性的细胞有了更大的转移潜能。Chen 等研究表明 nm23-H1 mRNA 的表达与转移呈负相关，与病灶的大小和肝硬化等肝脏病变无关。nm23 基因为转移抑制基因，其基因突变和基因表达产物减少使其抑癌作用减弱或消失，对其他肝癌相关基因失调控，从而促进肝癌的发生以及肝癌侵袭性的增加。

肝癌发生转移时，nm23-H1 基因有低表达的趋势。但肝癌发生淋巴结转移与 nm23-H1 的关系未见明确报道，这主要与肝细胞性肝癌发生淋巴结转移的比例较低有关。

c-erbB-2 基因：c-erbB-2 基因是一种癌基因，由 Semba 等（1985）研究发现，它位于染色体 17q21 上，其表达产物是一种具有酪氨酸激酶活性的糖蛋白，称 p185。它由细胞外区、跨膜区，又包括两个富含半胱氨酸的重复序列和细胞内的酪氨酸激酶区组成。pl85 分布于红细胞生成系统和成人的神经系统中，以及皮肤、胃肠、肺等脏器中，它对细胞和组织的增殖与分化可起一定的调节作用。p185 的结构和功能与表皮生长因子受体蛋白有高度的相似性（Bargmann 等，1986）。

目前认为是表皮生长因子等肽类激素一方面通过与 p185 形成异源二聚体，刺激 p185 酪氨酸磷酸化后可激活 c-erbB-2；也可通过激活表皮生长因子受体的激酶活性，然后通过受体磷酸化而激活 c-erbB-2。c-erbB-2 对一系列激活因子的应答、细胞和组织的增殖分化可获得一定的调控。若异常激活后，则导致其失常表达。c-erbB-2 是通过转化并由点突变激活的癌基因。胃癌等肿瘤则主要是通过基因扩增和 RNA 及蛋白的过度表达。c-erbB-2 基因与肝细胞性肝癌的发生及病人的预后有关，Heinze 等（1999）研究表明，c-erbB-2 表达高的肝细胞性肝癌者 1 年和 2 年生存率低于表达低者。因此，c-erbB-2 可成为一有价值的肝细胞性肝癌预后检测因子。有报道称 c-erbB-2 基因表达与 nm23-H1 的表达减少有关。c-erbB-2 基因异常扩增和基因产物过度表达，使细胞和组织异常增殖，呈现恶性特征，其表达程度与肿瘤病理分级相关，与肝癌的发生和预后有关。

CD44 基因：CD44 基因编码的 CD44 蛋白是一种跨膜透明质酸受体，是在淋巴细胞成熟和归巢过程中起重要作用的表面黏附分子。标准型 CD44 蛋白（CD44s）几乎存在于所有正常细胞，它至少由 19 个外显子组合而成，在转录过程中，只有 9 个外显子固定表达，其余外显子可一个或多个通过组合插入相应的 mRNA 链中，由此指导合成一系列结构相似但功能有别的 CD44 蛋白，即选择性拼接变异体（CD44v）。

CD44v 存在组织特异性，且某些类型可能与肿瘤的浸润转移有关，其中尤为重要的是 CD44v6。含有 CD44v6 的外显子的拼接变异体能使癌细胞发生以淋巴系统为途径的扩散转移，而且可能是肿瘤预后的独立判断指标。CD44 基因产物不但在淋巴细胞功能及细胞间质相互作用中，而且在肿瘤的生长和转移中起重要作用，在肝细胞性肝癌中，CD44 的表达与肝细胞性肝癌转移有正相关性，CD44 的高表达对肝癌发生淋巴途径的转移有重要作用。

近几年 CD44 基因与肝细胞性肝癌的关系未见有新的报道。目前的研究表明，CD44 的表达与肝癌转移有正性相关趋势。

N- ras 和 C-myc 基因：N-ras 与 C-myc 是两种原癌基因。N- ras 基因是通过 G 结合蛋白信号转导系统发生作用的原癌基因，其表达产物 p21 蛋白具有 GTP 酶活性。人类恶性肿瘤中 N-ras 基因的突变多在 12、16 或 61 密码子突变，但有学者研究的一组肝细胞性肝癌病例显示，N-ras 的 12、13 密码子突变达到 79.31%，同时提示突变不局限于 12 或 13 密码子。该基因发生突变时，p21 水解 GTP 为 GDP 的能力以及 p21 与 GTP 酶活化蛋白和 C-myc 基因的异常，主要是使细胞增殖失调（ras-GAP）的结合能力降低，导致 p21 持续结合 GTP，处于激活状态，使细胞内 IP3 和 DAG 增多，而 IP3 和 DAG 是细胞增生的细胞内第 2 信使，结果是细胞持续增殖，形成肿瘤。

C-myc 基因，编码 47KD 的蛋白，与配对蛋白 Max 构成异二聚体。Myc/max 异二聚体可以有效的与特异性 DNA 序列 GACGTG 结合，从而影响转录功能，引起系列反应，促进细胞进入 DNA 合成期（S 期）。

正常细胞 C-myc 基因表达低，且短暂；在某些情况下，如部分肝切除时，可表达增高，如伴某些生长因子如 IL-2，表皮生长因子等存在时，促进细胞增殖，否则促进细胞凋亡。

在恶性肿瘤中，常见其基因扩增，染色体易位，低甲基化等而活化，改变了 myc 基因

正常的表达调控机制。在肝细胞性肝癌中，C-myc 基因扩增在病灶较大、年龄偏低和癌细胞低分化的病例中更常见一些。C-myc 基因扩增时，肝细胞性肝癌中的癌细胞有高的增殖活性，其生存率低于无 C-myc 基因扩增的病人。因此，C-myc 基因扩增是肝细胞性肝癌的恶性程度和预后差的指标（Kawate 等，1999）。Challen 等报道 1 组肝细胞性肝癌病例，约 30.5% 有 N- ras 和 C-myc mRNA 阳性表达，而在正常肝组织中无 N- ras 和 C-myc mRNA 的同时表达。

多数学者认为，N- ras 基因主要在肝细胞性肝癌发生时有作用，而 C-myc 基因在肝细胞性肝癌的发展过程中起重要作用。因此，N-ras 基因和 C-myc 基因的异常，主要是使细胞增殖失调控，从而促使肝癌的发生和发展，表现出恶性病理特征。

肿瘤的发生是环境与遗传相互作用、多基因参与的多步骤的过程，是癌基因激活和抑癌基因失活的复杂过程的结果。基因的表达程度与肝癌的病理表现关系密切。肝癌 CT 表现及其增强方式与其病理学密切相关，而肝癌的病理学特征是由肝癌相关基因的不同表达决定的。当多种肝癌侵袭性相关的癌基因异常表达或抑癌基因突变时，肝癌表现出较多的恶性特征。目前肝癌相关基因的表达与肝癌病理学特征研究较明确，可以认为肝癌 CT 表现与肝癌相关基因的表达存在某种必然的联系。CT 检查是一种无创伤、快捷的方法，研究肝癌 CT 表现与肝癌相关基因表达的相关性，间接反映肝癌相关基因的分子生物学特征的内涵，为术前判断肝癌的恶性程度提供了更多信息，同时为肝细胞性肝癌治疗方案的选择以及疗效的判断等方面提供重要依据。

第五章　透明细胞型肝癌

第一节　原发性透明细胞型肝癌

透明细胞型肝癌是肝细胞癌的一种特殊细胞类型，癌细胞胞质内因富含糖原而呈透明状。当癌细胞中50%以上为透明细胞时，应诊断为透明细胞型肝癌。临床较为少见，发生率约占肝癌的0.9%~8.8%。其发生机制推测是由于门静脉血供减少和肿瘤的供血动脉不足所致的代谢紊乱和糖代谢异常。PAS染色几乎均为阳性。病理组织学上要与肝转移性透明细胞癌，尤其是肾透明细胞癌肝转移相鉴别。

透明细胞型肝癌的临床表现并无特异性，往往以腹痛和乏力等症状就诊；性别上以男性较多（12/19）；可有乙型肝炎表面抗原阳性（9/19）和甲胎蛋白增高（5/19）。一般认为透明细胞型肝癌的预后要优于普通型肝癌，但是也有人持相反观点。本病术前容易误诊，主要原因是对该病的认识不足。因此，熟悉该病的影像表现非常重要。

一组病例均为单发病灶，肿瘤直径大多<3.0cm（14/19）。CT平扫显示肿瘤实质密度明显低于正常肝组织，部分病灶密度不均匀，内部可见更低密度区。在MR见T_1WI上病灶多为稍高信号，加用脂肪抑制后病灶内的高信号有不同程度的下降。这可能与透明细胞富含糖原和存在一定的脂质成分有关。

此外，透明细胞也可以缩短组织的T_1值，从而使肿瘤的T_1信号增高。少数病灶在T_1WI上为等、低信号，可能与肿瘤内坏死有关。病灶在MR T_2WI上多为混杂高信号，则是由于肿瘤细胞胞质丰富，液性成分增多所致。该组病例中部分病灶（3/8）抑脂T_2WI为等、低信号，可能由于肿瘤细胞内含有较多的脂质成分有关。

增强CT和MRI上，动脉期病灶均呈现不同程度强化，门静脉期多数病灶为相对低密度或低信号，少数病灶呈等密度或等信号。该项研究中，部分病灶门静脉期还可见强化的环形包膜（5/19），这些表现均为肝癌的影像特征，有助于诊断。也有研究认为，透明细胞型肝癌动脉期无明显强化或轻微强化，门静脉期轻度持续强化，延迟期缓慢退出，呈慢进慢出的强化特点，原因可能与肿瘤分化较好有关。该组尚未发现。

误诊与鉴别诊断：该组19例患者术前仅8例诊断为肝细胞肝癌，其余均误诊为其他疾病，主要是因为对透明细胞型肝癌的影像表现缺乏认识，应注意与肝脏其他肿瘤或肿瘤性病变进行鉴别。

血管平滑肌脂肪瘤：透明细胞型肝癌CT平扫密度很低，MR T_1WI上信号较高，容易与含脂肪成分的良性肿瘤如血管平滑肌脂肪瘤相混淆。该组有6/19例误诊为血管平滑肌脂肪瘤。但是血管平滑肌脂肪瘤很少有包膜，并且病灶常见到中心血管影，特别是脂肪成分中见到血管影更具诊断意义。

炎性假瘤或再生结节：部分透明细胞型肝癌在MR T_2WI上表现为等、低信号，容易误诊为炎性假瘤或再生结节。一般炎性假瘤无肝动脉直接供血，在增强动脉期无强化表现，常为增强晚期环形或分隔强化；而肝脏增生结节以门静脉供血为主，增强后动脉期也无明显强化，门静脉期同周边肝实质强化一致，结合动态增强特征可资鉴别。

海绵状血管瘤：有文献报道肝透明细胞癌的影像表现介于普通型肝细胞癌与海绵状血管瘤之间，CT平扫肿瘤实质的密度明显低于正常肝组织，在T_2WI上信号明显增高，且与肝实质的信号对比度随回波时间延长而逐渐递增，此点类似海绵状血管瘤的信号特征，而不同于常见的肝癌信号，因此也需要与肝血管瘤鉴别。血管瘤在动态增强后一般都呈向心性充填,是其特征性的强化模式,而肝透明细胞癌多数仍具备"快进快出"的强化特点,两者不难鉴别。

其他脏器的转移性病灶:诊断肝透明细胞癌还需要排除其他脏器的转移性病灶,如肾脏、肾上腺以及卵巢来源的透明细胞癌。找到原发肿瘤则有助于明确转移灶的诊断。

总之,透明细胞型肝癌的影像表现较普通型肝细胞癌相对不典型,但又有其内在规律。由于肿瘤细胞含有较多糖原和一定的脂质成分, CT 和 MRI 检查可显示其一定的特征性表现,有助于识别该病。

第二节　原发性肝细胞性肝癌(透明细胞型)

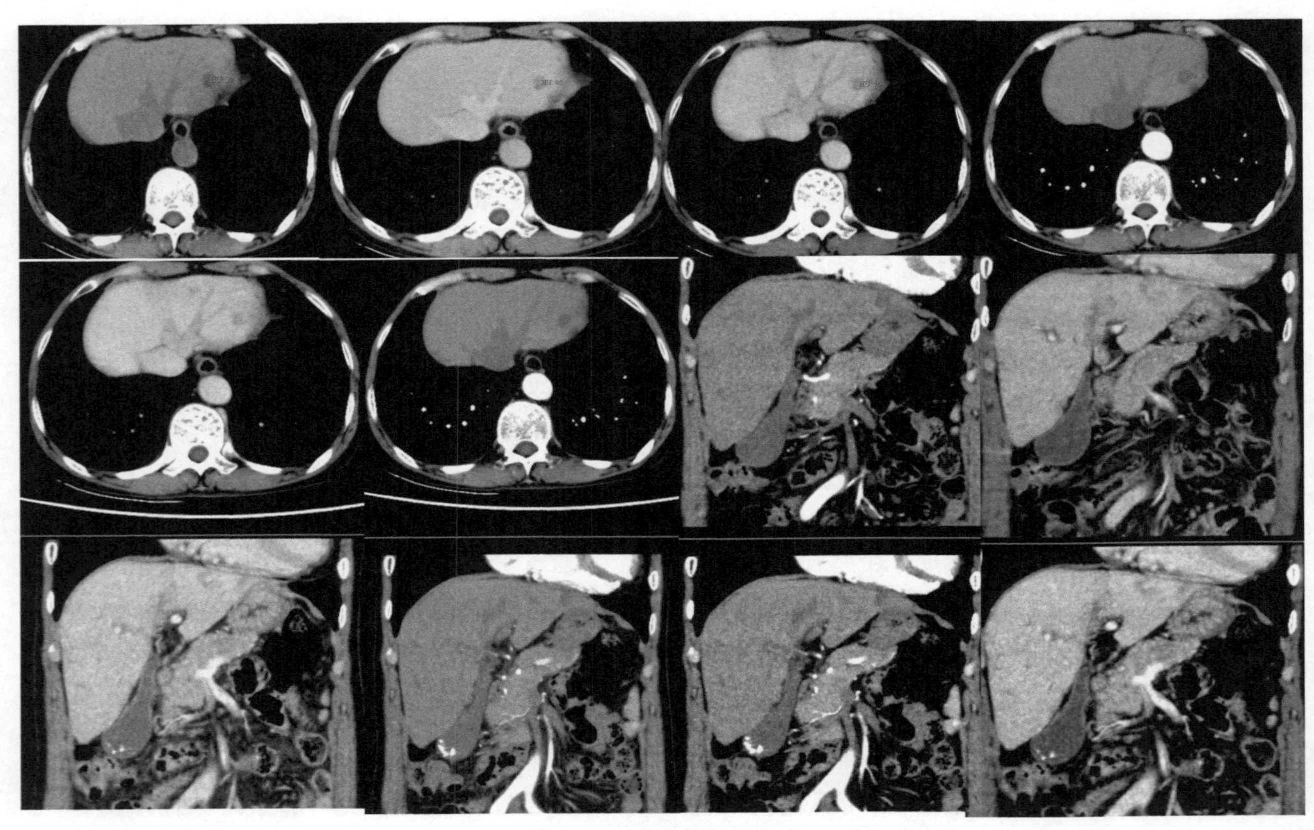

图 3-5-1　原发性肝细胞癌

患者,女, 68 岁。发现肝占位性病变 1 月余入院。患者缘于 1 月前在外院行腹部 CT 检查发现肝占位性病变,无明显腹痛腹胀不适,大小便正常,查甲胎蛋白 130.79ng/ml。口服中药治疗,之后定期复查 AFP 逐渐升高。 手术所见:腹腔网膜与腹壁严重粘连,肝脏被网膜包绕,分离网膜粘连后见肝右前叶上段一大小约 3.0cm × 2.5cm 的肿块突出肝表面,形态欠规律,边界欠清,腹腔内无积液,余肝脏表面光滑,无结节状状增生病灶。病理检查:肝左外叶肿物:肝组织一块,大小 4.5cm × 2.8cm × 1.5cm,切面见两个灰白色结节,直径 0.6~1cm,与周围界限尚清,其余切面土黄,质中。胆囊:胆囊大小 7.5cm × 4cm × 3.3cm,浆膜面光滑,黏膜呈细网状,内含灰黑色结石及墨绿色胆汁,胆囊壁厚 0.1cm。常规病理诊断:肝左外叶肿物切除标本:初步诊断原发性肝细胞性肝癌,待做免疫组化检测进一步证实。胆囊切除标本:慢性结石性胆囊炎,未见肝癌组织累及。免疫组化检测:阳性:CK18,CK8, AFP(灶+), CD34(肝窦内皮+), Hepatocyte(灶+), Villin(灶+), CK(P), HBsAg, Ki-67(+,约 30%);阴性: EMA, CEA,CD10,Vimentin,CK19,CK7,CK20,HBcAg。免疫组化诊断:肝左外叶肿物切除标本:原发性肝细胞性肝癌(透明细胞型)(图 3-5-1)。

第三节　肝脏原发性透明细胞癌

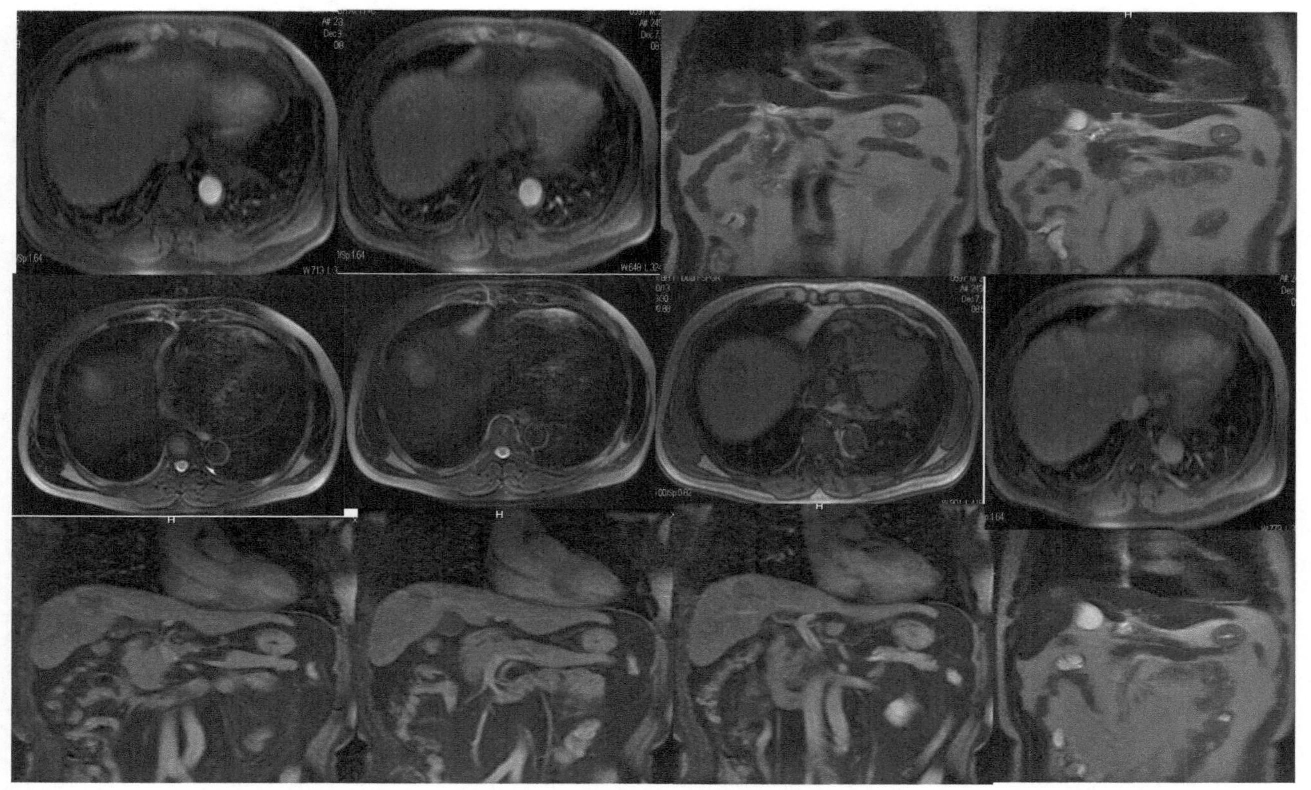

图 3-5-2　肝脏原发性透明细胞癌

患者，男，59 岁。体检发现右肝占位，无明显阳性体征。

病理检查：肝肿物切除标本：灰褐色组织一块，临床已剖开，大小 7.5cm × 5cm × 4.5cm，剖面可见一灰白结节，面积 4cm × 3cm，结节与周边组织界限较清，质中。胆囊切除标本：胆囊一具，临床已剖开，大小约 7cm × 3.5cm × 0.8cm，未见明显异常，壁厚 0.3cm。常规病理诊断：肝脏透明细胞癌，4cm × 3cm，合并结节性肝硬化。胆囊慢性炎症伴腺肌病。建议免疫组化标记排除转移性癌。

免疫组化检测：阳性：Hepatocyte，CK18（局灶），CK（L）（局灶），CK20（散在）；阴性：AFP，CD10，TTF-1，CK7，Villin，CK8，CK19，Vimentin。免疫组化诊断：免疫组化检测结果支持肝脏原发性透明细胞癌（图 3-5-2）。

第六章 纤维板层型肝细胞癌

纤维板层型肝细胞癌是肝细胞癌的一种特殊类型，其发病，临床表现，病理，预后，均与普通型肝细胞癌不同。此型肝细胞癌可切除率高达 58%，生存期亦较其他类型肝细胞癌为长。本病又称瘤囊型肝细胞癌，由 Edmundson（1965）首次报道。病因不明，为肝细胞癌的变异，无基础肝脏疾病。

病理学：本病 75% 以上发生于正常肝脏，左叶远较右叶为多，常为单发分叶状病灶，质地较硬，呈膨胀性生长，与正常肝组织分界清楚，可以有包膜，呈巨块型，直径通常大于 10cm。大体标本可见分界清楚的肿块，多有分叶。肿瘤增大时有出血坏死。肿瘤中心纤维瘢痕是其特点之一。纤维板层型肝细胞癌瘤体中央有星状纤维瘢痕向周围放射并将肿瘤分隔是其重要特征。另一特点是出现位于肿瘤中心瘢痕中央的不规则非特异性钙化。显微镜下，肿瘤细胞呈多边形，嗜伊红染色，细胞核大。纤维基质成分较多，有时排列较整齐，将肿瘤细胞分割成条带状或团状，有一定特征性。

病理组织学特点有三：含嗜酸性胞浆的多边形恶性肝细胞；围绕的纤维基质呈平行的纵行条束状；常见类似局灶性结节增生的图像。镜下表现，以被层状纤维束分割的嗜伊红肿瘤细胞为特征。多数纤维板层型肝细胞癌组织结构均匀，可见梁索状排列的肿瘤细胞与层状纤维混杂。大量纤维呈平行条束状或层状排列，包绕嗜伊红染色的多边形肿瘤细胞，其核仁较大，核有丝分裂相稀少。25% 病例有不典型区，可有典型的梁索状肝细胞癌。

临床表现：纤维板层型肝细胞癌发生于无肝硬化背景的青年患者，年龄范围 20~30 岁，患者中 35 岁以下者比例达 15%~40%，有作者认为纤维板层型肝细胞癌在 35 岁以下无基础肝脏病变的肝细胞癌中占 43%。男女发病率相近，有报告女性：男性 =（1~2）:1。

临床症状无特征性，有时偶然发现；以腹部肿块和上腹部不适为主，可有体重下降、厌食、腹痛、肝肿大，男性乳房发育也曾见报道，并被认为系继发于肝脏肿瘤引起的雄性激素芳香化过程增强。绝大多数患者无肝硬化基础、少有乙型肝炎病毒感染，肝炎血清学检查大多阴性。甲胎蛋白多阴性。纤维板层型肝细胞癌虽然肿块较大，但手术切除率高，有较好的预后。即使术后复发，也可再切除，术后生存期 32~68 个月，甚至更高。

影像学研究：超声成像可表现为低 - 高回声强度肿块，边界多较清楚。伴有出血，坏死及瘢痕形成时，表现为病灶中心回声密度不均匀。约 30% 肿瘤发生不均匀的非特异性钙化则可见伴有声影的强回声区。

CT：纤维板层型肝细胞癌的典型表现为平扫时呈低 - 等密度病灶，边缘清晰，可有分叶，中央瘢痕呈边界清楚星状或不规则低密度，30% 病灶中心可见斑点状钙化，肝门内淋巴结增大。增强扫描时，动脉期肿瘤实质均匀或弥散性早期强化，门静脉期肿瘤实质强化消退快，密度较周围的肝组织低。中央瘢痕在动脉期及门静脉期大多无明确强化。少数（25%）纤维板层型肝细胞癌在延时期出现强化。是由于这些中央瘢痕内含有血管间质成分所致。肝门部淋巴结转移率高于普通型肝细胞癌。纤维板层型肝细胞癌在 CT 图像上无明显特异性，但在年轻和无肝硬化的患者中，若发现肝内巨大肿块，除外海绵状血管瘤后，应考虑到纤维板层型肝细胞癌的可能性，但应注意与局灶性结节增生鉴别。

MRI：纤维板层型肝细胞癌的影像学表现以 MRI 较具特征。MR 扫描时，肿瘤 T_1WI 86% 为低信号，14% 为等信号，80% 的病例信号均匀；T_2WI 上肿瘤信号不均匀，多为高信号。中心瘢痕，在所有序列上基本都为低信号，这反映着瘢痕的高度胶原化性质，是一个很重要的鉴别点；然而还是有少数为高信号（类似局灶性结节增生的中央瘢痕——在 T_2WI 上高信号）。

纤维板层型肝细胞癌的 MRI 影像有以下特点：

不均匀信号强度，T_2WI 肿块内有低信号区；增强后肿瘤立即出现弥漫不均匀强化，并迅速变为与肝脏等密度；中心瘢痕即使在动态增强延迟像上也无强化。中心瘢痕同样可见于普通型肝细胞癌和巨大肝血管瘤，但是，普通型肝细胞癌钙化相当少见，而血管瘤则在血管造影中表现出血供更为丰富的影像学特点。局灶性结节状增生和少数高分化肝细胞癌的中央瘢痕与纤维板层型肝细胞癌不同，在SE序列 T_2WI 中呈高信号，并可在注入对比剂后出现强化。局灶性结节状增生的中央瘢痕增强仅见于延迟像中。

X线血管造影：纤维板层型肝细胞癌大多呈富血状态，可有大量肿瘤血管形成。偶有动-静脉短路。

核医学：肝胆连续闪烁照相为“冷病灶”，可与局灶性结节增生鉴别。

鉴别诊断：纤维板层型肝细胞癌的影像学表现与发生于肝脏的其他肿瘤（如：局灶性结节状增生，普通型肝细胞癌，肝腺瘤，巨大肝血管瘤，转移瘤等）有许多相互重迭之处。MRI对于鉴别诊断甚为重要。局灶性结节状增生、肝腺瘤、普通型肝细胞癌以及富血性肝转移瘤，在增强MRI中也可在注入对比剂后立即增强，并迅速变为同正常肝脏的等密度，但其强化多较均匀。

另外，年轻患者肿瘤内部见不规则钙化，肝内并见卫星灶存在，有利于纤维板层型肝细胞癌的诊断。但是，对于小的肿瘤，这些特征不一定适用。小的纤维板层型肝细胞癌可以在 T_2WI 和动态增强像中表现比较均匀；局灶性结节增生常可与纤维板层型肝细胞癌有相同的表现，但钙化发生率较低。因此，为获得正确诊断，取得足够量的活检标本常属必要。

普通型肝细胞癌：普通型肝细胞癌内可以出现纤维瘢痕，但是一般数量较少，罕见有钙化，临床常有肝硬化和甲胎蛋白升高。

肝海绵状血管瘤：肝海绵状血管瘤在动脉期可见边缘早期团状或点状强化，并由周边向中央蔓延，延时期肿瘤内强化消退慢，呈等密度或稍高于周围肝组织密度。

局灶性结节增生：形态上与本病相似，但钙化发生率低，强化较本病均匀。一些作者指出，务必注意！纤维层板型肝细胞癌不仅在影像诊断上与局灶性结节增生相似，而且活检时还可出现假阴性结果。

肝细胞腺瘤：肝细胞腺瘤常为单发圆形病灶，有包膜及瘤内出血，动脉期均匀强化，门静脉期为等密度或低密度，临床特点为青年女性患者，有的有长期口服避孕药史。

支持纤维层板型肝细胞癌的诊断标准：年轻病人，无预先存在的肝脏疾病，肿瘤内钙化，“中央”瘢痕，T_2 图像呈低信号，用Hepatobida后无浓集现象。

第七章　外生型肝癌

第一节　外生型肝癌

外生型肝癌,是指向肝外生长、增殖的原发性肝细胞癌,是原发性肝细胞癌在生长方式和外观形态上的一种特殊类型,肿瘤带蒂或主要向肝外突出生长,而且肝外部分最大横径应大于肝内部分。本病由 Roux(1897)首先报道并命名。成年人多见,50~60 岁为发病高峰,男性多于女性,其发生率约为 4.2%,容易误诊。

根据外生型肝癌肿块附着于肝脏的情况可分为带蒂型和无蒂型两类:带蒂型指肿瘤有明确的蒂带与肝脏连接,瘤体完全位于肝外,通过瘤带与肝脏相连并获取营养。可侵犯周围组织器官并与周围组织建立新的血液循环。因此只要观察到其带,影像诊断病灶来源相对容易;无蒂型也称为突出型,肿瘤主要向肝外突出,少部分仍位于肝内或病灶仅部分与肝缘相连,肿瘤也可以侵犯周围组织器官。带蒂型罕见,突出型相对多见。

外生型肝癌多膨胀性生长,病灶常常较大,压迫甚至侵犯周围组织,因此无蒂型外生肝癌影像诊断其来源定位较困难,容易误诊为周围其他脏器(如胃、十二指肠、胰头、肾上腺、腹膜后等)的肿瘤。螺旋 CT 多期增强扫描及多平面重建技术对无蒂型外生型肝癌的诊断有重要价值。按照 Eggel(1901)的分类,肝细胞癌分为巨块型、结节型和弥漫型。带蒂的肝细胞癌以它的蒂与肝相连接,基本上不侵入肝脏。Goldberg 和 Wallerstein(1934)报告一例出现于肝左叶的下表面,其蒂粗约 1.5cm。Okuda(1980)统计日本 1968—1977 年 4 031 例肝癌中,本型肝癌有 10 例,占 0.3%。Horie 等(1983)统计日本 Tottori 大学医院等单位 1977—1980 年 123 例肝癌中发现本型肝癌 3 例,占 2.4%。Horie 等(1999)报道,外生型肝癌的发病率约占原发性肝癌的 0.24%~3.00%。

Horie 等(1983)复习 1934—1981 年英文与日文文献报告共 15 例,其中男性占 11 例,年龄分布为 33~80 岁(平均 60 岁),15 例中只有 4 例是术前作出诊断的。肿瘤大小变化较大,最小者直径仅 3cm。发生于右叶者有 11 例。15 例均出现于肝的下表面或肝的边缘。文献有描述的 13 例中,有 10 例为肝硬化病人。带蒂的肝细胞癌还可出现在异位的肝组织。异位的肝组织已发现可发生于不同的部位,包括肝的三角韧带、脾脏、脐凹、网膜、腹膜后腔、腹腔干周围、胆囊及其附近。完全相同的病理改变出现于肝和异位肝组织。由于肝癌病例已有报告见于胸腔和腹膜后腔,可能都是源自于异位肝组织。

病理学:该病发病原因目前尚不十分清楚,可能与下列因素有关:①先天畸形的肝叶病变;②副肝叶病变;③异位肝组织癌变;④肝硬化,再生结节超出肝外并发生癌变。外生型肝癌符合肝炎、肝硬化、肝癌的一般发展规律,病情进展较缓慢,以肝内转移为主,可侵犯周围器官,腹腔转移少见。

外生型肝癌多分化较好,以中高分化为主。外生型肝癌患者甲胎蛋白增高多不明显,绝对数值较一般原发性肝癌低,可能与外生型肝癌病理类型多为高分化肝细胞性肝癌有关;同时由于病灶向肝外膨胀性生长,出现转移及周围侵犯较晚,引起症状而被发现时常常体积较大,推压周围组织,在临床中多误诊为胃、十二指肠、肾上腺、胰头、腹膜后等病变,其中以无蒂型误诊率最高,因为有蒂者当发现蒂带与肝脏相连,多能引起注意,较容易想象肝脏来源。一般认为外生型肝癌预后比肝内原发性肝癌好,其 1、3、5 年生存率明显优于肝内肝细胞性肝癌,可能瘤体膨胀性向外生长,包膜完好,有足够的切除范围,少有血管侵犯和组织分化较好等因素有关。但

Horie 等（1983）认为，由于外生型肝癌具有迅速生长及恶性侵犯的本性，如果不能早发现及时进行手术（特别是在肿瘤侵犯血管之前），其生存率与肝内肝细胞性肝癌无明显差异。因此，认识和正确诊断外生型肝癌的重要意义就是为手术争取机会，避免因肿瘤巨大的表象而放弃治疗。

临床表现：外生型肝癌是指肿瘤主要向肝外生长，肝实质较少累及或基本不累及，有蒂与肝脏相连或直接贴附于肝脏，属原发性肝癌的特殊类型，临床较为少见。Horie 等（1999）报道，外生型肝癌的发病率约占原发性肝癌的 0.24%~3.00%。一些作者报道的外生型肝癌占原发性肝癌的 3.7%（7/190）。该院同期收治原发性肝癌 575 例，其中外生型肝癌仅 17 例，占 2.96%。外生型肝癌以中老年男性发病居多，男：女＝ 3：1，50~60 岁为发病高峰。

外生型肝癌以向肝外生长为主，生长空间相对较大，早期不易发现，当出现腹部胀痛或扪及腹部包块时，瘤体往往已经较大，一组病例最大直径均已达到巨块型肝癌的诊断标准，平均直径超过 11 cm；如果肿瘤自肝脏膈面向膈下生长，由于空间相对较小，膈面易受侵犯而较早出现右侧肩背部放射痛，此时肿瘤可能相对较小，该组 2 例患者即具有此特点。该组外生型肝癌的乙型肝炎表面抗原和甲胎蛋白阳性率都较高，分别为 82.35%、76.47%，与肝内原发性肝癌相当。甲胎蛋白阳性率与一些作者的报道相似，但与国外文献报道外生型肝癌乙型肝炎表面抗原阳性率较低的特点有所不同，可能与我国的乙肝高发病率有关。该组病例合并肝硬化的占 58.82%（10/17），略低于肝内原发性肝癌，且肝功能代偿良好，Child 分级 14 例为 A 级，考虑可能是因为外生型肝癌主要向肝外生长，肝脏受损相对较轻的缘故。有作者认为，无肝硬化的外生型肝癌可能是先天畸形的肝叶或副叶癌。由于外生型肝癌主要向肝外生长，极少对胆系造成侵犯或压迫，故极少出现梗阻性黄疸。

外生型肝癌好发于肝脏的脏面，呈膨胀性生长，多有包膜，因较少侵犯肝组织及门静脉系统，患者多无临床症状，常因体检或肿瘤破裂而发现，瘤体巨大且有完整包膜，少有门脉癌栓和淋巴转移，是外生型肝癌的另一重要特点，其中包膜在 CT 上难以直接显示，仅表现为瘤体境界清楚，边缘光整。

影像学研究：目前 CT 检查在肝癌的监测和诊断中起着举足轻重的作用，特别是 MSCT，扫描速度更快、范围更大，可行多期扫描等优点，更提高了诊断的准确率。同样，螺旋 CT 多期扫描和多平面重建技术，对外生型肝癌的诊断有重要价值，更有利于全面观察了解病灶的血供、内部情况及周围关系。经过多平面重建处理，从多角度观察和了解病变的形态及解剖关系，并能更好地显示肿块局部向肝外突出，且与肝脏相连，与周围器官分界清楚，有助于进一步明确判断肿块的起源。

无蒂型外生型肝癌螺旋 CT 表现在许多个方面和肝内肝细胞性肝癌基本一致：①肿瘤一般显示低密度，少数显示等密度或稍高密度，密度的差别主要取决于肿瘤的分化和成分；②在低密度的肿块内，可见更低密度的不规则坏死区，在增强扫描时更明显，病灶内的更低密度区无强化，多位于病灶中心呈不规则斑点状、条片状，甚至是蟹足状或星茫状，并可见于多个层面，这种“更低密度区”是肝细胞性肝癌有别于肝其他肿瘤的 CT 特征之一；③增强扫描对比剂在肿瘤内多表现为“快进快出”，即病灶在动脉期肿瘤不均匀强化，以周边强化明显，且可见扭曲、增粗的血管影，门静脉期开始排空，部分有门脉供血或以门脉供血为主的肿块可呈继续强化，延时期病灶强化必然进一步减退，低于肝实质密度；④“晕圈征”：肿瘤多显类圆形，周围可见完全或不完全的环状带，“晕圈征”的病理基础为“假包膜”，增强检查“假包膜”强化以门脉期较明显；⑤伴有肝硬化（脾大）、门静脉癌栓、肝内转移、肝动脉与门静脉分流、肝门及肝内胆管压迫性扩张、腹水等征象。发现门静脉癌栓可以提示诊断。部分外生型肝癌是由于肝硬化再生结节突出肝外恶变而来，因此，发现肝硬化基础及肝内子灶可以提示诊断。

无蒂型外生型肝癌，除了具有上述肝细胞癌的 CT 特征表现外，尚具有其他的特点：如肿瘤于肝边缘向外膨胀性生长，肿块一般较大，内部多数密度不均，“更低密度区”更常见，且更容易出血、破裂，肿块除了肝动脉供血外，还可以有周围肝外动脉供血，更能体现“快进快出”的特点；病灶与肝缘连接处边界不清及并可见“鸟嘴征”，强烈提示病灶来源于肝脏、向外生长。

肿瘤与肝脏以宽基底或窄颈接触，肿瘤呈弧形不同程度压迫肝组织并向肝内突入，与正常肝组织分界清楚，两者交界区在不同层面和不同角度上可有不同表现，部分层面显示肝组织呈喇叭口样包绕部分肿瘤，是判断肿瘤起源于肝脏的较特征性的征象,由于肿瘤与正常肝组织强化不一致,在增强扫描图像上此征象更容易识别。部分层面显示肿瘤与肝缘呈锐角,类似肿瘤外压性改变,易造成肿瘤起源误判。

无蒂型外生型肝癌的特殊性在于其生长位置,CT 诊断的难点也就在于定位,因此,当在临床工作中遇见腹部肿块与肝脏相邻或有密切关系时,要提高警惕,考虑是否有外生型肝癌可能,应认真观察病灶内部及周围特点,如果 CT 平扫及增强多方面符合肝细胞性肝癌的表现,行 CT 多平面重建进一步确认肿块与肝脏的关系,再结合临床资料(病史、症状、实验室检查等)综合分析,诊断起来就更有把握,就能进一步提高诊断的正确性。

肿瘤血供一般来自于起源器官的供血动脉,显示肿瘤供血动脉是判断其起源的直接征象,外生型肝癌与肝内肝细胞性肝癌具有相同的血供特点,主要由肝动脉供血。外生型肝癌瘤体大部分位于肝外, MSCTA 上显示其扩张的供血动脉近段于正常肝内走行,于交界区伸入瘤体内分支供血,窄颈或蒂带连接者常为一支供血动脉,广基底者可有 2~3 支供血动脉进入瘤体供血。MSCTA 能通过显示肝动脉及其分支供血而准确判断肿瘤起源,是一种简单、可靠的定位诊断方法。由于外生型肝癌较大,向外生长过程中推挤周围组织,部分可与周围组织形成丰富的侧支循环,所以部分外生型肝癌可能会有肝动脉外的血供,有的病例即见胃十二指肠动脉的分支参与供血。

肝左叶与胃、胰腺、脾脏及左侧膈肌等紧邻,局部空间狭小,左叶源性外生型肝癌周围器官受压明显,肿瘤与器官间的脂肪组织因慢性压迫而吸收,间隙狭小甚至消失,一旦肿瘤穿破包膜,容易造成周围器官侵犯。

横结肠及结肠肝曲移动范围大,向下空间相对开阔,右叶及尾状叶源性外生型肝癌容易向腹盆腔方向生长,较少受到脏器阻挡,与周围器官间隙多较清楚。

该组外生型肝癌中经手术病理证实的 4 例 5 个病灶周围器官侵犯均为左叶源性外生型肝癌,CT 平扫和增强扫描仅 1 处胰腺侵犯得到准确诊断, 4 处漏诊,其中 1 例与胃壁间隙较清楚而漏诊胃壁侵犯,3 例肿瘤与周围器官间隙不清而过度诊断为侵犯,因此,单纯依靠肿瘤与器官间隙变化判断有无侵犯,可能造成误诊。

无血供联系的周围器官动脉出现向肿瘤侧支供血,是 MSCTA 诊断器官受侵犯的依据和可靠征象,但多出现在较晚期一项中 2 例胃壁、1 例网膜侵犯,显示胃左、胃右动脉及胃网膜右动脉侧支供血肿瘤,肿瘤侵犯周围器官侧支供血动脉显影率和诊断敏感度较高。

Longmaid 等(1986)指出,在 CT 检查时,肝细胞癌可表现为原发性肝外包块,他们报告 7 例肝癌均如此误诊,全部病例皆经皮穿刺活检、手术切除或尸检证实。这些病例在临床资料与 X 线检查发现的基础上事前无一怀疑为肝癌,其中 3 例起初疑及肝癌,但因其病史、胎甲球阴性、CT 扫描示包块位于肝外而考虑为其他疾病。该作者强调,尽管此类情况并不多见,但在怀疑肝癌的诊断时应想到它的可能性。

鉴别诊断:外生型肝癌起源于肝右叶后段者,应与胰头癌、右肾上腺及右肾肿块、腹膜后肿块等鉴别;起源于尾状叶的外生型肝癌应与胰腺内分泌肿瘤鉴别;起源于右叶前段的外生型肝癌应与胆囊癌相鉴别;起源于左叶外侧段的外生型肝癌应与肝左叶变异、肝门肿块、胃及十二指肠肿块等鉴别。

外生型肝癌侵犯周围器官后,可能出现肝动脉和受侵犯器官动脉双重供血,有时会造成定位诊断上的困难,一般情况下,肝动脉于肝脏内走行,于肿瘤与肝脏交界区伸入瘤体内,供血肿瘤的绝大部分区域,而侧支动脉主干走行于肝脏和肿瘤之外,供血受侵犯区域旁少部分肿瘤组织,亦可见细小分支供血受侵器官,仔细追踪观察动脉供血区域和范围,多可做出鉴别诊断。

无蒂型外生型肝癌有时诊断困难,但进行肝脏动态多期扫描,还是具备肝癌的平扫及增强特点,还可以找到肿瘤起源于某一肝叶的证据,尤其应用三维重建,可更好地显示肿块与肝脏的关系,从而明确诊断。有作者报告 1 例左叶外段巨大无蒂型外生型肝癌,外院 CT 误诊为胃间质瘤,但仔细分析病灶平扫及强化特点,仍然符合典型的肝癌表现,从而确诊。

外生型肝癌往往具有典型的临床及 CT 表现特征,综合运用临床表现、瘤蒂、肝动脉供血、“速升速降”型强化等特点将能提高外生型肝癌的诊断准确率。

第二节　误诊病例简介：外生性肝癌，低分化肝细胞性肝癌淋巴转移

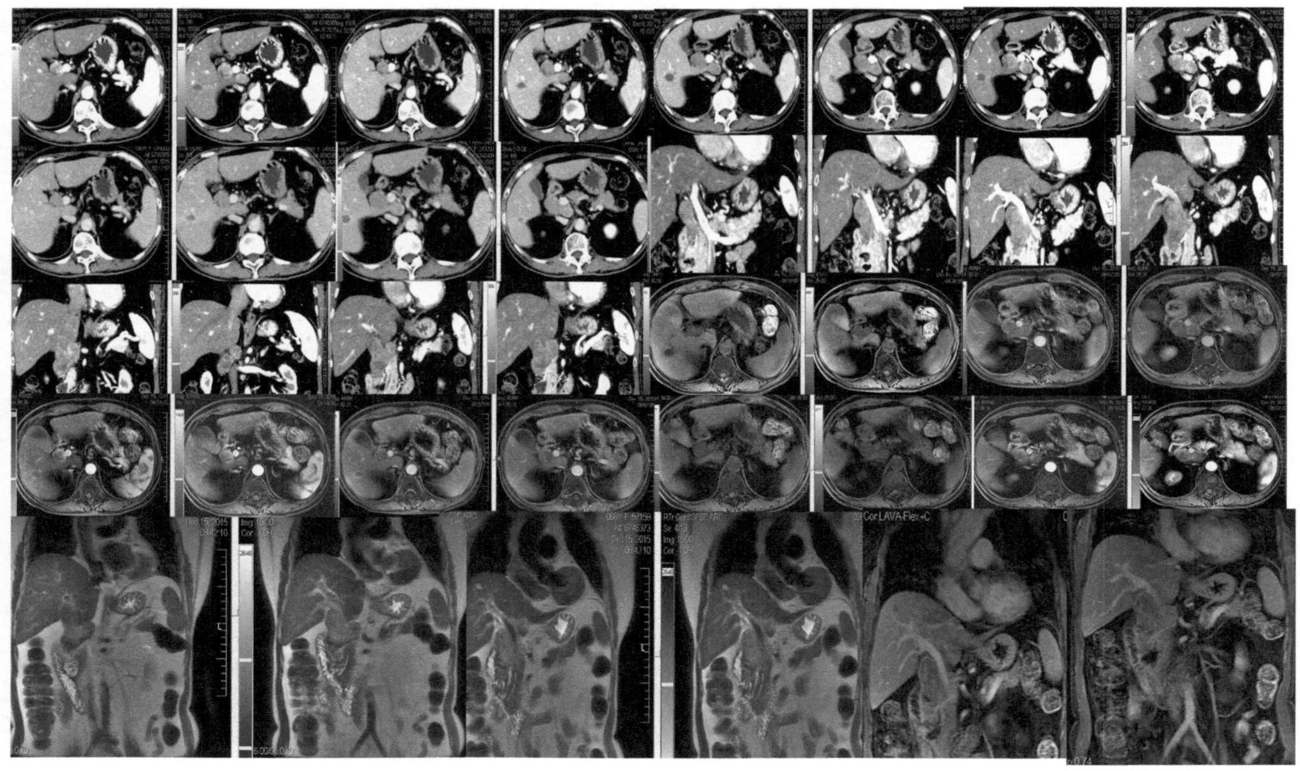

图 3-7-1　外生性肝癌

患者，女，68 岁。腰背酸痛不适 2 月入院。患者缘于 2 月前无明显诱因出现腰背部酸痛不适，活动后减轻，1 周前在街道卫生服务中心体检示甲胎蛋白 >500IU/ml，后就诊于院甲胎蛋白 >3000IU/ml，彩超示腹膜后实性肿物，考虑恶性肿瘤。今日 CT 增强扫描示肝门部胰十二指肠后部占位，与邻近肝尾叶、胰腺、门静脉分界欠清，考虑恶性肿瘤。

手术所见：肝十二指肠韧带内未触及肿大淋巴结，胆总管直径约 6mm，管壁无水肿增厚；切开十二指肠侧腹膜探查，可扪及一直径约 6.0cm × 5.0cm × 2.0cm 的肿块，肿瘤组织包膜完整，与十二指肠及胆总管右侧壁粘连，胰头组织无侵犯，肿瘤组织与肝尾状叶未见组织相连。Kocher 手法扩大十二指肠外侧后腹膜切口，将十二指肠第二、三段从腹膜后向前游离至腹主动脉前面，见十二指肠后方、胰头右侧缘一直径约 6.0cm × 5.0cm × 2.0cm 的肿块，下腔静脉和腹主动脉、门静脉、胰腺未见肿瘤侵犯；切开肝十二指肠韧带，清扫肝十二指肠韧带内脂肪组织，骨骼化显露肝总动脉、门静脉、胆总管，将肝总动脉、门静脉、胆总管予以红色导尿管牵向左侧，沿瘤体包膜逐步分离，完整切除瘤体组织。

病理检查：冰冻病理：腹腔肿瘤：灰红色肿物一块，大小 5.5cm × 4.5cm × 2cm，切面呈模糊结节状，可见出血及坏死，灰黄、灰红、暗褐相间，质偏软。冰冻病理诊断：腹腔肿瘤切除标本：镜下示淋巴纤维间质中可见异型的上皮样细胞巢，伴出血及坏死，结合临床病史，首选考虑肝细胞癌，待做常规石蜡切片及免疫组化检测进一步证实。常规病理诊断：腹腔肿瘤切除标本：镜下示淋巴纤维间质中可见异型的上皮样细胞巢，伴出血及坏死，结合临床病史，首选考虑肝细胞性肝癌，待做免疫组化检测进一步证实。

免疫组化检测：阳性：Hepatocyte，AFP，CD34（肝窦内皮血管化 +），CK8，CK18，CD10（散在 +），Villin，Vimentin（肝窦内皮血管化 +），P53（+，<1%），Ki-67（+，约 60%）；阴性：CK19，CK7，CK20，WT-1，CK5/6，CEA，EMA，P63，CA19-9。免疫组化诊断：腹腔肿瘤切除标本：镜下所见的异型上皮样细胞巢，伴明显出血及坏死，经做免疫组化检测，证实为低分化肝细胞性肝癌。同时，癌巢周围可见淋巴组织结构，结合临床及影像学检查，不排除淋巴结肝癌转移。肝穿刺活检标本：示结节性肝硬化伴肝细胞异型增生（图 3-7-1）。

第八章　硬化型肝癌

硬化型肝癌是肝细胞癌中的一种少见亚型。临床上,硬化型肝癌常被误诊为其他富含纤维结缔组织的肝脏原发或继发性恶性肿瘤,术前正确诊断困难。WHO 定义硬化型肝癌的特征为瘤内存在显著的纤维化,肝内存在多发肿瘤时,硬化型肝癌与普通类型肝癌可能并存。组织病理上,肿瘤细胞呈束状或巢状被纤维结缔组织所包绕,内部呈血窦样增生结构,周边可有放射样纤维瘢痕束向肿瘤中心延伸,部分伴有透明样变,瘤内纤维化 3 种类型常并存。组织病理学上,硬化型肝癌比较容易和肝内胆管细胞癌、混合型肝癌和纤维板层样肝癌区别。硬化型肝癌患者年龄、性别、肝炎病毒阳性率、甲胎蛋白水平、Child-Pugh 分级和肿瘤 TNM 分期和普通类型肝细胞癌差异无统计学意义,但硬化型肝癌患者整体存活率高于普通类型肝细胞癌。

一项 32 例研究中,30 例有肝炎病史,17 例合并肝硬化,和文献报道结果不符,分析其原因可能与肝炎肝硬化患者合并肝癌时往往因为肝储备功能不佳而无法进行手术有关,该项研究中手术切除及肝移植者仅 7 例,其余 25 例由穿刺活检病理证实。

影像学研究:一些作者对 7 例硬化型肝癌的研究显示,其动脉期及门静脉期强化方式多样,肝实质期表现为边缘强化和 / 或中心分隔样强化。Kim 等(2007)对 4 例硬化型肝癌研究显示,其影像表现主要为动脉期薄厚不均的边缘环状强化,门静脉期及肝实质期病灶呈同心圆形或不规则形向心性强化。该项研究中,硬化型肝癌的影像表现可分为下述三种:

(1)动脉期边缘厚薄不均的环状强化,门静脉期及肝实质期肿瘤出现向心性强化,向心性强化方式可为同心圆性或不规则性,此种表现具有一定特征性。Kim 等(2007)认为此影像表现的机制是在肿瘤边缘以瘤细胞为主,伴随少量富血管的纤维组织,肿瘤内部含有丰富的纤维间质和少量的瘤细胞。

(2)动脉期肿瘤无明显强化或不同程度的不均匀强化,门静脉期及肝实质期肿瘤边缘环状强化及内部分隔样强化。此种影像表现类似于大多数富含纤维间质的恶性肿瘤,如胆管细胞癌、转移性腺癌等的强化方式。

(3)动脉期肿瘤轻度不均匀强化,门静脉期及肝实质期对比剂流出,肿瘤呈明显低密度改变,类似于典型的结节型肝细胞癌的影像表现,影像鉴别困难,文献中也有个案报道。考虑其原因可能是瘤体较小所致,该项研究中 2 例及文献报道 1 例的病灶直径均 <15 mm,病理结果显示瘤体内部纤维化程度与前 2 种无明显区别,病灶内部无出血及坏死。2 例 MR 检查平扫 T_1WI 为均匀低信号, T_2WI 为不均匀高信号,不同 b 值时 DWI 均为明显不均匀高信号表现,增强扫描强化方式类似于 CT 扫描第一种强化方式,动脉期病灶呈边缘环状强化,门静脉期及肝实质期进行性不规则向心性强化,瘤体较小者平衡期对比剂完全填充,呈不均匀高信号改变,瘤体较大者延迟 50 min 行肝胆期扫描可见对比剂进一步向病灶中心区填充。

鉴别诊断:硬化型肝癌应与肝脏良性病变(如海绵状血管瘤)、富含纤维间质成分的肝脏原发及继发恶性肿瘤(如肝内胆管细胞癌、转移癌、混合型肝癌、纤维板层型肝癌、肉瘤样癌等)相鉴别。

肝内胆管细胞癌:肝内胆管细胞癌增强扫描动脉期病变周边正常肝组织可见带状强化,肿瘤本身可见边缘少许强化或无明显强化,门静脉期及肝实质期病变持久强化,并可见内部分隔样强化,病灶区常可见扩张的胆管。

纤维板层型肝癌:纤维板层型肝癌多见于无肝硬化基础的年轻人,肿瘤多有完整或不完整包膜,中央可见星状纤维瘢痕,瘢痕内有时可见钙化,增强扫描动脉期至门静脉期肿瘤实质呈持续性强化,肝实质期中心瘢痕组织可见强化,其中央瘢痕组织在 T_1WI、T_2WI 均为低信号。

混合型肝癌:混合型肝癌影像表现多样,强化方式取决于肿瘤成分的比例和分布。

该项研究的不足之处在于,手术切除患者较少,对病变的影像表现和病理的对照研究尚不全面;行MR检查的患者较少,不能对硬化型肝癌的MR影像特征进行总结,有待今后积累更多患者。

第九章　肉瘤样肝细胞癌

肉瘤样肝细胞癌，是指肿瘤的大部分或全部被肉瘤样梭形细胞替代，又称肝细胞癌肉瘤样变、梭形细胞型肝癌，约占肝癌尸检的3.9%~9.4%，占肝癌外科手术切除的1.8%。肿瘤好发于50~60岁，男性发病率明显高于女性，约为5倍。据统计，约46%患者可见甲胎蛋白升高，但多数不超过400μg/ml。病变生长快，恶性度高，边缘不规则，无明确的包膜，易侵犯周围组织、发生肝内播散、肝外转移和腹膜种植等。原发性肉瘤样肝细胞癌CT表现较普通型肝细胞癌相对不典型，术前容易误诊。与肝细胞癌的高发生率相反，肝细胞癌肉瘤样变发生率低。但经动脉化疗栓塞治疗肝细胞癌后，肉瘤样变的发生率呈上升趋势。肉瘤样变的肝细胞癌转移率高于普通型肝细胞癌，淋巴结转移和肝内转移亦明显多于普通型肝细胞癌，预后差，故对其正确诊断具有重要的临床意义。

病理学：肝细胞癌发生肉瘤样变后，呈侵袭性窦状生长无纤维包膜，故易于发生肝内转移、门脉侵犯和肝外转移。肉瘤样肝细胞肝癌由分化很差的细胞组成，生长快，由于血供不充分容易导致中间坏死。肉瘤样肝细胞癌的一部分或大部分被肉瘤样“纺锤”形或“梭”形肿瘤细胞替代，其内不含明确的横纹肌肉瘤、骨肉瘤成分，因此而区别于癌肉瘤。

文献报道癌瘤内肉瘤样成分占多少比例时称肉瘤样癌尚无明确的定义，但一般认为肉瘤样成分>50%者称为肉瘤样癌，<50%者称为小区或灶性肉瘤样变。

梭形细胞呈编织状或腺泡状排列，除与癌肉瘤鉴别外，还需与肌源性肉瘤、纤维源性肉瘤以及软骨肉瘤等鉴别。梭形细胞与典型的肝细胞肝癌常同时出现，免疫组织化学染色显示，梭形细胞可同时呈甲胎蛋白、Hep、肝组织细胞角蛋白（CK）和Vimentin阳性，提示来自肝细胞肝癌细胞的间叶性化生或肉瘤样变。

关于具有肉瘤样变表现和典型肝细胞癌特征的肝脏原发肿瘤，是肝细胞癌与肉瘤同时存在，抑或是肝细胞癌发生了肉瘤样变，既往曾有争论。由于真正意义的肝脏肉瘤发病率极低，而具有肉瘤样表现的肝脏原发肿瘤在免疫组化检查中常出现倾向于肝细胞癌的结果，目前一般认为，其本质系肝细胞癌部分发生肉瘤样变。

Kakizoe等（1987）曾认为发生肉瘤样变的肝细胞癌与普通型肝细胞癌在临床进程如生存期等方面并无明显差异，唯前者出现肝外转移的概率较高；但较后的研究认为肝细胞癌肉瘤样变使肿瘤的恶性程度增高，病变进展速度加快，故与普通型肝细胞癌的预后相比更差。因此，肝细胞癌肉瘤样变的及时和准确诊断具有重要临床意义。肿瘤切面可见瘤内灰白色固化和/或暗红色液化区，主要为凝固坏死与出血。组织学检查在肝细胞癌梁索状结构的基础上，常出现多种组织学表现，可见多形性梭状细胞。肿瘤外周有松散的共生连接和纤维基质，部分病变中见无纤维基质的变形细胞；中心部坏死不明显时，有散在的梁索状结构。

临床表现：患者多为男性，中年居多；乙型肝炎病毒的乙型肝炎三系阳性指标可能与该肿瘤有一定的关系，但常无肝硬化史及肝功能损害，此有别于一般的肝细胞肝癌；临床早期症状主要是腹痛和发热，缺乏特征性，但癌瘤生长速度快、侵袭力强，临床进展迅速。

影像学研究：CT平扫示原发性肉瘤样肝细胞癌病灶普遍较大，呈巨块型。病灶直径普遍较大的原因可能与其内的肉瘤样成分生长较快有关。肿瘤多为单发。Koo等（2008）认为较大肿瘤常伴有周围转移灶，较普通肝细胞癌更易发生转移，但门静脉癌栓相对少见。病灶发生部位以肝右叶为多。病灶边界及内部坏死区边缘清楚或比较清楚居多，边界不清者恶性程度较高，容易发生转移。病灶内密度不均匀，其内更低密度且不强化影与瘤内坏死及玻璃样变有关，多位于病灶的非中央区，与普通肝癌坏死常位于中心不同，也较普通型肝细胞癌坏死更常见，容易发生坏死的原因是由于肿瘤细胞分化差，生长迅速，肿瘤血管难以供应快速生长的肿瘤组织所致。所有病灶密度均低于正常肝组织，病灶密度不均匀，内部见不规则更低密度，位于病灶非中央区域，部分低密度区并见较厚分隔。病灶边界清楚或不清楚。

增强扫描：所有病灶动脉期均有强化，呈斑片状不均匀强化，内部更低密度区未见强化，门静脉期显示原动脉期强化区密度减低。延迟期部分病灶边缘及内部实性区或分隔有轻度延迟强化，部分病灶周围动脉期呈片状强化，门静脉期呈等密度。延迟期病灶边缘及内部实性区有轻度强化，表明活跃的癌组织内可能含有纤维间质等成分。

一般认为肿瘤低血供，影像表现缺乏特异性，与转移瘤不易鉴别。肿瘤CT平扫呈囊性低密度，中心可见不规则分隔，边缘部可见乳头状或结节状软组织密度影，但描述更类似未分化肉瘤。肝细胞癌肉瘤样变表现为不规则边界的肝内肿块，多呈完全低密度，少数亦可表现为中心低密度而外周高密度；有延迟或持续周边强化；常见肝内转移和淋巴结肿大。

由于肝细胞癌肉瘤样变后肿瘤细胞分化差，生长迅速，肿瘤血管难以为快速生长的肿瘤细胞提供足够的营养，故易出现坏死，使肉瘤样变的肝细胞癌中心坏死出血多于普通型肝细胞癌。这一特点在CT图像上得到明确显示。肿瘤周边环状强化表示含有纤维的多形肿瘤组织，中心不增强区域为凝固坏死和出血。延迟或持续增强与肿瘤的纤维基质有关。增大的间质腔隙以及造影剂进入血管和间质腔隙缓慢是强化延迟的主要原因。

一组两例肉瘤样肝细胞癌表现相似：动脉期及静脉期均为相对低密度，边缘不清，可累及肝被膜及周围组织。肿瘤内可见大片低密度坏死区。

在动态增强CT/MRI中，肿瘤表现为巨块膨胀型生长或多个结节融合而成，可伴有不完整的包膜。增强扫描显示病灶周边实质部分强化，中间不强化，分别对应于外周存活肿瘤组织和纤维间质，中间是坏死成分，实质成分强化表现可多种多样。由于周边肿瘤部分有延迟强化的表现，因此和肝内胆管细胞癌、混合型肝癌的表现有交叉重叠，有时不易鉴别。

本病需与以下病变相鉴别：

肝脓肿：因为原发性肉瘤样肝细胞癌的低密度病灶内可见条状分隔影，且动脉期部分病灶周围可见少许高灌注，有时与不典型肝脓肿不易鉴别。但肉瘤样肝细胞癌的低密度CT值较脓肿CT值高，且变化幅度大。肉瘤样肝细胞癌病灶周围无肝脓肿的环形低密度，同时也无白细胞计数增高表现。

转移性肿瘤：原发性肉瘤样肝细胞癌增强扫描常有病灶边缘及其内实性部分的延迟强化，与转移性肿瘤有相似之处，尤其当病灶多发或为转移性肉瘤时更难鉴别。

非血管性肝肉瘤：肝肉瘤一般也较大，增强扫描实性部分有强化，单发、囊实性居多，与本病较难鉴别，但肝肉瘤患者多无乙型肝炎病史，甲胎蛋白阴性，增强扫描并不同时具有肝癌“快进快退”的影像表现，可资鉴别。

延迟期周边强化在肝细胞癌肉瘤样变中通常远较其他肿瘤常见。延迟扫描中环形强化应与炎性假瘤相鉴别。部分肝细胞癌肉瘤样变可伴有发热，需行其他X线检查或活检以明确诊断。发现肝内边界不规则的肿块，延迟期或持续周边强化，同时伴有肝内转移和淋巴结转移，尤其是在既往曾诊断肝细胞癌，并施行经动脉化疗栓塞的情况下，应考虑肝细胞癌肉瘤样变的可能。

第十章 混合型肝癌

第一节 混合型肝细胞癌-胆管细胞癌

病理学:人们对混合型肝癌的认识已长达半个世纪之久，Allen 和 Lisa(1949)首次对其进行报道并将其分为3种类型。A型:肝细胞肝癌和胆管细胞癌在肝脏不同部位,不接触。B型:肝细胞肝癌和胆管细胞癌相邻,互相混合生长。C型:肝细胞肝癌与胆管细胞癌混合,在同一肿瘤中生长,相互移行,密不可分。Goodman(1985)提出不同的分型:Ⅰ型,碰撞型肿瘤;Ⅱ型,移行型肿瘤;Ⅲ型,纤维板层样肿瘤。Goodman Ⅰ型相当于 Allen A 型和 B 型。

目前 WHO 对混合型肝癌进行了重新定义,将在同一部位发生包含肝细胞癌与胆管细胞癌2种成分且相互混杂或移行者,称为混合型肝细胞癌-胆管癌,因此部分学者认为仅 Allen C 型属于真正组织学意义上的混合型肝癌。按此定义,一组18例均属于混合型肝癌。混合型肝细胞癌-胆管细胞癌组织来源目前尚无一致意见。

Cazals-Hatem 等(2004)进行的基因遗传学方面的研究发现混合型肝细胞癌-胆管细胞癌的组织来源更接近于胆管细胞癌。也有作者提出可能来源于更原始的肝祖细胞。因为肝细胞肝癌与胆管细胞癌2种成分混杂,比例不一,且临床和影像学表现不典型,混合型肝细胞癌-胆管细胞癌患者的术前诊断率很低。该组18例患者,多数在术前被误诊为肝细胞癌成胆管细胞癌。

混合型肝细胞癌-胆管细胞癌的恶性程度高,侵袭性强,同时具有肝细胞肝癌门脉侵犯及胆管细胞癌淋巴结转移的特征。也有报道称其生物学行为更接近于胆管细胞癌,其血管浸润及淋巴结转移率均明显高于肝细胞肝癌。混合型肝细胞癌-胆管细胞癌中的胆管细胞癌成分使其较单纯肝细胞肝癌更易发生转移,其预后也决定于病灶中的胆管细胞癌成分。

混合型肝细胞癌-胆管细胞癌切除术后3年、5年生存率分别为10%~50%、24%~30%;如不进行治疗,其生存率很低,分别为15%、6%,中位生存期为10~52个月,术后复发率高达81%~95%。其中,肿瘤大小、TNM分期、CA19-9水平、病灶数目以及淋巴结转移和血管侵犯情况均是影响混合型肝细胞癌-胆管细胞癌预后的重要因素。

对混合型肝细胞癌-胆管细胞癌的治疗方法仍以手术切除为主,并尽量施行广泛的淋巴结清扫,所以术前全面、准确的影像学评估具有重要意义,同时有利于指导穿刺活检在肿瘤内部不同部位取材,以便做出正确的诊断。

临床表现:混合型肝细胞癌-胆管细胞癌的临床特点报道不一,一方面可能与部分研究纳入病例数少,存在统计学偏倚有关,另一方面与混合型肝细胞癌-胆管细胞癌的概念不统一、病例选择标准不同有关。既往报道多是中老年起病,男性好发,亚洲人群多伴有肝炎病毒的感染及肝硬化。该组资料中,混合型肝细胞癌-胆管细胞癌的患者平均发病年龄为50.9岁,男性居多(94.4%),超过80%的患者具有乙型及丙型肝炎病毒的感染，72.2%的患者术前甲胎蛋白升高,其临床特征接近于肝细胞肝癌,而与胆管细胞癌差异较大。

有报道指出甲胎蛋白和CA19-9反映了病灶中的组织学成分,甲胎蛋白在肝细胞肝癌为主型中较高,CA19-9在胆管细胞癌为主型较高。该组因病例数较少,无法对其诊断价值进行评估。但该组资料发现67%的病例合并CA19-9升高,对于富血供的病灶,此指标有助于提示其内的胆管细胞癌成分。

影像学研究:有关混合型肝细胞癌-胆管细胞

癌的影像学表现报道较少，Sanada 等（2005）认为本病的 CT 表现和病理学特征相符，CT 动态增强扫描可以识别肿瘤中的肝细胞肝癌成分和胆管细胞癌成分。他们将 CT 增强方式分为 3 种类型：Ⅰ型以肝细胞肝癌成分为主，早期某区域显著强化，晚期对比剂廓清；Ⅱ型早期和晚期均呈现边缘强化；Ⅲ型肝细胞肝癌优势区对应于早期强化区域，胆管细胞癌优势区对应于晚期强化区域，并认为仅第 3 种类型可以术前明确诊断。该组资料的影像学表现和上述报道相似，大部分瘤灶或表现为肝细胞肝癌或胆管细胞癌为主的强化方式。其中 5 例表现出的增强方式和 Sanada 等（2005）报道的Ⅲ型强化方式相似，呈肝细胞肝癌和胆管细胞癌相混杂的增强方式，即动脉期呈片状或不规则，明显不均匀强化，随时间延长强化程度减低，强化范围逐渐向瘤体内部延伸，延迟期肿瘤局部仍可见对比剂滞留，表现为向心性延迟强化。该组研究认为该征象对于该病的诊断有一定的帮助。该组 8 例肝细胞肝癌为主的病灶中，4 例表现为胆管细胞癌常见的环形强化方式；10 例胆管细胞癌为主的病灶中，4 例表现为肝细胞肝癌快进快出的强化方式。所以该组作者认为增强 CT 及 MRI 检查能否确定病灶中的主要成分还有待于收集更多病例进行进一步研究。

此外，该组作者发现尽管胆管细胞癌为主型多表现为近似胆管细胞癌的增强方式，但胆管细胞癌的易患因素肝内胆管结石及胆管炎仅见于 2 例，这在混合型肝细胞癌 - 胆管细胞癌与胆管细胞癌的鉴别诊断中具有重要的提示作用。

该项研究的局限性：首先，因本病发病率低，该项研究的病例数目较少。其次，该项研究为回顾性分析，未能对各病例相对应的病理结构进行更详细的分析研究。

混合型肝细胞癌 - 胆管细胞癌是原发性肝癌中的一种少见类型，具有男性发病率、肝炎及肝硬化合并率、癌栓发生率、淋巴结转移率高等特点。临床特征不典型，术前诊断较困难，确诊需病理学检查。但是结合临床特征和影像学表现，以下三种情况存在时需要考虑混合型肝细胞癌 - 胆管细胞癌的可能：

病灶呈肝细胞肝癌和胆管细胞癌相混杂的增强方式，即动脉期呈片状或不规则，明显不均匀强化，随时间延长强化程度减低，强化范围逐渐向瘤体内部延伸，延迟期肿瘤局部仍可见对比剂滞留，表现为向心性延迟强化。肿瘤表现为胆管细胞癌的增强方式，但不伴有肝内胆管扩张和结石，同时伴有血清甲胎蛋白水平增高。肿瘤表现为肝细胞肝癌的增强方式，同时伴有 CA19-9 升高。

第二节　肝内混合型肝癌（胆管细胞癌 + 肝细胞癌）病例

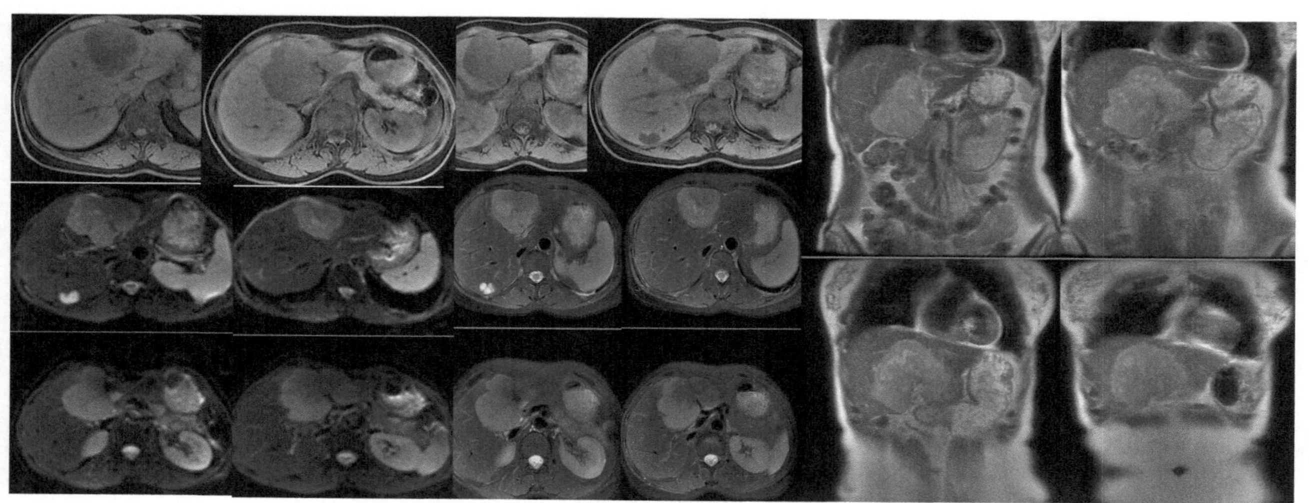

图 3-10-1　肝内混合型肝癌

患者，女，51 岁。缘于半年前无明显诱因出现右上腹疼痛不适，呈胀痛性质，无他处放射痛，疼痛持续约半小时左右自行缓解,未予重视及治疗。查血甲胎蛋白不升高。

手术所见:左半肝脏见一巨大肿瘤,大小约:10 cm×10cm质硬,边界尚清,部分瘤体突出于肝表面。

病理检查:左半肝:肝组织一块,大小14cm×8.5cm×6.5cm,切面见一结节样肿物,大小7.5cm×7cm×6.3cm,结节切面灰白,质硬,与周围肝组织界限尚清,其余切面灰黄、质中。第12A淋巴结:淡黄色组织一块,大小2 cm×1.5 cm×0.3 cm。常规病理诊断:左半肝切除标本:恶性肿瘤,大小7.5cm×7cm×6.3cm,周围肝组织呈轻度慢性炎症。肿瘤类型、预后及耐药待免疫组化检测报告。第12组淋巴结可疑癌转移,待免疫组化进一步鉴定。

免疫组化检测:切片A:阳性:CK(L),CK8,CK18,CK7,CK19,CA19-9,Villin,Vimentin,CD34(内皮细胞+),EGFR(+++),VEGF(+++),P-gp(+++),Topo-Ⅱ(+),Ki-67(+,约30%);阴性:CK(H),CK20,CEA,AFP,hepatocyte,F8,HBcAg,HBsAg,ERCC-1,5-Fu,Tubulin-β。切片B:阳性:上皮细胞CK(P),CK(L),组织细胞CD68,CD163。免疫组化诊断;左半肝切除标本:肝内混合型肝癌(胆管细胞癌+肝细胞癌),大小7.5cm×7cm×6.3cm,周围肝组织呈轻度慢性炎症。肿瘤预后及耐药免疫组化检测结果供临床参考。第12组淋巴结经免疫组化检测证实癌转移,1/2;伴窦组织细胞增生(图3-10-1)。

第十一章　肝细胞癌的扩散和转移

第一节　肝细胞性肝癌伴有胆管癌栓

肝细胞性肝癌伴有胆管癌栓而引起阻塞性黄疸的患者仅占肝细胞性肝癌患者的1.66%~13.00%，这个类型的肝癌也被称为黄疸型肝细胞性肝癌或淤胆型肝细胞性肝癌。

随着对该类型肝细胞性肝癌的深入了解和影像诊断技术的提高，临床上发现的肝细胞性肝癌合并胆管癌栓病例逐渐增多。肝细胞性肝癌合并胆管癌栓并不是手术的禁忌证，通过切除肿瘤、清除癌栓等手术治疗或进行综合治疗仍可获得较好的疗效。

胆管癌栓主要是由于原发性肿瘤的直接侵犯，肿瘤直接长入胆管内，胆管内充满肿瘤组织或侵入胆管的肿瘤发生溃破、出血，肿瘤组织及血凝块延伸至下游胆管，并可向下掉入肝外胆管而导致梗阻，另外，邻近胆管的门静脉癌栓直接侵犯也可导致胆管癌栓，一组13例中有1例肿瘤破溃入胆囊，胆囊受到侵犯，肿瘤组织通过胆囊管进入胆总管形成胆总管癌栓，这可能是胆囊窝附近的肝细胞性肝癌引起胆管癌栓的一种途径。

肝细胞性肝癌合并胆管癌栓的影像学研究：该研究结果显示，肝细胞性肝癌合并胆管癌栓在CT和MRI上有两个特征：肝内肝细胞性肝癌具有典型肝细胞性肝癌的CT和MRI表现，如CT平扫为低密度，边界不清，增强扫描肿瘤具有“快进快出”的特点等；癌栓表现为胆管内软组织块影，胆管壁无增厚，梗阻上方胆管扩张。

CT上软组织块为等或稍低密度，在动脉期有轻度强化，门静脉期及肝实质期呈低密度。在MR T_1WI上癌栓为稍低信号，T_2WI为稍高信号，在常规增强扫描图像上呈轻、中度强化。

Gabata等（2007）报道的6例癌栓在MRI动态增强的早期均可见癌栓强化，而在Tseng等（2001）报道的13例癌栓中有6例在MRI动态增强的动脉期均可见癌栓强化，因而动脉早期强化可能是胆管癌栓的一个重要特征。

胆管癌栓在MRCP上呈现恶性胆管梗阻的征象，表现为肝门部胆管或胆总管阻塞中断、狭窄或充盈缺损伴有梗阻上方胆管扩张，胆管突然截断或呈“鼠尾”状。胆总管内癌栓充填，周围缺乏胆汁，可仅仅显示肝内胆管扩张，而胆总管不显示。MRCP检查能立体、直观地观察癌栓的部位及癌栓在胆管系统的延伸范围，这对确定治疗方式及规划手术范围有重要的意义。虽然超声检查与CT和MR检查诊断胆管癌栓的准确率差异无统计学意义（P=0.270），但由于超声图像的对比分辨率和空间分辨率不如CT和MRI高，而且胆管癌栓的显示易受操作者技术熟练程度的影响，超声检查显示胆管癌栓的蔓延范围不及CT、MR检查清晰。因而超声检查仅仅只能作为胆管癌栓的一种筛查手段，胆管癌栓的诊断以及癌栓部位的显示仍有赖于CT和MR检查。

鉴别诊断：由于对该病的认识不足，对解剖结构不熟悉或对影像观察不仔细，胆管癌栓易误诊为胆管结石、胆管癌和门静脉癌栓等。

胆管结石：胆管阳性结石在CT上易与胆管癌栓鉴别。胆管阴性结石（多为胆固醇结石）在CT上呈软组织密度影，两者的鉴别可借助CT增强扫描，胆管癌栓可有强化，而结石无强化。胆管结石在MRI上具有一定的特征性，在T_1WI上为低或高信号，T_2WI上为低信号影，无强化，在MRCP图像上具有良性梗阻性病变的形态特点，因此，在MRI上结石不难与胆管癌栓鉴别。

胆管癌：胆管癌一般多见于肝门部以及胆总管

下端，胆管壁可见增厚、侵犯，在增强扫描上可呈现"快进慢出"的表现，延迟扫描图像上大部分肿瘤可轻度或明显强化。而胆管癌栓很少侵犯胆管壁，胆管壁无增厚，仅仅动脉期可出现早期强化，无延迟强化表现，另外胆管癌栓患者常见肝内典型的肝细胞性肝癌征象。

肝细胞性肝癌合并胆管癌栓患者如果肝内的肿瘤很小，则很难与胆管癌鉴别。该组中有2例由于肝细胞性肝癌病灶小（直径分别为2.0和2.5 cm）、肿瘤与胆管内癌栓紧密相连而误诊为胆管癌。因此，肝内肿瘤的清楚显示是诊断胆管癌栓的关键之一。

门静脉癌栓：单纯门静脉癌栓一般不伴有胆管扩张，在伴有胆管扩张的病例中应该注意是否合并有胆管癌栓的存在。在肝细胞性肝癌合并胆管癌栓的病例中有部分还可合并门静脉或肝静脉癌栓，因而，在诊断肝细胞性肝癌时要全面观察图像，以免造成胆管癌栓或门静脉癌栓的漏诊或误诊。

肝门转移淋巴结：转移淋巴结位于门静脉以及胆管周围，仅仅引起局限性肝门部胆管狭窄，狭窄部较短，边缘光滑，另外，MRCP显示胆管呈外压性改变也有助于鉴别。

总之，肝细胞性肝癌患者如出现黄疸应注意除外有无合并胆管癌栓。肝细胞性肝癌合并胆管癌栓的CT、MRI表现具有一定的特征性，表现为肝内出现典型肝细胞性肝癌病灶，胆管内出现软组织块影，增强后可有强化。

第二节　肝脏肿瘤侵犯胆管的MRI楔形征

Yukio（1997）为澄清 T_1WI 中和肝肿瘤相关联的楔形高信号对于诊断的重要性，研究了4例肝的直结肠转移癌，1例胆管癌。2例女性3例男性，41~65岁。肝肿瘤大小（直径0.8~6.5cm）由肝部分切除术确定。全部病人的MR影像均和病理学检查进行对照。

1.5 T扫描仪，在注入马根维显前，已得到横断面或矢状位快速SE T_2WI、SE T_1WI和FE序列MR影像。对比剂经静脉快速手推注入，（2ml/秒，0.1 mmo1/kg）。在注射开始后20秒（动脉期），60秒（门脉期）和2~3分钟（静脉期）采集影像。层厚8~10mm，层间距0~2mm。在 T_2WI 快速SE成像，4例的楔形区为高信号，1例为等信号强度。2例的楔形区在FE序列比SE序列更清楚。4例具有楔形区的肝肿瘤（3例转移瘤，1例胆管癌）的快速SE成像在 T_1WI 为低信号，在 T_2WI 为高信号。1例转移瘤在 T_1WI、T_2WI 均为低信号。此外，在FE成像上，肿瘤周围可见环形高信号强度。在增强后的动脉期，于SE、FE成像的 T_1WI 像显示高信号楔形区的相同区域可见清晰的楔形增强。

所有患者的增强由动脉期持续至静脉期。在快速SE和增强FE的 T_2WI 的楔形区内可识别出扩张的肝内胆管。3例的扩张胆管在远离肝门的肿瘤外侧被发现，而楔形区主要见于扩大的胆管周围，胆管腔内肿瘤扩展邻接肿瘤外侧。另2例肿瘤近于肝表面，在肿瘤中部可见局限性扩张胆管，也可识别出肝肿瘤周围的楔形区。在快速SE的 T_2WI，扩张胆管很难与门脉分支相区别。然而在增强MR像，这些胆管表现为中等低信号强度。

肉眼检查，5例和肝肿瘤有关的楔形区均为暗红棕色。1例转移瘤的周围也可见相同颜色区域。这些楔形区内的毗邻胆管内有肿瘤扩展。3例胆管内肿瘤扩展在肿瘤旁侧，2例位于中央。镜下检查发现楔形区内肝细胞萎缩，窦状隙扩张，血管周围纤维区炎症和胆管内来自母肿瘤的乳头状肿瘤扩展。镜检证实，3例门脉分支内有瘤栓。在环形或楔形区内均没有出血、脂肪变和铁沉积。然而，3例楔形区萎缩的肝细胞内可见胆色素和脂褐质的中度到重度沉积。该作者指出，在 T_1WI 和肝肿瘤相关的高信号楔形区提示肝内胆管腔内的肿瘤扩展，其 T_1 缩短可能是萎缩的肝细胞内脂褐质沉积所致。

第三节 肝细胞癌侵犯胆管

原发性肝细胞癌侵犯血管,形成血管内癌栓(如门静脉癌栓),在临床上相当常见。而原发性肝细胞癌侵犯胆管,则相对少见,常常被临床忽略。自Mallory首例报告以来,才逐渐被人们注意。以梗阻性黄疸为主要表现者占肝细胞癌病人的2%~8%肝细胞癌引起黄疸者约10%~40%为肝细胞癌直接侵犯胆管所致。

自Mallory首例起,到1979年为止,世界英文文献中共报告22例,van Sonnenberg和Ferrucci(1979)报告6例,Kojiro等(1982)搜集几所医院10年期间临床病理报告24例,含22例尸检和2例手术。Lee等(1984)报告22例中,17例经手术(10例)及尸检(7例)证实,其中8例为癌栓。Lau等(1990)在340例肝细胞癌中,发现11例伴梗阻性黄疸,其中8例为胆管内癌栓,3例为胆管内癌块的碎片。Lai等(1992)报告5例肝细胞癌引起黄疸和侵犯胆系,其中4例为癌栓,1例为凝血块。Roslyn等(1984)报告6例胆管内肿瘤碎块引起的间歇性黄疸中,有1例为肝细胞癌。

Shiina等(1992)报告1例超声检查,CT和血管造影发现左外叶肝癌,但未见到胆管内癌栓,经左肝动脉和右肝动脉注入2ml碘油,27天后ERCP见总肝管和右肝胆管内有5cm长的充盈缺损,伴肝胆管扩张,碘油正沉积于充盈缺损组织内,肝实质内碘油已清除干净,故认为碘油沉积有助于胆管内癌栓的诊断。

笔者在1996年报告19例肝细胞癌侵犯胆管的影像学资料。从我们当时搜集的资料看出,截至1996年为止,经40多年时间,国外英语文献共报告89例。认识和了解此型肝细胞癌在临床上有一定意义。此型肿瘤通常为浸润性生长,或浸润加结节性生长,有侵犯血管的倾向。与其他类型肝癌相比,在确诊以后,此型肿瘤的生存期较短,而且可有较特征性的临床表现。

命名:原发性肝细胞癌侵犯胆管,因其可引起黄疸,故又称为胆管型肝细胞癌,黄疸型肝细胞癌,黄疸型肝癌,淤胆型肝细胞癌等。

发生率:胆管内癌栓的临床发现率为1.3%~2.5%,尸检发现率为10.1%~10.8%。

发病的机制:肝细胞癌侵犯胆管的机制,大致包括四点:带蒂的肿瘤侵犯和延伸;肿瘤坏死与出血,导致血凝块和癌肿碎块的阻塞;肿瘤结节直接侵犯和挤压肝内胆管系统;肝门内转移性淋巴结肿大压迫大的胆管。胆管内癌栓的原因,可以为肝细胞癌的直接侵犯,也可以是门静脉癌栓同时向门静脉和肝胆管侵犯。显微镜下观察,可见肝胆管周围的毛细血管丛和/或淋巴管内,常有小的肿瘤栓子侵及附近的胆管。

有作者发现肝内的肝细胞癌与肝胆管内的癌栓位置有1厘米以上的距离,难以用肝细胞癌直接侵犯肝胆管来解释,而可能多为远处转移,推论可能有下述三种情况:由门静脉癌栓侵犯与门静脉并行的肝胆管,并在肝胆管腔内继续生长;肝内肝细胞癌侵犯穿破其附近的小胆管,肿瘤栓子可随胆汁流至肝门部或/和肝外胆管;肝内肝细胞癌侵犯血管并转移至胆管壁上的营养血管,穿破胆管上皮进入胆管腔内。

在后两种情况,当栓子到达肝门时,管壁上可能已有血块和结石的碎渣,癌栓与之结合,并逐渐增大;或可能为癌栓以近侧穿破的胆管为起点,逐渐向肝门部增大伸延,其机制可能与血管内血栓形成的机制相似;同时,当肝细胞癌较小而影像学尚不能检出时,即可能已有胆管内的转移,也可能为一发病机制。

病理学表现:从病理学看,肝细胞癌侵犯胆管的一般病理学特征为肝内癌灶、胆管内癌栓和胆管扩张共存。病理检查可见大多数病例胆管内肿瘤生长都是肝细胞癌直接侵犯的结果。胆管内的癌栓多数位于肝门(约占78%),阻塞以上的胆管有不同程度的扩张,胆管内癌栓与胆管壁无连接,或黏附不紧密,在手术和活检中相对较易移动和吸出,绝大多数病例中胆管上皮健存,可见不同程度的胆系出血,个别病例因大量出血而死亡。肉眼观察肿瘤碎块柔软,易碎,且呈浅白色,类似雏鸡脂肪。

肿瘤侵犯肝内胆管系统的分支,能以下述方式之一引起大的胆管的机械性梗阻:肿瘤向远侧继续生长,肿瘤实质脱落可充满整个肝外胆管;坏死肿瘤碎块可与近侧侵犯胆管的肿瘤分离;坏死肿瘤碎块可下移至胆管下端引起下端梗阻。

在大多数病例，同时还可见门静脉癌栓和肝硬化。

临床表现：可有三点特征性的临床表现：无显著肝细胞损伤情况下的进行性梗阻性黄疸；波动的梗阻性黄疸，可能由于坏死的胆管内肿瘤碎块间歇性脱落的缘故；少见的胆系出血。临床表现也可分为三类：胆管炎的表现；进行性或发作性梗阻性黄疸；少见的胆系出血和梗阻性黄疸。

影像学研究：一些作者归纳本症的主要影像学表现为四类：肝门结构紊乱，肝门胆管充盈缺损，凝絮征，网球拍征；部分或全部肝胆管扩张；肝实质占位性病变；肝脾肿大，门静脉癌栓。

超声：超声检查属断面成象，检查实质脏器甚优，但检查本症时，大多数病例都只诊断为肝癌，要明确肝癌是否侵犯胆管，超声检查确有一定困难。在超声扫描时，扫描者的操作技巧很重要。笔者曾见 1 例声像图上，清晰可见左肝实质包块紧贴扩大的总肝管，总肝管腔内清楚可见不规则不均匀团块，超声既可观察肝实质，又可了解胆管内的情况，所获信息远比直接胆系造影所见更为全面。本症部分病例，超声检查时可显示胆管内癌栓呈低回声或高回声病灶，其边缘可清晰，也可模糊不清。有的病例，超声可显示胆管内有絮状回声。目前，在大多数病例，一般的实时超声尚难以明确显示胆管内块状物是癌栓还是血凝块，内镜超声和高分辨率的超声对此有一定优势。本症大多数病例，超声都可发现肝胆管扩张，其程度和范围各异。

CT：在部分病例，可显示胆管内有低密度结节影，其边缘可清楚或不清楚。对于肝胆管扩张的情况，CT 图像上常可清楚显示。有的病例在肝实质与肝胆管内可显示密度相同的低密度病灶。我们总结本症病例时发现，CT 诊断时，常常对其以前的门诊超声检查结果，或他院的超声检查结果重视不够，只根据 CT 平扫图像即下结论，往往导致误诊。对于怀疑肝细胞癌的病人，在 CT 扫描时，不仅只作平扫，还应常规进行增强扫描，同时，对此前超声检查怀疑的区域宜再行薄层扫描，或认真调整窗技术，这对减少误诊实为有益。

MRI：有的病例，在肝实质和肝胆管内，可发现相同信号的病灶，单独显示肝胆管内癌栓者较少。可显示肝胆管扩张的情况。如今，MRCP 在临床上用得越来越广泛，它不仅可清楚观察活体胆胰管的形态学表现，而且其源图像是断面图像，观察肝实质十分清楚，这对于发现与诊断肝细胞癌侵犯胆管十分有用，从我们的点滴经验看，重要的是要知道和熟悉肝细胞癌侵犯胆管这种情况，思路开阔，才能做出正确的诊断。

直接法胆系造影

胆管的充盈缺损（胆管内癌栓）：此征象是肝细胞癌侵犯胆管的特异性征象，颇有诊断价值。当胆管内癌栓较小时，胆管无扩张，呈现为边缘清楚，密度均匀的卵圆形充盈缺损。

凝絮征：当胆管内癌栓较多时，胆管扩张，但无局限性膨胀表现。我们见到，癌栓充满肝门以下整个肝外胆管：当对比剂浓度较高，且量较多时，只见肝外胆管扩张，其密度略感不匀；当对比剂浓度较低，而量又较少（如 PTC）时，则见肝外胆管呈壳状显示，表现为管壁光滑完整的轮廓，而管腔中空；当对比剂浓度和剂量适中时，则见肝外胆管内充满大小不一的絮团影，它们的密度不匀，边缘不规则且感模糊，对比剂充填于各絮团之间的缝隙，呈线状，条片状，导致肝外胆管全呈斑驳状，犹如一试管内盛满含固态乳酪凝絮软团，我们称之为凝絮征（图 3-11-1）。

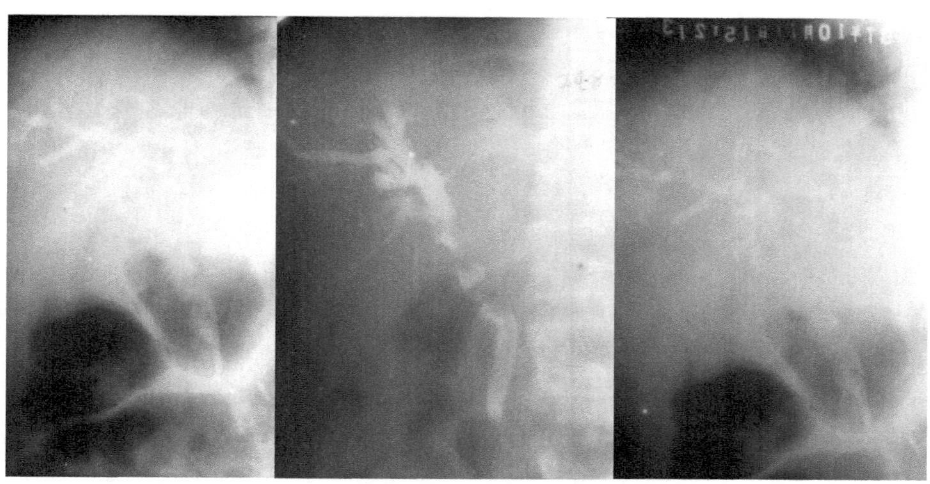

图 3-11-1　ERCP：肝癌侵犯肝外胆管的凝絮征

肝外胆管均匀性扩张，无明显胆管炎表现，各絮团影边缘模糊，它们浮于管中，而不是沉（堆砌）于胆管下端，这与胆管结石完全不同。肝外胆管尽管装满凝絮软团，但管壁光滑完整柔软，而又不同于胆管癌。

网球拍征：当胆管内癌栓大于胆管内径时，胆管呈局限性膨胀，其轮廓清晰可见，癌栓所造成充盈缺损的形状各异，可有分叶、分节、偏心性移位等。有的肝外胆管局限性膨大，轮廓清楚，位于肝外胆管中段，其内挤满癌栓，少许对比剂从癌栓缝隙中渗入，状似分叶，肝外胆管胰腺段不扩张。从形态上看，颇似网球拍，呈卵圆形的膨大处为球拍，其下方正常的细而长的肝外胆管胰腺段酷似球拍把，我们将之称为网球拍征，国外有作者又称之为高脚酒杯征。

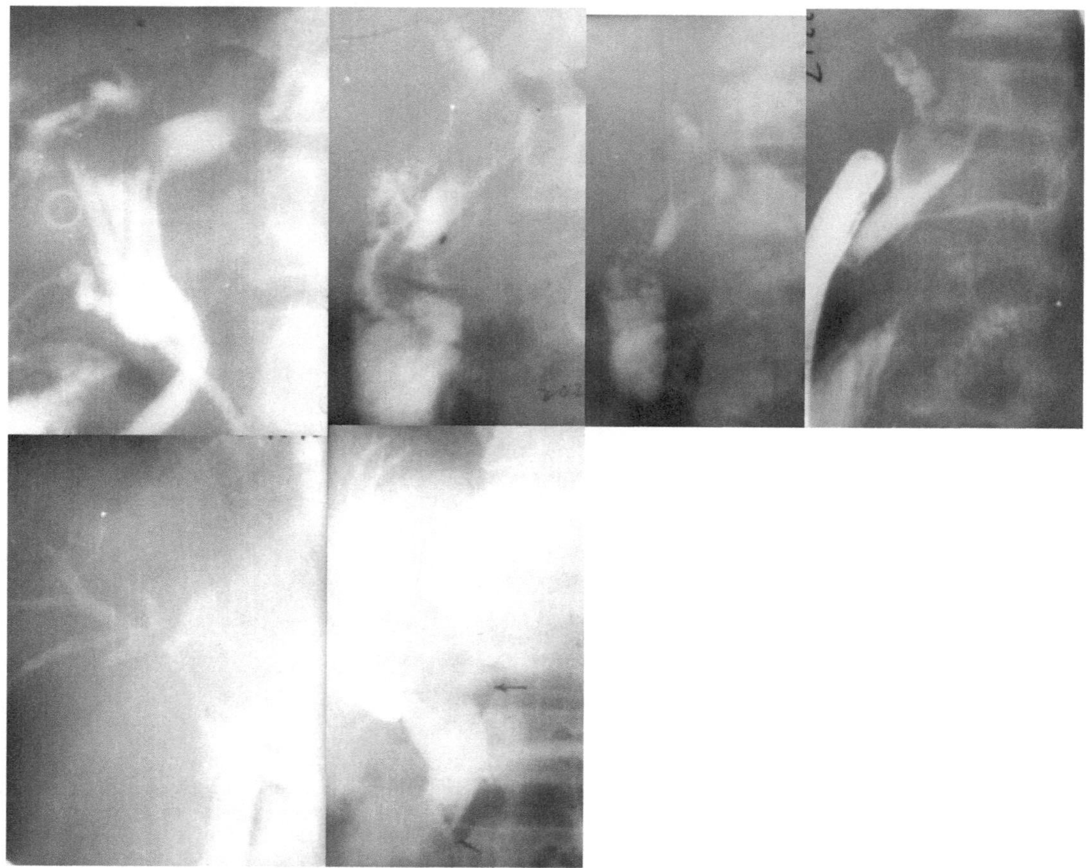

图 3-11-2　ERCP：肝细胞癌组织从肝内向下方肝外胆管坠落，癌块形成扩张的肝外胆管上方的充盈缺损，酷似网球拍，我们称之为网球拍征

胆管结石胆管炎,可使肝外胆管扩张,一般为全程性扩张,少数局限性扩张也是狭窄与扩张并存,而且,结石常常下坠,并从胆管下端向上方胡乱堆砌,与此征不同;胆管癌由胆管上皮产生,引起肝外胆管局限性扩张时,胆管壁早已破坏,其轮廓不可能光滑完整,而且,其下方胰腺段胆管也多受侵犯,也与此征相异。因此,我们认为,网球拍征可作为本症的较特异性征象。有的大的充盈缺损附近,另见一些细碎的充盈缺损,为肿瘤碎块和/或小血块所致。

肝门结构紊乱:直接法胆系造影时,肝细胞癌侵犯胆管病人的肝门结构,大多数都不像

正常肝门结构那样呈树支样显示,而是杂乱无章地呈现,或分散,或聚拢,或扭曲,或扩张,或狭窄;有的肝胆管分支无异常且显示清楚;有的肝胆管走行变化,其内部密度不匀或显示不清;有的肝胆管或/和总肝管内有不规则充盈缺损;有的肝胆管壁或总肝管壁不甚完整。

其他的征象:其他的征象有:偏心性狭窄(肿瘤侵犯和压迫胆管),跳跃性狭窄和多弧状狭窄(淋巴结压迫),以及胆管伸展,移位和狭窄等。

鉴别诊断:胆管内血栓:呈贯通整条胆管,边缘清楚的充盈缺损影,胆管不膨胀或轻度膨胀,ERCP检查时乳头部可有血液流出。

胆管结石:形态较规则,可呈卵圆形,方形和多边形,边缘清晰锐利,其密度较癌栓略低,少有分叶,超声可见其后方有声影,ERCP插管时可能阻力较大,而癌栓则较软。

分叶的胆管癌:呈现分叶状胆管内充盈缺损,但胆管壁不可能完整,这是其特点。

胆管内息肉:十分少见,一般较小,造成胆管局限性膨大者更为少见。

胰腺、胆囊、胆管等处的恶性肿瘤侵犯胆管时,也可有相似的充盈缺损表现,但常有其他部位脏器的原发病灶和病史。

笔者曾见一例肝门大块充盈缺损,胆管下端也见大块充盈缺损,二者的边缘轮廓均不规则,二者之间的胆管均匀性扩张且充满对比剂,结合以往临床经验考虑为胆管下端癌向肝门转移,实际上恰恰相反。该例病人胰腺头部也肿大,被误诊为胰头癌向肝门转移。从临床发病率看,肝门部胆管肿瘤以胆管癌多见,其次为胰腺癌及胆管下端癌转移到肝门,肝细胞癌侵犯肝门且有癌栓下降至胆管下端,淋巴转移到胰周,实属少见案例。该例病人肝门包块明显大于胆管下端者,理应想到后者源于前者,但是,当时却未曾考虑到这一点(图3-11-2)。

第四节 关于浸润型肝癌

详见本书 本卷 本篇 第二章 第十节 关于浸润型肝癌。

第十二章　肝癌与门静脉

原发性肝癌门静脉癌栓

门静脉内栓塞（血栓、癌栓）最常见于伴有肝细胞癌或不伴肝细胞癌的肝硬化门静脉高压病人，其次见于胰腺癌、胰腺炎、胆管炎及凝血功能障碍等。此外，还可见于腹部手术后，如脾切除术后可见到脾静脉栓塞向门静脉延伸形成门静脉主干栓塞。门静脉癌栓在肝癌中的发生率为 33.8%~90.2%，被认为是肝癌在肝内广泛转移的根源，是晚期肝癌的重要合并症。因此，早期确诊癌栓及其位置，对病变分期，治疗方案的选择和预后评估都具有重要意义。

病理病因学：门静脉癌栓的形成多为肝细胞癌侵犯门静脉的小分支，在其内形成微小癌栓，继而生长、伸延、扩展到段、叶以及门静脉主干。门静脉主干的癌栓进一步生长蔓延，形成肠系膜上静脉或/和脾静脉的癌栓。

肝细胞癌合并门静脉主干癌栓，其腹腔积液出现率很高，可达 80% 以上。一方面是由于肝硬化及门静脉高压的结果，另一方面肝细胞癌导致肝功能和全身情况恶化，门静脉主干癌栓的形成又加剧了门静脉高压，这样，腹腔积液很快出现或急剧增加，个别病例还出现肠道水肿。

门静脉主干癌栓的出现与肝细胞癌的类型有一定关系，一般统计认为，弥漫型最高，巨块结节型次之，再次为巨块型，结节型出现概率最低。通常是，病灶越大（直径大于 10cm），病灶数目越多，主干内癌栓形成的概率亦越高，弥漫型癌栓形成的机会尤其为多。

影像学研究：门静脉癌栓在 CT、DSA 和 B 型超声检查时呈现多种表现，部分征象具有一定的特征性。在 CT 增强扫描时，门静脉内出现低密度影或充盈缺损，经手术病理证实，为门静脉癌栓的可靠而具特征性的征象。

CT：在 CT 平扫，门静脉主干内癌栓的密度与门静脉本身的密度并无明显差异，仅显示门静脉直径增粗。增强扫描时，主要的 CT 表现为门静脉主干内低密度影，与增强前影像比较无明显变化，少数可轻度增强，而形成管腔内低密度充盈缺损。这一类低密度影常延伸至门静脉左支和右支或其中一个分支内。很难见到单纯门静脉主干内癌栓而分支不受累的病例。

门静脉主干旁多出现代偿性增粗的侧支静脉，向肝门伸延分布，部分病例可见胆囊周围静脉增粗呈网格状。侧支血管形成的多少与门静脉癌栓形成的速度和门静脉高压的程度有关。一般门静脉癌栓的形成较为缓慢，且有不同程度的肝硬化和门静脉高压，因此，绝大多数病例都有此类表现。门静脉主干癌栓形成后，对门静脉壁增强的表现的认识，各学者意见不同。有的发现癌栓形成后，管壁增强的程度较其他静脉壁明显，认为是供应管壁的滋养血管代偿性扩张的结果。由于管腔内癌栓无增强，管壁相对呈较明显的增强，称之为管壁的环形增强表现。在主干尚未完全形成癌栓时，或癌栓的末端可见到癌栓表现为新月状的低密度影。增强扫描的少见表现是门静脉主干的癌栓延续到肠系膜上静脉和脾静脉，此外，偶尔还可见到肠道水肿。

在 CT 平扫时，有的门静脉癌栓可偶尔表现为密度不均或高密度影，增强后，门静脉内呈充盈缺损，这可能是由于癌栓由肿瘤细胞和血栓混合形成所致。Mori 等（1987）认为，CT 平扫所示门静脉内高密度影，若 B 型超声诊断门静脉癌栓，则可确诊，不必再做 CT 增强扫描和 X 线血管造影。

X 线血管造影：在 X 线血管造影时，大多数门静脉癌栓表现为门静脉内结节状充盈缺损，经手术病理证实，这是一个常见而可靠的特异性征象。

门静脉内癌栓依其生长方式不同而有相应的 X 线表现。索状型：肝动脉造影时，在动脉期 3~5 秒就可见门静脉内显示数条线状影，提示门静脉主干内癌栓形成，称作“线样征”。Okuda 等（1975）认为，“线样征”是由于对比剂进入癌栓的供血动脉，或对比剂逆流到癌栓和门静脉壁间的腔隙所致。有作者认为，这些线条状透光影是癌栓内有多数与管径平行生长的新生血管所致。Marks 等(1979)报道,在67 例肝癌病人中, 17 例出现“线样征”的患者,经组织病理学检查,门静脉和肝静脉内均有癌栓形成。假腺管型:癌栓呈密度不均匀的充盈缺损。坚实型和硬化型:癌栓呈局限性生长,为圆形或椭圆形边缘清晰的充盈缺损。

当门静脉存在癌栓时,门静脉常有明显增粗,最粗的直径可达 3~4cm。在团块状充盈缺损出现时,缺损边缘有的可形成明显的弧形影,常出现于动脉造影早期,是诊断门静脉主干癌栓的可靠征象,有作者称之为杯口征。门静脉不显影,并不表示一定有门静脉癌栓形成,这是值得注意的。

肝静脉内的癌栓与门静脉内癌栓表现相似,其部位多在横膈与脊柱连接处的肝静脉内。

影响门静脉癌栓影像诊断的因素: CT、DSA、B 型超声作为门静脉癌栓的常规检查方法各有优缺点。CT 诊断门静脉癌栓,若以增强扫描所见门静脉内显示低密度影作为诊断标准,则其诊断特异性高。但是,在下列因素存在时,CT 的诊断敏感性则较低。一是增强扫描图像质量差,如患者耐受性差,对比剂量少,或注入速度慢,增强扫描效果不良,则可造成癌栓显示不清;二是 CT 扫描未扫到癌栓所在层面,如病人呼吸配合不佳,或扫描层距较大,或有癌栓的门静脉走向与扫描层面平行,导致未能显示有癌栓的平面,造成误诊或漏诊;三是癌栓位于门静脉三级分支。

有作者指出,CT 扫描主要用于诊断门静脉主干或一级分支内的癌栓。训练病人良好屏气,采用薄层扫描或重叠扫描,可减少误诊和漏诊。

X 线血管造影在门静脉癌栓诊断敏感性方面,较 CT 为高,但是,血管造影也受呼吸、减影质量等因素的影响。血管造影在特异性方面较 CT 为差,主要因为将“门静脉不显影”作为诊断门静脉癌栓的征象特异性低。因为,除门静脉癌栓外,还有多种因素可引起门静脉不显影,而在血管造影上却难以鉴别。

B 型超声可多层面灵活探查,且癌栓与血液界面间声阻抗差大,故对门静脉癌栓诊断的敏感性高于 CT 和 DSA。B 型超声可根据门静脉内血流信号和血液内异常强回声光团来判断门静脉内癌栓和门静脉高压是否存在。因此,对 DSA 不能鉴别是癌栓阻塞门静脉,还是门静脉高压引起的门静脉不显影的病例,B 型超声可协助诊断。然而,B 型超声也存在诊断的局限性,由于受腹腔积液、影像重叠等因素的影响,其特异性远不如 CT。

Okuda(1987)认为 B 型超声对门静脉内癌栓的检出率最高,其次是血管造影,CT 最次,它们对三级门静脉内癌栓的发现率分别是 71.4%、28.6%、14.5%

在门静脉癌栓的三种常规检查方法中,CT 和 B 型超声为非损伤性的,若以 B 型超声作为筛选手段,以 CT 作为辅助确诊,则可望提高门静脉癌栓影像诊断的准确性。

第十三章　肝癌与 CT

第一节　肝的 CT 扫描技巧点滴

CT 发现肝癌诊断的正确性仰赖于扫描技术和扫描仪的分辨力。大部分报导均称正确率高于80%，Takashima 等（1982）评价 7 例 <2cm 的肝癌，发现 CT 正确率为 1 例（14%）而血管造影为 6 例（86%），其错误的源泉盖因他们的 CT 扫描只用对比剂增强，而这些较小病灶则正好可变为等密度。理想的 CT 扫描技术利用团注对比剂前、后扫描将发现大部分小于 1cm 或更小的肝细胞癌。Inamoto 等（1980）基于强化前、后的特点将肝癌 CT 表现分为四类：①40% 强化前后扫描均为阳性，均显示清楚，大部分孤立包块属于此类；②30% 强化后可见而强化前未能发现；③25% 强化前可见肿瘤，而强化后肿瘤呈等密度或变得更小；④5% 强化前、后扫描均为阴性。其中，后三类以多发结节型或弥漫型居多。肝的 CT 扫描技巧每个单位都有不同，如扫描仪的效力和病人的负担常造成简化检查。

早在 20 世纪 70 年代，约翰霍普金医院对于怀疑肝脏包块的病人都规定作详尽 CT 扫描。当时，首先作一次层距 10mm 平扫，连续扫描整个肝脏。如果发现一个或更多病灶，则将扫描仪放归该层面，再以每公斤体重 1ml 泛影葡胺团注，迅速连续扫描以便评价病灶的血管情况。在团注后如此连续扫描，有助于区别肝新生物和肝血管瘤。肝的其余部分再用层距 10mm 扫描，以强化显示再力图发现其他病变。

第二节　肝癌内 CT 所见钙化

肝癌内 CT 所见钙化的发生率尚有争论。成功治疗（放疗或 / 和化疗）的病灶常有钙化。文献上许多资料不强调区分肝内胆管癌，混合型胆管肝细胞癌与肝细胞癌。少数资料将纤维层板型癌与硬化型肝细胞癌分开，前者已知倾向钙化，后者也怀疑如此。有作者认为，粗沙状、短而厚的、小梁状中心性钙化出现于肿瘤的小部分，它们是纤维层板型肝细胞癌、胆管癌或混合性肿瘤。而纤细的、斑点状的、沙样的钙化分布于肿瘤的大部分多提示转移性疾病或肝细胞癌的硬化型变态。通常肝细胞癌伴存硬化者在治疗前少有钙化，当其有钙化时也多为斑点样钙化。

表 3-13-1　美国约翰霍普金医院 117 例肝癌 CT 评价

病人情况：男性 81 例，女性 36 例，平均年龄 50.3 岁（范围 11~79 岁）
CT 表现　孤立性病变：26 例。（大小范围：2cm × 3 × 1cm~18cm × 18cm × 15cm）
多发性病灶：32 例。　<5cm：11 例；>5cm，<10cm：6 例；>10cm：15 例。
弥漫性实质侵犯：59 例。<50% 肝：44 例；>50% 肝：15 例。
肿瘤内钙化：27 例（23%）。
肝硬化为基础者：13 例。

表 3-13-1 示细心检查钙化发生率较高（与此类似文献不少），可解释为：①年青病人伴纤维层板型多；②已知肝硬化发生少；③硬化性变态或混合性胆管细胞 - 肝细胞癌病例数目不明，因为活检所获资料有限。从上述资料也说明，肝癌以肝硬化为基础

者的比例,国内外资料差异确实较大。

第三节 左肝内段低分化肝细胞性肝癌伴坏死

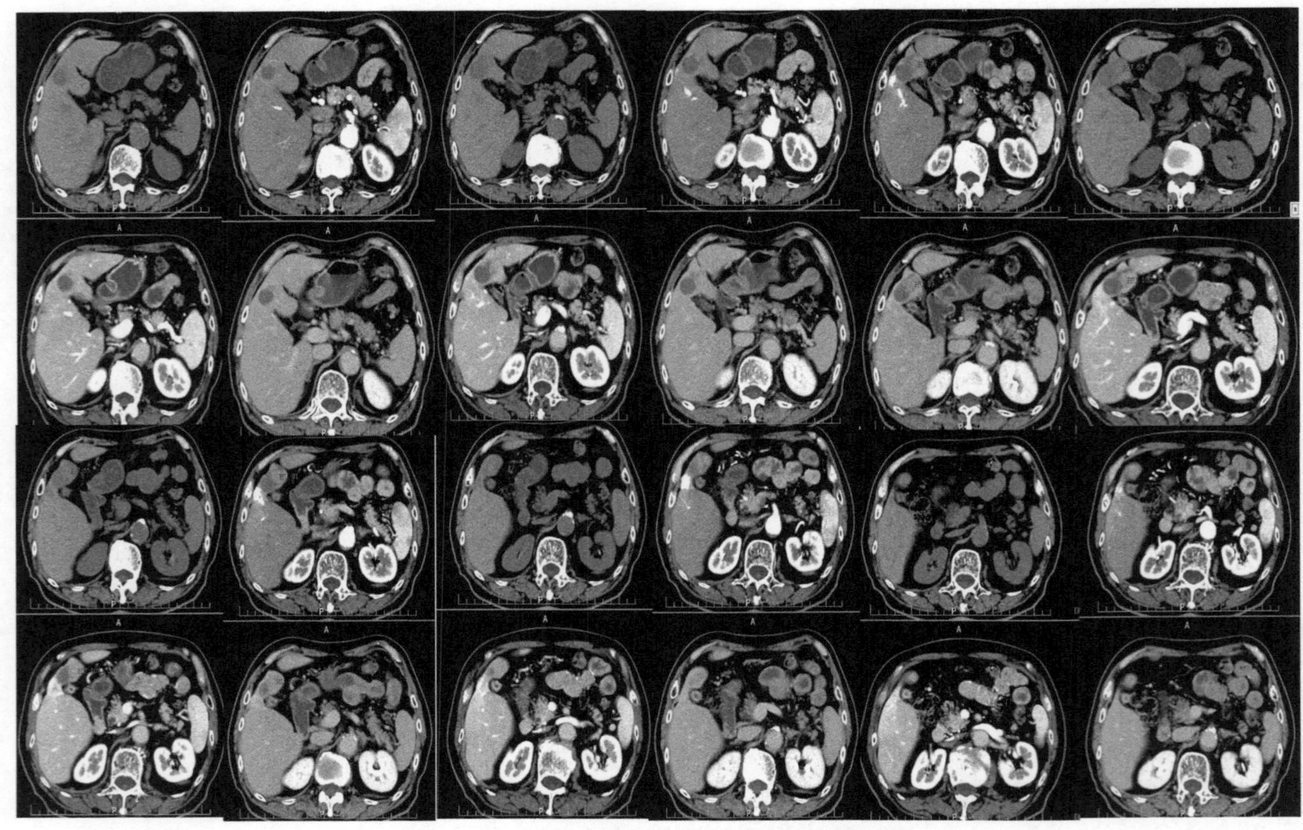

图 3-13-1 左肝内段低分化肝细胞性肝癌伴坏死

患者,男,82 岁。发现肝占位 3 周入院。

病理检查:左肝肿瘤及胆囊切除标本:灰褐色不规则肝组织二块,大小分别为 5.5cm × 5.0 cm × 3.5 cm 和 5.0 cm × 4.0 cm × 2.5 cm,断面可见一结节样肿物,大小约 3.5 cm × 2 cm,切面灰褐灰黄,质中,肿物邻近肝被膜最薄处约 0.1 cm,与周边肝组织界限尚清;其中较大块肝组织附有胆囊一具,大小 7 cm × 3.5 cm × 2 cm,腔内充满墨绿色液体,浆膜面光滑,黏膜面呈细网状,壁厚 0.1~0.2 cm。常规病理诊断:左肝肿瘤及胆囊切除标本:①初步考虑肝细胞性肝癌伴坏死,待做免疫组化检测进一步证实并分级,其肝组织断端切缘为阴性;②胆囊组织呈慢性炎,未见癌组织累及。

免疫组化诊断:左肝肿瘤切除标本:免疫组化检测结果支持低分化肝细胞性肝癌伴坏死,其余内容详见常规报告(图 3-13-1)。

第四节 MSCT 双动脉期与门脉期增强扫描对原发性肝癌检出比较

MSCT 扫描速度快,在较短的时间内完成全肝扫描,一般将对比剂在肝脏内的动态循环过程分为动脉期、门静脉期和平衡期 3 期,并可根据诊断需要进行不同时期的延迟期扫描。由于肝脏特殊的双重血供及肝细胞肝癌主要为动脉供血的特点,如何准确把握住动脉期的影像表现是提高肝细胞肝癌检出率的关键。对比剂从肝动脉进入肝脏到对比剂从门静脉流入肝脏之间的时间为准确的肝动脉期,MSCT 的快速扫描使肝脏在真正的动脉期显示成为可能。MSCT 使单层螺旋 CT 的动脉期可被分为动脉早期（20~22s）与动脉晚期（34~37s），有利于显示有丰富动脉供血的肝细胞肝癌病灶，因而使得肝细胞肝癌病灶的检出率和定性诊断准确率有明显提高。

双动脉期：有作者研究表明，如果采用双动脉期，对高密度病灶的检出率可达94%，明显优于动脉晚期（87%）。一项研究结果显示，对于小的肝细胞肝癌，动脉早期（39.5%）、动脉晚期（67.4%）和门静脉期（44.2%）的敏感度普遍较低，动脉晚期的敏感度高于动脉早期和门静脉期。这可能与肝细胞肝癌主要由肝动脉供血有关，小肝细胞肝癌供血血管较小，动脉早期病灶强化不明显，检出病灶较困难，动脉晚期时对比剂从肝动脉分布到肿瘤动脉并扩散至肿瘤间隙，大部分病灶可见不同程度的强化，表现为密度高于周围肝实质，因此比较容易检出；但病灶峰值停留时间大多数很短，然后迅速下降。伴随肝实质CT值的上升，两者密度接近，又可出现等密度交叉；此后病灶CT值下降，正常肝实质继续上升，病灶又成为低密度。当肝实质也处于峰值时（门静脉期），两者密度可形成明显差异。但由于扫描时间及对比剂在肝实质内进出的量与速度影响着癌灶的显示，部分病灶可表现为等密度，影响病灶的检出。因此，对于小肝细胞肝癌来说，动脉晚期的扫描相当重要，是显示富血供肝脏肿瘤的最有价值的期相，可以显著提高病灶的检出率，动脉早期则可用于CTA。

肿瘤的大小：从该研究的结果可以看出，对于最大径线≤3 cm的病灶，动脉早期、动脉晚期和门静脉期的阳性预测值均较低（51.5%~57.5%），可能是由于肝硬化存在动静脉短路或肿瘤细胞分泌肿瘤血管生成因子引起局部血管增多、血供增加，表现为肝动脉期呈叶、段或小的亚段分布的均匀高密度强化影，在门静脉期转变为等密度或稍高密度，少数病例因门静脉瘤栓出现肝叶、段或亚段的低强化，易当成病灶而过度诊断。对于最大径线>3 cm的肝细胞肝癌病灶，动脉早期的敏感度（89.6%）稍低，动脉晚期（99.6%）和门静脉期（99.1%）的敏感度较高，三者差异有统计学意义，阳性预测值均为100%，因此双动脉期增强扫描几乎不存在漏检大肝细胞肝癌的概率。

关于动脉晚期：对于所有病灶，动脉早期、动脉晚期和门静脉期的敏感度及阳性预测值差异均有统计学意义，动脉晚期的敏感度最高（90.9%），门静脉期（84.3%）次之，动脉早期最低（76.1%），而阳性预测值则门静脉期最高（93.7%），可能是由于动脉晚期病灶强化较明显，但由于肝硬化患者存在动静脉分流，有时造成假阳性，门静脉期由于动静脉分流多呈等密度改变，而真正的肝细胞肝癌结节由于主要由肝动脉供血，多表现为低密度，因此，病灶检出的阳性预测值较高。

影响因素：肝脏增强扫描对肝细胞癌的强化和显示受患者本身的因素和扫描技术的影响。患者因素包括心输出量、体重和肿瘤灶的血供情况（癌灶内的微血管数、周围肝实质的硬化情况等）；技术因素涉及扫描的技术参数、增强扫描的方法，后者包括对比剂用量、注射流率、对比剂碘浓度和各期数据采集的时间。因此上述因素影响对比剂进入癌灶的时间、浓度和滞留的时间，从而影响癌灶在采集时间点的强化程度。另外，双动脉期扫描难免会增加患者的辐射剂量，但如果目的在于提高病灶的检出率，双动脉期扫描应该作为首选方法。

综上所述，MSCT的临床应用优化了动脉期的扫描方案，使全肝扫描落在真正的动脉期内，并能进行动脉双期的扫描，3期表现的综合分析有利于提高病灶的显示，特别是对于小肝细胞肝癌，动脉晚期的扫描显得尤其重要。

第十四章 肝癌与MRI

第一节 关于原发性肝癌的动态增强MRI

多数原发性肝癌平扫 T_1WI 表现为低信号，部分可表现为高信号或等信号。动态增强时，早期病灶即刻出现强化，一般肿瘤实体全部强化，较大的瘤体有时仅见周边强化或不均匀强化。动物实验及病理组织学研究表明，原发性肝癌的血管含量丰富，而且其解剖结构不完整，难以辨认，有大量血管湖存在。动态增强早期，由肝动脉进入的对比剂大量地灌注于丰富的瘤血管和血管湖，因此，在增强检查早期，原发性肝癌即可出现强化。大肝癌的坏死区和少血管区由于缺乏对比剂的灌注，在增强早期不出现强化。

随着检查时间的延续，对比剂由肝动脉和门静脉同时进入肝，并由血管内向血管外扩散而进入组织细胞间隙(达到平衡的时间大约为 2 分钟)，使正常肝实质逐渐强化，肿瘤和正常肝组织之间的信号差异逐渐缩小，大约在注射对比剂后 8 分钟变为等信号。

部分病例由于肝组织的强化程度超过瘤体的强化，肝癌病灶可表现为稍低信号。肿瘤内的对比剂滞留时间一般比正常肝组织内的时间长一些，因此延迟扫描的某一阶段(大约在 10~15 分钟)瘤体可呈高信号表现。但是，如果扫描时间继续延长(如：延续到 60 分钟成像)，正常肝组织及肿瘤内的对比剂完全清除，此时的 MRI 征象又恢复到增强前表现。

增强晚期和延迟期肝癌的强化形式多为斑片状不均匀强化，有时可见肿块周边强化逐渐向中心发展，而最终表现为瘤体全部强化。较大的肝癌常有坏死区和囊变区存在，囊壁由内皮构成，内含清亮的囊液，外周无毛细血管包绕，动态增强检查一般不出现强化。

坏死区内常有少量的瘤血管穿过，瘤血管周围有结缔组织鞘包绕，在增强早期坏死区一般不出现强化，但在延迟期扫描(注药后 30 分钟)可出现不同程度的强化。

肝癌包膜形成是原发性结节性肝细胞癌的特征性表现，对肿瘤的治疗和预后有显著影响，病理学上肝癌包膜由纤维结缔组织构成，细胞外间隙较大，在病灶周边被挤压的肝实质内有大量的血管湖存在。MRI 发现肝包膜的敏感性明显优于 CT，在 SE T_1WI 上表现为环状低信号，动态增强 MRI 延迟期常表现为环状或月晕状强化，与动态增强 CT 表现类似。在 MRI 动态增强早期，肝癌包膜不出现强化。

第二节 MRI 动态增强误诊

MRI 动态增强扫描是诊断肝脏疾病的重要检查方法，但可能出现以下几种误诊：肝叶、段、亚段及包膜下过度灌注异常；早期强化的假性病变，尤其易发生在肝左叶内侧段；全肝的不均匀过度灌注异常；由血管伪影、不增强的肝血管、部分容积伪影、磁敏感性伪影和肝硬化再生结节等所致的低信号假病变。

在动态 MRI 增强动脉期，这些异常表现有时类似于真正的病变或类似于肿瘤向周围肝实质的侵犯。然而，多数情况下，在其他序列或延迟期 MRI

增强时没有相应的异常改变，而且，过度灌注异常的特定部位有助于同真正的肿瘤鉴别。

第三节　误诊病例简介：高分化肝细胞性肝癌与血管平滑肌脂肪瘤

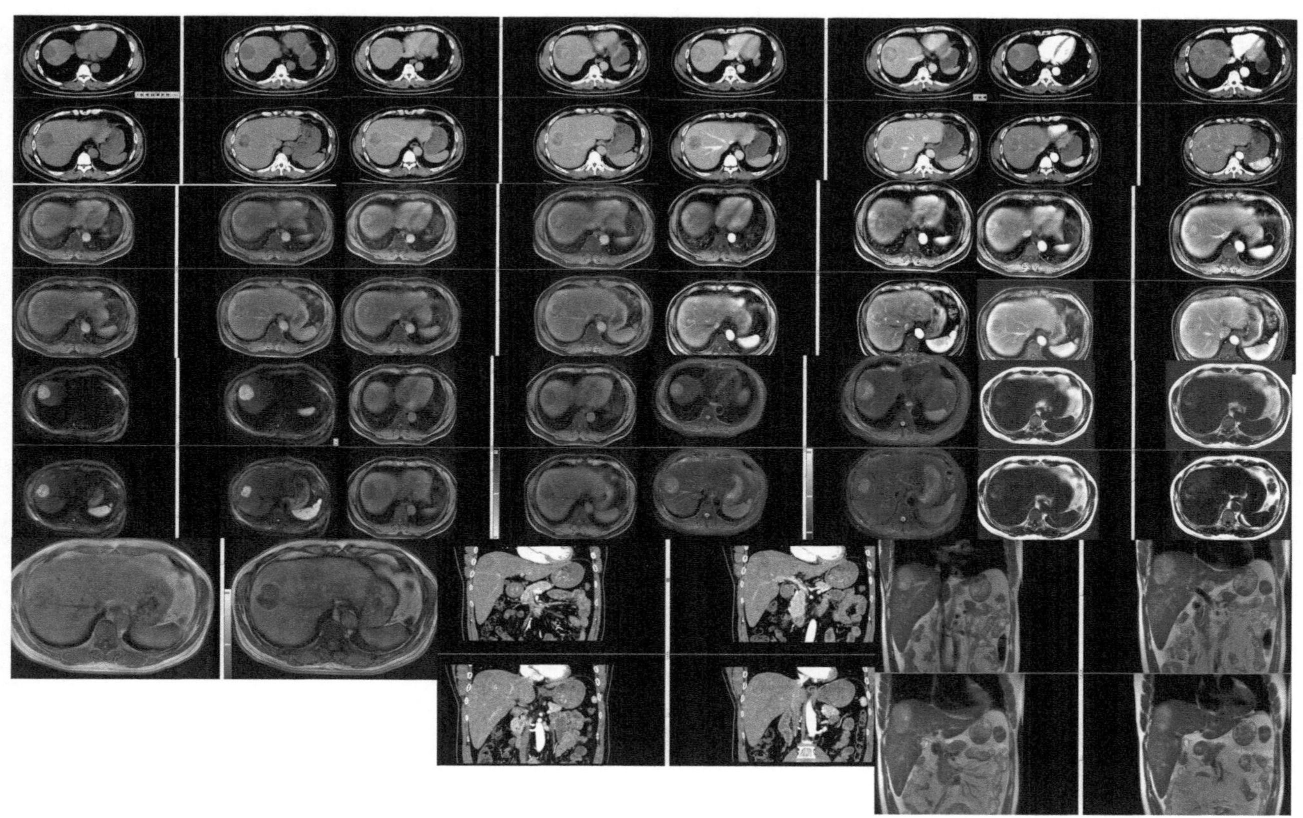

图 3-14-1　高分化肝细胞性肝癌与血管平滑肌脂肪瘤

患者，男，54 岁。体检发现肝占位性病变 3 天入院。患者缘于 3 天前在本院体检行 CT 检查示：肝Ⅶ段占位，考虑不典型肝癌可能，肝腺瘤或肝血管平滑肌脂肪瘤待排，建议 MRI 检查；胆囊结石。同日下午 MRI 示：肝右前叶上段占位，考虑：错构瘤，肝癌待排。

病理检查：肝肿物：肝组织两块，总体积 8.5cm × 7.5cm × 7cm，送检前已切开，切面可见一土黄色结节，大小 5.3 cm × 5 cm × 4.5 cm，质中，境界尚清，肿物紧邻肝被膜，距肝组织断端切缘 0.7 cm，周围肝组织切面呈黄褐色，质中。第 12 组淋巴结：灰黄色组织一块，大小 1.7cm × 1.7cm × 0.5cm。胆囊：胆囊一具，大小 8.8cm × 3.5cm × 3cm，浆膜面光滑，囊内充满墨绿色胆汁，黏膜面可见十余枚淡黄色息肉样物，最大径针尖大至 0.5 cm，壁厚 0.2~0.4 cm，囊内可见墨绿色结石一枚，最大径 0.6 cm。常规病理诊断：肝肿物切除标本：初步诊断肝细胞性肝癌，待做免疫组化检测进一步证实并分级，肿物紧邻肝被膜，肝组织断端切缘为阴性；第 12 组淋巴结切除标本：检出淋巴结 1 枚，未见癌转移；胆囊切除标本：未见癌组织累及，为慢性结石性胆囊炎伴多发胆固醇性息肉。

免疫组化检测：阳性：GPC3（灶 +），Hepatocyte，CD34（肝窦内皮血管转化 +），CK18，CK8，CD10（丛管状 +），Ki-67（+，<5%）；阴性：AFP，CK19，PAX-8，CK7，CK20，pCEA，CEA，HMB45，MelanA。免疫组化诊断：肝肿物切除标本：免疫组化检测结果支持高分化肝细胞性肝癌（大小约 5.3 cm × 5 cm × 4.5 cm），未见血管侵犯，其余内容详见常规报告。

误诊分析：右肝病灶，CT 平扫低密度，T_1 低信号，T_2 及 DWI 高信号，MRI 脂相显示病灶局部高信号，正反相位信号下降，增强后动脉期明显强化，静脉期及延迟期病灶大部分强化减弱，低于正常肝组织强化；结合病人有肝炎病史，需考虑肝癌可能；但是，本例病灶 MRI 脂相显示病灶局部高信号，正反相位信号下降，增强后静脉期及延迟期病灶部分仍强化呈高信号，手术切除标本免疫组化检测时，甲胎蛋白检测为阴性。术前 MRI 误诊为肝脏血管平滑肌脂肪瘤，值得我们认真总结、分析研究和学习（图 3-14-1）。

第十五章　肝癌与超声

肝脏术中超声

肝脏术中超声检查作为手术治疗（如肝段或叶切除、转移瘤的切除以及成年人活体肝右叶移植）的辅助方法，其应用越来越广泛。对于无经验的操作者，在开放式手术中进行超声操作最初是比较困难的。但随着放射科医师对该技术所需设备、操作要求的了解以及技术的熟练掌握，已经能够对实时影像做出解释，从而为外科医师提供有用的信息，有利于手术决策。

设备：肝脏术中超声检查需要专用的探头，常应用侧方发射 5~10 MHz 的“T”形线型或曲线型排列的导体。对于肝脏成像，探头应合适地放置于手掌和手指之间，使肝穹隆顶部和右外侧各段均可成像。也可应用端扫式探头，但因其不易插入右膈下间隙而作用受限。探头应具有彩色多普勒血流和脉冲多普勒成像的能力，而且应具有很好的近扫描野分辨力。

肝脏超声检查技术：放射科医师要进行消毒（包括对探头的消毒），穿手术衣，戴口罩和帽子，在适当的位置站好（一般在病人的右侧）以利于术中操作，将影像监视器放在易于观察的位置，同时要求光线稍暗些。术前应熟悉肝脏的断层影像，了解术中观察目的以及外科医师的特定要求。在手术开始时就应确定此次检查是全面探查肝转移灶，还是只希望确定不能触及的肝内深在病灶的位置。由于肝脏具有自然的湿性表面，因此术中检查通常不需使用耦合乳化液。对于肝脏的成像，须将探头保持横向位置，作连续叠加的矢状走行的探测，从肝左叶外侧段（第Ⅱ段）的最外缘向右侧延伸扫描全肝。

但是肝脏扫描的范围取决于影像研究的目的以及肝脏松动术和韧带切开术的范围。距离最近的病灶可能难以成像，将探测野用无菌的盐水浸泡可能有帮助，或者自肝的相反表面探测成像。必须恰当地将探头放置在病灶区，对第Ⅳ、Ⅴ、Ⅷ段成像时，要求距离近或远的区域均能够显示。最具挑战性的成像区域为肝穹隆后部以及盲区。有时可能需要自肝的下表面进行扫描，应注意在探头倒转时也要将影像翻转过来。

相关的术中解剖：放射科医师应熟悉肝段的解剖，在探头横向放置于肝脏中线区并向搏动的心脏成角时，只需轻压肝表面就能很容易地识别头侧方向的肝静脉。将探头下移放置于肝的下表面、第Ⅳ段之上以及向肝门方向成角能最佳显示门静脉，识别肝静脉和门静脉后即可确定肝脏的分段解剖。经常与术者有关的特殊动脉包括起自肠系膜上动脉并走行于门静脉后部的肝右动脉以及起自胃左动脉并穿过静脉韧带的肝左动脉或肝左副动脉。代表静脉韧带的强回声带的缺失或部分性消失可能提示有一等回声的病灶邻近肝尾状叶。根据手术方式，有时还要向外科医师提供有关肝副静脉的管径和位置。

肝脏盲区：术中对肝脏某些区域的成像特别具有挑战性，这些区域包括肝右叶外侧穹隆区，接近此区常需切开镰状韧带或三角韧带。肝后部膈下裸区的成像可能也很困难，其表面性病变常常为错构瘤，但有时也难以识别，特别是当探头与病变的距离很近而超出其分辨能力，或病变位于肝脏深部及局部区域使探头不能准确放置时，操作者应考虑使用水性介质，或自肝表面相反的方向扫描。

肝脏的假性病变：肝脏术中超声检查的影像分辨力远高于经皮检查，所以肝硬化病人或化疗病人的脂肪浸润灶在术中超声下可能表现得较分散。

脂肪灶一般较软，且在探头下易变形，常可见到血管在其中心通过。在肝脏的裸区以及邻近肝门区域常有少量脂肪，并可产生声影。脂肪的局部聚集也可继发于因病变而产生的灌注受限区。脂肪灶一般不会引起肝包膜的任何膨出或突出。

当识别出脂肪灶时，对其邻近肝实质的成像就显得非常重要，因为其他良性病变，如血管平滑肌脂肪瘤可有相同的表现，但需行手术切除。

在肝脏术中超声检查时，某些可能出现的表现应引起放射科医师的注意。

(1)肝段切除的边缘区常由于烧灼或声处理(常用于分段切除)后进入肝实质和窦状小管的少量气体而产生回声。

(2)在部分切除的肿瘤,其手术切缘处也可因残余肿瘤灶内的气泡而表现为产生回声区。

(3)烧灼处理时的影像可形成带状伪影。

(4)邻近下腔静脉或胆囊窝内的气体聚积,及外科填充材料,可类似于静脉内气体或产生声影。

(5)为更好地进行成像而常用的肝后触诊,也可形成类似黏液性转移瘤的声影。

另外,为定位紧靠肝表面下部的病变而常施行的肝表面烧灼处理产生的声影,必须与表浅性肿瘤的声影相区分。

肝脏术中超声检查的应用:原发性或转移性病变的检测:检查肝脏时,放射科医师应通过一整套方法对肝脏近、中、远各区肝段进行成像,以获得对原发性或转移性病变的满意识别。目前超声探头的分辨力允许识别大于 2 mm 的病变。文献报道肝脏术中超声对于肝脏病变的敏感度大于 90%,阳性或阴性预测值分别为 90% 或 78%,比术前超声检查的病变显示率增加 25%~35%,能检出更多的病变。能够在两个平面对病变成像也很重要,因为有些结直肠转移瘤可能类似于邻近的血管。

病变特点:虽然许多肝脏肿瘤在术中超声检查时的表现类似于经腹超声检查,但也有些肿瘤具有不同的表现。

血管瘤的表现各异,典型者较软,不显示丰富的血流或血流不比邻近的肝实质增加。术前成像方法不能检出的小血管瘤常可在术中超声检查中被识别出来。纤维性血管瘤可因其产回声边缘而被识别。

呈牛眼样或靶形的病变可能为来自结肠癌的转移瘤,或为类癌、局灶性结节性增生及肉瘤。这些病变可含有特征性地出现于黏液样结直肠癌转移瘤的钙化。结肠癌转移瘤与邻近的肝实质相比较常常呈等回声,可因血管闭塞或移位而被检出,也常被边界不清的低回声边缘所包绕。

黏液性肿瘤内的细小钙化如不伴声影则可能类似于血管瘤,但与血管瘤不同的是,转移瘤常产生声影。

良、恶性肿瘤常同时存在。放射科医师应注意的是,起自于单一的原发肿瘤且大小相近的转移瘤其超声学表现基本相似,而大小不同的转移瘤可能在超声检查时表现各异。因此,如果两个或多个大小相似的病灶具有不同的超声学表现,很可能其中一个是转移瘤,而另一个是其他肿瘤(如血管瘤)。

肿瘤切除或转移瘤切除术注意事项:为最好地评估肿瘤的可切除性,放射科医师须全面评价肝内病变,包括有无血管的闭塞或侵犯。如发现病变具有不典型的特点,可根据需要进行超声引导下的活检。

寻找转移性病灶时,放射科医师应注意肝脏的各个叶和段,特别是对于较小的肝段,如尾状叶。肝细胞癌常侵犯大血管,偶尔结直肠癌转移瘤也可有此表现。

另外,还要注意观察肝静脉和门静脉系统,注意肝门区有无增大的淋巴结。根据计划实施的手术方式显示病灶与邻近血管的关系,因为一般病灶周围 1~2 cm 的范围均需切除。

如发现一病灶在肝内,许多外科医师则烧灼病灶的肝包膜以标记计划手术的路径,特别是当进行非肝段式的楔形切除法时,此种烧灼操作可产生声影。

有时放射科医师还会被请回手术室以帮助确定切除范围,判断是否有残余肿瘤灶。有些肿瘤(常是那些难以接触到的或位于具有挑战性部位的,如肝静脉汇合处)可能会有少量的残留灶,术中超声检查可为指导进一步的切除步骤提供信息。

血管开放情况的评价:彩色多普勒血流及脉冲多普勒超声常常被用于区分扩张的胆管与血管。放射科医师须熟悉肝血管的正常解剖及变异,并且对肝表面不能有不必要的压迫,因为加压可导致血管受压,特别是腔静脉。当明确血管内存在栓子时,区分其为血栓还是瘤栓是非常重要的,前者为乏血管,而后者在脉冲多普勒评估时有动脉波形。瘤栓倾向于具有不可切除性,为达到诊断的目的可能需要进行术中超声引导下的活检。

排除危险区(如肝静脉汇合处、右心房及肝内、外门静脉)是否存在栓子是非常重要的。肝外肿瘤,尤其是肾细胞癌可能延伸进入下腔静脉,这在术中超声检查时能够被发现。

良恶性肿瘤均可侵犯血管,因此区分血管是受压移位还是受侵闭塞是很重要的,后者是肿瘤切除的禁忌证。术中多普勒超声检查可用于判断手术形成的门体分流通道的开放情况和血流方向,以及布加综合征病人的病变特点并有助于制定手术计划。根据手术的性质,可能需要应用多普勒超声评价肝外门静脉系统,并指导实施静脉切开和血凝块取出术。

肝移植术:在尸体肝移植中,术中超声有助于评价血管的开放情况和解剖学上的吻合情况,判断肝动脉的不易引起注意的损伤(如切割伤)及有助于在供、受体内血管间进行血管搭桥时准确置入移植物。还可用来判断留存血管(如留存腔静脉)中是否存在血栓,血栓很可能会延伸进入邻近的肝静脉,此时术中超声检查可用于指导血栓切除术。在成人肝右叶劈裂式肝移植中对供体肝脏进行切除时,常需要术中超声帮助识别肝中静脉右侧 1~2 cm 相对乏血管的切除层面。

同时术中超声检查还可用于识别和定位引流第Ⅴ、Ⅷ肝段的肝静脉,并对移植术中需进行单独吻合的肝副静脉进行定位并显示其特点。肝移植术中血管吻合后可立即行术中超声检查,测量血流速度、加速度时间,计算肝动脉阻力指数、搏动指数,及时评价移植肝的血供情况。如发现血流异常,可立即提示手术医师寻找原因并及时处理。

肿瘤消融:在进行间质性消融治疗(如低温消融法、乙醇消融术、微波烧灼法、射频消融术以及激光消融术)时,要求术中超声检查的导引。放射科医师应熟悉滴注或消融术时出现的变化及相应的在超声检查中出现的特点。因治疗时可形成声影,所以在监测穿刺针或电极的位置以及治疗效果时,探头需在探针插入的对侧进行成像。

胆系病变:术中超声检查可用于肝外胆管病变(包括结石)的成像,并定位囊性管道插入物的位置。另外,许多的肝内胆管病变可由超声检查进行全面的评价。对患有可切除性胆管癌的病人行术中超声检查,能够显示胆管的解剖关系以及确定左、右肝管汇合部;对胆管狭窄部位进行定位并显示其特点;在慢性炎性病变、先天性肝胆管囊肿或复发性化脓性胆管肝炎病人中确定肝段的累及范围。彩色多普勒成像可用于区分扩张性胆管与血管、胆管泥沙样结石与肿瘤。尽管术中超声检查难以区分胆囊及胆管的慢性炎性改变与恶性病变,但在指导切除术时会发挥重要作用,当对胆管癌病人进行三段切除术时,它可除外转移性病灶。

肝外病变:术中超声对肝脏成像时,邻近结构中的异常影像也可被识别。例如:肝门区常可见淋巴结,肿瘤可延伸进入膈肌、右心房或腔静脉。

术中超声检查的临床作用:术中超声检查对肝内病变的检出率较常规断面成像法(包括经腹超声检查)高,它可区分实性与囊性肿瘤。因其能够确定病变与血管的关系而有可能提供一种安全的肝大部分切除术式。当行切除术后的结直肠癌病人需辅助疗法而进行病变分期时,它能提供更加完整的临床信息。结直肠癌转移瘤病人术中超声检查的价值可能取决于操作者的经验以及相应肝脏病变的范围。

有研究表明术中超声对结直肠癌转移瘤检出的敏感度和特异度分别为 98% 和 95%,但也有作者提出其对隐匿性结直肠癌肝转移瘤的检出相对不敏感,不支持其应用于所有患结直肠癌的病人。将其应用于 T_3 或 T_4 期的病变,或出现复发癌肿的病人时可增加检出率。肝脏术中增强超声检查对结直肠癌肝脏转移瘤的敏感性更高,通过中心静脉注入对比剂后,转移瘤表现为“快进快出”,在门静脉期和延迟期呈低回声,从而提高了对隐匿性转移瘤的检出率。术前肝脏成像技术水平已明显提高,术中超声检查法与增强 MRI 检查对肝脏病变检出率分别为 94.3% 及 86.7%。

术中超声为术前进行肝脏 3 期增强 CT 扫描中 50% 的病人提供了额外有用的信息,如可检出 CT 不能发现的病灶,对 CT 不能确定的病变进行定性,还可以更清楚地显示肝脏解剖,这些信息使得 15% 的病人改变了手术方案,而即使术中超声检查未改变手术治疗方案,也会对 11% 的病人的病变分期进行修正,从而改变术后的治疗方法。

术中超声检查可为术中的外科医师提供关于病变诊断和分期的关键信息。此项技术已证明在看护病人、手术计划的制定以及判断临床转归方面具有积极作用。随着肝脏手术操作方式的进一步改进,转移性病变手术切除的机会增加,术中超声检查的进一步需求和应用将逐渐加大。

第十六章　肝癌与DSA

一、腹部DSA不同参数造影对肝癌病灶检出的影响

肝癌病灶的检出是选择治疗方案或提高手术成功率的关键。随着数字减影血管造影（DSA）技术及高压注射器智能化的发展，肝癌病灶的检出有了很大提高。但对于直径2 cm以下的肿块及血供不丰富的病灶显示不佳，有时甚至遗漏，有报道漏诊率达到74%，影响了患者的治疗。一些作者通过对220例肝癌患者进行肝总动脉常规造影与长时间低流率造影，发现肝总动脉常规造影与长时间低流率造影对肝癌病灶的检出有较大差别。

DSA技术下肝动脉造影及介入栓塞对肝癌的诊断及治疗得到了广大病人及医学界的公认，然而，介入治疗术的关键技术——肝动脉造影（诊断必须）却一直是局限于肝动脉常规造影（RA），这种造影法对于2 cm以下的肿块及血供不丰富的病灶显示不佳。通过改变造影参数对220例肝癌患者行长时间低流率造影（肝总动脉常规造影与长时间低流率造影），在病灶检出方面取得了很好的效果。

肝癌的血流动力学、DSA在诊断肝癌中的作用：学者们发现，当肝脏良性结节向恶性发展的过程中，存在一个血流动力学上的明显改变，即门静脉的血流逐步减少或截断，动脉的血流逐步增多或完全动脉供血。正常肝脏由肝动脉注入的对比剂在动脉期受到肝内门静脉血流的稀释作用，DSA动脉期中看不到异常染色；而在肝癌，动脉期由肝动脉注入的对比剂优先灌注肝肿瘤，瘤内无门静脉血流稀释，DSA表现为肿瘤血管和肿瘤染色。

已有研究表明，肝动脉造影较CT扫描、B超、核素扫描发现复发病灶的准确性和敏感性更高，肝动脉造影可显示0.2 cm的细小动脉及0.5 cm以下的小病灶。DSA是诊断小肝癌准确而有效的方法。

造影参数及造影方法的选择：造影参数的选择应根据造影部位和病情综合考虑。对比剂流率应与造影血管处血液流动的速度相同或略大，对比剂在该处流率过高而形成膨大可造成伪影，流率过低则造成对比不足，血管充盈不佳，使对比剂注入后取代血流而不被稀释或少稀释，同时又不致引起对比剂的返流，故造影中流率的选择必须恰当准确。

对比剂浓度及用量：在DSA检查中，不同的造影方式需要不同的对比剂浓度和用量，浓度随着观察病变的细致程度不同而不同，过高过低的对比剂浓度对血管的显示均不利，实际应用中，对比剂的每次用量应根据造影方式、造影部位和病情状况等全面考虑。

对于造影方法，有作者提出了慢注射血管造影技术的应用：行靶向血管超选择插管后，以缓慢的注射速度（1~2 ml/s）、较长的注射时间（10 s以上）行靶向血管造影，可使肝内小病灶得到充分的对比剂充盈，从而得以清晰显示。

也有学者提出灌注性肝动脉造影（IHA）可更多地显示肝癌病灶。肝总动脉常规造影、长时间低流率造影与“行靶向血管超选择插管后慢注射血管造影技术”相比，肝动脉常规造影与长时间低流率造影是在肝总动脉进行造影，而非靶向血管，这样可在全局上观察肝癌血供的变化，确定供血动脉分支和供血区域，有时还可显示引流静脉，显示的血管范围要大；与灌注性肝动脉造影相比，肝动脉常规造影与长时间低流率造影可很大程度地减少对比剂的用量，从而减少了对比剂的不良反应和患者的经济负担及肾脏负担。

各个地区、不同医院采用的造影参数各不相同，造影导管位于肝总动脉时注射流率一般为3~8 ml/s，注射量为15~40 ml。在对该组病例的造影中采用的参数为：肝动脉常规造影，流率为4~6 ml/s，注射量20~25 ml；长时间低流率造影，流率为1~2 ml/s，注射量15~20 ml，观察发现，在肝总动脉用5F导管造影，流率>4 ml/s，便可出现对比剂返流，某些少血管性肝癌病灶可不显示肿瘤血管或肿瘤染色。

该组通过对 220 例患者行肝动脉常规造影、长时间低流率造影，肝动脉常规造影共检出病灶 562 个，直径 1~3 cm 的 210 个，≤ 1 cm 的 148 个，病灶直径最小者 0.8 cm；行长时间低流率造影共检出病灶 691 个，直径 1~3 cm 的 225 个，≤ 1 cm 的 162 个，直径最小的 0.3 cm。220 例中 140 例在 2 种参数下造影检出病灶数相同，80 例出现长时间低流率造影较肝动脉常规造影检出病灶数多 129 个，并且有 4 例患者经 CT 扫描、超声探查显示为单发病灶，准备做病灶局部切除，手术前在 DSA 下行长时间低流率造影显示为多个病灶，便改变了手术方案，从而避免了不必要的手术治疗。

结果表明，肝动脉常规造影与长时间低流率造影相比，长时间低流率造影可明显提高病灶检出率，特别是对血供不丰富及较小病灶的检出更敏感，长时间低流率造影对肝癌治疗方案的选择有指导定位作用。

肝动脉常规造影与长时间低流率造影的造影效果：对于肝动脉常规造影，对比剂注射流率为 4~6 ml/s，注射量 20~25 ml，灌注时间 5 s 左右，由于流率太大，对比剂返流明显，肝脏血管持续灌注不充分，导致部分肿瘤血管显示不佳，染色征象不明显，该组病例肝动脉常规造影显示的最小病灶直径为 0.8 cm；对于长时间低流率造影，对比剂注射流率为 1~2 ml/s，注射量 15~20 ml，灌注时间 10 s 左右，其流率适中，对比剂返流不明显，肝脏血管持续灌注充分，无论是正常血管还是肿瘤血管均显示清楚，较小的肿瘤也能染色充分，长时间低流率造影显示的最小病灶直径为 0.3 cm。

对于同一病灶的显示，该组病例中有 8 例患者的病灶出现肝动脉常规造影较长时间低流率造影染色充分，说明肿瘤血供丰富程度与造影的染色程度成正比，在病灶的染色程度方面肝动脉常规造影与长时间低流率造影存在差异，肝动脉常规造影对显示血供丰富的病灶更明显；有 9 例患者肝动脉常规造影显示肿瘤周边无肿瘤染色征象，而长时间低流率造影显示肿瘤周边片状染色，说明如果肿瘤周边血管较细，则长时间低流率造影染色效果好，这对于在肝癌介入治疗后评价肿瘤血管的栓塞效果有重要意义。

肝动脉常规造影一般较易显示较大病灶或血管较丰富的病灶，较小病灶如复发子灶、转移灶易漏诊，但长时间低流率造影显示效果好，因其保证了动脉血管对比剂的持续灌注，其染色时间一般在 8 s 左右。

二、DSA 图像质量控制对病灶的检出有着重要的作用

减少或消除运动性伪影是 DSA 的关键：DSA 检查前要了解病史，包括病人的性别、年龄、临床诊断、碘过敏试验情况，术中造影及介入治疗的目的、方法、范围等。要耐心细致地做好病人的解释工作，做好对病人的心理护理，争取病人的配合。如不易合作、呼吸难以控制的病人，可以选择 DSA 超脉冲方式采集成像，可避免运动性伪影的产生，获得高清晰的 DSA 图像。

术者、技术人员的密切配合是 DSA 质量控制的根本；操作者在造影前要透视定位，减影部位位于图像中心，调节好球管、增强器与病人之间的距离，在肝动脉造影时，肺底与肝膈面处密度反差很大，使膈下肝血管不易显示，为了使照射部位密度趋于一致，减少饱和状伪影，要在肺底部用附加软滤过板的方法，或调节视野大小，使肺底与膈面处密度趋于一致。靶器官透视定位，DSA 连续采集至出现动脉期、毛细血管期、实质期、静脉期的图像，一般须延迟采集 10 s 左右。

技术人员严格执行各项操作规程及造影程序，配合医生于术前术中做好各项质控工作，根据造影部位和医生的要求进行造影参数的选择。护士在做好术前准备工作后，术中严密观察病人情况，并训练病人屏气，配合技师进行图像采集。

对比剂的选择及减影方式、帧频：由于对比剂的渗透压、黏稠度，对比剂的毒性以及给药时的浓度、剂量、流速和注入部位均可导致病人不同程度的过敏反应甚至危及生命，同时这些因素也影响着显影部位的清晰度。因此正确选择对比剂类型、流速及注射方式很重要，特别是病情严重、高龄、高敏、难以合作的患者应首选非离子型对比剂。

腹部 DSA 一般采用脉冲（PI）方式采集图像，摄像系列 Duration 为 5 s、5 s、30 s 3 个时间段，帧率（frame rate）分别为 6.3 F/s、3.1 F/s、1.6 F/s。因为整个系列如果用同一种帧率，太高容易增加辐射剂量，太低又不能很好地显示动脉期的血管像。

曝射参数的设定及图像后处理：除机器本身的自动曝光功能外，手动设定时应考虑：①影像增强器尽量靠近病人；②合理应用视野调节及胶片距

(SID)调节以改变放大率;③合理确定病人体型。曝光前充分应用曝光测试功能,使兴趣区(ROI)获得优化的曝光条件。合理应用 DSA 的后处理功能也尤为重要。

综上所述,肝总动脉长时间低流率造影较常规参数造影可大大提高病灶检出率,特别是对血供不丰富及较小病灶的检出更有意义。有效的图像质量控制是提高病灶检出率的保证。另外,X 线的质和量、DSA 机的分辨率、肝脏的体积也影响着图像质量和病灶检出效果。

第十七章　肝癌破裂出血

肝细胞癌自发破裂出血

肝细胞癌自发破裂出血是中晚期肝癌最严重的并发症之一，该并发症多见于亚洲及非洲，罕见于欧美国家，临床发生率为 12%~14%，一旦破裂而不采取有效措施几乎 100% 死亡。肝细胞癌自发性破裂出血作为一种急腹症，应该十分重视。

一、肝细胞癌自发性破裂的机制

肿瘤血管生成中的缺陷：肿瘤大多血供丰富，容易出血。而肿瘤血管生成过程非常复杂，主要包括宿主毛细血管受血管刺激因子作用，初期发生扩张，通透性增高；纤维蛋白外渗至血管周围的细胞外基质，导致其环境改变；蛋白酶和胶原酶激活，使毛细血管基底膜降解；血管内皮细胞增生、迁移；内皮细胞重排并贯通形成功能性血管。Hanahan 等（1996）提出了血管生成开关平衡学说，认为血管生成过程中正负调节因子浓度改变相当于一种开关，正调节因子，如血管内皮生长因子（VEGF）等，负调节因子，如血管抑素。正负调节因子可由肿瘤细胞、炎症细胞和基底细胞分泌。

新生的肿瘤血管在组织结构上具有如下特点：缺乏平滑肌细胞和神经末梢，故肿瘤血管无舒缩功能；内皮细胞基底膜不完整导致血管壁不成熟，外周间隙增大，通透性增高；血管数量明显增多，血管形态扭曲增粗，不规则分支，异常的血管网状结构。肿瘤血管的这种组织结构特点，很难适应内外环境的变化，极易导致破裂出血。

血液流变学异常及肿瘤内压升高：有研究证明，肝细胞癌病人的全血黏滞度、血浆黏度、纤维蛋白原、红细胞硬度及血沉等血液流变学指标明显高于正常值，主要是由于肝癌组织的生长导致机体产生了一系列变化。因肝癌病人大多合并肝硬化，病人红细胞中胆固醇含量增高，使红细胞变形能力下降，因表面负电荷减少，电泳率下降，血沉加快。同时，血液的高黏及高凝状态易产生微小的附壁血栓，肿瘤细胞被血栓包裹，逃避了机体的免疫系统攻击，在血流较慢的静脉形成癌栓。Yuki 等（1990）报道肝细胞癌病人门静脉和肝静脉形成癌栓的发生率可达 57.9% 和 21.3%。另外，门静脉癌栓常易形成动脉 - 门静脉瘘。肝静脉及其分支阻塞、静脉回流受阻时，肿瘤静脉可能经包膜下侧支循环引流或门静脉引流。当合并肝硬化或门脉癌栓或动 - 静脉瘘时，这种引流可能失败而导致肿瘤内血流淤滞、压力升高。

此外，肿瘤特别是带有包膜的巨块型肿瘤呈膨胀性生长时，快速增生的肿瘤细胞直接或间接地对血管压迫致肿瘤内的毛细血管压力高于正常毛细血管压力。肿瘤细胞间质中含有大量富含胶原的基质，以及伴随大量的肿瘤血管生成而有大量的液体渗漏到细胞间质，肿瘤组织又缺乏功能性淋巴系统，致使液体不能有效地被清除。肿瘤内压升高，当肿瘤位于肝脏边缘并凸出于肝脏轮廓外尤其凸向膈顶或腹腔时，呼吸运动的影响或轻微的外伤可导致破裂出血。

血管病变及抗原抗体复合物的血管壁沉积：肝细胞癌自发性破裂是一种出血性并发症，与血管损伤有一定关系。Zhu 等（1996，2001）通过 23 例肝细胞癌自发破裂的标本与 30 例非破裂的肝细胞癌标本对比，应用免疫组化方法检测与血管病变有关的因素，结果发现，与非破裂组相比较，肝细胞癌破裂组血管的 vWF 表达量明显下降，血管壁中弹性蛋白酶分布异常，弹性硬蛋白变性或增生过度，血管周壁胶原蛋白酶分泌量增加，Ⅳ型胶原蛋白被分解退化。vWF 为血管受损标志之一并参与凝血过程，低表达量的 vWF 说明肝癌破裂前血管壁即有病变存在，并伴有凝血功能下降。血管受损后，随即释放的细胞因子刺激血管壁细胞合成过量的弹性硬蛋白和胶原蛋白酶，导致弹性硬蛋白过度增生，血管弹性消失。胶原蛋白酶可分解胶原蛋白层，使血管壁支撑力下降。另外，中性粒细胞浸润受损的血管壁，释放弹性蛋白酶，使血管的弹力膜断裂，血管脆性增加。此时肝细胞癌病人在外力或肿瘤内压增高的作用下,极易发生血管壁破裂现象,导致肿瘤破裂出血。血管损伤现象仅发生于小动脉,与由乙型肝炎病毒e抗原HbeAg/L、免疫球蛋白和补体C1q所组成的抗原抗体复合物在血管壁上的沉积率有关。大动脉虽亦有抗原抗体复合物的沉积,但因其血小板衍生生长因子(PDGF)受体不表达,故抗原抗体复合物可沉积于大动脉却无病理损伤出现。

其他:肝左叶较易发生自发性破裂出血,与肝左叶体积较小,肿瘤易于向肝表面生长,并易于突破肝被膜侵犯肝外固有组织有关。当肿瘤侵犯肝外邻近组织并伴有腹水时,由于腹水进入肿瘤与被侵犯的组织之间而导致肿瘤滋养动脉撕裂出血。另外,由于解剖位置关系,肝左叶更易受外力作用及呼吸运动影响。

经导管动脉栓塞(TAE)后肝细胞癌自发性破裂已有报道,而经导管动脉栓塞是否是肿瘤破裂出血的一种诱因或一种机制,有待进一步研究,这可能与肿瘤内大量坏死,产生张力有关。

二、影像学研究

肝细胞癌自发性破裂出血临床诊断的敏感性、特异性不如影像学检查。

超声:其敏感性虽不如CT,但因其简便、灵活的特点可作为首选。通过发现腹水中出现不断移动性回声点而提示活动性出血。出血早期,可见肿瘤病变低回声区内出现高回声区,提示肿瘤内出血,60%的病人肿瘤周围有强回声的出血灶。超声还可显示肿瘤向肝表面突出且轮廓欠清,边缘不规则,结合临床及腹水异常可进行诊断。对于向膈顶凸出或腹腔凸出的肝细胞癌自发破裂出血病灶的诊断,超声较CT横断面扫描有优越性。

近来,高频多普勒超声可测量微血管血流和形态,从而揭示了肿瘤血管生成的独特方式。靶向性对比剂增强超声是通过把特定配体-对比剂复合物结合到相应的靶点而实现肿瘤强化。选择VEGF、组织生长因子等作为靶点,可监测肿瘤的血管生成,预测肿瘤的侵袭性,有望在肝细胞癌自发破裂的研究中得到应用。

CT:CT对肝细胞癌自发性破裂出血诊断的敏感度达100%。CT平扫可发现肿瘤大小、部位,也能通过发现肝脏边缘不规则提示肝硬化,还可显示肿瘤内高密度的出血灶、肝包膜下积血、肝脏表面的不连续性,并通过检测腹水CT值判断血性腹水。增强CT动脉期可表现为不强化的低密度病灶自强化但不连续的破溃的肿瘤边缘突入肝周间隙或腹膜腔,典型的表现为肿瘤内容物从强化不连续的肿瘤边缘破入腹膜腔,如同摘除了眼球内容物留下巩膜的眼眶,称之为“摘除征”(enuclcation sign)。增强CT还可发现对比剂外溢等活动性出血征象。位于肝尾叶的肝细胞癌自发破裂出血往往还可表现为突出的肿块中坏死的小囊内出现高密度的血肿。

最早,Kanematsu等(1992)即做了依据形态学对肝细胞癌自发破裂进行预测的研究,通过对23例肝细胞癌破裂前3个月内的CT影像与20例肝细胞癌无破裂而死亡前3个月内的CT影像比较,发现肿瘤的大小、肿瘤的外凸程度、肿瘤表面肝组织最小厚度及肿瘤是否突破肝脏表面并侵犯至邻近结构是肿瘤自发破裂的危险因素,对预测肝细胞癌自发性破裂有重要意义。

形态结构的不同虽可预测肝细胞癌自发破裂,但并不是肿瘤自发破裂的根本原因,肿瘤血管生成伴发肿瘤组织的血流量、血流速度、微血管通透性、血管外组织液体积及肿瘤内压的变化等CT可监测分析的指标可提示肿瘤自发破裂的内因。

运用动态增强CT,依据CT强化的组织生理学基础与肿瘤新生血管组织病理学基础的相似性,通过组织衰减系数建立的时间-浓度曲线、平均通过时间(MTT)等数学分布模型,分析相应的变化,会对肝细胞癌自发破裂的可能性做进一步的预测。

DSA:此方法可显示不同程度的肝动脉增粗,异常扭曲团块状的肿瘤血管及肿瘤染色。透视下可见到膈下积液并在注入对比剂后积液密度逐渐升高。如出血速度快可见到小动脉内对比剂向外喷洒现象。DSA对肝细胞癌自发破裂诊断的假阴性率较高,Ngan等(1998)报道的33例肝细胞癌自发性破裂出血中仅6例显示对比剂外溢,可能与造影时出血已停止,对比剂被稀释,或少量对比剂外溢与不规则肿瘤血管及肿瘤染色混杂难以鉴别有关。

MRI:MRI依据形态学特点预测肝细胞癌自发破裂并不是MRI的优势所在。MRI采用1.5T以上MR设备的动态增强检查,扫描速度进一步提高。在组织强化中可获得更精确的时间-信号强度曲线(TIC),可用来评价肿瘤的血管生成状态。其检测的指标有组织的血容量或血浆容量,血管内皮对水或溶质的通透性以及特异的血管生成因子相对浓度等,依据这些指标的变化会对肝细胞癌自发破裂的预测提供帮助。

大分子对比剂(MMCM)及靶向性对比剂的出现使动态增强MR可提供更为精确的组织灌注信息。大分子对比剂增强MRI可成功检测肿瘤微血管特性,包括跨内皮通透性及部分血浆容积。由于易自发破裂的肝细胞癌存在着以大分子跨血管内皮流量差的变化为前提的血管病变及肿瘤间质大分子的高渗性所致的肿瘤内压变化,因而大分子对比剂很适合监测大分子的血管内皮通透性及大分子的肿瘤血管内外分布。

靶向性对比剂通过对比剂与特异受体结合,可定量检测肿瘤新生血管结构及其功能特征。随着新的成像技术和方法的应用(包括对比剂、脉冲序列、分析方法和动力学模型等),MRI在肝细胞癌自发破裂中会有广阔的应用前景。

第十八章　关于肝占位性病变的鉴别诊断

肝癌和局灶性结节增生是肝脏常见的富血供病变。传统 CT 检查主要依靠病变的影像特征，包括形态、密度、增强后强化方式等进行鉴别诊断。其影像特征以前文献报道较多，大多仅为定性研究，很少进行定量分析。MSCT 仍是目前临床上诊断肝脏疾病最常用的影像检查技术。然而，传统 CT 采用的是单参数(CT 值)和混合能量(kVp)成像，此 CT 值不能准确反映物质对 X 线的衰减。64 层能谱 CT 是近年来开发的一项崭新技术，在优化图像质量及对比噪声比、物质定量分析和能谱综合分析等方面较传统 CT 均有重大突破。能谱 CT 的单能量成像突破了以往仅依靠 CT 值的单参数成像的诊断模式，能提供 40~140 keV 间一系列连续能量的图像，选取最佳的单能量图像，优化病灶与肝脏的对比度，从而更清楚地显示微小病灶。

单能量图像还能够有效规避射线硬化伪影，从而获得更准确的 CT 值。能谱成像不仅能够观察人体解剖的形态学信息，而且还能够通过综合混合能量图像、单能量图像、碘基图、水基图和钙基图等物质分离图像，对病变进行定量定性分析，了解其组织病理学信息。

一些作者利用能谱 CT 获得肝癌和局灶性结节增生病变的能谱系列图像，并对其进行定性、定量分析，比较两者不同能谱定量参数值的差异，旨在探讨能谱 CT 的能谱成像模式和能谱分析功能对肝癌和局灶性结节增生检出及鉴别诊断的价值。

CT 能谱成像可以获得常规混合能量图像、40~140 keV 内共 101 种单能量图像及多种基础物质对图像。常规混合能量图像与传统 CT 得到的图像相似，对一些小病变的检出敏感度不高，病变的显示也欠佳。不同能量水平的单能量图像可以满足不同疾病诊断的需要，应用最佳病灶 - 正常肝组织对比噪声比曲线得到最佳单能量，在此能量下所得到的单能量图像对病变的检出和显示最佳。此外，碘基图像有效抑制了背景 CT 值及容积效应的影响，对碘剂的沉积敏感，真实体现肝实质和病灶内碘剂的分布，有利于肝脏富血供病变的检出。该研究显示，单能量图像和碘基图像对肝癌的显示明显优于常规混合能量图像，因此有利于小肝癌的检出。

HU 衰减曲线反映了 X 线束穿过某种物质的衰减情况，是由组成物质的化学分子结构决定的，不同化学构成的组织具有不同的衰减曲线，可以用 HU 衰减曲线的差异来区分人体内不同化学成分。该项研究中，肝癌和局灶性结节增生的 HU 衰减曲线在两期中不平行也不重合，说明两者的组成成分不同。这种差别深层的原因在于肿块病理组织学、化学性质或代谢产物的差别。应用 HU 衰减曲线可以定性分析两种病变是否同源。

一般来说，高能量的图像组织对比度较小，低能量的图像组织对比度较大。肝癌和局灶性结节增生在不同能量水平下的病灶 - 正常肝组织对比噪声比呈现出一定的规律性，总的来说，病灶 - 正常肝组织对比噪声比随着单光子能量的增加而减小，但在部分能量点除外。

肝癌和局灶性结节增生的动脉期最佳单能量均为 50 keV，门静脉期最佳单能量分别为 70 keV 和 50 keV，此 2 种病变的最佳单能量位于低能量水平(50~70 keV)。低能量图像组织对比度较大，可以更好地显示小病灶，有利于小病灶如小肝癌的检出。

肝癌的动脉期和门静脉期标准化碘浓度、病灶与周围正常肝组织碘浓度比值及动脉期和门静脉期病灶碘浓度的差异值均低于局灶性结节增生，其差异均有统计学意义，这可能与肝癌的血供类型和分化程度有关。

一些学者对原发性肝癌血供特点的研究表明肝癌不仅由肝动脉供血，部分存在门静脉供血或少血供，肝癌血供方式与其癌细胞分化程度和组织学类型有关。

Asayama 等(2008)研究表明：肝癌中不成对肝动脉的数量随着高分化肝癌向中等分化肝癌发展而

逐渐增加，随着中等分化肝癌向低分化肝癌发展而逐渐减少。由此得知，部分存在门静脉供血的肝癌和低分化肝癌的肝动脉血供较差，导致了反映血供变化的碘浓度定量参数标准化碘浓度、病灶与周围正常肝组织碘浓度比值及动脉期和门静脉期病灶碘浓度的差异等值的下降。

而局灶性结节增生含有正常的肝细胞，其中央瘢痕及周边常可见增粗迂曲的供血动脉，血供丰富，因此其动脉期和门静脉期的标准化碘浓度、病灶与周围正常肝组织碘浓度比值及动脉期和门静脉期病灶碘浓度的差异值均较高。

此外，肝癌的脂肪（钙）浓度在两期中均比局灶性结节增生高，这可能与小肝癌易发生脂肪变性有关，尤其在直径 1.5 cm 左右的癌结节中最为常见，随着肿瘤的生长逐渐消失。2 组间的水（碘）浓度在动脉期和门脉期差异均无统计学意义，所以，水（碘）浓度对两者的鉴别无实用价值。

所有能谱定量参数值曲线均在参考线之上，说明其对鉴别肝癌和局灶性结节增生均有一定的价值。ROC 曲线下面积越大，诊断的准确性越高。

鉴别肝癌和局灶性结节增生的最佳能谱定量参数值是动脉期病灶与周围正常肝组织碘浓度比值，其阈值 4.33 鉴别两者的准确度、敏感度和特异度均为 100%；其次为门静脉期标准化碘浓度，其阈值 0.58 鉴别两者的准确度、敏感度和特异度分别为 90%、70%、100%；动脉期和门静脉期病灶碘浓度的差异值鉴别两者的准确度和敏感度均较其他定量参数值低。该项研究结果表明碘浓度定量分析在鉴别肝癌和局灶性结节增生中具有较高的敏感度和特异度，有助于提高鉴别诊断的准确性。Lv 等（2011）利用 CT 能谱成像研究了碘浓度定量分析在小肝癌和小血管瘤的鉴别诊断中的价值，其敏感度和特异度可分别高达 97% 和 100%，其研究结果也证实了碘浓度定量分析在鉴别肝脏富血供病变中的可行性。

该项研究的局限性：①病例数相对较少；②对于不同分化程度的肝癌未分类进行研究；③未对肝癌和局灶性结节增生的形态学特征及强化方式进行研究，因为这不是该研究的重点；④仅研究了肝癌和局灶性结节增生，以后的研究将进一步扩大研究范围，包括肝腺瘤、不典型血管瘤等；⑤该项研究为回顾性分析，未来将进行前瞻性研究来进一步完善研究结果。

综上所述，能谱成像的单能量图像和碘基图像有利于肝脏富血供病变的检出。碘浓度定量分析对肝癌和局灶性结节增生的鉴别有较大价值，能提高诊断准确性。

附：具体研究资料：所需测量和计算的数据包括：①病灶的 CT 值、碘（水）浓度、水（碘）浓度、钙（脂肪）浓度、脂肪（钙）浓度及正常肝组织和腹主动脉的碘（水）浓度；②病灶 - 正常肝组织对比噪声比（CNR），CNR=（CT 病灶 - CT 肝脏）/SD 噪声，CT 病灶为病灶 CT 值的平均值，CT 肝脏为正常肝组织 CT 值的平均值，SD 噪声为正常肝脏 CT 值的标准差，在该研究中以肝脏为背景；③标准化碘浓度（NIC），NIC=IC 病灶 /IC 腹主，IC 病灶为病灶的碘（水）浓度，IC 腹主为腹主动脉的碘（水）浓度；④病灶与周围正常肝组织碘浓度比值（LNR），LNR= IC 病灶 /IC 肝脏，IC 肝脏为正常肝组织的碘（水）浓度；⑤动脉期和门静脉期病灶碘浓度的差异（ICD），ICD=|IC 动脉期 - IC 门脉期 |，所有数据均测量 3 次，取其平均值。

第十九章 关于肝癌的误诊

第一节 螺旋CT三期增强扫描误诊或漏诊肝细胞性肝癌

癌的早期诊断和治疗是提高患者5年生存率的重要途径,也是临床不断探索的课题。经过长期的临床实践,螺旋CT双期或多期增强扫描已成为肝癌的首选检查方法之一,其诊断符合率可达90%以上。但在日常工作中,仍有少数病例被误诊或漏诊,特别是小肝癌。

一些作者回顾性分析一组20例经手术病理证实而螺旋CT三期增强扫描误诊或漏诊的肝细胞性肝癌病例,以进一步提高肝癌的诊断正确性。肝癌是肝脏的常见肿瘤,腹部B超及CT平扫、多期增强扫描均可发现病灶,做出定性诊断。但由于肝癌病理基础复杂,故注射对比剂后的表现呈多样化。大多数肝癌在注射对比剂后,肝动脉期明显强化,门静脉期密度减低即所谓"速升速降"征,诊断较为肯定。但少数肝癌表现不典型,容易误诊。

特殊部位肝细胞肝癌及CT扫描参数选择对较小肝细胞肝癌检出的影响

该组漏诊的3个病灶虽然在三期增强扫描中有典型的表现,但由于病灶位于肝门区及肝脏的边缘部,阅片不仔细误认为血管影或胃泡伪影而漏诊。这3个病灶中有2个病灶由于伴有肝硬化且为微小肝癌,CT平扫、门静脉期及延迟期时肝实质强化不均匀,致低密度结节未能观察到。肝动脉期对这些病灶的检出有重要意义,应予重视。但由于患者因年龄、心率、血压和一般情况等因素不同,其血液循环速度也不同,单层螺旋CT未必能准确获得肝动脉期、门脉期图像,有可能提前或落后,不能真实反映病灶的血供情况而导致漏检。随着MSCT技术的发展,扫描速度的提高大大减少了因呼吸运动伪影的干扰,而且MSCT借助示踪技术和自动触发扫描软件可获得理想的肝动脉期图像,对病灶检出率有较大提高。

另外,扫描参数优化组合尤其是扫描层厚、螺距选择,对小病灶检出影响较大。螺距改变时,噪声也有一定程度的变化,当螺距小于1时噪声较小,当螺距等于1时噪声增加,当螺距等于1.5时,噪声又有一定程度的下降,当螺距增大到2时,图像噪声明显增大,因此在临床中一般不选用螺距大于2的参数条件。层厚对图像的Z轴空间分辨力起决定性作用,层厚越大,部分容积效应增加,降低了Z轴空间分辨力,若层厚大于病灶上下径,则有可能因为部分容积效应而漏检。该组病例有2个病灶虽然甲胎蛋白持续明显增高,临床上肝癌诊断明确,但螺旋CT扫描未能发现,可能因为病灶较小,采用层厚8~10mm扫描,由于部分容积效应而漏检。近年来,随着多层螺旋CT的发展和推广,多排探测器的应用,扫描层厚可进一步变薄,最薄层厚可达0.5mm以下,可以更好地显示肝内微小的病灶,大大提高小肝癌的检出率。

病灶的定性,病灶的不典型强化方式是误诊的主要原因。对于呈典型表现的肝癌,很容易做出定性诊断,而对呈不典型表现的肝癌,如未经仔细分析,容易误诊为其他肝脏病变。此处主要探讨4种容易误诊的不典型强化方式。

第一种不典型强化方式:动脉期边缘有环形或点状强化,门静脉期强化程度和范围较动脉期大,延迟期强化范围进一步扩大,容易误诊为血管瘤或肝炎性假瘤。该组病灶中有5个病灶误诊为血管瘤,2个病灶误诊为炎性假瘤。手术病理证实均为硬化型肝癌,分化Ⅲ~Ⅳ级。这种肝癌少见,而且临床、病理和影像学表现均与其他类型的肝细胞肝癌有所不同,因此,熟悉其CT表现对临床诊断和治疗均有重要意义。在病理上,硬化型肝癌表现为细条状的癌细胞索被致密的结缔组织分隔。大量纤维组织的存在使对比剂在病灶内的滞留时间长,排泄慢,从而出现延迟强化的表现。以下征象有助于和血管瘤鉴别:①硬化型肝细胞肝癌虽在肝动脉期有边缘环形或结节状强化,但强化的程度不及血管瘤高,血管瘤在肝动脉期时的强化程度高,其密度和主动脉的密度接近或一致;②在门静脉期和/或延迟期时,病灶强化范围扩大,但始终无充填改变。肝炎性假瘤病理特点是中心凝固性坏死,周边有纤维包膜形成,在肝动脉期强化不明显,大部分门静脉期和延迟期病灶周边可见环形强化。较为有特征性的征象:病灶内可有纤维间隔、病灶在延迟扫描中可出现高密度强化(高于肝实质),而中心凝固性坏死区始终无强化。

第二种不典型强化方式:肝动脉期边缘部呈不规则环形强化,门静脉期和延迟期此强化环呈等密度,容易误诊为肝脓肿。该组4个病灶手术病理证实为中央大范围的坏死,其环形强化病理基础为病灶边缘残存癌组织,由于类似于不典型肝脓肿表现而误诊。

鉴别要点:肝癌坏死区域CT值一般高于脓液,病灶边缘明显高低不平,腔壁可见结节;病灶边缘部未坏死癌组织强化呈速升速降型,与肝脓肿的边缘逐渐强化征不同;不典型肝脓肿可有段性强化征、肿块缩小征、周边多囊征、花瓣征等征象。阅片时还应注意有无门脉增粗、充盈缺损等门脉癌栓表现及肝门区有无淋巴结肿大等支持肝癌的诊断。

第三种不典型强化方式:病灶始终无强化表现,呈低密度,容易误诊为肝硬化结节,该组有3个病灶,均为小肝癌,肿瘤分化为Ⅱ级2个,Ⅲ级1个,均误诊为肝硬化结节。

这类小肝癌的动脉和门脉血供都少于正常肝,属少血供的小肝细胞肝癌。增强后瘤灶肝动脉期、门静脉期及延迟期均呈低密度的原因是多方面的,其一是瘤灶的病理基础,瘤灶内有坏死和脂肪变是造成小肝癌在动脉期无明显强化或不强化的主要原因;其二是瘤灶的血供减少,Takayasu等(1995)报道有许多分化较好的或早期肝细胞癌是少血供的。

该组3个病灶均未见坏死,其中2个病灶内有脂肪变。这类小肝细胞肝癌属少见的CT表现,但仍有其特征性表现。①病灶边缘部的CT表现:平扫病灶边界模糊,增强病灶边界清楚且轻度不规整,小肝癌病灶边缘部多数缺乏纤维假包膜,以及肿瘤呈浸润性生长,边缘部的肿瘤细胞与正常肝细胞交错存在是此特征表现的病理基础。②病灶内部的CT表现:增强后仍呈低密度的小肝癌瘤体内密度不均匀,出现多个小斑点状密度更低区。

根据这些特点,可以与肝脏其他表现为低密度的病变进行鉴别,但与肝硬化结节鉴别相当困难,MRI检查在二者的鉴别上更有优势。

第四种不典型强化方式:肝动脉期呈高密度,门静脉期呈等密度,延迟期仍呈等密度,这种不典型表现的肝癌和局灶性结节增生不易鉴别,该组2个病灶为CT导引下穿刺活检后病理证实,无手术切除标本病理对照。这种表现的肝癌病灶血供相当丰富,可能存在肝动脉与门静脉双重供血,或者肿瘤的细胞外间隙较大,对比剂滞留时间较长,病灶可以持续强化。

另外,在病理分型上有一类血管扩张型肝癌,因有异常丰富的血管,门静脉期和延迟期可持续强化。局灶性结节增生较为特征性的CT表现有以下几点:①局灶性结节增生平扫呈略低密度或等密度,中央可见低密度瘢痕;②动脉期除瘢痕外明显均匀强化,门脉期呈等或略高密度,延迟后呈等或略低密度;③在病灶的中央或周边有时可见明显增粗扭曲的供血动脉。小肝细胞肝癌动脉期虽有明显强化但不如局灶性结节增生均匀一致,强化程度也低于局灶性结节增生。但是较小的局灶性结节增生中心星芒状瘢痕出现率低,应引起注意。

综上所述,三期增强扫描中强化方式不典型是肝细胞肝癌误诊的主要原因,而这种不典型强化方式是肝细胞肝癌的病理基础和生长方式所造成的。熟悉肝细胞肝癌的病理基础和生长方式,细致阅片和分析可进一步提高肝细胞肝癌的诊断准确性。

附:具体研究资料:该组20例共21个病灶,其中19例为单发,有1例为2个病灶,病灶直径为5~80mm,平均44mm。5个病灶漏诊,16个病灶误诊为其他肝脏病变,分别误诊为肝血管瘤(5个),肝脓肿(4个),肝硬化结节(3个),局灶性结节增生(2个),肝炎性假瘤(2个)。该组漏诊病灶5个,直径均小于10mm,其中2个病灶在三期扫描中均未能发现,但临床上AFP持续明显增高,后经肝动脉造影CT(CTHA)发现。其余3个病灶,2个位于肝门区血管旁,1个位于肝左叶外段肝脏边缘部,在三期增强扫描中有典型的强化表现(即肝动脉期呈高密度,门静脉期、延迟期呈低密度,呈“速升速降”型)。

该组误诊病灶 16 个,病灶增强扫描不典型 CT 表现为:①肝动脉期边缘有环形或点状强化,门静脉期强化程度和范围较动脉期大,延迟期强化范围进一步扩大,表现出延迟强化的特点, 5 个病灶误诊为血管瘤, 2 个病灶误诊为炎性假瘤;②肝动脉期边缘部呈不规则环形强化,门静脉期和延迟期此强化环呈等密度,内见壁结节影, 4 个病灶误诊为肝脓肿;③病灶始终无强化表现,呈低密度影, 3 个病灶误诊为肝硬化结节;④肝动脉期呈高密度,门静脉期和延迟期呈等密度,2 个病灶误诊为局灶性结节增生。

第二节 乏血供型肝细胞癌

肝细胞肝癌典型的 CT 征象为平扫显示(稍)低密度影,增强扫描呈"速升速降"型强化,其病理生理学基础为肝细胞肝癌由肝动脉供血且血供丰富。而乏血供型肝细胞肝癌较为少见,增强扫描强化形式多样,容易导致误诊。

螺旋 CT 尤其是 MSCT 扫描速度快,可做多期动态增强扫描检查,能充分反映病灶的血供特点,有利于病灶的检出和定性。正常肝脏的血供约 3/4 由门静脉供应, 1/4 来自肝动脉,而大部分的肝细胞肝癌由肝动脉供血,因此在 CT 增强扫描动脉期,主要由门静脉供血的正常肝组织尚未出现明显强化,而主要由肝动脉供血的肝细胞肝癌出现明显强化(高密度),但到了门静脉期,正常肝组织强化明显,肝细胞肝癌则因为没有门静脉供血,强化迅速减退,表现为低密度影,整个强化过程呈"速升速降"改变,这是典型富血供肝细胞肝癌动态增强表现的基础。乏血供肝细胞肝癌伴发肝炎、肝硬化及甲胎蛋白增高的概率虽然与典型富血供肝细胞肝癌相似,但是由于病灶的血供方式和病理成分等与后者有所不同,故 CT 表现可能会不典型,再加上经验不足,易导致误诊,因此,有必要加深对此类肝细胞肝癌的认识。

乏血供肝细胞肝癌的表现之一(3/12)是 CT 平扫及增强均呈稍低密度影,但增强扫描略有强化,且动脉期 CT 值稍高于门脉期和 / 或延迟期,说明病灶血供较差而且以肝动脉供血为主,CT 灌注成像显示癌灶的肝动脉灌注分数明显高于其他肝实质的肝动脉灌注分数,亦印证了病灶肝动脉供血比重增大的特点,符合肝细胞肝癌不典型"速升速降"型强化的曲线特征,因此肝硬化背景下的低密度影,需要详细分析 CT 平扫及增强 CT 值的变化特点,只要符合不典型"速升速降"型强化的趋势,就得警惕肝细胞肝癌的可能。如果合并有门静脉栓塞,诊断的把握性更大,CT 灌注成像能为肝细胞肝癌提供重要的诊断信息。

乏血供型肝细胞肝癌的表现之二是 CT 平扫及增强动脉期均表现为等密度,门脉期及延迟期迅速减退为低密度影。该组 4/12 例肝细胞肝癌呈此表现,动脉期仍为等密度的原因可能是此类病灶属低血供型肝细胞肝癌且为肝动脉供血,病灶的肝动脉血供有轻度增加,但不足以使病灶在动脉期呈高密度,因此仅见轻度强化(与周边肝实质强化效果相当而呈等密度影),但在门脉期和延迟期强化下降,观察其强化曲线仍属于不典型"速升速降"型改变。值得注意的是该型肝细胞肝癌单纯 CT 平扫会漏诊病灶,疑诊病例需行 CT 增强扫描检查;另外,与典型肝细胞肝癌不同,此类肝细胞肝癌的动脉期检出率极低。

乏血供肝细胞肝癌的表现之三(2/12)是肝细胞肝癌边缘不规则并形成壁结节,增强动脉期边缘可见多发点状强化,门脉期则减退为等密度,仍然具有"速升速降"型强化的特征,至于病灶内部增强扫描始终无强化的原因,考虑可能是由于癌灶中部坏死液化较为彻底所致。此类肝细胞肝癌需与肝脓肿鉴别,要点为:肝细胞肝癌的坏死区形状不规则,CT 值一般高于脓液,呈软组织密度影,病变边缘明显高低不平,强化持续时间很短,增强后病变与正常组织分界反而较清楚,而典型肝脓肿则具有环靶征、簇集征和脓腔内气体等 CT 诊断的特征性征象。该组 2 例 CT 平扫边缘模糊且不规则,其内无强化的低密度坏死区 CT 值较高(30 HU),动脉期所示的边缘点状强化于门脉期迅速减退(肝脓肿的边缘及分隔则多为延迟强化),增强后边界较清楚,这些征象均与上述研究结果相似,边缘壁结节的出现可能会对坏死较为彻底的肝细胞肝癌具有诊断价值,但有待于进一步研究;另外,甲胎蛋白增高、肝硬化背景及门静脉癌栓等征象有助于肝细胞肝癌的诊断和鉴别诊断。

乏血供型肝细胞肝癌的表现之四(2/12)是CT平扫为等密度，增强扫描各期均表现为低密度影，提示其动脉和门静脉供血均少于正常肝实质，属于少血供的肝细胞肝癌。多数文献赞成是瘤灶内有坏死和脂肪变以及癌细胞透明细胞变等病理基础造成的。该组2例虽然动态增强扫描均显示为低密度，但增强后CT值均高于平扫的CT值，说明病灶内是有血供的，只是由于病灶的强化程度始终低于同层面肝实质密度，所以各期均显示为低密度影。Lim等(2002)报道肿瘤的强化程度决定于肝动脉供血的程度，而肿瘤周围肝实质的强化决定于门静脉的供血，当肿瘤内的动脉供血不足以使肿瘤强化多于周围肝实质酌时候，肿瘤就呈低密度改变。

乏血供型肝细胞肝癌的表现之五是增强扫描呈“慢进快出”型强化，即增强动脉期、门脉期均有强化且门脉期密度更高，延迟期的病灶密度则迅速减退。该组该例CT平扫为低密度，增强动脉、门脉期均有强化且呈等密度，如果不做延迟扫描极易误诊为肝血管瘤，由此可见延迟扫描对于此类肝细胞肝癌的定性诊断极为必要。T_2WI及T_2WI脂肪抑制序列显示病灶为稍高信号影，并非肝血管瘤极高信号的“灯泡征”，因此MRI检查有助于这类肝细胞肝癌的诊断与鉴别诊断。“慢进快出”型强化的肝细胞肝癌考虑可能存在着肝动脉和门静脉双重供血，故门静脉期病灶密度不减退反而继续增高，该病例门脉期CT值达到113 HU，明显高于动脉期的53 HU，至延迟期则减退为低密度影。

研究显示，随着肝内病灶良、恶性成分的变化，供血比例也相应地发生改变，由正常的门静脉供血为主逐渐转变为肝动脉供血为主。肿瘤细胞分化好时可接受肝动脉、门静脉或双重供血；随着肿瘤细胞分化程度降低则以肝动脉供血为主。该病例手术病理为高～中度分化肝细胞肝癌，未见相关淋巴结转移，符合门静脉参与供血、恶性程度较低的肝细胞肝癌的特点。总之，乏血供型肝细胞肝癌的CT表现多种多样，增强扫描主要表现为：①极轻度强化，此时仍能反映肝动脉供血比重增大的特点，可称之为不典型“速升速降”型强化；②肝动脉、门静脉双重供血的“慢进快出”型强化；③不强化，此类肝细胞肝癌坏死较为彻底，其中动脉期病灶边缘多发点状强化于门脉期迅速减退以及边缘壁结节可能会对此类肝细胞肝癌具有诊断价值。CT多期增强扫描对乏血供型肝细胞肝癌的定性诊断极为必要，甲胎蛋白增高、肝硬化背景、门静脉癌栓等征象可协助诊断。

第三节　CT平扫为等密度的肝癌

CT平扫为等密度的肝癌较为少见，增强扫描强化形式多样，容易导致漏诊或误诊。等密度肝癌是指肝癌的密度与肝实质密度相等，CT平扫不易被发现，一组14例等密度肝癌螺旋CT平扫均未能显示即全部为假阴性，如果无增强扫描检查就会漏诊。

一些作者认为肝癌平扫呈等密度的原因有：①直径太小，10 mm以下受部分容积效应的影响；②肿瘤细胞分化较好，与正常肝实质密度相近；③肿瘤周围的肝组织发生脂肪变、肝硬化时，周围肝组织密度降低与肿块相近；④扫描技术原因，管电流太低及窗宽窗位不当。

亦有作者分析认为肝硬化脂肪浸润使肝实质本身的密度较低，与病灶之间的密度差减小，以及癌细胞分化较好致病灶本身密度较高是肝癌呈等密度的主要原因。该组14例中肝细胞肝癌中，有11例为小肝细胞癌，且多见于肝硬化合并脂肪肝患者(占71.43%)，病理学分级以中、高分化肝细胞肝癌居多(10例)，这与上述分析结果相符。

螺旋CT扫描速度快，可做多期动态扫描，能充分反映病灶的血供特点，有利于病灶的检出和定性。正常肝脏的血供约75%由门静脉供应，25%由肝动脉供应，而大部分的肝细胞肝癌由肝动脉供血，因此在螺旋CT增强扫描动脉期，主要由门静脉供血的正常肝组织尚未出现明显强化，而主要由肝动脉供血的肝细胞肝癌病灶出现明显强化(呈高密度)，但到了门脉期，正常肝组织强化明显，肝细胞肝癌病灶则因为没有门静脉供血，强化迅速减退，表现为低密度影，整个强化过程呈“速升速降”改变，这是典型肝细胞肝癌动态强化表现的基础，常被归为肝动脉供血型肝细胞肝癌。

该组有4例病灶具有典型肝细胞肝癌的强化方式，而且3例可见肿瘤假包膜征象，即使平扫表现为等密度，但螺旋CT增强扫描后不难做出定性诊断。由于肝细胞肝癌病灶血供方式、肝实质背景和病灶病理成分等的不同，使得少数病灶呈不典型表现，再加上经验不足，可造成定性困难或误诊，充分了解这些特殊的病理基础和CT表现，有助于提高小肝细胞肝癌的诊断准确性。

4例癌灶螺旋CT增强动脉期仍表现为等密度，门脉期及延迟期迅速减退为低密度影，动脉期仍为等密度的原因可能是此类病灶属低血供型肝细胞肝癌且为肝动脉供血，病灶的肝动脉血供有轻度增加，但不足以使病灶在动脉期扫描呈高密度，因此仅见轻度强化（与周边肝实质强化效果相当而呈等密度影），但在门脉期和延迟期强化下降，观察其强化曲线仍属于不典型“速升速降”型肝细胞肝癌。与典型肝细胞肝癌有所不同，此类肝细胞肝癌的动脉期检出率极低。

有2例病灶动态增强扫描各期均表现为低密度影，提示其动脉和门静脉供血均少于正常肝实质，属于少血供的小肝细胞肝癌。多数文献赞成是瘤灶内有坏死和脂肪变以及癌细胞透明细胞变等病理基础造成的，还有学者认为瘤灶内的血窦被肿瘤压迫、迂曲，血流通过缓慢，或者瘤灶内或瘤灶周围的血管内癌栓阻塞供应瘤灶的血管，也可能是增强扫描肿瘤呈低密度改变的原因。此类肝细胞肝癌容易误诊为其他病变。

该2例病灶虽然动态增强扫描各期均显示为低密度，但CT值均高于平扫的CT值，说明病灶内是有血供的，只是由于病灶的强化程度始终低于同期肝实质密度，所以各期均显示为低密度影，这与一些作者的研究结果相似。

Lim等（2002）报道肿瘤的强化程度决定于肝动脉供血的程度，而肿瘤周围肝实质的强化决定于门静脉的供血，当肿瘤内的动脉供血不足以使肿瘤强化多于周围肝实质的时候，肿瘤就呈低密度改变。

另外，值得注意的是增强后呈低密度的这2例小肝细胞肝癌瘤体内密度不均匀，出现多个小点状密度更低区，病灶内坏死、出血和囊性变、脂肪变以及透明细胞变等是这一征象的病理基础，有文献认为这也是低密度小肝细胞肝癌的瘤内CT特征，CT平扫难以显示此征象是因为小肝细胞肝癌的瘤内更低密度区较小，与邻近的肿瘤及肝实质密度差不大，同时由于部分容积效应的影响，导致小的低密度区显示不清，增强后这些低密度区不强化或强化不明显而得以显示。

该组3例肝细胞肝癌增强后动脉期呈高密度，门脉期及延迟期均呈等密度，可能的原因有：①此类病灶血供相当丰富，可能存在肝动脉和门静脉双重供血（可视为肝动脉-门静脉双重供血型肝细胞肝癌）；②肝硬化的产生使肝脏的血流动力学发生改变，门静脉灌注量的下降使得肝实质的强化效果减弱，病灶和肝实质之间密度差减小而呈等密度；③肝细胞肝癌病灶密度下降与肝实质密度增加的曲线处于交叉点附近及病灶内纤维组织较多等也可能是门脉期及延迟期癌灶呈等密度的原因。

有1例肝癌4月后复查改变为“速升速降”型强化，呈典型肝动脉供血型小肝细胞肝癌，病理诊断为低分化肝细胞肝癌，反映了癌灶分化程度的改变。

研究显示，随着肝内病灶良恶性成分的变化，供血比例也相应地发生改变，由正常的门静脉供血为主逐渐转变为肝动脉供血为主。原发性肝细胞肝癌分化程度高者主要为门静脉供血，分化程度低者门静脉参与供血的比例也相应减少，肝细胞肝癌血供变化的过程也就是其恶性特征形成的过程，病理形态学研究发现，从良性普通型腺瘤样增生经非典型腺瘤样增生到肝细胞肝癌形成，随恶性程度增加，门静脉血供不断减少而肝动脉血供不断增加。此类肝细胞肝癌需与肝血管瘤鉴别，后者MRI T_2WI表现为明显高信号即“灯泡征”，肝细胞肝癌则无此征象。

1例弥漫型肝癌CT平扫几乎呈等密度，考虑是由于肝硬化弥漫性脂肪浸润，肝实质本身的密度较低，与病灶之间的密度差减小，因而呈等密度改变。但动态增强扫描动脉期显示动静脉瘘，门脉期可见门静脉癌栓，加之具有典型肝硬化背景及甲胎蛋白阳性，不难做出定性诊断，可见多期增强扫描对于CT诊断肝细胞肝癌的重要意义所在。

总之，肝细胞肝癌的显示取决于病灶与肝实质之间的密度差异，单纯CT平扫极易漏诊等密度的肝细胞肝癌，增强扫描各期亦存在等密度的现象，因此，在临床工作中，对临床实验室检查或B超强烈提示有肝脏占位，尤其是小肝细胞肝癌或高危患者，均应采用CT平扫加多期增强扫描检查并做综合分析，从而反映出平扫为等密度的肝细胞肝癌的血供特点，可以有效地减少漏诊和误诊。

第四节　慢进快出型肝细胞肝癌

肝细胞肝癌的螺旋CT特征性增强扫描表现是动脉期病灶明显强化，门静脉期病灶强化密度迅速下降，称为“快进快出”或“速升速降”。但有部分肝细胞性肝癌的CT增强表现与之不同，表现为动脉期病灶强化，门静脉期病灶密度不下降，反而进一步升高，延迟期强化密度迅速下降，被称之为“慢进快出”型。有作者搜集手术病理证实的50例肝细胞性肝癌，其中18例CT增强扫描呈“慢进快出”型的强化特点。

肝脏螺旋CT多期增强扫描反映病灶的血供情况。正常肝脏的血供75%~80%由门静脉供应，20%~25%由肝动脉供应，而肝细胞性肝癌多由肝动脉供血，因此在螺旋CT增强扫描动脉期，主要由门静脉供血的正常肝组织尚未出现明显强化，而主要由肝动脉供血的肝细胞性肝癌病灶出现明显强化，但到了门静脉期，门静脉和正常肝组织明显强化，肝细胞性肝癌病灶因为没有门静脉供血，所以密度不再升高，反而迅速下降，整个强化过程呈“速升速降”或“快进快出”改变，这是典型肝细胞性肝癌动态强化表现的基础。

该组病例在门静脉期病灶密度不下降，反而继续进一步强化，与典型肝细胞性肝癌表现不同，说明病灶存在门静脉供血，但动脉期病灶也有强化，说明肝动脉对病灶也有供血，所以这种“慢进快出”型肝细胞性肝癌是由肝动脉和门静脉双重供血，与部分文献报道的肝细胞性肝癌血供可由门静脉参与相一致。

多项研究发现，肝细胞性肝癌的血供形式不仅只有肝动脉供血一种，还有肝动脉-门静脉供血型、门静脉供血型和少血供型。其中肝动脉供血型强化表现为“快进快出”改变，肝动脉-门静脉供血型强化呈“慢进快出”改变，门静脉供血型动脉期不强化，门静脉期出现明显强化，少血供型表现为动脉期和门静脉期病灶实质均强化不明显。

各型所占比例目前文献报道不一。Matsui等（1991）发现肝细胞性肝癌肝动脉供血型占94%，而门静脉参与供血仅占6%。另有作者报道，肝动脉供血型占72%，肝动脉-门静脉供血型占12%，门静脉供血型占8%，少供血型占8%。还有一些作者报道肝动脉供血型占60%，肝动脉-门静脉供血型占20%，门静脉供血型占6.7%，少供血型占13.3%。

一些作者报道的病例中肝动脉供血型占64.9%，肝动脉-门静脉供血型占35.1%。另有作者采用经腹腔动脉或肠系膜上动脉行间接门静脉DSA，观察肝细胞性肝癌门静脉供血情况，发现肝细胞性肝癌肝动脉供血型占89.7%，肝动脉-门静脉供血型占10.3%。一组50例肝细胞性肝癌，肝动脉供血型占64%，肝动脉-门静脉供血型占36%。此3组研究均没有门静脉供血型和少供血型报道。

一般认为，DSA应是观察肝细胞性肝癌血供的金标准，因为螺旋CT多期扫描受到扫描时相的影响，用对比剂示踪技术进行多期增强扫描可能会更接近DSA结果。有学者用DSA与CT增强扫描表现进行对照观察，证实CT增强扫描多期强化表现与肿瘤血供的关系，表明CT增强扫描多期强化表现可以反映肿瘤的血供情况，对肝细胞性肝癌介入化疗及栓塞治疗方案的制定有很好的临床指导作用。

有学者研究发现，肝细胞性肝癌血供形式与肿瘤的分化程度相关，随着分化程度的下降，病灶门静脉血供逐渐减少，而肝动脉血供增加，即肝动脉供血型肝细胞性肝癌分化程度要较门静脉供血型和肝动脉-门静脉供血型差。

但该组病例没有反映这一现象，该组50例中，肝动脉-门静脉供血型肝细胞性肝癌高中分化占72.2%（13/18），而肝动脉供血型肝细胞性肝癌高中分化占71.9%（23/32），两者差异无统计学意义，这与一些学者研究结果相一致。表明肝细胞性肝癌血供形式与肿瘤分化程度的相关性尚无定论，有待进一步研究。也有学者发现肝细胞性肝癌血供的形式与癌细胞的组织学类型有关。

鉴别诊断：“慢进快出”型肝细胞性肝癌要与肝血管瘤、周围型胆管细胞癌、肝局灶性结节增生等相鉴别。

肝血管瘤：多期动态增强扫描肝血管瘤动脉期病灶周围结节状强化，门静脉期病灶向心性强化，延迟期病灶持续强化呈等密度，而“慢进快出”型肝细胞性肝癌动脉期和门静脉期均为不规则强化，延迟期病灶呈低密度，仔细分析其强化表现，可以与肝血管瘤鉴别。一些作者报道 24 例类似肝血管瘤的不典型肝癌，认为进行 10 min 及 20min 的延迟扫描有利于两者的鉴别。

周围型胆管细胞癌：周围型胆管细胞癌强化表现为"慢进慢出"型，动脉期多为轻度强化，门静脉期继续强化，延迟期持续强化，强化也都不规则，与肝血管瘤周边向中心发展的强化方式和肝细胞性肝癌"慢进快出"的强化方式不同，此外周围型胆管细胞癌内部和／或周边可见扩张的胆管，病灶周围可见收缩性表现，无明显占位，也与肝细胞性肝癌不同。

局灶性结节增生：局灶性结节增生动脉期病灶明显强化，其中的放射状瘢痕不强化，门静脉期病灶继续呈强化状态，但密度有下降，延迟期病灶中心瘢痕可强化呈高密度，与肝细胞性肝癌强化方式不同。另外，肝细胞性肝癌多伴有肝硬化，甲胎蛋白多升高。

总之，螺旋 CT 多期增强扫描出现"慢进快出"型表现是肝细胞性肝癌除"快进快出"型外一种较常见的强化形式，与其肝动脉和门静脉的双重血供有关，是否与肿瘤分化程度相关有待进一步研究。仔细分析其强化的特点，可以与肝血管瘤、周围型胆管细胞癌和局灶性结节增生等疾病相鉴别。

附：具体研究资料：一组 18 例手术后病理诊断为原发性肝细胞性肝癌，其中位于肝右叶 13 例（72.7%），肝左叶 5 例（27.3%）。高分化 3 例（16.7%），中分化 10 例（55.6%），低分化 5 例（27.7%）。

CT 表现：18 例肝细胞性肝癌术前 CT 增强扫描均表现为动脉期病灶强化，密度增高，门静脉期病灶密度不下降，反而进一步升高，延迟期病灶密度均明显下降，成为低密度灶，即"慢进快出"型。其中动脉期轻度强化 5 例，CT 值平均增高 14 HU（10~18 HU），明显强化 13 例，CT 值平均增高 46 HU（28~75 HU）；均匀强化 4 例，不均匀强化 14 例；门静脉期病灶均有明显强化，CT 值平均增高 65 HU（46~89 HU），较动脉期平均增高 28 HU（14~56 HU），其中均匀强化 3 例，不均匀强化 15 例；延迟期病灶密度下降，较门静脉期平均 CT 值下降 49 HU（37~68 HU）。18 例病灶平扫呈等密度者 7 例，低密度者 11 例，病灶形态规则呈圆形类圆形 14 例，不规则形 4 例。无包膜者 10 例，有完整包膜者 2 例，有不完整包膜者 6 例。境界清楚 9 例，境界不清 9 例。5 例病灶直径 <3 cm（小肝癌），7 例病灶直径 3~5cm（结节型），6 例病灶直径 >5 cm（巨块型）；15 例伴肝硬化，无一例远处转移或肝内转移灶。

第五节　肝占位性病变 CT 误诊为原发性肝癌

原发性肝癌是我国常见的恶性肿瘤之一，在广西，肝癌发病率超过 30/10 万的就有 9 个县市，原发性肝癌是广西第一位的癌症杀手。而 CT 是其重要的诊断方法之一。肝癌治疗方法首选为手术切除，肝脏良性病变及部分恶性病变，如转移性癌误诊为肝癌，会导致不必要的手术及选择错误的手术方式。

误诊原因分析：病变与肝癌 CT 表现相似点较多，不易鉴别：肝细胞性肝癌约 2/3 为肝动脉供血或为双重供血。典型的肝细胞肝癌有假包膜，增强扫描呈"快进快出"改变，肿瘤较大时常伴有门脉癌栓。肝腺瘤是富血管肿瘤，动脉期明显均匀强化，有假包膜，但门静脉期病灶密度下降较肝癌慢，该组 4 例肝腺瘤中有 2 例 CT 表现与文献报道相符，与肝动脉供血的肝细胞肝癌混淆。

肝脏神经内分泌癌是非常少见的肝脏占位性病变，影像学表现为肝内边界清楚、密度不均匀肿块，病灶较大时可发生出血、坏死、囊变，动态增强扫描早期为不均匀强化，晚期肿瘤逐步转变为等密度及低密度，有假包膜形成。与该组病例表现一致，其表现与巨块型肝癌类似，因该组作者对该病的认识不足或从未见过此种病例而误诊。

未分化胚胎性肉瘤一般认为是原发于儿童的恶性肿瘤，发生于肝原始间叶组织。但该组 2 例均为成人，Nishio 等（2003）报道表明 40 岁以上患者仅见 10 例报道。有作者总结其 CT 表现为肝实质内巨大肿块，囊实性，可见明显假包膜，内可有出血坏死，强化方式多为"快进快出"型，与该组 2 例表现相符。成人未分化胚胎性肉瘤与肝癌 CT 表现极相似。

病变表现不典型，导致误诊：4 例局灶性结节增生中，有 1 例病理结果显示结节内伴有显著坏死、脂肪变及水肿，因此，其门脉期及平衡期强化减退，呈低密度改变，从而与肝癌"快进快出"的强化方式相似，而难以鉴别。该组 4 例肝腺瘤病史均不典型，均非育龄期妇女，其中2例病理成分不典型，肿瘤局部有出血，瘤周肝组织有结节性肝硬化，导致增强扫描动脉期病灶强化不均匀，CT表现不典型而误诊。

肝转移癌的形态各异，血流灌注及增强类型复杂多样，在不知道有原发癌存在的情况下，易造成误诊。该组11例转移性肿瘤中有8例为单发，其中有5例CT表现与原发性肝癌的CT表现类似，且均未见典型“牛眼征”改变。

原发性肝癌在CT上的不典型表现多，无法排除：原发性肝癌因其病灶大小、血供多少、生长方式、肝实质背景和病理成分的不同等，造成其在CT扫描中强化方式不典型。

一些学者将其分为以下3型：第一型，坏死及脂肪变较多的少血管型，动态增强扫描三期均表理为低密度。此类病灶易和其他少血供病灶混淆。本组5例肝硬化再生结节在增强扫描的三期中均呈略低密度，在肝硬化背景下，类似于少血供的肝细胞肝癌，其中2例多发肝硬化再生结节患者甲胎蛋白增高，可能与肝硬化肝功能损害有关。本组肝转移瘤有6例为少血管型，动态扫描的三期均表现低密度，为避免漏诊而无法排除为少血供型肝癌。

第二型，动脉和门脉双重供血型，病灶在门脉期和延迟期仍有持续强化，为等密度甚至高密度。本组2例局灶性结节增生符合其典型的CT表现：平扫低密度或等密度，强化特点是“快进慢出”，即动脉期为均匀高密度，门脉期和延迟扫描期病灶呈等密度，但病灶内未见其典型的中心瘢痕，而与富血供肝细胞肝癌混淆。

第三型，部分纤维硬化型，肝癌因纤维组织的存在使对比剂在病灶内滞留时间长，而表现为边缘延迟强化的特点，与炎性假瘤表现相似。炎性假瘤是门静脉供血，病理上其中心为凝固性坏死，周边有纤维包膜形成，故增强扫描早期强化不明显，而静脉期和平衡期可有边缘强化，病灶周围肝组织强化。

减少误诊的方法：加深对易误诊为肝癌的肝占位性病变的了解和认识，是减少误诊的关键。对性质不明的肝占位性病变应想到上述病变的可能，了解上述病变的特征性的病理改变和生长方式，掌握其CT表现，进行仔细分析和阅片可进一步提高CT肝占位性病变的诊断准确性。

对于CT表现相似、鉴别困难的病变，应结合其他先进的影像检查技术综合诊断：目前影像有很多新技术，当常规CT平扫及增强扫描无法定性诊断时，可做CTA、CTAP、MRI或DSA检查。Floriani等（2010）对肝胃肠道转移癌CT及CTAP的诊断准确率进行了Meta分析，结果显示CTAP的灵敏度较CT明显增高（94.8% vs. 80.1%；P<0.0001），MRI较CT的诊断准确率也有很大优势（OR=0.54；95%CI：0.42~0.70；P<0.00001）。另有作者研究得出CT诊断肝癌的确诊率为87.2%，MRI的确诊率为95.6%，均表明MRI优于CT。

该组30例CT误诊的病人中6例同时行MRI检查，诊断正确的有4例。此外，一些新的MRI技术不断涌现，包括DWI、化学位移成像、MRS、SWI、3D-DCE MRI以及MRI细胞靶向性对比剂的应用，为肝局灶性病变的诊断提供更有价值的信息。随着MRI技术的不断完善，在肝癌鉴别诊断方面将会有新的突破。Kim等（2004）经过统计，得出联合多种影像检查，可以优势互补，提高确诊率。

诊断应结合临床病史和甲胎蛋白等肿瘤标志物的检查进行综合分析：该组30例中，甲胎蛋白阳性者仅6例，均为轻度增高，如能结合上述检查结果做出CT诊断，可减少误诊的发生。11例转移性腺癌中，有3例CA125升高，有5例检查前已有其他部位恶性病变征象，而临床均未提供相应病史，再次说明详细询问病史对肝癌的鉴别诊断有重要意义。对于影像结合临床仍无法排除肝癌的，应谨慎而大胆地应用肝细针穿刺活检，避免误诊的发生。而对于有肝硬化背景的肝占位，穿刺活检无恶性证据时，先定期观察，病情有变时再考虑手术，从而既避免盲目手术，又避免漏诊肝癌而延误治疗。

第六节　误诊病例简介:高分化肝细胞性肝癌与肝结核

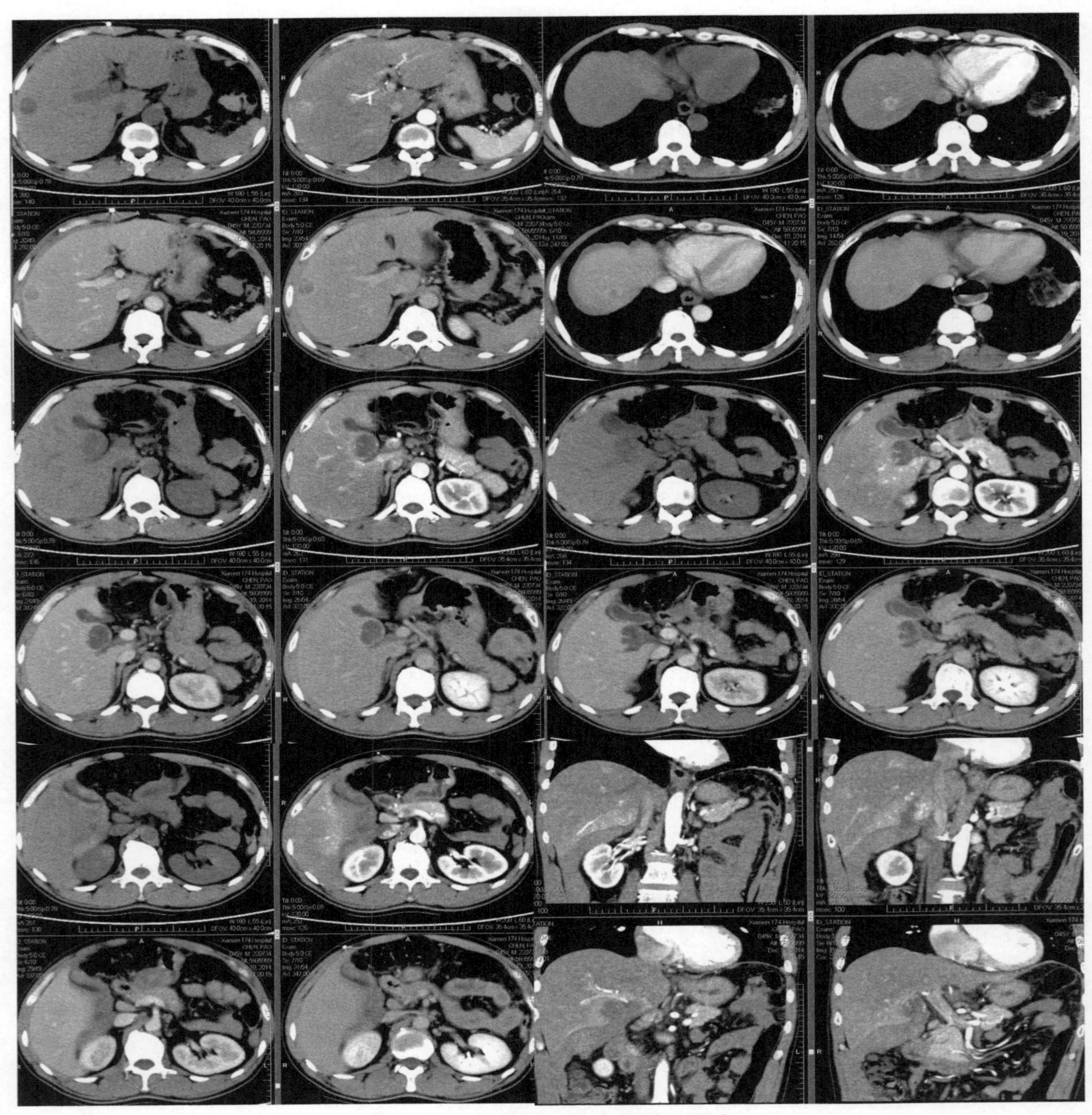

图 3-19-1　高分化肝细胞性肝癌与肝结核

病例,男,53 岁。患者因右上腹痛 2 天就诊于外院,甲胎蛋白提示正常,彩超提示:“肝内多发低回声结节及等回声结节,胆囊多发小息肉,胰体部低回声结节,左肾囊实性包块”。

检查时间:12-18CT 检查, 12-31MRI 检查,次年 1-15CT 复查。肺部 CT 平扫,肝脏平扫 + 增强:双肺透亮度减低,肺纹理增多,肺野内广泛分布密集磨玻璃密度结节;肝右叶见两枚低密度结节,直径在 20~30mm 之间, CT 值约 40HU,增强后边缘强化。内侧结节见破口,内容物沿腹腔间隙流注至腹、盆腔，密度略高，CT 值：66~70HU。肝、脾包膜下少量弧形液体密度影。右肾中极见一小点状高密度影；腹膜后见多发肿大淋巴结。CT 诊断：双肺广泛病变，考虑急性粟粒性肺结核，肿瘤待排；请结合临床进一步确诊；右肝占位，考虑肝结核脓肿破溃，伴腹腔内流注；心腔内密度减低，考虑为贫血；胆囊炎；腹腔淋巴结肿大；右肾小结石（图 3-19-1）。

MRI 平扫 + 增强：肝表面略不平整，肝前后叶可见 3 个大小不等的类圆形异常信号影，大小分别为 1.4cm × 1.4cm、2.6cm × 2.2cm 和 5.5cm × 7.0cm，以右前叶下段病灶较大呈多房状并向外下突起，T_1WI 高低混杂信号，T_2WI 不均匀稍高信号，DWI 内容物呈高信号，增强扫描囊壁环形强化呈高信号，边界清楚。腹膜后可见多个肿大淋巴结影。肝包膜下及右侧胸腔可见少量液体影。肝肾间隙、右侧结肠旁沟及盆腔可见异常信号液体影聚集，以盆腔较多主要位于膀胱直肠间隙，T_1WI 高低混杂信号，T_2WI 高或低信号，增强无强化，膀胱向前下推移，回肠向前上推移，直肠向后推移。MRI 诊断：肝右叶多发占位，考虑脓肿，结核待排？以右前叶下段病灶较大，且脓液经结肠旁沟流注到盆腔。右侧胸腔及腹腔少量积液。

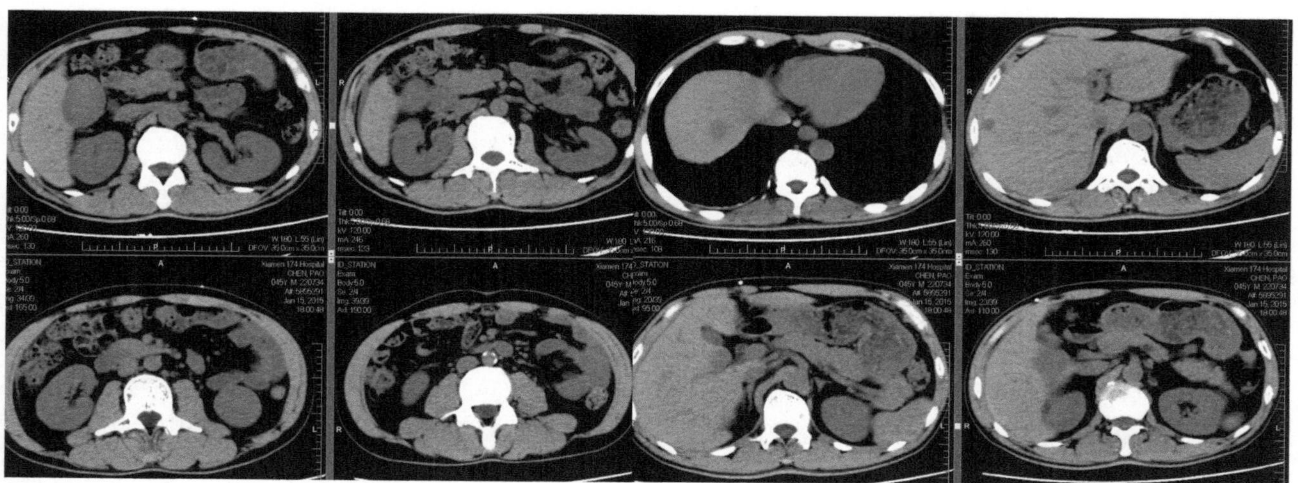

图 3-19-2　2015-1-15CT 复查肝脏平扫：肝右叶见两枚低密度结节，与前片相近，腹腔积液吸收。CT 诊断：右肝多发占位，与一月前 CT 图像比较密度减低，性质？考虑肝结核可能，其他病变待排，建议进一步检查；肝包膜下少量积液；慢性胆囊炎；胆总管轻度扩张

手术所见：腹腔内见陈旧性血性液，量约 300ml，肝Ⅳ段胆囊旁可见一大小约 5cm × 6cm 肿物，突出于肝脏表面，呈黄白色，包膜尚完整；肝Ⅷ段表面可见一大小约 2cm × 3cm 肿物，边界尚清；决定行肝部分切除 + 胆囊切除 + 肝肿物射频消融术。

病理检查：冰冻病理检查：肝肿物：结节样肿物一块，大小 1.8cm × 1.7cm × 1.5cm，切面见一囊腔，壁厚 0.2cm，囊内含淡黄色样物，切面淡黄、质中。冰冻病理诊断：肝肿物切除标本：高分化肝癌。常规病理诊断：肝肿物切除标本：初步诊断高分化肝细胞肝癌伴大量坏死，待做免疫组化检测进一步明确诊断。

免疫组化检测：阳性：Hepatocyte，CK8，CK18，Villin（灶 +），EGFR（4+），TOPO Ⅱ（2+），PgP（2+），5-FU（+），Ki-67（+，约 40%）；阴性：CK7，CK19，CK20，CDX-2，PSA，CD10，Mucin-2，VEGF，ERCC1，Tubulinβ。免疫组化诊断：肝肿物切除标本：高分化肝细胞肝癌。

术前 CT 及 MRI 本例均误诊为肝结核，腹盆腔脓肿流注；误诊原因主要为肺部病灶所误导，仔细分析肺部 CT 表现，肺部病灶表现为磨玻璃样结节、斑片状改变，与急性血型播散型肺结核的三均匀表现存在差异；患者无呼吸道及发热等结核中毒症状，从临床过程及目前检查情况分析，无结核病依据。追问病史，患者有长期大量粉尘接触史，肺部 CT 提示双肺门及纵隔见高密度淋巴结，符合尘肺表现；回顾本例肝癌伴肿瘤破裂、腹盆腔积血影像表现尚比较典型，因肺部病变干扰诊断思路，值得今后工作借鉴学习（图 3-19-2）。

第七节 误诊病例简介:不典型肝癌误诊为囊腺瘤

肝细胞癌的CT表现多种多样,大部分符合典型原发性肝细胞癌的CT表现:假包膜征、动态增强扫描强化呈快进快出特征等,而极少部分没有这些典型征象。

一例肝癌CT表现呈囊性,无常见肝癌之典型影像学表现,属于不典型肝癌,术前误诊为囊腺瘤,分析其原因如下。患者年龄较轻,无肝癌相关基础疾病,甲胎蛋白阴性;影像学表现特殊,病灶呈囊性,边缘光整,增强扫描囊内可见细小的肝动脉分支穿行似分隔强化,囊壁亦强化。

肝脏囊腺瘤起源于异位形成胆囊的胚胎组织或迷走错构瘤样胆管,CT表现为肝内低密度囊性肿块,囊内可有分隔及壁结节,增强扫描囊壁及分隔有强化,但囊内不会出现细小的肝动脉分支穿行。

当肝细胞癌中心发生坏死囊变时,可表现为囊性肿瘤,其病理基础可能是肝癌组织相对供血不足或继发感染后液化坏死,而未完全液化坏死的肿瘤组织可表现为"壁结节"。该例增强扫描肿瘤内动脉期可见细小的肝动脉分支穿行,门脉期及平衡期未见强化灶,提示肿瘤主要由肝动脉供血,而强化的囊壁可能为假包膜。

一些学者对肝细胞癌动脉期强化特点进行分析,发现随着肿瘤分化程度的降低,动脉期肿瘤血管增加,这些血管位于肿瘤周围或深入内部。

该病例的经验教训是,在肝脏CT上表现为囊性的肿瘤,即使边缘光整,病理上也有可能为实性,若囊内出现细小的肝动脉分支穿行,就不能排除恶性肿瘤,即便诊断不明也应尽早手术切除,以免延误病情。

我们还有一个体会,一些病灶密度较低,有的医生的诊断印象立即就是"囊性病变",事实上其CT值常常是30HU左右,并不支持为"水样密度",实际上在病理解剖时,也是实性病变,而非囊性病变,在临床上,这是值得我们注意的问题。

胆管囊腺类肿瘤是少见的肝内囊性肿瘤,占全部肝脏囊性病变的5%,患者多为中年女性。随着影像技术的发展,越来越多的囊腺瘤和囊腺癌被检出。本病可以发生在肝内或肝外胆管,85%发生在肝内胆管,其中又有55%发生在肝脏右叶,29%发生在肝脏左叶,16%为两叶同时发生。

囊腺瘤多为多房,仅有少数囊腺癌为单房。囊腺瘤衬以单层立方至高柱状黏液细胞,而囊腺癌多衬以小肠型上皮(含杯状细胞和潘氏细胞),伴有不同程度的异形及核分裂。有些女性病例其上皮下的结缔组织层内富含细胞,且类似于卵巢基质,这类患者病程进展缓慢,缺乏这种特殊基质的女性囊腺癌患者及所有男性囊腺癌患者病程进展较快。

在CT上病变主要表现为肝内或肝门区低密度、囊性肿块,边界清楚、光滑,最大径1.5~35.0cm,其内囊液密度均匀,CT值为0~30HU。囊腺瘤多为薄壁、多房,囊壁及囊内分隔厚薄一致,强化均匀;囊腺癌多为单房,囊壁多可见乳头状结节或软组织肿块,增强扫描明显强化,部分囊腺癌内可以出现不规则钙化。

囊壁乳头状结节及不规则钙化,被认为是囊腺癌区别于囊腺瘤的特征性表现,但在一些良性囊腺瘤中也可检出囊壁或分隔的纤细、规则钙化。

囊壁上有强化的乳头状结节是鉴别囊腺癌与囊腺瘤较为特异的征象,虽然既往文献也将囊壁的不规则钙化作为两者主要鉴别点,但因其在囊腺癌中的出现率并不高且同时在囊腺瘤中也可检出,故可以将其列为两者鉴别时的参考因素。偶有良性囊腺瘤囊内出现胆固醇结晶,增强CT上形似强化壁结节,进行CT平扫有助于两者的鉴别。

不典型肝细胞肝癌没有"快进快出"的表现,具体表现各异,无统一特征。肝癌坏死囊性变不少见,其表现与原发囊性病变包括囊性类肿瘤不同。就该病例而言需要注意的CT表现有:增强扫描动脉期肿瘤内可见细小的肝动脉分支供血,动脉期部分区域有强化,门脉期和延迟期部分区域少部分区域密度略有减低,门脉期和延迟期病变边缘可见包膜样强化,提示原发肝细胞肝癌的可能。

另外,引起本病例误诊的一个原因就是病变是否为囊性,通过仔细对比病变增强前后的密度,不难发现增强扫描动脉期部分区域比平扫密度增高,说明病变有强化,而且这种强化呈片状分布,边界不清,而不是具体的壁结节状,说明此病变是实性病变有囊变,不是原发囊性病变,诊断方向完全不同。

此外，将病变误认为是囊性，此病变也是单房、囊内有强化灶，应诊断囊腺癌而不是囊腺瘤。

综上所述，胆管囊腺类肿瘤是少见疾病，充分掌握其影像表现和肝癌的基本、特征性及特殊表现，在术前可以通过多期增强 CT 检查做出正确的诊断。

第八节　肝癌误诊与漏诊

漏诊病例：有作者报告 1 例肝脓肿患者，外院 CT 诊断为肝癌，经血管造影未见肿瘤血管而否定诊断；1 例肝细胞癌患者，CT 和超声检查均未见异常，而因其甲胎蛋白高达 11340μg/L 而作血管造影，发现肝左叶有一低密度病灶，术中见该病灶为 7mm × 16mm × 16mm 大小。

4/14 例小肝癌的误诊分析：一些作者报告 14 例直径在 30mm 以下的小肝癌，其中有 4 例常规 CT 扫描未见异常：1 例因外院 CT 机分辨力较差，1 例可能系病灶太小（仅 10mm × 10mm），也可能因病人每次扫描时屏气状态不一致而遗漏，此二例均因甲胎蛋白值升高后为血管造影和 / 或 CTAP 所检出和确诊；1 例因平扫时病灶呈等密度，且病灶较小（直径为 26mm）和较深在，肝局部轮廓无异常，增强扫描自上而下进行，仍呈等密度表现，因超声检查疑肝细胞癌故及时做双期 CT 发现异常，后经血管造影和 CTA 确诊；1 例漏诊的原因是增强扫描技术不当，尽管 CT 平扫已发现低密度病灶，注射对比剂后未首先对病灶层实施扫描，而是按自上而下的顺序扫描，在首层扫描后 73 秒才扫描病灶区，早已错过了显示肝细胞癌特点的血管期。

由此看来，在这些病例防止漏检的措施，主要应改进扫描技术，如平扫时已发现病变，增强时要在血管期（即 40 秒内）对病灶层实施扫描；如临床疑有肝细胞癌（甲胎蛋白值升高，或超声检查疑有肝细胞癌等）而常规 CT 扫描又无异常时，应不失时机地实施三期 CT 增强扫描、X 线血管造影、CTA 以及 CTAP 等检查。

该组作者还报告 1 例甲胎蛋白正常，作了常规 CT、X 线血管造影和 CTA 等检查，虽发现其自内向外顺序染色征象有别于典型的血管瘤表现，但未引起足够注意，再次就诊时，肿瘤直径已从 2cm 增至 8cm，正是由于此例误诊教训，才使他们特别重视有自内向外顺序染色这一有价值的征象。

第九节　肝细胞性肝癌强化表现

在对比剂团注强化后，病变可或不可更好描绘。由于大多数肝细胞性肝癌富有血管，故可强化，但比之于正常肝实质强化要低些。大病灶的更周围部分和小的肿瘤结节可为对比剂强化所遮掩，使之变成与周围肝实质等密度。

尽管在静脉侵犯的观察肝细胞性肝癌比转移瘤更为明显，孤立的肝细胞性肝癌不能只靠 CT 检查与肝转移瘤或其他原发性肝肿瘤可靠地区分开来。强化有助于发现肿瘤对门静脉或下腔静脉的侵犯。

在 CT 图像上肝细胞性肝癌表现为多发性散在包块也可与转移瘤所类似。大多数肿瘤包块在 2~4cm 范围内。

CT 第三种表现是弥漫性肿瘤侵犯和广泛性多灶性包块，在肝硬化基础上的弥漫性肝细胞性肝癌难以发现。

最后，在肝脂肪浸润病人，肝细胞性肝癌能表现为相当高密度的包块。

Itai 等（1979）报告 CT 评价肝脏包块 225 例中，下述情况提示肝癌：平扫时包块或是等密度或是略微低密度；围绕包块有透 X 线环状带（包膜）；肿瘤从肝表面外凸；整叶密度降低伴团注对比剂后有一强烈弥漫性不均匀染色。CT 发现和怀疑肝硬化，在肝细胞性肝癌为 62%，少于肝转移瘤 10%。

第十节 假肝癌

肝再生中的动静脉瘘类似肝癌：肝癌常表现为多血管性病变，而无血管性肝癌的继发征象(诸如动静脉瘘、染色区域与不规则的血管等)有助于诊断。Farrell 等(1972)报道一例经剖腹探查肝楔形切除证实的活动性肝硬化的再生结节误诊为无血管性肝癌。该病例在硬化的肝脏中有一显著的动静脉瘘，核素扫描时在肝右叶外侧缘上可见明显充盈缺损，而导致诊断为无血管的肝癌。

血管瘤伪似肝癌：在肝超声检查时，常可见到小的回声增强的局灶区，当单发的小灶回声增强区出现于无症状的病人时，几乎总是血管瘤。但当它们邻近横膈时，扫描可在膈上发现它的镜面像，而伪似肝癌。这类病变可用超声或其他影像检查技术(如 CT)追踪观察和确定性质。

肝硬化病人的假肝癌血管造影表现：肝硬化的血管造影表现常与其病变的阶段有关，在进展期，血管造影的征象有时类似于肝癌，或是原发性或是继发性肝癌。

Passariello 等(1978)指出这些异常血管造影表现包括：①肝动脉 - 门静脉瘘；②肝门的狭窄或实质内血管分支的狭窄；③富血管区的增加或减少；④实质内肝动脉分支走行的变化。这些异常表现出现于 154 例肝硬化中的 12 例病人，其中 8 例类似原发性肝癌，4 例为弥漫性而颇似肝转移癌。

超声技术不当与假肝癌：不适当的超声检查技巧可使肝的某部出现回声增强区而类似于肝癌，但此类人工伪影的本质可借助于下述因素加以确定：①极难见到肝癌不引起肝的动、静脉和门脉走行变化，而此类病例血管走行分布均属正常；②此回声增强区常常延伸超越肝的周界，更说明系伪影所致；③此类回声增强区可能与换能器固有的局灶带有关。

第十一节 肝细胞癌误为脾肿瘤

一般说来，肝细胞癌影像学诊断并不困难，但是，有作者报告一例患者经多次、多项影像学检查均误诊为脾肿瘤，回顾性分析其特点有：①肝脏形态特殊，肝左叶上缘向脾区异常延伸，即“獭尾肝”，其肿块与脾重叠形成类似增大之“脾脏”；②腹腔积液密度较高，平扫时从 CT 值上无法区分肝与脾，造成肿块与脾结合紧密之假象；③肝、脾强化的程度几乎一致，以至于难以将部分形态异常之肝左叶与脾区分开来。

经过认真地回顾分析，发现该患者误诊为脾肿瘤的影像学表现仍有一些可疑之处：①肿块组织无论平扫或增强均与典型巨块型肝癌表现一致；②增强扫描可见肿块后缘与相邻脾成锐角，提示该肿块位于脾之外。但是，在临床工作中，当时却未注意到这一点。

第十二节 肝癌的不典型表现和少见 CT 表现

不典型表现：肝细胞肝癌主要由肝动脉供血，动脉期 CT 值迅速上升达到峰值，由于肝脏实质主要由门静脉供血，动脉期增强不明显，平扫时为低密度的病灶此时明显高于正常肝实质，出现早期高密度强化征象；病灶增强峰值停留时间很短，迅速下降，与浓密显影的主动脉下降速度几乎一致。门静脉期肝脏实质明显强化，而肝细胞癌密度降低，表现为明显低密度影，即表现为“快进快出”的特点。采用螺旋 CT 机，其出现率可高达 90%，意味着大部分肝癌血供是比较丰富的。

少见 CT 表现：①动脉期和门静脉期均强化，密度高于肝脏：有作者报告一组肝癌病例，27% 表现为动脉期和门静脉期均强化，密度高于肝脏。可能与病人的血液循环较慢，门静脉期时肝动脉内碘浓度较高有关。发生于肝脏顶部的肝癌出现这种表现可能与门静脉期扫描先扫查肝脏顶部有关。脂肪肝背景下的肝癌可有此种表现。此时必须加扫延迟期，这些病灶在延迟期为低密度，即可诊断为肝癌。应注意与肝脏血管瘤和局灶性结节增生鉴别。②动脉期和门静脉期均为低密度：这类肝癌血供较少，动脉期和门静脉期不强化或轻度强化，均表现为低密度。可能与病灶脂肪变性或纤维组织较多有关。应注意与肝脏转移瘤、炎性病变及淋巴瘤等鉴别。③动脉期或门静脉期或动、门静脉双期呈等密度：肝癌病灶的密度从低到高再到低早于肝脏实质密度的变化，但两者有密度相等的交汇点，如果扫描时间恰好碰上此交汇点，病灶表现为等密度。这也与患者血液循环的个体差异有关。重要的是病灶在延迟期若表现为低密度，即可诊断为肝癌。可见延迟扫描在肝癌定性诊断中的重要性。疑难病例应结合临床资料，大部分肝癌病例甲胎蛋白增高或明显增高以及乙型肝炎表面抗原（HbsAg）阳性，30%左右甲胎蛋白正常。有研究认为，甲胎蛋白 >200μg/L，可诊断为肝癌。

第十三节　肝癌影像诊断误诊研究点滴体会（基层医院讲课提纲）

一般与疑难：临床影像诊断工作概分两类，一为一般的常规诊断工作，相对说来较为单纯和容易，占临床工作的大部分，不能轻视和粗心大意；一为疑难病人的诊断，尽管只占临床工作的小部分，但却相当费时费神，甚至还可能出现严重的错误。

提高放射科工作人员的素质，是提高诊断水平和减少误诊与漏诊的重要措施。提高素质不是一句空话，而是要不断地学习、研究和积累经验。医学服务的对象的是病人的生命，是十分宝贵的，切不可大意，因此医学本身就是需要不断学习和研究的学科，是需要我们付出终生的努力去学习和钻研的。

尊重知识，尊重科学：提高诊断报告的质量，一个重要的问题是给足医生诊断的必要的时间，要做好一个病人的诊断，既要观察、分析、思考、可能还要研究、讨论，甚至还要查资料，找文献，行政不宜干预太多，不宜硬性规定多少分钟一定要出报告，要尊重知识，尊重科学。还有本单位朋友及熟人，要提高技师和护士对书写报告的认识，不要以为写报告为“一键式”的操作？刚扫描就要诊断报告，碍于人情，不能不给，既打乱工作程序，又难以保证诊断质量，这太随意，太仓促，太不规范，容易误诊和漏诊。

手术病理后，需不需要再修改术前的诊断报告？要尊重知识，尊重科学，实事求是，不宜修改术前报告，这样有利于总结经验，吸取教训，提高诊断的能力。

自己的诊断被手术病理证实后，常常可能产生一种欣慰感，但切记不要沾沾自喜，要总结经验，再深入学习和钻研，对该疾病提高认识，争取以后诊断水平更高。如手术病理资料否认了自己的诊断，也不要气馁，要结合临床资料及病理资料，仔细地对照和研究影像学资料，找出其中的矛盾之处，吸取教训，进一步避免误诊与漏诊。

病例 1：男，53 岁，含脂肪肝癌，肝占位，动脉期强化，门脉期下降几呈等密度，周围有低密度环，脂肪密度？延迟期接近平扫密度时为 -7HU。手术病理：原发性肝细胞性肝癌，小癌型；门脉性肝硬化。肝组织切面见一直径 2cm 结节状肿物，切面灰白，质韧。光镜所见：肿块内肝小叶结构消失，细胞胞浆丰富，核大，核膜厚，核仁明显，脂变明显，伴粗大纤维增生。纤维包膜分隔肿块内癌细胞及肿块外肝组织。紧邻包膜外见少数几团癌细胞浸润灶。肿块外肝组织被增生纤维分隔包裹呈结节状。结节内中央静脉偏位，纤维中大量淋巴细胞浸润。

比较影像学：充分利用现代科学技术和诊断的手段，相互支持，优势互补，扬长避短，不要对立，不闹独立。超声、CT 与 MRI 三者更应如此。三者联合起来，与临床科室及病理科一块研究、讨论疑难病案，对于提高整个医院诊断的水平至关重要。重视 MRI 对软组织病变发现的敏感性，CT 无能时，或未见异常时，应充分考虑应用 MRI，互补！尽管扫描层稍厚，但对软组织病变敏感，不失为一大优点，大可利用之。

病例 2：女，70 岁，发现漏诊的过程：因病人对碘剂过敏反应而未再做 CT 三期增强，改为 MR 增强，MR 增强才发现右上后段病灶，再做平扫。肝右后上段结节影，呈长 T_1 稍长 T_2 信号，呈不规则不均匀强化，怀疑肝癌。右前段平扫低密度区，动脉期动脉分支清楚，MRI 见为异常血供。肝硬化结节多个，分析和诊断有一定难度。门脉栓塞清楚可见。08-31,检查后做脾切除术,术后09-26CT三期见门静脉瘤栓以后消失,证明并非瘤栓。门静脉主干及脾静脉栓塞三期表现不一样,与脾切除关系究竟如何?左前腹壁团块影,CT值52~68HU,周围低密度晕影,有稍高密度絮网影及含气窦道与腹壁外相通,多为脾切除术后所致血肿。腹水,包裹积液。心包积液伴心包增厚。

病例3:男,48岁,病理证实(肝右后叶)肝细胞性肝癌,分化型。直径2cm结节,呈淡黄色与周边分界清楚。(右后叶)门脉性肝硬化。(超声四次诊断均为增生结节,一次提到大的不排除肝癌,如何正确评价超声的诊断,应认真考虑),慎重对待,不可轻易否认。

病例4:男,52岁,10-07超声:肝右前叶类圆形实性低回声结节,12×11mm,边界欠清,内回声不均匀。诊断增生结节。超声见三期未见,9月后超声与三期都证实。某些结节超声早见,有些三期多见,与其性质有关。次年7-23手术病理证实肝细胞型肝癌。CK(+),EMA部分(+),CD31血管(+),AFP(±)。

尊重科学,尊重前人的经验:上腹部三期增强之前务必进行平扫,这对提高诊断质量十分重要,也是前人经验的总结,不要随意去掉。肝胆管结石的有无,胆囊壁及胆囊内有无钙化,肝内低密度区的表现?这些征象的发现都与平扫有关。

病例5:女,70岁,教训:无CT平扫,后补扫平扫见为等密度团块周围以一圈低密度带影,不是单纯低密度区;三期增强仅动脉期见略微强化,被忽略!门脉期见数小粒状低密度区,平衡期为等密度。术后病理诊断:肝细胞癌。

病例6:男,48岁,肝硬化结节平扫表现为各种稍高密度大小不等结节,第二天三期增强扫描全部见不到,只见到肝癌的低密度灶。弥漫性肝硬化更是一致性细小结节,以前曾见到;再做三期增强三维重建,见肝癌血管供应清楚。术后病理诊断:(右)肝(上叶上、下段)肝细胞性肝癌,中度分化;肝硬化;慢性胆囊炎。(胆管内赘生物)为部分肝细胞癌结节及凝血块。

上腹部CT三期增强的时间和范围应规范化,千万不要随意乱变,自作主张,准确三期扫描是诊断经验的总结,对于一些病灶的定性分析相当重要。制订规范后,一定要执行,不能只停留于纸上,要落实到行动上,才能真正起到规范的作用。

病例7:男,21岁,手术病理证实为肝细胞癌,Ⅱ-Ⅲ级;CT诊断为“不典型肝癌可能性大”

病例8:男,55岁,手术病理证实为中-低分化肝细胞癌,CT诊断为不除外不典型肝癌。

怀疑胰腺癌病人的扫描范围如何确定,至少应包括上腹,至少应包括膈顶,可就有不包括膈顶而造成肝顶肝癌漏诊的情况。

病例9:男,81岁,直肠癌切除术后一年余,怀疑复发和转移,初超声见胰腺稍大,遂行胰腺CT,肝顶被不正规的CT扫描漏掉,再做肝三期方发现肝顶转移性肝癌。

肝脏与其周围器官和组织的关系:肝脏与其周围器官和组织关系十分密切,都互相拥挤在腹腔内,它们的疾病可以互相影响,病变可以互相侵犯,如病变范围较大,常常分不清是谁侵犯谁,病变究竟来源于何处。

病例10:男,68岁,CT发现胃窦癌,未注意到肝脏的病变,手术发现肝结节1×1×1cm,病理证实为腺癌,中分化。

病例11:男,60岁,外生型肝癌,动脉期表现尤其明显。

病例12:男,67岁,小肝癌,高分化肝细胞型肝癌。

病例13:女,69岁,肝脓肿与肝癌。肝内乳头状腺癌(灰红色肝组织一块1×1×0.5cm),(腹壁组织黑红色5×3.5×2cm)乳头状腺癌浸润。

病例14:女,70岁,肝外型与肝内型肝癌同存。

病例15:男,42岁,手术病理:(左上腹)上皮性恶性肿瘤,考虑肝癌;(左上腹腔)癌结节。(左上腹腔)灰红灰白色肿物一块,5.5×3×1cm;(左上腹)灰白色肿物一块,10×10×12cm,切面红黄相间,有出血坏死;(左上腹肿物)灰白灰红色不整形肿物一块,12×11×9cm,切面灰白,质脆,可见部分包膜,另见凝血样组织一堆,12×9×1cm,其中见一灰白、灰黄结节。手术见肿块与肝有一蒂相连接,腹腔内可见约800ml出血,肿块内一半都是出血。

关于肝转移癌:时时刻刻都要注意提高对肝转移癌的高度警惕!

病例16:男,38岁,病理为左眼球恶性黑色素瘤,2-03CT发现后手术,同年10-19出现肝转移。

直肠癌病人,只扫下腹?或盆腔?忽略上腹肝脏转移。这又涉及到CT扫描的部位收费问题。直肠癌病人，直肠远端及肛管未进入扫描范围，也须注意，提高技师的素质，不要自作主张，而要执行规范。

病例 17：男，63 岁，直肠腺癌，中分化，侵及浆膜层，伴左肝外叶转移。（第一次扫描，直肠远端及肛管区均未进入扫描范围）。

第十四节　MRI 误诊为肝细胞癌的肝巨淋巴结增生症

巨淋巴结增生症，又称 Castleman 病、血管滤泡性淋巴组织增生，是一种少见的淋巴细胞增生性疾病，由 Castleman 等（1956）首次报道，其发病机制除了与较为明确的人类疱疹病毒 -8 和白细胞介素 -6 有关外，可能尚有其他细胞因子和病毒感染参与发病。其病理分为透明血管型、浆细胞型和混合型，临床上根据发病的范围分为局限型与弥漫型。局限型病变好发于胸部（70%），发生于腹部相对较少（10%~15%），而发生于肝脏罕见，搜索文献偶有报道；弥漫型病变可累及全身多组淋巴结。

巨淋巴结增生症的影像表现与病理类型密切相关。局限型病变主要为透明血管型，表现为沿中轴淋巴链分布的单发软组织肿块，边界清晰，周围组织受压推移改变无或轻中度，病变特征之一是瘤灶中央放射状或簇状钙化，特征之二是病灶内可见裂隙状低密度影或 T_2WI 低信号影，增强扫描动脉期病变明显强化，门脉期强化减退；弥漫型病变主要为浆细胞型，表现为全身多组淋巴结多发肿大，密度 / 信号较均匀，增强扫描多表现为均匀中度强化。

一例 MRI 误诊原因如下：影像表现与肝细胞癌存在重叠，均表现为稍长 T_1 稍长 T_2 信号改变，增强扫描动脉期明显强化，门脉期强化减退；既往乙肝病史 12 年，MRI 观察提示存在肝硬化、脾大、门脉期高压伴侧支循环背景；巨淋巴结增生症临床少见，影像医师对其认识不足且主观上未想到本病发生的可能。

目前 DWI 和 ADC 值广泛应用于肿瘤病变的鉴别诊断，有作者指出肝良性病变 ADC 值明显高于恶性肿瘤，肝细胞癌 ADC 值为（1.0 ± 0.13）$\times 10^3$mm²/s。一些作者观察 10 例行 DWI 检查的巨淋巴结增生症患者得出其 ADC 值为（1.78 ± 0.14）$\times 10^{-3}$mm²/s，提示 DWI 及 ADC 值有可能为鉴别两者的有效方法，但巨淋巴结增生症的相关研究较少，还需更多的病例去观察总结，该病例和 Jang 等（2012）报道的病例提示在肝脏富血供病变的诊断中，即使是存在乙肝肝炎病史及肝硬化背景的患者，尽管肝巨淋巴结增生症发生率极低，也需纳入鉴别诊断中。

局限型巨淋巴结增生症需要与相应部位常见病种相鉴别，该例病变发生部位于肝脏. 需要与以下肝脏富血供病变鉴别：

（1）肝细胞癌：肝癌患者多有肝炎、肝硬化背景，甲胎蛋白水平升高，增强扫描呈快进快出特点，可有肝内外浸润、播散及门脉癌栓表现，巨淋巴结增生症患者甲胎蛋白不高，DWI 及 ADC 图有可能作为鉴别两者的有效办法。

（2）肝局灶性结节增生：动脉期明显强化，门脉期、延迟期强化减退密度接近肝实质密度，病灶内可见 T_2WI 高信号的中央瘢痕. 而巨淋巴结增生症病灶内为 T_2WI 低信号的裂隙样改变可资鉴别。

（3）肝腺瘤：与口服避孕药和性激素治疗关系密切，动脉期明显强化，门脉期、延迟期强化减退，密度接近或稍高于肝实质密度，病灶可有包膜，病变易出血、坏死及脂肪变，而巨淋巴结增生症较少出现脂肪变的报道。

（4）肝血管瘤：增强扫描呈早出晚归特点，强化方式有从边缘向中央渐近强化趋势，两者不同的强化方式将有助于鉴别诊断。

（5）目前手术切除被认为是局限型病变最合适的治疗方法. 部分无法完整切除者可选择放化疗：弥漫型病变治疗方法包括化疗、受体拮抗剂治疗、免疫调节剂治疗、抗病毒药物治疗等：但对其治疗的标准方法仍未达成共识。

第二十章　关于肝癌的治疗与复发

第一节　肝癌的复发

肝细胞肝癌是最常见的肝脏恶性肿瘤,新患肝细胞性肝癌中 55% 发生在中国,中国的肝癌诊治形势十分严峻。肝癌恶性程度高,就诊时多数已属于中晚期,未能早期发现是肝癌治疗效果差的最主要原因。原发性肝癌术后复发与转移是影响肝癌远期疗效的重要因素,肝癌的复发多发生在术后 1~2 年,有资料表明,肝癌术后 1 年复发率达 20%~64%,3 年复发率可高达 57%~81%。一些作者报道肝癌切除术后 5 年复发率为 61.5%,小肝癌术后复发率为 43.5%。Ezaki 等(1996)报道 <4cm 肝癌根治性切除术后 5 年复发率可达 61%。

有作者相继报道术后超过 10 年出现复发的病例,这些后期复发的病例一般合并慢性肝炎,复发前的血清学检查出现转氨酶及甲胎蛋白升高。肝癌术后部分患者仍然会出现肿瘤复发的情况,如对此进行有效监测并早期发现肿瘤复发迹象,有利于肝癌术后肿瘤复发的治疗。

监测肝癌复发的方法包括磁共振扩散加权成像(DWI)及血清肿瘤标志物检测。DWI 能显示明显的肿块,但对于少数患者 DWI 可能漏诊,结合肿瘤标记物检测能显著提高肝癌转移复发早期的诊断符合率。肿瘤标志物是指存在于肿瘤细胞内或肿瘤细胞表达及脱落的物质,或是宿主对于体内肿瘤反应而产生的物质。特异性的肿瘤标志物对于疾病的筛查、早期诊断、疗效监测、预后判断都具有重要意义。甲胎蛋白是诊断肝癌的首选肿瘤标志物,作为普查、诊断及判断疗效的手段已广泛应用于临床。由于高分化和低分化的肝癌细胞均不合成甲胎蛋白,只有中分化的肝癌细胞才能合成,因此阳性率仅为 50%~70%,假阳性率较高,易受其他因素影响,其敏感性远远不能满足疾病诊断的要求。

在肝细胞性肝癌的早期诊断中,甲胎蛋白 -L3 是非常有效的。临床研究发现甲胎蛋白 -L3 的检测能够在慢性乙肝患者、慢性丙肝患者和肝硬化等高危人群中提示直径 <2 cm 肝细胞性肝癌的存在。研究发现甲胎蛋白 -L3 比影像学检查可以提前 9~12 个月发现肝细胞性肝癌的存在。肝细胞性肝癌的早期发现可以为患者争取更多的治疗机会,用甲胎蛋白 -L3 占总甲胎蛋白的比例来检测肝细胞性肝癌不依赖总甲胎蛋白量的增多。甲胎蛋白 -L3 对肝细胞性肝癌检测的特异度高达 95% 以上且费用低,高特异度的甲胎蛋白 -L3 对肝细胞性肝癌的早期鉴别诊断非常有效,对肝细胞性肝癌的诊治具有重要价值。

甲胎蛋白 -L3 的诊断敏感度与肝细胞性肝癌的临床分期相关,甲胎蛋白 -L3 检测肝细胞性肝癌总的敏感度为 50%~60%,在直径 <2 cm 肝癌中,其敏感度只有 35%~45%,随着肝细胞性肝癌的增大,甲胎蛋白 -L3 的诊断敏感度也随之升高,当肝细胞性肝癌的直径≥ 5 cm 时,甲胎蛋白 -L3 的诊断敏感度可高达 80%~90%。血清中总甲胎蛋白和甲胎蛋白 -L3 可以提供关于肝癌的不同信息,总甲胎蛋白升高可能提示肝癌患者肝脏有大的瘤块存在,甲胎蛋白 -L3 可以预测肝癌的恶性程度。

总甲胎蛋白的诊断敏感度与肿瘤的临床分期尤其是肿瘤的分化程度相关,而甲胎蛋白 -L3 的诊断敏感度主要与肝癌的生物学特性有关(如恶性程度),因此,甲胎蛋白 -L3 的诊断敏感度与肝癌的肿瘤学特性密切相关。在临床检测中,血清中总甲胎蛋白和甲胎蛋白 -L3 是被同时检测的,这是为了估算甲胎蛋白 -L3 占血清总甲胎蛋白的比例。甲胎蛋白 -L3 检测能够用于恶性肝癌的早期发现和治疗后患者随访。

应该注意的是，直径小的肝细胞性肝癌并不一定是早期的肝细胞性肝癌，如果甲胎蛋白-L3在总甲胎蛋白中的比例升高，即使直径<2 cm的肝细胞性肝癌在临床中也可能表现为高度恶性，其生长速度很快且可发生早期转移。相反，甲胎蛋白-L3阴性的小肝细胞性肝癌与甲胎蛋白-L3阳性相比通常其恶性程度低得多，这些患者预后通常较好。由于甲胎蛋白-L3具有较高的特异度，因此可用于肝癌患者治疗后的随访。甲胎蛋白-L3由阳性转为阴性提示临床治疗效果较好；而甲胎蛋白-L3持续阳性或者由阴性转为阳性的治疗后肝癌患者可能为肿瘤淋巴结或者其他器官的转移，也有可能是肿瘤复发。

多项指标联合检测能明显提高原发性肝癌诊断的敏感度，有助于肝癌的临床筛查。有作者发现在单个血清肿瘤标志物中甲胎蛋白灵敏度最高，癌胚抗原最低，同时观察到诊断敏感度随结节增大而增高。由此可见，多项指标联合检测能明显提高原发性肝癌的诊断敏感度，且结节大小也可影响肝癌的诊断敏感度。

因此，一些作者主张甲胎蛋白、甲胎蛋白-L3、CA199、CA125及癌胚抗原联合检测，有利于提高原发性肝癌及肝癌术后转移复发检测的敏感度。

DWI可通过检测活体组织内水分子的微观扩散运动状态来反映机体组织结构的生理、病理特点，对病理条件下活体内水分子的运动加以分析。不同正常组织、生理组织与病理组织间由于水的分布状态的不同，因而具有不同的ADC值，由于水分子的运动受诸多因素影响，因此难以测得精确的扩散系数D，在临床实践中，常用ADC值来代替真正的扩散系数。腹部DWI受心脏搏动、呼吸运动、脉搏、血流灌注、胃肠蠕动等多因素影响，要求成像速度快。EPI技术成像速度极快，基本可消除生理活动等伪影的影响，为最常用并较为成熟的扩散成像序列。一项研究选用SE EPI序列，虽然其图像易产生伪影，但其伪影位置相对固定，易鉴别，通过匀场、薄层扫描、短TE及抑脂技术可减少伪影的影响。b值的选择对于DWI成像非常重要，它是决定ADC值大小的决定因素之一。小b值及b值差反映组织血流灌注，大b值及b值差则反映组织内水分子的扩散远动，但大b值使DWI的TE时间延长，而TE过长则肝信号强度过低，影响图像质量，降低病灶的检出率。

有研究显示，肝脏DWI采用b值为500 s/mm^{2}时能得到较稳定的DWI图像，因此该项研究采用b值为100 s/mm^2、500 s/mm^{2}和800 s/mm^2。肝脏扩散为各向同性，其内各种局灶性病变的含水量、细胞密度、组织内液体流动及黏滞性不同，其扩散就各不相同，ADC值亦有差异，因此使用ADC值判断其良恶性成为可能。

肝囊肿内为运动相对自由的水分子囊液，因而扩散的信号衰减最大，测得的ADC值也最大，ADC图上表现为“灯泡征”。该组没有囊肿合并感染或出血病例，这种情况下水分子扩散运动受到限制，理论上ADC值降低，但降低程度如何以及能否与恶性局灶性病变相鉴别还有待于进一步研究。

肝血管瘤虽然也主要由液体成分组成，但常含有纤维间隔、瘢痕及出血，血窦内的血液黏度较高，分子运动受到一定限制，所以ADC值低于肝囊肿。

肝恶性局灶性病变内自由水相对较少，分子运动明显受限，因此ADC值明显低于肝囊肿及肝血管瘤。

一项研究说明DWI联合4项肿瘤标志物的诊断敏感度及特异度较4项肿瘤标志物联合检测升高，且随着肿块的增大而增高，诊断敏感度及特异度在肿块>5 cm时为最高，分别为98.4%、95.0%，说明DWI联合肿瘤标志物可明显提高诊断敏感度及特异度。

另外，该项研究中DWI联合肿瘤标志物检测的漏诊率低，但误诊率较高，这就要求影像诊断应联合肿瘤标志物检测，对具有转移复发倾向的肝癌患者进行有效干预，进一步提高肝癌患者的治疗效果，改善预后。

第二节　原发性肝癌术后复发的肝动脉造影表现

原发性肝癌（尤其是早期肝癌）的治疗，目前仍首选外科手术切除，但复发率高。有作者报告复发率为：一年17.1%，二年32.5%，五年61.5%。

如何处理好术后复发病人，是提高肝癌远期疗效的关键。由于复发病灶的位置、数目等因素的影响，复发性肝癌再行手术切除的机会甚少，而部分病人也不愿再行手术。近年经肝动脉化疗栓塞治疗肝癌发展较快,疗效亦较为满意,是治疗复发性肝癌的主要治疗方法之一。

X线肝动脉造影表现的特点:肝癌术后复发的肝动脉造影表现,除可具有原发性肝癌的造影表现外,尚有如下特点:复发病灶相对于未经手术切除时肝癌病灶,血供不丰富,供血的肝动脉及分支增粗不明显,肿瘤结节染色相对浅淡;复发病灶常呈多发性,单个病灶极少;小病灶(直径小于2cm)多见。有作者指出,复发病灶多为供血动脉增粗,迂曲,及细小网状的肿瘤血管;而供血动脉拉直,推移,肿瘤血管粗大紊乱,及动-静脉瘘较少见。

X线肝动脉造影分型的病理基础:根据肝动脉造影的结果,造影表现可分为三种类型。

边缘复发型:复发病灶主要局限于手术边缘,表现为多个小结节状影,直径约3~5mm,沿手术切缘浸润分布或聚集成团;由于血供不丰富,肝动脉及分支增粗不明显,或是正常粗细,不见血管或仅见少许肿瘤血管,实质期呈浅淡的结节染色;少数伴手术残腔病例可见沿腔缘分布的条状不规则浅半环状或环状染色。此型造影表现可能与几个因素(即:肿块巨大,未能行根治手术,门静脉内癌栓,肿块周围癌细胞残留等)有关。

肝内播散型:复发病灶散布于肝内,表现为数目及大小不等的结节状影,大多数病灶直径大于10mm,或者表现为巨块状伴结节状影。血供比较丰富,类似于原发性小肝癌或巨块型肝癌的造影表现,动脉期见扭曲,僵直,粗细不均的细小肿瘤血管影,部分病例见肝动脉分支增粗,小的动-静脉瘘,门静脉癌栓,实质期为浓密的结节状或巨块状肿瘤染色。此型X线肝动脉造影表现可能与下述因素有关,即:肝硬化基础上肝癌的多中心起源,门静脉癌栓扩散,手术过程中对肿瘤的挤压等。

隐匿复发型:肝内未见确切的复发病灶,X线肝动脉造影表现无异常,或表现为某一区域的小血管增多,轻度扭曲,拉直,或见小的动-静脉瘘。实质期无明确的肿瘤结节染色,但在碘油CT,或CTA、CTAP扫描图像上可见到明确的肿瘤结节影。此型复发病灶甚为微小,供应血管亦较纤细,因而有如上血管造影表现。

肝癌术后早期行肝动脉造影的意义:X线肝动脉造影较普通CT扫描,B型超声,常规核素扫描发现肝内复发病灶的准确性和敏感性高。肝动脉造影可显示直径为2mm的末梢动脉及直径小于5mm的小病灶,采用超选择交流速肝动脉造影还可以进一步提高显示病灶的准确率。一些作者报告在血管造影前有5例CT和B型超声检查均未见明显占位,14例甲胎蛋白小于20ng/ml,经肝动脉造影或碘油CT扫描都证实为肿瘤复发。因此,该作者建议,对于肝癌术后患者应该早期(术后2~4个月)行肝动脉插管化疗以预防复发。其目的为:通过肝动脉造影,可以提高肝癌术后复发的早期发现率;可以使部分患者经介入治疗后获得第二次手术切除的机会;可行预防性经肝动脉灌注和化疗栓塞治疗,有效地控制复发和转移,提高患者的生存期。

第三节 肝癌治疗中的CT观察

一些作者分析165例肝癌患者经肝动脉化疗栓塞术后再次血管造影复查的X线表现和重复治疗方面的有关问题,描述了肿瘤血管在治疗过程中的减少、消失、不变、增多、新病灶形成、侧支供血、血管推压征、动-静脉分流等改变;评价了血管造影在观察肿瘤变化和分析疗效中的重要作用;认为根据肿瘤血管的变化,相应地调整治疗药物剂量和剂型,对于保护肝,胃,胰等正常器官,减少合并症是非常必要的。

在治疗期间,肿瘤由多血管向少血管或无血管转变,对评价疗效具有重要临床意义。

肿瘤体积的变化对评价疗效是必不可少的,但肿瘤大小的变化不能反映其组织学的变化,假如一个实体瘤的肿瘤细胞已全部死亡,它仍然会在超声,CT检查中表现为占位。

而血管造影能明确地显示治疗期间肿瘤血管、侧支供血、动-静脉分流等有关肿瘤血供方面的动态变化,这种变化实质上反映了肿瘤组织学和病理解剖学的改变,这是其他方法不能代替的。就此而言,血管造影对肿瘤变化的观察和疗效的评价优于超声和CT,是评价疗效的最敏感和特异的方法。

第四节　肝癌射频消融术后特殊征象

经皮射频消融术目前广泛用于肝癌的治疗中，已有研究显示其治疗小肝癌疗效可媲美手术切除，且具有创伤小，恢复快等优点。但影响经皮射频消融术疗效主要为高局部复发率，据报道经皮射频消融术后局部复发率为 14.1%~58.1%，这很大程度归因于消融范围未能足够包围目标肿瘤引起。对于这些未能完全消融的所谓"复发灶"，若能早期发现并作经皮射频消融术补充治疗，可使完全消融率由原来的 77% 提升至 99.7%。由此可见，经皮射频消融术术后正确的疗效评价对于提高经皮射频消融术疗效意义重大。增强 CT 是目前评价经皮射频消融术疗效的主要手段。一项研究对具有完整随访 CT 资料的经皮射频消融术 630 例进行回顾性分析，特别通过对一些经皮射频消融术后特殊 CT 征象的解释，从而提高增强 CT 评价经皮射频消融术疗效的准确率。

增强 CT 评价经皮射频消融术疗效的依据；评价经皮射频消融术疗效关键在于判断射频消融灶能否完全包围整个目标肿瘤并取得安全消融边界。通过测量与对比消融灶与肿瘤径值的大小可有助于判断疗效。但是，单凭径值的测量不足以判断疗效的彻底性，目前被认为较可靠的影像学诊断应以病灶增强信息作判断。肿瘤在经皮射频消融术前的增强影像上显示有肿瘤血供强化表现，而完全消融灶一直表现为无强化。但一些经皮射频消融术术后的特殊征象往往影响疗效的正确评价。

经皮射频消融术术后特殊征象 CT 表现的解释：一项研究发现了 7 种比较特殊的经皮射频消融术相关影像学表现，其中部分构成对正确评价经皮射频消融术疗效的影响。

（1）肝脓肿：特别是早期肝脓肿，中央未见明显液化者，较易与肝内复发灶相混淆。鉴别上除症状与血象异常外，肝脓肿一般有典型的"二环征"或"三环征"，无"快进快退"征象，经抗感染治疗后缩小或消失。

（2）假性动脉瘤：极易与早期原位复发或残留相混淆，均表现为动脉期消融灶周边局部强化灶。有报道认为假性动脉瘤的出现可能为射频热损伤动脉壁导致局部去痉挛膨胀引起。该项研究中发现 8 例，虽没经过 DSA 血管造影证实，但随访过程中强化影相对稳定，且局部强化灶与肝内动脉明显相连接，无明显"快进快退"征象。

（3）胆汁湖：表现为局部低密度影，呈水样密度，边缘清晰，呈局部扩张样或"串珠"样，可位于消融灶内、周边或远离消融灶。目前一般认为是经皮射频消融术时热损伤胆管或损伤了胆管的供血小动脉，从而导致局部胆管受损膨胀，部分可能由于射频针直接穿透胆管引起肝内胆汁漏引起。

一般来说，胆汁湖的出现不会影响到消融灶在 CT 上的疗效判断，但在 MRI 上，由于胆汁湖液性成分较多，在 T_2WI 图像上表现为极高信号，类似于肝囊肿，而残留灶多表现为中等高信号，因而胆汁湖的存在，在一定程度上掩盖残留灶的信号，从而造成错误评价。此时增强 T_1WI 和超声造影有助于鉴别两者。

（4）异常灌注：其发生一般认为与经皮射频消融术引起机械性动脉门静脉瘘或动静脉瘘有关，并沿针道发生，在进行肝穿活检与 PEI 治疗时同样可以发生。增强 CT 上多表现为动脉期形状规则的片状均匀强化区域，非动脉期时与正常肝实质密度一样。可位于消融灶周边或远离消融灶区域。但位于消融灶周边的异常灌注病灶在一定程度上干扰了残留灶的判断。

由于异常灌注区域在动脉期同样表现为强化影，极易将可能存在的存活肿瘤强化灶掩盖，从而导致假阴性的发生。鉴别上应注意强化区域的强化特点和随复查时间的变化。异常灌注区域一般不随时间的推移而增大，并且会有突然消失的情况，国外报道由经皮射频消融术引起的异常灌注发生率为 10% 左右，大部分会在 4 个月内消失；而残留肿瘤灶一般随时间推移而增大。有"快进快退"征象。1~3 个月复查 CT 会有助于鉴别两者。

（5）中央高密度：表现为在消融低密度区中央局部高密度灶，与增强剂无关系。同样的发现在微波治疗中也会出现，国内外文献亦见报道。中央高密度影一般不会造成对经皮射频消融术疗效判断的影响。其出现的原因说法不一，Goldberg 等（2000）认为是经皮射频消融术后中央区域细胞裂解物堆积引起，Tsuda 等(2001)则认为是经皮射频消融术后中央区域高温脱水碳化引起局部密度增高引起,而 Raman 等(2000)认为是中央治疗区域由于射频针的破坏导致出血引起。

(6)良性反应带:亦称炎性反应带,由热介导的周边组织炎性水肿或肉芽增生引起。多表现为消融灶周边均匀、壁薄的强化带。该项研究发生率为 4.3%(27/630),较国外报道低(1 个月时 89%、1~3 个月时 56%、3~6 个月时 22%),这可能与其判断标准不一和增强 CT 检查时间不同有关。良性反应带的存在,在一定程度上会影响疗效的判断,增强的反应带有可能遮盖残留灶的强化信息。但炎性反应带强化一般较均匀,并随时间延长而逐渐减少,与残留灶呈结节样强化并随时间而增大不同。国外报道经皮射频消融术治疗结直肠癌肝转移瘤时炎性反应带的出现率很低,这可能与转移瘤本身呈乏血管有关;原发性肝癌在行 PEI 治疗时亦较少出现炎性反应带,可能与无水酒精对局部微血管床的损害导致炎性反应降低有关。因而在经皮射频消融术时结合不含碘化油的 PEI 治疗,可能在提高疗效的同时,亦可以降低炎性反应带的发生率,提高疗效判断准确率。

(7)中央气体影:一般在经皮射频消融术后极早期检查中发现,不会造成对经皮射频消融术疗效判断的影响。其出现主要是由于射频高温导致瘤内液体气化引起。在以超声作引导的经皮射频消融术实时监测上可以看到,局部液体气化在超声上呈高回声影,经皮射频消融术结束后 2~5 min,高回声团开始逐渐消退,消退从外周开始,而中央区域高回声可持续时间较长。该项研究 2 例在经皮射频消融术后 1 周内作 CT 检查发现中央气体影,而在随后的检查中消失。

经皮射频消融术术后增强 CT 检查时间的探讨:经皮射频消融术复查大致建议分三个时间段:经皮射频消融术后第 1 个月内,由于 1 个月内消融病灶未发生收缩,此时应以平扫 CT 测量径值与消融面积是否覆盖整个肿瘤作为主要的疗效评价途径,而 1 个月内的增强 CT 往往存在较多的炎性反应与异常灌注干扰;经皮射频消融术后 3 个月,此时炎性反应带基本消失,消融灶与周边组织界限分明,增强 CT 可发现大部分残留病灶;经皮射频消融术术后 12 个月,一般认为在经皮射频消融术术后 12 个月未见局部复发者,肿瘤基本得到彻底消融。

总而言之,在实际的临床工作中应具体情况具体分析,对未能确定的病灶应密切随访追踪避免延误诊断。

第五节 误诊病例简介:布加综合征合并原发性肝癌

一般认为淤血性肝硬化与原发性肝癌的发生无关,但布 - 加综合征引起的淤血性肝损伤导致肝细胞再生的慢性病理过程与其他致癌诱因导致肝癌发生的病理过程十分相似,因此两者之间并非毫无关联。

在布 - 加综合征病例中约 0.7%的患者,尤其是患有慢性病毒性肝炎、白塞病和长期烟酒史的患者,可在 4.5~24 年的病程中进展为具有多中心起源、结节状生长、增长迅速等特点的肝癌, TACE 序贯治疗后平均生存期为 9~29.3 个月,而无明显致癌诱因合并原发性肝癌的患者则十分罕见。

该例肝静脉与下腔静脉同时受累,属复合型布 - 加综合征,合并的原发性肝癌特征较上述特点有明显差异:单发团块状病灶; TACE 序贯治疗后肿瘤消失;患者首诊后随访至今已 38 个月仍无进展征象,疗效明显优于相关文献报道结果。

其良好疗效可能与以下因素有关:病灶单发,肝内无其他病灶,范围局限,血管造影无动 - 静脉瘘及门静脉侵犯征象,对介入治疗敏感;患者无其他常见致癌诱因,侧支循环建立充分,淤血性肝损伤相对较轻,肝脏储备及代偿功能较强(Child-Pugh A 级)。因此能耐受多次序贯治疗而具有较好的预后生存期。

分析该例前期漏诊布 - 加综合征的原因:首诊时已有肝硬化门静脉高压征象,但无引起肝硬化常见的病史;肝内原发块状型肝癌的“干扰”;患者体内侧支循环建立较为充分,未出现明显腹腔积液及双下肢水肿典型症状等。直至发生消化道出血才最终确诊。

第四篇　肝细胞性肝癌以外的肝恶性肿瘤

第一章　胆管细胞型肝癌

（请结合本书 本卷 第十六篇 第六章 肝内胆管细胞癌研究）

第一节　误诊病例简介：肝内胆管细胞癌与肝结核瘤

患者，女，57 岁。体检发现肝占位一月余入院。MRI 诊断：肝左内叶占位伴肝门部淋巴结肿大，考虑结核瘤，肿瘤待排？请结合临床。胸部 CT 提示：肝左内叶见一 5.4cm × 5.1cm 稍低密度影，CT 值 33HU，边界尚清。CT 诊断：肝左内叶稍低密度影，性质？炎性假瘤？请结合 MRI 检查。

病理检查：冰冻病理与常规病理：右肝肿物：红褐色碎组织一堆，总体积 1.8cm × 1.5cm × 1.5cm，其中一切面见一结节，直径 0.6cm，结节切面灰白质中；第 8 组淋巴结：结节一个，大小 2.8 cm × 1.8 cm × 1.8 cm，切面灰红灰白，质中；12L 淋巴结：灰红色组织三块，大小 2.8 cm × 1.6 cm × 0.8 cm，切面灰红，质中。

冰冻病理诊断：右肝肿物：腺癌；第 8 组淋巴结：转移性腺癌；12L 淋巴结：未见癌转移。常规病理诊断：右肝肿物：腺癌；第 8 组淋巴结：转移性腺癌；12L 淋巴结：转移性腺癌。建议免疫组化标记探讨其来源。

免疫组化诊断：第 8 组淋巴结：转移性腺癌，可能来自肝内外胆管系统或胰腺。建议临床进一步检查胆管胰腺，并注意肾脏、子宫内膜情况，明确原发灶。

病理检查：左肝内叶及胆囊切除标本：肝组织一块，大小 6.5 cm × 6.0 cm × 5.5 cm，切面见一不规则结节，大小 6.5 cm × 5.0 cm，呈灰白、棕绿色，质中，与周围界限不清。肝组织一侧附胆囊组织，胆囊大小 5.5 cm × 2.0 cm × 1.5 cm，黏膜呈粗网状，囊壁厚 0.2 cm；门静脉旁淋巴结清扫标本：结节样组织一块，大小，2.5 cm × 1.5 cm × 1.0 cm，切面灰白，质中。常规病理诊断：左肝内叶及胆囊切除标本：镜下可见腺癌样癌组织侵犯周围正常肝组织，待做免疫组化检测进一步明确癌肿类型。胆囊组织呈慢性炎，未受癌组织累及。门静脉旁淋巴结清扫标本：检出淋巴结一枚，可见癌转移。

免疫组化诊断：左肝内叶切除标本：结合临床病史、影像学检查、免疫组化检测结果及组织学图像，诊断为中低分化腺癌，癌组织侵犯周围正常肝组织，并可见脉管内癌栓，考虑来源于肝内胆管系统（胆管细胞癌）。

第二节　误诊病例简介:肝内胆管细胞癌与肝脓肿

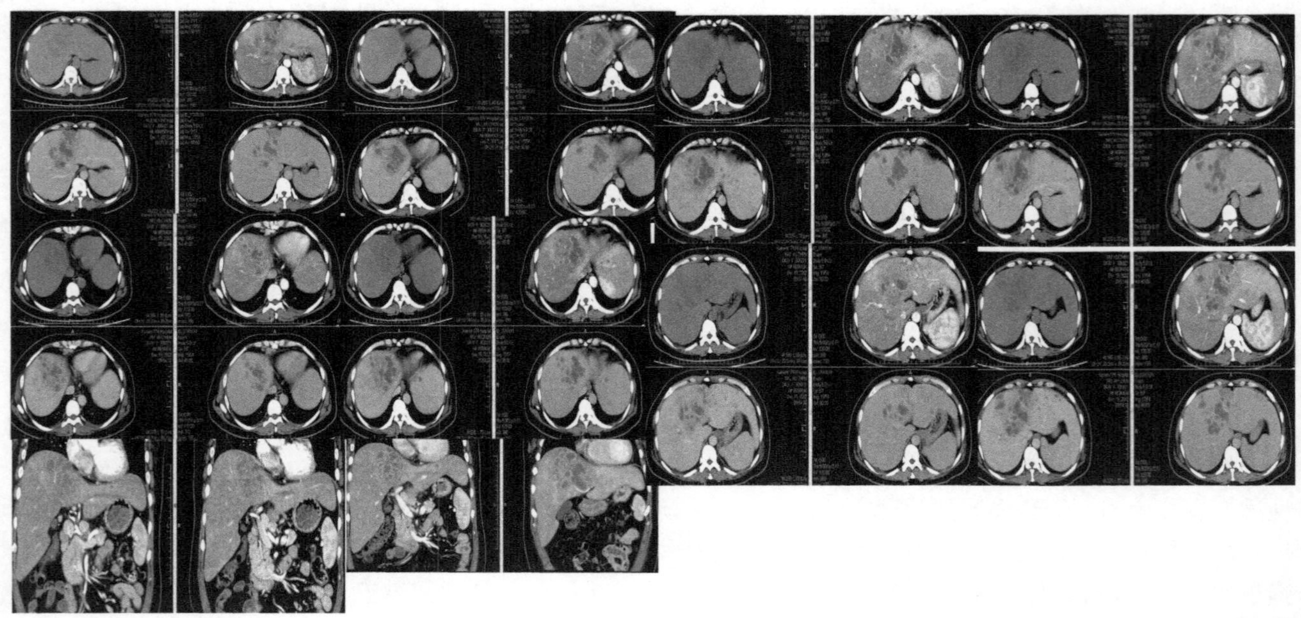

图 4-1-1　肝内胆管细胞癌与肝脓肿

患者,女, 43 岁。反复发热 1 月,伴腹痛 20 天入院。缘于 1 月前无明显诱因出现发热,体温最高达 38~39℃,伴有畏冷、寒战,全腹部闷痛,呈阵发性,休息后可缓解,曾于当地诊所予抗炎治疗后,仍反复发热。

病理检查:肝占位穿刺活检标本:灰白灰褐色细针穿刺组织三条,最长者 1.6cm,最短者 1.2cm,直径均为 0.1cm。常规病理诊断:肝占位穿刺活检标本:初步考虑恶性肿瘤伴坏死,待做免疫组化检测进一步探讨肿瘤类型。

免疫组化检测:阳性: CK19, CK7(部分 +), CK8, CK18, Vimentin, Villin(小灶 +), CA19-9(散在 +), Ki-67(+,约 25%):阴性: Hepatocyte, GPC3, CD34, AFP, CK20, CK5/6, P63, S-100, HMB45, Melan-A, CgA, Syn, TTF-1, NapsinA, PAX-8, GATA-3, CD10。免疫组化诊断:肝占位穿刺活检标本:结合免疫组化检测结果及组织学图像,符合胆管细胞癌。

误诊分析:本病例从影像表现结合临床症状上看,极易考虑肝脓肿,术前两次 CT 增强扫描均报告肝内混杂密度影,考虑肝脓肿;回顾性分析发现,尽管增强扫描延迟期病灶未见明显的填充式强化,但增强扫描动脉期病灶边缘呈"花环状"明显强化,静脉期及延迟期强化迅速减低与肝实质相仿,尤其是第二次复查 CT 增强扫描时,发现病灶有所增多,并且腹膜后可见多发肿大的淋巴结,肝恶性肿瘤的诊断不能排除(图 4-1-1)。

第三节　不典型的肝内胆管细胞癌

肝内胆管细胞癌典型的 CT 征象为平扫(稍)低密度影,边缘模糊不清,动态增强扫描呈渐进性延迟强化是其重要特征,灶周和 / 或瘤灶内包埋扩张的胆管,相应肝叶萎缩,可合并有肝内胆管结石。而不典型肝内胆管细胞癌的 CT 表现较为特殊,稍有不慎就可误诊或漏诊。

病理学:肝内胆管细胞癌是一种起源于肝内末梢胆管到肝门部胆管上皮细胞的腺癌,占肝原发恶性肿瘤的 5%~15%,居肝内原发性恶性肿瘤的第 2 位。依其生长方式和大体形态可分为肿块型、胆管周围浸润型和胆管内生长型,其中肿块型多见。肝内胆管细胞癌病因尚不清楚,但常与华支睾吸虫感染、慢性胆管炎及肝内胆管结石、胆总管囊肿、原发性硬化性胆管炎等合并存在，因此推测其可能与肝内胆管系统的长期慢性炎症和理化因素刺激有关。

临床表现：肝内胆管细胞癌多发生于40~70岁的中老年人，女性比例偏高，患者多无慢性肝炎、肝硬化病史，甲胎蛋白多为阴性。一组14例的CT表现虽然不典型，但临床特点仍与此相符，且仅有1例乙型肝炎表面抗原阳性，阳性率为7.14%，与文献报道中国人群乙肝病毒感染率基本一致，可见肝内胆管细胞癌与乙肝病毒感染没有明确的因果关系。

肝内胆管细胞癌缺乏特异性临床症状和体征，容易与肝细胞肝癌、肝胆管结石、肝脓肿发生混淆，而肝内胆管细胞癌的治疗与肝细胞肝癌不尽相同，提高术前诊断准确率，制订合适的治疗方案对改善预后有重要意义。

影像学研究：表现为"延迟强化"但无肝内胆管结石和扩张的肝内胆管细胞癌：此类肝内胆管细胞癌的强化方式与肝血管瘤相似，且均具有不合并乙型肝炎、肝硬化以及甲胎蛋白增高的特点，因此两者的鉴别诊断至关重要。肝血管瘤增强扫描主要表现为动脉期边缘结节样明显强化，其密度和主动脉的密度接近或一致，门脉期强化范围呈向心性扩大，延迟期呈等密度。

该组3例肝内胆管细胞癌增强动脉期边缘同时出现花环状强化而非结节样强化，强化程度亦达不到同层腹主动脉的水平，门脉、延迟期强化范围虽然向病灶中心扩展，但中心始终未能完全填充，而且延迟期肿瘤边缘环状密度减低，仔细分析这些差异有助于与肝血管瘤进行鉴别。MRI检查对肝内胆管细胞癌与肝血管瘤的鉴别诊断有重要价值。T_2WI图像上肝内胆管细胞癌表现为稍高信号影，并非肝血管瘤极高信号的"灯泡征"，显示实质性病灶的特点；肝血管瘤主要由液体成分组成，而肝内胆管细胞癌的主要成分为实性肿瘤组织，自由水相对较少，其分子运动明显受限，因此表观弥散系数（ADC）值明显低于肝血管瘤，在高b值的DWI图像上表现为不均匀高信号。该组1例在T_2WI及高b值DWI图像上均具有实质性病灶的特点，可避免误诊为肝血管瘤。

肝内胆管显著扩张但无明确占位的肝内胆管细胞癌：此类肝内胆管细胞癌属于胆管壁浸润型，肿瘤组织沿着胆管壁浸润性生长，胆管壁可因肿瘤浸润增厚而致其远端肝内胆管扩张，如果肿瘤沿胆管浸润至肝门水平，则可引起肝门侧的受侵，胆管壁出现不规则狭窄，甚至引起对侧肝叶内胆管扩张。周围胆管呈显著不均匀软藤状扩张为其重要征象。由于肝内胆管细胞癌不形成肿块，CT不易显示癌灶，周围胆管扩张可能为唯一的征象，认识不足极易漏诊。该组2例术前CT检查即因认识不足而未能给出肝内胆管细胞癌的诊断，由此可见慎重认真观察细微影像学征象对于正确诊断的重要性。另外，值得注意的是，此肝内胆管细胞癌伴有扩张胆管周围血供异常，即动脉期片状明显强化影，门脉期、延迟期则与周围正常肝组织呈等密度改变，这可能是由于肿瘤本身使肝动脉血供增加或者扩张胆管压迫相邻的门脉而使肝动脉血供呈代偿性增加所致，此征象可能对肝内胆管细胞癌的诊断具有一定的参考价值。

动脉期边缘花环状强化、门脉期强化减退且边缘毛糙的肝内胆管细胞癌：此型肝内胆管细胞癌动脉期呈较明显的薄边样环形强化，考虑是由于肿瘤的周边存在较多的肿瘤实质细胞，而纤维结缔组织较少的缘故。如果不合并肝内胆管扩张及相应肝叶萎缩等表现时，需警惕误诊为肝脓肿，肝脓肿常可见延迟强化的环形脓肿壁，这与毛糙且不规则的肝内胆管细胞癌边缘有所不同，而且肝脓肿坏死脓腔的腔内缘多表现规整，无肝内胆管细胞癌的条索状或不完全分隔状强化，外缘尚可见水肿引起的低密度环，临床多有发热及白细胞计数升高等表现。仔细观察CT所见并结合临床病史不难进行鉴别诊断。

发生于胆总管囊肿的肝内胆管细胞癌：此类肝内胆管细胞癌常可见肝内胆管扩张，但癌灶往往显示不清。有学者指出：成人的胆总管囊肿并发胆系肿瘤的可能性较高。因此，进行影像学检查时，不能仅仅满足于发现和诊断胆总管囊肿，还要注意排除胆总管囊肿有无恶变或合并肿瘤的可能，尤其是发生于成人的胆总管囊肿。

"速升速降"型强化的肝内胆管细胞癌增强动脉期可显示增粗迂曲的供血肝动脉和瘤灶内病理血管影，稍有不慎极易误诊为肝细胞肝癌，尤其是合并有肝硬化的病例，而肝内胆管细胞癌与肝细胞肝癌的治疗不尽相同，有必要对患者进行准确的定性诊断。表现为"速升速降"型强化考虑是由于此类肝内胆管细胞癌的组织学成分与常规不同，无论是肿瘤的外周还是中央区域都是由大量的恶性肿瘤细胞组成，纤维组织成分较少，因而恶性程度也较高，该组一例术前即误诊为肝细胞肝癌，且术后3个月就发生了肝内多发转移灶。

但是“速升速降”型强化的肝内胆管细胞癌可见伴有肝内胆管结石和扩张，这些肿瘤周围的胆管扩张是由于肝内胆管细胞癌起源于胆管上皮，引起相应部位胆管狭窄闭塞所致，此征象较少见于肝细胞肝癌及转移瘤，是肝内胆管细胞癌的一个重要表现，可作为一个具有重要鉴别诊断价值的影像学征象。总之，不典型肝内胆管细胞癌的CT表现较为特殊，考虑可能与癌灶的生长方式、病理特点以及血供等因素有关，仔细观察和分析其CT的细微征象可避免误诊或漏诊，提高术前影像诊断准确性。

第四节　不同生长方式肝内胆管细胞癌

肝内胆管细胞癌相对肝细胞癌少见，仅占原发性肝癌的3.25%~8.2%。生长方式的不同，影像学表现也不尽相同。

1. 病理学　肝内胆管细胞癌起源于肝内一、二级胆管或更大胆管的上皮细胞。按其生长方式可以分为肿块形成型、管壁浸润型和腔内生长型，生长方式不同，影像学表现各异。一组34例肝内胆管细胞癌中，表现为肿块形成型27例，管壁浸润型5例，腔内生长型2例。

2. 影像学研究　肿块形成型：CT表现肿块形成型胆管细胞癌起源于肝脏外围胆管分支或肝门部胆管黏膜，侵犯和穿透胆管壁，在肝细胞板间播散，沿肝窦间隙生长形成肿块，肿瘤有侵犯门脉小分支的倾向，于邻近肝实质形成子灶。CT表现为肝内低密度肿块，其内可包埋高密度结石，中央可出现不规则单发或多发更低密度区域。该组资料27例肿块形成型肝内胆管细胞癌中，24例表现为低密度肿块，3例因合并有脂肪肝而表现为等或高密度。远段胆管可有扩张，邻近肝实质萎缩。若肿块位于肝门部可阻塞左右肝管，骑跨和分隔胆管。位于外围肿块邻近肝包膜可有凹陷。动态增强肿块早期周边环形强化，门脉期强化程度逐渐增加，延迟期强化明显；肿块中央更低密度区可始终无强化，若更低密度为多发，表现为分隔强化的所谓“网状强化”。该组资料27例肿块形成型肝内胆管细胞癌，动脉期表现为周边强化，门脉期逐渐向肿块中央强化。延迟期16例表现为较周围肝实质密度略高或等均匀强化，11例表现为周边的延迟强化中央不规则低密度区。延迟强化主要是由于胆管细胞癌富含纤维结缔组织，对比剂弥散至细胞外组织间隙，结缔组织灌注较差，因此对比剂较难被廓清而滞留于肿瘤内呈现延迟强化。另外，纤维结缔组织收缩可以使肝包膜凹陷以及远段扩张的胆管向肿块处纠集。

管壁浸润型：管壁浸润型胆管细胞癌起源于肝内胆管黏膜，穿透浆膜，通过神经和神经周围Glisson包膜沿胆管向肝门播散，因此，肿瘤纵向生长，沿胆管轴像树枝一样伸展而不形成可见的肿块。CT表现为肝内胆管壁增厚，伴或不伴胆管梗阻。一组5例管壁浸润型胆管细胞癌2例表现为胆管不规则增厚狭窄，另外3例表现为胆管壁增厚及管腔闭塞。

腔内生长型：腔内生长型胆管细胞癌主要为乳头状腺癌，肿瘤细胞局限于黏膜层，并不侵犯黏膜下层。腔内乳头状突起细长易碎，有时可自发脱落，脱落的肿瘤细胞可以种植于邻近胆管内形成多发肿瘤。CT表现为扩张的胆管内软组织结节，增强后结节有强化。该组资料中2例腔内生长型胆管细胞癌均表现为扩张胆管腔内强化结节。

此外，该组资料有6例肝内胆管细胞癌周围观察到一过性强化，考虑为异常灌注。该征象主要见于肝脓肿和富血供肿瘤，肝内胆管细胞癌仅见数例报道，推测可能与门脉受累肝动脉代偿性供血或合并胆管炎有关。

3. 鉴别诊断　肝内肿块形成型胆管细胞癌常需和原发性肝细胞癌、转移瘤、肝脓肿相鉴别。

原发性肝细胞癌：原发性肝细胞癌远较胆管细胞癌常见，临床上常有肝炎肝硬化病史，实验室检查常有甲胎蛋白升高，动态CT表现为动脉期强化，门脉期低于周围肝实质的“快进快出”的特点，肿块周围胆管扩张少见，容易侵犯门脉形成门脉癌栓以及血行转移至肺。

转移瘤：转移瘤患者常有原发肿瘤病史，特别是消化道肿瘤，常为多发，CT表现为肿块轮廓光整低密度肿块，中央常见更低密度坏死区域，增厚后周边强化表现出“牛眼征”，另外结肠黏液腺癌肝内转移灶内可有不定形钙化需与胆管细胞癌包埋结石相鉴别。

肝脓肿：肝脓肿临床上常有感染症状和体征，CT 可表现出“簇征”或“靶征”，但有时两者鉴别需依赖超声或 CT 引导下穿刺活检。

原发性硬化型胆管炎：肝内管壁浸润型胆管细胞癌中表现为管壁增厚者需与原发性硬化型胆管炎相鉴别，后者影像学上表现为胆管串珠样扩张与狭窄相间，而且常合并胆管细胞癌。在动脉期和门脉期扩张的胆管可能也表现为周边环样强化，Lacomis 等（1997）报道延迟扫描可以鉴别扩张的胆管和胆管细胞癌，后者表现为延迟强化。

肝细胞癌脱落胆管癌栓形式生长：肝内腔内生长型胆管细胞癌有时需要和肝细胞癌可脱落到胆管内并以癌栓形式生长相鉴别，后者常有肝内动脉期强化门脉期呈低密度肿块以及其他肝细胞癌的临床和实验室检查特征。

第五节　肝内胆管细胞癌淋巴结转移

肝内胆管细胞癌发生隐匿，其恶性程度较高，发展迅速，临床预后较差，有作者认为，其主要原因是由于肝内胆管细胞癌常发生中上腹部淋巴结转移。淋巴结转移是影响肿瘤预后的重要因素，术前对肝内胆管细胞癌患者中上腹部淋巴结转移进行准确评价，对临床判断能否手术、手术方式的选择及估计预后具有重要意义。

肝内胆管细胞癌淋巴结转移观察：一组 46 例肝内胆管细胞癌患者中，22 例发生淋巴结转移，淋巴结转移阳性率为 47.8%。22 例发生淋巴结转移的病例中，19 例（86%）表现为分离结节影，3 例（14%）有淋巴结融合现象。转移淋巴结基本呈等或略低密度，边缘多较模糊，短径 1~4.5 cm。9 例（40.9%）出现了Ⅱ级淋巴结增大（短径 ≥ 2.5 cm）。10 例（45.4%）有 1 个或多个淋巴结中出现坏死，主要见于Ⅱ级增大的淋巴结。增强扫描淋巴结呈均匀轻度或中度强化，坏死部分不强化。

淋巴结转移判断：结合文献，设定淋巴结的短径 >1cm 为淋巴结阳性的影像表现。统计阳性淋巴结的出现率，并根据各区域淋巴结短径的大小分为 2 级，Ⅰ级淋巴结短径在 1.0~2.5 cm 之间，Ⅱ级淋巴结短径 ≥ 2.5 cm。

淋巴结分组：按解剖分布，结合淋巴引流范围将其分为以下 6 组：①肝十二指肠韧带淋巴结组（包括肝门）；②腹主动脉旁淋巴结组；③胰后淋巴结组；④肝总动脉淋巴结组；⑤腹腔干淋巴结组；⑥贲门 - 胃小弯 - 胃左淋巴结组。

肝内胆管细胞癌转移淋巴结的分组

22 例转移病例中，以肝十二指肠韧带淋巴结组转移发生率最高，其次为贲门 - 胃小弯 - 胃左淋巴结组、胰头后方淋巴结组、腹主动脉旁组、肝总动脉组、腹腔干周围淋巴结组。转移淋巴结分布比较集中，且常为多组同时受累。在 22 例中共观察到 49 组淋巴结转移，平均每例有 2.2 组淋巴结受累。2 例肝左叶肝内胆管细胞癌患者未出现肝十二指肠韧带组淋巴结受累，仅表现为胃小弯 - 贲门 - 胃左淋巴结组及以远淋巴结转移（表 4-1-1）。

表 4-1-1　肝内胆管细胞癌局部淋巴结转移分布（22/46 例）

淋巴结转移分组	例数	所占比例（%）	Ⅰ级（枚）	Ⅱ级（枚）
肝十二指肠韧带淋巴结组	20	90.9	23	8
贲门 - 胃小弯 - 胃左组	8	36.4	12	5
胰后淋巴结组	8	36.4	10	3
腹主动脉淋巴结组	6	27.3	8	1
肝总动脉淋巴结组	4	18.2	5	0
腹腔干淋巴结组	3	13.6	6	0

淋巴结转移影像学研究：和肝细胞型肝癌相比，肝内胆管细胞癌甚至在行手术切除后，临床预后仍然很差，其主要与该肿瘤局部侵犯与否和肝外转移（包括淋巴结转移）有很大的关系。因此，使用影像学的方法判断肝内胆管细胞癌的淋巴结转移对临床的分级、分期及预后的判断有十分重要的临床价值。一组 46 例肝内胆管细胞癌患者中，共有 22 例出现淋巴结转移，占 47.8%。该组 22 例肝内胆管细胞癌患者出现淋巴结转移，短径为 1~4.5 cm，与同侧膈肌

脚相比，转移淋巴结基本呈等或略低密度表现。该组中短径 <2.5 cm 的淋巴结密度多较均匀，短径 ≥ 2.5 cm 的淋巴结中央可出现坏死，以不完全坏死为主。转移淋巴结融合较少，多表现为分离结节影，其边缘欠清晰，分析原因可能是因为转移淋巴结多呈浸润生长，侵犯被膜及周围组织，故边缘显示欠清晰。该组淋巴结转移的病例中，以肝十二指肠韧带组淋巴结转移发生率最高，其次为贲门 - 胃小弯 - 胃左淋巴结组、胰后淋巴结组，腹主动脉旁、肝总动脉旁、腹腔干周围淋巴结组相对较少。转移淋巴结分布比较集中，且常出现多组淋巴结受累，平均每例有 2.2 个部位淋巴结肿大。之所以肝十二指肠韧带组淋巴结转移发生率最高，是因为它是肝内胆管细胞癌淋巴引流的最主要途径。

肝左、右叶的淋巴引流途径有所不同，肝右叶肝内胆管细胞癌以肝十二指肠韧带组淋巴结向远处引流，左叶由于有部分淋巴管从左半肝的尾侧面引流入胃左淋巴结和贲门周围淋巴结，因此，左叶肝内胆管细胞癌是以肝十二指肠韧带组和贲门 - 胃小弯 - 胃左淋巴结组 2 种方式向远处淋巴结转移。但是，不管肝内胆管细胞癌的位置如何（左肝或右肝），其最主要的淋巴转移途径都是先转移到肝十二指肠韧带淋巴结组，然后向胰后、腹主动脉旁、肝总动脉以及腹腔干动脉旁等淋巴结组引流。该项研究中，各组淋巴结受累情况与一些作者的报道略有不同，可能是由于纳入样本量小、入组病例分期不同、累及部位不同等原因所致，尚需大的样本进一步研究。有作者指出，肝十二指肠韧带淋巴结可能是肝内胆管细胞癌的前哨淋巴结，防止肝十二指肠韧带组的淋巴结转移，就有可能阻断远处淋巴结的转移。事实并非如此，根据肝脏的表浅淋巴引流，肝存在迷走血管时淋巴引流可直接汇入主动脉旁右侧淋巴结组。因此，肝内胆管细胞癌淋巴结转移并不一定逐级发生，可表现为跳跃性转移。

该研究发现，36 例高 ~ 中分化癌中，有 15 例出现淋巴结转移；而 10 例低分化癌中，7 例出现了转移，说明肿瘤的分化程度与淋巴结转移发生率有明显相关性。

第六节　无胆管扩张的肝内胆管细胞癌

周围型肝内胆管细胞癌病灶常较大，直径可达 5~20 cm，质地较硬，切面常有硬化表现，中心可有致密的纤维条索。直径≤ 3 cm 的无胆管扩张的周围型肝内胆管细胞癌少见，肿瘤起源于毛细胆管，临床表现、体征及实验室检查表现无特异性，诊断主要依靠影像检查。以往对无胆管扩张的肝内小胆管细胞癌的诊断主要依靠 CT 检查，但对表现不典型者误诊率高。

周围型肝内胆管细胞癌的 MRI 特征及其病理基础：周围型肝内胆管细胞癌组织学上肿块主要由纤维组织、恶性肿瘤细胞和坏死组织构成，不同组织类型和区域肿瘤的各种成分所占比例和分布特点明显不同。一项 12 例研究结果显示，在 MRI 平扫图像上，恶性肿瘤细胞、纤维组织呈 T_1WI 低信号、T_2WI 低信号；凝固性坏死可呈 T_1WI 低或混杂信号、T_2WI 高或混杂信号；当肿瘤囊变、出血、坏死时也可呈混杂信号；当肿瘤以出血、坏死为主时，T_1WI 可呈低、高或混杂信号，T_2WI 为高、低或混杂信号。该项研究中的混杂信号主要以坏死、囊变、黏液湖为主。MRI 增强扫描的强化方式也与纤维组织、恶性肿瘤细胞、坏死组织的成分有关，动脉期强化与恶性肿瘤细胞的区域、分布特点有关，延迟期强化与纤维组织的成分所占的比例有关，不强化与坏死组织有关。当肿瘤细胞分布在病灶边缘，中心以纤维组织为主，坏死不明显，病灶边缘可呈线样、细条状、均匀一致的完整或不完整环形强化，即表现出周边薄环强化型，延迟后纤维组织强化呈等信号。当肿瘤细胞分布在病灶边缘，中心以坏死组织为主，有少量或无纤维组织，病灶边缘呈厚薄不均、粗细不一的完整或不完整环形强化，中心有少量或无纤维组织，即表现出周边厚环强化型，延迟后强化不明显。

当有极少量至散在、不均匀或中等量肿瘤细胞分布在病灶内，病灶以坏死为主，部分纤维组织，病灶可呈岛状强化型或不均匀强化型，部分轻度延迟强化。当肿瘤细胞分布在病灶边缘，但因整个肿瘤呈明显囊性扩张，显著出血、坏死，肿瘤细胞成分所占的比例少，MRI 无法显示，只有在显微镜下可见排列成实性片状、梁索状、腺管样及矮乳头状瘤细胞，瘤细胞异型明显，细胞多形，核分裂象多见，即表现出全瘤灶无强化型。

当肿瘤细胞均匀分布在病灶内，肿瘤呈小至中等大小，均匀一致，未见明显坏死，即表现出全瘤灶明显强化型。而其中见散在均匀纤维间质，延迟后呈等信号。该项研究中的 1 例表现少见，呈全瘤灶明显强化型，肝内周围型小胆管细胞癌以中分化为主，低分化少见。

鉴别诊断：炎症坏死期炎性假瘤：增强扫描动脉期未见明显强化，门静脉及延迟扫描呈轻度强化，其内见少许网格状强化，病理显示肿瘤纤维组织多，活性肿瘤含量少，与周围型肝内胆管细胞癌强化相似。部分感染性病变具有不规则的边界、渐进性延迟强化等共性特征。此外，周围型肝内胆管细胞癌外周可继发炎性改变，周围型肝内胆管细胞癌无局灶胆管受侵扩张时，易误诊为炎性病变，两者重叠时，诊断难度更大。影像表现上感染性病变可见残留组织形成的分隔，壁及分隔强化规整，而炎性肿块可见延迟强化的纤维包膜，上述特征不同于周围型肝内胆管细胞癌。

原发性肝细胞癌：周围型肝内胆管细胞癌需与含纤维成分较多的硬化型肝细胞癌鉴别。硬化型肝细胞癌一般有包膜，且境界相对清楚，肝细胞癌与胆管细胞癌混合存在时，影像诊断困难。当发现肝内肿块，兼具两者影像特征，影像特征与血清肿瘤标记物结果不符时，应考虑两者混合存在的可能。部分肝细胞癌肿瘤边缘存在肝动脉、门静脉双重血供及肝动脉、门静脉分流，这种双重血供也可能深入到瘤内，导致延迟期瘤内和边缘部都产生延迟强化，但这种延迟强化常低于同层肝内血管的强化信号，而周围型肝内胆管细胞癌延迟强化常等于同层肝内血管的强化信号。

来源于胃肠道转移性腺癌：特别是瘤内含丰富纤维和胶原等间质成分且为单发肿块时，与周围型肝内胆管细胞癌鉴别困难。此时，需要结合病理、免疫组织化学检查。

该研究的局限性：该研究为回顾性研究，患者例数较少，只定性描述了周围型肝内胆管细胞癌的 MRI 表现与其病理基础的关系。今后还需扩大样本量，进行疾病早期发现方面的研究。综上所述，无胆管扩张的周围型小肝内胆管细胞癌临床症状、体征及实验室检查缺乏特异性，但 MRI 表现具有一定特征性。病灶的信号由纤维组织、恶性细胞、囊变、出血、坏死组织构成决定，病灶的强化方式与纤维组织、恶性肿瘤细胞、坏死组织构成有关：对于病变表现不典型的患着，尤其在肿瘤富含血供，合并炎症或 3 期均不强化时，需要排除早期胆管细胞癌的可能。

第七节　肝内胆管细胞癌与转移性肝癌的鉴别

详见本书 本卷 第二篇 第三章 第二节　肝内胆管细胞癌与转移性肝癌的鉴别。

第二章 肝脏恶性纤维组织细胞瘤

肝脏恶性纤维组织细胞瘤及误诊分析

恶性纤维组织细胞瘤,又称为恶性纤维黄色瘤、纤维黄色肉瘤等,最早由 Orien 等(1964)首次报道。该瘤以老年人多见,主要好发于四肢和躯干深部软组织内,其次为腹膜后,原发于肝脏的恶性纤维组织细胞瘤临床罕见,Conran 等(1985)首次报道。原发于肝脏的恶性纤维组织细胞瘤少见,临床及影像科医师对该肿瘤常常认识不够充分,又因其缺乏特征性的影像学表现,在术前的影像诊断上往往未能有所发现。

病理学:原发于肝脏的恶性纤维组织细胞瘤与其他恶性纤维组织细胞瘤有相似的组织学特性,主要由排列成"席纹"状、"车辐"状的梭形细胞及炎性细胞、多核巨细胞构成,该瘤属于软组织肉瘤性质,组织来源目前有两种不确定学说,一种认为起源于原始的间叶细胞;另一种认为来源于组织细胞。在组织学上又分 5 种亚型:席纹状多形性型、黏液型、巨细胞型、炎症型、血管瘤型。以席纹状多形性型最为多见,其中前 2 型为高度恶性,后 3 型为低度恶性。外科手术治疗为肝脏恶性纤维组织细胞瘤的首选及最有效的治疗方法。

临床表现:肝脏恶性纤维组织细胞瘤临床主要表现为右上腹疼痛,可伴有发热、厌食及消瘦。甲胎蛋白及 CA19-9 等肿瘤标记物通常为阴性。

影像学研究:CT 表现为:平扫呈不规则的低密度占位性病灶,中心伴大面积的坏死,病灶呈浸润性或膨胀性生长,左右叶均可发生。增强后以周边的实性部分强化为明显,动、静脉期均有中等度强化,周边实质部分可呈"伪足"状、间隔样突向中心部分坏死区。据 Anagnostopoulos 等(2005)统计的 28 例肝脏恶性纤维组织细胞瘤显示,无 1 例瘤体内有钙化,局部淋巴结无肿大,11 例侵犯邻近器官,2 例出现肺部远处转移。

肝脏恶性纤维组织细胞瘤临床症状与肝癌极其相似,而原发于肝脏的恶性纤维组织细胞瘤又较罕见,因此当发现肝脏肿瘤性病变时,容易对肝脏恶性纤维组织细胞瘤的诊断缺乏足够的预知性。实验室检查甲胎蛋白、CEA、CA19-9 和 CA125 等为阴性。

误诊分析:该组 3 例肝脏恶性纤维组织细胞瘤,术前 CT 拟诊 1 例肝内胆管细胞癌、2 例肝细胞肝癌。例 1 误诊为胆管细胞癌,主要是基于肝内胆管伴有扩张而做出的诊断,忽略了肿瘤对胆管压迫梗阻的原因,一些作者曾报道 1 例肝脏恶性纤维组织细胞瘤并肝内转移,此组中例 1 也同样出现肝脏的结节性转移灶,而且还合并有肝内胆管癌栓形成,因恶性纤维组织细胞瘤具有极高的浸润性生长病理组织特性,推测可能是肿瘤直接侵犯胆管所造成的。

例 2、3 误诊为肝细胞癌的主要原因,是对肿瘤的坏死液化及动静脉期强化特点未能细致地评估,另外对患者具有乙型肝炎、肝硬化病史的佐证依赖性过强。肝脏恶性纤维组织细胞瘤除了易误诊为肝细胞肝癌外,还应注意与肝脓肿、肝转移相鉴别,当肿瘤大部分坏死伴液化明显,仅边缘少部分实性强化时,与肝脓肿、肝转移的鉴别就显得尤为重要。

肝脏恶性纤维组织细胞瘤具备很多肝癌和类似肝癌的 CT 特征,仅在程度上有一定差异。肿瘤较大,对邻近组织器官侵犯较常见,坏死液化、出血比肝癌常见,动静脉期均有强化,强化的程度不如肝癌,强化过程相对于肝癌呈"快进慢出"表现,但实验室检查甲胎蛋白为阴性,临床可有乙型肝炎及肝硬化的病史,所以,特别是对甲胎蛋白阴性的肝癌诊断时,应该考虑肝脏恶性纤维组织细胞瘤的可能性。

第三章 肝血管源性恶性肿瘤

第一节 肝脏原发性血管肉瘤

肝原发肉瘤:肝原发肉瘤发生率极低,是肝脏较少见的恶性间叶组织肿瘤。临床上进展迅速,预后差。肝肉瘤主要起源于肝脏间叶组织,其原因不明,来源较广泛,可源于肝内的血管、淋巴管、胆管周围的结缔组织及囊肿、囊肿壁和肝硬变的再生结节等。由于来源不同,其分类繁杂,临床较常见的有血管肉瘤、平滑肌肉瘤、纤维肉瘤、脂肪肉瘤等,其中血管肉瘤多见,约占40%。按免疫组织学可分为血管肉瘤(相对多见)、纤维肉瘤、平滑肌肉瘤、脂肪肉瘤及恶性纤维组织细胞瘤等;可发生于任何年龄,但以小儿及50~60岁多见。

肝脏原发性血管肉瘤:肝脏原发性血管肉瘤,又称血管内皮肉瘤、枯否细胞肉瘤、恶性血管内皮瘤,是一种罕见的间质性肝脏恶性肿瘤。以往报道的肝血管肉瘤常因接触环境致癌物而发生,常见的环境致癌物有二氧化钍,氯乙烯和砷;然而,现在临床发现的血管肉瘤常缺乏这些已知的危险因素。

病理学:肝血管肉瘤起源于血窦内皮细胞,镜下肿瘤组织呈有瘤细胞衬覆的海绵状血管腔样。瘤细胞沿血窦、终末肝静脉和门静脉分支扩散,边界不清,可累及整个肝脏。组织病理上的特点是存在显著的坏死和出血。肿瘤内可见纤维化和含铁血黄素沉积。此病恶性程度较高,该病肝外转移很常见。

分型:血管肉瘤按其生长方式可分为四种类型:多发结节型、单发肿块型、巨块结节混合型以及很少见的弥漫浸润型。Nakashima等(2001)按其生长方式肿瘤形态将其分为4种类型:弥漫微小结节型、弥漫多结节型、巨块型和混合型。

临床表现:该病临床无特异表现,早期瘤体较小可无任何临床症状,当瘤体增大时可出现上腹部不适或右上腹部可扪及肿块,伴消瘦、乏力、发热等症状。一组资料中7例患者中有3例发现腹部隐痛不适而就诊,其余4例患者均为体检发现肝占位。肿瘤可以单发或多发,患者通常无肝炎病史。当病灶为单发且无转移时,手术可以切除。肝脏血管肉瘤属于富血供的肿瘤,经肝动脉栓塞化疗可作为一种很好的姑息性治疗手段。

影像学研究:肝血管肉瘤的影像学表现为单发或多发肿块。CT平扫与周围肝实质相比呈低密度,但也可以为混杂有高密度(新鲜出血)或更低密度影(囊变坏死)。动脉期病灶边缘或中央明显强化,形态不规则,随时间延长有充填趋势,但充填速度较慢。

MRI上的肝血管肉瘤信号强度特征可与血管瘤相似,可见出血,和类似肝细胞癌的混杂信号。主要鉴别诊断包括转移,血管瘤,和肝细胞癌等。由于血管肉瘤含有丰富的血窦,MRI增强扫描对其病理特征的显示有重要意义。单发肿块或巨块结节型的主灶增强后动脉期常呈明显不均匀强化,强化的区域分布于病灶中心,部分位于周边,形态很不规则,强化的程度明显高于肝实质,略低于主动脉,且随着时间推移可有充填,但充填的速度较慢。

另组3例中有2例属于单发巨块型,周缘均伴有少量子病灶,1例属于弥漫多结节型。

肝脏原发性血管肉瘤的肿瘤细胞沿血管腔隙生长,侵入中央静脉和门静脉分支,阻塞管腔,因此常导致出血和坏死,其中以巨块型多见,该组2例巨块型在CT平扫中,其肿瘤内可见部分呈“岛屿”状的密度增高影,为瘤内出血所致。

肝脏原发性血管肉瘤血窦丰富,因此CT增强扫描对其病理特征的显示有重要意义。巨块型病灶增强后,动脉期显示病灶中心及周边均可见明显不均匀强化,周边强化常呈花边状,病灶内部强化形态多呈粗条、小团状,强化的程度高于肝实质而低于腹主动脉,门脉期及延迟期可见强化区域不断增大,向病灶中心充填,但充填的速度较慢。该组 2 例巨块型血管肉瘤呈此种强化方式。

血管肉瘤表现为弥漫多结节型时,动脉期呈不规则局灶性强化,部分结节可见周缘不完整的环形强化。该组 1 例弥漫多结节型在动脉期强化程度较 2 例巨块结节型的卫星灶强化明显,而门脉期及延迟期的表现与巨块型主灶不同,强化区的强化程度较动脉期减弱,但均可见向病灶内部填充的趋势。弥漫微小结节型由于坏死区域比较局限,强化相对均匀。混合型可出现以上三种分型的强化方式。当病灶出现三期增强扫描均无明显强化时,可能是由于坏死、纤维化成分过多引起。

鉴别诊断:肝细胞性肝癌:由于本病患者大多无肝炎肝硬化,脾大等病史,且甲胎蛋白为阴性,影像学与肝细胞性肝癌快进快出的强化特征相比,肝血管肉瘤表现为连续渐进的向心性强化,因此很容易和肝细胞性肝癌进行鉴别。

肝血管瘤:与肝血管瘤相比,肝血管肉瘤的强化充填速度较慢,病灶中心常合并出血坏死,增强后出血坏死区始终无强化。

肝囊性病变:由于肝肉瘤多较大,常因肿瘤血供减少合并有中心部组织坏死、液化,形成囊腔,腔内液体可达数百至数千毫升,酷似囊肿,而瘤体坏死或合并感染可致发热,又难与囊肿合并感染或肝脓肿鉴别,是肝肉瘤误诊的最常见原因。肝囊肿囊壁薄而光滑,囊内呈均匀水样密度,增强后并无强化,易与本病鉴别。肝脓肿也可有类似表现,但多数伴有实验室化验白细胞增多及发热症状,不难鉴别。

虽然原发性肝血管肉瘤罕见,但进展较快,预后差。因此,对于肝内巨块占位性病变,甲胎蛋白为阴性,伴有出血坏死,影像学表现有缓慢渐进性强化时,应考虑到本病的可能,以提高诊断率,及早发现,提高患者的生存率。

第二节　肝脏上皮样血管内皮瘤

肝脏上皮样血管内皮瘤是少见的血管源性恶性肿瘤,一般进展缓慢,经积极治疗 5 年生存率可达 43%~55%,高于其他肝脏恶性肿瘤,肝脏移植可明显提高其生存率。肝脏上皮样血管内皮瘤患病率低,临床上常被误诊为其他疾病,提高对肝脏上皮样血管内皮瘤影像表现的认识,早期诊断,对确定治疗方案和改善患者预后具有重要意义。

病理学:上皮样血管内皮细胞瘤是少见的血管源性肿瘤,是由上皮样细胞、内皮细胞和树突细胞组成的具有独特边界特征的肿瘤,病因学及病原学不明。多发生于骨、软组织、脑、小肠、脾脏等器官,原发于肝脏者少见。肝脏上皮样血管内皮瘤的病理重要特征为具有细胞内血管腔的上皮样瘤细胞和血管内皮标志物染色阳性、免疫组织化学 CD34、CD31 和因子Ⅷ相关抗原阳性。肿瘤细胞由不同比例上皮样细胞和树突样细胞组成,并易侵及肝静脉和门静脉的末梢。该项研究中,4 例累及肝静脉或门静脉。

临床表现:肝脏上皮样血管内皮瘤男女患者比例为(1.6~2.0):1,好发年龄为 30~40 岁,发病原因与口服避孕药、暴露于聚乙烯下、肝外伤或病毒性肝炎有关。肝脏上皮样血管内皮瘤的临床症状常不典型,表现多样,一般从发病到确诊历时数月到数年。实验室检查血清胆红素、碱性磷酸酶、天冬氨酸转氨酶可升高,肿瘤标记物甲胎蛋白、CA199 多正常,少数患者癌胚抗原轻度升高。一项 14 例研究中,仅 1 例癌胚抗原升高, 1 例 CA125 升高,其余未见异常。肝脏上皮样血管内皮瘤的治疗方法包括手术切除、肝脏移植、经导管动脉栓塞治疗及姑息疗法。对于不能手术的患者,肝脏移植是最好的选择,可使患者的 5 年生存率达到 82%。因本病常为多发,故手术切除的机会不多。放疗和化疗对此病生存率的提高影响不大。

影像学研究:肝脏上皮样血管内皮瘤的不同进程影像表现不同,结节型为其早期表现,弥漫型为病变进展肿瘤增大融合所致,该项研究中 1 例术前诊断为融合性肝纤维化的患者表现为位于肝缘下的多结节不全融合,形成带状,提示其可能为病变进展、结节融合所致。该项研究的 14 例中,多发型 11 例,单发型 1 例,弥漫型 2 例,后 2 型患者较少可能与这 2 种类型表现缺乏特异性,诊断困难有关。

多发型病变在 CT 平扫上表现为低密度结节或肿块, T_2WI 上呈均匀高信号或靶征,与 Paolantonio

等(2014)的报道相符,可表现为三环或双环靶征。该项研究结果显示,增强扫描病灶呈现多种强化方式,可为均匀轻度渐进性强化、动脉期周边结节样强化、门静脉期向内填充类似血管瘤样的强化,还可表现为黑靶征或白靶征,与 Kim 等(2014)报道的表现相符。黑靶征病灶自内向外信号(密度)呈低、高、低改变,白靶征病灶自内向外信号(密度)呈高、低、高改变。

Paolantonio 等(2014)认为组织学上肿瘤中心的凝固性坏死、出血区域与 T_2WI 上中心高信号和增强中心无强化区有关,而周边肿瘤细胞胞质内出现充盈着红细胞的管腔结构与 T_2WI 稍高信号的晕环和环状增强有关。但是,该项研究发现, T_2WI 呈三环或双环靶征的病灶与增强后的黑靶征并不对应,增强后的黑靶征在 T_2WI 上可表现为均匀一致稍高信号结节,也可表现为三环或双环样靶征。

门静脉期出现的白靶征其他疾病中均未见,对提示肝脏上皮样血管内皮瘤的诊断具有一定意义。该组作者认为白靶征和黑靶征的表现可能与肿瘤中出现黏液变性和富有细胞区交替出现有关。该项研究中弥漫型肝脏上皮样血管内皮瘤征象与 Barton 等(2014)的报道一致。

该项研究中,多发型肝脏上皮样血管内皮瘤共发现 228 个病灶,多数位于肝脏边缘。4.4% 病灶肝门侧可见与一血管分支关联,即“棒棒糖征”,与 Aloman(2006)的报道相符。4 例血管受侵,以肝静脉及门静脉受侵为主。该组未见钙化征象出现,与其他学者报道的 20% 钙化的结果不符,还需扩大样本量进行更深入的研究。

鉴别诊断:单发型肝脏上皮样血管内皮瘤易被误诊为胆管细胞癌或血管肉瘤,多发型肝脏上皮样血管内皮瘤易被误诊为转移瘤。

转移瘤:转移瘤亦可表现为被膜回缩、肝内弥漫分布及增强后黑靶征,但肝脏上皮样血管内皮瘤患者 MRI 延迟期的渐进性向心强化、白靶征、棒棒糖征、侵及静脉特征转移瘤不具备,可资鉴别。

胆管细胞癌:胆管细胞癌多数可出现对应胆管的扩张,未见胆管扩张时需要考虑到肝脏上皮样血管内皮瘤的可能。

血管肉瘤:血管肉瘤与肝脏上皮样血管内皮瘤均为血管源性肿瘤,影像鉴别困难,此时需结合临床体征及检查资料协助诊断。

综上所述,肝脏上皮样血管内皮瘤虽为少见恶性肿瘤,但其影像表现具有一定的特征。对于多发结节或合并单发肿块的患者,当出现病变渐进性强化,平扫见靶征及被膜回缩征,增强后出现黑靶征、白靶征、棒棒糖征或类血管瘤样结节样强化时,应考虑到此病。

第四章 成人肝未分化肉瘤

成人肝脏未分化胚胎性肉瘤

关于成人肝脏未分化胚胎性肉瘤的国内外相关报道多为个案，Yedibela 等(2000)报道表明 50 年来全球报道成人未分化胚胎性肉瘤仅 15 例，Nishio 等(2003)报道表明 40 岁以上患者仅见 10 例报道。既往文献报道绝大多数病例术前未能明确诊断，往往误认为是肝脏良性肿瘤，如囊肿或肝癌等，其原因有二：一是由于成人肝脏未分化胚胎性肉瘤实属少见，医务人员对本病认识不够；二是目前尚未发现有特异性肿瘤标志物能提示本病。

临床表现：成人肝脏未分化胚胎性肉瘤发病年龄分布无特殊性，各个年龄段均可发生，文献报道的年龄最大者为 1 例 86 岁女性；但一般认为成人肝脏未分化胚胎性肉瘤女性稍多于男性，而儿童肝脏未分化胚胎性肉瘤男性多见，男女之比约 1∶0.65；患者的临床特征无特异性。主要表现为与肿瘤相关的症状，包括腹部肿块、上腹部疼痛或饱胀、发热等，但值得注意的是肝脏未分化胚胎性肉瘤患者发热的发生率较高，如一组 6 例中就有 5 例，可能与多数肝脏未分化胚胎性肉瘤中存在出血和坏死有关；另一主要特点是肝脏未分化胚胎性肉瘤患者即使肿瘤巨大，病情进展到晚期，也多无腹水、黄疸及脾大、肿瘤破裂等。

一般情况下，患者无肝硬化病史，无乙型肝炎病毒感染，血清学肿瘤标记物检查无阳性发现，肝功能正常或轻度异常，但与儿童肝脏未分化胚胎性肉瘤不同的是成人肝脏未分化胚胎性肉瘤可合并肝细胞肝癌存在。1 例 46 岁男性肝右叶肝脏未分化胚胎性肉瘤患者，肝左叶同时存在中分化型肝细胞癌，且合并结节性肝硬化，查血乙型肝炎表面抗原(HbsAg)阴性、HBeAb 及 HBcAb 阳性。

影像学研究：表现为肝实质内单发巨大肿块，文献报道肿块直径一般为 10 cm，最大径可达 30cm，该组有 1 例肝脏未分化胚胎性肉瘤直径约 6 cm，明显小于文献报道，可能与该患者同时合并肝细胞癌，因后者症状较明显而被发现有关；肿块多发生于肝右叶，如该组 6 例中有 4 例位于肝右叶；肿块性质为囊性或囊实混合性，其中囊性成分病例较大，实性成分病例小，CT 平扫表现为不均质低密度肿块，实质性成分多位于病灶的边缘，呈散在的结节状分布；CT 增强扫描示病灶内囊性成分无强化，实性成分强化方式多样，可为“快进快退”型(动脉期明显强化，静脉期强化消退)及延迟强化型(动脉期轻中度强化，静脉期或延迟扫描强化更加明显)，但肝脏未分化胚胎性肉瘤总体上仍被认为是少血供肿瘤；肿块内出血较常见，有文献报道一组 13 例肝脏未分化胚胎性肉瘤均存在出血，该组 6 例中有 4 例存在大量不规则出血，甚至于肿块内出血掩盖了实性成分的存在，如文献中所提到肝脏未分化胚胎性肉瘤的病灶内可见条状、强化的分隔影；肝脏未分化胚胎性肉瘤的出血灶在肿块内呈散在不规则分布，而一般肝癌出血坏死灶多位于肿瘤中心；肿块多呈类圆形，边界清晰，多数文献报道病灶边缘可见较完整假包膜存在，即在肿瘤与正常组织间有薄层纤维分隔，但肝脏未分化胚胎性肉瘤亦可轻微侵犯邻近正常肝组织(包括血管)，如该组有 1 例肝脏未分化胚胎性肉瘤与下腔静脉分界不清。

鉴别诊断：肝囊腺瘤或囊腺癌：该病亦是成人少见的以囊性成分为主的肝脏囊实性肿瘤之一，多发生于女性。CT 亦可表现为巨大囊实性肿块，边界清楚，可见壁结节和纤维分隔，恶性者壁较厚而不规则。由于该病起源于胆管，故可合并肝内胆管扩张，但成人肝脏未分化胚胎性肉瘤极少有黄疸症状，同时前者少见肿块出血报道，后者肿块内出血较常见。肝囊腺癌患者血清学检查多有 CA125 和 CA19-9 升高。

肝囊肿、肝脓肿等肝脏良性病变：巨大肝肉瘤合并中心部组织坏死、液化、形成囊腔，腔内液体可多达数百甚至上千毫升，酷似囊肿；而瘤体坏死或合并感染可导致发热，又难与肝脓肿鉴别。但成人肝脏未分化胚胎性肉瘤肿块内出血明显。呈散在不规则分布，而上述病变极少见到出血。

鉴别诊断时一定要求患者行 CT 或 MRI 增强扫描。仔细寻找病灶周边的实性成分，成人肝脏未分化胚胎性肉瘤表现为向囊腔内呈乳头状突入的特点，单纯囊肿无壁结节存在；并观察其强化过程，如成人肝脏未分化胚胎性肉瘤的实性成分强化方式可呈快进快退型及缓慢强化型，肝脓肿的强化方式为缓慢强化型；同时观察病灶对血管的侵犯情况，成人肝脏未分化胚胎性肉瘤可存在对血管的侵犯。

肝细胞腺瘤：肝细胞腺瘤也是一种有出血倾向的肿瘤，边缘亦清楚，当成人肝脏未分化胚胎性肉瘤出血时易与肝细胞腺瘤混淆；但肝细胞腺瘤周围正常肝细胞常含较多脂质，其 CT 表现为一围绕肝细胞腺瘤的低密度环，病理基础一般认为是由瘤周被挤压的肝细胞内脂肪空泡增加所致，是肝细胞腺瘤极为特征的 CT 表现；而成人肝脏未分化胚胎性肉瘤边缘有时也可见到假包膜，为纤维成分，可见强化；同时肝细胞腺瘤多发生于年轻女性，与口服避孕药有关，结合病史资料可进一步鉴别。

其他肝脏恶性肿瘤：包括其他类型肉瘤和少见类型肝癌，如肝平滑肌肉瘤、肉瘤样肝癌等，这些均为发生于成人少见的恶性肿瘤，与成人肝脏未分化胚胎性肉瘤一样可呈囊实性改变，CT、MRI 影像学区别往往不明显，鉴别诊断时需结合临床，肝癌患者常有明确的乙肝病史，肝硬化病史，甲胎蛋白多升高，出血较肝脏未分化胚胎性肉瘤少见且量较少，最终的确诊依赖于病理检查结果。

总之，成人肝脏未分化胚胎性肉瘤的临床特征与 CT 影像学特征有一定的特征性，即病灶巨大、边界清楚，患者发热多见而黄疸少见，少有乙型肝炎病毒感染，肿瘤标记物检查阴性。肝功能正常或轻度异常；病灶囊性成分病例较高，病灶内不规则出血较多见，实性成分较少，位于边缘，可有强化，病灶周围肝组织基本无肝硬化病史。

第五章 癌肉瘤

第一节 肝脏原发性癌肉瘤

病理学:癌肉瘤是指在同一肿瘤内既有肯定的癌成分,又有肯定的肉瘤成分,常见的发病部位有肺、食管、乳腺、喉、胆囊等。原发于肝脏的癌肉瘤十分罕见。WHO(2000)将肝癌肉瘤单列为肝脏间叶源性肿瘤的一种,并定义为由癌样成分(既可是肝细胞源性也可是胆管细胞源性)和肉瘤样成分细胞混杂在一起的恶性肿瘤,因此肝癌肉瘤也属于肝脏恶性混合瘤范畴。癌肉瘤的组织起源尚不清楚,多数学者认为来自多潜能胚胎干细胞,可同时分化为癌组织和肉瘤组织,也有学者认为癌性成分通过化生的机制转化为肉瘤性成分。

临床表现:肝癌肉瘤患者多为中老年人,发病年龄46~84岁,平均60岁,男性明显多于女性,男女之比为15:6,多继发于肝硬化且乙型肝炎表面抗原阳性,肿瘤较大,直径4~23 cm,平均约12.3 cm。癌肉瘤的临床症状以非特异性消化道症状为主,如腹部隐痛、腹胀、厌食和体重下降等;肿瘤标记物甲胎蛋白正常或轻度升高,肝功能损害较轻;即使肿瘤巨大,病情进展到晚期,患者也多无腹水、黄疸及脾大等。肝癌肉瘤为高度恶性肿瘤,发展迅速,预后非常差,患者从出现症状至死亡的平均生存时间为4~7个月,常于手术后发生远处转移,最常见的部位是肺和腹腔淋巴结。

影像学研究:肝癌肉瘤的主要影像学表现:肿瘤多单发,体积往往较大,平均直径约12 cm左右;肿瘤边界多清楚、光滑,密度不均,甚至以囊性密度为主,极少出现钙化;少数可见瘤周子灶、门静脉癌栓以及局部组织器官侵犯。

CT平扫表现为肝实质内巨大囊实混合性肿块,肿块实性部分呈条索状分隔或结节状散在分布,偶可形成蜂窝样结构。

MRI平扫T_1WI上肿瘤以低信号为主、T_2WI上呈高信号为主的混杂信号。CT及MRI动态增强扫描示肿块实性成分早期呈不均匀强化,门脉期强化减低,囊性区域始终无强化。

关于癌肉瘤的影像学表现报道较少,并多缺乏特征性,因此术前诊断困难,误诊率极高。

鉴别诊断:肝癌肉瘤在影像学上与肉瘤样肝细胞癌、肝脏非血管源性肉瘤、囊性肝癌、肝囊腺癌、不典型肝脓肿等表现相似,影像上鉴别较为困难,应结合临床表现和实验室检查结果综合判断,最终确诊依靠组织病理学检查。

第二节 误诊病例简介:肝肉瘤样癌(梭形细胞癌)与腹膜后占位

患者,女,67岁。纳差、乏力1月余入院。患者缘于1个月前无明显诱因出现纳差、乏力,无畏寒、发热,无恶心、呕吐,无黄疸、尿黄等不适,未予重视,5天前就诊外院彩超示:肝右叶实质性占位;右肝内胆管结石;腹膜后实质性占位。今门诊拟“腹膜后占位性病变”收住入院。

常规病理诊断:肝脏肿物切除标本:肝脏恶性肿瘤伴显著坏死,待做免疫组化检测进一步确诊。免疫组化诊断:肝脏肿物切除标本:肝肉瘤样癌(梭形细胞癌)。注:肿瘤细胞异型明显,大多呈梭形,弥漫分布,呈肉瘤样表现,表达上皮与间叶性标记,符合肉瘤样癌(图4-5-1)。

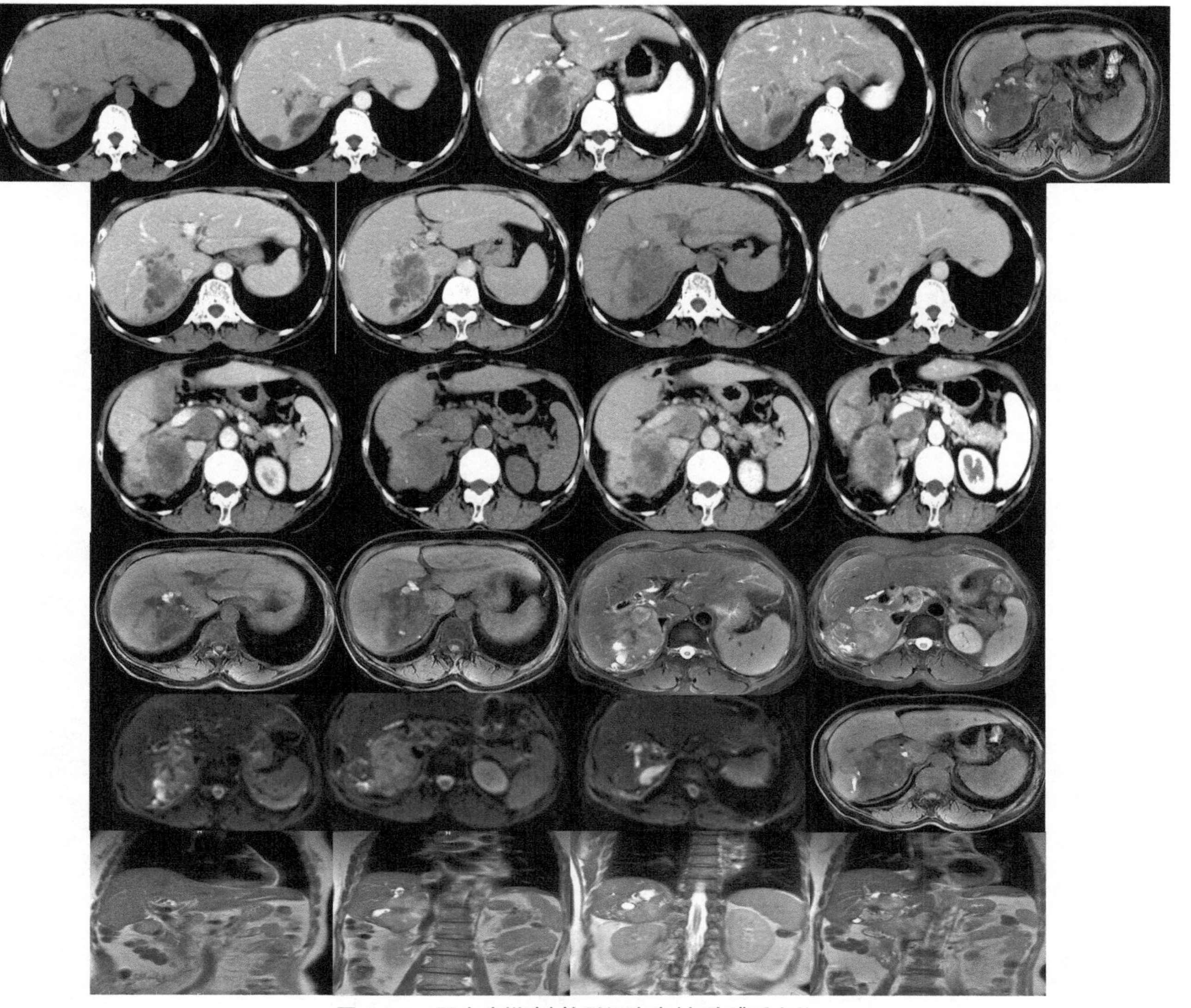

图 4-5-1　肝肉瘤样癌（梭形细胞癌）与腹膜后占位

第三节　肝肉瘤样癌肝门淋巴转移

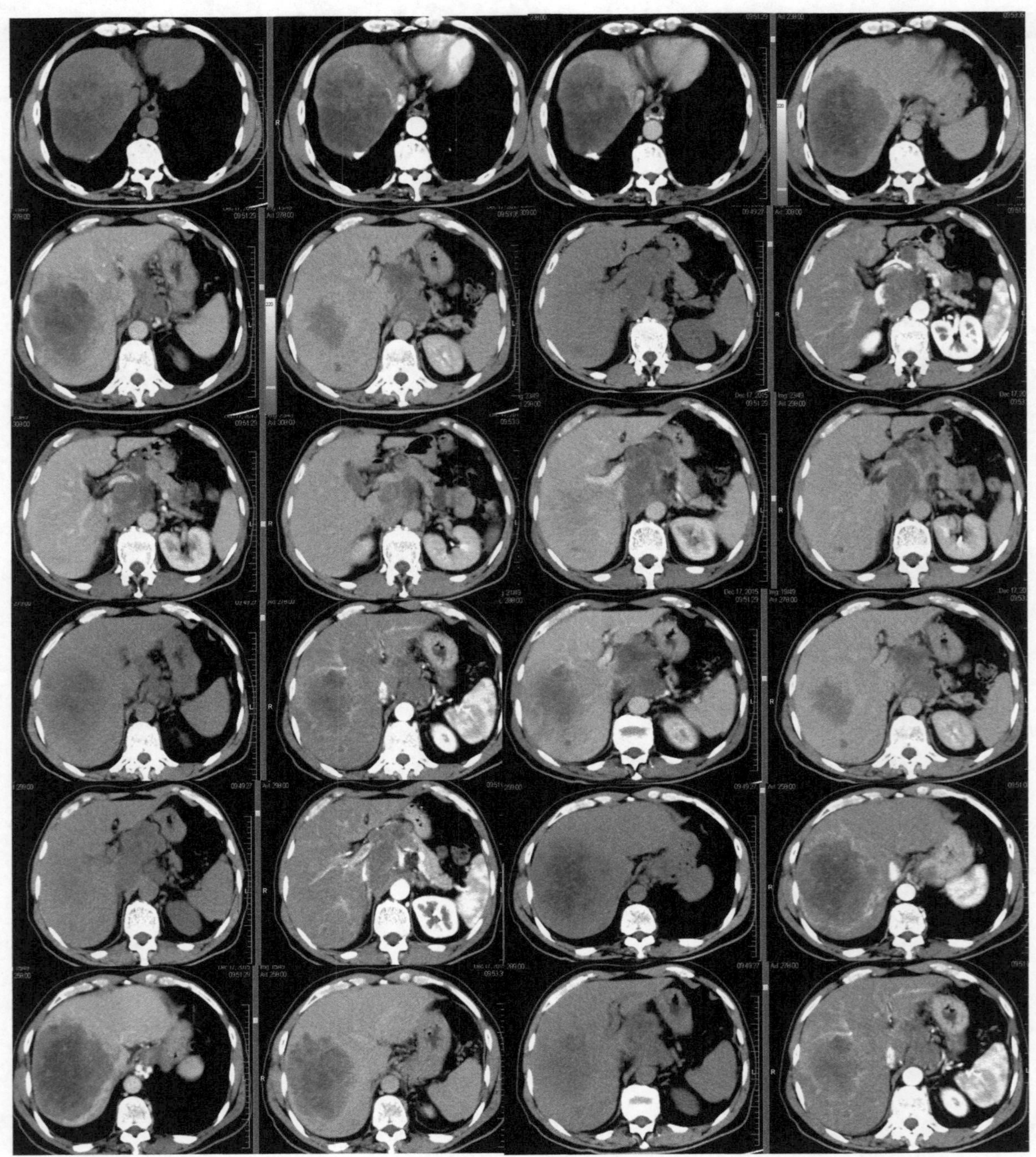

图 4-5-2　肝肉瘤样癌肝门淋巴转移

患者,男,58 岁。病理检查:肝穿刺组织一堆,长 0.1~0.7 ㎝,直径 0.1 ㎝。常规病理诊断:肝脏肿物穿刺活检标本:恶性肿瘤,待做免疫组化检测进一步明确诊断。

免疫组化检测:阳性: CK18, Vimentin, CK(P)(弱+), Ki-67(+,约 70%);阴性: CK8, CK7, CK20, Villin, CK19, P63, EMA, CgA, Syn, CD56, CEA, CA19-9, AFP, Hepatocyte, CD34, Calponin, SMA, H-caldesmon, Desmin, S-100, CR, MC, CD99。免疫组化诊断:肝脏肿物穿刺活检标本:肝恶性肿瘤,免疫组化结果提示肉瘤样癌(图 4-5-2)。

第六章　其他肝肉瘤

第一节　误诊病例简介:膈下腹膜间皮肉瘤与血管瘤

生长于膈下而且局限性压迫至肝内的间皮肉瘤十分少见,以致定位、定性都错,尤其是定位的错误。由于定位错误,没有进一步向上多扫几个层面,加上CT表现特殊,病变呈肝脏左叶内局限性软组织块状影,增强扫描病变周围晕状强化,且有延迟征象,以致误诊。

误诊教训:上腹部扫描未扫到膈顶为一大的失误。对双侧肺底、膈肌及膈下一点信息都未获得,令人遗憾。肝脏表现为肿瘤压迫所致凹陷性改变,却对肝周围未行观察。对任何病变的邻近部位都应该尽量设法观察,收集信息,这对于分析病变实为必要。观察范围应该到病变周围器官和组织完全正常的区域为止。

附:具体病例资料:患者女性,48岁。无明显诱因右肩背部疼痛后出现上腹疼痛2周。无恶心、呕吐,无黄疸、发热,无肝炎病史,轻度贫血貌,体重近期下降5公斤余入院。体检:全身淋巴结无肿大,腹平坦,右上腹肋下缘与腋前线交界处压痛,无肌紧张、反跳痛,肝区叩痛,肝、脾无肿大,右肾区叩痛,莫菲征阳性。影像学检查:X线胸片正常。腹部B超检查提示:肝内血管瘤,考虑肝内海绵状血管瘤。CT平扫:于肝左叶内显示5cm×4cm大小边界欠清楚之低于肝脏密度之实质结节状影,该低密度影轮廓呈分叶状,且边缘不规则,周围无血管瘤的典型强化出现,CT值40 HU,脾无肿大。增强扫描动脉期:病灶周围可见晕状强化,病灶较平扫范围有所缩小,其内无明显强化。门脉期:病灶内仍无明显强化。延迟期:病灶内可见强化征象,CT值50 HU。肝脏边缘显示较光滑整齐,肝周及胸腹腔内无积液征象。CT诊断:肝左叶内占位病变,考虑为肝左叶血管瘤。

手术所见:腹腔无积液,左膈肌近心脏底部一5cm×4cm大小肿物,表面凹凸不平,青紫色,肝脏被压呈凹陷性改变,与下腔静脉距离约2cm。自膈肌切除肿物,膈肌未破裂。

病理所见:镜下示有包膜,瘤体含胶原纤维,成纤维细胞、瘤细胞异形。病理诊断:间皮细胞肉瘤。

第二节　误诊病例简介:左肝外叶平滑肌肉瘤与肝血管平滑肌脂肪瘤

病例,男,32岁。体检发现肝占位2天入院。缘于2日前行全身PET/CT检查提示左肝团块状影,代谢轻度升高,提示原发性肝癌可能。CT诊断:肝血管平滑肌脂肪瘤。

手术所见:腹腔无腹水,肝脏表面光滑,未扪及肝硬化结节及结石,左肝第1、2、3段可见一大小约6cm×5cm肿物,血供丰富,突出肝脏表面,与周围膈肌、网膜无明显粘连。腹腔淋巴结无肿大。

病理检查:部分肝组织一块,总体积13.5cm×7.5cm×4.5cm,切面见一结节,直径4.5cm,切面灰白,夹杂坏死组织,质中,与周围交界尚清,其余切面暗褐色,质中。常规病理诊断:左肝外叶梭形细胞肿瘤,直径4.5cm,待免疫组化协助分型。周围组织肝细胞轻度水肿及脂肪变性,肝小叶内外散在小灶性淋巴细胞浸润。免疫组化检测:阳性:SMA(+++),Calponin(+++),H-caldesmon(+++),Desmin(+),ERCC-1(++),VEGF(+),Vimentin(+);阴性:CK-P,EMA,Hepatocyte,AFP,CK8,CK18,CK19,CA19-9,CK-L,S-100,CD34,CD117,DOG1,CD31,F8,HBsAg,HBcAg,EGFR,5-FU,Ki67,TOPO-II,P-gp,Tubulin,Myoglobin,Myo-D1。免疫组化诊断:左肝外叶平滑肌肉瘤(图4-6-1)。

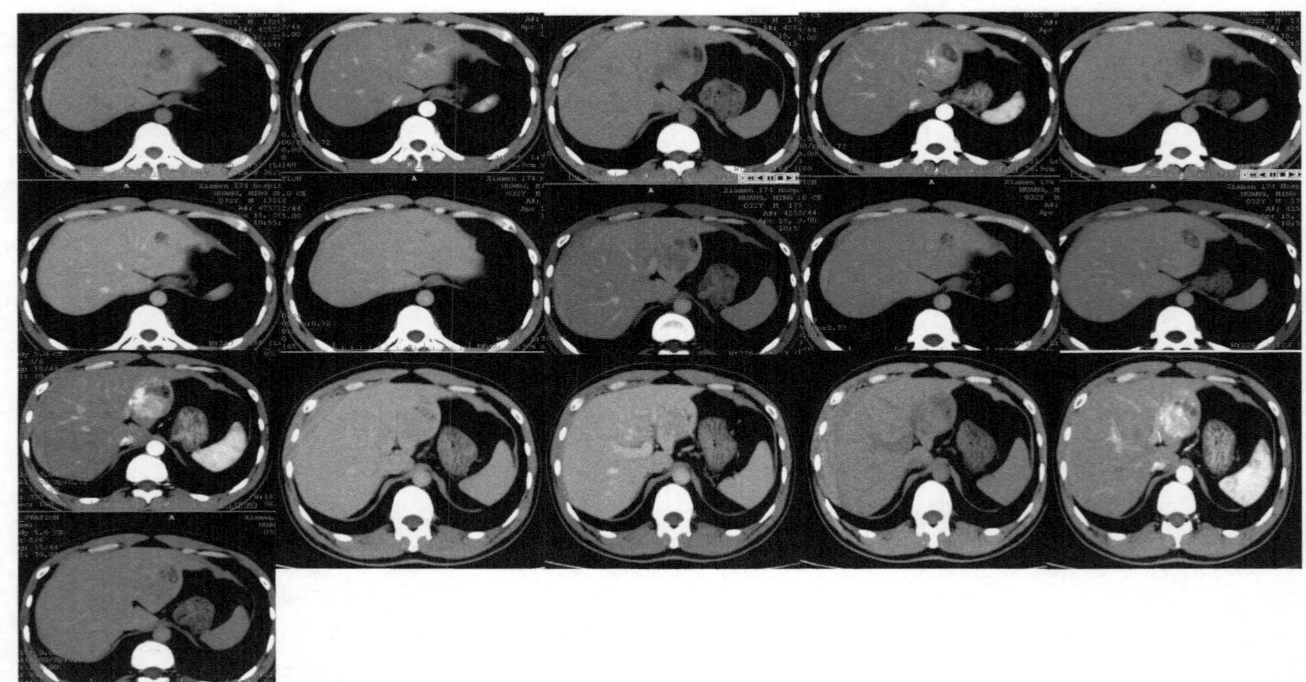

图 4-6-1 左肝外叶平滑肌肉瘤与肝血管平滑肌脂肪瘤

第三节 误诊病例简介:肝平滑肌肉瘤与肝血管平滑肌脂肪瘤

患者,男,33 岁。体检发现肝脏占位 2 天入院。CT:左肝外叶见大小约 4cm × 4.5cm 低密度肿块影,平扫 CT 值 46~60HU,病灶前部见斑片状更低密度影,CT 值 -14~26HU,边界较清楚;增强扫描动脉期病灶呈不均匀明显强化,CT 值 110~160HU,静脉期及延迟期强化减低,CT 值 70~107HU,病灶前部更低密度区呈渐进强化,CT 值 76HU。肝内外胆管无扩张,胆囊如常。CT 诊断:左肝外叶占位性质待定,肝血管平滑肌脂肪瘤?恶性肿瘤待排。

病理检查:左肝肿瘤切除标本:肝组织一块,总体积 13.5cm × 7.5cm × 4.5cm,切面见一结节,直径 4.5cm,切面灰白,夹杂坏死组织,质中,与周围交界尚清,其余切面暗褐色,质中。常规病理诊断:左肝肿瘤切除标本:左肝外叶梭形细胞肿瘤,直径 4.5cm,待免疫组化协助分型。周围组织肝细胞轻度水肿及脂肪变性,肝小叶内外散在小灶性淋巴细胞浸润。

免疫组化检测:阳性:SMA(+++),Calponin(+++),H-caldesmon(+++),Desmin(+),ERCC-1(++),VEGF(+),Vim;阴性:CK-P,EMA,Hepatocyte,AFP,CK8,CK18,CK19,CA19-9,CK-L,S-100,CD34,CD117,DOG1。免疫组化诊断:左肝肿瘤切除标本:左肝外叶平滑肌肉瘤。

误诊回顾分析发现,病灶前部更低密度区的存在对诊断影响甚大,除考虑肿瘤含脂以外,从肿瘤的病理标本检查看,还应考虑肿瘤周围肝细胞的脂肪变性。病灶的不均匀富血管强化表现已提示病变可能为恶性肿瘤,但却未被诊断者重视。

第七章　肝淋巴瘤

第一节　肝淋巴瘤

病理学：原发性肝淋巴瘤少见，继发性肝的受累不难见，一组尸检报告霍奇金病患者60%有肝的侵犯，非霍奇金病有50%受侵。适当的肝活检是确定肝淋巴瘤的可靠方法。有报告经皮穿刺活检假阴性高达50%，腹腔镜假阴性20%，剖腹术假阴性15%。霍奇金病肝内侵犯最常见类型是整个肝实质的弥漫性分布。霍奇金病病灶发自于肝实质内的枯否细胞，而产生肉芽肿，它可以生长或融合形成结节而变成尸检时大体表现。胆管通常未犯。虽然肝的一定程度肿大不难见及，但大块肿大少见，而且肝肿大是非特异性的临床表现，在霍奇金病和非霍奇金病对肝的侵犯上，都不是好兆头。门静脉周围淋巴结常常肿大，但它们可挤压胆管系统立刻引起黄疸。局灶性结节性病变比之于浸润少见，弥漫性加上结节性病变，只占霍奇金病犯肝的3%。非霍奇金淋巴瘤的尸检显示，弥漫性肝侵犯，常见为不同大小的肿瘤结节，可类似转移癌。恶性淋巴瘤在肾移植后恶性肿瘤中高达20%。

影像学研究：在大多数肝淋巴瘤病人，肝门都有淋巴瘤组织弥漫性浸润。他们可有肝功异常，肝可肿大或不肿大。影像学检查常有明显的局灶性团块。确定诊断仰赖于肝内病灶核心组织活检材料。肝淋巴瘤的不同超声表现已有报告。低回声相对边界清楚包块，无透声，最为常见。虽然大多数病灶是低回声，此种回声包块类似于转移性疾病或原发性肝细胞癌，或偶尔发现于肝硬化病人中。在超声发现本症以前，必定已存在大体疾病，因此，阴性的肝超声表现并不意味着肝内无病变，而超声阳性则示肝已明显受犯。

在获得性免疫缺陷综合征的本症患者，CT扫描可见肝、脾和肾呈现明显的多灶性结节状包块，均为恶性淋巴瘤所累，包块大小从几毫米到几厘米。在淋巴瘤，这是少见的情况，它更多见于非霍奇金淋巴瘤之获得性免疫缺陷综合征患者。这些包块为低密度块，且可有边缘强化。鉴别诊断包括条件性感染的肝脓肿，或已存的原发性恶瘤（含卡波西肉瘤）的肝内转移。本症病人硫胶扫描时肝大和脾大是非特异性的，它们可能或不可能确定为肝和脾的新生物。肝和脾内放射性示踪剂不均匀分布伴脾吸收降低也可能见到，亦非特异。偶尔，散在的光子减低区可见，相当可靠地指出为新生物侵犯。

突出的肝门常提示病人肝门淋巴结肿大。由于淋巴瘤常是镓的热聚点，镓核素扫描可用于确定淋巴瘤病人胶体扫描光子减少区的性质。

肝淋巴瘤大多数病例的CT表现是非特异性的，可能伪似转移性病变和原发性肝新生物。淋巴瘤的弥漫性浸润型能产生整个肝脏的不规则斑状衰减值降低，而难与肝硬化和脂肪肝区别。钙化不常见，如出现多提示为非淋巴瘤疾病，诸如转移性黏液腺癌。CT最常见是相当均匀的衰减降低区，某些伴不规则边缘，意味并存有少量正常肝实质。

淋巴瘤性肝病变在静脉给予对比剂后少有强化到正常肝实质程度，尤如弥漫性病变较局限性病变更为常见一样，肝淋巴瘤CT诊断的相对用处较小是可以理解的，而且微小病变还难以发现。在肾移植后病人淋巴瘤的肝侵犯有其特点：迅速生长的孤立或多发性肝内包块，伴腹膜腔内及腹膜后包块，以及相关于中心坏死的低密度中心区。

乙碘油乳剂-13（EOE-13）是一选择性肝脾影像药物，是碘化的婴粟子油的脂肪酸的乙基酯，此剂的静脉内滴注产生肝脾衰减值上升。此药副作用轻微。此药最初观察的结果，是明显改善了对肝脾受淋巴瘤侵犯的评估。大于5mm的病灶是恒定显示。当肝脾淋巴瘤病灶与正常实质组织之间衰减值差异相当微小时,应用此药常可有助于病灶的发现。一次正常的EOE-13检查不能除外小病变的存在(直径小于5mm),对于弥漫性镜下病变,此对比剂也难以发现。在肝淋巴瘤,血管造影是少有表示需要,也少有应用。其征象包括主要动脉的移位,围绕肝内单个或多个包块。有时可见中等数目的肿瘤血管,但供养动脉并不扩张。在肝相照片包块显示为充盈缺损,当淋巴瘤弥漫性侵犯肝时,唯一的非特异征象是肝肿大和血管分散。

第二节 肝脏弥漫大B细胞淋巴瘤病例

患者,女,80岁。

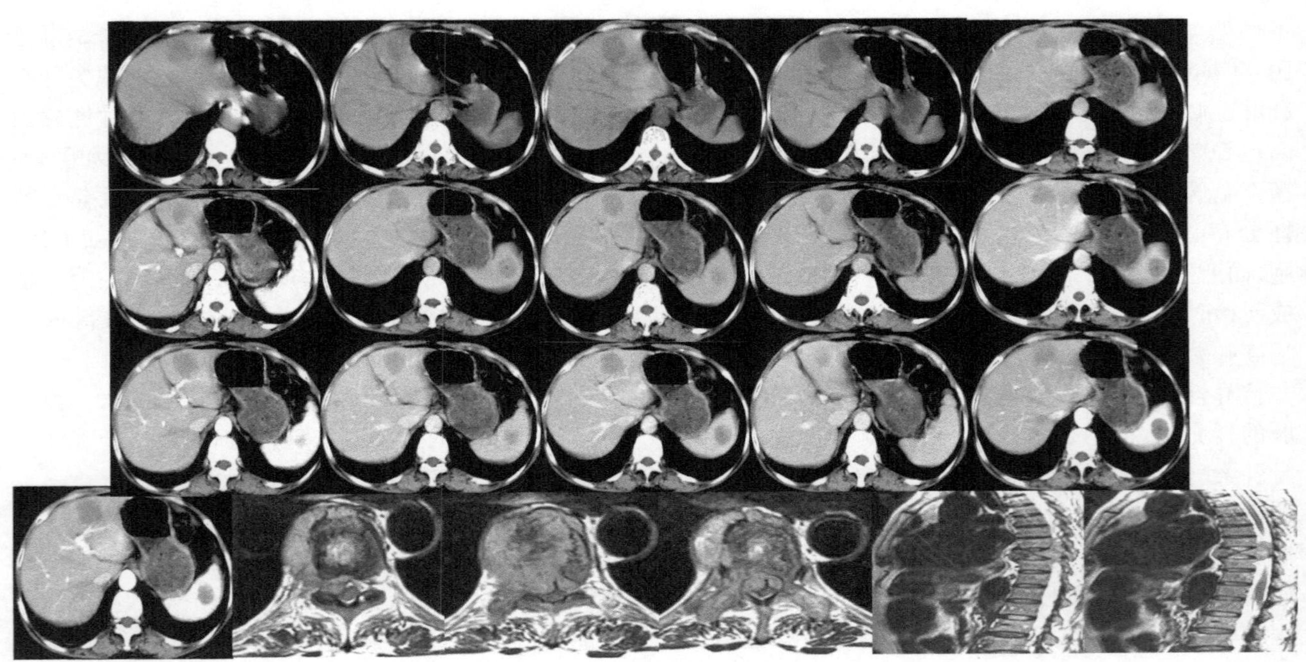

图4-7-1 肝脏弥漫大B细胞淋巴瘤

病理检查:肝穿刺标本:免疫组化检测:阳性:CD20(+),CD79α(+),Ki-67(80%),Bcl-6(+)MuM-1(+),CD43(+);阴性:CD10,CyclinD1,TDT,Bcl-2,CD23,CD3,CD45RO,CD56,CD30,ALK,EMA,Muc-2,CDX-2,CD5,CK7,CK20,Villin,CK(L),CK(P),AFP,TTF-1,EBV,TiA-1,端粒酶。免疫组化诊断:(肝脏穿刺)弥漫大B细胞淋巴瘤(活化B细胞淋巴瘤)(图4-7-1)。

第八章　肝恶性肿瘤的一些检查方法和影像学表现

CT 能谱单能量成像对肝脏肿瘤检出的影响

MSCT 具有空间分辨率高、采集层厚薄、数据各向同性以及图像后处理功能强大等优点，是目前临床上发现和诊断肝脏肿瘤最常用的一种影像检查方法。CT 对肝脏肿瘤的检出率主要取决于肿瘤的大小、肿瘤与肝实质之间的密度差别，因此 CT 图像质量对于肝脏肿瘤的检出非常重要。传统 CT 设备采用混合能量成像，线束硬化效应导致 CT 值不准确和产生硬化伪影，影响图像质量和病灶检出。能谱 CT 采用不同的成像模式，快速转换双 kVp 技术实现两组数据的瞬时同时采样，经投影数据空间的双能量解析，在基物质密度图像的基础上得到不同能量水平的单能量图像，单能量图像能有效减除硬化效应，得到准确 CT 值并消除硬化伪影，改善图像质量和病灶检出。

有作者对一组肝脏肿瘤患者采用能谱成像模式扫描，比较同一患者的 140 kVp 混合能量图像和 70 keV 单能量图像，旨在探讨能谱 CT 单能量成像对肝脏肿瘤检出的影响。

混合能量成像与单能量成像的比较：CT 扫描是通过测量 X 线在物质中的衰减来进行成像的，CT 图像精确重建的基本原则是同一物质的衰减系数在任何测量方法和方向中必须保持恒定。传统 CT 设备采用混合能量成像，X 线中包含不同能量水平的光子，线束硬化效应导致 CT 值不准确和硬化伪影产生，影响图像质量和病灶检出。

单能量图像是指处于某一能量水平的 X 线穿过物体后产生的衰减图像，它能有效减除硬化效应，得到准确 CT 值并消除硬化伪影，改善图像质量和病灶检出，但目前的 CT 设备尚不能提供真正单一能量水平的 X 线。

CT 能谱成像的理论基础为基础物质分解原理，当 X 线光子能量处于 30~140keV 时，任何一种物质的衰减系数都可以用两种基础物质的衰减系数的加权和来表示，从而将求解 CT 值转化为求解基物质对的密度值，而这个密度值和 X 线能量无关，能谱 CT 就是通过双能量成像获得的基物质密度数据来演算出不同能量水平的单能量图像。

70 keV 图像与 80 kVp 图像表现的异同：该研究结果显示，与 140 kVp 图像相比，70 keV 图像上不同肝脏肿瘤在不同期相的对比噪声比均有不同程度的增高，病灶检出率提高，同时肝实质噪声明显降低，图像质量改善。这与以往双能量成像中 80 kVp 图像的表现有所不同。

Marin 等（2009）报道，与 140 kVp 图像比较，80 kVp 图像上动脉晚期肝脏富血供肿瘤的对比噪声比、病灶显著性和病灶检出率均有显著性提高，但图像噪声亦增高一倍，图像质量降低。70 keV 图像和 80 kVp 图像均能提高肝脏肿瘤的对比噪声比和病灶检出率，这是由于物质的衰减系数与物质的密度和 X 线的能量有关，低能量水平的 X 线对物质穿透力减低，光电吸收效应增加，使同一物质的衰减系数增高，不同物质间衰减系数的差别增大。

但 70 keV 图像和 80 kVp 图像的成像原理并不相同，70 keV 图像是通过基物质密度数据演算得到的单能量图像，其图像性质与 70 keV 能量水平的 X 线穿过物体后产生的单能量图像相似，同一物质的衰减系数保持一致，因此图像噪声主要来源于 X 线的穿透力降低。而 80 kVp 图像采用依然是混合能量的 X 线，光子能量水平的不同使同一物质的衰减系数不一致，加上 X 线穿透力降低所导致光子量不足，因此图像噪声大大增加，硬化伪影加剧，图像质量明显降低。

70keV 图像对不同肝脏肿瘤检出的影响：该研究结果显示，除动脉期的肝转移瘤和肝血管瘤外，不同大小、不同性质肝脏肿瘤在不同期相的 70 keV 图像上病灶检出率均较 140 kVp 图像增高，尤其是 1 cm 以下的小病灶。这是由于 CT 对肝脏肿瘤的检出率与肿瘤的大小、肿瘤与肝实质之间的密度差别密切相关，对于体积、密度差别较大的肿瘤，140kVp 图像相对易于检出，与 70keV 图像的病灶检出率差异不明显,而对于体积、密度差别较小的肿瘤, 140 kVp 图像由于噪声和硬化伪影较大,会影响到病灶的检出, 70 keV 图像则通过改善图像质量,增大肿瘤与肝实质之间的对比,从而提高小病灶的检出。

选择 70 keV 图像的原因:能谱 CT 通过双能量成像获得的基物质密度数据能演算出 40~140 keV 不同能量水平的单能量图像,该研究中的病例肝脏肿瘤的最佳对比噪声比处于 50~70keV 能量水平,但图像噪声在 65~70keV 能量水平时相对较低,综合考虑图像质量和病灶对比,选择 70 keV 图像与 140kVp 图像进行比较。此外,在 50~70keV 的单能量图像中, 70keV 图像的物质衰减与 140 kVp 图像最为接近,有利于二者间采用相同的观察窗进行观察。

该研究的局限性:首先,在病灶检出率的分析中,以 3 个期相两组图像上所能显示的病灶数为参照,假阴性的存在会导致两组图像上病灶检出率增高,但该组研究的目的是比较两组图像病灶检出率的差别,而并非 CT 检出肿瘤的敏感度,因此采用本方法。其次,在 40~140keV 图像上,不同肿瘤在不同期相的检出情况不同,最佳对比噪声比图像并不一定噪声最小,某一病变的最佳对比噪声比图像是否同样有利于其他病变的检出,对于能谱 CT 单能量成像,是单纯追求最佳对比噪声比,还是兼顾对比噪声比和图像质量,有待于进一步研究。第三,病例数较少。

综上所述,能谱 CT 70 keV 单能量图像通过改善图像质量并增加肿瘤与肝实质的对比,有利于肝脏肿瘤的检出,对小病灶的检出更为敏感。

第九章　原发性肝脏神经内分泌肿瘤

第一节　原发性肝脏神经内分泌癌

神经内分泌肿瘤多发生于胃、肠及胰腺，胰腺最为常见，原发于肝脏的非常少见，国内外仅有一些个案报道。

神经内分泌癌，也称类癌或嗜银细胞瘤，属于胺前体摄取脱羧系统肿瘤的范畴，是一种极为罕见、生长缓慢的上皮细胞性肿瘤，具有恶变倾向。肝脏是神经内分泌肿瘤最常转移的部位，而原发于肝脏者非常少见。原发性肝脏神经内分泌癌的来源一般认为起源于肝内毛细胆管的神经内分泌细胞（Kulchitsky 细胞），或起源于肝内异位的胰腺或肾上腺组织。诊断神经内分泌癌必须严格满足两个条件：组织病理学证实为神经内分泌癌和无肝外原发病灶。病理学表现为低分化、中分化或者混合分化，肿瘤细胞排列成腺管状、团状、不规则网状或者片状，核异型性明显，核有丝分裂可见。免疫组织化学分析显示 Syn、CgA、CD56、神经原特异性烯醇化酶（NSE）为阳性染色，这是特异性较高的神经内分泌标记物，对该病的诊断有很高的价值。

临床表现：原发性肝脏神经内分泌癌临床表现缺乏特征性，多数患者无症状，体检时偶然发现。部分患者有右上腹胀痛不适、纳差、乏力等症状，患者通常不伴有慢性肝炎及肝硬化病史，且甲胎蛋白正常。该病预后较肝细胞肝癌好，转移至骨及淋巴结较肺更常见。

原发性肝脏神经内分泌癌发病率约占消化系各种粪癌的 0.2%~2%，男女之比约为 0.77：1，发病年龄多在 8~83 岁，平均年龄 49.5 岁。

在一组 7 例中，患者平均年龄 60.3 岁，其中女性 4 例，男性 3 例，这和文献报道基本相同。该组病例其中 4 例为无诱因中上腹胀痛就诊发现，另外 3 例偶然体检发现，6 个病灶位于肝右叶（60%），2 个位于肝左叶（20%），2 个病灶于左右叶交界区（20%），肝右叶较左叶好发，与文献报道一致。该组病例仅有 1 例患者有慢性肝炎病史，1 例患者甲胎蛋白轻度升高。

影像学研究：原发性肝脏神经内分泌癌影像学表现仅有少量个案报道，肝脏往往无肝硬化背景，CT 多表现为肝脏内单发或多发低密度结节或不均质肿块，病灶内常有囊变或液化坏死区，动态增强后病变在动脉期厚壁不均匀强化，内壁不规则，门脉期持续强化，中心呈不规则无强化低密度。超声表现为肝实质内可见结节状肿物或包块，肿瘤多表现为强回声或高回声，肿物边界尚清楚，未见确切包膜，较大的肿瘤内部多伴有囊性改变，囊内透声好；彩色多普勒血流显像示结节囊壁上血流信号丰富。

MRI 表现为 T_1WI 低信号，T_2WI 及 DWI 高信号，病灶中心存在 T_1WI 更低信号和 T_2WI 更高信号影，提示部分囊变或坏死液化，DWI 扩散受限为高信号，ADC 值介于肝癌与肝良性肿瘤之间，增强扫描实性部分动脉期不均匀明显强化，门脉期持续强化，延迟扫描为相对低信号，较小病灶实质部分可以均匀强化，囊性部分或中心坏死液化部分不强化。

PET 或 PET/CT 表现为病灶内核素的浓集，不具有特异性。

CT 和 MRI 对诊断原发性肝脏神经内分泌癌的比较：CT 和 MRI 对原发性肝脏神经内分泌癌诊断具有重要价值，主要在于它们能很好地显示肿瘤的生长方式，确定肿瘤的发生部位，清楚显示肿瘤的形态、大小及范围，很好地显示肿瘤内部的坏死、囊变、出血等情况，增强后强化幅度及方式及与周围组织器官的关系。该组有 2 例同时行 CT 和 MRI 检查，2 例 CT 增强后对病灶周边的细小血管显示均优于

MRI,这给临床提供有治疗价值的信息，CT对病灶钙化的显示优于MRI,同时CT扫描时间较MRI短,对于年老和不能耐受长时间检查的患者较有优势。MRI优势在于软组织分辨率高及多方位成像,对肿瘤内部囊变、血管流空信号及肿瘤浸润范围优于CT，MRI对判断肿瘤囊变或坏死的显示强于CT，T2WI较其他MRI序列对显示肿瘤囊变及液化坏死好，MRI在确定肿瘤的发生部位、与周围结构的关系以及对于肝脏、淋巴结转移的显示方面更具优势,同时多期动态增强扫描更可以全面地了解肿瘤的强化方式和性质。所以CT、MRI优势互补更有利于原发性肝脏神经内分泌癌的诊断。

误诊分析:全组7例中，2例结合影像学表现及病史,术前诊断考虑为原发性肝脏神经内分泌癌。5例误诊，3例误诊为肝细胞肝癌,其中1例病灶较小直径约1.5 cm,增强后动脉期实质部分强化均匀,静脉期为均匀等信号,内见小片低密度不强化区,原发性肝脏神经内分泌癌征象不典型,误诊为肝细胞肝癌,后病理证实为神经内分泌癌；1例肝右叶巨大包块伴肝内多发结节,包块中央为大片坏死低密度区,误诊巨块结节型肝癌;另外1例甲胎蛋白轻度升高,误诊为肝癌。

1例位于肝门区,肿块较大引起肝门区胆管扩张,增强后肿块厚壁明显强化,内壁不规则增厚,故与肝门胆管细胞癌混淆,造成误诊；1例位于肝左内叶,动脉早期明显强化,门脉期为等信号、延迟期为低信号,中央见小片不强化低信号,误诊为肝局灶性结节增生,病理证实为原发性肝脏神经内分泌癌。故原发性肝脏神经内分泌癌需要与上述疾病进行鉴别。

鉴别诊断:肝细胞性肝癌患者往往有肝炎、肝硬化病史,甲胎蛋白阳性,动态增强早期多数肝细胞肝癌呈显著结节状或团块状强化,门脉期迅速下降为低密度或低信号,强化方式呈“快进快出”,可见假包膜。胆管细胞性肝癌的病变胆管壁不规则增厚或形成结节、肿块影,管腔不规则狭窄或闭塞,病变近段肝内胆管扩张,胆管细胞性肝癌增强早期轻度强化,延迟扫描持续强化,较典型的为“花环样”强化。肝局灶性结节增生的病灶动态增强早期明显强化,门脉期病灶的密度或信号仍高于肝实质,约50%可见肿瘤中心星芒状瘢痕。

综上所述,原发性肝脏神经内分泌癌症状多不典型,多数无症状或体检发现,部分患者无诱因中上腹持续胀痛,常无肝硬化、慢性肝炎病史,影像学检查在术前诊断中发挥重要作用。CT及MRI在观察肿瘤形态、大小、位置、有无坏死及囊变、增强后强化幅度及方式及对周边邻近结构的侵犯都有较大的优势,从而对准确判断肿瘤有较大的帮助。原发性肝脏神经内分泌癌与其他肝脏相关肿瘤在组织起源、临床及影像学表现均不尽相同。因此,提高对影像学特点的认识有助于原发性肝脏神经内分泌癌的术前诊断及鉴别诊断。

第二节　原发性肝胆神经内分泌肿瘤

详见本书 本卷 第十七篇 第二章　原发性肝胆神经内分泌肿瘤。

第十章　肝其他恶性肿瘤

第一节　误诊病例简介：肝左外叶导管内乳头状腺癌

肝导管内乳头状腺癌是肝内胆管细胞癌的一种亚型，即导管内生长型肝内胆管细胞癌，是一种胆管上皮分化的肝内恶性肿瘤。

肝内胆管乳头状腺癌极罕见。本病的病因及发病机制尚不清楚，有文献报道该病与胆管结石、炎症、先天性胆总管囊肿、胆胰管合流异常等有关。一例亦合并多发肝内胆管结石。该病缺乏特异性临床表现，临床上多表现为结石引起的梗阻性黄疸、胆管炎、腹痛等，且胆管内大量黏液潴留使肝内、外胆管明显扩张而呈先天性肝内、外胆管囊肿改变，T_1WI上呈低信号，T_2WI上呈高信号，故需准确诊断很困难；且因肿瘤生长较小，常规影像学检查，如B超、CT、MRI、MRCP等仅能提示肝内、外胆管扩张。胆管内即使充满黏液，也因黏液与正常胆汁有相近密度而不能被MRCP发现，多误诊；该例术前亦误诊为胆石胆囊炎及先天性胆总管囊肿。

如ERCP检查发现十二指肠乳头有“胶冻”状黏液流出，且DWI上发现呈稍高信号的小病灶应考虑本病可能。术中纤维胆道镜检查和活检是诊断本病的最佳方法。经口胆管镜检查可以成为一种诊断调查以评估肝内胆管乳头状肿瘤患者的方法。肝内胆管乳头状腺癌如病变局限于半肝或肝脏的一叶，手术切除是最好的治疗方法且预后较好；如病变分布广泛，行大口径胆肠引流，可暂时缓解黄疸情况。

第二节　肝上皮样血管内皮瘤

病例，男，36岁。体检发现肝脏多发占位2周入院。

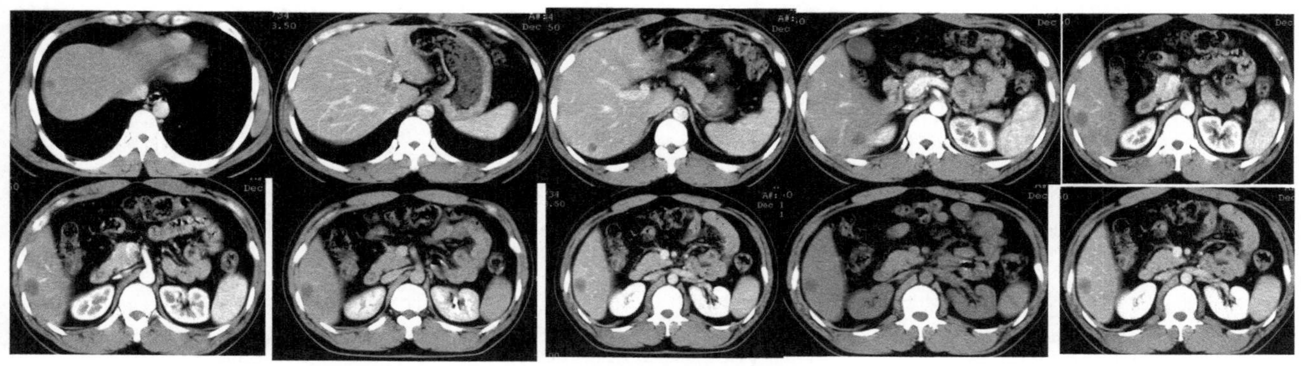

图4-10-1　肝上皮样血管内皮瘤

CT诊断：右肝多个低密度影，边缘轻度环形强化，中心无明显强化，考虑多发肝囊肿可能，请结合临床研究，并请复查。

手术所见：腹腔无腹水，盆腔、胃肠道未触及肿瘤；肝脏大小正常,肝脏Ⅵ～Ⅶ段可见大小不等肿物相互融合,大小约 7 cm × 5cm,质软,包膜较完整,左肝表面可见大小不等肿物,最大直径约 1.5cm。

病理检查:免疫组化检测:阳性:Vimentin, CD34, F8, CD31, SMA, D2-40(灶+), Actin(血管壁平滑肌+), CK(P)(散在+), EMA(散在+), S-100(散在+), Hepatocyte(肝细胞+), Ki-67(+,约 10%), PAS 染色, 网状纤维染色;阴性:AFP, HMB45, Desmin。免疫组化诊断:肝上皮样血管内皮瘤。

肝上皮样血管内皮细胞瘤极为少见,医师对其认识不足,不能很好的分析其特征性影像学表现,容易造成误诊(图 4-10-1)。

第三节 误诊病例简介:原发性肝间质瘤并多发性转移与多发性巨大血管瘤

发病机制:间质瘤是起源于间叶组织的肿瘤,是一个随着病理临床技术发展而逐渐被认识的诊断概念。近年来胃肠道间质瘤作为一种新近发现的肿瘤逐步为国内外学者所认识和熟悉,相关研究也较多,大量研究证明,以往诊断的胃肠道平滑肌瘤、平滑肌肉瘤及神经鞘瘤大多属于间质瘤,但间质瘤患者的临床表现及影像学表现各异,发生机制尚不明确。

胃肠道间质瘤的概念最早由 Mazur 和 Clark(1983)提出,以区别胃肠道间质瘤与平滑肌瘤,以区分一组既不是平滑肌来源也不是神经源性的消化道肿瘤。日本学者 Hirota(1998)提出胃肠道间质瘤可能起源于胃肠道 Cajal 细胞。胃肠道 Cajal 细胞与胃肠道间质瘤肿瘤细胞有共同特征,即均表达 KIT 受体酪氨酸激酶 CD117, CD117 阳性从而成为胃肠道间质瘤诊断的重要标准。早期发现的间质瘤多起源于胃肠道,研究发现胃肠道间质瘤与胃黏膜的 Cajal 细胞关系密切,推测胃肠道间质瘤来源于 Cajal 细胞,但这种说法无法解释原发于胃肠道外间质瘤的发病原因。

病理学:组织学上富于梭形细胞、上皮样细胞,偶或多形性细胞,呈束状、弥漫状排列,免疫表型上表达 c2kit 蛋白(CD117)、巢蛋白以及功能未知蛋白、遗传学上存在频发性 c2kit 基因以及血小板源生长因子受体。基因突变、具有广谱生物学行为、可能起源于幼稚间充质细胞向 Cajal 间质细胞分化的消化道最常见的间叶源性肿瘤。

2001 年美国国立卫生院会议的共识是胃肠道间质瘤肿块直径 <2cm 伴细胞有丝分裂 <5 个 /50 高倍视野,为极低危;肿块 2~5 cm 伴有丝分裂 <5 个 /50 高倍视野为低危;肿块 >5cm 伴细胞有丝分裂 >5 个 /50 高倍视野,肿块 >10 cm,或 >10 个 /50 高倍视野有丝分裂,有三项之一者都属高危。胃肠道间质瘤可发生于食管到肛门的任何部位,以胃和小肠最多见。

胃肠外间质瘤:胃肠外间质瘤是指组织形态、免疫表型等与胃肠道间质瘤相似,但起源于腹腔或腹膜后,且与肠壁或内脏浆膜面无关的一类肿瘤,发病率较低,有病例报道发生于肠系膜、大网膜、后腹膜及女性生殖系统,原发于肝脏的少有报道,然而,无论是胃肠道间质瘤还是胃肠外间质瘤,肝脏都是常见转移部位。

由于胃肠道内间质瘤病例和研究较多,而胃肠道外间质瘤病例报道较少,且胃肠道外病灶与胃肠道内病灶生物学性质及免疫组化检查及临床表现等相近,胃肠道外病例多参考胃肠道内病例标准。但有学者认为根据是否可切除、体积是否超过 10cm、处于分裂期细胞多少、明显核分裂相细胞数、异型性大小及分化程度判断腹腔内胃肠外间质瘤预后更为合理,认为可完全手术切除且无转移浸润的病例 5 年生存率较高,否则一般预后较差。

胃肠外间质瘤多数体积巨大超过 5 cm。间质瘤可为囊性,也可为实性,可原发于肠道外的多种脏器,包括大网膜、腹膜、肠系膜。原发于大网膜的巨大间质瘤易自发性破裂,迫使外科手术治疗。

具有不同恶性潜能的肿瘤:既往认为间质瘤具有良、恶性之分,但随着对该病的不断认识发现,认为即便未发生复发或转移时,不同的间质瘤仅侵袭危险性不同,并没有绝对的“良性”肿瘤,因此该病是一类具有不同恶性潜能的肿瘤。评估其恶性潜能的因素较多,目前较公认的标准是综合肿瘤大小和核分裂数计数将其危险程度进行分级。

临床表现:间质瘤临床表现无特异性,肿瘤小则通常无症状,肿瘤大时,胃肠道间质瘤主要表现为消化道出血、中上腹部不适、腹痛、腹部肿块等,与常见消化道疾病类似的症状;胃肠外间质瘤的主要表现为腹部包块、胀痛不适等非特异性症状。内镜和消化道造影检查是胃肠道间质瘤术前主要的检查手段，B超或CT检查主要用于胃肠道间质瘤的定位诊断，可显示肿块与周围组织和血管的关系。影像学检查是胃肠外间质瘤术前诊断的主要手段，但定性诊断困难。最终确诊目前仍依赖于组织病理学和免疫组化的结果。

外科切除被认为是治疗间质瘤的最主要手段，适用于原发、较局限者，完整的肿瘤切除是外科手术治疗的基本原则，术中应轻柔操作，防止肿瘤脱落种植，避免增加术后复发的危险。间质瘤对放化疗均不敏感，由于属富血管肿瘤，在肝脏的转移瘤可经导管肝动脉栓塞或栓塞化疗。甲磺酸伊马替尼现已成为治疗间质瘤的一线治疗药物，该药是一种酪氨酸激酶抑制剂，可选择性作用于胃肠道间质瘤的c-Kit酪氨酸激酶，阻断与细胞生长有关的信号传导通路，从而抑制肿瘤的生长，达到治疗作用。

原发和转移：原发于肝脏的间质瘤少有报道，文献报道多为胃肠间质瘤，偶可见肝内转移。该病例经手术探查证实原发于肝脏并肠系膜多处转移，病理检查和免疫组化确诊为间质瘤。病理诊断为梭形细胞瘤；免疫组化示Vimentin(+)、CD34(-)、CD117(+)、Actin(部分+)、S-100(-)、Desmin(-)；临床表现患者仅有轻度腹部不适、饱胀感，并没有消化道疾病症状，手术探查时未发现肿瘤浸润消化道管壁；在发病过程中曾出现过腹痛，根据影像学检查及手术探查推测为肝内肿瘤破裂引起疼痛，后手术探查发现肠系膜转移，考虑为肿瘤破裂后瘤细胞落入腹腔发生种植转移。

鉴别诊断：原发性肝细胞肝癌：CT检查平扫示肝内单个或多个边缘模糊的圆形、类圆形、分叶状或不规则形的低密度病灶，少数可为等密度或混合密度，高密度者少见；增强扫描成呈特征性的“快进快出”的特点。巨块型肝癌增强后密度不均匀，呈网格状、蜂窝状极不规则增强，但其增强程度多不如正常肝，病变区还可出现密度稍高的结节或分隔，这与肿瘤局部坏死、肿瘤细胞脂肪变性、胆管内胆红素栓形成以及瘤内间隔强化等有关。肝癌较大时易侵犯肝门生成静脉癌栓，或转移至肝门附近淋巴结而引起阻塞性黄疸。

肝血管瘤：肝脏最常见的良性间叶细胞肿瘤，肿瘤大小从不到1cm到超过20cm，当病变大于4cm时就直接称为巨大血管瘤，常见于女性。一些学术研究表明，雌激素可能在其病因学上有一定作用。小血管瘤一般无症状，病变较大者主要引起腹部不适、疼痛、腹胀和压迫症状，包括较早饱满、食欲减退和反胃。螺旋CT平扫示低密度灶，增强扫描示早期周边强化，随后在连续的图像上呈进行性向心性充填。典型表现为病变经过3min或更长时间延迟后变得完全强化。病变越大，CT诊断的敏感性和特异性越高。

肝肉芽肿：肉芽肿是一种独特的病理学表现，代表着单核巨噬细胞系统(网状内皮细胞系统)对存在的异物所采取的一种易于识别的炎症反应类型。其特异的组织学表现是一种结节性反应，后者含有被称为上皮样细胞转化了的巨噬细胞；其他类型的炎症细胞还包括淋巴细胞和嗜酸性粒细胞，这两种细胞居于肉芽肿内部或其周围，多数肉芽肿内可见到多核巨细胞。肝肉芽肿很少引起临床上明显的肝脏损害。肝肉芽肿患者血清碱性磷酸酶(ALT)升高最常见。肝脏可能增大，右上腹痛有时会很严重。若大量肉芽肿弥漫地分布于肝小叶及肉芽肿周围炎性反应活跃，这些患者可有血清转氨酶升高。多数患者仅表现为发热、疲乏无力和血清碱性磷酸酶升高三联征，因此肝活检的结果就成为诊断性评估的重要依据；影像学检查可无异常发现，或表现为弥漫性的肝脏质地不均一。

第四节　肝门部肿瘤MRI误诊分析

肝门部肿瘤按其生长形态可分为外生肿块型、浸润型和管内生长型。

有研究显示平扫中T_2WI对于显示病变及淋巴结肿大、腹水等伴随征象方面敏感性不亚于增强扫描。一组资料单发于肝门区的转移性病变，多来自邻近器官(特别是消化系统肿瘤)，以直接蔓延方式转移者居多。

有作者认为，MRCP加梗阻部位薄层扫描或增强显示胆管梗阻的准确率高于内镜逆行胰胆管造影(ERCP)和经皮肝穿胆管造影(PTC)。该研究显示MRCP对肝门部肿瘤致胆管梗阻水平定位准确率达93.3%，由于空间分辨力相对低，MRCP难以区分完全梗阻与高度狭窄,两者均表现为阻塞性改变。动态增强扫描对于肝门部肿瘤鉴别诊断具有重要价值。该组肿块型肝细胞性肝癌动态增强扫描以延迟期强化为主,体现了癌组织动脉供血不丰富及富含纤维组织、细胞外间隙大的病理组织学基础。

胆管癌:该组资料胆管癌组术前定性诊断错误4例,其中2例于动脉期、门脉期表现为轻度强化,加上并发肝内多发转移灶而误诊为肝门转移性病变,2例浸润型胆管癌胆管壁增厚、强化而误诊为胆管炎性改变。

肝细胞性肝癌:该组肝细胞性肝癌三期均未见明显强化2例而误诊为良性病变,产生病理基础为瘤内血供较少,该组作者认为结合患者症状、体征及甲胎蛋白检查非常重要。肝细胞性肝癌动脉期开始强化,门脉期信号仍高于肝组织2例,产生原因主要是肿瘤为动脉和门脉双重供血。

肝门转移性病变:肝门转移性病变误诊为胆管癌3例、误诊为肝细胞性肝癌2例,其中2例为富血供性转移性病变。分析这5例误诊的主要原因为原发肿瘤病史不详,肿瘤单发且强化方式与肝细胞性肝癌、胆管癌类似所致。

肝门区肿瘤术前评估及术中所见:肝门区肿瘤术前评估需了解肿瘤大小、范围、胆管及血管受侵及淋巴结转移情况等。MRCP整体感强,有利于病变的定位;T_2WI及增强扫描可以更准确地观察肿瘤边界,3D DCE-MRA显示的血管改变同血管造影有很高的一致性,3D DCE-MRA在显示门静脉瘤栓及动-静脉瘘方面有独特的优势,但对于血管局部的轻微浸润方面显示欠佳。

该组资料胆管癌组术前评估认为可切除的9例中。有3例分别因术中见病变侵犯2级胆管,对侧肝内转移及门静脉浸润而行姑息治疗,术前有2例认为病变侵犯2级胆管,术中见病变局限肝总管分叉处及左、右肝管予以完全切除,分析这5例评估错误的主要原因有:①MRCP的最大信号强度投影重建图像上扩张的胆管互相重叠,二级分支受累显示欠清,因而影响了病灶范围的判断;②肝门区胆管解剖结构复杂、变异,导致对病变是否累及二级分支的定位出现偏差。

该组资料中的肝细胞性肝癌组术前评估认为可手术切除、无包膜的肝细胞性肝癌2例,因MRI术前未显示门静脉左支受侵而行手术,术中见肿块与门静脉左支侧壁粘连,左肝管与门静脉间部分肿瘤组织未能完全切除,提示肝癌包膜可能是肝门血管受侵的保护性因素。

肝门转移性病变术前未能定性而手术探查者不在少数,该组有4例术前误诊为胆管癌、肝细胞性肝癌而行手术,术中均未能完全切除。

总之,该研究建议肝门区肿瘤欲行手术者均应行MRI平扫联合动态增强扫描、MRCP及3D DCE-MRA等无创性检查,以提供给临床最全面的、较准确的诊断和术前评估信息。

第五篇　肝的其他局灶性疾病

第一章　关于肝局灶性病变

肝局灶性病变的各种分类

1. 肝局灶性病变的组织学分类　按照组织病理学的标准，肝局灶性病变可依其分化程度分成若干类别，原发性肿瘤可再分成间质型、上皮型或混合型；继发性肿瘤主要是由转移癌及寄生性疾病所构成。表5-1-1列举了与临床密切相关的肝原发性、继发性肿瘤，以及肿瘤样病变，后者必须与真正的肿瘤相区别。

表 5-1-1　肝局灶性病变组织病理学分类

	肝的良性肿瘤	肝的恶性肿瘤
原发性肿瘤		
上皮型肿瘤		
肝细胞性	肝细胞性腺瘤	肝细胞性癌
		纤维板层癌
胆管细胞性	胆管腺瘤	胆管细胞性癌
	胆管乳头状瘤	胆管囊腺癌
间质型肿瘤		
血管性肿瘤	血管瘤	血管肉瘤
	血管内皮瘤(儿童)	恶性上皮样血管内皮瘤
	血管肌脂瘤	胚胎性肉瘤
		平滑肌肉瘤
		非霍奇金淋巴瘤及霍奇金病
		肝母细胞瘤
混合型		
继发性肿瘤		
	寄生虫感染	转移瘤
肿瘤样病变		
	囊肿	
	局灶性结节增生	
	结节再生性增生	
	间质错构瘤	
	肝性紫癜	
	炎性假瘤	

2. 肝局灶性病变的放射学分类　肝的局灶性病变可依据动态增强MR成像，特别是动脉期时病灶的血供程度分成以下三个类别：在动脉期时，病变部位与正常肝实质相比，呈富血供，因而在动脉期时表现为高信号；病变呈乏血供，在成像的血管期时不强化；在动脉期的后期，病变信号增强，在平衡期时仍持续为高信号。此一放射学分类并没有考虑肝肿瘤在组织病理学上的区别，因为它是基于血管化程度的不同，而不是组织学的表现，但这对于在动脉MR成像中鉴别肝局灶性病变的性质却是必需的。

肝的局灶性病变的动态增强MR成像三种类别的典型病变分别是①富血供—肝腺瘤；②乏血供—囊性转移瘤；③血管瘤。

（1）常规MRI表现按血供分类：富血供的肝局灶性病变：①中央瘢痕：中央瘢痕，T_2WI呈高信号——局灶性结节增生；在延迟期成像中，中央瘢痕无增强信号，T_1WI及T_2WI均呈低信号——纤维板层样肝癌；②有出血征象，无中央瘢痕，退行性变化——肝细胞性腺瘤；③肝硬化征象，内部病变呈不规则形状：均匀或非均匀的富血供病灶，T_2WI呈高信号——肝细胞性肝癌(假包膜，弥漫型或小结节型)；均匀的富血供病灶，T_2WI呈低信号——再生性结节；④轻度但均匀的富血供：经对比剂增强5分钟后，呈等信号或稍高信号，T_2WI呈均匀的稍高信号——平滑肌肉瘤的转移；⑤已知为原发性肿瘤，动脉期呈高血供：在动脉期时，由于血供丰富，T_2WI呈极高信号，在门脉期时，T_1WI通常为等信号——神经内分泌肿瘤(如：胰岛素瘤、胃泌素瘤类癌瘤)的转移；T_2WI呈高信号，中央部分呈更高信号为坏死区——各种原发肿瘤的转移，如肾上腺样瘤、嗜铬细胞瘤、胰胚细胞瘤、黑色素瘤(亦可为低信号)、乳癌(通常亦为低信号)；⑥局部区域高血供：在动脉期，见有不规则的高信号区，在相应的平扫T_1WI及T_2WI无异常信号，静脉期为等信号——focal attenuation difference(FAD)。

（2）乏血供的肝局灶性病变：①囊性病变：边界

锐利,无富血供外环——囊肿(单发或多发),肝胆管囊肿,多囊肾;低信号环,囊内有分隔,子囊——肝包虫病;②有富血供外环:注射对比剂5分钟后有对比剂清除现象;T_2WI图像中呈饼圈征、晕环征——腺癌的转移(胰腺、结肠、胃及其他原发性肿瘤);囊性表现,囊壁不规则伴局部增厚,囊内有分隔与实质性部分——囊性转移瘤;③动脉期及门脉期呈高信号,对比剂注射5分钟后呈等信号:平扫T_1WI上呈不规则的低信号区,T_2WI为高信号——非霍奇金淋巴瘤,霍奇金病;④富血供的边缘环状强化,中央部分无对比剂的摄入:T_2WI,中央部分为高信号强度,偶见气体的形成——肝脓肿;⑤富血供的边缘呈持续环状强化,中央部分无对比剂的摄入:囊样表现,血管移位,T_2WI为高信号——胆汁瘤;边缘不规则;T_1WI及T_2WI为不均匀信号强度;细胞外正铁血红蛋白使边缘呈环状高信号,随着时间延长,中央信号也增高——血肿破裂。

(3)延迟期持续增强的肝局灶性病变:①沿门脉通路浸润,节段性胆管梗阻,常在延迟期呈均匀强化:动脉期为低信号伴周边高信号强化,平扫T_1WI呈低信号——胆管细胞癌;②已知原发肿瘤,延迟期有均匀信号强化:动脉期时为低信号或高信号,T_1WI呈低信号,T_2WI呈高信号,部分病例有周边对比剂清除征象——平滑肌瘤及胃肠道间质瘤(GIST);③均一性增强(可显示依赖血流的均匀性富血供的特点):T_2WI为高信号(相当于血管瘤的信号),平扫;T_1WI呈低信号,延迟期呈等信号或高信号,常态不规则——肝性紫癜;④周边结节状增强:均一的向心性充盈,在较大的病灶内,中心区可无增强,此乃由于血栓形成/纤维化所致——血管瘤;⑤不规则部分性结节状增强:离心性或不规则充盈;在中央部位,早期未见增强;边缘不规则;T_2WI高强信号,可与血管瘤相仿——血管肉瘤。

肝脏局灶性病变以CT动脉期强化类型分类:Nino-Murcia等(2000)对100例患局灶性肝脏病变的病人(女性42例,男性58例,年龄25~84岁,平均57岁)的CT动脉期图像进行了回顾性分析,不包括单纯肝囊肿的病人,每例病人只分析1个病灶。

其中40例有1个病灶:23例肝细胞癌,7例转移瘤,5例局灶性结节增生(FNH),5例海绵状血管瘤。60例有多个病灶:46例转移瘤,8例肝细胞癌,4例海绵状血管瘤,1例胆管癌,1例肝脓肿。转移瘤直径1.0~16.5cm(平均4.9cm),肝细胞癌直径1.0~14.3(平均5.2cm),海绵状血管瘤直径2~10cm(平均4.6cm),局灶性结节增生直径2.2~7.7cm(平均4.9cm)。

最后确诊依靠手术后组织病理学检查或经皮活检标本或根据临床病程及影像学随访结果。应用螺旋CT,行全肝平扫检查:层厚10mm,间隔20mm,然后以4~5ml/秒的速度静注含300mg/m1碘的非离子型对比剂150ml,注药后25秒获取屏气动脉期图像,层厚7mm,螺距1.0~1.6;注药后60~70秒获取屏气门静脉期图像。

将病灶的动脉期强化方式分为5种类型:“均一”型是指病灶弥漫均匀强化,中心有不超过10%的管腔结构清楚的低密度区;23例病灶呈均一型强化:13例(57%)肝细胞癌,5例(22%)局灶性结节增生,4例(17%)转移瘤,1例(4%)海绵状血管瘤。

“异常肝内管腔或不均匀强化”型是指内部管腔轮廓不规则和分支扭曲或无规则分布的高、低密度区;10例病灶呈异常肝内管腔或不均匀强化型;9例(90%)肝细胞癌,1例(10%)转移瘤。

“周边结节状强化”型是指分散的、边界清楚的强化结节,其密度与强化的动脉相等;7例病灶呈周边结节状强化型:6例(86%)海绵状血管瘤,1例转移瘤。

“环状强化”型是指以低密度区为主,周围环绕强化区;49例病灶呈环状强化型:40例(82%)转移瘤,7例(14%)肝细胞癌,1例(2%)胆管癌,1例(2%)脓肿。

“不完整环状强化”型是指非环状周边强化。3例病灶呈不完整环状强化型:2例(67%)海绵状血管瘤,1例(33%)转移瘤。

此外,8例病灶没有强化:6例(75%)转移瘤,2例(25%)肝细胞癌。

以下3种强化类型的阳性预测值大于或等于82%:肝细胞癌的异常肝内管腔或不均匀强化;海绵状血管瘤的周边结节状强化;转移瘤的环状强化。

肝细胞癌有两种强化类型:均一型和异常肝内管腔或不均匀强化型,前者敏感性高。海绵状血管瘤的周边结节状强化特异性很高,但敏感性较低。

所有的局灶性结节增生均表现为均一型,这使其敏感度很高,而特异度不高。

53例转移瘤中有13例表现为富血供病灶,其最多见的强化类型为环状强化(6个)和均一型(3个);其余40例转移瘤的原发灶均为乏血供病灶,强化类型多为环状强化(34 个)。

研究表明,肝脏局灶性病变的 CT 动脉期强化类型对确定特定的诊断有潜在作用,同时作者提出的分类方案可作为肝脏 CT 动脉期研究的有效工具。

第二章 肝血管瘤

第一节 不典型血管瘤

不典型血管瘤及其伴随病变：不典型血管瘤，包括：大的、不均质血管瘤；对比剂快速充填的血管瘤、钙化血管瘤、玻璃样变血管瘤、血管瘤伴随液－液平面、外生性的血管瘤。

不常见的强化及其他异常包括肝动脉门静脉分流、包膜缩进，血管瘤也可以发生于局部脂肪肝浸润中。不典型血管瘤还包括血管瘤进行性的增大，及妊娠期间出现血管瘤。血管瘤的伴随病变包括多发血管瘤、肝细胞腺瘤病、肝局灶性结节增生，伴随异常包括动静脉瘘、包膜缩进，血管瘤也可以发生于局部脂肪肝浸润。

不典型血管瘤的影像学表现：巨大血管瘤：大的，不均质的血管瘤——巨大血管瘤，一般直径大于4cm。但也有作者以大于6cm或者大于12cm作为标准。CT平扫为低密度，中心可见更低密度区，动脉期则可见到边缘的早期、结节状、粗斑点状的典型强化表现。在门静脉期及延迟期则向心性充填，但不会完全充填。大的血管瘤常常表现不均匀，有中心瘢痕存在，增强后期不强化，病理成分可以是黏液变性组织、血栓、纤维和坏死组织，常规T_2WI往往不能区分其内部成分，因为中心T_2高信号在黏液变性组织中也可见到。内部分隔是另外一不典型表现，表现为长T_1、短T_2信号特征，其主要是纤维组织，增强后强化不明显。

对比剂快速填充的血管瘤：随着影像设备时间分辨力的明显提高，血管瘤少见的强化表现越来越多地被发现，所谓"闪现充填"，即表现为快速、均匀一致动脉期强化，典型地表现为与主动脉同步强化，多见于2 cm以下血管瘤。与其他动脉期强化病灶相鉴别的关键点在于动态增强后期病灶仍有持续强化呈高密度或高信号。对比剂快速填充的血管瘤并不常见，大约占所有血管瘤的16%。最常见于小的血管瘤，特别是直径小于1cm的血管瘤。CT、MRI表现为立即均匀的强化。与其他富血供的肿瘤鉴别较困难，T_2WI对鉴别诊断有所帮助，但富血供的胰岛细胞瘤肝转移也可以有类似的表现。准确的诊断依赖于延迟期扫描，因为延迟扫描血管瘤持续强化，而富血供的转移瘤没有这样的表现。另外一个征象是血管瘤在所有的增强期都和主动脉密度相一致。

钙化的血管瘤：体内其他部位的血管瘤如软组织、胃肠道、腹膜后腔，以及纵隔，也会出现钙化(静脉石——诊断血管瘤的特异征象)。肝血管瘤较少出现钙化，但在临床上也会发现。肝血管瘤的钙化发生于病变的边缘或者中心，可以是多发点状的钙化——静脉石，也可以是大的钙化灶。一些钙化血管瘤也许强化较轻，特别在CT图像上。肝内发现非强化的钙化的病变，并不能排除血管瘤可能。在T_2WI上非钙化区域的高信号中表现为低信号结节，提示血管瘤的诊断。

玻璃样变或透明样变或硬化性血管瘤：玻璃样变或透明样变或硬化性血管瘤，一般认为其代表血管瘤进展的终末期，其血窦被透明样变的纤维组织所代替，从而失去典型强化特征和MRI T_2WI高信号的特点，在T_2WI仅为轻微高信号。实际工作中，对此种病例做出明确诊断相当困难，病理检查是必要的，其可表现为广泛纤维组织和血窦的闭塞。鉴别诊断应该包括乏血供肿瘤，尤其是转移瘤。玻璃样变的血管瘤的影像表现与典型血管瘤完全不一样。病理检查显示病变的弥漫性纤维组织形成及血管腔的闭塞。典型血管瘤T_2WI明显高信号，而此种血管瘤在T_2WI仅为轻微高信号。另外，缺乏早期强化的表现。在晚期才会出现外围的轻度强化。MRI 不能区分此类血管瘤与其他的恶性肿瘤。

瘤内有液 - 液平面的血管瘤：超声常不能发现液—液平面。上层液性成分为非凝固状态的血清——CT 上为低密度，T_1WI 与肌肉等信号，T_2WI 明显高信号；下层为红细胞——CT 上为高密度，T_1WI 高于肌肉信号，T_2WI 上轻度的高信号。液 - 液平面并不是血管瘤的特异性的诊断。有些作者认为，如果 CT、MRI 能够发现液 - 液平面，而超声不能发现的话，可以提示血管瘤的诊断。肿瘤内出血 CT 一般表现为高密度，MRI 对识别肿瘤内出血有其独到优势，表现为 T_1WI 高信号，T_2WI 上的表现是变化多样的，依赖于其血红蛋白降解产物的成分，没有出血的区域通常仍保持典型血管瘤的信号特征和增强特点。但是液 - 液平不是血管瘤的特征表现，其还可见于其他肿瘤如囊腺瘤、慢性血肿、伴有出血和坏死的肿瘤和坏死性转移。一般而言，在鉴别诊断有困难时，组织病理活检是非常必要的。

外生性的或有蒂的血管瘤：外生性的血管瘤确实较少见。可以是无症状的，但可以由于扭转或者梗死引起症状。多平面重建可以帮助诊断。强化方式同典型血管瘤。部分大血管瘤中心位于肝脏，尤其是第Ⅳ段和肝门周围可导致胆管扩张，在此情况下，容易误诊为胆管细胞癌，应仔细鉴别。

有肝动脉 - 门静脉瘘的血管瘤：动 - 静脉瘘通常伴随恶性肿瘤，但是在良性肿瘤也可见到。表现为动脉期病变的早期强化伴随着门静脉早显。

伴有包膜皱缩的血管瘤：包膜皱缩通常见于恶性肿瘤，如胆管细胞瘤、血管内皮瘤和少见含纤维成分的转移瘤。血管瘤也可伴随包膜皱缩，但甚为少见，其原因可能是继发于外周纤维化。一项研究中，血管瘤伴随包膜皱缩仅见到一例。

发生于脂肪肝背景的血管瘤：在脂肪肝存在的情况下，血管瘤的 CT 表现应重新认识，特别是中度和重度脂肪肝。平扫 CT，病变可以高于邻近肝脏的密度，或者见不到明确的病变。对比增强则可见血管瘤的典型强化表现。要注意，在动脉期，血管瘤可以表现为等密度。在这种情况下，MRI 更有帮助。由于肝脏实质密度的降低，在平扫时血管瘤表现为等密度，或呈高密度病灶，给显示病灶和诊断带来一定困难。但增强后的表现多与一般血管瘤一致，对比剂由周边向中央扩展，最后将病灶充填，而延迟扫描血管瘤表现为高密度。或增强早期明显强化呈高密度，持续至门脉期和延迟期。此时血管瘤的密度不应与存在脂肪肝的肝实质密度相比较，可以密度相对恒定的脾脏作为参考。要注意，在动脉期，血管瘤可以表现为等密度。部分病灶于 CT 上外周有一圈致密环，是由于病灶压迫所致的动脉血供增加，门脉血供减少而致肝组织没有发生脂肪变。和肝细胞性肝癌包膜区别在于增强后没有明显强化，与周围肝实质趋于一致。在这种情况下，MRI 可更好显示其影像特征，尤其在正反相位成像可以消除脂肪肝背景影响，同时 T_2WI 高信号和动态增强特征可以显示。

多发的血管瘤：有作者报告，10% 的血管瘤呈现多发。肝内散在分布的多发血管瘤有典型表现。T_2WI 显示肝内多发高信号病变。

血管瘤病：血管瘤，即使巨大的血管瘤，边界也是清楚的。但是，有很少的病例，病变较大且边界不清，代替大部分肝脏实质。在幼儿常见，可伴随心力衰竭，有高的死亡率。成年人的血管瘤病常无症状。CT 上没有典型的表现，但是延迟扫描可以提示诊断。MRI 有较为典型的表现。

血管瘤与局灶性结节增生的并存：血管瘤与局灶性结节增生的并存较常见，概率为 23%。目前认为，并存并不是偶然发生的。在多发的局灶性结节增生病例中，并存血管瘤更加常见，有 33% 的多发局灶性结节增生伴有血管瘤。一般认为局灶性结节增生是由于肝脏局部动脉血流的增加引起的增生反应，因此局灶性结节增生类似血管瘤，都是血管源性的。有作者报告，口服避孕药的年轻女性血管瘤和局灶性结节增生并存的发生率为 100%。

血管瘤的进行性增大：大部分血管瘤大小保持不变，或者随时间增大很少。有文献报道血管瘤的进行性增大：1 例在妊娠期，2 例发生于应用雌激素患者。影像表现同典型血管瘤的表现。进行性增大的机制可能是由于血管的扩张，应用雌激素也可能起作用，但未得到证实。文献也报道，妊娠期间出现血管瘤——也证实血管瘤与雌激素有关。

第二节 误诊病例简介:肝外生性海绵状血管瘤与胃肠间质瘤

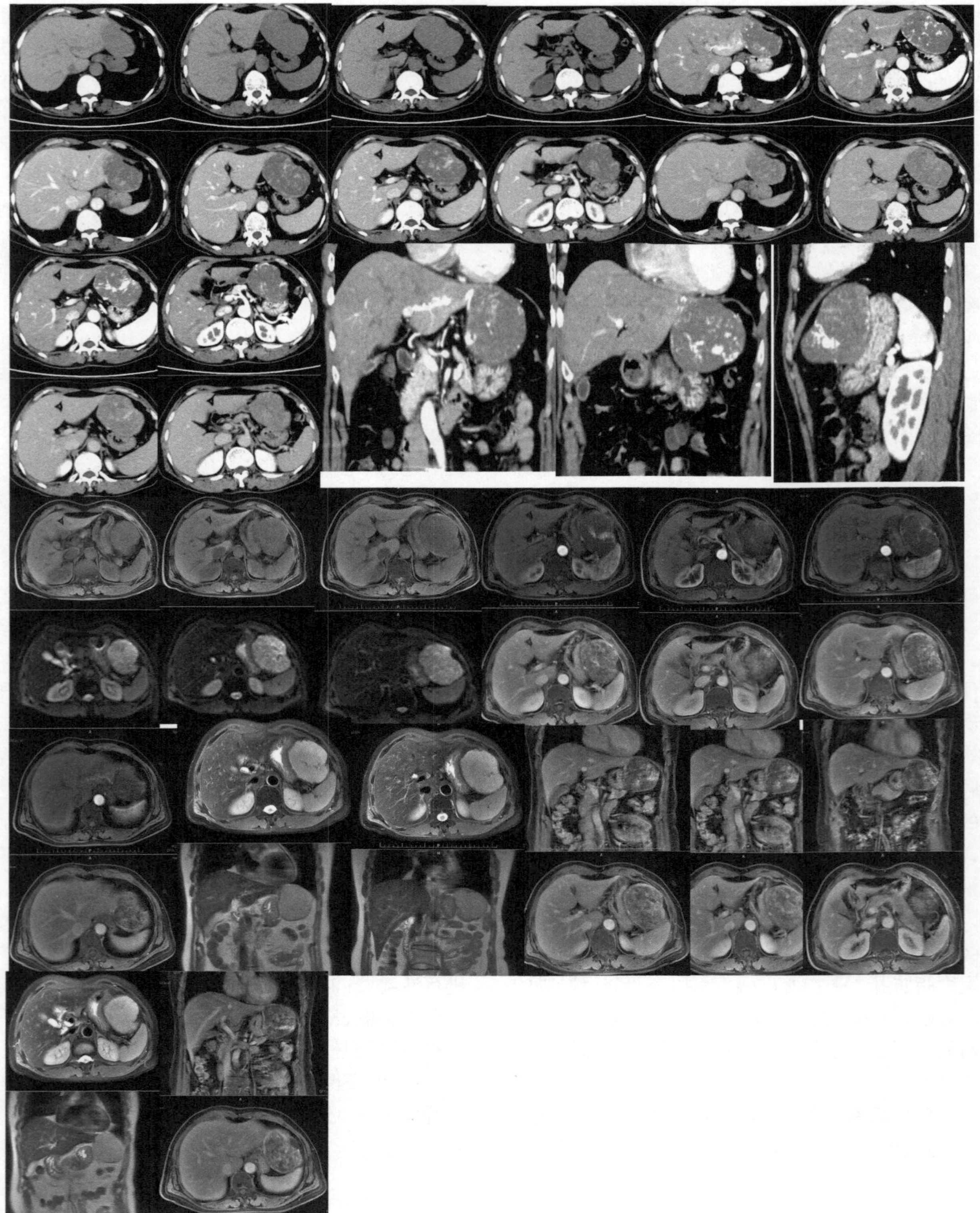

图 5-2-1 肝外生性海绵状血管瘤与胃肠间质瘤

患者，女，57岁。CT：肝胃间隙占位，考虑胃来源可能性大，胃肠道间质瘤？胃其他性质恶性肿瘤？部分血液供应来自于肝动脉，不排除病灶来源于胃和肝，建议结合临床分析研究；肝囊肿。MRI：肝左外叶外生性肝癌可能性大，请结合临床；肝内多发囊肿，肝内外胆管轻度扩张。

手术所见：左肝外叶下缘可见一大小约7cm×5cm肿物，突出肝脏表面，胃大弯侧受推挤移位，与周围膈肌、网膜无粘连，胆囊大小约5cm×4cm，与周边无粘连。

病理检查：肝左外叶肿物切除标本：灰褐色不规则组织一块，大小8.5cm×8cm×5cm，切面暗红，质中偏软。病理诊断：肝左外叶肿物切除标本：海绵状血管瘤。

误诊分析：术前对肿瘤部分血供来自于肝脏重视不够，对血管瘤的动静脉短路没有认识，只是不除外肿瘤来自于肝；反过来，术前却将肿物与胃的关系太过重视，思维陷入盲目性，一直考虑为胃的肿瘤，自然想到胃肠间质瘤，导致误诊；在肿瘤来源的考虑上，我们体会到，不只是看肿瘤与该器官关系密切与否，有的关系密切是由于肿瘤挤压所致而非真正起源于该器官，本例即如此；还要看肿瘤的血液供应情况，通过此例的总结，肿瘤的血供来源在确定肿瘤来源于该器官与否实际上更为重要。

术前思路太窄，对病变与肝的关系考虑太少，未考虑到肝的外生性肿瘤，MRI考虑到肝的外生性肿瘤，但也只是考虑外生性肝癌，而未想到外生性的海绵状血管瘤，从文献看，肝的外生性海绵状血管瘤确实少见；回顾性分析，血供研究尤其重要，增强表现不典型，但三期表现仍有血管瘤的特点，慢进慢出，延迟期强化明显增加；应观察肿物大部分与周围器官的关系，而不要只看少部位邻近情况。从影像表现特点看，用海绵状血管瘤解释还相当典型，只是它不在肝内而在肝外，术前未仔细认真地分析影像表现特点，这也是我们临床诊断工作中的一个思维缺陷，值得总结的经验教训（图5-2-1）。

第三节　肝脏血管瘤不常见CT和MRI表现

随着影像技术的发展，空间分辨力大大提高，对于小的肝脏局灶性病变检出率有很大提高，偶然发现的肝脏局灶性病变越来越多，同时也提出对所谓偶发病灶的定性问题。

对于肝脏偶发病灶定性，有几个因素可能影响诊断，如病变的典型或不典型影像表现，以前有无肿瘤病史存在，随访中病灶影像表现和大小的变化等。而病变的影像学表现是影响判断的重要因素。在肝脏偶发病灶中，血管瘤是其中常见的病变。

病理学：肝脏血管瘤尸检发现率估计在0.4%~20.0%，中年女性多见。多发者也不少见。在形态上，境界往往比较清晰，圆形或卵圆形，可以发生在肝实质的任何部位，但更常见于外周和包膜下，肝脏右叶后段最常见，镜下可见病灶为多发的血窦，窦腔内面被覆单层的内皮细胞，窦腔之间见薄的纤维结缔组织间隔。一般而言，在这些血窦中的血液流动缓慢。

血管瘤大小一般稳定，可以从数毫米到超过20cm大小，依据大小可以分为小（小于15 mm）、中（15~50 mm）和大血管瘤（大于50 mm）。大的血管瘤可以引起并发症，如出血，对邻近组织的压迫和扭转等。

肝脏血管瘤的常见CT和MRI表现：平扫一般表现为境界清晰的低密度灶，T_1WI低信号，在T_2WI由于血窦的长T_2弛豫时间呈现明显均匀高信号，表现为“亮灯征”，小的病灶信号均匀，大病灶信号欠均匀。增强扫描早期显示边缘结节样或云絮状强化，范围大小差别较大，其密度（信号）等于或接近于腹主动脉。

随着时间延长，后期（门脉期和平衡期甚至延迟期）显示病灶缓慢的进行性向心性填充，表现为高密度（信号），有时病灶也可以呈等密度（信号）充填。后期病灶内对比剂的聚集可以用血窦的缓慢血流来解释，然而，延迟充填表现均匀等或高密度不能常常见到，尤其对于大的病灶，中心往往伴有瘢痕、坏死、囊变等而不能被充填。

肝脏血管瘤不常见CT和MRI表现：肝脏血管瘤不典型影像表现主要有三方面：形态和结构的改变，不典型的强化特征，或伴有肝脏实质的异常。对于有恶性肿瘤病史和以前有正常检查结果，病灶表现为非典型的影像表现时，诊断需要综合可能的检查结果，甚至包括侵袭性检查技术。这些不典型表现在诊断中有误导作用，因此，放射科医生应该熟悉和了解这些方面以避免在诊断中错误判断和应用更多的检查，包括侵袭性检查技术。

不常见的形态/结构表现：大的血管瘤常常表

现不均匀,有中心瘢痕存在,增强后期不强化,病理成分可以是黏液变性组织、血栓、纤维和坏死组织,常规 T_2WI 往往不能区分其内部成分,因为中心 T_2 高信号在黏液变性组织中也可见到。内部分隔是另外一个不典型表现,表现为长 T_1、短 T_2 信号特征,其主要是纤维组织,增强后强化不明显。

包膜皱缩是血管瘤不常见的表现,但不应排除血管瘤的诊断,其往往继发于外周纤维化,在这种情况下,其他诊断应予排除包括肝内胆管细胞癌,上皮样血管内皮瘤或者少见含纤维成分的转移瘤。

有蒂的血管瘤罕见,一般根据其信号特征和强化特点可做出诊断,可发生扭转和坏死,应用多平面重建可清晰显示其肝脏来源。部分大血管瘤中心位于肝脏,尤其是第Ⅳ段和肝门周围可导致胆管扩张,在此情况下,容易误诊为胆管细胞癌,应仔细鉴别。

血管瘤钙化较为少见,可见于中央和外周部分,多发小钙化常常是静脉石, CT 可较好的显示钙化,表现为条状或结节高密度影,在 T_2WI 高信号的肿瘤中表现为低信号结节。

肿瘤内出血 CT 一般表现为高密度, MRI 对识别肿瘤内出血有其独到优势,表现为 T_1WI 高信号,T_2WI 上的表现是变化多样的,依赖于其血红蛋白降解产物的成分,没有出血的区域通常仍保持典型血管瘤的信号特征和增强特点。

腹腔内出血极度罕见,在大的表浅血管瘤合并腹部创伤时易发生。

囊性和多房性血管瘤极度少见,此种非典型特征表现为单发或多发瘤内空腔,表现为长 T_1、长 T_2 信号特点,但是外周强化仍可出现。

在罕见病例中,病灶内可见到液 - 液平,其代表静止或缓慢流动血液伴红细胞沉积,上层液体含有血浆,下层含有没有凝固沉积的红细胞。CT 上表现为上层是液体密度,下层为高密度, MRI T_2WI 上层表现为高信号,下层信号略低。但是液 - 液平不是血管瘤的特征表现,它还可见于其他肿瘤如囊腺瘤,慢性血肿,伴有出血和坏死的肿瘤和坏死性转移。一般而言,在鉴别诊断有困难时,组织病理活检是非常必要的。

不常见的强化特征:随着影像设备时间分辨力的明显提高,血管瘤少见的强化表现越来越多地被发现,所谓“闪现充填”,即表现为快速、均匀一致动脉期强化,典型地表现为与主动脉同步强化,多见于 2 cm 以下血管瘤。与其他动脉期强化病灶相鉴别的关键点在于动态增强后期病灶仍有持续强化呈高密度或高信号。

与这种高血流量高动力的血管瘤相反,慢血流低动力血管瘤则表现为延迟充填,这类病例需要延长检查时间以观察到向心性强化和对比剂在病灶内滞留的表现。这种血流动力学差异可能与构成血管瘤的血窦大小有关系,大血窦为慢血流,小血窦内为高动力血流。

在 19%~25% 的病例可见病灶周围肝实质的强化,表现为一过性肝脏密度差异,对应于动脉期肝实质强化,后期呈等密度或等信号,其病理基础在于与高血流动力相关的动静脉分流或早期引流静脉显影。尽管一过性肝脏密度差异绝大数见于小的“闪现充填”特征的血管瘤,大血管瘤由于门脉压迫和代偿性的动脉血供增加也可出现此种表现。值得注意的是病灶周围一过性肝脏密度差异可以出现于许多局灶性肝脏病变如转移,脓肿和肝癌等。

也有少数血管瘤在增强早期表现为中心强化,在病理上表现为病灶中心为血窦,外周主要是纤维成分。

透明样变或硬化性血管瘤,一般认为其代表血管瘤进展的终末期,其血窦被透明样变的纤维组织所代替,从而失去典型强化特征和 MRI T_2WI 高信号的特点。实际工作中,对此种病例做出明确诊断相当困难,病理检查是必要的,其可表现为广泛纤维组织和血窦的闭塞。鉴别诊断应该包括乏血供肿瘤,尤其是转移瘤。

伴有肝脏实质的异常:脂肪肝背景上的血管瘤,由于病灶与肝脏之间密度对比发生变化。在 CT 平扫上血管瘤可以表现为等密度,甚至高密度,动态增强 CT 能显示特征性强化表现, MRI 可更好显示其影像特征,尤其在正、反相位成像可以消除脂肪肝背景影响,同时 T_2WI 高信号和动态增强特征可以显示。

部分病灶于 CT 上外周有一圈致密环,是由于病灶压迫所致的动脉血供增加,门脉血供减少而致肝组织没有发生脂肪变。和肝细胞肝癌包膜区别在于增强后没有明显强化,与周围肝实质趋于一致。

肝硬化背景上的血管瘤,在病理检查中发生率约为 1.7%。尽管肝实质发生硬化,血管瘤通常保持其特征性表现。在部分进展期肝硬化病例中,由于纤维化的影响,其可失去典型影像特征, MRI 对于肝硬化背景上血管瘤定性比 CT 有优势,由于其内

在高组织分辨力和 T_2Wl 所提供的补充信息。

血管瘤伴存局灶性结节增生，报道发生率约20%，比一般人群发生率要高。一般病理生理机制可以解释此种高相关性，即由于局灶性肝脏血供紊乱，促使肝脏增生性反应和随后发展成良性肿瘤样变。

总之，肝脏血管瘤有其特征性CT、MRI影像特征表现，CT和MRI对其检出率和定性准确性都非常高。然而，由于病灶结构/形态的多样性和血流动力学变化，其有不典型表现的方面，认识这些不典型表现可以帮助放射科医生增加对于偶发肝脏血管瘤诊断的信心。

第四节　肝不典型海绵状血管瘤

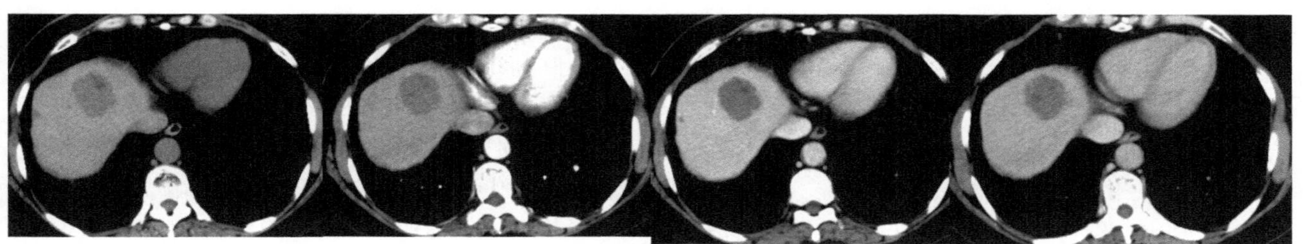

图 5-2-2　肝不典型海绵状血管瘤

病例，女，52岁。手术所见：右肋缘下取长约15cm斜切口，术中探查见右肝Ⅳ a段大小约3cm×2.5cm血管瘤，部分稍高出于肝脏表面，边界清楚，包膜完整；右肝Ⅴ段表面大小约0.5cm×1cm血管瘤，肝脏表面光滑。病理检查：红色组织一块，大小3.3cm×2.5cm×1cm，切面见一海绵状区域，大小2.5cm×2cm，部分灰白，质中偏软。病理诊断：海绵状血管瘤，周围肝细胞水肿较明显。

本病例CT增强扫描病灶轻度强化，边缘无结节状明显强化，与典型的肝血管瘤强化特点有一定的差异，由于对典型肝血管瘤影像特点具有较深的印象，诊断医师思维较固定，容易造成误诊。仔细分析本病例影像图像，病灶动脉早期既有强化，虽然强化较轻，但延迟期病灶强化仍无减退，符合肝血管瘤“早出晚归”的特点，因此考虑到不典型血管瘤（图5-2-2）。

第五节　不典型和不常见的血管瘤

肝海绵状血管瘤是最常见的肝脏良性肿瘤。CT平扫常呈均匀低密度，与邻近血管密度相仿。在脂肪肝背景下可呈相对高密度。在增强扫描时，一般早期（动脉期）呈周边结节状或弧形强化，其密度与同层面的血管密度相仿，随着时间延迟向中央渐进性充填，注药后5~7分钟，逐渐扩大至全瘤强化，强化密度逐渐降至稍高于或等于正常肝脏。

大的血管瘤往往中央有星形、大的低密度区，可以为纤维化或囊性变所致，纤维化成分可在延迟20分钟时完全充填，呈等密度，但囊变区则不会强化。

不典型和不常见的血管瘤一般表现在三个方面：不典型的形态/结构表现；不常见的强化特征；伴有肝脏实质的异常。在19%~25%的病例可见病灶周围肝实质的强化，表现为一过性肝实质强化。其他不典型的CT表现有：增强扫描强化不明显，呈点状较轻程度的强化，充填慢，可能与供血动脉较细和较大的血管间隙有关；以及中央先强化等。

小血管瘤动脉期全部强化：不典型CT表现常见于直径≤3cm的小血管瘤。小的壁薄腔大的血管瘤可以在动脉期即呈全部致密的均匀强化，不呈典型的周边结节状强化表现，但其密度往往较高，和肝细胞癌的表现相似，但两者不同的是血管瘤的强化密度更高，有作者统计，血管瘤强化后的CT值比肝细胞癌高50HU左右。有的强化与主动脉相仿，在延迟期呈高密度或等密度。另外血管瘤强化持续的时间较长，可从动脉期持续到门脉期和/或延迟期。故螺旋CT多期动态扫描是必要的，可充分显示血管瘤的强化特征，其时间-密度曲线为“快进慢出”，和肝细胞癌的“快进快出”完全不同，因此对增强早期均匀强化的血管瘤的诊断是容易的。

增强扫描强化不明显的血管瘤：慢血流低动力血管瘤表现为延迟充填，这类病例需要延长检查时间以观察到向心性强化和对比剂在病灶内滞留的表现。这种血流动力学差异可能与构成血管瘤的血窦大小有关系，大血窦为慢血流，小血窦内为高动力血流。

有的血管瘤增强扫描强化不明显，仅呈点状较轻程度的强化，充填相当慢，可能与其供血动脉较细和具有较大的血管间隙有关。这类血管瘤管壁厚腔小，对比剂进入慢，有些病灶在增强后 5 分钟才出现强化表现，但目前多数单位均使用螺旋 CT，扫描速度很快，在一般的检查过程中极少会长时间的等待，因此对这部分血管瘤的诊断有一些困难。在临床工作中，这是十分值得注意的问题。另外，罕见的是纤维性血管瘤，病灶内有大量的纤维组织增生使对比剂也难以进入。

中央先强化的血管瘤：个别小的血管瘤也可早期出现中央强化，与典型的血管瘤完全不一样，非常容易引起误诊。此类病灶在病理上表现为病灶中心为血窦，外周主要是纤维成分。

增强动脉期病灶均匀强化，门脉期和 / 或延迟期呈等密度。此种表现的血管瘤和肝细胞癌及局灶性结节样增生易于混淆，属真正意义上的不典型血管瘤。动脉期病灶强化的程度对鉴别有一定的帮助，但还需结合其他检查。

囊性和多房性血管瘤：囊性和多房性血管瘤极度少见，此种非典型特征表现为单发或多发瘤内空腔，表现为长 T_1、长 T_2 信号特点，但是外周强化仍可出现。

肝硬化背景上的血管瘤：肝硬化背景上的血管瘤，在病理检查中发生率约为 1.7%。尽管肝实质发生硬化，血管瘤通常保持其特征性表现。在部分进展期肝硬化病例中，由于纤维化的影响，其可失去典型影像特征，由于其内在高组织分辨力和 T_2WI 所提供的补充信息，MRI 对于肝硬化背景上血管瘤定性比 CT 有优势。

在上述情况下，血管瘤表现不典型，容易误诊。此时，MRI 是非常有价值的补充手段。

第六节　肝左右叶多发性巨大外生型海绵状血管瘤

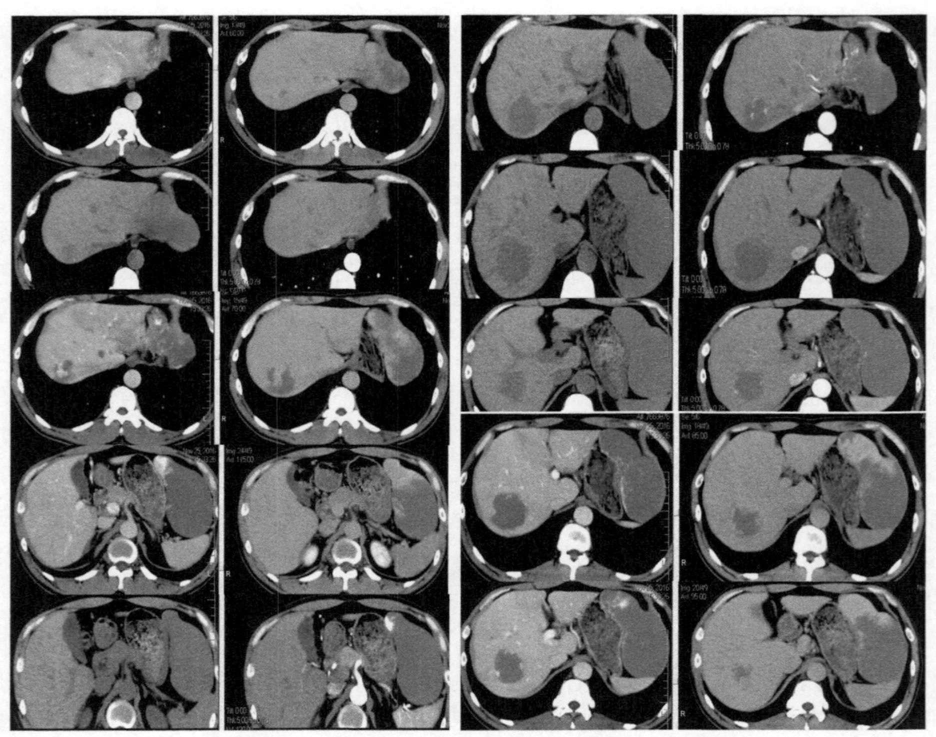

图 5-2-3　肝左右叶多发性巨大外生型海绵状血管瘤

患者，男，36 岁。体检发现肝占位性病变 3 周入院。

手术所见：腹腔内无积液，肝脏表面光滑；左肝外叶一外生性肿物，大小约 15 × 8cm，边界清楚，质软，包膜完整，与周围无明显粘连；肝右叶上段包膜下一大小约 5 × 4cm 的肿物，边界清楚，质软，包膜完整。

病理检查：左肝肿物：肝组织两块，大小分别为 8.5cm × 6cm × 2cm 和 5cm × 2cm × 1.5cm，表面呈棕黄色，大者切面见一灰白灰红色结节，直径 2.5 ㎝，呈海绵状，质软，与周围界限欠清，周围组织切面深棕，质软。右肝肿物：肝组织一块，大小 15.9cm × 10.5cm × 5cm，表面呈紫红色，光滑，切面见一灰白灰红色结节，大小 9cm × 8cm，呈海绵状，质软，与周围界限欠清，周围组织切面深棕，质软。病理诊断：左侧及右侧肝肿物切除标本：多发性海绵状血管瘤（图 5-2-3）。

第三章　肝脏局灶性结节增生

第一节　误诊病例简介:右肝炎性肌纤维细胞瘤被误诊为局灶结节性增生

病例,男,35岁。厌食、发热,尿黄近一个月入院。胸部CT发现右肝多发小斑片状稍低密度影,边界欠清楚,CT考虑右肝多发小斑片状低密度影性质待定,建议肝CT平扫+增强扫描。MRI:肝脏体积增大,表面略不平整,肝左内叶及右前叶散在多个大小不等的类圆形异常信号结节影,以右叶为主,最大者约2.4 cm×1.9 cm,T_1WI稍低信号,T_2WI压脂不均匀高信号,中央点状更高信号,边界清楚。增强扫描早期结节呈斑片状强化,内见裂隙状无强化影,静脉期及延迟期强化趋于均匀,强化程度稍减低,与周围血管分界清楚。肝门结构清楚,门脉无增宽。MRI诊断:肝内多发病灶,考虑局灶结节性增生,转移瘤待排?请结合临床。手术所见:腹腔无腹水,肝脏表面无硬化结节,肝内多发性肿瘤,最大一个肿物位于右肝Ⅵ段,大小约3.0 cm×2.0 cm,质中,边界清楚,包膜完整;胆囊无肿大。肠管、脾脏、胰腺、盆腔未见肿瘤转移。

病理检查:冰冻病理与常规病理:右肝肿物取材标本:灰红色组织一块,大小4 cm×3 cm×2 cm,切面灰红;另一肿物,大小2.0 cm×1.5 cm×1.0 cm,质软。冰冻病理诊断:右肝肿物取材标本:右肝肿物为梭形细胞病变,性质类型待定,部分切缘可见少量病变。常规病理诊断:右肝肿物取材标本:初步考虑间叶源性肿瘤,待做免疫组化检测进一步明确诊断。

免疫组化检测:阳性:Vimentin,LCA,CD68,CD163,CD31,Actin,Calponin,SMA,CD34(血管内皮+),Ki-67(+,约10%);阴性:CK(L),CK(P),CK19,CK18,CK8,P63,AFP,CD21,CD35,CD117,DOG1,Desmin,ALKP80,S-100,CD1α,PAS染色。免疫组化诊断:右肝肿物取材标本:炎性肌纤维母细胞瘤。

第二节　误诊病例简介:局灶性结节性增生与肝癌

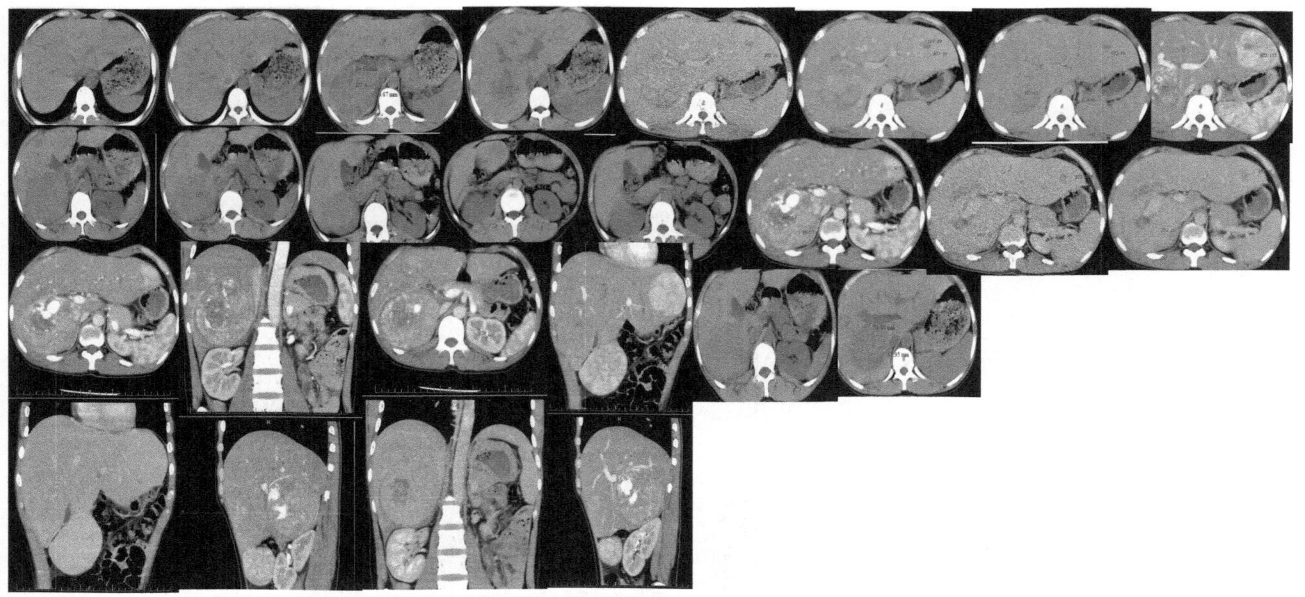

图 5-3-1　局灶性结节性增生与肝癌

患者,男性, 26 岁,车祸致右小腿疼痛畸形一小时入院。急诊 CT 示:肝内多发占位,性质待定。CT 增强扫描:右肝后下段及左肝外叶上段及内叶下段可见多发类圆形稍低密度影,密度较均匀,平扫 CT 值 36~46HU,以肝右叶明显,约 8.4 cm×9.7 cm× 11.2cm,边界清楚。增强肿块不均匀弥漫性强化, CT 值 75~86HU,内可见斑点状低密度影, CT 值 25~44HU;静脉期强化稍减低, CT 值 75~86HU,延迟期 CT 值 66~70HU,动脉期右肝病灶内可见数枚类圆形稍高密度影, CT 值 85~104HU,静脉期强化退去,最大直径约 2cm,边缘清楚。CT 诊断:原发性肝癌,多发肿块,肝内多发转移;肝硬化,脾肿大;右肾上极与肝肿瘤粘连。

病理检查:淡黄色条索状物一条,大小 1cm× 0.1 cm×0.1 cm。第一次肝占位穿刺标本:肝细胞广泛浊肿,脂肪变性,局部可见肝血窦扩张及不典型肝细胞,点状坏死。建议重取。灰白条索组织 3 条,长分别为 1.2 cm、1.2 cm、0.6 cm,直径 0.1 cm。第二次肝占位穿刺标本:结合临床甲胎蛋白血清学检测, CT 检查及第二次肝穿刺组织与第一次肝穿刺组织学图像相似,肝细胞腺瘤可能性大,免疫组化待报。(注:因标本小,即使免疫组化结果,也较难确诊)

免疫组化检测:阳性:网染、Masson、VG、CD34(血管内皮)、CD31(血管内皮)、P53(40%)、ki-67(5%);阴性: HBsAg、HBcAg、AFP、CEA、F8。免疫组化诊断:两次肝占位穿刺标本图像相似,肝小叶结构不明显,肝细胞排列不规则呈结节状,肝细胞增大、浊肿及脂肪变,有散在异型性,结合血清学甲胎蛋白、CT 及免疫组化检测结果,最终诊断为肝脏局灶性结节性增生。注:肝局灶性结节性增生、肝细胞腺瘤、高分化肝细胞癌影像学图像相似,仅靠肝穿刺活检往往很难鉴别,供参考。

该病例 4 年后来院复查 CT:肝脏体积增大,表面欠光滑,肝内可见多个大小不一肿块影,边界欠清,最大位于左肝外叶,约 9.2cm×9.7cm,平扫 CT 值 37~51HU,右肝后叶病灶内见斑片状高密度影,与右肾上极分界欠清;余肝实质颗粒稍增粗,肝内外胆管不扩张,肝门结构清楚;胆囊及脾脏未见异常。CT 诊断:肝内多发占位,局灶性结节性增生可能性大,恶性肿瘤待排,与 4 年前 CT 图像对比,右肝后叶病灶有变小,请结合临床分析研究(图 5-3-1)。

第三节　肝左外段局灶性结节性增生

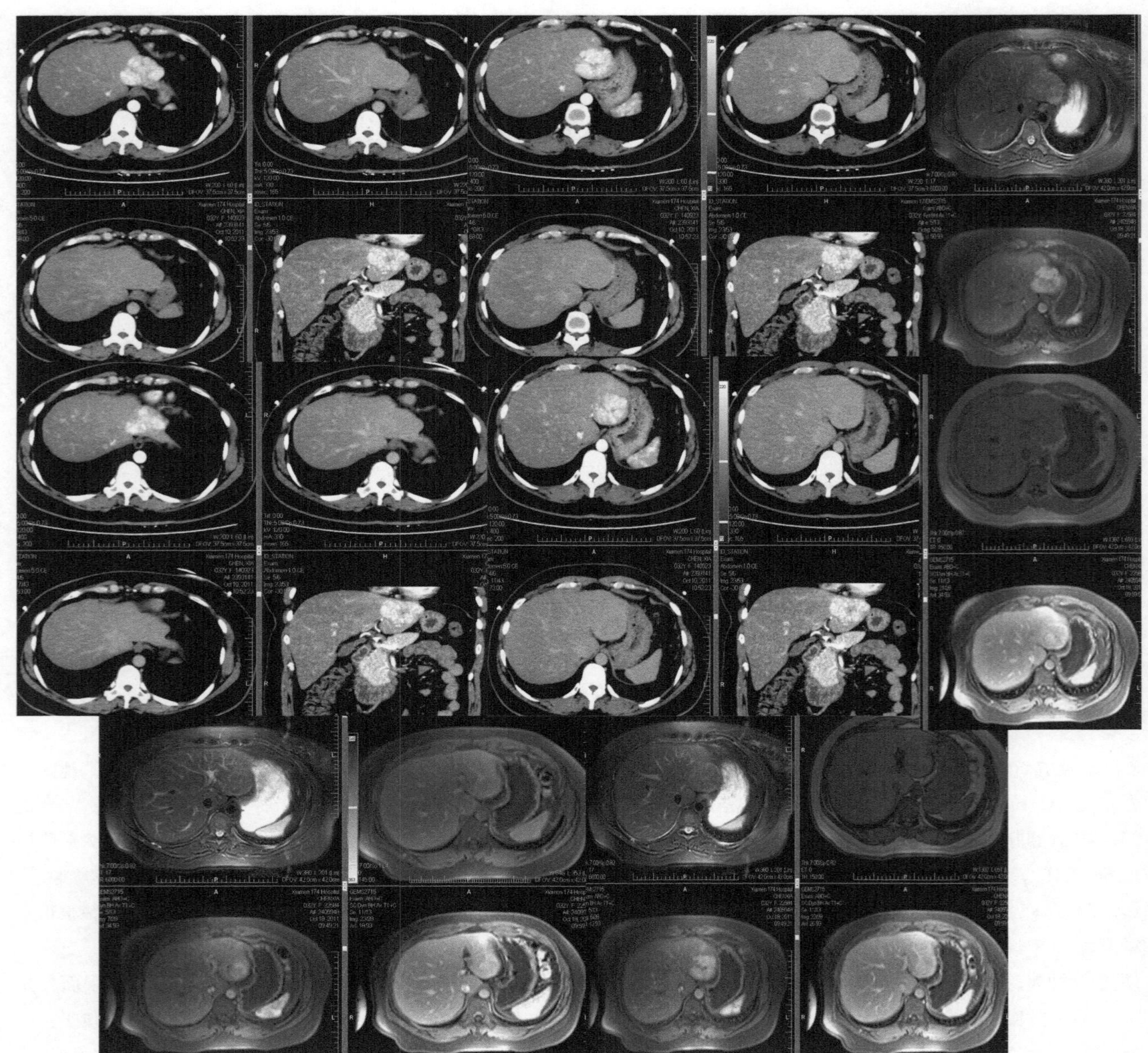

图 5-3-2　肝左外段局灶性结节性增生

患者，女，31 岁。因急性腹痛到我院急诊科就诊，平素无异常。

CT 增强扫描：左肝外侧叶 5cm × 6.5cm 肿块影，增强动脉期明显强化，CT 值 155HU，静脉期及延迟扫描强化明显减低，呈等密度改变，CT 值 85~96HU，边界不清。MRI：左肝外侧叶肿块影，T_2WI 呈不均匀稍高信号，T_1WI 呈低信号，增强动脉期呈不均匀明显强化呈高信号，静脉期及延迟扫描强化均匀，强化程度减低。

手术切除后病理诊断：局灶性结节性增生（图 5-3-2）。

第四节　肝局灶性结节性增生

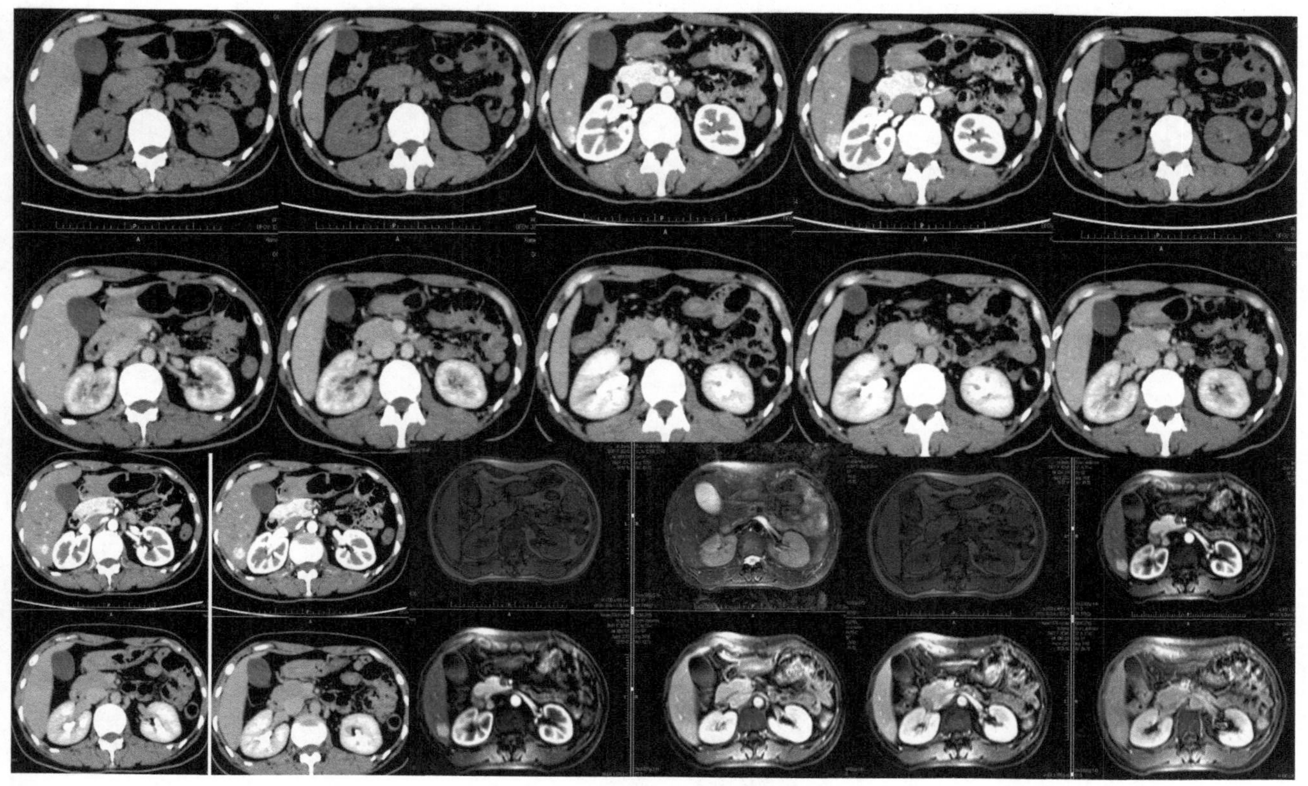

图 5-3-3　肝局灶性结节性增生

患者，女，44 岁。CT 诊断：肝右后叶结节影性质难定，小肝癌？肝腺瘤？血管瘤？肝内多发囊肿。

病理检查：灰褐色组织一块，体积 1cm × 0.7cm × 0.4cm，切面灰褐，质中。病理诊断：肝右后叶局灶性结节性再生（图 5-3-3）。

第五节　左肝局灶性结节增生

病例，男，33 岁。发现左肝占位半年入院。手术所见：腹腔无腹水，肝脏大小正常，包膜光滑，肝左外叶可见大小约 32mm × 33mm 肿块，部分呈外生性生长，边界清晰，形态规则，胆囊、胃未见明显异常。

病理检查：灰红色肝组织一块，大小 5cm × 5cm × 3cm，切面灰黄，中央见一灰红区，大小 4.5cm × 1.5cm × 1cm，质软。常规病理诊断：肝脏结节状病变，初步考虑为局灶性结节性增生。建议做免疫组化标记进一步诊断。免疫组化检测：阳性：Hepatocyte，CK18，CK8，Ki-67（+，约 1%）；阴性：CK19，CA19-9，AFP，HBsAg，HBcAg。免疫组化诊断：左肝肿物切除标本：结合免疫组化检测结果及组织学图像，符合局灶性结节性增生，伴局灶性肝细胞固缩，轻度水肿，脂肪变性。请注意复查（图 5-3-4）。

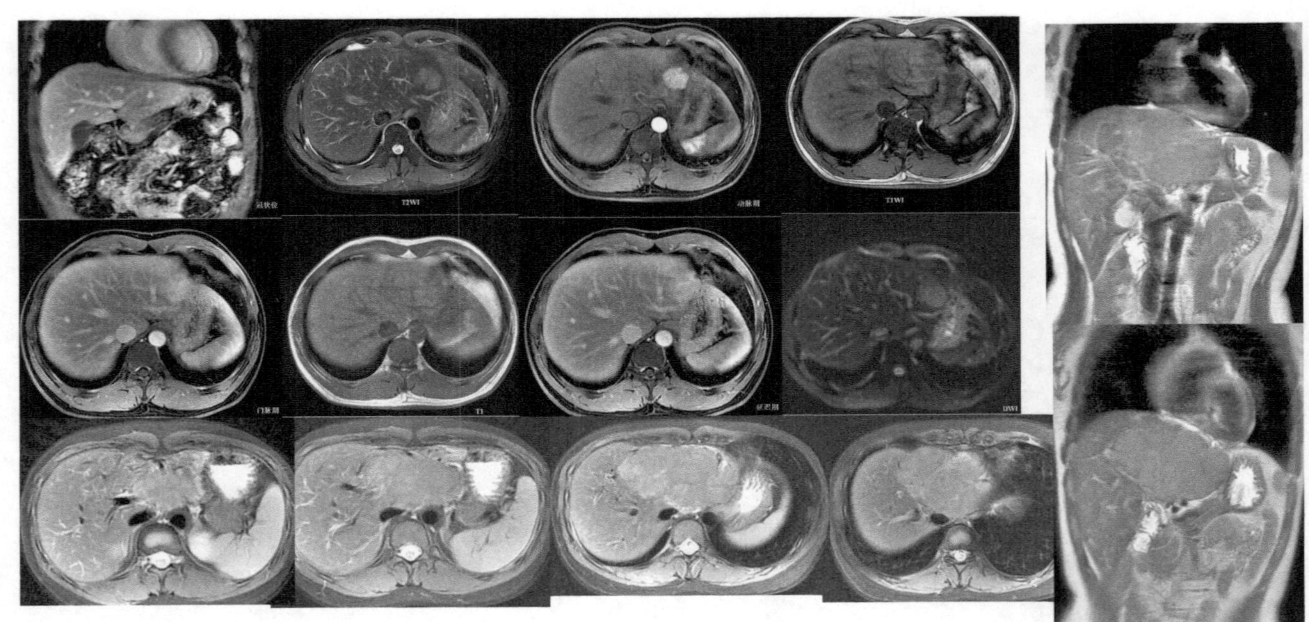

图 5-3-4　左肝局灶性结节增生

第六节　局灶性结节增生合并局灶性海绵状淋巴管瘤

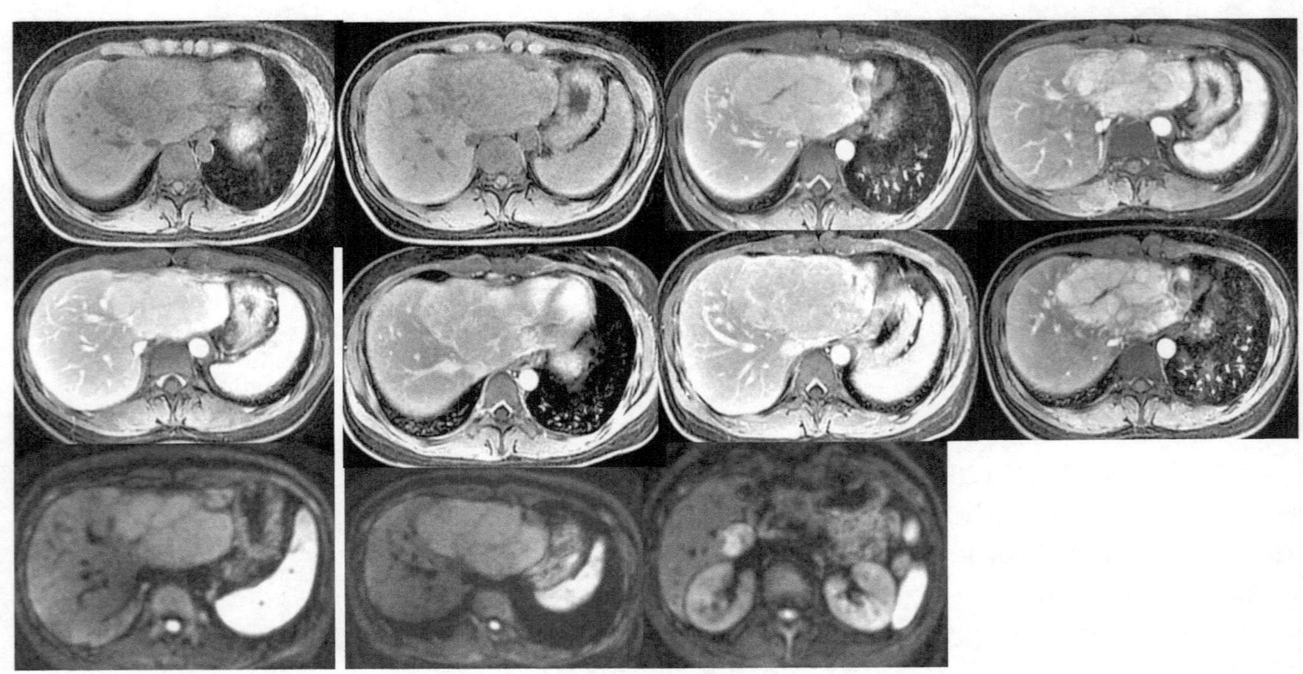

图 5-3-5　局灶性结节增生合并局灶性海绵状淋巴管瘤

患者,女,27 岁。体检发现肝占位性病变 2 天入院。

手术所见:腹腔内无腹水,肝脏质地及颜色无明显异常,胆囊未见明显异常,左半肝近膈面见一大小约 11cm × 8cm 的肿块,累及右半肝内侧约 1cm,肿块部分突出于肝表面,质中,边界清楚,右肝前叶下段脏面见一大小约 3cm × 2cm 的血管瘤,突出于肝脏表面、尾状叶萎缩。

病理检查：肝左叶：肝组织一块，大小 11.5cm × 9.5cm × 5.5cm，切面见一巨大结节，9cm × 6cm × 5cm。边界清楚，灰黄质中，呈分叶状，由多个小结节融合而成，最大者大小 3.3 × 3cm，最小者大小 2.2cm × 1.3cm，局部见灰白条索。肝脏一侧见一紫红色结节，大小 3cm × 2.2cm × 1.5cm。病理诊断：局灶性结节增生合并局灶性海绵状淋巴管瘤（图 5-3-5）。

第七节　肝局灶结节性增生

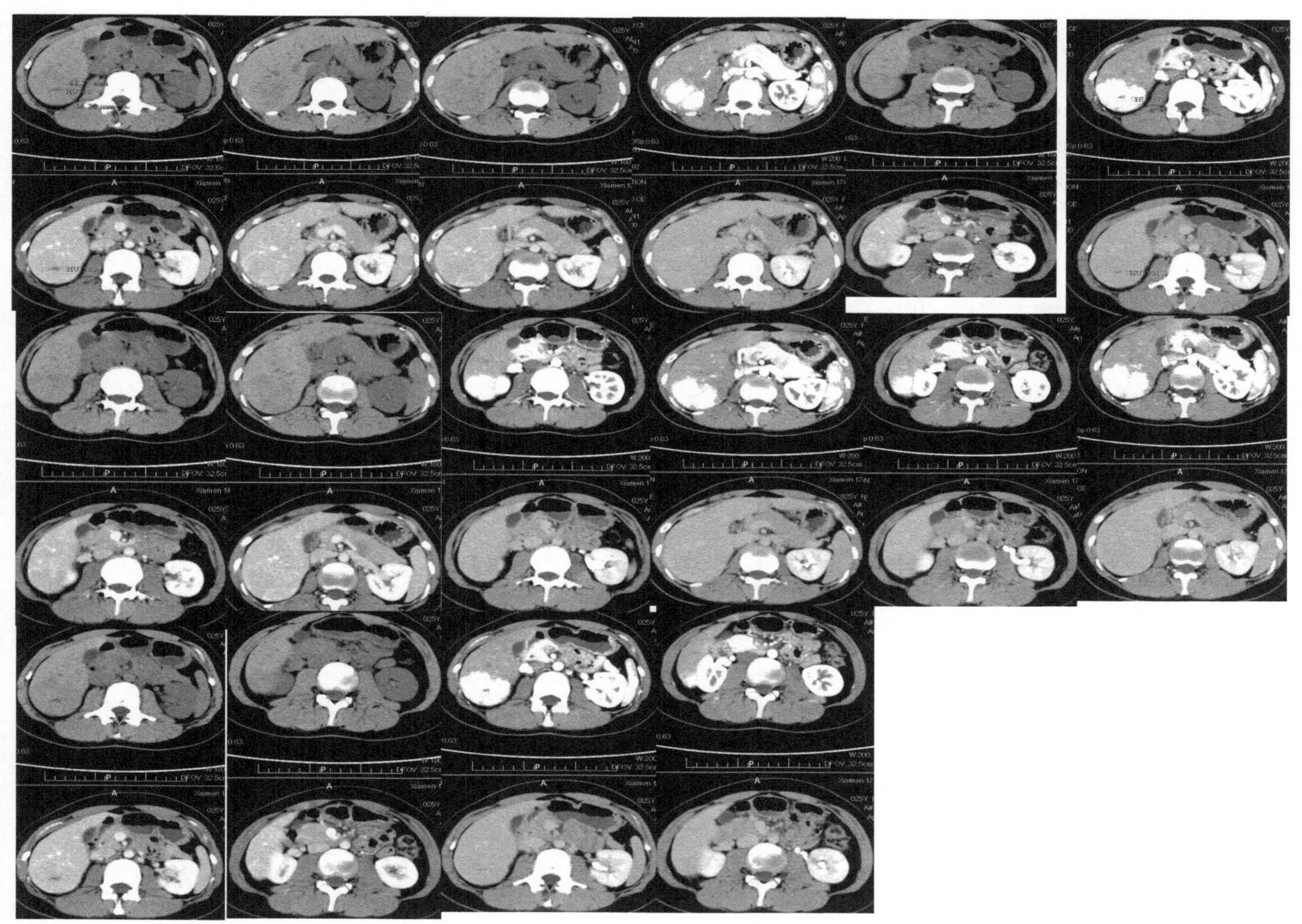

图 5-3-6　肝局灶结节性增生

患者，女，25 岁。因发现肝占位性病变半年余入院。手术所见：腹腔无腹水，肝脏表面无硬化结节，肿瘤位于右肝后叶第 6 段外侧，大小约 6 cm × 4cm，质软，红润，边界清楚，包膜完整；余肝脏未扪及明显肿物，腹腔淋巴结未触及明显肿大。肠管、脾脏、胰腺、盆腔未见明显异常。 病理检查：右肝肿物切除标本：灰黄色组织两块，总体积 7.5cm × 6.5cm × 4.5cm，切面灰黄，质软，境界不清。常规病理诊断：右肝肿物切除标本：肝组织结节状增生，具体类型待做免疫组化检测进一步明确诊断。免疫组化检测：阳性：Hepatocyte，CK18，CK8，CD34，Ki-67（+，约 2%）；阴性：CK19，CA19-9，AFP，HBcAg，HBsAg。免疫组化诊断：右肝肿物切除标本：结合免疫组化结果，符合肝局灶结节性增生（FNH）（图 5-3-6）。

第八节 局灶性结节增生之不典型表现

肝脏局灶性结节增生是肝内少见的肿瘤样病变,并非真正的肿瘤。它属于少见的良性局灶性富血供肝实质占位性病变,无潜在恶变。自从 Edmondson(1958)在病理学明确以来,欧美报告较多,日本及中国报告较少。目前发病机制尚不清楚,有学者认为先天性血管畸形导致肝细胞结节增生可能是原因之一。

局灶性结节增生多见于女性,可能与雌激素刺激血管畸形发展和肝细胞的增生有关,但与口服避孕药和其他类固醇类无密切关系,也可发生于小儿,在儿童(0~16 岁),局灶性结节增生仅占肝脏肿瘤的 0.02%。常为单发,约 20% 为多发,易发生于肝被膜下,深部少见,边界大多清楚,其病理特征为肿块内部有放射状纤维瘢痕组织由内向外分布构成辐条状纤维分隔,隔内含动脉、静脉及增生的胆管,但无包膜。临床上多见于 30~50 岁女性,无特异性症状,多偶然发现,可表现为腹痛、腹部肿块,少数病例可自发性破裂而大出血,约占 2.5%。

局灶性结节增生于 1975 年被 WHO 使用,并在 1976 年被国际肝脏研究协会采纳,沿用至今。影像学诊断的关键在于病灶的特征,近年来多种影像方法诊断局灶性结节增生的研究较多。B 超检查无特异性,既往 CT 对局灶性结节增生术前定性诊断符合率较低,主要是以前常规 CT 成像速度慢,其次是此病少见,对其认识不足。随着 CT 技术的改进,双期或三期增强扫描可充分反映肝内病灶的血供特点和强化特征,从而大大提高了该病的术前诊断符合率,避免不必要的外科手术。

局灶性结节增生的病理特点:局灶性结节增生的病因现在尚未了解清楚,先天性血管畸形或血管损伤可能是肝细胞增生的潜在机制。体内或体外的雌激素对病灶生长有一定作用。局灶性结节增生是富血供实质性肿块,其内部结构均匀,出血和坏死少见。局灶性结节增生由肝细胞、胆管、枯否细胞及血管组成。病灶中心有星状瘢痕及辐射状纤维分隔,瘢痕内有厚壁供血动脉。镜下局灶性结节增生可见纤维分隔和增生的肝细胞区,在局灶性结节增生中心缺乏正常的中央静脉和门静脉。瘢痕内也可见到胆管但不和胆管树相连。有时可见急、慢性炎性细胞。

局灶性结节增生的血流动力学特征:离心性血液供应,局灶性结节增生有 1 条或多条供血动脉由病灶中心向周围呈辐射状分布。血管造影时,大的局灶性结节增生 57%~90% 可显示离心性血供,但小局灶性结节增生很难显示这些血管。

血液引流途径:显微镜下,在邻近病灶的正常肝组织内、病灶与肝组织连接区及大的星状瘢痕内,均可见到大的同心或偏心性厚壁静脉。一些作者报道用胶凝剂注射到尸体的肝动脉和门静脉内,证实局灶性结节增生的血液引流途径有两条:①血液直接引流到病灶周围肝组织的中心静脉或肝静脉。②局灶性结节增生内血窦直接引流到周围肝窦。

多期增强扫描常规显示病灶血管:评价局灶性结节增生理想的 CT 扫描技术是动脉、门静脉双期螺旋 CT 扫描,延迟扫描(2~5 分钟)有利于显示中心瘢痕的强化和肿瘤周围包膜样强化环。

(1)肿瘤强化特征:早期肿块呈快速明显的均匀强化(动脉期和门静脉早期),在门静脉后期或延迟扫描可见对比剂迅速退出呈等密度。这种强化特征是由于局灶性结节增生有丰富的动脉血供及大的引流静脉和血窦。

(2)肿瘤周围血管影:在门静脉晚期和延迟扫描图像上,局灶性结节增生周围可见血管影,这与肿瘤周围扩大的血管、血窦有关。这些大的引流血管已被彩色多普勒证实。通常,这些血管围绕肿块呈不完整的强化环,易误认为是包膜强化。

(3)增粗的供血动脉:有作者认为局灶性结节增生是一种先天性血管畸形,动脉血流灌注增加导致肝细胞增生。血管造影可显示这些肿瘤异常增粗的供血肝动脉,在动脉期螺旋 CT 扫描也常能显示异常动脉。

(4)瘢痕和分隔:显微镜下几乎所有的局灶性结节增生均可见中心瘢痕。然而在 CT 上仅有 1/3 可以显示。瘢痕在平扫时呈低密度,增强扫描动脉期,瘢痕内可显示供血动脉,在门静脉期和延迟扫描时可见瘢痕逐渐强化呈等或高密度。有时在增强时可显示辐射状纤维分隔。Carlson 等报道 45 例中,可显示瘢痕 27 例(60%),17 例延迟扫描中 12 例呈低密度（12%），显示辐射状分隔5例（11%）。

多期增强扫描反映病灶的内部结构：多期增强扫描CT扫描检查能很好反映病灶的内部结构。从一组资料来看，大部分局灶性结节增生的CT表现具有一定的特征性，中央见星状延迟强化的瘢痕和病灶明显强化且呈"快进慢出"的典型者较易诊断。Procacci等（1992）认为局灶性结节增生的CT诊断敏感度约70%，特异度91.5%。一般CT平扫表现为低密度或等密度的肝内占位，少有钙化；动脉期多呈均匀高密度明显强化。目前，动脉期病灶的中央或周边出现明显增粗迂曲的血管（供血动脉）亦认为是局灶性结节增生的一个特征征象，但该组仅有6例可见到这种特征表现，动脉期病灶中央的瘢痕组织一般无强化；门脉期及延迟期病灶多呈略高密度或等密度，少数呈低密度，但中央瘢痕延迟强化呈星芒状高密度，具有较特征性表现。

多期增强扫描与细小的中央瘢痕：据统计约有31%的局灶性结节增生病灶可见中央瘢痕。该组平扫显示7个伴有中央星状瘢痕者，多期增强扫描CT显示15个病灶有中央瘢痕，两者显示率有显著性差异（$\chi^2=6.125$，$P=0.0133<0.05$），提示多期增强扫描扫描的瘢痕显示率明显高于平扫，尤其是动脉期在局灶性结节增生病灶明显强化的衬托下，相对低密度的星芒状瘢痕易于识别。由此可见多期增强扫描对细小的中央瘢痕显示率较高，因此，对怀疑局灶性结节增生病灶进行多期增强薄层扫描在其诊断与鉴别诊断显得尤为重要；同时该组资料结果亦提示与直径<3.0cm病灶比，直径>3.0cm病灶的中央瘢痕结构出现率明显较高，两者的瘢痕出现率有显著性差异（$\chi^2=6.2391$，$P=0.0125<0.05$）。但中央瘢痕也并非局灶性结节增生特有，纤维板层肝细胞癌、海绵状血管瘤及肝腺瘤也可见，但多表现为相对不规则的星芒状形态结构。

一些作者指出不典型的局灶性结节样增生有以下几点表现：年龄：80%~95%的局灶性结节样增生发生于30~40岁的妇女，而在儿童期（0~16岁），其发病率仅占肝脏肿瘤的2%。肿瘤大小：85%的局灶性结节样增生直径<5cm，12%在5~10cm之间，而3%的局灶性结节样增生病灶的直径>10cm。大的病灶可引起症状，如腹部疼痛，可扪及肿块。病灶多发。病灶内出血、坏死和脂肪堆积。是极为少见的表现，因多数局灶性结节样增生呈密度均匀的实质性肿块。无中心瘢痕。有些病例其中心瘢痕特别小，在CT上无法显示，约占16%~40%。这类病例有时和肝实质的密度一致甚至不能发现，仅表现为肝脏轮廓的改变和邻近血管的受压。假包膜样强化。以往认为局灶性结节样增生无包膜，而且这是和肝细胞癌鉴别的一个重要特征。但也有文献报道，局灶性结节样增生可以有假包膜，不过概率很低。包膜的出现表明病灶的生长缓慢，使周围正常肝实质受压。包膜由增厚的、透明的纤维组织构成。须注意勿将正常受压的血管或增粗的、病灶周围的滋养血管误认为包膜。部分中心瘢痕无强化。此类瘢痕为胶原性的，和腺瘤、纤维板层样肝细胞癌等的瘢痕一样缺乏血管，因此增强扫描后无强化表现。以上列举的几点局灶性结节样增生不典型表现，从局部看虽为不典型，但从整体分析也许仍较典型，不影响诊断。如病灶的大小，年龄并非关键因素。中心瘢痕显示高度提示诊断，延迟强化则更为可靠。

不典型影像学表现：部分局灶性结节增生血供特点不典型、无瘢痕显示或瘢痕强化的非特异性造成一组病例中2例误诊为原发性肝癌，另1例未明确定性的主要原因是对CT增强三期扫描时间掌握不准，造成动脉期、门脉期时相有误，影响对病灶血供特点的分析。

局灶性结节增生不典型CT主要表现如下：

（1）血供特点不典型：该组病例局灶性结节增生的非典型表现有：动脉期强化不显著；或出现动脉-门脉、动脉-静脉分流出现对比剂早退，在门脉期及延迟期呈低密度；延迟期出现包膜样强化等。

（2）病灶密度不均匀和/或钙化：由于局灶性结节增生血供非常丰富，除中央瘢痕外，病灶密度多较均匀，其内很少见到出血、坏死和钙化，该组有2个见钙化，1个见不规则坏死；有作者报道3例妇女局灶性结节增生中有局灶性梗死，她们均有口服避孕药史，CT扫描示密度不均。

（3）脂肪积累：局灶性结节增生的脂肪积累很少见。该组资料见1例经二次肝穿病理证实伴脂肪变性和坏死。文献一般认为局灶性结节增生中的脂肪是患者基础疾病所致，即肝脏脂肪变性。常见的基础疾病有肥胖、酒精中毒、糖尿病、蛋白质吸收障碍、营养不良等。

（4）局灶性结节增生内未见中央瘢痕：有文献报道有部分病例在病理上确实未能找到中央瘢痕，但有部分病例仅因中央瘢痕过于细小，CT扫描未能明确显示（16%~40%）。在这些病例，病灶常很难显示,仅表现为肝脏边缘膨隆、变形或肝脏血管移位。

(5)中央瘢痕不强化或动脉期就出现强化:少数病例中央瘢痕在CT增强扫描时未见强化,可能与瘢痕中增生血管腔的闭塞有关,而动脉期强化主要因为部分病灶的瘢痕内含有较粗大的滋养动脉血管,易与肝细胞腺瘤、肝纤维板层样癌、肝细胞癌或肝内胆管细胞癌等中见到的胶原瘢痕相混淆。

不典型的MRI表现与分析:另组11例中有少数病例表现不典型,导致在诊断上误诊为肝恶性肿瘤和与血管瘤。该组4个病灶信号不均匀,结节内见杂乱的条片状长T_1、长T_2信号,同时见小囊变区。增强扫描表现为动脉期轻中度不均匀强化,延迟期病灶大部分低于正常肝组织,且信号不均匀,病理证实为局灶性结节增生。病理可见脂肪变性、坏死灶,并有血窦明显扩张。Alltal等(2003)报道13例毛细血管扩张型局灶性结节增生的影像学表现,指出影像学的不均匀在对应的病理上也表现为不均匀,主要原因是灶内有出血、脂肪变性、坏死灶,并有血窦明显扩张。

关于假包膜,Hussain等(2004)认为受压的肝实质、绕行的血管与炎性反应等因素所致。该组2例患者出现包膜样改变,为局灶性结节增生不常见的表现,病理表现为局灶性结节增生周围纤维组织增生所形成的假包膜,说明局灶性结节增生也可有假包膜的存在。随着影像诊断水平提高,观察逐渐细致,假包膜出现率也可提高,因此,应该认识到假包膜不单为恶性肿瘤的征象。

该组病例中3例患者可见占位效应,周围可见胆管受压、移位,其中1例患者结节压迫肝门区,可见肝左叶胆管明显扩张,类似恶性肿瘤生物学行为。

1例患者病灶体积较小,最大径仅为2 cm,呈明显长T_1、长T_2改变,增强扫描于动脉期与延迟期呈结节样强化,信号均匀。表现类似肝脏海绵状血管瘤。但在延迟期于病灶中央见点状高信号强化灶,考虑为瘢痕组织。通过此病例体会到应细致观察病变特点,综合分析才可得出正确诊断。对于不典型局灶性结节增生,需要综合分析其MRI平扫及动态增强表现,结合临床资料多数可以作出正确诊断。

关于枯否细胞:局灶性结节样增生含有枯否细胞,因此可以反映枯否细胞活动的影像学技术均可用于局灶性结节样增生的诊断。80%的局灶性结节样增生可吸收^{99m}Tc,但腺瘤和肝细胞癌也可吸收^{99m}Tc,但吸收量不如局灶性结节样增生多,因此^{99m}Tc的浓聚可提示局灶性结节样增生的诊断,但并非病理诊断。

肝细胞特异性对比剂如Gd-EOB-DTPA或Mn-DPDP等也可用于诊断,局灶性结节样增生含正常肝细胞因而可以吸收Gd-EOB-DTPA或Mn-DPDP而明显强化,表明病灶为肝细胞性,其强化的程度高,峰值持续的时间长,和肝细胞癌有别,但和高分化的肝细胞癌相似。而且中心瘢痕的显示率提高。网状内皮细胞特异性对比剂如SPIO也可被局灶性结节样增生中的枯否细胞吞噬,病灶的信号在T_2WI上受到抑制。该项检查同样可与肝细胞癌、转移灶等区分,但高分化肝细胞癌也可枯否细胞,须结合其他资料综合分析。

鉴别诊断:肝细胞癌主要由肝动脉供血,大多呈"快进快出"强化特征;局灶性结节增生多呈"快进慢出"强化特征。肝细胞癌部分病灶有假包膜,边界清楚;局灶性结节增生无包膜,平扫大部分病灶边界不清。临床甲胎蛋白增高者,则提示肝细胞癌可能。肝细胞癌常有裂隙状低密度坏死区,增强后无强化;而局灶性结节增生往往仅中央有低密度瘢痕区,且多有延迟强化。肝细胞癌常可见门脉癌栓及淋巴结转移等恶性肿瘤的表现,而局灶性结节增生为良性病变。

血管瘤:局灶性结节增生还需和血管瘤鉴别。局灶性结节增生与肝血管瘤的鉴别关键在于两者的强化方式。典型的血管瘤其增强方式为早期从周边开始呈结节状或环形强化,逐渐向中心推进,延迟期呈等密度或高密度充填,而局灶性结节增生从病灶中心开始强化并向周边迅速推进,除中央瘢痕外呈均匀强化;其次血管瘤平扫边界大多清楚,而局灶性结节增生多边界模糊。部分不典型小血管瘤动脉期病灶亦可全部充填,门脉期、延迟期呈略高密度或等密度,与局灶性结节增生鉴别困难,此时MRI的检查有利于两者的鉴别,血管瘤在T_2WI上呈"灯泡征"。此外,还应注意与肝腺瘤、纤维板层肝细胞癌等相鉴别。

总之,CT平扫及多期增强扫描检查能较全面显示局灶性结节增生的病理特征和血供特点,明显提高与其他富血管恶性肿瘤的鉴别诊断能力,对部分不典型者,必要时做穿刺活检以明确诊断。

第九节　右肝局灶性结节性增生

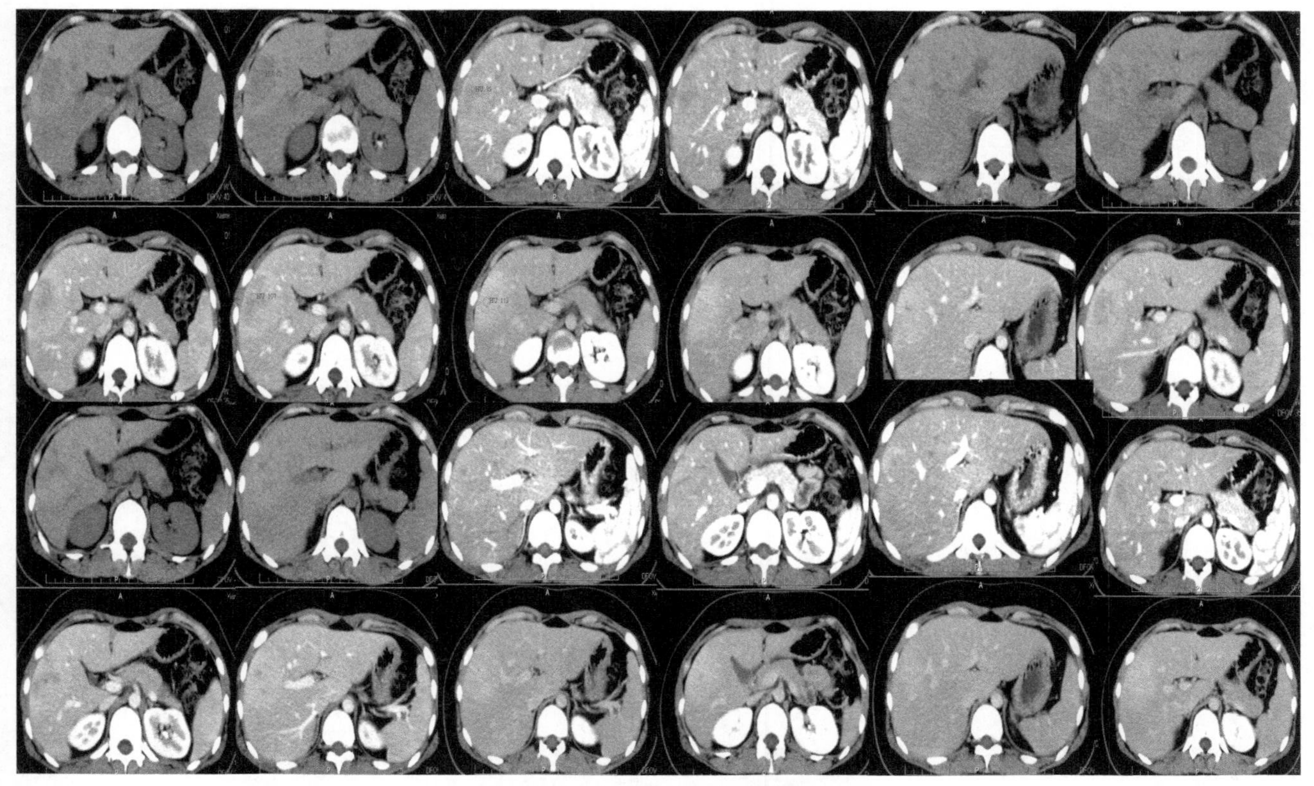

图 5-3-7　右肝局灶性结节性增生

患者,女，15 岁。体检发现肝占位性病变 1 周入院。病理检查:肝脏肿物穿刺活检标本:穿刺组织两条,长分别为 1.5cm 和 1.6cm,直径均为 0.1cm。常规病理诊断:肝脏肿物穿刺活检标本:镜下示送检肝组织肝小叶及汇管区结构存在,汇管区纤维组织增生,倾向良性病变,待做免疫组化及组织化学特染检测进一步协助诊断。免疫组化检测:阳性:CK18，Hepatocyte(小灶+)，Masson 染色，CK19(小胆管+)，CK8，CK7(小胆管+),网染，Ki-67(+，<2%);阴性:CK20,GPC3,CD34,CD10,CEA,Vimentin,AFP。免疫组化诊断:肝脏肿物穿刺活检标本:结合免疫组化及组织化学特染检测结果,符合肝良性病变,结合影像学提示,倾向于肝局灶性结节性增生,请结合临床(图 5-3-7)。

第十节　肝脏局灶结节增生不典型 CT 表现

肝脏局灶结节增生在西方国家发病率较高,我国近几年发病率也明显增高,目前局灶性结节样增生在肝脏良性肿瘤中的发病率仅次于血管瘤居第二位。中青年女性多见。

早期文献认为局灶性结节样增生的发生与使用避孕药有关,目前的研究认为雌激素与局灶性结节样增生的发病机制无关。

目前认为局灶性结节样增生是肝脏细胞对血管发育异常或损伤的一种增生性反应,由正常形态的肝细胞围绕富于胆管和血管的纤维结缔组织间隔生长,间隔中有枯否细胞等。

大体病理特点为无包膜、轮廓光整的良性肝脏肿物。中央为“星状瘢痕”,瘢痕内有一条或数条较大的动脉,也可以有门静脉,但动脉与静脉的关系与正常门脉汇管区者不同。瘢痕内有增生的胆管，其管径较动脉小，还有结缔组织及炎性细胞。

局灶性结节样增生多为单发实性肿物，约7%~20% 为多灶，好发于肝脏的游离缘。局灶性结节样增生无特征性的临床症状、体征及实验室检查异常，常由影像检查偶然发现。

CT 平扫局灶性结节样增生表现为等密度或略低密度影。局灶性结节样增生血供丰富，并由肝动脉供血，增强扫描动脉期表现为均匀的明显强化影。门静脉期密度下降表现为高密度或略高密度，延迟后平衡期扫描表现为高密度、略高密度或等密度，可能与局灶性结节样增生的结构异常、对比剂的排泄及廓清较慢有关，与肝癌的“快进快出”不同，表现为“快进慢出”。

19%~78% 的病灶内有纤维分隔或瘢痕，动脉期和门静脉期为低密度，延迟扫描纤维分隔或瘢痕可表现为高密度或仍为低密度。文献报道 1.4% 的局灶性结节样增生含有钙化。

局灶性结节样增生的不典型影像表现并不少见，可能与其细胞增生及不典型增生等有关。局灶性结节样增生不典型表现有：CT 平扫呈不均匀的低密度，增强扫描呈低血供，有假包膜及钙化等，无中心瘢痕和纤维分隔等。

不典型的局灶性结节样增生也需与肝腺瘤、肝细胞癌鉴别，用 ^{99m}Tc 硫胶做核素显像，由于局灶性结节样增生内有枯否细胞，可浓聚核素，而肝细胞癌及肝腺瘤无浓聚。

第十一节 肝局灶结节性增生

患者，男，21 岁。体检发现肝内占位 5 月入院。

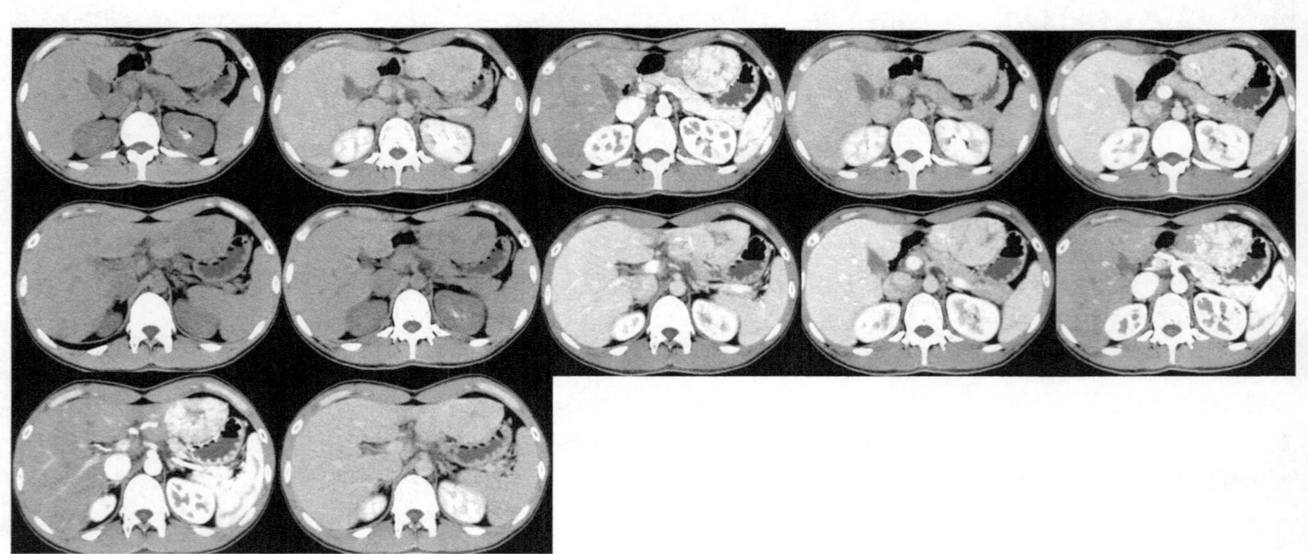

图 5-3-8 肝局灶结节性增生

手术所见：腹腔无腹水，左肝外叶下缘可见一大小约 7cm × 5cm 肿物，突出肝脏表面，胃大弯侧受推挤移位，与周围膈肌、网膜无粘连，胆囊大小约 5cm × 4cm，与周边无粘连。病理检查：左肝肿瘤切除标本：肝组织一块，大小 7.5cm × 7.5cm × 4.5cm，肝被膜完整，表面凹凸不平，切面灰褐，可见瘢痕样纤维间隔，呈分叶状，质中。常规病理诊断：左肝肿瘤切除标本：初步考虑肝局灶结节性增生，待做免疫组化检测及组织化学特染进一步证实。免疫组化检测：阳性：Hepatocyte（肝细胞 +），CK19（小胆管 +），Vimentin（纤维间隔 +），CD34（肝窦 +），网染，Nasson 染色，CK18（肝细胞 +），CK8（肝细胞 +），AAT（肝细胞 +），AACT（肝细胞 +），Ki-67（+，约 3%）；阴性：CD10，CEA，AFP。免疫组化诊断：左肝肿瘤切除标本：免疫组化检测及组织化学特染结果支持肝局灶结节性增生（图 5-3-8）。

第十二节　关于肝脏局灶性结节增生的鉴别诊断

按照 WHO 的病理学诊断标准，是指肝实质增生并被星形纤维瘢痕间隔成结节状，很少并发出血，也无肯定恶变。

局灶性结节增生与恶性肿瘤的鉴别：原发性肝细胞癌：本症主要是与甲胎蛋白阴性的原发性肝细胞癌鉴别。①局灶性结节增生以青壮年多见，肝细胞癌以中老年多见；局灶性结节增生大多没有肝炎、肝硬化病史，且肝功能基本正常，而肝细胞癌患者则相反。②局灶性结节增生多呈“快进慢出”的增强方式，肝细胞癌多呈“快进快出”的增强方式；局灶性结节增生及肝细胞癌均由肝动脉供血，但局灶性结节增生内动脉呈由中央向四周放射状，肝细胞癌内血管纡曲不规则，常伴动 - 静脉瘘及动 - 门脉瘘。③多数局灶性结节增生中央见低密度瘢痕区，瘢痕延迟增强，肝细胞癌内多见片状不规则低密度坏死区，无增强。④由于局灶性结节增生的假包膜为压迫周围正常组织以及一些灶周血管和炎性浸润，因此在 T_2 上为高信号（特征性），而且可能会有延迟强化。而肝细胞癌的假包膜主要为纤维成分在 T_1，T_2 上为低信号，增强扫描的延迟期呈持续强化。⑤肝细胞癌可见门脉癌栓及淋巴结转移的恶性肿瘤征象，而局灶性结节增生无此征象。

纤维板层型肝癌：局灶性结节增生一般发生于年轻及中年女性；局灶性结节增生病灶最大径很少超过 5cm；局灶性结节增生钙化少见，有文献报道少于 2%；两者中心瘢痕信号的不同及强化表现的不同；两者包膜信号的不同。纤维板层型肝癌约 68% 的患者有钙化，可为星状或结节状，并且常伴有其他恶性指征，如淋巴结肿大、转移、胆管、血管侵犯。

肝转移瘤：有原发灶病史，常为多发，增强特点为动脉期周边环状增强，逐渐向中央充填，呈典型的“牛眼征”。

局灶性结节增生与良性肿瘤的鉴别：①肝腺瘤：局灶性结节增生比肝腺瘤更常见，发病率约为腺瘤的 2 倍，且与口服避孕药无关。约 80%~95% 为单发。肝腺瘤多见于长期口服避孕药的育龄期妇女，是比较少见的富血供良性肿瘤，其与肝局灶性结节增生的造影表现相似。肝腺瘤影像表现为，动脉期病灶内部可迅速出现较均匀增强改变，门脉期上病灶仍可保持强化状态，最后表现为低密度，其边界不清。对于肝内出现生长缓慢、信号均匀、有包膜、不侵犯血管的肿块，结合患者的病史特点，应考虑本病可能（见表 5-3-2）。

表 5-3-2　局灶性结节增生与肝腺瘤的影像学鉴别要点

病变类型	中央瘢痕	不均质*	强化不均匀	被膜下供血动脉	动脉期强化程度	门脉期瘤体强化程度	出血	T_1WI 高信号	Gd-BOPTA** 延迟摄取
FNH	+	-	-	-	>	+	-	+/-	+
腺瘤	-	+	+	+	<	++	+/-	+/-	-

注：动脉期局灶性结节增生强化程度远高于腺瘤；局灶性结节增生强化率 >1.6（动脉期衰减值与平扫时衰减值比）；腺瘤强化率 <1.6。在门静脉期局灶性结节增生常为等密度，而腺瘤则为高密度；*：含 CT 密度与 MRI 信号强度；**：中译名为钆贝葡胺莫迪司

②肝海绵状血管瘤 CT 平扫密度为低密度，以均匀多见，诊断难度较大。而 MRI 平扫时，肝脏血管瘤在 T_1WI 呈均匀等信号或稍低信号，但在 T_2WI 呈均匀的高信号并随回波时间延长而信号强度增高，且病变边界清楚，称为“灯泡征”，诊断的准确性较高。CT 和 MRI 的血管瘤增强所见相一致，动脉期病灶内部无明显增强改变，在门静脉期或实质期，病灶出现环球状或周边增强，呈向心性填充，充填时间常需 2min，持续达数分钟。因此 CT 和 MRI 综合分析对大多数肝脏血管瘤可作出定性诊断。

MSCTA 三维重建可以更加充分显示局灶性结节增生增粗的供血动脉、引流静脉、假包膜、中心瘢痕、纤维间隔及网格状强化，这些特征性表现可以在不需要病理及其他检查的情况下正确诊断局灶性结节增生，具有重要价值。

肝细胞癌、肝血管瘤、肝腺瘤均无网格状强化方式、无独立的引流静脉，病灶中心低密度区无强化可与局灶性结节增生鉴别。

总之，CT 和 MRI 平扫及三期增强扫描检查能较全面地显示局灶性结节增生的病理特征及血供特点，提高与肝内其他富血供肿瘤的鉴别诊断能力，对于部分不典型病例，肝脏穿刺活检是确诊的主要手

段，对有乙型肝炎病毒感染证据、甲胎蛋白阴性的肝脏实质性占位者，应特别慎重做出“肝癌”的诊断，此时应作穿刺进行细胞学检查，有利于提高局灶性结节增生诊断率。

第十三节　肝脏多发性局灶性结节增生

肝脏局灶性结节增生以前普遍认为是一种少见的肿瘤样病变，近年来，由于腹部动态增强扫描检查能够发现在 MRI 平扫上呈等信号的病灶，从而使局灶性结节增生的检出率大幅上升。局灶性结节增生是继血管瘤后，第二种常见的良性局灶性肝实质性病变，由肝细胞、发育不良的小胆管和枯否细胞构成，发病率约为 0.7%~1.2%，其病因是肝动静脉血管畸形，肝血流持续增加引起周围肝组织假瘤样增生。

由 3 名经验丰富的 MR 医师分析每例多发局灶性结节增生的 MR 影像表现与诊断。多发局灶性结节增生按如下 MR 表现诊断：无瘢痕的病灶 T_1WI 常为稍低或等信号、T_2WI 呈稍高或等信号。注射 Gd-DTPA 后，动脉期中度至显著均匀强化、门静脉期和延迟期逐渐呈等或稍高信号。

病灶内出现中心或偏心瘢痕则病灶表现为 T_1WI 不均匀低或等信号、T_2WI 不均匀稍高或等信号。病灶内瘢痕在 T_1WI 上呈低信号、T_2WI 上呈高信号。注射 Gd-DTPA 后，动脉期病灶呈中度至明显不均匀强化，门静脉及延迟期逐渐廓清，病灶内瘢痕动脉期未见强化、门静脉期和延迟期瘢痕逐渐强化。中央瘢痕是局灶性结节增生的特征性表现，如果病灶内出现中央瘢痕有利于局灶性结节增生的诊断。

局灶性结节增生多见于年轻女性，2~5 个局灶性结节增生的病例可高达 20%~30%，5 个以上局灶性结节增生少见。多发局灶性结节增生同时伴有血管瘤，血管畸形和（或）颅内肿瘤则称之为多发局灶性结节增生综合征。该组 9 例均符合多发局灶性结节增生综合征定义。

局灶性结节增生的发病机制未明，目前普遍认为与血管畸形或血管损伤有关。病理上局灶性结节增生由异常排列的肝细胞组成，根据其内部表现的不同被分为典型局灶性结节增生和不典型局灶性结节增生。此外瘢痕是局灶性结节增生的特征性表现，该组中 16 个病灶出现瘢痕，瘢痕 T_2WI 呈稍高信号，其形成机制为病灶中心瘢痕内的结构如（血管、胆管）及其周边的炎性反应等。

Grazioli 等（2001）认为在直径 >30 mm 的局灶性结节增生中瘢痕的出现是典型局灶性结节增生的重要特征。该组 12 个病灶 T_1WI 呈高信号，光学显微镜下可见局灶出血，故认为出血可能是 T_1WI 高信号的主要原因。

脂肪抑制技术对检测中等或大量的脂肪组织敏感而且特异度高，对少量或微量的细胞内脂质不敏感；化学位移成像（反相位图像）对少量或微量细胞内脂质敏感、特异度高。该组 1 个病灶局部含少量脂质，病理组织学切片发现病灶局部少量脂肪变性，但脂肪变性的程度和分布显著小于 T_1WI 高信号的范围，因此在少数情况下脂肪变性可能是 T_1WI 高信号的部分原因。

鉴别诊断：多发肝腺瘤：典型多发局灶性结节增生诊断较为容易，不典型多发局灶性结节增生常需要与多发肝腺瘤相鉴别，尤其以局灶性结节增生在 T_1WI 高信号的情况下鉴别较困难。30%~66% 的肝腺瘤有假包膜，而局灶性结节增生假包膜罕见文献报道。25%~40% 的肝腺瘤有出血，约 35%~90% 的肝腺瘤在 T_1WI 上呈高信号，因此 T_2WI 上肝腺瘤信号常不均匀也无中心瘢痕的出现，此外，肝腺瘤虽然含有肝细胞但通常功能不全，延迟 1 h 后常为低信号。临床上多发肝腺瘤较多发局灶性结节增生少见，肝腺瘤内常可含大量脂质及脂肪，而局灶性结节增生含脂质及脂肪者少见。

无肝硬化背景的多灶性肝细胞癌：多发局灶性结节增生还需与无肝硬化背景的多灶性肝细胞癌鉴别，纤维板层型肝癌中央瘢痕 T_2WI 通常为低信号，增强延迟期一般无强化，而局灶性结节增生中央瘢痕 T_2WI 为高信号，增强后延迟期强化。

第十四节　几个问题的讨论

发病机制:局灶性结节增生是一种发生于正常肝脏结构的增生性疾病,并非真正肿瘤,有自发性消退倾向。Wanless 等(1985)报道,形态学上血管畸形在局灶性结节增生形成之前出现,肝细胞异常增生可能是由肝血窦内高压和高速的血流造成的。其病理特点为含有大量具有正常功能的肝细胞、增生结缔组织、枯否细胞、畸形胆管、巨噬细胞及异常血管。病变中心存在畸形血管和纤维组织,表现为中心瘢痕。典型的局灶性结节增生中心瘢痕组织向边缘呈放射状延伸,将病灶分隔为多个结节。局灶性结节增生中可见急、慢性炎细胞,缺乏正常的中心静脉和门静脉。

显微镜下,在邻近病灶的正常肝组织内、病灶与肝组织连接区及大的星状瘢痕内均可见大的中心性或偏心性厚壁静脉。动静脉畸形引起肝实质周围的假瘤增生、放射状血管结构和中心瘢痕内的供养动脉是局灶性结节增生的特征性表现。

合并病变: Brancatelli 和 Federle(2001)报道 78 例局灶性结节增生患者中 18 例(23%)合并血管性病变。一组 18 例局灶性结节增生患者, 5 例(27%)合并良性血管病变。Nguyen 等(1999)报道行外科手术的 168 例局灶性结节增生患者中,肝腺瘤发生率为 3.6%,肝海绵状血管瘤发病率为 6.5%,低于该组的发病率。

局灶性结节增生患者中血管性肿瘤样疾病的高发病率,证明肝血管功能不全导致了局灶性结节增生的发生。Mathieu 等(1998)报道口服避孕药不会增加局灶性结节增生的发病率,但可促进局灶性结节增生的生长,也有停服避孕药病灶会消退的报道。

局灶性结节增生在 CT 平扫呈等密度或略低密度肿块,境界清楚,密度均匀,如同时合并脂肪肝或布 - 加综合征等病变时,可表现为相对高密度,0.8%~1.4% 可见钙化,但很少见脂肪密度,该组病例有 1 例见钙化灶。

星状瘢痕:部分病例可以显示瘢痕组织,在平扫时呈低密度,增强扫描动脉期,瘢痕内可显示供血动脉,在门静脉期和延迟扫描时可见瘢痕逐渐强化呈等或高密度。有时在增强时可显示辐射状纤维分隔。一组多数病灶中心可见星状瘢痕(55%),此为与其他富血供肿块的鉴别点。

增强扫描病灶动脉期呈快速明显均匀强化,门静脉期及延迟期对比剂快速退出呈稍高或等密度,这种强化特征是由于局灶性结节增生有丰富的动脉供血及增粗的引流静脉和血窦。中心星状瘢痕平扫呈低密度,增强扫描动脉期多为低密度,但瘢痕内可见供血动脉,门静脉期、延迟期可见瘢痕逐渐强化呈等或高密度,瘢痕面积减少或消失,也有延迟后仍为低密度,可能与瘢痕中增生血管腔闭塞有关。

该组中心瘢痕显示率为 55%,与一些文献报道相近,但直径≤ 3 cm 的病灶显示率仅为 33%,而直径 >3 cm 的病灶显示率为 69%,充分说明了中心瘢痕的显示与病灶的大小明显相关。病灶的均匀强化、肝脏轮廓的改变、病灶周围血管的推移及扩张程度亦与病灶的大小密切相关。

假包膜:局灶性结节增生是没有纤维包膜的,但是有假包膜。假包膜的组成:局灶性结节增生压迫周围正常的肝实质;周围的血管;炎性的反应。

假包膜作为局灶性结节增生的一个特征性表现,在许多文献中都已报道。该组病例假包膜的显示率为 36%,高出相关文献报道,考虑与该组大病灶较多有关。其原因可能为病灶边缘压迫的肝实质轻度纤维化、扩张的血管及肝血窦所致,脂肪肝表现为高密度,假包膜的存在不应该视为恶性肿瘤的一个征象。

增强扫描和 MSCTA:肿瘤强化特征:早期肿块呈快速明显的均匀强化(动脉期和门静脉早期),在门静脉后期或延迟扫描可见对比剂迅速退出呈等密度。这种强化特征是由于局灶性结节增生有丰富的动脉血供及大的引流静脉和血窦。

肿瘤周围血管影:在门静脉晚期和延迟扫描图像上,局灶性结节增生周围可见血管影,这与肿瘤周围有扩大的血管、血窦有关。

增粗的供血动脉:一些作者认为局灶性结节增生是一种先天性血管畸形,动脉血流灌注增加导致肝细胞增生。在动脉期螺旋 CT 扫描常常能显示异常动脉。

MSCTA 的三维重建可清楚显示供血动脉和引流静脉,为影像学诊断局灶性结节增生提供了依据。

局灶性结节增生绝大多数为富血供病变,周边和中央见一支或数支增粗迂曲的供血动脉,其内分成多个穿支血管,形成了病灶特征性的网格状强化。

MSCTA 的三维重建上肿块内见多条血管影呈轮辐状,这是由于供血动脉分支似蜘蛛样结构,由中央向外周辐射状伸入结节内或表面,并形成了典型的离心式强化方式。

供血动脉的增粗与病灶的大小明显相关,有学者报道病灶直径 <2 cm 未发现异常供血动脉。这可能由于随着病灶的增大,营养需求增多,供血动脉随之增粗扭曲。

门静脉期和延迟早期局灶性结节增生周围可见引流血管,与病灶周围扩大的血管、血窦有关,有时这些血管围绕肿块呈不完整的强化环,易被误认为包膜强化。

延迟后粗大的静脉直接流入肝静脉或扩张的肝窦,较大肿瘤可见数支引流静脉,并可清晰显示占位效应,肝静脉、门静脉受推压移位。

门静脉不参与局灶性结节增生血供及引流,此点可与肝细胞癌鉴别。

误诊病例简介:有时,小的局灶性结节增生在 MSCT 平扫和增强扫描时,可误诊为其他疾病,我们曾遇见一例:女，44 岁。体检发现右肝小结节影，MSCT 平扫与增强提示，1.0cm × 0.7cm × 0.4cm,考虑小肝癌？肝腺瘤？血管瘤;手术病理证实为局灶性结节增生。

第四章　肝肉芽肿性疾病

肝脏的肉芽肿性疾病，表示肝内存在着伴有肉芽肿组织学特点的局灶性炎症。肉芽肿性肝炎这一名词，已用于描述此类情况，但是它并不正确，因为这些病变不是肝炎，而且不常出现肝细胞的功能障碍。

肝脏肉芽肿性疾病，包括炎性肉芽肿、非炎性肉芽肿和特发性肉芽肿三大类：炎性肉芽肿由细菌、霉菌、寄生虫、病毒等引起，其中结核、寄生虫感染是常见病因，常见的为肝结核、组织胞浆菌病、布鲁氏菌病、钩端螺旋体病；非炎性肉芽肿病变主要包括结节病等非感染因素引起者；不能查明原因的肝脏肉芽肿，称为特发性肉芽肿，至少有 20% 的肝脏肉芽肿性疾病无特别的病因可寻。

病理学：肝脏肉芽肿性疾病的病因的宿主已经比较清楚，包括病毒、细菌、霉菌以及寄生虫性感染，儿童的慢性肉芽肿病、类肉瘤病、韦格纳肉芽肿病，多种药物及化学试剂（磺胺类药物、保泰松、用作吸入性麻醉的氟烷、别嘌呤醇、降血压的联胺嗪、奎尼丁、铍）的中毒性反应。肉芽肿呈结节状，通常边界锐利，与周围正常肝组织分界清楚。它们由组织细胞和肥大的成纤维细胞的血管性的积聚组成，形成圆形或卵圆形的形状。

肉芽肿可以保持完整，或经历干酪样坏死、化脓性坏死、肉芽肿性坏死。肝脏肉芽肿性疾病的特异性的诊断，以组织学的征象研究肝内的肉芽肿性反应，常常不可能。然而，在某些疾病，可产生相当特异性的肉芽肿性反应。类肉瘤病可有轻微的或中央性坏死，而结核病则引起干酪样坏死。至少有 20% 的肝脏肉芽肿性疾病无特别的病因可寻。

临床表现：肝脏的肉芽肿，可见于任何年龄的病人，性别差异和种族差异都不大。症状常常是非特异性的：发热、体重下降、身体不适、以及厌食等。体征包括：肝肿大、脾肿大、黄疸、淋巴结肿大、以及皮肤病变。深入了解病史是重要的，诸如同结核病、梅毒或其他炎症接触或以前曾经治疗过，接触药物或化学试剂，接触动物或扁虱，或曾经旅游于难见的地方性寄生虫的热带地区等。

第五章　肝细胞腺瘤

第一节　误诊病例简介:老年男性肝细胞腺瘤与肝癌

肝细胞腺瘤是少见的肝脏良性肿瘤。多见于中青年女性(99%),偶尔见于儿童或男性,平均发病年龄为31岁或34岁。病因不明,除少数病例外均有长期服用避孕药和激素类药物史。服药常作为鉴别诊断依据之一。但并发Ⅰa型糖原贮积病或Von Gierke病的肝细胞腺瘤常有家族性,男性占67%,发病年龄也较小。

影像学研究:B超检查肿瘤较小时为较均匀的低回声或较高回声,也可不均匀,较大的腺瘤内常有出血、坏死和液化。表现为混合回声,即瘤体出现不规则的高回声团和/或无回声团。CT上主要表现为平扫时低密度或等密度占位性病变,出血、钙化部位可为高密度,边缘光滑,周围可见"透亮环"影,动态扫描早期可见均匀性强化,之后密度下降与正常肝组织呈等密度,晚期呈低密度。

肝细胞腺瘤的单一影像与综合影像表现与肝癌相似(假包膜出现率高,强化方式与肝癌相似),缺乏典型征象,确诊仍然需要手术或穿刺病理诊断。

一例误诊原因为,该患者为老年男性,行CT检查时作为门诊患者,没有完整的实验室检查资料和详细的病史,而且该患者的CT表现虽然有肝细胞腺瘤的典型的"包膜",但是与原发性肝癌十分相似。

鉴别诊断:局灶性结节增生:临床很少有症状,无出血和恶变,CT可见肿块内强化的较低密度瘢痕,坏死少见,无瘤周透亮影;而肝细胞腺瘤可见瘤周透亮环,常见坏死、出血。病理学上肝细胞腺瘤常有空泡变性,无胆管和枯否细胞;

巨块型肝癌:巨块型肝癌CT影像未见瘤周透亮环影,甲胎蛋白值升高,选择性肝动脉造影和^{99m}Tc-PMT有助于鉴别两者。

对于不典型病例应及时行CT引导下肝脏穿刺活检获取病理证实。

第二节　多发性肝细胞腺瘤与先天性Ⅰ型糖原累积症

患者,女性,27岁,患者缘于8年前于外院体检发现肝占位性病变,具体不详,无畏寒、发热,无恶心、呕吐,无腹痛、腹胀,无黄疸、尿黄等不适,未行处理。定期复查示肝占位性病变逐渐增大,体重未见明显增减。既往患先天性Ⅰ型糖原累积症。手术所见:腹腔无腹水,肝脏体积增大,表面无硬化结节,肝左叶一肿物向肝下方膨胀性生长,大小约10cm×9cm;肝左外叶可见一大小约3.0cm×4.0cm肿物,质中,边界清楚,包膜完整;右肝后叶可见一大小约6cm×5cm肿物,质中,边界清楚,包膜完整;腹腔淋巴结未触及明显肿大;肠管、脾脏、胰腺、盆腔未见肿瘤转移。病理检查:左肝肿物切除标本:结节状肿物一块,大小9cm×8.5cm×7cm,表面呈灰褐色,尚光滑,切面灰褐墨绿,质软,界清;周围附少许肝组织,大小8cm×5cm×1.5cm,切面灰黄,质软。常规病理诊断:左肝肿物切除标本:肝细胞肿瘤伴大片梗死,待做免疫组化检测进一步明确诊断。免疫组化检测:阳性:Hepatocyte,CD34,CK(P),CK18,CK8,Masson,PAS,网染,Ki-67(+,<5%);阴性:Vimentin,CK19,AFP,SMA,H-cal desmon。免疫组化诊断:左肝肿物切除标本:肝细胞肿瘤伴大片梗死,肝细胞腺瘤(图5-5-1)。

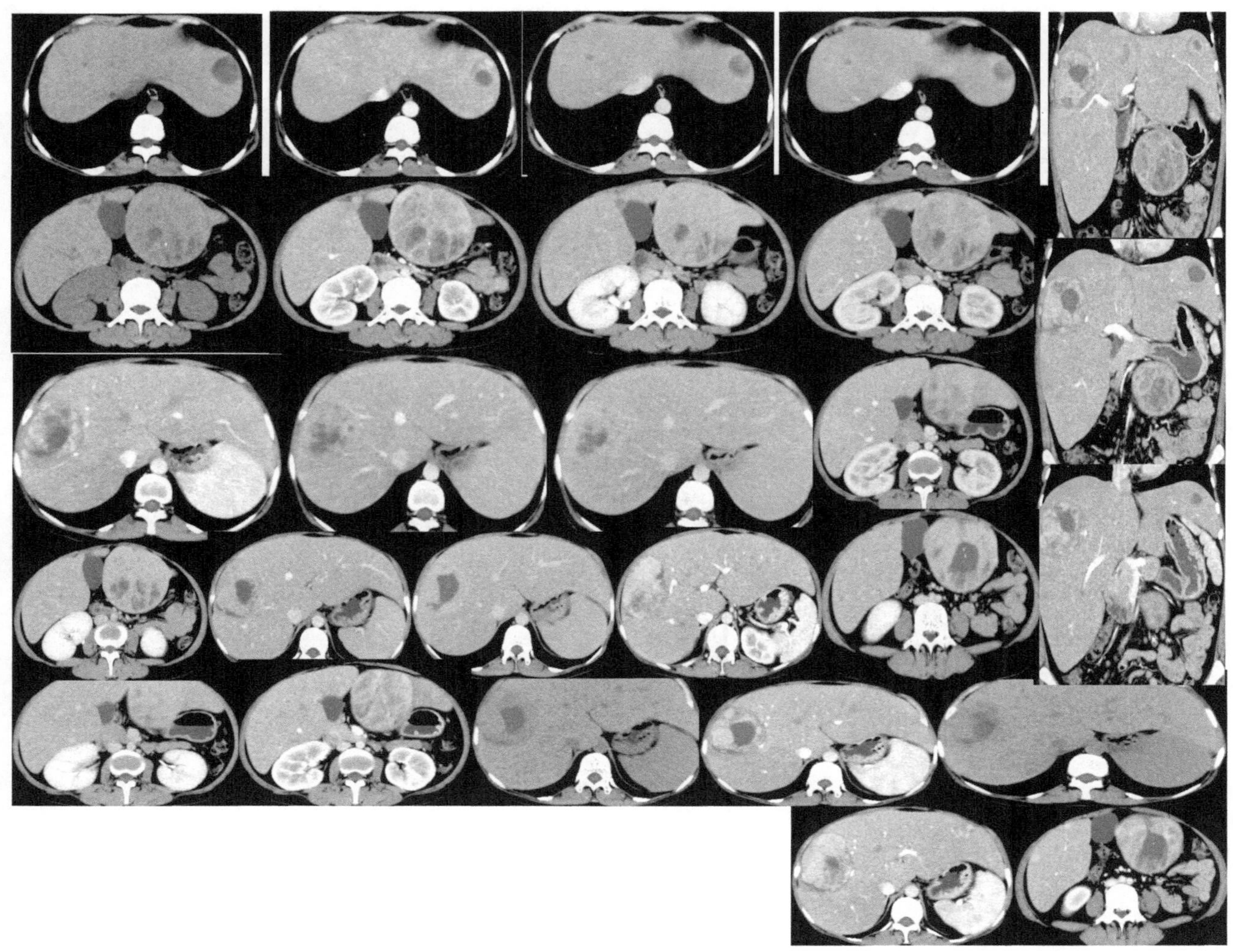

图 5-5-1 多发性肝细胞腺瘤与先天性Ⅰ型糖原累积症

第三节 肝细胞腺瘤

患者，女，64 岁。外伤致腰部剧烈疼痛，不能活动。PET/CT：肝右后叶巨大软组织肿块，大小 9.6 cm × 9.7cm，代谢增高，考虑肝癌。病理检查：第一次肝穿刺活检物：见少量可疑的肝细胞性肝癌细胞。第二次肝穿刺活检物：灰褐色软组织一堆，体积 0.3cm × 0.2cm × 0.1cm。

免疫组化检测：阳性：Villin、CK8（散在）、CK18（散在）、CD34（血窦）、Ki-67（3%）；阴性：CK7、CK20、Hepatocyte、CD10、CK19、CEA。免疫组化诊断：肝穿刺活检标本：肝小叶结构不清，肝索存在，肝细胞浊肿，呈轻度不典型增生，肝血窦扩张，未见汇管区，局部见肝细胞片状坏死。肝细胞腺瘤可能性大（图 5-5-2）。

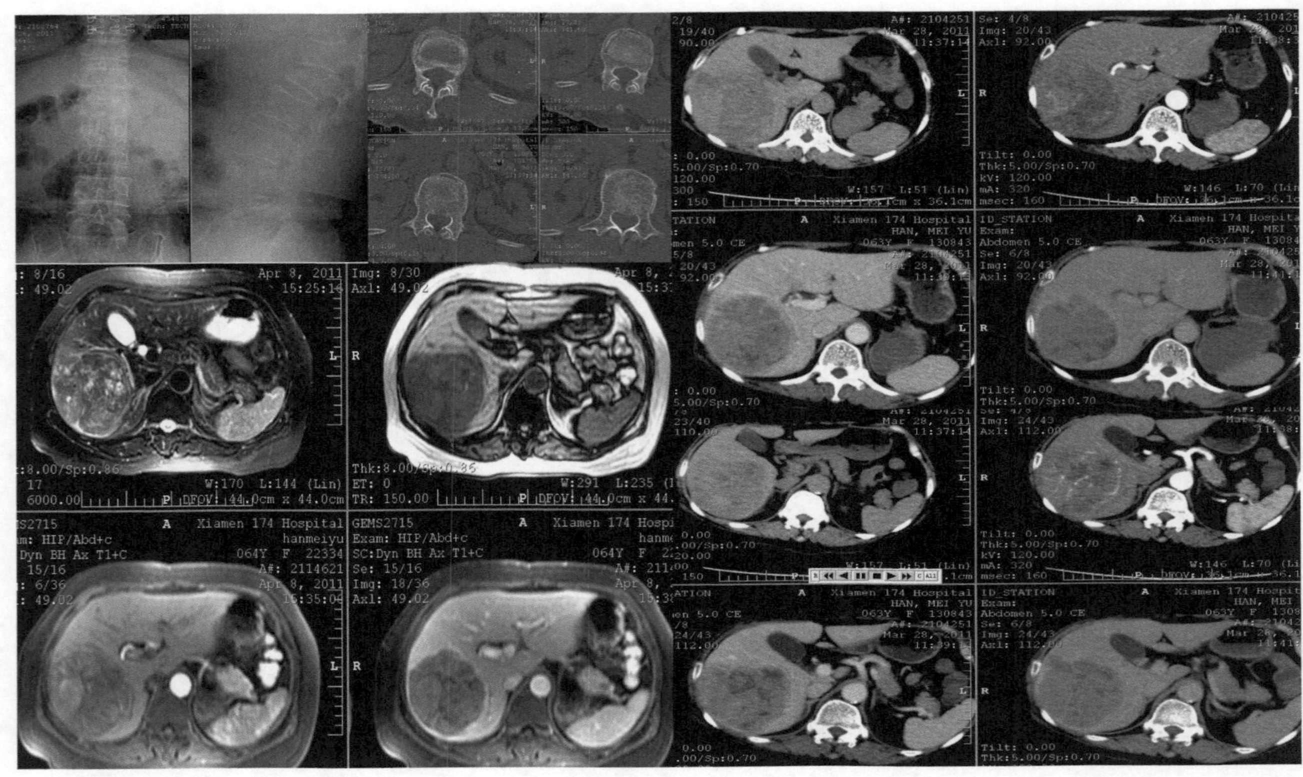

图 5-5-2 肝细胞腺瘤

第四节 肝腺瘤

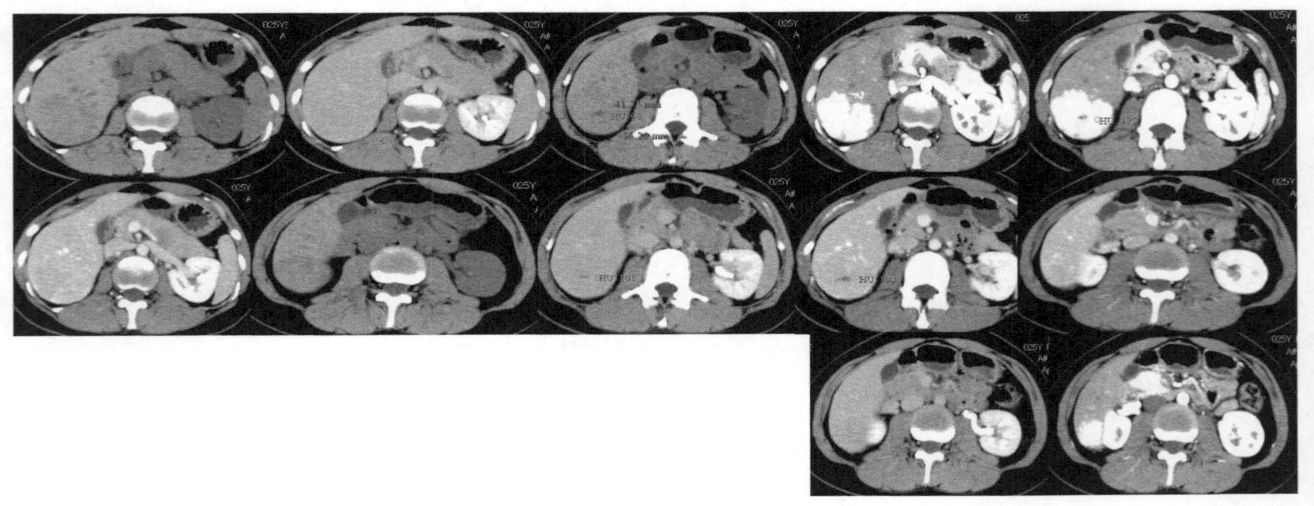

图 5-5-3 肝腺瘤

患者,女，25 岁。因发现肝占位性病变半年余入院。半年前无明显诱因出现右上腹胀痛不适,无畏寒、发热、恶性、呕吐、黄疸等不适,在外院检查行 CT 示:肝右后下叶富血供占位,考虑局灶性结节性增生可能性大。病理检查:灰黄色组织两块，总体积 7.5cm × 6.5cm × 4.5cm，切面灰黄，质软，境界不清。常规病理诊断：右肝肿物切除标本：肝组织结节状增生，具体类型待做免疫组化检测进一步明确诊断。免疫组化检测：阳性：Hepatocyte，CK18，CK8，Ki-67（+，约 2%）；阴性：CK19，CA19-9，AFP，CD34，HBcAg，HBsAg。免疫组化诊断：右肝肿物切除标本：初步考虑肝腺瘤，待进一步分析（图 5-5-3）。

第六章 肝脏间叶性肿瘤

第一节 移动性肝副叶上皮样血管平滑肌脂肪瘤

肝副叶是一种罕见的先天发育畸形,多见于肝脏下方,且与正常肝组织间呈蒂状连接,也有发生于肝脏上方,甚至胸腔的文献报道。而位于其他器官或部位的肝组织,且与正常肝脏无任何连接者,称之为异位肝。

一例肿块与肝脏左叶有一蒂状结构连接,其MRI表现得到手术证实,符合左肝副叶的诊断。术后病理学进一步证实该例左肝副叶内存在一上皮样血管平滑肌脂肪瘤,且MRI和CT显示病变具有移动性,实属罕见。

肝副叶通常是在尸检、腹腔镜检查、剖腹手术或腹部影像学检查时偶然发现,部分肝副叶也可以具有临床症状,如反复的腹部不适、疼痛,甚至肝功能损害等。该例左肝副叶上皮样血管平滑肌脂肪瘤也有类似临床表现,可能与肿块体积较大,对邻近胃、肝或胆囊产生压迫有关,而肝脏上皮样血管平滑肌脂肪瘤本身少有临床症状。

该例肝副叶CT和第2次MRI检查显示位于肝裂区域,而第1次MRI检查发现其位于左上腹,提示病变具有移动性,这与肝副叶本身的解剖结构有关。由于肝副叶仅有一蒂状结构与正常肝脏连接,其余部分均与邻近组织无任何联系,在变换体位或邻近活动性器官的推动下容易发生位置的改变。肝副叶这种解剖结构也使得它容易发生扭转,导致急性缺血性坏死,出现较重的临床症状。目前MSCT和MRI多平面重建对肝副叶的定位、定性诊断均能取得很好的效果,可以清晰显示肝副叶与正常肝脏之间的蒂状连接,从而明确肝副叶的诊断。

第二节 肝血管平滑肌脂肪瘤不典型CT表现

肝血管平滑肌脂肪瘤(AML)多见于肾脏,发生在肝脏者仅占5%~10%,为罕见的肝良性肿瘤。组织学特点为含有血管、平滑肌及成熟脂肪成分。

Tsui把血管平滑肌脂肪瘤病理分为4型:混合型、脂肪型(脂肪≥70%)、平滑肌型(脂肪≤10%)和血管型,其中混合型最常见。

血管平滑肌脂肪瘤病理组成不同决定其影像学表现存在多样性,加之扫描技术使用是否合理和肿块大小等因素的影响,使血管平滑肌脂肪瘤的影像诊断有一定困难。

CT检查中发现脂肪成分是提示血管平滑肌脂肪瘤的关键,脂肪成分的CT值呈负值(-20HU以下)。平滑肌型和血管型脂肪成分较少或不含脂肪成分影像诊断困难,肿瘤在CT表现为混杂密度,平滑肌成分动脉期一般中度或明显强化,血管主要由扭曲的动脉、静脉构成,强化程度与同层主动脉相仿,两者对比剂廓清慢,在门静脉期仍为高密度。巨大的血管平滑肌脂肪瘤,由于其内含有较大的不成熟血管可形成“假性动脉瘤”。

肝癌、肝转移瘤、肝腺瘤和局灶性结节样增生等也可有脂肪成分,含有较少的脂肪成分而有较丰富血供的血管平滑肌脂肪瘤与上述肿瘤鉴别有困难时,超声引导下的穿刺活检有助于明确诊断。

第三节　肝脏炎性肌纤维母细胞瘤

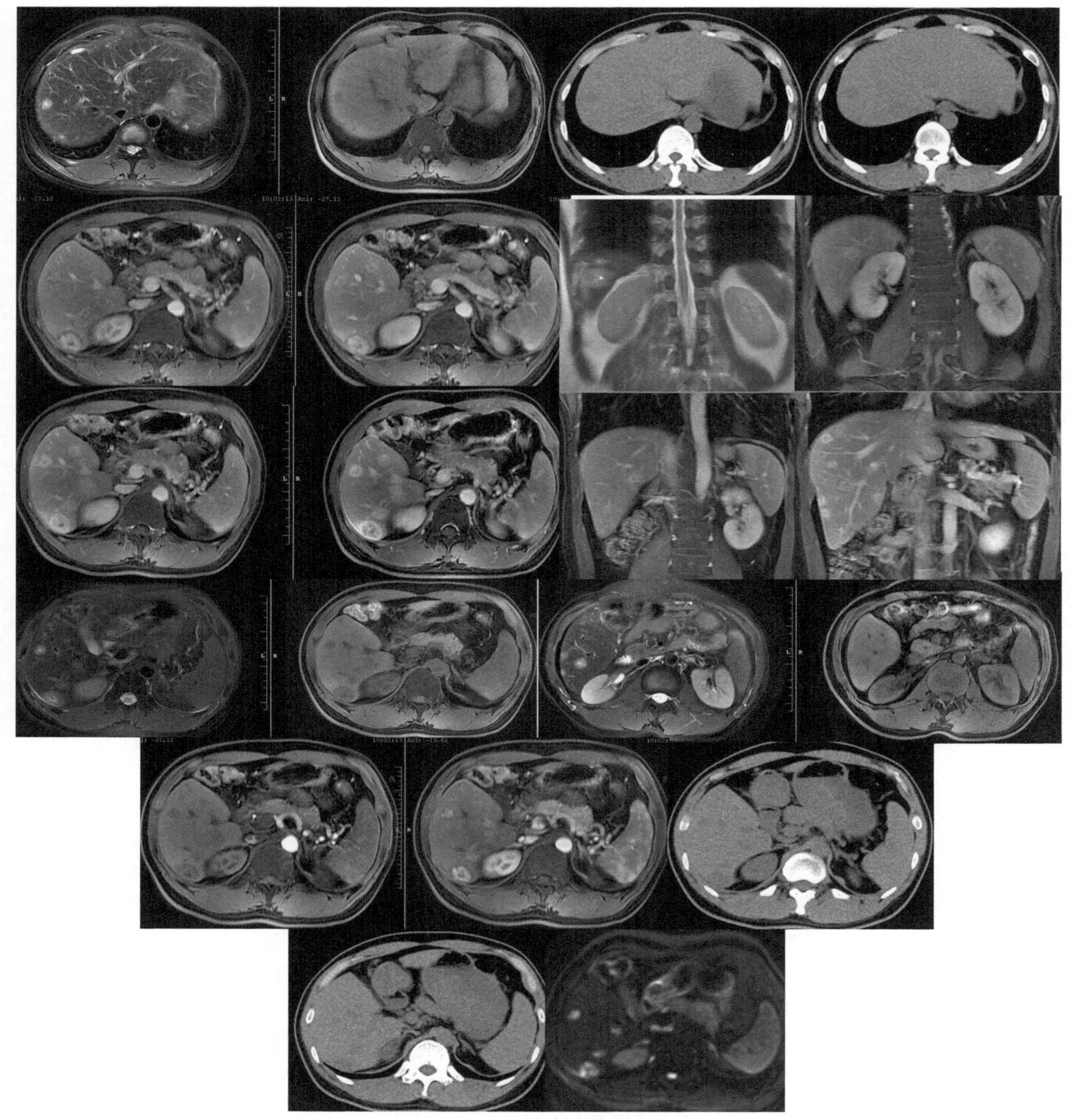

图 5-6-1　肝脏炎性肌纤维母细胞瘤

患者，男，35 岁。厌食、发热、尿黄近 1 月入院。患者因厌食伴乏力、发热、小便色黄，体温最高近 39℃，先后就诊于外院，超声及 CT 平扫提示肝内多发占位。

手术所见：腹腔无腹水，肝脏表面无硬化结节，肝内多发性肿瘤,最大一个肿物主要位于右肝第Ⅵ段,大小约3.0cm×2.0cm,质中,边界清楚,包膜完整。

病理检查:冰冻病理:右肝肿物:灰红色组织一块,大小4cm×3cm×2cm,切面灰红,见一肿物,大小2cm×1.5cm×1cm,质软。冰冻病理诊断:右肝肿物为梭形细胞病变,性质类型待定,部分切缘可见少量病变。常规病理诊断:右肝肿物取材标本:初步考虑间叶源性肿瘤,待做免疫组化检测进一步明确诊断。

免疫组化检测:阳性:Vimentin,LCA,CD68,CD163,CD31,Actin,Calponin,SMA,CD34(血管内皮+),Ki-67(+,约10%);阴性:CK(L),CK(P),CK19,CK18,CK8,P63,AFP,CD21,CD35,CD117,DOG1,Desmin,ALKP80,S-100,CD1α,PAS染色。免疫组化诊断:右肝肿物取材标本:炎性肌纤维母细胞瘤(图5-6-1)。

第四节 误诊病例简介:肝脏上皮样血管内皮细胞瘤与血管瘤及转移瘤

肝脏上皮样血管内皮细胞瘤是一种罕见的血管源性肿瘤,临床及影像诊断很容易误诊。

上皮样血管内皮细胞瘤是一种罕见的血管源性肿瘤,多发生于软组织、肺、骨、脑和小肠等脏器,原发于肝脏的非常罕见,其发病率约为0. 1/10万,男女患病比例2:3,平均发病年龄为41岁。一组5例中,男1例、女4例,2例年龄较小,为3~4岁,3例年龄为40~50岁,且多为中年妇女。患者临床无典型症状。

病理特征主要为肿瘤细胞由上皮样细胞组成,呈巢状或短条索状不规则排列,可见梭形(树突状)细胞,并含有大片黏液性或致密纤维性间质,少数患者可出现钙化;免疫组化瘤细胞对Vim表达阳性,对内皮细胞标记物CD31、CD34及FⅧRag因子至少一种表达阳性。该项研究中有1例患者为出生前即发现肝脏肿块,这也提示肝脏上皮样血管内皮细胞瘤是否和先天发育有关,值得进一步研究。

影像学研究:肝脏上皮样血管内皮细胞瘤在不同时期有2种不同表现形式:结节型:表现为各自独立的结节,直径0.5~12.0 cm,多为早期表现;弥散型:随着疾病的进展,肿瘤逐渐增大和融合,同时常伴有肝血管浸润,多数病灶分布于肝脏外周,延伸到肝包膜,为结节型的晚期表现。本组中,结节型4例,弥散型1例。CT平扫示肿块均呈类圆形稍低密度影,境界较清,密度不均匀;可伴有斑片状、类网形更低密度区,这与瘤体组织成分复杂有关,如果病灶体积较大,病灶中心供血不足或者黏液变性则继发坏死、囊变。多发性病灶瘤体大小差异很大,直径2.0~9.9 cm,平均6.5 cm.且多分布在肝周近包膜下,考虑可能因为肿瘤伴有肝血管浸润,通过门静脉和肝静脉分支蔓延。未见纤维间隔及斑点状钙化影。

肝脏上皮样血管内皮细胞瘤增强扫描强化方式大致有2种表现:一种为动脉期病灶实质部分强化不明显或轻微强化,门静脉期及延迟期周边向中心递进强化,坏死区不强化,各期扫描强化程度不超过平扫CT值的50%,呈“慢进慢出”和向心性强化模式;一种是动脉期周边显著强化,静脉期及延迟期对比剂不消退,且由边缘向中央递进强化,各期扫描强化程度在平扫CT值的50%~100%之间,与肝脏多发血管瘤表现类似,表现“快进慢出”和向心性强化模式。

该项研究中3个病灶,动脉期边缘强化明显,静脉期及延迟期病灶由边缘部分向中央递进强化,类似于血管瘤的强化特点。2个病灶动脉期强化不明显,中心有坏死低密度区,类似于转移瘤的“牛眼征”,静脉期及延迟期病灶周边向中心递进式持续性强化,与中心坏死区密度差加大,显示病灶缩小。

该组作者认为显微镜下病理证实病灶内富含纤维组织及纤维硬化区与肝脏上皮样血管内皮细胞瘤强化特点密切相关。当肿瘤实质内含有的纤维组织间质及纤维硬化区较少时,病灶呈逐步向心性强化:即动脉期病灶边缘部分富含瘤细胞血管,强化明显,但是病灶中心部分含有的纤维组织间质及纤维硬化区,对比剂扩散受限,呈逐渐填充的特点。当瘤体富含纤维组织间质及纤维硬化区时,对比剂进入困难,即表现为类似转移瘤的强化特点。

MRI信号的改变直接反映肿瘤的组织特征。肝脏上皮样血管内皮细胞瘤典型表现为在T_1WI序列上病灶实质部分呈均匀的稍低信号,T_2WI上呈均匀中、高信号,病灶周围见不规则低信号环。肝脏上皮样血管内皮细胞瘤瘤体实质内含有树枝状和上皮样细胞,而且由于肿瘤增殖较快,富含水分,在T_1WI上常表现为稍低信号,T_2WI上常表现为稍高信号;病灶中央的液化坏死区,呈长T_1、长T_2信号改变;如果液化坏死区内合并出血，则信号高低混杂；

1 例病灶边缘出现的不规则低信号环，可能与瘤体生长压迫周围组织、邻近组织继发纤维增生有关，手术大体病理也证实了这种推断，病理检查中可见明确的不完整包膜，但这种包膜为纤维性包膜，这也可以解释在 CT 平扫及增强时未能显示假包膜的原因。

该组中 5 例患者，只有 2 例进行了 MR 检查，其中有 1 例病灶存在包膜回缩的情况。由于患者数量太少，尚不能确定“肝包膜回缩征”发生的概率：该组作者认为此征象出现是由于肿瘤富含纤维组织及纤维硬化区，随着纤维组织的累积，纤维成分继发收缩、牵拉；如果这种纤维收缩性反应邻近肝包膜，则出现“包膜回缩征”。此征象不同于其他肝脏恶性肿瘤的假包膜向外膨胀的表现，是肝脏上皮样血管内皮细胞瘤较为特征性的表现。

鉴别诊断：由于本病罕见，影像表现缺乏特异性，60%~80% 的肝脏上皮样血管内皮细胞瘤患者初诊时被误诊为其他疾病，最常见误诊为血管瘤、血管肉瘤以及转移瘤。该组 5 例中，3 例误诊为血管瘤，2 例误诊为转移瘤。

如果病灶为多发，则需要同以下疾病鉴别：①转移瘤，瘤体在肝内分布散在，位于肝包膜附近的，肝包膜常局限性突出，一般不会有“包膜回缩征”，增强后同样可有周边环形强化，中心坏死区不强化，呈“牛眼征”，但无周边向中心递进强化的特征，临床上常有发热、消瘦等恶病质的表现，如果临床上能找到原发灶，对诊断更有帮助，②肝多发海绵状血管瘤，肝脏血管瘤患者多无明显临床症状，短期内复查病灶增大不明显，但血管瘤无肝周边区域分布的特点，且不会相互融合，无肝包膜凹陷。

如果肝脏上皮样血管内皮细胞瘤为单发，则需要同以下疾病鉴别：①硬化性胆管癌可有胆管扩张的表现，部分患者会有不同程度黄疸；②血管肉瘤病灶增大迅速，常有明显的恶性临床体征；③单发血管瘤与单发的肝脏上皮样血管内皮细胞瘤鉴别困难，但典型的海绵状血管瘤早期一般为周围结节状强化，较大病灶一般不会出现瘤体实质部分显著强化，而且无肝包膜凹陷征。

综上所述，如果发现肝脏多发病灶，病灶多位于肝包膜下，密度不均，边缘清晰，增强早期边缘轻微或显著强化，门静脉期、延迟期由周边向中心递进持续性强化，应考虑到该肿瘤可能性，若见包膜回缩征，则进一步支持该病诊断。最终确诊须依靠病理学和免疫组化检查。

第五节　误诊病例简介：肝脏上皮样血管内皮瘤与多发肝囊肿

病例，男，37 岁。因体检发现肝占位 4 个月余入院。4 年前 CT：肝脏平扫 + 增强：右肝前后叶可见多个大小不等的类圆形低密度影，最大者约 1819，边界较清楚，CT 值 1642HU，增强各期病灶边缘轻度环形强化，CT 值 53HU，中心无明显强化，CT 值 3846HU。CT 诊断：右肝多个低密度影，边缘轻度环状强化，中心无明显强化，考虑多发肝囊肿可能，请结合临床研究，并请复查。

入院后第一次 CT 诊断：直肠壁不规则稍增厚，性质？恶性肿瘤待排，建议结合肠镜检查；双肺多发结节影，性质待定，转移瘤待排；双侧腋下多发肿大淋巴结；肝内多发大小不一稍低密度灶，性质？转移瘤待排，与四年前 CT 图像比较，病灶有所增大。

入院后第二次 CT：肝内多发大小不一稍低密度灶，边界欠清，部分病灶相互融合，较大者 7.0cm × 4.5cm，CT 值约 26~32HU，部分病灶内可见更低密度影，肝内外胆管无扩张。CT 诊断：肝内多发大小不一稍低密度灶，性质？转移瘤待排，与三月前入院第一次 CT 图像比较，部分病灶增大。

手术所见：肝脏Ⅵ～Ⅶ段可见大小不等肿物相互融合，大小约 7cm × 5cm，质软，包膜较完整；左肝表面可见大小不等肿物，最大直径约 1.5cm。病理检查：肝脏穿刺组织标本：穿刺组织一条，长 1.3cm，直径 0.1cm。常规病理诊断：肝脏穿刺组织标本：可见散在的异性细胞及腺管样结构，考虑恶性肿瘤，需作免疫组化进一步分型。

肝脏Ⅵ～Ⅶ段肿瘤切除标本：肝组织两块，大小分别为 13 cm × 7.5 cm × 5.8 cm 和 10.5 cm × 7.0 cm × 4.5 cm，切面均见多个灰白色结节，最小者大小为 1.7 cm × 1.5 cm × 0.8 cm，最大者为 9.0 cm × 5.0 cm × 5.0 cm，结节切面灰白质韧，与周围边界欠清。常规病理诊断：肝脏Ⅵ～Ⅶ段肿瘤切除标本：初步诊断为肝脏恶性间叶性肿瘤,局部区可见肿瘤组织向周围肝组织内浸润,待做免疫组化检测进一步明确肿瘤类型。

膈肌肿瘤切除标本:灰褐色组织一块,大小2.0 cm×1.5 cm×0.6 cm。常规病理诊断:膈肌肿瘤切除标本:送检少量膈肌组织,局灶区可见单核及多核组织细胞样细胞聚集,待做免疫组化检测进一步协助诊断。

免疫组化检测:①阳性:Vimentin,CD34,F8,CD31,SMA,D2-40(灶+),Actin(血管壁平滑肌+),CK(P)(散在+),EMA(散在+),S-100(散在+),Hepatocyte(肝细胞+),Ki-67(+,约10%),PAS染色,网状纤维染色;阴性:AFP,HMB45,Desmin。②阳性:CD68(组织细胞+),CD163(组织细胞+),CD31(血管内皮+),CD34(血管内皮+),LCA(淋巴细胞+),Ki-67(+,约2%)。免疫组化诊断:肝脏Ⅵ~Ⅶ段肿瘤切除标本:肝脏上皮样血管内皮瘤,局部区可见肿瘤组织向周围肝组织浸润。膈肌肿瘤切除标本:送检少量膈肌组织,局灶区可见单核及多核组织细胞样细胞聚集,未见肿瘤组织累及。

第六节 肝血管周上皮样细胞肿瘤

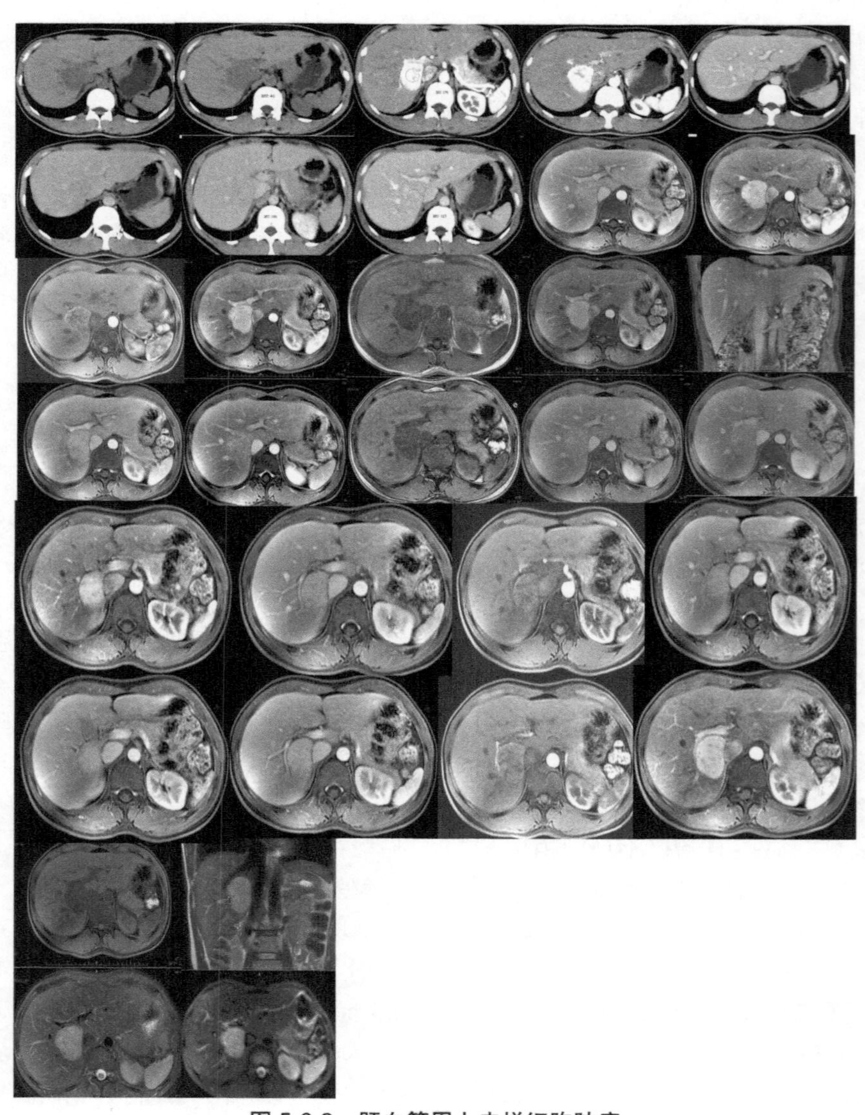

图 5-6-2 肝血管周上皮样细胞肿瘤

患者,女，42岁。体检发现肝占位性病变3月入院。手术所见:腹腔无腹水,盆腔、胃肠道未触及肿瘤;肝脏大小正常,右肝后叶下段肝尾状叶可见一肿物大小约6 cm×5cm,质软,包膜较完整,余肝未触及异常。病理检查:肝组织一块,大小14cm× 8.5cm×7cm,切面见一结节,大小约4cm×3.5cm,结节切面灰黄灰褐相间,质中,与周围境界尚清,其余切面灰红,质软。常规病理诊断:右半肝切除标本:初步诊断肝细胞癌,大小4cm×3.5cm,待做免疫组化检测进一步明确诊断。免疫组化诊断:右半肝切除标本:结合免疫组化检测结果及组织学图像,诊断为血管周上皮样细胞肿瘤(简称PEComa),大小4cm×3.5cm(图5-6-2)。

第七节　肝脏血管平滑肌脂肪瘤不同表现

Martignoni等(1998)报道3例不同表现的肝脏血管平滑肌脂肪瘤,1例CT表现类似局灶性纤维结节增生,1例类似原发性肝细胞性肝癌(HCC),还有1例典型的血管平滑肌脂肪瘤。

第七章 肝脏炎性疾病

第一节 误诊病例简介:肝炎性肌成纤维细胞瘤与局灶性结节增生

患者,男,35岁。厌食、发热、尿黄近一个月入院。临床初步诊断:肝囊肿。门诊MRI:肝脏体积稍增大,表面略不平整,肝左内叶及右叶散在多个大小不等的类圆形异常信号结节影,以右叶为主,最大者约2.4cm×1.9cm,T_1WI稍低信号,T_2WI为不均匀高信号,中央点状更高信号,边界清楚;增强扫描早期结节呈斑片状强化,内见裂隙状无强化影,静脉期及延迟期强化趋于均匀,强化程度稍减低,与周边血管分界清晰。胆囊增大,壁略厚,其内可见分隔。MRI诊断:肝内多发病灶,考虑局灶性结节性增生,转移瘤待排?请结合临床;慢性胆囊炎。

胸部CT发现:右肝多发小斑片状低密度影,建议肝平扫+增强扫描。

病理检查:灰黄色穿刺组织一条,长1cm,直径0.1cm,另见灰白色组织两块,大小均为0.2cm×0.2cm×0.2cm。病理诊断:肝穿刺组织:镜下描述(HE和网状纤维染色、VG染色、Masson染色)(病变范围-~++++,25%为+)。肝小叶:结构存在,中央静脉2个,肝细胞水肿(++),毛玻璃样变(-),脂肪变性(+),点状/灶性坏死(+),碎屑样坏死(-),桥接坏死(-),网状纤维支架塌陷(-)枯否细胞增生(+),肝细胞/毛细胆管淤胆(-)。汇管区:(4)个,扩大(+),纤维组织增生(+),淋巴细胞单核细胞浸润(+),小胆管增生(-)。慢性肝炎分级G、分期S:炎症活动度(G0~4):1级,纤维化分期(S0~4):1期。

免疫组化染色(阳性范围+~++++,25%为+):肝细胞HBsAg阴性,肝细胞HBcAg阴性,胆管上皮细胞CK19阳性,枯否细胞CD163阳性,内皮细胞CD34阳性。免疫组化诊断:慢性轻型肝炎G1S1,伴轻度脂肪变性,未见肿瘤性改变,如考虑肿瘤,请再次送检。注:另见微量皮肤、纤维、肌肉及软骨组织。

手术所见:腹腔无腹水,肝脏表现无硬化结节,肝内多发性肿瘤,最大一个肿物主要位于右肝第Ⅵ段,大小约3.0cm×2.0cm,质中,边界清楚,包膜完整;胆囊无肿大。肠管、脾脏、胰腺、盆腔未见肿瘤转移。

病理检查:右肝肿物取材标本:冰冻病理与常规病理:灰红色组织一块,大小4cm×3cm×2cm,切面灰红,见一肿物,大小2cm×1.5cm×1cm,质软。冰冻病理诊断:右肝肿物取材标本:为梭形细胞病变,性质类型待定,部分切缘可见少量病变。常规病理诊断:右肝肿物取材标本:初步考虑间叶源性肿瘤,待做免疫组化检测进一步明确诊断。

免疫组化检查:阳性:Vimentin,LCA,CD68,CD163,CD31,Actin,Calponin,SMA,CD34(血管内皮+),Ki-67(+,约10%);阴性:CK(L),CK(P),CK19,CK18,CK8,P63,AFP,CD21,CD35,CD117,DOG1,Desmin,ALKP80,S-100,CD1α,PAS染色。免疫组化诊断(右肝肿物取材标本):炎性肌成纤维细胞瘤。

第二节 肝脏炎性假瘤

患者,男,37岁。体检发现肝占位半天入院。

病理检查:肝脏组织2块,大者大小8cm×6.5 cm×

5cm，小者 6 cm × 5.5 cm × 2 cm，一侧光滑，另一侧粗糙，附少量血凝块，切面灰红紫红，质软，均未见局限性占位病变。病理诊断：右肝组织标本：可见肝细胞广泛水肿及脂肪变性，局部见散在肝细胞点状坏死，汇管区较多慢性炎细胞浸润（图 5-7-1）。

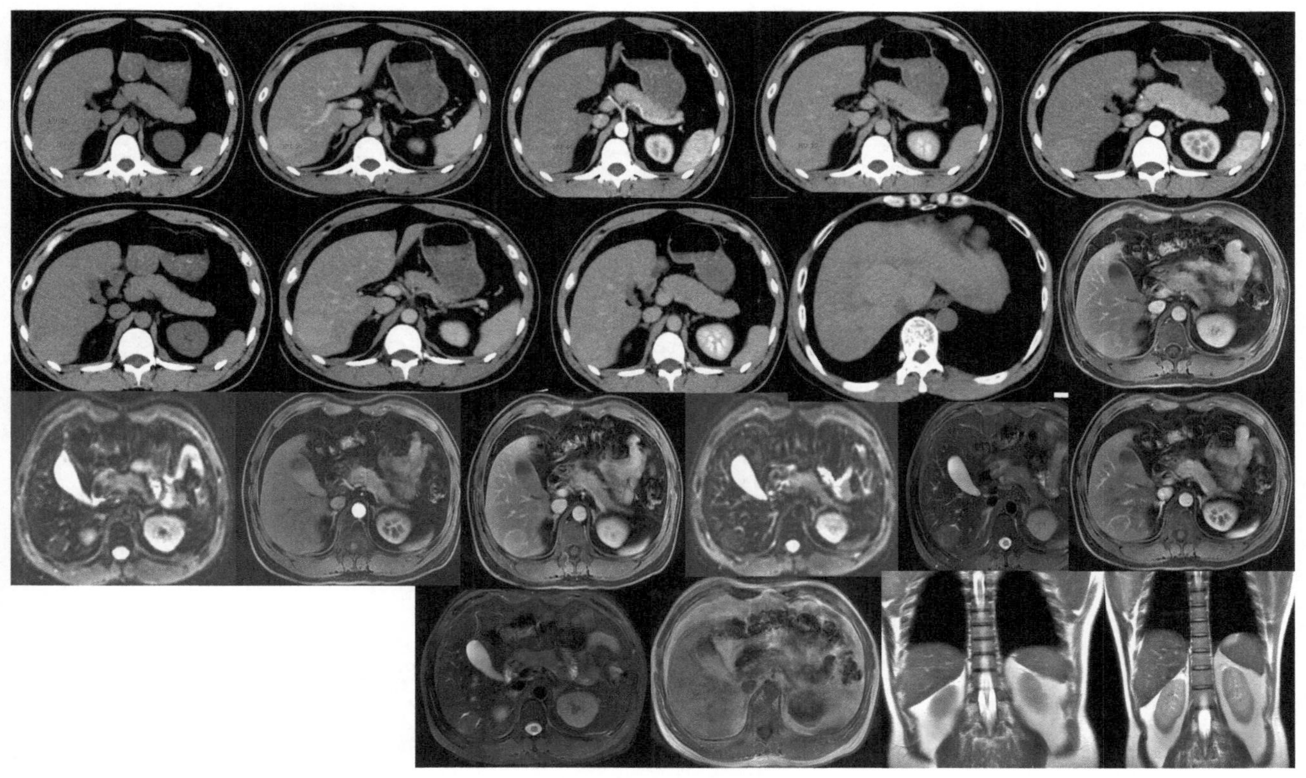

图 5-7-1　肝脏炎性假瘤

第三节　误诊病例简介：肝脏孤立性坏死性结节被误诊为炎性假瘤

病例，男，57 岁。体检发现肝占位 6 天入院。MRI：肝右后叶下段见一类圆形结节影，大小约 1.6cm × 1.8cm，T_1WI 低信号，T_2WI 略高信号，中间囊变区呈更高信号；DWI 实性部分信号稍高；增强扫描结节边缘环形强化呈稍高信号，中间无强化仍呈低信号，边界变清楚。MRI 诊断：肝右后叶下段结节影，考虑炎性假瘤可能，请结合临床。

手术所见：肝脏表面无硬化结节，肿物位于右肝第 6 段，大小约 2.0cm × 2.0cm，质中，边界清楚，包膜完整。腹腔淋巴结未触及明显肿大。

病理检查：右肝肿物切除标本：灰褐色组织一块，大小 2.3cm × 2.0cm × 2.0cm，切面见一黄色坏死样结节，大小 1.8cm × 1.5cm，与周围界限清楚。常规病理诊断：右肝肿物切除标本：镜下见肝组织中央有一凝固性坏死结节，结节与周围界限清楚，周围肝小叶及汇管区存在，小叶内肝细胞浊肿，汇管区可见少量慢性炎细胞浸润，待做免疫组化检测进一步协助诊断。

免疫组化检测：阳性：Hepatocyte（肝细胞 +），CK19（胆小管 +），CK18（肝细胞及胆小管 +），CK8（肝细胞及胆小管 +），CD34（血管内皮 +），Ki-67（+，约 5%，主要为炎细胞）；阴性：HBsAg，HBcAg，CEA，AFP。免疫组化诊断：右肝肿物切除标本：结合临床病史，HE 组织学图像及免疫组化检测结果，符合肝脏孤立性坏死性结节（solitary necrotic nodule），属一种少见的良性病变，病因尚不明确，建议治疗后复查。

第四节 中度慢性肝炎(肝脏假性占位)

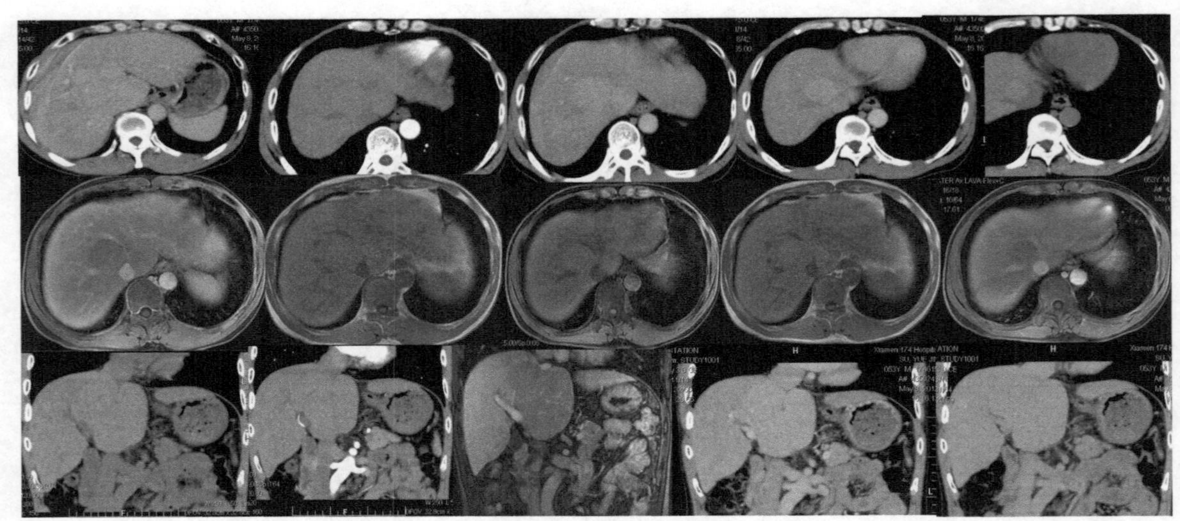

图 5-7-2 中度慢性肝炎(肝脏假性占位)

病例，男性，53岁。体检发现肝内占位性病变2个月余入院。

手术所见：探查见肝脏表面呈结节状改变，大小不等，肝方叶及肝尾状叶增生明显，质地较硬。肝脏Ⅷ段可见一局限性隆起，质地较硬。腹腔内未见明显腹水，胃、十二指肠、小肠、胰腺、结肠及直肠未见明显异常。

病理检查：肝活检组织冰冻病理：红褐色组织一块，大小2.8cm×2.0cm×0.8cm，切面黄褐，质中偏软。方叶肝活检组织：红褐色组织一块，大小2.4cm×1.6cm×1.2cm，切面黄褐质中。右肝占位：红褐色组织一块，大小5.0cm×3.5cm×3.0cm，切面黄褐质中。

冰冻病理诊断：肝组织先后送检三次，第一次为肝组织，第二次为方叶组织，第三次为肝占位组织。三次送检病变基本一致，其中以肝占位活检块较明显。肝小叶存在，肝细胞肿胀，肝索部分可分辨。肝界板有破坏，汇管区扩大，可见较多淋巴细胞和一些中性粒细胞浸润，肝小叶中可见小点状炎细胞浸润。综上，初步诊断为中度慢性肝炎。病理诊断：中度慢性肝炎(图5-7-2)。

第五节 肝脓肿

患者，男，61岁。患者20天前无明显诱因出现发热，体温最高达38.6°。10天前就诊于外院，行彩超示右肝前叶不均匀低回声团块。今门诊收治入院。

CT：肝右前叶下段见一不规则混杂低密度灶，大小约8.1×5.8×8.2cm，局部向肝包膜外稍突出肝轮廓，与膈肌分界欠清，其内见多发坏死区，边界模糊，平扫CT值6~34HU，增强后动脉期实性部分及周围强化，CT值45~60HU，静脉期及延迟期逐渐填充，CT值42~52HU，中心液化坏死区未强化。临床穿刺抽吸病理证实为细菌性肝脓肿(图5-7-3)。

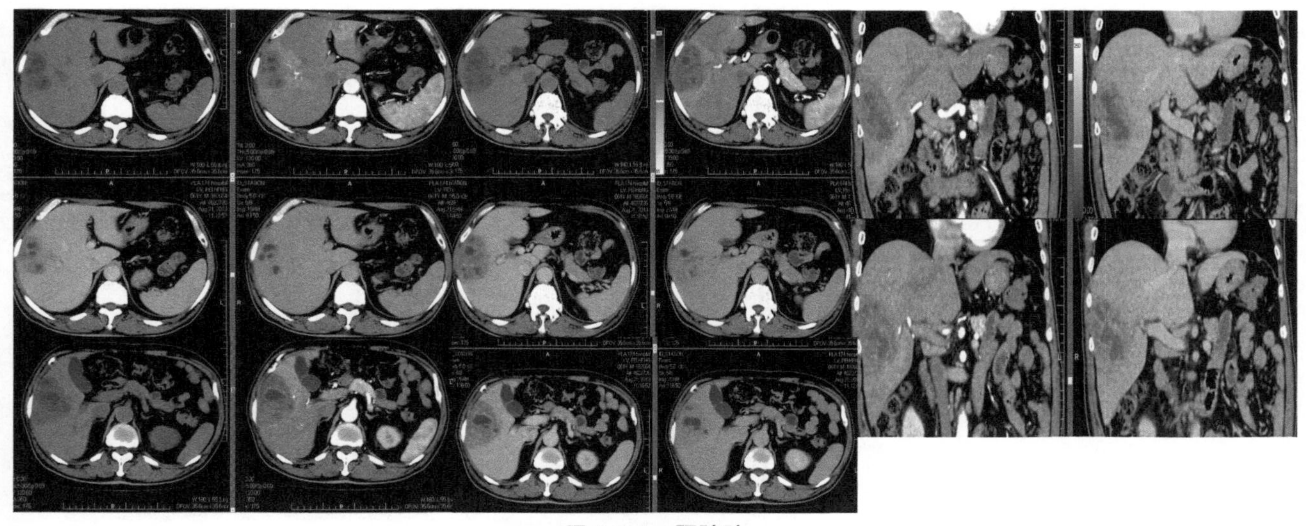

图 5-7-3　肝脓肿

第六节　容易误诊的含气肝脓肿破裂

产气性细菌感染引起的肝脓肿可见气体，CT 诊断含气肝脓肿的报道较少，肝脓肿的死亡率现仍然高达 30%，含气肝脓肿破裂引起的游离气体及腹膜炎是严重急腹症，危及患者生命，因此及时准确诊断有利于处理治疗。

由于患者症状和体征及 X 线片表现与胃肠穿孔有相似之处，极易误诊；立位腹部片对腹腔膈下游离气体显示率并不高，约 70%~80%，有报道仅有 48%。腹部立位片上很难鉴别是含气肝脓肿破裂所致的膈下游离气体还是胃肠穿孔所致。

另外由于脓肿含气量少和肝脏实质和肝包膜的阻隔，气体和液体游离到腹腔量较少，不易发现膈下游离气体。而 CT 对腹腔游离气体显示率高，可达 95.6%，能清晰显示腹腔少量游离气体和腹膜腔积液，腹腔积液少见，对肝脏实质及肝脓肿气 - 液平显示更是立位腹部片所不能及的，因此 CT 扫描有利于找到更多诊断依据。一组 2 例病例均明确显示肝组织前缘的小的新月形气体密度影及腹膜腔积液和肝实质内大小不一的低密度影和气 - 液平，从而易于与胃肠穿孔鉴别。由于含气肝脓肿破裂临床工作中较少见，当立位腹部片出现右侧膈下肝区气 - 液平时易误诊为右侧膈下肠曲积气（如间位结肠），即使合并膈下游离气体，而且有明显临床症状和体征也易惯性思维考虑为胃肠穿孔以致于误诊。该组 1 例 X 线片上见少量膈下游离气体，右侧肝区见一 3 cm 长液平仍然误诊为胃肠穿孔，将液平解释为肠管反应性扩张或者郁张，另 1 例 X 线片无明显膈下游离气体仅肝区气液平征象诊断为不排除为产气菌引起的肝脓肿。

以上 2 例诊断的经验和教训认识到当腹部立位片发现右侧肝区膈下气液平和膈下少量游离气体，特别当患者有明显腹痛，腹膜炎体征时要怀疑本病行 CT 检查。由于 CT 能较好显示腹腔积液和游离气体，而且患者明显寒战，高热，白细胞明显升高，肝右叶多发低密度影，多个气液平，肝前缘见小的新月形游离气体，容易考虑到肝脓肿，不易误诊。

与右侧膈下肠曲积气鉴别不难，右侧膈下肠曲积气以间位结肠多见，多能看到结肠带，症状和体征亦可帮助鉴别。含气肝脓肿破裂腹腔积气和积液量一般较少，CT 检查更敏感，有利于了解破裂情况发现少量游离气体与胃肠穿孔鉴别。由于患者病情紧急未行增强扫描。

第七节 左肝外段肝脓肿

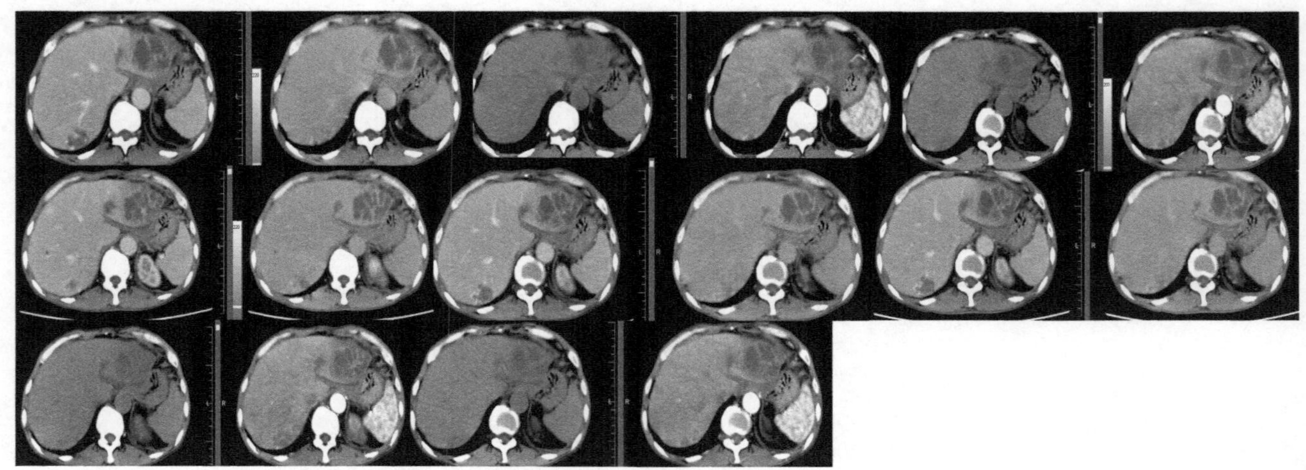

图 5-7-4 左肝外段肝脓肿

患者,男,67 岁。

病理检查:肝左外叶:肝组织一块,大小 12cm × 7.5cm × 4cm,表面呈暗褐色,切面灰红灰褐,质中偏软,其中见一灰白灰红区域,大小 4.5cm × 3cm,与周围界限不清。胆囊:胆囊切除标本一具,大小 8.5cm × 3.5cm × 2cm,表面光滑,剖开胆囊腔内含大量黑褐色结石,黏膜粗糙,壁厚 0.7cm。常规:肝左外叶切除标本:病理诊断镜下可见正常肝小叶结构被破坏甚至消失,残存肝细胞团间纤维组织增生伴坏死及脓肿形成,纤维间质可见散在的受压扭曲的腺管样结构,待做免疫组化检测进一步协助诊断。胆囊切除标本示慢性结石性胆囊炎伴罗 - 阿窦形成。

免疫组化检测:阳性:Hepatocyte(肝细胞 +),CK19(胆小管 +),CK18(肝细胞及胆小管 +),CK8(肝细胞及胆小管 +),CK(P)(肝细胞及胆小管 +),CK(L)(肝细胞及胆小管 +),CK7(胆小管 +),CD10(胆小管 +),Villin(肝细胞及胆小管 +),Actin(纤维间质及血管壁平滑肌 +),SMA(纤维间质及血管壁平滑肌弱 +),Desmin(灶区纤维间质 +),CD34(血管内皮 +),Ki-67(+,约 15%,主要为肝细胞);阴性:CK20,CEA,AFP,ALKP80。肝左外叶切除标本免疫组化诊断:结合临床、影像学检测、免疫组化检测及组织学图像,符合肝脓肿形成(图 5-7-4)。

第八节 误诊病例简介:嗜酸性肝脓肿与肝的恶性肿瘤

肝脓肿常见有 3 种类型,其中细菌性肝脓肿常为多种细菌所致的混合感染,占 80%;阿米巴性肝脓肿约占 10%;而真菌性肝脓肿低于 10%。肝脓肿常见的临床表现包括高热、寒战、肝区疼痛、乏力、食欲不振、恶心和呕吐等。

鉴别诊断:随着抗生素的广泛应用,不典型肝脓肿渐趋增多,不少被误诊为其他占位性病变,特别是早期肝脓肿,与肝内其他病变鉴别有一定困难。

硬化型肝癌:是肝细胞性肝癌的一个特殊病理类型,平扫为片状低密度影,增强动脉期病灶强化程度不一,可仅轻度强化或不强化,门静脉期和延迟期强化反而明显,可见边缘环形强化或病灶内点状强化,有持续强化特点。

胆管细胞癌:多位于肝左叶及汇管区,常伴有肝内胆管扩张及邻近肝包膜凹陷、回缩,CT 增强主要表现为轻度不均匀强化,以边缘为主,邻近肝实质无一过性异常强化。

炎性假瘤:平扫为低密度或等密度而不易发现,

由于缺少肝动脉供血,故在动脉期无明显强化表现,门静脉期或延迟期病灶边缘环状强化,分隔增强,中心或壁结节强化,中心可有更低密度区为凝固性坏死,病灶中的分隔增强及增强后病灶相对缩小对炎性假瘤有重要诊断意义。

该例误诊的主要原因:患者无发热病史;病灶内脓腔不明显, CT 值约 30 HU,部分与正常的肝组织相似;病变较小,单发,内部无蜂房样改变;无典型的晕环征; MRI 信号及 CT 增强特点不典型;自身对不典型肝脓肿认识不足。另外,该例可能是肝脓肿的过渡阶段或吸收好转的方式之一,以肝纤维组织增生、肉芽组织形成和凝固性坏死为主,液化坏死的相对较少,故无明显的液体成分,可能亦是导致误诊的主要原因。

第九节　细菌性肝脓肿的误诊与置管引流

细菌性肝脓肿是临床常见严重疾病,CT 引导下经皮穿刺置管引流已成为首选治疗方法。然而在实际工作中,有时却面临这样一个尴尬的局面:临床和影像学表现上高度怀疑肝脓肿,在经皮穿刺病灶后却不能抽出典型的脓液,很难判断是脓液黏稠还是术前诊断错误所致,以致难以决定是否继续置管治疗。

多数肝脓肿的 CT 表现为中央均匀液化坏死区、边缘有“双靶征”、病灶内有积气等 CT 征象,少数肝脓肿可表现为“簇状征”、“蝴蛛征”、“蜂窝征”、“周边多囊征”等。大多数肝脓肿容易诊断,但少数肝脓肿与肝细胞癌、胆管细胞癌、肝转移瘤的临床和 CT 表现存在重叠,容易造成误诊。

一组有 1 例肝细胞癌和 1 例胆管细胞癌病灶内积气,术前误诊为肝脓肿,而肝细胞癌容易发生肿瘤卒中,病灶内积气可能是氧气与血红蛋白分离所致。该组有 2 例肝转移瘤和 1 例肝细胞癌 CT 增强边缘有“双靶征”改变,术前误诊为肝脓肿,活检组织病理证实肿瘤中央凝固性坏死,周边残存的肿瘤强化形成内靶,肝细胞癌周围的纤维组织和被压缩的肝组织、转移瘤周围水肿带形成外靶。

该组 14 例肝脓肿,病理镜下可以发现多处脓细胞聚集,脓腔之间为部分坏死肝组织、较多成纤维细胞及小血管增生、大量中性粒细胞浸润。这揭示了该组肝脓肿属于脓肿壁形成早期,而脓肿壁形成后期将出现较多的胶原纤维。

该组肝脓肿病灶造影均表现为对比剂迅速均匀分布到在病灶各个区域,形成集簇或蜂窝状对比剂充盈,比较直观显示出脓腔,也印证了组织液化性坏死。病灶造影显示脓腔细小,加上脓液黏稠,故往往难以抽出脓液。

值得一提的是,该组肝脓肿的小脓腔大多相通,在一处注射,整个病灶轮廓全部显示,是否可以推测脓肿早期,细菌毒素使组织坏死,继而大量嗜中性粒细胞浸润崩解释放出蛋白溶解酶,使坏死组织液化形成脓液,脓液沿着肝组织间隙向四周附近流动蔓延,如果细菌毒力相对较弱而人体抵抗力相对恢复的情况下,肝组织残存的地方迅速展开组织修复形成局部脓肿壁,以致形成这些相互连通的蜂窝状脓腔。

该组肝转移瘤中央均为凝固性坏死,缺乏流动性,故对比剂只能在针尖局部聚集,不能向病灶各个区域流动。而存活肿瘤组织致密,对比剂仅能在针尖附近肿瘤间质中渗透。该组 1 例肝细胞癌对比剂相对弥散范围较大,且在病灶后缘形成新月形潴留,可能与肿瘤间质丰富有关。

该组 14 例肝脓肿通过术前病灶造影获得了明确的诊断,均成功置管引流,取得了满意的效果。关于置管引流适应证,文献报道中存在分歧,部分作者认为脓腔较大时才适合置管引流,而另外作者认为即使脓肿液化不全亦可穿刺抽吸引流,认为这样可以清除已坏死组织,减轻脓腔压力,同时向脓腔内注射一定量的抗菌药和糜蛋白酶,有助于周围坏死组织的液化及炎症吸收好转。该组作者同意后者观点,该组病例通过引流管以抗菌药生理盐水冲洗病灶,可以增强抗菌效果,稀释黏稠脓液,带走坏死组织碎片,有利于病灶的修复。该组没有使用糜蛋白酶或尿激酶腔内注入,主要是考虑到病灶造影时脓腔是相通的,事实证明通过生理盐水稀释脓液,可以达到彻底引流的目的。综上所述,病灶内造影能够直观显示出脓腔,可以协助明确肝脓肿的诊断。对于诊断不明确的肝脓肿,如果经皮穿刺抽不出脓液,建议先行病灶造影,不宜盲目置管。

第十节 误诊病例简介：肝脏 IgG4 相关性炎性假瘤

炎性假瘤是一种以纤维结缔组织增生伴有大量炎性细胞浸润为特征的良性非肿瘤性病变，肺脏是最好发部位。肝脏炎性假瘤少见，仅占全身炎性假瘤的 7%~8%。部分肝脏炎性假瘤与 IgG4 密切相关，属于 IgG4 相关性疾病。

肝脏 IgG4 相关炎性假瘤的 MRI 特征：肝脏 IgG4 相关炎性假瘤以中老年男性患者多见，临床症状缺乏特征性，MRI 在术前诊断中发挥着重要作用。本病病理表现为大量淋巴细胞及 IgG4 阳性浆细胞浸润、纤维组织增生和闭塞性静脉炎，其 MRI 表现与病灶内炎性细胞、纤维组织、坏死等成分的构成、分布以及病变的进程密切相关。

一项研究结果显示，典型病例呈渐进性或持续强化，伴延迟包膜样强化及中央无强化区。这主要由于病灶中央富含炎性细胞，而周边以聚集的纤维组织为主；且此种包膜样强化往往较厚，需要与肝细胞癌中薄包膜强化（≤2 mm）相鉴别。病灶中央无强化区则与凝固性坏死、微脓肿形成、小胆管扩张及致密的细胞成分等相关。该项研究中 1 例患者的 2 个病灶呈不典型廓清表现，与肝细胞癌难以鉴别，Kong 等（2014）认为可能与闭塞性静脉炎所致的病灶门静脉供血不足有关。DWI 可提供组织细胞微结构信息。肝脏 IgG4 相关炎性假瘤在 DWI 上均呈高信号，ADC 图上呈相对稍低信号，这与病灶中大量密集淋巴细胞浆细胞浸润有关。但由于 DWI 图像信噪比及分辨率较低，且 ADC 值受多种因素影响，诊断还需结合其他序列进行综合考虑。

肝脏 IgG4 相关炎性假瘤的诊断要点：肝脏 IgG4 相关炎性假瘤除需与肝内胆管细胞癌、乏血供肝细胞癌、转移性肝癌、淋巴瘤等恶性病变鉴别外，还需要与孤立性坏死结节、肝脓肿、不典型血管瘤、肝腺瘤等良性病变鉴别。根据该项研究结果，结合文献，该组作者认为以下特点有助于诊断。中老年男性患者多见，临床表现缺乏特征性，实验室检查可呈炎性改变，肿瘤标志物常无异常。病灶多单发，肝包膜下分布，边界清楚。T_1WI 上病灶呈相对低信号，T_2WI 上呈相对稍高信号，DWI 上呈不同程度高信号，ADC 图上呈稍低信号，增强扫描多为渐进性强化及持续强化，可伴随延迟包膜样强化、灶中无强化区等征象。

该项研究的局限性：①样本量小；②回顾性分析可能造成选择偏倚；③ IgG4 相关炎性假瘤及非 IgG4 相关炎性假瘤的影像表现有无差异尚有待进一步研究。

综上所述，肝脏 IgG4 相关炎性假瘤的 MRI 表现具有一定特征性，病灶于肝包膜下分布，边界清楚，T_1WI 为低信号、T_2WI 稍高信号，DWI 呈高信号，ADC 图上为稍低信号，增强后呈渐进性或持续高信号，伴延迟包膜样强化及中央无强化区。

第八章　肝寄生虫病

第一节　肝泡性包虫病与肝癌的鉴别

常规 MRI：泡球蚴与肝癌在肝内均呈浸润性生长，形成实质性肿块，病灶呈不规则的实性占位，磁共振的鉴别诊断：①泡状棘球蚴在 T_1WI 和 T_2WI 上以低信号为主，感染的病灶在信号强度上有变化，而肿瘤富含水分故绝大部分肝癌多为长 T_1 长 T_2 信号（在 T_1WI 上为低信号，在 T_2WI 上为高信号）；②泡球蚴病变境界较清，无灶边水肿，而肝癌病灶边界欠清，多有灶边水肿；③泡球蚴的坏死液化区不规整，为具有特征性的“溶岩状”或“地图状”，肝癌病灶的坏死形态多位于中心部；④注射顺磁性对比剂后泡球蚴病灶不强化，而肝癌病灶多明显强化，其动态强化过程呈“快进快出”表现；⑤水成像对包虫小囊泡显示更清楚，还可显示泡状棘球蚴病灶侵蚀破坏肝门部胆管，引起胆管梗阻，病变区内胆管破坏、邻近胆管受压移位等情况。

功能性 MRI：肝泡状棘球蚴在肝内呈浸润性生长，形成实质性肿块，在 B 超及 CT、MRI 常规扫描上可显示为肝脏内高密度或稍长 T_1、稍长 T_2 信号占位病灶，不规则坏死液化腔及散在或不规则片状钙化灶为其典型的影像学特征。当肝泡状棘球蚴内缺乏典型钙化或合并感染时，与肝癌鉴别较难。肝癌是由密集的肝癌细胞组成，水分子运动受限，ADC 值较低；但泡状棘球蚴由无数密集微小的囊泡组成，其内为豆腐渣样或胶冻状蚴体碎屑和小泡，水分子运动相对实性肿瘤要自由，因此其 ADC 值高于肝癌。肝泡状棘球蚴中心液化坏死区的 ADC 值大小不一，大部分 ADC 值较高，少数 ADC 值很低且接近肝脓肿的 ADC 值，这是因为肝泡状棘球蚴在肝内浸润性生长破坏了肝内胆管并继发感染所致，因此通过 ADC 图来判断病灶内是否合并感染，可为肝泡状棘球蚴的合理治疗提供依据。

第二节　不典型的肝血吸虫病表现

血吸虫病是热带地区分布最广的寄生虫病之一，全球每年大约有 500 万 ~600 万易感人群，其中超过 200 万人感染血吸虫病，包括 120 万人显性感染，20 万危重病例。血吸虫，也称裂体吸虫，是寄生在宿主静脉中的扁形动物。寄生于人体的血吸虫种类较多，主要包括日本血吸虫、曼氏血吸虫和埃及血吸虫 3 种。其中在亚洲主要是日本血吸虫，被认为是致病性最强、感染最难控制种系，可能与其人畜共患特点有关。中国长江流域及日本、菲律宾及印度尼西亚少部分地区是日本血吸虫病高发地区，每年有数百万人饱受日本血吸虫病困扰与折磨。在 3 种血吸虫中，埃及血吸虫易于寄生在盆腔静脉内，尤其是前列腺 - 膀胱静脉丛，虫卵穿过静脉壁进入膀胱，随尿排出。日本血吸虫和曼氏血吸虫主要寄生在大、小肠静脉中，向肠腔内排卵，随粪便排出体外。

血吸虫成虫主要寄生在门脉系统，引起门脉系统栓塞。且虫卵可随门脉血流进入肝脏，引起慢性肉芽肿性改变，从而继发肝脏纤维化及门脉高压等。虽然，日本血吸虫及曼氏血吸虫均易引起汇管区纤维化，然而，小叶间隔纤维化却是日本血吸虫的特征性表现。晚期血吸虫病病人可并发各种胃肠道、肝脾及神经系统严重并发症，严重者可导致死亡。并且血吸虫病患者结直肠癌、肝癌及胆管细胞癌的发病率明显增加。尽管有文献报道曼氏血吸虫与肝脓肿发生和发展相关(包括单源性和多源性病原微生物感染),但到目前为止,由日本血吸虫感染引起类似改变病例未见文献报道。

有作者报道1例肝血吸虫患者以肝脓肿为主要临床和影像学表现。研究发现病原菌对血吸虫诱发的慢性肉芽肿内胶原蛋白、纤维粘连蛋白及蛋白多糖等细胞外基质有高度亲和性,认为血吸虫病患者易继发感染,伴发肝脓肿;且由血吸虫虫卵导致慢性肉芽肿内细胞外基质及层粘连蛋白形成和降解本身也可导致脓肿形成。因此,上述观点有可能解释该病例仅行经皮穿刺引流疗效不佳而必须经手术切开排脓才能获得最终根治的原因。

肝血吸虫病典型超声和CT表现常在感染数年后出现,其中以何种表现为主,取决于其病理类型,包括汇管区纤维化、坏死后性纤维化以及虫卵钙化等。

超声典型表现肝脏形态大小异常,轮廓不规整,实质内可见线形分隔,围成大小不一的多边形或不规则形,联合其间相对正常肝实质,呈大小不一网格状改变,即"马赛克"征;少数患者还可出现斑点状、结节状及筛网状改变,提示部分小叶间隔纤维化和钙化。该组2例超声表现为肝脏不均匀低回声肿块,与典型肝血吸虫病表现不同。

小叶间隔钙化是肝血吸虫病最具特征的CT表现,钙化通常呈线形,与肝脏包膜垂直,表现为"龟背"、"蟹足"及"地图"样改变。肝血吸虫病其他CT表现还包括肝脏大小异常、轮廓不规整、周边出现压迹,以及因肝纤维化、实质回缩引起肝门区脂肪向肝实质内蔓延等。CT增强上肝血吸虫病通常表现为分隔状、不规则形及包模样强化。

该组第2例CT表现为单发密度不均匀性肿块,其间夹杂小片状低密度区,未见明显钙化;增强病灶呈轻度强化,与肝脏炎性假瘤的表现相识,容易误诊为肝脏肿瘤。虽然Rodrigues等(2009)曾报道肺血吸虫病可表现为炎性假瘤样改变,但肝血吸虫病未曾有类似改变报道。磁共振成像对钙化显示不佳,因此对肝血吸虫病诊断价值受限,仅提示非特异性肝小叶间隔的纤维化,表现为长T_1/稍长T_2信号改变。

总之,该组报告的病例1旨在提示疫区肝血吸虫病患者有继发双重感染,伴发肝脓肿的高度风险,而对此类患者给予肝脓肿常规治疗,通常会效果不佳。病例2旨在说明肝脏血吸虫病可呈炎性假瘤样改变,即非典型地表现为肝实质内不均匀性肿块,呈轻度强化,没有钙化。此类患者极易误诊为肝脏肿瘤,给诊断带来很大困难,鉴别诊断有赖于病理学检查。而且,本身慢性疾病通常就与恶性病变程度相关,因此准确诊断及彻底的治疗至关重要。

第三节 误诊病例简介:肝肺吸虫病误诊为肝癌并腹腔多发转移

肝肺吸虫病是一种有一定区域性分布的肺外型吸虫病,临床少见,潜伏期长,起病缓慢,常无特异性症状,临床诊断比较困难。有作者报告1例误诊为原发性肝癌并腹腔多发转移、经病理活检证实及吡喹酮治疗有效的肝肺吸虫病。肺吸虫病是一种人兽共患的自然疫源性寄生虫传染病,其病原为肺吸虫,广泛分布于东南亚国家,我国仅在少数山区流行,人类感染肺吸虫病主要是通过进食带有后期囊幼虫的生的或未煮熟的石蟹、蝲蛄、河蟹和小龙虾等。

肺是其最常感染的器官,中枢神经系统亦常受累,临床上肝脏受牵连的情况比较少见。但肝脏实际被牵连的情况远远比想象中的要多,主要原因与该病误诊率极高有关。

该例患者虽未进食过生的或不熟的鱼、蟹等食物,但居住在肺吸虫病发病率较高区域,血中嗜酸性粒细胞比例明显升高,仔细观察其CT表现,肝右叶和左叶内病灶为多发囊状、分叶状低密度影,囊腔内无强化,囊壁强化,符合Kim等(2004)、Rha等(1999)报道的肝肺吸虫病的影像学特点。但因该病临床少见,很多医生对其认识不够,忽视嗜酸性粒细胞升高的意义,尽管该患者既往无肝病史,甲胎蛋白正常,在肝病疾患高发,肝脏的实性占位极易诊断为肝癌,尤其是在影像学诊断肝癌有95%的特异性的影响下,故可能误诊为肝癌。

病理检查是诊断肝肺吸虫病最可靠的手段。一些作者认为只要在病变组织中查见肺吸虫体或虫卵,即可确诊,如未见虫体或虫卵,只要具备以下特点亦可明确诊断:①含有凝固性坏死的多房性小囊腔或坏死腔穴形成；②在坏死物中查见多量夏科-登（Chareot-Leyden）晶体；③大量嗜酸性粒细胞浸润。

该病例病灶中虽未查见肺吸虫体和虫卵，但病理见大片坏死伴嗜酸性粒细胞浸润，嗜酸性脓肿形成，并可见夏科-登晶体，结合肺吸虫血清学检查阳性，给予吡喹酮治疗后症状消失病灶吸收，诊断肝肺吸虫病成立。

肝肺吸虫病具有一定区域性，临床少见，很多医生不了解，且其临床表现不典型，诊断标准不易获得，误诊率极高，加强对该病的宣传和教育，使广大医生对该病保持高度的警惕性是减少该病误诊的关键；另外提高医生对该病影像学特点的认识、尽早行活组织病理学检查亦可大大减少误诊。

第九章 肝脏孤立性坏死结节

第一节 误诊病例简介:肝孤立性坏死结节与肝炎性假瘤

患者,男, 57 岁。体检发现肝占位 6 天入院。MRI:肝右后叶下段见一类圆形结节影,大小约 1.6cm × 1.8cm, T_1WI 低信号, T_2WI 略高信号,中间囊变区呈更高信号,扩散成像实性部分信号稍高;增强扫描结节边缘环状强化呈稍高信号,中间无强化仍呈低信号,边界变清楚。肝内外胆管无明显扩张,肝门结构清楚。MRI 诊断:肝右后叶下段结节影,考虑炎性假瘤可能,请结合临床。

手术所见:肝脏表面无硬化结节,肿物位于右肝第 6 段,大小约 2.0 cm × 2.0 cm,质中,边界清楚,包膜完整。余肝未扪及明显肿物,腹腔淋巴结未触及明显肿大。无腹水。

病理检查:右肝肿物切除标本:灰褐色组织一块,大小 2.3cm × 2cm × 2cm,切面见一黄色坏死样结节,大小 1.8cm × 1.5cm,与周围界限清楚。常规病理诊断:右肝肿物切除标本镜下见肝组织中央有一凝固性坏死结节,结节与周围界限清楚,周围肝小叶及汇管区存在,小叶内肝细胞浊肿,汇管区可见少量慢性炎细胞浸润,待做免疫组化检测进一步协助诊断。免疫组化检测:阳性:Hepatocyte(肝细胞 +),CK19(胆小管 +),CK18(肝细胞及胆小管 +),CK8(肝细胞及胆小管 +), CD34(血管内皮 +), Ki-67(+,约 5%,主要为炎细胞);阴性: HBsAg, HBcAg, CEA, AFP。右肝肿物切除标本:免疫组化诊断:结合临床病史、HE 组织学图像及免疫组化检测结果,符合肝脏孤立性坏死结节(solitary necrotic module,据文献,属一种少见的良性病变,病因尚不明确,建议治疗后复查)。

第二节 误诊病例简介:肝脏孤立性坏死性结节与肝脓肿

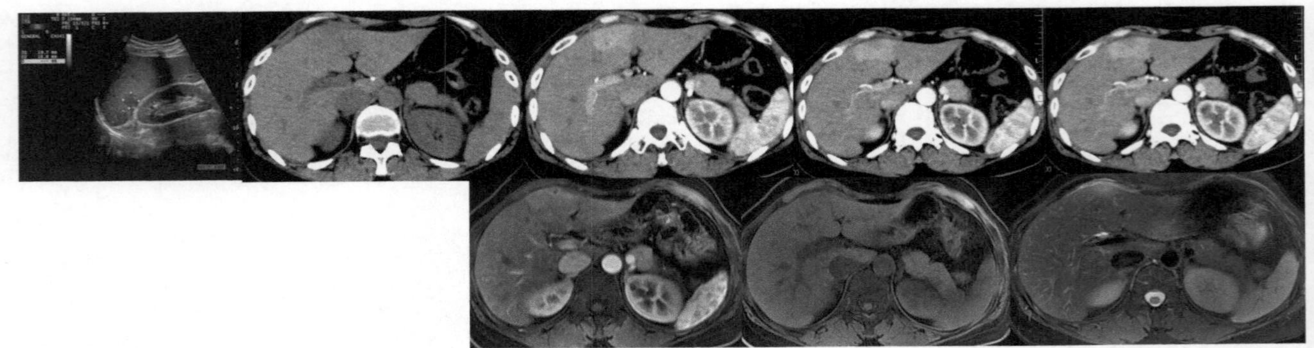

图 5-9-1 肝脏孤立性坏死性结节与肝脓肿

病例,女, 43 岁。反复上腹部疼痛不适 1 年加重 4 天入院。MRI 诊断:肝脓肿。

手术所见:上腹部正中 15cm 手术切口。腹腔无腹水,肝脏表面无硬化结节,肿物位于肝第 4 段,大小约

1.0cm × 1.0cm，质中，边界清楚，包膜完整；余肝脏未扪及明显肿物，腹腔淋巴结未触及明显肿大。肠管、脾脏、胰腺、盆腔未见肿瘤转移。病理检查：左肝肿物：肝组织一块，大小 6.0cm × 4.5cm × 3.5cm，切面暗褐、质中，可见一灰白结节，直径 0.8cm。病理诊断：左肝肿物切除标本：肝脏孤立性坏死性结节（图 5-9-1）。

第三节　误诊病例简介：肝脏孤立性坏死结节与炎性假瘤

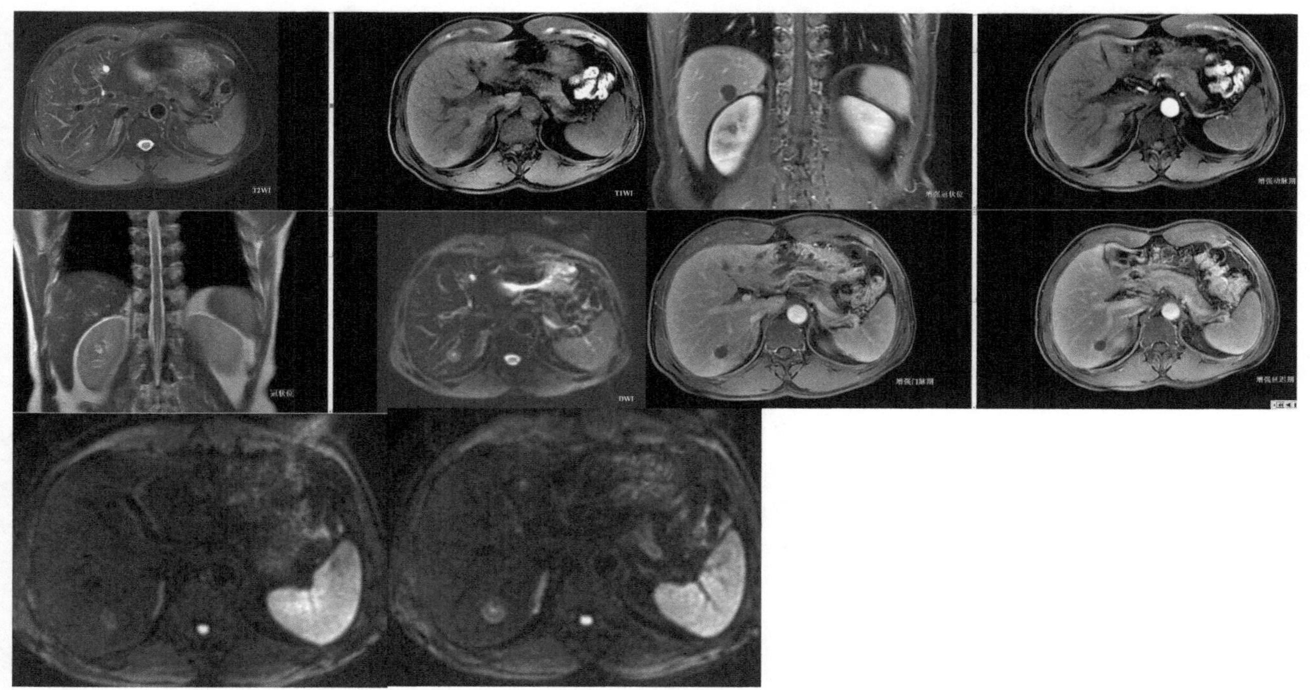

图 5-9-2　肝脏孤立性坏死结节与炎性假瘤

病例，男，57 岁。体检发现左肝占位六天入院。

MRI 诊断：肝内多发囊肿，左肾囊肿；肝右后叶下段结节影，考虑炎性假瘤可能，请结合临床。

手术所见：腹腔无腹水，肝脏表面无硬化结节，肿物位于右肝第 6 段，大小约 2.0cm × 2.0cm，质中，边界清楚，包膜完整；余肝脏未扪及明显肿物，腹腔淋巴结未触及明显肿大。肠管、脾脏、胰腺、盆腔未见肿瘤转移。病理检查：灰褐色组织一块，大小 2.3cm × 2cm × 2cm，切面见一黄色坏死样结节，大小 1.8cm × 1.5cm，与周围界限清楚。常规病理诊断：右肝肿物切除标本：镜下见肝组织中央可见一凝固性坏死结节，结节与周围界限清楚，周围肝小叶及汇管区存在，小叶内肝细胞浊肿，汇管区可见少量慢性炎细胞浸润，待做免疫组化检测进一步协助诊断。

免疫组化检测：阳性：Hepatocyte（肝细胞 +），CK19（胆小管 +），CK18（肝细胞及胆小管 +），CK8（肝细胞及胆小管 +），CD34（血管内皮 +），Ki-67（+，约 5%，主要为炎细胞）；阴性：HBsAg，HBcAg，CEA，AFP。免疫组化诊断：右肝肿物切除标本：结合临床病史、HE 组织学图像及免疫组化检测结果，符合肝脏孤立性坏死性结节，属一种少见的良性病变，病因尚不明确（图 5-9-2）。

第四节　肝脏孤立性坏死性结节与海绵状血管瘤同存

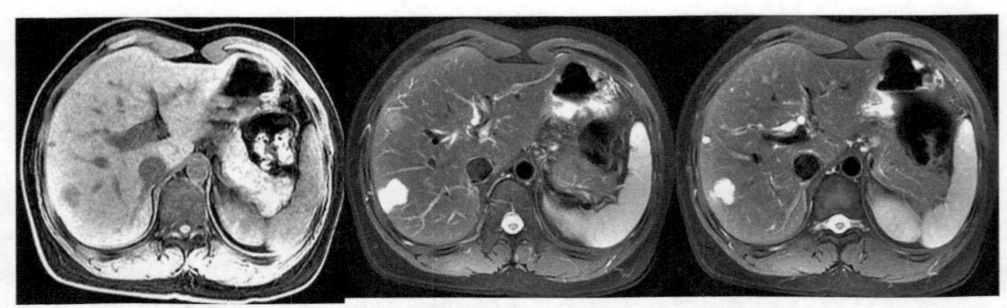

图 5-9-3　肝脏孤立性坏死性结节与海绵状血管瘤同存

患者，女，45 岁。因反复右上腹胀痛不适 17 年，再发 2 个月入院。肝胆脾胰彩超示：肝内实性占位病变、肝血管瘤、胆囊泥沙样结石，胰、脾未见明显异常。实验室检查：乙肝病毒核心抗体 2.300S/C.O.（+）、乙肝病毒表面抗体 >1000.00mIU/ml（+），甲胎蛋白 19.59ng/ml ↑，凝血指标示活化部分凝血活酶时间 25.6 秒↓、国际标准化比值 0.80 ↓、凝血酶原时间 9.1 秒↓。

病理检查（右肝前叶病灶）：冰冻病理：右肝前叶肿物：淡黄色组织一块，大小 4.5cm×4.5cm× 2.0cm，中央可见一淡黄色肿物，直径 1.7cm，质中与周围组织界限清楚。冰冻病理诊断：右肝前叶肿物切除标本：初步诊断肝脏孤立性坏死结节，待作石腊常规切片进一步证实。常规病理检查：肝肿物切除标本：镜下见病变大片坏死，周边纤维组织明显增生，并形成包裹，与正常肝组织分界明显；肝组织浊肿，部分汇管区纤维组织增生，炎细胞灶区浸润。病理诊断：肝脏孤立性坏死性结节。附：本例有血管瘤记录，文献上记载，该病与肝血管瘤硬化后，肝中央发生坏死有关。

病理检查（右肝后叶病灶）：A“血管瘤”：肝组织两块，大小分别为 6cm×3.3cm×1.5cm 和 2cm× 1.2cm×0.7cm，切面灰黄质中，局灶灰红面积 1.5cm×1.1cm。B“胆囊”：胆囊一具，大小 10.5cm× 4.5cm×4cm，剖开内含透明液体及泥沙样结石，内壁光滑，壁厚 0.2cm，胆囊颈见一结石，大小 1.5cm×1.3cm×1cm，另见游离的结石一个。病理诊断：右肝后叶海绵状血管瘤，肝细胞水肿。慢性胆囊炎伴结石形成（图 5-9-3）。

第十章　肝神经源性肿瘤

第一节　误诊病例简介:神经纤维瘤病侵犯肝脏与肝脏多发占位病变

神经纤维瘤病属于斑痔性错构瘤病。其特征为皮肤色素沉着,伴全身多器官和多系统的神经纤维结节性病变,病理为神经鞘瘤和神经纤维瘤,多属良性病变,少数可恶变。神经纤维瘤病常为广泛的腹部及腹膜后侵犯,侵犯肝脏极其少见。

有作者报告一例误诊病例,其临床表现为:年轻女性,右上腹部胀痛不适为主要临床表现;既往有先天性神经纤维瘤病;无家族史;肝脏病变病史较长,由5年前体检B超发现;肝功能正常,甲胎蛋白、癌胚抗原及癌抗原检查均正常;入院后根据病史、体检及辅助检查发现为肝脏多发占位病变。

腹部影像学表现:B超发现肝左叶病灶,回声不均匀,形态不规则,低血供;CT平扫见肝左叶多发不规则均匀低密度病灶,增强动脉期、门静脉期及延迟期(3 min),病灶未见明显强化,相对于正常肝组织保持为均匀低密度。病灶边界清晰,主要位于门静脉周围,包绕门静脉左支及肝动脉,未见门静脉内栓子形成及左侧肝门分支的变形。由于肝脏神经纤维瘤病罕见,为误诊的主要原因。但该患者既往有先天性神经纤维瘤病,应该考虑到肝脏神经纤维瘤病的可能性。本病需与肝内占位病变,如血管瘤、转移瘤等鉴别,根据病史和CT表现可以区别。

第二节　误诊病例简介:肝脏副神经节瘤

病理学:副神经节由数量众多的神经上皮细胞组成,形态学具有共同的特征,即具有大量富含儿茶酚胺的神经分泌颗粒。副神经节瘤是一类发生于副神经节体上肿瘤的总称。肾上腺髓质的副神经节瘤就是我们所熟悉的嗜铬细胞瘤。发生于肾上腺外的其他部位的副神经瘤,按解剖位置和功能命名,具有儿茶酚胺分泌功能的肿瘤称为功能性副神经节瘤。副神经节瘤的发生部位以腹膜后较常见,其次是纵隔、颈部、颅底等,发生于肝脏的极其少见,相关文献报道甚少。

副神经节瘤根据与交感神经系统相关性分两类:前者常位于头颈部,包括颈动脉体、迷走神经内的及纵隔和主动脉、肺动脉之间的不含嗜铬细胞的副神经节;后者为位于交感神经周围,可以反应性分泌儿茶酚胺的富含嗜铬细胞的副神经节。副神经节多位于中轴线附近(脊柱旁和椎前神经节)或者邻近骨盆的结缔组织内,在颈胸段的后腹膜腔占优势。

肾上腺外、腹部的副神经节瘤分为三组:主动脉弓上、主动脉弓下和膀胱的副神经节瘤。还有报道发生于罕见部位的副神经节瘤如:胆囊、肠系膜、肾脏、前列腺和卵巢等。发生于肝脏的副神经瘤少见,国内外文献鲜见。有作者猜测发生于肝脏的副神经节瘤是否为通过肝动脉迁移而来的副神经节细胞形成的。

组织学上,副神经节主要由主细胞和支持细胞构成,前者细胞聚集形成特征性的“zellballen”结构,胞质内富含神经内分泌颗粒;后者位于主细胞周围。电镜下,这两种成分排列呈巢状或腺泡状,构成特征性的副神经节组织的图像。

免疫组织化学检查:神经特异性烯醇化酶、CgA、Syn和一些神经肽阳性为诊断副神经节瘤诊断的敏感性指标, S-100阳性亦有助于诊断,该例

CgA(+)、Syn(+),提示副神经瘤诊断;而上皮膜抗原(-)、平滑肌肌动蛋白(-)可与上皮源性及肌源性肿瘤相鉴别。

副神经节瘤的良、恶性鉴别比较困难,恶性副神经节瘤的特征包括发病部位、肿瘤的坏死、血管侵犯、局部侵犯及透明小体的缺失等。神经肽的低表达、尤其是生长抑素和 VIP 的负染色与肿瘤的恶性有关。该病例可见肿瘤内部呈类圆形坏死,与周围边缘正常肝脏组织分界不清,提示为恶性。

临床表现:副神经节瘤可能具有遗传性,常与家族性副神经瘤、神经纤维瘤病Ⅰ型、脑视网膜血管瘤病、Carney 三联征(肺软骨瘤、胃平滑肌肉瘤和肾上腺外副神经节瘤)和多发性内分泌腺瘤病等有关。因此,当患者有副神经节瘤应行遗传学检查。大部分肾上腺外的副神经节瘤常表现为腹部疼痛或可触及的腹部包块;但是有时当肿瘤很大时患者仍无症状,常因其他原因的检查中偶然发现。

腹部副神经节瘤临床症状包括:恶心、呕吐、腹泻、腹胀和体质量减轻。在一些功能性副神经节瘤,因分泌儿茶酚胺可表现为高血压、出汗、头痛、焦虑、心动过速和心悸等。

手术完整切除肿瘤是副神经节瘤的唯一有效的治疗手段,传统手术方法为剖腹探查及肿瘤完整切除术,但随着腹腔镜技术的不断提高及术前影像诊断水平的提高,腹腔镜越来越多得到运用。本病例因肿物巨大而未行腹腔镜切除。当肿瘤切除过程中可因肿瘤受到挤压、牵拉,引起儿茶酚胺的大量释放,从而引起急性肺水肿、心脑血管意外以及心功能衰竭等发生,因此术前明确诊断很重要。副神经节瘤对放、化疗不是很敏感,但放、化疗作为术后辅助治疗手段,对预防患者术后复发转移及提高术后生存率有一定的帮助。

影像学研究:文献报道的副神经节瘤影像表现多为圆形或卵圆形,通常直径大于 5 cm,实性或囊实性,边缘清楚、锐利,密度均匀或不均匀(伴有坏死、囊变)。CT 增强表现为强化明显,坏死囊变区不强化,这与副神经节瘤富血供有关,仅有少数病例强化不明显。该病例 CT 增强后强化明显,中心可见不强化的囊变坏死区。

第十一章　肝脏淋巴动力学异常

详见本书 本卷 第九篇 第七章 肝脏淋巴动力学　　异常。

第十二章 朗格汉斯细胞组织细胞增生症

朗格汉斯细胞组织细胞增生症在肝脏

朗格汉斯细胞组织细胞增生症是一组发病原因不明的可造成局限性或广泛性多脏器损害的多系统疾病,发病率约为 4.5~9/1 000 000,最常见的受累部位为骨骼和皮肤,其他受累部位包括淋巴结、耳、眼眶、骨髓、脾、肺、胃肠道和肝脏。朗格汉斯细胞组织细胞增生症,过去称为组织细胞增生症 X,是一组发病机制未明的全身多系统疾病,目前认为本病是局部或全身的朗格汉斯组织细胞异常增生所致;国际组织细胞协会按照是否累及多系统器官,将朗格汉斯细胞组织细胞增生症分为单系统及多系统型,一组 17 例患儿均为多系统受累型。

病理学:朗格汉斯细胞组织细胞增生症的诊断金标准的主要依据为具有特征性的朗格汉斯组织细胞形态,且细胞内必须 CD1a 和/或 CD207 呈阳性。因为 CD207 呈阳性可证实 Birbeck 小体的存在,因此,现在朗格汉斯细胞组织细胞增生症的确诊并不必须依赖电镜检查来发现 Birbeck 小体。该组所有行活检的病例的免疫组织化学结果均为 CD1a 呈阳性。

临床表现:临床上,以肝脏受损为主要表现的朗格汉斯细胞组织细胞增生症较罕见,其诊断及鉴别诊断也较困难。然而,明确有无肝脏受累并与其他肝脏病灶的鉴别对于儿童朗格汉斯细胞组织细胞增生症患者的预后判断及治疗措施制订非常重要。

据文献报道,有肝脏累及者的 3 年存活率仅 51.8%,而无肝累及者 3 年存活率为 96.7%,

因此,朗格汉斯细胞组织细胞增生症患者肝脏有无受累对于朗格汉斯细胞组织细胞增生症的预后及治疗具有重要意义。肝脏朗格汉斯细胞组织细胞增生症通常具有以下临床表现:肝大、梗阻性黄疸、继发于门静脉高压的脾大、肝功能异常、胆管浸润导致的碱性磷酸酶增高。该组病例中有 14 例患儿表现为肝功能异常,有 5 例出现皮肤巩膜黄染。

影像学研究:朗格汉斯细胞组织细胞增生症肝脏受累的影像学表现与其病理分期密切相关,朗格汉斯细胞组织细胞增生症肝脏损伤的病理改变主要为异常增生的组织细胞浸润门静脉周围的结缔组织,常选择性地侵犯胆管而导致胆管破坏和损伤,进而导致硬化性胆管炎,最终发展为胆汁性肝硬化及肝功能衰竭。

肝脏朗格汉斯细胞组织细胞增生症在组织病理学上通常分为四个阶段:增殖期、肉芽肿期、黄色瘤期、肝纤维化期。增殖期、肉芽肿期出现门静脉周围组织炎性浸润、水肿,相应地在 B 超上呈门静脉血管周围相对界限清楚的低回声病灶,在 CT 上呈低密度,MRI 上呈 T_1WI 低信号、T_2WI 高信号;在黄色瘤期,门静脉周围病灶富含脂肪,在 B 超上呈高回声,在 CT 上呈低密度,MRI T_1WI 上呈低信号,T_2WI 呈高信号;纤维化期以胆管周围纤维化和小结性胆管硬化为特征,并出现硬化性胆管炎表现,在这个阶段,B 超显示门静脉周围边界清楚的低回声灶,其内可有点状高回声灶, CT 及 MRI 的影像学表现除上述表现外,还可表现为肝脏形态异常,肝表面凹凸不平,MRCP 还可表现肝内外胆管不规则扩张。

该组资料基本支持上述观点,但是该组作者在 MRI 上并没有发现明确的黄色瘤期病变,即 MRI T_1WI 上低信号,T_2WI 呈高信号的病灶,考虑与病例数较少有关。

Henter 等(2004)认为肝脏肿大是肝脏朗格汉斯细胞组织细胞增生症最重要的表现之一,主要为朗格汉斯组织细胞的直接浸润或由于全身免疫系统活化导致枯否细胞增殖所致,影像学改变主要为肝脏上下径超过正常范围,肝叶边缘膨隆,肝脏周围间隙变窄,肝下角变钝。

肝内弥漫性小结节灶及门静脉周围间隙分布的软组织灶考虑为朗格汉斯细胞组织细胞增生症浸润肝实质所致,病理上朗格汉斯细胞组织细胞增生症浸润有选择性侵犯门静脉周围间隙为主的特点,在早期表现为弥漫性分布的结节,在晚期结节灶融合,CT 增强扫描显示为门静脉周围树枝样异常密度灶或者“门静脉晕征”，而MRI增强扫描“门静脉晕征”不明显。在CT扫描的患儿中，有4例仅表现为肝内弥漫性结节灶而无“门静脉晕征”及肝内胆管扩张改变，这4例患儿病程较短（为5天~2个月），且有3例肝功能正常，其中2例显示肝稍大，另1例肝形态正常，出现该种表现可能是病变处于早期阶段，病灶较小尚未融合所致，同时也提示影像学在肝功能出现异常之前即可显示病灶。

朗格汉斯细胞组织细胞增生症肝脏受累后导致胆管不规则扩张，这和病变侵犯胆管，胆管壁增生及纤维化，进展为硬化性胆管炎有关。胆管周围广泛性纤维化、胆管硬化以及继发性门静脉高压所致，CT和MRI均表现为肝脏形态异常，边缘凸凹不平，肝叶段比例失调，肝裂增宽，门静脉主干直径增宽，脾肿大。此征象和常见的病毒性肝炎等所致肝硬化不同的是，其肝脏的萎缩并不明显，甚至可见肝脏肿大。晚期肝门区和/或腹膜后淋巴结肿大考虑为朗格汉斯组织细胞浸润所致。

CT和MRI均可显示朗格汉斯细胞组织细胞增生症各期肝脏受累的改变，但是各有优势。CT的优势在于：扫描速度快，可以进行任意方向的三维成像。但是CT让患儿不可避免地接触了射线，况且，单凭CT仍难以在增殖期、肉芽肿期、黄色瘤期之间准确区分，尽管病理上黄色瘤期病灶内出现脂肪浸润，但CT难以区分其内的微量脂质成分。因此要判断病灶内脂质成分的有无，MRI可能更有帮助。MRI的优势在于对于软组织的分辨率较CT高，更有利于微小病灶的检出，而且可进一步行MRCP了解胆管情况，明确有无硬化性胆管炎。因此，对于怀疑肝脏朗格汉斯细胞组织细胞增生症的患者，建议行MRI及MRCP检查。

鉴别诊断：当肝脏朗格汉斯细胞组织细胞增生症表现为门静脉周围树枝样病变及“门静脉晕征”时，则需要与淋巴瘤、肝淤血、肝先天性囊性纤维化鉴别；当表现为弥漫性小结节灶时，需要与肝结核、肝脏真菌感染等鉴别；当表现为胆管扩张及肝硬化时，则主要需与原发性硬化性胆管炎或其他原因所致肝硬化鉴别。尽管有时单纯影像学表现与上述疾病鉴别仍有一定的难度，但由于肝内病变多为朗格汉斯细胞组织细胞增生症多系统受累的表现之一，很少有朗格汉斯细胞组织细胞增生症单独侵犯肝脏的病例，故仔细询问病史，体格检查全身皮肤有无皮疹或浅表淋巴结肿大，进一步行颅脑MRI检查了解有无垂体柄病变，X线或CT检查有无骨骼病变或肺内病变，可有助于鉴别诊断。

从该组病例中可以初步总结出以下结论：当朗格汉斯细胞组织细胞增生症患者肝脏在CT上出现弥漫性分布的小结节灶或门静脉周围树枝样低密度灶及门静脉晕征时，或者在MRI上出现弥漫性分布的稍长T_1、长T_2结节灶或门静脉周围树枝样稍长T_1、长T_2信号灶时，高度提示肝脏受累，预示朗格汉斯细胞组织细胞增生症患儿的预后欠佳，有必要采取积极的治疗控制病变的发展。

第十三章　肝脏真菌感染

第一节　免疫抑制状态下并发肝脏真菌感染

血液系统肿瘤化疗后,导致外周血中性粒细胞数目渐少、功能下降,细胞免疫力低下,易诱发真菌感染。血液系统肿瘤化疗后发生真菌感染的概率约7%。然而真菌引起的肝脓肿,仅凭临床症状很难诊断。

发病机制:血液系统肿瘤化疗可以引起机体免疫抑制,器官移植后、恶性肿瘤化疗后、慢性消耗性疾病、不合理使用抗生素、长期静脉插管、大量激素或免疫抑制剂应用也可以引起机体免疫抑制,这些都易导致机体深部真菌感染。近年来,随着局灶性肝脾真菌感染发病率的升高,而逐渐认识。引起机体深部真菌感染最常见的病原菌为白色念珠菌,还有其他一些自然界普遍存在的真菌,如曲霉菌、组织胞浆菌、球孢子菌和放线菌也较常见。血液系统恶性肿瘤的病人深部真菌感染的诊断决定治疗方案,对预后有重大影响。

如果误诊为白血病肝脾浸润,而继续加大化疗药物的剂量,将导致严重的后果,使深部真菌感染难于控制,甚至引起病人死亡。因此,深部真菌感染的早期诊断有及其重要的意义。

影像学研究:影像学检查对于肝脏真菌感染的诊断和随访观察有重要的意义。在临床上,常用超声、CT 和 MR 来诊断和观察肝脏真菌感染。肝脏真菌感染在 CT 上表现为弥漫性低密度影,边界清楚,大小约 0.5cm~2.0cm,增强扫描轻度强化或无强化,在急性期可以是双环征、牛眼征,但是这些征象很少在 CT 上表现出来。一组病例中有一例纯红系再生障碍性贫血患者的一个病灶较大,直经大于4.0cm,该病灶在平扫和多期增强扫描表现双环征。

该组病例强化程度与文献报道的结果一致。该组病例均是多发病灶(>2 个)。Metser 等(2005)研究了肝脏真菌感染的 CT 多期增强扫描,动脉期病灶的发现率为 100%,而门静脉期病灶的显示率为69%。CT 动态扫描有助于肝脏真菌感染的发现,动脉期最有利于对病灶的发现。超声对肝脏真菌感染的发现率与 CT 扫描静脉期的发现率接近,然而 CT 比超声更易发现微小肝脓肿。Anttila 等(1996)研究了 CT 静脉期对肝脏真菌感染的显示,与 MR 动态扫描对比,发现 CT 对病灶的发现率只有 MR 的60%。所以对肝脏真菌感染病灶的显示, MR 能显示更多病灶,是最好的检查方法。肝脏真菌感染的影像表现与其病理变化有密切的关系。免疫抑制病人由于机体白细胞数目降低或缺乏、功能低下,对侵入机体的病菌的炎症反应较轻或几乎没有,而脓肿的形成有待于一定中性粒细胞在炎症部位的聚集。所以在病人白细胞数目降低缺乏或功能低下时,机体内即使有真菌感染,却不能形成脓肿,所以在肝脏真菌感染只有到机体和中性粒细胞数量上升到一定程度时,在 CT 才可以显示。所以机体的炎症反应对于肝脏真菌感染的 CT 显示有着重要的意义,同时提示在没有形成脓肿时,CT 动脉期扫描对肝脏真菌感染发现具有重要的价值。

鉴别诊断:①细菌性肝脓肿在 CT 表现为典型的“环靶征”,中心的坏死,肉芽组织增生形成脓肿壁,脓肿壁外围组织环形水肿,脓腔内可见气体影,平扫病灶边缘模糊,增强扫描病灶境界相对清晰,脓肿壁明显强化;真菌感染的病灶周围无水肿,与细菌性肝脓肿比较,细菌性肝脓肿的病灶比较大,周围有水肿,全身感染症状明显,没有导致免疫抑制的病因;真菌性肝脏感染病灶均为多发,病灶最大直径较小,大部分伴有肺部真菌感染(8/9),有导致免疫抑制的病因。近年来由于抗生素早期使用,使得一些肝脓肿表现不典型，形成蜂窝状或簇状，中间分隔是由于没有完全液化残留组织，如果脓肿进一步发展，分隔则可以液化。

②白血病肝脾浸润：白血病肝、脾、肾浸润时，常表现为异常结节影，多单发，也可多发，病灶大小不一，常伴全身多脏器侵犯和后腹膜淋巴结的增大，肝脏病灶常有明显的强化，一般无全身感染症状。

③肝脏结核：结核性肝脓肿的CT表现与本病比较相似，但是二者的临床表现差异较大，一般没有高热，同时伴有肺部结核病史；深部真菌感染常常是多个器官同时累及，而且脾脏也是多发病灶，有报道经常是肝、脾、肾同时累及。

④肝转移瘤：肝转移瘤平扫为圆形、椭圆形、类圆形或不规则形低密度灶，边缘清楚，密度可以均匀或不均匀，可以单发、多发或弥漫于全肝，大小不等。由于多来自于胃和结肠，缺乏血供，增强时无明显强化，极少数为血供丰富。又因是门静脉供血，故动脉期强化改变少见，在门静脉期时出现的强化，主要为周边强化，中心不强化，即“牛眼征”，一般有原发病史。CT不仅在肝脏真菌感染的检出上有很大的优势，同时对肝脏真菌感染抗真菌药物疗效的观察有重要意义。对于免疫抑制病人，如果临床怀疑感染的发生，而抗生素治疗无效，同时CT显示肝内多发性低密度灶，增强后无或轻中度环形强化，则首先应该考虑到真菌感染的可能。

第二节 原发性肝脏隐球菌病

新型隐球菌是广泛存在于某些动物消化道内的真菌，鸽粪被认为是最重要的感染源，正常人的胃肠道有时也能分离出该菌，因此为条件致病菌，是真菌感染中重要的致病菌。隐球菌病常发生于细胞免疫功能低下患者，如获得性免疫缺陷综合征、血液病、器官移植等患者，而免疫正常者的发病率仅为0.2%。由于病菌常通过呼吸道进入人体，首先引起肺部病变，同时对脑膜和脑具有特殊亲和力，因此肺和中枢神经系统是最常受累部位，严重者也可表现为多个器官系统播散受累。

一例患儿无免疫抑制病史，并且仅以发热和肝功能不全作为首发症状，在隐球菌病相关文献报道中少见，多为个案报道，因此给诊断带来困难。回顾性分析患儿有长期农村生活史，可能是通过食用不洁带菌食物、肠道感染后经门静脉系统累及肝、脾。由于患儿免疫功能正常，菌体引起的组织病理反应是非干酪样肉芽肿形成，这种病理状态是影像学基础。

该例多期相CT扫描主要特征是：①肝、脾病灶边缘动脉期强化明显，可能代表肉芽组织边缘炎症反应活跃，血供丰富；②病灶边缘与周围实质分界欠清晰，反映病变的侵袭性质，这是与淋巴瘤重要的鉴别点；③随采集时间延长，低强化病灶体积渐缩小，内部呈低度均匀强化，中心未见非强化坏死区，这可能与患儿免疫力正常相关，因为目前文献研究显示真菌引起的弥散性肝脾小脓肿往往发生于免疫抑制患者，尤其是使用细胞毒性药物的血液病患者；④肝门区、胰头区及腹膜后淋巴结肿大，反映了病变的播散特性；淋巴结低度强化是坏死性淋巴结炎的常见表现，而后者目前被认为是真菌或分枝杆菌感染性肉芽肿的特征性改变，本例患者淋巴结虽然低度强化，但未见明显坏死区；⑤肝内外胆管系统未见明显受累，未见胆管炎症或梗阻性胆管扩张征象，这与以往文献中胆管受累为主明显不同。

鉴别诊断：本病需与淋巴瘤、腹腔内结核、转移瘤、原发肝脏恶性肿瘤等鉴别诊断。

（1）恶性淋巴瘤：恶性淋巴瘤多见于中、青年，淋巴瘤多数不发生坏死，因此受累淋巴结密度均匀。由于大多数为少或无血供病变，增强后呈低度均匀强化，即使少数增大淋巴结有坏死灶，但坏死灶周围增大淋巴结亦呈均匀强化，不似坏死性淋巴结炎普遍环状强化，且其与周围实质分界更清晰，同时淋巴结受累范围更广，纵隔内淋巴结常增大，而新型隐球菌所致淋巴结炎累及纵隔或颈部淋巴结报道较少，并且主要发生于人类免疫缺陷病毒患者。

（2）腹腔内结核：分枝杆菌组织病理反应亦是肉芽肿形成，但其内为干酪样坏死物并容易发生钙质沉着；因此结节型肝结核增强扫描形成环状或花边状强化、中心为粉末状钙化的特征性改变；而脾脏病灶内出现散在点状钙化灶则基本可诊断为结核；肿大淋巴结部分钙化亦是常见表现。

（3）转移瘤：转移瘤可找到原发病灶，增强扫描后病灶中心低密度、边缘高密度、最外层低于实质的“牛眼征”改变,转移淋巴结多发生坏死,增强扫描后环状强化。

(4)原发性肝脏恶性肿瘤:原发性肝脏恶性肿瘤(多中心型肝母细胞瘤和肝细胞癌)甲胎蛋白大多增高明显;肝细胞癌动脉期明显强化具有特征性,肿瘤虽可淋巴结转移,但同时门脉常有受累。

第十四章　肝紫癜

误诊病例简介:肝紫癜

肝紫癜是一种罕见的肝脏血管源性良性病变,多见于成人。国内外报道大多为个案报告,临床及影像上误诊率高。

病理学:肝紫癜是肝窦腔隙呈多灶性囊状充血改变,病变可呈弥漫性或局限性。该病病理表现按形态学分为2种类型:①充血的囊腔内表面布满内皮细胞,形成源于中央静脉瘤,称为静脉扩张型;②囊腔内表面无内皮细胞,常伴有肝实质的出血坏死,称为实质型。一组收集的病例属于实质型。肝紫癜发病机制尚不清楚,多数学者认为可能与长期慢性消耗性疾病如结核、恶性肿瘤、肾移植、血液病有关,也有报道称与激素、免疫抑制剂、避孕药物有关,并且近年来服用雌激素的女性患者增多。Zafrani等(1984)认为发病机制可能有3种:肝静脉会合处的肝窦流出道梗阻;某种毒性物质对肝窦壁的影响;肝细胞坏死导致囊腔形成。

临床表现:肝紫癜患者多无明显临床症状,部分患者可有乏力、黄疸、腹水等症状,也可合并肝功能不全,但这些表现没有特异性,临床诊断较为困难。一例感染乙肝病毒4年,肝炎病毒对肝细胞的侵害能否致紫癜发生值得商榷。

影像学研究:肝紫癜影像学检查可以提供鉴别诊断线索,影像学表现因病变腔隙大小、病灶与肝窦相通与否、腔隙内血栓是否存在而不同。

Kim等(2007)对8例局灶性肝紫癜影像资料进行回顾性分析后认为:局灶性肝紫癜在增强CT和MRI上可以有不同增强模式。具体表现方式如下:①向中心性强化,4例;②持续性低强化,2例,同时分析①、②可能是由于扩大肝窦充满淤血所致;③持续性强化,可能由于肝窦内充满的血液是新鲜血液所致。

该组作者收集国内外关于肝紫癜文献报道25篇,具有完整影像学资料15篇,共15例,其中弥漫性病变5例,局限性病变10例。弥漫性病变强化方式表现为:肝实质内弥漫分布大小不等结节,增强部分结节呈边缘轻度环形强化。局灶性病变多表现为动脉期轻度环形强化,门脉期及延迟期有持续强化的特点(8/10)。1例患者(编号3)行超声造影检查具体表现为:动脉相病灶增强,信号高于肝实质;门脉相及实质相增强信号减退并且低于肝实质;实质相病灶回声低于肝实质。

该组作者总结归纳的15例病例中局限性病灶10例,平扫病灶多为低密度,低或混杂信号影;增强有8例表现为动脉期轻度环形强化,门脉期及延迟期持续强化,但是相对于肝实质仍为低密度或低信号影;表现类似上述②所述。

另2例患者(编号10,14)影像表现同肝脏海绵状血管瘤,表现类似上述①所述。该组作者分析①、②表现可能是肝窦淤血所致,由于窦腔相通与否导致强化程度有所不同。窦腔大且相通时对比剂弥散快,表现同①;窦腔小且不相通时如②。该组5例弥漫性肝紫癜表现为肝实质内弥漫多个结节,一般呈低密度,低或混杂信号,增强示部分结节轻度环形强化,部分不强化;与肝实质相比,结节在增强图像上表现为低密度或低信号结节。由于肝紫癜病变的病理学基础是肝血管病变,因此在MRI上所显示信号强度多变,若出血处于亚急性期,在T1WI和T2WI上为高强度信号,这时比较有特异性,然而在实际工作中很难遇到。

鉴别诊断:转移瘤:患者发病年龄较大,且有原发肿瘤病史,增强扫描呈周边环形强化,无渐进性强化特点。弥漫性结节性肝紫癜易与肝脏转移瘤混淆。转移瘤患者多提供相关肿瘤病史;没有发现原发肿瘤时,应注意肿瘤标记物的观察,肝紫癜患者肿瘤标记物为阴性。

原发性肝细胞肝癌:典型的影像表现为“快进快出”,诊断容易,且肝癌患者常伴有肝炎、肝硬化病史并且甲胎蛋白增高等。

肝脓肿:典型表现为出现“三环”征。临床工作中肝脓肿多数表现为环形强化,仔细辨别可以发现肝紫癜多为轻度环形强化,肝脓肿外周的“环”是肉芽组织成分,强化较肝紫癜明显。肝脓肿病人多数伴有高热、白细胞增多等感染症状,而肝紫癜很少出现感染相关症状。

肝紫癜发病率低,局限性肝紫癜病变平扫多为低密度,低或混杂信号;增强表现为:动脉期多为轻度环形或不均匀强化,门脉期具有持续性强化的特征。无论病灶体积大小,均无明显占位效应。弥漫性病变多为轻度低强化结节。结合病人相关病史、症状、体征及实验室检查可以提高早期诊断的准确性。

第十五章　肝平滑肌瘤

第一节　肝脏良性转移性平滑肌瘤

良性转移性平滑肌瘤是有子宫平滑肌瘤病史的妇女，在远离部位如肺、肝、腹膜后等脏器出现良性平滑肌瘤。良性转移性平滑肌瘤中多数为肺转移的良性平滑肌瘤，其他部位罕见，其来源和性质尚不十分清楚。良性转移性平滑肌瘤呈良性经过，预后较好。

良性转移性平滑肌瘤的影像表现缺乏特异性，以转移瘤所发生的部位不同而有所不同，发生在肺的良性转移性平滑肌瘤，可为肺内多发结节，也可为单发结节，大多呈圆形，也可有分叶，密度比较均匀；发生在腹膜的良性转移性平滑肌瘤，多为实质性的肿块或结节，边界清楚，可呈分叶状，增强有不同程度强化。

一例肝良性转移性平滑肌瘤影像以肝脏肿块为主要表现，CT 平扫显示病变体积较大，形态规则，边界清晰，密度均匀，肿块内未见囊变、坏死及出血，肿块血供丰富；增强扫描动脉期、门静脉期以及延迟期均有明显强化。

肝良性转移性平滑肌瘤诊断困难，术前基本上难以明确诊断，多由术后病理确诊。

本病需要与腹膜播散性平滑肌瘤和肝脏原发性平滑肌瘤相鉴别。

第二节　原发性肝脏平滑肌瘤

Damel 等（1926）首先报道原发性肝脏平滑肌瘤，随后更多的是个案报道。

发病机制：Prevot 等（1994）报道获得性免疫缺陷综合征（AIDS）并发平滑肌瘤患者 EB 病毒呈阳性，Lee 等（1995）发现 EB 病毒与肝脏平滑肌瘤相关。这些初步结论提示 EB 病毒在免疫缺陷患者中发生肝脏平滑肌瘤的可能性。在无免疫缺陷的患者中发生原发性肝脏平滑肌瘤极其少见。平滑肌瘤常见于子宫及胃肠道等含有平滑肌成分的脏器中。肝脏平滑肌瘤是起源于肝脏间叶组织的良性肿瘤。Hawkins 等（1980）提出诊断原发性肝平滑肌瘤的两个标准：①肿瘤由平滑肌构成；②术前诊断和术中显示无肝外平滑肌瘤和转移性肿瘤存在的依据。

病理学：在病理上，平滑肌瘤与胃肠道间质瘤的组织学鉴别较困难。胃肠道间质瘤对 c-kit 表达阳性，而平滑肌瘤对 c-kit 和 S-100 不表达，对 α-SMA 表达呈阳性，几乎无核分裂象，借此可以明确肝脏平滑肌瘤的诊断。

临床表现：肝脏平滑肌瘤以肝脏肿块为主要表现。疾病早期无任何不适，当肿瘤长到一定大小，对邻近器官产生压迫和牵拉时才出现症状。一例无肝病病史，肝功能正常，病灶不大，术前未能明确诊断。

影像学研究：CT 平扫为低密度，注射对比剂后为明显团状均一强化；MR T1WI 呈低信号，T2WI 高信号，增强早期显示与 CT 增强相同特征，延迟期增强病灶信号快速消退，并有完整包膜。尽管这些表现缺乏典型性，但提示肿瘤为富血管性，与肝细胞癌、肝腺瘤等鉴别有一定困难。肝脏平滑肌瘤常因无特殊临床症状，影像学表现亦不典型，故难以与其他肝脏肿瘤相鉴别，确诊依靠活检。

第十六章　肝横纹肌样瘤和肝门区横纹肌母细胞瘤

第一节　误诊病例简介:肝横纹肌样瘤

横纹肌样瘤最初以“预后不良的横纹肌肉瘤样Wilm瘤”被Beckwith和Paimer(1978)报道,Rorke等(1996)给予正式命名,WHO(2007)将此类肿瘤归为胚胎性肿瘤。位于肝脏的鲜有报道。横纹肌样瘤病程长短不一,多数表现为无痛性结节,形态上类似横纹肌母细胞,但电镜及免疫组化未发现横纹肌分化的证据。横纹肌样瘤其组织上多种多样,可见上皮细胞、组织细胞、神经外胚层,偶可见黑色素细胞、间叶细胞等,目前病理学尚未获得一致的意见。

鉴别诊断:横纹肌肉瘤:横纹肌肉瘤含有横纹肌样细胞、原始神经外胚层细胞及多向分化成分,与畸胎瘤类似,其在CT平扫多表现为混杂密度病变,内多有囊变及坏死,增强扫描肿瘤呈不均匀强化,瘤周可见低密度水肿带,在临床诊断中与肝血管肉瘤较难鉴别。

肝血管肉瘤由于肿瘤细胞沿血管腔隙生长,可阻塞中央静脉及门静脉分支导致瘤内出血。CT平扫时病灶内呈混杂密度影;由于含有丰富的血窦,增强CT动脉期常明显不均匀强化,强化的幅度明显高于肝实质并略低于主动脉,随着时间推移病变可有不同程度的充填,延迟期病灶很不均匀,病灶中心的大片低密度常提示肿瘤的坏死,在病灶中心有时还会看到条状或分隔状强化。静脉期及延迟期无明显增强与该例病变非常类似。

另外,本病还需与上皮样肉瘤、软骨肉瘤、恶性间皮瘤、滑膜肉瘤、Wilm瘤等相鉴别。

第二节　肝门区横纹肌母细胞瘤

胆管树横纹肌母细胞瘤常发生于肝门区,胆管扩张较为常见。在CT图像上,此症表现为边缘几乎与囊肿一样光整或欠光整的低密度区,钙化不常见。

第十七章　其他肝局灶疾病

第一节　类似肝脏肿瘤的肝内异位脾组织植入

异位脾组织可分为先天性和获得性两大类，即副脾和脾组织植入。前者来自胚胎发育阶段背侧胃系膜的左侧，常发生于残余部或其附近，后者是由脾组织自体移植，这常由于脾破裂后行脾切除所产生。脾组织植入结节常见于腹腔，但胸内和皮下发生的亦有报道。

Yoshimitsu(1993)报道1例53岁女性患者，23年前由于患Banti综合征行全脾切除，CT扫描示肿大的肝左叶外侧段内一边界清楚，直径约2.5cm的低密度肿块，增强扫描示早期周边强化，在动态CT扫描晚期仍呈低密度；在MRI，病变于T_1WI呈均匀低信号强度，在质子密度象上呈高信号强度，T_2WI未获得。X线血管造影显示肿块由肝左动脉供血，并见轻度对比剂聚集。由于不能完全排除肝癌的可能性而行手术摘除。手术病理标本显示肿块邻近肝表面，并完全位于肝组织内，由含纤维包膜的正常脾组织构成，外周绕以硬变的肝实质。

该例23年前行全脾切除，手术记录，术中曾行肝组织活检，在记录中没有描述活检的部位，手术过程虽为典型的全脾切除，然而该作者推测，脾组织已种植于肝实质内，特别容易种植于活检处。该例异位脾组织的放射学特征几乎是非特异性的，病变的MRI信号强度与正常脾相似，与其他肝肿瘤（例如：小肝细胞癌，局灶性结节状增生，和血管瘤等）几乎无法区别。X线血管造影表现为动脉期缺乏新生血管形成，毛细血管期呈轻度对比剂聚集并伴以透亮环，这仍不具备足够的诊断意义。动态CT可能稍有价值，在早期肿块从外围向心性强化，在延迟期肿块呈均匀略低密度，这种早期外周强化可能是由于特征性血供所致，即多个小动脉穿过病变包膜，此表现还需求进一步进行评估。

第二节　猫抓伤病

猫抓伤病是由于皮肤抓破而受微生物感染产生的感冒和淋巴结发炎，Rocco等(1985)报告一例难见的病例，不仅有上述症状体征，而且还有肝的大块充盈缺损。这是1例平素健康的16岁少年，出现颈部包块、肝脾肿大及感冒症状，颈块病理检查为慢性炎症和局灶性坏死的淋巴结。腹部CT扫描示肝有大块低密度病灶且为腹腔镜证实。猫抓伤病皮肤试验阳性。

第三节　肝包膜下血肿误诊

肝包膜下血肿是肝脏损伤的常见征象，多发生于肝外伤患者，也可发生于肿瘤、肝硬化、血管瘤甚至脂肪浸润等肝脏疾病患者，并可见于妊娠合并高血压疾患的妇女，尤其是子痫前期——子痫并有溶血、肝酯升高及血小板减少（HELLP综合征）者。

肝包膜下血肿CT表现为肝周包膜下新月形或

双凸形低密度或等密度区，CT 值约 20~47 HU，伴有局部肝实质受压变平，部分表现为葱皮样混杂密度影，肝包膜下血肿密度取决于出血量及出血时间，若血肿新鲜，CT 值接近于肝实质，随着时间延长，可转化为低密度或水样密度。肝破裂出血临床诊断常根据病史、临床表现、体征、腹腔穿刺及超声检查等。

一例术前误诊考虑有以下几种原因：患者外伤史不明确；术前彩超提示肝海绵状血管瘤可能；未行腹腔穿刺；肝包膜下血肿边缘不规则伴结节状稍高密度影，血肿内密度不均匀，酷似囊实性占位病变，诊断医师经验不够。

术后分析该病例出血可能因为：患者曾有过外伤史而未注意，导致肝损伤慢性出血，

血液积聚于肝包膜下，压迫肝实质致肝脏部分坏死及纤维化，因活动后再发出血而发病；肝边缘血管畸形（血管瘤）破裂后出血。该例独特的影像表现可能与病变区有新鲜出血有关。该例病变需与肝边缘的血管瘤鉴别，CT 增强扫描有助于鉴别诊断。

第四节 镰状韧带脂肪瘤

Kakitsubata（1993）报道 1 例 56 岁男性患者，超声检查偶于上腹部前方见一 7cm × 3cm × 9cm 不均质实质性肿块，呈相对低回声，边缘光滑，对胃有挤压。肿瘤形状压之能变。CT 平扫示一脂肪密度实质性肿块，CT 值为 -95HU，无强化，肿瘤内有少量软组织。MRI 为不均质强信号，在 T_1WI 和 T_2WI 图像上为均匀且边界清晰的肿块，其信号强度同皮下脂肪组织。血管造影为少血管性，无肿瘤染色，考虑起源于大网膜。手术见腹前部有一黄色分叶状肿块，有完整包膜，肿瘤血管起源于镰状韧带。该作者认为，脂肪瘤是最常见的实质性肿瘤之一，广泛分布于全身各部，但位于镰状韧带者罕见，其报道甚少。

第五节 肝脏多灶性结节状脂肪浸润

详见本书 本卷 第一篇 第三章 第九节 肝脏多灶性结节状脂肪浸润。

第六节 肝的不规则局灶性脂肪浸润

Scott 等（1980）报告 5 例肝的不规则脂肪浸润，主要表现为肝右叶内脂肪的不一致分布，给超声图像的解释带来严重的困难，超声曾解释为转移性病变或原发性肝新生物。

CT 扫描能清楚地了解脂肪蓄积区的低密度灶，然而在某些病例，脂肪、正常肝组织和转移灶的同时并存则可能产生混淆。肝、脾的放射性核素显像可有助于显示正常吸收区，澄清超声和 CT 所示图像。该作者 5 例的病因盖为：1 例为用药（ACTH 等）后；1 例为滥饮酒精；3 例为营养缺乏，其中 1 例脂肪变出现十分迅速，其时间进程宛如转移病变的迅猛发展。

在 CT 图像上，肝的局灶性脂肪浸润可与肝转移混淆，Halvorsen 等（1982）报告 16 例，其中 3 例同时并存肝转移。局灶性脂肪浸润通常不呈球形，也不是块状的缺损，其 CT 值接近于水；而肝转移灶除非囊性变或坏死，常为圆形或卵圆形，CT 值接近正常肝实质 而超过水。放射性核素肝显像几乎总可以澄清任何混淆于灶性脂肪肝的区别诊断，由于新生物而产生的光子欠缺的边界清楚的病灶与局灶性脂肪浸润完全不同。

第七节　肝裂中的脂肪

肝裂内的脂肪是X线平片上不常见到的组织结构，它可引起急腹症X线诊断的混淆。肝裂内脂肪表现为肝影背景上竖行的透光线影，一般见于卧位片上，而立位片上无腹腔内游离气体可见。CT扫描可清楚看见此透光线影适位于左、右叶之间，为肝圆韧带的脂肪，它常常与肝组织之一舌状突起重叠，称这为肝桥（pons hepatis）。Halber和Daffner（1979）报告1例肝裂内脂肪就是在急腹症病人X线照片时发现的，它可误为胆管内积气或门静脉积气。Haswell（1975），Hillman等（1979）都有类似的报告。另外，在超声扫描时，肝左、右叶相连处可发现一回声区，横行扫描时容易看见，其频率不一致，这即是肝镰状韧带。此正常的组织结构应和肝内肿块区别，镰状韧带影的恒定位置，在扫描时改变换能器的轴可使它的回声结构发生变化，均是镰状韧带的特征性表现，有利于鉴别。

第八节　局灶性肝脂肪浸润

CT表现：局灶性肝脂肪浸润主要见于肝裂周围，表现为孤立的或多发的球形、扇弧形或大片状不规则形低密度病灶，CT值约为0~30HU，对其周围血管无推移，无占位效应。增强扫描如动态CT扫描，病灶不强化或轻微强化，其动态增强曲线与正常肝组织相似。MRI表现：在常规SE序列T_1WI及T_2WI像上局灶性肝脂肪浸润呈略高信号，脂肪抑制序列扫描，该病灶表现为低信号。正常肝岛：弥散型脂肪肝中有时可见无脂肪化的正常肝岛，多见于左内叶后部Ⅳ段和胆囊窝周围，有时不易与肝肿瘤区别。

第九节　肝脏假性淋巴瘤

肝脏假性淋巴瘤是临床上一种极为少见的良性肿瘤。假性淋巴瘤，又称反应性淋巴组织增生，或结节样淋巴组织增生，常见于皮肤、眼眶、胃肠道及肺等，发生于肝脏者罕见，Snover等（1981）首次报道了此病。以往报道的患者中，女性患者多于男性（29∶3），平均年龄为54岁（15~85岁）。一项研究4例中，女3例，男1例，平均年龄50岁。

目前此病的病因仍未明确，可能与全身或局部免疫异常有关。该项研究中的2例合并乙型病毒性肝炎，肝炎病毒感染与此病的发生是否有关尚不清楚，Grouls（1987）认为持续的细胞因子刺激及肝炎病毒感染可能导致假性淋巴瘤的发生。

肝脏假性淋巴瘤病理主要表现为由较为单一的淋巴细胞组成，无异型，有淋巴滤泡形成，中央为生发中心，另有数量不等的免疫母细胞、浆细胞和组织细胞。组织中可有残留的肝细胞索和小胆管，病灶边界清楚，对周围肝组织无侵犯。免疫组织化学，B细胞和T细胞数量相同呈多克隆性。IgH和TCR-γ基因重排分析显示无重排，呈多克隆性。该项研究病理结果与之相符。

肝脏假性淋巴瘤是良性肿瘤，但也有可能转变为恶性淋巴瘤，手术治疗是目前唯一有效的方法，放疗或化疗可能加快疾病向淋巴瘤转变。1例干燥综合征患者发生假性淋巴瘤未作治疗，随访2年变为低度恶性的B细胞淋巴瘤。该项研究中的4例患者均通过手术切除治疗，随访未见肿瘤复发及转变为恶性淋巴瘤。

影像学研究：根据该项研究结果，该组作者小结肝脏假性淋巴瘤的影像特点为：肝脏单发病灶，边界清楚，可合并肝炎或肝硬化背景，左右叶均可发生，病灶最大径约13~53 mm，平均28 mm。CT平扫为均匀的低密度灶，增强后动脉期病灶轻度强化，门静脉期、延迟期强化减退，低于正常肝实质。T_1WI上病灶呈不均匀低信号，与肌肉相仿，T_2WI上呈不均匀稍高信号，稍高于肝组织，强化方式与 CT 增强扫描基本一致。无肝静脉及门静脉的侵犯，无肝门部及腹膜后淋巴结转移。

Ookubo 等（2001）报道肝脏假性淋巴瘤病灶大小为 4~23 mm，单发或多发，增强扫描无强化或轻度强化，与原发性肝癌影像特征相似。该项研究结果与之符合，增强扫描病灶动脉期轻度强化，门静脉期、延迟期强化减退低于正常肝实质强化程度，该组作者推测可能是因为假性淋巴瘤为淋巴组织增生，缺乏血管组织，为乏血供肿瘤，故强化不明显或不强化。

该项研究中 2 例在 CT 增强扫描动脉期见微小血管影进入病灶内，提示病灶内有小的毛细血管通过，病理结果未提及，但与推测其为乏血供肿瘤并不矛盾。2 例行 MR 检查的患者，其病灶在 T_1WI、T_2WI 为不均匀信号，提示为出血坏死灶，与病理结果相符。另外该组病灶最大径为 13~53 mm，较文献报道结果偏大，可能与肝脏假性淋巴瘤常无临床症状及患者不定期体检有关。

鉴别诊断：在影像表现上主要需与原发性肝癌、转移瘤等恶性肿瘤及局灶性结节性增生（FNH）和炎性假瘤等良性肿瘤相鉴别。

原发性肝癌：原发性肝癌发展较快，主要是肝动脉供血，因此在动脉期出现明显均匀或不均匀强化，门静脉期强化程度迅速减低，呈典型的“快进快出”表现，常有假包膜，可有肝内、外转移或门静脉癌栓，且 60%~70% 的原发性肝癌甲胎蛋白（AFP）阳性。而肝脏假性淋巴瘤发展缓慢，女性常见，常合并自身免疫性疾病，增强扫描在动脉期仅有轻度强化，且肿瘤指标常为阴性，因此结合临床病史可鉴别。

肝脏转移瘤：肝脏假性淋巴瘤可合并其他器官的恶性肿瘤，因此需与肝脏转移瘤鉴别，前者常单发，可有轻度均匀或不均匀强化，短期随访病灶无明显变化。而转移瘤常多发，增强扫描呈环状强化，或与原发肿瘤强化方式一致，短期随访病灶增大或进展。

局灶性结节性增生：局灶性结节性增生为肝脏少见的良性病变，病灶一般为 4~7 cm，甚至更大，较肝脏假性淋巴瘤大，增强扫描动脉期明显强化，门静脉期强化逐渐减低，中央的星状瘢痕组织表现为延迟强化，为特征性表现。而肝脏假性淋巴瘤强化程度较弱，亦无星状瘢痕组织。

肝脏炎性假瘤：肝脏炎性假瘤是致炎因子引起的肝局部以组织炎性细胞浸润和纤维增生为特征的瘤样病变，较常见的影像表现是增强扫描周边呈环形强化，当鉴别困难时，可短期复查，经抗炎治疗后肿块变小或消失时，提示为肝脏炎性假瘤，短期无变化，增强扫描呈轻度强化者为肝脏假性淋巴瘤。

综上所述，当肝脏内出现单发较小病灶，边界清楚，增强扫描呈轻度强化，肿瘤指标为阴性，且为合并有自身免疫性疾病的女性，短期随访无明显变化，应当考虑肝脏假性淋巴瘤的可能，认识肝脏假性淋巴瘤的影像特征，有利于提高临床诊断及鉴别诊断的能力。

第十节　局灶性脂肪变和局灶性肝岛

详见本书 本卷 第一篇 第三章 第八节　局灶性脂肪变和局灶性肝岛。

第六篇　肝结节性病变

第一章　肝结节性病变

肝内少见结节性病变

1. 外生性肝癌　外生型肝细胞癌（EG-HCC）是指向肝外生长的肝细胞癌。多见于成人，50~60 岁为发病率高峰。男性多于女性。外生型肝癌的肝外部分最大横径应大于肝内部分，以此可以区别于常见的巨块型肝癌。

分型：带蒂型，有明确的瘤蒂，瘤体完全位于肝外，通过瘤蒂与肝脏相连病获取营养，可侵犯周围组织器官并与周围组织建立新的血液循环；突出型，肿瘤主要向肝外突出，少部分仍然位于肝内，肿瘤也可以侵犯周围组织器官。带蒂型罕见，突出型相对多见。

影像学研究：影像学表现同普通的肝细胞癌。须与腹膜后肿瘤及胃肠道肿瘤相鉴别。发现门静脉癌栓可以提示诊断。部分外生型肝癌是由于肝硬化再生结节突出肝外恶变而来，因此，发现肝硬化基础及肝内子灶可以提示诊断。

2. 纤维板层型肝细胞癌　纤维板层型肝细胞癌（FL-HCC）多见于左叶，常为单发分叶状病灶，质地较硬，呈膨胀性生长，与正常肝组织分界清楚，可以有包膜，呈巨块型，直径通常大于 10cm。瘤体中央有星状纤维瘢痕向周围放射并将肿瘤分隔是其重要特征。另一特点是瘢痕中央可有斑点状钙化。

病理学：镜下，肿瘤细胞呈多边形，嗜伊红染色，细胞核大。纤维基质成分较多，有时排列较整齐，将肿瘤细胞分割成条带状或团状，有一定特征性。

临床表现：纤维板层型肝细胞癌是一种罕见的肝细胞癌类型，仅占总发生率的 1%~2%。男女发病率相近，以青少年好发，患者中 35 岁以下者比例达 15%~40%。临床症状无特征性，以腹块和上腹部不适为主。绝大多数患者无肝硬化基础、少有乙型肝炎病毒感染，甲胎蛋白多阴性。 纤维板层型肝细胞癌虽然肿块较大，但手术切除率高，有较好的预后。即使术后复发，也可再切除，术后生存期 32~68 个月，甚至更高。

影像学研究：CT 平扫为低密度肿块影，边缘清晰，可有分叶。中央瘢痕呈边界清楚星状或不规则更低密度影，可见斑点状钙化。动脉期肿瘤实质均匀或弥散性早期强化，门静脉期肿瘤实质强化消退快，密度较周围的肝组织低。中央瘢痕在动脉期及门静脉期大多无明确强化。少数 25% 纤维板层型肝细胞癌在延时期出现强化。是由于这些少数中央瘢痕内含有血管间质成分所致。肝门部淋巴结转移率高于普通型肝细胞癌。

MRI：肿瘤 T_1WI 86% 为低信号，14% 为等信号，80% 的病例信号均匀；T_2WI 上肿瘤信号不均匀，多为高信号。中心瘢痕，在所有序列上基本都为低信号，这是一个很重要的鉴别点；然而还是有少数为高信号。（类似局灶性结节增生的中央瘢痕在 T_2WI 上高信号）

鉴别诊断：普通型肝细胞癌内可以出现纤维瘢痕，但是一般数量较少，罕见有钙化，临床常有肝硬化和甲胎蛋白升高；肝海绵状血管瘤在动脉期可见边缘早期团状或点状强化，并由周边向中央蔓延，延时扫描肿瘤内强化消退慢，呈等密度或稍高于周围肝组织密度；肝细胞腺瘤常为单发圆形病灶，有包膜及瘤内出血，动脉期均匀强化，门静脉期为等密度或低密度，临床特点为青年女性患者，有的有长期口服避孕药史。

纤维板层型肝细胞癌在 CT 图像上无明显特异性，但在年轻和无肝硬化的患者中，若发现肝内巨大肿块，除外海绵状血管瘤后，应考虑到纤维板层型肝细胞癌的可能性，但应注意与局灶性结节增生鉴别。

3. 局灶性结节增生　病理学：局灶性结节增生是多血供实质性肿块，其内部结构均匀，出血和坏死少见。局灶性结节增生由正常排列成结节的肝细胞、纤维间隔、增生的胆管、浸润的炎性细胞、血管组成。特点是病灶中心有星状瘢痕及辐射状纤维分隔，瘢痕内有厚壁供血动脉。肿瘤内出血、坏死及梗死均罕见，这与肝细胞腺瘤不同。局灶性结节增生比肝腺瘤更常见，约为腺瘤的 2 倍，且与口服避孕药无关。约 80%~95% 为单发。临床表现：肝脏局灶性结节增生为肝细胞良性再生结节，属肿瘤样病变。多见于中青年女性。临床上一般无症状，多偶然发现。

影像学研究：CT 平扫：多数呈孤立的等密度或略低密度肿块，境界清楚，密度均匀，很少有钙化。少数在病灶中可见低密度瘢痕。当肿块呈等密度时，仅表现占位效应或中心之低密度瘢痕。增强：①肿瘤强化特征：早期肿块呈快速明显的均匀强化（动脉期和门静脉早期），在门静脉后期或延迟扫描可见对比剂迅速退出呈等密度。这种强化特征是由于局灶性结节增生有丰富的动脉血供及大的引流静脉和血窦。②肿瘤周围血管影：在门静脉晚期和延迟扫描图像上，局灶性结节增生周围可见血管影，这与肿瘤周围有扩大的血管、血窦有关。③增粗的供血动脉：有作者认为局灶性结节增生是一种先天性血管畸形，动脉血流灌注增加导致肝细胞增生。在动脉期螺旋 CT 扫描常常能显示异常动脉。④瘢痕和分隔：部分可以显示瘢痕组织，在平扫时呈低密度，增强扫描动脉期，瘢痕内可显示供血动脉，在门静脉期和延迟扫描时可见瘢痕逐渐强化呈等或高密度。有时在增强时可显示辐射状纤维分隔。

MRI：MRI 平扫：T_1WI 和 T_2WI 可表现为四种情况：①都为等信号（典型）；②相对低信号和高信号；③等信号和相对高信号；④相对低信号和等信号。典型者中央或偏心瘢痕在 T_1WI 和 T_2WI 分别为低信号和高信号，不典型者 T_2WI 上可表现为低信号等。

局灶性结节增生的假包膜：局灶性结节增生是没有纤维包膜的，但是有假包膜。假包膜的组成是：局灶性结节增生压迫周围正常的肝实质；周围的血管；炎性的反应。由于局灶性结节增生的假包膜为压迫周围正常组织以及一些灶周血管和炎性浸润，因此在 T_2 上为高信号（特征性），而且可能会有延迟强化。肝细胞性肝癌的假包膜主要为纤维成分在 T_1，T_2 上为低信号，增强扫描的延迟期呈持续强化。

纤维板层型肝细胞癌与局灶性结节增生的鉴别诊断：局灶性结节增生一般发生于年轻及中年女性；局灶性结节增生病灶最大径很少超过 5cm；局灶性结节增生钙化少见，有文献报道少于 2%；中心瘢痕信号的不同及强化表现的不同；包膜信号的不同。

4. 肝细胞腺瘤　病因及发病机制：好发于生育年龄年轻女性。如果不应用合成代谢类固醇，男性不会发生。口服避孕药及应用合成代谢类固醇药物导致发病危险性增高。妊娠可能加速肿瘤的生长以及导致肿瘤破裂。另外一个危险因素是 I 型糖原累积症患者，常为多发，且易恶变。病理学：70%~80% 腺瘤为单发，但是多发者并不少见，I 型糖原累积症患者常多发腺瘤，且易发生恶变。大体病理——边界清晰、质地较软、灰白色或者黄褐色，常染有胆汁的结节。组织学类似正常肝细胞，体积较大，富含脂肪和糖原，细胞内外均可见脂肪沉积，细胞间隔有扩大的血窦，由动脉供血，缺乏门静脉供血，血供丰富。缺乏结缔组织，无中央瘢痕，易于出血，有恶变倾向。腺瘤与高分化的肝细胞性肝癌有类似的病理表现，有时组织学上鉴别困难。肿瘤内无中央静脉、汇管区、缺乏小胆管结构——可以与局灶性结节增生鉴别。腺瘤内可见枯否细胞，但数目少且功能差。腺瘤可以有或无包膜。腺瘤细胞体积大，内富含脂肪及糖原，胞质苍白。

影像学研究：CT：平扫：边界清晰、圆形等密度或低密度肿物，部分可见出血及脂肪成分，少数可见钙化。增强：动脉期，不均匀高密度强化；门静脉期，密度相对均匀，可以是高、等或低密度；延迟期，均匀低密度。有时可见包膜的延迟强化。MRI：T_1WI：信号强度不均匀；信号强度增高——脂肪或者新近出血；信号强度下降——坏死、钙化或者陈旧出血。T_2WI：信号强度不均匀；信号强度增高——陈旧出血或坏死；信号强度下降——脂肪或者新近出血。增强 MRI：Gd-DTPA——与 CT 增强类似；超顺磁性氧化铁——腺瘤不摄取。

5. 不典型血管瘤　请详见本书 本卷 第五篇 第二章 第一节 不典型血管瘤。

6. 肝血管平滑肌脂肪瘤　肝血管平滑肌脂肪瘤是一种少见的良性肿瘤。它是由不同含量的脂肪组织、平滑肌和异常血管组成，具有一定特征性影像学表现。肝脏血管平滑肌脂肪瘤可与肾脏血管平滑肌脂肪瘤伴发。发生于肾脏的血管平滑肌脂肪瘤有 20% 患者合并结节性硬化。发生于肝脏的血管平滑肌脂肪瘤有 6% 的患者合并有结节性硬化。在影像学上，肝血管平滑肌脂肪瘤因含脂肪，术前可做出定性诊断，但因瘤内所含脂肪、平滑肌及异常血管的比例不同，具有不同的影像学表现。病理学：大体病理通常见肿块为球形，质较软，呈淡黄色或灰色，可伴有灶性出血坏死，多无包膜。光镜下，典型血管平滑肌脂肪瘤由异常厚壁血管、平滑肌细胞和成熟脂肪组织构成，可伴有髓外造血组织。其中平滑肌细胞可呈梭形或上皮样细胞形态，常以上皮样细胞为主，呈多边形，胞浆丰富，伊红色或透明，有时含有色素颗粒。细胞核可出现显著的异型性，并见多核巨细胞，核仁明显。瘤细胞可成片或成团分布或形成梁索状，并有血窦分隔。多形性上皮平滑肌细胞是病理诊断上的难点，常误诊为肝细胞癌或腺癌。根据瘤内脂肪含量的不同分为四型：混合型、脂肪瘤型（≥ 70% 脂肪）、肌瘤型（≤ 10% 脂肪）、血管瘤型。

影像学研究：肝血管平滑肌脂肪瘤的影像学特点主要取决于肿瘤内脂肪的含量及异常血管所占的比例。肿瘤内存在脂肪是肝血管平滑肌脂肪瘤的特征性表现之一。肝血管平滑肌脂肪瘤的三种组成部分在肿瘤中有的可明确区分。通常，当脂肪含量稍多时，影像上可显示其特征。以脂肪为主（脂瘤型）的血管平滑肌脂肪瘤，应注意与脂肪瘤或脂肪肉瘤相鉴别。当以异常血管为主时，影像学表现与肝血管瘤有些类似之处。50% 的肝血管平滑肌脂肪瘤在影像学上因缺乏脂肪而无特征性表现。对缺乏此特征者，CT 动态增强扫描对诊断有重要价值。肝血管平滑肌脂肪瘤易误诊，应与肝内其他含脂肪的病变相鉴别。

第二章　肝再生性结节

肝内结节性病变的分类和命名：众所周知，肝癌的发生与肝脏的慢性疾病，特别是肝硬化的改变关系密切，尤其在亚洲国家，肝癌多是在乙型肝炎引起的肝硬化的基础上发生。肝内结节性病变多种多样，命名也很多。按照国际胃肠病学会 1995 年对肝内结节进行的统一命名方法，肝实质的结节性病变首先分为再生性结节（RN）和非典型增生结节或肿瘤性结节（DN）两大类。

病理学：再生性结节是肝实质对组织坏死、循环改变及其他刺激所引起的结节状的增生，根据其解剖特点，又分为单腺泡再生结节、多腺泡再生结节、硬化结节、肝段或肝叶的增生、局灶性结节增生等。

当结节的周围没有纤维基质包绕时称为结节再生性增生，常合并有结缔组织病；当周围有纤维间隔分隔时称为硬化结节，在乙型肝炎病毒、丙型肝炎病毒感染或酒精性肝硬化时常见，因此，它代表了通常所称的再生性结节。部分再生性结节内有铁离子沉积时，又称为铁质沉着性结节。目前认为，慢性肝病基础上发生的退变结节是第一步，随后通过腺瘤样增生、不典型腺瘤样增生，最后发展到早期小肝癌进而到进展期肝癌。按照现在的命名法，即从再生性结节到低度非典型增生结节到高度非典型增生结节再到小肝细胞性肝癌，最后到进展期肝癌，在这个过程中，影像学监控非常重要。

影像学研究：肝硬化的再生结节依其大小可分为小结节、大结节和混合型结节，多数属于混合型。按照是否有铁离子的沉积又分为铁质沉着型和非铁质沉着型两种。

病理上再生性结节是在肝硬化基础上增生而形成的肝实质小岛，复制的肝细胞被纤维基质分隔，并压迫周围的基质和胶质，从而导致假小叶的形成。结节大部分或全部被纤维基质包绕。小再生性结节直径多在 0.3 cm 以下。大的再生性结节直径一般在 0.5~2.0 cm，一般不超过 2.0 cm，超过时通常为非典型增生结节。

弥漫分布的小结节型再生性结节（包括铁质沉着型和非铁质沉着型）MRI 上表现比较典型，如果为铁质沉着性结节，在 T_1WI 和 T_2WI 上均为低信号，被中等信号的网状分布的纤维组织所分隔，动态及延迟增强扫描结节本身无强化，后期由于纤维组织的强化而使分隔更加清楚；非铁质沉着性结节在 T_1WI 上和 T_2WI 上均为中等信号，周围纤维间隔为偏低信号，动态及延迟增强扫描结节轻度强化，较纤维组织的强化稍低。

在大结节中，大多数再生性结节在 T_1WI 和 T_2WI 上表现为与肝实质相同的信号，其动态增强模式亦相同，诊断并不困难，该研究的大量病理切片也证实了这点。

该组所选取的再生性结节其信号与周围的肝组织有所不同，需要和其他性质的肝结节病变进行鉴别，特别是与非典型增生结节和小肝细胞性肝癌等鉴别。Murakami 等（1990）认为，再生性结节一般在 T_1WI 上呈高信号，T_2WI 上为低信号。该组所选择分析的再生性结节表现基本上与之相符，即 94.1%（16/17）的病灶 T_1WI 为偏高信号，T_2WI 为低信号。

再生性结节在 T_1WI 上高信号在再生性结节的总体中毕竟是少数，该作者发现其中 62.5% 的病灶在 T_1WI 压脂序列上信号较 IP 序列更高，其机制考虑可能是由于 T_1WI 压脂序列具有完全抑制脂肪的功能，肝脏运用该技术时信号明显提高，与其他的脂肪抑制技术不同，推测可能再生性结节病灶与周围肝组织的信号同时提高，也说明再生性结节的性质与周围肝组织类似。另外，胰腺在 T_1WI 压脂序列上信号也明显增高，其原因是由于含有的水蛋白物质成分，可能再生性结节也有类似的因素影响。由于样本量的关系，其增高的程度未作统计学分析，尚需进一步的统计学和病理方面的证实。

再生性结节在 T_2WI 为低信号的原因不明，Murakami 等（1990）认为可能与含铁血黄素沉着有关，含铁血黄素能有效缩短 T_2，降低 T_2 信号。Kita 等（1996）认为可能病灶周围大量纤维组织的存在也是原因之一，纤维间隔的炎症反应或扩张的血管含水量增加，形成小环形或网状高信号影，从而使结节呈现低信号。再生性结节与正常肝组织相似，都是门静脉供血占优势，因此，在动态增强过程中，非铁质沉着性结节也存在着轻度的强化，虽然其强化程度始终低于周围肝组织。时间信号强度曲线也显示这一变化，呈持续轻度强化，与周围组织的强化趋势一致。但由于病灶 T_1WI 本身信号较高，容易误解成病灶无强化。至于有铁质沉着的结节是否癌变的发生率高，还存在着一些争论。

鉴别诊断：弥漫分布的再生性结节在诊断上并不困难，但孤立性的大结节型再生性结节需与肝脏的其他结节性病变进行鉴别。由于大结节的再生性结节绝少在 T_2WI 上呈现高信号，且在动态增强中不会出现动脉和门脉的高峰期强化，因此和多数小肝癌比较容易鉴别。非典型增生结节直径一般大于 2 cm，其 MRI 信号改变亦有所不同，但再生性结节与部分非典型增生结节之间的鉴别尚有一定困难。

第三章　肝硬化结节

肝硬化中的结节性病变

肝细胞癌常并有肝硬化。一些作者报告 41 例经 MRI 诊断经手术病理证实的肝细胞癌,其中合并肝硬化者 73.2%,由此可见,肝硬化是导致肝细胞癌的重要原因之一。

在 MRI 的 T_1WI 上肝硬化显示有弥漫性等信号或高信号结节,在切除的标本中,除了肝细胞癌主癌外,其他伴随的结节并没有明确的癌细胞,故辨认肝硬化中的结节是重要的。因为,将良性的结节误为肝细胞癌而行手术,对肝硬化病人极为不利。有作者提出,慢性肝脏疾病形成肝细胞癌时,再生结节是第一步,然后经过腺瘤性增生结节(AHN),含有非典型肝细胞或恶性病灶的腺瘤性增生结节,最后发展成肝细胞癌。肝硬化再生结节(RN)在 MRI 的 T_1WI 显示为等信号或稍高信号,直径小于 10mm 的结节;在 T_2WI 为低信号结节。

有作者认为,T_2WI 上的低信号是由于其内有铁质沉着,但是 Matsui 等对 4 例结节用普鲁蓝染色,仅有 1 例有轻度铁质沉着,因此,在 T_2WI 显示低信号的原因并不明确。

腺瘤性增生结节比再生结节大,直径大于10mm,无真正的包膜,但内有血管及胆管,组织变异大。Matsui 将之分为两型,即不含非典型肝细胞的腺瘤性增生结节和含有非典型肝细胞或恶性病灶的腺瘤性增生结节。

在 Matsui 的病例中,所有不含非典型肝细胞的腺瘤性增生结节(n=5)在 T_1WI 为高信号结节,而在 T_2WI 为低信号;含有非典型肝细胞的腺瘤性增生结节(n=2)在 T_1WI 为高信号,而在 T_2WI 也为高信号,与肝细胞癌相似。一些作者报告 1 例重度肝硬化病人,在 T_2WI 肝内有弥漫性高信号的小结节,在 T_2WI 均显示为低信号,其中只有一个直径 10mm 的结节在 T_1WI 为低信号,而在 T_2WI 为高信号,符合肝细胞癌的特点,后经手术证实。另 2 例肝硬化病人,其中 1 例在肝左叶内段有一直径 25mm 结节,T_1WI 显示为高信号,T_2WI 为等信号,经增强 MRI 扫描也未见强化,不符合恶性病变,经手术病理证实为肝硬化腺瘤性增生结节不含非典型肝细胞。另 1 例在肝右叶前段有一直径 20mm 结节,T_1WI 为低信号,T_2WI 为等信号,两个月后复查 MRI,该结节直径已为 30mm,在 T_1WI 仍为稍低信号,而 T_2WI 结节周边有高信号,根据病变信号特点及增长速度认为此结节符合含有非典型肝细胞或恶性病灶的腺瘤性增生结节。

表 6-3-1　肝硬化结节性病变的 MRI 表现

MRI 技术	肝硬化再生结节	腺瘤性增生结节	腺瘤性增生结节	小肝细胞肝癌
		不含非典型肝细胞	含非典型肝细胞	
SE				
T_1WI	低,等或高信号	高或等信号	等或高信号	低或稍高信号
T_2WI	低信号	低信号	稍高信号	稍高信号

第七篇　肝囊性病变

第一章　肝脏囊性病变

第一节　肝囊肿CT诊断的陷阱

Barnes等(1981)认为，CT扫描不能确切地区别良性肝脓肿与其他肝内和肝外的囊性病变,单纯肝囊肿的CT值与感染及新生物有些类似,它们均可出现光滑的边缘,在某些病例不可能看见,也不可能区别病变壁与周围的正常肝实质。有作者认为,在区别良性囊肿和其他病变上,CT检查的特异性在肝脏比肾脏等器官为低,如诊断难以确定,应尽力施予活检。

肝囊肿可为一弧立的病变,或伴发肝的先天性囊性病变。在病理学上,良性肝囊肿考虑为先天性的,它大概出现于胆系形成中的发育缺陷,这些囊肿中可含有胆汁染色或为清沏的液体。肝囊肿通常无症状,除非它加杂一些进行性疾病(如出血或/和感染)。如果囊肿达到足够大,常规体检时也可扪及。更常见肝囊肿可表现为一占位性病变,而在肝转移的搜寻中被发现,由于肝转移大都影响生存,所以区别良性囊肿与肝转移变得极为重要。CT与核素显像比较,在区别诊断中CT特异性较高，CT诊断肝囊肿的标准包括:衰减系数接近于零,边缘光滑,壁薄,增强扫描缺乏对比。

囊性肝包块常见诊断应考虑有:坏死性的肝转移灶和脓肿等。肝转移病灶坏死的CT表现为:比周围正常肝实质密度略低的厚边缘;病灶中心衰减系数接近于零;边缘不规则;壁上结节;液-液平面(流动的平面)等。同样,肝脓肿在CT图像上表现为一密度减低区,其衰减值介于囊肿与新生物之间,而脓肿的密度可因脓肿发展阶段不同而迥异。偶尔，CT以发现病变内有气体而提示为肝脓肿，然在脓肿的区别诊断上临床资料比CT征象更具重要价值。一个病变的囊性可为它的密度的肉眼所见提示,更具特异性者可以测其CT值,典型肝囊肿CT值为0~10HU,而新生物的CT值通常仅稍低于正常肝实质,不幸的是坏死性肝转移、晚期肝脓肿以及慢性血肿之CT值皆可接近于零。相反，CT值稍高于10HU也可见于良性肝囊肿,技术因素(含体积平均或偏斜校准)能虚假地提高囊肿的CT值,加之新近的出血、碎屑或感染皆可使囊肿密度增高。比之于脓肿或坏死性转移,囊肿典型的有一较薄的壁。当囊肿位于肝的边缘时,囊肿的壁能为CT观察到,此刻,有一足够的密度差异来区别囊肿壁与邻近的腹膜后脂肪或壁上可见的腹内脂肪;然而,当囊肿边缘邻接正常肝组织而密度类似时,不应将囊肿与肝轮廓之间的肝实质误为囊肿的厚壁。

关于液-液平面,有作者报告见于肝转移灶坏死,可用以区别于其他病变,事实上此征属非特异性,既可见于肿瘤,也可见于良性肝囊肿。钙化也是非特异征象,周围性钙化常出现于包虫囊肿和淋巴管瘤,也可出现于单纯肝囊肿,并可在动脉内化疗后出现于恶性病灶的周围边缘,所以此征存在并不能完全除外恶性。在某些情况,可能难以确定一个囊性病变是位于肝内或肝外。如果囊性包块壁的密度类似于肝的密度,除非有足够的腹膜后脂肪或腹内脂肪介于肝与该包块之间,CT扫描将难以看清其界面如何,此刻一些征象(如下腔静脉移位)可以有所帮助,但它们又并非绝对可靠。超声对辨别组织密度差异有时可给予帮助。自然,当肿块极大时则更难确定其起源于何处了。

第二节　误诊病例简介:肝囊肿与肝胆管囊腺瘤

患者,女,40 岁。体检超声发现肝囊肿 2 个月入院。CT:肝内多发(约 9 个)大小不等类圆形低密度影,左内叶前缘病灶较大,约 3cm × 5.4cm × 4.1cm,边界清楚,CT 值 9~17HU,增强各期病灶无明显强化,CT 值 11~19HU,肝内外胆管无扩张。CT 诊断:肝脏多发囊肿。术后病理检查:肝脏囊性病变切除标本:灰白色囊壁样组织一块,体积 2.5cm × 1.5cm × 0.2cm,壁光滑。肝脏囊性病变切除标本病理诊断:肝脏囊状病变,纤维性囊壁内衬单层立方和柱状上皮,考虑为肝胆管囊腺瘤。

误诊病例回顾分析体会:回顾认真阅片发现,部分囊壁有强化,但术前被忽略;不少囊壁可见多个小的壁结节,大者约为 0.5cm × 0.4cm,术前观察时也未看见;体检超声发现肝囊肿,误导 CT 诊断未认真仔细观察,这也是一条教训。对待任何囊性病变,都要认真仔细地观察各个囊壁的情况,寻找壁结节之类病变,才能减少和避免误诊。

第二章　肝脏肿瘤性囊性病变

第一节　肝脏肿瘤性囊性病变 CT 诊断

肝脏囊性病变分类：肝脏囊性病变可分为 5 类：①发育性囊性病变，包括肝囊肿，多囊肝，肝胆管错钩瘤，肝内胆管囊肿等；②肿瘤性囊性病变，如肝胆管囊腺瘤、胆管囊腺癌、胆管黏液乳头状瘤、囊性肝细胞癌、囊性肝转移瘤等；③炎性囊性病变，如肝脓肿、肝结核等；④寄生虫性囊性病变，如肝包虫囊肿；⑤其他囊性病变，如肝血肿、肝胆汁瘤、肝表面的假性胰腺囊肿等。肝脏肿瘤性囊性肿瘤性病变少见，随着检查方法的增多及检查技术的提高，对此类疾病的认识在不断提高。

肝脏肿瘤性囊性病变：肝脏肿瘤性囊性病变不多见，临床易误诊。

肝脏的转移性肿瘤是全身脏器中发生率最高的器官之一，多数为实质性，真正原发囊性转移性肿瘤比较少见。文献报道肝脏转移性肿瘤的囊变发生率为 3.3%。囊性肝转移瘤在肝转移性肿瘤中虽不常见，然而它在肝囊性肿瘤中最为常见。肝脏的转移瘤在 CT 上表现多种多样，考虑到肝脏囊性肿瘤时，首先要考虑到转移瘤。肝脏囊性转移瘤常见于：富血供肿瘤快速生长造成坏死和囊变（胰岛细胞瘤、肉瘤、黑色素瘤等）、肿块较大者或黏液腺癌转移（结肠 - 直肠癌、卵巢癌）。囊性转移瘤形成的病理基础为肿瘤的严重液化坏死。肿瘤囊壁边缘不规则结节状或乳头状增厚增粗的房隔等均为恶性囊性病变的征象。该组 18 例中有 6 例为转移瘤，最多的原发肿瘤来源于胃肠道，特别是大肠的恶性肿瘤，该组 3 例（占 50%），CT 表现病灶囊壁可薄可厚，厚壁者需与囊腺类肿瘤鉴别，条状间隔和壁结节以及肿瘤病史可资鉴别，薄壁者囊壁可显示不清，需与肝囊肿鉴别，该组 1 例单发的薄壁转移瘤类似肝囊肿，仅囊内密度较单纯性肝囊肿高，边缘稍欠锐利，结合肠道肿瘤病史及多次检查随访病灶的进行性坏死演变过程得以诊断。

1. 肝转移瘤　该组 6 例肝转移瘤的 CT 表现为：①形态为类圆形或类椭圆形，大小约 2.2~10.5 cm，单发 1 例，多发 5 例；②囊壁单发者为薄壁，多发者为厚壁，未见壁结节；③囊内均为水样密度，CT 值 18~37 HU。增强扫描可见囊壁强化。

2. 肝脏胆管囊腺类肿瘤　肝脏胆管囊腺瘤是罕见的肝脏肿瘤，约占胆管源性囊性肿块的 5%，85% 发生于肝内胆管，肿瘤生长缓慢，但属癌前病变，好发于中年女性，平均年龄 38 岁。临床表现与肿块占位效应有关（间隙性腹痛、黄疸）。病理学特点：肿块大小不定（1.5~35 cm）；边界清楚，有厚层纤维包膜；囊壁内衬单层黏液分泌细胞；囊内液体可为蛋白性或黏液性，偶可胶样、脓性或血性（外伤）；囊内有纤维间隔。胆管囊腺癌与胆管囊腺瘤为同源性肿瘤，可能由囊腺瘤发展而来，有时鉴别困难，与囊腺瘤的不同点：①年龄偏大；②密度更不均匀；③囊壁厚薄不一，实性肿块部分更多；④间隔厚或明显厚薄不一；⑤囊壁息肉样或带蒂肿块多见、明显；⑥囊壁结节强化更为明显。

肝胆管囊腺类肿瘤 CT 特点是：孤立性多房性囊性肿块，边界清楚，有纤维包膜，囊液呈低密度，有纤维间隔和壁结节，偶有包膜钙化，多房性囊腔的密度不均匀，各腔之间的 CT 值可有较大差异，包膜、间隔及壁结节有轻 - 中度强化。囊腺瘤有潜在的恶变可能，可恶变为囊腺癌。

囊腺癌的 CT 特征为：单房或多房囊性肿块，多有壁结节，囊壁大部分清晰，小部分壁厚毛糙，伴有钙化，可见卫星灶，远端胆管常有扩张。囊腺癌与囊腺瘤相比，其囊壁和间隔厚薄明显不均匀，实质性成分更多,实质部分强化更明显。另外,囊腺癌发病年龄较囊腺瘤大。该组2例囊腺癌均为囊腺瘤恶变而来,因为病史中10年前均有B超发现肝脏相应部位“肝囊肿”的历史。囊腺类肿瘤误诊为其他病变较少。

该组3例肝脏囊腺瘤均为类椭圆形薄壁囊性病灶,大小约3.3~11.7 cm.,内见条状薄间隔及小的壁结节,囊内为水样密度,增强扫描为囊壁和间隔及壁结节均明显强化。该组中1例肝囊腺癌巨大,约18cm × 11 cm × 13 cm,边界清楚,大部分囊壁较薄,实质部分为多发壁结节呈肿块样突向腔内,增强扫描实质部分显著强化。另1例向肝包膜突起,约12 cm × 9 cm × 10 cm,边界清楚,囊壁较厚,内见多条实性较厚间隔形成多房,多房内密度不均,增强后壁及间隔明显强化。

3. 囊性肝癌　原发性肝癌为肝脏最常见的恶性肿瘤,但囊性肝癌却非常少见,囊变多为继发的坏死。肝癌细胞可排列成小梁状、实性巢状或假腺样结构,有时可有乳头状结构。瘤细胞间有丰富的血窦,某些窦状隙由瘤细胞衬覆。瘤细胞之间有毛细血管形成是肝细胞性肝癌的重要特征之一。肝脏原发性恶性肿瘤,不论何种细胞类型,其肿瘤坏死所形成的囊肿,均表现为囊肿不规则,囊壁厚薄不均匀,并见壁结节突入囊内,增强检查肿瘤实质成分明显强化。肝细胞癌经局部介入治疗常造成局部组织的凝固性坏死。该组3例均体检发现并未经治疗,其中1例可见多发壁结节,增强后壁结节强化呈花边样,病灶中部有较高密度出血并未见强化, DSA显示了病灶中的肿瘤血管及中部无血管的坏死区,手术也证明病灶中有大片坏死。另有1例病理检查并未发现大片坏死,而提示肿瘤细胞排列呈滤泡状,同时可见透明细胞型肝癌细胞,可谓比较特殊。囊性肝癌虽然也有壁结节,但与囊腺类肿瘤不同,它常常没有完整的可强化的囊壁,壁结节强化仍是肝细胞癌快进快出的特点。囊性肝癌常有肝硬化背景、肿块实性部分仍具有肝细胞癌的影像学特征、治疗史,部分并有甲胎蛋白升高。

该组3例原发性肝细胞性肝癌均为肿块型,类圆形,大小5.0~6.8 cm,均有壁结节样改变,均为体检发现,其中1例壁结节呈花边样强化,中部有较高密度出血,数字减影血管造影(DSA)显示了肿块内的肿瘤血管及中部无血管的坏死区。1例仅乙肝表面抗原阳性,其余化验检查均正常,肿块约5 cm,壁薄,可见分叶,增强扫描见明显强化的壁结节,术前误诊为肝脏囊腺类肿瘤,术后病理为原发性肝细胞肝癌。

4. 肝癌肉瘤　肝癌肉瘤少见甚至罕见,病理学检查可见肝癌肿瘤细胞同时有肉瘤样细胞分化,癌细胞分化和肉瘤细胞分化多少比例可不同。影像表现肝癌肉瘤与肝细胞性肝癌却相去甚远。该组的2个病理诊断为肝脏癌肉瘤的病例临床均无肝炎及肝硬化病史,仅其中1例乙肝表面抗原阳性,甲胎蛋白均阴性。1例因发热就诊,化验血白细胞总数及中性均高, B超提示“肝脓肿”,临床以肝脓肿治疗,但经多种抗生素治疗无显效,CT表现肿块巨大,分叶状,多中心坏死,包膜显示不清,更无典型肝脓肿的环形强化的壁结构,内部也不是早期肝脓肿的蜂窝状,而是火焰状强化灶向腔内延伸。剖腹探查时肿块较软,呈鱼肉状,并可触及坏死灶,坏死腔内穿刺未能抽出脓液,肿块周围见灰白色肿瘤结节,质硬。肝癌肉瘤虽存在肝细胞癌成分,但是发病基础、临床及影像表现均不同于肝细胞肝癌,鉴别诊断方面除肝脓肿外,还需与肝脏囊腺类肿瘤和肝脏平滑肌肉瘤等鉴别。

该组2例肝癌肉瘤肿块均巨大,呈分叶状不规则,内见多发囊性灶,增强扫描实质部分强化明显,囊内不全坏死区呈火焰状。2例均无肝硬化病史,甲胎蛋白均阴性,其中1例因伴有发热和血白细胞计数增高,术前被误诊为肝脓肿。

5. 肝胆管黏液乳头状瘤　肝胆管黏液乳头状瘤是肝胆管乳头状肿瘤中黏液高分泌一类,病理学上类似于胰腺的乳头状囊性肿瘤,肿瘤或呈乳头状生长,或呈实性细胞巢,可有小囊形成。CT影像常表现为肝内囊性肿块,边界清楚,无明显的壁,囊内软组织肿块(结节)影,轻至中度强化,壁无强化,邻近胆管非梗阻性扩张,上下游胆管均可扩张,因黏液高分泌所致,胆管内可有黏液栓,除非出现转移征象,良恶性难以区别,该肿瘤良性可恶变,恶性程度低,预后明显好于胆管细胞癌。胆管黏液乳头状瘤与胆管囊腺类肿瘤不同,它的囊是扩张的胆管,由于肿瘤膨胀生长和黏液的张力形成,囊壁即胆管壁,当然也不是肿瘤上皮和纤维组织。该组中2例均见囊性病灶中有实性结节呈乳头状突向腔内,囊壁薄而显示不清,增强后突起结节呈中度强化。病灶较大者约5cm × 5cm,周围胆管可见非梗阻性扩张;病灶较小约3.0 cm × 1.5 cm,周围胆管改变不明显。

综上所述，肝脏肿瘤性囊性病变以转移瘤最常见，各种病理类型的肿瘤性囊性病灶有其相似和不同的CT征象，典型的CT特征结合临床，多数肿瘤术前可作出正确诊断，并与肝脏非肿瘤性囊性病变有鉴别意义。

第二节　横纹肌母细胞瘤

一些作者指出，胆管树横纹肌母细胞瘤，常发生于肝门区，胆管扩张较为常见。在CT图像上，此症表现为边缘几乎与囊肿一样光整或欠光整的低密度区，钙化不常见。

第三章 其他肝囊性病变

肝脏非肿瘤囊性病变

当肝内发现占位性病灶时,首先要区分实质性和囊性。目前应用影像学手段区分病灶的囊、实性已较简单,但要明确其囊性病变的性质仍存在一定的困难,需要以病理形态学为基础并认真观察、分析CT和MRI中的每个征象,如病变的大小、形态、部位、密度、信号特点等,可对大部分病变做出准确的诊断。

1. 肝囊肿　CT图像上的密度反映人体组织X线吸收量的差异,水的CT值为0,肝实质的CT值为40~50HU。单纯性肝囊肿CT值一般比肝实质低,CT平扫表现为清楚的低密度灶,通过测量CT值可以推断囊肿内容物的性状,但灵敏性不及超声。囊肿与周围肝实质密度相差不大时,CT平扫可表现为稍低密度、等密度甚至高密度,这种密度的差异考虑是囊液含有不同程度的蛋白质和脂质等成分所致。由于CT扫描存在部分容积效应,当囊肿小于扫描层厚时,其CT值实际是囊肿本身和周边肝组织的平均值,在识别病灶及判断囊肿的内容成分时应予以考虑。多房性肝囊肿在间隔很薄的情况下,CT平扫囊肿和血管瘤等都可以表现为相近的低密度影。另外,微小肝脓肿、肝胆管微小错构瘤、肝紫斑病及肝胆管周围囊肿等多发性小囊肿,在相互重叠交错囊壁或囊腔不能分辨的情况下,所测的CT值一定要考虑部分容积效应的因素,因病灶越小所测得的CT值相对越高,故对肝内小的病灶要尽量采用薄层CT扫描,以获得高分辨力影像;增强CT和动态增强CT扫描对诊断帮助较大,可显示囊壁的环状强化及多房性囊肿间隔的线形强化。

肝囊肿的MRI表现主要取决于内容物的成分。蛋白质和脂质等高分子化合物可使结合水的比例增加,内容物的黏稠度上升,T_1、T_2缩短以致影响信号强度。当囊肿内为低黏稠度的液体时,T_1WI、T_2W1分别表现为低信号和高信号,随着高分子化合物含量的增加,MRI信号渐渐发生变化,表现为T_1WI上低~高信号和T_2WI上高~低信号的变化过程。

MRI的空间分辨力低,受部分容积效应的影响比CT大,不能显示小的囊性病变内部间隔和囊壁。另外,小的血管瘤和胆管微小错构瘤等病变,腔内的血液和内容液决定着信号强度,因此在T_2WI上表现为高信号,酷似单房性肝囊肿。

2. 肝胆管周围囊肿　本病的尸检发现率为20.20%,影像学检查发现本病合并肝硬化者占9.09%,不合并肝硬化的发生率仅占3.3%。组织学研究证实,本病是胆管壁外腺的囊状扩张,由于本病常并发成人多囊肾、肝硬化、门脉高压症、胆系感染及全身感染等疾病,故推测其发病机制可能与炎性感染、缺血性变化、胆管周围血管丛异常及先天性因素等有关。病变局限于门脉分布区的1~5级比较粗大的胆管分支是本病的特点,再结合囊肿的大小、数目及原发疾病等征象一般不难确诊。CT扫描病变大部分位于肝门区,多与门脉并行且呈低密度影,少数情况下沿门脉分支呈树枝状分布,随着病灶数量的增加可连成串珠状甚至索状,严重的病变从肝门至末梢部门脉的两侧均可受累。囊肿直径1~10mm,直径也可超过20mm;病变数目在数个至数十个不等,而囊肿本身无其他特征性。

在胆管的全周发生囊肿时,由于病变的推压使胆管和门静脉不能并行,二者分开或交叉,看起来似乎在门脉的两侧都有胆管和病变的存在。基于胆管和囊肿的这种密切关系,CT平扫和静脉胆系造影术并用可使病变显示得更清楚,表现为对比剂不能进行囊肿腔内。根据病变位于门脉区域在胆管周围分布的特点,磁共振胆胰管造影(MRCP)可使病变显示得更好,但从治疗角度并不适用,显示囊肿的数目和大小仍以多平面重建(MPR)效果为佳。

3. 纤毛前肠性肝囊肿(CHFC)　本病最早报道于1896年,因囊肿的内面结构与食管囊肿和支气管囊肿一样都衬有纤毛上皮,同时,肝脏的本身也和食管、支气管一样都发生于前肠,故命名为纤毛前肠性肝囊肿。Chatelain等(2000)经过7例组织学研究提出，纤毛前肠性肝囊肿来源胸腹膜管迷走于肝组织内发生细支气管的前肠遗迹。囊壁的结构在组织学上有特征性，即从囊腔内向外分别由上皮层、纤维结缔组织、发达的平滑肌和纤维性包膜4层结构组成，但通过影像学检查来区分这些结构往往比较困难。本病的影像学表现取决于囊肿内容液的性状和量的多少，根据囊液蛋白质和脂质成分等含量不同，影像学表现各异。CT平扫表现为明显的密度减低区，与孤立性肝囊肿无任何区别，当密度与周围的肝实质相近或略低时易误诊为实质性肿瘤，有时囊肿甚至与周围肝实质的密度完全一致，表现为等密度影，以至于CT平扫不能显示病变，须通过增强CT才能诊断。

在MRI，囊腔内容液黏稠度决定其信号强度的变化，这在T_1WI表现得比较明显。当囊肿大小一定、囊腔内为低黏稠度的液体时，则T_1WI上表现为低信号，而高黏稠度的液体呈等信号甚至高信号；但在T_2WI中，囊腔内容液的黏稠度对信号强度的影响较小，多数病变与肝囊肿相同，表现为明显的高信号。另外，囊肿内出血对MRI的信号强度影响较大，T_1WI和T_2W1分别表现为高信号和低信号。可见，MRI对本病的诊断价值明显优于CT，不仅能根据T_1WI和T_2WI中的信号强度变化区分病变的囊、实性，而且大致可以判断囊肿内容液的性状。由于纤毛前肠性肝囊肿的特征是单房性囊肿，故增强CT和增强MRI往往必不可少，特别是较小的病灶。大量研究显示，仅仅依靠平扫的CT值和MRI信号强度很容易将其误诊为少血供实质性肿瘤，另外在合并脂肪的情况下，要根据增强前、后的CT值和MRI信号强度的变化等进行定量对比分析。

4. 肝内胆汁瘤　肝内胆汁瘤，又称胆汁漏、肝内胆汁性假囊肿，系肝内胆管系统破裂、胆汁漏出并局限包裹在肝内形成的囊性病变。综合文献报道，本病的病因可归纳为三大类：①外伤性肝内胆管系统损伤；②医源性肝内胆管系统损伤，如胆囊手术后、肝切除术后及肝癌经动脉栓塞治疗术（TAE）等；③自发性，不明原因。

本病的诊断首选超声和CT扫描，前者可显示囊性病变、内部无回声、多为多房性和边界清楚等特征性表现，后者主要表现为大小不一的圆形或类圆形、边缘清楚且大部分光整、紧邻胆管系统的低密度病灶，测得CT值20HU左右。增强CT扫描囊内无强化，CT值几乎不变和无明显的囊壁视为本病的特征。

MRI是诊断本病的重要手段，能显示病变的大小、内容物性状、形态和部位等征象，尤其是MRI的信号表现具有特征性，即T_1WI和T_2W1分别表现为低信号和高信号。增强MRI上显示囊内无强化和无明显或无完整的囊壁，均有助于本病的诊断。在CT和MRI中本病与肝囊肿、血管瘤、肝脓肿及肝肿瘤坏死等病变有很多类似之处，需密切结合临床表现，对超声等各种检查做认真分析以进行鉴别诊断，必要时可行穿刺检查，如穿刺内容液中含胆汁成分即可确诊。

5. 肝脓肿　是指病原体侵入肝内引起肝组织损害，发生液化坏死，使脓液在肝内聚集形成脓腔。根据病原体的不同可将肝脓肿分为细菌性和真菌性两大类。CT和MRI的价值除对囊肿的定性诊断外，还可了解病灶的大小、数目、部位及与血管和胆系的解剖关系等，为临床进一步治疗提供信息。当病灶累及到肝外时，提示阿米巴性肝脓肿的可能性大，而真菌性的肝脓肿往往很小。

CT和MRI检查要重点观察肝脓肿的腔内结构和边缘情况：①脓肿腔内结构：首先明确有无液体和气体、液体的性状。当脓肿腔内容为黏稠液体时，CT平扫表现为比水高的CT值，而MRI的T_1WI、T_2WI上分别表现为低信号和不均匀高信号；早期小的肝脓肿可显示为清楚的蜂窝状和分房状特征性表现，随着脓腔的进一步扩大，可形成多房性或单房性大脓腔，此时较容易诊断。真菌性肝脓肿在MRI T_2WI中，其中心部呈明显的低信号，周边即中间层呈高信号，最外边缘层为低信号，形成典型的3层分界的特征。另外，真菌性肝脓肿的脓腔有多房性倾向，其房隔通过增强CT和MRI可以显示得很清楚。当脓腔内含有气体时，CT扫描呈低密度影，而MRI上则表现为无信号。

②脓肿的边缘情况：肝脓肿的边缘总是伴有不同程度的水肿、肉芽组织增生、纤维化和血管炎等。CT平扫脓肿周围炎性水肿表现为境界不清的低密度区，动态增强CT扫描的早期具有特异性，约30%病例可见脓腔内部呈边缘环状强化，经组织学证实为脓肿的内膜；有时脓肿周围可见楔形和斑片状强化，其机制可能与炎性细胞浸润而导致门静脉变细和肝动脉代偿性扩张有关。MRI可以显示脓肿周围肝实质水肿，表现为T_1WI低信号和T_2WI高信号，增强MRI可清楚地显示脓肿的内膜和周围水肿

的程度，动态增强 MRI 能够达到与 CT 相同的效果。

6. 肝紫癜症　肝紫癜症，又称肝紫斑病。病理解剖学研究显示，本病在肝实质内可见多发性直径 1~5mm 大小囊样扩张的血液滞留腔，呈圆形或不规则形，其内壁无囊肿样上皮结构。本病由 Wangner 等（1986）最早报道，多见于成人，临床可无任何明显症状，尸检的发现率 0.02%~1.00%。随着腹腔镜的广泛应用，其发现率呈上升趋势，文献报道其发病率为 0.19%~6.89%。CT 扫描对本病的诊断价值尚有争议，过去认为 CT 平扫缺乏特征性，多表现为低密度影，脂肪肝时反而表现为密度增高影。增强 CT 可见病灶不规则形强化或边缘性强化，研究证明这种强化表现实际上是血液滞留腔和血窦的直接交通，导致对比剂进入而显影的结果。Gouya 等（2001）通过动态增强 CT 研究发现，本病的强化特点是从病变的中心向边缘部渐进扩展，至于有些病灶不出现强化，是因为病变被机化的血栓堵塞所致。

近年来，有关 MRI 在本病应用的报道日益增多，常在 T_2WI 中表现为较高信号或明显的高信号，而在 T_1WI 中的信号变化较大，可以呈高信号，也可呈等信号或中低信号。即使同一病灶的不同部位，由于其内部血栓机化的程度等因素，仍可表现为各种不同的信号。

另外，T_1WI 的信号强度的变化反映了出血和血肿的病理过程，亚急性期在 T_1WI 中应呈高信号，增强 MR 检查时，于注入对比剂 60 分钟后的脂肪抑制 T_1WI 上，可见特征性明显强化的“分支状”血管影，动态增强 MR 可见病灶从中心向边缘逐渐强化，平衡期整个病灶呈均匀性强化。

第八篇　儿童肝占位性病变

第一章　肝恶性肿瘤

第一节　儿童肝母细胞瘤

病理学：该病病因不清，母亲职业性接触某些环境因素（金属、石油产物、油漆、色素）可能为重要原因。另外，Beckwith-Wiedemann 综合征、胎儿酒精综合征、偏身肥大的病儿发生肝母细胞瘤的危险增高。肝母细胞瘤大体表现典型的为绿色单发肿物，可为光滑或分叶状、实性和 / 或囊性；最常发生于右叶，瘤体一般较大，巨型肿瘤可侵犯全肝。可有包膜，肿瘤可发生出血、坏死、斑条或大片钙化。镜下肝母细胞瘤可分为上皮型和混合性上皮间叶型：上皮型以不同程度的上皮细胞为主，上皮成分常被胶原性间隔分为不规则叶状，上皮型又可分为胎儿型、胚胎型、巨梁型、小细胞未分化型；混合性上皮间叶型以上皮和间叶细胞类型的不同程度混合为特征，混合型又可分为非畸胎瘤样、畸胎瘤样。

不同的组织类型预后不同，以胎儿型、混合型预后相对较好。肿瘤增长迅速，肝外转移多见于肝门淋巴结、横膈、肾上腺，血行转移易至肺、中枢神经系统、骨骼等处。

临床表现：肝母细胞瘤是原发于肝脏的恶性胚胎原性上皮组织的肿瘤，多见于 3 岁以下婴幼儿，男性占优势，一组男女比例为 3：1。临床多以肝大、右上腹包块就诊，晚期则有发热、纳差、体重下降、贫血、黄疸、腹水等。5.5% 病人伴发先天性异常，偶尔可出现与肿瘤所产生的人类绒毛膜促性腺激素有关的青春期早熟。高达 80%~90% 的病例血清甲胎蛋白升高，且滴度常很高。

影像学研究：肿瘤多为单个巨大分叶状低密度肿块，多见于右叶，该组肿瘤位于右叶 5 例（41.67%），平扫边缘清楚或不清，内可见多发散在更低密度区，巨型或肝下部肿瘤常突入腹腔，边缘性外生性肿瘤呈哑铃状，约半数病例肿瘤内可见散在或聚集状钙化灶，多呈点状、弧线状、圆形或大块状，该组 6 例（50%）。

增强扫描病灶周围呈结节状、片状明显强化，密度高于肝脏，门脉期呈低密度，该组 9 例（75%）；部分病例动脉期、门脉期肿瘤强化均低于正常肝实质，该组 3 例（25%）；可见假包膜强化，该组 4 例（33.33%），包膜完整或不完整，瘤区内更低密度坏死区增强后显示更清楚，一些病例肿瘤内可见迂曲血管，该组 3 例（25%），部分病例可见下腔静脉瘤栓形成。

多发结节型、弥漫型及囊性肝母细胞瘤均属罕见，CT 表现缺乏特异性。

CT 随访的价值：以往肝母细胞瘤手术切除率低，短期内易复发，但同时应用化疗的切除率明显增高，超过 90%，而且 60%~70% 的病人长期存活，CT 检查对肿瘤化疗后疗效的评价有重要意义，一般治疗 1~2 个月后，肿瘤可见明显缩小，为手术切除创造了条件；术后 CT 随访可检出复发、转移等病灶，为临床进一步治疗提供依据。该组 6 例行 1~4 次随访复查，其中 1 例进行了 5 年随访，未见肿瘤复发、转移。

鉴别诊断：儿童特别是 3 岁以下出现肝脏巨大肿瘤伴甲胎蛋白升高，应首先考虑为肝母细胞瘤，但需与下列疾病鉴别。

原发性肝癌：甲胎蛋白亦可显著升高，但该病儿童少见，发病年龄多 >5 岁，瘤灶内钙化少见，呈小点状，肝炎病史和抗原抗体反应有助于本病诊断。

肝内转移瘤：肝转移瘤通常为多个或单个大小不一低密度结节，主要分布于肝的外围部，增强扫描周围常有环形强化，临床一般表现有原发癌症状，甲胎蛋白一般不高。

海绵状血管瘤:儿童罕见,具特征性 CT 表现,平扫为边缘清楚的类圆形低密度病变,增强扫描病变边缘呈点状、小结节状增强,密度与腹主动脉接近,强化从末梢部向中心部扩散,延迟扫描,中心部被填充,与肝实质呈等密度;此外,无假包膜,甲胎蛋白不高均有助于鉴别。

肝脏未分化胚胎性肉瘤:本病为儿童期后发病,血清甲胎球蛋白(AFP)阴性,年龄大多 6~10 岁,幼童少见,肿瘤钙化少见。

第二节 非分化性(胚胎性)肉瘤

肝的恶性间叶性肿瘤相当难见到。非分化性形态单一的肉瘤,诸如:横纹肌肉瘤、平滑肌肉瘤、纤维肉瘤、以及脂肪肉瘤,在老年人中少见,且通常不能切除。在病理学上,它们都是较大的,有出血的,且有部分坏死。圆韧带的肉瘤偶尔出现于较年青的病人,常可切除。

非分化性(胚胎性)肉瘤,虽然一直不甚常见,但为儿童年龄组中第四个最常见的肝肿瘤。

病理学:非分化性肉瘤有 75% 位于肝右叶,10% 位于肝左叶,从右叶生长进入左叶者占 15%。带蒂的肿瘤少见。肿瘤从肝脏向外扩展蔓延和转移都可以见到。肿瘤最大的直径一般在 10~20cm。大体观,非分化性肉瘤是球形的、边界清楚的和软的。切面呈黄灰色到黄褐色。超过 50% 有多囊性区域伴存坏死碎屑、凝血块或胶状物质。一个不同厚薄的纤维性假性包囊通常围绕着肿瘤,部分地分隔肿瘤与正常肝组织及受压的肝实质。散布于整个肿瘤的是多数血管,其中大多为薄壁静脉。

镜下观察主要内容是星状或梭形的肉瘤细胞紧密包裹和排列成螺旋状和薄片状,或散存于一个富于黏多醣酸的实质背景中。网蛋白和胶原纤维是存在于细胞之间。大约有 50% 可见造血的病灶。少许上皮成分见于肿瘤的周边。肉瘤细胞有圆形的、细长的或极不规则的核,与众多的丝状分裂的图像。某些细胞有嗜伊红的对氨基水杨酸(PAS)阳性小球,它既不是 α-1- 抗胰蛋白酶也不是甲胎蛋白。无交叉条纹出现。非分化性肉瘤与间叶错构瘤有着相同的组织学起源——间叶组织。间叶错构瘤是一种发育的先天性异常,无恶性潜在性,它通常见于婴儿。而非分化性(胚胎性)肉瘤是真正的肿瘤,最常出现于较大的儿童。

临床表现:大约 90% 的病例在 15 岁以下,余下的 10% 出现在 15 岁到 30 岁之间。52% 出现于 6 到 10 岁,只有 5% 出现在出生后 2 个月内。病人一般均有腹部肿块,伴有或不伴有腹部疼痛。发热大概由于出血和坏死引起,大约 5% 的病人发热明显。自发性破裂可导致急腹症。一般无黄疸。出现症状期间,通常为几天到一月,但也有长达两年的报告。

物理检查时,可触及右上腹或上腹包块。实验室资料包括,50% 的病人可有轻微的白细胞增多和贫血,甲胎蛋白测定无异常,大约 30% 左右的病人可有肝酶的升高。

如果可能,应行手术切除治疗。纵使进行切除治疗、化疗以及放射治疗,大多数病人都在诊断做出后 12 个月内死亡。已有 1 例在手术切除后生存 52 个月,尚未见有复发征象的病例。

影像学研究:胸部平片和腹部平片可显示肝肿大和膈肌移位,但无钙化。胃肠道的造影检查常常显示胃、十二指肠、升结肠或横结肠的移位。排泄性尿系造影可显示右肾的下移。硫胶肝脾显像不变地显示一个缺损。超声和 CT 可显示大的肝内包块,常可见有大的囊状区域及低密度区域,相当于出血和坏死区。血管造影可显示肿瘤血管化的程度,它变化于多血管性到少血管性之间,这依赖于出血和坏死的程度。肝内血管被肿瘤拉直和分离,可见散存的新生血管病灶,而没有延迟出现的对比剂湖。

鉴别诊断:只靠影像学表现难以区别非分化性肉瘤与间叶错构瘤,这个鉴别诊断也不能只靠大体观察做出。

间叶错构瘤:间叶错构瘤更好发于 3 岁以下儿童,而非分化性(胚胎性)肉瘤则多见于较大的儿童。此瘤虽可发生于任何年龄,但 5 岁以下儿童罕见,6~10 岁儿童最常见。病理学上,肿瘤常倾向于囊性变,CT 图像上则常可能表现出不同的实质内容,其中亦可能包含钙化,病灶亦可呈周围环状增强。

恶性间叶瘤:恶性间叶瘤以 6~10 岁多见,CT 表现多为囊性,有不同程度的实性部分,呈壁上结节或条块影突起，可有钙化，边缘假包膜可强化。手术切除标本剖面见囊内为出血，坏死和胶冻样物，囊壁不规则。

转移性病变：神经母细胞瘤、肾胚胎瘤、横纹肌肉瘤和淋巴瘤均喜转移至肝，为常见的肝转移性肿瘤。转移性病变最常见的表现为界限清楚低密度单发或多发性病灶，神经母细胞瘤和恶性胃肠道肿瘤可发生钙化。一些在平扫未显示的病例仅可见于增强扫描中，偶尔，某些病变增强后与相邻的肝实质呈等密度。中心坏死灶则构成牛眼样表现。

当CT主要表现为实性病灶时，诊断上应多考虑肝母细胞瘤和肝细胞癌，甲胎蛋白显著升高者，诊断可更明确；如病灶中出现钙化，尤其是多数性或大块钙化的，诊断上则应首选肝母细胞瘤。另外，年龄在鉴别此两种肿瘤上也有一定意义。

间叶性错构瘤也可以实性为主，但病灶内有多个囊，无钙化，甲胎蛋白阴性。当CT主要表现为囊性时，诊断上应多考虑恶性间叶瘤和间叶性错构瘤，恶性间叶瘤为巨大单囊，囊壁有结节或条块状软组织影突起，而间叶性错构瘤则为多囊，囊壁光整，囊内密度可不一致。当CT增强扫描，病灶周边明显强化，且强化向病灶内发展，使病灶缩小时，则应考虑为血管内皮瘤。

横纹肌母细胞瘤：胆管树横纹肌母细胞瘤常发生于肝门区，胆管扩张比其他肿瘤更为常见。CT图像上，本症表现为边缘几乎与囊肿一样光整或欠光整的低密度区，钙化不常见。

第三节　丛状纤维组织细胞瘤侵犯肝脏

丛状纤维组织细胞瘤是一种罕见的主要发生于儿童和青少年体表呈局部浸润生长的低度恶性间质肿瘤，属于中间型（交界性）纤维组织细胞瘤。Enzinger（1988）首先报告本瘤，目前国内病理及影像学报道较少。发病年龄30岁以前占90%，女性多于男性，约为7∶3。常见于肢体，近65%见于上肢（其中45%见于手和腕部），头和颈部少见。有作者报告个案发生于下胸壁累及肝脏，病理诊断为此病，表现为低度恶性肉瘤，较为少见。临床上通常表现为无痛性、生长缓慢的皮下结节，局部复发率高，局部切除复发率约为40%，偶见局部淋巴结转移，直至目前本瘤未发现有远处转移。该瘤大多位于真皮深部，向上可延伸至真皮浅层，但不累及表皮，向下浸润皮下层，甚至肌肉层，侵犯肝脏者少见。文献报道瘤体直径很少超过3cm，但该例直径达到10cm，并出现坏死，非常罕见。

该瘤组织学特点为瘤组织有相似于单核和多核的组织细胞样细胞及分化好的成纤维细胞样细胞组成的结节状或丛状的结构。免疫组织化学和超微结构特点为波形蛋白和平滑肌肌动蛋白免疫反应呈阳性（主要是多核巨细胞和单核组织细胞样细胞）；CD68阳性（主要是成纤维细胞样细胞）。一例CD68和肌动蛋白（actin）均为阳性。关于该瘤的组织发生仍未有定论，可能起源于成肌纤维细胞。

该例螺旋CT虽然能凭借其很高的密度分辨率清楚显示病变的位置、大小、形状、密度和毗邻关系，三期扫描进一步明确了肿块的强化方式，但表现不具有特异性，难以判断肿瘤的起源和性质。其影像学特点还需要更多病例进行总结，其最终确诊仍需病理检查。需要鉴别的疾病包括胸壁结核、肝脏恶性间叶组织肿瘤等。

第二章 肝良性肿瘤

第一节 婴儿血管内皮瘤

婴儿血管内皮瘤是婴儿期最常见的有症状的血管性肝肿瘤。一般考虑此肿瘤为良性肿瘤,但是,肿瘤细胞向周围的侵犯行为偶尔可见于镜下,有报告还见到此肿瘤出现远距离的转移。85% 以上的肝血管内皮瘤病例出现于半岁之前,65% 以上患儿可见有高输出量充血性心力衰竭。男女发病率之比约为 1/2。没有种族的偏爱或先天性遗传。在发现以后,肿瘤趋向于迅速生长,而且,如果患儿能够支持而未行手术处理,肿瘤在几个月时间内逐渐退变。很少见到肿瘤持续存留至青年时代。婴儿血管内皮瘤的准确的发病率难以确定,因为在文献上,它常被误诊或误称为海绵状血管瘤。海绵状血管瘤是老年组最常见原发性肝肿瘤,然而作为有临床重要意义的肿瘤它在婴儿期实为罕见。当在婴儿期发现它时,它一般表现为尸解中偶然发现的一个小病灶。

病理学:血管内皮瘤可以是圆形光滑的,或多叶状和不规则状。虽然它们无真性包膜,但它们趋向于与周围正常肝组织分界清楚,因为它们的生长是压迫性生长而不是侵蚀性生长。带蒂的病变不常见。肿瘤呈粉红棕色或白色,相当柔软,尤如海绵。大的肿瘤的中心区域趋向于显示梗死、出血、纤维化和营养不良性钙化病灶。钙化常常只见于镜下,它不总是出现于影像诊断的图像上。虽然小的肿瘤在理论上少有并存充血性心衰,但是,在肿瘤大小与充血性心衰之间并无明显相关;局限性或多中心性肿瘤可以伴存充血性心衰。

婴儿血管内皮瘤可有两个组织学亚型。1 型为不同大小的血管间隙组成,它被覆以相对未成熟的簇状的内皮细胞,有时是多层,且伴有一定特色的丛状或芽状表现。这些内皮细胞是支持在突起的网蛋白网上。此支持基质是纤维性的,可偶尔见到少许小灶状的分化良好的黏液瘤性组织。胆管散存于血管性间隙之间,后者可含有某些造血细胞。2 型有更不成熟的更大的多形的细胞,伴有更多色素过深的核,反映此类病变活动状态中的更具侵袭性的一面。在大的肿瘤的中心区,可发现类似于海绵状血管瘤的病灶,这就导致命名学的混淆。

在组织学上,2 型血管内皮瘤可伪似血管内皮肉瘤,但是后者一般是老年人的疾病。除了年龄的差异外,成人的肉瘤典型地可观察到血管窦内的扩展,与中央静脉和门静脉的受侵,这些都不见于婴儿血管内皮瘤。虽然如此,婴儿血管内皮瘤可能有某些限局性的恶性潜在性;它可能表现具有侵袭性,而且已有转移的病例报告,尽管确切研究这些是真正的转移或多灶性肿瘤还有一定的困难。与此相反,血管瘤的特征是不同大小的血管性间隙,被覆以单层成熟的扁平内皮细胞。其支持的基质不足,常由成熟的纤维组织组成,虽然更广泛的纤维化区域和少见的营养不良性钙化偶尔可以见到。通常见于老年病人。胆管缺如。

临床表现:肝血管内皮瘤最多见于婴幼儿,女孩的发病率是男孩的 2 倍,是新生儿期最常见的能引起症状的血管性病变之一,85% 的病例在 6 个月之前出现症状,腹部肿块伴有杂音和充血性心力衰竭,可导致消耗性凝血病(血小板减少症)。经过几个月或者几年有无需治疗自然消退的可能,约有一半的婴幼儿伴有皮肤血管瘤。

最常见的表现为可扪及的包块,肝肿大或弥漫性腹部肿大。Levick 和 Rubie(1953)首先发现肝的血管内皮瘤与充血性心力衰竭同时并存,继后不少作者证实了这种同存现象。然而,Dachman 等(1983)回顾 27 例肝血管内皮瘤病人中,只 1 例同存充血性心衰，在住院期间有 3 例出现充血性心衰。因此，一般认为，在婴儿血管内皮瘤病人中，充血性心衰并不像以往所认为的那样常见。超过 45% 的病儿伴存皮肤血管瘤。罕见情况下，可在肝区听见血管杂音，也可出现黄疸。血浆甲胎蛋白测定通常无异常，但有的病例也有中度增高。此类增高大概是由于在这些年幼病人甲胎蛋白的持续存在，而不是肿瘤的产物。如果随访，它将逐渐降低。

影像学研究：腹部 X 线平片可能显示一个软组织包块，肝肿大，或斑点状钙化。钙化是提示一岁以下幼儿可能存在血管内皮瘤，它是非特异性，也可见于肝母细胞瘤（主要的鉴别诊断应予考虑），以及错构瘤与转移性神经母细胞瘤。如果存在充血性心衰，胸部 X 线片可显示心影增大与肺静脉高压。

超声显像用于肝内包块的定位，在血管内皮瘤可以显示为一个低回声的，混声的或高回声病灶。病变可以是单个或多个，分离的或难以画出轮廓。个别病例的低回声病变接近于无回声而伪似于囊肿。如果发现大的囊性组成内容，那么，少见的间叶错构瘤则变成首先考虑的诊断。超声可用于血管内皮瘤的随访。病变趋向于慢慢地退变，在几个月的时期内，变成渐增的高回声和皱缩。

血管内皮瘤的 CT 平扫，可显示一个或多个比周围肝组织密度为低的包块。用团注增强，动态扫描及延迟扫描可显示低衰减值的局灶性区域，在团注对比剂后早期周边性强化，伴不同延迟时间的中央性强化。此类表现颇类似于成人的海绵状血管瘤。这被认为是血管内皮瘤的血流动力学活动较少的缘故。目前尚无足够的资料确定这些征象的可靠性和特异性。

肝的核素显像偶尔用于超声和 CT 的辅助手段，观察病变的肝的起源。放射性核素血管显像合并血池检查能显示出包块的血管性质。

X 线血管造影可证实包块的血管性质，当肝受侵犯呈弥漫性时，它可以部分用于勾画病变的范围，为术前准备重要的步骤。可以见到肝动脉起点以远的主动脉直径的缩小，肿瘤供养血管的扩张与扭曲，不如正常那样逐步变尖。常常出现肿瘤内的血管湖或大片区域的对比剂延长淤滞。早期动 - 静脉短路与扩张扭曲的供养血管一块可能与少数高输出充血性心衰病例的血管造影 - 病理生理变化相关。（与此相反，海绵状血管瘤通常有正常大小的供养血管且动 - 静脉短路少见）。如果进行排泄性尿系造影，在全身不透光化期间可以观察肝内的相当于肿瘤内的血管性区域的致密影，而在 X 线血管造影时，则见该区实为扩张的血管湖。

肝血管内皮瘤 CT 平扫为低密度，可有钙化。增强扫描早期外围强化，随着时间推移，对比剂逐渐进入中心部分，肿瘤呈不均匀的高度强化，病灶内可见粗大的血管。CT 随访可见肿块明显减小并可发生钙化。磁共振表现为 T_2WI 高信号，T_1WI 低信号，肿块的内部及外围可见粗大的滋养 / 引流血管流空表现。肝血管内皮瘤血管造影表现为肝动脉扩张、扭曲，早期肝静脉显影，病灶部位对比剂异常聚积，降主动脉在腹腔干水平以上粗大，腹腔干水平以下相对细小。

第二节　误诊病例简介：肝脏间叶错构瘤与多房性肝囊肿

肝脏间叶错构瘤多发生于 2 岁以下儿童，成人较少见，男女发病率无明显差异。根据组织来源不同分为内胚层性、中胚层性、内中外胚层性和混合性 4 种，混合性错构瘤主要表现为肝脏间叶错构瘤。镜下主要由杂乱的结缔组织、脂肪、平滑肌及异常增生的血管、扩张的胆管等间叶性成分构成，肝细胞分化成熟，肝细胞单个散在或成簇排列，但无正常的肝小叶。研究表明肝脏间叶错构瘤与染色体 19q 13.4 位点的异位有关。

肝脏间叶错构瘤早期症状轻或无，但随着肿瘤的增长，邻近脏器出现受压表现。B 超多为肝内多个类圆形或椭圆形无回声液性暗区，大小不一；部分囊壁内有不规则乳头状突起，边界清晰。CT 示肝内多房囊性肿物，囊腔内密度均匀，囊腔由于出血、感染等使部分囊腔密度增高，CT 值在 12~24 HU 之间；囊壁及分隔厚薄较均匀，边界清楚，少数囊壁有壁结节。MRI 上囊腔呈长 T_1、长 T_2 信号，囊壁、分隔为稍长 T_1、稍长 T_2 信号。增强扫描囊腔无强化，囊壁与分隔轻、中度强化。

一例术前误诊为肝囊肿，究其原因主要是对该病认识不足。肝脏间叶错构瘤一般单发、多房，囊壁可辨认，囊壁有轻、中度强化；肝囊肿一般壁菲薄，但继发感染囊壁可增厚(一般有感染症状)、周围肝实质有低密度水肿。

肝脏间叶错构瘤还需与肝包囊虫病、肝母细胞瘤、淋巴管瘤等疾病相鉴别。肝包囊虫病常有流行病学病史,病变有“囊内囊”“水上浮莲”等特征性表现,鉴别不难。肝母细胞瘤常发生于小儿,多数为实性肿物,少数液化坏死类似囊状,病灶内常有钙化。淋巴管瘤囊壁菲薄,与肝脏间叶错构瘤不同。肝脏间叶错构瘤不常见,但当发现小儿肝右叶多房囊性肿物时应考虑到肝脏间叶错构瘤的可能。肝脏间叶错构瘤发展缓慢,因有恶变的可能,所以仍需定期随访。手术为治疗本病首选,一般预后良好。

第三章 先天性囊性疾病

第一节 先天性囊肿

先天性囊肿在儿童罕见，多见于30~50岁成人。CT图像上囊肿表现为圆形或卵圆形，带有光滑的薄壁边缘，接近水密度的病变。偶尔中间出现分隔，增强后囊肿密度不改变。罕见的情况下，少数其他病变可与囊肿相似，包括包囊虫病，陈旧性肝血肿和脓肿。在这些病变中，临床表现可有助于诊断。

第二节 间叶性错构瘤

本症是一种非肿瘤性的发育异常，但一般学者都把它与良性肿瘤相提并论。多发于2岁以内儿童。Stanley等(1986)报道9例间叶性错构瘤中，8例为囊性，1例为实性。有作者报道3例均以实性为主。CT表现为病灶内含多数大小不等的囊，囊壁光整，无钙化。病理所见囊腔由增生扩张的胆管、血管、淋巴管或囊壁无上皮内衬的退变积液区组成，囊内可以是胆汁、血液或浆液。由于囊内容物不同，CT检查各囊内密度也就可以不一致。

关于本病，请详见本书 本卷 本篇 第二章 第二节 误诊病例简介：肝脏间叶错构瘤与多房性肝囊肿。

第三节 先天性肝内胆管囊肿

本症的特征为肝内胆管非阻塞性扩张，它可以伴发或不伴发先天性肝纤维化。CT图像上，表现为圆形或卵圆形的局限性低密度多发性囊状区，可见或不见沿肝内胆管分支走行的扩张胆管。多发性囊状区可显现一细小的逐渐增强的局灶性囊壁隆起影，代表扩张胆管区的门静脉分支。

请详见本书 本卷 第十六篇 第四章 胆管囊肿。

第四节 肝外胆管囊肿

先天性肝外胆管囊肿或先天性肝外胆管梭形扩张，可能扩展至肝门及其分支，进入肝实质内，也可能伴存左、右肝内胆管的中心部的扩张。如果胆管扩张仅在肝外，则其他诊断的可能性应考虑，如十二指肠重复性囊肿，肠系膜囊肿以及肝外周型囊肿。

请详见本书 本卷 第十六篇 第四章 胆管囊肿。

第四章　后天性囊性疾病

第一节　包囊虫病

包囊虫病的CT表现多样,它可能与先天性单发性肝囊肿完全一样,或含有分隔、子囊、钙化和由于出血感染或包囊虫病种植而引起的非匀质性密度改变。

第二节　感染性疾病

化脓性脓肿:肝脓肿好发于右叶表层。CT表现各异,与肝囊肿及肝实质性肿瘤均可非常相似。最常见为边缘锐利的低密度区,其CT值介于水密度和实质性肿块之间。少于半数的肝脓肿可发生边缘性强化,则需与其他病变(如:肿瘤和血管瘤)鉴别。双靶征,即低密度的中心区周围为内层高密度环和外层低密度环所包绕。

联想到脓肿的更多的特征性表现,有近1/3的病例的诊断是根据动态扫描提供资料做出的。脓肿内出现气体并不常见(约占20%),但当发现气体时,则非常支持脓肿的诊断。

第五章　肉芽肿性病变

第一节　慢性肉芽肿性疾病

儿童的慢性肉芽肿性疾病的特点，是白细胞在完成正常杀菌的活动中吞噬细菌的能力降低。此种情况是由于烟草酰胺-腺嘌呤二核苷酸氧化酶的先天性缺如，在正常情况下，它转变辅酶1的还原型成为氧化型，产生过氧化氢。过氧化氢形成的缺乏，致使白细胞杀死细菌的能力受到损害。这个特性通常见于男性，属X链隐性遗传，虽然偶尔它也见于女性，在这些病人，它为常染色体隐性遗传。

此病在临床上的特点是反复地感染，主要侵犯鼻副窦、肺、骨、淋巴结和肝脏。典型的细菌种类是金黄色葡萄球菌，或表皮葡萄球菌、沙雷菌属、产气杆菌属。曲菌属微生物有时也可出现。病人对慢性肉芽肿病的病理反应类似于正常人对抗酸杆菌、布鲁菌属或李斯德菌属的肉芽肿的应。淋巴结肿大，肝脾肿大和肝门淋巴结肿大，伴同肺的实变即刻出现于病势加重抗生素治疗中止以后。葡萄球菌脓肿可以累及肝脏，骨髓炎可出现于双侧手和脚的短骨，或长骨。慢性肉芽肿病中，肝脏的受累的范围可从界限不明确的肉芽肿组织到明显的脓肿形成。陈旧的已经愈合的肉芽肿能以多发性肝内钙化的表现而被发现，而且，在任何男孩伴有多发性肝内钙化，都可能提示为慢性肉芽肿病。

在这些病人，肝受侵犯的类型和范围都可用超声显像来确定。肉芽肿组织是低回声病灶，且伴与正常肝组织之间的边缘不清楚。增强扫描时病灶无强化。另外，一个明显的脓肿显示为边界清楚的，充满液体的透声良好的病灶。在肉芽肿组织与明显的脓肿之间，受累及的肝脏可显示这些征象的不同组合。肉芽肿病的早期识别将有利于即刻的早期治疗。以超声或CT导引行经皮穿刺活检或抽吸，对于肝内以往未发现的疾病的证实，引流任何存在的脓肿，确定微生物的种类以选择适当的抗生素治疗，都是非常有用的。

第二节　霉菌和肉芽肿性病变

霉菌和肉芽肿性病变最常见为多发性，细小的（直径约1~2cm）低密度区。孤立性单发或多数性霉菌性脓肿与化脓性脓肿相似。肝硬化中的退变结节：退变结节的直径常小于2cm，可见低密度和高密度区并存。高密度表现特别，可见于遗传性酪氨酸贫血。退变结节表现与邻近低密度脂肪肝衬托有关。

第六章 儿童肝占位的误诊

第一节 化疗后继发肝、脾、肾霉菌感染

儿童非霍奇金淋巴瘤或白血病易引起肝、脾、肾的浸润已逐渐为广大临床医生所认识,但是对于儿童运用抗肿瘤药物化疗后引起弥漫性的肝、脾、肾霉菌感染却往往认识不足,而后者的发病率有升高的趋势。如果将两者混淆,可能导致延误病情甚至危及生命。

Chen 等(2003)曾报道 500 例接受化疗的白血病患者中,有 37 例发生肝、脾的霉菌感染,约占 7.4%。有作者报告一组 106 例非霍奇金淋巴瘤或白血病病例,发生化疗后继发弥漫性肝、脾、肾霉菌感染者有 8 例,占 7.54%。由于样本有限,随访时间较短,因此儿童运用抗肿瘤药物化疗后继发弥漫性的肝、脾、肾霉菌感染的发生率将有待进一步的研究。

致病因素:在儿童非霍奇金淋巴瘤或白血病引起的深部霉菌感染中,易感因素包括使用强烈的化疗药物和免疫抑制剂、广谱抗生素和静脉插管等。病原菌最常见的为白色念珠菌,但其他一些自然界普遍存在的真菌,如曲霉菌、组织胞浆菌、球孢子菌和放线菌也较常见。但本病仅依靠实验室检查确诊却相当困难, Lin 等(2003)曾报道 5 例儿童白血病伴有肝、脾、肾霉菌感染的病例,仅有 2 例血或大便培养为阳性。该组 8 例依靠皮下结节穿刺、皮疹培养和血培养确诊 4 例。而要通过肝脏活检确诊也有相当大的难度,因此 CT 的表现对本病的认识就显得尤为重要。

影像学研究:化疗后继发肝、脾、肾霉菌感染的 CT 表现一般为肝、脾、肾内多发性低密度灶,伴或不伴肝、脾、肾体积增大,病灶形态多呈规则的圆形或椭圆形,大小可均匀一致或大小不一,但直径多 <2.0cm,增强后无强化或呈轻度环行强化,其中以肝和脾的受累最常见。Chen 等(2003)报道 CT 显示肝、脾、肾有上述表现的比例为 89%、70% 和 27%。

该组 8 例中 3 个脏器的累及程度与之相接近。值得注意的是,该组病例在未做增强前,肝、脾、肾霉菌感染表现与浸润很难区别,均表现为等或略低密度病灶,如果仅做腹部平扫则很容易将病灶遗漏,所以应对所有的病例进行增强扫描,并且应包括上述 3 个脏器,以免误诊或漏诊。另外,该组病例在抗霉菌治疗后的随访中,有 2 例病例临床症状已经恢复正常,但肝、脾、肾仍可见少许病灶残留,考虑为局部病灶治疗后的退化,局部愈合形成肉芽肿或纤维化。该组 1 例脾、肾霉菌感染在随访 10 个月时肝脏发现有点状钙化灶,考虑为肝脏曾经有过真菌感染。另 1 例病例伴有肺部的霉菌感染。

诊断与鉴别诊断:如上所述,儿童应用抗肿瘤药物化疗后继发弥漫性的肝、脾、肾霉菌感染的 CT 诊断并不困难。当临床上正在运用抗肿瘤药物进行化疗的患儿出现抗生素治疗无效的发热、腹痛或者肝、脾肿大,而 CT 显示肝、脾、肾内多发性直径 <2.0cm 低密度灶,增强后无或呈轻度环行强化,则首先应该考虑到霉菌感染的可能。其特殊的“牛眼征”能区别于其他病原体感染。

①非霍奇金:非霍奇金淋巴瘤或白血病肝、脾、肾浸润时,平扫可显示病变部位异常结节影,为单发或多发,病灶大小不一,常伴全身多脏器侵犯和后腹膜淋巴结的增大,其 CT 强化方式与霉菌感染也不尽相同,一般均有较明显的强化,可根据这些特征进行鉴别。②另外,结核性肝脓肿的 CT 表现与本病比较相似,需结合临床甚至病理确诊。由于儿童运用抗肿瘤药物化疗后继发弥漫性的肝脾肾霉菌感染的发病率较高,CT 不仅在检出肝、脾、肾霉菌感染上有很大的优势,同时对抗真菌药物疗效的观察有重

要意义。因此，一般认为临床如果怀疑感染的发生，则腹部 CT（包括平扫和增强）是不能缺少的。

第二节　可能误诊为肝肿块的病变

局灶性脂肪增生症：本症可误诊为低密度肿块。寻求正确的诊断包括病变与正常肝轮廓的一致性和在异常肝区中呈现正常的肝血管纹理。

肝坏死：肝坏死可由于感染、外伤、血管梗死或肝中毒引起。坏死区可呈局灶性或弥漫性低密度区。出血则呈高密度表现。增强后可形成血管性充血。肝坏死在 CT 图像上可与肿块及增殖性病变相混淆。

肝外肿块：在 CT 图像上，邻近肝的肿块偶可表现像肝内原发性肿块。利用多方位性诊断技术（如超声检查、MRI）可做出鉴别。

第三节　新生儿特发性肝内巨大血肿的误诊

Singer 等（1999）和 Amodio 等（2004）认为肝包膜下和肝内血肿病因可能与产伤、脓毒血症、缺氧和凝血机制异常有关，与母亲疾病如妊娠高血压综合征、凝血机制异常与胎盘后期出血也有一定的关系。有作者报告一例早产低体重儿，胎膜早破，脐带绕颈、臀位，经催产后经阴道分娩，凝血机制未见异常。其母亲体健无妊高征、凝血机制异常和胎盘后期出血史，该作者认为其发病可能与产伤、缺氧与败血症等多种因素有关。至于其黄疸，因出生后 3 d 出现，12d 后于手术前消退，该作者认为可能是生理性黄疸与血肿没有直接关联。

肝实质内血肿在 CT 下密度改变依出血时间的长短不同而不同，最初 24~72 h CT 平扫表现为高密度，增强后血肿 CT 值低于正常肝脏，随着血液的溶解，密度逐渐减低，CT 值减少，变成等密度，最后成为低密度，边缘光滑或不规则，增强扫描无强化。MRI 对亚急性期和慢性血肿检查有绝对优势。

该例出生后 8 d，CT 平扫为低密度改变，内见少量略高密度影，代表血肿进入亚急性期，尚未完全溶解液化且破入肝包膜下。而单纯肝包膜下血肿往往呈梭形，肝脏推移，边缘光整，与腹壁交角呈钝角，最大径位于包膜下。

该例术前超声和 CT 检查诊断为肝囊肿并出血。对新生儿肝内血肿认识不足，片面强调无明显引起肝内血肿危险因素，未行 MRI 检查是术前主要误诊原因。

Amodio 等（2004）报道的 1 例新生儿肝内血肿 CT 最初考虑为新生物，后经 MRI 检查和超声随访吸收后证实，因此应注意与新生儿肝脏肿瘤如间质错构瘤、肝血管内皮瘤、肝母细胞瘤、神经母细胞瘤肝内转移灶并出血等鉴别。

总之，新生儿肝实质内血肿的病因多为特发性，往往找不到明显引起血肿的危险因素，其诊断主要依靠影像学检查，一旦发现肝实质血肿建议临床采用保守治疗并超声随访动态观察血肿的吸收。

第九篇　肝脏弥漫性病变

第一章　肝脏弥漫性病变简介

肝弥漫性疾病分型

肝弥漫性疾病根据病灶分布及其信号强弱可分为4种类型：弥漫均匀型、节段型、弥漫结节型和血管周围型。MRI在T_1WI、T_2WI及增强后各具特征性表现。

弥漫均匀型包括肝细胞及网状内皮细胞病变，肝实质信号可表现为T_1WI或T_2WI上均匀增高或均匀降低；节段型包括节段型脂肪肝和亚急性肝炎局灶性纤维化融合；弥漫结节型特征为肝内多发性结节状异常信号灶，它包括肝硬化、Willson病、肝结节病和布-加综合征等；血管周围型见于门静脉周围淋巴管及肝纤维囊的病变，肝淤血常引起门静脉周围肝组织信号增高，日本血吸虫可影响肝纤维囊，导致纤维囊和分隔在T_2WI上高信号。

（一）弥漫均匀型

1. 血色素沉着症　血色素沉着症是一种因铁质过多导致肝实质或网状内皮细胞内铁沉积的病变。在T_2WI上，由于铁的强顺磁效应引起肝实质信号低于脊柱旁肌肉信号。梯度回波序列T_2WI对磁敏感效应较敏感。因T_2缩短效应，在T_1WI上肝实质信号示降低。

2. 脂肪肝　非酒精性脂肪肝有炎症反应引起，无酗酒史，无肥胖、糖尿病、高脂血症及神经性厌食。该病有时与急性肝衰竭相关，少数发展为肝硬化病人其肝组织学表现为弥漫性脂肪浸润、肝实质炎症伴纤维化和Mallory’s小体。该病在T_1WI信号均一增高，在脂肪抑制像上表现为信号均匀降低，炎性病理改变并不影响MRI表现。

3. 糖原沉积症　Ⅰ型糖原沉积症其特征是6-磷酸葡萄糖脱氢酶不能发挥转变糖的功能，但病人能产生内源性糖。糖原沉积症在超声图像上表现为回声增强，CT图像上密度异常，MRI T_1WI信号高于骨髓。病人常伴有肝细胞腺瘤，CT表现为低密度肿瘤，MRI T_1WI、T_2WI均表现为高信号。

（二）节段型

1. 脂肪肝　肝细胞脂肪变出现在糖尿病、肥胖、营养过剩、肝移植、酗酒及化学中毒病人。节段性脂肪肝特点是脂肪浸润呈节段性分布，与肝灌注有关。SE序列T_1WI上，由于脂肪浸润，信号轻度增高。相位MRI上正常肝实质和脂肪变信号相似，用脂肪抑制观察脂肪变引起的低信号最为有效。

2. 亚急性肝炎　亚急性肝炎主要是由乙肝病毒或丙肝病毒感染或药物引起的，预后较差，死亡率高。肝损害严重时，肝实质信号在T1WI上减低，在T_2WI上增高。另外，节段性萎缩可表现为信号轻度异常。

（三）弥漫结节型

1. 病毒感染后的肝硬化　肝硬化是肝细胞反复损害的一种慢性反应，以再生纤维化为特征。肝硬化常见病因有酗酒及乙型、丙型肝炎病毒感染。肝细胞再生表现为肝内满布结节，T_2WI呈低信号，梯度回波序列上更清晰，这缘于再生结节内的含铁血黄素沉积。CT增强门脉期因结节的门脉血供而表现为再生结节强化，而肝细胞癌表现为灌注缺损区。

2. 肝豆状核变性（Willson病）　肝豆状核变性病人中，铜经胆汁排泌减少，导致铜在肝脏、大脑、角膜蓄积中毒发病。铜在肝内门脉周围区域及沿着肝血窦沉积引起炎性反应导致肝硬化。因为铜在肝细胞内与蛋白质结合，所以无顺磁性效应。肝豆状核变性最常见的表现是肝硬化改变。T_2WI上因再生结节内铁沉积，表现为全肝弥漫分布的无数小结节影，信号与病毒感染引起的肝硬化相似。

3. 结节病　为一种常见的系统性肉芽肿性病变。偶见于肝、脾和膈下淋巴结。周边纤维化的非干酪性上皮样肉芽肿发生于门脉及其周围区域。已有肝脾结节病的CT报道，表现为肝脾肿大，伴有或不伴有大量低密度微小结节。T_2WI上此结节信号低于肝实质，注射Gd-DTPA后强化。

4. 布-加综合征　布-加综合征可致肝弥漫性结节性再生性增生（NRH）。于超声图像上较大结节表现为强回声、均质、周边清晰。典型CT表现为低密度结节,增强后表现为动脉期、门脉期明显强化。MRI 表现为 T_1WI 高信号,T_2WI 表现为等信号或低信号结节,与腺瘤病信号强度类似。因结节的组织成分类似于正常肝细胞和枯否细胞,故 MRI 常难发现。布 - 加综合征所致肝弥漫性结节性再生性增生须与肝细胞癌鉴别。肝细胞癌 MRI 表现为 T_1WI 低信号,T_2WI 为高信号,增强门脉期对比剂迅速退出。

(四)血管周围型

1. 肝淤血　肝淤血是由于肝实质内静脉血淤滞而致静脉引流代偿。它是充血性心力衰竭、缩窄性心包炎及由于肺癌肺动脉栓塞的常见并发症导致的右心衰竭的表现。增强 CT 肝实质表现为斑片状网状交织相间,密度不均匀。门脉周围低密度 T_2WI 上表现为门脉周围高信号,血管周围明显低密度带可能因血管周围淋巴水肿所致。

2. 日本血吸虫病　日本血吸虫感染可导致严重的肝疾病。血吸虫生活在肠腔,并在肠系膜内产卵,虫卵钻进静脉内,随血流致门静脉内并堵塞门静脉末支,引起血管压力增高并激发肉芽肿反应。炎性反应导致虫卵的纤维化及肝脏的弥漫性纤维化。虫卵死亡后钙化,表现为门脉周围及肝囊周围分隔的特征性钙化,即所谓"龟背"样钙化,钙化及非钙化区均可强化。MRI 显示的钙化的分隔在 CT 上为线样异常密度,常见于肝右叶的膈下部。分隔表现为 T_1WI 低信号,T_2WI 高信号。因氧化铁超磁性效应,纤维隔于 T_1WI、T_2WI 可显示为高信号。

第二章　肝弥漫均匀型病变——密度升高

第一节　弥漫均匀型病变

肝弥漫均匀型病变，包括肝细胞及网状内皮细胞病变，肝实质信号可表现为 T_1WI 或 T_2WI 上均匀增高或均匀降低。它包括：血色素沉着症、脂肪肝、糖原贮积症等。

肝脏弥漫性密度升高的疾病包括：肝脏铁过载，如多次输血；血色素沉着症；含铁血黄素沉着症；肝豆状核变性，即威尔逊病；糖原贮积症；胺碘酮、顺铂等药物引起的疾病及金、慢性砷中毒等。

肝脏弥漫性密度降低的疾病包括：弥漫性脂肪变性，如弥漫性肝脂肪浸润；急性酒精性肝硬化；非酒精性肝脂肪变性；弥漫性恶性病变（原发性或转移性）；肝充血（心力衰竭、缩窄性心包炎引起）；肝淀粉样变；布加综合征（Budd-Chiari 综合征）；血吸虫病；多发性囊肿，如包虫病、多囊性肝脏疾病、先天性肝内胆管囊肿（卡罗利病）。

第二节　不典型原发性血色素沉着症

原发性血色素沉着症是因为铁吸收过多形成体内铁贮存过量而导致以肝实质损害为主要特征的遗传性疾病，欧美国家常见，通常在 40~50 岁发病，我国少见。原发性血色素沉着症Ⅰ～Ⅲ型属常染色体隐性遗传性疾病，Ⅳ型为常染色体显性遗传性疾病，是位于第 6 号染色体短臂上的基因突变而导致的铁代谢障碍；患者肠黏膜细胞及肝细胞表面的膜铁结合蛋白增加，每天铁吸收量稍多于正常人，而人体每天铁排出量极少，致使体内贮存铁逐渐增多。

而继发性血色素沉着症是铁利用障碍或摄入过多、溶血性贫血、多次大量输血、肝病和转铁蛋白缺乏等导致铁在组织器官过度沉积所引起。而沉积于组织器官的游离铁参与过氧化反应、氧自由基产物聚集，引起组织器官损伤、功能障碍。血色素沉着症与 HFE 基因有关，非 HFE 基因相关性血色素沉着症分布于世界各地，我国存在非 HFE 基因相关性血色素沉着症和血红蛋白病引起的继发性血色素沉着症。

临床表现：原发性血色素沉着症典型的临床特点：90% 患者有皮肤色素沉着，一般全身呈铁灰色或古铜色，尤其是面、颈、手背面等；95% 患者有肝肿大、肝硬化，且常发生于临床症状及肝功能异常之前；65% 患者有糖尿病；15% 患者有心脏病变、心律失常、心脏扩大等；其他症状如性欲降低、甲状腺机能减退症等。

原发性血色素沉着症常有血清铁、铁蛋白、转铁蛋白饱和度的升高，在排除导致转铁蛋白合成减少的肝脏疾病时，若转铁蛋白饱和度重复检查超过 0.62，则此病概率超过 90%。

肝穿刺活组织病理学检查为该病诊断的金标准，肝细胞内可见大量含铁血黄素沉积。

影像学研究：CT 平扫表现为肝脏密度普遍增高，CT 值大于 72 HU，而肝血管密度相对减低，特异性可达 96%。而 MRI 则表现为肝脏极低信号。

一组作者报告一例患者因黄疸住院检查，而无临床常见表现，如皮肤色素沉着、肝肿大、性功能障碍、糖尿病、心脏疾病等，临床表现极不典型，而依靠影像学及病理学检查确诊，临床上极为少见。另一方面也提醒我们临床医师:若患者肝功能表现为黄疸,尤其是以间接胆红素升高为主而无常见血色素沉着症表现的患者在排除常见疾病的情况下,也需考虑此病,可行CT、肝穿刺等检查来明确。

第三节 肝豆状核变性

请详见本书 颅脑和脊髓卷 第七篇 第八章 肝豆状核变性。

第四节 CT平扫呈弥漫性高密度的肝脏疾病

见表9-2-1。

表9-2-1 CT平扫呈弥漫性高密度的肝脏疾病及其临床特征

呈高密度的肝脏疾病	临床特征
原发性血色素沉着病(primary hemochromatosis)	常染色体隐性(autosomal recessive),肝细胞性肝癌危险增加,糖尿病,青铜色皮肤(bronze skin),心肌病(cardiomyopathy)
含铁血黄素沉着症(hemosiderosis)	多次输血史(numerous blood transfusions)
碘沉积(iodine deposition)	抗心律失常药物:胺碘酮(amiodarone),常有肺基底浸润或纤维化
贮积病(storage disease)	可引起肝脏高密度改变,但糖原贮积症更常见为低密度改变
肝豆状核变性(Wilson's disease)	常染色体隐性(autosomal recessive),铜沉积(copper deposition)
金沉积(gold deposition)	治疗类风湿关节炎药物:硫代苹果酸金钠(gold sodium thiomalate)

第三章　肝弥漫性病变——密度降低

第一节　脂肪肝背景导致的漏诊

脂肪肝是常见的肝脏弥漫性病变，当脂肪肝合并肝局灶性病变时，由于多数局灶性病变的影像学表现与肝脏背景之间的对比度变小甚至消失，可导致一些局灶性病变难以被发现而造成漏诊。有作者曾遇到直径约 3 cm 大小的血管瘤，先后经超声和 CT 平扫检查，由于病灶与肝背景的对比度甚微以致被漏诊，随后经 MRI 检出该病灶。但上述情况对肝局灶性病变的漏诊概率究竟有多大？超声、CT、MRI 3 种检查方法各自受影响的程度如何？

超声、CT 和 MRI 对脂肪肝的诊断价值：脂肪肝是指由于各种原因引起的脂肪在肝细胞中蓄积过多的一种病理状态，是指当肝细胞内脂质蓄积超过肝湿重的 5%，脂肪肝已成为肝纤维化和肝硬化重要的前期病变之一。因此，对脂肪肝的认识正不断引起人们的重视。

活组织病理检查虽为诊断本病的金标准，但因其创伤性和患者依从性差而无法普及。按 2003 年全国脂肪肝会议制定的诊断标准，各种影像学检查是诊断脂肪肝的重要方法，甚至是独立的诊断标准。但是超声诊断易受患者个体差异、检查仪器性能及参数选择、操作经验等诸多因素影响，因此超声定量诊断脂肪肝仍存在局限性。CT 诊断脂肪肝是比较可靠的方法，肝脏细胞内脂肪含量越高，CT 值越低，或肝 / 脾 CT 值之比 <0. 85，则诊断为脂肪肝。

由于 MRI 本身有较强的组织分辨率和快速抑脂技术，它可以较容易地确定脂肪肝的存在。MRI 根据双回波化学位移成像诊断脂肪肝：(Sip-Sop)/ Sip ≥ 0.135 或 Sip-Sop ≥ 29.0(Sip 正相位信号强度， Sop 反相位信号强度)。Rinella 等(2003)采用双梯度回波和化学位移梯度回波成像定量测定肝脏捐献者肝脏的脂肪含量及其脂肪变程度，并与病理活检对照，发现 MRI 脂肪变指标与病理活检脂肪变分级呈正相关，相关系数为 0.84。

Lee 等(2010)前瞻性比较 CT、双梯度回波 MRI(DGE-MRI)、质子磁共振波谱成像(^{1}H-MRS)和超声用于诊断和定量评估脂肪肝的准确性，结果显示诊断肝细胞内脂质蓄积超过肝湿重≥ 5% 脂肪肝，DGE-MRI 和 ^{1}H-MRS 明显优于 CT 和超声。

诊断肝细胞内脂质蓄积超过肝湿重≥ 30% 脂肪肝，增强 MRI 比其他影像学方法表现出更高的准确性，它在最佳分界值的有效敏感性和特异性分别为 90.9% 和 94%，相比之下，其诊断肝细胞内脂质蓄积超过肝湿重≥ 5% 的脂肪肝的准确性分别为 76.7% 和 87.1%。

双回波化学位移成像可能成为无创性评估脂肪肝的首选影像检查方法。Qayyum 等(2005)初步研究结果显示，对肝脏脂肪含量的测量，脂肪抑制成像比梯度回波成像更准确，尤其是对于有肝硬化背景的患者。因此，一项研究脂肪肝的诊断主要参考 3 种检查技术中的两种，特别是 CT 和 MRI 有脂肪肝表现者，即计入脂肪肝组，应是可信的。

超声、CT 和 MRI 对肝局灶性病变的诊断价值：肝局灶性病变主要包括：肝细胞癌、转移性肝癌、胆管细胞癌、局灶性结节性增生、肝硬化再生结节、血管瘤、坏死结节等，上述病变早期高能力检出，一直是医学界追求的目标。而肝囊肿和肝脓肿由于影像学检查方法容易检出，就未列入该研究。该研究检出率采用以病变数目统计，当一个病例的病变数 >4 个时，也以 4 个计算，两组病例 3 种检查技术同样用这一方式统计有可比性。肝局灶性病变的超声可以表现为低回声、等回声、高回声或混杂回声团块，境界清楚或不清楚，其回声特点与肝脏背景有关。肝局灶性病变在CT平扫上多数表现为单发或多发圆形、类圆形低密度或等密度肿块，如肝癌、肝血管瘤等，CT值介于水与正常肝之间，也是以肝脏背景作为参照判断其密度。CT增强扫描多数病变都会出现不同程度和不同特点的强化，更有利于病变的检出和定性。MRI对显示局灶性病变的大小、形态、数目、边缘等表现与CT所见相似，肿块的MRI信号则表现为低信号、等信号、高信号和混杂信号，也是以肝脏背景作为参照确定其信号特征。大多数病变在T_1WI上表现为低信号，T_2WI表现为高信号或稍高信号。静脉注射对比剂后行快速多期扫描，肿块的对比增强表现与CT多期扫描表现相似。

随着影像学设备分辨率的不断提高以及增强技术的普遍使用，超声、CT、MRI 3种影像检查方法对肝局灶性病变的检出能力逐步提高，但三者的检出能力还是有差别的。由于MRI是多种序列和多种切面成像，加之其软组织分辨率在3种检查方法中最高，因此，其对肝局灶性病变的检出率高于超声和CT平扫。该组88例非脂肪肝患者中，肝局灶性病变的检出率超声为70.97%，CT为85.71%，MRI为87.56%，超声检出率明显低于CT和MRI，与超声均为平扫，且以图文报告回顾性分析可能也有关系，而CT检查的增强率占83%，MRI增强率仅占51.1%，所以CT和MRI在非脂肪肝组的检出率才是相似的。

超声、CT、MRI对脂肪肝背景下肝局灶性病变的检出能力的比较：当脂肪肝与肝局灶性病变同时存在时，脂肪肝背景常导致局灶性病变与肝脏背景在影像学上的对比度变小，易漏诊。但这种漏诊的风险有多大？并无确切的文献报道。该项研究结果表明，脂肪肝背景明显降低了超声和CT对肝局灶性病变的检出能力，且降低的程度分别达到18.4%和15.7%，这足以让我们对脂肪肝患者要提高警惕了。这个结果与3种检查技术的成像原理和特点不同有关。由于脂肪肝在超声检查中表现为回声增强，而肝局灶性病变也多表现为高回声。当脂肪肝与肝局灶性病变同时存在时，两者之间的对比度变小，对肝局灶性病变的检出会有一定的影响。目前，常规彩色多普勒超声对脂肪肝背景下合并实性占位病变的诊断和鉴别诊断较困难，有文献报道其在肝脏局灶性病变中的正确诊断率为30%~60%。

一些作者对经病理证实的脂肪肝伴实性占位70例（91个病灶）采用超声造影技术实时观察，并与增强CT进行对照分析，得出超声造影对脂肪肝背景下的肝占位诊断的敏感性和特异性均较高，与螺旋CT的敏感性和特异性基本相似，可见超声造影可提高其检出率。

肝脂肪性变在CT平扫时表现为低密度，肝局灶性病变也多以低密度为主，导致与病变间的密度差异变小，这是CT平扫对伴脂肪肝时肝局灶性病变漏诊的主要原因。同时，也有将脂肪肝背景下的肝局灶性病变误诊为肝岛的情况。一项在脂肪肝背景下肝转移瘤的CT诊断研究课题中将CT平扫时8个肝转移瘤误诊为肝岛，其研究结果显示，肝岛发生于肝脏周边部位的比率较高，因此对于肝脏周边区域分布的局灶性病变应注意与肝岛鉴别。

脂肪肝在MRI T_1WI双回波相上具有特征性表现，表现为正反相位的信号异常和差异化，而局灶性病变一般没有这样的差异化表现；在T_2WI抑脂序列上，脂肪肝肝脏信号强度衰减，而局灶性病变则以稍高信号或高信号表现为主，正好形成更良好的对比度。因此，脂肪肝的存在并没有影响MRI对肝局灶性病变的检出。

该项研究结果还表明，任何一种检查技术都不可能检出所有病变。这对临床评价各种影像技术的价值与限度很有临床意义。

该项研究不足之处就是CT平扫的病例较少，所选病例多是CT直接增强，所以和非增强超声比较，结果肯定占有优势，均未增强的3种检查对脂肪肝背景下肝局灶性病变的检出率的结果如何，还有待于以后进一步研究。

该项研究表明，MRI对肝局灶性病变的检出不受脂肪肝的影响，明显优于CT和超声。在非脂肪肝背景下，CT和MRI对肝局灶性病变的检出无明显差异，都优于常规超声。对肝局灶性病变的检出，脂肪肝背景下超声的检出能力受到限制，可造成较高的假阴性，对怀疑有肝局灶性病变患者的影像检查，要重视脂肪肝背景对病灶检出的影响，并结合临床和多种影像检查方法综合诊断，尤其是MRI检查，可以提高病变的检出率。

第二节　脂肪肝背景

详见本书 本卷 第一篇 第三章 第五节　关于脂肪肝背景。

第三节　弥漫性脂肪肝与占位病变同时存在

在弥漫性脂肪肝的病人，肝内的恶性或良性占位病变的诊断可能十分困难。衰减值大于周围脂肪肝的球形病变，可能认为是一明显的包块，也可简单地认为是未受侵犯的正常肝中的一个小岛。如果这包块（或多个包块）具有低的类似于周围脂肪肝的衰减值，这包块则可能被低估或不被发现而漏诊。

在这种情况下，更具有损伤性的检查，诸如经皮穿刺活检、选择性肝动脉造影、以及 CT 血管造影可能都是必需的。

第四节　肝弥漫性病变——密度降低

CT 平扫显示肝脏密度改变：正常人肝细胞内糖原含量较高，致肝脏 CT 值要高于腹腔内其他实质性脏器（胰腺、肾和脾）。平扫时肝实质的平均 CT 值在 40~80HU 之间，较脾高 7~8 HU。

但肝脏的背景密度并不等同或固定，有些情况下改变很大。脂肪肝病人由于肝细胞内脂肪的堆积使肝密度降低，严重脂肪弥漫浸润者肝实质的密度甚至低于血液密度，使肝内血管成为相对高密度的分支状影。

反之，肝实质密度也可因某些原因（如肝脏贮积性疾病和重金属药物的使用）而升高。在这种情况下肝脏内所呈现的低或高密度病变，只能称之为相对低密度或相对高密度。因此，阅读 CT 影像判断肝内病变密度时，首先需留意背景肝情况。

CT 平扫呈弥漫性低密度的肝脏疾病及其 CT 增强后表现详见表 9-3-1。

表 9-3-1　CT 平扫呈弥漫性低密度的肝脏疾病及其 CT 增强后表现

呈低密度的肝脏疾病	增强后表现
脂肪浸润（弥漫性、局灶性、多结节性）	无改变；肝内血管无肿块效应
恶性浸润（弥漫性肝转移）	呈不均质强化
肝充血	
心力衰竭	下腔静脉 / 肝静脉扩张、肉豆蔻肝伴斑状强化
三尖瓣狭窄 / 闭锁不全	下腔静脉 / 肝静脉扩张、肉豆蔻肝伴斑状强化
缩窄性心包炎	心包增厚、钙化，下腔静脉 / 肝静脉扩张，肉豆蔻肝伴斑状强化
布 - 加综合征	肝静脉和（或）腔静脉不显示；肝门部可见多数侧支
	急性期：肝肿大；慢性期：肝脏缩小，尾叶增大，呈高 CT 值
淀粉样变	增强前后无变化；其他器官同时受累
贮积性疾病	
糖原贮积症（von Gierke）	肝细胞性肝癌 / 肝细胞腺瘤危险性增加
葡糖脑苷脂酶不足（Gaucher）	
神经鞘脂贮积症（Niemann-Pick）	

第四章　密度下降——肝弥漫性节段型病变

第一节　局灶性脂肪变和局灶性肝岛

详见本书 本卷 第一篇 第三章 第八节　局灶性脂肪变和局灶性肝岛。

第二节　脂肪肝迅速地出现和消失

CT 能显示肝的脂肪内容物的弥漫性或局灶性变化可以迅速出现。在淋巴母细胞性淋巴瘤用 L-天门冬素酶治疗后随访观察，在 2 周时间内出现显著的脂肪性变化。在肠外营养的初期也有类似的发现。

脂肪浸润也可迅速消退。Bashist 等（1982）报告 2 例嗜酒者的肝的局灶性和弥漫性脂肪浸润，在住院和改善营养状况后观察，分别在 6 天和 19 天内戏剧性地减少。Sawada 等（1983）发现在 3 个月的间隔期后，局灶性的脂肪改变完全消退。

第三节　局灶性脂肪肝与更重要的占位病变的区别

尽管局灶性脂肪肝的 CT 诊断标准一般都能使人做出正确诊断，但是，偶尔当脓肿或肿瘤不能排除时则可出现区别困难。在这些病人，CT 的异常表现，结合 ^{99m}Tc- 硫胶或 ^{133}Xe 肝的核素显像，有助于解决这问题。实在区别有困难的病例或十分可疑的病例，还可用 22 号针或更可取的 18 号针经皮穿刺活检证实诊断。超声诊断局灶性脂肪肝有一定困难，它是有回声的包块，其回声稍大于正常超声的衰减。由于操作不当，可以把弥漫性脂肪浸润的肝内的局灶性的正常肝实质，常常错误地描写为一个透声包块。

第四节　诊断陷阱：肝的局灶性脂肪浸润

详见本书 本卷 第一篇 第三章 第六节　肝的脂肪浸润与诊断陷阱。

第五节　肝的脂肪浸润与超声：脂肪变性中的局灶性跳跃区

详见本书 本卷 第一篇 第三章 第七节　肝的脂肪浸润与超声的跳跃区。

第六节　弥漫性脂肪肝的局部未受累区域

弥漫性脂肪肝病例中常可见局部未受累区域，应与脂肪肝合并肿瘤相鉴别，其常见部位为肝门部及胆囊窝周围的肝实质。病因学方面的解释为非门脉性内脏静脉供血所致，更普遍的观点认为，病因为富含甘油三酯和脂肪酸等营养物质的门静脉血供缺失，因而在增强扫描章节里讨论的缺乏门静脉供血的区域会形成脂肪肝中的未受累区。

另外，还发现肿瘤周围的肝实质在脂肪肝时可不发生脂肪变，而脂肪肝的成因正是营养过剩。局部未受累区域偶尔可发生于肝被膜下的肝实质，但诊断较发生于常见部位者困难。

第七节　肝弥漫性节段型病变

肝弥漫性节段型病变，一般指呈节段形分布的病变，含节段型脂肪肝和亚急性肝炎局灶性纤维化融合，及其他引起节段形影像学表现的病变。它包括：脂肪肝，亚急性肝炎等。

亚急性肝炎：亚急性肝炎主要是由乙型肝炎病毒或丙型肝炎病毒感染或药物引起的，预后较差，死亡率高。肝损害严重时，肝实质信号在 T_1WI 上减低，在 T_2WI 上增高。

另外，节段性萎缩可表现为信号轻度异常。

第五章　布 - 加综合征

请详见本书 本卷 第十篇 第一章　布 - 加综　　合征。

第六章　肝结节状再生性增生

影像诊断困难的肝脏结节状再生性增生

肝脏结节状再生性增生是一种非常少见的肝细胞结节性弥漫性增生而不伴有纤维化为特征的病变。病因还不十分明确，可能与口服避孕药、类风湿性关节炎、结节性多动脉炎、布-加综合征、系统性红斑狼疮、自身免疫性疾病有关。

1. 发病机制　目前认为结节状再生性增生发病机制与肝实质内微循环障碍有关，是肝脏对血流分布异常的一种非特异性适应性改变，病理改变的基础是肝动脉或门静脉的末级分支弥漫性狭窄或闭塞，形成局部缺血，导致血供减少部位肝细胞萎缩，而那些血供正常的部位肝细胞则代偿性增生，形成再生性结节，这是肝组织对肝内血流变化异常的一种继发性代偿性改变。

2. 临床表现　临床上多数病人无症状，少数出现上腹部不适，病程后期可以出现非特异性的门静脉高压甚至肝衰竭。

3. 影像学研究　在影像上，结节状再生性增生表现为弥漫性和局灶性，弥漫性以肝内广泛分布的小结节为主，局灶性病变表现为散在分布的肝内结节，大者可达数厘米。局灶性结节状再生性增生多出现在布-加综合征和自身免疫性肝炎患者，弥漫性结节状再生性增生多见于非肝硬化的门静脉高压患者，可出现静脉曲张破裂出血和脾功能亢进。

结节状再生性增生的影像表现依赖于结节的大小，弥漫的细小病变不易检出，当结节较大或有融合倾向时，可表现为肝内占位。可能伴随的影像表现包括食管-胃底的静脉曲张、腹水和脾大等。结节状再生性增生的超声表现无特异性，显示为正常肝实质或低/等回声结节灶。CT平扫多为低或等密度，增强后强化少见或仅表现轻度强化，但病变的弥漫性强化或周围环状强化也有报道。

一例患者的超声检查提示肝硬化，CT平扫肝内可见多个小的类圆形低密度病变，增强后表现为延迟强化，出现病变中央强化而周围低密度环围绕的独特表现。

结节状再生性增生的MRI影像表现不具特异性，仅有个案报道且差异较大，在T_1WI和T_2WI上均可出现高至低信号改变。结节在DWI序列上为等信号，Gd-DTPA增强后动脉期病灶出现强化，门脉期及平衡期表现等信号，与肝癌的快速流出不同，增强后的1~3 h仍表现为高或等信号。也有研究发现增强后肝内结节倾向于静脉期强化。

该例患者的MRI影像显示T_1WI上低信号，T_2WI和DWI上高信号；增强后病变倾向于延迟强化，出现类似于CT表现的中央强化而周围低密度环围绕改变。患者DSA表现未见肿瘤染色。

结节状再生性增生影像诊断困难，主要因为表现不特异，但结合临床表现（如特发性门脉高压）及延迟强化的影像特征应考虑到本病的可能。

4. 鉴别诊断　结节状再生性增生与局灶性结节增生和肝腺瘤的影像表现存在重叠，如果结节为多发，还应与转移瘤鉴别，肝细胞腺瘤年轻女性多见，无肝硬化背景，常有口服避孕药史。动脉期病灶均匀强化，有时伴出血坏死。局灶结节性增生患者多无慢性肝炎或肝硬化病史，影像检查显示血管丰富，结节境界清楚，中央放射状纤维化，组织学上肝细胞形态与正常肝细胞基本相同，主要改变是结节内出现许多不规则的血管。

本病的预后主要取决于门静脉高压的严重程度、诊治疗效以及合并的系统性疾病。结节状再生性增生的影像报道很少，影像特征还需大样本总结。

第七章 肝脏淋巴动力学异常

第一节 肝脏淋巴异常动力学改变的CT研究

肝脏淋巴管是除门静脉、肝动脉、肝静脉和胆系以外的重要引流系统，在排出肝组织内过量水分中起重要作用。许多疾病可致肝脏淋巴动力学的异常改变。常规放射学方法显示肝内淋巴管困难，随着肝移植和CT的发展，肝脏淋巴动力学异常改变的CT研究逐渐受到重视。

肝脏淋巴系统的解剖和生理基础：肝组织液起于毛细血管周围间隙，液体沿微静脉周围间隙进入门静脉周围间隙，由此穿过肝内淋巴管的内皮细胞进入肝脏淋巴管，形成淋巴液。肝内淋巴系统由包膜(表面)淋巴管和肝内淋巴管组成，肝内淋巴管又分为门静脉、胆管周围系统和肝静脉周围系统两部分。显微镜下，肝内淋巴管位于围绕门静脉、胆管和肝静脉周围的结缔组织内。正常情况下，显微镜下不能显示肝内淋巴管，当有淋巴管阻塞和淋巴液生成过多时，显微镜下才能显示肝内淋巴管，并可由X线检查和腹腔镜发现。

经皮肝造影显示，大多数病例肝内淋巴管，皆以一条或数条不规则纡曲管状致密影向肝门引流，淋巴管与胆管及门静脉分支伴行，然后与胆管和门静脉的主支一起出肝，出肝后与肝外胆管并行且吻合成不规则的网状，最后引流到乳糜池。80%以上的肝淋巴液经此路径引流出肝，并且主要位于肝十二指肠韧带内。

在肝外，淋巴管也可以分为一个或几个管状结构，形成脊柱旁较大的交织成网状的不规则淋巴丛。部分病例可见肝内淋巴管向左侧头端引流，这是伴行于肝静脉的淋巴管，它经膈裂孔进入胸腔，20%的淋巴液由此路径引流。

用兔和鼠结扎肝门淋巴管后，显微镜下可见到肝内淋巴管扩张和结缔组织增生，Disse间隙(分隔肝窦状隙与肝细胞的小间隙，肝淋巴液由此运送)内淋巴水肿，结扎后3~4天最明显，4~6周后恢复正常，原因是肝内淋巴管的再生。

肝脏淋巴液来源有三：大部分来源于肝血窦，部分来源于胆管，少量来源于肝动脉。正常成人肝淋巴引流量1~3L/24小时，由液体和蛋白质组成。血窦壁对血浆蛋白具有高渗透性，无胶体渗透压存在，跨血窦壁的液体流动直接受到流体静压改变的影响，任何原因致肝静脉压增加，均可导致肝内间质液增加，肝内淋巴液生成增多。胆管壁内淋巴管紧贴胆管上皮细胞，完全结扎总胆管可致肝淋巴液增加三倍。

门静脉内毛细血管由肝动脉供血，毛细血管压力增加或血浆胶体渗透压降低，使血管内液外渗增加，产生大量含蛋白的间质液，使肝淋巴管的引流增加。

经肝实质造影后，见肝内淋巴管的引流速度相对加快，但仍比肝静脉内对比剂流速慢。用狗和羊经淋巴管插管，以肝淋巴管流出液压力与淋巴液流速的关系来分析肝脏的淋巴引流，当淋巴管流出液压力小于19±4cm水柱时，增加下腔静脉压力并不改变淋巴液流速，当此压力大于19±4cm水柱时，流速与压力之间呈线性正相关。

肝淋巴液对肝静脉压力增加非常敏感，下腔静脉压力增加后，肝淋巴液流出量迅速增加，几分钟即可产生反应，而肺淋巴液对左心房压力改变的反应时间可达30~90分钟。下腔静脉压力增加后，肝淋巴液产生增多，是由于肝内淋巴管有效阻力减低和有效淋巴液驱动压增加，其中以淋巴管有效阻力减低作用更明显。肝内淋巴管有效阻力减低，是由于肝内淋巴管的扩张，和关闭状态的淋巴管开放；有效淋巴液驱动压增加，是由于淋巴管收缩，被动受压的泵机制，以及肝间质内液体压增加所致。

一、影像学研究

检查方法：Moreno 等（1963）首次报道肝实质内注射对比剂显示肝脏淋巴管的非手术方法，在局麻下，用 18 号针，于右腋中线第 9 肋间隙穿刺肝实质，深度约 3~4cm，针吸负压肯定针尖不在胆管和血管内后，注入 50% 对比剂 20ml，速度为 2ml/s，于注射后 0s、2s、4s、6s、10s、20s、30s、60s 分别摄 X 线片，肝内淋巴管为条状的致密影，由注射处向肝门扩散。随后，Clain 和 Mcnalty 证明肝内淋巴管可经肝实质内注射对比剂而显示，在电视引导下经右季肋部第 7~8 肋间隙向肝门胆管分叉稍上方进针，最深可达脊柱旁数厘米，缓慢拔针同时以中等压力推注对比剂，当有条状淋巴管显示后，在照片的同时推入 5~10ml 对比剂。此法称为经皮肝造影，其并发症为胆汁漏和出血，发生率为 0.6%。

我们在进行经皮肝穿胆系造影检查时发现，梗阻性黄疸病人（尤其是肝门胆管癌）有时对比剂进入肝实质内显示成网篮状的细线条影，每一线条影粗细相近，一般难分出其为上游或下游淋巴管，它们常常表现有轻微的弯曲而不呈直线，但其走行都向着肝门方向，它们与显影的胆管的伴行关系不明确。有的病例，它们表现呈抱球状，我们用它来诊断肝内占位病变的所在。

随着肝移植和 CT 技术的进步，肝移植后 CT 扫描时，发现增强后有不同于胆管扩张的，肝内门静脉分支和肝内下腔静脉等血管周围低密度影，经病理和实验研究证实主要与肝内淋巴管的异常扩张有关。CT 图像上，血管周围低密度影，作为反映异常的肝内淋巴动力学改变的指标已被肯定。CT 扫描与常规肝脏扫描相同，层厚 8~10mm，自膈顶连续扫描至肝下缘，静脉团注或团注加滴注增强，对比剂为 60~100ml。血管周围低密度影增强 CT 图像上的表现是：围绕门静脉主干及其分支，和 / 或肝内下腔静脉周围的条状或环状低密度区，不伴存梗阻性黄疸征象。增强扫描，使用足量对比剂，高分辨 CT 和快速扫描技术等，皆有利于 CT 显示血管周围低密度影。有学者认为，血管周围低密度影应于门静脉和肝内下腔静脉周围同时出现。

一些学者将肝外缘到肝门外的门静脉主干之间，以门静脉为圆心，分成三等分的同心圆，靠近肝门区的内 1/3 的血管周围低密度影称为中心性血管周围低密度影；其余为外周性血管周围低密度影，外周性血管周围低密度影中弥漫于全肝的又称为弥漫性血管周围低密度影，仅局限于肝叶或肝段者称为局灶性血管周围低密度影，并认为中心性血管周围低密度影对疾病诊断的提示不如外周性血管周围低密度影。

二、肝脏淋巴动力学异常的病因

肝移植：肝移植病人手术后 CT 增强扫描时间可出现血管周围的低密度影，部分学者试图将其作为肝移植后急性排斥的一种征象。肝移植后 CT 图像有血管周围低密度影者，7 天内活检组织学均证实血管周围低密度影，为位于肝内血管周围扩张的肝内淋巴管，原因是手术完全阻断了肝脏淋巴管，致使肝正常淋巴引流受到破坏。血管周围低密度影与急性排斥反应同时存在，且肝脏生化指标异常，血管周围低密度影提示肝移植急性排斥反应的敏感性为 50%，特异性为 80%，准确性为 73%。血管周围低密度影与活检的排斥证据之间相关显著（$P<0.05$）。当肝脏生化指标正常后，血管周围的低密度影亦随之消失，这与肝脏淋巴引流重建有关。

肝癌和肝转移性肿瘤：肝脏的肿瘤转移有两种基本形式，常见的是肝实质内形成结节灶的血性转移，其次是淋巴转移。晚期肝癌淋巴转移并不少见，一组 439 例肝癌尸解资料，25% 有淋巴转移，表现为 CT 图像上门静脉分支扩大，胆管扩张，增强扫描见血管周围低密度影出现。组织学上表现为病灶周围肝内淋巴管扩张，其内有瘤栓，扩张的淋巴管和肿瘤细胞致门静脉分支、胆管和肝动脉受压阻塞。结肠癌肝转移中 41%CT 扫描时可见血管周围低密度影，肝内肿瘤浸润程度与血管周围低密度影出现有相关关系。尸解发现肝转移癌组织学表现为灶性静脉阻塞和肝淤血，疏松结缔组织内膜增厚和毛细淋巴管扩张，癌细胞位于淋巴管内，由于淋巴管对癌细胞侵犯的反应，可导致肝内淋巴管阻塞，回流受阻。原发和继发肝肿瘤造成血窦阻力增加，液体渗入组织间隙内，肝淋巴液生成增多，均是肝内淋巴管扩张的发生机制的重要因素。

胆系梗阻：一组 32 例胆系梗阻病人中，12%CT 扫描时出现血管周围低密度影，在梗阻性黄疸病人，小淋巴管在 X 线直接法胆管造影时的反流显示，提示肝内淋巴管液体流动是双向的，与阻力和压力有关。胆系梗阻致胆系内压引流受阻,作为补偿机制肝淋巴液生成增多,实验性结扎胆总管可致肝淋巴液较正常增加 3 倍,肝淋巴液的增多则致肝内淋巴管扩张。血管周围低密度影是扩张的肝内淋巴管,此征象在鉴别肝内淋巴管扩张和胆管扩张中有重要的临床意义。胆管扩张仅是伴随血管,常位于血管前方,不环绕血管,淋巴管则围绕血管形成弧形或环状低密度区,尤其在血管呈横断面时更为明显。另外,需鉴别的是血管周围脂肪,尤其在近肝门处,这有赖于对 CT 值的仔细分析。

感染:严重外伤病人尸解时可见肝内多发灶性淋巴管扩张,是继发于急性或/和慢性小毛细胆管或/和细毛细胆管感染的外伤并发症。动物实验证实,炎性改变而无肝静脉或下腔静脉梗阻时,肝淋巴液生成增多,可致肝内淋巴管扩张。胆管扩张也可造成感染,使淋巴液产生增多及周围淋巴管的阻塞,产生淋巴管扩张。Siegel 等(1992)报道急性肝炎和慢性肝炎 CT 扫描时的血管周围低密度影,其原因为肝淋巴引流受影响和门静脉及胆管周围的炎性浸润等。

心衰和下腔静脉压力升高:心衰病人静脉团注对比剂增强时, CT 表现为肝实质内斑片状增强,血管周围低密度影,腹腔积液和心影增大。此时,血管周围低密度影为肝血管周围淋巴水肿所致。三尖瓣功能不全者 52%CT 扫描时有血管周围低密度影,血管周围低密度影与动脉高压、心输出减少、心脏指数间无相关性,但有血管周围低密度影者 90% 肝静脉的反向性增强,反映了三尖瓣功能不全的程度。这类病人 CT 图像上出现的血管周围低密度影是由于肝静脉回流受阻,压力增高,静脉淤血,肝淋巴液生成增多,致使肝内淋巴管扩张。

外伤:有作者报告 1 例死于严重颅脑伤后 7 天的病人尸解发现肝内多灶性淋巴管扩张,原因是继发于严重外伤后的并发症(感染和炎性渗出)。外伤病人 CT 图像上有血管周围低密度影者, 80% 有可致肝内淋巴回流受阻和肝内淋巴液生成增多的原因,包括:肝挫伤、腹腔血肿(血肿位于可致肝脏淋巴系统受压的部位,血肿清除后, CT 图像上的血管周围低密度影可消失)。Patrick 等(1992)和 Siegel 等(1992)分别报道的外伤后 CT 图像上的血管周围低密度影发生率为 21.9% 和 65.2%,尸解时均发现相当于血管周围低密度影处有明显的淋巴管扩张。外伤时发生血管周围低密度影的原因有:淋巴引流阻塞(尤其有门脉周围血肿时);大量液体回流所致的容量过大;腹部受压致使门脉压力升高;淋巴管由于外伤刺激的相应损伤。血管周围低密度影与外伤的严重程度有关,有血管周围低密度影者较无血管周围低密度影者伤势严重。

其他原因:其他可致肝内淋巴管扩张的原因有:良性或恶性肝门淋巴结肿大、先天性异常、淋巴瘤、血管内皮损伤等。其机制也与肝内淋巴液生成增多或/和淋巴回流受阻有关。

综上所述,肝脏淋巴系统对于肝脏内过多组织液的引流致关重要,常规 X 线造影方法复杂,且有一定创伤性。CT 图像上出现的血管周围低密度影为无创性评估肝内淋巴引流提供了一种实用而简便的影像学方法,其作为评价肝内异常淋巴动力学的指标已被肯定,但其对于各种疾病的敏感性、特异性和准确性还有待于更进一步的研究。

第二节　门静脉周围晕:肝病的一个 CT 征象

门静脉周围晕,是指增强 CT 影像中门静脉或亚段门静脉周围的环形低密度区。Lawson(1993)复习 3 777 例腹部增强 CT 图像,并对照临床与实验室检查、经皮或手术活检结果等资料后指出,门静脉周围晕可能是肝门三管道(门静脉、肝动脉、胆管)周围疏松结缔组织内增多的液体或扩张的淋巴管。

由于约 80% 的肝内淋巴经肝段淋巴管引流至肝门区,肝门肿物可能阻塞肝脏淋巴引流,造成远侧门静脉周围淋巴水肿,最常见于恶性淋巴结肿大,也可见于炎症与良性肿瘤。肝外伤患者可见出血引起的门静脉周围晕征。充血性心力衰竭所致肝淤血,重度肝炎或小静脉阻塞性病变可造成肝脏淋巴生成过多,超过淋巴引流能力,继发门静脉周围水肿,形成门静脉晕征。肝移植后的门静脉晕征可能与术后淋巴管紊乱,淋巴向心性引流障碍有关。

该作者认为,门静脉周围晕虽然无特异性,但确为一病理征象,应提示临床对肝脏全面检查,以找到可能存在的病因。

第八章　自身免疫性肝病和 IgG4 相关性疾病（IgG4–RD）

第一节　自身免疫性肝炎、原发性胆汁性肝硬化、原发性硬化性胆管炎重叠综合征

自身免疫性肝病是自身抗体介导的慢性肝胆系统疾病的总称，AIH-PBC-PSC 重叠综合征指患者同时具有 AIH、PBC 和 PSC 三种疾病的临床表现、血清学和组织学特征，其中 AIH、PBC 确诊主要靠病理结果，而 PSC 确诊需结合病理和影像表现，MR 胆胰管成像具有较大诊断价值。一组作者报告一例 AIH-PBC-PSC 重叠综合征患者 MRI 平扫主要表现为肝脏体积增大，有别于病毒性肝硬化的肝脏体积减小表现。肝实质内见多发肝硬化结节，结节间可见长 T_2 信号纤维间隔网，此征象可能与肝纤维增生及炎性渗出有关。

门静脉周围可见异常长 T_2 信号，门静脉增粗，脾脏明显增大，门静脉增粗及脾脏体积增大与肝硬化门静脉高压、自身免疫功能紊乱有关。有研究显示 AIH 患者表现为肝外门静脉周围异常信号，与门静脉周围水肿有关；PBC 患者表现为肝内门静脉周围异常信号，与炎性细胞浸润有关。

MR 胆胰管成像示胆总管尚可显示，肝总管、左右肝管显影淡，走行僵硬，粗细不均，局部可见狭窄，肝内 2、3 级胆管显示不清，肝内胆管周围可见条状、网状高信号。肝总管、左右肝管显影淡，肝内 2、3 级胆管显示不清与 PBC 肝脏淤胆或胆汁分泌减少有关；肝内胆管周围的异常网状高信号与肝内纤维增生及炎性渗出有关。有学者报道，PSC 患者 MR 胆胰管成像主要表现为肝外胆管粗细不均，呈串珠样改变，该例表现与之相符。

第二节　免疫球蛋白 G4 相关肝胆疾病的诊断和鉴别诊断

免疫球蛋白 G4 相关疾病（IgG4-RD）是一类具有共同特定病理学、血清学和临床特征的免疫介导性疾病。IgG4-RD 可能包含炎性假瘤、IgG4 相关自身免疫性肝炎、1 型自身免疫性胰腺炎累及肝脏三种临床类型。IgG4 相关硬化性胆管炎罕见单独发病，多与 1 型自身免疫性胰腺炎同时存在，需要与原发性硬化性胆管炎相鉴别。近十几年来，免疫球蛋白 G4 相关疾病（IgG4-RD）作为一种新的慢性、累及多器官或组织炎症纤维化的自身免疫性疾病，引起了越来越多临床和基础研究者的关注。

一、IgG4 相关肝病或肝炎

IgG4-RD 可涉及近 40 个器官，迄今研究最多的器官是胰腺、唾液或泪腺以及胆管树等。与硬化性胆管炎不同，只有少数文献是关于 IgG4-RD 累及肝脏的报道，主要有炎性假瘤、IgG4 相关自身免疫性肝炎（AIH）及 IgG4 相关胰腺炎累及肝脏三种类型。

1.IgG4 相关肝病与 IgG4 相关 AIH 的诊断　有报道在 AIP 患者中经常见到肝功能障碍，且几乎所有 AIP 患者肝活组织检查均显示出 IgG4+ 浆细胞浸润的证据：HPF 下肝实质内可见平均 2~60 个 lgG4+ 浆细胞广泛浸润。Umemura 等（2007）以 5 种模式对 AIP 的肝组织学进行了分类：①门静脉炎症模式：门静脉炎症明显，有或无界面性炎症；②大胆管损伤模式：由胆管增生、中性粒细胞浸润和门静脉区域水肿；③门静脉硬化模式：表现出密集的门静脉硬化，门静脉炎症瘢痕；④小叶型肝炎的模式：显

示小叶内水肿,肝细胞坏死类似病毒性肝炎;⑤胆汁淤积型:主要以小叶中心区的小管型胆汁淤积为主,这种 IgG4+ 浸润 AIP 的肝脏病理学模式被称为“IgG4 相关肝病”。

AIP 中 IgG4+ 浆细胞的数量明显高于其他自身免疫性肝病,且与血清 IgG4 浓度显著相关。因此,当怀疑 AIP 的诊断时,组织学研究和肝活组织检查的 IgG4 免疫染色可提供支持性证据。肝活组织检查可以提供 AIP 诊断的重要信息。

IgG4-RD 另一种可能的肝脏相关表现是淋巴浆细胞性炎性假瘤,表现为 IgG4+ 浆细胞高度浸润、纤维化和闭塞性静脉炎。该实体类似原发性恶性肝肿瘤。

Chung 等(2010)描述了一种新型的 AIH 亚型:IgG4 相关 AIH。其特征在于 IgG4+ 浆细胞 >5 个 /HPF,称为“IgG4 相关 AIH”。与 IgG4 非相关患者相比,IgG4 相关 AIH 患者的总血清 IgG 水平更高。但 IgG4 相关 AIH 和 IgG4 非相关 AIH 患者的血清 IgG4 水平无明显差异,泼尼松龙治疗非常有效。

2. IgG4 相关肝病与 IgG4 相关 AIH 的鉴别诊断　对 AIP 患者的肝功能检查和病理性肝活组织检查的结果可以提示 IgG4 相关肝病,AIP 的肝内 IgG4+ 浆细胞浸润的数量及范围很广,平均值为 2~60 个 /HPF。IgG4+ 浆细胞 10 个 /HPF 以上的病例发生率约为 24%。泼尼松龙治疗 4 周后肝脏小叶型肝炎的病理学改变明显好转。

AIH 的特征是:肝脏慢性炎症、氨基转移酶水平升高、高丙种球蛋白血症、血清自身抗体水平升高、界面性肝炎的组织学证据以及对免疫抑制治疗的有利反应。根据临床、血清学和 / 或组织学标准,临床上仍有一些患者不能确定特定的 AIH 亚组,此时需要考虑 IgG4 相关 AIH 的可能。有报道 1 例 AIH 患者治疗前血清 IgG4 浓度高于 5 000 mg/L、肝脏广泛的 IgG4+ 浆细胞浸润,该病例不仅满足了 AIH 的诊断标准,而且具有 IgG4 相关疾病的特征,可以诊断 IgG4 相关 AIH。日本 60 例 AIH 患者的队列研究结果显示有 2 例血清 IgG4 升高和肝内 IgG4+ 浆细胞浸润,IgG4-AIH 的发病率为 3.3%(2/60),并提出了 IgG4-AIH 的临时诊断标准:血清 IgG4 浓度升高(1350 mg/L)、明显的 IgG4+ 浆细胞浸润肝脏(10 个 /HPF)是本病的标志性特征,并且在肝外胆管或胰腺中未见明显异常表现。

总之,通过对 AIP 和 AIH 的肝实质研究证实了一种新的肝病存在,肝实质病灶主要由浸润的 IgG4+ 细胞组成。IgG4 相关肝病包括一些胆管炎和 AIH 特征,需要更多了解 AIH 与 IgG4 的关系和长期应用皮质类固醇的预后。现有数据表明 IgG4 相关肝病治疗比 AIH 更有效,最重要的是要认识到这种疾病,并设计出最合适的治疗方案。

二、IgG4 相关硬化性胆管炎(IgG4-SC)

硬化性胆管炎有三种临床类型,包括 IgG4-SC、原发性硬化性胆管炎(PSC)和 PSC/AIH 重叠综合征。

1.IgG4-SC 的诊断:IgG4-SC 的疾病特点与 IgG4-RD 相似:临床方面,它是最常见的 1 型 AIP 的胰腺外病变,在此类患者中的发生率超过 70%。表现为局灶性占位或弥漫性胆管组织肿胀;实验室指标胆红素升高,以直接胆红素升高为主,皮肤瘙痒、腹痛、胆管炎、食欲减退、体质量下降等。

诊断要点如下:IgG4-SC 极少单独发生,最常见为 1 型 AIP 的胰腺外病变;多同时累及下颌腺、腮腺、胰腺等其他脏器,单独发生的 IgG4-SC 病例罕见;血清学方面为 IgG4 和 IgE 明显升高;病理方面可表现为胆管周围席纹状纤维化,淋巴细胞和浆细胞浸润,胆管管壁环形增厚及闭塞性静脉炎,典型的病理表现包括肝门大胆管周围炎症和席纹状纤维化、大量浆细胞浸润的慢性炎症以及可见 IgG4+ 浆细胞浸润。

IgG4-SC 分型:Ⅰ型:胆总管下端狭窄;Ⅱ型:肝内胆管狭窄伴狭窄远端扩张,伴胆总管下端狭窄;Ⅲ型:肝门及胆总管下端狭窄;Ⅳ型:肝门部胆管狭窄。

IgG4-SC 的诊断应基于组织学、影像学、血清学和其他器官受累,及对类固醇治疗有反应。可应用为诊断 AIP 而开发的 HISORt 标准。

2.IgG4-SC 的鉴别诊断　IgG4-SC 和 1 型 AIP 同时存在时诊断 IgG4-SC 较容易,但是临床没有明显胰腺累及时,需与 PSC、胰腺癌、胆管癌鉴别。

IgG4-SC 与 PSC:临床上两者均好发于男性,但 IgG4-SC 好发于老年,与 AIP 或其他器官相关,血清 IgG4 水平升高,与胆管细胞癌罕见相关;PSC 好发于青少年或老年,与炎症性肠病相关,血清 IgG4 一般正常,4% 与胆管细胞癌相关。病理学上 IgG4-SC 为局灶透壁性病变,可见 IgG4+ 细胞浸润、闭塞性静脉炎,胆管黏膜一般正常,常见假性囊肿。PSC 为弥漫性黏膜糜烂或溃疡病变,无或轻度 IgG+ 细胞浸润，罕见闭塞性静脉炎，无假性囊肿。IgG4-SC 患者常见节段性胆管狭窄、长段狭窄伴狭窄前扩张，以及胆总管远端狭窄，PSC 则多见带状狭窄、串珠状、枯树枝状或憩室状扩张（表 9-8-1）。IgG4 相关疾病通常对皮质类固醇有反应，但在 PSC 中不常见。血清 IgG4 水平在 1.4~2.8 g/L 的患者，IgG4/IgG1 的比值 <0.24 可诊断为 PSC，而非 IgG4-SC。

表 9-8-1　PSC 与 IgG4-SC 的鉴别诊断

临床特点	PSC	IgG4-SC
年龄	青少年或老年	老年
性别	男 > 女	男 > 女
炎症性肠病相关	有	无
血清 IgG4 水平	正常	升高
胆管细胞癌相关	4%	罕见
病理特点		
分布	弥漫性	局灶性
炎症部位	黏膜层	透壁性
$IgG4^+$ 细胞浸润	无	轻度
闭塞性静脉炎	罕见	多见
胆管黏膜	糜烂 - 溃疡	正常
假性囊肿形成	无	有
影像学	1. 带状狭窄	1. 节段性狭窄
	2. 串珠状	2. 下端共同胆管通道狭窄
	3. 枯树枝状	
	4. 憩室状外翻	

注：IgG4-SC：免疫球蛋白 G4 相关硬化性胆管炎；PSC：原发性硬化性胆管炎

日本学者对 527 例 IgG4-SC 患者进行回顾性分析，其中 449 例（85.2%）患者同时合并 AIP，有 15% 合并泪道炎和口腔涎腺炎，7% 合并后腹膜病变，另有 4 例患者因反复炎症刺激而进展为胆管癌。

Lian 等（2017）为澄清 IgG4-SC、PSC/AIH 重叠综合征和 PSC 的区别，回顾性分析了血清 IgG4 对 IgG4-SC 的诊断价值和用作预测硬化性胆管炎预后生物标志物的价值。结果显示免疫球蛋白水平在各组间的差异有统计学意义，并且所有患者均有胆汁淤积表现；在 57 例 IgG4-SC 中，20 例有肝硬化表现，36 例 PSC/AIH 重叠综合征中 15 例有肝硬化表现，55 例 PSC 患者中 18 例有肝硬化表现。血清 IgG4 水平在 92.65% IgG4-SC 患者中升高，灵敏度 86%，特异度 98%。总之，血清 IgG4 ≥ 1.25 倍正常值上限倾向诊断为 IgG4-SC。IgG4-SC 主要是免疫介导的炎症过程，而 PSC/AIH 重叠综合征更倾向于胆汁淤积性疾病。

综上所述，IgG4-SC 是 IgG4-RD 系统性疾病的胆管表现，罕见单独发病，多与 1 型 AIP 同时存在，血清学上表现为 IgG4 水平升高，组织学上可有大量 IgG4+ 浆细胞浸润、席纹状纤维化和闭塞性静脉炎；本病为一系统性疾病，需同时检测系统性器官损伤，治疗方面激素效果佳，预后好，但易复发，需要排除胰腺癌、胆管癌。

总之，IgG4 相关性肝胆疾病是一种正在不断得到更多认识但病因未明确的综合征，最常见于中老年男性，通常数种表现，具有受累器官中亚急性包块形成或器官弥漫性肿大和淋巴结肿大、血清学 IgG4 水平升高和肝脏及胆系的炎症。

诊断主要依靠特征性组织病理学的检查结果，单纯血清学检查结果不具有诊断性，但具有重要的辅助诊断作用。详细病史、体格检查、常规实验室检查和选择性影像学检查可能会发现额外器官受累。糖皮质激素初始治疗效果良好也是特征之一，治疗自然病程和预后并不明确，停止治疗后常见复发，需进一步研究患者的恶性肿瘤风险。

第九章 肝炎

第一节 肝炎

病理学:肝炎是肝脏的弥漫性炎症,它可分为急性和慢性两型。慢性肝炎又可分为活动性和非活动性两种。急性肝炎显示肝细胞的坏死和弥漫性紊乱,无肝门及肝门周围异常。在慢性非活动性肝炎,有肝门周围的炎症,但保存小叶结构。慢性活动性肝炎则有更广泛的炎症,零碎的坏死,常常还有纤维化。

影像学研究:超声检查:急性肝炎,当其足够严重时,可引起肝实质回声降低,清楚可见门静脉分支壁的光亮度增加。确切的征象已报告见于中毒性休克综合征、白血病、糖尿病性酮症。肝门周围回声增加可见于巨细胞病毒性感染、胆系闭锁、胰岛母细胞增殖、α- 胰蛋白酶抑制素缺陷、微脓肿以及特发性新生儿黄疸。超声的表现可源于肝细胞的肿胀,或肝实质的声学特性某些因素的改变。慢性肝炎,当其严重达到一定程度时,可引起肝实质结构变为粗糙,门静脉分支壁的'侧面影像'导致回声有某些增强。这些征象能以炎症浸润和肝小叶周围纤维组织增多来解释。脂肪浸润、慢性充血性心力衰竭、弥漫性肝细胞癌、淋巴瘤、弥漫性转移性疾病、胆系闭锁、胰岛母细胞增殖、以及上升性胆管炎等疾病都有报告出现与此相同的征象,其中,脂肪浸润大概是最常见的。在急性或慢性肝炎,进行超声检查的目的主要是在肝脏疾病的病因中,除外胆系梗阻。CT 扫描:除非有脂肪浸润存在,在急性肝炎和慢性肝炎时,肝的衰减值一般无改变,所以肝的大小的改变可能是唯一的发现。

核素显像:轻度肝炎的病人,核素显像多为正常或有轻度肝肿大,伴有或不伴有轻度的斑驳状吸收。这些改变是间质性水肿的结果,而且在疾病好转后将恢复正常。脾肿大有时见于病毒性肝炎,而且偶尔还可见到其内有局灶性缺损伪似包块性病变。

在急性病毒性肝炎,肝的大小可以是肿大、正常、或缩小,而且核素的吸收将减少。肝脏如缩小,与出现肺的吸收一样,则提示预后不良。急性肝炎病人多有明显的胶体再分布,核素清除减少,以及一定程度的脾肿大。

第二节 急性戊型肝炎致肝内淋巴淤滞

戊型肝炎是由戊型肝炎病毒引起的急性传染病,经粪、口途径传播。临床表现与甲型肝炎相似,但黄疸型多见,病情较重,常见于中青年人。其 CT 表现无特异性,主要为肝脏增大,肝内胆管壁增厚,脾大及肝门部淋巴结轻度肿大。部分患者可见肝内门静脉分支和 / 或下腔静脉周围环形低密度影,是由于肝细胞炎性肿胀、静脉压增高,淋巴回流受阻,引起肝内淋巴管淤滞扩张和肝血管周围浸润性淋巴水肿所致。此征象提示肝功能损害较重。

一例在门静脉左右支两侧可见条状低密度影,在肝下部门静脉及下腔静脉肝内段周围可见环状低密度影,具有典型肝内淋巴淤滞的影像表现。

第三节　病毒感染后的肝硬化

肝硬化是肝细胞反复损害的一种慢性反应，以再生纤维化为特征。肝硬化常见病因有酗酒及乙型、丙型肝炎病毒感染。肝细胞再生表现为肝内满布结节，T_2WI 呈低信号，梯度回波序列上更清晰，这缘于再生结节内的含铁血黄素沉积。

CT 增强门脉期因结节的门脉血供而表现为再生结节强化，而肝细胞癌表现为灌注缺损区。

第十章 肝脏体积和形态变化

第一节 肝脏肿大

肝脏或全身性疾病都可导致肝脏体积增大,包括肝脏原发和来自肝外的转移性肿瘤、全身性代谢/贮积性病变、肝血管以及心源性疾病造成的肝充(郁)血、肝感染/炎症等(表9-10-1)。

表 9-10-1 引起肝脏肿大的疾病及其临床特征

引起肝脏肿大的疾病	临床特征
肝脏肿瘤	
弥漫性肝转移	原发灶见于肺、乳腺、结肠及其他
肝细胞癌(弥漫性)	局灶性、多结节性或弥漫性,25%侵犯门静脉、肝硬化
血管瘤	大多是良性肝肿瘤,>5cm者称巨大血管瘤
肝母细胞瘤	最常见于儿童的肝脏恶性肿瘤
婴儿血管内皮细胞瘤	见于儿童,呈混合密度、增强后强化,可有肝动脉扩张/高输出量充血性心力衰竭(CHF)
血管肉瘤	有接触钍、砷或聚乙烯氯化物(PVC)史,具侵袭性和富血管性特征
淋巴瘤	50%的霍奇金淋巴瘤/非霍奇金淋巴瘤(NHL)可继发肝淋巴瘤病,但影像学少有描述
代谢/贮积性	
脂肪浸润	肥胖、乙醇、肾上腺皮质素、糖尿病、化疗、营养过度等可引发
淀粉样变	肝脏CT值通常减低,常伴有其他器官受侵犯
Wilson disease	铜积聚、肝脏CT值增高
血色素沉着病	CT值增加,致肝细胞癌(HCC)危险性增加
贮积病(storage disease)	有神经鞘脂贮积症、糖原贮积病、葡糖脑苷脂酶不足(戈谢病)
肝充(郁)血	
心力衰竭	下腔静脉(IVC)/肝静脉扩张,豆蔻样肝脏伴有斑片状强化
缩窄性心包炎	心包增厚、钙化,ⅣC/肝静脉扩张,豆蔻样肝伴斑片状强化
三尖瓣关闭不全或狭窄	扩大的ⅣC/肝静脉,豆蔻样肝伴斑片状强化
Budd-Chiari综合征	肝静脉无对比剂充盈,肝斑片状强化、腹水
静脉-阻塞病变	常见于骨髓移植术后
感染/炎症	
病毒性	感染和血清性肝炎、单核细胞增多症(Epstein-Barr virus)
细菌	脓肿:细菌、阿米巴;结核:包括局部病变和淋巴结增大

续表

引起肝脏肿大的疾病	临床特征
真菌	组织胞浆菌病
原虫	疟疾、阿米巴
寄生虫	包虫病;血吸虫病;门静脉周围纤维化、间隔钙化
其他疾病	
肝硬化	通常肝右叶萎缩,肝尾叶与左叶增大
儿童慢性肉芽肿疾病	有遗传性免疫缺陷、继发化脓性感染、脓肿、淋巴结炎
骨髓增生性疾病	骨髓纤维化(myelofibrosis)、红细胞增多(polycythemia vera)
结节病(sarcoidosis)	全部或近半数结节病人有肝脏肿大、局部肉芽肿
多囊性疾病	多发囊肿
髓外造血	脾肿大,骨髓扩展,其他造血部位:后纵隔

第二节　淀粉样变性

淀粉样变性是由一些不溶性淀粉样蛋白和纤维沉积于细胞间和/或血管壁内导致器官和组织损害的一种非常少见的疾病,可分为原发性、继发性和家族性等几类,往往累及多种组织器官而造成多系统损害,主要累及心、肝、肾、脾、胃肠、舌、肌肉及皮肤等多系统多器官。临床表现复杂多样,极易误、漏诊。肝、脾是常见的受累脏器。

病理学:病理上,淀粉样物质在肝窦周间隙大量沉积,肝细胞严重受压、萎缩,门静脉可由于大量淀粉样物沉积受累而扭曲。临床上可出现肝功能衰竭、门脉高压。当淀粉样物质大量浸润时肝质地变为橡胶样弹性的质地,肝切面大体上呈“淀粉样肝(1ardaceous liver)”。

临床表现:原发性淀粉样变病常累及肝,95%的病人尸体解剖时有肝淀粉样物质沉积,有肝淀粉样变者,约60%~81%有肝肿大,只有不到20%的病人因为肝脏肿大而就诊。肝淀粉样变性多表现肝、脾肿大,可出现腹水、肝功能轻度异常、黄疸等,临床上易误诊为肝炎、肝硬化、脂肪肝、肝癌等。体重下降和肝肿大是肝受累的临床特征,其他可有蛋白尿、碱性磷酸酶增高等。由于实验室检查缺乏特异性指标,其确诊需要肝组织活检。

由于临床表现无特异性,确诊依赖于病理活检。但由于淀粉样物质在血管周围沉积而致血管脆性增加、X因子缺乏、凝血酶时间受抑制而延长,肝可以发生自发性破裂和大出血。因此,细针穿刺应非常小心。直肠黏膜和脐周脂肪活检有利于避免严重出血并发症。

影像学研究:CT显示局灶或弥漫性肝实质密度下降,有或无钙化。不均匀局灶或弥漫性实质密度下降,不对称和以镰状韧带为顶点三角形肝肿大是肝淀粉样变特征性的轮廓异常,即尽管肝肿大,2个肝叶前外侧缘镰状韧带两侧轻度萎缩的改变,这在其他浸润性疾病少见。这些表明由于淀粉样物质在肝Disse间隙窦或在血管壁沉积,肝细胞受到淀粉样物质挤压而萎缩,甚至消失,大量血管受累和肝实质受浸润导致血流灌注下降。左叶显著增大,延迟期显示不均匀强化,这些结果提示淀粉样物质浸润的同时有部分肝细胞代偿性肥大。

淀粉样物质常浸润脾而在脾红髓或血管沉积,83%的病人尸体解剖时有脾受累,然而只有4%~13%病人有脾肿大。淀粉样纤维蛋白常在脾红髓或血管沉积,从而导致脾肿大和变硬、变脆,大量浸润时,在脾切面上呈淀粉样脾(bacon spleen)。常常是无症状的,但可因脆性增加而发生自发脾破裂或脾功能减退而增加感染的危险。

脾肿大、钙化、增强强化差是原发性淀粉样变病脾受累的特点。脾增强强化差和弥漫性低灌注,这可能和淀粉样物弥漫性浸润脾实质和脾血管受累有关。延迟相,正常脾均匀强化,病变脾不均匀增强,因此延迟相CT有助于观察脾受累。

在肝淀粉样变性,肝的核素显像能提供有用的资料。在含有淀粉样蛋白的器官,骨的扫描放射性药物的浓度与 ^{99m}Tc 焦磷酸盐的浓度,较 ^{99m}Tc 甲烯二磷酸效果为佳。镓扫描给予不一致的结果,硫胶扫描对于肝淀粉样变性的诊断已令人失望。在肝功能试验与肝淀粉样蛋白之间相关微弱,而且在正常肝功试验的病人,焦磷酸盐扫描能出现阳性。在淀粉样变性,焦磷酸盐吸收的机制尚了解甚少。

鉴别诊断:本病须和局灶或弥漫性浸润疾病相鉴别,如不规则脂肪浸润、肝硬化、恶性肿瘤等。原发淀粉样变 CT 上一个表现为脾受累,脾弥漫性低灌注伴脾肿大或脾正常大小是原发性淀粉样变的一个重要特征。不均匀的密度降低和不对称的以镰状韧带作为顶点三角形肝肿大,有助于和其他浸润性疾病鉴别。

第三节 Niemann-Pick 病和 Gaucher 病

1.Niemann-Pick 病 Niemann-Pick 病是全身脏器(特别是网状内皮系统和中枢神经系统)发生神经鞘髓磷脂蓄积的先天性代谢性疾病,常染色体隐性遗传,可引起肝脾肿大。Niemann-Pick 病由于缺乏神经鞘髓磷脂酶,不能将不断产生的神经鞘髓磷脂降解,于是便蓄积在网状内皮组织中。

根据 Grunebaum(1976)报告 Niemann-Pick 病的组织学和组织化学检查结果,桥脑、延髓、肝、脾、淋巴结、骨髓、肺、肾、肾上腺、Meisner 神经节和肠道的 Auerbach 丛均有含磷脂物质的细胞浸润。Niemann-Pick 病是一种遗传性疾病,由于鞘磷脂酶缺乏及鞘磷脂积集于网状内皮系统而引起鞘脂沉积。

根据起病年龄、累及中枢神经系统的范围和鞘磷脂酶的活性可分为五型:①型为急性神经元病型,为其经典型,占病人总数 85%,起病于婴儿早期,中枢神经系统损害严重,4 岁左右死亡;肝脾肿大在此型病例十分严重,它并使肠袢向腹部中间移位,有的病人还可见肝钙化。②型为慢性非神经元病型,起病于婴儿早期,但不侵犯中枢神经系统或智力,可能寿命正常;中枢神经系统无神经鞘髓磷脂蓄积,而在内脏和骨骼有蓄积。此型骨骼表现为普遍性骨质稀疏,以手骨为明显;掌骨骨干增粗,腕骨骨化延迟;耻骨联合缘不光整,腰椎生理曲度消失。肺部实质与间质均可有改变,诸如:粟粒状影、小片影、肺纹粗乱等;肺部病变的轻重与肝脾肿大程度一致,当肝脾肿大显著时,肺部病变多较重。③型为慢性神经元病型,起病年龄(2 岁以上)和死亡年龄(5 岁至成年)不等,侵犯中枢神经系统的范围也不等。④型为新斯科舍(Nova Scotia)的变异型,类似 3 型。⑤型为成年型非神经元病型,可能是 3 型的起病较迟的变异型。

3.Gaucher 病 Gaucher 病一种脂沉积病,由葡糖脑苷脂酶(葡糖苷酰鞘氨醇酶)缺乏引起,葡糖脑苷(葡糖脑苷鞘氨醇)在肝、脾、淋巴结、肺毛细血管和骨髓内的储藏细胞(细胞)内贮积。临床上可分三型:①型为慢性非神经元病型或成人型,或出现于任何年龄,有脾功能亢进、血小板减少、贫血、黄疸及骨损害;②型为急性神经元病型或婴儿型,发作于婴儿期,有肝脾肿大和严重中枢神经系统损害,通常死于 1 岁以内;③型为亚急性神经元病型或少年型,差异最大,临床表现与 1、2 型相同,但病程较长。

第四节 肝肾淀粉样变性

患者,女,64 岁。患者因反复腰部酸痛 3 年余,浮肿 2 月余入院。查体:血压 153/96mmHg,颜面轻度水肿,心肺检查未见明显异常。腹部饱满,肝脏右肋下 9cm、剑突下 17cm 可触及,表面平,质中偏硬,无压痛,未触及胆囊, Murphy 征阴性;脾脏左肋下约 2cm 可触及。无移动性浊音。肠鸣音正常,双下肢重度指凹性水肿。B 超示:肝脾肿大,肝脏、双肾弥漫性损害改变。肝肾穿刺病理诊断:肝肾淀粉样变性。

肝淀粉样变性常被误诊为许多其他疾病:因血清碱性磷酸酶、γ- 谷氨酰基转移酶明显升高,肝脏影像学显示肝脏增大,肝实质密度低,回声细密,可能被临床误诊为酒精性肝病;因血清碱性磷酸酶、γ- 谷氨酰基转移酶明显升高,肝脏增大,体重明显下降,可能被临床误诊为肝癌;因患者有腹水、CT 或 MRI 显示肝脏血管变细,而可能被误诊为布 - 加综合征,血管造影或增强检查可排除布 - 加综合征,其血管变细只是因为肝脏肿大压迫血管所致；兼有肾脏淀粉样变性的患者，则因大量蛋白尿，严重低蛋白血症，可能被临床误诊为肾病综合征。

故对于临床上有不明原因的肝大，血清碱性磷酸酶、γ-谷氨酰基转移酶明显升高，低蛋白血症、高脂血症、腹水、肝血管变细、大量蛋白尿，影像上表现为肝脾肿大，密度减低，血管变细的患者，应考虑肝淀粉样变性，作肝脏、肾脏的活体组织病理检查及特异性组织学染色（刚果红染色），以明确诊断（图 9-10-1）。

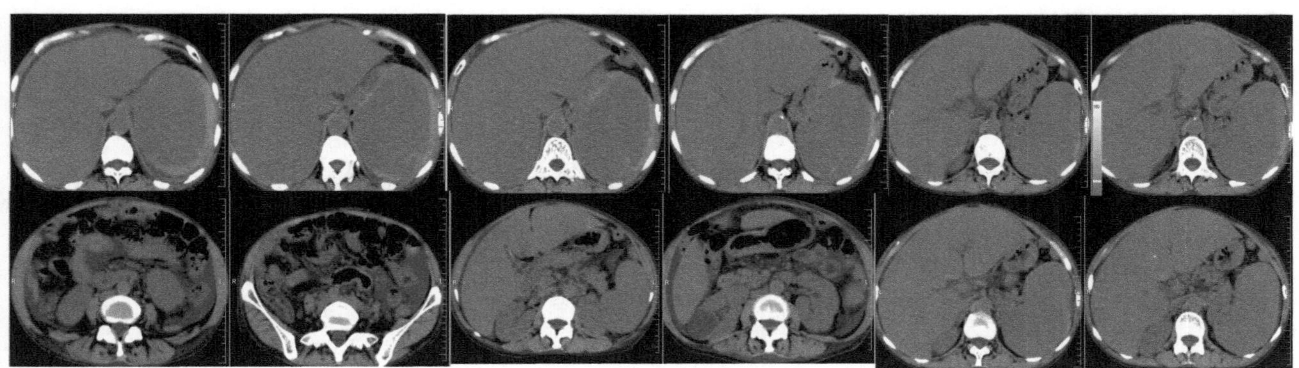

图 9-10-1　肝肾淀粉样变性

第十一章 肝纤维化形态学研究

第一节 肝纤维化程度的诊断

对肝纤维化程度的影像学判断,是目前研究的一个热点和难点问题。也是减缓肝纤维化进程的重要环节。我国是肝病高发区,重视影像学的肝纤维化和肝硬化程度的评估对治疗有重要价值。从目前研究看,影像学对肝纤维化的 S3、S4 期确有诊断价值,对 S2 有诊断可能。

主要的影像学检查方法有彩色多普勒超声的血流观察、超声实时弹性成像、CT 灌注成像、MR 扩散加权成像和 ADC 值测定、肝 MR 弹性成像以及 MR 灌注成像。主要表现为肝灌注血流量下降、扩散受限及弹性降低。

其中超声弹性成像和肝 MR 弹性成像和扩散加权成像无需使用对比剂,更有研究前景和实用价值。超声弹性成像对Ⅳ期肝纤维化显示的敏感度为 87%,特异度为 91%;对 S2~S4 期肝纤维化显示的敏感度为 70%,特异度为 84%。

MR 弹性成像对 S4 期肝纤维化显示的敏感度可达 98%,特异性可达 99%;对 S2~S4 期肝纤维化显示的敏感度为 86%,特异性为 85%。ADC 值测定时,有报道 b 值在 200 或 400 较为合适,也有报道 b 值在 600 或 1 000 较合适;肝硬化 Child C 级 ADC 值降低明显,Child A、B 级也有降低,提示对肝硬化有一定的诊断价值,但对早期肝纤维化分级病理对照的研究尚无大宗报道。

第二节 融合性肝纤维化

融合性肝纤维化常见于肝硬化的后期,有 14%。多为楔形,自肝门向外放射,常伴有肝包膜的内陷和肝段实质的收缩,有时纤维化病灶位于肝脏的外围不伸向肝门。增强 CT 扫描融合纤维化区的密度可有等、低、高三种密度差别。

第十二章　肝纤维化功能代谢研究

肝纤维化与磁共振扩散加权成像

磁共振扩散加权成像（DWI）是一种能够无创性反映活体组织内水分子扩散运动的功能影像学检查方法，其对神经系统缺血性病变及占位性病变的诊断价值已得到认可。随着快速成像技术的发展，DWI 应用于腹部器官疾病（尤其是肝脏疾病）的诊断研究逐渐增多并渐趋成熟。

肝纤维化检查中 b 值选择：理论上，b 值的改变主要是改变了 DWI 对探测组织中水分子扩散运动的敏感性。由于 DWI 反映的是体素内水分子的运动，当水分子的运动幅度在施加运动敏感梯度场期间超过 1 个体素的范围，DWI 则不能反映其超出体素后的那部分运动。

组织内血流灌注的运动速度明显快于水分子的扩散运动，因此，当 DWI 的敏感性较低时（采用小 b 值），测得的主要是运动速度较快的血流运动，此时如果不考虑血流灌注因素的影响，测得的 ADC 值实际上过高地估计了扩散系数。由于低 b 值受血流灌注影响大，所以采用的 b 值越小，得到的 ADC 值越大。因此认为，应用高 b 值是获得接近真实 ADC 值最有效的方法。对于肝脏的 DWI 检查，大多数研究者认为应选取较大的 b 值。但随着选取 b 值的增大，影像的信噪比却逐渐下降，尤其采用高 b 值（b=1 000s/mm^2）时，肝脏信号衰减非常明显，影像伪影严重，很难保证测量的准确性。有作者对 85 例肝纤维化病人及 22 名健康志愿者行 DWI 检查，b 值取 100s/mm^2、300s/mm^2、500s/mm^2、800s/mm^2、1000s/mm^2，采用肝穿刺活检确定肝纤维化分期及肝实质炎症的分级，结果显示 ADC 值与肝纤维化的严重程度呈负相关，尤其是当 b=800s/mm^2 时相关性最佳（r=-0.697，P=0.000），因此认为 DWI 检查可用于肝纤维化程度的判定。另有作者对 49 例慢性病毒性肝炎病人及 10 例健康志愿者在 3.0T MR 设备上行 DWI 检查，b 值分别取 100s/mm^2、200s/mm^2、400s/mm^2、600s/mm^2、800/mm^2，结果表明当 b 值取 400s/mm^2、600s/mm^2、800s/mm^2 时，肝纤维化组与非肝纤维化组的 ADC 值差异具有统计学意义，且当 b=800s/mm^2 时，ADC 值可以区分不同程度的肝纤维化。

Taouli 等（2007）对 23 例肝纤维化病人和 7 名正常人的肝脏进行 DWI 定量分析研究，取 b 值为 50s/mm^2、300s/mm^2、500s/mm^2、700s/mm^2、1000s/mm^2，结果表明，b ≥ 500s/mm^2 时对肝纤维化的定量分析更有意义且能获得较稳定的 DWI 影像。

但有些研究者认为较小 b 值对于肝纤维化的判定更适合，如 Aube 等（2004）对 14 例健康志愿者和 13 例肝纤维化病人用多个 b 值（200s/mm^2、400s/mm^2、600s/mm^2、800s/mm^2）行 DWI 检查后认为，b 值取 200s/mm^2 和 400s/mm^2 时更有助于判定肝纤维化；Koinuma 等（2005）对 163 例检查者采用小 b 值进行 DWI 检查，b 值分别取值为 0.01s/mm^2 和 128.01/mm^2，结果表明 ADC 值的变化同肝纤维化病变程度呈负相关；一些作者利用兔肝纤维化模型行 DWI 检查，b 值取 300、600、1000s/mm^2，结果显示当 b 值取 300s/mm^2 时，ADC 值可以有效地将轻、中度纤维化从无纤维化和重度纤维化中鉴别出来。

每位研究者对肝纤维化时所选择的 b 值结果并不统一，如果认为导致 ADC 值减低的各种因素中以肝纤维化时肝实质内血流灌注减少最为关键，那么是否可以认为采用小 b 值对肝纤维化进行 DWI 检查得出的结果更为准确，这还需要大量的实验研究来逐步证实。

应用 DWI 评价肝纤维化：多数研究报道认为 DWI 用于评价肝纤维化的程度是可行的，且是针对肝纤维化的极具发展前景的一种无创性功能影像学检查方法。

Aube 等（2004）在证实肝纤维化病人 ADC 值减低的基础上，发现 ADC 值的变化与 Child-Pugh 分级和血清透明质酸含量的变化存在显著相关性。Koinuma 等（2005）对 63 例慢性肝炎、66 例肝硬化病人及 34 例肝功能正常者进行 DWI 检查，测量

ADC 值结果表明，慢性肝炎和肝硬化组肝实质 ADC 值随着肝纤维化积分及 Child-Pugh 级别的升高而降低，且肝病组肝实质 ADC 值与肝纤维化积分及 Child-Pugh 级别显著相关（$P<0.0001$），但与肝实质的炎症积分却无明显相关性，据此认为肝实质 ADC 值测量可有效评估肝纤维化的程度。

Girometti 等（2007）对 29 名健康志愿者及 28 例肝病病人进行 DWI 检查，结果显示利用 ADC 值判定肝纤维化的特异度及敏感度分别达 100%、92.9%，阳性预测值、阴性预测值及总体准确度分别为 100%、99.9% 及 96.4%，因此认为 ADC 值可以作为判定肝纤维化程度的指标，并且得出肝纤维化时其 ADC 值的上限值为 $1.31\times10^{-3}mm^2/s$。

Sandrasegaran 等（2009）对 78 例经肝穿刺活检确定为不同时期的肝纤维化病人进行 DWI 检查，结果表明 ADC 值的变化与肝纤维化的程度具有相关性，但却不能根据 ADC 值的范围明确区分各期纤维化。Lewin 等（2007）对 54 例慢性丙型肝炎所致肝纤维化病人及 20 名健康志愿者行 DWI 扫描，结果显示中重度（F_2~F_4）纤维化的 ADC 值 [$(1.10\pm0.11)\times10^{-3}mm^2/s$] 要明显低于无纤维化或轻度（$F_0$~$F_1$）纤维化时的 ADC 值 [$(1.30\pm0.12)\times10^{-3}mm^2/s$]，特异度、敏感度、阳性预测值、阴性预测值分别为 87%、87%、72%、94%，结果表明，DWI 作为无创性检查肝纤维化的一种手段具有发展前景。

Taouli 等（2008）又进一步对肝纤维化病人行传统 DWI 及 DTI 扫描，通过测量 ADC 值来判定肝纤维化程度分期及肝脏炎症分级，结果表明肝纤维化伴炎症者的 ADC 值较无肝纤维化或肝脏炎症者的 ADC 值明显减低，对于肝纤维化程度≥ 1 级者与≥ 2 级者，其各自的 ROC 曲线下面积（AUC）分别为 0.848 和 0.783，敏感度分别为 88.5% 和 73.7%，特异度分别为 73.3% 和 72.7%，ADC 值分别 $\leq1.40\times10^{-3}mm^2/s$ 和 $\leq1.30\times10^{-3}mm^2/s$；肝脏炎性程度≥ 1 级者的 AUC 为 0.825，敏感度为 75.0%，特异度为 78.6%，ADC 值 $\leq1.30\times10^{-3}mm^2/s$，因此认为肝脏的 ADC 值可以用来对肝纤维化及肝脏炎症程度进行评估。

近年来，国内外对 DWI 应用于肝纤维化的研究不断增多，主要是探讨 DWI 是否能对肝纤维化程度进行分级，是否可根据不同 ADC 值的范围确定肝纤维化的发展程度。但可能由于设备条件、选取扫描序列参数的不同以及不同的临床诊断要求等原因，尚未能确定合适的 ADC 值范围用于肝纤维化的分级，这也是未来研究的一个重要方向。

DWI 应用于肝纤维化检查时的影响因素：DWI 用于肝纤维化的研究也存在许多影响因素。一方面，形成肝纤维化的各种病因不同，例如病毒性肝炎所致肝纤维化、酒精性肝纤维化、毒素和药物所致肝纤维化、遗传代谢性疾病所致肝纤维化以及淤血所致的肝纤维化等。病因不同则组织内的变化也不尽相同，因此 DWI 检查时可能对 ADC 值有一定的影响。

Taouli 等（2003）认为，肝组织内铁的沉积可引起磁场的不均匀，显著缩短了横向弛豫时间，进而干扰水分子的扩散运动，对 ADC 值测量的影响较大。还应考虑到肝内脂肪浸润及肝组织炎症等改变能够增加肝实质内水分子的数量，从而使测量的 ADC 值增加。

另一方面，还需注意肝纤维化 ADC 值测量时感兴趣区（ROI）的选择，有研究认为 ROI 面积 >100 个像素时所得出的结论更为准确，但也有研究者认为 ROI 取值的差异对实验结果的影响并无统计学意义。ROI 的选择具有一定的主观性，可能会导致研究者意见不统一，因此，ROI 的选择还需要经过大量可重复性的数据来验证。

DWI 应用于肝脏疾病的检查时还需要注意心跳及呼吸运动的影响，DWI 对运动高度敏感，虽然目前多采用单次激发自旋回波（EPI）进行 DWI 扫描，其速度之快可以在影像采集过程中冻结许多的生理性运动，但 EPI 极易产生磁敏感性伪影，使影像局部结构扭曲、失真。为使 DWI 广泛地应用于肝脏疾病，许多研究者仍在不断实验探索新的解决办法。

目前的研究趋势表明，虽然 DWI 在肝纤维化等弥漫性肝脏疾病的应用中仍处于研究探讨阶段，但 DWI 较传统的形态学影像检查方法确实能更早地反映肝纤维化的情况。相信随着 MR 技术的不断发展以及 DWI 临床应用经验的不断积累，DWI 有望成为早期、无创性发现肝纤维化可行的方法之一。

第十三章　肝弥漫性病变中的血管疾病

第一节　肝窦阻塞综合征

详见本书 本卷 第十篇 第一章 第三节　肝窦阻塞综合征。

第二节　肝淤血

肝淤血是由于肝实质内静脉血淤滞而致静脉引流代偿。它是充血性心力衰竭、缩窄性心包炎及由于肺癌肺动脉栓塞的常见并发症导致的右心衰竭的表现。慢性肝淤血，继发于心肌病，三尖瓣闭锁不全，布 - 加综合征，可导致心源性肝硬化。这种情况下，肝发生肿大，肿胀，呈现小结节性肝硬化。腹腔积液，脾肿大，门静脉系统静脉曲张与显示在其他类型肝硬化一样。增强 CT 肝实质表现为斑片状网状交织相间，密度不均匀。肝脏肿大。门脉周围低密度 T_2WI 上表现为门脉周围高信号，血管周围明显低密度带可为血管周围淋巴水肿所致。

第三节　日本血吸虫病

日本血吸虫感染可导致严重的肝疾病。血吸虫生活在肠腔中，并在肠系膜内产卵，虫卵钻进静脉血管内，随血流致门静脉内并堵塞门静脉末支，引起血管压力增高并激发肉芽肿反应。炎性反应导致虫卵的纤维化及肝脏的弥漫性纤维化。虫卵死亡后钙化，表现为门脉周围及肝囊周围分隔的特征性钙化，即所谓“龟背”样钙化，钙化及非钙化区均可强化。

MRI 显示的钙化的分隔在 CT 上为线样异常密度，常见于肝右叶的膈下部。分隔表现为 T_1WI 低信号，T_2WI 高信号。因氧化铁超磁性效应，纤维隔于 T_1WI、T_2WI 可显示为高信号。

第十四章 肝弥漫性病变中胆管疾病

第一节 胆管微小错构瘤

胆管微小错构瘤属于先天性胆管板发育畸形，非常少见。病理特征是一个 von Meyenburg 复合体包含数个扩张的胆管,有不同程度的肝纤维化。影像学可以显示遍及全肝的多发的小囊性错构瘤病灶或形成的肿块。MRCP 很具特征,可见伴有胆管扩张。

第二节 继发性肝内胆汁淤滞

胆管结石、慢性胆管炎、胆管结石术后是继发性肝内胆汁淤滞最常见病因。各种影像学检查都可以看到肝内外胆管的原发病变和继发的胆管扩张,病理表现为肝内外胆管狭窄,管壁弥漫性增厚、硬韧、呈条索状,病理诊断为慢性炎症,即继发性硬化性胆管炎。

该病容易诊断,但肝实质纤维化和肝硬化的征象不容忽视。MRI 对该病具有良好的应用和研究前景。

第三节 肝弥漫性病变的胆管造影表现

MRCP 和直接法胆系造影(通常为 ERCP)有时在肝硬化病人排除机械性胆管梗阻起决定性作用。当脂肪浸润在疾病的早期显得突出时,可以看见肝胆管变直、伸长及互相分离。这些征象出现于任何肝内浸润性疾病(如弥漫性淋巴瘤)。在轻度脂肪浸润病人,胆管造影表现一般无异常。肝纤维化加剧导致肝萎缩时,肝胆管变得挤在一块。弯曲靠近的、扭曲的、以及肝胆管直径轻度改变可出现,也可不出现。较大的再生结节圆滑地推挤和弄斜邻近肝胆管。

第四节 先天性肝内胆管囊性扩张症(Caroli 病)

先天性肝内胆管囊性扩张症表现为肝内胆管的先天性异常扩张,胆汁排泄不畅,容易继发胆管炎症与胆系结石,晚期导致胆汁性肝硬化,甚至癌变。

根据有无肝纤维化、门静脉高压分为Ⅰ型(单纯型)和Ⅱ型(伴肝纤维化和门静脉高压)。

超声、CT、MRI 和 ERCP 均可显示囊状扩张的肝内胆管,及其伴发的结石情况和肝硬化情况。CT 增强的中心点征,提示门静脉被扩张的胆管包绕,较有特征。ERCP 与 PTC 最具诊断价值。但为有创性检查,而 MRCP 可以立体直观显示囊肿与胆管的关系,是目前最常用的检查技术。

有关本章介绍胆系疾病的内容,请详见本书 本卷 第十五篇 胆系疾病及第十六篇 胆管疾病。

第十五章 肝脏弥漫性病变与MR扩散加权成像

MR 扩散加权成像（DWI）是目前活体进行水分子扩散测量与成像的唯一方法，是一种无创性反映组织功能状态的检查技术。随着 MRI 硬软件技术的进步，特别是超快速 MRI 技术，如回波平面成像（EPI）序列的广泛应用，DWI 在全身各部位的应用越加广泛，尤其是肝脏的研究近年来倍受关注，体现出良好的应用前景。

DWI 在诊断肝脏局灶性病变中的应用：通过病变 DWI 的信号特征及表观扩散系数（ADC）值的定量测量可以提高肝脏局灶性病变的检出率。扩散成像主要反映的是组织内水分子活动的自由度，能够反映组织内部的生理状态和结构特点；通过 ADC 值的测定可以对病变内水分子的活动度进行量化分析。不同性质病变的 ADC 值各不相同，因此有助于病变性质的确定。常见的肝脏局灶性病变有肝囊肿、海绵状血管瘤、原发性肝癌、肝转移瘤和肝脓肿。

DWI 可以均匀地抑制肝脏背景信号（如血管、胆管），有利于肝脏局灶性病变，尤其是小病灶的显示。Yuan 等（2008）在 40 只新西兰兔 VX-2 肿瘤模型动物实验中，肿瘤种植后不同时间内，DWI 肿块检出率均高于 T_1WI 和 T_2WI，并可鉴别肿瘤坏死、囊变或液化。Zech 等（2008）对 20 例确诊或怀疑肝占位的患者进行腹部扫描，显示 DWI（b=50s/mm^2）图像质量优于脂肪抑制 T_2WI，检出病灶的敏感性高（敏感性分别为 83% 和 61%）。Parikh 等（2008）也得出相似的结论，通过对 53 例肝脏至少有一个病灶的患者（共 211 个病灶）检查比较，认为 DWI 检测肝内小病灶的能力明显优于 T_2WI；临床研究证明取小 b 值（50 s/mm^2）时，肝脏局灶性病变的检出率高于 T_2WI，尤其是小病灶（直径 1~3cm）且 DWI 检出肝脏左叶病变具有优势。

与常规增强 MRI 序列相比，Vandecaveye 等（2009）发现 DWI 在检测直径 <2 cm 的肝癌有优势，但对直径 >2 cm 的肝癌诊断没有特异性。另外，在常规 MRI 基础上增加 DWI 也可以使病灶检出率提高。

Koh 等（2008）的研究发现，DWI、锰福地吡三钠增强 MRI 以及两者结合诊断结肠肝转移瘤的准确性分别为 83%~90%、88%~92% 及 94%、96%。

Nishie 等（2010）采用 1.5 T MRI 对 30 例患者 50 个肝癌结节灶扫描，通过 DWI 和超顺磁性氧化铁动态增强 MRI 结合与超顺磁性氧化铁动态增强 MRI 比较，发现虽然二者结合可以提高病灶的检出敏感性，但对于直径 <1 cm 病灶的检出率并没有明显增加，可能与病灶太小、空间分辨率低及生理运动的干扰有关。

肝脏局灶性病变的定性诊断一直是影像学研究的重点。常规 MRI 凭借病灶的形态、信号特点及强化方式鉴别其良、恶性，虽然动态增强扫描可以反映病灶的强化方式，但是，当同一类型病灶的血供状况不同或发展阶段不同引起血供形式变化等都会导致其强化方式不同，从而使诊断困难。DWI 及 ADC 值能在微观水平反映组织的结构特点，有助于肝脏局灶性病变的定性诊断。

一般认为，肝囊肿与肝血管瘤主要由液体成分构成，水分子运动相对自由，因此其 ADC 值明显高于肝脏恶性肿瘤，并随 b 值增加其信号强度衰减也很明显；肝血管瘤内部主要含血液，并有纤维间隔、瘢痕及出血，且血窦中所含的血液较囊肿的液体黏度高，因而其 ADC 值又低于肝囊肿；局灶性结节增生和腺瘤的 ADC 值介于恶性病变与正常肝实质之间；恶性肿瘤（肝细胞癌和肝转移瘤）由实性肿瘤细胞组成，水分子运动相对受限，在高 b 值的 DWI 图像仍呈高信号，ADC 值降低，肝细胞癌的 ADC 值又低于肝转移瘤；肝脓肿病灶内含有大量炎性细胞、细菌、黏蛋白，同时伴有较多的坏死、变性的细胞成分，黏稠性高的脓液明显限制了水分子的运动，因而其 ADC 值明显低于其他占位性病变，在高 b 值的 DWI 图像上呈高信号，其信号高于其他实性肿瘤；恶性肿瘤的坏死、囊变，也表现为高 ADC 值。

有些学者在应用不同 b 值测得 ADC 值分析也得到相同结论，肝脏良性肿瘤的 ADC 值大于恶性肿瘤，肝脏局灶性病变的 ADC 值从大到小依次为肝囊肿、肝血管瘤、局灶性结节增生、转移瘤、原发性肝癌、肝脓肿。很多研究用 ADC 值作为鉴别肝脏良恶性病变的量化指标，而 ADC 值随着 b 值的增加逐渐下降。ADC 值不仅受水分子扩散影响，还与血流灌注有关。当取小 b 值时，测得的水分子运动主要来自运动较快的血液流动，当增大 b 值到一定程度，水分子的扩散运动对 DWI 的信号影响逐渐加重，这时 DWI 所反映的主要是组织内水分子的扩散情况，因此，采用小 b 值（≤ 200 s/mm²）得到的 ADC 值大于采用大 b 值（≥ 200 s/mm²）。尽管肝脏良性病变的 ADC 值高于恶性病变，但二者之间有一些重叠。

诊断肝脏恶性病变的阈值为（1.4~1.6）× 10^{-3}mm²/s 的敏感性、特异性分别为 74%~100%、77%~100%。DWI 不能单独用于肝脏局灶性病变的鉴别诊断，良性病变也会出现扩散受限，表现为低 ADC 值，而恶性肿瘤的囊变、坏死也可表现为高 ADC 值。

Xu 等（2009）对 37 例患者行腹部 MRI 检查，结果发现虽然 DWI 与动态增强 MRI 结合提高了小肝癌的检出率，但在肝硬化背景下，ADC 值不能用来鉴别病变的良恶性，因为肝硬化和肝实性良性肿瘤都表现为低 ADC 值，肿瘤的坏死及血管再生也改变了水分子的扩散特征，故常会出现假阳性。

肝脏病变与正常肝实质的 ADC 值有一定重叠，肝转移瘤的 ADC 值范围是（0.94~2.85）× 10^{-3}mm²/s，而正常肝实质的 ADC 值范围是（0.69~2.28）× 10^{-3}mm²/s。

此外，通过 ADC 定量参数还可以反映肿瘤组织的分化程度，但目前此方面的研究还比较少。Heo 等（2010）通过对 27 例原发性肝细胞癌的 DWI 表现与组织学分化程度及血管内皮生长因子表达的比较发现，低分化的原发性肝细胞癌的平均 ADC 值为（0.9 ± 0.13）× 10^{-3}mm²/s，高分化肝癌平均 ADC 值为（1.2 ± 0.22）× 10^{-3}mm²/s，中度分化肝癌为（1.1 ± 0.01）× 10^{-3}mm²/s；原发性肝细胞癌的 ADC 值与组织学分化程度有明显相关性，但是与血管内皮生长因子的表达没有相关性。

DWI 在肝硬化、纤维化诊断中的应用：肝硬化、肝纤维化是临床上常见的肝脏弥漫性疾病，确诊主要依赖穿刺活检，但其为有创性检查，另外肝纤维化的分布不均匀也会造成假阴性结果。常规 MRI 很难诊断肝纤维化，采用影像学手段对肝纤维化肝储备功能评价的研究较少。ADC 值可以客观量化反映组织的病理变化。很多研究发现肝纤维化、肝硬化时肝脏的 ADC 值比正常肝脏低，其机制目前还不完全清楚，可能原因为肝组织内不同程度的胶原纤维增生，细胞间隙和细胞内外水分子的扩散受限，在 DWI 上表现为高信号，ADC 值低于正常肝脏。

也有研究认为肝硬化组织的 ADC 值降低可能是增生的纤维破坏了微循环，造成肝实质血流灌注的下降所致。Mwangi 等（2010）利用 ADC 值在活体及离体鉴别肝硬化基础上的纤维化和再生结节，并提出肝硬化的低 ADC 值是肝再生结节形成引起的，而不是肝组织纤维化的结果。肝纤维化常伴有炎症反应、脂肪变性及铁沉积等病理改变，因此在证明肝纤维化的扩散机制时，还要将这部分的 ADC 值变化计算进去。Koinuma 等（2005）实验结果发现，ADC 值与肝纤维化分期有相关性，而与肝炎活动没有相关性。

研究发现以肝功能实验室检查指标及临床表现为基础的 Child-Pugh 分级与所测 ADC 值有明显的相关性。肝纤维化时，胶原纤维沉积，含水量减少，测得的 ADC 值较正常肝脏实质低，通过检测肝脏组织的 ADC 值，能够探测出肝脏组织内胶原纤维的沉积情况和细胞外间隙内水分子含量的变化，并可根据 ADC 值的高低进行肝纤维化分级和分期的评估。

Lewin 等（2007）对 20 名正常人和 54 例丙型肝炎（HCV）患者肝脏分析发现，中重度纤维化的患者肝脏 ADC 值低于轻度纤维化患者，以 ADC 值 ≤ 1.2 × 10^{-3}mm²/s 作为诊断严重纤维化阈值的敏感性、特异性分别为 87%、87%，并发现 ADC 值与肝炎活动有明显的相关性，推测可能与肝脏脂肪变性有关。

Girometti 等（2008）分别对 29 例肝硬化患者及 29 名正常人行 DWI，测量不同 b 值下（b=0 s/mm²、150s/mm²、250 s/mm²、400 s/mm²）的 ADC 值并做比较研究，发现肝硬化的 ADC 值 [（1.11 ± 0.16）× 10^{-3}mm²/s] 低于正常肝组织 [（1.54 ± 0.12）× 10^{-3}mm²/s]，阈值为 1.31 × 10^{-3}mm²/s 的敏感性、特异性、阳性预测值、阴性预测值、准确性分别为 92%、100%、100%、99%、96%。DWI 在肝脏的应用主要是如何有效地避免伪影，提高病灶肝脏的对比噪声比，增加检出率以及如何优化 b 值对局灶性肝脏病变进行定性。

DWI 对运动高度敏感，心跳、呼吸、胃肠蠕动均可影响图像质量。EPI 序列的固有特点是图像容易产生各种伪影，如磁敏感伪影，表现为膈面与肺组织交界及肝脏与邻近肠道气体交界区解剖结构的扭曲变形，会掩盖病灶，尤其当病灶位于肝左叶时；化学位移伪影，表现为腹壁脂肪重叠于肝脏，会遮盖病变，图像信噪比低，空间分辨率低，病灶检出率较低。选择合适的 b 值对提高 DWI 图像质量和 ADC 值测量的准确性至关重要。

在生物组织内，DWI 图像上的信号强度变化取决于两个主要因素，即水分子的扩散效应和毛细血管微循环的灌注作用。低 b 值（$<200\ s/mm^2$）时，血流灌注的影响较大，不利于病变的诊断准确性，高 b 值时，图像的信噪比下降，采用 $<100\sim150\ s/mm^2$ 的 b 值有助于肝内病灶的检出，而采用 b 值，$500\ s/mm^2$ 可帮助病灶性质的诊断。

一些作者分别对 41 例肝脏良性病变和 62 例恶性病变采用低（$100\ s/mm^2$、$200\ s/mm^2$、$300\ s/mm^2$）、中（$400\ s/mm^2$、$600\ s/mm^2$）和高（$800\ s/mm^2$、$1\ 000\ s/mm^2$、$1\ 200\ s/mm^2$）3 种不同 b 值组行 MR DWI 扫描，结果发现，肝脏良、恶性病变的 ADC 值随着 b 值的增加逐渐下降，而指数化表观扩散系数（eADC）值相反，低 b 值组病变的 ADC 值受血流灌注的影响很大，随着 b 值的增加，血流的影响逐渐减弱。随着高场强 MR 的广泛应用，如何有效降低高场强 DWI 的伪影，提高病灶检出仍是目前的一个挑战。一项研究发现，3.0 T DWI 以低的特异吸收率可取代常规 T_2WI 序列，但有待于积累更多的资料。

总之，DWI 在肝脏病变的检出和定性以及疗效评估中具有一定作用，其价值还有待于临床进一步评价，但将 DWI 与其他 MR 技术，如动态增强 MRI 等结合起来，可为肝脏局灶性病灶、肝纤维化、肝硬化的诊断和鉴别诊断及治疗疗效的评价提供有用的信息，具有很好的应用前景。

第十六章 肝弥漫性病变与灌注成像

CT 灌注成像在弥漫性肝病方面的应用

在弥漫性肝病的 CT 灌注成像研究方面,目前已有较多的报道,主要集中在肝硬化相关问题上。由于临床发现,肝血流动力学的改变与肝硬化门脉高压的治疗方式的选择和预后有关。现行的肝功能检测法判断肝硬化病人对手术的耐受性。手术方案的选择及预后往往不甚准确,致使某些肝功能 Child A 级的患者术后出现肝性脑病。肝功能进行性恶化,而某些 Child C 级的患者又失去了手术治疗的机会。研究认为,当门静脉入肝血流量维持在全肝血流量的 40% 以上,肝脏对高摄取物如氨。胆汁酸。利多卡因等的摄取率接近正常时,分流手术,尤其是分流量较大的术式,必将导致肝性脑病和肝功能的持续恶化,此时以断流术或分流量小的术式为佳。同样,门静脉入肝血流量趋于零,全肝血流量几乎完全由肝动脉所提供,又无肝性脑病表现时,门体分流术式对肝功能的影响不大。因此,血流动力学检测对可手术患者在术式的选择及预后的判断方面,远较现行的肝功能检查法准确可信。了解其血流动力学改变情况,对分析病情。指导制订治疗方案,评价疗效及估计预后等有重要的临床意义。

Myers 和 Taylar(1951)首次提出嵌塞肝静脉测定法测定肝静脉楔压(WHVP)。数十年来,此项技术一直是门脉高压症经典检查方法,但这一技术为创伤性的,一般病人很难接受,更难重复测定,阻碍了其在临床的广泛运用。Tsushima 等使用 CT 灌注成像研究肝硬化时发现:肝脏门静脉灌注量与凝血酶原(可作为肝实质损害的一个指标)之间存在正相关(r=0.662),而脾脏灌注量与肝静脉楔压负相关(r=-0.741)。他们认为门静脉灌注量降低可作为肝实质损伤的标志。利用动态 CT 对肝脏灌注进行定量将来有可能用于评价肝硬化治疗的效果和判断病人的预后。近年来,通过大鼠肝硬化病理模型的动物实验,对比大鼠肝硬化病理——血流动力学指标——CT 灌注成像的灌注参数,研究发现,随着病理上肝硬化程度的加重,肝脏灌注量呈动态变化过程。在早期表现为肝动脉灌注量、门脉灌注量下降,全肝血流量已有较大幅度的降低;中期,门脉灌注量继续下降,但肝动脉灌注量开始上升,全肝血流量进一步下降;晚期,肝动脉灌注量加大上升的幅度,但并不足以代偿门脉灌注量的降低,全肝血流量继续下降;平均通过时间和表观分布容积呈持续性延长和增加。这一特征提示:CT 灌注成像对于肝硬化早期诊断和判断肝硬化程度有较高的临床价值。

另外,门静脉自由压与门脉灌注量呈显著性负相关性,根据门静脉灌注量,运用直线回归方程能较准确地推算出肝硬化大鼠的门静脉压力,这提示 CT 灌注成像今后可以作为一种无创。迅速的间接测量门脉压力的有效手段。在测定肝脏灌注参数方面,另一个具有较大研究空间的领域就是肝移植后肝脏血流动力学的评价。既往的研究都表明肝移植后血流动力学存在一个动态变化和渐进性转归的过程,但对于血流灌注量方面仍缺乏直接的依据。研究这种动态变化过程有利于早期诊断肝移植后一些与血流动力学相关的并发症。其中由于动脉和胆系并发症的早期诊断与预后关系密切,功能影像是解决早期诊断的希望所在。最早探讨肝移植后 CT 灌注成像的是 Bader 等人,他们对肝移植术后 7~14 天的病人进行灌注成像的研究,虽然其研究结果目前尚存在一定的争议,但 CT 灌注成像在该方面的应用价值并没被人否认。通过严格筛选术前肝硬化病例,深入探讨肝移植早期血流动力学变化规律,发现终末期肝病肝移植后早期存在肝动脉和门静脉灌注量均增加的现象。并根据这一变化对肝移植后早期血管并发症病例进行诊断,显示出 CT 灌注成像相对其他影像手段在诊断灵敏度。阳性预测价值上的优势,提示其可用于肝移植后并发症的早期诊断。

第十七章　肝硬化相关结节

第一节　早期肝癌(不典型增生伴恶性灶)

早期肝癌平均直径小于15mm,因此发现困难。有报道总体敏感性是:超声检查为64%, CT为58%, CT血管成像为50%, CT动脉性门脉造影为71%,X线血管造影为31%,术中超声为88%。早期肝癌的精确诊断并非总是容易。超声检查常表现无包膜或镶嵌征的一个低回声占位,很像不典型增生。但是,彩色多普勒血流成像已在直径小于25mm的肝癌显示有搏动的肿瘤供血血管或恒定流动的肿瘤引流血管,或两者都有。这些表现不见于不典型增生。

早期肝癌通常是少血管的,与不典型增生不同,几乎所有Edmondson 2级或以上的肝癌在动脉性门脉造影CT扫描上都有明确的结节内门脉供血减少。在中间性病变(如早期肝癌和高分化肝癌),结节内门脉供血可随恶性等级的增加而逐渐减少,但结节内的肝动脉供血增加。与早期肝癌不同,不典型增生因有门脉血流而在动脉性门脉造影CT扫描上不显示。CT血管成像与动脉性门脉造影CT的结合,在确定与肝硬化有关的结节性病变的性质上较单独应用其中一项更为准确。在MRI,早期肝癌在T_1WI主要呈高或等强度表现,在T_2WI表现为等强度信号。有时,早期肝癌有一个独特的MR表现:T_2WI一个低强度信号为主的结节伴有一个中等或高强度信号的小病灶。

成像技术在治疗计划中的作用:超声和CT在肝癌筛查中的作用是互补的,但是,超声因其高敏感性和实时性已成为亚洲人群中的一种主要筛查技术。而且实时超声的简单和灵便性使其成为肝癌导向诊断性抽吸和治疗的一种主要工具。

CT也是一种用于评价肝癌的准确而相对无创伤性的技术。当超声不能回答临床的问题时,CT是一个补充性筛查技术。CT不仅能更准确地确定肝癌的范围,还可以确定疾病的肝外扩散。当影像学筛查表明为多发性结节,血管侵犯或肝外转移不能手术时,使用超声引导经皮活检通过组织学表现可获得最后诊断。若结节是可以手术的, MRI用于进一步显示其特征。若结节小且在MRI呈良性(如再生性结节或不典型增生),隔期复查是目前随访的唯一实用方法。若影像表现提示结节恶性,有必要用动脉性门脉造影CT,碘油CT或超声血管造影给结节分期。若结节有可能切除,术中超声对证实和确定最佳术式是必要的。

第二节　肝硬化结节

详见本书 本卷 第六篇 第三章　肝硬化结节。

第三节　弥漫性结节性肝硬化,伴局灶结节性增生

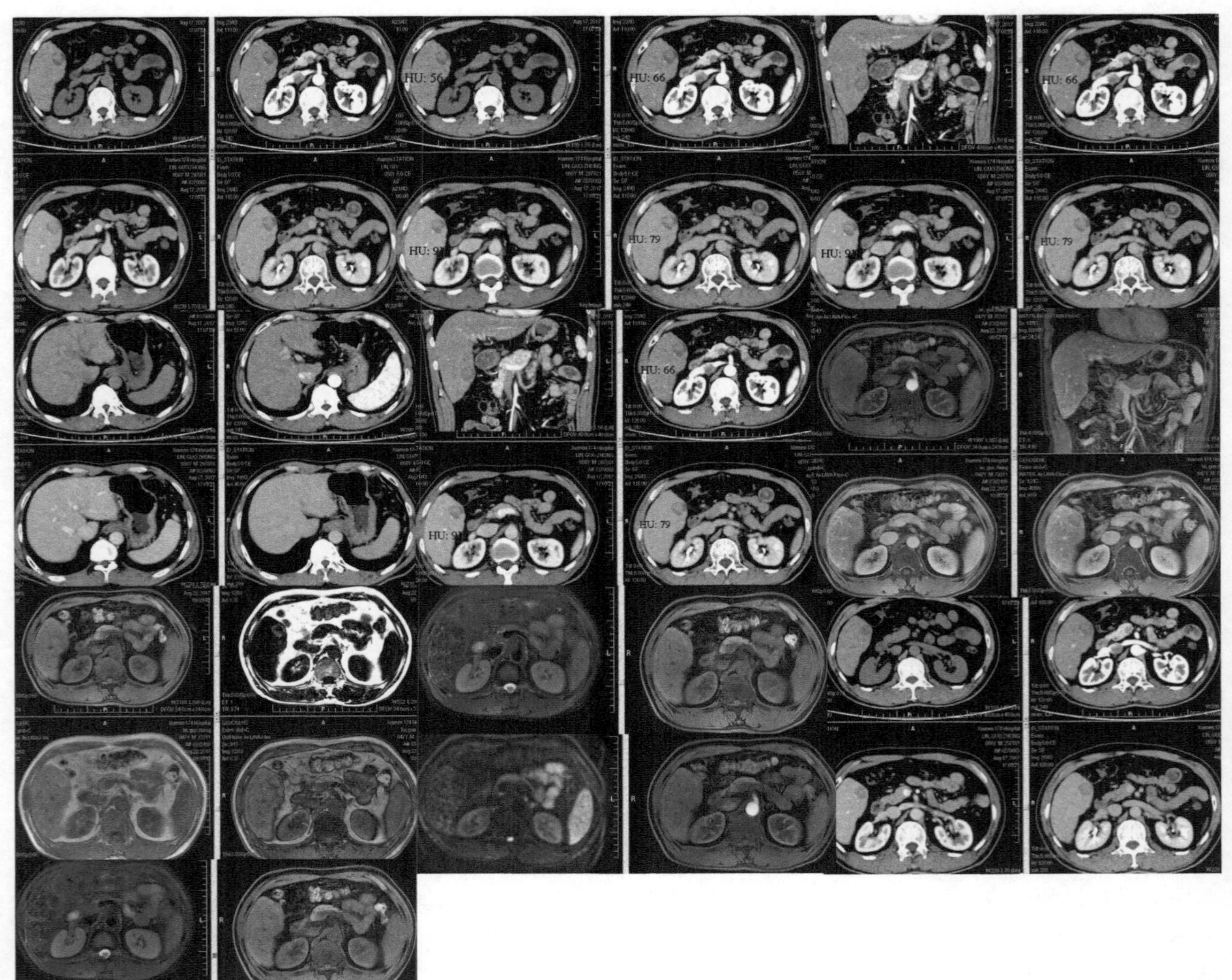

图 9-17-1　弥漫性结节性肝硬化,伴局灶结节性增生

患者,男, 57 岁。手术所见:探查见左肝萎缩,肝表面可及大小不一结节状改变,肝叶Ⅴ段近包膜处可及一大小约 4cm×3cm 肿物,质软,边界尚清,活动度可。

病理检查:肝组织一块,大小 6.5cm×4.7cm× 2.3cm,被膜光滑,呈结节状隆起,切面灰黄,呈多结节状,质中,其中最大结节直径 2.3 ㎝,紧邻断端切缘。另见脂肪组织一堆,总体积 8cm×4cm× 0.7cm。未检出淋巴结。常规病理诊断:右肝肿瘤切除标本:初步诊断结节性肝硬化,伴中度脂肪变性,待做免疫组化检测进一步排除肿瘤性病变,送检脂肪组织中未检出淋巴结。

免疫组化诊断:右肝肿瘤切除标本:弥漫性结节性肝硬化,伴局灶结节性增生(FNH),并肝细胞中 - 重度脂肪变性(图 9-17-1)。

第四节　肝硬化与癌前病变

表 9-17-1　肝硬化中肝细胞结节新旧名词对照

新名词	旧名词
1. 再生结节(regenerative nodule, RN)	再生结节(regenerative nodule)
2. 发育不良性结节(dysplastic nodules, DNs)	巨再生结节，Ⅰ型 普通腺瘤样增生(AH，低级 adenomatous hyperplasia)
3. 发育不良性结节(DNs)，高级	巨再生结节，Ⅱ型 腺瘤样增生，非典型(adenomatoid hyperplasia with atypia, AAH)
4. 发育不良性结节伴癌亚灶(dysplastic nodules with subfocus of HCC)	早癌(early HCC)，腺瘤样增生伴镜检肝细胞性肝癌
5. 小癌(small HCC)<2cm	腺瘤样增生伴可视癌灶(adenomatoid hyperplasia with macroscopic HCC)

再生结节(RN)：肝硬化的再生结节是由再生的肝细胞为纤维间隔包绕所形成，结节的直径多在3mm以下，但可融合成为较大的结节，进一步发展为发育不良结节(DN)。

CT 表现：在 CT 平扫不易发现，偶尔显示为稍高密度病灶。少数大的再生结节平扫呈等密度；增强 CT 的动脉期、门静脉期和平衡期均显示为低密度病灶。此外，在肝硬化的肝脏中，还可见到坏死结节，不易与小肝癌鉴别。

肝脏发育不良性结节(DN)：肝脏发育不良性结节属于癌前病变，在肝硬化中15%~25%，肝脏发育不良性结节的直径常为1mm~10mm，但也有达20mm者。

CT 表现：在 CT 上检出率不高，平扫上可呈高或低密度，在增强扫描上呈等或高密度。96%的肝脏发育不良性结节主要由门静脉供血，而94%的肝细胞性肝癌由主要肝动脉供血，当肝硬化患者的肝脏有多结节时，其中较大的结节可考虑为肝脏发育不良性结节。

MR 表现：典型肝脏发育不良性结节在 T_1 为略高信号，T_2 低信号。增强扫描动脉期无强化或轻度强化，门静脉期轻度强化，延迟期呈等信号；肿块都呈均质性，边缘清楚，无包膜。

布 - 加综合征与大再生结节：近年来由于 CT、MRI 等先进技术的发展，能发现布 - 加综合征的多发性结节表现，由于肝静脉的血流量的减少或闭塞，引致多灶性肝动脉扩张，久之则形成结节状肝细胞增生，被称为“大再生结节”，这种结节需与癌前病变的“发育不良结节”相鉴别。大再生结节多见于慢性布 - 加综合征，数目较多，常在10个以上，大小在数 mm 至 4cm。CT 平扫呈高密度，增强扫描密度更高或呈外低中高的结节。极少数大再生结节向肝外生长，易误诊为肝外肿瘤(表 9-17-1)。

第十八章 肝硬化与脑

肝硬化患者大脑基底节 MRI 观察

肝硬化患者 T_1WI 可见大脑基底节区尤其苍白球呈对称性高信号，但是 T_2WI 无异常改变。有作者对上述部位及大脑白质进行 T_1 值测量，并应用 ROC 曲线对比分析患者与正常对照组的测量值。ROC 曲线下面积表示阳性和阴性诊断结果分布的重叠程度，曲线下面积越接近于 1.0，说明其诊断效果越好；若曲线下面积为 0.5，则表示该方法不能将患者组和正常对照组区分开来，无诊断价值。

该项研究 ROC 曲线图显示肝硬化患者苍白球、壳核、尾状核头、丘脑与皮层下白质的 T_1 值曲线下面积均接近于 1，说明苍白球、壳核、尾状核头、丘脑与皮层下白质的 T_1 值对肝硬化累及脑的诊断有一定价值。

该研究结果表明肝硬化患者基底节区 T_1 值明显缩短，T_2 值无显著变化，而且 T_1 值缩短与肝硬化严重程度和血氨水平明显相关。这与一些作者的研究结果相符合。此外，Genovese 等(2000)认为有 MRI 信号异常者的病程较无信号异常者短，而且 T_1WI 信号增高程度与肝硬化的严重程度有相关关系($P = 0.008$)。所以，他认为基底节区 MRI 信号异常可能是与肝硬化病情程度有关的某种代谢异常有关。该研究加大样本量，使研究结果更为可信。

肝硬化引起肝性脑病至少有肝细胞功能受损和门 - 体静脉分流 2 个原因，有学者认为肝硬化患者大脑基底节区 T_1WI 信号强度增加与肝硬化程度和门体静脉分流有关。由于肝细胞功能受损或门 - 体静脉分流，导致氨不能转化为尿素而排出体外，可能是肝硬化患者血氨异常升高的原因。该研究结果证明患者基底节区 T_1 值缩短与血氨升高呈显著相关。

Kulisevsky 等(1992)认为患者的血氨水平与脑组织受累呈显著正相关，因此进行基底节区弛豫时间测量可能是诊断与高血氨症相关脑损害的有效方法之一。

肝硬化患者大脑基底节区出现信号异常的机制尚不完全清楚，通常认为是顺磁性物质(尤其是锰)的异常沉积所至。Maeda 等(1997)对 4 例肝硬化患者行 MRI 扫描，结果其中 3 例在 T_1WI 上苍白球呈高信号，他们对这些患者进行脑金属浓度测定和组织病理学检查，3 例患者的苍白球、壳核和皮层下白质的锰浓度分别为正常人的 4~10 倍，其中 2 例患者的铜浓度亦高于正常值 50% 左右，而其他金属元素(如：钙、铁和锌)含量正常。第 4 例 MRI 信号正常者的各种金属浓度均在正常范围。病理检查发现，有 T_1WI 基底节高信号者，均出现神经胶质细胞和小胶质细胞坏疽和脱落，与慢性锰中毒所见相符，提示局部锰浓度增加可能与 MRI 信号异常和神经细胞坏死有关，而铜对 T_1WI 信号强度无明显影响。Lucchini 等(2000)也发现肝性脑病患者脑 MRI 表现与有锰过量接触史的工人相同。

应该指出，虽然 MRI 对肝硬化累及大脑的诊断敏感度很高，但是特异度却不佳，确诊肝性脑病或亚临床肝性脑病还需结合其他检查(如：智力测验或脑诱发电位检查)的结果进行综合分析。总之，T_1WI 上苍白球、壳核、尾状核头等部位出现高信号是肝硬化累及大脑较为特征性的 MRI 征象。应用 MRI 进行头颅扫描并测量这些部位的 T_1 值，有助于肝性脑病的早期发现、预防和治疗。

第十九章　肝硬化与骨

肝性骨营养不良

慢性肝脏疾病患者中出现骨矿物质密度整体改变的一种代谢性骨骼疾病，称为肝性骨营养不良，或称肝性骨病，表现为骨软化症和骨质疏松症，是慢性肝脏疾病患者常见而又经常被忽视的并发症。肝性骨营养不良可严重影响患者的生活质量和长期预后。

病因及发病机制：肝性骨营养不良的病因是多因素的，根据基础肝脏疾病的不同，其病因和严重程度也不同。肝性骨营养不良在慢性肝脏疾病患者中的发病率约为 20%~50%，可发生于慢性胆汁淤积性肝病、慢性病毒性肝炎和肝硬化、酒精性肝病、血色素沉积症、肝脏良恶性肿瘤及肝移植等患者中。其中慢性胆汁淤积性肝病、慢性病毒性肝炎和病毒性肝硬化的平均患病率约为 13%~60%、20% 和 55%，酒精性肝病与骨质疏松的关系尚不十分明确。

慢性肝脏疾病患者骨质疏松症的发病机制尚未完全清楚。正常的骨代谢是骨组织不断进行改建活动的一个复杂过程，主要包括破骨细胞介导的骨吸收和成骨细胞介导的骨形成。在骨代谢过程中，每天都有一定量的骨组织被重吸收，又有相当数量的骨组织合成，两者保持动态的平衡。当骨吸收增加或骨形成减少，则可引起骨质的丢失和骨质疏松症。所有可导致破骨细胞活性增加或成骨细胞功能受损的因素均可引起骨质疏松。

肝性骨营养不良的发生大多数被认为是由于成骨细胞功能受损，导致骨形成率降低。以下原因可能增加肝性骨营养不良的发生。

性别和激素：睾酮与成骨细胞表面的睾酮受体结合，参与成骨细胞增生、生长因子及骨基质蛋白形成等一系列代谢过程，对正常骨生长、代谢、骨量维持起到重要的调节作用。

男性慢性肝脏疾病患者由于雌激素的灭活能力下降及雄激素转化为雌激素能力增加，使血中雌激素水平相对升高，后者通过反馈作用抑制下丘脑 - 垂体 - 性腺轴导致促性腺激素和促肾上腺皮质激素分泌减少，最终导致性腺功能低下，睾酮水平下降；女性慢性肝脏疾病患者除促卵泡成熟素和促黄体生成素水平显着降低外，睾酮水平比男性降低更明显。睾酮水平低下使成骨细胞功能受损，引起骨质流失。慢性肝脏疾病患者自身雌激素高于雄激素，但明显低于正常水平。雌激素对骨代谢的作用主要表现为抑制破骨细胞活性，减少骨吸收。低水平的雌激素使破骨细胞活性增加，引起骨转化降低，骨形成减少，特别是女性慢性肝脏疾病患者绝经后会加速骨质流失。

遗传因素：已经有研究证明某些基因的遗传多态性可促使慢性胆汁淤积性肝病患者发展为骨质疏松症，包括 I 型胶原蛋白 α1 基因，维生素 D 受体和雌激素受体基因，低密度脂蛋白受体结合蛋白 5 基因，胰岛素样生长因子基因等，但基因多态性尚未证明与具体骨折风险的增加相关。

细胞因子：慢性肝脏疾病患者血清中细胞因子水平增加也会引起肝性骨营养不良。酒精性肝炎和肝硬化组与其年龄匹配的对照组相比，血清白细胞介素 -1、白细胞介素 -6 和肿瘤坏死因子 -α 的水平较高，后者是强大的骨吸收刺激因子，并可直接抑制成骨细胞功能且增加其他细胞因子的形成，并可刺激培养的成骨细胞合成 RNA 和前列腺素 E2，抑制胶原和骨钙素的合成以及 1，25(OH)维生素 D3 刺激的碱性磷酸酶活性。但也有报道认为细胞因子不是引起肝性骨营养不良的直接原因。

维生素 K 缺乏：除肠道细菌合成的维生素 K 外，脂溶性维生素 K 的吸收需要胆汁协助。由于慢性肝脏疾病患者肝细胞功能受损，胆汁合成减少，肠道菌群失调，导致维生素 K 合成和吸收减少。除参与凝血外，维生素 K 的重要功能之一是成骨细胞合成骨钙素——骨软骨蛋白的一个重要辅助因子。骨钙素是骨组织中 3 种维生素 K 依赖蛋白之一，具有调节破骨细胞活性，偶联骨吸收和骨形成的作用。维生素 K 还可通过调节钙代谢影响骨代谢，可抑制成骨细胞凋亡和破骨细胞活性。因此当维生素 K 缺乏时,骨钙素活性下降,破骨细胞活性增加,骨形成减少。

钙和维生素 D 代谢异常:维生素 D3 可促进小肠黏膜和肾小管上皮细胞对钙、磷的重吸收,并能通过增加破骨细胞的数量使钙、磷释放入血,使血钙升高。慢性肝脏疾病患者体内 25-OH-D3 水平降低,使血钙降低,继发性甲状旁腺功能亢进,增加骨转换并加快骨量丢失。引起慢性肝脏疾病患者维生素 D 缺乏的主要因素是有限的紫外线照射和营养不良或肠道吸收不良。然而,在慢性胆汁淤积性肝病患者中骨质疏松和维生素 D 水平减少之间并没有显著的联系。

高胆红素血症:动物实验证明非结合型胆红素的增加会损害成骨细胞的功能,这种作用是剂量依赖性且是可逆的。临床研究结果显示,血清胆红素水平与骨破坏之间呈正相关,即原发性胆汁性肝硬化和原发性硬化性胆管炎患者中骨质疏松与黄疸以同样的速度进展。但也有认为高胆红素血症不是慢性肝病患者骨密度改变的主要因素,两者关系还有待研究。

核因子 κB:核因子 κB 受体活化因子配体和护骨素(RANKL/OPG)系统通过调节破骨细胞活性调节骨代谢。破骨细胞的活性受患者护骨素 / 核因子 κB 受体活化因子配体比值的调控,即核因子 κB 受体活化因子配体对破骨细胞具有激活作用,而护骨素起抑制作用。慢性肝脏疾病患者的护骨素 / 核因子 κB 受体活化因子配体比值较高,表明在激活破骨细胞活性时有配体的消耗,并为防止骨量丢失代偿性的产生过量的护骨素。

胰岛素样生长因子 1 缺乏:胰岛素样生长因子 1 是调节成骨细胞增殖和功能的旁分泌及自主分泌细胞因子。胰岛素样生长因子 1 可刺激 I 型胶原合成,提高基质沉积速率,抑制胶原降解,对于形成新骨和维持骨基质具有重要作用。肝硬化患者肝脏合成胰岛素样生长因子 1 显著减少,导致成骨细胞数目和功能受损,引起骨质流失。

药物:糖皮质激素(治疗 >3 个月或长疗程),利尿剂,消胆胺,免疫抑制剂等均可导致肝性骨营养不良。类固醇激素直接作用于骨细胞,通过增加破骨细胞活性,提高白细胞介素 -1 和白细胞介素 -6 水平,减少成骨细胞分化、生成及寿命。

乙醇:饮酒是肝性骨营养不良的一个独立危险因素。它既是导致患者骨矿物质密度降低的独立危险因素,又与患者的年龄、低体质量指数和消极的生活方式有关。酒精直接抑制成骨细胞的活性,增加骨质流失,即使不酗酒的长期持续饮酒的酒精性肝病患者也有较低的骨矿物质密度,尤其是年轻的患者,骨矿物质密度甚至低于比其年长 10 岁的正常人。

诊断　慢性肝脏疾病的患者出现骨痛、背痛、身高变矮、脆性骨折、脊柱后凸 / 脊柱侧弯时应警惕肝性骨营养不良的发生,应及时检测血常规和基本的生物化学指标,包括肝功能、钙磷代谢、性腺激素和甲状腺功能等,有条件时应进行骨代谢标志物和骨矿物质密度检测。

双能 X 线骨密度仪是测量和评估骨矿物质密度的最好方法。T 积分表示受检者骨矿物质密度与同性别骨峰值的差别, Z 积分表示受检者骨矿物质密度在同性别同年龄组平均值的差别,当 T 积分和 / 或 Z 积分低于正常参考值 -1 个标准差时称为骨质疏松,低于正常参考值 -2.5 个标准差以上时称为骨质疏松症(WHO 标准)。

第二十章　肝铁过载

第一节　肝铁质沉积病

血色素沉积症是一种肠道铁质吸收先天性缺陷症，它造成肝、脾、胰和心脏的铁质沉积。未治疗的血色素沉积症导致进行性肝硬化、门脉高压、胰功能不全、心肌病，偶尔可并发肝细胞癌。输血性含铁血黄素沉积症伴发于先天性溶血性贫血、获得性无成形的贫血和其他的骨髓紊乱。过度的铁质沉积能导致肝硬化。

血色素沉积症和含铁血黄素沉积症造成肝衰减值上升。在CT平扫，肝的衰减值通常为55~60HU。在铁质沉积病，肝的衰减值可高达70~100HU之间。肝的铁质含量以使用双能CT技术进行测定，在动物模型的实验研究中，用双能CT测定铁质含量与活检标本直接测量之间有着正相关。在血色素沉积症和输血性含铁血黄素沉积症病人，可用双能CT测定肝的铁质含量。肝衰减值增加的另外原因有继发于amiodarone治疗和糖原贮积症。后者是一种先天性代谢紊乱，它常伴存相当高发病率的肝腺瘤。此种情况少见，目前只见于儿科人群中。继发于糖原贮积症的肝衰减值增加可能被同时存在肝脂肪浸润所修改，从而导致衰减值为正常或稍低于正常。

人体内贮存铁，主要以铁蛋白及含铁血黄素形式存在，肝脏是铁贮存的主要器官，因此，当铁含量过多时，肝最易受到影响。从病因学看，铁质过度沉积可分为两类：肝细胞内铁质过度沉积；网状内皮细胞内铁质过度沉积。由于受累细胞不同，在治疗和预后方面亦不相同。

肝细胞内铁质过度沉积的主要病变为原发性（或称特发性、遗传性）血色素沉积症，系常染色体隐性遗传性疾病，因肠道铁吸收增多，导致肝、胰、心脏等细胞内铁质过度沉积，能够引起肝细胞受损、肝功能异常、肝硬化，乃至肝细胞性肝癌，也可引起糖尿病或心肌受损，若治疗不当则预后较差；其他原发性病变，如病毒性肝硬化、酒精性肝硬化及血管内溶血等病变，虽然也能造成肝细胞内铁含量增高，但程度较轻。

网状内皮细胞铁质过度沉积，主要原因是血液病或肾功能衰竭等治疗过程中反复大量输血，导致铁在肝、脾及骨髓的网状内皮细胞内过度沉积（在肝脏内则沉积在枯否细胞内），也称为继发性铁质过度沉积。此类铁质沉积一般不会造成器官功能损害，故临床意义不大。

铁并不直接产生MR低信号，但它的顺磁性作用能明显地缩短其周围氢质子的T_2弛豫时间，从而产生T_2WI低信号。Stark等（1985）推测低分子量铁缩短T_2弛豫时间的作用，可能较铁蛋白或含铁血黄素更大。由于T_2弛豫时间较T_1弛豫时间缩短更显著，可采用对铁沉积更为敏感的T_2WI来进行观察。MR不受脂肪肝的影响，较CT更适合对肝脏铁质沉积进行评价。骨骼肌由于在T_1WI和T_2WI均较正常肝脏等器官信号低，并且受铁沉积的影响很小，因此，可作为参照物。将肝脏等器官的信号强度与其比较，可作为判断铁沉积是否存在的简便方法。无论原发性或继发性肝脏铁质过度沉积，在T_2WI均表现为弥漫均匀的低信号。因此，仅根据肝脏MR信号改变，虽然能提示铁质过度沉积，却无法区分类别，而结合胰腺和脾脏的信号改变及临床资料，则有助于鉴别原发性和继发性铁质过度沉积。

原发性肝脏铁质过度沉积可合并原发性肝细胞癌，其发病率较高。因此，对于疑为原发性肝脏铁质过度沉积症者，应给予积极治疗并密切随访，而对诊断为继发性肝脏铁质过度沉积症者，则不需特殊处理。肝脏铁质过度沉积的MR定量测定已有一些报道。应用肝脏/肌肉信号强度比,肝脏 T_2 值等与血清铁或肝组织铁含量进行相关性研究表明, MR 在定量研究方面有一定意义,是目前较为理想的无创性检查方法,可用于追踪观察和评估预后。

第二节 MR 磁敏感加权成像检出肝硬化铁沉积结节

约 45% 的肝硬化结节中会有选择性铁沉积,称为铁沉积结节。MRI 是无创性检测肝脏铁沉积的最佳影像学方法,以梯度回波序列(GRE)序列最为敏感。磁敏感加权成像(SWI)是一种新兴的 MRI 序列,对磁敏感物质(如铁、出血、脱氧血红蛋白等)的显示极具优势,目前已用于帕金森病、阿尔茨海默病等患者的脑内铁沉积评价。

SWI 腹部应用挑战及技术优化:常规 SWI 采用高分辨、长回波时间、3D GRE 序列进行扫描,采集时间达数分钟,在腹部的应用仍有许多技术难题尚需解决。最大的挑战是呼吸运动和胃肠道蠕动伪影的影响;另外,在磁化率差异特别大的区域(如空气-肠袢界面)存在有明显的磁敏感伪影,尚需通过相位优化技术予以去除。

一个研究小组在 Siemens 公司科研人员协助下将 SWI 技术优化用于肝脏成像,应用 2D 序列联合并行采集技术将采集时间缩短至 49s,通过多次屏气采集减轻呼吸运动伪影;将多个采集通道中的数据单独处理再加权融合以减轻了多通道所致局部磁场不均匀伪影;应用高通滤过去除磁敏感伪影,所得 SWI 图像可以满足诊断需求。

SWI 检出肝脏铁沉积的优势:正常肝脏铁含量较低,常规影像技术难以显示,该项研究中 40 例健康志愿者在 SWI 图像上均未见肝脏铁沉积检出。T_2^* 序列是目前显示肝脏铁沉积的最敏感序列,其检出能力优于 T_1WI 和 T_2WI,该项研究中 T_2^* 检出肝硬化铁沉积的能力分别是 T_1WI 和 T_2WI 的 9.4 倍和 2.9 倍,与既往研究结论相符。该项研究显示 SWI 对肝硬化铁沉积的显示能力优于 T_2^*,检出铁沉积结节总数目和微小铁沉积结节的数目分别是 T_2^* 的 1.5 倍和 2.2 倍,而且 SWI 能够显示 5 例 T_2^* 漏诊的微小铁沉积结节病例。SWI 的本质是 T_2^* 序列,通过利用相位信息可以大大增加磁敏感物质的对比。

肝硬化铁沉积通常以两种形式存在,肝细胞内铁沉积多为铁蛋白,网状内皮系统内铁沉积多为含铁血黄素,二者均为强顺磁性物质,可导致质子失相位,这种相位信息为 SWI 所利用,有助于铁沉积的检出。另外, SWI 的模糊效应较 T_2^* 更为显著,小于 1 个像素的磁敏感物质会放大到 1 个像素大小而得以显示,这可能也是有更多微小铁沉积结节得以检出的原因。该项研究在 3.0T 机型上进行, T_2^* 和 SWI 序列选用相同回波时间(10ms),理论上其磁敏感效应为 1. 5T 机型的 2 倍。Krinsky 等(2001)的 1 组肝移植病理对照标本分析显示在 1. 5T 场强,选用 10ms 的回波时间检出铁沉积结节的敏感性为 80%。

该项研究尽管无病理对照,但结合 Krinsky 等(2001)的研究,若以 SWI 为检出铁沉积结节的“金标准”, T_2* 检出 5mm 以上铁沉积结节的敏感性为 85%,与 Krinsky 等(2001)的报道基本相符,提示 SWI 检出铁沉积结节的敏感性可能接近于病理金标准。

肝硬化铁沉积结节的临床意义:较多的循证医学证据显示了铁沉积与肝细胞癌生成的密切关系。铁可以影响干扰素抗病毒疗效,导致肝炎病毒的持续感染状态,诱发氧自由基的产生、对细胞功能、蛋白合成和 DNA 造成损害。另外,铁还会降低肝脏局部免疫微环境,间接促使结节癌变。对于伴铁沉积肝硬化病例,可能需要更为严格的随访监测。

该项研究显示 SWI 能够清晰显示常规序列不能检出的铁沉积结节,有望避免不必要的肝穿刺活检,而且因其无创性可用于肝脏铁沉积动态随访。另一方面,结节内的铁分布可能有助于肝细胞癌与癌前结节的鉴别,早期研究即发现铁沉积结节内部可出现局灶性的增生活跃的亚结节-“结中结”,这些亚结节几乎都是恶性的,发生于铁沉积结节者,新生的亚结节常呈乏铁改变。

铁沉积结节内铁摄取下降高度提示肝细胞癌,弥漫性铁沉积背景中出现局灶性乏铁区域也应高度怀疑肝细胞癌。SWI 有望从铁沉积角度为肝细胞癌的诊断提供额外信息。

该项研究尚有一些不足之处。首先,研究选用 2D 序列,分辨率尚待提高;其次,磁敏感效应在肝脏周边区域仍然较为明显，主要源于肋骨、椎体、心脏搏动等，尚需对后处理技术进行优化，进一步改善图像质量；最后，无组织病理学证据是研究的最大不足，尚需进行精确的影像病理对照研究进一步证实研究结论。另外，SWI 定量评价肝硬化铁沉积程度的价值尚需进一步研究。

总之，SWI 能够较常规序列更敏感的检出肝硬化铁沉积结节，并且具有更好的图像对比，有望成为肝脏铁过载无创性评价的新方法。

第二十一章　药物性和放射性肝损伤

第一节　药物性肝病

药物性肝病是指由于药物及其代谢产物引起的肝脏损害。近年来随着用于临床的药物种类日益增加，药物性肝病的发生率逐渐增加，目前报道已有1 000余种药物可引起药物性肝病，几乎涉及各类药物。药物性肝病是药物不良反应中较为严重、病死率较高的一种，占所有药物损害的10%~15%，因此药物性肝病已经成为世界的一个重大公共卫生问题。但是由于药物性肝病缺乏特异的临床表现和检测指标，尤其是特异性体质引起的药物性肝损害，故临床上容易漏诊或误诊。

发病机制：目前药物的肝毒性机制尚未完全明确。可能机制包括代谢物调节毒性、超敏反应、胆汁分泌受阻、小胆管的自身免疫性破坏、脂蛋白分泌减少、脂肪酸线粒体β氧化受阻、溶酶体磷酸酶阻滞、动脉缺损引起胆道缺血、肝星状细胞激活等。总体来说，药物损伤肝脏的机制包括药物对肝脏的毒性损害、机体对药物的特异质反应两个方面。药物的肝毒性表现可从无症状、轻微、非特异性的生化改变到急性肝炎、慢性肝炎、急性肝功能衰竭、胆汁淤积，甚至肝硬化、肝脏肿瘤等。

临床分析：由于药物性肝病的发病较为隐蔽，与原发疾病相重叠，发病初期症状和体征缺乏特异性等，在临床上难以明确诊断。虽然诊断标准的准确性和可操作性都取得了一定的突破，但目前仍无特异性诊断方法，主要根据用药史、临床表现、化验检查以及停药后的效应做出综合诊断。各类药物引起肝损伤的比例在国内外报道不一致，国外有报道以抗生素为主，也有报道以抗结核药物和抗肿瘤药物为主；国内多以抗结核药物和抗肿瘤药物为主，也有以抗生素为首的报道。中药制剂引起的肝损害近年来也日益增多，一组病例21例(42%)患者服用中药制剂，在用药种类中排在首位。

该组资料中，女性多于男性，男女比例1∶1.5，30岁以上占大多数(88%)，考虑由于男性肝微粒体内的药酶活性略高于女性，因此女性对药物的敏感性高；随着年龄的增长，中老年的基础疾病的比例增大，用药概率增高，且生理功能逐渐减退，肝血流减少，微粒体酶系活性降低，机体对药物的生物转化和排泄能力减弱，以致中老年发病人数增多。以往多数文献强调，药物性肝病常伴有发热、皮疹、关节疼痛等变态反应性改变，但该组资料中仅16%发热，6%皮疹，2%关节痛，提示以上指标作为诊断药物性肝病意义似乎不大。至少70%以上患者出现乏力、纳差、尿黄、黄疸，但不具有特异性，与病毒性肝病的临床表现类似，临床上易被诊断为“急性黄疸性肝炎(病原未定)”收入院，故在遇到有乏力、纳差、发热、尿黄等症状，化验转氨酶和/或胆红素升高的患者，应注意排除药物性肝病的可能。

病理分析：药物性肝病在血清学结果及临床症状、体征上无特异性，主要依靠用药史及排除其他各种肝病，故需结合病理组织学改变，才能做出正确的诊断。因此在有明确用药史，存在肝功损害，排除其他各种肝病的患者，如出现以中央静脉周围为主的肝细胞坏死，富含中性粒细胞和嗜酸性粒细胞的炎细胞浸润，肝细胞和毛细胆管淤胆，混合性脂肪变性，上皮样肉芽肿结构出现以及空泡核肝细胞易见等病理改变，有助于药物性肝病的诊断。

该组病例肝穿病理发现中央静脉周围肝细胞肿胀35例(70%)，肝细胞缺失、坏死24例(48%)，点灶状坏死25例(50%)，肝细胞及毛细胆管淤胆15例(30%)，混合性细胞浸润32例(64%)，嗜酸性粒细胞增多16例(32%)，出现局灶性再生结节10例

(20%),说明以上这些病理表现具有一定诊断意义。在该组病例中有6例患者因为未能提供服药史,最后能够确诊得益于病理诊断,所以应重视肝穿刺活检在诊断药物性肝病中的作用。也有文献报道慢性药物性肝病以慢性胆汁淤积型为主,占47.1%,与本组10例慢性药物性肝病中出现5例(50%)胆汁淤积的比例比较相符。

影像学研究:该组50例患者影像有异常变化的有48例,其中局灶性肝损害29例(58%),CT平扫及增强可见多发小斑片状低密度改变,其病理基础可能与大量肝细胞缺失、坏死有关;弥漫性肝脏损害14例(28%),5例CT平扫肝脏密度均匀性减低,其病理机制可能是病变区的炎性细胞浸润、动脉血供增加、细胞间隙增大、细胞间隙和血管间隙间的扩散速率降低所致;9例平扫肝内可见弥漫分布的稍高密度结节,增强后动脉期病灶明显强化,病理表现可见弥漫性再生结节。当药物导致肝脏损害严重,不可逆转时可形成坏死后肝硬化,从影像学上不难诊断。由于药物损伤造成肝细胞大量点灶状坏死,中央静脉周围肝细胞的缺失、坏死,以及汇管区水肿扩大,局灶性纤维组织增生和纤维化,正常组织与坏死组织共存,这些病理改变在影像上则表现为肝脏表面欠光整,左、右叶比例失调,而且可见弥漫存在的点状低密度影。当坏死区域比较大,左、右叶失调严重时,便会造成肝裂增宽。

该组29例(58%)存在脾大,可能是因为肝细胞及毛细胆管淤胆,及窦周纤维化,阻塞或压迫肝窦,使门脉压力升高,最终造成脾脏静脉回流受阻,出现脾大。影像诊断脂肪肝7例(14%),病理证实均有脂肪沉积,目前多数学者认为某些药物会抑制蛋白质的合成,从而导致药物性脂肪肝,但具体机制有待深入研究。

鉴别诊断:弥漫性肝癌:弥漫性肝癌CT平扫见全肝广泛性低密度区,呈密集斑点状或结节状,或融合成块状。肝内血供丰富,CT动态增强扫描典型的表现为对比剂快进快出,即肿瘤动脉期呈浓染灶,门静脉期对比剂移出较快,平衡期为低密度病灶。可以有肝脏体积增大,左、右叶比例失调,门静脉瘤栓形成,表现为门静脉主干及分支内充盈缺损或不成像。而药物性肝病虽肝体积增大,左、右叶比例失调,但增强扫描动脉期可见小片状异常强化,静脉期呈低密度影,延迟期仍不均匀。

弥漫性脂肪肝:脂肪肝血液循环障碍,肝内缺血,CT平扫肝脏密度普遍降低,严重病例肝CT值呈明显负值。根据脂肪浸润程度的不同,肝内血管影变得模糊不清或血管呈相对高密度。增强扫描肝实质仍保持相对低密度,同样低于增强后的脾脏,低密度区内血管影显示完整。

肝脏灌注不均:肝移植术后、肝射频术后等由于血流灌注再分布,出现肝脏灌注不均,平扫呈斑片状低密度或等密度,增强扫描动脉期出现斑片状异常强化区,静脉期和延迟期等密度均匀。而药物性肝病由于弥漫性点灶状坏死,动脉期可见弥漫点状强化,静脉期为低密度,延迟期仍不均匀。

综上所述,药物性肝病影像表现主要为肝脏局灶性损伤和弥漫性损伤,肝表面欠光滑,肝叶比例失调,可以合并脂肪肝、脾大等,有一定特征性,但缺乏特异性,结合病理可做出明确诊断。

第二节　放射性肝损伤

接受放射治疗后的病人肝脏出现异常的影像学表现,病理上出现肝细胞肿胀、肝静脉闭塞,晚期可出现肝硬化。CT表现较具特征,可见与照射野一致的肝密度减低区,增强后出现延迟强化:在肝硬化基础上的放射损伤表现为该区域过度强化;在脂肪肝基础上的放射损伤则表现为照射野的高密度。结合放射治疗史,诊断不难。其他影像学检查的报道较少。

随着我国放射治疗,尤其是适形治疗的增多,对该病的认识也应提高。如何早期诊断该病,也是值得研究的课题。

第二十二章　部分肝弥漫性肿瘤

第一节　弥漫型肝脏上皮样血管内皮细胞瘤

上皮样血管内皮细胞瘤是一种起源于血管的少见的低度恶性肿瘤，约占肝脏原发恶性肿瘤的1%~2%，属于中间型血管来源的肿瘤，其恶性程度介于血管瘤与血管肉瘤之间，远处转移率较低，好发于成年人，女性多见，也可见于婴幼儿。可发生于皮肤、四肢、深部软组织、甲状腺、骨等多个器官，而肝原发性上皮样血管内皮细胞瘤少见。

肿瘤细胞虽然有上皮形态，但免疫组化上皮表达（如CK19、CK20）与上皮类癌表达（如第Ⅷ因子相关抗原）及CEA却为阴性，而内皮表达（如CD34、CD31）为阳性，故称之为上皮样血管内皮细胞瘤。Weiss和Enzinger（1982）首次报道上皮样血管内皮细胞瘤。

肝上皮样血管内皮细胞瘤的影像表现可分为2型：多病灶型与弥漫型，有学者认为多病灶型为弥漫型的早期改变。肿瘤常肝脏左、右叶多发（77.4%~82.0%），单发病变罕见，病变多分布于肝脏周边，相互融合，常呈菜花状，肝门处的肝脏多无肿瘤，常见萎缩，而肝脏外形大致保持正常或不同程度肿大为病变的特点。

一例病变以右叶为主，无瘤肝脏极少，但除体积增大外，肝外形改变不明显，左叶病变较少，多位于肝脏被膜下。肿瘤少血供，该例病变CT平扫呈相对肝实质低密度，动脉期强化不明显，静脉期及延迟期病灶边缘有所强化，左叶部分病灶内部呈结节样明显强化，与以往一些文献报道强化明显的特点不同。该例MR T_1WI表现为相对肌肉低信号，部分病灶内可见更低信号，代表肿瘤内的硬化性坏死，T_2WI及FLAIR像呈稍高及高信号。与CT相仿，MRI可很好显示肿瘤的大体形态特点。

鉴别诊断：①上皮样血管肉瘤和本病都属于血管源性肿瘤，可出现上皮样结构，见到不规则的窦样血管网，但是一般没有典型的细胞质内管腔结构，并具有明显的异型性、核分裂象及出血坏死多见。恶性度高，预后差，病死率高，影像鉴别尚无明确的特征性，部分患者初诊易误诊为肝细胞癌。②在肝脏转移瘤，影像增强动脉期与静脉期多呈环形强化或边缘强化，该例上皮样血管内皮细胞瘤动脉期强化不明显，静脉期可见明显强化的结节。

多数文献认为上皮样血管内皮细胞瘤属于低度恶性肿瘤，Deyrup等（2008）认为根据组织学特征（核分裂率和肿瘤大小）其可分为高危险组与低危险组，两者生存率和转移率差异明显，所以，也有部分患者病情进展迅速，病死率高。但是肝上皮样血管内皮细胞瘤患者的预后要好于肝血管肉瘤，由于上皮样血管内皮细胞瘤具有多中心性起源并呈多结节性生长，且对放、化疗均不敏感，部分患者发现不及时，延误了早期手术治疗的时机。部分患者也可出现多脏器的转移。虽然最终诊断要依病理与免疫组化，然而肝脏原发性上皮样血管内皮细胞瘤具有一定影像特征，正确认识这些特征有助于及时正确诊断病变，为临床治疗与预后提供帮助。

第二节　恶性组织细胞病

恶性组织细胞病是组织细胞及其前体细胞呈系统性、进行性浸润的恶性疾病，较为罕见，而病情进展迅速，常常在6个月内导致病人死亡（Friedman等，1965）。主要临床表现有发热、乏力、肝脾及淋巴结肿大。病理上主要表现为肝、脾增大，肝、脾淋巴结、骨髓等造血组织及一些非造血器官和组织中有分化不同阶段的异常组织细胞呈灶性或弥漫性浸润。脾脏、淋巴结和肝脏是最易累及的器官。受累组织可以部分或全部被破坏，浸润也可以出现粟粒样和小的肉芽肿，但形成巨大肿块的少见（Yang等，1988）。

脾脏的病变也可由于主要脾动脉或其分支动脉阻塞所致，脾脏动脉是终末供血动脉，所以病变通常发生在脾脏的周围部分，在CT检查中通常表现为脾脏周围的低密度病灶（Yang等，1988）。本病CT表现缺乏特异性征象，与常见的脾淋巴瘤等恶性肿瘤很难鉴别，确诊要靠病理学检查，但CT检查能确定病灶大小，了解病变的范围、周围脏器受累的情况和有无远处转移，为治疗提供重要信息。

第三节　弥漫型的肝细胞癌与胆管癌合并存在

Yoshida等（1985）报告1例弥漫型的肝细胞癌与胆管癌合并存在，最初在临床上和影像诊断上皆只表现一小的局灶结节，它生长十分迅速，血清癌胚抗原水平极高，最后在2个月期间内肝重量增加约4倍。此病人死于肝功能衰竭伴出血，尸体检查见肝内转移性病灶内有多数小结节存在。

第二十三章 关于肝富血管性疾病

第一节 肝富血管性疾病

肝脏疾病中存在着许多相似的病理改变,可呈现一些类似的影像学表现,给影像学诊断和鉴别诊断带来困难。肝脏富血管性病变分为原发于肝脏的富血管性疾病和继发的肝脏转移性富血管肿瘤。肾细胞癌、乳腺癌、甲状腺癌、黑色素瘤、类癌、胰岛细胞癌和肉瘤等是最常见的富血管性肝转移的来源。

最常见的原发于肝脏的单个较大的富血管性肿块是局灶性结节增生、肝腺瘤和肝细胞性肝癌,较小的肝血管瘤在早期增强影像上有时亦可表现为一小富血管病变。

肝脏的富血管性病变主要包括:肝细胞性肝癌、富血管性肝转移、(上皮样)血管内皮细胞瘤、血管肉瘤、纤维板层肝细胞癌、肝内胆管癌(罕见)、血管瘤(小)、肝腺瘤、血管平滑肌脂肪瘤、局灶性结节增生、布-加综合征中再生结节(和其他血管性疾病中的再生结节)、肝紫癜症、肝硬化发育不良结节(罕见)、肝硬化再生结节(罕见)、动静脉畸形:先天性或介入手术后、肝动脉动脉瘤:创伤性或炎症性。

大多数肝细胞性肝癌可依据其侵袭特性和临床背景做出鉴别。但伴有中央瘢痕的局灶性结节增生难以与纤维板层肝细胞癌鉴别,肝腺瘤也常难与低度恶性肝细胞性肝癌鉴别。

第二节 局灶性结节增生与肝腺瘤的鉴别

两者都可发生于中青年女性,肝腺瘤可有服用避孕药的病史。影像学检查有助于两者鉴别(表9-23-1)。应用特殊MRI对比剂会对鉴别更有帮助。与常规钆剂不同,3%~5%钆贝葡胺莫迪司(Gd-BOPTA)是通过肝胆管路径排出,由于肝腺瘤内无胆管结构,Gd-BOPTA增强时,延迟(1~3h)影像上呈低信号。而局灶性结节增生含有畸形的胆小管,故在延迟影像上几乎都呈高信号或与肝脏呈等信号。此外,因局灶性结节增生和肝腺瘤对超顺磁性氧化铁颗粒(SPIO)摄取类似,故对局灶性结节增生的定性诊断,Gd-BOPTA优于SPIO。

表 9-23-1 局灶性结节增生(FNH)与肝腺瘤的影像学鉴别

病变类型	中央瘢痕	不均质*	强化不均匀	被膜下供血动脉	动脉期强化程度	门脉期瘤体强化程度	出血	T_1WI 高信号	Gd-BOPTA** 延迟摄取
FNH	+	-	-	-	>	+	-	+/-	+
腺瘤	-	+	+	+	<	++	+/-	+/-	-

注:动脉期局灶性结节增生强化程度远高于腺瘤;局灶性结节增生强化率 >1.6(动脉期衰减值与平扫时衰减值比);腺瘤强化率 <1.6。在门静脉期局灶性结节增生常为等密度,而腺瘤则为高密度;*:含CT密度与MRI信号强度;**:中译名为钆贝葡胺莫迪司

关于肝脏局灶性结节增生,请详见本书 本卷 第五篇 第三章 肝脏局灶性结节增生。

关于肝腺瘤,请详见本书 本卷 第五篇 第五章 肝腺瘤。

第三节　肝血管瘤与肝富血管肿瘤鉴别

依据血管瘤的球形、周围性、进行性强化特点，很容易与其他病变进行鉴别。然而，小血管瘤可以在动脉期或门静脉期呈均匀性强化，难以与其他富血管性病变进行鉴别。有些方法可协助区别。下述四点可供参考：①强化程度：血管瘤的强化程度在动脉期与主动脉相当；而在门静脉期则与血管湖相当；而其他富血管性病变则强化程度稍低。②强化延长：在延迟影像上，血管瘤持续存在着相当于血管湖的衰减值，而其他病变则已被洗脱，成为相对于肝脏的低密度。③MRI T_2WI：在重 T_2WI 上，血管瘤较其他富血管性病变有更高的高信号。④病灶周围强化：在动脉期，血管瘤有时可在病变周围显示有一过性衰减差（THAD）。但这一现象也见于肝细胞性肝癌。

关于肝血管瘤，请详见本书 本卷 第五篇 第二章　肝血管瘤。

第四节　肝硬化中的肝脏富血管病变

在肝硬化背景下，如显示一富血管性病变应首先考虑为肝细胞性肝癌。但有些富血管性的假病变、再生性结节和非典型增生结节也难以与肝细胞性肝癌鉴别。

肝细胞性肝癌：肝细胞性肝癌是富血管性的，在 MRI T_2WI 上常能与再生结节和非典型增生结节鉴别。然而，极少数的再生和非典型增生结节也可为富血管性的。在这些不典型病例中，肝细胞性肝癌的有些特性有助于与再生或非典型增生结节进行鉴别：①病变的不均质性；②在门静脉期和延迟期影像上的低衰减（CT 值）或低信号强度；③周围强化的被膜；④MRI T_2WI 上呈高信号。关于肝细胞性肝癌，请详见本书 本卷 第三篇　肝细胞性肝癌。

假病变：在肝硬化或慢性肝炎病人中，能见到一些不明原因（动脉 - 门静脉分流可以是一个原因）的富血管性小的假病变。这些病变难以与小肝细胞性肝癌鉴别。然而肝细胞性肝癌有些特性有助于鉴别两者：①中心部位快速洗脱，小肝细胞性肝癌具早期强化与中心快速洗脱特点，而假病变常强化较晚，且强化持续较久；②围绕病变（肝细胞性肝癌）的“花冠状”强化，这一表现在假病变中见不到；③圆形轮廓的病变更可能是肝细胞性肝癌；④隆起凸出的被膜只见于肝细胞性肝癌；⑤在 MRI T_1WI 和 T_2WI 上，假病变与背景肝呈等信号。

融合性肝纤维化：在肝硬化中所见的其他潜在的富血管性病变是融合性肝纤维化。而融合性肝纤维化在动脉期极少见强化，通常是延迟强化。融合性肝纤维化常在 MRI T_2WI 上呈高信号，但若它也是富血管性，则易与肝细胞性肝癌相混淆。

以下的特征可使两者易于鉴别：①融合性肝纤维化特征性部位是肝右前叶和左叶内段；②融合性肝纤维化呈楔形；③融合性肝纤维化可见被膜回缩；④融合性肝纤维化时，可见血管纹直接穿过病变，而无血管受侵。

关于肝纤维化，请详见本书 本卷 本篇 第十一章　肝纤维化形态学研究，第十二章 肝纤维化功能代谢研究。

第五节　不常见的肝脏富血管病变的诊断与鉴别诊断

布 - 加综合征中的结节状再生性增生结节：这类再生结节常较小，多发且富血管。可能是由于肝血供不足区发生萎缩，而有适当血供的区域发生代偿性结节增生的结果。这类结节也在造成肝血供损害（减少）的其他全身性疾病中被报道，如自身免疫性疾病、淋巴 - 骨髓增生性疾病和类固醇与抗肿瘤药物治疗后。相似的结节也见于自身免疫性肝炎中。这些再生结节是来自结节状再生性增生。结节之间没有纤维变性。如结节直径 >1cm,则可见有中央瘢痕。有时结节在 MR T_1WI 上呈高信号,通常在 T_2WI 呈等信号到低信号。同局灶性结节增生一样,它们也可延迟摄取 Gd-BOPTA。结节的多样性特征有助于它们与其他的肝脏富血管病变鉴别。发生于布 - 加综合征的再生结节,在这些方面不同于继发于肝硬化中的再生结节。

布 - 加综合征中的再生结节的鉴别特征:MR T_1WI 呈高信号;动脉期常强化;直径 >1cm 的病变常有中央瘢痕。很重要的一点是,这些结节性病变不是孤立出现的,而是出现于布 - 加综合征的病人的肝脏中。

关于布 - 加综合征中的结节状再生性增生结节,请详见本书 本卷 第十篇 第一章 布 - 加综合征,本书 本卷 本篇 第六章 肝结节状再生性增生。

肝血管肉瘤:肝血管肉瘤的强化并不同于血管瘤。肝血管肉瘤可表现为不规则形、中心或环形局部强化,强化程度低于主动脉。通常延迟期还呈进行性强化,这有助于血管瘤与肝细胞性肝癌鉴别。此外,在肝血管肉瘤中,有脾转移时可与肝细胞性肝癌鉴别。

关于肝血管肉瘤,请详见本书 本卷 第四篇 第三章 肝血管源性恶性肿瘤。

肝紫癜症:肝紫癜症的特征是肝内多发性、不同大小的充有血液的囊肿。它常伴同恶性病变、慢性感染、获得性免疫缺陷综合征(AIDS)和各种药物(如口服避孕药和蛋白同化甾体药物)引起。其增强模式有从周围向中央扩展(模拟血管瘤),以及从中央向周围扩展(更常见)。典型的表现为病变缺乏占位效应,这有助于与其他肝脏病变进行鉴别;病变在延迟期强化延长,这有助于与其他富血管性肝脏病变进行鉴别。

肝内胆管(腺)癌;富血管性肝内胆管癌极罕见。它们在延迟期强化延长,可与肝细胞性肝癌进行鉴别。

关于肝内胆管癌,请详见本书 本卷 第十六篇 第六章 肝内胆管细胞癌。

第二十四章　肝弥漫性病变的其他情况

第一节　肝衰竭CT表现

肝衰竭是指由多种因素引起的严重肝脏损害，导致肝脏本身合成、解毒、排泄和生物转化等功能发生严重障碍或失代偿，临床上出现以凝血机制障碍、黄疸、肝性脑病、脱水等表现的一组症候群。在肝移植技术推广之前，肝衰竭的生存率不足15%；肝移植后，短期生存率可达65%，肝脏移植已经成为其最有效的治疗方法。

病理学：病理标本全部来源于肝移植。病理特点是肝内存在大块状肝细胞坏死、桥接坏死、融合状坏死、炎性细胞浸润、红细胞填充坏死区等。亚急性肝衰竭可见肝细胞的结节样再生；慢性和亚急性肝衰竭可见肝硬化基础上的大块状新鲜的肝细胞坏死。

一项5例研究中，患者的病理特点为大范围的肝细胞坏死、桥接坏死、炎性细胞浸润等。亚急性肝衰竭肝内出现典型的结节样肝细胞再生。

肝衰竭数日内就可形成大块状的肝细胞坏死，病程进展1周以上时，坏死部位出现收缩，导致肝叶或全肝的体积缩小。病程超过数周，肝内可形成结节样再生，整个过程可能很迅速，甚至发生在病程的第2周，这一病理变化过程构成了肝衰竭的影像改变基础。

临床表现：根据我国2006年的《肝衰竭诊疗指南》，肝衰竭分为急性、亚急性、慢加急性（亚急性）和慢性肝衰竭。国内外引起肝衰竭的病因不同，国外多由药物、酒精等肝毒性物质引起，特别是对乙酰氨基酚类解热镇痛药。国内则以乙型肝炎导致的肝衰竭为主，其次中草药导致的肝衰竭报道也在增加。

该研究的5例中，乙酰氨基酚和乙型肝炎导致的肝衰竭各2例，尼美舒利导致者1例。

肝衰竭的临床表现包括极度乏力、精神萎靡、严重的消化道症状、重度黄疸（短期内黄疸呈进行性加重）和明显的出血倾向。随着病情进展，出现大量腹水和肝性脑病，实验室检查凝血酶原活动度<40%。该研究中的5例患者均出现肝性脑病，4例凝血酶原活动度<40%，1例未凝集。急性肝衰竭以肝细胞的一次性大块状坏死为特点，显微镜下见广泛的肝细胞坏死，炎性细胞浸润等。亚急性肝衰竭不仅存在大片状肝细胞坏死，还可出现肝细胞再生，显微镜下可见新旧不等的大片坏死和肝细胞再生。慢加亚急性肝衰竭是在慢性肝病病理损害的基础上，出现大块或亚大块的新鲜坏死。

影像学研究：肝衰竭CT影像与病理对照研究的国内外文献报道较少，国外只是个案。肝衰竭发生的大块状肝细胞坏死在CT平扫表现为地图样分布的低密度影，增强后坏死区明显强化并高于周围的肝组织。这种强化机制主要与肝脏内病变区的炎性细胞浸润、动脉血供增加、细胞间隙增大、细胞间隙和血管间隙间的扩散速率改变有关。

坏死后的结节样再生在平扫CT上表现为稍高密度，增强后中等强化，强化程度低于坏死区域的密度。病灶分布上，肝细胞大块状坏死多位于肝脏中央部，结节样再生多出现在肝脏外周区域。其他异常表现包括肝脏体积缩小、门静脉增粗、肝静脉狭窄等。

该研究中，肝细胞坏死的影像表现特点包括大灶性融合病变、弥漫性的结节样病灶、多发小片状病灶3种形态。通过与肝脏标本的对照，发现肝坏死的CT平扫呈低密度改变；增强扫描肝内坏死区域的强化以静脉期表现显著，与平扫图像比较呈“反转”表现。

2例亚急性肝衰竭出现肝细胞再生的表现形态

不同，分别为弥漫的小结节样再生和大块状融合的结节样再生，CT 表现具有特征性，平扫为稍高密度，增强后动脉期出现强化，静脉期及延迟期近似于等密度改变，与文献报道相符。另 1 例慢加亚急性肝衰竭的弥漫性结节样坏死的 CT 平扫表现为稍高密度，动脉期强化明显，静脉期及延迟期呈低密度表现，具有一定的特征。该研究中 3 例肝内出现大面积坏死的患者，肝脏体积缩小，肝包膜皱缩；2 例肝脏内出现多发小结节状改变的患者，肝脏体积无明显缩小。5 例患者脾脏体积则与病情无明显关联。

CT 检查能否准确地反映肝衰竭患者的肝脏病理动态变化，取决于影像检查与获得病理标本的间隔时间。该组患者的间隔时间在 0~8 d，比较接近实际的病理表现，也短于以往的文献报道。该研究中患者的肝内坏死灶在增强后的强化突出表现在静脉期，这种与平扫图像呈"反转"的现象，在过去文献中未明确报道，这可能与该组病例使用螺旋 CT 扫描机的快速扫描有关。该研究结果显示，肝坏死与随后出现的结节样再生的 CT 影像表现不同，这种再生可表现为弥漫的结节样或融合状，平扫及增强扫描均与肝细胞的块状坏死不同。慢加亚急性肝衰竭的结节状坏死与结节型肝癌增强扫描的影像表现相似，二者鉴别还应结合临床病史、实验室检查，避免错误诊断。

该研究的局限性在于病例数目较少，还有待于今后更多病例的研究。CT 增强扫描及 3D 血管重组有助于外科明确患者的肝脏血管解剖及腹腔内其他脏器状况，可以提供准确的供、受体的全肝和各肝叶体积，避免术后供体或受体由于肝体积不足引起的并发症。

第二节　结节病侵犯肝脏

结节病为多系统肉芽肿病变，主要累及胸部、眼、皮肤、腹部内脏、中枢神经系统和骨骼。结节病侵犯肝脏时，表现为肝内不规则团块状低密度阴影，伴有后腹膜淋巴结、纵隔淋巴结多处淋巴结肿大，及结节病的其他表现。

Farman（1995）报告 4 例腹部结节病的 CT 表现。男性 3 例，女性 1 例，年龄分别为 53 岁、32 岁、53 岁、30 岁。3 例与肺部结节病有关，1 例胰岛素依赖性糖尿病患者结节病病变仅限于腹部。临床表现发热，不适 2 例，支气管炎反复发作 1 例，下肢深静脉血栓 1 例。体检可触及脾脏 2 例；化验检查见碱性磷酸酶升高 3 例，天门冬氨酸转氨酶和丙谷氨酰转肽酶升高 1 例。腹部 CT 发现肝肿大伴多发性低密度区 2 例；脾肿大 4 例，伴存多发性低密度区 3 例；腹膜后淋巴结肿大 4 例，其中广泛性肿大 3 例。经组织活检证实 3 例，另 1 例鉴于支气管镜检确诊为结节病，腹部病变临床诊断为结节病，并随访 2 年其症状及血液生化无变化。

结节病患者尸检发现腹腔和盆腔淋巴结肿大高达 90%，肝肉芽肿高达 70%，而临床上肝脾肿大仅 20%。

腹部 CT 扫描结节病表现为淋巴结肿大、脾肿大和肝肿大。肿大的淋巴结最常见于主动脉旁、腔静脉旁和胰腺周围区域；较少区域是胃肝韧带、肠系膜、骨盆及膈脚后淋巴结。

肺部和腹部结节病两者之间受累及的范围常无关联。

肝脾最常见的 CT 表现是肝脾肿大，实质弥漫性密度不均匀，其肉芽肿的直径常小于 2mm，使用高分辨 CT 作腹部扫描可以发现更多的、更小的肉芽肿。

第三节　弥漫性病变中的部分局灶性病变

详见本书 本卷 本篇 第二十三章 第四节　肝硬化中的肝脏富血管病变。

第十篇　肝血管性疾病

第一章　布 – 加综合征

第一节　误诊病例简介：布 - 加综合征合并原发性肝癌

有作者报告布 - 加综合征合并原发性肝癌一例。该病例最初诊断肝癌，给予介入治疗，疗效甚佳，然后才发现布 - 加综合征。一般认为淤血性肝硬化与原发性肝癌的发生无关，但布 - 加综合征引起的淤血性肝损伤导致肝细胞再生的慢性病理过程与其他致癌诱因导致肝癌发生的病理过程十分相似，因此两者之间并非毫无关联。

在布 - 加综合征病例中约 0.7% 的患者，尤其是患有慢性病毒性肝炎、白塞氏病和长期烟酒史的患者，可在 4.5~24 年的病程中进展为具有多中心起源、结节状生长、增长迅速等特点的肝癌，肝动脉化疗栓塞术序贯治疗后平均生存期为 9~29.3 个月，而无明显致癌诱因合并原发性肝癌的患者则十分罕见。

该例肝静脉与下腔静脉同时受累，属复合型布 - 加综合征，合并的原发性肝癌特征较上述特点有明显差异：单发团块状病灶；肝动脉化疗栓塞术序贯治疗后肿瘤消失；患者首诊后随访 38 个月仍无进展征象，疗效明显优于相关文献报道结果。

其良好疗效可能与以下因素有关：病灶单发，肝内无其他病灶，范围局限，血管造影无动 - 静脉瘘及门静脉侵犯征象，对介入治疗敏感；患者无其他常见致癌诱因，侧支循环建立充分，淤血性肝损伤相对较轻，肝脏储备及代偿功能较强（Child-PughA 级）。因此能耐受多次序贯治疗而具有较好的预后生存期。

分析该例前期漏诊布 - 加综合征的原因：首诊时已有肝硬化门静脉高压征象，但无引起肝硬化常见的病史；肝内原发块状型肝癌的“干扰”；患者体内侧支循环建立较为充分，未出现明显腹腔积液及双下肢水肿典型症状等。直至发生消化道出血才最终确诊。

第二节　布 - 加综合征与结节性再生性增生

布 - 加综合征可致肝弥漫性结节性再生性增生。于超声图像上较大结节表现为强回声、均质、周边清晰。结节性再生性增生的典型 CT 表现为低密度结节，增强后表现为动脉期、门静脉期明显强化。

MR 表现为 T_1WI 高信号，T_2WI 表现为等信号或低信号结节，与肝腺瘤信号强度类似。因结节的组织成分类似于正常肝细胞和枯否细胞，故 MRI 常难发现。

布 - 加综合征所致肝弥漫性结节性再生性增生须与肝细胞癌鉴别。肝细胞癌 MRI 表现为 T_1WI 低信号，T_2WI 为高信号，增强门脉期对比剂迅速退出。

第三节　肝窦阻塞综合征

肝窦阻塞综合征，又称为肝小静脉闭塞症，是以肝中央小叶区肝窦和小静脉闭塞性内膜炎及肝细胞损害为特征性病理改变和以肝脏肿大、黄疸、腹腔积液、肝区疼痛和体重增加为主要症状和体征的临床综合征。

1. 病理学　近年实验和病理研究表明肝窦阻塞综合征起源于肝窦内皮细胞损伤，由此引起一系列病理变化最终导致肝窦血流阻塞，因此 DeLeve 等（2002）学者将肝小静脉闭塞症更名为肝窦阻塞综合征。肝穿刺活检是本病诊断的金标准，但患者往往存在血小板减少、凝血功能障碍及大量腹腔积液等穿刺禁忌证。临床诊断通常参照 Seattle 标准、Baltimore 标准或修订后的 Seattle 标准，这些标准多依据临床症状和体征等间接征象，不够客观或缺乏特异性。

2. 临床表现　肝窦阻塞综合征在西欧和北美绝大多数发生在干细胞移植、恶性肿瘤放化疗后，在我国主要是食用了含肝毒性吡咯双烷生物碱的中草药而发病，最常见于外伤后服用土三七。其组织病理学特点为：急性期首先发生肝窦内皮细胞损伤和脱落，纤维沉积，继而肝窦扩张淤血，肝索受压，胆汁淤积，肝细胞发生缺血、变性和坏死。亚急性期肝中央静脉及小叶静脉内皮下纤维化，管腔狭窄、闭塞。慢性期可形成小结节性肝硬化。

3. 影像学研究　一组 25 例 CT 及 MRI 表现为肝脏密度 / 信号不均，显示以第二肝门为中心环绕三支肝静脉和下腔静脉分布的“爪”形稍高密度或 T_1WI 稍高信号、T_2WI 稍低信号灶，部分病例另有散在斑片灶，并且增强扫描门静脉期明显强化。其病理基础为肝窦状隙的阻塞，肝窦血流受阻或缓慢，小叶静脉管腔狭窄、闭塞、引流不畅，相应肝实质出现淤血、水肿和坏死等；而肝静脉和下腔静脉周围为相对正常肝实质，这是因为局部有较多细小引流静脉使血流动力学改变相对较小。增强扫描延迟期呈渐进性强化，即强化范围增大，强化更加明显，这是肝脏血流减慢、延迟灌注所致。

该组病例 CT 和 MRI 表现与 Dumont 等（2004）描述的 1 例 MRI 表现相同，与一些作者所描述的超声表现基本一致。有的作者认为肝窦阻塞综合征的强化方式为“地图”状或“花斑”样强化，仅少数病例表现为沿肝静脉和下腔静脉的“爪”形强化，与该研究的表述不完全一致，其原因可能是患者病变严重程度的不同或没有从整体上观察强化区域的分布特点。

肝窦阻塞综合征患者的病变程度不同，其影像学表现有差异：病变越严重，残留相对正常肝实质越少，“爪”形强化灶越细窄，该组病例多数病变严重，“爪”形形态明显；相反病变程度越轻，残留相对正常肝组织越多，“爪”形强化灶越粗大，融合越明显，散在强化灶越多，导致第二肝门以下层面或者延迟期部分层面表现为“地图”状或“花斑”样强化，但此表述没有从整体上体现强化区域的分布特点和肝窦阻塞综合征的血流动力学特征性改变，而通过认真观察可以发现以第二肝门为中心沿肝静脉和下腔静脉分布的强化特征，因此可以用“爪”形强化统一描述，即病变程度较轻的患者表现为在粗大的“爪”形强化灶基础上散在斑片状强化灶。

CT 和 MRI 增强扫描肝静脉未见对比剂充填、或模糊显示或较细，是由于肝窦受阻、肝小静脉壁增厚、管腔狭窄、血流减慢以及肝实质肿胀压迫所致。门静脉增粗、侧支开放、脾肿大、腹腔积液、胆囊壁水肿、小肠壁增厚这些是门静脉血流受阻及肝功能受损的征象。沿门静脉走行的“晕环征”，是门静脉周围水肿的表现，与肝淋巴回流受阻和 / 或腹腔积液有关。

CTA 及 MRA 肝静脉不能显示或较细；肝动脉因受压可有轻度扭曲改变。肝脏肿胀使下腔静脉轻度受压，但其血流依然通畅，远段无扩张，相应侧支静脉无增粗曲张。

临床上肝窦阻塞综合征与布 - 加综合征常难以区分，但 CT 和 MRI 表现有助于鉴别，布 - 加综合征可有以下征象：肝静脉型布 - 加综合征表现为第一肝门周围肝实质的“扇”形强化；下腔静脉型及混合型布 - 加综合征因下腔静脉梗阻常出现相应侧支循环开放，如腰静脉、腰升静脉、奇静脉、半奇静脉增粗迂曲及下肢静脉曲张等；布 - 加综合征晚期可出现尾状叶代偿性增大；CTA 及 MRA 可以显示引起布 - 加综合征的膜状分隔、血栓及受压等征象。

肝穿刺活检是肝窦阻塞综合征诊断的金标准，但患者往往存在诸多穿刺禁忌证，而国际上常用的临床诊断标准多依据症状和体征等间接征象，不够客观或缺乏特异性。随着对肝窦阻塞综合征病理生理认识的深入，CT、MRI 及超声等影像学检查发挥着更大的作用。

肝窦阻塞综合征的病理基础决定了在疾病的早期就出现肝脏血流动力学的特异性改变，而动态增强 CT 及 MRI 检查能敏感地反映肝脏血流灌注的改变及其继发的病理改变，对该病诊断具有重要意义。该组病例 CT 及 MRI 检查均有以第二肝门为中心环绕三支肝静脉和下腔静脉的“爪”形肝实质渐进性强化及肝静脉不强化或显影差的表现。

该组患者中 4 例在治疗后进行了复查，其中 3 例出现强化灶增大或肝实质密度 / 信号由不均匀变得较为均匀，肝静脉由不强化变为较清晰显示，因此认为 CT 及 MRI 检查有助于治疗前后患者肝脏血流灌注及其继发病理改变的比较，有助于疗效的评价。

总之，肝窦阻塞综合征动态增强 CT 及 MRI 表现具有一定的特征，尤其是以第二肝门为中心环绕三支肝静脉和下腔静脉的“爪”形肝实质渐进性强化及肝静脉不强化或显影较差的表现，有助于准确诊断肝窦阻塞综合征，并且 CT 及 MRI 检查有助于疗效的随访观察。

附：具体研究资料：一组 25 例中，1 例肝移植患者经手术病理证实，其余 24 例根据土三七服用史和典型临床表现及影像学表现综合诊断为肝窦阻塞综合征，其中参考了修订后的 Seattle 标准：①其他原因无法解释的高胆红素血症，血清总胆红素 >34.2μmol/L（2mg/dl）；②肝脏肿大或右上腹肝区痛；③不明原因的体重增加 2% 以上；以上 3 项出现 2 项。

第四节　诊断陷阱：脾肺固定术后

布 - 加综合征患者做脾肺固定术后，有的在左下肺出现类圆形致密包块影，X 线正侧位胸片上都可显示。在正位片上可见左膈稍升高，包块经左侧膈顶中心部凸入下肺野，其上缘呈半圆形，光滑规整，高约 3~5cm，左右宽约 4~6cm；下部与膈肌相连，两侧缘与膈肌成钝角，密度高于肺部而低于腹部。侧位胸片显示包块位于后纵隔，与脊柱相重叠，前后缘稍现模糊。在透视下，深呼吸时左侧膈肌与包块同时上下移动，但较右侧膈肌动度弱。

脾肺固定术是外科治疗布 - 加综合征所选用的多种术式的一种，其目的是通过脾肺间毛细血管的产生，建立起侧支循环回流。为使脾肺接触，术中要在左膈顶开窗，并将脾脏上极的包膜切开，然后再将脾上极与肺底部磨擦后互相吻合，使再生毛细血管形成新的侧支循环。术后脾脏仍位于膈下，当膈顶开窗过大或腹腔压力增加时，脾上极可向膈上移位，造成脾疝，在左下肺野显示出包块样影。

此包块内毛细血管丰富，血液经增粗的肺静脉回流，包块下部也有致密的血管网络。一般认为，出现此包块是一种正常的术后 X 线表现，对手术效果无不良影响。

X 线检查时易将此包块误为占位性病变，此刻，需要熟悉布 - 加综合征的发病史和治疗方法，并注意以下几点：①询问有否布 - 加综合征病史及手术史；②胸透时嘱患者深吸气，见包块与膈肌分不开而且有同步运动，左侧膈肌活动度减弱或有胸膜粘连改变；③较高电压（85~90kV）胸部透视，显示左膈下有与包块紧密相连的密度增高影（此为手术后正常上移的脾下极），正常胃泡向内侧推移或消失；④随访检查，包块无增大或缩小变化。

第五节　关于布 - 加综合征的误诊

布 - 加综合征是由于肝静脉和 / 或下腔静脉狭窄，甚至闭塞导致的肝静脉回流障碍性肝病，晚期表现为肝硬化，许多病人被临床长期误诊为肝硬化而失去了最佳治疗时机。因此，提高对该病的认识至关重要。

影像学表现极具特征，是诊断该病的主要手段。超声、CT 和 MRI 均可显示肝静脉或下腔静脉肝段狭窄或闭塞，继发肝脏淤血增大，CT 出现肝脏花斑样强化，肝静脉不强化、下腔静脉缺如，以及体静脉侧支循环形成，结合临床下肢水肿等表现可提示该病的诊断。

但检查时忽略对肝静脉与下腔静脉的观察是导致误诊的关键。超声、CT 和 MRI 有时对狭窄静脉显示不清，也是造成误诊的主要原因。

第六节 布-加综合征误诊为肝癌

布-加综合征(BCS)是由于各种原因所致的肝静脉和邻近的下腔静脉狭窄闭塞,肝静脉和下腔静脉血液回流障碍,产生肝大及疼痛、腹水、肝脏功能障碍等系列临床表现。该病误诊率高。布-加综合征是由于各种原因(如血液高凝状态、长期口服避孕药、血管及血液疾病等)所致的肝静脉和邻近的下腔静脉狭窄闭塞,肝静脉和下腔静脉血液回流障碍,产生肝大及疼痛、腹水、肝脏功能障碍等系列临床表现。可发生于任何年龄, 10岁以后多发,最常发生在30岁左右,在我国男性稍高于女性,在西方国家因口服避孕药,女性发病率有上升趋势。

诊断标准:急性布-加综合征大多有腹痛、肝脏肿大压痛和腹水三联征,慢性患者有肝大、门体侧支循环和腹水三联征。实时超声和多普勒超声可以对85%以上的患者提示布-加综合征的诊断,确诊仍有赖于肝静脉和/或下腔静脉造影及肝穿刺活组织检查。

病例突出特点是腹胀、腹水、肝脏肿大、侧支循环形成及实验室检查有高胆红素血症等类似肝硬化表现;B型超声显示肝脏肿大、脾大、腹水;CT显示有肝内占位,并且呈低密度影,边界欠清,类似肝癌表现,这种情况下很容易误诊为肝癌。误诊原因主要是急性期或者亚急性期有肝脏内淤血及出血,影像学观察有不规则低密度影,类似肝癌影像学诊断。

分析这种病例有几个特点不符合肝癌:①患者往往年龄较小,虽然目前癌症年轻化,但不是癌症高发人群,且没有肝病基础及引起肝细胞肝癌的因素;②患者有脑梗死病史,也不符合发病人群流行病学,脑梗死也均为年龄较大患者,患者之所以引起脑梗原因是自身免疫性血管炎;血管炎不但可以引起脑血管狭窄或阻塞,亦可以引起全身血管狭窄或阻塞,包括肝静脉及下腔静脉。故高度怀疑该患者为布-加综合征。

其诊断有几个特点可以遵循:一方面布-加综合征类似肝硬化失代偿期及肝脏肿瘤临床表现和体征,但一般没有严重肝硬化低蛋白血症及转氨酶变化,即“症状重,化验轻”的特点;另一方面有类似肝硬化失代偿期的表现,但没有明显引起肝硬化的基础病变,如酒精性肝炎、病毒性肝炎、药物性肝炎、自身免疫性肝病等;其次,年龄也是诊断疾病的主要因素。上述情况如果出现肝脏肿大、腹水等,在没有禁忌证情况下,尽量做肝静脉造影及/或肝穿刺活组织检查,以免误诊。

第二章　肝动脉

第一节　肝动脉变异影像学研究

肝动脉变异对于肝癌化疗药物灌注及栓塞治疗、肝脏部分外科切除、全肝或部分肝移植和肝脏疾病的诊疗等有重要意义。为了避免诊治中严重并发症的发生和有助肝脏疾病的诊疗，全面了解肝动脉发育变异非常必要。除数字减影血管造影（DSA）外，CT 血管成像（CTA）、磁共振血管成像（MRA）、彩色多普勒超声（CDF）等新技术的应用又开辟了肝动脉变异认识的新方法。

肝动脉变异及分型：Haller（1756）首先描述并报告迷走肝动脉。1958 年开始在放射专业文献上有副肝动脉选择性血管造影的报告。国内外分型研究主要有以下几种，其中最经典的是 Michels 分型，以后的研究多在此基础上进行。

Michels（1955）通过 200 例尸体解剖的仔细研究，将变异肝动脉分为替代肝动脉和副肝动脉两大类共十种类型。

所谓替代肝动脉指替代了同名正常肝动脉供血的变异肝动脉；而副肝动脉指正常肝动脉仍然存在，只参与正常同名肝动脉分布区域内的一部分血供的变异肝动脉。

10 种类型是：1 型，正常型，即肝固有动脉分出肝左动脉、肝中动脉与肝右动脉；2 型，替代肝左动脉来自胃左动脉；3 型，替代肝右动脉来自肠系膜上动脉；4 型，替代肝右动脉来自肠系膜上动脉 + 替代肝左动脉来自胃左动脉；5 型，副肝左动脉来自胃左动脉；6 型，副肝右动脉来自肠系膜上动脉；7 型，副肝右动脉来自肠系膜上动脉，且副肝左动脉来自胃左动脉；8 型，替代肝右动脉和副肝左动脉或替代肝左动脉和副肝右动脉；9 型，肝总动脉来自肠系膜上动脉；10 型，肝总动脉来自胃左动脉。

这种肝动脉起源的分型法较全面地概括了肝动脉的变异情况，至今仍被国际学术界视为研究肝动脉发育变异分型的主要标准。

Michels 还提出了肝脏侧支循环的三个主要类型，共 26 条途径。

（1）10 条基本途径，即他描述的迷走肝动脉（替代或副肝动脉）起源于肠系膜上动脉、胃左动脉或其他途径。

（2）与肝动脉相连的 6 条非肝途径：①胃下动脉（胃网膜左动脉和胃网膜右动脉）；②胃上动脉（胃左动脉和胃右动脉）；③结肠下动脉（在横结肠下大网膜后层大的 Barkow 弓）；④食管周围或肝胃动脉（来自于胃左动脉和脾动脉与肝左动脉相连的心食管分支）；⑤食管后动脉（经心食管动脉分支与肝左动脉相连的左隔下动脉的返支）；⑥胰横动脉。

（3）10 条基本途径以外途径：①肠系膜上动脉经胰十二指肠下动脉；②肠系膜上动脉经胰横动脉分支；③膈下动脉在膈肌处与肝动脉分支的交通；④来自于内乳动脉的膈上动脉在膈肌处到肝动脉分支；⑤内乳动脉的剑形分支经镰状韧带和肝圆韧带与肝中动脉和肝左动脉相连；⑥行走于冠状、左、右三角韧带的动脉；⑦肋间动脉；⑧后腹壁动脉；⑨肝静脉、门静脉和下腔静脉的滋养血管；⑩沿胆管走行的纤细的动脉。

这些途径的认识可帮助临床医生更全面地理解肝脏供血的复杂性和多样性。

Hitta（1994）分析了 1 000 例肝移植手术患者的肝动脉，将起源于胃左动脉替代或副肝左动脉分为一类，将起源于肠系膜上动脉的替代或副肝右动脉分为另一类。从而将 Michels 分型简化为 6 型：1 型，正常解剖结构，肝总动脉起源于腹腔干，分成肝固有动脉及胃十二指肠动脉，前者向远端分为肝左右动脉；2型，替代或副肝左动脉起源于胃左动脉；3型，替代或副肝右动脉起源于肠系膜上动脉；4型，双替代型，肝右动脉起源于肠系膜上动脉+肝左动脉是胃左动脉分支；5型，肝总动脉起源于肠系膜上动脉；6型，肝总动脉起源于腹主动脉。此种分型至今也是经常被国际学术界作为研究肝动脉发育变异分型标准之一。

Ruzicka（1970）把腹部肿瘤的动脉供血分为规则性、变异性和寄生性三类。他的研究特点是基于腹部肿瘤的供血进行的研究。规则性血供是指肝脏和其病变的血供均来自正常的肝动脉；变异性血供是指肝脏或其病变存在起源异常的肝动脉供血；寄生性血供主要是指肝脏的病变除了接受肝动脉本身的血供外，还可通过浸润肝脏邻近组织结构或病变的末梢小血管与邻近组织器官的小血管末梢吻合形成侧支，继而从其获取血供。

国内的一些学者基于肝动脉DSA检查也进行了一些研究。2002年有作者分析了1 000例肝动脉DSA资料，对Michels的分型浓缩和修订，从而将肝动脉分为6种类型。也有学者在Ruzicka的分类基础上根据肝动脉起源部位不同又将变异性供血进一步分为5个亚型，即：腹腔动脉-肝右动脉供血型、肠系膜上动脉供血型、胃十二指肠动脉供血型、胃左动脉供血型、肠系膜-胃左动脉供血型。

近年文献报告了Michels分型中尚未列出的少见的肝动脉变异的类型：①双肝动脉，无肝总动脉，肝右动脉和肝左动脉分别起源于腹腔干，胃十二指肠动脉可以起源于肝左、右动脉；②四分叉肝动脉，肝左、中、右动脉和胃十二指肠动脉分别起自肝总动脉；③3支副肝动脉，肝固有动脉如常，发自肝总动脉，分出肝左动脉和肝右动脉，一支副肝右动脉发自胃十二指肠动脉，一支副肝左动脉发自胃左动脉，另一支副肝左动脉发自胃右动脉；④副肝右动脉起自胃左动脉，副肝左动脉起自腹腔干动脉，副肝左动脉起自肝总动脉；⑤肝总动脉起源于腹腔干；⑥替代肝固有动脉起自肠系膜上动脉；⑦替代肝固有动脉起自腹腔干；⑧替代肝固有动脉起自胃左动脉；⑨替代肝右动脉起源于腹腔干；⑩肝动脉起源于胃十二指肠动脉。

这类变异又分为以下几种情况：副肝右动脉起源于胃十二指肠动脉；副肝左动脉起源于胃十二指肠动脉+副肝右动脉起源于肠系膜上动脉：替代肝左动脉起源于胃十二指肠动脉+替代肝右动脉起源于肠系膜上动脉。

肝动脉发育变异包括起源分支走行的变异，其发生率较高，各家报道不一，约占6%~24%。鉴于肝动脉变异的发生率较高，变异类型多样复杂，且近年又有一些新的变异被报道，刻意简化分型会遗漏一些变异，不利于指导具体临床工作，所以对Michels的10类分型进一步补充，将肝动脉变异分为肝动脉分叉异常、替代肝动脉、副肝动脉、替代肝动脉+副肝动脉、肝总动脉起源异常、肝固有动脉起源异常和多种变异共有7大类，再分为24种类型。如临床再配合使用其26条侧支循环途径，则可全面包括肝动脉的变异供血及侧支供血情况。

肝动脉变异影像学研究：CT在腹部应用最有影响力发展就是多探测器螺旋CT（MSCT）薄层扫描结合三维重建，经该技术处理后可清晰显示变异肝动脉的起源及肝内走行，所显示的血管图像在某些方面可与血管造影相媲美。图像后处理使用最大密度投影、容积再现、表面遮盖显示。但是目前CTA还有含碘对比剂的副作用和放射线辐射作用等不足之处。

受饱和伪影、相位弥散、采集时间长等因素的限制，以往常规MRA技术很少被应用于肝动脉的评价。Prince等（1995）使用快速对比三维增强MRA技术显示腹主动脉、肠系膜上动脉和肾动脉。肝脏三维对比增强磁共振血管造影（3D CE MRA）技术可显示腹腔干肝总肝固有和肝右动脉以及一些肝动脉变异。但有关肝动脉发育变异的MRA和DSA的对照研究较少。MRA图像质量与DSA相关性最好的是：肝总动脉、脾动脉、肠系膜上动脉；相关性较好的是：肝固有动脉、胃十二指肠动脉、肝左动脉、胃左动脉；相关性较差的是：胃右动脉、肝右动脉。MRA的不足是不能显示直径小于1mm肝脏动脉，如胃右动脉、肝右动脉分支、替代和副肝动脉。克服这些不足的方法是未来新技术的发展，如：小于1mm的薄层扫描、轴位高分辨率和快速扫描时间等。

有关肝动脉发育变异的超声研究较少。彩色多普勒可显示肝左动脉主干和副肝左动脉。但对左段的动脉供血显示不准确，且不能正确显示左肝动脉的直径和长度，特别是远端分支。 彩色多普勒的优势是可动态观察肝移植和肝癌栓塞化疗术后肝脏动脉血流。

数字减影血管成像（DSA）研究肝动脉变异自然是金标准。它不但可以清晰显示各种肝动脉变异的起源及走行，还能清晰显示正常或异常起源的CTA、MRA无法显示的肝动脉细小分支，并且可用DSA的特殊功能，如岁差运动、旋转功能及C臂CT等，立体清晰显示异常起源肝动脉主干或其中的一个分支。还可作腹主动脉造影、肾动脉造影等。更为重要的是具有引导血管内介入治疗的独特功能。

肝动脉变异的临床意义：肝动脉化学性栓塞或放置化疗泵前应全面了解肝动脉有无变异，以及肝肿瘤的供血动脉，可避免医师误入歧途，预防并发症的发生，或放置不当而影响治疗效果。肝胃间动脉的发现有利于提高TACE的治疗效果，减少并发症的发生，且在胃黏膜动脉出血和胃肿瘤的诊断中有重要意义。利于肝脏外科手术切除前的手术方案选择和制定，以增加手术的准确性，缩短手术时间取得了良好的治疗效果。肝移植手术前了解肝动脉变异为外科医师制定手术方式提供依据。可避免因估计不足等造成术中忙乱及其他一些特殊情况。

了解肝脏病变的动脉三维表现特征：肝硬化CTA图像表现与肝脏体积缩小的程度有关，明显肝硬化患者，肝动脉与门静脉之间的平衡被改变，动脉血液的灌注量增加，而门静脉血流量减少，导致了肝动脉肝内分支显示特征性的螺旋样改变。同时，脾动脉也增粗延长迂曲。

肝癌CTA，尤其是富血供肝癌表现为肿瘤的染色，肿瘤供血动脉明显充盈、增粗、边缘不整齐，伸入瘤灶内，可出现肝动脉-门静脉分流。

肝脏局灶性结节增生不良CTA容积显示法可以显示局灶性结节增生异常的蜘蛛样供血动脉和引流肝静脉，有助于鉴别局灶性结节增生不良和其他病变。

肝脓肿CTA可见周围血管被推压，未见肝内动脉伸入其内，在相邻部位的肝动脉可出现侧支循环充盈。

胰腺癌侵及血管预示肿瘤不能进行手术切除治疗，腹腔动脉及其分支的显示可评价胰腺癌可切除性，尤其是肿瘤比较大且位于胰头部的肿瘤，可显示对肝动脉侵犯情况。

总之，在肝癌化疗药物灌注栓塞治疗、肝脏部分外科切除、全肝或部分肝移植和肝脏疾病的诊疗时，为提高肝脏疾病的诊疗水平和避免严重并发症的发生，全面了解肝动脉变异非常有必要。在各种影像检查手段中，对于肝动脉变异的显示效果方面，DSA是金标准，CTA优于3D CE MRA，3D CE MRA优于超声。这些检查方法各有优点和不足，且都可从不同角度为临床提供肝动脉供血和变异情况。临床了解肝动脉变异并正确选择影像检查手段对各自的实际工作有重要意义。

第二节 关于肝动脉的发育变异

肝动脉的经典型解剖表现仅见于55%的病人中。至少有10种肝动脉发育变异在尸检材料中已有描述。随着螺旋CT与CT血管造影的发展，对肝动脉及其变异成像已成常规。

部分肝动脉发育变异：有些变异与肝中动脉有关。肝中动脉通常来源于肝左或肝右动脉，供应肝左叶的内侧段。大约10%的病人，肝固有动脉直接分成左、中、右三支肝动脉。另一种常见的变异为肝右动脉起源于肠系膜上动脉。

除肝动脉的正常起源外，还有副肝动脉。这些副肝动脉包括起源于胃左动脉的左副肝动脉和起源于肠系膜上动脉的右副肝动脉。副肝动脉为其所属的特定区域单独供血。其他小分支和副肝动脉也可同时参与供血。肝动脉不起自腹腔动脉而起自肠系膜上动脉或胃左动脉者十分少见。肝动脉还可以直接起源于主动脉，与脾动脉的起源相邻。

肝动脉不仅变异常见，而且变异的种类也很多典型分布的肝动脉解剖是指，左、中、右三支肝动脉均发自腹腔-肝总动脉干，否则视为发育变异。

一般将变异动脉分为副动脉和替代动脉。副动脉是指正常动脉之外的一支动脉，它参与通常由正常动脉供血区域中的部分供血。替代动脉是指起源异常的动脉，它供血于通常由正常动脉供血的区域。

肝动脉有相当多的发育变异，其变异发生率高达24.5%~46.5%，变异肝动脉中，发自肠系膜上动脉者最为常见，其次是发自胃左动脉者，此外，还可发自于腹主动脉、肾动脉、胰背动脉等，肝动脉不仅变异常见，而且变异的种类也很多。

一些作者根据 211 例血管造影资料,初步提出将肝动脉解剖分为四大类:腹腔动脉供血型、胃左动脉供血型、肠系膜上动脉供血型和其他动脉供血型,其中后三型为变异。

有关肝动脉的一些发育变异,还可参见巫北海总主编《活体形态学》腹盆上卷, 2006 年第一版,科学出版社。

第三节　肝总动脉变异

目前对于腹部大血管,包括腹腔干和肝总动脉的显示,MSCT 血管造影 CTA 几乎代替了传统的血管造影。DSA 和 CTA 检查对全身大血管显影的对比研究表明, CTA 同样能清晰显示血管走行,并且在判断与邻近器官的解剖关系上优于 DSA。传统的肝总动脉是指从腹腔干发出后到胃十二指肠动脉之间的动脉段。但实际工作中常会遇到不同起源和不同的解剖路径,使肝总动脉的准确识别与定位出现困难。

为更清晰地描述这些发育变异,Song 等(2010)认为肝总动脉应包括一段肝动脉和胃十二指肠动脉,不论它的起源及解剖路径如何。如果胃十二指肠动脉独立起源,而没有任何肝动脉成分,则认为肝总动脉缺如。这种观点不仅能够较完善地评估和解释各种腹腔干及肝总动脉的发育变异,同时也使肝总动脉的正常走行得到准确描述。

腹部大血管来源于胚胎早期 4 支腹主动脉的原始腹支,腹支之间以腹侧纵向吻合支相互连接,肝总动脉作为重要的腹腔血管,发生变异往往与其他血管相关联。

目前肝动脉解剖分型的标准多采用 Michels 分型,这种分型将肝动脉变异分为 10 种类型, Ⅰ ~ Ⅷ型可见正常起源的肝总动脉,即起源于腹腔干,其中Ⅱ ~ Ⅷ型因为肝动脉的变异而出现不同的替代性肝动脉和 / 或副肝动脉参与肝脏的血供,Ⅸ型为肝总动脉起自肠系膜上动脉, Ⅹ型为肝总动脉起自胃左动脉。

这种分型尽管对肝动脉的大部分变异进行了概括,但对肝总动脉的其他不同起源类型(如腹主动脉起源)和解剖路径的变异未进行描述。

肝总动脉是指从腹腔干发出到胃十二指肠和肝固有动脉分支的动脉段,但在工作中会遇到胃十二指肠动脉和肝固有动脉分别独立起源的变异情况,使得肝总动脉的确认存在困难。Michels 分型未考虑肝总动脉的构成,特别是在胃十二指肠动脉独立起源的情况下,这将给肝脏外科手术或肝移植手术增加难度。

为了更准确地评价肝总动脉变异,首先确定其解剖学特征是必要的。Song 等(2010)提出肝总动脉应包括胃十二指肠和肝动脉这 2 个分支,并对肝总动脉缺如的情形也作了说明,即胃十二指肠动脉是肝总动脉的第一分支动脉,是构成肝总动脉的重要条件,当它独立起源时则认定为肝总动脉缺如。这种分型能够较客观地评估和描述各种肝总动脉变异,同时也弥补了 Michels 分型的不足。

正常情况下,肝总动脉从腹腔干发出后,从左至右沿胰头上缘到达幽门部或十二指肠升段水平走行。发出胃十二指肠动脉之前,其末段位于门静脉主干前方。由此可见,肝总动脉作为一个动脉段可能在起源及路径行程这 2 方面出现变异。有作者通过对 1 129 例肝总动脉变异的观察,并结合相关文献将肝总动脉变异分为起源变异、路径变异和肝总动脉缺如 3 种类型,路径变异以胰腺和门静脉主干或肠系膜上静脉为参照、肝总动脉起源变异:肝总动脉可以有 4 种不同位置的起源。即腹腔干、肠系膜上动脉、胃左动脉及腹主动脉,通常将腹腔干以外起源的肝总动脉称为起源变异。Song 等(2010)通过 5 002 例受检者的研究发现肝总动脉起源变异的发生率为 3.5%(176/5002),其中肠系膜上动脉起源变异占 84. 1%,胃左动脉起源变异占 4.5%,腹主动脉起源变异占 11.4%。

Michels 在 200 例尸检中发现肝总动脉起源变异占 5%(10/200),其中肝总动脉起源于肠系膜上动脉 9 例(90%),胃左动脉起源 1 例(10%),但未见腹主动脉起源变异。

一些作者在 180 例患者的 CTA 中发现肠系膜上动脉起源变异和腹主动脉起源变异各 2 例。一组肝总动脉起源变异共 31 例,占 2.7%(31/1129),包括肠系膜上动脉起源 23 例,腹主动脉起源 6 例,胃左动脉起源 2 例。其中肠系膜上动脉起源变异最多见，占该组肝总动脉起源变异的 74%（23/31）。

路径变异：肝总动脉起源于腹腔干，但走行路径不是常规的胰腺上方、门静脉主干前方，而是经过 3 条变异路径，分别为：①经胰腺上方、门静脉后方走行；②经胰腺下方、在肠系膜上静脉前方走行；③穿过胰腺、在肠系膜上静脉前方走行。Song 等（2010）报道此类变异 7 例，占 0.14%（7/5002）。其他文献中也有个案报道。该项研究发现此变异 4 例，全部为经过胰腺上方、门静脉后方变异。

肝总动脉缺如：是指胃十二指肠动脉与肝动脉不共干且二者均独立起源。Song 等（2010）报道 5002 例中胃十二指肠动脉独立起源 55 例，其中 41 例起源于肠系膜上动脉；50 例受检者中 34 例的肝动脉起源于腹腔干，替代肝动脉 21 例。Covey 等（2002）报道在 600 例的肝动脉 DSA 检查中，发现类似于 Song 等报道的肝总动脉缺如 2 例，2 例均是肝动脉起自肠系膜上动脉，胃十二指肠动脉单独起源于腹主动脉。

该项研究此种变异 11 例，其胃十二指肠动脉均起源于腹腔干，肝动脉独立起源肠系膜上动脉 4 例，相当于 Michels 分型中的Ⅸ型；以替代右肝动脉及替代左肝动脉的形式分别独立起源 7 例，类似于 Michels 分型中的Ⅳ型。

随着肝脏外科手术和肝脏介入治疗的不断发展，Michcls 分型的局限性逐渐显示出来。该研究采用 CTA 技术对肝总动脉变异进行了较大样本的研究，并参考 Michels 和 Song 等分型，将肝总动脉变异分为起源变异、路径变异和肝总动脉缺如 3 种类型，能够为临床医生提供可靠的、较全面的解剖学参考。同时对于肝总动脉的下级动脉分支、替代性或副肝动脉的描述也将变得更简便。随着肝脏外科手术和肝移植的进步，术前对腹部大血管及肝动脉的影像评价变得非常重要。传统的血管造影检查操作复杂，风险大，目前多被 CTA 取代。64 层 MSCT 的各向同性，为多方位显示各部位活体形态学奠定了基础，结合后处理技术，可清晰显示肝总动脉走行路径及与周围脏器的解剖关系，为手术提供快捷和清晰的影像资料。

第四节　肝动脉的假性动脉瘤

肝假性动脉瘤是钝伤或穿通伤少见的并发症。假性动脉瘤可引起胆系梗阻，自发性肝内或肝周出血，动 - 静脉瘘或胆系出血。假性动脉瘤能为团注对比剂动态 CT 扫描诊断，并为彩色多普勒超声证实。选择性动脉造影用以确诊和进行治疗性栓塞。Andersen（1971）报告左肝动脉假性动脉瘤继发于胆囊切除术，指出本症病因学除手术创伤外，还有：腹部钝伤、胆管结石压迫右肝动脉、系统性感染、动脉硬化等，不常见病因为梅毒和肝脓肿。该作者回顾文献共 26 例，22 例死亡，其中 12 例一直到去世也未能认识本症。单纯剖腹术容易漏掉单个的动脉瘤，故术前动脉造影是诊断的必要措施。经皮肝穿胆汁引流通常是安全和有效的，然可出现一些并发症，诸如败血症、出血和胆汁性腹膜炎等。

引流时出血进入胆管并不少见，但几乎总是可以自行停止或保守治疗痊愈。不过也可出现危及生命的出血，有的立即发生于引流术后，有的作为迟发的并发症，有的却见于常规更换导管时。经肝胆汁引流时，途经导管或围绕导管出血是肝内假性动脉瘤、动脉 - 门静脉瘘以及血肿最常见的临床表现，此刻手术治疗甚为困难，因其损害通常深藏于肝实质之中，且多位于浸润性病变或肝门附近肿瘤中，经肝内途径进行介入放射学的栓塞治疗常可成功地控制出血。

第五节　肝动脉成像中的误诊

为最佳显示肝动脉，CT 扫描必须在动脉期进行，采用薄层及窄间隔扫描。这种检查最好不要口服阳性对比剂，三维 CT 血管造影有助于评价肝动脉及其变异。

肝动脉血栓形成：肝动脉血栓形成可以导致肝脏不均匀强化或散在的肝梗死，这是最常见的外科手术包括腹腔镜胆囊切除术并发症之一，但也可以发生于腹部外伤。

肝动脉瘤:肝动脉瘤很少见,它通常是动脉粥样硬化的结果,肝动脉钙化的显示有助于肝动脉瘤的诊断。肝动脉瘤也可发生于静脉吸毒者或继发于外伤。肝动脉瘤常很小(小于2cm),在CT图像上显示为富血管性病变,似血管瘤改变。要注意的是必须确认血管的走向,以避免严重错误。假性动脉瘤与真性动脉瘤CT表现相同,但前者常继发于胆管导管放置或动脉内化疗和活检后。

另外,罕见的肝动脉-门静脉瘘也可以发生,这常常继发于外伤、活检或外科手术,需要在动脉期扫描才能达到最佳观察效果。

第三章　一过性肝实质强化

第一节　一过性肝实质强化

肝灌注异常，是一种局限性或弥漫性的肝脏血流动力学异常改变，由Itai等在进行团注动态CT研究时首先发现，并称之为一过性肝实质强化或称一过性肝实质强化差异，是指螺旋CT动态增强扫描时于动脉期出现局部肝内以叶、段或亚段分布的高密度影，典型CT表现为肝动脉期一过性楔形或三角形高密度强化区，边缘平直，常位于肝脏边缘部位，其中血管走行正常，而门静脉期恢复正常肝脏密度。造成一过性肝实质强化的因素多种多样。

诊断标准：一过性肝实质强化按Chen等（1999）执行的标准判断：①异常灌注区域在动脉期表现为高密度，而门静脉期恢复到正常等密度或接近等密度，延迟期均表现为等密度；②异常灌注区域呈楔形、节段性、叶性分布；③异常灌注区域有正常血管通过；④对有争议或表现不典型者，运用其他影像学检查手段结合临床资料未能发现器质性病变的证据。

一过性肝实质强化形成的病理生理基础：肝脏具有独特的肝动脉和门静脉双重供血系统。门静脉血流量占70%~75%，肝动脉血流量占25%~30%。这种独特的双重供血是进行肝脏双期螺旋CT（SCT）增强扫描诊断疾病的解剖学基础。

肝脏肿瘤以肝动脉血供的多少分为富血供、中等血供和少血供病变。以肝动脉供血为主的富血供病变，在肝动脉期表现为高于肝实质密度；而此期由于对比剂尚未到达门静脉，以门静脉供血为主的肝实质则呈相对低密度表现。门静脉期正常肝实质强化明显，而上述多血供病变呈等或稍低密度影，与明显强化的肝实质密度差异小，容易漏诊。显然，门静脉期是少血供肿瘤最佳显示期。和传统CT相比，螺旋CT具有快速容积采集数据、无运动伪影、便于双期增强扫描等优势。

正常肝脏的双重血供并非2个独立系统，两者之间有许多交通吻合，包括：肝窦间通路；脉管间途径；血管丛途径，即胆管周围血管丛途径。甚至在某些病理情况下，肝动脉和门静脉可以通过跨肿瘤途径相交通。当肝脏发生血供障碍时，通过神经-体液因素的调节这些交通吻合支开放，双重供血发生血流量的变化甚至血流方向的改变。

一过性肝实质强化反映了局部肝脏双重血供的重新分布，即局部肝实质门静脉或肝静脉血流量减少及伴随的肝动脉门静脉分流或局部肝脏的变异或迷走血供所致。一过性肝实质强化发生率占肝脏双期螺旋CT扫描的13%。影像科医师认识一过性肝实质强化的CT表现有利于肝脏疾病的准确诊断。

分类：根据一过性肝实质强化形态学表现分为4种。

（1）肝叶、多段型：一个肝叶或一叶几乎所有肝段均表现一过性肝实质强化。常常由于原发性肝动脉血流量增加所致，因此其形态和肝动脉分布区相一致。

（2）扇形：表现为三角形或扇形一过性肝实质强化，和正常肝实质有一个清楚的分界线，形成一个平直边缘，又称之为“平直边缘征”。

（3）多形态型：一过性肝实质强化表现为多种形态和大小，无“平直边缘征”的表现。

（4）弥漫型：弥漫分布的斑片状一过性肝实质强化或沿胆管周围分布。

引起一过性肝实质强化常见的原因及机制：根据病因病理和血流动力学改变将肝动脉血流增多所致的一过性肝实质强化分为原发性和继发性。

引起一过性肝实质强化常见下述原因：

(1)肝动脉门静脉分流:肝动脉门静脉分流是形成一过性肝实质强化最常见的原因之一。它是肝动脉分支和门静脉系统之间的一种器质性或功能性的交通,最终导致局部血流重新分布,肝动脉血流进入门静脉分布区。当门静脉阻塞或受压时,肝动脉门静脉分流起重要作用。

引起肝动脉门静脉分流的途径有:明显的肝动脉门静脉瘘,常为医源性所致;肝窦间通路,小的小叶间动脉和门静脉分支之间的吻合途径;脉管间吻合途径,由于肿瘤栓塞所致;经肿瘤途径,通过来自富血供肿瘤的引流静脉途径;血管丛途径或胆管周围血管丛途径。

引起肝动脉门静脉分流的原因包括:肝脏肿瘤,如肝细胞癌、肝血管瘤和胆管细胞癌;肝外伤或肝脏穿刺活检、脓肿引流、无水乙醇注射等介入治疗;肝硬化;其他少见的功能性肝动脉门静脉分流;肝转移瘤、肝动脉瘤破裂、先天畸形也可出现肝动脉门静脉分流。

该组有1例不明原因一过性肝实质强化,临床无任何异常发现,于动脉期可见肝动脉与门静脉相应分支吻合,考虑为先天发育变异。肝动脉门静脉分流的螺旋CT征象不仅表现为肝动脉期门静脉分支早显,还可表现一过性、肝脏周边部位楔形或三角形肝实质强化,常有一平直的边缘。当一过性肝实质强化为唯一发现时,肝动脉门静脉分流引起的一过性肝实质强化有时与肝脏结节样病灶很相像,因而难以鉴别。

(2)门静脉阻塞:门静脉阻塞是形成一过性肝实质强化另一常见原因。门静脉由于栓塞(血栓、菌栓或癌栓)、肿瘤的直接侵犯、压迫或手术结扎等原因而阻塞时,其血流量减少,肝动脉通过以下途径使血流量代偿性增多,即肝窦间通路、脉管间的吻合途径、经肿瘤途径尤其是血管丛途径,亦即胆管周围血管丛途径形成的功能性肝动脉门静脉分流(此时门静脉变成引流静脉)起重要的代偿作用,同时继发性肝淋巴管扩张,容量增大,典型动脉期表现弥漫性不均匀性网格状强化,维持到门静脉期。双期螺旋CT中的表现为:平扫受累肝实质由于水肿、纤维化的原因密度减低;增强扫描动脉期常见呈大片状、三角形一过性肝实质强化;显示门静脉内低密度充盈缺损或门静脉受压迫的直接征象。当门静脉主干发生栓塞时,以尾叶和左叶内侧段为主的中央部位的肝组织,由门静脉的侧支静脉代偿供血;而以右叶为主的周边部位肝脏则门静脉血流供应明显减少,肝动脉代偿性血流增多,肝动脉期可见肝脏周边部位散在分布的一过性肝实质强化,又称为“中心-边缘现象”。

(3)肝硬化:肝硬化是引起肝实质坏死的主要原因,肝实质内结缔组织增生、纤维化、肝细胞再生结节和假小叶的形成等均可导致肝内脉管系统扭曲,门静脉高压。众所周知,肝硬化时正常肝脏的血流动力学发生改变,肝动脉血流增多,门静脉血流减少。

肝硬化病人肝动脉期出现高密度强化灶时通常诊断肝细胞性肝癌,然而一过性肝实质强化在肝动脉期也表现为高密度区,与肝细胞癌有相似表现。一过性肝实质强化表现为肝动脉期楔形、平直边缘征、其内有正常的血管走行、门静脉期呈等密度表现等有利于鉴别。鉴别诊断困难时可行MR检查,一过性肝实质强化在T_1WI和T_2WI中均表现正常。

(4)肝肿瘤:常见肝细胞癌,有时合并门静脉受压,但很少合并肝静脉受压。肝细胞癌时,可通过脉管间途径(由于门静脉栓塞)、肿瘤途径或肝窦间途径形成肝动脉门静脉分流。63%的肝细胞癌具有肝动脉门静脉分流。此外,门静脉受阻时胆管周围血管丛也起重要的代偿作用。对于肝细胞癌病人,明确门静脉内有无癌栓是很重要的,因为这直接关系到病人的治疗和预后。位于肝门部的胆管癌肝动脉期常表现为肝叶分布的一过性肝实质强化,这是血管受侵犯的一个重要指征。周边部位的胆管癌发生一过性肝实质强化概率为29%~45%。

(5)肝脏外伤:腹部外伤和肝脏的多种介入诊疗有时可致肝动脉和门静脉系统之间器质性交通,或由于门静脉的损伤产生功能性的肝动脉门静脉分流。肝脏的穿刺活检、胆管或脓肿的引流可产生医源性动脉门静脉瘘。肝动脉假性动脉瘤在CT增强的肝动脉期表现为局灶性、圆形、强化病灶,类似富血供肿瘤。

(6)肝静脉阻塞:肝静脉阻塞可继发于右心衰、心包疾患、布-加综合征或纵隔纤维化。肝静脉阻塞时肝血窦内压力增高,肝窦和门静脉之间的压力梯度反转,此时门静脉成为肝脏的引流静脉,肝动脉血流增多,同肝硬化时一样导致功能性肝动脉门静脉分流。

CT表现为受阻肝静脉分布区一过性肝实质强化,其形态表现与门静脉阻塞时相似,均为楔形,但前者尖端指向下腔静脉的特点有利于和门静脉受阻所致的楔形尖端指向肝门部的一过性肝实质强化鉴别。通常肝静脉阻塞表现不均匀、网状或马赛克样一过性肝实质强化可延续于门静脉期，而在延迟扫描时方变成等密度。布-加综合征病人的肝脏尾叶不受影响，因其有独立的引流静脉。

（7）遗传性出血性毛细血管扩张症：即Osler-Weber-Rendu病，是一种常染色体显性遗传性血管疾病。病理改变以多发毛细血管扩张、动静脉畸形为特征。人体任何部位均可受累，以皮肤黏膜受累最常见，肝脏也可受累。在肝脏常见肝动脉分支与肝静脉、门静脉分支间的动静脉分流。由于病人常无症状，所以临床上无准确发生率的统计。遗传性出血性毛细血管扩张症肝脏病理改变包括：肝动脉扩张、扭曲；肝脏毛细血管扩张；肝动静脉或肝动门脉肝动脉门静脉分流或动静脉瘘。遗传性出血性毛细血管扩张症肝脏受累及可导致肝脏纤维结缔组织增生和不典型肝硬化、高心排出量和由于心脏左至右分流导致的充血性心力衰竭；而门体循环分流可导致门静脉高压、胃肠道出血、腹水及门体循环性脑病。螺旋CT增强扫描的肝动脉期见扭曲、扩张的肝动脉，肝脏显示增大，肝静脉可见扩张；当有肝动脉门静脉分流发生时，扩张的肝动脉和肝静脉同时显影，同时可见多发、不均匀且周边部位呈楔形的一过性肝实质强化灌注区。

（8）富血供肿瘤的“盗血现象”：肝脏富血供肿瘤及肿瘤样病变，如肝细胞癌、局灶性结节性增生、血管瘤、肝腺瘤及富血供的转移瘤，一方面所在肝段或肝叶的肝动脉血流量较正常肝组织明显增多，另一方面由于局部肝实质动脉血流增加，产生虹吸效应，对周围肝实质产生“盗血现象”，使邻近肝组织代偿性获得较多的肝动脉血流，也可出现一过性肝实质强化。

（9）炎性病灶：常见于肝脓肿、胆管炎、胆囊炎和急性胰腺炎等。急性炎症病变常常引起局部组织充血、水肿及炎性细胞浸润，局部动脉血流量增加；此外炎症所致的局部水肿可致门静脉血流障碍，使门静脉血流明显减少，肝动脉血流量代偿性增多。

肝脓肿发生一过性肝实质强化概率为30%~67%。CT上表现肝动脉期局部肝脏一过性肝实质强化，门静脉恢复正常肝脏密度。一过性肝实质强化可围绕在炎性病灶的周围。此外，肝脓肿还可导致门静脉血流阻滞。

（10）肝脏变异血供或称作迷走血供：肝脏的迷走血供，如胆囊静脉、副胆囊静脉、包膜静脉或迷走胃右静脉等构成“肝的第三流入道”，静脉血流可引流至肝窦内。局部静脉回流过早，于肝动脉期可将含有对比剂的血液引流入局部肝窦，形成一过性肝实质强化。常见于胆囊窝附近、肝门前方（第Ⅳ肝段后缘）、镰状韧带附近及肝包膜下区的肝组织。肝脏变异血供往往需血管造影最终确立诊断。

有作者报告3例急性胆囊炎患者呈半环状强化，其产生的原因之一可能是胆囊周围肝实质接受了胆囊异常引流的静脉血流。这些含对比剂的静脉血流由于路径短而早于来源于门静脉的血流进入局部肝实质引起一过性肝实质强化，而门静脉期这种强化差别消失。

（11）肝实质受压迫：正常肝脏血流动力学状态下，门静脉系统呈低压状态，肝动脉系统为高压状态。肝内或肝外病灶的压迫使肝实质压力增高，低压状态的门静脉系统更容易受影响，门静脉血流量减少，受累肝段的肝动脉血流代偿性增加；但肝动脉血流量降低时则不引起门静脉血流的增加。肝外脏器或病变，如肋骨、肝脏周围腹膜种植性肿瘤、肝包膜下积液等的压迫同样可导致局部肝实质压力升高，受压部位出现一过性肝实质强化，但当这些外压因素被解除时，血流动力学恢复正常。

（12）其他原因：除上述原因外，肝外门静脉主干及肠系膜上静脉受阻引起一过性肝实质强化，或下腔静脉阻塞后血流经胸廓静脉、腹壁上静脉引流肝圆韧带进入门静脉左支，引起肝左叶内侧段一过性肝实质强化。

局部肝动脉血流增加：富血供肿瘤和炎性充血可引起局部病灶周围肝动脉血流增加，从而出现一过性肝实质强化现象。有作者报告2例胆囊炎术后患者，术前增强检查未出现一过性肝实质强化，故考虑为术后炎性充血出现此征象。

上腔静脉阻塞也可导致楔形一过性肝实质强化，常见于左内叶。肝转移性肿瘤早期也可出现，我们就曾见下咽癌肝转移性肿瘤的病例。

此外，临床上还有一些原因不明的一过性肝实质强化。

一过性肝实质强化与肝脏实质性病灶的鉴别诊断：肝细胞癌、血管瘤一般由于其有典型的CT强化特征，故不难与一过性肝实质强化相区别。一些肝转移瘤（尤其是来源于神经内分泌性肿瘤）、肝腺瘤、肝局灶性结节增生在动脉期也可呈均匀强化,但在延迟扫描时一般都是低密度,有别于一过性肝实质强化。

部分肝血管瘤、肝岛容易与一过性肝实质强化混淆,这些病灶动脉期可表现出明显结节状或斑片状强化,此时主要观察静脉期及延长期病灶特点,血管瘤有其强化特点,具有延迟向心性强化特点;弥漫性脂肪肝中的肝岛平扫呈相对低密度影,多位于胆囊或肝包膜下,其动态增强扫描曲线与脂肪变肝实质大致相符,借此可资鉴别。肝硬化结节、小肝癌等,尤其位于肝包膜下区域时,有时鉴别诊断困难。

此外,一过性肝实质强化还需与弥漫性脂肪肝中的肝岛相鉴别。正常肝岛在平扫时呈相对高密度,多位于胆囊、叶间裂附近或肝包膜下,注射对比剂后其时间 - 密度曲线与脂肪变的肝组织相一致,由此易与一过性肝实质强化鉴别。

正确识别一过性肝实质强化的临床意义:一过性肝实质强化是肝脏团注动态增强检查肝动脉期局部肝密度异常强化,既非伪影亦非病灶本身,但它反映了潜在的肝脏异常,反映肝脏血流动力学改变的重要信息,并可能是多种肝脏疾病伴随的特征性改变。

正确识别一过性肝实质强化,有助于寻找或区分可能与一过性肝实质强化伴随的肝内或肝外病灶,尤其是恶性病灶。有助于消除诊断带来的困惑,同时能够避免肝脏肿瘤和其他病变的假阳性或假阴性诊断及其过高估计肝脏病变的范围。对于一些部位或形态不典型的灌注异常,应密切结合临床和实验室指标等检查进行追踪随访。

对不明原因的一过性肝实质强化,应密切结合临床和实验室指标及其他检查进行随访。由此,可以避免肝脏病灶的漏诊、假阳性诊断或对病变范围的过多估计。

第二节 一过性(暂时性)肝实质强化

一过性(暂时性)肝实质强化在双期 CT 上所见为一过性肝脏密度(衰减)差异,在双期 MRI 上所见为一过性肝脏信号强度差异,在实时超声上所见为一过性回波差异。

其发生机制有:动脉供血增加、门静脉分支阻塞、异常肝脏血供和动脉门静脉分流。

病因 一过性(暂时性)肝实质强化是指某个无肿瘤区域在增强动脉期的 CT 密度、MR 信号或超声回波分别增加,而到门静脉期即成为等密度、等信号或等回波。典型的一过性肝脏密度差异表现为边缘锐直的楔形区内无肿块和血管穿过。一旦出现一过性肝脏密度差异,应寻找其伴同的病变,即足以引起一过性密度增高的动脉 - 门静脉分流和门静脉阻塞的原因。门静脉阻塞可引起相应的动脉血流增加和门静脉血流减少。相似的现象也见于肝实质受压导致的门静脉血流减少(表 10-3-1)。

表 10-3-1 一过性肝脏密度差异的病因及其对应疾病

病因	疾病
动脉 - 门静脉分流	伴存病变:肝细胞癌、血管瘤、胆管癌、富血管性转移;医源性:介入手术;先天性:动脉 - 门静脉分流;肝硬化
肝内血管(门静脉)受压或阻塞	肿瘤:良性(血管瘤、局灶性结节性增生),恶性(肝细胞癌、胆管癌、肝转移);炎症:继发于胆囊炎、肝脓肿、胆管炎
血管异常:迷走血管供应	变异血管:副胆囊静脉、异位胃右静脉;遗传性出血性毛细血管扩张症;心血管病变:右心衰竭、心包病变、布 - 加综合征、纵隔纤维化
富血管(供)的窃血现象	肝细胞癌;富血管的肝转移:胰岛细胞瘤、类癌、肾细胞癌和乳腺癌

肝硬化肝脏中一过性肝脏密度差异的形成原因可能有:硬化肝脏内包含有很小的非肿瘤性动脉 - 门静脉分流;也可能是由继发的伴有动脉 - 门静脉分流的肝细胞性肝癌所引起。因此,在肝硬化病人中见有一过性肝脏密度差异时都需深入探索其原因。

2. 影像学研究:一过性(暂时性)肝实质强化在 CT、MRI 以及超声动态增强成像中出现时,仅于动脉期呈现或不呈现肝叶、段或亚段分布的强化灶，部分一过性（暂时性）肝实质强化在其内或邻近可见局限性炎性或良、恶性肿瘤性病变，它们可能就是一过性（暂时性）肝实质强化的原因。

增强CT动脉期，一过性（暂时性）肝实质强化表现为单个（或多个）三角形、楔形或不规则形的暂时性等高密度区；门静脉期则表现为等或轻度高密度区。MRI平扫T_1WI和T_2WI影像上均呈现肝段或亚段等信号强度，MRI动态增强表现与增强CT表现相似。

一过性（暂时性）肝实质强化（一过性肝脏密度差异或一过性肝脏信号强度差异）可有3个表现型：①扇形，由门静脉低灌注区与动脉高灌注区之间界线为缘的三角形区；②多形态强化差异，具有不同形状和范围，常没有一条直线的边；③弥漫性强度差异，分布的多样表现，通常是多个相等大小的暂时性强化病灶，血流阻塞于窦状隙前、后或窦状隙水平。

3. 鉴别诊断　累及肝叶或亚段的一过性（暂时性）肝实质强化在影像学上大多表现典型。而较小（<1.0cm）且形态规则者，则需与小肝细胞癌进行鉴别。在肝硬化或慢性肝炎病人中，一过性（暂时性）肝实质强化大多为伴或不伴局限性病变的动脉门静脉分流所致，不伴肝脏局限性病变的一过性（暂时性）肝实质强化需与小肝细胞癌的鉴别（表10-3-2）。鉴别有困难时，可行穿刺活检；伴有肝脏局限病变的一过性（暂时性）肝实质强化，即使为小肝细胞癌伴有一过性（暂时性）肝实质强化，往往不难鉴别，可根据同时显示的小肝细胞癌影像学特征做出定性诊断。

表10-3-2　不伴肝局限性病灶的一过性（暂时性）肝实质强化与小肝细胞癌的鉴别诊断

疾病	鉴别诊断			
	三期动态增强CT或MRI	MRI T_2WI SPIO* 肝脏成像	CT或MRI随访	超声检查
不伴肝局限性病灶的一过性肝实质强化	仅动脉期强化，少数可伴门静脉分支显影	不能显示	可能消失	不能显示
小肝细胞性肝癌	动脉期强化；部分门静脉延迟期呈低密度或低信号强度；有假包膜显影	能显示（高分化者可不显示）	不消失，并可能长大	能显示

第三节　肝外胆管细胞癌所致肝实质一过性密度差异

详见本书 本卷 第十六篇 第十三章 第一节　肝外胆管细胞癌所致肝实质一过性密度差异。

第四章　肝脏血流灌注异常

第一节　多层面动态 MRI 中肝左叶内段早期增强的假病灶

Ito（1993）采用多层面动态 MRI 诊断肝脏肿瘤或肝硬化时，在动脉期影像上偶尔发现一个早期增强的假病灶，他为探讨引起这种现象的机制及其临床意义，特意回顾分析了 185 例怀疑肝脏疾患的多层面动态 MRI 图像，包括 93 例肝细胞癌，肝硬化 35 例，肝海绵状血管瘤 26 例，转移瘤 14 例，囊肿 9 例，脂肪肝 4 例，胆管癌和恶性淋巴瘤各 2 例。

使用 1.5T 超导机，首先应用常规自旋回波 T_1WI（500/15）和 T_2WI（2000/90）横断扫描，然后进行梯度回波的屏气多层面动态 MRI 扫描（150/6），偏转角 60°，屏一口气采集 10 幅图像，平扫后静脉注射 Gd-DTPA，在 20~46 秒时扫描获得动脉期图像，3 分钟时行延迟扫描。6 例疑假病灶的患者在行 MRI 的前和后两周都作了超声和 CT 检查，4 例作了血管造影，此 6 例均进行了 6 个月的超声和 CT 随访。

该项研究结果发现，185 例患者中，6 例在动脉期时可见肝左叶内段早期增强的假病灶，4 例肝硬化，1 例肝细胞癌，1 例脂肪肝，病灶都位于肝左叶内段靠近肝门处的包膜下，病灶直径为 10~25mm，5 例为卵圆形，1 例为三角形。

在 T_1 和 T_2WI，除 1 例脂肪肝患者外，其余 5 例在早期增强假病灶的相应位置处未见异常，在增强前及延迟的多层面动态扫描 MRI 图像上假病灶与周围肝脏组织呈等信号；超声、CT 及血管造影上均未见相应的病灶。1 例脂肪肝患者，CT 平扫假病灶呈高密度，MRI T_1WI 呈低信号，增强前快速小角度激发成像呈稍高信号区。

该作者推测，引起早期增强假病灶的原因可能是由于肝左叶内段近肝门处包膜下区接受胆囊动脉和肝动脉的供血，使该区较周围肝实质有较丰富的血液供应；胆囊的引流静脉系统亦与门静脉周围小支有交通，通过此门 - 体交通，胆囊静脉血供较门脉系统血液更快地进入肝窦，在动脉期造成假病灶出现。

在延迟期，门脉血进入肝窦使得病灶与周围肝脏实质呈等信号。在多层面动态 MRI 图像上，富血管肿瘤在动脉期显示增强，肝左叶内段早期增强的假病灶可误认为肿瘤，所以在多层面动态 MR 成像上出现典型部位的早期增强病灶应考虑到假病灶的可能。

第二节　肝脏的高灌注异常

正常肝脏的血供 25% 来源于肝动脉，75% 来自门静脉。在 CT 动态增强时，两者均携对比剂进入肝脏。

肝动脉血流带来的对比剂较随门静脉内到来者早 20~30s；此时（即动态增强动脉早期）主要是由肝动脉提供对比剂对肝脏起增强作用，而同时流入的门静脉血流中尚不含对比剂，因此具有稀释对比剂的效用，CT 影像上显示为肝实质强化不明显或仅获得轻微强化，主动脉和肝动脉强化、明亮，而门静脉系统和肝静脉未被强化。

在注射对比剂 20~30s 后（门静脉期），才由门静脉为主带有大量对比剂进入肝内，使肝脏呈现明显强化。

由门静脉血管栓塞或血栓形成，以及肝内恶性肿瘤或炎症等浸润、压迫和/或阻塞邻近门静脉造成门静脉血流减少，引发肝内动脉-门静脉分流及通过肝静脉的异常回流增加。导致肝内病变部位（肝叶、肝段或亚段、肝包膜下）在动态增强扫描动脉期的动脉血流（含较多对比剂）增加，显示为早期强化区出现范围大小不等的高灌注异常（表10-4-1）。

表 10-4-1　肝脏的高灌注异常发生部位及原因

部位及特征	原因
肝叶/肝段	门静脉血栓形成，由恶性肿瘤阻塞造成，动脉门静脉分流的结扎，富血管的胆囊疾病
亚段	外周门静脉分支阻塞，急性胆囊炎，细针抽吸活检
全肝、异质性	肝硬化
包膜下	特发性
其他	胃或胆囊静脉的异位引流

第三节　肝脏的第三供血血管与“假性病变”

人们对肝脏的双重血供已熟知，却很少注意到部分肝组织还有一些其他的供血血管，Yoshimitsu等（2001）称之为肝脏的第3供血血管，它常由体循环的一些正常或迷走的静脉不经门静脉系统直接进入肝脏而形成。由于这些血管常对肝脏的第Ⅰ、Ⅳ段供血，故在该区易形成这种独特的血流动力学状况，并由此导致该区门静脉血供的减少或缺失，在动脉性门静脉造影CT（CTAP）上形成灌注缺损区。

所谓“假性病变”，是指能够在CTAP图像上形成的灌注缺损区，而其本身并不是一种有临床意义的真性病变。多种因素均可导致假性病变形成，如因肝硬化或明显的肝内血管受压而致的侧支循环开放，各种原因所致的肝内肝动脉-门静脉瘘等，均可在CTAP图像上形成灌注缺损区而形成假性病变。

此处所描述的肝脏第Ⅰ、Ⅳ段假性病变仅限于上述独特的血流动力学所致者，其在CT平扫和经静脉动态增强CT扫描中可有两种类型的表现。第1种类型为CT平扫上无异常发现，而在动态增强CT图像上，Ⅰ、Ⅳ段肝实质可出现一过性的异常灌注区。第2种类型为在CT平扫上，该区出现相对的低或高密度灶，在动态增强CT图像上亦有明显的异常灌注表现。两者的区别在于CT平扫上假性病变是否出现密度的异常。

若这种独特的血流动力学状况已持续很久，那么就有可能造成局部肝实质的代谢发生变化，形成局灶性脂肪肝，或在肝实质代谢改变而出现脂肪浸润时，该区则形成弥漫性脂肪肝中所谓的正常“肝岛”，此两者在CT平扫上均有密度的异常，即为第2种类型的假性病变表现。

一、胆囊静脉

胆囊静脉可以分成两组，第1组为一些细小的分支，直接进入肝脏第Ⅳ、Ⅴ段，这些分支向胆囊体和底部周围的肝实质供血，其在肝内与门静脉的周围分支相交通，从而稀释了该区的门静脉血流，为假性病变的形成提供了基础。

这种血供特点可在胆囊旁区形成动态增强扫描中的一过性异常灌注表现（即第1种类型的假性病变），也可形成弥漫性脂肪肝中的正常“肝岛”，而目前尚未见到该区可形成局灶性脂肪浸润的报道，其原因可能是胆囊静脉血成分中各种营养物质、激素及其他因子对局部肝组织的作用，使之不会产生脂肪浸润。

CT平扫表现：第1种类型假性病变无密度异常，而“肝岛”则表现为在周围相对密度较低的肝组织衬托下，围绕胆囊周围的薄层相对高密度区，其他典型表现还包括非结节样的外形、不清楚的边界和无定形的形态。

动态增强CT扫描：由于解剖关系的邻近，流经该组静脉的血液快速进入肝脏，故在动脉期有可能出现胆囊旁区的肝实质提早强化的表现,类似于肿瘤的早期强化。尤其在急性胆囊炎以及胆囊癌时,胆囊的血供异常增加,这种早期强化的假性病变可能更加明显,因而在胆囊癌中不应将这种提早强化区与胆囊癌的局部肝实质侵犯相混淆。

在门静脉期,第1种假性病变基本呈等密度,即仅在动脉期出现一过性高灌注表现。而"肝岛"并不是想当然的表现为等密度或相对低密度区,其原因有以下两方面:假性病变区只是门静脉血供被稀释,并不是完全被替代,故该区在门脉期仍有一定程度的强化;周围受脂肪浸润的肝组织,其强化程度较正常时略低,故多数病例中,假性病变区在门静脉期仍表现为相对高密度。由于这组胆囊静脉较短小,故它们在静脉性增强CT扫描中大多不显示。

CT血管成像(CTA)和CTAP表现:在经导管选择性胆囊动脉造影的CTA图像上,这两种类型的假性病变均表现为浓密的高密度区,而在CTAP图像上则表现为局部的灌注缺损区。结合CTA和CTAP的灌注表现,常能将假性病变与肿瘤鉴别开。

第2组胆囊静脉穿过胆囊三角汇入肝门区的胆管旁静脉丛,并构成该静脉丛的前上部分,再引流入肝脏的第Ⅰ、Ⅳ段,亦可形成假性病变,见下述胆管旁静脉系统节。

二、胆管旁静脉系统

该静脉丛走行于肝十二指肠韧带中,主要由3组静脉汇成,即包括上述第2组胆囊静脉,收集胰头区静脉血的胰十二指肠静脉和收集胃远端小网膜囊侧静脉血的胃右静脉(或称幽门静脉),并分别构成该静脉丛的前上、下外侧和内侧部分。多数情况下,这些静脉引流入门静脉主干或门静脉系统的较大分支。但偶尔它们在肝门附近汇合形成静脉网并附着于胆管壁上,沿着胆管直接进入肝脏,该静脉系统由此得名。

入肝后,该静脉系统或与门静脉系统的小分支汇合,或继续分支形成一支向某个肝段单独灌注的血管。胆管旁静脉丛进入肝内可以与除Ⅷ段外的所有肝段内的门静脉分支相交通,其中交通频率最大的是第Ⅰ、Ⅳ段内的门静脉分支。而且,由胆管旁静脉丛向肝段的供血中,不经与门静脉小分支的广泛交通,而直接以较大分支形式向肝段供血的情况仅发生在第Ⅰ、Ⅳ段。

其向第Ⅳ段的供血包括以下两种形式:一种是一个较大的胆管旁静脉分支独立于门静脉左支,直接进入Ⅳ段;另一种形式是与门静脉左支的分支相汇合后向Ⅳ段供血。以上述方式向肝脏Ⅳ段供血的血管多来自于胃右静脉,且在Ⅳ段背侧假性病变的研究中,有关迷走胃右静脉的报道也最多。但各家报道的迷走胃右静脉的影像学检出率不尽相同,Takayasu等(1990)统计的血管造影检出率为1.5%,Fernandez和Bernardino(1991)在其50例研究中,检出率为14%,而Matsui等(1994)在其300例研究中,检出率为6%。

由于胆管旁静脉丛的血管分支间有着丰富的交通,故在三组中,何组静脉在形成假性病变中成为主要因素,是由这些交通血管中的血流方向和血流量来决定,也有可能假性病变是由多根静脉共同形成。

至于形成的假性病变是局灶性脂肪肝,还是弥漫性脂肪肝中的正常"肝岛",有作者提出可能与迷走血管中的血液成分有关,由胰十二指肠静脉灌注Ⅳ段形成的假性病变多为局灶性脂肪肝,其原因可能与该血管中富含胰岛素有关,而由第2组胆囊静脉和迷走的胃右静脉灌注形成的假性病变中,两者均可发生,但以弥漫性脂肪肝中的正常"肝岛"为多,出现这种同样部位、同样的血供变异为什么在某些病例中形成局灶性脂肪肝,而在另一些病例中却形成弥漫性脂肪肝中的正常"肝岛",其具体机制目前尚不明确。

CT平扫表现:第1种类型的假性病变无异常密度,局灶性脂肪肝表现为局限性低密度,而"肝岛"则为局限性相对高密度区。

动态增强CT表现:第1种类型的假性病变并不一定都显示出异常灌注的特点,因为胆管旁静脉丛常在Ⅰ、Ⅳ段肝内与门静脉的分支相交通,故含对比剂的血液经门静脉血液的稀释后对肝实质的强化作用已明显下降;只有在胆管旁静脉丛的分支向Ⅰ、Ⅳ段单独供血的情况下,假性病变区才有可能出现一过性高灌注表现。

局灶性脂肪肝和"肝岛"在CT动态增强扫描的动脉晚期均有强化表现,因为含对比剂的血液经胆管旁静脉丛流入Ⅳ段假性病变区的时间要短于经肠系膜上静脉回流至肝脏的血流。故在门静脉期肝实质增强之前,假性病变区先发生强化。但局灶性脂肪肝仍表现为相对低密度区,只是与周围肝实质的密度差有所缩小;而弥漫性脂肪肝中的正常"肝岛"仍为相对高密度区,但与周围肝实质的密度差进一步加大。门静脉期由于周围肝实质明显强化，故两种假性病变与周围肝实质的密度差分别增大和缩小，但仍为相对低和高密度区。

由胆管旁静脉丛供血引起的假性病变中，Ⅳ段背侧的典型部位非常关键，对诊断的确立有很大的价值。另外，假性病变的边界可以不清晰，也可较清晰，这取决于胆管旁静脉丛在肝内是否与门脉分支有丰富的交通，若有，则假性病变区有这两种静脉共同供血，其间无明确分界，故常显示边界不清晰；反之，则边界清晰。由通过胆囊三角的胆囊静脉和迷走的胰十二指肠静脉向Ⅳ段供血形成的假性病变中，在静脉性对比增强的CT扫描中一般很难发现这些静脉，因为胆囊静脉较短小，而胰十二指肠静脉也因为太小，且走行与肝动脉较靠近而不易区分；而在高质量的动态增强CT扫描上，有时可以显示迷走的胃右静脉，表现为动脉晚期一条由肝门区向Ⅳ段背侧引流的细小血管影，同时可见该区肝实质的强化。

CTA和CTAP表现：在选择性胆囊动脉、胰十二指肠动脉和胃右动脉成像的CTA上，无论是局灶性脂肪肝还是弥漫性脂肪肝中的正常“肝岛”，假性病变区都会出现浓密的强化，证实有迷走静脉的灌注；在CTAP图像上，假性病变区均显示为对比剂的灌注缺损区，表明局部门静脉血流的减少或缺失。

三、腹壁-附脐静脉系统

该静脉系统由镰状韧带旁的小静脉组成，引流腹壁前部的静脉血直接进入肝脏，稀释局部的门静脉血液，形成假性病变。该系统由3组静脉构成：Sappey上、下静脉（即附脐静脉）和Burow静脉。

Sappey上静脉引流镰状韧带上部和膈肌内侧的静脉血进入肝左叶，并与门静脉的周围分支相汇合，它也与腹壁上静脉或胸廓内静脉的分支相交通。

Sappey下静脉引流镰状韧带下部的静脉血进入肝左叶的门静脉分支，它沿着圆韧带下行与脐周的腹壁下静脉的分支相交通。

Burow静脉是由两条腹壁下静脉和一条发自膀胱的静脉汇合而成，它终止于闭锁的脐静脉的中部，并不直接进入门静脉。它引流腹壁前部和部分膀胱的静脉血。Burow静脉与Sappey下静脉之间也有一些小的交通支，称为插入静脉。

所有这些静脉在出现腔静脉梗阻时，向肝内的血流量则加大。而在门静脉高压时，这些血管内的血液会反向流动，成为离肝的血流。由该静脉系统形成的假性病变可以为局灶性脂肪肝和弥漫性脂肪肝中的正常“肝岛”。

CT平扫表现：多在Ⅳ段前缘的镰状韧带及肝圆韧带旁出现相对的低和高密度区，边界常不清晰，分别代表局灶性脂肪肝和“肝岛”。而第1种类型的假性病变则无异常密度。

CT动态增强扫描：局灶性脂肪肝和“肝岛”的表现与胆管旁静脉丛形成的假性病变的表现一致，而第1种假性病变在动脉期常无强化表现，这可能是由于血液从腹壁回流到假性病变区的解剖距离较远所致。

然而，在腔静脉梗阻的情况下，则其CT增强表现要根据梗阻的血管是上或下腔静脉以及注药部位而有所不同。若上腔静脉阻塞，而从上肢注药扫描时，早期对比剂经胸廓内静脉、腹壁上静脉和Sappey上静脉进入肝脏，可在Ⅳ段前缘出现浓密的增强表现，而门静脉期转为低密度区；若从下肢静脉注药，由于对比剂到达肝脏的时间要晚，故不能表现出早期的增强。在下腔静脉梗阻的病例中会出现上述现象的镜像表现，即从下肢注药后扫描，对比剂早期即经腹壁下静脉、Sappey下静脉以及Burow静脉进入肝脏形成明显的强化区，若从上肢注药则无早期强化表现。在这些情况下，沿着胸、腹壁走行的相关侧支血管的显影也有助于假性病变的诊断。

CTA和CTAP表现：很少行选择性胸廓内动脉或腹壁上、下动脉插管的CTA及CTAP，若行肠系膜上动脉插管的CTAP，则假性病变区形成灌注缺损。

总之，肝脏第Ⅰ、Ⅳ段独特的血流动力学是形成假性病变的重要因素。肝脏第Ⅰ、Ⅳ段易于发生这些血管变异主要是胚胎发育所造成。肝动脉、胆管、胆管旁静脉系统及肝脏的第Ⅰ、Ⅳ段发育较晚（约在妊娠第32~34天，而大部分的肝组织和门静脉系统发育较早（约在妊娠第26~28天），故第Ⅰ、Ⅳ段形成时，这两段可由胆管旁静脉系统等血管供血。了解这些供血血管的有关情况，有助于理解假性病变形成的基础及相关的CT表现，以减少其对诊断的干扰。

第五章 肝血管性疾病

第一节 肝动脉瘤

肝动脉瘤是一种少见的血管性病变,约占内脏动脉瘤的20%,仅次于脾动脉瘤居第二位。第一例肝动脉瘤的尸检报告是在1809年,Erskine(1973)统计文献报告大约有250例。

肝动脉瘤的发生原因按其发生率从高到低排列是:系统性炎症、动脉硬化、胆囊炎、创伤(含医源性损伤)、结核、真菌性感染、多发性结节性动脉炎、马凡综合征、胰腺炎症、肝脓肿、囊性内膜坏死、以及先天性。当代,则以创伤与动脉硬化为最多见。

创伤性肝动脉瘤多为假性动脉瘤,近年来其发病率有上升趋势,一方面与工业交通事故损伤增加有关,另一方面可能与胆系手术、肝动脉滴注化疗及经皮经肝介入放射学技术的广泛应用产生的损伤增多有关,后者即医源性肝动脉瘤。

有作者指出,源于胆囊切除术后的肝动脉瘤多数系在手术过程中遇到顽固性出血,为竭力控制其出血损伤了胆管与附近肝动脉所致。术后引流的T管对胆管的机械性损伤也可引起假性肝动脉瘤。

肝动脉瘤破裂是最严重和最常见的并发症,多数在术后数周或数月后发生,破裂多与胆系相通从而引起胆血症,少数亦可破入腹腔、门静脉或T管窦道。导致破裂的诱因不明。一些作者报告一例是在拔T管时发生的,提示在动脉瘤形成后,拔除T管时任何粗暴操作均有可能成为诱因导致动脉瘤破裂。

在肝动脉瘤,肝外肝动脉受累,大约是肝内肝动脉的4倍,而肝总动脉又是最常受到侵犯的部位。肝外肝动脉瘤比肝内肝动脉瘤大。肝动脉瘤周围结构常见有纤维性粘连。

1. 临床表现 发病年龄范围为10~83岁,平均38岁,男女之比大约为(2~3):1。在手术或尸解以前做出诊断是不常见的。肝动脉瘤在没有破裂时,由于无明显临床症状或症状无特异性而不易被发现,因此,多数是在破裂后才得到诊断。疼痛,不在上腹部就在右上腹,是最常见的症状,大约出现在2/3的病例。破裂引起胆系大出血的典型临床表现,包括上腹疼痛(胆绞痛)、消化道出血(提示胆系出血)、及阻塞性黄疸,但是,有此三联征者仅占1/3病例。当上述表现并存腹部杂音或有搏动的包块,则更应怀疑有肝动脉瘤。由于临床表现明显,结合胆系手术史,对合并大量胆系出血的病例诊断不难。

但有些病例呈小量间歇性出血,则临床表现可能不明显,或仅出现大便潜血阳性,慢性贫血等症状时,则易被忽略。因此,有作者指出,凡是有胆系手术史,出现消化道出血的病例,均应考虑有胆系出血的可能,应进一步检查以明确诊断。

肝动脉瘤破裂,按其发生率高低次序为:能进入腹膜腔、肝外胆管、十二指肠、胆囊、门静脉或胃。如果破裂以后未行治疗或治疗不当,肝动脉瘤常可危及生命。黄疸可以源自于胆系内的血凝块梗阻或胆系外的挤压。胃镜检查对辨别消化道出血是否来自胆系,有重要价值,但须在出血期间才能检出,因此,阳性率仅有50%左右。

2. 影像诊断研究 X线平片检查:当右上腹见到环状钙化,不在胆囊,也不在肾脏,则应怀疑肝动脉瘤的存在。然而,这类钙化并不多见。钡餐检查:可观察到大的肝动脉瘤对邻近脏器的推挤和压迫。

超声与CT扫描:观察到的肝动脉瘤的征象,类似于见于主动脉或其他部位的动脉瘤。近侧肝动脉的肝动脉瘤,其走行十分邻近胰腺,可伪似囊性胰腺肿块。为避免误诊,大剂量对比剂团注的动态扫描是有必要的。超声与CT对确定肝内有无占位性病变有一定价值，但定性常有一定困难，对较小的病变尤其如此。

肝动脉瘤通常是动脉粥样硬化的结果，肝动脉钙化的显示有助于肝动脉瘤的诊断。肝动脉瘤也可发生于静脉吸毒者或继发于外伤。肝动脉瘤常很小（直径小于2cm），在CT图像上显示为富血管性病变，似血管瘤改变。要注意的是必须确认血管的走向，以避免严重错误。假性动脉瘤与真性动脉瘤CT表现相同，但前者常继发于胆管导管放置或动脉内化疗和活检后。另外，罕见的肝动脉-门静脉瘘也可以发生，这常常继发于外伤、活检或外科手术，需要在动脉期扫描才能达到最佳观察效果。

血管造影：是能确诊肝动脉瘤的方法，除MRA和CTA外，当首推X线选择性肝动脉造影，完全的肝动脉造影应包括腹腔动脉造影和肠系膜上动脉造影，必要时还应作选择性胃左动脉造影，以免因肝动脉起源变异导致病变遗漏。肝动脉造影，不仅能明确动脉瘤的有无，大小，分布，在出血时造影有时还能显示胆系出血的征象，而且，在诊断确立后，随即可经导管作肝动脉栓塞治疗。因此，建议对疑为胆系出血的病例，应首先考虑使用肝动脉造影检查。多发性结节性动脉炎及其他血管炎患者的肝动脉瘤，通常是小的、多发性的、肝内的，常伴存血管的不规则。

第二节　肝动脉的假性动脉瘤

详见本书 本卷 本篇 第二章 第四节　肝动脉的假性动脉瘤。

第三节　肝脏遗传性出血性毛细血管扩张症

遗传性出血性毛细血管扩张症，也称Rendu-Osler-Weber病，是一种少见的常染色体显性遗传血管发育异常疾病，以出血和血管扩张为主要表现，可累及皮肤黏膜、胃肠道、肺、脑、脊髓及肝脏等部位，肝脏受累更为少见，其在遗传性出血性毛细血管扩张症中的发病率约为8%~31%，检索近年来国内外肝脏遗传性出血性毛细血管扩张症影像研究多为中晚期的典型表现，早期表现介绍很少。

遗传性出血性毛细血管扩张症的发病机制及临床表现：遗传性出血性毛细血管扩张症是一种少见的常染色体显性遗传性疾病，目前认为遗传性出血性毛细血管扩张症的发生主要与9号染色体Endoglin基因和12号染色体上的活化素受体样激酶1（ALK-1）基因位点突变有关，其分别引起1型遗传性出血性毛细血管扩张症（遗传性出血性毛细血管扩张症1）和2型遗传性出血性毛细血管扩张症（遗传性出血性毛细血管扩张症2）。

患者出生时并没有遗传性出血性毛细血管扩张症相关临床表现，而是随着年龄的增长逐渐显现，例如通常最早发生的鼻出血一般在儿童时期发生，其他临床症状在40岁以后逐渐出现。一组患者也表现出随年龄增长，其临床症状逐渐增多、加重。

遗传性出血性毛细血管扩张症的主要临床表现是皮肤黏膜或者内脏血管发育不良性病变。多发性皮肤黏膜毛细血管扩张、反复鼻出血及阳性家族史被称为遗传性出血性毛细血管扩张症三联征。病变主要累及毛细血管、小静脉及小动脉，表现为毛细血管扩张、动-静脉畸形及动-静脉瘘。毛细血管扩张多发生于口、鼻、胃肠道、皮肤及手指等部位，血管异常多发生于胃肠道、肺、脑及肝脏等部位，轻微病变表现为毛细血管后静脉局部出现扩张，严重者病变血管出现显著扩张和扭曲，扩张的动、静脉常相通。

2000年国际遗传性出血性毛细血管扩张症基金科学顾问委员会对临床诊断标准规定如下：反复发作的自发性鼻出血；多个特征部位出现毛细血管扩张，如唇、鼻、手指和口腔黏膜等；内脏受累，如消化道的毛细血管扩张，肺、肝、脑的动静脉畸形；阳性家族史，直系亲属中有遗传性出血性毛细血管扩张症患者。

符合2条以上条件者可确诊为遗传性出血性毛细血管扩张症，符合2条者为疑似病例。

早期肝遗传性出血性毛细血管扩张症的病理、临床和CT表现：肝遗传性出血性毛细血管扩张症镜下观察:肝实质和汇管区内扩张的毛细血管和小静脉呈瘤样增生,较大的门静脉分支显著扩张、扭曲,血管周围纤维组织增生并有纤维间隔形成和慢性炎细胞浸润(主要是淋巴细胞和浆细胞),汇管区内胆管增生;肝实质区内可见肝细胞增生,肝细胞脂肪变性和空泡变性,无肝细胞坏死和炎细胞浸润;肝小叶结构正常,无假小叶形成。

肝遗传性出血性毛细血管扩张症患者女性较多,有家族史,典型临床表现有腹痛、高排量心力衰竭、门静脉高压、胆系疾病等;实验室检查肝功能可正常或出现碱性磷酸酶、γ-转氨酶升高。肝损害主因是血液在肝内短路,肝脏长期缺血、缺氧造成肝脏纤维化,继而出现非典型性肝硬化及食管静脉曲张和肝性脑病。一组4例患者属早期,临床症状相对较轻,除鼻出血及部分消化道症状外,尚未出现明显心功能损害、肝损害和门静脉高压等表现,实验室检查也仅1例提示轻微肝功能异常,尚无肝硬化等相关症状及体征。本组未发现门静脉增粗和门静脉高压改变,但门静脉早显提示肝动脉-门静脉瘘是广泛存在的。

影像学研究:早期肝遗传性出血性毛细血管扩张症CT平扫多为阴性,动态增强检查具有很高的诊断价值:动脉期肝实质染色不均,见弥漫分布的点状、小斑片状及结节状明显强化影,肝动脉及分支明显增粗、迂曲、延长,呈细小弹簧状,肝静脉及门静脉动脉期早显,可以出现门静脉、肝静脉增粗及门静脉高压征象,实质期、延迟期肝实质染色未见异常。

文献报道,和肝内不同类型的血管异常一样,多发性结节状、小斑片状再生性结节性病变在肝遗传性出血性毛细血管扩张症中有很高的发生率,是肝实质对血管瘘引起的低灌注的反应性改变,动脉期明显强化。

与典型的中晚期肝遗传性出血性毛细血管扩张症不同,本组并未发现明显的门静脉高压和肝硬化征象。推测肝动脉-门静脉瘘可能较肝动-静脉瘘晚发生,随病程的慢性进展,门静脉高压和肝硬化等表现才出现。同样,该组没有发现肝内胆管受累的表现,例如局限性的肝内胆管坏死引起的类似肝囊肿样的改变和肝内胆管扩张等,CT上与肝内胆管囊性扩张症和硬化性胆管炎表现类似。这些胆管病变与肝内血管异常,胆管供血不足有关。

鉴别诊断:本病需与动脉期同样表现为弥漫分布结节状明显强化病变进行鉴别,如肝感染性病变、不典型海绵状血管瘤及转移瘤,结合临床与动态增强扫描门静脉期及延时期影像特点鉴别不难。

肝遗传性出血性毛细血管扩张症诊断的金标准为血管造影,但此方法有创且操作复杂,不适用于患者的追踪观察及大范围的家族性筛查。超声在此病的筛查、诊断及追踪观察等方面亦具有重要作用,但超声受操作者个人技术水平影响较大。MR血管造影技术与CTA有一样的诊断价值,而且不必担心电离辐射。

总之,肝遗传性出血性毛细血管扩张症罕见,早期临床症状更不典型,对其认识不足是临床漏诊与误诊的主要原因,只有提高对本病的认识,才能为其早诊断、早治疗、改善预后提供帮助。本病属于家族性遗传性疾病,预防性筛查和随访是必要的,以减少潜在并发症的发生。CT多期动态增强扫描对早期肝遗传性出血性毛细血管扩张症的诊断有重要的帮助。

第六章　肝动静脉分流

第一节　肝脏动静脉短路的病因和分类

肝脏的动静脉短路以肝动脉-门静脉短路多见,肝动脉-肝静脉短路较少见。这与肝动脉和门静脉分支紧密相邻、并列走行的解剖结构有一定关系。肝脏动静脉短路的病因可分为肿瘤性和非肿瘤性两大类。

(1)肿瘤性动静脉短路:肿瘤性动静脉短路最常见于原发性肝癌,也可见于肝血管肉瘤、多血性肝转移瘤(如源自平滑肌肉瘤或肾癌的转移)等;但是,肝良性肿瘤(除婴幼儿的肝血管内皮瘤和肝血管平滑肌脂肪瘤以外)罕见并发动静脉短路;成人多见的肝脏海绵状血管瘤不像肌肉软组织海绵状血管瘤(95%可并发动静脉短路),一直认为其很少并发动静脉短路,既往文献中仅报道过数例。

(2)非肿瘤性动静脉短路:肝脏非肿瘤性动静脉短路可见于下列疾病:包括肝硬化、肝再生性结节、先天性肝血管畸形和布-加综合征等;也可作为肝脏钝器伤或穿通伤的一个结果,包括医源性肝损伤,例如经皮经肝活检、乙醇注射治疗(PEI)、经导管动脉化疗栓塞(TACE)和肝胆外科手术等。有作者报告一组筛选出的30例皆已除外上述肝肿瘤和非肿瘤性疾患。

肝脏动静脉短路的形成机制可分为经肝窦性、经血管性和经血管丛性等3种动静脉短路形成途径。肝硬化病例出现的细小肝动脉-门静脉短路属典型的经肝窦性动静脉短路,主要是由于肝静脉小支闭塞引起肝窦腔压力升高,肝窦和门静脉小支间的腔内压力梯度倒置,从而使病变区肝窦只有肝动脉小支供血以及肝窦腔内动脉血逆流入门静脉小支(似导出静脉)。另外,一些潜在的动静脉吻合,如肝动脉终末支与门静脉小支间的吻合、胆管周围小动脉丛与门静脉小支间的吻合,此时也可开放而形成肝动脉-门静脉短路;肝窦的渗透性改变可能也与肝硬化的肝动脉-门静脉短路形成有关。类似肝硬化一样的动静脉短路形成途径也可见于肝再生结节和布-加综合征等。

恶性肝肿瘤并发的动静脉短路已证实是经血管性途径,可以是由于肝内静脉受肿瘤组织侵蚀而形成直接的动静脉短路,也可以是经过肿瘤血管间或通过门静脉的滋养小动脉而形成。先天性肝血管畸形和肝损伤(包括医源性)所引起的动静脉瘘(即直接的动静脉间短路),血管造影可清晰显示。然而,经导管动脉化疗栓塞术后的肝动脉-门静脉短路形成机制尚不清楚,有人认为与采用的化疗药物、导管和导丝对血管的损伤有关。

第二节　少见的肝动脉-门静脉瘘

肝动脉-门静脉瘘少见,它们可出现在肝动脉与入肝处门静脉主干之间,也可见于肝动脉分支和肝实质内门静脉分支之间。

Foley等(1971)报告5例肝内的肝动脉-门静脉瘘,其中4例临床未曾怀疑为此症,只是血管造影才揭露本症的存在。2例为腹部钝伤所致,2例为针刺活检引起,1例为肝硬化自发形成瘘。与系统性的动-静脉瘘相比较,本症不引起心排出量的增加,这考虑是由于肝血管窦内阻力改变的缘故。

Trinez等(1973)介绍一例30岁男性患者,有胃肠出血和进食后疼痛,且以进食食物较多而加重,血管造影发现从左肝动脉分支到门静脉系统有一较大的动-静脉瘘,从而存在腹腔内血液的偷窃现象,瘘的血液来自肠系膜上动脉,故造成该动脉供应区域的小肠局部贫血;同时,门静脉压的动脉化伴存门脉高压,出现静脉曲张。该作者认为此类系膜动脉的局部贫血是这种难见的动-静脉瘘的少见并发症。

第七章　肝静脉

第一节　肝静脉发育变异

在CTAP和超声上肝静脉在肝内的变异偶可见到，而在螺旋CT上更常见到。肝静脉的经典型解剖表现仅见于70%的病人中。在CTAP上最常见的变异是额外的下肝静脉，它引流第5及第6肝段的血液，在三条肝静脉的尾侧水平进入下腔静脉。其他变异如肝静脉共干也有发生。

在肝脏增强的动脉期，肝静脉和下腔静脉正常时不发生强化。然而，在心功能障碍者中，对比剂能够从右心房逆流到肝段下腔静脉和肝静脉内。充血性心力衰竭和缩窄性心包炎引起右心房压力升高和肝静脉回流障碍，导致肝淤血。这种情况可随着心功能的改善而改善，但长期严重病例，可导致称为心源性肝硬化的永久性肝损伤。

在肝淤血病例中，静脉给予对比剂后肝脏实质呈花斑样强化，下腔静脉和肝静脉扩张，并可见对比剂从右心房逆流入下腔静脉和肝静脉等改变。此时，也可见到门静脉周围的水肿。除了充血性心力衰竭，缩窄性心包炎也可导致上述肝淤血的类似表现。

第二节　肝窦阻塞综合征

详见本书 本卷 本篇 第一章 第三节　肝窦阻塞综合征。

第三节　副肝静脉

肝静脉血液回流除了三大主肝静脉外，尚有数支直接汇入下腔静脉的细小肝静脉，统称为副肝静脉或肝短静脉，其数目较多，形态和分布变异较大，影像学检查具有较高的临床价值。正常人群中副肝静脉多数细小，且不是肝脏的主要回流静脉，以往未引起足够的重视，随着医学影像学、肝胆外科的迅速发展及布 - 加综合征介入治疗的深入开展，在3支主肝静脉阻塞时副肝静脉起到的代偿作用以及如何利用与保护副肝静脉的功能逐步受到关注。

第三肝门范围：第三肝门范围是从主肝静脉开口的第二肝门以下第一支细小肝静脉至最下一支肝静脉汇入下腔静脉处，即第二肝门以下凡是有肝静脉开口处均应属于第三肝门的范围，而不仅是口径较大的肝静脉汇入下腔静脉处。在这段距离内有右后上静脉、右后下静脉、右后中静脉、尾状叶静脉、左右膈下静脉及右肾上腺静脉汇入，而膈下静脉及右肾上腺静脉不属于肝静脉支，可视为单个情况处理。

以上除膈下静脉及右肾上腺静脉开口在下腔静脉肝段的后壁外，其他4组细小肝静脉均开口在右壁、前壁及左壁，此处应为第三肝门。有作者观察56例尸肝标本，根据直径 >0.5 cm的肝静脉的分布规律，结合临床意义，将肝后下腔静脉分为上、中、下三段，第三肝门位于下段，长（3.6 ± 1.0）cm，第二肝门位于上段，长（2.1 ± 0.4）cm，肝门间段长

（1.7 ± 0.9）cm。

肝脏尾状叶：全尾状叶于肝后下腔静脉前，第一肝门的后方，三支主肝静脉的下方。Yanaga 等（1994）基于 23 例尸体肝铸型标本的研究，将肝的全尾状叶分成三部分，即 Spigel 叶（固有尾状叶）、腔静脉旁部和尾状突。Couinaud（1989）将 Spigel 叶称为Ⅰ L（Ⅰ段左部），腔静脉旁部和尾状突合称为Ⅰ R（Ⅰ段右部）。

多数布 - 加综合征的尾状叶明显增大，尾状叶静脉明显扩张，血流量明显增大，即引流尾状叶的静脉血流，也与其他肝静脉相互沟通，从而引流肝右叶甚至于肝左叶部分的静脉血液至体循环。尾状叶代偿性增大，副肝静脉代偿性增粗是布 - 加综合征的特征性表现之一，无论超声、CT 或是 MRI 几乎在布 - 加综合征患者中都可以见到此征象。

尾状叶为肝脏的一个自主段，不仅有单独的肝动脉、门静脉血供，而且静脉血液直接回流至下腔静脉，而其他肝段均由肝段静脉汇成肝静脉主干后，再汇入下腔静脉。因此，布 - 加综合征主肝静脉阻塞后，尾状叶由于尾叶静脉直接汇入下腔静脉，受病变的影响小，静脉直径代偿性增粗，尾状叶体积代偿性增大，对于缓解病情有重要意义。

肝后间隙：Couinaudt（1989）发现肝脏的尾状叶和下腔静脉之间有一疏松结缔组织间隙，此间隙中有一缺少副肝静脉的无血管区，称为 Couinaud 间隙。主要指第Ⅰ、Ⅸ肝段，甚至Ⅵ、Ⅶ和Ⅷ肝段与下腔静脉之间的间隙，其前壁为肝尾状叶的腔静脉窝，后壁为肝后下腔静脉，左侧为尾状叶的左侧部及尾状叶静脉，右侧为尾状叶的腔静脉旁部的右侧部、尾状突起及其发出的尾状叶静脉和右叶的肝右后下静脉，下口为肝右后下静脉左侧尾状叶后下腔静脉前的裂隙，上口为肝上静脉窝。有学者分别测定此无血管区宽 0.5~1.5cm，长 4.1~7.8 cm。

副肝静脉；副肝静脉的应用研究起源于 20 世纪 50 年代。Elias 和 Petty（1952）认为存在第二肝门以外的低位肝静脉，Goldsmith 等（1957）对除第二肝门以外直接进入下腔静脉的肝静脉进行解剖后，称这些静脉为肝小静脉，并将其分为右侧组和左侧组两组，右侧组在右前方进入下腔静脉，较短粗，左侧组在左前方及左侧壁进入下腔静脉，数目较多且纤细。

Nakamura 等（1981）明确了两组各自的引流区域：右侧组主要引流Ⅶ段上部、Ⅶ段中部、肝裸区深面近下腔静脉区域的静脉血以及Ⅵ、Ⅶ段下部肾压迹处的静脉血；左侧组主要引流尾状叶的静脉血。左、右两组之间以及两组静脉与肝静脉、门静脉之间通过侧支相互吻合，当肝静脉有阻塞时，该两组静脉是直接联系门、腔静脉的“桥梁”。

Willams（1995）将肝静脉分为上、下两组，上组肝静脉由肝左、中、右 3 支组成，经第二肝门汇入下腔静脉；下组的肝静脉统称为副肝静脉，包括主要引流肝右后部段Ⅵ段、Ⅶ段静脉血的肝右后下静脉和主要引流尾状叶静脉血的尾状叶静脉，经第三肝门汇入下腔静脉。

另有作者通过 200 余例下腔静脉和肝静脉造影资料分析认为，使用副肝静脉这一名词能够比较全面地反映下组肝静脉的分布与功能，同时也使三大主肝静脉分支以外出肝的静脉血管的命名得以统一。

副肝静脉的数量各家报道不尽相同，有作者认为副肝静脉有 3~32 支，其内径为 0.10~3.43cm，内径 >0.5cm 的静脉占 9.6%~40.7%，>1.0cm 的静脉占 2.6%~25.4%。Camargo 等（1996）报道平均每例肝有 14.7 个副肝静脉开口，分为大、中、小及微小 4 种类型。

Goldsmith 等（1957）认为副肝静脉有 3~27 支。Nakamura 等（1981）认为具有临床意义的副肝静脉有 3~11 支，平均（7 ± 2）支，内径 0.2~1.4 cm，平均（0.32 ± 0.18）cm。另有作者报道副肝静脉的内径在 0.1~0.5 cm 者占 40.47%，0.5~1.0 cm 者占 42.86%，1.0~2.0 cm 者占 16.67%。

Nakamura 等（1981）进一步解剖证实右侧组为肝右后下静脉，主要引流肝右后部段Ⅵ、Ⅶ段静脉血，左侧组为尾状叶静脉，主要引流尾状叶静脉血，右侧组分布于下腔静脉右侧壁下段居多（55.9%~72.6%），左侧组分布于下腔静脉左侧壁（27.4%~44.1%）。

肝右后下静脉变异也较大，其中肝右后静脉直径常较粗大，位于肝的脏面肾压迹处，开口位置较低，常有 1~2 mm 的肝外行程，构成肝静脉的下开口。有作者观察成人组肝右后下静脉出现率为 87.2%，支数范围为 1~8 支；新生儿组出现率为 88.89%，支数范围为 1~5 支。两组肝右后下静脉总的发生率为 88%，支数范围为 1~8 支。

一些作者研究人体尸肝 156 个，肝右后下静脉出现率为 84%。肝右后下静脉与肝右静脉间呈彼消此长的关系。依据肝右后下静脉汇入下腔静脉肝后段的位置，可分为上、中、下 3 组，分别称之为肝右后上、中、下静脉。

肝右后下静脉较粗大时主要引流段Ⅵ和Ⅶ段下部肾压迹处的静脉血，较细时则仅引流段Ⅴ下部的血液。肝右后静脉越靠近下腔静脉则越表浅，41.82% 成人肝上发现肝右后下静脉在肝裸区右侧即将汇入下腔静脉处有一半或全部管壁裸露于肝外。

在影像上，若发现患者存在粗大的肝右后下静脉时，应考虑有原发性布 - 加综合征的可能性。粗大的肝右后下静脉常与门静脉右后叶支平行而呈现"假平行管征"，因此易将粗大的肝右后下静脉误诊为扩张的肝管；粗大的肝右后下静脉也极易与肝右静脉混淆而造成肝脏分叶分段的错误。

一、副肝静脉在布 - 加综合征中的临床应用

副肝静脉在布 - 加综合征中的代偿性变化：布 - 加综合征是因肝段下腔静脉和 / 或肝静脉部分或完全性狭窄、闭塞导致静脉血液回流受阻，血液淤滞而产生的一系列肝后性门静脉高压和下腔静脉高压两大症候群。副肝静脉是 3 支主肝静脉之外重要的肝引流血管，当 3 支主肝静脉引流不畅时，肝内侧支血流即可经开放的副肝静脉引流到下腔静脉，起到减轻肝窦压力作用。

布 - 加综合征的静脉血管类型复杂而繁多，但副肝静脉的显示无论在诊断还是治疗中均有重要的意义。国人布 - 加综合征虽然以下腔静脉病变为主，但合并主肝静脉阻塞者并非鲜见，平均累及 2~3 支，此时正常情况下存在于尾叶静脉与主肝静脉之间的交通支扩张增粗，形成大量肝内交通支，同时副肝静脉也代偿性增粗，以代偿主肝静脉的血液回流功能。

在节段性下腔静脉型和混合型布 - 加综合征的介入治疗中，三大主肝静脉血液经由肝内交通支、副肝静脉，而后进入下腔静脉。副肝静脉成为沟通门 - 腔静脉的重要"桥梁"。此时了解副肝静脉汇入下腔静脉的位置，避免或减少介入治疗时下腔静脉支架与副肝静脉接触尤其是跨越副肝静脉，防止下腔静脉内支架长期置入而横跨副肝静脉，继发副肝静脉阻塞，这对于介入治疗成功与否、特别是长期疗效极其重要。因而在其介入治疗前，通过各种影像学检查尤其静脉血管造影提供下腔静脉形态结构，3 支主肝静脉阻塞的部位、程度、范围和交通支形成情况，代偿性增粗的副肝静脉开口部位等，是必不可少的步骤之一。

副肝静脉在布 - 加综合征的分型中具有重要作用。以往布 - 加综合征主要根据下腔静脉和肝静脉的闭塞及狭窄情况分型，副肝静脉的被认识使布 - 加综合征的分型更有利于治疗，无疑副肝静脉的代偿性增粗极大地缓解了主肝静脉阻塞而引发的门静脉高压，减缓了淤血性肝硬化的病理过程。不少作者在他们的分型中均以有无副肝静脉作为亚型的标准。有作者在布 - 加综合征肝静脉病变的超声分型中直接将副肝静脉作为分型标准。另有作者主张以肝静脉和肝小静脉为核心分型，并单独将肝小静脉闭塞作为一型，并发现此型病例 2 例。

人肝的副肝静脉数量多，管径自数毫米至 1 厘米不等，部分管径粗大，在肝静脉血引流中起着重要的作用。值得注意的是，布 - 加综合征病变不仅累及下腔静脉和肝静脉，还可累及部分副肝静脉，甚至仅表现为副肝静脉狭窄、闭塞，诊断过程中要避免惯性思维，全面检查，防止误诊、漏诊。

影像学研究：近年来，随着影像诊断的发展和对布 - 加综合征临床认识的提高，其发现率明显提高，超声检查对布 - 加综合征的诊断价值已得到临床的一致公认。它既能观察病变的形态结构，又能了解血流动力学情况，可明确判断血管阻塞部位、程度、范围及侧支循环情况，并可对病情分型，术后随访和疗效判断，可作为布 - 加综合征诊断的首选检查方法，亦可作为术后随防的主要检查手段。

另有作者报道，超声观察 31 例布 - 加综合征患者中，28 例超声检测到代偿性增粗的副肝静脉，显示率为 90.3%(28/31)。其汇入部位大多位于第二肝门 1.5 cm 下方的肝后段下腔静脉管壁上；典型的副肝静脉表现为与下腔静脉相通的异常迂曲的管道，并通过交通支与 3 支肝静脉相通；肝右后叶内走行无明显迂曲或稍迂曲的副肝静脉主要分布于肝段Ⅵ及邻近肝组织内，与三大肝静脉较少形成交通支。

有作者报道，超声观察 214 名正常成人肝右后下静脉的显示率为 24%，平均管径为(0.43 ± 0.12) cm；布 - 加综合征患者肝右后下静脉的显示率为 74%，平均管径为(0.78 ± 0.16)cm，两组之间的差异具有显著统计学意义。布 - 加综合征患者尾状叶静脉的显示率为 79%，平均管径为(0.52 ± 0.17)cm。

有作者报道 14 例布 - 加综合征患者 MSCT 检查发现副肝静脉增粗 11 例,与 DSA 相比,副肝静脉的准确率为 85.71%。还有作者观察 24 例布 - 加综合征患者的 CT、MRI 表现, 20 例检测到副肝静脉,显示率 83.3%。

副肝静脉的 CT、MRI 表现分为两类:主干直径 <0.5 cm 的副肝静脉常表现为多支细小、走行迂曲的管道,开口于下腔静脉的右侧壁或左前壁,以锐角或钝角汇入下腔静脉;主干直径≥ 0.5cm 的副肝静脉多表现为走行无明显迂曲或稍显迂曲的管道,多开口于下腔静脉的右侧壁,以直角或近似直角汇入下腔静脉。

第四节 肝静脉发育变异与诊断陷阱

肝静脉是肝内静脉血进入下腔静脉的通道,典型的有三条肝静脉干(左、中、右肝静脉),三者向下腔静脉方向集中并进入下腔静脉,呈“W”样,这在 CT 轴面图像上常可见到。有时可看到两支肝右静脉在进入下腔静脉之前汇合形成一条主干。

约 70% 的人有肝左、中、右三支肝静脉,并注入下腔静脉。其中 65%~85% 的人肝左静脉和肝中静脉形成一共同主干后汇入下腔静脉;其余 15%~35% 的人三支肝静脉分别独立汇入下腔静脉。

约 30% 的人有三支以上肝静脉,但一支或多支肝静脉的缺失很少见。约 30% 的人有肝左静脉或肝右静脉的边缘分支。虽然术前有关肝静脉解剖知识的掌握不如肝动脉解剖那么关键,但也是十分重要的信息。

5%~18% 的人有一支副肝右静脉。其中最常见的是肝右后下静脉,见于 10%~18% 的人群中。副肝右静脉收集回流第 6 肝段的肝静脉血并注入到下腔静脉内,其注入口在肝静脉主支入口水平以下、下腔静脉的背侧。

此外,据报道肝右中静脉见于 5.5% 的人群,其回流肝脏第 5 肝段的静脉血,并在肝右静脉主支与右后下静脉之间注入下腔静脉。这两支肝静脉副支可以比肝右静脉主支还粗大。

第八章　肝血管其他疾病

CTA 与肝移植

（一）CTA 在肝移植术前的临床应用价值

CTA 是一项无创性检查，病人易于接受，并且减少了医患双方的辐射剂量。更重要的是，CTA 能对肝移植病人进行全面而准确的评价，在术前准确回答临床关注的许多问题。有研究表明，CTA 与传统的血管造影（CA）对肝移植血管评价的准确性一致，可为外科手术计划提供可靠的信息。CTA 还能提供肝实质和腹腔内改变的信息，为病人的选择提供必要的信息。而 MRA 扫描时间长，最佳扫描参数仍不确定，空间分辨力相对低，这些缺点使其应用受到一定限制。在对 30 例病人的对比研究中，15 例 MSCTA 的影像质量优于 MRA，CTA 显示了 8 例重要的肝动脉变异，而 MRA 未能显示这些变异，因此认为 MSCTA 影像质量和对肝动脉的显示均优于 MRA，CT 可以取代 MRI 成为肝移植术前评价的一部分。

（二）CTA 对受体血管的评价

肝动脉变异：肝动脉的起源和分支变异是常见的。Michel 于 1966 年的最初研究显示 200 例尸解中肝动脉变异占 45%。在后来的 1 000 例肝切除术中显示了 75.7% 的肝动脉解剖正常，24.3% 存在肝动脉变异。常见的肝动脉变异是肝右动脉起自肠系膜上动脉，而肝左动脉起自胃左动脉。有研究认为，最常见的肝动脉变异是肝右动脉变异，发生率为 13%~18%。

肝动脉重建在肝移植中是一个关键的步骤，必须保证受体能对移植后的肝有足够的血供，血供不足往往是因为受体血管直径小，这种情况常见于有多个不同起源的肝动脉。这样的病例须采用另外的血供通道，最常见的是主动脉 - 肝动脉搭桥术。此外，肝动脉变异对外科手术还存在其他影响。例如，受体的替代或副肝左动脉起自胃左动脉，在受体肝切除过程中，这支动脉须从胃左动脉的起始处结扎。

腹腔干狭窄：腹腔干狭窄的原因有动脉粥样硬化和正中弓状韧带综合征。正中弓状韧带由主动脉裂孔两侧的膈肌脚融合而成，该韧带可能会压迫起自主动脉的腹腔干和其他内脏动脉。肝动脉重建时受体侧支循环常常被阻断，包括结扎胃十二指肠动脉，使得腹腔干成为移植肝唯一的供血动脉。如果存在腹腔干狭窄却未被发现，仍采用标准的肝动脉端端吻合，肝脏将面临血供不足的问题，有可能导致肝动脉栓塞。因此，手术时应避免这种狭窄而可能带来的问题，如果狭窄继发于动脉粥样硬化，可更换肝脏供血动脉，常用供体血管在受体腹腔干上方或肾动脉下方或右髂总动脉与供体肝动脉间进行搭桥；如果狭窄是由于弓状韧带压迫所致，手术时松解该韧带即可。

脾动脉瘤：肝硬化和门静脉高压病人脾动脉血流增加导致脾动脉瘤形成，发病率占该类病人的 7%~10%，尸检中发现率更高。脾动脉瘤缺乏症状和体征，可突然破裂引起致命后果，发生率为 2% 左右。有研究者报道，肝移植后脾动脉瘤破裂呈增大趋势。因随着肝移植门静脉压力下降，脾血流增加可使脾动脉瘤破裂，因此，必须在移植时结扎脾动脉瘤。这一区域手术时不属于常规暴露的术野，故术前影像学诊断是重要的。

门静脉和肠系膜上静脉通畅性：在肝硬化时可逐渐形成门静脉血栓，其病因学尚不清楚，可能与肝内阻力增加而致门静脉血流降低或呈双向性有关。有研究显示，门静脉血栓的发生率在肝硬化的自然病程中是 2.1%~13.8%。当门静脉血栓形成后，会产生丰富的侧支静脉回流，临床表现不明显，但在手术前必须明确，否则对肝移植和移植物存活产生不利影响。尽管目前门静脉血栓已不再是肝移植的绝对禁忌证，但门静脉和肠系膜上静脉弥漫性血栓形成仍是肝移植的绝对禁忌证。

（三）CTA 对供体血管的评价

供体肝动脉变异：1/3 的潜在供体因肝动脉发育变异而不适合作供体。肝动脉血供充足才能够保证移植物存活并且避免胆道结构坏死。有研究显示，只有55%的人有正常的肝动脉解剖,即肝固有动脉分肝左、右动脉2支,其余的人存在各种动脉的发育变异。普通人群中,肠系膜上动脉发出的替代肝右动脉占11%,胃左动脉发出的替代肝左动脉占10%,副肝右或肝左动脉占8%。供体肝叶存在副动脉,在受体需要进行至少2次动脉吻合,多个动脉供应1个肝叶的供体更容易发生动脉管径细小。如果动脉直径小于2 mm,受体术后血栓形成的危险性增加。为了降低这种危险性,外科医生用显微外科技术行动脉吻合。存在多个细小动脉的供体一般不予采用。

供体左内叶动脉:保证肝左内叶的血供对维持供体该段肝功能非常重要,因此了解肝左内叶动脉起源和走行对肝右叶或左叶切除均具有重要意义。肝左内动脉可起自肝左或肝右动脉。当肝左内叶动脉起自肝右动脉时,肝右叶切除受到限制,反之左外叶切除受限。另外,肝左内叶动脉起自肝右动脉时,左内叶动脉起点和肝右动脉起点间距离是重要的,因为这个信息能为外科肝切除提供参考。CTA的容积再现和最大密度投影后处理方法均可用于肝左内叶动脉的显示,有研究比较了容积再现和最大密度投影显示肝左内叶动脉的能力,认为最大密度投影优于容积再现。

供体门静脉变异:与肝动脉和肝静脉相比,门静脉发育变异相对较少。Erbay等(2003)对107例病人的研究中发现,26例门静脉变异中有13例是门静脉在肝门处分为3支(即门静脉在肝门处直接分为左支、右前支和右后支)。如果肝右叶有2个门静脉主干分支,肝右叶移植至受体时需要2次吻合。如果用左叶或左外叶作为供肝,详细估计门静脉左干的长度和直径是非常重要的。门静脉左干的肝外长度也因人而异。水平段缺如这种少见的变异,在活体供肝移植(LRLT)是最关心的问题,因为它事关供肝采集(左叶或左外叶)策略和供肝门静脉的重建。也有报道认为CTA对门静脉显示的准确度与手术结果之间无显著性差异。

肝静脉解剖:肝静脉解剖知识对于移植外科医生是必不可少的。当行右半肝切取时,肝中静脉的取舍就成为关键的技术问题。有报道进行包括肝中静脉的右半肝切取,其优点是扩大静脉流出道,保证供肝植入后肝静脉回流通畅。北美的多数医疗中心则采用不包括肝中静脉的右半肝以减少供体危险。肝右后下静脉是最常见的肝静脉变异,约占67%,大于0.5cm的肝右后下静脉应保留供受体吻合用,以确保移植后静脉回流通畅。如果肝右静脉较小,又有较粗大的Ⅴ段和Ⅷ段肝静脉回流至肝中静脉,这种供体应考虑捐献扩大右半肝(Ⅳ ~ Ⅷ段)。

如果左外叶作为供肝则切取肝左静脉,如果左叶作为供肝,则切取肝中静脉和肝左静脉,所以主要是肝中和肝左静脉的变异。肝中和肝左静脉合干占65%~85%。引流肝Ⅷ段的前上肝静脉常汇入肝中静脉。这种情况下,如果肝中和肝左静脉均需切取,这支静脉常会被结扎掉。10%的受检者显示靠近肝圆韧带的左外叶下段引流入肝中静脉,此时如需左外叶供肝,则须进行较复杂的静脉吻合。CTA对正常和变异的肝静脉解剖显示也是满意的。

由于肝血管解剖的复杂性及正常血管发育变异的发生率高,术前为移植外科医生提供供受体肝血管路径,对手术成功是非常重要的。目前,CTA作为一项无创性检查得到普遍的认可,逐渐取代了传统的血管造影而成为肝移植术前评价供受体肝血管的首选方法。

第十一篇　肝的先天异常和发育变异

第一章　肝的先天性异常

第一节　糖原蓄积病

糖原蓄积病是一组遗传性代谢性紊乱，大多数都有肝糖原转变为葡萄糖过程的异常，反映为肝糖原结构或浓度的异常。此病分型仰赖于特殊酶的缺陷和/或确切的临床表现。

1. 临床表现　在1型（von Gierke病），为肝和肾内的葡萄糖-6-磷酸酶缺如或缺少，导致糖原蓄积转变的损害，从而引起糖原贮存在肝细胞内和肾的近曲小管内。葡萄糖合成如受损害，可出现低血糖症，高胰高血糖素症及甘油三酯、胆固醇和尿酸的血浆内水平升高。肝腺瘤和肝细胞癌均可出现于1型。后者考虑为前者恶性变的结果，它至少已出现于3例1型病人。

肝肿大能出现于1、3、4和6型，而脾肿大能出现于1、4和6型。肝硬化只累及3和4型。肝腺瘤考虑为继发于慢性低血糖症与胰岛素降低和糖原水平的升高引起的慢性激素刺激所致。它们出现于小儿或青少年。

1型的治疗，是连续地经鼻胃管的夜间的高碳水化合物的补充营养，或胃造瘘术后在一天时间内多次餐饮和小吃。如果高的血浆葡萄糖水平能够保持，生长可改善，化学成分恢复正常，腺瘤可以退变，病人能生活于相当正常的情况下。

2. 影像学研究　X线腹部平片可以发现肝肿大。

在放射性核素显像检查中，^{99m}Tc硫胶肝脾显像的最早发现是肝肿大，紧随着的是胶体转移到脾伴斑状肝吸收。此时，轻微的到显著的脾肿大甚为常见，但是骨髓蓄积增加却少见。腺瘤通常是光子聚集区，有时它可被一吸收增加的边缘围绕，这可能反映实质部分受到挤压。罕见地，腺瘤表现为小的相对吸收增加的区域。光子聚集区的迅速扩大，多提示为恶性变。

超声检查，肝肿大伴存回声增强，声束的衰减大概是由于脂肪浸润所致，然而可以理解的，广泛的糖原蓄积也是一个因素。与肾脏比较，肝是高回声，肾肿大也可出现。腺瘤，当其较小时，是均质的边界清楚实质性回声包块，比较于异常回声的肝来说，腺瘤可以是高回声，也可以是低回声。较大的腺瘤是不均质的，而且伴有低回声区，这大概反映肿瘤内的出血或/和坏死。某些作者报告，它有一薄的低回声边缘（可能是压迫实质或有一包囊形成）。

在1型糖原蓄积症的肝腺瘤，没有发现透声增强的肿瘤的边缘有折射影的其他的肝腺瘤。这能用比较于无腺瘤的肝实质部分来说，腺瘤内的脂肪和糖原相对缺乏来解释。

在随访检查中，腺瘤是稳定的，生长很慢。一个生长迅速的腺瘤，或者腺瘤边缘欠光滑或不清楚，都提示恶性变。定时的超声随访检查对于观察1型糖原蓄积病是可行的措施。

肝脏CT扫描是相当独特的，能发现低密度的，正常密度的，或高密度的病灶，这依赖于糖原与脂肪相对含量的比例。前者趋向于升高CT值，后者趋向于降低CT值。

此外，对于肝脾肿大，肾肿大伴糖原蓄积所致的皮质变浓密，均可由CT扫描发现。

1型糖原蓄积病的肝腺瘤有着与其他肝腺瘤类似的CT特征性表现（在CT平扫时，为正常肝内的低密度病灶），除了在有脂肪浸润存在时它们可以表现为假性的高密度以外。在个别病例可有环状增强的表现。1型糖原蓄积病的腺瘤的血管造影表现与其他的肝腺瘤一样。

第二节　囊性纤维化

肝和胆系异常约占囊性纤维化病人的 20%~50%，但在临床上并不是经常引起人们的注意。胆汁性肝硬化约占有症状的病人的 2%~3%，但不见于胰腺未受侵犯的病人。胆系结石是一不常见的发病的原因。罕见地，胆系梗阻表现类似于胆系闭锁可出现于新生儿时期。

病理学：在尸检时，脂肪浸润，血色素沉积和胆汁性肝硬化的局灶区域是最常见的组织学发现。在 15% 的病人中，脂肪浸润是大量的。在年长的儿童，肝硬化的局灶区域可能融合，有 5% 的儿童可出现多小叶性胆汁性肝硬化和纤维化。由于右心衰竭所致的组织学的小叶中心性萎缩有时可同时呈现。

在新生儿可显示下述表现：弥漫性胆汁淤滞；门脉周围的感染，纤维化和胆小管的增生；不伴存肝内胆汁淤滞的门脉周围的改变。这些改变可以由于伴发的梗阻性胃肠疾病的影响，或禁食和营养过度的影响而出现某些变化。一个不常见但却很确定表现，是大的肝内胆管上皮和腔内的过量胆性黏液的局灶性区域的出现。罕见地，黏液能梗阻肝外胆管。

胆囊管可以狭窄或闭锁，伴同黏膜的增生和残存腔内黏液的浓缩。胆囊可能萎缩，也可能含有胆泥和结石。

临床表现：胆汁性肝硬化可能少有为囊性纤维化的临床表现，症状有黄疸、腹腔积液、呕血和脾功能亢进。胆囊炎和胆系结石可出现于 10 岁到 20 岁之间的病人。新生婴儿病人可出现难以解释的持续的新生儿黄疸。

影像学研究：分析一组 24 例青年与成年囊性纤维化病例发现，一半的病人肝脏有异常的超声表现：不规则的回声增强。其中 3 个病例可见门静脉扩张和脾肿大。15 个病例有一个小的胆囊（其中大多数都有结石）或一个不确切的胆囊，8 个病例属于无异常。

逆行性胆管造影可以观察到多发性充盈缺损，胆管不规则，甚或某些肝内胆管局灶性扩张。

伴存肝内胆管的广泛的黏液栓的新生儿，在放射性核素 ^{99m}Tc-IDA 肝胆扫描时可见到完全性胆系梗阻，颇为类似于胆管闭锁。当黏液和胆汁充盈胆管树出现时，在胆管内容物吸出后术中胆系造影可显示胆管树开放，手术即可做出正确的诊断。

在囊性纤维化的小儿和青少年病人，CT 扫描可以显示肝脏的异常，甚至在临床尚未疑及肝脏疾病时也能如此。已报告的异常征象包括：大小、形态的异常，与肝硬化相符合的轮廓变化，与脂肪浸润相一致的异常低的密度，和 / 或门静脉高压的表现，诸如脾肿大、脾静脉或肠系膜上静脉的扩张等。当肝脏疾病在 CT 发现时，胰腺的脂肪替换则可能是一伴随征象。

第三节　肝发育不全和发育不良

正常人肝脏的大小和形态各有不同。肝发育不全（agenesis）和发育不良（hypoplasia）可波及肝脏的左、右两叶。肝脏左叶的先天缺如是一种少见的变异，这种变异被限定为胆囊窝左侧的肝组织缺失。它通常合并有肝右叶增大、肝副叶和尾叶肥大。肝右叶的发育不全也有报道，但更为少见，它通常被认为是发育异常，可能伴有右半膈缺失。

这些肝叶的发育不全与肝叶萎缩有着本质的区别，后者可在肝硬化基础上或放疗后发生。

在影像学研究中，除了需要了解先天性肝脏过度发育所致的异常外，尚有肝发育不全引起的肝脏变异，累及一个肝段甚至一个肝叶。

与医源性肝部分缺如的鉴别点是，发育不全无外科手术史，也无银夹所致的磁敏感性伪影。

肝位置反转：肝位置反转是一种明显的发育变异。肝脏与脾脏的位置关系与正常相反，根据大小、形态、内部血管及早期强化的特点易于鉴别两者。正常肝脏呈均匀一致性强化，而脾脏增强早期呈多样化强化。这些病人常伴有心血管、呼吸系统及胃肠道的先天性异常。

第二章　肝的发育与活体形态学简介

第一节　腹腔动脉与肠系膜上动脉的发育变异

腹腔动脉与肠系膜上动脉及其分支有着众多的变异，Tandler(1903)对腹侧内脏血管和纵行吻合动脉的胚胎发育变化的观察作了较为满意的解释。Michels(1956)也描述了腹腔动脉与肠系膜上动脉的最终成人型的详细情况，随后，不少作者通过标本与血管造影资料补充了他们的研究。

Michels 报告最常见的表现是肝脾胃干。在大约 55%~65% 的标本，第 11 和第 12 腹侧支和纵行吻合血管退化，而第 10 和第 13 腹侧支分别变成腹腔动脉与肠系膜上动脉。肝动脉可为单一动脉干(总肝动脉)，也可从腹腔动脉分别发出两支形成肝左动脉与肝右动脉。在后面这种情况，胃十二指肠动脉通常为肝左动脉的一条分支。在 10% 病例，肝左动脉可发自于胃左动脉。在 3.5% 病例，胃左动脉直接以一独立支发自于主动脉。此时，腹腔动脉则归属于肝脾干。肝脾系膜干是一少见的变异，只出现在 0.5% 的病例。第 10 节段支持续存在成为胃左动脉，第 11、12 支退化，而腹侧吻合血管保留连接于肝动脉和脾动脉到肠系膜上动脉。肝胃干形成于 1.5% 的病例。第 10 节段支保留成为腹腔动脉，发出胃左动脉与肝总动脉。第 11、12 节段支退化，而腹侧吻合血管持续存在，连接脾动脉与肠系膜上动脉。由于脾动脉发自于腹腔动脉(第 10 节段支)者占 95% 以上的病例，所以此型十分少见。

第 10 节段支持续存在成为脾胃干者占 5.5% 的病例。肝动脉被持续存留的腹侧吻合血管之肠系膜上动脉所替代。胃十二指肠动脉可发自于腹腔动脉(96%)或来自于替代肝动脉(4%)。肝动脉的其他六种变异也可出现，仰赖于腹侧吻合血管持续存在的程度，或肝左动脉的发育，或副肝左动脉为胃左动脉的一条分支。

腹腔系膜干的形成出现于 0.5% 以下的病例，第 10、11、12 节段血管退化，而腹侧纵行吻合动脉持续存在，所以胃左动脉、脾动脉和肝总动脉都发自于肠系膜上动脉。

腹侧吻合动脉完好地持续存在，伴存一正常的肝脾胃干，导致腹腔动脉和肠系膜上动脉直接连接，称之为 Buhler 弓。

Marchal 等(1981)与 Ralls(1981)在研究肝动脉的超声表现时，发现肠系膜上动脉与腹腔动脉可共同起源于腹主动脉的一处，此发育变异见于人群的 15% 左右。替代的右肝动脉发自于肠系膜上动脉的变异，可见于大约 20% 的人群。Hausdorf(1984)在研究小儿尾肝静脉的超声图像时，发现尾肝静脉此类变异可出现于人群中，约占 30%。

第二节　腹腔动脉发育变异

1. 腹腔动脉分型　Brown 将腹腔动脉分支分为六型：肝脾胃共干型；胃左动脉独立及肝脾动脉共干型；胃左动脉独立，肝脾肠系膜上动脉共干型；腹腔动脉与肠系膜上动脉共干型；胃脾动脉共干及肝肠系膜上动脉共干型；胃脾动脉共干，肝动脉缺如及肠系膜上动脉独立型。

2. 腹腔动脉及其分支　主要分支：腹腔动脉发自于主动脉的前部，位于第 12 胸椎～第 1 腰椎平面,正好在胰颈的上方,主动脉横膈裂孔之下,介于两膈脚之间。腹腔动脉的走行,或向腹侧,或向颅腹侧,或向尾腹侧。它的主要分支是肝动脉、脾动脉、以及胃左动脉,它也可发出背胰动脉和下膈动脉。下膈动脉可作为一独立分支,或作一共干发自腹腔动脉上缘。约有 22% 的病例,背胰动脉发自于腹腔动脉近侧的下部。

肝动脉有许多变异。Michels 报告有十种基本类型,其中有四种类型出现在 90% 以上的病例。最常见的类型是肝脾胃干(占 55%~65%),从腹腔发出肝总动脉,然后分出胃十二指肠动脉、肝左动脉与肝右动脉。肝左动脉与肝右动脉极少成为腹腔动脉的直接分支,如果成为直接分支,胃十二指肠动脉通常为肝左动脉的一条分支。

脾动脉在 95% 以上的病例,发自于腹腔动脉,它也可独自发源于主动脉,或为肠系膜上动脉所替代。脾动脉由 4 段组成。

胃左动脉发自于腹腔动脉近侧上部者,约占 90%。大约 3.5% 的病例,它作为一独立支发自于主动脉,正好在腹腔动脉的上方。在其余的病例,它或作为一附属的侧支,或为肝左动脉或为脾动脉所替代。

熟悉腹腔动脉活体形态学的意义能提高造影的成功率。在腹腔动脉与肠系膜上动脉共干者,常常导管极易插入肠系膜上动脉而不能插入腹腔动脉。无经验时可认为这是插管失败,当了解此类型后,作肠系膜上动脉造影,腹腔动脉同时显影,造影获得成功。

作为相应区域血管造影诊断的解剖基础。如胃十二指肠动脉正常多沿脊柱右缘下行,但有少数可偏向内侧,不要误认为外侧肿瘤压迫所致。中肝动脉上方有时血管稀少,分支又常弯向下方,不要误认为该处有占位性病变。

有助于对造影中出现的一些问题的解释。如肝动脉可有一支,多支或整个肝动脉起源异常。因此,作腹腔动脉造影时,右肝动脉一部或全部可不显影。如了解这种变异,继续作肠系膜上动脉造影,可使变异的肝动脉显影。

又如,作超选择性肝总动脉造影,为何胃左动脉和肠系膜上动脉上部分支也相继显影,只有了解变异的副胃左动脉的起源,与胃左动脉的通路,及胰十二指肠动脉前后弓在腹腔动脉与肠系膜上动脉之间的吻合支情况,才能阐明上述影像。

第三节 肝动脉的发育变异

详见本书 本卷 第十篇 第二章 肝动脉。

第四节 误诊与诊断陷阱

脂肪浸润:肝脏脂肪浸润与肥胖、饮酒、糖尿病、使用类固醇、营养过剩或营养不良有关。在螺旋 CT 增强的早期,因为肝脏没有完全强化而表现为低密度。在这种情况下,很难对比肝/脾的密度差异,因此有必要将肌肉作为参考标准。CT 上脂肪肝表现为均匀或不均匀的低密度。由于低密度病变与脂肪肝密度的对比度降低,CT 在脂肪肝基础上检出肝内病变常有困难。由于灌注差异,肝脏脂肪浸润偶尔呈区域或局灶性改变,不应误认为是肝脏肿块或梗死。如果有脂肪浸润,在脂肪浸润区域内可见到正常血管影像,而无占位效应。然而,当局灶性脂肪肝表现为一小团块时,可与肝脏肿块或转移混淆。局灶性脂肪肝常发生在镰状韧带邻近区域,即肝动脉供血的分水岭区域。

局限性脂肪浸润所致的非均匀性脂肪肝偶可误诊为肝脏占位病变,这种改变在门静脉周围区域最为常见。为鉴别局灶性脂肪浸润抑或肝脏肿块,进一步的影像学检查是必要的,其中超声与 MRI 检查有助于区别二者。偶尔需要经皮活检。

有作者发现大的回声包块位于肝前方,CT 证实为肝周的膈下脂肪,而起初却曾被误认为新生物包块。肝周、脾周脂肪,超声检查可误认为腹腔积液。腹膜前脂肪可有变异,它可以下伸几乎抵达盆腔,如不注意也可误诊。

Thickman 等（1983）指出，肝的前方和上方的脂肪蓄积产生回声区，由于肝下方的气体多重反射，在声像图上可出现慧星尾伪影，妨碍观察且导致误诊。

局灶性脂肪变和局灶性肝岛：肝脂肪浸润既可为均匀的，又可为不均匀的；既可呈局灶性，又可弥漫分布于全肝，其边界清楚或模糊。偶尔，肝内脂肪灶可类似于病变，通过比较同相位与异相位 T1WI 可鉴别脂肪灶与病变。

利用化学位移选择抑制技术（脂肪饱和技术）诊断脂肪浸润并不可靠。当一个体素内脂肪和水含量大致相等如肝脂肪浸润时，异相位成像显示最大的信号丢失。当脂肪成分接近 100% 时，脂肪饱和抑制成像则显示最大的信号丢失，后者常出现于局灶性脂肪病变，包括脂肪瘤和血管平滑肌脂肪瘤。肝脏假性病变常发生于镰状韧带周围，应与脂肪浸润相鉴别。

肝弥漫性脂肪浸润时可伴有正常不含脂肪的肝组织，即肝岛。肝岛常见于胆囊窝、镰状韧带周围及第 4 肝段。异相位成像可鉴别残留的局灶性正常肝实质与局灶性肿块。

冗长的肝左叶：偶尔肝左叶很大，向腹部左上象限延伸，形成所谓的包围肝，类似于正常脾脏或来自脾脏或肝左叶的外生性肿块。该发育变异的特点是增强扫描时与正常肝脏增强同步。正常肝脏信号 T_1WI 较脾脏高，T_2WI 较脾脏低。

肝脏放射性损伤：在治疗原发性肝脏肿块（例如肝癌）或是肝脏邻近器官肿瘤（例如下肺肿块或胰腺肿块）时，肝脏可能被包括在放疗区域内。这种情况下有可能发生误诊。在 CT 增强扫描早期，放疗区域内的肝脏强化程度可低于邻近没有受射线照射的肝脏，其 CT 表现与局灶性脂肪肝或肝脏肿块相似。如果仅做 CT 平扫及平衡期（延迟）扫描，则难以显示这种密度差别。在肝脏受到轻微放疗损伤的病人中，肝脏酶可能轻度升高，肝脏放疗的慢性期变化包括肝脂肪浸润和萎缩。

放疗后肝脏信号的变化与治疗和 MR 扫描的间隔时间有关。放疗后立即行 MR 扫描，受累肝脏表现为水肿改变，T_1WI 呈低信号，T_2WI 呈高信号。之后，由于受累肝脏发生慢性纤维化，则 T_1WI 和 T_2WI 均呈低信号。

在放疗照射野肝实质内甘油三酯沉积常常减少，因此，在脂肪抑制技术及异相位成像技术中，相对于含有脂肪的正常肝组织而言，照射区肝组织信号维持正常。照射区出现的放射诱导的急性血管炎或慢性肉芽组织形成，在延时增强扫描时出现强化。放疗后改变常沿照射野有一个区域性的清楚边界，即异常信号区与照射野一致而与肝段分布不一致。

局限性积液：局限于肝裂或隐窝内的液体和门静脉周围的水肿可能被误认为肝内病变。放射学工作者必须知道这些可能出现的误诊情况。肝圆韧带裂与大网膜囊相通，偶尔会有积液。液体也可以聚集在静脉韧带裂中，此裂隙与大小网膜囊均相通。液体可以聚集在胆囊窝内，成为胆囊切除术的一种并发症。腹膜腔内的液体能聚集在由横裂形成的潜在间隙内。必须注意不要将这些改变误认为肝内肿瘤或脓肿。

聚集在肝右叶附近的液体可能位于三个不同的间隙：胸膜腔、肝被膜下或肝周。当病人仰卧位扫描时，右侧胸腔积液将位于胸腔后部，并聚集在后肋膈角内。腹部 CT 扫描，若液体出现在肝裸区，可确定右侧胸腔积液而非腹水，因腹水不会聚集在此处。肝被膜下积液可压迫邻近的肝实质。肝周积液常见于腹水病人，实际上就是位于肝脏周围的游离性积液，它常呈新月形，对肝脏不产生占位效应。

部分容积效应：因为每一 CT 像素值代表相应体素的平均密度，当两个相邻组织具有明显的密度差别时均可发生部分容积效应，因此，部分容积效应可以在体内任何一部分发生。如果一个像素包含着具有不同衰减系数的组织，那么组合成的像素就有一个中间的衰减值，使不同组织的界限模糊。在普通 CT 上，可以通过减小层厚来降低或防止发生部分容积效应。尽管螺旋 CT 的部分容积效应比普通 CT 更明显，但它可用重叠重建来减小。研究表明，利用螺旋 CT 检出肝脏局灶性病变，可以通过减小层间距提高检出率。螺旋 CT 可对兴趣区进行额外的后处理，而不需要再行扫描，这种后处理避免了病人的额外再次照射，并可基本消除部分容积效应的影响。

部分容积效应还导致将肝外结构误诊为肝内病变，常遇见的问题是增大的右肾上腺、肾脏包块或门静脉周围淋巴结与原发肝肿瘤的鉴别。这一问题在儿童或腹部脂肪少的消瘦成年人中尤其多见。减小扫描层厚和进行三维重建有助于疑难病例的鉴别。

线束状伪影：当 X 线束穿透骨质和坚硬物体时，可能产生线束状伪影。这种伪影可见于肋骨附近的肝组织内，导致邻近右侧下位肋骨的肝组织内出现边缘不清的低密度伪影；这种伪影也可见于高密度导管或手术银夹的周围。不应将线束状伪影误认为肝内肿块或肝破裂。在特定病例中，采用高电流进行延迟或重复 CT 扫描有助于克服这种潜在的误诊。

膈肌附着点：膈肌由外周的肌肉和中心的腱膜构成，外周肌纤维向中心腱呈放射状集中，肌肉部分依其起源不同分为胸骨部、肋骨部和腰椎部。

偶尔，沿肋缘走行的宽大的肌肉附着处在肝内可引起信号强度变化，最常见于肝右叶。T_1WI 多表现为沿肝顶外周部纵行条带状低信号，或沿肝边缘出现局限性，圆形假性病变；T_2WI 常表现为膈肌附着处呈线形低信号，而多数肝脏局限性肿块呈高信号，可资鉴别。

肝位置反转：肝位置反转是一种明显的发育变异。肝脏与脾脏的位置关系与正常相反，根据大小、形态、内部血管及早期强化的特点易于鉴别两者。正常肝脏呈均匀一致性强化，而脾脏增强早期呈多样化强化。这些病人常伴有心血管、呼吸系统及胃肠道的先天性异常。

部分肝切除术后：肝脏手术后可导致肝脏变形。肝叶或肝段切除术后，肝脏轮廓可出现各种变形。切除术后 6~12 个月出现肝组织再生，沿肝脏手术切缘可出现信号强度的改变以及强化，类似于病变复发。此外，常可见手术银夹产生的金属伪影，这种“礼花”状的低信号伪影可类似于圆形局灶性病变。在毁损梯度回波序列或其他 T_2WI 上，伪影更加明显，以此可与真正的病变鉴别。

活检通道：由穿刺针、导管及低温消融后所致的通道也可改变受累区肝脏的信号强度。T_1WI 上水肿为局限性低信号，T_2WI 为高信号。出血 T_1WI 和 T_2WI 信号多种多样。反应性炎症表现为相邻组织的强化，常呈线状分布，根据临床病史可排除病变。

第三章　肝发育变异与诊断陷阱

第一节　肝脏形态发育变异

常见的肝形态学的发育变异，包括：里德尔叶、右肝叶后段副裂、肝右叶或肝左叶的先天性萎缩。先天性肝叶萎缩大概继发于宫内肝脏血液供应的发育异常。

肝脏形态发育变异并非少见，但真正的畸形则不多见。

肝脏的一叶可以增大或缩小（一侧肝萎缩时，另一侧肝可代偿性肥大）：①左外叶可萎缩，或仅成一扁平的带状组织。有作者指出，先天性萎缩大概继发于宫内期肝血液供应的发育异常。有的人在新生儿时期有较大的左外叶，以后逐渐萎缩而成一薄膜组织，其中仍遗留有残余的血管及胆管等，称为纤维附件。②左外叶缺如，很少见。CT 图像上于胆囊外侧无肝实质，也应结合超声诊断。③肝左叶内段发育不全：CT 图像上显示左叶内段发育小，肝轮廓出现凹陷部，结肠肝曲上升占据此凹陷。肝左叶内侧区发育不全为 Chilaiditi 症候群的原因之一。④肝左外叶也可很发达，其左端细长，甚至伸达脾脏，称獭尾肝。肝左叶也可稍大而略呈圆形。⑤右侧肝也可出现萎缩，但比较少见。

网膜隆起：CT 图像上，于肝左叶外侧段后面有时可见限局性突出，称之为网膜隆起。

分叶：肝的右叶的后段可显示分叶，为正常发育的变异，在 CT 检查或核素显像时不应将右叶后段外侧表面的分叶误认为一包块或一断裂。

肝的叶及段的大小与形态有相当变异，这些变异在放射性核素扫描上可能是误诊的根源，但在 CT 图像上却很易辨认。

肝副叶：人类肝脏很少发现多叶肝，文献曾报道有 16 个肝叶者，但并非真正的多叶肝。肝副叶均较小，且多位于肝的后面，常常只是在手术或尸检时才被发现。肝副叶也可发生于膈的上面，突向肺部，与肝脏没有任何联系，它有自己的独立的门静脉、肝动脉、胆管和肝静脉结构，这是因为在胚胎期，肝脏与膈一道由横膈发育而来，如一部分肝组织分居于膈上，就构成独立的肝副叶。

肝副叶通常附着于肝表面的下方，由具有血管与胆管的肝实质组成。它们无症状，通常是偶尔发现，但如果有蒂，则似肿块或肿大淋巴结。在先天性前腹壁缺损的病人（如脐疝病人）中，肝副叶的发生增多。

如附加肝叶（副叶肝）的体积较大或位于肝脏上方时，常规 X 线检查可见右膈呈局限性隆起或右下胸内包块影，因而引起临床注意，除了用超声、CT、MRI、人工气腹及 X 线照片以明确包块与膈、肝关系外，更直接准确的诊断方法是肝的核素检查。

黑岩俊郎等（1984）报告 1 例类似左膈肿瘤的肝副叶，当时指出气腹是鉴别膈、胸内及肝脏病变的基本方法，但欲鉴别肿瘤与肝副叶，只能靠大体和 / 或镜下检查。肝核素显像对确定里德尔叶及其他变异肝叶有用，但该例位于左侧，实难与脾上移区别。而肝胆核素显像的优点是脾不显像，肝却特异吸收核素，在该例鉴别诊断中起了重要作用。

有作者认为，肝副叶主要是肝右叶的变异副叶，为正常肝组织，有功能，有完整的血管、胆管和肝包膜，与肝右叶相连。通常肝副叶发生于肝下缘腹面，即里德尔叶。

里德尔叶（Riedel 叶）：此变异出现于大约 4% 的正常人，常见于女性。德国外科大夫 Riedel 首先报告。里德尔叶通常表现为舌状向下伸延，也可出现显著的分叶，甚至可伸长进入右髂窝，有时可直达盆腔，肝左叶、尾叶变小或基本见不到。反之，也可为肝左叶呈舌状伸延至脾外侧,伴横膈松弛,肝上升。胆囊窝和肋骨压痕以及右肾上极和肝内脏面之间的压迹变大。

里德尔叶是一种常见的发育变异,即肝右叶副叶,从肝右叶下方沿结肠旁沟向下延伸到髂窝。这种变异在瘦长体形的女性中多见,通常无症状,但在体检时易被误诊为肝肿大。

里德尔叶是肝右叶外侧部分增大,且向下呈舌状突出,有肝实质、胆管血管蒂与右叶相通连,少数的二者连接处只是由增厚的腹膜所包围的胆管血管蒂。胆囊可以附着于里德尔叶的下面。它不是一分离的肝叶,而是肝右叶的解剖上的下伸。

查体时,一个肥大的里德尔叶可错误解释为肝大或一异常的腹部包块或右肾下垂。里德尔叶可发生局部的病理改变,如扭转、结石、感染及肿瘤等,也可发生与肝脏相同的病变,如肝硬化等。核素显像如不注意也可导致误诊。

肝右叶相对于肝脏其他部分也可出现延长增大。与肝左叶的横向延长不同,里德尔叶增加了肝右叶的上下径。如仅以肝右叶的上下径来确定肝脏大小,一个正常的肝脏可能由于里德尔叶的存在而误诊为肝脏肿大。延长的肝右叶的轮廓有助于鉴别正常肝和病理性肿大的肝脏。冠状面成像里德尔叶呈向下逐渐变细的锥形,而获得性肝肿大常表现为肝横径和上下径同时增大,肝下缘呈圆形。

里德尔叶的信号强度与其邻近的正常肝脏呈等信号,以此可与肝右叶下缘的外生性肿块相鉴别。在腹部 X 线照片上,有时可见肝里德尔叶类似腹部肿块,偶尔在排泄性尿系造影照片上也可见到。

第二节　肝动脉诸分支起源变异、形态变化

一项研究 260 例血管造影所示的肝动脉诸分支起源变异、形态变化情况如下:

肝总动脉:260 例中, 256 例起自腹腔动脉,占 98.5%。仅 4 例(1.5%)起源变异,其中 3 例起始于肠系膜上动脉,由该处,肠系膜上动脉 - 肝总动脉再分出胃十二指肠动脉和肝固有动脉;另 1 例整个腹腔动脉与肠系膜上动脉共干发自腹主动脉。肝总动脉呈水平向右或微向上、下方走行者 219 例(84.2%);肝总动脉本身迂曲或肝总动脉与肝固有动脉两者间明显曲折成角者 41 例(15.8%),其中两者间夹角小于 45° 者 19 例,占 7.3%。

肝固有动脉:共 256 例发自肝总动脉,占 98.5%,其中 237 例(92.6%)为肝总动脉本干的直接延续。变异起源于肠系膜上动脉 - 肝总动脉者 4 例(1.5%)。肝总动脉由腹腔动脉分支后,右行大致呈水平走向,近脊柱右侧旁分为升、降两支,上升支即为肝固有动脉,下行支为胃十二指肠动脉。

肝右动脉:260 例中,有 236 例为肝固有动脉的直接延续,占 88.7%。异位起始于其他动脉者,占 11.3%。其中起于肠系膜上动脉者最多,占 8.3%,此时肝左动脉源自腹腔动脉 - 肝总动脉或腹腔动脉 - 胃左动脉;其次是起自腹腔动脉干和肝总动脉者,各占 1.2%;始于胃十二指肠动脉及腹主动脉者最少,各占 0.4%。肝右动脉由本干向肝右叶内延伸,主要分为肝右动脉前支和后支,由粗渐细, 1 支再分成 2 支,分布在肝脏右叶。

肝中动脉:一组肝中动脉显影者 246 例。始于肝固有动脉者 20 例(8.1%);发自肝右动脉者 73 例,占 29.7%;而占优势的是发自肝左动脉占 62.2%(153/246)。有时亦可见从肝左、右动脉各发出一小支肝中动脉的情况。肝中动脉较短,分支较少,向头侧行走。

肝左动脉:一组肝左动脉显影者 234 例。其中源自肝固有动脉者 221 例(94.4%);发自肝总动脉者 8 例(3.4%);而异位起源于胃左动脉者 5 例(2.1%)。肝左动脉起始后向左走行,一般分尾状叶动脉、左内叶动脉、左外叶动脉上段支和下段支。

胃十二指肠动脉:胃十二指肠动脉与肝总动脉两者之间呈钝角者 226 例(86.9%);锐角者 34 例(13.1%)。肝总动脉与肝固有动脉间曲折成角,其夹角小于 45° 者 19 例,占 7.3%。肝总动脉、肝固有动脉和胃十二指肠动脉三者可相互成角。

肝动脉起源的发育变异十分常见,文献报告许多,此处从略。熟悉肝动脉的起源,走行及其与病灶和邻近脏器的关系,对放射科和外科医生进行肝脏及其附近病变的诊断、介入性治疗和手术切除均有重大价值。

在按常规作腹腔动脉插管造影,而肝内动脉未

显影或部分未显影时，应考虑有迷走肝动脉的存在，需根据情况加作肠系膜上动脉甚至腹主动脉造影。作超选择性肝动脉造影前，宜常规首先作腹腔动脉造影，阅片时，对一些较少见的迷走肝动脉应进行仔细辨认，不可误认为其他血管，引起误诊。

因欧美人肝动脉变异率较高，故有的医院已将肝、胰大手术前进行腹部动脉造影作为常规。国人肝动脉变异的发生率虽然较低（这是否与我们研究欠缺有关，尚待分析），但在诊断和治疗时也应引起重视。

第三节　镰状韧带及镰状韧带周围的假性病灶

镰状韧带的大小及形状可出现不少的变异。在X线腹腔充气造影仰卧位照片时，可以见到镰状韧带，Han（1980）分析91例腹腔充气造影病人（成人11例，新生儿6例及儿童4例），皆清楚见到此韧带。在成人，其长度为6~14cm，宽约0.1~1.lcm；其最大伸展范围是从第9胸椎下缘平面到第3腰推下缘平面；韧带表现笔直者7例，凹向脊柱者4例。在儿童和婴儿，长为1.5~7.0cm，宽0.1~0.2cm；最大伸展范围从第8胸椎下缘平面到第3腰椎下缘平面；韧带笔直8例，凹向脊柱2例。横膈的右叶的膈脚和结肠袋的阴影有时可伪似镰状韧带，值得注意。

在CTAP检查时，镰状韧带周围的假性病灶是附脐静脉血流注入门脉左干，稀释了来自门脉主干的对比剂。肝硬化患者由于门脉高压，附脐静脉形成离肝血流，所以镰状韧带周围的假性病灶正常人比肝硬化者出现率高。Matsui通过选择性胃左、右动脉造影证实肝段IV（肝左叶内侧段）后缘的假性病灶与胃静脉引流变异有关。另外，被膜下的灌注缺损系指小的、扁平或楔形低密度区，位于被膜下，它们大多数与门脉灌注的变异或肋骨压迫有关。

在CTAP，产生这些假阳性表现的原因很多，包括肝纤维化、局灶性脂肪浸润、变性结节、肝静脉未强化、肝内胆管扩张、解剖变异（如副裂的发生），位于肝门附近的肿瘤压迫门静脉分支，肠系膜上静脉及脾静脉血流的非等量混合、肝门静脉栓塞以及穿刺后肝包膜下出血等。诸如起源于肠系膜上动脉的肝右动脉可以解释肝右叶后段过分强化；胃静脉的异常引流常可发生Ⅳ段的假阳性病灶；肝硬化伴门静脉高压的患者改变了肝脏的血流动力学，可造成肝脏的局灶性灌注缺损，引起假阳性病变；值得注意的是，尽管变性结节在组织学上属于分化良好的肝细胞肿瘤，但据统计，约96%的变性结节，门静脉参与其供血，因此，变性结节的CT衰减值接近于周围的肝实质。但在肝硬化或门静脉高压的患者，退变性结节在CTAP图像上的表现可与肝细胞癌结节相似。

在CTAP、CTHA影像中，可依据低密度、高密度的灌注异常区来判断肿瘤的存在。但灌注异常区并不都意味着肿瘤，它可能是良性或恶性肿瘤，也可能是非肿瘤的灌注异常。造成非肿瘤灌注异常的原因很多，包括病理性的（如再生结节、不典型腺瘤样增生、局限性纤维化、局部脂肪浸润、动-门脉分流、门脉高压等）和非病理性的（如血供变异、层流及技术因素等）。镰状韧带周围的假病灶是附脐静脉血流注入门脉左干，稀释了来自门脉主干的对比剂。肝硬化患者由于门脉高压，附脐静脉形成离肝血流，所以镰状韧带周围的假灶正常人比肝硬化者出现率高。Matsui等（1994）通过选择性胃左、右动脉造影证实段Ⅳ（肝左叶内侧段）后缘的假性病灶与胃静脉引流变异有关。Irie等（1996）认为并非所有的这类假灶均如此，也有因为胆囊静脉形成的肝外胆管静脉丛进入了段Ⅳ。胆囊周围的假灶是由于胆囊静脉汇入门脉分支，稀释了对比剂。

上述假灶在CTHA上有时表现为低密度（脂肪浸润），有时为高密度（与胆囊静脉引流或肝动脉生理性优先灌注有关），有时为等密度。被膜下的灌注缺损系指小的、扁平或楔形低密度区，位于被膜下，它们大多数与门脉灌注的变异或肋骨压迫有关。

腹腔充气造影仰卧位照片可见镰状韧带，Han（1980）分析91例腹腔充气造影病人（成人11例，新生儿6例及儿童4例），皆清楚见到此韧带。在成人其长度为6~14cm，宽约0.1~1.1cm，其最大伸展范围是从第9胸椎下缘平面到第3腰椎下缘平面；韧带表现笔直者7例，凹向脊柱者4例。在儿童和婴儿，长为1.5~7.0cm，宽0.1~0.2cm；最大伸展范围从第8胸椎下缘平面到第3腰椎下缘平面；韧带笔直8例，凹向脊柱2例。

横膈右叶的膈脚和结肠袋的阴影有时可伪似镰

状韧带,值得注意。

第四节 病人的体位和肝脏的位置

肝脏的大小、形状的变化,大概超过任何一个实质脏器。Friedell 等(1957)与 McAfee 等(1965)至少在前方正位扫描图像上确定了正常肝的表现及其变化的范围。Covington(1970)再次强调解剖学的变化以及前方观察的偏差。侧方扫描,虽长期以来已认识其良好的诊断价值,并知晓此摄像位置上正常形状变异较小,但这些大概皆源于只在左侧卧位上进行侧方观察。随着医学进步,改变病人体位进行核素扫描已有可能,坐位、站立、仰卧、俯卧或侧卧,常只做其中某一体位。

Winston 等(1972)指出,病人体位的变更引起肝脏形状的变化却很少为人注意。从诊断角度看,右肝扫描最麻烦的地方是仰卧位时的前下切迹,在左侧卧位或坐位扫描时很少看到此切迹,俯卧位时则一般见不到它。此种因体位不同而引起的形状的变化的范围各人互不相同,在某些人变化较小,而在另一些人则十分明显,且类似肿块占位。

右肝的前下切迹大概为叶间分离所致。仰卧位时它比较恒定,此刻,体积较大的右叶移向体积较小的左叶的后方或背侧。

一般大体解剖皆称左右二叶比较,右叶更靠前方,这与上述发现有矛盾。有作者解释此矛盾称,正常活体肝脏相当柔软,仰卧位时重力可产生一较大的扭转力,加之右叶固定不甚佳良,导致右叶转向背侧。在左侧卧位(即左侧靠床面的侧卧位)此类旋转不出现,右叶更为完全地重叠于左叶,很少见到右前下切迹。

Custer 与 Shafer(1975)专门著文讨论脾切除术后引起的肝扫描的变化时指出,脾切除术后可产生肝的移动或变位。手术后左肝叶的移动十分常见,此移动的范围仰赖于肝脏的柔软性、病人的年龄、切除脾脏的大小,以及病人的肥胖程度。肝脏的此种移动导致正常的左右肝叶之间的分界增宽。核素显像时务需注意。

肝位置反转是一种明显的发育变异。肝脏与脾脏的位置关系与正常相反,根据大小、形态、内部血管及早期强化的特点易于鉴别两者。正常肝脏呈均匀一致性强化,而脾脏增强早期呈多样化强化。这些病人常伴有心血管、呼吸系统及胃肠道的先天性异常。

第五节 肝核素显像与肝脏实质的柔软性

在肝核素显像中清楚可见肝的轮廓,值得注意的是,由于肝脏是一柔软的实质性脏器,肝的邻近结构的变化常可使肝的轮廓发生改变,从而造成肝影形状的变迁。

肝脏上部分正常上凸至横膈,呈穹隆状。在肝右叶和左叶之间出现内凹,乃为膈脚所致。横膈的变化常常造成肝上面轮廓的改变。膈的抬高,部分性或完全性右肺叶切除可导致肝右叶向上凸出。

慢性梗阻性肺部疾病可使肝上缘变平,由于肺叶的过度膨胀,致使肝脏向下移位,从而临床可在肋下扪及肝脏,造成临床上肝脏增大的误诊,然而肝脾核素显像却见肝为正常大小。肝上缘变平与肝脏位置下移也出现于任何原因所致的胸膜渗出或胸腔积液,此时,如行肝与肺的核素扫描,则可见右肺与肝之间出现分离,乃为胸腔积液所致。

膈下脓肿、纤维胸以及胸膜反应还造成右肝边缘显著变直。

肝脏实质的柔软性,允许邻近病变改变肝的形状或放射性药物的分布,有时这些假性缺损可错误解释为肝内包块。

右侧肾上腺肿块可使右肝叶前后径缩短,前面肝扫描见肝变薄,后方肝扫描则几乎不见右肝叶影像。皮质样肾瘤改变右肾的正常光滑的对肝的压迹,而使右肝叶后方明显受压推移。Covington(1970)与 Chaudhuri(1975)分别讨论了此类易引起误诊的情况。

左叶在形态学上的变异很大,左叶的外段可以向左伸延直达腹壁,也可很短,不超过中线,这种肝脏形态学的变异在放射性核素扫描时常造成诊断上的困难，但在超声和 CT 影像中容易识别。

第六节　肝胃韧带及肝的毗邻关系

通常认为肝胃韧带是连于肝和胃小弯之间的双层腹膜，食管腹段和胃均属于腹膜内位器官；一些教材的图显示小网膜囊上隐窝的前界为肝左叶，左肝上后间隙与小网膜囊相通。但是，有作者在解剖断层标本和 CT 观察时发现：肝胃韧带后层在近胃小弯处反折至膈，形成内侧胃膈韧带；肝胃韧带构成小网膜囊上隐窝的前界并将其与左肝上后间隙隔开。

肝之胃小弯面，于 CT 平扫及增强扫描时，与周围肝组织均为等密度，有病变存在时，鉴别不困难。但当胃蠕动产生干扰时，此部分肝组织的密度评价较为困难。有时需结合超声检查判断。

研究发现，在活体，肝的毗邻关系的变异相当大，而体位与呼吸运动是其部分的原因。

第七节　动态扫描

准确的动态扫描概念应该是对比剂在动脉期至平衡期间的扫描，而以往将团注对比剂后 1~3 分钟期间的快速扫描认为是动态扫描。一般 CT 机扫描速度可在 2~3 分钟内扫 15~20 个层面，这是由于解决了 X 线管快速冷却问题和扩大了计算机的存贮量之故。再有，肝扫描至肝下缘时，最好能扫到肾脏非平衡期至平衡期到来时的图像。

对比剂注入后 3~4 小时的延迟扫描时，正常肝细胞可以将 1%~2% 的对比剂分泌入胆管系统，而肿瘤组织内已无对比剂，此时，相对低密度的肿瘤区域呈现在中度强化的正常肝实质背景上。为了准确率，延迟扫描前要做动态扫描，这样将有助于血管的观察。应用 EOE-I3（碘化脂类物质）对比剂增强与 MRI 扫描对肝癌的敏感性已达 85%~90%，延迟扫描因此受到了挑战。

第八节　肝脏大小的变异

肝右叶几乎占据肝影右半，肝左叶延伸向前，镰状韧带在其间形成一裂隙。

肝脏的大小对于诊断胃肠疾病等常有一定关系。Niederau 等（1983）用超声对 915 例健康人测量肝之大小，指出肝在瘦削的人纵径较长，在重体重者则横径较大，因此肝的纵径与前后径均必须测量，这样才比较准确，不然，只测纵径则可使测量值变得过高或过低。在超声检查肝时，有作者发现肝的左叶内段有时可相当小，而肝的右叶后段又可显示分叶，这些都是发育变异。

冗长的肝左叶：偶尔肝左叶很大，向腹部左上象限延伸，形成所谓的包围肝（wraparound liver），类似于正常脾脏或来自脾脏或肝左叶的外性性肿块。该发育变异的特点是增强扫描时与正常肝脏强化同步。正常肝脏信号 T_1WI 较脾脏高，T_2WI 较脾脏低。

肝发育不全：除了先天性肝脏过度发育所致的异常外，尚有肝发育不全引起的肝脏变异，累及一个肝段甚至一个肝叶。与医源性肝部分缺如的鉴别点是，发育不全无外科手术史，也无银夹所致的磁敏感性伪影。

第九节　肝右叶发育不良

影像学研究：影像学上诊断肝右叶发育不良必须满足 3 个条件，即肝右叶门静脉或分支、右叶静脉或分支不可见,以及肝右叶胆管扩张,如果可见肝静脉或门静脉右支完整,则可以排除肝右叶发育不良的诊断。

目前国内外文献及个案报道归纳分析,肝右叶发育不良在影像上的主要征象有:肝右叶体积减小甚至不可见,肝脏门静脉右支或其分支不可见,肝内胆管扩张,肝左叶及尾状叶的体积代偿性增大。这些征象均可以通过 CT 及 MRI 扫描发现。

一组 18 例均可见肝右叶体积的明显减小,门静脉右支不可见,肝内胆管扩张等征象。一般可引起肝左叶及尾状叶体积代偿性增大,该组病例中 1 例出现尾状叶体积的减小,且尾状叶内多发结石并胆管扩张,考虑多是由于尾状叶长期胆汁淤滞而引起萎缩。这些表现通过 CT 增强扫描及 MRI 非对比剂成像可以清晰的显示门静脉的形态及走行。

肝右叶发育不良常常合并有胆囊异位,包括肝上胆囊及肝后胆囊,但以右后方异位最为常见。文献报道 1 例肝上胆囊。胆囊异位致使胆囊管变长扭曲,胆汁排泄障碍,肝内分泌的胆汁淤积导致肝内外胆管结石及胆囊结石形成。该组病例中 1 例胆囊与十二指肠形成内漏,胆囊萎缩并伴有炎症,这可能也是肝右叶发育不良伴有胆囊结构的先天异常所造成的。

该组病例中曾因为胆系结石而切除胆囊 9 例,考虑这些患者同样合并胆囊结构的异位,因为胆囊异位而极易形成胆囊结石而最终手术切除。Hisatomi 等(2004)报道 1 例肝右叶发育不良合并腹膜后纤维化的病例,其排除了其他导致腹膜后纤维化的原因,但其发生机制并不明确。Suh 等(2008)报道 1 例肝右叶发育不良合并下腔静脉发育不良。

肝右叶发育不良的并发症多是由于胆系及门静脉系统的阻塞而引起。胆管系统的阻塞常常引起胆囊结石、肝内胆管及胆总管结石及胆系感染等。门脉系统的异常常常引起门脉高压的表现,该组病例中脾脏增大者有 11 例, 1 例曾经因出现脾亢进行过治疗。

一些作者报道 1 例肝右叶发育不良并发布加综合征,其形成机制认为是肝右叶发育不良,导致左叶代偿性增大,因此肝左静脉相对狭窄,增大的左叶压迫下腔静脉所致。

此外,先天性肝右叶发育不良患者由于长期的胆汁淤滞及胆管结石并感染,易引起肝硬化及肝实质恶变,此为预后最差的并发症,肝实质恶变多为胆管细胞癌,目前已经有个案报道肝右叶发育不良合并胆管细胞癌。

CT 及 MRI 平扫可以探测到右叶体积缩小,左叶及尾状叶体积增大,肝内外胆管扩张、肝内外胆管结石及胆囊的位置形态等均可得到较好的显示,但 CT 平扫对静脉及门静脉的显影欠佳,采用上腹部 CT 三期增强扫描,可以清晰的显示静脉及门静脉,有较高的诊断价值。

MRI T_2WI 序列亦可以较清晰的显示门静脉系统, MRCP 序列对胆管系统的显影。尤其是现今 MRI 不使用对比剂血管成像序列的使用,如 SLEEK 序列的使用,使得肝脏静脉及门静脉成像更简便更清晰。

鉴别诊断:肝右叶萎缩的原因主要有各种原因导致的肝硬化,肝门部胆管细胞癌所致门脉右支狭窄。CT 增强扫描及 MRI T_2 压脂序列上均可以较清晰的显示门静脉的分支及走行。此外,诊断分析时明确病史同样非常重要,有无肝炎、血吸虫及长期酗酒等病史。一组病例中所有患者均无此类病史。

肝门部胆管细胞癌侵犯肝门脉右支导致右支狭窄甚至闭塞引起肝右叶血流供应减少,动脉供血代偿不足引起右叶萎缩,门脉左支受累及时,左叶及尾状叶代偿性肥大,但对于肝右叶发育不良并发肿瘤性病变时,到底是肿瘤性病变累及肝门静脉右支引起右支狭窄甚至闭塞,继发肝脏右叶萎缩,还是肝右叶发育不良并发肿瘤性病变,仍然可以通过探测肝右叶门静脉及肝静脉系统是否存在来进行鉴别。

第十二篇　肝与肝外

第一章　肝外疾病侵犯肝脏和诊断陷阱

第一节　肺癌直接侵犯肝脏

临床上，原发于肺底部的癌肿比较少见，而肺癌直接穿破膈肌，侵犯肝脏的病例更为少见。

右肺底肺癌可向下浸润，破坏膈肌致膈神经麻痹，膈肌升高；侵犯胸膜和肝脏，引起胸腔积液或胸腔积脓，肝脏占位病变，以及癌性肺段性肺不张，肺内淋巴结转移。

有时，因胸部照片未能显示肺癌肿块，只见右肺下野大片阴影或密度增高，肋膈角不清，或膈肌上升遮掩病变的显示，而只考虑为肺部及胸部炎症，或肺脓肿伴胸腔积液，抗炎治疗效果甚差。再用超声显像或 / 和 CT 扫描则可能见到邻近肺底的膈肌和肝脏的病变，从而做出正确诊断。问题是，在这样的情况下，应广开思路，想到肝脏被侵犯的可能性，再进一步进行检查。

第二节　误诊病例简介：神经纤维瘤病侵犯肝脏

详见本书 本卷 第五篇 第十章 第一节　误诊病例简介：神经纤维瘤病侵犯肝脏与肝脏多发占位病变。

第三节　腹膜后、肝尾叶炎性假瘤与肝尾叶肝癌

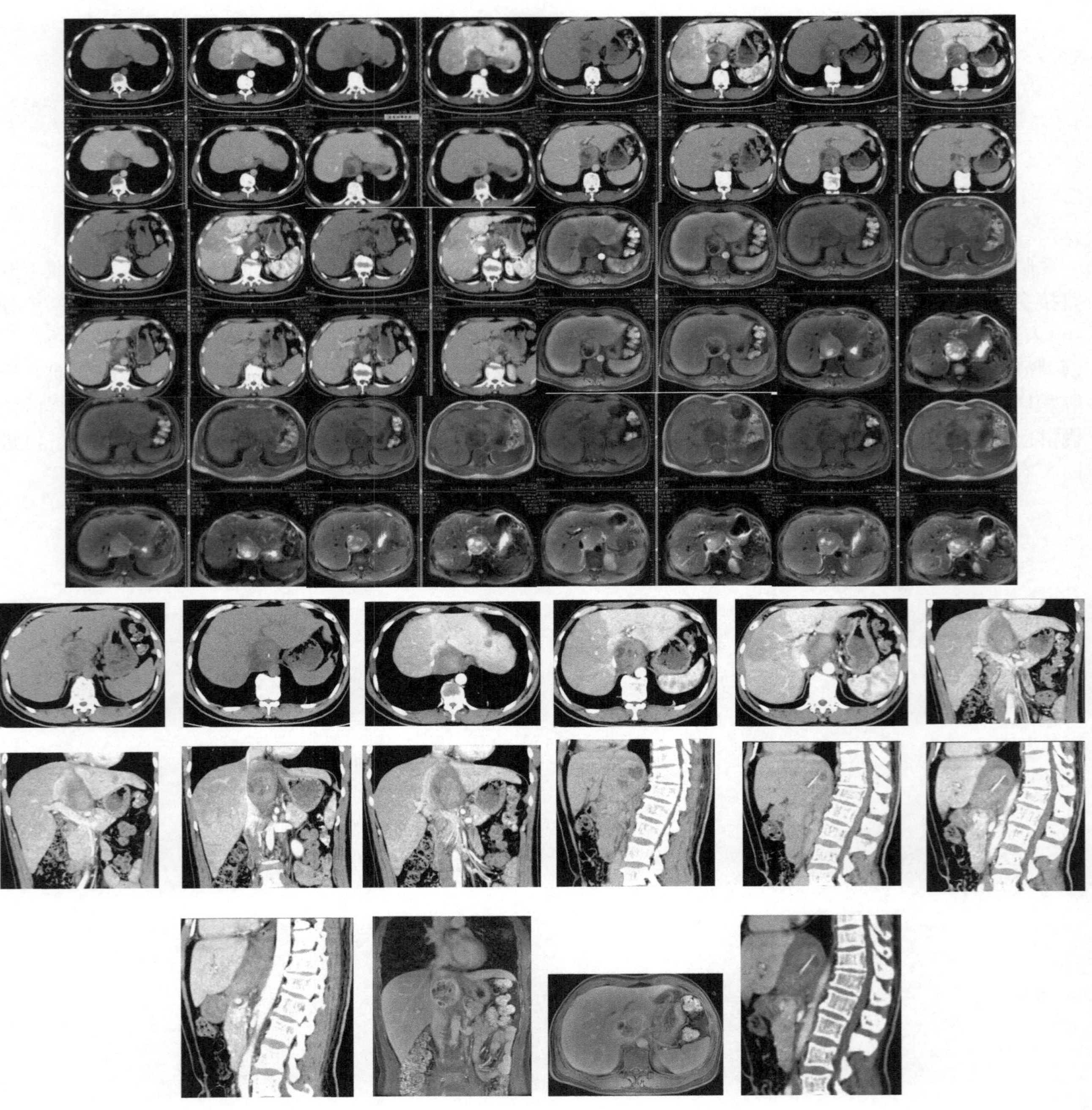

图 12-1-1　腹膜后、肝尾叶炎性假瘤与肝尾叶肝癌

患者,男，47 岁。反复纳差乏力 10 余天入院。患者于 10 天前无明显诱因出现全身乏力、纳差,伴头晕、畏寒,发热、上腹部持续性闷痛不适,程度较剧烈,难以难受,就诊于当地诊所,予对症治疗,症状不能缓解。近 10 天来体重下降 5kg。

CT 拟诊:第二、第三肝门区占位性病变性质待定,恶性肿瘤可能性大,生物学行为侵犯周围组织不明显,来源于肝？腹膜后？建议 MR 检查;左肝、右肝下极小结节低强化

影,性质待定;肝血液灌注异常;腹膜后多发淋巴结。MRI 拟诊:肝尾状叶占位伴内部囊变、坏死,考虑肝癌可能,请结合临床;双肾囊肿。

手术所见:肝尾状叶可见一肿瘤,大小约 4 cm × 5cm,包膜较完整;决定行肝尾状叶切除术。

病理检查:肝尾状叶肿物:肝组织一块,大小 8.0cm × 4.5cm × 4.0cm,切面见一结节,直径 4.0cm,淡黄、质中,与周围界清。12L 淋巴结:灰白色组织一块,大小 3.5cm × 2.5cm × 1.0cm,切面灰白质中。常规病理诊断:肝尾状叶肿物切除标本:增生性病变,细胞形态一致,初步考虑恶性肿瘤,待免疫组化进一步明确诊断。12L 淋巴结切除标本:检出淋巴结(1/2)可见肿瘤转移。

免疫组化检测:阳性:CD68, CD163, LCA, Vimentin, PAS, VEGF(+), 5-FU(+), TOPO Ⅱ(+), Ki-67(+,约 20%);阴性:CK(P),CK7,CK8,CK18,CK19,CK20,TTF-1,Villin,PSA,AFP,Hepatocyte,HMB45, CD20,CD21,CD23,CD35,CD79a,CD5,ALK80,P63,CyclinD1,BCL-2,BCL-6,CD1a,CD10,TDT,AB,S-100,SMA,Calponin,Desmin,Actin,CD34(血管内皮+),EGFR,PgP,Tubulinβ,ERCC1。

免疫组化诊断:肝尾状叶肿物切除标本:经免疫组化证实,常规病理图像下所见的一致增生的细胞为组织细胞,并伴有小脓肿形成,符合炎性假瘤改变,考虑瘤块较大,且形态不典型,建议外院进一步会诊。外院会诊结果:肝尾状叶:结节状病变主要由显著的组织细胞、泡沫细胞、淋巴浆细胞增生构成,中央可见小脓肿,病变周围见广泛的纤维化及残余或增生胆管及肝组织,结合原单位免疫组化结果,考虑炎性假瘤,建议定期随访。

误诊分析:术前考虑鉴别诊断有三:肝癌;胆管细胞癌;腹膜后淋巴源性肿瘤。本例病灶系炎性假瘤,病灶内条状高密度影手术后证实为鱼刺影,系误食鱼刺后,鱼刺穿破食管进入食管肝间隙,局部慢性炎症形成包裹,与肝尾状叶紧密粘连。该病例炎性肉芽肿较大,与肝尾状叶分界不清,术前误以为来源于肝尾状叶肿瘤,导致误诊为肝脏来源肿瘤, CT 与 MRI 均将肝癌作为首选诊断;该例误诊与 CT 常规横断扫描也有一定关系,如当时接诊医生能够及时再做三维重建,鱼刺的影像一定能够发现,此类误诊即可避免。CT 常规横断扫描图像上看见了小点状高密度影,但却完全被忽略,未进一步分析,误以为病灶钙化,术后回顾再行多平面重建显示为一针状规则的长条状高密度影,清楚显示为鱼刺,如果术前观察图像认真一些,在诊断时思路开阔一些,再带着问题与病人直接交流病情进展情况,此类误诊也可能避免。腹膜后异物极为少见,食管异物穿破食管进入周围组织,与肝尾叶紧密粘连,导致炎性假瘤形成,术前诊断困难(图 12-1-1)。

第四节　白血病肝浸润

虽然肝的白血病侵犯不常见,它通常见于急性髓性白血病或淋巴细胞性白血病,常形成镜下浸润。在这些病例,肝超声显示正常,或可能示非特异性肝脏肿大,或正常肝回声结构的非特异性改变。局灶性肝的白血病浸润(绿色瘤)表现为多数性边界清楚的几乎无回声包块,无透声,侵犯两肝叶。此类病变许多均含有中心性斑点高回声区而产生一种“牛眼”征。

第五节　丛状纤维组织细胞瘤侵犯肝脏

详见本书 本卷 第八篇 第一章 第三节　丛状纤维组织细胞瘤侵犯肝脏。

第六节　急性胰腺炎对肝脏损害的 CT 观察

急性胰腺炎是临床常见急腹症,因产生酶血症及胰腺解剖位置关系,常有多脏器损害,肝脏损害较常见。

急性胰腺炎肝损害 CT 表现:重症胰腺炎肝损害时,肝实质密度普遍降低,平均 CT 值为 35.8 HU,肝、脾密度比值倒置明显,肝血管影明显显示,增强扫描时肝实质动静脉期均为均匀一致强化改变。

轻型胰腺炎肝损害时,肝实质密度亦普遍降低,

2 例肝脏密度明显降低，肝、脾密度比值倒置，平均 CT 值为 41 HU，强化亦呈均匀一致增强。

轻型和重型胰腺炎肝损害时，随着胰腺炎病情的治疗好转，肝脏密度亦随着逐渐恢复至正常 CT 值，一组 30 例平均时间为 23 d。

急性胰腺炎肝损害发生机制及肝脏病理改变：其机制较为复杂，胰腺水肿造成胆管梗阻是肝功能受损的重要原因，且急性胰腺炎时从炎症胰腺组织内释放各种破坏因子如胰腺的细胞色素 P450 和自身活化代谢产物——溶血卵磷脂、弹力蛋白酶 E、激肽 E、组织胺等通过静脉回流肝脏，在肝脏损害中起重要作用。

急性胰腺炎肝脏病理改变主要为：肝窦充血，肝细胞发生颗粒变性，水肿坏死，炎性细胞浸润，肝组织以小叶中心性凝固性坏死为主，在重症胰腺炎时可发生片状肝细胞坏死，而肝细胞的线粒体及溶酶体破坏最明显，其发生也最早，因而导致肝脏在 CT 上表现为均匀一致密度降低影。

而重症胰腺炎肝损害时肝脏密度降低发生率高，约为 80.8%，轻型胰腺炎肝损害时肝脏密度降低发生率低不如前者，约为 58.9%，与肝细胞的损害程度与胰腺炎的程度呈正相关。

随着急性胰腺炎病情的治疗好转，肝脏密度逐渐升高，其可能原因为从炎症胰腺组织内释放的各种破坏因子亦明显减少，肝损害减少，肝功能逐渐恢复，肝脏密度亦逐渐恢复至正常。文献报道急性胰腺炎病人肝脏损害随着原发病好转可恢复正常，均为可逆性，急性胰腺炎肝脏损害时肝脏 CT 表现与此一致。

急性胰腺炎肝损害与弥漫性脂肪肝区别和联系：在 CT 表现上两者均为肝实质密度普遍降低，强化表现亦一致。前者在发生急性胰腺炎时均排除有脂肪肝、肝炎、肝硬化等疾病；后者发生机制虽尚未完全明确，大多认为是由各种原因引起的脂肪代谢障碍，是肝细胞内甘油三酯超过正常生理范围的过度蓄积所致，通常与酗酒、糖尿病、慢性肝病及营养不良有关，虽通过饮食及原发病治疗，肝脏密度在 CT 上可恢复正常，也是可逆的。但时间大多较前者长。

在临床工作中，我们还发现一些原来有脂肪肝的病人，在患急性胰腺炎治疗中，或急性胰腺炎治愈后，CT 检查随访观察中，脂肪肝的表现逐渐好转，甚至脂肪肝完全消失，其机制尚有待进一步研究。总之，在急性胰腺炎时，特别是重症急性胰腺炎时，容易发生肝脏损害，虽然 CT 不如肝功能敏感，可通过其 CT 表现对急性胰腺炎作更全面的了解和认识。

第七节　膈肌附着点与假性病变

膈肌由外周的肌肉和中心的腱膜构成，外周肌纤维向中心腱呈放射状集中，肌肉部分依其起源不同分为胸骨部、肋骨部和腰椎部。偶尔，在 MRI 扫描中，沿肋缘走行的宽大的肌肉附着处在肝内可引起信号强度变化，最常见于肝右叶。T_1WI 多表现为沿肝顶外周部纵行条带状低信号，或沿肝边缘出现局限性、圆形假性病变；T_2WI 常表现为膈肌附着处呈线形低信号，而多数肝脏局限性肿块呈高信号，可资鉴别。

第八节　肝外的假性病变

在 CT 图像上，邻近肝脏的其他脏器或组织的肿块，偶尔可表现伪似肝内原发性肿块，此刻，应用多方位性的影像诊断技术（如超声、磁共振成像及其他）常有助于正确地鉴别诊断。

上腹部 X 线平片上的肝影中，肝圆韧带周围脂肪可产生肝双叶影像，或形成似肿瘤。

在正位腹部平片上，婴儿的皮肤皱褶在肝影处产生特殊的影像，可表现为肝影上重叠一圆弧形的更高密度影。有作者报告，在正位腹部平片上，右季肋部出现假肿瘤征，表现为胁腹线的脂肪密度影向内呈圆弧状凸出，事实上是由右侧肌肉挤压所致。

有腹部照片上，肺后下缘重叠于上腹部，可类似腹部肿块。

第二章　其他疾病影响肝脏

第一节　肝脏多发脾种植

肝内脾种植临床上罕见。Buchbinder(1939)首次报道7例外伤后脾种植，此后文献陆续出现个案报道。脾种植是自身脾组织在异位生长而形成的占位性病变，一般继发于脾外伤，由于破裂的脾组织碎屑种植于腹腔并逐渐建立血液循环供给促进脾组织发育，形成具有脾功能的自体异位脾组织。

脾组织种植灶外观呈淡红色，形态多样，呈椭圆形、颗粒状或分叶状，其直径小至几毫米，最大至12 cm，但多小于3 cm。其好发部位依次为小肠浆膜面、大网膜、壁层腹膜、大肠表面、肠系膜、膈肌的腹侧面和胸部。

在脾破裂、脾切除的患者中，发生脾种植的可能性高达67%，文献报道，种植灶数目与脾损伤严重程度以及播散的脾组织多少有关。

脾破裂发生到异位脾组织诊断的间隔时间5个月至32年不等，平均确诊时间约为10年。由于肝内脾种植少见，难以与其他肝脏肿瘤或肿瘤性病变鉴别，容易误诊、漏诊。

肝内脾组织植入的机制不是很清楚，可能有两种：脾破裂或脾切除时，脾细胞种植到肝脏浆膜表面并向肝内陷入；也可能脾细胞通过脾静脉血行播散而种植于肝脏，一例患者因有脾破裂后自体血回输病史，故以后者方式种植可能性大。

脾种植易发生于膈与肝Ⅱ段之间，因其邻近脾组织，并且在脾切除术时碎裂脾组织容易转移到此部位。由于膈的慢性挤压作用易导致脾组织侵入肝实质。

自体脾种植一般术前很难发现和诊断，患者一般无任何临床症状，无需特殊处理。但少数患者由于脾种植部位特殊，易被误诊为恶性肿瘤而行手术治疗。

一例患者起初在外院误诊为肝结核或炎性假瘤，主要因诊断时未结合脾切除术史，忽略了异位脾组织植入的可能。因此对于有脾切除病史的患者，在出现新的腹部病变时应该考虑到脾种植的可能。

超顺磁氧化铁(SPIO)增强MRI检查有助于脾种植的术前诊断，核素检查、细针穿刺活检可以术前确诊，避免不必要的手术。肝内脾种植在注射SPIO增强后于T_2WI呈低信号，但与肝实质相比，其信号偏高，具有鉴别意义。

当难以区分恶性肿瘤病变与肝内脾种植时，可以采取核素检查、细针穿刺活检等方法。最为特异的方法是放射性核素^{99m}Tc-DRBC扫描，因其能特异性地被脾摄取，其摄取率为50%~90%，可达到选择性脾显像的目的，对于诊断脾种植是特别有效的方法。CT引导下穿刺活检，虽具有细微的创伤性，但具有确诊作用，一些患者选择了CT引导下穿刺活检，避免了开腹探查创伤性更大的手术。

脾种植结节需与副脾鉴别，首先前者为外伤或手术后天所致，后者为先天性。其次脾种植结节可发生在腹腔任何部位，副脾则一般发生在脾区周围的系膜上；脾种植结节网状脾小梁结构明显减少，无脾门，血供来自穿透结节包膜的数支小血管，而副脾有脾门，血供来自脾动脉分支。种植的脾组织具有部分代偿脾功能，降低爆发感染性发生率，因此，无临床症状者不建议切除。但对于出现临床症状，如出血、梗死造成急腹症，压迫性肠梗阻，以及造成慢性盆腔痛时，应予以手术切除。

综上所述，异位脾种植一般由外伤或脾切除术所引起的脾组织自体种植，肝内脾种植罕见。CT、MRI增强扫描等影像学方法有助于诊断与鉴别诊断，诊断困难时可考虑^{99m}Tc-DRBC或细针活检。异位脾种植无临床症状者一般不需要特殊治疗,可定期观察,对于出现临床症状者应予以手术切除。

第二节 上腔静脉阻塞综合征肝内异常强化灶

肝脏血供来源广泛、途径多样,它接受门静脉和肝动脉的双重供血,此外还有许多其他脏器血管侧支直接供应肝脏,这一特点决定了邻近脏器病变时可能导致肝脏血供出现异常。

上腔静脉阻塞综合征患者肝脏可出现体静脉供血现象,主要经由胸部或上腹部开放的侧支血管,通过 Sappey 静脉系统引流而来,部分在肝内形成局限性强化灶,容易误诊。

上腔静脉阻塞综合征肝内异常强化灶的血流动力学基础:肝脏具有独特的血供,它接受门静脉和肝动脉的双重血供,此外还有许多其他血管供应肝脏。Sappey 等(1883)首先描述了位于肝悬吊韧带内的“副门脉”系统——位于镰状韧带内,沟通体壁前静脉和门静脉左支的静脉血管,后被命名为 Sappey 静脉。

随着影像学技术的发展,人们对该血管的认识逐渐加深,并将其进一步分为 Sappey 上静脉和 Sappey 下静脉。Sappey 上静脉位于镰状韧带上部,接受来自胸内和膈下血管的供血; Sappey 下静脉位于镰状韧带下部,接受腹部和脐旁静脉的供血。

由于该静脉的存在,导致了两种病理学现象的产生,一是门静脉高压时,出现门体分流,门静脉血液通过 Sappey 静脉进入体循环;二是腔静脉阻塞时,侧支血管开放,通过 Sappey 静脉引流进入肝脏。后者是上腔静脉阻塞综合征,CT 增强扫描肝内出现异常强化灶的血流动力学基础。生理状态下,体循环静脉血也可通过 Sappey 静脉进入肝 S_4 段前中部的小范围区域,表现为平扫或增强 CT 的局灶性低密度区,或表现为 CT 肝动脉造影的灌注缺损区。

Ohashi 等(1995)曾报道一组通过内乳静脉供血的肝 S4 段局部强化灶,但在非上腔静脉阻塞综合征时动态增强 CT 很少观察到此类现象。

相关研究以 Sappey 下静脉多见,用以解释门静脉高压或闭塞时的血流动力学改变。

关于 Sappey 上静脉的影像学研究较为少见,主要是由于非上腔静脉阻塞综合征增强 CT 扫描时,Sappey 上静脉基本不显示;少量血流过早抵达肝脏(动脉前期),早于动态增强时的动脉期,或血液呈少量缓慢通过,而无法显示肝脏的局灶强化现象。

影像学研究:根据上腔静脉阻塞综合征的血流动力学, CT 增强扫描时,经肘静脉注入的对比剂在动脉前期即可通过体静脉侧支,经由 Sappey 静脉引流入肝脏。文献报道为局灶性高强化区。强化灶出现部位根据供血侧支的不同而有差异:经过 Sappey 下静脉供血时,高强化区多出现在 S_3S_4 的前中部;经过 Sappey 上静脉供血时,高强化区出现在 S_2 S_4 的顶部。

该组病例中供血血管均来自内乳静脉或 / 和下段食管静脉,经由 Sappey 上静脉引流,故强化灶出现在 S_2 S_4。Itai 和 Parisi(2002)称肝内门静脉和体静脉之间存在着生理性静脉通路,当上腔静脉阻塞综合征发生时,门体静脉侧支开放,在肝裸区可出现异常强化区,该组研究未发现此类病例。

肝内强化灶以单发多见,该组共计 7 例;多发者 5 例,检出强化灶数目最多者 4 个。强化灶形态呈不规则片状或类圆形结节状,10 例病灶边缘清晰锐利,2 例边缘稍模糊。直径 1.0~4.5 cm 不等,结节状强化灶多在 2 cm 以下,范围大者多呈片状强化。

该组病例均表现为早期高强化特征,除 1 例边缘受强化侧支影响,1 例呈多发均匀强化结节外,余 10 例均呈现中心高、周边稍低的强化特点,可与血管瘤鉴别。通过调整窗宽、窗位观察可显示,高强化区均邻近侧支血管分布,可与肝内占位病变鉴别。多数强化灶 CT 值可高达 300 HU 以上,易与占位病变鉴别。

但该组中 1 例肝 S_2 S_4 多发结节状强化灶,部分 CT 值约为 120 HU,需与肝内占位病变鉴别。上腔静脉明显狭窄,显示供血侧支及引流静脉可作为依据,另外随访观察也具有一定价值。

文献报道上腔静脉阻塞时,其远端血管可经由奇静脉 - 半奇静脉通路、内乳静脉通路、胸腹壁表浅静脉通路以及椎体静脉弓通路 4 条路径回流至右心房。该研究通过追踪发现,12 例肝内异常强化灶周围均可见到供血的侧支通路显影,并借助 PACS 软阅读(Soft-copy Reading)电影回放的手段追踪到其胸内属支,结果发现内乳静脉供血者居多,占 75.0%

(9/12),另有 22.2%(2/12)通过下段食管静脉供血,仅 1 例为内乳静脉和下段食管静脉联合供血。多数强化灶可显示通过肝内开放的血管回流入下腔静脉(83.3%,10/12)。

该组共有 6 例复诊,初诊与复诊间隔 14~82 天。发现肝内异常强化灶与上腔静脉受压及侧支血管开放程度存在一定关系。2 例经治疗(包括 1 例上腔静脉内支架术)后原发瘤灶缩小,上腔静脉狭窄减轻,侧支血管减少,其中 1 例肝内异常强化灶消失,1 例体积缩小;2 例复查发现原发瘤灶范围扩大,上腔静脉受压加重,侧支血管增多,肝内出现强化灶或原有强化灶范围略扩大;其余 2 例原发瘤体积变化不大,1 例肝内异常强化灶消失,另 1 例未见明显变化。肝内强化灶的出现及范围随上腔静脉受压及侧支血管开放的程度大小而有增减,可作为追踪定性的重要依据。

PACS 工作站电影回放在肝内异常强化灶检出的应用:研究表明,PACS 工作站软阅读综合各种软硬件手段,可以提高结节病灶的检出率。该作者将 PACS 工作站电影回放的方法应用于此类研究,并对其应用优势进行了总结,认为:动态调窗有利于肝内异常强化灶形态及分层强化特征的显示,3 例强化灶通过 PACS 工作站窄窗处理清晰显示中心高、周边低的强化特征;电影回放有利于连续追踪血管走行,该组病例供血侧支全部得到清晰显示,并顺利追踪到其来源的静脉属支;采用兴趣区(ROI)内多点测值法,可对病变的强化特征进行更细致、精确的了解。

鉴别诊断:上腔静脉阻塞综合征肝内异常强化灶有时需要与肝血管瘤、转移瘤及原发肝肿瘤进行鉴别。肝血管瘤:上腔静脉阻塞综合征肝脏 CT 异常强化灶多数强化幅度较高,需要与血管瘤进行鉴别。

肝细胞性肝癌、肝细胞腺瘤及肝脏局灶性结节增生:上腔静脉阻塞综合征肝脏 CT 异常强化灶强化幅度较低且为多发时,需要与富血供转移瘤鉴别,有时还需要与肝细胞性肝癌、肝细胞腺瘤及肝脏局灶性结节增生等鉴别。

显示异常供血侧支及引流血管是重要鉴别点之一,上腔静脉阻塞综合征肝内异常强化灶形态常不规则而边缘清晰锐利可作为另一鉴别点。另外,发生位置也具有一定的提示意义,上腔静脉阻塞综合征肝脏 CT 异常强化灶绝大多数位于肝左叶,其中又以 S_2 S_4 段最为常见。肝细胞性肝癌、肝细胞腺瘤及肝脏局灶性结节增生虽具有动脉期高强化的特点,但幅度多达不到异常强化灶的程度。

总之,在上腔静脉阻塞综合征患者胸部 CT 检查时若见到肝内高强化灶时,应考虑到异常强化灶的可能性;若病灶不典型而鉴别困难时,可结合复诊或腹部 CT 等相关检查以进一步明确。作为回顾性分析,该研究存在难以避免的缺憾,其一所用资料多为胸部 CT 图像,部分未包括全肝而影响对肝脏血供情况的全面分析;其二扫描时相单一,无法得到肝脏多期动态图像;另外,作为一种良性改变,本征象也很难获得病理支持。

希望通过该研究提高对上腔静脉阻塞综合征胸部 CT 增强扫描时出现肝脏异常强化灶相关征象的认识,以减少误诊。

第三节　误诊病例简介:CT 诊断不典型药物性肝损害与肝内多发肿瘤

药物性肝损害是指由于药物及其代谢产物引起的肝脏损害。近年来药物性肝损害的发生率逐渐增加,引起药物性肝损害的药物达 1 000 余种。国外文献报道,药物引起肝脏损害以抗生素类最多见,国内报道多以抗结核药和抗肿瘤药为主,抗生素及中草药为主的报道亦可见。药物的肝毒性表现可从无症状、轻微、非特异性的生化改变到急(慢)性肝炎、肝功能衰竭、胆汁淤积,甚至肝硬化、肝脏肿瘤等。本病目前仍无特异性诊断方法,主要根据用药史、临床表现、化验检查以及停药后的效应做出综合诊断。病理改变包括肝细胞变性、局灶性或大块的肝细胞坏死、脂肪变性、胆汁淤积等。近几年来随着 MSCT 的临床应用,已有多名学者对药物性肝损害的 CT 表现进行归纳总结,如弥漫性肝脏损害;灶性肝脏损害(包括大片融合病灶、多发小片状病灶、多发小结节灶);肝硬化表现等。其不同表现缺乏相对特异性,但部分灶性肝脏损害病例 CT 平扫表现为大片融合或多发小片状低密度病灶,动脉期病灶可见强化,静脉期持续明显强化,与平扫图像呈“反转”表现者,具有一定特征性,其病理改变以肝细胞炎性坏死为主。

该例患儿1个月时即有肺部真菌感染病史，CT检查无明显肝脏异常发现;外院痰培养曲霉菌阳性，抗真菌治疗1~2个月即发现肝脏多发病灶;其他因素所致肝内损害均为阴性,停抗真菌药数月至1年后肝内病变逐渐好转,符合相应诊断标准。

该病例特点:年龄小，3~4个月时发病,明显小于以往报道年龄;无明显临床症状及体征,患儿发病期间除因肺部真菌感染所致临床症状外,无明显肝脏损害所对应临床征象,多次肝功能检查阴性;病灶影像表现较为特殊,病灶多、分布广且较大,部分呈较大类圆形病灶,与肿瘤相似,但平扫为低密度影,增强早期呈团状或厚壁环状强化,延迟扫描持续强化,并高于正常肝实质,呈“反转”现象;引起肝损害药物为抗真菌药;转归,患儿未行特殊护肝及肝移植等治疗,停用抗真菌药数月至1年后,肝内病灶即呈明显逐步好转趋势。

第三章　肝周

第一节　HELLP 综合征相关肝脏并发症

HELLP 综合征，又称为溶血、肝酶升高及血小板减少综合征，是一种与妊娠有关的血栓性微血管病变，Pritchard（1954）首次报道，Weinstein（1982）首次以这三个特征性表现命名，可发生于 0.5%~0.9% 的妊娠期妇女，但在合并先兆子痫或子痫患者中发病率达 20%。

HELLP 综合征约 80% 发生于孕 37 周前，1/3 发生于产后，其中大多发生于产前合并重度子痫患者。临床上除有水肿、蛋白尿及高血压等妊娠高血压综合征的表现外，还表现为恶心、呕吐、右上腹和上腹部疼痛，实验室检查白蛋白及胆红素升高，血小板减少，天门冬氨酸及乳酸脱氢酶升高。

目前临床上完全性 HELLP 综合征的诊断标准为在确诊妊娠高血压综合征的基础上血管内溶血，血涂片 RBC 变形、破碎、网织红细胞增多，总胆红素 >20.5 mol/L，乳酸脱氢酶 >600 U/L；肝酶异常，丙氨酸转氨酶（ALT）>70 U/l，血小板减少，<100. 000/mm^3。

肝包膜下血肿是 HELLP 综合征罕见的严重并发症，在所有并发症中约占 0.9%，但其病因和发病机制尚不清楚，研究认为可能为血管内皮细胞受损，胶原组织暴露，血小板与之接触、黏附并激活，导致患者的肝脏血管痉挛、血管内皮损伤和纤维素沉积使肝窦内血流受阻，肝细胞肿胀灶性坏死，细胞内酶释放至血液循环导致肝酶升高，肝血管痉挛加重，血管本身受损严重可发生肝被膜下出血形成血肿，血肿破裂可导致肝破裂甚至死亡。

一些学者报道 90% 孕妇会出现腹部或右上象限疼痛，且右上腹疼痛是 HELLP 综合征最先出现的症状，但因其无特异性，常被延误诊断，因此对于出现右上腹、颈部及肩部疼痛的孕妇应及早行肝脏影像学检查，及时排除其他胃肠疾病，正确诊断 HELLP 综合征。

但目前关于超声、CT、MRI 对 HELLP 综合征肝脏并发症的报道较少。有学者认为，超声诊断在 HELLP 综合征生化指标改变前即可提示妊娠相关肝病的局灶性强回声病灶。在病变早期连续超声声谱仪即可发现肝包膜强回声，与肝实质间出现边界清楚的梭形无回声区，血肿机化时呈强回声；另可见肝实质内楔形、境界清楚的高回声梗死区；但 B 超检查并不作为常规和首选，CT 和 MRI 具有更高的分辨力，能更准确地判断血肿的位置和程度。

CT 可发现肝包膜下界限清楚的新月形低密度带和肝实质内楔形低密度区，增强扫描无强化；MRI 平扫在出血早期表现为肝包膜下的条状液性高信号带，局部肝表面受压内陷，随着血肿的形成，信号强度可升高或降低，梗死则表现为肝实质内楔形低信号影，增强扫描无强化。

HELLP 综合征肝脏并发症患者往往合并腹水，CT 表现为肝脾周水样低密度带；MRI 表现为肝脾周围条状液性信号影。

经过积极有效治疗后 MRI 检查可发现肝包膜下血肿和腹水逐渐消失，但肝脏梗死的表现依然存在。

另外，在诊断 HELLP 综合征所致的肝包膜下血肿和肝脏破裂出血时需注意与肝挫裂伤出血、肝脏肿瘤破裂出血、肝穿或介入射频治疗出血相鉴别。

第二节　误诊病例简介:肝包膜下血肿误诊为囊实性占位病变

肝包膜下血肿是肝脏损伤的常见征象,多发生于肝外伤患者,也可发生于肿瘤、肝硬化、血管瘤甚至脂肪浸润等肝脏疾病患者,并可见于妊娠合并高血压疾患的妇女,尤其是子痫前期——子痫并有溶血、肝酶升高及血小板减少(HELLP 综合征)者。

肝包膜下血肿 CT 表现为肝周包膜下新月形或双凸形低密度或等密度区,CT 值约 20~47 HU,伴有局部肝实质受压变平,部分表现为葱皮样混杂密度影,肝包膜下血肿密度取决于出血量及出血时间,若血肿新鲜,CT 值接近于肝实质,随着时间延长,可转化为低密度或水样密度。

肝破裂出血临床诊断常根据病史、临床表现、体征、腹腔穿刺及超声检查等。

该例术前 CT 误诊为囊实性占位病变,考虑有以下几种原因:患者外伤史不明确;术前彩超提示肝海绵状血管瘤可能;未行腹腔穿刺;肝包膜下血肿边缘不规则伴结节状稍高密度影,血肿内密度不均匀,酷似囊实性占位病变,诊断医师经验不够。

术后分析该例出血可能因为:患者曾有过外伤史而未注意,导致肝损伤慢性出血,血液积聚于肝包膜下,压迫肝实质致肝脏部分坏死及纤维化,因活动后再发出血而发病;肝边缘血管畸形(血管瘤)破裂后出血。该例独特的影像表现可能与病变区有新鲜出血有关。

该例病变需与肝边缘的血管瘤鉴别,CT 增强扫描有助于鉴别诊断。

第三节　肝裂或隐窝内局限性积液可误为肝内病变

局限于肝裂或隐窝内的液体和门静脉周围的水肿可能被误认为肝内病变,影像诊断工作者必须知道这些可能的误诊。

肝圆韧带裂与大网膜囊相通,偶尔会有积液。液体也可以聚集在静脉韧带裂中,此裂隙与大、小网膜囊均相通。液体还可以聚集在胆囊窝内,成为胆囊切除术的一种并发症。

腹膜腔内的液体也能聚集在由横裂形成的潜在间隙内。必须注意,不要把这些改变误认为肝内肿瘤或脓肿。

聚集在肝右叶附近的液体可能位于三个不同的间隙:胸膜腔、肝被膜下或肝周间隙。当病人仰卧位扫描时,右侧胸腔积液将位于胸腔后部,并聚集在后肋膈角内。

腹部 CT 扫描,若液体出现在肝裸区,可确定右侧胸腔积液而非腹腔积液,因腹腔积液不会聚集在此处。肝被膜下积液可压迫相邻的肝实质。

肝周积液常见于腹腔积液病人,实际上就是位于肝脏周围的游离性积液,它常呈新月形,对肝脏不产生占位效应。

第四节　肝周超声检查的一些情况

Rao 和 Woodlief(1981)发现大的回声包块位于肝前方,CT 证实为肝周的膈下脂肪,而起初却曾被误认为新生物包块。肝周、脾周脂肪,超声检查可误认为腹水。腹膜前脂肪可有变异,它可以下伸几乎达到盆腔,如不注意也可误诊。Thickman 等(1983)指出,肝的前方和上方的脂肪蓄积产生回声区,由于肝下方的气体多重反射,在声像图上可出现慧星尾伪影,妨碍观察且导至误诊。Gardner 等(1980)在研究超声检查中肝的镜面伪影时发现,明显的左膈上方的胸膜渗出可表现为脾和左半膈的镜面影像。横膈上方的回声可伪似横膈下方的回声,这是一种声学的伪影,该区并无真实的结构,称此为膈上方的镜面伪影。由于超声的镜面伪影,有时显示横膈为双重轮廓,考虑这是因为一些回声延迟回转到换能器所致。

第五节　关于腹水

液体充盈的十二指肠伪似右前肝下间隙积液：有作者报告，在超声检查时右上腹的纵断和横断图像发现右前肝下间隙有液体积聚时，不要忘记可能是液体充盈的十二指肠肠袢，为区别二者，可让病人饮水，饮入水中的微小气泡通过十二指肠的蠕动运动在声象图上清楚可见，从而有助于鉴别。

环形伪影类似腹水：Jolles 和 Coulam（1980）在讨论腹水的 CT 鉴别诊断时提到环形伪影可佯似腹水。他们发现沿着肝的外侧缘有一低密度带状影，类似腹水表现，究其原因方了解到此低密度带实为一环形伪影，乃由于 CT 扫描器中的 X 线探测器口径不当所致。

腹水病人肝脏的假性病变：Sommer 等（1979）报告 1 例腹水病人在肝的右上前部分出现一回声区，类似转移性病变。改变超声换能器倾斜的角度常常可立刻澄清其肝脏是否为正常的肝组织的问题。

膈下脂肪过多类似腹水：肝 - 肺核素显像是发现右膈下腹水的一种敏感的检查方法。

但许多原因均可产生肝 - 肺分离，Pozderac 等（1979）报告 1 例类似腹水的右膈下脂肪增多。膈下脓肿、肺灌注溢入右肺底、肝脏顶部局限性缺损以及肺下积液可引起核素显像上肝 - 肺分离。

Yeh 等证明腹水可引起核素显像异常，且在前方观察时可能与膈下脓肿混淆。Briggs 提出要注意右侧观察对评价膈下腹水的重要性，他描述一个提示腹水的征象，即肝、肺的间隔由前向后逐渐变窄，这是因为液体在肝和右膈之间流动，后方受到冠状韧带的限制。

第四章 肝脏疾病与肝外

第一节 肝肾综合征(HRS)

定义:肝肾综合征是严重肝病患者病程后期出现的功能性肾衰竭,肾脏无明显器质性病变,是以肾功能损伤、血流动力学改变和内源性血管活性物质明显异常为特征的一种综合征。

肝肾综合征是急性肾损伤的一种特殊形式,由极度血管舒张引起,且对扩容治疗无反应。肝硬化腹水患者合并急性肾功能衰竭,即出现肾小球滤过率急性显著下降,血肌酐 >1.5 mg/dl(133μmol/L)可诊断急性肾损伤,排除其他引起急性肾损伤的病因,结合肾脏无明显器质性病变等可做出肝肾综合征的诊断。

根据患者病情进展及预后,肝肾综合征分为两型:Ⅰ型肝肾综合征:快速进展性肾功能损害,2 周内血肌酐成倍上升,超过基础水平 2 倍或 > 226 μmol/L(2.5 mg/dl),或 eGFR 下降 50% 以上 <20 ml/min。2 型肝肾综合征:缓慢进展性肾功能损害,中度肾功能衰竭,血肌酐水平 133~226 μmol/L(1.5~2.5 mg/dl),常伴有顽固型腹水,肾功能下降过程缓慢;多为自发的过程,有时也有诱因,预后相对Ⅰ型较好,但中位生存期较无氮质血症的肝硬化腹水短。

发病机制;肝硬化肝肾综合征的发病机制目前尚未完全清楚。一般认为主要是由于严重的肝功能障碍导致的血流动力学改变进而影响到肾功能。严重的肝功能障碍使得血管活性介质灭活减少,如半胱氨酰白三烯、血栓素 A2 等,在门脉高压时经门体分流进入体循环,使内脏血管舒张导致有效动脉血容量减少和平均动脉压下降。有效血容量减少,通过神经体液系统反射性地引起肾内血管收缩和水钠潴留。交感神经系统和 RAAS 激活导致肾血管收缩和肾血管自动调节功能改变,致使肾血流对平均动脉压变化更加敏感。

此外,内毒素血症也是严重肝病患者发生肝肾综合征的重要因素。严重肝病时由于肝细胞解毒功能降低,由肠道吸收的内毒素可通过肝脏或侧支循环大量进入体循环。内毒素可引起肾内血管的强烈收缩,肾血流减少,肾小球滤过率降低,导致少尿和氮质血症。

近年,临床上发现并不是所有肝功能严重异常的患者均会发展成肝肾综合征。因此,有学者提出“二次打击”学说,认为窦性门脉高压和肝功能失代偿作为“第一次打击”,引起全身外周血管扩张,有效循环血容量减少,在此基础上,任何加重血流动力学异常的诱因(如上消化道出血、过度利尿、自发性细菌性腹膜炎、大量抽取腹水等),即“第二次打击”,可促进肝肾综合征的形成。

诊断:肝肾综合征的诊断标准:①肝硬化合并腹水;②无休克;③血肌酐升高大于基线水平 50% 以上,>1.5 mg/dl(133μmol/L);④至少停用 2d 利尿剂(如使用利尿剂)并且使用人血白蛋白 $1g \cdot kg^{-1} \cdot d^{-1}$,直到最大 100 g/d 扩容后肾功能无持续性改善(血肌酐 <133 μmol/L);⑤近期无肾毒性药物使用史(NSAIDs、氨基糖苷类抗菌药物、对比剂等);⑥无肾实质疾病。

尿量在肝硬化合并腹水的肝肾综合征的诊断意义存在争议,原因是肝硬化腹水患者常合并尿少及严重钠潴留却维持相对正常的肾小球滤过率,有些患者可能由于使用利尿剂而造成尿量增加。2015 年国际腹水俱乐部提出动态监测血肌酐更能准确反映肝肾综合征患者急性肾损伤的过程,即 48 h 内血肌酐急性升高并超过基线水平的 50%,并最终≥ 1.5 mg/dl(133μmol/L)。并对急性肾损伤进行分期:1

期：血肌酐升高≥ 0.3 mg/dl（26.5μmol/L），或血肌酐升高至 1.5~2.0 倍基线值；2 期：或血肌酐升高≥ 2.5 mg/dl（226μmol/L），或血肌酐升高 >2.0~3.0 倍基线值；3 期：血肌酐升高至 >3.0 倍基线值，或血肌酐升高≥ 4.0 mg/dl（353.6μmol/L）并且急性升高≥ 0.3 mg/dl（26.5μmol/L），或开始连续性血液滤过（RRT）。

与肝肾综合征相比，其他因素导致的急性肾损伤往往更容易缓解，且损伤持续时间较短，短期（30 d）病死率较肝肾综合征低。而肝肾综合征患者的非移植生存率更低、预后更差。因此，即使是血肌酐的轻微升高，都要及早发现并给予尽可能的早期干预，以防止肝肾综合征发生。如患者存在上消化道出血、电解质紊乱、腹水感染控制不佳、大量放腹水、大量利尿及严重呕吐、腹泻等情况，且肾功能快速减退，要考虑肝肾综合征：①了解患者近期用药情况，将利尿剂减量或停用，停用具有潜在肾毒性药物、血管扩张药或 NSAIDs；②对可疑低血容量患者进行扩容治疗（根据临床判断可采用晶体液、人血白蛋白或血制品）；③如确诊或高度怀疑合并细菌感染，应进行细菌鉴定并给予早期抗感染治疗；④经上述措施无效，且血肌酐继续升高 > 基线水平 50%，>1.5 mg/dl（133 μmol/L）可诊断肝肾综合征。

第二节　获得性肝脑变性：一种少见的肝病相关神经系统病变

严重慢性肝脏疾病可并发神经系统病变，包括肝性脑病、获得性肝脑变性（AHCD）和肝性脊髓病。获得性肝脑变性是一类少见的而且不可逆性神经功能损害的临床综合征，其发病是由于反复发生肝性脑病，或长期多次代谢紊乱所引起。获得性肝脑变性起病一般隐匿，多以精神异常、认知能力下降、帕金森病样症候群为主要表现，极易误诊为神经系统变性疾病。

流行病学与临床表现：获得性肝脑变性由 Van Woerkom（1914）首次提出，随后 Victor 等（1965）学者发表了具有里程碑意义的文章。目前约有 550 万美国人患肝硬化，其中等待肝移植的约 17 000 例患者中运动障碍的发生率高达 20%~90%。获得性肝脑变性在肝硬化患者中的发病率为 0.8%~2%。

获得性肝脑变性的症状通常发生在 50 至 60 岁的成年人中，然而，少数可见于儿童，因此发病年龄无法区分获得性肝脑变性与肝豆状核变性。获得性肝脑变性发生于肝功能失代偿后数周或数年后，病程具有可变性，可能出现突然加重。生存期从发病后数周至超过 30 年不等。大多数患者死于肝硬化的晚期并发症如感染、凝血功能障碍、肝肾综合征、肝细胞癌、肝性脑病等。

获得性肝脑变性是慢性肝病引起的一种不可逆性锥体外系综合征。临床主要表现为帕金森综合征、共济失调、意向性震颤、舞蹈症等运动障碍以及精神行为异常和智能障碍等神经心理学改变。神经精神症状可表现为淡漠、嗜睡、过度嗜睡、继发性痴呆等；锥体外系症状常见为局限性肌张力障碍、体位性震颤、肌阵挛、强直、构音障碍、舞蹈手足徐动等；小脑症状如构音障碍、共济失调、眼球震颤等。上述症状可以仅有其一，也可兼有之。获得性肝脑变性通常发病隐匿，最先出现的症状通常由患者的亲属发现。最常见的症状为运动迟缓、肌强直、姿势性震颤。

1. 发病机制　获得性肝脑变性的发病机制迄今为止尚未完全阐明。有研究结果显示获得性肝脑变性是与多种代谢异常有关，如氨、芳香族氨基酸、锰等，伴有某些特定大脑区域异常敏感性低灌注。锰的毒性作用可能是一个重要的致病因素。已证明锰是在肝胆系统被清除，获得性肝脑变性患者的血清及脑脊液中锰浓度高于正常范围数倍。获得性肝脑变性患者大脑中锰的沉积可能会引起脑实质弥漫性变性。锰的神经毒性机制包括与多巴胺受体结合、干扰神经递质摄取、改变细胞膜受体表达以及多巴胺受体功能，引起多巴胺的自动氧化作用，形成儿茶酚胺的毒性。获得性肝脑变性病理的特征性表现为神经元的缺失、Alzheimer Ⅱ型星形胶质细胞、基底节区细胞质内糖原颗粒。组织学表现为大脑皮质及基底节区发生弥漫性脑萎缩和半透明变色，光镜下可见多发性微泡样变性。微泡样变性起源于深皮质层和基底节，且延伸至相邻的白质纤维束。Alzheimer Ⅱ型星形胶质细胞存在过量线粒体、粗面内质网和含有脂褐素颗粒的空泡，或者是细胞内存在过量的顺磁性物质（可能为过量的锰元素）。

此外,Kleinschmidt-DeMasters 等(2006)研究观察到获得性肝脑变性患者可能存在与脑桥中央髓鞘溶解症相同的渗透机制。

2. 早期诊断方法:

(1)实验室检查:有研究结果显示获得性肝脑变性患者空腹状态下测量血锰水平升高,脑脊液中锰浓度可升高。铜蓝蛋白水平和血清铜均在正常范围内。血氨水平可正常或升高。

(2)影像学表现:MRI 已被广泛用于检查与慢性肝病有关的神经系统并发症,获得性肝脑变性其影像学特征在双侧基底节及脑干出现 MRI T_1WI 高信号。MRI 的 T_1WI 像通常显示在基底核的高信号,以及额顶叶和小脑萎缩是常见的。文献中报道的部位还有:垂体、下丘脑、红核。MRI 的 T_1WI 像高信号区域的强度和延伸与肝病的严重程度之间可能存在相关性。然而,这种相关性在异常信号区域与神经系统症状之间不存在。虽然这种异常信号的起源尚不清楚,有研究结果显示,这种损害是可逆的,可能由于门-腔静脉分流术或肝功能障碍所致的顺磁性物质的沉积引起的代谢改变。

有研究报道某些患者 MRI 的 T_2WI 序列在基底节、中脑、脑桥臂、双侧小脑齿状核显示信号强度的增加。获得性肝脑变性患者中苍白球的 T1 高信号可能与锰沉积有关。Maffeo 等(2014)认为获得性肝脑变性与肝硬化的原因、急性肝性脑病的发作、MRI 信号强度无相关性,血锰浓度不能反映 MRI 信号或获得性肝脑变性。MRI 苍白球 T_1 高信号是获得性肝脑变性临床表现的先决条件而不是充分条件。

3. 鉴别诊断:

(1)肝豆状核变性是一种常染色体隐性遗传的铜代谢障碍引起的疾病,主要的神经系统症状为帕金森综合征、肌张力障碍、小脑病变、锥体束征、舞蹈病、手足徐动症、肌阵挛、行为异常。获得性肝脑变性的典型临床表现与之相似,因此鉴别主要依靠实验室检查。肝豆状核变性患者由于铜代谢障碍,可引起血清铜蓝蛋白和总铜量减少,血清游离铜和尿铜增加,并且过多的铜可在肝、脑、肾、角膜等部位沉积,使相应部位发生病变,常见角膜色素环(K-F 环)形成。获得性肝脑变性患者上述检查则无明显异常。此外,两者影像学检查也存在差异。肝豆状核变性的头颅 CT 可发现基底节区的异常,可先于症状出现,常见为双侧豆状核区对称性低密度或异常信号。MRI 表现更敏感,除基底节区外,还可见丘脑、脑干、齿状核的 T_2WI 高信号、T_1WI 低信号。这与获得性肝脑变性的 MRI 表现截然不同(表 12-4-1)。

表 12-4-1 获得性肝脑变性鉴别诊断

鉴别诊断	肝性脑病	肝豆状核变性	肝性脊髓病
临床表现	意识障碍、行为失常和昏迷	锥体外系症状	慢性、进行性双下肢运动受累的痉挛性截瘫
体征及检查	扑翼样震颤,血氨可升高	K-F 环(+),血清铜蓝蛋白和总铜量减少,血清游离铜和尿铜增加	多为对称性,近端较远端明显,肌力下降,肌张力升高,腱反射亢进,阵挛及锥体束阳性,运动诱发电位异常
影像学表现	无临床表现时即可出现苍白球的对称性 T_1W1 高信号;可出现脑萎缩或少数 MRI 显示广泛异常,如额叶、岛叶、脑白质 T_2Wl 及 DWI 高信号	头颅 CT 示双侧豆状核区异常低密度影;MRI 表现为双侧基底节、丘脑、脑干和齿状核的 T_2Wl 高信号、T_1W1 低信号	MRI 无特征性表现

(2)肝性脑病(HE):肝性脑病是指发生于肝脏功能严重障碍或失调且排除其他已知脑病的神经心理异常综合征,其主要临床表现是意识障碍、行为失常和昏迷,是急性肝衰竭及慢性终末期肝病相关的常见并发症,脑部的病理改变主要是弥漫性脑水肿。获得性肝脑变性主要与 C 型肝性脑病鉴别,C 型肝性脑病以慢性反复发作的性格、行为改变、甚至木僵、昏迷为特征,常伴有肌张力增高、腱反射亢进、扑翼征、踝阵挛阳性,或巴宾斯基征阳性等神经系统异常,发作时可伴有血氨升高。获得性肝脑变性与肝性脑病不同,它存在典型的大脑器质性改变,表现为 Alzheimer Ⅱ型星形胶质细胞增生和神经元的缺失。

肝性脑病的 MRI 表现较早,在无临床表现时即可出现苍白球的对称性 T1WI 高信号,进一步可见白质和其他锥体外系结构信号都增强。但 MRI 的表现无特异性,也可见于其他脑部疾病。

（3）肝性脊髓病:肝性脊髓病是由多种急慢性肝脏疾病引起的一种少见的神经系统并发症,临床上以慢性、进行性双下肢痉挛性截瘫为特征性表现。主要病理改变为脊髓侧索对称性脱髓鞘。肝性脊髓病多在长期肝病的基础上隐袭起病,除特征性痉挛性截瘫外,偶有感觉障碍、肌肉萎缩、括约肌功能障碍。一般多为对称性,近端较远端明显,肌力下降,肌张力升高,腱反射亢进,阵挛及锥体束阳性。获得性肝脑变性则以神经精神症状和锥体外系综合征为主。运动诱发电位测量可表现为严重的神经生理学异常。部分患者头、脊髓 MRI 可以表现为完全正常。

关于肝脏疾病与肝外的部分内容,请详见本书本卷 第九篇　肝弥漫性病变:第十八章　肝硬化与脑;第十九章　肝硬化与骨。

第十三篇　肝创伤和肝手术后

第一章　肝创伤

第一节　肝创伤

腹部钝性创伤引起的器官受损 20% 发生于肝脏。肝损伤包括撕裂伤、包膜下血肿、肝实质挫伤、肝静脉损伤、肝动脉损伤以及肝脏胆系的破裂。钝性创伤通常产生肝实质的撕裂伤，该损伤引起的腹腔内出血很显著，可能与肝脏的双重供血有关。肝脏的包膜下血肿通常是由于穿透性创伤产生的，无论是钝性或是穿透性创伤均可引起活动性出血。

肝脏的撕裂伤常常累及肝右叶的后段，因这部分肝与肋骨和脊柱相邻。肝左叶的损伤往往是垂直方向上的，是由于自肝左叶向脊柱从前向后的压力所致。这些可能与其他的压力性损伤相关，如胰腺、小肠、十二指肠和横结肠。撕裂可以累及重要的肝血管结构，例如大的肝静脉和门静脉的分支，在 CT 上显示为血管邻近撕裂处有活动性出血的征象。

肝脏裸区是位于肝脏后表面的不受腹膜覆盖的不规则菱形区。肝脏裸区的肝撕裂伤延伸至肝脏表面，导致腹腔内出血进入腹膜后，而不形成腹腔出血。体格检查通常不能发现典型的腹膜刺激征象，但腹腔检查可能是阳性的。CT 扫描能显示肝撕裂伤，通常累及肝右后叶并常伴有腹膜后出血。

Patten 等报道的 185 例肝脏创伤病人的 CT 表现，有 25 例是包膜下血肿限于肝裸区的（约占 16%）。25 例中的 22 例（约 88%）可见右侧腹膜后出血，5 例（20%）有腹腔内出血。肝脏裸区损伤的病人保守治疗效果非常好。对于累及肝裸区的肝撕裂伤，CT 扫描可诊断出无腹膜后损伤的腹膜后出血。

第二节　肝、脾动脉破裂出血

肝脏、脾脏在腹部外伤中最容易受到伤及。肝脏外伤的发生率为 1%~8%，严重肝外伤死亡率为 50%~80%。目前，钝性肝损伤明显增加，每年肝严重损伤的发生率为 16%。

对于血流动力学稳定的病人，非外科处理为标准的治疗措施。技术成功率为 88%~94%。选择性肝动脉结扎现很少应用；大部分肝切除用于肝广泛裂伤或有大段失活肝组织时，现为 3%~6%；网膜片修复现使用率 10%；填充压迫和再手术为控制损伤策略；近年有大于 80% 的病人采用非外科手术治疗。

第三节　肝内胆汁肿与亚急性血肿 MRI 鉴别诊断

Shigemura（1995）报道 2 例肝钝伤，伴发远端小胆管破裂致胆汁肿的 MRI 表现，并讨论它与亚急性血肿的鉴别。

例 1 为 62 岁男性伤员，因交通事故腹部钝伤伴肋骨骨折。MRI 见肝右叶前段大的撕裂伤及肝周间隙轻度腹腔积血。CT 只见腹腔积血。伤后 13 天出现发热，白细胞增高，MRA 见右肝 3 个病灶，前段 2 个，后段 1 个。前段上方病灶在 T_1WI 上为不均质信号，下方及后段病灶在 T_1WI 和 T_2WI 均为高信号，CT 皆为低密度。遂行右肝前段 2 个病灶经皮经肝引流，结果见上方病灶为胆汁肿，下方病灶为亚急性血肿，造影检查见胆汁肿腔与肝内胆管和肝外胆管相通。引流后，体温及血象均恢复正常。胆汁肿逐渐缩小，60 天后全部病灶痊愈，无复发。

例 2 为 28 岁男性伤员。腹部钝伤，CT 见腹腔积血，未见肝裂伤。急诊手术证实为肝撕裂伤及腹腔积血，遂作肝缝合术。术后 6 天在 T_1WI 见一等信号强度的撕裂周围出现高信号，在 T_2WI 上撕裂为高信号；16 天后，T_1WI 及 T_2WI 均为高信号；25 天后撕裂增大，原术后 16 天发现的高信号几乎全部消失，T_1WI 出现低信号，T_2WI 皆为高信号，经皮经肝引流见病灶前部为胆汁肿，造影检查见其与肝内胆管相通，25 天后痊愈，无复发。

亚急性血肿在 T_1WI 和 T_2WI 均为高信号，而肝内胆汁肿在 T_1WI 为低信号，T_2WI 为高信号，此可解释胆汁肿在 T1WI 的不均质信号。因此，在亚急性肝裂伤者，在 T_1WI 出现边界不规则的低信号，提示有胆汁肿。

血肿可以自愈，而胆汁肿痊愈缓慢，或不易痊愈，经皮引流可以促进治愈，所以早期区别两者甚为重要。

第四节　肝损伤的其他情况

任何原因引起的门静脉血流衰竭都可导致肝实质损伤，T_2WI 呈高信号，偶尔在 CT 平扫上呈低密度。脓肿形成或其他炎症过程中的充血在 T_2WI 上也呈高信号。肝硬化引起的纤维化和暴发型肝炎所致的肝损伤，在 CT 平扫上呈低密度，T_2WI 上呈高信号，需与肝脏肿瘤鉴别。肝损伤病例可见呈解剖分布或非解剖分布的局灶性的铁沉积，尤其常见于肝硬化再生结节，在梯度回波 MRI 表现较明显。肝损伤时，梗阻性黄疸病人可见沿解剖分布的异常密度，但与肝肿瘤易于鉴别。另外，在肝损伤病例，一些肝囊肿难以与囊性肿瘤（复合型囊肿）或液性肿瘤（肝纤毛前肠囊肿）鉴别。

第二章　肝的放射性损伤

放射性肝损伤的发生正随着腹部肿瘤的放疗、骨髓移植及肝脏恶性肿瘤三维适形放疗的开展而越来越受到重视。准确判断并评价肝脏放射性损伤的有无及其程度，对临床药物学治疗和/或肿瘤放疗方案的制定与修正均显得尤为重要。MRI 虽然最近才被应用于该领域，却已显露出其令人瞩目的优越性。

接受放射治疗后的病人肝脏出现异常的影像学表现，病理上出现肝细胞肿胀、肝静脉闭塞，晚期可出现肝硬化。CT 表现较具特征，可见与照射野一致的肝密度减低区增强后出现延迟强化：在肝硬化基础上的放射损伤表现为该区域过度强化；在脂肪肝基础上的放射损伤则表现为照射野的高密度。结合放射治疗史，诊断不难。其他影像学检查的报道较少。随着我国放射治疗，尤其是适形治疗的增多，对该病的认识也应提高。如何早期诊断该病，也是值得研究的课题。

在治疗原发性肝脏肿块（例如肝癌）或是肝脏邻近器官肿瘤（例如下肺肿块或胰腺肿块）时，肝脏可能被包括在放疗区域内。这种情况下有可能发生诊断陷阱。在 CT 增强扫描早期，放疗区域内的肝脏强化程度可低于邻近没有受射线照射的肝脏，其 CT 表现与局灶性脂肪肝或肝脏肿块相似。如果仅做 CT 平扫及平衡期（延迟）扫描，则难以显示这种密度差别。在肝脏受到轻微放疗损伤的病人中，肝脏酶可能轻度升高，肝脏放疗的慢性期变化包括肝脂肪浸润和萎缩。

放疗后肝脏信号的变化与治疗和 MR 扫描的间隔时间有关。放疗后立即行 MR 扫描，受累肝脏表现为水肿改变，T_1WI 呈低信号，T_2WI 呈高信号。之后，由于受累肝脏发生慢性纤维化，则 T_1WI 和 T_2WI 均呈低信号。

在放疗照射野肝实质内甘油三酯沉积常常减少，因此，在脂肪抑制技术及异相位成像技术中，相对于含有脂肪的正常肝组织而言，照射区肝组织信号维持正常。

照射区出现的放射诱导的急性血管炎或慢性肉芽组织形成，在延时增强扫描时出现强化。放疗后改变常沿照射野有一个区域性的清楚边界，即异常信号区与照射野一致而与肝段分布不一致。

第三章 肝手术后

第一节 部分肝切除术后

肝脏手术后可导致肝脏变形。肝叶或肝段切除术后,肝脏轮廓可出现各种变形。

切除术后 6~12 个月出现肝组织再生,沿肝脏手术切缘可出现信号强度的改变以及强化,类似于病变复发。此外,常可见手术银夹产生的金属伪影,这种“礼花”状的低信号伪影可类似于圆形局灶性病变。在毁损梯度回波序列或其他 T_2WI 上,伪影更加明显,以此可与真正的病变鉴别。

第二节 活检通道

由穿刺针、导管及低温消融(cryoablation)后所致的通道也可改变受累区肝脏的信号强度。T_1WI 图像上水肿为局限性低信号,T_2WI 上为高信号。出血 T_1WI 和 T_2WI 信号多种多样。反应性炎症表现为相邻组织的强化,常呈线状分布,根据临床病史可排除病变。

第三节 肝叶切除术后的误诊

根据肝动脉解剖,肝脏被分为左、右两叶。尾叶则由左、右肝动脉双重供血。每一肝叶又被分为两段:肝右叶被分为前段和后段,而肝左叶被分为内段和外段。每一段又被分为上、下两个亚段。肝脏部分切除术往往改变了肝脏的解剖形态,多种诊断方法尤其是 CT 检查,都可以显示这些变化。残留肝组织通过肥大和/或增生的方式而再生。这种再生在肝叶或肝段切除后很快就会发生,有时甚至在术前即有肝脏再生。其再生情况取决于病变累及肝组织量的多少及残留肝组织的功能状况。如果残留肝组织功能正常,只要保留 10%~15% 的肝组织,人体即可存活。

一些作者在动物实验中发现,肝脏切除 80%~85% 的体积后,肝组织不断再生,至恢复全肝体积大约需 4 个多月时间。外科手术 6 个月至 1 年后,CT 图像可以显示肝脏的再生,表现为肝脏体积进行性增大以及肝实质轮廓的改变。肝叶切除后,随着残留肝组织的再生和塑形,胆囊常移位至别处而类似病变。

第十四篇　关于肝移植

第一章　肝移植

第一节　CTA 与肝移植

详见本书 本卷 第十篇 第八章　肝血管其他　疾病。

第二节　活体供肝者肝血管与胆管发育变异之间的关系

由于尸体肝匮乏，活体家属肝移植已成为尸体肝移植替代方法。肝右叶移植可为受者提供充足的肝脏体积，但肝右叶血管和胆管的发育变异常见，虽然这些变异不是绝对禁忌，却常需要矫正。如果外科医生不能充分了解对肝动脉、门静脉分布以及胆管回流情况，就会增加供者肝右叶切除后并发症的发病风险。

Macdonald 等（2005）报告 39 例成人活体肝移植供者，其研究目的是确定门静脉和 / 或肝动脉分支与胆管发育变异是否有关联。

活体肝移植手术方法需根据胆管分支类型而变化。虽然目前关于术前胆管分支成像的作用尚有争议，但在术前计划时仍在使用。研究表明，门静脉异常和胆管异常之间、肝动脉异常和胆管异常之间以及任何一个动脉或门静脉异常与胆管异常之间没有显著相关性。

有可能某一特定的血管分支亚型变异与某一特定的胆管分支亚型变异相关，但是该研究样本大小不足以确定。门静脉和肝动脉分支类型与胆管分支变异之间相关性不佳，肝血管正常的病人中常见胆管变异，因此依据已知肝血管分支类型不能可靠地预测胆管发育变异。

第二章 肝移植术后

第一节 肝移植术后并发症

肝移植是治疗终末期肝脏疾病的一种有效手段。然而,肝移植的术后并发症是阻碍进一步提高移植肝存活率及受体存活率的重要因素。CT 和 MRI 检查可以较早发现肝移植术后并发症,在一定程度上提高了肝移植的成功率。

一、血管并发症

肝移植术后血管源性并发症的病理基础包括肝动脉吻合口狭窄和血栓形成、门静脉狭窄和血栓形成、肝静脉 - 下腔静脉吻合口狭窄。各种并发症可单独或同时发生,多出现在术后数月内。其中肝动脉狭窄或血栓形成是肝移植术后较常见的一种并发症。一组资料 78 例肝移植术后并发症中,有血管并发症 8 例,其中肝动脉狭窄 3 例。肝动脉狭窄多发生于血管吻合口,常于 2 个月以内出现。可能由于外科手术操作中损伤血管所致,是导致移植失败的重要原因之一,早期诊断是治疗成功的关键。

门静脉并发症 2 例,门静脉狭窄原因是术中静脉排列不良或残段过长导致扭曲狭窄、吻合口紧张、痉挛、扭曲及外压所致,临床上呈门静脉高压,目前一般认为肝移植术后门静脉直径至少应 >3.5mm。下腔静脉狭窄 3 例,下腔静脉狭窄可发生于肝上或肝下段吻合口,主要见于术后早期。常由于脏器旋转引起下腔静脉肝上段扭曲或吻合口不符引起,纤维化、慢性栓塞或新生血管内膜增殖可引起迟发性下腔静脉吻合口狭窄。

MSCTA 在肝移植术后血管源性并发症中的应用:DSA 是诊断肝移植术后肝动脉并发症的"金标准",但由于此检查的有创性,往往不宜用于刚施行了大手术的患者。

彩色多普勒超声检查虽简便、无创,但由于其敏感性及特异性稍差,如当探头投射角度接近 90º 或存在发育变异等时有一定的假阳性,当肝内肝动脉侧支循环建立时有一定的假阴性,而且受操作者主观影响较大,故而可作为肝移植术后血管源性并发症的主要随访工具,但不能作为最终确诊手段。MSCTA 由于扫描速度快,覆盖范围大,能满足肝动脉、门静脉以及下腔静脉成像的需要,属无创性检查,且准确性非常高。MSCTA 可以作为显示移植肝血管有无闭塞的首选。8 例血管并发症中肝动脉狭窄、门静脉狭窄患者在 MSCTA 通过三维重组技术可清楚显示狭窄的部位。MSCTA 不仅能为外科手术提供足够的解剖信息,能显示腔内、外情况,还可了解此时肝实质缺血改变及程度,显示肝脏血流灌注情况。

总之 MSCTA 作为 CT 技术的进展,为 CTA 的检查又提供了一种更具潜力的检查方法,在对肝移植术后血管腔内病变进行安全、无创、准确诊断的同时,MSCT 还可对移植肝实质的情况进行观察。MSCTA 为肝移植术后血管源性并发症的下一步治疗提供依据。

3D-CE-MRA 技术在肝移植术后血管源性并发症中的应用价值:3D-CE-MRA 很好地显示腹主动脉的主要分支动脉和门静脉的形态,为了解术后患者的血管吻合情况,有无肝动脉血栓形成、狭窄或闭塞等情况提供重要信息,为临床上采取预防和治疗的措施提出必要的证据。通过统计学分析,MRI 和 MSCTA 在诊断肝移植术后并发症方面均具有重要价值,两者诊断肝移植术后血管并发症无显著差异。

二、胆管并发症

肝移植术后胆管并发症病理:胆管并发症是肝

移植术后的常见并发症之一，包括胆总管扩张、吻合口狭窄、非吻合口狭窄、胆漏和胆泥形成等，是造成肝移植失败及影响存活的重要原因。该组中胆管并发症共 12 例，其中 8 例为吻合口狭窄，致使胆汁引流不畅淤积，最终导致胆总管及肝内胆管扩张，胆管并发症中 4 例术后肝总管狭窄（非吻合口狭窄）发生的部分是左右肝管汇合处，其左肝管较右肝管扩张明显。

由于影像检查尤其是 MRI 能直观地了解其形态学的改变，所以越来越受到人们的重视，胆漏绝大多数见于胆总管端吻合口，主要是吻合口有张力或缝合技术不完善所致，另一原因是胆管血供不足引起的胆管坏死所致。任何原因引起肝动脉供血不足、肝动脉吻合口狭窄、血栓形成、受体肝动脉过细或异常等，均可以引起胆管黏膜缺血性损伤，最终发生胆漏或胆管梗阻，其表现为产生胆汁湖或者胆汁性腹膜炎。胆泥形成是由于胆汁浓缩、变稠或胶原组织在受损的胆管壁积聚所致，主要发生在胆总管和大的肝内分支。

肝移植术后胆管并发症 MSCT 胆管成像的表现：可分为吻合口狭窄和非吻合口狭窄，CT 表现为肝内胆管扩张，胆漏的 CT 表现表现为肝门胆囊窝内水样密度影，边界清晰、光滑增强扫描未见强化。

肝移植术后胆管并发症 MRCP 的表现：胆总管吻合口部位狭窄胆管吻合口部位狭窄 MRCP 显示胆总管吻合口局限性狭窄，吻合口以上胆总管明显扩张。胆总管非吻合口部位狭窄和胆总管吻合口部位狭窄 MRCP 均显示胆总管及肝内胆管管径变窄，管壁不光滑。胆漏表现为 T_2 高信号。该组结果显示，MRI 和 CT 检查相结合可以明显提高肝移植术后胆管并发症的诊断准确性。

三、肝排斥反应

1. 病理　急性排斥反应常发生在术后 4 天至 2 周。主要病理表现为汇管区水肿，伴汇管区和终末肝小静脉的内膜炎。慢性排斥反应一般发生在移植后 60 天或数年后，特征性病理表现为胆管减少或消失及闭塞性血管病变。

2. 临床表现　缺乏特异性表现，急性排斥反应多发生在 4~10d，主要表现为畏寒、发热、肝区胀痛、黄疸，需于肝动脉栓塞与术后胆管并发症鉴别。

CT 与 MRI 表现：①静脉与下腔静脉周围袖套征，在 CT 表现为围绕门静脉主干及其分支和下腔静脉的低密度环，出现在门静脉主干及左右支为多见，门静脉末端和下腔静脉周围相对少见，其 MRI 信号特点为 T_1WI 上低于邻近的肝实质，但又高于肝血管的信号，多回波成像第一回波像上其信号强度进一步增高；②肝门周围可见液体积聚 CT 上表现为低密度，MRI 信号特点为 T_1WI 上为低信号，多回波相上为高信号；③3D-DCE-MRI 可借助于软件测量肝动脉、静脉内血流速度来反映肝血管阻力变化情况；④MRCP 显示肝内胆管僵直、变细。

3. 排斥反应的诊断与鉴别诊断

（1）供肝失活：由于肝质量不佳或缺血、灌洗损伤，术后患者常出现黄疸及肝功能损害，一般较急性排异反应为早。

（2）感染：尤其是胆管与肝脏感染，可出现肝脏肿大与胆管扩张。胆汁培养及经 T 管造影有助于鉴别。

（3）血管栓塞：肝移植术后高凝状态或手术失误所致的门脉及肝动脉阻塞可发生肝脏肿大，类似急性排异反应，MSCT、MRI 动态增强扫描有较大的鉴别诊断价值。

四、肝脏移植术后的其他肝内并发症

（1）肝脓肿：主要由于缺血区或继发于胆管梗阻、上行性胆管炎，MRI 表现为片状异常信号影，T_1WI 为等低信号，T_2WI 及脂肪抑制像为略等高信号。增强后动脉期呈不均匀强化，门脉及延迟其余肝实质强化程度近乎一致。

（2）肝局灶性坏死：其原因可能是供体与受体大小不成比例，肝实质受压，与肝动脉血栓形成无关。MSCT 表现为肝内多发大小不等类圆形病变，平扫呈低密度，增强扫描延迟强化。

（3）胆管炎：CT 表现为肝内胆管扩张，肝内胆管壁增厚，肝内胆管积气。

总之，随着 MSCT 及 MRI 技术的不断发展，能更加清晰准确地显示肝移植术后影像表现及血管、胆管并发症，尤其是两者结合，能提高肝移植术后胆管及血管并发症的诊断准确率，从而能为临床提供有价值的信息，利于临床及时治疗。

第二节 肝移植术后排斥反应

急性排斥是肝移植出现排斥中最常见的一种,通常发生在移植后 5~30 d。其发生率因免疫抑制剂的用量不同而异,在 30%~70% 之间。

两类排斥:大量临床经验证明,肝移植后 7d 的活检标本经常可见急性排斥反应的形态变化,但多数患者无临床症状和体征,称为生物性排斥。生物性排斥无需增加免疫抑制剂的用量,患者可自行恢复。而对于临床上有发热、黄疸、腹痛等非特异性症状和体征,又具有形态学改变的急性排斥,称为临床排斥,需要调整免疫抑制剂的用量。急性排斥反应的临床表现无特异性,病理活检是判断急性排斥的可靠依据。

超声:彩色多普勒超声判断肝移植术后急性排斥反应标准:①肝移植术后,肝静脉形态变钝,呈低沉的单相波;②术后最初诊断正常者,继后出现频谱变钝对急性排斥反应诊断敏感度高达 92%。经抗排斥药物有效治疗后,静脉波形可恢复原有的三相波,峰值速度增高;③肝内胆管及胆总管扩张;④肝动脉阻力明显降低。

在超声表现上,肝静脉血流模式从三相到单相的变化,可以提示急性排斥反应的存在,敏感性较高,但无特征性。该组观察有 1 例患者肝静脉波形变钝,呈低沉的单相波,但是临床无急性排斥反应表现,跟踪观察逐渐恢复到三相波。另外,移植术后,由于各种引流管道、敷料及手术切口的影响,为操作带来一定的困难,肝静脉波形有时显示不够理想。所以,单纯依靠肝静脉波形变化判断急性排斥反应有一定局限性。

MRI:总结该组病例中肝移植术后排斥反应的 MRI 表现,排斥反应患者均有肝脏体积增大、饱满,但多数排斥反应患者肝脏信号强度无明显变化。

该组中仅 1 例重度急性排斥反应患者肝脏右叶呈稍长 T_1、短 T_2 信号,增强扫描肝右叶信号强度较左叶低,考虑为肝实质缺血表现可能。文献报道其发生原因是因为肝脏原来存在的肝外供血动脉在肝移植后被破坏。因此,当移植肝动脉供血不足或发生胆管坏死时,就可能导致肝实质梗死。肝梗死在 CT 上表现为不规则或边界清楚的低密度灶,增强扫描不强化或不均匀强化,通常位于肝脏边缘。

回顾性分析该病例,可见其同时合并肝右门静脉明显变细,肝右叶血管分支亦见减少,符合肝梗死的成因,但认为此病例尚未达到不可逆梗死的程度,仅是肝供血不足,T_2WI 低信号与缺血过程中发生血管通透性增高、慢性渗血、含铁血黄素沉着有关,一旦供血改善是可以恢复的。在其后追踪复查过程中,肝右叶异常信号区范围逐渐缩小,边界模糊。

一、排斥反应血管异常

该组病例中血管异常表现包括:肝静脉末梢分支杵状扩张;肝动脉串珠样改变;供体段门静脉变细。1 例急性排斥反应患者肝静脉末梢分支杵状扩张,而观察另外 1 例肝静脉末梢分支杵状扩张患者肝组织活检病理结果正常。所以肝静脉末梢分支杵状扩张不是急性排斥反应的特征性表现。

肝动脉串珠样改变与血管附壁血栓形成有关。肝动脉血栓形成是最常见的肝移植血管并发症,在成人中发生率为 4%~12%,常发生于吻合口或供体肝动脉,与供体肝缺血时间长有关。MRA 清楚显示了血管形态及狭窄部位。肝动脉血栓形成对移植肝的长期存活率有重要影响,因此早期发现可挽救移植肝。

1 例患者供体肝门静脉变细,但对比剂充盈好,因此认为该病例为门静脉狭窄而非血栓形成,另外肝内门静脉分支亦减少,肝右叶明显,且肝实质亦有信号改变,可见此狭窄并非因个体差异所致的假性狭窄,而是病理性狭窄,考虑与供体肝缺血时间过长有关。

二、排斥反应胆管异常

急性排斥反应典型的 MRCP 表现为肝内胆管纤细稀疏或者未显影。急性排斥反应病理变化:①汇管区混合炎性细胞浸润;②小胆管上皮细胞炎症和损伤;③血管内皮炎。而汇管区混合炎性细胞浸润和血管内皮炎又会加重胆管缺血性损伤,所以急性排斥反应胆管异常出现的早而且病变程度严重。肝内胆管纤细稀疏或者未显影可以理解为弥漫性的胆管狭窄或者功能不良。

慢性排斥反应特征性的 MRCP 表现为肝内胆

管串珠样改变或者分支稀疏；胆总管胆泥形成而肝内胆管未见扩张。慢性排斥反应病理变化：①小胆管和中等大小胆管消失；②泡沫细胞性动脉炎或动脉病。慢性排斥反应胆总管胆泥形成而肝内胆管未见扩张可能与胆管缺血及灌注损伤有关，胆管功能不良导致没有正常的胆汁分泌和排泄，所以肝内胆管不能正常显影，即使有胆总管胆泥形成。排斥反应造成的胆管黏膜损伤也是胆泥形成的原因。这些胆管异常表现是其他肝病及肝脏手术后所没有的胆管表现。

总之，肝移植术后排斥反应有一些特征性的血管和胆管 MR 表现。磁共振血管造影和胆管造影作为一种非侵袭性影像检查方法，可以辅助临床诊断肝移植术后排斥反应。

第三章　肝移植后的胆系并发症

一、原位肝移植术后胆系并发症的影像学检查与评价

自 Starzl(1963)开展首例原位肝移植以来,原位肝移植现已成为终末期肝病和急性肝功能衰竭的有效治疗手段。近年,原位肝移植的生存率较前明显提高,但移植后并发症的发生率也随之升高。胆系并发症、血管并发症及移植排斥反应是术后移植肝脏无功能的主要原因,尤其是胆系相关并发症具有高发病率、早期诊断困难及预后不良的特点,成为移植界一直关注的焦点。在尸体全肝移植中,胆系并发症的发生率为 10%~15%,甚至有研究者统计高达 10%~30%。发生率因移植的术式、供体的选择及胆系吻合方式的不同而有所差异。

目前,由于胆系并发症临床表现的隐匿性及相关实验室检查缺乏特异性,因此各种影像学检查方法及肝脏穿刺活检成为了临床获得诊断依据的主要手段,如何选择和评价不同影像学检查方法,使之更合理地用于肝移植围手术期的监护和处理,是临床关注的热点之一。

1. 胆系造影术　胆系造影术是诊断胆系并发症的金标准,可以准确显示胆管的解剖形态与分布以及病理改变等,包括经 T 形管胆汁引流术、内窥镜逆行性胆胰管造影术(ERCP)、经皮穿刺肝胆系造影术(PTC)。目前,部分移植中心于肝移植病人术中在吻合口受体端留置胆汁引流管,放置时间 3~6 个月,所以留置 T 管的病人疑有胆系并发症时通过 T 管可以方便快捷地进行胆管造影,密切观察胆管系统的变化。ERCP 作为诊断技术及后续治疗手段一直被国内外肝移植界广泛采用。

Mata 等(2004)认为, ERCP 应作为原位肝移植术后胆系并发症的一线治疗措施。但是, ERCP 属于有创性检查,而且可能诱发急性胰腺炎、胆系感染、出血等并发症,其成功率与操作者的技术水平密切相关。一直以来,人们对于 ERCP 的诊断准确性存有置疑。在一项前瞻性对照研究中,对 23 例原位肝移植术后 3~6 个月肝功能异常而无胆系症状的病人采用 ERCP 及经皮肝穿刺活检技术进行研究。结果表明,仅 1 例(4%)的 ERCP 是异常的,而穿刺病理的阳性发现为 13 例(57%)。有些研究者认为,对于肝移植术后病人, ERCP 的主要用途在于治疗胆系并发症,而非诊断。ERCP 对于肝移植术后胆系并发症的治疗应该遵循个体化的原则。ERCP 治疗 T 管拔出后出现的轻中度胆管狭窄、胆瘘及胆管结石效果很好;对于重度胆管狭窄、弥漫性肝内胆管狭窄则 ERCP 效果不佳;胆肠吻合手术影响十二指肠乳头的正常解剖,故无法行 ERCP。PTC 影像清晰,能够为胆系疾病的诊断提供可靠信息,临床上怀疑术后合并胆系并发症时,如果超声及 MRCP 诊断不明或显示不清,应考虑通过 PTC 来确诊。原位肝移植术后胆管梗阻、胆系感染及胆汁湖形成需胆汁引流者则为经皮穿刺肝胆管胆汁引流术(PTCD)的最佳适应证。合并肝内胆管扩张的病人 PTC 成功率高达 99%~100%,并发症发生率 3%~4%,主要包括败血症、胆瘘和腹腔出血等。

2. 磁共振胆胰管成像(MRCP)　MRCP 是利用重 T_2 加权技术将体内近似静止状态的液体(胆汁、胰液和胃肠液等)清晰地成像,对于没有留置 T 管或 T 管已经拔出的肝移植术后病人,如果可疑合并胆系并发症,影像学检查方法中通常首选 MRCP 检查。

其优势在于 4 点:避免了胆系造影所引起的并发症;能清楚显示狭窄或梗阻近端、远端的情况;节省时间;如有需要可方便地加做肝脏增强扫描及血管成像,同时可观察肝实质及血管吻合的情况。有文献报道, MRCP 诊断肝移植术后胆系并发症的敏感度达 93%,特异度为 97.6%,准确度为 95.6%。但如果病人有胆汁瘤或出现大量腹水、极度虚弱、神志不清、呼吸不能配合等情况,对 MRCP 影像质量的影响仍然很大。近年来,随着 MRCP 逐渐广泛使

用，一些研究者普遍认为肝移植术后并发症的诊断、治疗应该向无创和微创的方向发展。

3. MSCT　MSCT 对于诊断肝移植术后的血管并发症具有重要意义，同时也可以为胆系并发症的诊断提供一定的影像依据。MSCT 多期增强扫描对于胆系结石、胆汁湖、胆汁囊肿、胆管狭窄远端的胆管扩张以及胆源性肝脓肿有一定的诊断价值。但对于胆管狭窄的部位和程度显示存在局限性，不能显示胆泥、胆管坏死，也没有 MRCP 和胆系造影的图像直观、形象，信息量较小，故需要结合 MRCP、胆道造影综合分析。

4. 超声　灰阶及彩色多普勒超声包括彩色多普勒血流成像（CDFI），对于原位肝移植后血管并发症及胆石、胆汁湖、腹腔积液、胆管狭窄远端的胆管扩张具有重要的诊断意义，并可在超声引导下穿刺引流局部的胆汁漏出液，放置引流管等，但很难显示胆管狭窄、胆瘘的具体部位及胆泥。此外，超声诊断存在着较高的假阳性率与假阴性率，易受胃肠道气体干扰及操作者人为因素的影响。超声诊断可以作为肝移植术后胆系并发症的粗筛方法，对于超声结果为阴性而临床可疑胆系并发症的需结合胆系造影或 MRCP 才能作出准确的诊断。

二、肝移植术后胆系并发症的影像学表现

早在 1976 年，Calne 就指出胆系重建技术是肝移植的“阿喀流斯之踵（Achilles heel）”，这一说法沿用至今。胆管重建技术的水平直接影响胆系并发症的发生。此外，肝动脉血供不良、冷缺血和热缺血的时间、供肝获取及保存条件、巨细胞病毒感染、ABO 血型是否相符等也是胆系并发症的影响因素。大约有 2/3 的胆系并发症发生在 3 个月以内，大约有 1/3 的胆系并发症发生于 1 个月以内，80% 发生在 6 个月以内，有报道称移植后 1 年后胆系并发症的发生率 <4%。胆系并发症包括胆系狭窄和扩张、胆系结石和胆瘘等，这些并发症不是完全孤立的，并且发病机制也有部分相似之处，如非吻合口狭窄常伴有胆管坏死、胆泥及胆瘘存在等。

1. 胆管狭窄　胆管狭窄是最常见的胆系并发症，按照发生部位分为吻合口狭窄和非吻合口狭窄；按发生的时间可分为早期狭窄和晚期狭窄。早期狭窄主要是因为技术原因，如胆管断端对合欠佳，胆管断端周围毛细血管网被破坏使吻合口局部缺血狭窄及胆管吻合时缝合针距过密，缝线收拢过紧等。晚期的狭窄常常是因为各种原因引起的胆管血供不足，包括肝动脉栓塞、胆系感染、慢性排斥反应、硬化性胆管炎等基础疾病的复发以及胆管的缺血再灌注损伤等。

2. 吻合口狭窄　吻合口狭窄是发生于受体胆管与供体胆管吻合口处的狭窄，据统计在各种胆系并发症中发病率最高，占 36.4%，多发生在肝移植术后晚期，常与胆石、胆泥等合并症共同存在，其形成与手术后瘢痕形成、外科吻合技术有关。需要注意，肝移植后梗阻性黄疸的病人未必伴有梗阻近端胆管的扩张，大多数（61%）吻合口狭窄的病人并无明显的近端胆管扩张，这可能与冷保存再灌注损伤的移植肝胆管顺应性下降有关。

T 管留置的病人可以通过直接的 T 管造影发现吻合口的胆管狭窄及狭窄远端的胆管扩张。T 管拔出或无 T 管引流的病人可选择 MRCP。

CT 对于狭窄部位显示不清，仅能通过胆管扩张这一间接征象来判断狭窄存在，对于可疑胆管狭窄而 CT 未见胆管扩张者，并不能排除胆管狭窄（因为即使存在胆管的重度狭窄，远端胆管也可以不扩张）。由此可见，CT 诊断胆管狭窄不可避免地存在假阴性的可能。同样，超声诊断也存在着与 CT 相似的假阴性问题。

MRCP 能够清楚地显示吻合口狭窄及肝内胆管扩张的程度，诊断吻合口狭窄的敏感度、特异度及准确度均可达 95% 以上，但是近年临床上发现 MRCP 诊断吻合口狭窄存在一些问题，如较低的空间分辨力导致漏诊轻度的吻合口狭窄，夸大吻合口的狭窄程度，不能明确区分吻合口周围局限性的腹水和胆汁瘤等。

胆管吻合口狭窄得到确诊后可采用内镜球囊扩张、内置支架等技术微创治疗，通过 ERCP 和 PTC 行胆管气囊扩张和支架置入对约 70% 的吻合口狭窄和 60% 的肝内胆管狭窄有效，但往往需反复多次施行。若内镜介入治疗失败，则需改行外科修补吻合口或胆肠吻合术。肝内胆管弥漫性狭窄或重度吻合口狭窄时，主张尽早积极进行再次肝移植。

有文献报道，肝移植术中放置胆管吻合口塑料支架内支撑，能够明显减少吻合口狭窄等胆系并发症的发生。

3. 非吻合口狭窄　是移植肝的胆管树出现非吻合口性狭窄和扩张等胆管缺血的改变。大部分非吻合口狭窄是由于缺血引起的，所以非吻合口狭窄又

称为“缺血性胆管狭窄”,肝门部胆管分叉处是高发部位。

缺血性胆管狭窄最常见的诱因是肝动脉栓塞。肝移植术后早期阶段最常见、最严重的并发症是肝动脉栓塞,当发生肝动脉栓塞时,要注意合并缺血性胆管狭窄的可能。

值得注意的是,相当一部分非吻合口狭窄是无肝动脉栓塞的,这是一种相对更为严重的并发症,移植肝无功能的概率及死亡率较高,是近年研究的热点问题。其原因主要可分为缺血性损伤、免疫性损伤两方面。

缺血性损伤指由于供肝热缺血、冷缺血后缺血再灌注损伤导致的胆系微循环缺血性损伤。目前国内主要采用心跳停搏供体肝移植,其热缺血损伤对胆管的破坏更为严重,更容易造成肝内胆管的狭窄。存在热缺血损伤严重的尸体供肝,肝内胆管弥漫性狭窄的发生率显著高于脑死亡供体,并且供肝冷、热缺血时间均与缺血性胆管损伤的发生率及胆管损伤程度呈正相关。

免疫性损伤则包括巨细胞病毒(CMV)感染、ABO 血型不符以及慢性排斥反应等导致的动脉病变或直接的胆管上皮损伤,继而发生狭窄,还包括胆系的免疫性疾病,如原发性硬化性胆管炎的复发造成胆管上皮细胞破坏,炎性肉芽组织增生导致的肝内胆管的狭窄,也有研究者将后者单独列为感染性损伤。

硬化性胆管炎的肝移植病人与其他基础病(如肝癌、终末期肝硬化及巨大海绵状血管瘤等)病人比较,前者肝移植术后发生非吻合口狭窄的可能性几乎是后者的 2 倍,而且硬化性胆管炎肝移植术后复发率高达 20%。

非吻合口狭窄的临床表现为黄疸、发热,MRCP 及胆系造影检查(T 管造影、ERCP、PTC)可以发现肝内胆管僵直、不规则扩张,狭窄则多数位于肝门区周围的胆管,CT 及超声诊断非吻合口狭窄缺乏特异性。

Boraschi 等(2004)研究发现,28 例确诊的缺血性狭窄病人,其中 4 例手术重建胆管系统,7 例再移植,以病理结果和胆管造影结果作为对照标准,MRCP 发现并确诊了 26 例狭窄,同时清楚地显示了其中 16 例病人胆管内的胆泥和胆石,因而 MRCP 可以无创、准确地诊断移植肝非吻合口狭窄。

非吻合口狭窄与吻合口狭窄相比,一般预后不良并且传统的内镜和介入治疗效果较差。球囊扩张和放置支架治疗肝门部和肝内狭窄的成功率只有 28.6%,而治疗吻合口狭窄的成功率为 75%。尽管疗效不佳,但是非吻合口狭窄的治疗还是首选介入或内镜治疗。如果胆管缺血性狭窄的病人对非手术治疗无效,或经积极的抗炎治疗仍出现发热、血清胆红素水平进行性升高症状,特别是怀疑有原发性硬化性胆管炎复发的病人,其移植肝会在短时期内失去功能,应尽快接受再次肝移植手术,若不及时实行再次移植,死亡率可高达 100%。

三、胆瘘

胆瘘在肝移植术后早期发病率较高,多发生于术后 1~3 个月之间,晚期也可发生,但较为少见,仅有 7%,平均发生在术后 4 个月左右。早期胆瘘的发生与胆管吻合方式无关,供受体胆管端端吻合与侧侧吻合的胆瘘发病率的差异无统计学意义。胆瘘的临床症状中最常见的是腹痛,其次是发热、腹肌紧张等。约 1/3 的病人表现为急腹症,最直接的征象是腹腔引流管流出胆汁性液体或胆汁引流管引出的胆汁减少甚至无胆汁引出,按发生的不同部位分为 T 管瘘、吻合口瘘和非吻合口胆瘘,临床上以 T 管瘘最多见。

1. T 管瘘　大多数早期胆瘘为 T 管瘘,发生于 T 管放置处。在放置引流管和拔出引流管后,胆汁均可从 T 管引流口位置流出。早期的 T 管瘘常引起瘘口远端的胆管阻塞或胆胰管下端括约肌功能障碍等。T 管造影可以直观地发现对比剂外漏这一直接征象。T 管已拔出者可行 MRCP、超声等检查。MRCP 能够清楚显示胆汁积聚的部位、范围。超声可发现肝下、肝门部、腹腔内局部积聚的胆汁,并且可在超声引导下进行腹腔积液穿刺抽吸、放置引流管。

轻度的 T 管瘘,可以通过腹腔引流、原 T 管窦道放置引流管保守治疗而治愈。严重的 T 管瘘可通过经皮肝穿刺放置引流管或在内镜引导下瘘口处放置支架等措施得到治疗。对存在括约肌功能障碍的可采用内镜下括约肌切开术,24~48 h 非手术治疗不缓解的应予以手术治疗。目前,世界各地的移植中心正尝试采取各种方法来减少 T 管瘘的发生,其中对于胆系重建中的 T 管留置问题存在较多争议。Scatton 等(2001)在前瞻性随机对照研究中发现,90 例病人中留置 T 管的胆系并发症发生率为 33%,比未置 T 管的高 15.5%。然而，Tung 等（1999）总结了 1987—1996 年间的 2 645 例肝移植病例，发现未置 T 管者胆管狭窄的发病率较置 T 管者高。尽管留置引流管并不能降低胆管狭窄的发生率，但是 T 管有其独特的临床使用价值，本身能够抑制吻合口瘢痕组织增生，防止吻合口狭窄，同时通过 T 管观察移植术后肝脏分泌胆汁功能，进行胆系冲洗，降低胆系压力，可预防胆泥形成及胆管炎，故至今仍为一些移植中心采用。关于 T 管留置与否问题还需要有大样本多中心的前瞻性随机对照研究。

2. 吻合口瘘　即胆汁瘘口位于受体 - 供体胆管吻合口，通常是由于外科吻合胆管时操作不当造成。放置 T 管病人，T 管造影即可确诊吻合口瘘。保持 T 管通畅，1~2 周后通过胆系造影可以确定是否治愈。T 管已拔出的病人，MRCP 可以有效地帮助诊断吻合口瘘，95% 的吻合口瘘通过内镜放置塑料支架可以得到控制，术后 2~3 个月取出支架。

严重的吻合口瘘或胆汁大量外渗，大多数需要进行外科吻合口修补术，或改行胆肠吻合术。胆肠吻合术式的病人吻合口瘘较少见，推荐放置内外引流支架，经皮穿刺抽取腹腔积液、胆汁瘤，也可经超声引导下穿刺引流，必要时可同时注射抗生素。但是，很多时候在控制了腹腔感染之后，有必要手术修补吻合口或建立新的吻合口。

3. 非吻合口胆瘘　可能继发于缺血性胆管狭窄，常合并胆汁瘤或胆源性腹膜炎。病理表现为局限的胆管血管丛的微循环破坏、胆管细胞坏死。治疗此种胆瘘推荐经皮肝穿或内镜下放置塑料内引流支架，4 周至 3 个月后移除支架。若微创治疗效果不佳，尤其是继发于肝动脉栓塞的胆管胆瘘应在肝衰竭前及时进行再次肝移植术。

四、胆管坏死碎屑、胆泥以及胆管结石

胆管坏死碎屑、胆泥、胆石形成较胆管狭窄、胆瘘少见，大多数发生在肝移植术后晚期，多与吻合口或非吻合口狭窄等其他胆系并发症伴随存在。虽然发病率不高，但是同时合并移植物无功能或胆管炎的概率很高，不容忽视。这一组并发症中以胆石平均发生时间最长，距手术时间约 135 周；胆管坏死碎屑最短，约 17 周；胆泥居中，约 45 周。胆泥的形成明显早于胆石，这一发现提示持续存在的胆泥最终可能会形成胆石。

胆管细胞是一群高代谢、高氧耗、低缺氧耐受的细胞，对缺血的耐受能力低于肝细胞。大部分胆管坏死是胆管缺血所致，据 Sheng 等（1996）统计，供体与胆石和胆泥相比，胆管坏死病人的供肝冷缺血时间更长，冷缺血时胆管黏膜下血管丛的血管内皮细胞缺氧、肿胀引起胆管血液循环障碍，从而导致胆管上皮坏死、脱落。

胆泥的成分是浓稠的胆汁或是破坏的胆管壁脱落的结缔组织，形成主要与排斥反应、胆系感染、缺血等有关。胆泥的起病隐匿，直到晚期引起肝外胆管扩张或胆管炎时，病人才会有相应的临床表现，如发热、腹痛、黄疸及谷丙转氨酶、谷草转氨酶、γ- 谷氨酰转肽酶等升高，但以上表现均不典型，所以诊断主要依靠影像学及穿刺活检。

在胆管造影和 MRCP 上，胆泥主要征象为胆管腔内不规则形充盈缺损，边缘较为模糊，可以分布于单条或多条胆管，胆管木塞状闭塞，胆管壁粗细不均，多处狭窄，伴有肝内和 / 或肝外胆管的扩张。MRCP 与胆系造影均可清楚地显示胆泥及胆管碎屑的分布及肝内外胆管的扩张情况。超声诊断胆泥有一定的困难，直接征象为沿胆管分布的条索状或木塞状的中等回声，后方无明显声影。

Barton 等（1995）统计的 51 例经胆系造影确诊为胆泥的病人中，超声发现了 16 例（31%）胆管腔内中等回声的物质，其中的 6 例似木塞状，12 例伴有不同程度的胆管扩张。剩余的 35 例中的 10 例（20%）超声显示了胆管扩张但未能显示出胆泥，25 例（49%）超声提示胆管无异常。超声漏诊胆泥的原因可能为：胆泥为等回声，易与肝实质相混淆；肠道气体干扰了胆泥的显示。对 12 例胆泥病人进行 CT 增强扫描，遗憾的是 CT 均未能显示胆泥，可能与胆泥为等密度而不易区分有关，不过 CT 显示胆管扩张较为敏感而准确。

胆管结石常继发于胆管坏死、胆泥淤积，临床症状与胆泥类似，影像诊断并不困难。在胆系造影、MRCP 上表现为胆管腔内充盈缺损，边界清楚，诊断准确率达 89.9%。超声表现为胆管腔内强回声光团，后方伴明显的声影。当结石成分以胆红素结晶为主时，MSCT 表现为无强化的团块状、沙粒状高密度影；以胆固醇为主时，常为等或稍高密度影。

胆泥经确诊后首先采用保守治疗，口服鹅脱氧胆酸、熊脱氧胆酸等促进胆汁排泄的药物，同时推荐低脂饮食。当保守治疗无效，而胆泥主要局限于肝内大胆管或肝外胆管，同时不合并其他并发症时，进

一步采用经皮肝穿介入治疗或内镜介入治疗,包括放置胆管支架,网篮取泥等。需要注意如果肝内胆管有大量的胆汁淤积,介入治疗会相当费时且很难清除干净,这时应手术重建胆系。胆石的治疗包括手术、内镜或经皮肝穿刺放置胆管支架、网篮取石、引流胆汁、冲洗胆管等。内镜下括约肌切开术和取石术的成功率高达 88%~91%。手术重建胆管的适应证有二:肝外胆管的大范围梗阻或非吻合口的广泛狭窄;放射 / 内镜介入治疗失败。对于合并胆管严重狭窄、常规手术无效的病人应及时在移植肝无功能前果断实施再次肝移植术,以免贻误时机。

五、其他胆系并发症

在肝移植术后,少见的胆系并发症包括胆胰管下端括约肌功能障碍、供体与受体胆管比例失衡、胆管扭转等。

1. 胆胰管下端括约肌功能障碍　肝移植术后胆胰管下端括约肌功能障碍的原因不明,可能与胆胰管下端括约肌神经支配失调,移植前胆管的普遍扩张等有关,另外末梢胆管梗阻、巨细胞病毒等机会感染也可能与胆胰管下端括约肌功能障碍的发病有关。

胆胰管下端括约肌功能障碍表现为胆管内压升高,肝外胆管轻度扩张,典型胆胰管下端括约肌功能障碍的 ERCP 表现为,对比剂由十二指肠经大乳头向胆胰管返流。胆胰管下端括约肌功能障碍引起其上游的胆管压力增高,可能会引起吻合口的胆瘘。传统的处理方法是将胆管 - 胆管吻合改为胆管 - 空肠吻合,近年来逐步采用内镜下放置支架、括约肌切开术微创治疗或内镜治疗失败再手术治疗。

对于括约肌切开术目前还存在一些争论,因为移植术后胆管内压可以在 3~4 个月后趋于正常,因此有研究者主张短期放置十二指肠乳头支架,对于短期放置支架后胆管扩张、胆汁淤积仍然存在者再行括约肌切开术。

2. 供体与受体胆管不成比例　多数表现为供体胆管光滑、纤细,而受体的胆管由于基础病导致轻度的扩张。这种情况很容易误诊为肝内胆管狭窄,两者的区别是肝内胆管狭窄往往表现胆管僵直,狭窄也不均匀,胆管管腔粗细不均,常合并胆瘘。也有少数病人表现为受体胆管纤细而供体胆管轻度扩张。

3. 胆管扭转　胆管上两条透明的平行线为胆管造影或 MRCP 上的特征性表现,即为扭纹。一般见于吻合口水平。目前,肝移植术后胆管扭转的原因不明,尚需进一步的研究。

肝移植术后当可疑存在胆系并发症时,留置 T 管的病人可以方便地通过胆管造影得到诊断。对于未置或已拔出 T 管的病人,MRCP 检查可以作为无创性检查的首选,但是 MRCT 对于轻微胆管狭窄而不伴有远端胆管扩张的诊断存在一些困难,可能会夸大胆管吻合口狭窄的程度,不能明确区分吻合口周围局限性的腹水和胆汁瘤,这些是值得进一步探究的问题。

超声及 CT 对于非吻合口狭窄、胆泥、胆管坏死以及胆瘘等病变均不能直接显示或缺乏特异性,假阴性率高,适宜作为移植术后病人的粗筛检查方法。ERCP、PTC 作为胆系并发症的微创治疗手段,治疗效果值得肯定,但是应当注意各种治疗手段的禁忌证,因为任何一种方法都不是全能的。

肝移植术后胆系并发症及时有效的诊治有赖于多学科的共同努力,正确合理地选择影像学检查方法,早期、无创或微创地诊治肝移植术后胆系并发症,将进一步提高肝移植病人的围手术期生存质量和肝移植的成功率。

第十五篇　胆系疾病

第一章　胆系结石类疾病

第一节　误诊病例简介:非肝移植胆管铸型综合征

详见本书 本卷 第十六篇 第一章 第一节　误诊病例简介:非肝移植胆管铸型综合征。

第二节　黏稠胆汁和胆泥

胆泥,即胆汁淤泥,是由胆固醇和胆色素结晶浓缩形成,在进食和胆囊收缩时,胆囊可将其内胆泥排出。超声检查时,可见胆泥表现为胆囊腔内块状物的自由活动, Jeanty 等(1983)专门介绍这类情况。Reinig 和 Stanley(1984)在研究超声胆囊显像中胆囊不显示的原因时,发现黏稠胆汁充盈胆囊为一个原因,如再给予进食脂餐,可见黏稠胆汁在此刺激下从胆囊排出;如胆泥充盈胆囊,则不见胆囊的声影。Sanders 等(1983)在讨论高回声胆囊时也发现与此类似的情况。

第三节　误诊病例简介:黏胆症与黏液性乳头状癌

大量黏液积聚在肝内外胆管腔内,即黏胆症(mucobilia)。临床上少见报道。引起黏胆症的病因较多,常见的有产黏液(黏蛋白)的胆管癌、胆管囊腺瘤及囊腺癌、胆管乳头状瘤病、肝叶纤维化并胆管囊状扩张伴黏膜上皮增生等。黏胆症大多以黄疸、腹痛、发热等胆系炎症为临床表现,易与胆管下段肿瘤、结石及胆管炎等所致胆管梗阻性疾病相混淆, CT、MRI 不易鉴别。肝左外叶囊柱状扩张胆管内的黏液较稀薄,密度较低。因 CT 所示胆总管下段腔内见类似软组织样密度的占位性病变,从而被误诊为胆管下段肿瘤,而位于较高位置的肝内胆管内黏液样物质由于其密度与胆汁类似而不易被发现。

由于该例肝左外叶肿瘤为沿肝内胆管管壁生长,无明显肿块及结节, CT 所示胆管壁仅有轻度增厚、边缘毛糙,该征象与胆管炎极难鉴别。由于胆管内黏液样物质与正常胆汁的信号特点具有较明显的差异性,且 MRCP 为三维立体图像,并可不同视角观察,因此 MRI 相比 CT 对于胆管梗阻整体显示及病因诊断具有相对的优越性。

该例胆总管、肝管及肝左外叶胆管内稍短 T_1、长 T_2 信号物质与胆管管壁有缝隙存在,这说明它是单独存在并不与胆管管壁相连,从而可排除胆总管下段肿瘤,可能是炎性赘生物或者是黏稠的胆汁。经 ERCP 进行进一步检查,发现胆管内有可漂浮移动并可发生形变充盈缺损,胆总管下段未发现明确肿瘤样病变,于是想到粘胆症可能。如果经皮肝穿刺胆管引流(PTCD)引流出胶冻样液体,则有助于本病的诊断。但最终诊断仍有赖于开腹胆系探查及术中胆管镜的应用。

通常根据黏胆症病因及具体病变情况选择不同的外科治疗。肝内胆管黏液腺癌、管内型胆管癌、乳头状胆管癌,不同角度定义的胆管癌,与黏胆症产生密切相关,其最好的治疗方法就是行肝段、肝叶切除术,与其他类型胆管癌相比有着相对较好的预后。若术中诊断仍不明确,常只行胆总管切开探查T管引流或胆肠吻合术,一些学者报道2例肝内胆管黏液腺癌带瘤生存超过18个月,但这些姑息性手术后,因黏液不断分泌必将复发梗阻性黄疸和胆管炎,往往需多次手术,在首次手术时未发现或未能切除原发病灶,预后欠佳。因此,根治性切除产生黏液的病灶,彻底清除胆管内胶冻样物和胆管通畅引流是其治疗原则。

第四节　肺内胆石

Schwegier 和 Endrei(1975)报告1例70岁女性病人,她有数年胆囊疾病疼痛史,1966年手术见胆囊壁破裂,为瘢痕组织增厚,但未见结石。组织学示严重增生部分坏死的胆囊炎症,伴脓肿形成,炎症已蔓延至肝。3年后病人间断咯血,X线胸片示右下叶密度增加,其中央有一三角形致密影。2年后胸片见此影无变化。1972年咯血加重,伴呼吸困难及心跳过速入院。纤维支气管镜示出血源于右侧第8、9级支气管,未发现肿瘤。

X线胸片见右下叶三角影指向肺门,侧位断层片示该区硬币性病变被肺不张所包围,支气管造影发现外基底支气管背侧有一光滑压迹,遂手术切除右下叶。病检:外基底支气管内胆石伴支气管扩张和远侧肺不张。该支气管腔增宽,直径约3cm,且为胆石充盈。胆石化学分析见胆固醇钙(94%)和镁(6%),周围为胆色素钙。回顾1966年胸片未见异常,手术又未发现胆石,提示胆石可能已穿过胃肠道吸入肺内,但当时外科大夫与麻醉师均怀疑此假设。病人只出现咯血,第二次手术见右下叶与膈之间粘连特别严重。在支气管造影后5天,侧位断层片清楚可见支气管对比剂(dionosil)残余位于肺部病变的尾侧端,扩展至膈下,故推断结石可能来自膈下,致膈肌胸膜穿孔而吸入支气管内,右膈升高及严重的粘连也支持此种解释。

第五节　黏胆症

黏胆症(mucobilia)是由于胆管上皮肿瘤或肿瘤样病变分泌大量黏液积聚在肝内外胆管腔内,引起胆管的梗阻性扩张,进而导致梗阻性黄疸和胆管炎。黏胆症在临床上较少见,患者缺乏特异性临床表现,也无特异性肿瘤标志物,多数病例术前易误诊为胆总管末端炎性狭窄伴肝内外胆管炎性扩张或胆管内结石伴胆管炎性扩张,部分病例误诊为先天性胆管扩张。

1. 发病机制　黏胆症临床上较少见,以日本和我国中国台湾地区、香港地区较多,欧美地区也有个案报道,具体病因尚不明确,多数报道认为复发性肝内胆管结石或胆管炎症的长期慢性刺激导致胆管周围炎症、胆管上皮增生和不典型增生,胆管上皮增生和肠化形成胆管内的乳头状肿瘤,过度分泌黏液出现黏胆症,导致胆管梗阻性扩张,又进一步加剧胆管炎症,反复的胆管炎症又促进胆石及胆泥形成,胆石及胆泥又加剧胆系梗阻及胆管感染,胆石和炎症的长期刺激最终导致胆管内乳头状肿瘤癌变。一组11例患者中5例合并胆管结石,有8例患者既往有胆系手术病史。

2. 病理学　黏胆症病理类型较多,常见的有产生黏液(黏蛋白)的胆管囊腺瘤、胆管乳头状瘤、胆管乳头状瘤病以及不同病理类型的胆管恶性肿瘤(胆管囊腺癌、胆管乳头状癌、胆管黏液腺癌)、肝叶纤维化并胆管囊状扩张伴黏膜上皮增生等。

3. 临床表现　由于黏胆症临床表现缺乏特异性,无特异性肿瘤标志物,胆管内存在大量胶冻样黏液容易掩盖肿瘤本身,常规影像学检查难以术前诊断,加之临床医生对本病缺乏足够的认识,本病很少能在术前获得诊断,部分病人因发生恶变或累及范围扩大,失去了最佳的治疗机会。临床主要表现为波动性黄疸合并反复发热,右上腹部痛等胆管炎症状。黄疸主要由胆管梗阻所致,胆管梗阻一是肿瘤本身所致,梗阻可以是完全的,梗阻以远的肝内胆管扩张更为明显,黄疸为渐进性加深;二是肿瘤分泌的胶冻样黏液,分泌到胆管或对侧肝内胆管,对胆管的梗阻一般是不完全的，肝外胆管梗阻更为明显，对侧肝内胆管不扩张或较轻度扩张，表现为不对称性胆管扩张，临床以波动性黄疸为主。实际上黏胆症患者常并存两种梗阻方式，合并胆管感染时常表现为急性胆管炎。

4. 影像学研究　黏胆症 MRI 平扫表现为肝内外胆管非枯枝样扩张及不同程度的囊状或圆柱状扩张，胆管内附壁或胆管壁向腔内生长的结节状、乳头状、斑片状病灶，呈等或稍长 T_1、等或稍长 T_2 信号，增强扫描病灶呈轻～中度不均匀强化，部分黏胆症患者胆管内病灶强化不明显，单纯依靠 MRI 平扫胆管壁病灶易被胆管内分泌的黏液掩盖，导致病灶漏诊或误诊。2D 及 3D MRCP 能多方位显示肝内外胆管扩张情况，胆管内胆汁及黏液在 MRCP 重 T_2 水成像下显示为明显高信号，更有助于显示胆管壁病灶。MRCP 是术前黏胆症诊断的有效手段，其主要特征有：①肝内胆管扩张不对称性，可表现为病灶侧肝内胆管和肝外胆管同时扩张，但未受累肝内胆管不扩张或轻度扩张，除非肿块累及肝门部胆管或健侧肝内胆管；②远离肿瘤的远端或近端肝内胆管都扩张，未受累的肝内胆管亦可扩张，这是与先天性胆管囊状扩张相鉴别的主要特征；③肿瘤在 MRCP 高信号的胆汁衬托下呈结节状、乳头状、斑片状相对低信号，部分黏液与胆汁呈现分层征象；④无肝外胆管突然截断征象；⑤胆囊增大不明显，与胆胰管连接区肿瘤“大胆囊”的表现不同。

其中肝内胆管扩张不对称性，无肝外胆管的突然截断，这是黏胆症的 MRCP 检查最具特征表现。诊断上要与胆囊癌侵犯肝内胆管、肝内胆管癌以及胆胰管连接区肿瘤鉴别；胆囊癌侵犯肝门胆管或肝门部胆管癌可表现为肝内胆管一侧或双侧扩张，但胆总管无扩张；肝内胆管癌表现为局部胆管受侵、狭窄，梗阻远端胆管扩张；胆胰管连接区肿瘤表现为肝内外胆管的均匀性扩张及胆囊的显著增大。

5. 黏胆症治疗及手术可切除性评估　目前认为黏胆症首选手术治疗，由于肿瘤分泌的黏蛋白可引起胆管炎及胆系梗阻反复发作，所以无论肿瘤良、恶性均具有手术指征。对于可切除的黏胆症患者，手术主要目的是切除肿瘤病灶，术中可以采用多次灌洗胆管的方法清除胆管中的黏液及黏蛋白。术前 MRCP 能初步确定胆管内病灶累及范围，有助于手术方式的选择，根据扩张的胆管与相对正常的胆管之间的交界线，可以初步判断肿瘤累及范围及可切除性，如果扩张的胆管局限于某一肝段或肝叶，行肝段或肝叶切除，如果对侧胆管扩张明显，提示病灶累及肝门部胆管或对侧胆管，无法完整切除病灶，这类患者只能行姑息性切除或胆管引流，针对这类患者术中常规搔刮肿瘤后采用电刀烧灼肿瘤或行肿瘤黏膜剥脱术，术后长期 T 管引流，并定期冲洗维持引流管通畅，在一定程度上能延缓黄疸再次发生的时间。

综上所述，黏胆症的 MRCP 术前诊断的关键在于认真准确的阅片，如果符合上述 5 条 MRCP 征象，特别是同时有肝内胆管不对称性扩张、肝外胆管无截断、胆管内病变呈相对低信号 3 种征象，加上临床上有波动性黄疸病史，即可诊断本病。MRCP 可作为术前黏胆症的诊断与评估手术可切除性的有效手段。

第二章 胆系积气、胆系损伤和胆系出血

第一节 胆系积气

一般情况下,胆系内无气体存在。如果在胆系内发现气体,则应想到:自发性胆系肠道内瘘、产气菌引起的胆囊炎或胆管炎、胆胰管下端括约肌松弛。胆系内气体可由多种原因引起,在医源性方面的原因有:ERCP、胆管支架、胆管十二指肠吻合术后或胆胰管下端括约肌成形术后、胆胰下端括约肌开放状态;手术误伤形成的胆系肠道瘘等。在外科分流、括约肌切开术或ERCP后,看到胆管树内气体即胆管积气并非少见,胆管分支类型与胆管系统解剖一致。偶尔,进行胆总管结石排石时在胆管树内可见到气体。

一种潜在的诊断误区是气腹延伸到肝门而误认为是肝管积气。有作者报告,在腹腔镜胆囊切开术后2天。螺旋CT增强扫描显示气腹,游离的空气扩散至肝门部,亦呈管条状,与胆管积气十分相似。另一种潜在诊断误区是胆管积气与门静脉系统积气的混淆,此时鉴别二者甚为重要。门静脉积气通常是肠坏死的一个先兆征象。然而,门静脉积气的其他原因包括近期外科手术或是留置导管(包括G管)。门静脉积气通常有典型分支形状,可达到肝脏的周边,与胆管积气不同(胆管积气集中在肝脏的中央部位)。

在MRCP检查时,胆系内气体可误诊为结石,两者在所有序列中均表现为圆形无信号区。两者的鉴别点为:气体位于胆管的远地位置,而结石位于胆管的近地位置;气体可产生磁敏感性伪影,而结石则无伪影。MRCP对磁敏感性伪影不敏感,不易辨认。

第二节 假性胆系积气

在X线检查和CT扫描时,胆管周围脂肪、肝圆韧带周围脂肪、腹膜外脂肪延伸至肝门周围的脂肪、肝内裂隙内脂肪都可在右上腹出现树支状透光影或低密度影。高居于右上腹区的异位阑尾积气,有时也可伪似胆系积气。上述构成假性胆系积气的透亮阴影,从其形态、分布的特定位置看,不像右肾周围脂肪、右侧腰大肌上部脂肪层、肝区结肠周围脂肪线、肝下缘或网膜脂肪线、空肠内积气、门静脉内积气等。

第三节 有关胆系积气的诊断陷阱

有时,在右上腹部X线平片可见到密度均匀一致的肝区背景上有边缘清楚的透光带,它可为弓形,也可呈分支状,在不同位置多次摄片它表现形态恒定,颇似胆系积气,可导致误诊。右上腹部管状透光影的原因甚多,应考虑者至少有下述几项:①胆系积气:自发性或手术后的胆肠内瘘,胆管下端括约肌松弛,胆管下端括约肌强行扩张后,化脓性胆囊炎及胆管炎、胆系外伤、气性坏疽性胆囊炎、新生儿坏死性

肠结肠炎等。②门静脉内积气。③阑尾高位，位于肝下。④肝圆韧带周围脂肪沉积。⑤右肺下叶后基底段支气管充气。⑥腹膜外脂肪，可扩展到肝门并包绕胆管及其分支，表现如袖套状。⑦肝内裂隙内脂肪沉积。⑧肝区结肠周围脂肪、网膜脂肪沉积等。②～⑧可称作假性胆系积气。

它们与胆系积气颇有类似之处，这些透光影均投影于肝区，位于右肾前方，十二指肠球部之上，且可轻微外凸，其上段也可出现分支。但是，腹膜外脂肪常沿着肝下缘行走，在边缘有一结节状影伸向肝门，多呈一连续的管状透光影，一般在断层片中有时见到。变换病人的体位不能使这些透光带向胆管的深部肝管分支行走。而胆系积气或门静脉积气则可继续向分支充气，出现形态的变化。另外，有作者指出，在超声扫描时，胆管树内的空气可类似于钙化。在胆肠吻合术后，空气反流入胆系，肝内常见高振幅回声区，它位于门静脉的前面，常难以区别是胆管内的空气或是钙化，在区别时，病史甚为重要。

胆系积气：胆系内常出现气体即胆系积气，尤其常见于有胆系手术史者，如胆肠吻合术、括约肌切开术后。胆系积气可引起敏感性伪影，利用某一扫描序列可将伪影降低到最低限度，如这种伪影在快速自旋回波（turbo SE）序列中是稳定的。极少情况下，过量的气体在胆总管内可形成完全不均匀信号，降低了 MRCP 的诊断价值。

气泡：括约肌切开术后病人胆系内常见气泡。与常规胆管造影一样，在 MRCP 图像上气泡与结石表现相同，需要与小结石鉴别。鉴别小结石与气泡的有效方法是选择一个与胆总管长轴垂直的平面（通常为倾斜轴位平面）进行 MRCP 成像。

这一额外成像可通过三维序列扫描重建横轴位平面的容积数据获得，也可通过二维成像获得，后者可获得另一组图像。横轴位平面显示胆总管结石位于胆总管的下垂部位，而气泡则位于其非下垂部位。

第四节　十二指肠 - 胆系逆流的少见原因之一

在没有胆系 - 十二指肠瘘的情况下，总胆管下端开口异常可引起十二指肠 - 胆系返流。

Chermet 等（1975）统计以往法文文献中有 13 例总胆管开口于十二指肠球后部引起此类返流的报道。

该作者报告一例 67 岁老人有类似的表现，分析研究系因溃疡周围瘢痕化与收缩，导致总胆管高位开口，并有十二指肠乳头关闭不全，术中胆系造影证实诊断，并清楚见及总胆管远端呈鱼钩状开口进入十二指肠球后部。

第五节　胆囊腺鳞癌伴坏死，胆囊穿孔，腹膜炎

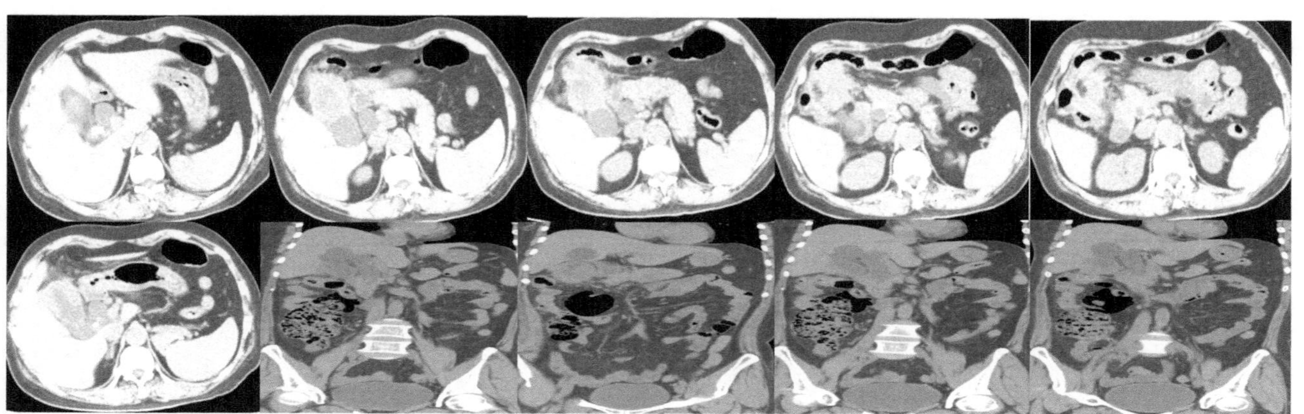

图 15-2-1　胆囊腺鳞癌伴坏死，胆囊穿孔，腹膜炎

患者，女，51岁，反复腹痛2年，复发并加重22小时。入院诊断：腹膜炎，胆囊穿孔，胆囊占位性病变的局限性腹膜炎？手术所见：腹腔有浑浊脓性渗液约200ml，胆囊被大网膜包裹，表面有脓苔附着，分开粘连后见胆囊大小约10cm × 5cm，胆囊底部大小约3.0cm × 2.5cm肿物，侵及全层并穿透囊体，侵及结肠系膜，与横结肠、胃、十二指肠粘连紧密，胆囊三角解剖结构不清，肝十二指肠韧带明显增厚，胆总管直径约0.9cm，胆囊颈部可见一大小约0.4cm结石。术中快速冰冻回报提示腺癌，向家属交代病情后行胆囊切除术姑息治疗。病理检查：冰冻及常规病理：胆囊切除标本：胆囊一具，大小8cm × 4cm × 3.3cm，送检前已剖开，浆膜面灰红光滑，黏膜面见一隆起型肿物，大小3cm × 2.5cm × 2cm，切面灰白灰红，质中，肉眼观侵及全层，胆囊壁厚0.1~0.3cm。冰冻病理诊断：胆囊切除标本：胆囊腺癌，侵及囊壁全层，分类待常规多块取材。常规病理诊断：胆囊切除标本：低分化癌伴坏死，侵及囊壁全层，待做免疫组化检测进一步确诊。免疫组化检测：阳性：CA19-9，CK19，CK7，CK（L），CK（H），CK5/6，P40，P63，CEA（散在+），MUC-5（散在+），Ki-67（+，约70%）；阴性：CK20，Villin，CDX2，MUC-2。免疫组化诊断：胆囊切除标本：结合免疫组化检测结果，诊断为腺鳞癌伴坏死，侵及胆囊壁全层（图15-2-1）。

第三章　胆系肿块

第一节　肝门部肿瘤 MRI 误诊分析

详见本书 本卷 第十六篇 第十二章 第一节　肝　　门部肿瘤 MRI 误诊分析。

第二节　误诊病例简介:胆系横纹肌肉瘤与胆总管囊肿合并感染

横纹肌肉瘤多发生于头颈、泌尿生殖系统及腹膜后、四肢,发生于胆系极为罕见,约占儿童横纹肌肉瘤的 0. 8%,且恶性程度高, 5 年内死亡率接近 80%。胆系的横纹肌肉瘤以胚胎性多见,大多发生于 1~6 岁的儿童,男性较女性多;发生部位多位于胆总管,当肿瘤生长在黏膜下时常形成葡萄串样息肉,因此也称为葡萄状肉瘤。临床表现多为梗阻性黄疸、消瘦、腹痛、发热及肝大,容易误诊为"黄疸型肝炎"延误治疗。

影像学检查可以提供重要的依据。腹部 B 超典型表现为扩张的胆总管内混杂回声团块,团块周围完全或不完全环形液性暗区且不伴声影。CT 表现为扩张的胆总管内囊实性或密度不均匀肿块,轮廓一般不清楚。肿块密度较低是由于其内富含疏松黏液基质,其中更低密度区域可能与葡萄状肿物间胆汁积聚有关,增强扫描肿块实性成分轻度强化。

典型病理表现为疏松黏液背景中可见星芒状细胞,细胞胞质少,胞浆极其丰富,因此 MRI 图像上与胆汁信号类似,然而仔细观察亦可发现信号不均匀,提示实性组织存在。

一例 CT 增强图像上表现出胆总管内部蜂窝状强化肿块,误诊为胆总管囊肿合并感染。

本病亦需与下列疾病进行鉴别:胆系蛔虫:胆总管扩张,亦可见其内条形肿块,但肿块无血供,增强没有强化。肝吸虫:肝吸虫多表现为胆管轻度扩张,胆壁增厚。若虫卵聚集形成肿块阻塞胆管时,类似胆管肿瘤表现;但增强没有强化。慢性胆系感染:多有胆系手术病史,胆管壁纤维化改变。

第四章 胆系炎症

胆系新型隐球菌感染

隐球菌病是新型隐球菌所引起的亚急性或慢性深部真菌病,正常人出现隐球菌感染较少,胆系的隐球菌病罕见。本病通常发生于获得性免疫缺陷综合征、恶性肿瘤、白血病、淋巴瘤等患者,但是也有一半以上病人并无基础疾病。其预后主要与患者的免疫状况、菌种的毒力及接种物的功能相关。

1. 临床表现　该病主要侵犯中枢神经系统和肺,但亦可侵犯骨髓、皮肤、黏膜和其他脏器。隐球菌病发生于肝胆系统少见。在免疫功能正常或相对正常的患者中,隐球菌感染常较局限。一些病变主要局限于胆总管和胆囊内,肝内未见明显感染灶。

2. 影像学研究　本病以胆系梗阻扩张、胆管内异常增生物为主要表现。分析影像学资料特征,病灶局限在胆系内增生,在胆系内散在分布,无管壁及周围组织破坏。

影像检查主要见肝内胆管不规则扩张,胆囊颈部囊壁及肝外胆管管壁增厚。CT 平扫可见肝外胆管管壁全长增厚(超声见为 4.1mm,手术时见最厚处约 10mm),呈环形低密度影,增强后有强化,且 MRI 显示增厚的胆管壁于 T_2WI 呈低信号,此表现较具有特异性,可能为胆系隐球菌感染较为特征的影像诊断表现。

3. 鉴别诊断　需要鉴别者包括原发性硬化性胆管炎和恶性肿瘤引起的梗阻性胆管病变。

(1)硬化性胆管炎:硬化性胆管炎临床发病年龄偏大,以梗阻性黄疸为主,糖皮质激素治疗有效,其 X 线特征主要为肝内胆管串珠样改变及肝外胆管不规则憩室样突出。该例却以肝内胆管由周围扩张至肝门逐渐变细,肝外胆管较长范围管壁增厚为主要表现。

(2)胆管癌或胆管邻近的恶性病变:胆管癌或胆管邻近的恶性病变侵犯胆管常表现为进行性黄疸,胆管扩张较明显,胆管病变较局限,胆管常为不规则增厚,与该例胆管呈均匀增厚、T_2WI 呈低信号改变且范围广泛有一定区别。

本病最终确诊尚需要依靠病理检查或胆汁的真菌培养及墨汁染色。

鉴别诊断可以考虑恶性肿瘤、阴性结石等,但是这些疾病在儿童比较罕见,蛔虫、先天性胆管扩张继发慢性炎性增生以及硬化性胆管炎可以导致类似改变,采用经皮肝穿刺活检并引流术对本病的检出和治疗有重要的临床意义。

结合 Kim 等(1994)的病例报道,本病的另一个特征为淋巴结的侵犯。由于感染新型隐球菌存在免疫低下或者缺陷的基础,或者感染时隐球菌多糖可以抑制人体吞噬细胞,因此在肺部的感染以及该例胆系感染中,其引流区域的淋巴结是一典型的特征性改变,可以为以后的鉴别诊断提供依据和参考。

第五章　胆系其他疾病

第一节　活体供肝者肝血管与胆管发育变异之间的关系

详见本书 本卷 第十四篇 第一章 第二节 活体供肝者肝血管与胆管发育变异之间的关系。

第二节　胆肠 Roux-Y 吻合术后空肠桥袢结石

胆肠 Roux-Y 吻合术后空肠桥袢结石少见，国内外文献少见影像专题报道，本病原因特殊，临床表现无特异性，易误诊。单凭临床表现对其诊断有一定难度，临床与影像结合分析，尤其是综合影像学检查能明确诊断。

一、胆肠 Roux-Y 吻合术后肠腔结石的形成机制及临床特点

胆肠 Roux-Y 吻合术是将距屈氏韧带约 15~20 cm 空肠切断，近端留作吻合，远侧空肠桥袢经结肠后及胃幽门后方上提至肝门部与已分离之胆管作吻合，根据胆管直径大小作胆管与空肠侧侧或端侧吻合，此段肠管又称输胆肠袢。于胆肠吻合口下方约 40~60 cm 空肠桥袢对系膜缘半周切开与近端空肠作端侧吻合，恢复消化道连续性。该手术适用于肝内外胆管结石、胆管狭窄畸形及不能切除的胆管肿瘤等，最常适用于肝内外胆管结石。一组病例均为胆管结石施行胆肠 Roux-Y 吻合术者。

术后输胆空肠结石形成原因主要有以下三个方面：

胆管空肠 Roux-Y 吻合术后消化道正常解剖关系发生改变而导致输胆空肠袢存在动力障碍，另外，胆肠 Roux-Y 吻合术后空肠内非结合胆酸及细菌含量增多高于其他胆系手术。上述两种因素均为输胆肠袢结石的形成、积聚及排出障碍创造了条件。

原发病灶如胆管结石及胆管狭窄在行胆管空肠 Roux-Y 吻合术时未能彻底清除和矫正，而致术后结石经胆肠吻合口排至空肠后瘀滞、增大。该组有 1 例发现合并肝胆管结石，原发性胆管结石经胆肠吻合口不断排出是形成胆肠吻合术后输胆肠袢结石的重要原因。

远端空肠穿横结肠系膜孔周围粘连狭窄、肠肠吻合口狭窄、输胆肠袢过长等均影响胆汁引流、形成结石并积聚。该组有 2 例肠肠吻合口狭窄，2 例为远端空肠穿横结肠系膜孔周围粘连狭窄。

胆肠 Roux-Y 吻合术后空肠肠袢结石病例较为少见，临床表现无特异性。该组 5 例术前均曾到多家医院就诊，误诊为胆管结石及再生胆囊结石、右上腹肿块等。临床表现主要有右上腹疼痛不适、畏寒发热、腹部包块、不全性肠梗阻等。

该组中主要表现为反复发作的右上腹痛，伴寒颤、高热，皮肤巩膜轻度黄染，右上腹可扪及坚硬肿块，虽有 1 例出现恶心、呕吐，但无肛门停止排便排气，考虑为肠道反射性改变，并非肠梗阻。

胆管空肠 Roux-Y 吻合术后空肠肠袢结石的治疗原则为再次手术，手术原则同一般胆石症手术，即取尽结石，解除狭窄，通畅引流。该组手术为肠袢切开取石，狭窄松解及肠袢内置管引流，1 例合并胆管结石者加以胆道镜胆管取石。

二、影像学研究

胆肠 Roux-Y 吻合术后空肠肠袢结石具有较为

典型的CT表现:肠腔结石;肠管扩张及肠梗阻征象;胆管内出现气体及结石。

肠腔结石一般位于胆肠吻合口与肠肠吻合口之间,呈圆形,通常较大,该组中结石最大径6 cm,结石密度以高密度为主,多分层呈"树轮"状改变,"树轮"状现象可能与病程较长、结石成分逐步沉积有关,该组5例中有4例结石呈"树轮"状改变。

如果肠腔结石距离胆肠吻合口较近,在横断面CT上需与胆囊结石或再生胆囊内结石鉴别,仔细询问原手术病史是否胆囊已切除、观察结石周围腔壁结构有无空肠黏膜皱襞、结合结石形态与密度("树轮"状)以及多平面重建技术进一步显示胆肠吻合口及胆肠关系可帮助鉴别。如果肠腔结石距离胆肠吻合口较远,而靠近肠肠吻合口,这样结石距离肠腔盲端较远,胆囊或再生胆囊都不可能太长,则无需鉴别。如果结石位于肠肠吻合口远侧,很容易引起肠梗阻,与一般胆石性肠梗阻表现相似且结石多位于远端回肠口,结石也相对较小。

该组中5例结石均位于肠肠吻合口近侧。虽然结石较大,肠腔结石区域及以上肠管扩张,但该组病例肠梗阻征象均不明显,究其原因与该组结石均位于肠肠吻合口近侧,而食物并不行经吻合口近侧,故消化道梗阻征象不明显。胆管内出现气体与结石并非胆肠Roux-Y吻合术后空肠肠袢结石的特有征象,但该征象会引导临床追问手术史及思考方向,从而得出正确结论。

早期MRI对肠道病变临床应用较少,随着MRI快速成像技术的出现和临床应用,现用于肠道疾病的诊断已逐渐增多,尤其是同时存在胆系与肠道病变的情况下,MRCP检查有着更为广泛的应用。

该组2例MRI对肠腔结石本身的显示虽不及CT直观,但MRCP更能立体地显示胆管树与肠管的关系,且显示胆肠吻合的肠管盲端也更清楚,这样对确认结石位于肠腔而非胆囊或再生胆囊较CT有优势。

MRI对胆管积气的显示不及CT,该组1例胆管内既有结石又有积气者误认为均是结石。

总之,胆肠Roux-Y吻合术后空肠肠袢结石CT与MRI检查均能明确诊断,对肠腔结石的显示和定位CT与MRI各有优势。密切结合临床,综合运用影像学检查,可提高本病术前诊断的正确率,为协助临床制定治疗方案提供重要线索。

第三节　门静脉性胆病

详见本书 本卷 第二十八篇 第四章 第二节 门静脉性胆病。

第六章 磁共振胆胰管成像(MRCP)

第一节 磁共振胆胰管成像误诊

目前,磁共振胆胰管成像(MRCP)已成为常规胆系成像方法中的组成部分。MRCP类似于常规胆管造影术,如静脉内、经皮或经内镜逆行胆管造影,但也存在误诊。因此,对选定的病人应采用特殊的诊断标准。为提高诊断正确率,减少假阳性和假阴性,需认识某些发育变异和误区。

1. 技术性误区

成像角度:成像角度不当可造成部分总胆管成像失败,不能显示胆管结石或狭窄,胆胰管成像不全者可将垂直起源的胰管误认为肝外胆管。

静态影像:胆管括约肌收缩呈现总胆管下段突然变细,似结石或肿瘤表现,但括约肌松弛后的成像或给予解痉药能消除这种误区。

进动后技术:虽然最大信号强度投影有助于显示胰胆管3D成像中的复杂性狭窄,但是过度表现狭窄,使胆系结石的充盈缺损藏匿而产生误区。

2. 认识上的误区

与病变相似的正常结构:MRCP的某些表现可将正常结构或伴随伪影误认为病变,如充满液体的十二指肠球部含有食物碎块极易误认为含有结石的胆囊。同样,因为胆管与胃、胰的毗邻关系,所以胃黏膜间的潴留液体在MRCP上易误认为异位的、不规则的胰管而诊断为慢性胰腺炎。但通过观察正常腹部冠状面的图像可避免这些误诊。有作者指出,经稀释的MRI对比剂Gd-DTPA可作为一种安全而有效的口服阴性对比剂,从而消除胃肠道液体的干扰,提高图像质量。

发育变异:胆系的发育变异与胚胎期发育异常密切相关,包括肝内和肝外胆管扩张以及胆总管和胆囊管异常。有作者将前者分为不同的亚型,包括胆总管憩室和肝内胆管囊状扩张即卡洛里病。MRCP可诊断卡洛里病,在原始图像和最大信号强度投影重建图像上表现为肝内多发的囊状扩张结构,并互相交通。这种起源于胆管的囊肿由此可与其他病变如多发的单纯肝囊肿和肝脓肿鉴别。

临床上特别感兴趣的其他发育变异为副胆管以及胆囊管的异常汇合,尤其是腹腔镜技术应用后更是如此。约18%的病人有异常副胆管,多见于右侧胆管系统。引流第7肝段或第8肝段胆汁的异常胆管,汇入胆总管或胆囊管的变异对手术十分重要,在腹腔镜的操作中,它很容易因疏忽而被切断。

胆囊管与胆总管汇合部的位置变异很大,最常见的汇合部位为胆总管中1/3外侧壁,此外还有低位汇合和高位汇合。低位汇合时,胆囊管较长,行走在胆总管内侧,并与之平行,类似于扩张的胆总管。应分析原始图像或斜位最大信号强度投影重建图像,以避免误诊。

总胆管扭曲和胆囊管重叠:扭曲的胆管可产生梗阻征象或正常变异表现,过度扭曲的胆管壁重叠部分影像,极似胆管内结石的充盈缺损,过多的胆管皱襞在高信号的胆汁中表现为低信号区。改变成像采集角度或轴位成像,可区别胆管扭曲与结石。

胆囊管重叠于总胆管上段的正位像,似胆管内结石的充盈缺损样表现,是MRCP的不同角度成像造成胆囊管内的高信号胆汁与总胆管之间的间隙,产生总胆管内的充盈缺损表现。如果胆囊管重叠发生在总胆管下段,这种发育变异极易被误认为总胆管下段结石,再次不同角度成像可显示缺损表现的真正原因。

总肝管的血管压迹:MRCP图像上的血管压迹可类似总肝管上段的结石或狭窄,是MRCP成像角度平行于肝动脉前后层面显示的缺损表现。这种血管压迹主要为右肝动脉通过总肝管所引起(约占21%)。MRA 有助于显示和判断该部位通过的血管影。

胆系手术折襞形成的缺损:即胆管吻合术发生的胆管折襞, MRCP 图像上可谬误地提示为结石或肿瘤的征象。MRCP 不能判断术后形成的缺损、结石或肿瘤的区别,但采用不同体位——仰卧位、俯卧位可见这种缺损是固定不变的,从而有助于支持胆系折襞缺损的诊断。

十二指肠降段乳头旁憩室的影响:充满液体的十二指肠降段乳头旁憩室可误认为胆囊或憩室内积气重叠于总胆管,易误认为总胆管结石的信号缺失,改变成像角度可予区别。

胃肠道内液体的干扰:一些作者指出,经稀释的 Gd-DTPA 可作为一种安全而有效的口服阴性对比剂,从而消除胃肠道液体的干扰,提高图像质量。另外,应用以 FerriSeltz 和 ferricannonium 为主要成分的对比剂及单次激发快速翻转序列(SSFIR)也可充分消除胃肠道伪影。

十二指肠憩室的影响:充满液体的十二指肠憩室可误认为胆囊,憩室内积气与肝外胆管重叠,易误认为肝外胆管结石的信号缺失,改变成像角度可予区别。

邻近血管搏动造成的压迹伪影:有作者指出,由于毗邻的肝动脉及胃十二指肠动脉的搏动可对左右肝管、肝总管及胆总管产生压迹,形成假性狭窄。结合源像、横断面的 T_2WI 的流空效应及 MRA 可明确诊断。

MRCP 上的血管压迹可似总肝管上段的结石或狭窄,是 MRCP 成像角度平行于肝动脉前后层面显示的缺损表现。这种血管压迹主要为右肝动脉通过总肝管所引起(约占 21%)。由于毗邻的肝动脉及胃十二指肠动脉的搏动可对左右肝管、肝外胆管产生压迹,可形成假性狭窄。结合源图像、横断面的 T_2WI 的流空效应及 MRA 可明确诊断。

主胰管的假性狭窄:禁食的病人胰液分泌减少,正常的胰管会出现阶段性的萎陷,而被误认为狭窄。利用促胰液分泌素促进胰液分泌,有助于鉴别。

总胆管扭曲:扭曲的胆管可产生阻塞征象或发育变异表现,过长扭曲的胆管壁重叠部分影像极似胆管内结石的充盈缺损,过多的胆管皱襞在高信号的胆汁中表现为低信号区。改变成像采集角度或横断面成像,可区别胆管扭曲与结石。

胆囊管重叠:胆囊管重叠于肝外胆管上段的正位像,似胆管内结石的充盈缺损样表现,是 MRCP 的不同角度成像造成胆囊管内的高信号胆汁与肝外胆管之间的间隙,产生肝外胆管内的充盈缺损表现。如果胆囊管重叠发生在肝外胆管下段,这种发育变异极易误认为肝外胆管下段结石,再次不同角度成像可显示缺损表现的原因。

3. 胆系 MRI 检查的诊断陷阱和伪影

(1)胆囊切除术后银夹:胆囊切除术留置的银夹与胆管靠得很近时,有时可类似于胆管结石。利用包括横断面成像在内的两个平面的 MR 胆系成像技术,可鉴别银夹与结石。多数情况下,横断面成像可显示银夹的无信号区位于胆管外,并可见来自于银夹的磁敏感性伪影。

(2)MRI 动态增强: MRI 动态增强扫描是诊断肝脏疾病的重要检查方法,但可能出现以下几种误诊:肝叶、段、亚段及包膜下过度灌注异常;早期强化的假性病变,尤其易发生在肝左叶内侧段;全肝的不均匀过度灌注异常;由血管伪影、不增强的肝血管、部分容积伪影、磁敏感性伪影和肝硬化再生结节等所致的低信号假病变。

(3)在动态 MRI 增强动脉期,这些异常表现有时类似于真正的病变或类似于肿瘤向周围肝实质的侵犯。然而,多数情况下,在其他序列或延迟期 MRI 增强时没有相应的异常改变,而且,过度灌注异常的特定部位有助于同真正的肿瘤鉴别。

肝胆成像中常见的 MRI 伪影:一般而言, MRI 伪影不是来自于被检体真正的解剖结构。

在肝脏的成像过程中,不仅显示了基本的解剖结构,同时还会显示某个部位实际上并不存在的假性信号。根据不同的来源伪影可分为三类:来自于扫描过程中病人有关的运动,包括血液的流动和由呼吸或胃肠蠕动引起的肝脏运动所产生的伪影;与扫描时间无关,而与特殊的扫描技术或特殊的扫描参数有关的伪影,包括化学位移伪影,相消伪影、磁敏感性伪影、折叠伪影及截断伪影;与系统相关的伪影,指在数据采集过程中由于一个或多个扫描仪部件出现故障或错误校准所引起的伪影,包括磁场的紊乱、系统不稳定性或错误校准、尖峰信号和噪声。总之,伪影与正常肝脏易于或不易于分辨,主要取决于伪影能否再现。讨论伪影的目的是认识肝脏 MRI 中常见的伪影,以采取措施减少或消除对最终图像的负面影响。

第二节　胆汁流动伪影的 MRCP

MRCP 在临床上应用越来越多，但是，作为天然对比剂的胆汁并不是静止的，而是间歇地缓慢流动的，可在 MRCP 图像上产生流动伪影。

MR 成像时，心脏血管搏动和血液、脑脊液、胆汁流动，以及胃肠蠕动等均会产生运动伪影。伪影严重者，会影响诊断，甚至导致误诊。Sugita 等（2003）制作模型模拟胆汁在正常和病理状态下在胆管中的流动状态，进行 MRCP 检查，认为肝外胆管在正常管径范围时，胆汁流动在 MRCP 图像上不产生流动伪影。

一项研究结果显示，肝外胆管直径≤ 4 mm 时，无胆汁流动伪影，但 4mm<φ ≤ 8mm 时可以有胆汁流动伪影，主要表现为单线征，少数为二线征。一些作者报道，在肝外胆管轻度扩张组中未见胆汁流动伪影。研究结果显示，肝外胆管轻度扩张组中，胆汁流动伪影多数表现为三线征，少数表现为多线征、单线征或无胆汁流动伪影。在中度扩张组中，多数表现为多线征，少数表现为三线征或无伪影。在重度胆管扩张组中，部分表现为多线征，部分表现为无伪影。

该研究结果显示，肝外胆管扩张组胆汁流动伪影发生率高于肝外胆管正常组，差异有统计学意义，与文献报道结果一致。同时该组还发现胆汁流动伪影的表现形式与肝外胆管直径有相关性。该研究中胆汁流动伪影的检出率较高，考虑与将 PACS 工作站上的原始薄层图像作为研究对象有关。

原始图像没有容积效应影响，同时在 PACS 上能够调节窗宽、窗位，因此，比阅读胶片更容易观察到伪影。该研究中，最大信号强度投影像上大部分流动伪影表现为条形低信号，与文献报道中 MRCP 上胆汁流动伪影为线状低信号相似，部分能分辨出单线征、三线征或多线征。该组认为，胆汁流动伪影的产生及不同表现，主要由流动胆汁的失相位及胆汁分层状流动引起。无胆汁流动伪影的患者，考虑为检查时胆汁处于静止状态，或流动伪影较轻微，肉眼不能分辨。

识别胆汁流动伪影的重要意义在于避免误诊。一些作者报道 9 例胆系蛔虫症在 MRCP 上表现为胆管内条状异常信号，在高信号的胆汁内可见 3 条平行的异常信号影，中间为条状高信号，两边为平行的低信号，呈三线征，且低信号线影间距离较一致，宽 3~6 mm，长 18~30 mm。该组曾根据这一表现特点拟诊 12 例胆系蛔虫，但是经手术肝外胆管切开或 ERCP 造影均未见蛔虫或蛔虫残体，临床上患者也无胆系蛔虫的钻顶样疼痛病史。由于这些误诊病例，该组开始对 MRCP 上胆汁流动伪影进行研究。

该组所示二线征与一些作者关于胆系蛔虫 MRCP 表现的描述一致。因此，一些作者将三线征作为 MRCP 诊断胆系蛔虫的可靠依据，该组认为不妥当，同时也对他们的诊断提出质疑。尽管胆系蛔虫已经少见，但偶有发生。

文献报道胆系蛔虫在 MRCP 上表现为高信号胆汁内长条形或长管状低信号，走行与胆管壁平行，当蛔虫自身的消化道因含有液体显影时，表现为在管状低信号中央出现细线样高信号，当扫描层面与虫体垂直时，表现为管腔内点状或圆环状低信号。

胆系蛔虫的 MRCP 表现，与表现为单线征或二线征的胆汁流动伪影相似，因此需要鉴别。胆汁流动伪影位于管腔中央，不同扫描序列或扫描时相，伪影可以消失，胆系蛔虫可位于管腔任何地方、在各个扫描序列上都能显示。文献报道的 4 例胆系蛔虫中 3 例偏于管腔一侧，1 例位于中央。1 例蛔虫卷曲，轴面 T_2WI 表现为并列环形断面，称眼镜征，而胆汁流动伪影在横断面上为单环状。

在轴面 T_2WI 上胆汁流动伪影表现为管腔中央点状低信号，还需要与管腔内小结石鉴别，轴面图像上胆管结石多位于靠近管腔下壁一侧，在冠状面 MRCP 上结石多表现为小结节状，伪影表现为细线状，位于管腔中央。有时肝外胆管内放置内引流管，表现为管状低信号，与流动伪影相似，但内置引流管的低信号更锐利、僵直，有明确病史。

该组主要探讨了 MRCP 原始薄层图像上胆汁流动伪影的表现规律，因为随着越来越多的医院应用 PACS 进行影像诊断，影像医师发现胆汁流动伪影的机会也随之增多，尤其是表现为单线征和三线征的伪影，特别提醒影像医师注意不要误诊为胆系蛔虫或结石。

第三节 磁共振胆胰管成像的误诊

目前,磁共振胆胰管成像(MRCP)已成为常规胆系成像方法中的组成部分。MRCP类似于常规胆管造影术,如静脉内、经皮或经内镜逆行胆管造影,但也存在误诊。因此,对选定的病人应采用特殊的诊断标准。为提高诊断正确率,减少假阳性和假阴性,需认识某些发育变异和误区。根据不同的临床情况,MRCP诊断中常见的误诊可分为三种:肝外胆管结石的误诊;胆管狭窄的误诊;十二指肠壁内段病变的误诊。

肝外胆管结石诊断中的误诊:MRCP诊断肝外胆管结石相对比较容易,与常规胆管造影的诊断标准一样,结石表现为卵圆形低信号区,周围由高信号胆汁环绕。MRCP诊断结石的准确性主要取决于对常见误诊原因的认识。最常见的误诊原因有四:最大信号强度投影重建图像未显示结石;肝外胆管内多发结石呈弥漫性低信号,类似于胆管狭窄;胆管内气体引起的敏感性伪影;酷似小结石的气泡。

小结石:与最大信号强度投影相关的伪影,并不影响诊断直径大于10mm的大结石,即使在最大信号强度投影重建图像上,也很容易分辨出充盈缺损及其周围环绕的高信号胆汁。但对小结石,有必要分析原始图像。

在最大信号强度投影图像上包围结石的高信号胆汁可掩盖小结石,出现与内窥镜逆行胆管造影相类似的误诊,后者由于肝外胆管过度充盈对比剂可掩盖小结石。在一组51例肝外胆管结石病人研究中,56.8%的结石在最大信号强度投影图像上显示,结石的显示主要依赖于结石大小,但即使比较大的结石(范围在5~10mm)在最大信号强度投影图像上也会漏诊(占54.2%)。因此,对所有的病例都应该同时观察最大信号强度投影图像和原始图像。

多发结石:多发结石完全充填肝外胆管时可出现误诊。由于在多发嵌顿的结石之间有很少量胆汁,结石表现为极不均匀低信号,同时伴近端胆管显著扩张,MRCP看起来像近端胆管双向狭窄,而原始图像可作出正确诊断。

胆管结石的伪影:冠状位上胆管内气体的充盈缺损会被误认为结石,联合横断面MRCP,可见气泡漂浮在胆汁的上方,形成气液平。有时在胆管的中心部位发现一个独立的圆形充盈缺损,可能为胆管的流空,时间飞越法MRI可发现流空的胆管呈高信号。

胆管积气:胆管内常出现气体即胆管积气,尤其常见于有胆系手术史者,如胆肠吻合术、括约肌切开术后。胆管气体可引起敏感性伪影,利用某一扫描序列可将伪影降低到最低限度,如这种伪影在快速自旋回波序列中是稳定的。极少情况下,过量的气体在肝外胆管内可形成完全不均匀信号,降低了MRCP的诊断价值。

在MRCP高信号胆汁中的气泡呈现低信号的充盈缺损,酷似结石,常出现在置胆管支架术,胆管空肠吻合术和ERCP胆管下端括约肌切开取石后不久的MRCP检查者,了解病史有助于鉴别诊断。胆管内血块、肿瘤亦可显示为低信号。冠状位上胆管内气体的充盈缺损会被误认为结石,结合横断面MRCP,可见气泡漂浮在胆汁的上方,形成气液平。有时在胆管的中心部位发现一个独立的圆形充盈缺损,可能为胆管的流空现象。

气泡:括约肌切开术后病人胆管内常见气泡。与常规胆管造影的情况一样,在MRCP图像上气泡和结石表现相同,需与小结石鉴别。鉴别小结石与气泡的有效方法是选择一个与肝外胆管长轴垂直的平面(通常为倾斜轴位平面)进行MRCP成像。这一额外成像可通过三维序列扫描重建横轴位平面的容积数据获得,也可通过二维成像获得,后者可获得另一组图像。横轴位平面显示肝外胆管结石位于肝外胆管的下垂部位,而气泡则位于其非下垂部位。

胆管狭窄的误诊:诊断胆管狭窄的同时,可能出现胆管狭窄性质和程度的误诊。伪影是由于MRI图像的矩阵较常规MRI图像小或与最大信号强度投影重建有关。仅仅利用MRCP成像来显示狭窄的形态特征不足以做出正确诊断。事实上,矩阵的减少限制了细微结构(如黏膜不规则性)的显示;不注射对比剂,一方面反映了生理状态下的狭窄,另一方面限制了其他特征(如胆管扩张性等)的显示。MRCP是完整腹部成像的一部分,将MRCP和常规成像联合使用,有助于显示狭窄的特征和性质。

另一误诊是狭窄的程度,最大信号强度投影重建图像常过度估计胆管狭窄。在最大信号强度投影图像上，重度狭窄处的少量胆汁不能显示，表现为完全性梗阻的假象。分析原始图像可减少误诊，因为即使很少量的胆汁也能在原始图像上显示；分析继发征象比如狭窄上方胆管扩张程度，也可减少误诊。诊断胆管狭窄的其他问题是不能显示远端萎陷的肝外胆管，无法确定肝外胆管狭窄的长度。

肝右动脉横过肝外胆管可造成肝外胆管假性狭窄。正常解剖中，肝右动脉行走在近端肝外胆管的后方，对肝外胆管可产生一种外压性改变，某些情况下，这种外压性改变可类似于一种轻度狭窄。除了同时分析原始图像和轴面 T_2WI 外，典型的部位也有助于鉴别真性和假性狭窄。嵌顿于肝段胆管的小结石，周围有极少量的胆汁包围，引起肝段胆管扩张，也可表现为肝内胆管假性狭窄。

十二指肠壁内段的误诊：胆胰连接区的肿瘤、结石及括约肌的收缩或痉挛之间常易混淆。有文献指出，口服脂肪餐及静脉注射促胰液分泌素后，用 RARE 序列单厚层采集，获得一系列括约肌部位的 MRCP 影像，再加上经此部位的横断面扫描，可有效鉴别连接区的病变。另外，使用低张药物也有助于连接区的显示。

肝外胆管远端解剖结构细小，含胆汁量少，产生的信号弱，MRCP 显示十二指肠壁内段十分困难。为提高该区域的显示，一种有效的方法是检查前饮水，以充盈和扩张十二指肠，这样乳头部炎症所致的小突起能被很好地显示出来。分析常规 T_1WI 有助于排除十二指肠壁内段和十二指肠壁内段周围肿块性病变。然而，鉴别十二指肠壁内段小肿瘤与炎症所致的乳头部狭窄在所有的病例中都较难做到。

其他误诊与嵌顿于乳头内的小结石有关（若结石周围无液体包围，则显示结石比较困难），也与肝外胆管远端不典型的形态结构有关，它可类似于嵌顿的结石。对于这两种情况，有必要结合原始图像的分析，这样，就可以明显地提高诊断的正确率。

胆胰共同管假结石征象：当胆管下端括约肌收缩时，MRCP 呈现似嵌入在总胆管下端的充盈缺损，易与结石相混淆，然而这种缺损影与结石的不同之处是只有上缘的高信号胆汁，且这种表现是暂时的，括约肌松弛时该影则会消逝。

有作者指出，口服脂肪餐及静脉注射促胰液分泌素后，获得一系列括约肌部位的 MRCP 影像，再加上经此部位的横断面扫描，可有效鉴别胆胰连接区的病变。另外，使用低张药物也有助于胆胰连接区的显示。

第七章 胆系MRI

第一节 肝胆成像中常见的MRI伪影

一般而言，MRI伪影不是来自于被检体真正的解剖结构。在肝脏的成像过程中,不仅显示了基本的解剖结构,同时还会显示某个部位实际上并不存在的假性信号。根据不同的来源伪影可分为三类:第一类伪影来自于扫描过程中病人有关的运动,包括血液的流动和由呼吸或胃肠蠕动引起的肝脏运动所产生的伪影;第二类伪影与扫描时间无关,而与特殊的扫描技术或特殊的扫描参数有关,包括化学位移伪影、相消伪影、磁敏感性伪影、折叠伪影及截断伪影;第三类是与系统相关的伪影,指在数据采集过程中由于一个或多个扫描仪部件出现故障或错误校准所引起的伪影,包括磁场的紊乱、系统不稳定性或错误校准、尖峰信号和噪声。总之,伪影与正常肝脏易于或不易于分辨,主要取决于伪影能不能再现。此处介绍伪影的目的是认识肝脏MRI中常见的伪影,以采取措施减少或消除对最终图像的负面影响。

第二节 MRI动态增强误诊

MRI动态增强扫描是诊断肝脏病变的重要检查方法,但可能出现以下几种误诊:肝叶、段、亚段及包膜下过度灌注异常;早期强化的假性病变,尤其易发生在肝左叶内侧段;全肝的不均匀过度灌注异常;由血管伪影、不增强的肝血管、部分容积伪影、磁敏感性伪影和肝硬化再生结节等所致的低信号假病变。

在动态MRI增强动脉期,这些异常表现有时类似于真正的病变或类似于肿瘤向周围肝实质的侵犯。然而,多数情况下,在其他序列或延迟期MRI增强时没有相应的异常改变,而且,过度灌注异常的特定部位有助于同真正的肿瘤鉴别。

第八章　胆系其他影像学检查技术

第一节　MRCP 与 ERCP 的比较

MRCP 可无创地显示生理状态下的正常胆管、胰管及其发育变异;可同时观察胆管与胰管周围组织结构的情况;全面准确地显示胆管、胰管与胆胰管十二指肠连接区及其周围的病理情况;为胆、胰疾病术前方案制订及术后评价疗效提供确切的依据;能准确判断胆管、胰管的梗阻部位,同时显示梗阻上游与下游的情况;结合梗阻端形态及原始图像对梗阻的性质做出推断;上消化道手术及改建后,或食管、十二指肠严重狭窄时难以插管,只能用 MRCP 检查。

在以前, MRCP 是 ERCP 检查失败或不能行 ERCP 检查者的最佳替代方法,而在当前,应用新技术所获得的 MRCP 图像是三维实时立体的,不仅完全可与 ERCP 相媲美,并在获得诊断信息方面远远超过 ERCP,基本已取代 ERCP,一般来说,临床医生已习惯地将 MRCP 作为观察胆、胰系统的首选方法,只在需要乳头活检和进行内镜治疗时才做 ERCP。

以往在诊断肝癌侵犯胆管、肝门胆管癌、胆胰共同管及其周围肿瘤、胰腺癌等疾病时,由于 ERCP 只能观察胆、胰管,难以了解管外的组织的情况,如不与 CT、超声及 MRI 结合分析,难免误诊。而目前, MRCP 不仅观察胆、胰管内情况,同时观察管外组织的变化,分析研究相当方便,深受临床医生的欢迎。

一、MRCP 与 ERCP 的对比

MRCP 是一种非介入性胆胰管成像技术,它不需要对比剂即能较好地全貌反映胆胰系统解剖关系和病理变化,诊断及分析原则基本与 ERCP 相同,还能结合 MRI 影像资料,较 ERCP 提供更多有价值的诊断参考信息。

相对于 ERCP 而言,MRCP 具有以下优势:胆管梗阻远、近端均可显示。对于胰腺有无病变显示清晰,并可显示胰管扩张情况;结合 MRI,易于全面观察肝门区梗阻及范围,有文献报道,对于高位梗阻、高度狭窄或由于外科手术造成的消化道狭窄等会影响 ERCP 检查的成功率,而 MRCP 不受这些限制。MRCP 在评价肿瘤侵犯范围、远处转移及手术可切除性等方面亦明显优于 ERCP;检查时间短,成功率、显影率高;无 ERCP 的并发症,如胆管感染、胰腺炎等。

尽管 MRCP、ERCP 各有所长,但就疾病定性方面,不存在显著性差异。MRCP 的局限性在于不具备介入治疗作用,并且对大量腹水和某些体内有金属内置物(如胆管支架、心脏起搏器、血管支架)的患者无法进行正常检查。

有作者指出 MRCP 对胆胰管十二指肠连接区的结构显示欠满意,但是,大多数学者认为,如果在 MRCP 检查时,有目的地对连接区进行扫描和观察,此问题则不复存在。在 MRCP,胆管狭窄长度往往因十二指肠降段不显影而难以准确判断。

ERCP 的优点则是对胆总管末端的观察不受近端结石或肿瘤造成梗阻的影响,并能直观显示十二指肠降部和乳头形态并取活检病理检查,在造影的同时可进行引流、乳头切开取石和放置胆管内支架等治疗。

第二节 术中胆系造影

术中胆系造影的必要性:一些作者指出,在条件许可时,对每例胆囊切除术的病人,均应进行术中胆系造影。因为,单凭临床症状来决定是否进行肝外胆管切开探查是不够确切的。经验告诉我们,术中胆系造影证实有胆系结石,而并无临床症状者并不在少数。因胆系结石而进行第二次手术者,有 95% 是在第一次手术时因未做术中胆系造影所致。术中胆系造影可以协助外科医生正确地了解结石是否已完全取出。术中胆系造影还可以了解非结石所致的肝外胆管梗阻,狭窄等其他原因。

一、术中胆系造影的质量控制

机器设备:将机器分擦拭干净,当手术室进行空气消毒时将机器一同消毒,并用一无菌巾将 X 线管包裹,避免照片时污染手术野。

放置胶片:首先,应定好位。一般胶片上缘包括横膈,即第 10 胸椎或剑突平面,下缘应包括髂嵴;但对肥胖或消瘦病人则有一定的差异:肥胖病人因横膈高于一般病人约一个肋间隙,因而胶片上缘应相应上移 5cm,对消瘦病人则相反;其次,在病人麻醉后,皮肤消毒前,将暗盒竖放于病人肝胆区背部手术台面床单下一特制的木盒内(或专用术中造影 X 线机的片盒内)。这样,即可不必术中搬动病人,照片与取片也较为方便。

病人体位:患者仰卧,两手臂自然放置于身体两侧。有的病例,需要加照头低足高 15° 位或头高足低 15° 位,才能清楚看见对比剂进入肝胆管或十二指肠的情况。

X 线中心线:对准欲照的肝胆区范围中心(一般在右季肋部与右锁骨中线交叉点处)垂直射入。投照方法:待手术医生将对比剂(30% 左右的泛影葡胺 40ml)注入肝外胆管仅剩下大约 5ml 时,在不停止注入对比剂的情况下,嘱病人在呼气末时屏住气曝光。

投照注意事项:投照前,一定要检查机器是否工作正常,避免重复投照。把握好曝光时机:对神志清醒的病人,嘱其呼气末屏住气曝光,此时,病人膈肌上升,肝脏及胆系等腹腔脏器处于相对静止的平稳状态,可避免因呼吸所致的影像模糊;对因手术麻醉而处于昏睡状态的病人,因其呼吸不能自行控制,则应注意其呼吸规律,寻找间隙时间曝光,以使腹部平稳。在基层单位,由于使用小型 X 线机,故应使用高速增感屏(它比中速增感屏效果好,如果有条件采用感绿屏,感绿片,更可减少辐射剂量,增加照片对比度与锐利度)。固定 mA,在机器容量允许范围内,尽量采用高 kV,短时间,以降低器官活动引起的运动模糊度,提高造影成功率。

注射对比剂的若干问题:术中胆系造影的对比剂注入速度甚为关键。手术医生在注入对比剂时要用力均匀,速度适中,以 10ml/ 分钟连续匀速注射为宜。速度太慢,对比剂会大量流入十二指肠,使胆管及肝胆管显影不佳;速度太快,将使胆系内压力增大,如压力超过 300mmHg(1mmHg=0.133kPa),胆汁可能出现返流,进入淋巴管,淋巴结和血液,而引起感染或诱发胆管壁出血,从而引起胆管下端括约肌痉挛,胆管扩张变形,甚至胆管破裂。尤其是,肝外胆管下端有明显梗阻时,不仅推注速度应适当放慢,对比剂用量亦应酌情减少。

要使胆系显影充分,注射前应回抽部分胆汁,排尽空气,以免出现假结石影。术中胆系造影有一个重要的观察项目,就是肝内外胆管残存结石。而肝内外胆管结石又以阴性结石居多,往往需要在对比剂衬托下才能显示。对比剂浓度高于 30%,可遮掩结石,影响结石的显示和观察;对比剂浓度低于 20%,则结石不易显示。最佳浓度为 25%~30%

关于左右肝胆管的显示:肝脏为实质性脏器,左右肝胆管分布于密度较高的肝区内。在术中胆系造影时,管电压采用较高的 kVp 值,可使照片层次丰富,胆管树阴影清晰。

二、术中胆系造影胆系正常表现

对比剂能顺利进入十二指肠;可清楚地看到肝外胆管下端胆胰管十二指肠连接区;肝外胆管最大直径小于或等于 15mm;肝内外胆管内对比剂充填良好,无充盈缺损可见;肝内胆管各支显影清晰,走向自然,分布匀称,无明显过量对比剂逆行充盈;胆囊各部及胆囊管全段显影清楚,无充盈缺损,胆囊无扩大,胆囊管无扩张。术中胆系造影简便易行,安全可靠，在胆系外科领域中的价值早已肯定，它对提高胆系手术效果，减少术后并发症，降低再次手术率和胆系阴性探查率起着积极的重要作用。据文献报道，不少的肝胆管囊肿及硬化性胆管炎病例在术前均未考虑到，而由术中胆系造影发现和确诊。有时造影可发现胆总管末端分叉，再度探查发现胆总管末端粘连，探针可从两个方向进入十二指肠，这种胆总管内瘘仅能借造影或十二指肠镜查见胆管下端双开口。Fork 等（1985）在 181 例术后胆系造影中发现 27 例，Bergner（1965）称它的发生率为 1%。术中胆系造影中肝外胆管正常宽度标准应该是多少？各作者意见不一，有作者认为不应超过 10mm，其他一些学者报告标准为 12mm~15mm 不等。

第九章 胆系手术后

第一节 手术损伤性胆管狭窄

详见本书 本卷 第十六篇 第十六章 第二节 手术损伤性胆管狭窄。

第二节 腹腔镜胆囊切除术后并发症

自 1980 年以来,作为对胆囊疾病治疗的首选技术,腹腔镜胆囊切除术已被外科医师和病人广泛接受。目前,美国每年完成胆囊切除手术超过 50 万例,其中绝大多数使用腹腔镜技术。与开腹胆囊切除术相比,腹腔镜的效果更受青睐,但腹腔镜造成的损伤并发症却略高,多发胆管损伤为 0.2%~0.8%,而开腹胆囊切除术为 0.1%~0.2%。因此,需要影像诊断和介入放射学治疗的胆管损伤有增加趋势。

总的并发症:腹腔镜胆囊切除术总的并发症发生率接近 3%,感染是与操作有关的最普遍并发症。胆囊窝内能发生感染,并且常与术中血肿或胆汁外溢以及残留结石所致有关。其他并发症主要与套管的放置有关,包括腹壁或网膜出血、腹部或腹膜后血管损伤、胃肠穿孔、肝或脾的损伤以及套管放置部位的疝伴有肠梗阻。与操作有关的并发症还包括心律不齐、深静脉血栓形成、纵隔积气、气胸以及二氧化碳栓塞等。

胆管并发症:胆管损伤是腹腔镜胆囊切除术最严重的并发症之一,可发生于 0.2%~0.8% 的病人,并与术者的操作程序和经验密切相关。

肝外胆管的异常,如异常的右肝胆管位于胆囊或肝外胆管后方,再如左右肝胆管低位汇合,可能导致术后胆管并发症。另外,右肝胆管也可能有异常的引流到胆囊,以及在 Luschka 管(胆囊腺管:胆囊壁内的管状结构,其中有些与胆管相连,但没有一条与胆囊腔相通,它们可能是迷走胆管)的小胆管也能直接通向胆囊。如果在 Luschka 管区横切肝脏,可导致胆漏;如果在远端切断胆囊管,可导致肝外胆管的损伤,肝外胆管处可发生胆汁漏。不正确的解剖标记的识别可导致完全性胆管切断或部分性肝胆管阻塞。

胆囊管残余部分完全阻塞和/或胆管残余部手术夹放置不当能导致胆汁肿或持续性胆汁漏。虽然可发生慢性胆漏,但异常引流管或异常胆管所致无症状的少量术后潴留能自行吸收。极少情况下,手术夹能从胆囊管残端处脱落,需外科手术处理,此类脱落能产生胆汁肿。偶尔,由于经验不足造成不完全性胆囊切除,导致持续性胆漏,胆汁性腹膜炎和/或脓肿形成。

在胆管和胆囊切除期间,如果发生供血动脉阻断和局部缺血,肝总管或胆管也可发生狭窄。同样,由于过量的激光或电灼,也可导致肝总管的热损伤,胆总管的部分损伤和胆管周围漏,造成胆管周围瘢痕,也可形成狭窄。胆管损伤初步手术修补后,也可在手术吻合处形成胆管狭窄。少数病人,胆总管内残留结石,是引起腹痛复发的原因。

影像学研究:超声检查:有作者指出,对胆管并发症的确诊,通常首选超声成象,它能显示肝内胆管系统并能评价由于胆漏、出血和感染在胆囊窝形成的积液。

X 线检查:腹腔镜胆囊切除术后可疑胆管损伤病人的影像学检查,对于确认损伤的类型和范围提供了重要依据，并直接影响到介入放射学和外科修补。

腹部X线平片可显示许多并发症，包括肺炎、肠穿孔引起的腹膜腔游离气体、腹腔内脓肿以及腹腔积液等。

CT扫描：能提供解剖细节，特别对于腹部、腹膜后的评价和确认术后积液的部位。

胆管阻塞和狭窄：超声和CT能发现由于胆管阻塞和狭窄继发的胆管扩张，如果超声或CT证实胆管阻塞，可采用PTC或/和ERCP进一步检查。虽然PTC和ERCP能帮助确定胆管狭窄的部位和范围，并允许放置内支架缓解阻塞，但许多单位都提出把ERCP作为诊断或处理胆管狭窄的首选方法。因为PTC的并发症比ERCP略高。对胆管狭窄的病例的筛选，ERCP难以显示胆管树的全貌，而胆管树全貌的观察对除外部分肝胆管的阻塞又是必需的。

胆漏：有症状的病人若可疑胆漏，特别是对治疗的选择，ERCP具有特征性，因为逆行推注对比剂能够明确胆漏的部位。另外，通过内镜能放置临时性支架，横跨在包括胆管残余部、胆总管至胆囊窝内异常胆管的小漏口处。介入治疗后漏口常被治愈，随后取出支架。如果漏口过大，ERCP能帮助明确解剖部位，因此有助于制定手术计划。有时，放射性核素也可用来证实胆漏的存在，由此可避免进一步损伤性诊断操作，如ERCP或PTC。

术后积液：除描述胆管横断或狭窄导致的继发性胆管扩张外，常应用超声或CT评价术后的积液、胆汁肿和脓肿。如果诊断确切，可同时用超声或CT导向，治疗性抽吸积液。大多数病例，术后少量积液可自行吸收，而不需介入性治疗。

残留胆管结石：虽然ERCP对特殊并发症的诊断和治疗仍为首选方法，偶尔胆总管内的残留结石也可由超声或CT发现。如果能发现残留结石，ERCP同时可行内镜取石。ERCP还适用于对乳头功能障碍的胆囊切除术后综合征病人进行评价，通过内镜乳头切开术也可缓解乳头的功能障碍。

第三节　胆管空肠吻合术后吻合口狭窄

胆管-空肠吻合术是治疗多种胆系良性疾病和胆系胰腺恶性肿瘤最基本术式，现广泛应用临床。吻合口狭窄是常见的术后并发症，患者多有发热、腹痛和黄疸，但部分患者无明显症状。诊断主要依据临床症状和影像学检查。及时发现吻合口的狭窄及引起的原因，对患者恢复和及时采取相应的治疗措施都至关重要。

胆管-空肠吻合术概况：胆管-空肠吻合术是治疗多种胆系良性疾病和胆系胰腺恶性肿瘤最基本术式，其疗效已经得到多数学者的证实。手术方法是将空肠切断，远侧上提，与需引流的器官（胃、肝、胆等）吻合。近侧与远侧空肠吻合，恢复消化道连续性。

胆总管与空肠的吻合方式主要有3种：端-端、端-侧和侧-侧吻合。由于端-端吻合时胆、肠断端口径不容易匹配且术后易导致吻合口狭窄，同时肠袢末端呈弯曲状态，若用其断端吻合，可增加其系膜的张力，故较少使用。目前临床上常用的主要是端-侧和侧-侧吻合，一项研究病例中，端-侧吻合27例（87.1%）、侧-侧吻合4例（12.9%）。其中，端-侧吻合病例数多，可能与患者的具体情况、术者的经验与手术习惯，以及为避免漏斗综合征的发生有关。胆管空肠吻合口的大小、是否通畅，是影响整个手术成败的关键；吻合口要足够大，不应 <1.5 cm。

MRI检查较其他影像学检查的优势：目前胆管空肠吻合术后的影像学检查方法较多。超声检查价格便宜，特别适用于以黄疸为首发症状者，对肝内残留或复发结石较为敏感。但术后空肠远端上提至肝门区，由于肠道气体的干扰，不利于吻合口狭窄的显示。

CT扫描可清楚地显示胆管扩张、积气，对胆管炎、结石有一定作用，但由于相当部分胆石、胆汁密度与吻合口区域组织接近，致使吻合口区结构显示不清，狭窄不易被检出。

ERCP虽被认为是胆胰管系统疾病诊断的金标准，但由于胆管-空肠吻合术后胆总管下端为盲端或已切除，对胆肠旁路插管极为困难，ERCP往往难以进行，且该方法为侵入性诊断方法。PTC同样为侵入性诊断方法，难以被患者接受，应用日渐减少。

MRI具有快速、无创、多角度、多参数扫描的优点,利于胆管-空肠吻合术后并发症的显示。MRI优势在于:①不受术后解剖结构的影响,技术操作无依赖,安全无创,无严重并发症;②能够提供详细的胆管树结构图,可清楚显示梗阻的远、近端,可全面、立体观察梗阻部位的形态,并为手术方案设计提供依据;③胆管扩张的形态为生理状态下的扩张,无注入对比剂时压力因素的影响,反映的空腔直径准确;④对原发疾病及胆管-空肠吻合术术式判别有一定的帮助,为制订再次手术方案提供依据。

胆管空肠吻合术后吻合口狭窄的MRI表现:虽然手术吻合的方式能一定程度减少吻合口狭窄的发生,但吻合口狭窄仍为胆管空肠吻合术后常见的并发症。在该项研究胆管-空肠吻合术后随访的病例中有8.1%发生吻合口的狭窄(31/382),比文献报道的发病率略低。

吻合口狭窄MRI表现为吻合口变细(8/31)或信号消失(23/31),吻合口部位信号消失可能与吻合口周围平滑肌压迫以及局部肠腔未被充盈有关。此外,还可能与肠道气体可占据胆肠吻合口有关。按狭窄的病因可以分成炎性狭窄、瘢痕性狭窄、肿瘤性狭窄。该组病例中有3例为肿瘤性狭窄,表现为吻合口区团状软组织影,且有相关原发病病史(1例为胰头中分化腺癌、2例为胆管癌)。1例炎性狭窄同样表现为吻合口区团状软组织影,经手术病理证实为慢性炎性增生。故询问胆管-空肠吻合术前的病史对吻合口狭窄性质的判定有一定的帮助。

28例为良性狭窄,可以通过吻合口区炎性或瘢痕性信号进行判断,如梗阻及肝损伤不严重,可通过短期抗感染治疗后复查MRI,比较吻合口区信号和上方胆管扩张程度来判断。该组病例中吻合口上方胆管均出现不同程度扩张(31/31),因此,吻合口上方胆管的扩张可作为诊断吻合口狭窄的一个重要的间接征象。该组作者曾尝试根据胆管的扩张程度来对吻合口狭窄程度进行判断,由于胆管扩张的程度与吻合口狭窄的程度、狭窄的时间、肝功能、术前胆系的病变等多种因素有关,致使判断失败。

值得注意的是,肝内胆管扩张形态以"枯树枝"扩张较为多见,这可能与2个因素有关:一是患者的术前病变所引起胆管的改变;二是胆肠吻合为非生理性手术,使胆汁引流永久性改道,放弃了胆胰管下端括约肌应有的正常生理功能。

胆管空肠吻合术后肠内容物容易通过吻合口返流入胆系,导致化学性细菌性损害,致吻合口、胆系急、慢性炎症改变和纤维组织增生,因此客易形成吻合口的狭窄和返流性胆管炎。

在吻合口及胆管狭窄和继发感染的基础上,部分病例在狭窄近端有继发结石的形成,并且在狭窄、感染和结石之间,会互为因果,形成恶性循环。在该组病例中74.2%(23/31)患者伴有吻合口或肝内外胆管结石,16.1%(5/31)合并胆管积气,16.1%(5/31)合并肝内感染,6.4%(2/31)胆汁淤积性肝硬化,提示后者可能是形成"枯树枝"状扩张的重要原因。

综上所述,MRI能显示胆管-空肠吻合术后吻合口狭窄、吻合口上方胆管的扩张及其他并发症征象,具有快速、准确、安全的特点,可用于胆管-空肠吻合术后患者的随访,对吻合口狭窄的诊断和制订进一步的治疗方案提供可靠依据。

第四节 术后引流管造影

检查方法:术后造影时间。胆汁清亮而无胆管严重感染及出血,全身情况尚佳者,一般在术后1~2周内进行。对比剂:以前曾用12.5%碘化钠溶液、碘油、钡胶浆等,目前多采用有机碘制剂,一般用20%~30%泛影葡胺。对比剂剂量。在T管造影,一般用10~20ml,如在电视透视监视下,则以肝胆管充盈满意时停止注药;如未透视监视,则当病人感觉右上腹发胀时停止注药。在胆囊引流管造影,剂量应增加,约为30~40ml。具体病人具体剂量还要看病人胆管有无扩张及扩张的程度来定。剂量过多过少都会影响造影的质量。

注入方法:用直接加压法注入对比剂,少数病人造影后可出现不良反应,如:寒战、发热、上腹剧痛等。冉瑞图(1977)介绍负压弥散造影法值得推广,经反复抽吸几次,使胆汁与对比剂混合,再缓慢注入,避免加压。由于胆管抽吸的负压作用及胆汁与对比剂之间的弥散作用,使胆管充盈更好,同时可避免术后反应的发生。注药前,应排出及抽出T管或引流管内的空气,以免干扰影像。造影结束后,即刻吸出胆管内对比剂,放松夹子,继续引流。

胆管内压力超过 2.94 kPa,即可出现胆汁逆流,甚至进入淋巴而流入血液内,故可引起逆行感染及诱发溃疡出血,亦可引起胆胰管下端括约肌痉挛,促使对比剂逆流入胰管。如压力过低,胆汁与对比剂进入十二指肠,导致肝胆管不易充盈。因此,在注入对比剂时一定要注意速度不能过快,压力不能过大,药量不能过多。

投照技术:一般取仰卧头低(15º~30º)位,曝光条件较腰椎正位条件略高。照片后,夹闭 T 管。如照片尚满意,可即刻再照一张,以便对比观察,同时看对比剂自然引流情况。如需重照,再根据情况决定。造影失败或不满意有多种原因。左侧肝胆管偏前,在仰卧位不易充盈至 2~3 级,可试行头低右侧抬高,或加照左侧卧位,亦可在电视透视观察下转动体位,使其充盈满意后再照片。杨竞飞(1964)指出,左肝胆管不显影或显影不良时,首先考虑有病变,可采用多种方法反复造影,以显示其病变。Strin(1962)介绍侧位照片有助于肝胆管的观察。

观察时须注意:肝内外胆管的内径情况;胆管的走行与分布;肝胆管各支显影情况;肝内外胆管内有无局限性狭窄、扩张、充盈缺损;对比剂下达十二指肠的量和速度;在总胆管切开探查术后,常难以彻底清除结石,尤其是肝胆管结石较多者更是如此。肝胆管结石,可下行至肝外胆管,亦可有结石再形成。又因术后胃肠道功能的紊乱,可使肠道蛔虫进入胆管。

杨竞飞(1964)报告 239 例术后 T 管造影,有阳性发现者 106 例,占 44.3%,其中结石 68 例,蛔虫 38 例,两者同时存在 10 例。据 Kakos 等(1972)统计,在作总胆管探查时,约有 9%~25% 病人的结石被忽视或残留有结石。Haenisch 分析 1 000 例胆管术后病例后认为,约有 1/3 因未做术中胆系造影而使结石被遗漏。Kakos 等指出,进行术中胆系造影再加胆管切开术,可使阳性发现从 28% 提高到 62% 因此,术中胆系造影实应推广应用。

有作者指出,术中有结石,术后造影可见肝外胆管均有不同程度的扩张;术中有结石而术后造影未见结石者,肝外胆管纵有扩张,也甚为轻微;术中无结石,术后造影肝外胆管常无明显扩张。胆管扩张的表现不一:在下端嵌顿性结石及多发性结石,肝内外胆管均有明显扩张;如系孤立性结石或少数结石,则呈局限性扩张及近侧肝胆管相应扩张;如系 1、2 级肝胆管结石,则所属分支扩张或充盈不良,或梗阻,而肝外胆管扩张不明显;如系肝外胆管下端瘢痕性狭窄,或胆胰管下端括约肌痉挛,胆管一般轻度扩张,下端局限性狭窄,但充盈良好,引流亦好,无结石;如系肝外胆管蛔虫,一般胆管轻度扩张。在肝内外胆管结石取出后,或梗阻病因解除后,扩张的胆管可逐渐恢复如常。一般术后造影所见的胆管内径均较术中造影所见为小。T 管造影时对比剂漏出与亚急性胆汁性腹膜炎的关系:Mosley(1992)报道 56 例胆囊切除术后(7~10 天)T 管造影,发现 28 例有对比剂外漏至 T 管周围,其中 4 例临床上表现为严重的胆汁性腹膜炎。在常规胆囊切除术,肝活组织检查及经皮肝穿胆系造影术后,可有少量至中等量的胆汁漏入腹腔,胆汁所致的化学性腹膜炎可以自愈,然而,含有细菌的胆汁能引起脓毒性腹膜炎。临床上 T 管拔出后有胆汁外漏的发生率为 7%~18%,在行 T 管造影时,不仅应注意是否有残留结石及对比剂是否顺利进入十二指肠,而且应注意观察 T 管周围是否有对比剂外漏,如果有外漏,T 管宜再保留 7~10 天,然后再行 T 管造影。这样,就有足够的时间在 T 管周围形成一道屏障,以防胆汁继续漏入腹腔。

第五节　黏胆症

详见本书 本卷 本篇 第一章 第五节　黏胆症。

第十六篇　胆管疾病

第一章　胆管梗阻一般情况

第一节　误诊病例简介：非肝移植胆管铸型综合征

胆管铸型是指肝内外胆管胆泥样凝固物形成，形似树干树枝，最早由 Waldram 等（1975）报道，胆管铸型综合征由 Starzl 等（1977）正式提出，可能的原因有胆系上皮缺血、排斥反应、理化因素、感染、手术因素等。

以往认为胆管铸型及胆管铸型综合征均为肝移植术后的一种并发症，但是 Byme 等（2003）报道了 1 例先天性胆管炎胆管铸型综合征及颅脑损伤患者经内窥镜、外科手术并最终行肝移植治疗。Katsinelos 等（2008）报道了 1 例非肝移植患者胆管铸型综合征的内窥镜治疗。

该例非肝移植患者，经胆囊切除、胆总管切开取石术治疗，术后患者恢复良好。由此可以认为，胆管铸型综合征并不只发生于肝移植患者，非肝移植胆管铸型综合征胆总管切开胆管铸型剥出对该例疗效肯定。

肝移植术后胆管铸型综合征需要临床表现、实验室肝功能监测、术后 T 管造影及胆道镜观察等综合诊断，其中术后 T 管胆系造影是诊断肝移植术后胆管铸型综合征乃至所有胆系并发症的金标准。

该例术前影像表现值得回顾性分析，B 超提示胆栓形成；CT 仅见肝内外胆管扩张，由于铸型物未含钙质，主要含胆红素成分，在 CT 上难以分辨，缺乏诊断依据。

MR 检查见肝门区及沿肝内胆管分布区域增宽，肝内胆管内未见典型液体长 T_2 信号，增强检查见胆管壁增厚，呈线状强化，肝内胆管见等 T_1 信号充盈缺损。MRCP 示肝内外胆管液体信号减低、粗细不均、边缘不清楚、胆管内信号不均匀，部分胆管断续扩张，其内可见斑点、线条状或铸形等 T_1、短 T_2 信号。

回顾该例影像表现，可以认为 MRI 尤其是 MRCP 的征象更具特异性，其表现与病理改变即胆管壁充血水肿、增厚，胆管内胆红素等凝集物铸型充填于管腔，致长 T_2 信号胆汁较少。铸型物表面不光整，即形成该例所见的 MRI 改变，故 MRCP 观察肝内外胆管内填充物更直观、清晰。

由于此病在临床上少见，对其影像表现认识不足，导致术前诊断欠缺。通过以上分析，影像检查，尤其是 MRI+MRCP 对非肝移植术后胆管铸型的诊断具有一定特异性，认识其 MRI 征象对本病术前正确诊断及评估治疗方案有较大帮助。

该例胆管铸型物光学显微镜下为胆汁凝集，病理为坏死性胆管炎，影像观察认为胆管铸型应有多种成分，这与以往在肝移植术后胆管铸型的患者标本有所不同，后者成分大部分为胆红素结晶，未见坏死胆管结构，两者之间是否存在明显差异及相同点还有待进一步相关研究。

附具体病例资料：患者，女，60 岁，受凉后畏寒、发热伴咳嗽、咳白痰 3 天入院。1 个月前曾患急性胰腺炎，既往有糖尿病、肾功能不全、胆囊及胆管结石、胆囊炎胆管炎病史。体检：体温 40℃，皮肤巩膜中度黄染，腹肌紧张，无压痛及反跳痛。实验室检查提示肝功能异常、梗阻性黄疸，血淀粉酶正常。

影像检查：B 超示胆总管炎、胆总管结石并胆栓形成，肝内胆管结石。CT 示胆管炎、胆囊多发结石。MRI 示肝实质未见病变，肝门区肝裂增宽，沿胆管分布向肝内延伸，呈长 T_1、稍长 T_2 信号，MR T_2WI 肝门区胆管及肝左右叶胆管近段少许液性长 T_2 信号，内见小颗粒状、条状短 T_2 信号。胆总管内未见液性长 T_2 信号，显示欠清。增强扫描肝左、右叶胆管壁呈线状强化，肝右叶胆管近侧见条状等信号。MRCP 见肝内外胆管轻度扩张，边缘不清楚，其内液体信号减弱、不均匀,未见明确结石样充盈缺损,胆总管内见不清晰的轨道状低信号。MRI 诊断为胆管炎、肝内胆管结石,胆总管结石不除外。

手术所见:胆总管粗糙,直径约 1.3 cm,质硬,切开见胆总管内褐黑色质硬物,呈柱状、条索状,向上进肝内,试行拔除,拉出树枝状物长约 11 cm,质硬,内有少许细粒状物,拔除后流出较混浊的胆汁,胆总管壁充血水肿。光学显微镜下见胆管表面黏膜大部分坏死、脱落,仅残留少量黏膜上皮,胆(囊)管纤维组织增生,血管扩张充血,其间炎细胞浸润,胆管内剥出物为凝集的胆汁,表面见纤维被膜包裹。病理诊断:胆囊慢性炎症急性发作,胆管坏死性炎,胆囊、胆管结石。

术后影像检查:MRI 示肝胆管部分扩张,程度较术前减轻,胆管壁仍呈线状强化,MRCP 示胆管内液体信号增强、清晰,胆管边缘清楚,信号均匀,原肝内外胆管内小条形异常信号影消失,仅见少许小点状影存留。T 管造影示左右肝管及肝左右叶内胆管管径变细、粗细欠匀称。

第二节 Mirizzi 综合征

详见本书 本卷 第十八篇 第三章 Mirizzi 综合征。

第二章　梗阻性黄疸

第一节　恶性胆管梗阻

引起恶性胆管梗阻的原因很多，主要有5种。

(1)胆管癌：胆管癌具有浸润型、息肉性、腔外型及混合型4种生长方式。根据病变累及的部位，胆管癌包括肝内性和肝门肝内性、肝外性胆管癌。不同部位的胆管癌有不同的生长方式。肝内性胆管癌发生于肝内小胆管，是原发性肝癌的一种，又称肝内胆管细胞癌。该肿瘤以肿块形成为主，远端肝内胆管阻塞、扩张，形成Ⅰ型MRCP改变。肝门肝内性和肝外性胆管癌则以浸润性生长方式为主，常规MRI难以发现肿块。肝门部胆管癌是指位于左、右肝管及其汇合部和肝总管，即胆总管起始部以上的肝外胆管癌，也称高位胆管癌、近端胆管癌、肝门胆管癌。肝门部胆管癌约占整个胆管癌56%，是胆系常见恶性肿瘤之一，以浸润型、外生型为主。表现为肝门胆管截断，形成肝门空虚征，近段胆管阻塞扩展，呈枯树枝状(Ⅱ型)。发生于中下段时，MRCP表现胆总管截断，肝内胆管及近段扩张(Ⅲ型)。由于肝外胆管癌浸润性生长的特点，研究表明52%(12/23例)常累及邻近的胰头、胰管，MRI形成胰头异常信号和胰管扩张表现。该组有60%(6/10)侵及胰管，引起胰管扩张。

(2)胆胰共同管癌：胆胰共同管癌常引起胆管及胰管扩张(Ⅳ型)，又称双管征；该组6例共同管癌中3例有此改变。共同管癌的双管征常互相平行。

(3)十二指肠乳头癌：十二指肠乳头癌是较少见的肿瘤，在所有消化系统恶性肿瘤中，十二指肠乳头癌不到1%。但是，在胆胰共同管周围恶性肿瘤中，十二指肠乳头癌占第2位，且有逐年增加趋势。十二指肠乳头癌可发生于任何年龄，但60~65岁年龄组更常见；男女发生比例约3:2。该组2例十二指肠癌单纯侵犯胆总管引起梗阻扩张，文献报道也可同时侵犯胆总管及胰管，引起梗阻扩张。MRCP示胆总管扩张或胰管扩张、梗阻的部位，有利于肿瘤分期，决定进行根治性的治疗或姑息性的治疗。

(4)胰头癌：胰头癌主要是由导管上方上皮细胞发生的导管腺癌。其浸润性极强，可通过胰内淋巴扩散至胰腺内的胆总管、神经组织、静脉、动脉、淋巴结和邻近器官。通常胰头癌常伴胆管梗阻、扩张，与肿瘤的大小、肿瘤的生长方向、胆胰管及主副胰管汇合的类型等有关。特异MRCP征象是胆总管胰头段及主胰管胰头段被癌瘤组织破坏中断，二者之残留近段均有扩张(Ⅳ型)，二者在正常情况下应相交，而在胰头癌时则不相交、相互分离。

(5)胆囊癌：胆囊癌也是常见的肿瘤，好发于老年人，该组平均年龄为62岁。文献报道50%以上的胆囊癌病例可见胆管阻塞。阻塞原因是胆管受肿块或肿大的淋巴结压迫，或肿瘤直接侵蚀胆管造成。胆囊癌导致的梗阻性黄疸迄今仍常常被当作“已丧失手术治疗机会”的标志之一。近年的国内外文献均表明，部分已有肝门胆管侵犯的晚期胆囊癌仍可得到根治性切除，远期疗效明显优于姑息治疗。MRCP尤其能清晰地显示肝内外胆管受累所致胆管梗阻征象，有利于临床对胆囊癌的治疗方案选择。

第二节　左肝外段低分化肝内胆管细胞癌

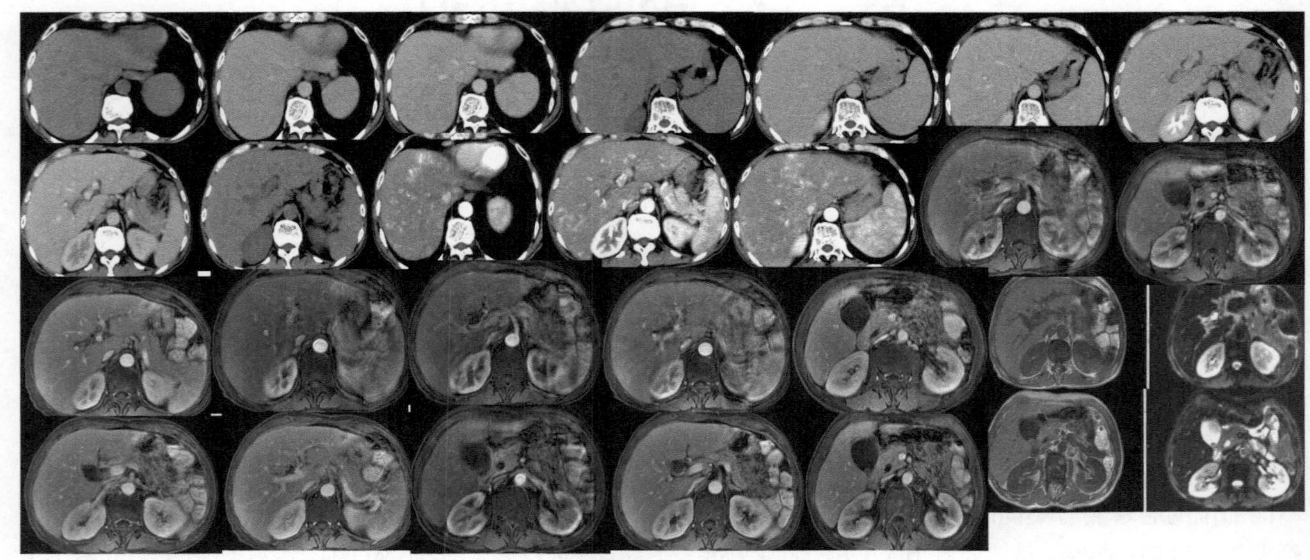

图 16-2-1　左肝外段低分化肝内胆管细胞癌

患者,男, 61 岁。反复咳嗽咳痰 10 余年伴乏力 1 个月入院。

病理检查:胆囊:标本为切除之胆囊,送检前未剖开,大小 9cm×4cm×2cm,表面光滑,腔内含大量黄褐色黏液,另见黑色结石一枚,大小 1.5cm×1cm× 0.5cm,壁厚 0.1~0.3cm。肝左外叶肿物:肝组织一块,大小 7cm×4cm×3.2cm,浆膜面粗糙,灰褐色,切面见一灰白色区域,大小 2.5cm× 2cm×2cm,切面质软。常规病理诊断:肝左外叶肿物切除标本:初步诊断肝内胆管细胞癌,待做免疫组化检测进一步证实。胆囊切除标本:慢性结石性胆囊炎伴罗 - 阿窦形成,未见癌组织累及。

免疫组化结果:阳性: CK19,CK7,CK18,CK8,CA19-9, Villin, Ki-67(+,约 30%);阴性: CK20, CEA, AFP, Hepatocyte, CD34。免疫组化诊断:肝左外叶肿物切除标本:低分化肝内胆管细胞癌(图 16-2-1)。

第三节　胆汁淤滞

胆汁淤滞是由于胆汁排泄障碍造成的胆汁成分在肝和血液中的淤滞。胆汁的排泄取决于不同的步骤。在考虑梗阻性胆汁淤滞的机制时,应将胆管梗阻的定位诊断作为第一步。因此, Phillips(1986)提出了胆汁淤滞的分型(见表 16-2-1)。从表中可以看出梗阻可发生在不同的部位,并且不同类型的胆汁淤滞都伴有各自的临床情况,提示每种胆汁淤滞都包含有许多原因。

胆汁淤滞的病理:无论非扩张性或扩张性胆管梗阻性胆汁淤滞,其病理特点如下:

胆汁淤滞常伴有上行性胆管炎:如果持续时间较长,则胆管增粗,纤维组织增生,胶原纤维沉着,小叶周围间隔形成和/或肝脓肿,以及偶见的梗阻性胆汁性肝硬化将会相继发生。始发于第三级胆小管的胆汁淤滞则在肝细胞和枯否细胞内出现胆汁。随后可见胆汁湖和胆汁性坏死的肝门脉部炎症和胆管病变。

表 16-2-1　梗阻性胆汁淤滞病理分类

梗阻部位	病理分类	常见原因
肝外胆管	胆管扩张、非扩张（约占 10%~30%）	结石、狭窄、闭锁、胆管囊肿、寄生虫、胆管或胰腺肿瘤、逆行性胆管炎、原发性或继发性胆管炎。
肝内胆管	肝门部和中央混合性改变	结石、寄生虫、硬化性胆管炎、复发性化脓性胆管炎、狭窄、闭锁、原发性胆汁性肝硬化、混合性胆汁淤滞、胆小管性肝炎、胆管癌。

胆汁返流通路：过去认为胆汁淤滞是胆汁从破裂的胆管"返流"入血。事实上胆管破裂非常少见，而且仅在长期胆管梗阻病例才能见到。因此，滞留胆汁的返流通路很可能是通过细胞通路，最可能是通过囊泡。结合复合体的功能，尤其是与胆小管相邻的紧密连接部一直是研究的课题。它们将胆小管与肝窦及肝窦周围间隙隔开。最初认为它们是相邻细胞的邻接细胞膜完全融合而成，是密封性结构。近来发现融合的部位不是相邻的细胞膜，而是插入相邻细胞膜之间的多排微粒所形成的一系列紧密接触的点和线。而且并不是所有的紧密连接部都是'紧密'的，而是存在漏隙，至少某些物质可以漏出。

急性局灶性肝细胞坏死：急性局灶性肝细胞坏死，特别是在肝门脉区周围可见到这种改变。它也是胆汁物质返流入血的一种原因，但不多见，除非是在梗阻的后期。

引起肝内胆汁淤积的原因大多为机械性梗阻。胆管结石、慢性胆管炎、胆管结石术后是最常见病因。各种影像学检查都可以看到肝内外胆管的原发病变和继发的胆管扩张，病理表现为肝内外胆管狭窄，管壁弥漫性增厚、硬韧、呈条索状，病理诊断为慢性炎症，即继发性硬化性胆管炎。该病容易诊断，但肝实质纤维化和肝硬化的征象不容忽视。MRI 对该病具有良好的应用和研究前景。

也有作者提出胆汁从损伤的胆管直接漏出。特别是在肝门小胆管损伤时。曾一时称之为'胆管溶解性肝炎'，但是除了光镜检查见到的明显的肝门部炎症反应外，没有明确证明。电镜下也未见胆管损伤，这种概念不再被人重视。然而，根据细胞旁路和肝细胞间紧密连接存在漏隙的新概念，应想到某些胆汁淤滞的情况中，胆汁经小胆管和细胆管返流的可能性。

占位性病变对邻近肝脏组织的影响：占位性病变可能造成邻近肝脏组织（包括肝血窦、胆小管、静脉和细胆管）的压迫和 / 或梗阻。在肿块周围，胆汁淤滞是常见的。其他病变有局限性胆管扩张、炎症、胆管上皮的多形性、肝窦扩张和小管胆汁淤滞等。

不完全性胆管阻塞："不完全性胆管梗阻"是一种特殊类型的胆管梗阻。梗阻可能具有节段性、不全性或间隙性。此类胆管梗阻无典型的胆汁淤滞的病理形态学改变，而血清碱性磷酸酶增高，血清胆红素正常。有报告在选择性胆管梗阻实验中，发现梗阻部位胆小管通常正常，而在非梗阻小叶中却扩张。且发现梗阻部位的高尔基体发育不良，在非梗阻部位高尔基体较大、较多，并含有嗜锇颗粒的囊泡。认为上述改变反映了非梗阻部位的功能增强。另一解释是认为肝门附近大的胆管存在丰富的吻合网，彼此交通，因此当一部位梗阻时，胆管经吻合支而减压。

胆管不扩张的胆管梗阻：一般认为，有胆管梗阻时，胆管就有扩张。但有些病例的肝胆管和肝外胆管并不扩张或仅有肝外胆管扩张，有作者报道这种有梗阻而胆管不扩张的矛盾现象，占经皮肝穿刺胆系造影检查患者的 9%，其他作者也有类似的报告，这说明，胆管不扩张也不能否认梗阻性黄疸的诊断。近年来，无胆管扩张的胆管梗阻的病例报告不断增多。这些病例，如果只根据超声测量胆管是否扩张来决定是否有胆管梗阻，就有可能会误诊。尽管胆管大小正常，如果临床仍疑有胆管梗阻，可用其他影像诊断手段进行确诊。

一些学者分析 9 例胆管不扩张的梗阻性黄疸，9 例肝内外胆管都无扩张。经经皮肝穿刺胆系造影或 / 和手术证实，其中 1 例为胰腺炎、胰头增大，2 例胆总管结石，2 例肝内转移性病变压迫肝内胆管根部变形；4 例为肝门部转移性病变压迫肝外胆管变形。

为什么有梗阻而没有胆管扩张？从流体力学 Laplace 定律和 Pascal 定律来看，肝外胆管急性梗阻的早期，在一定的时间内，肝胆管可能看不到扩张；肝外胆管内结石的球瓣机制可能是梗阻性黄疸无胆管扩张的另一因素，多见于圆形结石。关于胆管不扩张的机制尚不清楚，有学者认为胆总管结石不扩张的原因可能是由于结石的球形瓣性梗阻特征。这点应引起我们的注意，因为人们都认为超声和 CT 是鉴别梗阻与非梗阻性黄疸的筛选方法，而上述 9 例，超声和 CT 都未能做出梗阻性黄疸的正确诊断。

因此仅凭胆管不扩张这一间接征象来排除梗阻性黄疸是不适当的。

非梗阻性扩张:有胆管扩张不一定就有胆管梗阻存在,即所谓的非梗阻性扩张。这些病例,经皮肝穿刺胆系造影和经内镜逆行胆胰管造影都不能显示梗阻的依据,测胆系静止压正常,胆系灌注后压力也不增高。因此,胆管扩张不是判定梗阻的特征性征象。非梗阻性扩张的机制还不清楚,可能与老化,及过去曾有胆管梗阻,胆管炎症伴管壁弹性丧失或胆胰管下端括约肌功能异常有关。

关于胆管大小的研究:因为胆管的回声与其周围结构的不同,所以超声评价胆管系统比较理想。随着新的超声技术的出现,正常胆管树的微小结构都可显示,并可在解剖上与邻近的静脉和动脉区别。超声发现胆管扩张,是胆系疾病的一个重要提示;肝内胆管扩张的超声表现,描述为平行管征或枪管征。这征象的解释是:门静脉和肝胆管分支走行毗邻,门静脉进入肝实质后,胆管缠绕门静脉分支紧密伴行,轻度的肝胆管扩张可通过同行的门静脉分支的表现而易于发现,中度及重度肝胆管扩张则更易发现。

在静脉注射对比剂后,胆管在正常情况下不强化,这样就易与肝内血管区分。接受肝内小胆管胆汁的左、右肝管下行,在肝门处形成肝总管,在胆囊管并入后形成胆总管,胆总管继续下行进入胆胰共同管入十二指肠。

因为正常的肝内胆管在 CT 扫描上常不能显示,过去认为在 CT 上显示出肝内胆管即是胆管扩张和阻塞。然而,随着 CT 技术的发展,现在有高达 40% 的病人可见正常粗细(1~3mm)的肝内胆管,而无胆管疾病。认识上述表现对评价可疑的胆管阻塞非常重要。

在许多病人中,肝外胆管能够分辨。在对无胆管疾病的 100 例病人的研究中,66 例可以看到肝总管,平均直径 2.8mm;82 例可见到胆总管,平均直径 3.6mm。尽管胆总管直径 6~10mm 不能明确界定有无胆总管扩张,但是正常胆总管的直径通常小于 6mm。正常肝管自肝门向肝周逐渐变细。

肝外胆管壁厚度正常应小于 1.5mm。胆总管壁强化亦可发生在无胆管疾病的病人中,仅有胆管壁的强化并不是胆管病变的指征。

肝外胆管扩张的发现常常仰赖于肝外胆管管径正常值的确定。在超声检查,Williams 等(1977)将 8mm 作为正常上界,未见胆管扩张的假阳性,96% 病人诊断正确,假阴性为 7%。Sample 等(1978)对未行胆系手术者,用 6mm 作正常标准,6~8mm 为可疑扩张,以此区别内外科黄疸,敏感性为 85%~100%,特异性为 76%~100%。该作者以 5mm 作正常上界者,93% 诊断正确,假阳性为 4%,假阴性为 10%。Cooperberg 等(1980)对 170 例黄疸病例分析,以 4mm 作正常标准,来区别内外科黄疸,敏感性为 98.8%,特异性为 86.7%,假阳性至少 7%,假阴性 1%;而以 5mm 为标准,则敏感性降低到 94%,特异性不变。该作者认为以 4mm 作总肝管正常大小的上限值,5mm 为界限值,≥ 6mm 则需要作进一步的胆系造影。

胆管大小的测量颇受检查方法的影响。超声测量胆管管径,对人不施予任何干预,属于生理状态下。但由于管壁回声反射的影响,超声所测得的管内径数值较实际管内径约小 1.5mm。声象图中管壁的亮带占据了部分管腔,其数值因增益条件不同而变化,增益越高,管壁亮带越宽,而内径越窄。X 线检查口服胆囊造影时,胆管内径大小受胆胰管下端括约肌开闭状态和胆囊内压的影响,服脂餐后,十二指肠黏膜释放胆囊收缩素,使胆囊收缩,胆胰管下端括约肌松弛,胆管内庄下降,因此其管径小于非排泄状态下的管径。静脉胆系造影,对比剂的利胆作用,使胆汁流量增加,从而增高管内压,胆管被动扩张,所以,管径比生理状态下的管径为大。直接法造影(如经皮肝穿刺胆系造影和经内镜逆行胆胰管造影),对比剂直接注入胆管,管内压升高,胆管扩张,故管径比静脉胆系造影还要大。X 线照片的放大因素,肝外胆管为卵圆形,其横径与斜径的区别等因素也须考虑,X 线测量总胆管正常内径为 5~6mm,一般超过 7mm 为扩张。

胆管的大小与年龄有关:年龄增大胆管增宽,对 60 岁以上者,总胆管正常上限为 7mm。

胆囊切除后胆管大小的情况较复杂。有学者用超声研究了 67 例胆囊切除后正常总肝管的大小,结论为:①胆囊切除后,总肝管一般不扩张;②大多数病例(84%)总肝管内径之 4mm,5mm 为界限值;③少数病例(16%)总肝管增粗,可大至 10mm;④术前扩张的总肝管在术后可恢复正常大小。后来,他又研究了胆总管大小在胆囊切除前后的对比,40 例无症状病例,没有发现胆囊切除后胆总管扩张的证据,于是他得出结论:在胆囊切除后,原来正常的胆管依然正常,原有扩张的胆管可变小,非梗阻性扩张的胆管可持续存在。

一些学者指出，胆管不因胆囊切除而扩张，胆囊切除后胆管正常值标准应和未手术之正常人相同（即肝外胆管平均最大内径为 5mm，7mm 为正常最大值）。忽视胆囊切除者的肝外胆管扩张有一定的危险，在他的'非黄疸病人的胆管扩张'一文中，11 例胆囊切除者有 9 例存在新的部分梗阻性病变。但问题在于，由于过去长期梗阻，在胆囊切除后，胆管扩张一般都继续存在，因此很难确定胆囊切除后肝外胆管的正常平均值和最大值。理想的方法是对每人作预先的基线检查，如术前超声或术中胆管造影。对有症状的胆囊切除后患者，特别化验异常者，如肝外胆管大于 7mm，则需认真对待，梗阻的可能性随胆管管径增大而增加。

胆管扩张可以只发生在部分胆管。如只发生肝内或肝外胆管扩张。其原因，有的很好解释，如肝门部转移病变只引起肝内胆管扩张。但有的则不好解释。重要的是，只有肝内胆管扩张或只有肝外胆管扩张都有可能被忽视。因此，要强调作全面的整个胆系的检查。

另外，胆管大小可在很短期内发生变化。肝外胆管主要由弹性纤维和结缔组织组成，很少或无平滑肌，富有弹性。在急性梗阻或直接胆管内注射后，胆管可很快发生扩张。在胆管未发生不可逆性变化（如慢性炎症，纤维化）之前，一旦梗阻解除，扩张的胆管可很快缩小至正常大小。因此，多次超声检查胆管大小，并作前后对比，可明显提高诊断率。

对确诊胆管梗阻的研究：胆系压力测量对鉴别有无胆管梗阻很有价值，对不扩张的胆管梗阻或非梗阻性扩张病例尤为明显。多数作者认为，正常胆系压力为 0.5~2.0 kPa，无论胆管大小是否扩张，胆系压力增高则说明有胆管梗阻；压力正常则说明无梗阻。

超声显示肝外胆管内径甚优，除了解解剖结构外，可用脂餐后测量胆管大小的方法，来进一步获得关于胆系功能的信息。这种动力学的研究，对发现不扩张的胆管梗阻和评价胆管扩张的意义尤为有益。脂餐后，如原正常或轻度扩张的胆总管管径增大，则强烈提示有胆管梗阻存在；如管径变小，则提示动力正常，实际上排除胆管梗阻。有作者指出：脂餐后胆管直径无变化，提示胆管远端无梗阻。因为增加的胆汁流量由胆胰管下端括约肌松弛来平衡。脂餐后，胆管大小不变化的机制可能与胆管壁的弹性丧失有关。

非扩张型胆管梗阻性胆汁淤滞发病机制研究：胆管梗阻引起非扩张型胆汁淤滞的报告日渐增加。一些作者指出能被手术纠正的胆管梗阻性病例中，10% 以上表现为肝内、外胆管不扩张。另有作者观察到当胆管梗阻时，尤其是部分性或间隙性狭窄时，CT 和超声检查有 10%~30% 的病例表现为胆管大小正常。多数报告梗阻的主要原因为胆总管结石、胆胰管下端括约肌异常、硬化性胆管炎、良性狭窄、肝内肿瘤、肝门的转移肿瘤、胰癌、胆管癌等。

一些学者分析了 16 例结合胆红素水平在 1.5~27.1mg/dL 而无肝内胆管扩张的病例，发现肝门转移性病变、良性狭窄和胆石为三种最常见原因；梗阻平面可在肝门至胆总管的任何部位。其中 5 例，尽管肝内胆管无扩张，而肝穿刺胆管造影却发现胆总管扩张。在该作者观察的 32 个月中，采用肝穿刺胆管造影者，9% 有梗阻而无胆管扩张。

一般解释为：①按照 Laplace 定律，压力相同时，管道内压大小与管道（胆管树）的内径成正比。假定胆管内压力是相同的，则胆总管所承受的压力远大于肝内胆管。因此，远端梗阻时，胆总管的扩张先于肝内胆管。②同样，按照 Laplace 定律，胆管的扩张程度与梗阻的时间成正比。因此，总胆管结石引起的急性梗阻，胆管可无扩张。③胆管周围肿瘤的生长引起对胆管的侵蚀和包围，阻止了胆管的扩张，常见于肝胆系的淋巴瘤、胆管癌、转移癌等，硬化性胆管纤维化也是一原因。④有作者认为胆总管结石的球形瓣机制是非扩张性胆管梗阻引起黄疸的原因。⑤一些作者认为，胆汁淤积常伴有反流性胆管炎，如果持续时间较长，则可能发生胆管胶原化、纤维化，因而造成胆管僵硬，不易扩张。硬化性胆管炎的胆管及其周围的纤维化也是一个原因。我们报告 15 例病人中，梗阻原因达 10 种之多，因此，我们认为，发病机制可能是多种多样的，有待进一步探讨。

影像诊断与非扩张型胆管梗阻性胆汁淤滞：现将非直接性和直接性两类影像诊断方法在非扩张型胆管梗阻性胆汁淤滞中的作用作一对比，以期对其地位有一定认识。

非直接法胆管成像：多位作者对 CT 和超声在非扩张型胆管梗阻中的诊断作用，以及对于非扩张型与扩张型胆管梗阻的鉴别诊断的敏感性看法不一。有作者报导的 6 组病例超声确诊率为 83%~97%。一些作者报导的 4 组病例 CT 对非扩张型胆管梗阻的确诊率为97%~100%。另有作者对87例经手术证实为胆总管结石的病例进行分析,31例(36%)术前经超声和CT都没有发现胆总管扩张。

一些学者报导29例胆管梗阻病例中,9例为非扩张型胆管梗阻性黄疸。先行腹部超声检查,因未发现胆管扩张而确诊困难。9例中2例为胆总管结石,超声检查考虑为胆囊结石;1例急性胰腺炎,超声则表现为胰头增大;2例肝转移性病变和2例肝门肿块中各1例被怀疑。9例中仅2例行CT检查,也因未发现扩张胆管,未诊断为梗阻性黄疸。

有作者报导16例非扩张型胆总管梗阻性黄疸中,有5例在采用胆管造影前行超声检查:2例胆总管结石未能发现;1例胆管癌怀疑为胰腺炎或胰腺肿瘤;1例胆总管远端良性狭窄误为阴性;将1例胆总管腺癌误诊为胆囊扩张。该作者认为超声可能在3%~17%的病例不能显示胆管。失败的原因包括:胆管内充满胆汁衍生物的碎屑,肝内胆管的极小扩张,以及由于技术不熟练而致观察影像不确切等。

CT也会出现假象。所以超声和CT对于梗阻的部位和原因是相对不敏感的。此外,有作者报告仅18%~66%的胆管结石和30%~70%的胰腺癌被超声显示。另有报告梗阻的部位和原因仅有50%~66%的超声显示率。

一些学者认为超声和CT难发现梗阻的精确解剖部位和了解梗阻的原因。且对发现新生物者,梗阻近端常不能确切显示。明显的非扩张性功能性梗阻,还可见其他许多病变,尤其是胆胰管下端狭窄、硬化性胆管炎,偶尔也可见于早期胆管和胰腺肿瘤。

在这种情况下,尽管超声和CT结果是阴性的,引起临床上怀疑肝外胆管梗阻的异常肝功能结果,将引导进一步作直接胆管造影,如经皮肝穿刺胆系造影、经内镜逆行胆胰管造影等。一些作者认为超声和CT对于确定胆管的梗阻部位和原因比较敏感,而CT似乎更确切些。CT主要对确诊下列两类病例有作用:①检查结果似是而非,或尽管是正常,而临床高度怀疑胆管梗阻者;②对于那些肥胖型病例和胆肠吻合术后患者,超声检查效果不佳,而CT可作为优越诊断手段。总之,超声和CT可作为本症的初期诊断手段。然而,它们一般都需要一些补充检查方法。对于那些不能从初期估计做出肝内、外黄疸诊断的病例,这两种方法可为进一步的检查提供更多的借鉴。这些检查对于确定肝内新生物、囊肿和脓肿、胆管结石以及由于肝外胆汁淤滞所造成的胆管改变是有价值的。

随着MSCT在临床的广泛应用,比较于普通CT和常规超声来说,它在确定胆管的梗阻部位和原因方面已大有进步,加上MRI软件与硬件的不断发展,目前MSCT与MRI在临床上应用越来越广泛,已基本上能满足临床诊断的要求。

MRI在显示和测量肝外胆管方面,因不同的加权序列,其测量值可出现一定的差异。有作者利用MRI测量一组正常人总胆管的宽度,在T_1WI中,总胆管宽度为10mm,但在T_2WI中却达11.8mm。产生上述差别的原因可能有二:一是由于脉冲序列的不同,使肝外胆管与周围组织的对比度不同;二是不同脉冲序列图像的畸变效应不同。

在胆系的MRI检查中,胆囊内胆汁的MR信号与胆汁的浓度有关:禁食或空腹时,胆汁内富含胆酸、胆固醇和磷脂,水含量相对低,故在T_1WI中呈高信号;进食后,由于胆囊浓缩胆汁排空,大量低浓度的肝胆汁进入胆囊,致胆汁浓度降低,在T_1WI中表现为低信号。一些学者测量浓缩胆汁的T_1值为94ms,而稀释胆汁的T_1值长达2 646ms。

肝细胞分泌的"新鲜"肝胆汁进入胆囊后,因其比重较低,悬浮于残留浓缩胆囊胆汁上,T_1WI可见胆囊内分层现象:上层胆汁浓度低,呈低信号;下层浓度高,呈明显高信号。

MRI对肝内胆管的显示与所用的脉冲序列及肝胆汁的信号特征有关:①在常规SE序列中,肝胆汁由于未经浓缩过程故浓度较低,因此,肝内胆管在MRI的T_1WI中表现为低信号,与同样低信号的肝内血管不易区分;T_2WI成像时,因肝内胆管较细小,与肝组织间产生部分容积效应而不易显示。但有肝内胆管扩张时,肝内胆管在T_2WI中则呈明显条索状或圆形高信号,很容易与低信号的血管区分;②MRCP能清楚显示肝内胆管的分支,表现为树枝状高信号。

直接法胆管造影:经内镜逆行胆胰管造影(ERCP)、经皮肝穿刺胆管造影(PTC)和胆囊穿刺胆管造影(TCC)对于非扩张型胆管梗阻的显示,均为有效的诊断手段。

经内镜逆行胆胰管造影:一些作者提出在进一步了解梗阻性黄疸方面,经内镜逆行胆胰管造影对肝内胆汁淤滞和肝外梗阻的鉴别有重要作用。该作者认为对于非扩张型胆管梗阻的病例,经皮肝穿刺胆系造影和经内镜逆行胆胰管造影对于胆管树的直接显示都有突出的作用。而经内镜逆行胆胰管造影较经皮肝穿刺胆系造影具有下述优点：①可用于用经皮肝穿刺胆系造影受限的病例，如：继发于肝脏疾病的凝血性疾病，可疑肝脓肿等。②经内镜逆行胆胰管造影对于本症病例采用的成功率较经皮肝穿刺胆系造影为高，后者不高于 50%。③经内镜逆行胆胰管造影的禁忌证相对较少，而且并发症的发生率及其严重性均低于经皮肝穿刺胆系造影。最常见的并发症为胰腺炎，有报导这种并发症的发生率为 2%。④经内镜逆行胆胰管造影是非手术方式显示胰管的一种较好的方法。⑤对于十二指肠和胆胰管下端的观察，经内镜逆行胆胰管造影可提供更有价值的资料。⑥能直接对胆胰管下端狭窄和胆总管结石进行治疗。因此，它对胆汁淤滞的临床诊断和治疗两方面起着桥梁的作用。随着诊断技术和仪器的进步，经内镜逆行胆胰管造影的成功率比较稳定地提高到 95% 以上。

经皮肝穿刺胆系造影：有学者提出经皮肝穿刺胆系造影对非扩张型胆管梗阻的显示率为 82%~95%，与普通超声和传统 CT 相反，经皮肝穿刺胆系造影对梗阻的部位和原因的发现相当敏感。一些作者对 9 例本症病例进行了经皮肝穿刺胆系造影观察，发现非嵌顿结石位于胆总管远端造成部分梗阻 1 例、先天性胆总管囊肿十二指肠脱垂部内结石引起梗阻者 1 例、因胆总管远端漏斗改变和狭窄而提示胰腺炎者 1 例、由于肝内转移性病变而造成肝内胆管压迫和变形 2 例、因肝门部的转移性病灶而造成胆总管的外压性变形 4 例。该作者提出经皮肝穿刺胆系造影在下列三方面对诊断潜在性梗阻有作用：①梗阻性和非梗阻性黄疸的鉴别；②确定梗阻性病变的部位和原因；③确立手术的可能性。

一些作者在对比了超声、CT 和经皮肝穿刺胆系造影对本症的诊断作用后指出：经皮肝穿刺胆系造影能证实非扩张型胆管梗阻性黄疸的大多数病例，普通超声和 CT 尽管对于观察扩张型胆管有较高的敏感性，却不能证实非扩张胆管梗阻的部位和原因，容易导致此类病人的误诊。而经皮肝穿刺胆系造影对证实此类病例有较高的准确性。

另有作者提出，一般来说，经皮肝穿刺胆系造影对于揭示胆管梗阻的成功率几乎达 100%，穿刺进入正常大小的胆管的成功率为 50%~90%。但采用经皮肝穿刺胆系造影的病例中有 31% 出现并发症，其中 10% 为严重的并发症。

经皮肝穿刺胆系造影的采用受到下列因素的限制：①出血及过敏体质、败血症、严重黄疸、贫血和剧烈的疼痛等；②仅能显示胆管树，限制了对胰腺和胆胰管下端的确切诊断；③由于穿刺处的胆汁漏出，必要时须采取紧急手术；④为了诊断性胆管造影和继之的引流术，常需多次穿刺肝脏。

胆囊穿刺胆管造影：一些学者报导 20 例用胆囊穿刺胆管造影作检查方法的病例中，15 例在普通超声和 CT 检查中表现为正常形态的胆管，5 例为部分性胆总管梗阻。他提出对于临床怀疑梗阻性黄疸的病例，用经皮肝穿刺胆系造影和经内镜逆行胆胰管造影对显示胆管为一有价值的检查方法，但它必须由一熟练的内窥镜医生掌握，而且在上消化道因手术而致正常解剖改变时，常难以施行。

经皮肝穿刺胆系造影可以对所有扩张胆管显示，然而，在非扩张性胆管的显示率为 36%~90%。加之经皮肝穿刺胆系造影较高的失败率，可能需时间较长，而且需多次穿刺肝门部肝脏，因为这里的胆管较肝内胆管大。该作者认为，经肝进行胆管造影和减压与经胆囊穿刺胆管造影比较，前者技术上困难得多，而且需冒更大风险。胆囊穿刺胆管造影还可用于对正常和接近正常的肝内胆管经肝减压后的持续性造影。

MRI：在胆系的 MRI 检查中，胆囊内胆汁的 MR 信号与胆汁的浓度有关：禁食或空腹时，胆汁内富含胆酸、胆固醇和磷脂，水含量相对低，故在 T_1WI 中呈高信号；进食后，由于胆囊浓缩胆汁排空，大量低浓度的肝胆汁进入胆囊，致胆汁浓度降低，在 T_1WI 中表现为低信号。Hricak 等曾测量浓缩胆汁的 T_1 值为 94ms，而稀释胆汁的 T_1 值长达 2646ms。

肝细胞分泌的‘新鲜’肝胆汁进入胆囊后，因其比重较低，悬浮于残留浓缩胆囊胆汁上，T_1WI 可见胆囊内分层现象：上层胆汁浓度低，呈低信号；下层浓度高，呈明显高信号。

MRI 对肝内胆管的显示与所用的脉冲序列及肝胆汁的信号特征有关：①在常规 SE 序列中，肝胆汁由于未经浓缩过程故浓度较低，因此，肝内胆管在 MRI 的 T_1WI 中表现为低信号，与同样低信号的肝内血管不易区分；T_2WI 成像时，因肝内胆管较细小，与肝组织间产生部分容积效应而不易显示。但有肝内胆管扩张时，肝内胆管在 T_2WI 中则呈明显条索状或圆形高信号，很容易与低信号的血管区分。②MRCP 能清楚显示肝内胆管的分支，表现为树枝状高信号。MRI在显示和测量肝外胆管方面，因不同的加权序列，其测量值可出现一定的差异。Spritzer等利用MRI测量一组正常人总胆管的宽度，在T_1WI中，总胆管宽度为10mm，但在T_2WI中却达11.8mm。产生上述差别的原因可能有二：一是由于脉冲序列的不同，使肝外胆管与周围组织的对比度不同；二是不同脉冲序列图像的畸变效应不同。

第四节　梗阻性黄疸和门静脉钙化

门静脉的海绵状血管瘤变性时，在栓塞之中常可发现钙化，然而，此类钙化甚为轻微。一般只见于病理标本检查中，偶尔活体X线照片也有个别可以见到。诸如Haddow，Kemp-Harper（1967），Blendis等（1968），Losowky，Walker（1968）等学者报告所载。

Mackenzie等（1978）报告2例门静脉钙化伴存梗阻性黄疸的病人，为寻找梗阻性黄疸的病因，进行一系列影像学检查，发现肝外胆管为钙化的海绵状血管瘤所压迫，导致黄疸。

第五节　假性肝外胆管梗阻

Taylor等（1982）报告3例急性腹痛患者在^{99m}Tc-PIPIDA肝胆核素显像时，提示为部分总胆管梗阻，其中2例手术，1例为急性阑尾炎继发回肠末端梗死，2例胆管胆囊均无异常；第3例为吗啡治疗（吗啡可增加胆管内胆汁压，引起胆胰管下端括约肌收缩）。均为假性肝外胆管梗阻。

所有3例病人在核素显像前皆曾应用meperidine（一种麻醉镇痛剂），该作者认为，急腹症或给予吗啡或应用meperidine，能使扫描图像表现为总胆管远端部分性梗阻，而胆囊胆管均无病变。肝胆核素显像对胆系疾病（急性胆囊炎等）的诊断及鉴别诊断是高度敏感，特异性甚好，可发现肝管及胆管部分梗阻，而且可确定梗阻平面。扫描的结果仰赖于胆管实际大小与其内核素的浓度，已有报告核素浓度增加也可造成胆管假阳性扩张。

第六节　肝细胞性肝癌合并胆管癌栓

发病机制：肝细胞性肝癌引起阻塞性黄疸的原因有：肝细胞性肝癌侵犯胆系，导致胆管癌栓；转移淋巴结压迫肝外胆管；肿瘤引起胆系出血，形成胆管内凝血块；肿瘤广泛侵犯肝脏。肝细胞性肝癌合并胆管癌栓在临床上较为少见，胆管癌栓主要是由于肝内肿瘤直接侵入胆管，胆管内充满肿瘤组织，从而形成胆管内癌栓。侵入胆管的肿瘤可发生溃破，胆管内癌栓组织与原发灶脱离，胆管内癌栓组织下行至肝外胆管引起梗阻性黄疸。

临床表现：肝细胞性肝癌合并胆管癌栓患者通常在早期无特殊临床症状或体征，仅仅在胆管内癌栓延伸至肝总管或胆总管时才会出现阻塞性黄疸。实验室检查主要是甲胎蛋白及总胆红素升高。由于此类患者的临床缺乏特征性，发生率低以及对该病的临床、影像表现认识不足，不易与其他原因导致的阻塞性黄疸鉴别，因而此类患者很难在术前获得准确的诊断，常被误诊为胆管癌、胆系出血、胆管结石等。

影像学研究：肝内肿瘤较小可能是该种类型肝细胞性肝癌的一个特征。有些病例由于原发癌很小，即使手术探查肝表面亦不易触及到癌肿结节，仅有胆管癌栓所致的阻塞性黄疸的表现。胆管癌栓是其唯一的临床表现。因此仔细寻找肝内肿瘤灶对准确诊断该病及手术方案的选择非常重要。在Peng等（2005）报道的53例合并胆管癌栓的肝细胞性肝癌直径为（5.0 ± 2.6）cm，其中有7例未能发现肝内肿瘤，有25例肝细胞性肝癌的肿瘤直径 <5 cm。Yeh等（2004）也发现合并胆管癌栓的肝细胞性肝癌

的肿瘤直径为(3.8±2.1)cm，较不合并胆管癌栓的肝细胞性肝癌小，其可达(6.7±4.6)cm(P<0.05)。

一项9例研究结果显示合并胆管癌栓的肝细胞性肝癌具有典型的CT表现。在平扫呈低或等密度改变，在动态增强扫描时由于肿瘤由肝动脉及门静脉双重供血，增强后动脉期可见早期强化，门静脉期持续强化，而平衡期对比剂开始退出。

在Tseng等(2001)报道的13例合并阻塞性黄疸的肝细胞性肝癌中也发现，在MRI上有6例肝内肿瘤在动脉期强化，而且在平衡期所有肿瘤均呈低信号改变。在病理组织学上合并胆管癌栓的肝细胞性肝癌与不合并胆管癌栓的肝细胞性肝癌并无不同，均以低分化肝细胞性肝癌为主，可呈膨胀性生长或浸润性生长，可有包膜或无包膜。

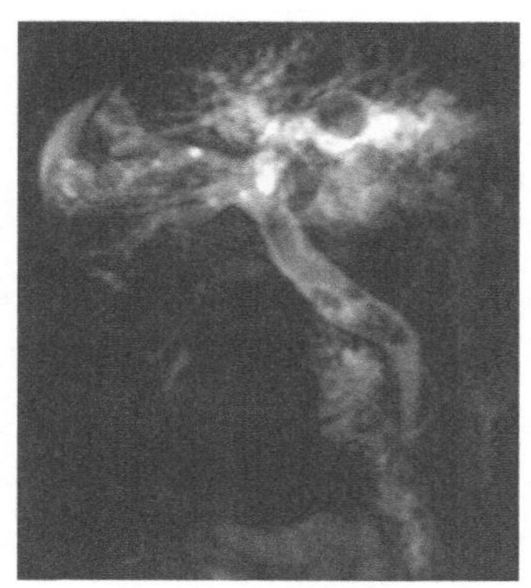

图16-2-2　ERCP：手术病理证实肝癌侵犯胆管

胆管内癌栓在CT上表现为胆管内软组织块影，梗阻上方胆管扩张。胆管内软组织块可与肝细胞性肝癌病灶相连或不相连。CT平扫为低密度或等密度。动脉期癌栓有不同程度强化(CT值增加约10~20 HU)，癌栓与周围正常肝实质比较可呈高、等或低密度改变，提示胆管癌栓有动脉参与供血，其供血动脉的来源可能是与肝内肿瘤相连的胆管癌栓通过供养肝内肿瘤的肝动脉同时滋养癌栓，而不与肝内肿瘤相连的胆管癌栓通过胆管壁上的滋养血管进行供血(肝动脉终末分支形成的胆管周围血管丛或支配肝外胆管壁的肝总动脉分支)。Gabata等(2007)报道的6例胆管癌栓也发现类似现象，6例癌栓在MRI动态增强的早期均见强化(图16-2-2)。

Jung等(2006)报道的14例胆管癌栓在CT增强的动脉期均见癌栓早期强化。因而早期强化是胆管癌栓的一个重要特征。该组5例癌栓在延迟期扫描上均呈低密度，无延迟强化表现，而胆管癌在延迟扫描上为轻度或明显强化，密度高于周围正常肝实质，这可能是与胆管癌的重要鉴别要点。

门静脉癌栓是肝细胞性肝癌晚期的重要合并症和转移方式，是肝细胞性肝癌肝内扩散最主要的形式。尽早明确门静脉癌栓的存在对肝细胞性肝癌的分期、选择适当的治疗方法和估计预后具有重要意义。由于门静脉及胆管被包绕在同一格氏鞘内，胆管癌栓很容易压迫或侵犯门静脉分支，胆管癌栓也可以是由于邻近的门静脉癌栓的侵犯所致。

肝细胞性肝癌合并胆管癌栓患者同时合并有门静脉癌栓的发生率学者报道不一。Gabata等(2007)报道的6例肝细胞性肝癌合并胆管癌栓的病例中有5例合并门静脉癌栓。而在Peng等(2005)报道的53例胆管癌栓的病例中仅有3例合并门静脉癌栓。在该组的9例患者中发现2例同时合并有门静脉癌栓。因而在诊断肝细胞性肝癌时要全面观察图像，以免造成胆管癌栓或门静脉癌栓的漏诊或误诊。

单纯门静脉癌栓一般不伴有胆管扩张，在伴有胆管扩张的病例中应该注意是否合并有胆管癌栓。胆管癌栓与门静脉癌栓不同，前者通过切除肝内肿瘤、清除胆管癌栓等手术治疗或进行综合治疗可获得较好的疗效，症状可得到缓解，能延长生存期，因而早期及准确诊断该类型肝细胞性肝癌非常重要；后者则提示全身性转移，预后较差，因为癌细胞随时都能脱落而向全身散播(图16-2-3)。

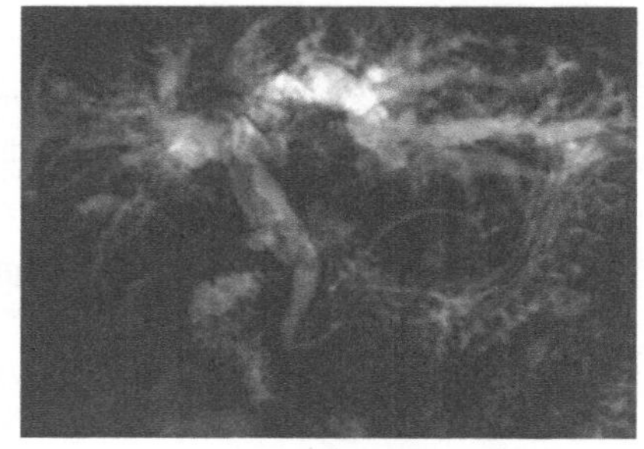

图16-2-3　ERCP：手术病理证实肝癌侵犯胆管↑

胆管癌栓易误诊为胆管结石、胆系出血、肝门部转移淋巴结、胆管癌。但肝细胞性肝癌合并胆管癌栓表现为胆管内软组织块影，呈条索状或柱状，胆管远段扩张，在动脉期胆管癌栓早期强化，同时肝实质内有肝肿瘤病灶，不难与胆管结石、胆系出血及肝门部转移淋巴结鉴别。

胆管癌一般容易侵犯胆管壁,并向壁外生长,肝内可见部分胆管扩张。在CT上胆管癌呈现“慢进慢出”的强化特点,延迟像上大部分肿瘤为可轻度或明显强化,呈相对高密度改变,密度高于周围正常肝实质,与典型肝细胞性肝癌的“快进快出”的强化方式明显不同,而且胆管内癌栓出现动脉早期强化,无延迟强化表现,胆管癌栓不侵犯胆管壁,胆管壁无增厚,这些是肝细胞性肝癌合并胆管癌栓与胆管癌的鉴别要点。但如果肝内的肿瘤很小,影像检查未能发现肝内病灶,仅仅有胆管癌栓的表现,则很难与息肉状生长的胆管癌鉴别。

总之,肝细胞性肝癌患者如合并出现阻塞性黄疸,应仔细寻找阻塞性黄疸的原因,注意除外有无合并胆管癌栓。肝细胞性肝癌合并胆管癌栓的CT表现具有一定的特征性,表现为肝内出现典型肝细胞性肝癌病灶,胆管内出现软组织块影,远端胆管扩张,胆管内癌栓动脉早期出现强化,无延迟强化表现。

第七节　误诊病例简介:胆管黏液性乳头状腺癌

一些作者认为,大量黏液充填在肝胆管内造成胆管梗阻扩张称为黏胆症。

一例胆管黏液性乳头状腺癌,在手术前未能做出正确诊断,其原因是肿瘤本身较小,影像检查中MRI、MRCP虽然发现胆总管扩张,但其中又未见明显软组织块影,胆总管下端没有发现可能梗阻物。

ERCP、经皮肝胆管造影(PTC)可见胆管腔内因大量黏液所形成的腔内边缘模糊的充盈缺损影。该例MRCP上左侧肝管支上端形态不规则,提示有渐进性的内压增高征象所致可能。ERCP检查虽在胆总管中上段发现有巨大充盈缺损影,但没有在内镜下发现有黏液从十二指肠乳头溢出,所以也未能做出准确诊断。

CT检查虽然从多方位看到了扩张的胆管,但没有能发现较小的肿瘤病灶,测量扩张胆管内的黏液和淤积的胆汁CT值相差无几,不能分辨肿瘤分泌的黏液或受阻的胆汁。

回顾分析该病例,如综合诸多影像检查未能确定胆总管内有新生物或结石而有胆总管扩张、出现梗阻性黄疸、胆管炎症表现时,应想到胆管黏液性乳头状腺癌引起黏胆症的可能。

本病还应注意结合临床情况与胆管内血块、胆管结石、胆管癌等病鉴别。

第八节　继发性肝内胆汁淤滞

胆管结石、慢性胆管炎、胆管结石术后是最常见病因。各种影像学检查都可以看到肝内外胆管的原发病变和继发的胆管扩张,病理表现为肝内外胆管狭窄,管壁弥漫性增厚、硬韧、呈条索状,病理诊断为慢性炎症,即继发性硬化性胆管炎。该病容易诊断,但肝实质纤维化和肝硬化的征象不容忽视。MRI对该病具有良好的应用和研究前景。

第九节　黏胆症

详见本书 本卷 第十五篇 第一章 第五节　黏胆症。

第三章　良、恶性胆管梗阻的鉴别

第一节　MRI、超声、CT对胆系良、恶性梗阻鉴别诊断的对比研究

相对良、恶性征象标准：较具特征性的良性征象有胆管腔内结石等；较具特征性的恶性征象有腔内外实性软组织肿块、淋巴结肿大等。

比较影像学：胆管梗阻性病变是临床、尤其是普外科常见病，在其良、恶性发病率中良性（尤其是胆系结石）占绝大多数，恶性仅占少数；因此，临床诊断中定性诊断的主要问题，是如何提高从良性中筛选出恶性病例的灵敏度，以及如何提高排除恶性的可信度。

诊断的依据除病史、体征、实验室检查等临床资料外，影像学检查已成为不可替代的主要方法。胆系的非侵入性影像学检查方法过去主要为超声，近来应用较多者有CT、MRI。

超声对梗阻定位的准确率较高，超声对胆囊和肝内胆管以及部分肝门区胆管结石诊断的敏感度、特异度均高；但超声因组织分辨率较低，对梗阻区域、尤其是肝外胆管下段的病变征象，如胆胰区肿块、邻近肠腔含气情况下胆总管下段或吻合口区结石、淋巴结肿大等往往分辨不清，故常不能做恶性肿瘤的定性诊断。

CT、MRI均有较高密度/信号分辨率，对梗阻定性具有较高价值。CT虽然对胰腺区肿块、淋巴结肿大等征象显示的敏感度与MRI近似，但对胆管结石的密度分辨率明显低于超声和MRI，对肝门区肿块的显示亦略低于MRI。

常规MRI T_1WI、T_2WI具有良好的信号对比，对病变组织和正常组织均有较高分辨力，可直接显示梗阻区软组织情况、可较好地显示肿块，对鉴别诊断很有帮助。

MRCP因其成像效果类似直接胆系造影，可直观显示胆胰管树的二维、三维解剖结构及其病变形态，故与常规MRI结合检查，对良、恶性鉴别准确率更有提高。

虽然胆管梗阻性病变通过CT、超声可作定位诊断，但它们定性诊断的效能均不及常规MRI结合MRCP。由于常规MRI结合MRCP能提供较这些检查更为丰富可靠的诊断信息，越来越多的病例被作为常规检查。一些作者建议，对临床怀疑胆系疾病的无痛性黄疸患者可首选MRI。

ROC曲线和7级信度诊断法：良、恶性诊断标准采用7级信度法对病变良、恶性进行诊断。诊断标准见表16-3-1。

表16-3-1　7级信度诊断法

7级信度法	
1分	肯定良性
2分	良性可能性大；或多系良性
3分	可能良性
4分	良、恶性不能确定
5分	可能恶性；或不排除恶性
6分	恶性可能性大；或多系恶性
7分	肯定恶性

注：良、恶混合性病变，在最后诊断中归为恶性病变类

影像诊断系统由诊断试验（影像学方法）和试验者（诊断医师）组成。由于各种干扰因素的影响（如图像质量，成像参数的选择，仪器空间、密度分辨率的差异等），均可影响诊断效果，造成假阳性或假阴性。对每个诊断系统而言，诊断某种疾病采用不同的诊断标准均会有不同的假阳性或假阴性（以敏感度和特异度来评价）。

受试者操作特性曲线（ROC曲线）分析的本质就是动态分析、比较不同诊断试验在多个诊断界值

的条件下,其相对应的敏感度 - 特异度曲线的差异。在实际临床工作中,影像科诊断医师面临的往往是多种可能的诊断,以多等级法的形式进行影像学定性诊断已越来越多地得到使用。7 级信度法即属该范畴。

受试者操作特性曲线的评价指标为曲线下面积(Az 值)的比较。通过受试者操作特性曲线可确定该类方法诊断的最佳临界分值,最佳敏感度、特异度、准确率等效能指标,从而更客观、高效地诊断病变的性质。在研究中,该方法可用于比较 MRI 和超声、CT 在鉴别胆系良、恶性病变中的诊断效能,结果提示前者优于超声和 CT,且有显著性差异。

综上所述, MRI 是鉴别胆管梗阻性病变良、恶性的一种准确的非侵入性检查方法。与超声、CT 相比, MRI 更适用于排除胆管梗阻病人恶性占位性病变。

良、恶性低位梗阻性黄疸胆管扩张特点:肝内胆管扩张的形态及程度:呈软藤状的重度扩张是恶性梗阻的重要征象,而竹节状轻度扩张则为良性梗阻的征象。

肝内、外胆管扩张是否成比例:肝内胆管扩张较轻,而肝外胆管扩张相对明显的内轻外重的征象提示良性梗阻;恶性梗阻胆道系统多成比例的扩张。

梗阻端肝外胆管壁的改变:肝外胆管壁弥漫环形增厚为良性梗阻较为可靠的征象,是由于肝外胆管壁炎性肥厚和纤维化所致。肝外胆管壁局部偏环形增厚,是肿瘤直接侵犯的可靠征象。

梗阻端肝外胆管形态的变化:恶性低位梗阻近梗阻端肝外胆管扩张明显且突然中断;良性低位梗阻则肝外胆管扩张较轻且逐渐变细后中断。

肝外胆管梗阻端的表现:梗阻端病变无强化,特别是“新月征”和“靶征”的出现是结石的特征,胆囊及肝内胆管内是否有结石有重要参考价值。肝外胆管炎性狭窄,胆管扩张较轻,肝外胆管逐渐变细呈漏斗状,管腔内外无软组织肿块,增强扫描管壁环状均匀强化,壁厚不超过 5 mm。而恶性低位梗阻可见肝外胆管腔内外软组织肿块,有强化,具有特征性。

第二节　胆管扩张的研究

良性与恶性疾病的胆管扩张程度:胆管扩张程度对良、恶性疾病的鉴别诊断也是临床上非常重要的问题。目前对不同性质梗阻所致的阻塞端形态特点已经有了比较一致的看法。但是对良、恶性梗阻所致的胆管扩张,在程度上究竟有无差别,还存在着不同的观点。

有作者认为胆管的扩张程度和阻塞的病因之间没有相互关系,肝内外胆管的扩张程度不是鉴别良、恶性梗阻的可靠征像。Suhod 用超声检查了 14 例肝外胆管结石病人,发现肝外胆管的平均直径为 15.1 mm,而 16 例胰腺癌所致的肝外胆管阻塞病人的肝外胆管平均直径为 15.7mm,他认为良、恶性梗阻所致的胆管扩张在程度上无差别,大多数作者认为良、恶性梗阻在肝肿大、胆囊肿大、肝内外胆管扩张程度上存在差异。一般良性病变多表现为胆管轻度扩张,而恶性病变则表现为胆管重度扩张。Sachs 观察到胰腺癌引起的胆管扩张可达 30mm,腔内压力超过 5.88 kPa。反之胰腺炎引起的胆管扩张一般在 20mm 以下,腔内压力在 2.45~5.88 kPa 水柱之间。

胆管扩张是胆管梗阻的反映,不同性质的病变引起不同程度的胆管扩张,说明梗阻程度和病因之间有一定的关系。一般良性病变多造成胆管轻度的不完全性梗阻,有缓解时机。在临床上可看到,结石一般不引起胆管完全性梗阻,造影时可见对比剂从结石周围包绕而过,呈分流征。肝外胆管结石病人的血中胆红素浓度是轻度升高,而且有波动,同时黄疸也是间歇性的。对这种间歇性不完全阻塞,大多数作者认为,是结石的球瓣效应造成的。

胆总管末端的结构特点是球瓣效应产生的解剖学基础。胆总管上段的壁较薄,由疏松结缔组织、弹力纤维和稀少分散的平滑肌构成。在胆总管末端接近十二指肠处,管壁的环形平滑肌突然增多,增厚,形成了一个完整的肌层包绕着胆总管。同时管壁的结缔组织和黏膜腺体也增加,使胆总管末端管壁增厚,增厚的环形肌延续到乳头,形成了胆总管末端括约肌。这种管壁突然增厚引起了管腔的骤然变窄,因此上段胆总管与胆总管末端的连接是骤然的,没有逐渐延续过程。结石往往不能通过这个管腔突然狭窄处,从而形成了球瓣形间歇性阻塞。

恶性病变如胆胰管连接区癌、胰腺癌、胆管癌等，其生长方式是进行性包裹和阻塞胆管。因此造成的梗阻多是渐进性的、完全性的，没有缓解时机。

胆管梗阻时，胆管内的压力升高。根据 Laplas 定律，肝内、外胆管对这种压力升高的反应程度是不同的。轻度阻塞的情况下，可能只发生肝外胆管扩张，或伴有轻度肝内胆管扩张。而重度阻塞，胆管内的压力可使肝内、外胆管都发生显著扩张。因此肝内胆管的扩张程度对于鉴别良、恶性疾病比肝外胆管扩张程度更可靠。

胆管扩张与超声诊断结石；Einstein 等（1984）分析了 138 例胆总管结石指出：肝外胆管扩张者 25% 超声能作出明确的诊断，而对肝外胆管不扩张的结石的诊断率仅为 12%。究其原因可能是：气体常使胆总管显示不清；肝外胆管不扩张；在结石周围需要一定量的胆汁将其衬托出来，超声才能有良好的对比，而胆管未扩张者这种衬托不佳；弯曲的胆管壁引起的声束的反射及折射干扰；胆总管可能在高频换能器需要显示结石的最佳焦点区以外等诸多因素，影响了对结石的诊断。该作者由此认为，超声对胆总管结石的诊断的敏感性较差。

胆管阻塞时肝内外胆管的非一致性扩张：近年来许多学者注意到，在早期和部分阻塞情况下，肝内、外胆管并非同时产生扩张的，肝外胆管可在肝内胆管扩张前就已发生扩张。这种现象目前有两种解释，一种认为是肝实质纤维化或肝内胆管炎使管壁纤维化，弹性降低，造成肝内胆管在早期和部分阻塞的情况下不扩张。这种解释显然是不够全面的，因为在有些肝内胆管不扩张的病例，并没有肝实质纤维化或肝内胆管炎发生。

大多数作者认为生理学上的 Laplas 定律可以应用于胆系，解释胆管阻塞时肝内、外胆管的非一致性扩张。根据 Laplas 定律，在圆柱体内流体的扩张力（F），与管内压力（P）、管腔直径（D）、管道长度（L）成正比，即 $F = PDL$。对于一定的压力，管腔的直径越大，所受的扩张力存在着一个梯度差，最大的扩张力将作用在肝外胆管而不是肝内胆管。当肝外胆管发生阻塞时，胆系内流体静压升高，肝外胆管将首先发生扩张，随着梗阻加重，腔内流体静压继续升高，肝内胆管最后才发生扩张。

动物实验证实，胆管阻塞发生后，整个胆系内不是同时发生扩张的。胆囊、胆总管在阻塞 24 小时后就发生扩张；而肝内胆管在阻塞一周后才发生扩张。由此可以看出，肝内外胆管对诊断胆管阻塞的作用是不同的。

肝外胆管扩张是诊断胆管阻塞的灵敏指标，在阻塞的早期就可表现出来。肝内胆管对诊断胆管阻塞，虽然缺乏灵敏性，但准确性高，肝内胆管扩张了，说明胆管肯定有阻塞，但目前关于肝内胆管各分支的管径正常值研究还很少。

第四章 胆管囊肿

第一节 肝外胆管憩室(Ⅱ型肝外胆管囊肿)

Ⅱ型肝外胆管囊肿是肝外胆管的先天性憩室,通常从它的侧壁凸出。这是一种少见的先天性异常,可在儿童及成人做出诊断。类似的憩室可出现于右肝内胆管主干的外侧缘。

临床表现:可为疼痛伴可扪及包块,也可为无任何症状。如同Ⅰ型肝外胆管囊肿,门静脉受囊肿挤压可导致门脉高压和静脉曲张。肝的酶学检查值可以升高,但少见出现黄疸。手术处理是通常的治疗方法。此憩室有纤维性壁,内衬以扁平的和萎缩的胆管上皮细胞。

影像学研究:超声可发现肝外胆管憩室为一透声性包块,邻接于肝外胆管或右肝管主干。连接囊肿与胆管的颈部实际上很难描绘出来。结石和胆泥可存在于憩室内。

由于肝外胆管憩室的颈可能不开放,直接法胆管造影与放射性核素肝胆显像可能充盈憩室,也可能未能充盈憩室。当憩室未显影时,在胆管造影时它可表现为邻近胆管的一个原因不明的圆形的光滑的外在性压迫。在普通CT,因为只有横断面表现的限制,在CT图像上区别肝外胆管憩室与肝囊肿或胆囊有一定困难。在MRCP和/或MSCT三维重建的图像上,则可清楚观察憩室与肝外胆管的关系。

少见的感染的肝外胆管憩室在临床上和影像学上的表现都颇似新生物。此类低度的慢性炎症,产生一个炎性包块可伪似肝外胆管癌,甚至在手术时也出现误诊。

第二节 总胆管壁内囊肿

总胆管壁内囊肿,又称为总胆管憩室、十二指肠内胆管囊肿、Vater乳头囊肿、十二指肠肠源性囊肿、十二指肠重复囊肿、Ⅲ型肝外胆管囊肿、总胆管壁内憩室、总胆管壁内膨出、总胆管壁内囊泡等,是一极为少见的、容易漏诊的、原因不明的先天性异常。类似于输尿管壁内囊肿,总胆管壁内囊肿是扩张的壁内段总胆管突出于十二指肠内。

病因学:十二指肠乳头炎症反应伴存壁内段胆管的梗阻性膨出;先天性十二指肠重复性囊肿接纳胆胰共同管;总胆管壁内段的胆管囊肿;先天性总胆管憩室。

病理学:总胆管壁内囊肿为胆汁充盈,且附着于胆胰管十二指肠连接区的十二指肠的后壁或后内壁。常可见到结石或胆泥。在影像学表现与手术所见方面可分成两种解剖学类型。一为总胆管终止于总胆管壁内囊肿内,在其壁内途经一个孔隙引流进入十二指肠,主胰管也可排空于总胆管壁内囊肿内。另一型是当总胆管壁内囊肿途经总胆管充盈和排空,而总胆管经正常乳头引流进入十二指肠,主胰管通常进入总胆管壁内囊肿的近侧总胆管内。

组织学上,总胆管壁内囊肿的外表面覆盖着十二指肠黏膜,内表面衬以十二指肠的、胆系的或非特异性肠上皮。

临床表现:总胆管壁内囊肿能出现于儿童或成人。长期的上腹疼痛、恶心、呕吐是最常见的临床表现。常见胆绞痛、发作性黄疸和胰腺炎。此类先天异常也可以是偶尔的意外发现。

影像学研究:十二指肠造影可见一边界清楚的

光滑的充盈缺损，凸出于腔内，或是宽基底，或是窄基底与带蒂。典型者，挤压或蠕动可使总胆管壁内囊肿形状发生改变。钡餐检查时，与腔内憩室相对比，总胆管壁内囊肿中不为钡剂所充盈。在静脉法胆系造影时，大多数总胆管壁内囊肿都可为对比剂充盈，然而征象可能是非特异性的，即总胆管扩张伴排泄延迟，甚或正常。直接法胆系造影观察总胆管壁内囊肿最好，可见它为总胆管壁内段的囊袋状扩张。对于显示总胆管壁内囊肿的薄壁，和除外肿瘤作为梗阻的原因，十二指肠的同时显影很重要。

超声成像、CT 扫描与放射性核素检查对于诊断总胆管壁内囊肿有一定困难。

第三节　先天性肝内胆管囊肿

详见本书 本卷 本篇 第九章 先天性肝内胆管囊肿。

第四节　胆总管囊肿破裂

胆总管囊肿，又称先天性胆总管扩张症，为临床上最常见的一种先天性胆总管畸形，其主要病理改变是胆总管的一部分呈囊状或梭状扩张，有时可伴有肝内胆管扩张。Vater（1793）首次报道 1 例胆总管囊肿病例。

临床分型目前采用日本学者户谷 Todani 分类方法，即分 5 型：Ⅰ型占 80%~90%，胆总管呈囊状或梭状扩张；Ⅱ型占 2%，胆总管形成单发憩室；Ⅲ型占 1.4%~5%，壁内段胆总管囊状膨出；Ⅳ型占 19%，为多发性胆管囊肿，位于肝外和肝内，或肝外多发；Ⅴ型为肝内胆管扩张，又称 Caroli 病。胆总管囊肿多见于女性，男女之比为 1:（3~4），婴幼儿多见，占 50%~80%。

临床主要表现为黄疸、腹痛、上腹部包块，婴幼儿以黄疸最常见，成年患者自幼出现间歇性发热、黄疸，部分在体检或其他疾病行 US 或 CT 检查时发现。成人胆总管囊肿易恶变，或合并其他消化道肿瘤。

胆总管囊肿破裂发生率低，但可导致严重并发症，如感染性休克。Yamaguchi（1980）分析 1 433 例胆总管囊肿病人，发现 26 例发生穿孔致胆汁性腹膜炎（占 1.8%），胆总管囊肿破裂原因包括外伤、腹内压增高（如呕吐、胆总管远段梗阻、妊娠等）、持续性胰液返流等，其原因不十分明确。术前诊断比较困难，Ando 等（1998）分析 13 例胆总管破裂术前正确诊断率只有 5 例（占 38%）。

Gan 等（2003）报道 1 例Ⅰ型胆总管囊肿破裂，认为 CT 上不仅清楚显示胆总管囊肿，而且可显示胆总管囊肿破裂缺口和囊肿周围胆汁漏出形成的积液，胆总管囊肿和囊肿周围积液显示为双腔影。另有作者报告一例为Ⅰ型胆总管囊肿破裂，破裂口显示模糊（考虑与 CT 扫描层厚较厚有关），并见胆总管囊肿和囊肿周围积液形成的双腔影。

CT 可作为胆总管囊肿破裂的有效检查方法，但需要与急性胰腺炎、后腹膜囊性肿瘤、胰腺囊肿等疾病鉴别。

第五章 胆管肿块

第一节 假胆管癌征

Bayraktar 等(1992)报道了内窥镜逆行性胆胰管造影(ERCP)检查时所见的“假胆管癌征”,是由于扩张、迂曲的胆管周围静脉压迫胆管,造成胆管狭窄,出现梗阻性黄疸。因此,在门脉海绵样变时出现梗阻性黄疸应想到此征。

第二节 原发性肝癌侵犯胆管

详见本书 本卷 第三篇 第十一章 第三节 肝细胞癌侵犯胆管。

第三节 肝细胞性肝癌伴有胆管癌栓

详见本书 本卷 第三篇 第十一章 第一节 肝细胞性肝癌伴有胆管癌栓。

第六章　肝内胆管细胞癌①

第一节　误诊病例简介:肝内胆管细胞癌与肝脓肿

患者,男，64 岁。右上腹疼痛不适 10 天入院。门诊彩色超声考虑结石性胆囊炎,门诊以胆囊结石伴胆囊炎收治住院。CT:肝胆脾 CT 平扫 + 增强:肝内可见多个类圆形稍低密度影,部分融合，CT 值 26HU,边界不清,周围见环状稍低密度影，CT 值 47HU;增强后病灶边缘强化,呈分隔状改变,边界不清,肝内胆管无扩张,肝门结构无异常;胆囊不大,壁厚,边缘模糊,内见多发结节状高密度影。CT 诊断:肝内多发占位病变,考虑肝脓肿,建议治疗后复查;胆囊结石,胆囊炎。

6 天后行彩色超声引导下肝脏穿刺引流术:通过正常肝组织至彩超所示肝脏液化腔,回抽见浑浊脓性液体流出,抽取 10ml 送细菌培养 + 药敏。经穿刺针侧孔导入导引钢丝,退出穿刺针,沿导引钢丝插入扩张管,扩张皮肤及皮下组织,退出扩张管,沿导引钢丝送入肝脓肿脓腔留置导管,插入长度约 10cm,退出导引钢丝,回抽导管通畅,共计抽出脓液 50ml。

10 天后 CT:肝内可见多发斑片状低密度影,边界模糊,最大者位于左肝内叶,大小约 6cm × 6.2cm × 3.9cm,内见高密度引流管置入影,密度不均匀,少许积气，CT 值 3~27HU。胆囊体积不大,壁增厚,毛糙,见絮状低密度影,胆囊内见多发小结节状致密影,较大者直径 0.8cm。胆总管下段内见小斑片状高密度影,大小 0.3cm × 0.4cm，CT 值 111HU。CT 诊断:肝内多发脓肿,左肝内叶脓肿引流术后改变;胆囊多发结石,胆囊炎;胆总管下段结石。

18 天后手术所见:肝Ⅵ b、Ⅴ段一大小约 5cm × 6cm 白色不规则肿物,质地较硬,胆囊萎缩,部分网膜组织与肝Ⅵ b、Ⅴ段粘连,质地较硬,肝门部见多个肿大淋巴结,融合成团,与血管、胆管粘连紧密;余肝脏表面可见弥漫性结节影,最大结节位于肝左外叶,直径约 0.5cm。胃、十二指肠、小肠、胰腺、余结肠及直肠未见明显异常。

病理检查:冰冻病理与常规病理:肝左叶肿物切除标本:灰白色组织一块，大小 2.5cm × 1.5cm × 1.0cm,切面灰白质中。冰冻病理诊断:肝左叶肿物切除标本:肝组织中可见癌组织浸润,待做常规石蜡切片及免疫组化检测进一步确定癌肿类型。常规病理诊断:肝左叶肿物切除标本:肝组织中可见癌组织浸润,待做免疫组化检测进一步确定癌肿类型。

免疫组化诊断:肝左叶肿物切除标本示肝胆管细胞癌。

误诊病例回顾分析:CT 平扫见多发斑片状低密度影,边界模糊,用“肝脓肿”解释有一定困难;在 CT 增强扫描图像上可见“母灶”周围出现多发“子灶”,是典型的肿瘤及向周围播散的征象,可是却被忽略,未认真分析研究;肿瘤与胆囊相邻,且边界欠清楚,也未引起诊断医生的重视;思路较为狭窄,只想到肝脓肿,一点不留余地,也是一条教训。

① （请结合本书 本卷 第四篇 第一章 胆管细胞型肝癌研究）

第二节 肝内胆管细胞癌,累及大网膜组织

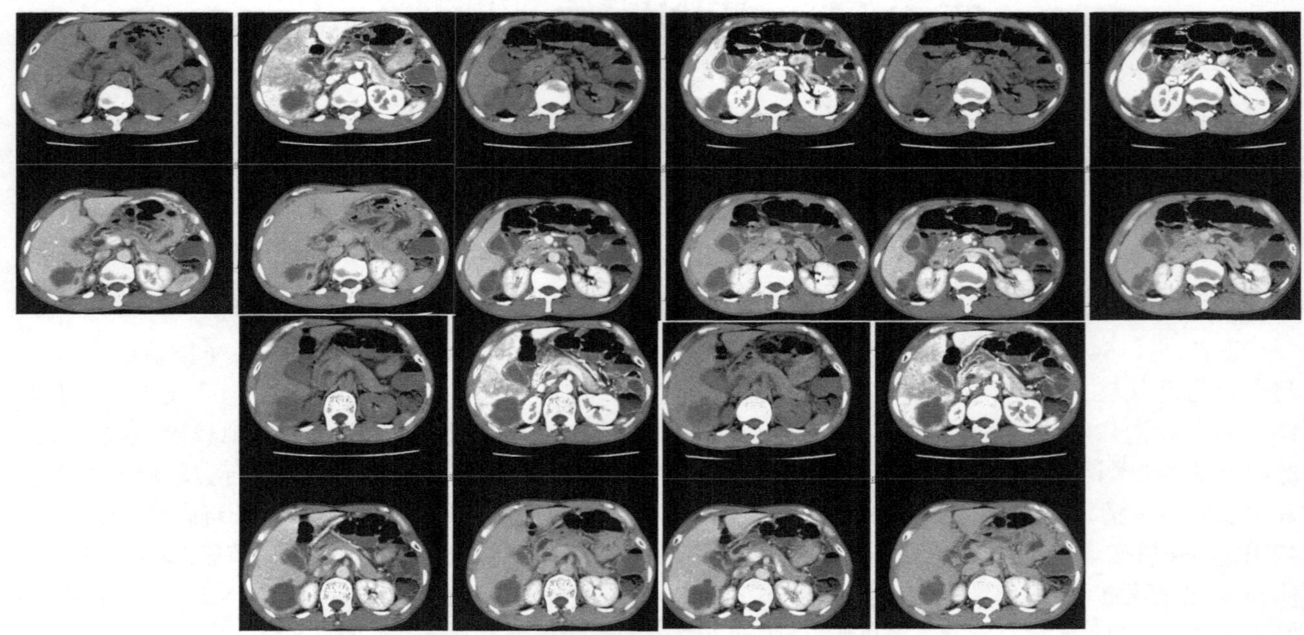

图 16-6-1 肝内胆管细胞癌,累及大网膜组织

患者,男,55 岁。上腹部闷痛 4 月余伴腹胀 7 天入院。

手术所见:腹腔内少量淡黄色腹水,大网膜及腹膜见多发散在结节,右肝后叶下端触及大小约为 4×4.5cm 肿物,质地软,边界不清。

病理检查:①肝组织:灰白灰褐色组织一块,大小 4.8cm×4.2cm×0.4cm,切面灰白灰褐,质中。②部分大网膜:网膜组织一堆,总体积 15cm× 13cm×2.5cm,其中散在分布多枚灰白色结节,直径 0.2cm~1.5cm,切面灰白,质中。免疫组化检测:①阳性:CA19-9,CK7,CK19,Villin(散在+),Ki-67(+,约 10%),CK(L),EMA,CK8,CK18,Vimentin;阴性:HBcAg,HBsAg。②阳性:CA19-9,CK7,CK19,Villin;阴性:CK20,CDX2。病理诊断:肝组织及部分大网膜标本:初步考虑胆管细胞癌,累及大网膜组织,待做免疫组化检测进一步明确诊断。免疫组化诊断示肝组织及部分大网膜标本:肝内胆管细胞癌,累及大网膜组织。注:肝组织及大网膜组织中的癌组织图像及免疫表型基本一致(图 16-6-1)。

第三节 肝细胞癌和肝内胆管细胞癌共存

有作者报道一组 6 例既有肝细胞癌又有肝内胆管细胞癌的混合癌。

在病理检查时,发现 3 例肿瘤显示肝细胞癌和肝内胆管细胞癌的成分密切混合;3 例肝细胞癌与肝内胆管细胞癌各有独立的块影,但二者是连续的。超声图像上肿瘤的回声或 CT 图像上肿瘤密度的差异与病理上肿瘤的不同组织无关。病理标本的肝细胞癌部分显示密集的碘油存留,而肝内胆管细胞癌部分则无密集的碘油存留。

临床表现:男性 5 例,女性 1 例,年龄 46~60 岁,平均 53 岁。6 例均有慢性肝炎。乙型肝炎表面抗原阳性 5 例,乙型肝炎表面抗体阳性 1 例,3 例甲胎蛋白异常(20~200μg/L),6 例癌胚抗原正常(<5μg/L),均有肝硬化。肿瘤最大径 0.9~7.5cm,平均 3.6cm。肿瘤位于肝右叶前段 3 例,肝右叶后段 2 例,肝左叶内段 1 例。

影像学研究:超声检查 6 例皆表现为圆形或椭圆形的低回声块影,其中央为高回声区(靶征)。5

例 CT 平扫,显示边界较清楚的低密度块影 1 例,低密度伴等密度块影 2 例,未显出块影 2 例; 5 例 CT 增强扫描,显示边界较清楚的低密度块影 2 例,低密度伴等密度块影 2 例, 1 例肿瘤最大径 9mm 者,未能显示。X 线血管造影 5 例中,显示少血管块影 4 例,其中 1 例中央为多血管区; 1 例 9mm 最大径者未能检出。碘油 CT 扫描,6 例均显示部分碘油在肿瘤内存留。肿瘤内碘油存留区与超声或常规 CT 表现无关。X 线血管造影发现肿瘤的多血管区显示密集的碘油存留,而肿瘤的少血管区也有一些碘油存留。

超声图像上的靶征, X 线血管造影表现为少血管块影内的多血管区,以及碘油 CT 图像显示肿瘤内碘油部分存留等影像学表现,有助于对这些罕见肿瘤做出正确诊断。

第四节　肝内混合型癌(肝细胞癌 - 胆管细胞癌)

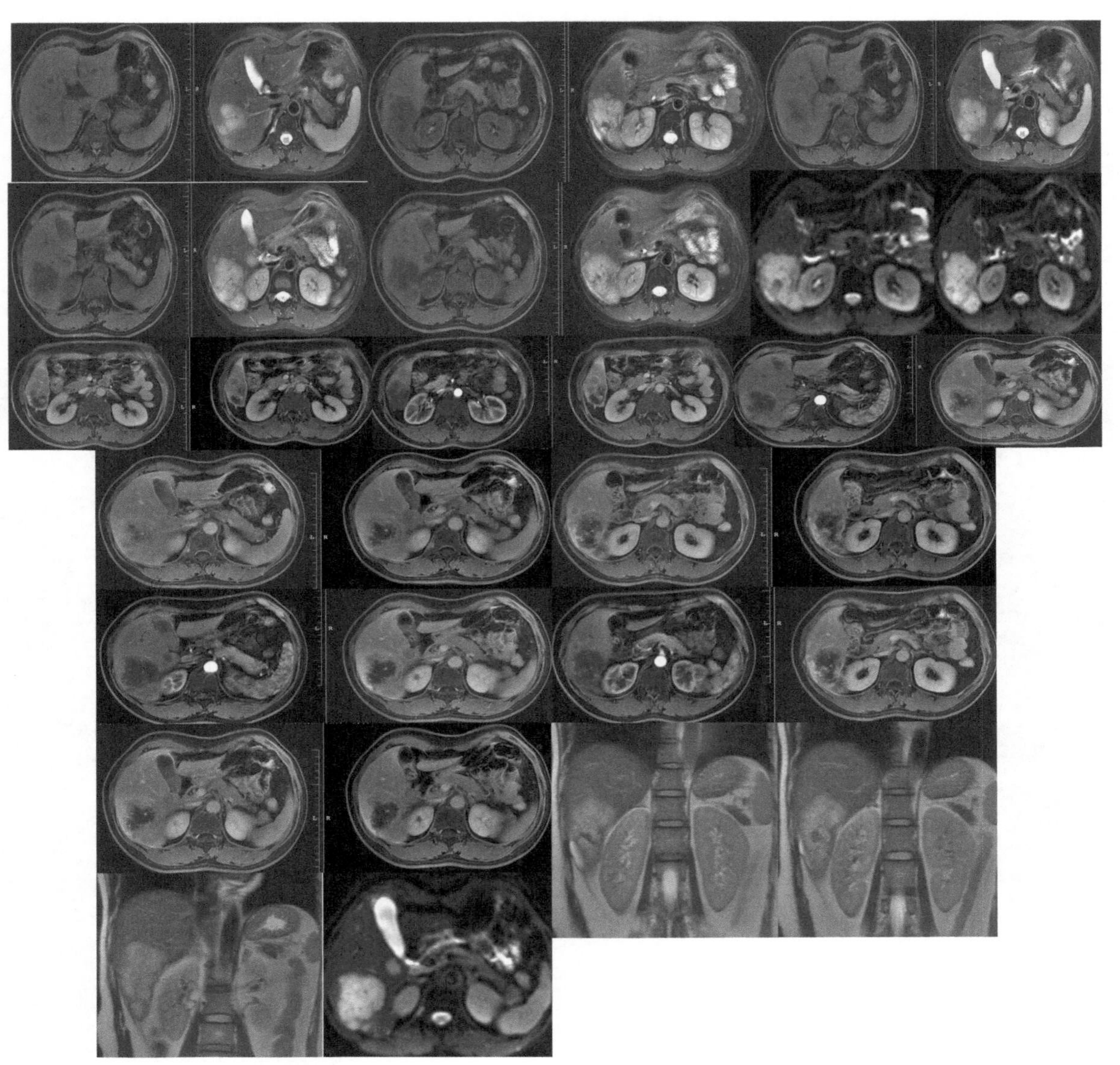

图 16-6-2　肝内混合型癌(肝细胞癌 - 胆管细胞癌)

患者，女，49 岁。

病理检查：冰冻病理：肝肿物：结节样肿物一块，大小 1.7cm × 1.5cm × 1.2cm，切面灰白，质中。冰冻病理诊断：肝肿物切除标本镜下示送检肝组织中可见癌组织浸润，待做常规石蜡切片及免疫组化检测进一步明确癌肿类型及探讨来源。常规病理诊断：肝肿物切除标本镜下示送检肝组织中可见癌组织浸润，伴坏死，待做免疫组化检测进一步明确癌肿类型及来源。

免疫组化检测：阳性：CK（L），CK18，CK19，CK7，CK8，CEA，CA19-9，Villin，Hepatocyte，CD31，CD34；阴性：CK20，AFP，TTF-1，Mucin-2，CDX-2。免疫组化诊断：肝肿物切除标本免疫组化结果支持肝内混合型癌（肝细胞癌 - 胆管细胞癌）。其他情况参见常规组织学报告。（图 16-6-2）

第五节　不同生长方式肝内胆管细胞癌的 CT 表现

请详见本书 本卷 第四篇 第一章 第四节 不同生长方式肝内胆管细胞癌。

第六节　原发性肝内胆管细胞癌与肝转移性肿瘤及胰腺癌

详见本书 本卷 第二篇 第二章 第五节　误诊病例简介：原发性肝内胆管细胞癌与肝转移性肿瘤及胰腺癌。

第七节　肝左内叶中分化肝内胆管细胞癌

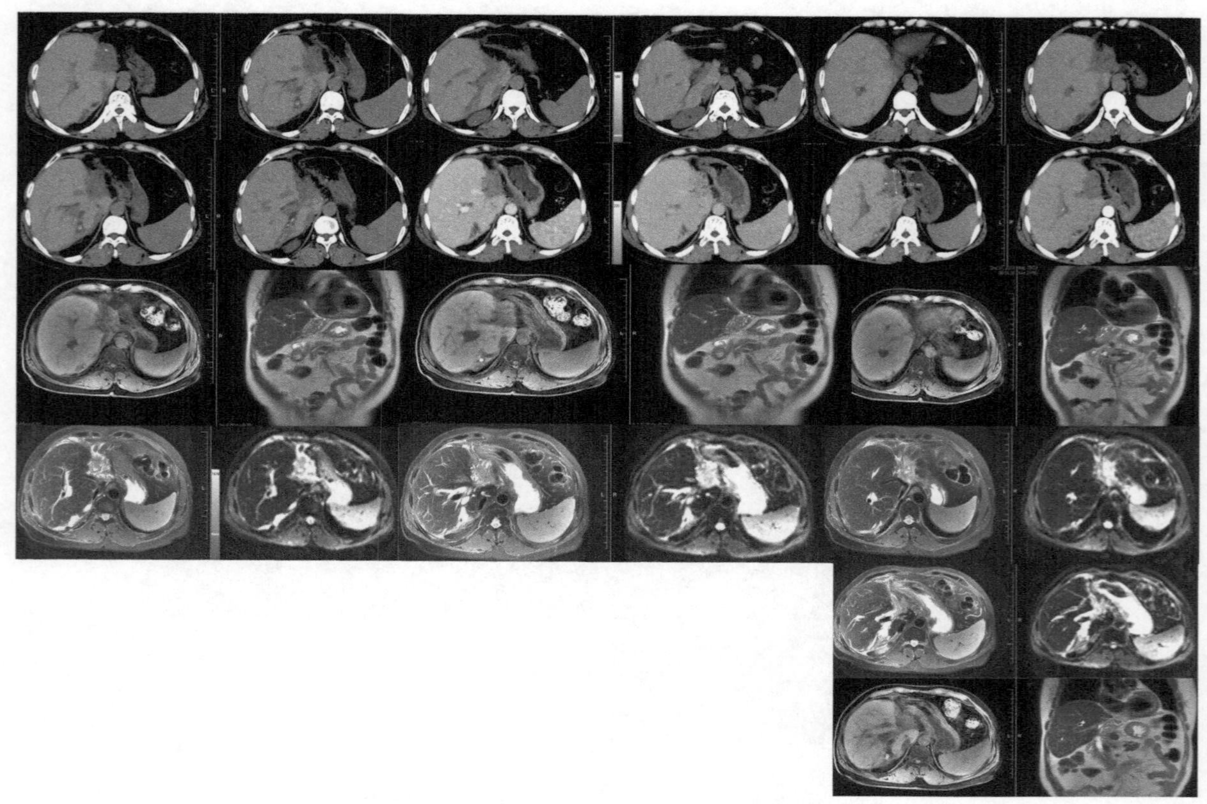

图 16-6-3　肝左内叶中分化肝内胆管细胞癌

患者，女，60 岁。因胆囊切除术后 4 年，右上腹闷痛 3 月入院。辅助检查：甲胎蛋白 5.56ng/ml、糖类抗原 125 42.00U/ml ↑、糖类抗原 19-9 6368.59U/ml ↑、癌胚抗原 3.39。肝功能：白蛋白 38.3g/L ↓、尿素 2.5mmol/L ↓、钙 2.16mmol/L ↓、γ- 谷氨酰基转移酶 68.4IU/L ↑、钾 2.97mmol/L ↓、总蛋白 59.5g/L ↓。

手术所见：进腹后见大网膜与右侧腹壁粘连，松解粘连后暴露肝脏，见胆囊缺如，左肝萎缩变硬，第一肝门粘连严重，胰头区可触及质硬肿物，与周围组织粘连成团，右肝后叶可触及结石，胃肠未见明异常。

病理检查：肝左内叶切除标本：不规则软组织一块，大小 8cm × 4cm × 2cm，切面灰黄灰白，质中偏韧。常规病理诊断：肝左内叶切除标本：中分化肝内胆管细胞癌，癌组织侵犯周围肝组织，肿瘤细胞耐药及预后检测免疫组化待报。

免疫组化检测：阳性：CK19，CD34（血管内皮 +），Hepatocyte（灶区正常肝组织 +），Tubulinβ（2+），EGFR（3+），P-gP（3+），TOPO Ⅱ（+），Ki-67（+，约 20%）；阴性：AFP，VEGF，ERCC1，5-FU。免疫组化诊断示肝左内叶切除标本：中分化肝内胆管细胞癌，癌组织侵犯周围肝组织（图 16-6-3）。

第八节　左肝高分化肝内胆管细胞癌

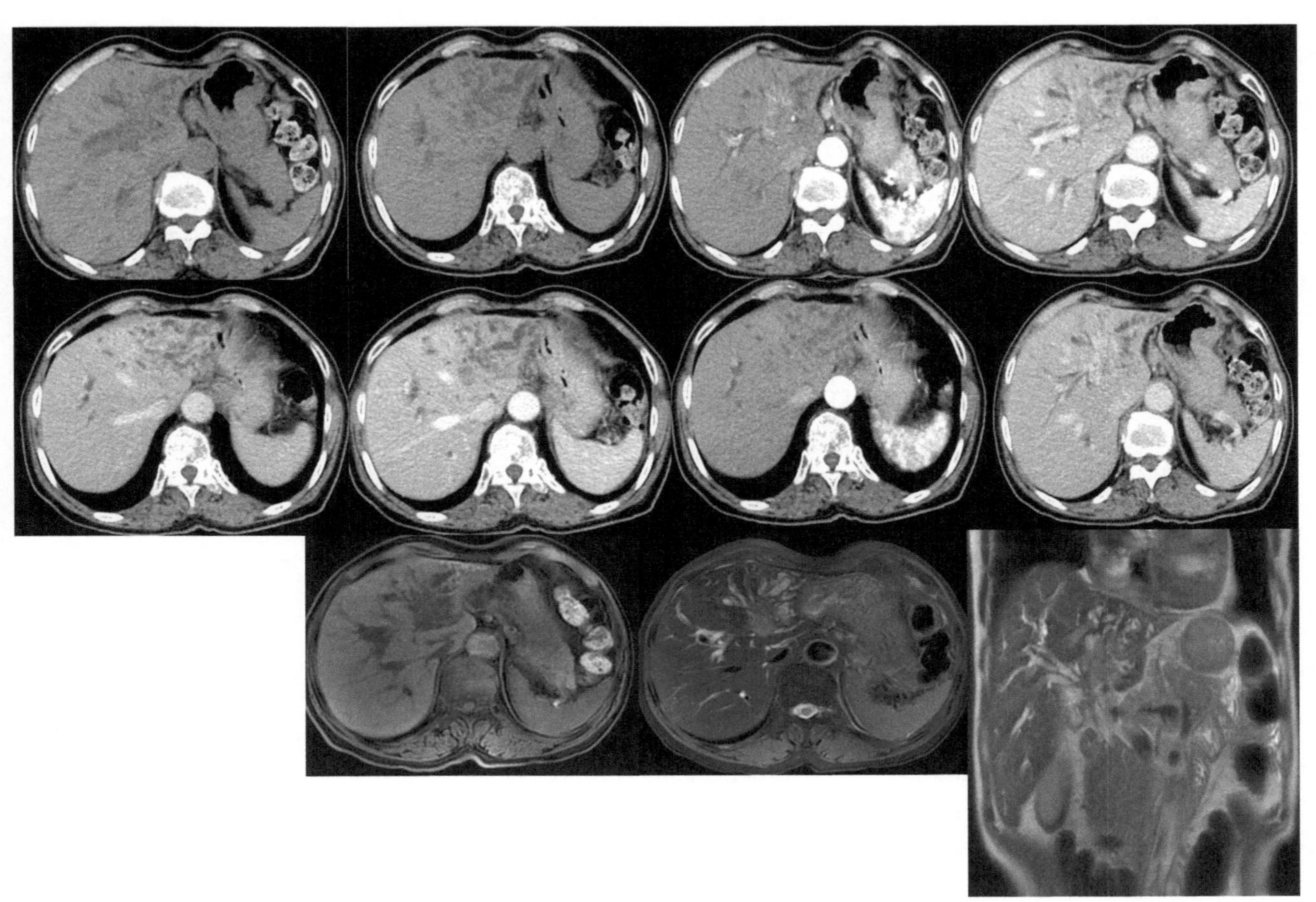

图 16-6-4　左肝高分化肝内胆管细胞癌

患者，女，75 岁。因无明显诱因出现中上腹肿痛不适，并皮肤巩膜进行性黄染，伴乏力、纳差，无畏寒、发热、腹胀、腹痛、返酸、嗳气等不适，体重进行性下降。

病理诊断：胆管癌根治标本：高分化肝内胆管细胞癌，7cm × 5 cm × 4.5 cm，侵犯神经，累及肝总管壁及胆囊管壁；合并慢性肝炎，肝细胞脂肪变性，送检的“胆管残端”内见少数不规则腺管，考虑为癌组织。肿瘤细胞预后及耐药性待免疫组化检测报告。胆囊慢性炎，未见癌组织累及；送检的“左尾状叶"未见癌组织累及。送检的第7组淋巴结和8P组淋巴结均为阴性,分别为0/1和0/3。免疫组化诊断:高分化肝内胆管细胞癌,免疫组化确定侵犯神经。其他情况参见常规组织学报告。肿瘤细胞预后及耐药性待免疫组化检测结果供临床参考。(图16-6-4)

第九节　囊性肝内胆管细胞癌与肝脓肿

肝内胆管细胞癌是较常见的肝脏原发性恶性肿瘤,其发病率仅次于肝细胞癌,起源于肝内小胆管或末梢胆管上皮的腺癌,预后较差。囊性肝内胆管细胞癌是肝内胆管细胞癌的一种特殊表现,是肿瘤内纤维基质坏死和黏液分泌所致。另一方面,由于抗生素的广泛应用等原因,肝脓肿越来越不典型,无论在临床和影像学上,与囊性肝内胆管细胞癌鉴别有时较为困难,常常导致相互误诊。

囊性肝内胆管细胞癌与肝脓肿鉴别诊断的临床意义:囊性肝内胆管细胞癌与肝脓肿无论是临床症状还是CT表现均有较多重叠,比较容易混淆,实验室检查结果常有交叉,年龄特征也不明显,因而容易相互误诊。但两者的治疗方法和预后截然不同,故鉴别诊断非常重要。

囊性肝内胆管细胞癌与肝脓肿CT表现相同点:①囊性肝内胆管细胞癌和肝脓肿CT平扫一般均呈低密度影,少部分呈等密度,边缘不清晰,病灶多为单发。增强后病灶边缘囊壁均可环状的强化,形成靶征。②两者均有灌注异常,正常或相对正常肝实质在动态增强扫描动脉期出现强化,其密度高于周围其他肝实质,到门脉期略高于周围其他肝实质,延迟期该区域的密度与周围其他肝实质相同或相近。肝脓肿周围的正常肝实质在增强早期出现楔形强化或圆形强化,而在晚期该表现消失。Gabata等(2001)对其病理基础进行了研究,发现围绕肝脓肿周围的门静脉分支有明显的炎性浸润,导致血管狭窄,从而引起了门静脉血液减少和动脉血代偿性增加。囊性肝内胆管细胞癌出现的异常灌注与肝脓肿CT表现相同,其病理基础是肿瘤引起肝动脉门静脉异常分流,由于肝动脉血液压力明显大于门静脉,对比剂动脉血提前通过瘘口进入门静脉灌注区。在一项研究中两组灌注异常发生率没有明显差异($P>0.05$),因此灌注异常对于两者无明显鉴别诊断意义。

囊性肝内胆管细胞癌与肝脓肿CT表现差异:囊性肝内胆管细胞癌好发部位以左肝叶多见,可能与左肝易感染及容易发生肝内胆管结石有关,该组21例病例中有13例位于左肝叶,占该组总数的59%。肝脓肿发生于肝右叶多见,这与门静脉分支走向有关,该组26例中有19例位于肝右叶,占该组总数的63%。

靶征:囊性肝内胆管细胞癌靶征出现率低,且多为单靶,即中央为低密度坏死区,边缘为囊壁形成的强化环。该组出现靶征的有2例,出现率为9.1%,明显低于肝脓肿组。其病理基础可能是病灶沿着胆管弥散浸润,侵及血管鞘周围结缔组织所致。而肝脓肿靶征出现率较高,常可见双靶,即在单靶囊壁外又环绕低密度水肿带。外环可延时增强为等密度,此被认为是其特征。该组肝脓肿靶征21例,出现率为72.41%,与文献报道相符。其病理基础为中心低密度区为坏死的脓腔,强化环为脓肿壁(为增生的纤维肉芽组织及炎症组织构成),周围低密度环为炎症周围的水肿带。

分隔状强化:又称为簇状征、花瓣征、蜂窝征等,多出现在动脉期、门脉期,呈多房或蜂窝状低密度区,增强扫描病灶内间隔可有强化。有文献报道CT检查患者肝脏发现簇状征和坏死区出现气-液平面,可作为肝脓肿诊断的重要线索。对于肝脓肿内出现的强化程度不均匀的细索条状间隔影,多为肉芽组织或残存的尚未坏死的炎性充血肝组织形成。而囊性肝内胆管细胞癌病灶内部呈线状、斑片样网格状强化,病理基础为索条状纤维间质带分隔部分癌巢,且部分纤维组织疏松,血管较多所致。该研究肝脓肿组分隔状强化的出现率为68.97%,囊性肝内胆管细胞癌的出现率为18.18%,两者间差异有统计学意义($P<0.05$)。因此,分隔状强化对于提示肝脓肿具有重要的参考价值。

边缘强化征:表现为病灶周围有环状或部分环状强化,动脉期明显强化,门脉期及延迟期与正常肝组织相同。肝脓肿边缘增强征的病理基础有3种:脓肿破坏灶周围的肉芽血管生成;肝动脉、门静脉异常通道形成;脓肿生长迅速,挤压周围肝细胞,使周围肝细胞密度增高。而囊性肝内胆管细胞癌的病理基础是肿瘤周围部分血供相对丰富，有大量的肿瘤细胞和少数纤维组织。

当肝脓肿与囊性肝内胆管细胞癌都表现为边缘环形强化时，对环形是否完整的观察和评价在两者的鉴别诊断中起重要作用。该项研究肝脓肿组中环形完整强化占 79.31%，而环形不完整强化占 17.24%。囊性肝内胆管细胞癌组中环形完整强化占 13.63%，环形不完整强化占 72.72%。结合卡方检验，环形完整强化在肝脓肿的出现率更高，环形不完整强化在囊性肝内胆管细胞癌的出现率更高，因此，对环形的完整强化与不完整强化的观察对两者的鉴别诊断有较大价值。

向心性延迟强化：向心性延迟强化被认为是囊性肝内胆管细胞癌特征性表现。表现为门脉期可见病灶边缘强化下降，强化向病灶内部延伸，但强化程度低于肝实质，延迟期进一步强化，其中央低密度无强化区随着时间延长而缩小，似“沙滩征”。病理上门脉期逐渐增强及延迟期强化区为大量纤维结缔组织，少量散在的癌组织。

对比剂在纤维组织间质与血管之间弥散慢，即经血管进入纤维间质内及从纤维间质与血管之间清除慢，这是肝内胆管细胞癌门脉期进一步强化及延迟期强化的病理基础。在囊性肝内胆管细胞癌组 19 例出现向心性延迟强化，其出现率为 86. 36%。将囊性肝内胆管细胞癌组和肝脓肿组出现向心性延迟强化的征象进行检验，二者差异有统计学意义（$P<0.05$），因此向心性延迟强化是囊性肝内胆管细胞癌的非常重要征象，具有诊断性意义。

肿块缩小征：多见于延迟期，表现为病灶同围延时强化为等密度，而病灶内间隔可见持续强化，低密度液化坏死区显示更清楚，病灶较平扫时缩小。肝脓肿肿块缩小征反映了化脓性炎症其或残留肝组织的炎症反应，机制是脓肿炎性肉芽组织内对比剂向外缓慢渗透而廓清较慢所致，其坏死区未见明显强化。该项研究肝脓肿组中肿块缩小征的出现率（72.41%）明显高于囊性肝内胆管细胞癌（13.16%），所以肿块缩小征在两者鉴别诊断中更能提示肝脓肿。

肝被膜回缩征：病灶区的局部肝被膜呈局限性凹陷。有研究认为该征象仅出现于恶性肿瘤，但近年来有文献报道良性病变也会出现此征。其病理基础为肿瘤内纤维组织丰富，肿瘤呈浸润性生长，富含纤维间质，造成肝被膜回缩。该项研究中囊性肝内胆管细胞癌组出现肝被膜回缩征 2 例，肝脓肿组未出现此征象。

综上所述，囊性肝内胆管细胞癌和肝脓肿在 CT 检查中征象复杂，二者容易混淆，通过对其征象仔细分析将有助于最后的诊断。该项研究发现通过比较各个征象在两种病变的出现率对于提示不同的诊断具有重要意义，但单个征象对于鉴别诊断的价值受到不同程度的限制，在鉴别诊断中应综合多个征象全面研究分析，更有利于得出正确诊断结论。

第十节　右肝内胆管癌（乳头状腺癌）

患者，男，63 岁。

手术所见：经术中 B 超及触摸发现肿物贴近右肝门静脉后支，超声显示肿物呈囊实性，大小约 3 cm × 3cm，质软。

病理检查：不规则组织一块，大小 4 cm × 2 cm × 1.5 cm，切面灰白，质中。常规病理诊断：肝肿物切除标本示肝脏乳头状肿瘤，性质类型待免疫组化进一步诊断。

免疫组化检测：阳性：CK（L），CK7，CK8，CK18，CK19，EMA，P504S，Hepatocyte，EGFR（+++），5-Fu（+++），VEGF（++），Topo Ⅱ（+），Ki-67（+，约 20%）；阴性：Villin，PSA，CEA，CK20，CDX2，TTF-1，TG，Mucin-2，CA19-9，HBsAg，HBcAg，AFP，CD10，Vimentin，ERCC-1，P-gp，Tubulinβ。免疫组化诊断：肝肿物切除标本示肝内胆管癌（乳头状腺癌），肿瘤耐药及预后检测结果供参考（图 16-6-5）。

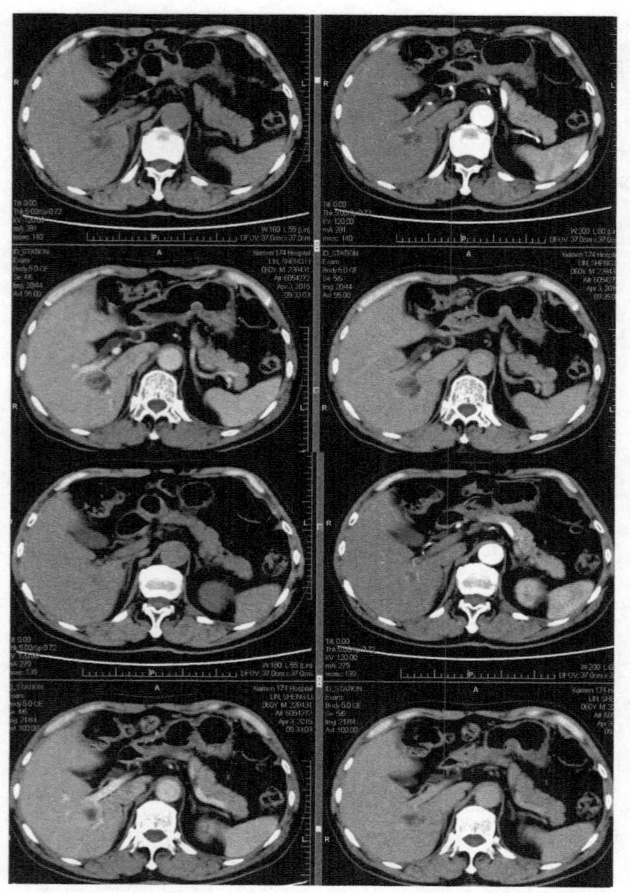

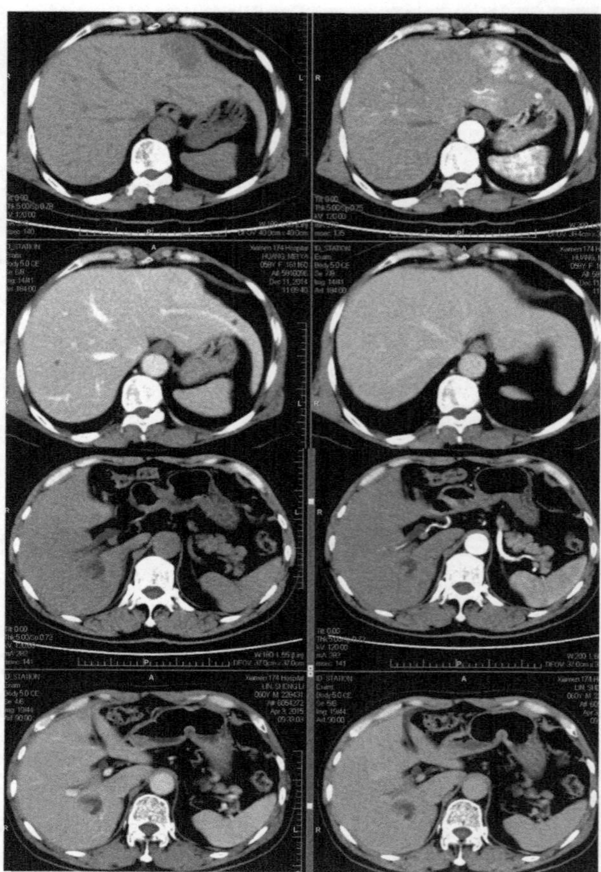

图 16-6-5 右肝内胆管癌(乳头状腺癌)

第十一节 肝内胆管细胞癌淋巴结转移

详见本书 本卷 第四篇 第一章 第五节 肝内胆管细胞癌淋巴结转移。

第十二节 左肝外段胆管细胞癌

患者,女,60 岁。2 年前在我院发现肝多发血管瘤,给予肝血管瘤栓塞介入治疗,术后恢复良好出院;近日外院复查彩超示肝左叶实性占位性病变,再就诊我院。

病理检查:部分肝组织一块,大小 10cm × 8cm × 5.5cm,切面见一肿物,大小 8.2cm × 7.5cm × 5.8cm,肿物切面灰白灰黄,质中。常规病理诊断:左肝恶性上皮性肿瘤,大小 10cm × 8cm × 5.5cm,伴轻度慢性肝炎。肿瘤细胞分型、预后及耐药检测待免疫组化报告。免疫组化检测:阳性:CK18,CK19,CK7(局灶 +),CK8,CK(L),CA19-9,Villin,EGFR(+++),Topo-Ⅱ(+),Ki67(+,约 10%);阴性:Vimentin,CK20,CD34,AFP,HBcAg,HBsAg,S-100,CA125,CEA,TTF-1,hepatocyte,CD10,P-gp,VEGF,ERCC-1,Tubulin-β,5-Fu。免疫组化诊断:左肝胆管细胞癌,大小 10cm × 8cm × 5.5cm,伴轻度慢性肝炎。耐药及预后检测结果供临床参考(图 16-6-6)。

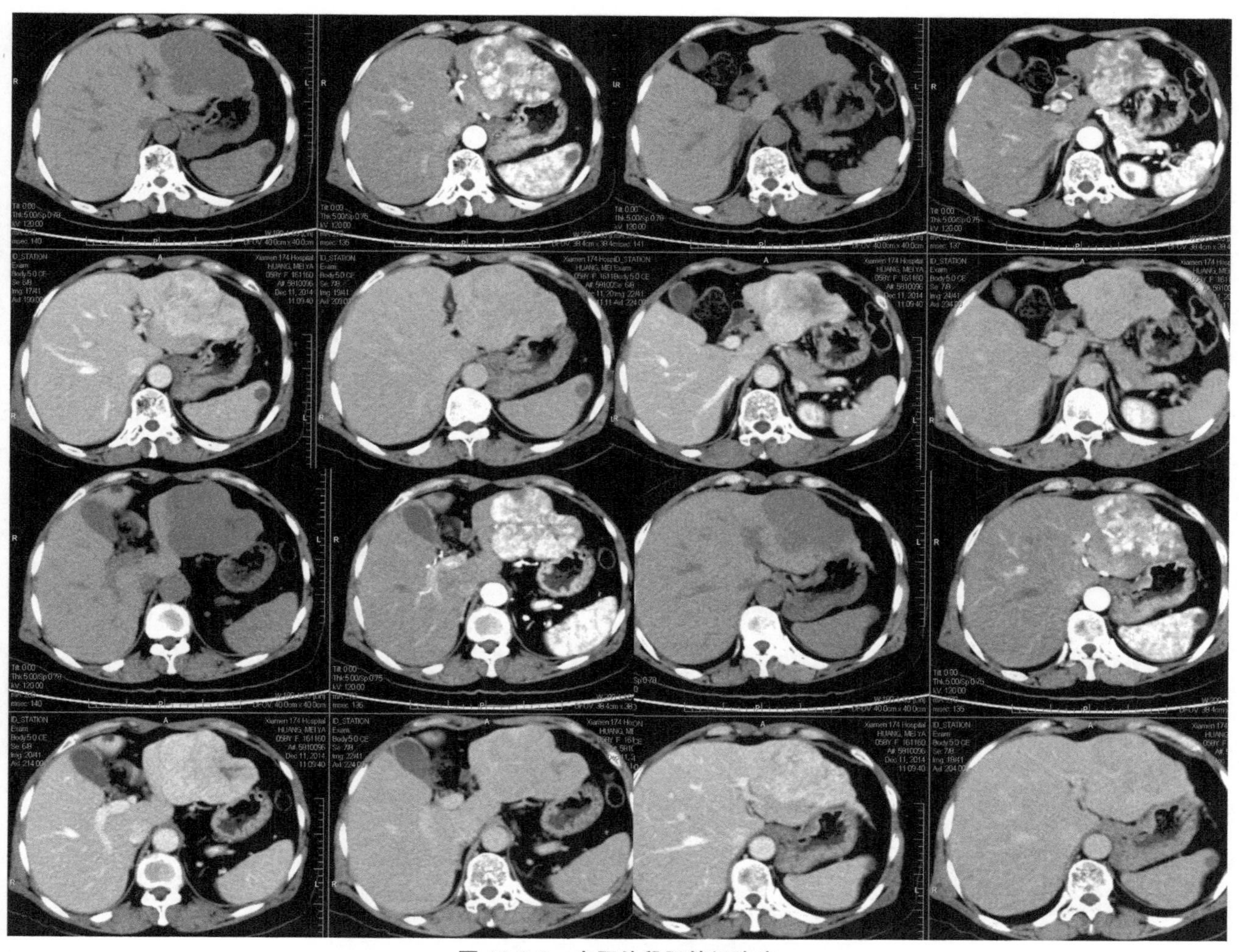

图 16-6-6　左肝外段胆管细胞癌

第十三节 左肝外叶肝内胆管腺癌，高分化，侵犯广泛

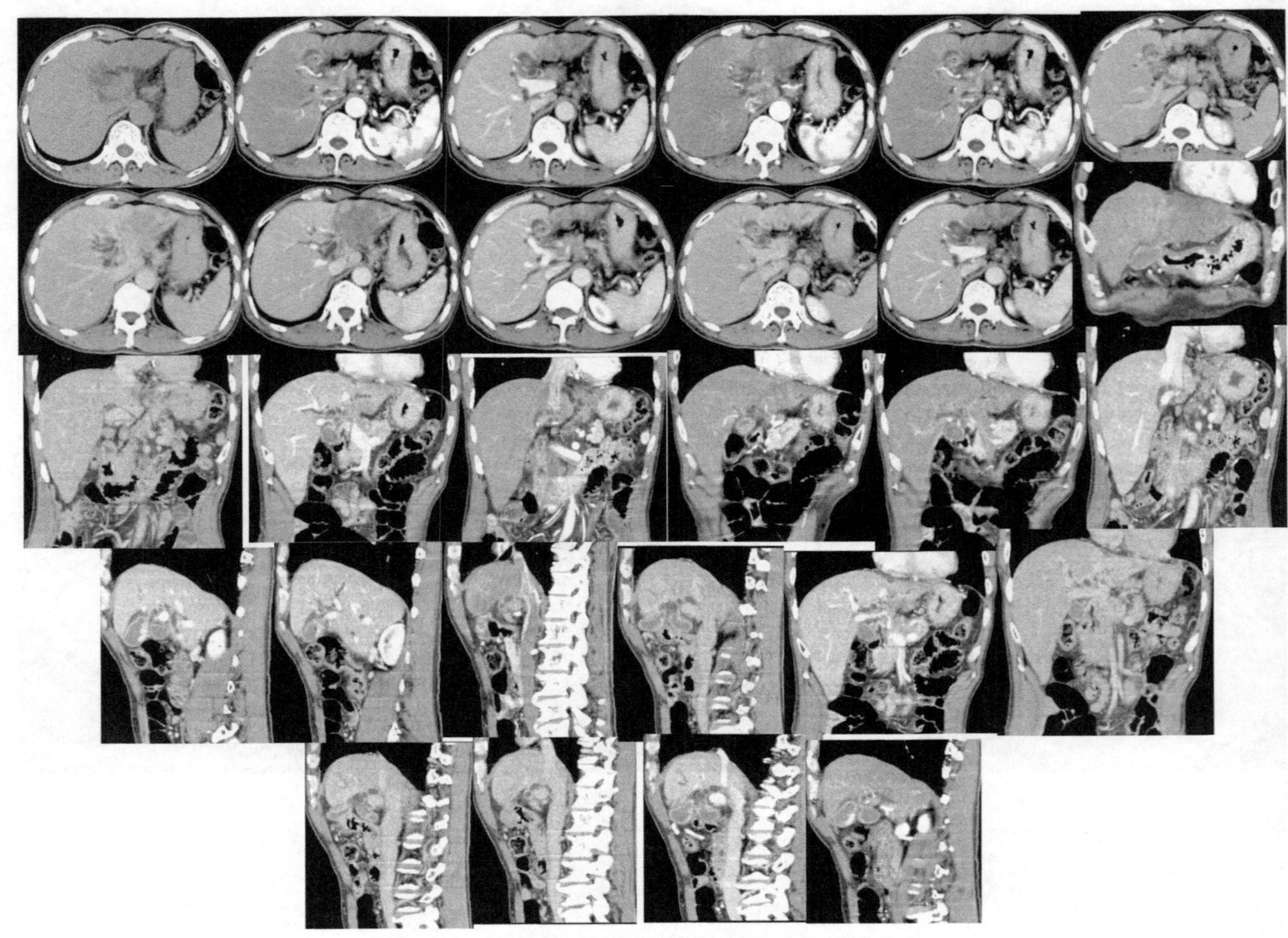

图 16-6-7 左肝外叶肝内胆管腺癌，高分化，侵犯广泛

患者，男，65 岁。术后病理免疫组化诊断：肝内胆管腺癌，高分化，大小 7cm × 6cm × 4cm，侵犯肝脏被膜及周围纤维脂肪组织，并可见脉管内癌栓。胆管壁与胆囊肌层及周围纤维脂肪组织内可见癌组织累及；淋巴结清扫 12 枚，其中 10 枚可见癌转移。最大一组为不规则块，大小为 4cm × 3.5cm × 2cm。手术见两个团块，为左肝外叶肝内团块及左肝门团块，病理证实后者主要为肿大融合淋巴结加上增厚的胆管壁。CT 增强扫描清楚可见左肝内胆管多处扩张，总肝管及左肝内胆管壁增厚，胆囊与病变分不开，说明已受累及（图 16-6-7）。

第十四节 肿块型胆管细胞癌

肝内胆管细胞癌是肝脏常见的原发恶性肿瘤，其患病率仅次于肝细胞癌。肿块型胆管细胞癌是肝内胆管细胞癌的最常见亚型，占 60%。影像检查在肿块型胆管细胞癌的诊断、分期及疗效评估中具有重要作用，影像表现典型的肿块型胆管细胞癌诊断不困难，呈不典型影像表现的肿块型胆管细胞癌临床上易造成误诊或漏诊。

肿块型胆管细胞癌的动态增强影像表现及其病

理基础：一项研究通过回顾性分析95例肿块型胆管细胞癌患者的CT及MRI动态增强表现，发现其强化方式大致分为5种类型。肿块型胆管细胞癌最多见的强化方式为动脉期边缘强化，平衡期渐进性强化，即类型1表现，与多数文献结果相符，称之为经典强化方式，相应的病理特征为肿瘤中心部位以纤维间质为主，边缘以瘤细胞为主。以往的文献中对肿块型胆管细胞癌不典型强化方式表现的报道较少。

研究结果显示，患者的强化方式和肿瘤细胞所占比例、分布、血供、纤维组织的致密性以及肿瘤内出血坏死范围有关。

强化类型2对应的病理表现为肿瘤中心纤维间质最为致密且血供丰富；强化类型4对应的病理特征为病灶内部肿瘤细胞成分所占比例较高且分布广泛，纤维间质成分含量相对较少；强化类型5对应的病理特征为肿瘤内部有大量纤维间质，但间质疏松、呈透明样变，血供较差，瘤细胞皱缩、脱失，嵌插在其内。

Kim等（2011）将肿块型胆管细胞癌的强化方式分为典型强化和不典型强化两种，二者总体预后差异无统计学意义，但后者无病生存率明显高于前者，而慢性肝炎患者更易出现不典型强化。Asayama等（2006）的研究显示，肿瘤内部纤维间质所占比例与患者预后相关，含量越高，预后越差，并据此将肿块型胆管细胞癌分为硬化型和非硬化型。因此，肿瘤强化方式与预后存在相关性。

该研究结果显示，肿块型胆管细胞癌的强化方式与肿瘤分化程度以及患者是否存在基础肝病无明显相关性，而和肿瘤大小有关，肿瘤越小出现不典型强化方式的概率越高。

Kim等（2007）报道，在肝硬化患者中，肿块型胆管细胞癌的影像表现与肿瘤大小有关，当肿瘤 < 3 cm时与肝细胞癌鉴别困难。因此，肿块型胆管细胞癌因常临床症状不明显，发现时肿瘤体积多较大，若慢性肝炎患者由于基础肝病定期检查而能更早发现肿瘤，则出现不典型强化方式的概率就会增加，鉴别诊断也更困难。

该项研究中，通过和病理结果对照，排除了因扫描技术原因所致肿瘤强化方式出现差异的患者。因为病变未出现典型的延迟强化可能与延迟时间不足有关，而非真正的不典型强化。因此，通过和病理结果对照，影像表现不同而病理表现基本一致时，不典型强化与扫描技术规范有差别相关，排除了此类患者。

鉴别诊断：根据强化方式不同，肿块型胆管细胞癌应与富含纤维间质成分的肝脏原发及继发良、恶性病变，如硬化型肝细胞癌、转移癌、硬化性血管瘤等鉴别。

（1）硬化型肝癌：硬化型肝癌的强化方式亦多表现为动脉期病灶边缘厚薄不均的环状强化，平衡期出现环状渐进性强化，与肿块型胆管细胞癌相似，但其环状渐进性强化多为同心圆形，而肿块型胆管细胞癌多表现为不规则形。

（2）肝转移癌：肝转移癌常为多发病灶，根据肿瘤内部成分不同，强化方式多样，影像诊断应密切结合病史，若肿块型胆管细胞癌患者既往存在恶性肿瘤病史，影像极易误诊。

（3）肝细胞癌：当肿块型胆管细胞癌出现对比剂“快进快出”的特殊强化方式时，若患者同时存在慢性肝炎肝硬化，在影像上则与普通类型的肝细胞癌很难鉴别。

该项研究的局限性：患者样本量较少，影像检查技术不够规范，有待今后在严格技术规范后进行更大宗研究。病理检查病例约2/3（/95）为穿刺活检标本，病理诊断的可靠性欠缺，仅39/95例为手术切除标本，与影像一对一地对照研究有一定困难。因此，该组作者得出结论是：肿块型胆管细胞癌的CT和MRI强化方式多样，影像表现与病理分化程度无相关性。我们认为，说相关性可能不明显似乎更合适一些。难以一对一地进行对照研究，要讨论肿瘤病灶强化表现与病理改变的相关性，真是谈何容易。

附具体研究资料：

纳入标准：经病理诊断为肿块型胆管细胞癌；手术或穿刺前行腹部多期动态增强CT和/或MRI检查，同时行CT及MRI检查者检查间隔不超过30 d。排除标准：同一病灶多发患者的病灶强化方式不同；通过和病理结果对照，因扫描技术原因所致肿瘤强化方式出现差异的患者。

95例患者纳入研究，男73例，女22例；年龄26~81岁，平均（57 ± 10）岁；59例经穿刺活检证实，36例经手术病理证实。既往有慢性肝炎病史患者56例，其中54例有乙型病毒性肝炎病史，2例有丙型病毒性肝炎病史；无肝病史患者39例，其中3例有恶性肿瘤病史（肺癌、子宫内膜癌及结肠癌各1例）。

肿块型胆管细胞癌患者的多期动态增强CT及MRI强化方式主要分以下5种：

类型 1：60 例（63.2%，60/95），表现为动脉期边缘厚薄不均的环状强化和 / 或内部分隔状强化，部分伴周围肝实质一过性高灌注，平衡期表现为同心圆形或不规则形（以后者为主）向心性强化和 / 或分隔状强化。

类型 2：11 例（11.6%，11/95），表现为动脉期呈边缘环状强化，部分伴周围肝实质一过性高灌注，平衡期肿瘤边缘对比剂流出，呈环状低密度（信号）改变，中心呈明显结节状强化，表现为“眼征”。

类型 3：15 例（15.8%，15/95），表现为动脉期无明显强化，平衡期肿瘤内部可见对比剂不均匀填充。

类型 4：6 例（6.3%，6/95），表现为动脉期肿瘤呈整体不均匀强化，平衡期对比剂流出，肿瘤呈低密度（信号）改变，内见少许索条状强化，表现为“快进快出”模式。

类型 5：3 例（3.2%，3/95），动脉期至平衡期肿瘤均无明显强化，始终呈低密度（信号）改变。

慢性肝炎组和无肝病组肿块型胆管细胞癌患者年龄、强化方式差异无统计学意义；无肝病组中女性患者数量多于慢性肝炎组，且病灶最大径大于慢性肝炎组。最大径 <3 cm 组、3~6 cm 组和 >6 cm 组肿块型胆管细胞癌患者的强化方式差异有统计学意义。

第十五节　肝内胆管细胞癌与转移性肝癌的鉴别

详见本书 本卷 第二篇 第三章 第二节 肝内胆管细胞癌与转移性肝癌的鉴别。

第十六节　左肝中分化胆管细胞癌

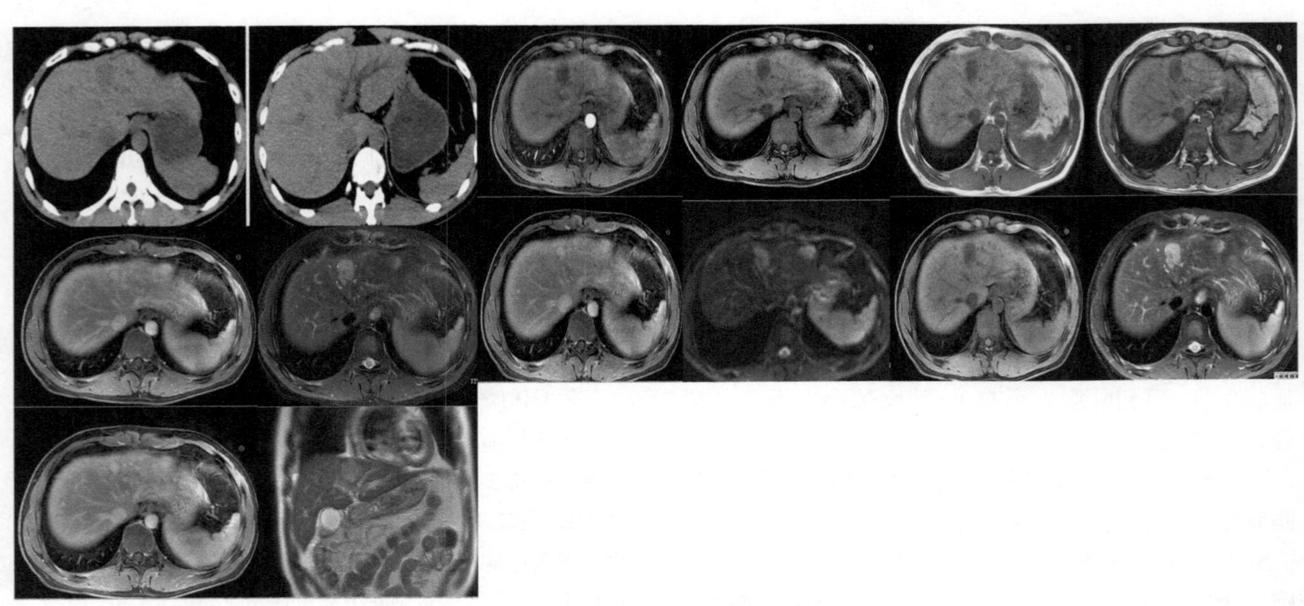

图 16-6-8　左肝中分化胆管细胞癌

患者，男，37 岁。腹痛 1 天入院。

乙肝病毒核心抗体、乙肝病毒 E 抗体、乙肝病毒表面抗原阳性，余阴性；今日复查肝功能：丙氨酸氨基转移酶 120IU/L、γ- 谷氨酰基转移酶 228.1IU/L、总胆汁酸 28.4μmol/L；肿瘤标志物：甲胎蛋白、糖类抗原 125、癌胚抗原正常；糖类抗原 19-9 40.09U/ml。

手术所见：腹腔内无腹水，左内叶近肝圆韧带可触及一大小约 3cm × 4cm 肿物，质硬，边界尚清楚，肝组织切开后可见左肝内胆管癌栓组织。胆囊大小约 7cm × 2cm，壁稍厚，约 3mm，未扪及结石，胆总管稍增粗，直径约 1.2cm，切开后见胆总管内癌栓，胆道镜探查右肝胆管未见明显异常，胆总管下段开口正常。胃、十二指肠等未见明显异常。

病理检查：左肝肿物切除标本：肝组织一块，大小 15cm × 8.5cm × 3cm，切面见一肿物，大小 2.5cm

×2.5cm×2cm，肿物切面灰白、质硬，与周围界限尚清，其余肝组织红褐、质软。常规病理诊断：左肝腺癌，大小2.5cm×2.5cm×2cm，合并轻度慢性肝炎（以汇管区淋巴细胞浸润为主）。肿瘤分型、耐药及预后检测结果待免疫组化报告。

免疫组化检测：阳性：Vimentin，CK18，CK19，CK7，CK8，CK（L），Villin，CA19-9，EGFR（+++），5-Fu（++），Topo-Ⅱ（+），Ki67（+，约70%），Tubulin-β（++）；阴性：CK20，hepatocyte，HBcAg，HBsAg，AFP，CEA，CD10，TTF-1，S-100，P-gp，VEGF，ERCC-1。免疫组化诊断：左肝中分化胆管细胞癌，大小2.5cm×2.5cm×2cm，合并轻度慢性乙型病毒性肝炎（以汇管区淋巴细胞浸润为主，HBsAg阳性）。耐药及预后检测结果供临床参考（图16-6-8）。

第七章　肝内胆管囊腺瘤和囊腺癌

第一节　肝内胆管囊腺癌

肝内胆管囊腺癌较为少见,其预后优于肝内胆管细胞癌。

1. 病理学　肝内胆管囊腺癌的来源,多数学者认同是起源于胆管上皮细胞,是胆管细胞癌的一种特殊类型。肝内胆管囊腺癌可能起源于囊腺瘤上皮的恶变。大体病理肿瘤呈圆形或卵圆形囊性肿物,与周围界限清楚。肿瘤直径 4~20 cm,单发单房或有间隔分隔成多房,壁可发生钙化。病灶切面可见囊内间隔,完整或不完整,内含灰白色或淡黄色半透明黏稠液体。

囊壁和间隔壁被覆分泌黏液的上皮细胞,异形性明显,癌细胞呈结节状或乳头状向囊内生长。囊腺癌有结节或乳头立方或扁平状组织突入囊腔内,囊壁和分隔可厚薄不均。腔内含黏液伴出血。囊液大多呈淡褐色,部分囊泡液体呈淡白色。囊内壁大部分外观光滑,有的囊壁较厚并有多个水泡样结节聚集。部分囊内壁毛糙并兼有灰白色实体区域,质地较硬。

镜下显示分散分布的扩张管腔,乳头及腺样结构。上皮呈立方形或高柱状,向腔内形成多数壁上结节和 / 或乳头样突起。细胞有明显的异型和核分裂,部分突破基底膜。癌变区域之间的邻近肝组织可见良性被覆上皮细胞。

胆管囊腺癌镜下见囊腔衬覆柱状、立方或扁平的分泌黏液细胞,多灶性上皮呈多层排列、特征性的乳头状结构并出现核分裂及间质内浸润,常见囊内壁被覆良性立方或扁平细胞过度至恶性区间。免疫组化显示其表型与胆管细胞癌类似。

病理上又把肝内胆管囊腺癌分成 2 个类型:一类为肿瘤内含有卵巢间质,仅见于女性,可由胆管细胞囊腺瘤发展而来;另一类为肿瘤内不含卵巢间质,男女均可见,与以往有无胆管细胞囊腺瘤无关。前者预后较后者好,但目前用影像学方法还不能鉴别此 2 种类型。

2. 临床表现　肝内胆管囊腺癌临床上没有特异性症状和体征,患者常以右上腹胀痛不适及波动性黄疸等就诊,主要体征是肝脏肿大,有囊性感。免疫组织化学:癌胚抗原、CA19-9 均可升高,甲胎蛋白正常。原发性肝内胆管囊腺癌,多见于男性,病情发展快、预后差;肝内胆管囊腺瘤或先天性肝囊肿恶变的胆管囊腺癌好发于女性,病程缓慢,预后较好。

影像学研究:一些作者提出,肝内一个界限明确的圆形囊性肿块伴有向内的乳头状突起,尤其同时出现肝内外胆管扩张似可看作肝内胆管囊腺癌是特征性 CT 表现。

CT 可显示肝内囊性低密度肿块。囊壁可有结节和粗大钙化斑块,多平面重建显示钙化与囊壁和乳头状突起密切相连。囊内有完整或不完整间隔分割成多房;囊壁、间隔壁薄厚不均,最厚可达 1 cm;囊内壁不光滑,有乳头状物向腔内突起。增强多期扫描囊壁、间隔壁和乳头样结节呈明显强化,门静脉期强化逐渐减退。囊内呈液体密度,伴有陈旧性出血者各房密度不等, CT 值为 8~20 HU,增强扫描囊内无强化。肝内外胆管明显扩张,窄窗显示管腔内密度不均,未见结石和肿瘤征象。

虽然 CT 表现无法完全鉴别良性胆管细胞囊腺瘤与恶性胆管细胞囊腺癌,但是有间隔增厚、壁上结节或乳头状突起、囊内出血以及伴粗大钙化者多考虑为恶性的肝内胆管囊腺癌。

胆总管黏液性阻塞与黄疸:手术证实或术后“T”形管引流或胆管镜发现,扩张的胆管腔内充填大量胶冻样黏液,是肝内胆管囊腺癌分泌大量含有黏蛋白的黏液，经囊腔 - 胆管通道进入胆管，黏液中黏蛋白凝聚成胶冻样物质，堆积在胆总管下端引起胆管阻塞和继发性扩张，临床出现波动性黄疸。

CT 表现为与囊腔相通连的肝内外胆管扩张明显，肝外胆管扩张直径达 87 mm，有的病例在“T”形管引流期间多次阻塞并出现黄疸，经冲洗抽出胶冻样黏液后黄疸减退。

这种胆总管的黏液性阻塞，密度一般略高于水，呈类圆形低密度环影，CT 值在 8~20 HU 之间，大小与病程长短正相关。扩张的胆管内壁呈“苦瓜皮”样，或有乳头样软组织影突向管腔，没有结石的直接征象。

CT 不能区别黏液或低密度结石，当临床出现波动性黄疸，CT 发现肝内囊性肿块、肝内外胆管明显扩张，没有低密度结石（“靶征”“半月征”）和肿瘤性阻塞（胆总管下段软组织肿块、管壁结节、管腔狭窄、截断征）的特异征象，应想到黏液性堵塞的可能性。

胆总管的黏液性阻塞和扩张是肝内胆管囊腺癌和囊腺瘤恶变的特有的并发征象。有作者提出术中胆管探查不管有无结石，只要有大量的黏液均应考虑有胆管黏液癌的可能。如在术后“T”形管引流出胶冻黏液，则应尽快行 CT 检查，及时发现肝内胆管囊腺癌存在。

3. 鉴别诊断　肝内胆管囊腺癌应与肝内胆管先天性囊性扩张鉴别，肝内胆管先天性囊性扩张沿胆管走行分布，相互分离，可见“中心点征”，青少年多见。肝内外胆管不扩张的病例应注意与以下疾病鉴别：

（1）肝内胆管囊腺瘤：本病与肝内胆管囊腺瘤难于鉴别，一般认为其与服用避孕药有关，好发于育龄妇女，为单发多囊性病灶，囊壁光整、厚薄一致。间隔壁增厚、壁结节和 / 或乳头状突起、囊内出血、粗大的钙化多考虑为恶性囊腺癌。一些作者认为，虽然部分胆管细胞囊腺瘤和囊腺癌在 CT 上能够区分，但是两者区分的意义不大，普遍认为胆管囊腺瘤是囊腺癌的癌前病变，治疗上均需外科手术切除，故鉴别诊断上最基本的是与肝内的囊性病变鉴别。

（2）肝包虫囊肿：肝包虫囊肿有流行区域，其 CT 特征为母囊中内含子囊，子囊小而规则，可有环形或半环形的钙化。

（3）肝囊腺癌：肝脏囊性占位内有分隔，囊壁厚薄不均伴乳头样物突出者鉴别困难，肝囊腺癌多为混杂密度肿块伴有囊变，增强扫描囊内强化的软组织密度成分较肝内胆管囊腺癌多。

（4）肝细胞性肝癌：肝细胞性肝癌表现为坏死为主时，可类似囊性肿瘤，而残留的癌组织可类似囊壁结节，病灶周边显示“晕圈征”。但胆管细胞囊腺癌的囊壁光滑、锐利，壁结节也规则，壁和结节内钙化，囊内为水样密度，不合并肝硬化，肝炎系列检查和甲胎蛋白阴性可以与肝细胞癌鉴别。

（5）囊性转移瘤：囊性肝内转移瘤非常少见，但是与胆管细胞囊腺瘤和囊腺癌表现相似，为具有壁结节的多房囊性病灶，囊壁厚而模糊，不规则间隔呈絮状，实性部分偏多，结合临床有原发癌病史即可明确诊断。如果未能找到原发病灶，经皮穿刺活检可予鉴别。

（6）肝囊肿：肝囊肿一般为单房，多发性囊肿各自独立或相邻的呈外切关系，囊壁极薄且均匀，边缘光滑锐利，没有乳头样结节，内部密度均一。

（7）胆管囊肿：先天性肝内胆管囊肿恶变表现为邻近胆管扩张，而本病仅见远端胆管扩张，而范围较局限，并有壁结节。

上述病变癌胚抗原及 CA19-9 值多无异常增高。经皮肝穿刺活检对诊断有帮助。

必须重视的一点是，拟诊肝内胆管囊腺癌者不宜轻易进行穿刺，以免引起种植性转移。

第二节　肝胆管囊腺瘤

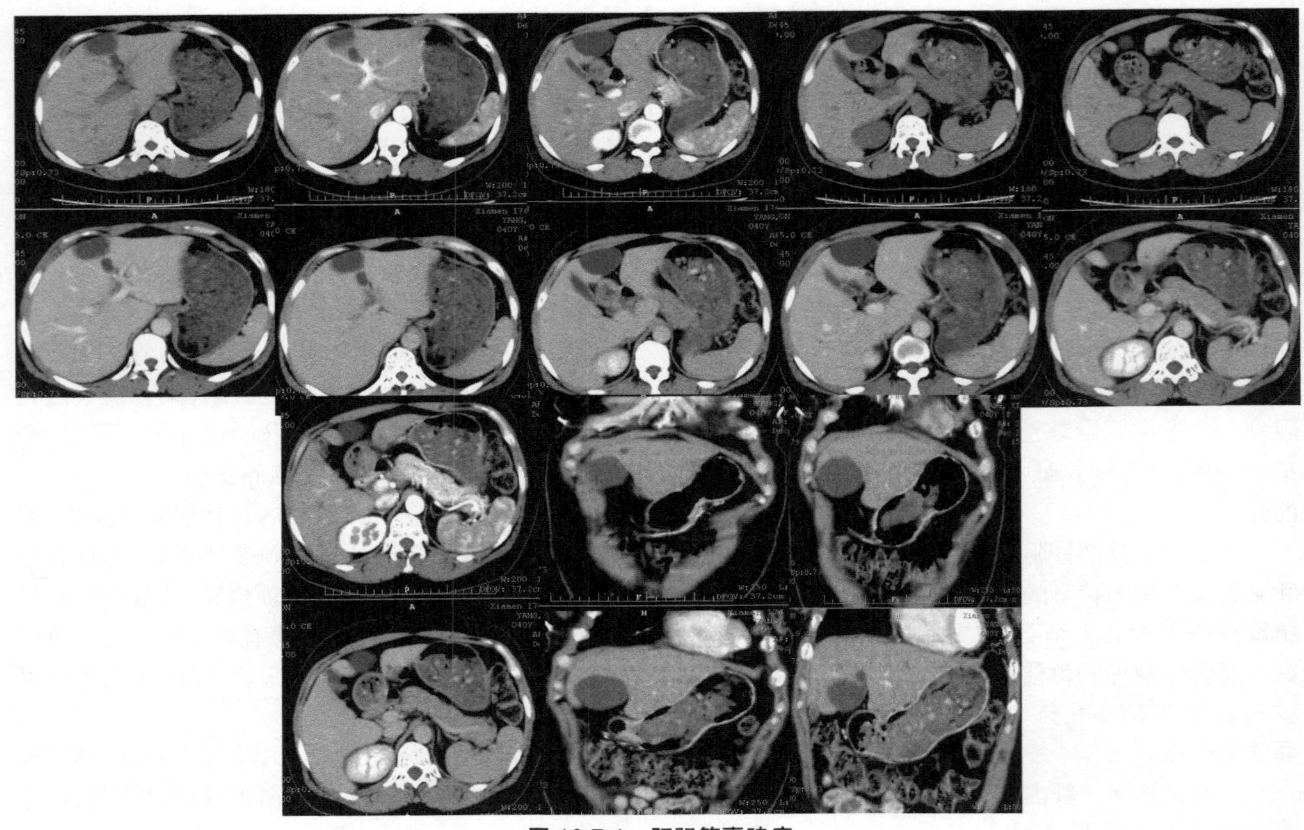

图 16-7-1　肝胆管囊腺瘤

患者，女，40 岁。体检发现肝囊肿 2 个月入院。

病理检查：灰白色囊壁样组织一样，体积 1.5 cm × 2.5 cm × 0.2cm，壁光滑。病理诊断：肝状囊性病变，纤维性囊壁内衬单层立方和柱状上皮，考虑为肝胆管囊腺瘤（图 16-7-1）。

第八章　肝内胆管乳头状肿瘤

1. 病理学　肝内胆管乳头状肿瘤可为良性、交界性或恶性。与胆管细胞来源的其他恶性肿瘤（如胆管壁外胆管细胞癌和管壁浸润性胆管细胞癌）恶性度高、容易出现淋巴转移不同，胆管内乳头状癌多为低度恶性，肿瘤生长缓慢，主要沿管壁黏膜层生长，晚期会侵犯胆管壁深层，向肝实质浸润；但是，胆管内乳头状癌很少出现淋巴结转移。

部分胆管内乳头状瘤只有一个蒂附着于胆管，肿瘤在胆管内爬行生长，尽管肿瘤范围较广，但手术时可以牵引出整个肿瘤。胆管内乳头状瘤容易恶变，文献报道其最高癌变率可达 64%。患者很少死于肿瘤浸润转移引起的恶液质，慢性胆汁淤积引起的胆汁性肝硬化和肝功能衰竭是主要致死原因，所以及早明确诊断和治疗能显著改善患者的预后。

胆管内乳头状瘤多位于胆总管，位于肝内胆管者少见。肿瘤起源于肝内胆管黏膜上皮，瘤体质地较软，呈分叶样的乳头状内折，倾向于沿胆管黏膜表面虫爬样播散。

2. 临床表现　肝内胆管乳头状肿瘤临床少见，容易误诊。肝内胆管乳头状肿瘤可以发生在胆系的任何位置，胆总管的发病率相对较高，肝内胆管发病者相对较少，通常不到 30%。

本病多见于中老年男性，发病机制尚不明确，一般认为与胆管结石、炎症的长期刺激有关，但一组 16 例中，多没有胆管结石和炎症长期刺激的病史，但部分病例伴有胆管囊肿。

3. 影像学研究　CT 平扫多表现为扩张胆管内形态多变的类圆形、扁平状或珊瑚状的低密度结节或肿块，有时由于肿瘤体积较小而无法显示，仅表现为肝内胆管扩张。该组病例中，7 例胆管乳头状腺瘤和 7 例乳头状腺癌表观为扩张的肝内胆管内结节或肿块，呈类圆形、扁平状、珊瑚状；2 例胆管乳头状腺瘤表现为胆管重度扩张，相应的胆管内壁毛糙，如绒毛状。

如果不注意观察，平扫很容易与肝内胆管结石混淆。肝内胆管结石境界清楚，多引起梗阻部位近侧胆管扩张，胆管内乳头状肿瘤境界不清，扩张胆管的远侧无梗阻，病灶位于梗阻的中间段。

胆管扩张：与其他肝内胆管占位病变一样，肝内胆管乳头状肿瘤会引起胆管扩张，但也有不同之处：肿瘤组织由多级分支排列的腺管组成，会分泌过多的黏液而阻碍胆管内胆汁的正常流动，引起胆管弥漫性或节段性中度至重度扩张，程度明显高于胆管结石，且与肿瘤大小不成比例。该组病例中，13 例胆管呈中度以上扩张，其中 4 例呈软藤状扩张，类似于胆管细胞癌；4 例伴有胆总管中重度扩张，十二指肠乳头部开口扩大，连同十二指肠乳头突出于十二指肠腔内，考虑与肿瘤分泌的黏液较多而黏稠，胆管内压力过大有关，对本病的诊断可能具有一定的提示作用。

无论肿瘤近端还是远端的胆管均有扩张，这与胆管癌或结石仅出现在病灶近端不同，有时给较小肿瘤的定位带来困难；胆管扩张往往以肿瘤所在位置最为明显，与其他肝叶、段的胆管扩张程度不成比例，该组 5 例肿瘤所在胆管出现动脉瘤样扩张，Lim 等（2004）认为这是肝内胆管乳头状肿瘤特征性表现，与肿瘤阻塞胆管，分泌出的黏液不易排出有关，有时 CT 表现类似于肝内胆管囊腺癌，病灶与扩张胆管是否相通是二者的重要鉴别点，囊腺癌与胆管相通少见，很少造成病变区域胆管扩张。部分囊腺癌也可分泌黏液，但黏液局限于肿瘤内不进入胆管。

MSCT 动态增强：关于肝内胆管乳头状肿瘤 MSCT 动态增强表现，该组资料显示其有一定的强化特点：

首先，肿瘤多为乏血供或少血供，动脉期多轻度强化，门静脉期呈轻度至中度持续强化，强化明显低于管壁外型胆管细胞癌和围管浸润型胆管细胞癌。该组 9 例胆管乳头状腺瘤动脉期轻度强化，强化幅度约 10.1 HU，门静脉期轻度至中度持续强化，CT 值较平扫增加约 29.9 HU；7 例胆管乳头状腺癌中，2

例类似乳头状腺瘤呈轻～中度强化，5 例血供较丰富，呈持续较明显强化，7 例癌动脉期强化幅度约 50.7 HU，门静脉期 CT 值较平扫增加约 62.3 HU。一些学者认为良恶性肝内胆管乳头状肿瘤在影像上无法鉴别，但通过该组 7 例胆管乳头状腺癌和 9 例胆管乳头状腺瘤的增强动脉期及门静脉期 CT 值对比发现，胆管乳头状腺癌多较胆管乳头状腺瘤强化明显（$P< 0.05$）。

其次，由于肿瘤内多有胆汁残留，病灶强化多不均匀。该组 9 例病灶内部见“芯样”强化，以门静脉期或延迟期强化明显，可能与乳头中含有纤维血管芯有关；其中 6 例瘤内呈筛孔状改变，可能与肿瘤内残留胆汁混杂分布有关。

第三，由于肿瘤纤维间质丰富，对比剂在肿瘤内弥散较缓慢，所以病灶强化峰值多出现在中后期，肿瘤轮廓更加清晰。增强后期大部分病例可见到较完整的胆管壁，也是鉴别于胆管细胞癌的重要征象，但是在良恶性的鉴别上，意义不大，该组 7 例乳头状腺癌中，2 例病灶周围仍可见到较完整的胆管壁，4 例肿瘤基底部胆管壁增厚，但外缘轮廓尚清楚，考虑肿瘤尚未突破胆管壁。

多数肝内胆管乳头状肿瘤为交界性肿瘤，较少出现远处转移，该组病例中，仅 1 例乳头状腺癌出现腹腔肿大淋巴结，所有病例均未见腹腔积液；该组 3 例肿瘤所在肝叶或段出现萎缩、肝包膜回缩征，考虑与肿瘤分泌过多的黏液，引起胆汁淤积，导致胆汁性肝硬化和血管受压，血供不足有关。

以下几点重要征象在肝内胆管乳头状肿瘤的 MSCT 诊断中具有重要的临床意义：

扩张肝内胆管内形态多变的类圆形、扁平状或珊瑚状的低密度结节或肿块，肿瘤密度低于肝脏，但高于胆汁；有时由于体积较小，仅表现为肝内胆管扩张或扩张胆管内壁毛糙如绒毛状；肝内胆管弥漫性或节段性扩张：无论肿瘤近端还是远端的胆管均有扩张，以肿瘤所在胆管扩张最为显著，与其他肝叶、段的扩张胆管不成比例；动态增强检查：肿瘤多为进行性持续强化，其中胆管乳头状腺瘤多为轻度至中度强化，部分胆管乳头状腺癌因血供较丰富，强化程度多较前者明显；肿瘤强化多不均匀，部分内部可见“芯样”强化征，与胆汁混杂分布，呈类似“筛孔”状改变；肿瘤强化峰值多出现在中后期，大部分病灶可见到完整的胆管壁，发现肿瘤穿透胆管壁向肝实质内扩散时，提示为恶变；部分肿瘤伴有胆管炎，胆管结石、肝叶萎缩或肝包膜回缩征等继发征象。

鉴别诊断如下：

（1）围管浸润型胆管细胞癌：胆管乳头状腺癌侵犯胆管壁引起管壁增厚时，要与围管浸润型胆管细胞癌鉴别，后者肿瘤多沿胆管壁纵向浸润生长，以肝内胆管壁不规则增厚、僵硬及管腔狭窄改变为主，强化更明显，腔内较少形成结节或肿块。

（2）肿块型肝内胆管细胞癌：胆管乳头状腺癌穿透胆管壁形成边界不清的肿块时，与肿块型肝内胆管细胞癌鉴别较困难，后者以胆管外肿块表现为主，并伴有局部胆管壁增厚及异常强化。围管浸润型与肿块型胆管细胞癌伴发肝内胆管扩张多局限在肿瘤近侧，远端胆管一般扩张不明显，同时易侵犯神经、血管及淋巴管，淋巴结转移较多见。

（3）肝内胆管囊腺癌：肝内胆管囊腺癌一般为肝内多房性囊实性肿瘤，囊壁及间隔较厚，壁上见结节或乳头状突起、囊内出血以及伴粗大钙化；病灶与胆管相通较少见，一般不会引起肝内外胆管明显扩张。

（4）肝内胆管结石：肝内胆管乳头状肿瘤强化极不明显时，易误诊为肝内胆管结石，结石多表现为胆管内类圆形、不规则充盈缺损，轮廓多较光滑，近端胆管扩张而远端及胆总管一般无扩张，不难鉴别。

第九章 先天性肝内胆管囊肿

第一节 先天性肝内胆管扩张(Caroli 病)

有作者指出,先天性肝内胆管扩张是介于先天性肝纤维化与先天性胆管囊肿之间的一种疾病,它常伴存于这两种疾病的报告中,而大多数先天性肝内胆管扩张病例则与之不同,有足够的临床经过与治疗证明,此病是与它们不一样的疾病。大多数病例是非家族性的。肝动脉闭塞和肝梗死能导致与胆管囊肿交通,有作者猜测出生前后的肝动脉闭塞可能是先天性肝内胆管扩张发生的因素之一。

1. 临床表现　尽管先天性肝内胆管扩张可出现于任何年龄的病人,但通常仍以儿童与青少年为多。腹痛、发热、革兰氏阴性败血症是其特征性表现。黄疸通常不出现或极轻微,但在胆管炎发作期间则常见黄疸。常可见到吸收不良,但肝功相当正常,而且不出现门脉高压。胆管结石、胆系结石、肝脓肿、以及胆管癌是其并发症。在炎症控制和/或结石通过以后,症状可以暂时消退,然而却经常复发。可以减轻症状而非治愈的治疗包括:抗生素、胆系引流以及结石的去除。先天性肝内胆管扩张的预后较差,而其病情经过通常随着败血症的发展而进展,甚至危及生命。

2. 病理学　先天性肝内胆管扩张的特点是主要的肝内胆管的囊状扩张。此类囊状扩张衬托以杯状上皮,且与大的肝内胆管分支相连续。肝活检可能发现伴存着先天性肝纤维化。肾脏囊性疾病与管状扩张可以出现,虽然这在临床上通常无重要性。

3. 影像学研究　X 线平片偶尔显示小的肝内结石或髓质性肾钙质沉着。生理性尿系造影能观察到常常伴存的肾的管状扩张和皮质性或髓质性囊肿。口服性胆囊造影或静脉性胆系造影可能显示结石,后者有时还可发现经肝排泄的造影剂的模糊的、不规则的斑状积聚。放射性核素检查时,硫胶肝显像显示相当于扩张肝内胆管的示踪剂吸收减少的分支状区域。虽然孟加拉玫瑰肝胆显像通常只显示肠曲显影延迟,^{99m}Tc-HIDA 及其类似物能成功地描绘肝内胆管的囊状扩张。超声成像观察到透声的肝内管状结构,齐向肝门积聚,为扩张的肝内胆管。如细心地应用换能器多角度地扫描,可能显示出囊状区与肝内胆管相交通。回声的胆泥的丛集,有时还见结石影,且偶尔可见与扩张的肝内胆管相通连。CT 扫描显示低密度的管状结构,伸向肝的周围,并与局限性扩张的区域相通。有时高密度物质位于肝内胆管内,乃为碎屑或非钙化性结石。平片所见的肝内钙化,CT 扫描可证实位于肝内胆管内。如果囊状区域为主要表现,它们与肝内胆管树的交通,能由经静脉注射胆影葡胺后的 CT 扫描图像证实。

直接法胆系造影可观察到肝内胆管系统与囊状区域相交通,先天性肝内胆管扩张几乎总是侵犯两个肝叶。在大多数先天性肝内胆管扩张病例,肝外胆管也见扩张,虽然它并不引起造影剂流向十二指肠的梗阻。区别诊断包括多发性肝内脓肿与肝内胆管树相交通。

X 线血管造影可见围绕大的囊状区的血管的移位。

第二节 先天性肝内胆管囊性扩张症

先天性肝内胆管囊性扩张症,即 Caroli 病,是一种先天性肝内胆管多发节段性囊性扩张病,由法国学者 Jaeclue Caroli(1958)首先描述、报道而得名。此病为一种少见病,发病率小于 1/10 万。先天性肝内胆管囊性扩张症的特征为肝内胆管多发性节段性或囊性扩张,是一种常染色体隐性遗传病;超过 60% 的患者伴有肾囊肿等囊性纤维化疾病。由于扩张仅存在于肝内胆管,不同于先天性肝外胆管扩张所继发的肝内胆管扩张,二者治疗和预后差异也较大,近年来倾向于将该病独立于先天性胆管扩张症之外,归属于先天性囊性纤维化疾病。

根据有无先天性肝纤维化和门静脉高压,又将先天性肝内胆管囊性扩张症分为单纯型与门静脉周围纤维化型两类。单纯型少见,而门静脉周围纤维化型除肝内胆管扩张外,还存在先天性肝纤维化,临床表现除发热、黄疸外,肝硬化、门静脉高压进行性进展,出现脾大,反复上消化道出血和门体分流性脑病。此病多在儿童和青少年时期发病,临床表现较复杂,早期缺乏特异性的症状、体征和实验室检查指标,容易误诊和漏诊。一例通过 MRCP 确诊,属于门静脉周围纤维化型,合并有肾脏囊性病变。患者幼年时反复发热,在基层卫生所输注抗生素后可暂时缓解,至 11 岁即出现门静脉高压、脾大、上消化道出血以及肝性脑病。

MRCP 不仅可以很好地显示胆管与囊肿的关系,对于判断侵及范围和明确肝实质、血管及胆管的改变都具有明确的意义,因其无创并具有特征性影像学表现,已逐步被认为是先天性肝内胆管囊性扩张症的首选检查方法;但应注意与肝内囊性病变、梗阻性肝内胆管扩张症、弥漫性肝癌、小错构瘤等疾病相鉴别。

本病确切的病因和发病机制目前尚不清楚。最近发现该病患者的胆管细胞中血管内皮生长因子(VEGF)、其受体(VEGFR-1、VEGFR-2)以及血管生成素 -2 表达上调,它们通过促进胆管周围微血管形成,促进胆管细胞的增生。VEGF 还可通过自分泌作用直接诱导胆管细胞增生导致胆管扩张。雷帕霉素靶点介导的信号通路也可能与该病胆管细胞的增生有关。除增生外,胆管细胞还通过过度表达纤溶酶原和组织纤溶酶激活物,使纤溶酶生成增加,从而使肝内胆管基底膜上表达的层黏连蛋白和Ⅳ型胶原被纤溶酶降解,促使胆管扩张。

对于青少年肝硬化患者,除了常见的肝炎病毒、酒精因素、遗传代谢因素、药物毒物肝损害、自身免疫性肝病、血吸虫等原因外,应当考虑到先天性肝内胆管囊性扩张症的可能, MRCP 有助于确诊。约有 8.8%~15% 的先天性肝内胆管囊性扩张症可能发生胆管细胞癌,必需引起重视。

在医学影像的误诊研究和学习中,我们深深地体会到,作为一个影像诊断工作者,在日常的临床工作中,应该提倡多向临床学习,多读临床的文献,多与临床医师交流,学习临床知识,学习临床经验,学习医学基础的研究,学会对疾病的比较全面的认识,这样才能更好地避免和减少误诊。

第十章　肝内胆管其他疾病

第一节　胆管性错构瘤

胆管性错构瘤，即胆管微小错构瘤，又称 Von Meyenburg 综合征，由 Von Meyeburg（1918）首先描述。胆管性错构瘤是一种少见的肝脏病变。

1. 发病机制　该病变系紊乱、畸形的胆管形成不同大小的囊状结构，发病率为 1%~3%，多发于肝内的毛细胆管和肝管之间，或胆管的分支，与先天性发育障碍有关。

胆管错构瘤的发病机制尚不清楚，该病在肝内胆管囊肿、先天性肝纤维化和多囊肾的患者中被频繁发现，它与这些先天性胆系疾病的关系提示其为遗传性疾病。有学者认为胆管错构瘤与胆系胚胎形成后期外周小叶间胆管畸形有关。一些作者认为本病属于先天性胆管板发育畸形，非常少见。它系畸形的胆管形成不同大小的囊状结构，常为多发。被认为是由于正常胆管的原始管板（胚胎胆管）发育阻滞或异常所致的错构性病变。

2. 病理学　本病常为多发，散在分布于肝实质内。切面表现为灰白色 0.1~1.5 cm 大小局限性坚硬结节，常在包膜下。本病单发更为少见，文献仅见个案报道。

本病镜下所见具有一定的特征：它们是小管状结构，为成熟结缔组织间质适量地分隔开。它们常含有中等大小的动脉和静脉。病灶由位于纤维间质中众多致密的导管形成，纤维间质可玻璃样变，导管轮廓常不规则，有时可见扩张或含有颗粒状浓缩的胆汁，与胆管树不交通。

有作者指出，本病的病理特征是一个 von Meyenburg 复合体包含数个扩张的胆管，有不同程度的肝纤维化。本病与肝脏间叶性错构瘤不是同一种病变，后者列儿童肝脏良性肿瘤第二位，需要认真鉴别。

3. 临床表现　本病一般见于中年人，通常为男性，剖腹术和尸检均如此。该病临床症状和体征不典型，部分病例表现为肝脏进行性肿大，压迫周围脏器引起胃肠道反应，成年人多因反复肝功能异常或疑为肝脏肿瘤而就诊。有作者指出，本病主要的临床表现是在大体视诊容易混淆为转移性癌。胆管性错构瘤多无临床表现，常在体检行影像学检查、手术探查或尸检时偶然发现，病灶生长缓慢，有的有轻度右上腹疼痛，甲胎蛋白、癌胚抗原一般正常。

影像学研究：磁共振成像检测胆管性错构瘤较超声和 CT 敏感，约 44% 的胆管性错构瘤在 CT 扫描时难以显示。胆管错构瘤的典型 MRI 表现为大小及分布一致，直径通常小于 1cm 的 T_1WI 低信号、T_2WI 高信号结节性病灶，此征象有助于与肝囊肿及肝转移癌鉴别。

多发胆管性错构瘤在影像学上有一定特征性的表现，表现为肝内散在分布不规则的直径 <1.5 cm 囊状影，轮廓不甚规整，与胆管树不交通，因 MRI 对水的敏感性较高，故比 CT 更有利于显示病灶。本病增强扫描无特征性的强化模式，多数报道病灶无强化、边缘强化或缓慢、均匀的强化，有病灶呈环形强化报道，认为系病灶压迫邻近肝组织或炎症细胞浸润所致，也有作者发现病灶呈均匀性强化。在其他脏器有恶性肿瘤的患者，多发胆管性错构瘤在有环状强化的病灶时需与转移灶相鉴别。本病影像学可以显示遍及全肝的多发的小囊性错构瘤病灶或形成的肿块。MRCP 很具特征，可见伴有胆管扩张。

一组 3 例均发生于成人，且均为单发，与多发病灶常为囊性不同，均呈囊实性或实性生长。该组肝脏胆管性错构瘤的病例数较少，其影像学表现不一致，但尚有一些相似的表现：

B 超上呈稍低或稍强回声,内部回声不均匀;CT 平扫呈较均匀或不均匀的较低密度,增强扫描呈较均匀或不均匀轻中度强化,有延迟强化。1 例 MRI 表现为:T_1WI 呈较低信号,T_2WI 呈较高信号,增强扫描呈环状强化。一例因上腹部不适 1 个月就诊,腹部检查未及肿大肝脏及肿物,结合病史及临床表现,入院诊断考虑为肝硬化活动性失代偿期,B 型超声检查亦未见特征性改变,最终经肝穿活组织检查得以确诊,提示对于常规检查难以确诊的罕见肝病,应行肝穿刺组织病理学检查以明确诊断。肝穿刺组织病理学检查为确诊本病的主要依据。

本病病灶如有足够大小,核素检查时,在硫胶扫描则表现为放射活性降低的边界清楚的病灶。本病的血管造影表现为异常血管的小区,呈现于晚期动脉相,持续至静脉相。染色可为环状。肿瘤血管、血管湖以及动 - 静脉瘘未见到。

4. 鉴别诊断　本病的临床和影像学表现缺乏特异性,术前多被误诊为肝转移瘤、肝脓肿、肝海绵状血管瘤等肝脏常见占位病变。

(1)肝转移瘤:增强扫描有环状强化或延迟强化者,有时与肝转移瘤不易鉴别,尤其是患者有其他脏器原发癌者,但本病的环状强化为厚环,而占多数肝转移瘤的腺癌多为薄环状强化,一时无法鉴别者可短期随访。

(2)肝脓肿:本病可合并炎症细胞浸润,此时临床和影像学表现有与肝脓肿相似之处,但后者病灶早期周围有水肿带,中晚期有明显的环状脓肿壁,而本病无此表现。

(3)肝海绵状血管瘤:病灶较小,增强扫描动脉期呈中度强化,并有延迟强化者,需与肝海绵状血管瘤相鉴别,典型的海绵状血管瘤增强扫描动脉期呈周边结节状强化,延迟扫描呈与门静脉等密度 / 信号的均匀强化,与本病不符。

在病理学上本病应与肝脏间叶性错构瘤和胆管腺瘤鉴别:

(1)肝脏间叶性错构瘤:本病与肝脏间叶性错构瘤不是同一种病变,肝脏间叶性错构瘤列儿童肝脏良性肿瘤第二位,其生物学和发病机制不明,细胞学发生研究表明,可能是一种肿瘤,而非错构瘤,多数肿瘤逐渐增大,其典型表现为肝脏大的良性多囊肿瘤,3 岁以下,应完全切除。

(2)胆管腺瘤:本病汇管区周围以结构紊乱的小胆管增生为主,并伴有胆管的囊状扩张,胆管分支状,内壁衬扁平单层上皮,细胞无异型,胆管间见疏松玻璃样胶原。而胆管腺瘤常为单发性结节,少数为多发性结节,病变界限清楚,没有包膜。

第二节　左肝内胆管腺癌,高分化

患者,男,66 岁。上腹胀痛 1 个月入院。

手术所见:腹腔内无腹水,肝脏明显淤胆性改变,左肝可见一大小 6cm × 5cm 肿物,边界不清,质硬,余肝内未扪及明显转移灶,肝门部胆管肿瘤上端累及左肝管,下端累及胆总管上段,未突破胆管浆膜,大小约 5.5cm × 2.5cm × 2.5cm,肝十二指肠韧带、腹腔干、及小肠系膜根部多发肿大淋巴结,胆囊大小约 6.5cm × 3.0cm,张力不高,内可触及多个大小不一结石。

病理检查:①左肝肿物:肝组织一块,大小 9cm × 8 cm × 5 cm,送检前已切开,切面见一灰黄色结节,大小 7 cm × 6 cm × 4 cm,质中偏硬,与周围组织界限不清,周围组织切面黄绿色,质中;②胆囊:胆囊一具,大小 7 cm × 3 cm × 2.3 cm,浆膜面光滑,腔内充满墨绿色黏液及泥沙样结石。黏膜面粗网状,壁厚 0.1 cm~0.3 cm;③胆管壁:灰褐色不规则组织一块,大小 2.5 cm × 1.7 cm × 1 cm,切面灰褐,质中;④ 7 组淋巴结:不规则组织一块,大小 4 cm × 3.5 cm × 2 cm,表面粗糙,切面灰白,灰褐,质中;⑤ 8P 组淋巴结:灰褐色碎组织一堆,总体积 2.4 cm × 2 cm × 1 cm;⑥ 9 组淋巴结:黄褐色组织一块,大小 1.8 cm × 1.5 cm × 0.8 cm,切面灰白灰黄,质中。

免疫组化检测:阳性:CK19,EP-CAM,CEA,CK18,CK8,CK7,Villin,Mucin-5,CA19-9,CK20(个别细胞 +),CD10(灶　+),EGFR(+++),P-gP(+++),VEGF(++),TOPO Ⅱ(+),Ki-67(+,约 20%),Tubulinβ(+);阴性:CDX2,Mucin-2,CgA,Syn,5-FU,ERCC1。

常规病理诊断:①左肝肿物切除标本:初步考虑肝内胆管腺癌,侵犯肝脏被膜及周围脂肪组织,并可见脉管内癌栓。待做免疫组化检测进一步分析;②胆囊切除标本:胆囊肌层及周围纤维脂肪组织内可见癌组织累及;③胆管壁切除标本:可见癌组织累及;④淋巴结清扫:"7 组淋巴结" 4/5,"8P 组淋巴结" 6/7,共检出淋巴结 12 枚,其中 10 枚可见癌转移,送检的"9 组淋巴结"为纤维脂肪组织及骨骼肌组织,可见癌组织累及。免疫组化诊断:左肝肿物切除标本:肝内胆管腺癌，高分化，大小 7 cm × 6 cm × 4 cm，侵犯肝脏被膜及周围纤维脂肪组织，并可见脉管内癌栓。注：肿瘤细胞预后及耐药检测结果供临床参考（图 16-10-1）。

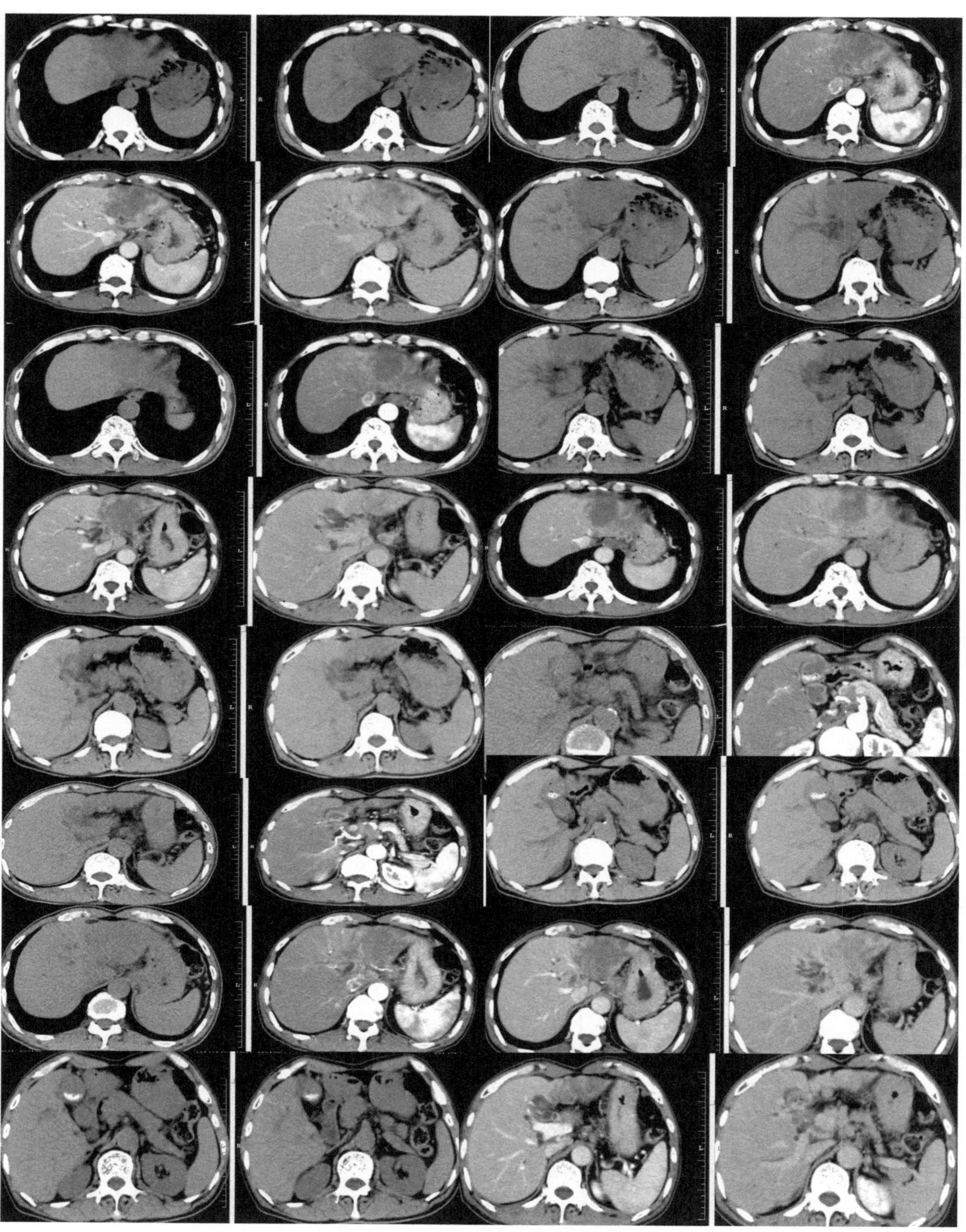

图 16-10-1　左肝内胆管腺癌，高分化

第三节　肝内胆管成像中的误诊和诊断陷阱

正常的肝内胆管位于对应的门静脉分支前方，二者均在肝门部汇聚。超声或增强 CT 可辨别出它们较大的肝门部分支，而正常管径的外周部肝内胆管很难由 CT 显示，当发生脂肪肝时，CT 更难显示。胆管闭锁的婴儿肝内胆管消失，影像检查技术上的局限性限制了对其显示。超声的作用是显示因纤维化所致肝实质回声改变和门静脉周围回声增加，排除其他原因所致的梗阻性黄疸，了解有无并存的其他异常，如胆总管囊肿、胆囊闭锁或发育不全。

迷走胆管和副肝管：胆管扩张时横断面成像能更好地显示肝内胆管的发育变异和异常。例如，高达 20% 的人群出现引流肝右叶后段或前段的迷走胆管，该胆管通常汇入肝门部主肝管或肝总管，胆囊切除术时易疏忽而结扎，术后影像检查可发现肝段性胆管梗阻。关于这种胆管异常的影像诊断和医源性损伤的治疗已有报道。发育变异中还包括来源于肝脏的细小副胆管沿胆囊窝走行，汇入胆囊三角(Calot 三角)内的肝外胆管，胆囊切除术时可能被切断，造成胆漏和腹膜炎。

CT 或超声能很好地显示这些并发症，但显示潜在的胆管异常则需借助于经 T 管、经皮或经内镜直接胆管造影。使用快速自旋回波序列(FSE)或半傅里叶快速采集弛豫增强(RARE)技术所获取的非侵袭性 MRCP，对多种胆管异常如迷走的右肝管和低位胆囊管有诊断价值。

胆管梗阻：成人胆管梗阻常为后天性因素，原因有嵌顿性结石、狭窄或肿瘤，而一些先天性异常表现为肝内胆管非梗阻性扩张，两者影像表现有类似之处，应加以鉴别。

先天性肝内胆管扩张是一典型的例子，它与胆管炎复发、结石形成、肝纤维化和肾小管扩张有关，表现为肝内胆管节段性或弥漫性海绵状扩张，CT 和超声上的主要特征为肝内胆管囊状扩张，位于门静脉分支周围，门静脉分支向囊腔内突入并形成桥状结构。

肝内胆管动脉瘤样扩张：孤立的肝内胆管动脉瘤样扩张少见，与先天性管壁薄弱、上皮隔膜所致的部分性梗阻有关，或继发于局部病变，CT 表现为肝内边界清楚的局限性低密度区，类似于肝内胆囊、肝囊肿、脂肪瘤或空洞性转移灶。胆管造影和其他影像学检查方法有助于确定胆管动脉瘤样扩张的性质，并进行鉴别诊断。

肝内胆管积气：在外科分流、括约肌切开术或 ERCP 后，看到胆管树内气体即胆管积气并非少见，胆管分支类型与胆管系统解剖一致。偶尔，进行胆总管结石排石时在胆管树内可见到气体。一种潜在的诊断误区是气腹延伸到肝门而误认为是肝内胆管积气。另一种潜在诊断误区是胆管积气与门静脉系统积气的鉴别。

门静脉积气的其他原因包括近期外科手术或是留置导管(包括 G 管)。门静脉积气通常有典型分支形状，可达到肝脏的周边，与胆管积气不同(胆管积气集中在肝脏的中央部位)。

第十一章　肝门胆管癌

第一节　肝门部浸润型胆管癌的早期诊断

近年来，随着医学影像学技术的进步，特别是MSCT及高场强MRI的应用，胆管癌的早期诊断成为可能。该病变的早期诊断对治疗方案的选择及患者的预后具有重要意义。

肝门部浸润型胆管癌的MSCT与高场MRI特点：肝门部浸润型胆管癌的CT及MRI表现有一定特点，具体表现在病变的强化方式方面，一组15例中12例病变于动脉期即见明显均匀强化，门静脉期强化达峰值，平衡期亦见明显强化，MRI扫描显示病灶于延迟期呈持续性明显强化。以前研究资料提示，胆管细胞癌具有延迟强化和强化方式从周边向中央区扩展的特点，但该组资料仅3例有此特点。学者推测，出现这种差别的原因可能有以下几个：

其一，早期的报道资料因受外科学技术及影像学技术的限制，发现的病变多为病灶相对较大的肿块型胆管癌，后者多见于肝内且肝内病变大多为此类型，该类病变具有延迟强化及强化由瘤周向中央区扩展的特点。而该组资料显示的多为肝门部浸润型胆管癌，该种病理类型的胆管癌可能大多数具有早期明显强化并持续强化的特点。

其二，该组资料发现的可能多为早期病变，尚未形成较明显的软组织肿块，病变血供相对较丰富，纤维化改变尚不明显，故而具有早期明显均匀强化的特点。

此外研究结果的差别可能还跟机器的扫描速度、扫描参数的选择、对比剂的类型及注射流率等有一定关系。该组资料标本数目有限，可能有一定的偶然因素，研究结果尚需进一步的资料积累来证实。

该组资料还提示，MSCT及高场MRI在肝门部浸润型胆管癌的诊断方面具有较高的敏感度及诊断符合率，且对肝门部浸润型胆管癌的术前分型具有较高的可靠性。有研究资料提示，薄层螺旋CT结合三维重建技术，对胆管癌诊断的符合率相当高，该组MSCT强化扫描的诊断符合率亦达到相当高。一些资料报道MRI特别是结合MRCP，对肝门部胆管癌术前分型诊断的符合率高达90%以上，该组MRI薄层强化扫描、冠状面扫描及MRCP的综合应用，对术前患者均进行了较准确的诊断及分型。

MSCT及高场MRI在肝门部浸润型胆管癌分期中的作用：若肝门部胆管癌的诊断已确立，肿瘤正确的局部分期对进一步的治疗将起到十分重要的作用。肝门部胆管癌的分期应以判断病变的范围以评价是否可切除为目的。影像学分析应包括肿瘤的范围、有无肝脏侵犯、血管受累情况（特别是肝动脉和门静脉）、淋巴结转移及远处转移（特别是肝内转移）。

胆管癌不可切除的标准包括：门静脉主干受累、门静脉左右支受累、一叶肝的门静脉受累伴另一叶肝的肝动脉受累、一叶肝的血管受累伴另一叶肝广泛的胆管受累、双侧肝内胆管段以下分支受累、肝内或淋巴结转移。

传统上，肝门胆管癌的影像学评估的最终诊断常依赖于直接法胆管造影，如ERCP及PTC，二者曾被认为是术前评价胆管癌沿纵轴侵犯范围的最佳方法。但众所周知，直接法胆管造影可导致严重的并发症，且不能评估肿瘤对胆管壁横轴的浸润程度。另外，对腔内生长型的病例，直接法胆管造影可因腔内坏死物质的存在而高估胆管的受累范围。

MSCT及高场强MRI，特别是MRI及MRCP，在评估肝门部胆管癌的可切除性方面具有重要意义。它们可以显示胆管、血管及附近肝实质的受侵情况。

首先,在胆管的侵犯方面:研究结果显示 PTC 效果优于 ERCP,但二者均不如 MRCP,后者评估胆系梗阻平面及胆管受累的准确率可达 88%~96%。MSCT 动态扫描结合多平面重建技术在该方面亦具有明显优势。但各影像学检查方法均存在以下问题:①高估病变沿纵轴的侵犯范围;②对病变黏膜下(即横轴)侵犯的评估都存在一定困难,容易低估病变的程度。有资料提示,在延迟扫描中,胆管壁的延迟强化的有无及其强化程度对估计病变沿胆管侵犯有一定帮助,但确切意义尚需进一步的研究。

其次,在血管的侵犯方面:术前对肝动脉及门静脉受累情况的精确评估十分重要。在评估肝门血管系统受累方面,动态增强 MRI 效果可与血管造影相媲美。在 MRI 血管造影,血管壁的狭窄、突然截断及局部不规则缺损清晰可见。

需要说明的是,MRCP 部分或完全抑制了背景组织的信号,故而在显示原发病变与血管的关系方面效果并不理想,因此,在行 MRCP 检查的同时,行轴面及冠状面常规强化扫描是十分必要的,这对显示肿瘤的浆膜面侵犯情况及肿瘤与周围结构的粘连情况很有帮助。

另外,据报道,冠状面或斜冠状面动态增强扫描对鉴别血管与胆管很有帮助,并能显示肿瘤与门静脉的关系,因为这种扫描方式能使门静脉在 1~2 幅图像上显示,肝门区病变容易定位,且冠状面成像的解剖效果与手术所见相似。

肝实质侵犯:附近肝实质的受侵情况对评估肿瘤的可切除性具有重要意义。CT 多平面成像能显示突破胆管并侵犯相邻肝实质的肿物。MRI 脂肪抑制的对比剂增强扫描对显示附近肝实质的侵犯及转移也很有帮助。脂肪抑制技术能抑制肝门区的脂肪,这能提高胆管癌的显示效果,并利于估测肿瘤的范围及其对周围组织、器官的浸润情况。

总之,MSCT 及高场 MRI 在肝门部浸润型胆管癌的诊断方面具有重要意义,并可对肿瘤的可切除性进行有效评估。

第二节 肝门部胆管癌 MR 3D-VIBE 序列和 MRCP

肝门部胆管癌的病理基础及临床表现:肝门部胆管癌,又称 Klatskin 瘤,是指发生于胆囊管开口近端的肝外胆管癌,其发生率居胆系肿瘤的第二位,男性多见,好发于 50~75 岁。近年来,其发病率呈逐渐上升趋势,病因不明,可能与胆管结石、硬化型胆管炎、胆系寄生虫及病毒性肝炎等诱发有关。病理上分为结节型、硬化型、乳头型及浸润型,以硬化型癌多见。组织病理学一般为高分化分泌黏液的腺癌,其次为低分化癌、未分化癌及鳞状细胞癌等。

肝门部胆管癌患者早期多无症状,或仅有上腹部不适、疼痛、乏力、食欲不振等不典型症状,易误诊为上消化道慢性炎症,随着病变的进展,可出现无痛性、渐进性黄疸,皮肤瘙痒,大便呈陶土色及腹痛等症状,合并胆管炎时可出现寒颤、高热,晚期患者多消瘦、贫血,并有腹腔积液、大便隐血等。

一、肝门部胆管癌的分型和分期

提高肝门部胆管癌患者的生存率有赖于肿瘤的早期发现和完整切除。肝门胆管癌起病隐匿,早期不易发现,又因解剖结构特殊,周围毗邻关系复杂,切除困难,预后较差。如果能早期发现,对临床制订手术方案,采取治疗措施具有重要指导意义。

目前,临床多以国际通用的改良 Bismuth-Corlette 分型标准对肝门胆管癌进行术前评估(表 16-11-1)。此分型对临床选择术式有一定帮助,对肿瘤在肝门胆管中的定位有一定价值,但不能反映出肿瘤与周围其他结构的关系,从而影响了临床术前对手术方案的评估。因此,Burke 等(1998)提出了一个新的改良 T- 分期系统用于肝门部胆管癌的术前评估(表 16-11-2)。

表 16-11-1 肝门部胆管癌 Bismuth-Corlette 分型标准

分型	标准
Ⅰ型	肿瘤位于肝总管,未侵犯汇合部
Ⅱ型	肿瘤位于左右肝内胆管汇合部,未侵犯左右肝内胆管
Ⅲ型	肿瘤位于左右肝内胆管汇合部,并侵犯右肝内胆管(Ⅲa)或侵犯左肝内胆管(Ⅲb)
Ⅳ型	肿瘤位于左右肝内胆管汇合部,并侵犯肝总管及左右肝内胆管

表 16-11-2　肝门部胆管癌的 T 分期标准

分期	标准
T_1 期	肿瘤侵及肝内胆管汇合部和/或单侧扩展至二级胆管
T_2 期	肿瘤侵及肝内胆管汇合部和/或单侧扩展至二级胆管的同时合并同侧门静脉受累和/或同侧肝叶萎缩
T_3 期	肿瘤侵及肝内胆管汇合部并且双侧都扩展至二级胆管；或肿瘤单侧扩展至二级胆管的同时合并对侧门静脉受累；或肿瘤单侧扩展至二级胆管的同时对侧肝叶萎缩；或肿瘤累及门静脉主干或者双侧门静脉均受累

该分期不但充分考虑到了肿瘤在胆管系统中的位置，而且对门静脉系统是否受累、肝叶是否萎缩等都有详细的说明，更有助于临床术前相对准确地预见肿瘤的可切除率，因此该分期系统目前已越来越多地被临床接受和应用。

二、MR 3D-VIBE 序列和 MRCP 的优点及在 T_1 期中的影像学表现

T_1 期肝门部胆管癌多数病灶较小、范围局限、症状不典型，漏、误诊率较高。因此，选择合理的检查序列很重要。磁共振三维容积式内插法屏气检查（3D-VIBE）序列联合 MRCP 检查可以明显提高诊断符合率。该组资料显示，两者的联合应用诊断肝门部胆管癌准确性高达 100%，T_1 期准确性达 94%（15/16），因而具有重要的临床应用价值。

MRCP 是一种观察胆管系统解剖和病理形态的 MR 技术，不需要特殊的插管技术，也不需要对比剂，安全、简便、适应证广、成功率高、并发症少，其诊断价值已得到肯定。MRCP 图像清晰，可以完全达到诊断要求，图像表现与直接胆管造影相似，能够显示胆系的整体观和连续性，可以明确肝门部梗阻情况，判断梗阻部位、范围、断端形态及邻近组织结构情况。

MRCP 对胆管梗阻定位诊断准确性达 85%~100%，定性诊断准确性达 64%~98%。

MRCP 在肝门胆管癌 T- 分期系统中对肿瘤的定位和梗阻范围能提供一定信息，结节型和乳头型肝门胆管癌主要呈结节样或乳头样软组织影向腔内外生长，MRCP 表现为肝门部胆管截断，管腔内充盈缺损，边缘欠光整，其上肝内外胆管呈"软藤"样扩张。肿瘤仅限于肝管汇合部时，双侧肝内外胆管多对称性扩张；单侧扩张至二级胆管时，表现为该叶胆管狭窄和病变以上肝内胆管扩张。

硬化型和浸润型肝门胆管癌主要沿胆管壁生长，肿块多不明显，以管壁增厚和管腔狭窄为主，MRCP 表现为病变处管腔不规则狭窄、变细、僵硬，肝左右叶扩张的肝管在肝门部不能汇合，胆管断端呈"鼠尾"状或"矛尖"状狭窄，可有肝叶萎缩。MRCP 对病变侵及范围也能很好地显示。

但是 MRCP 无法提供门静脉和肝动脉是否受侵、周围实质脏器有无转移、腹腔和腹膜后淋巴结是否增大等信息。同时 MRCP 因受空间分辨率限制，难以显示微小的狭窄和轻微的病变，对左侧二级胆管汇合部受累亦显示欠佳，因而也就影响了肿瘤的分期，这就需要 MRCP 和 MRI 其他序列联合应用才能给肿瘤划分出准确的分期，从而给临床提供更多的信息。

MR 3D-VIBE 序列可以很好地解决 MRCP 所不能解决的上述问题。3D-VIBE 成像技术因扫描层厚薄、间距窄，每次扫描时间短、可以行 Gd-DTPA 三期扫描及软组织分辨率高等特点，因而能够发现肝门部胆管内较小肿瘤，更有利于显示肿瘤的形态学及血供特征，对肝实质有无侵犯、肝动脉及门静脉有无受累、局部淋巴结有无增大也能够很好显示。

从该组资料上看，该扫描序列可以发现肝门胆管内 0.3~0.5 cm 小肿瘤，对门静脉和肝动脉也有较好地显示，进而更有助于肝门部胆管癌 T_1 期肿瘤的检出。

在肝门部胆管癌 T_1 期肿瘤中，结节型和乳头型肝门部胆管癌表现为管腔内充盈缺损，向腔内外生长，边缘欠光整；硬化型和浸润型表现为胆管弥漫增厚及管腔狭窄，内缘凸凹不平。增强扫描动脉早期肿瘤轻度强化，动脉晚期及门静脉期多数明显强化。文献报道肝门部胆管癌不仅会沿着胆管壁浸润生长，且易环绕整个格里申鞘，包绕、浸润大血管，而通常不侵犯腔内形成癌栓，CT 检查对此有一定局限性，MR 3D-VIBE 序列三期增强则可以明确提供门静脉及肝动脉受累的信息，对门静脉内癌栓也能较好显示。T_1 期肝门部胆管癌可有局部淋巴结增大。该组 16 例 T_1 期肝门部胆管癌中，有 5 例出现局部淋巴结增大。

三、鉴别诊断

肝门部胆管癌应与硬化型胆管炎、肝门部结石、胆囊癌及肝细胞癌伴胆道癌栓等鉴别。

1. 硬化型胆管炎　硬化型胆管炎好发于肝门左

右肝管汇合部,表现为肝内胆管弥漫性增厚,管腔狭窄,增强可强化,但其发病少见且肝内胆管不扩张或轻度扩张或局灶性扩张有利于和肝门部胆管癌鉴别。

2. 肝门部胆管结石　肝门部胆管结石表现为肝管内柱状、圆形或类圆形充盈缺损,呈低或无信号,增强不强化, T_2WI 周围环以高信号胆汁, MRCP 梗阻断端多呈倒“杯口”状,少数平直,梗阻以上胆管树呈“枯树”状扩张,结石可以引起胆管炎使管壁增厚,增强有强化,但管壁规则、光滑,这些特征有利于与肝门部胆管癌鉴别。

3. 胆囊癌　发生在胆囊颈部的胆囊癌常累及肝门部胆管引起胆管狭窄并肝内胆管扩张,但胆囊壁不规则增厚,胆囊体部明显胀大是两者的主要鉴别点。

4. 肝细胞癌伴胆管癌栓　肝细胞癌伴胆管癌栓可以引起肝门部胆管狭窄并腔内充盈缺损,但肝内一般可以发现原发灶,增强扫描呈“快进快出”征象,结合患者有肝硬化表现且甲胎蛋白明显增高有助于和肝门部胆管癌鉴别。

总之, MR 3D-VIBE 序列联合 MRCP 在肝门部胆管癌 T_1 期的诊断中具有一定的优势。MRCP 可以明确肝门部梗阻情况,判断梗阻部位、范围、断端形态及邻近组织结构情况。3D-VIBE 能够显示肝门部胆管内较小肿瘤,更有利于显示肿瘤的形态学及血供特征,可以提供肝实质有无受侵、肝动脉及门静脉有无受累、局部淋巴结有无增大等信息,两者的联合应用可以进一步提高肝门部胆管癌 T_1 期的检出率,有助于指导临床术前制定合理的手术方案。

第三节　肝门部胆管癌与肝门肿大淋巴结

一组肝门部胆管癌伴存肝门肿大淋巴结病例中, MRI 检出 8 例淋巴结,而 CT 仅为 6 例,可能与以下三个因素有关: MRI 中的 T_2WI+ 脂肪抑制,对肿大的淋巴结敏感,在该序列中淋巴结呈很亮的信号,与周围的组织、血管分辨率高而易被发现; FLASH T_1WI+ 脂肪抑制序列中,肿大淋巴结的信号明显低于肝实质,因而肝门淋巴结易被检出;有作者报道,肝门肿大淋巴结在 MRI 上易呈“古钱征”,因门静脉在 MRI 上呈流空现象,肝门部胆管癌的肝门肿大淋巴结易包绕门静脉而未侵入腔内形成此征象。因此,该组作者认为 MRI 的多序列扫描较 CT 更易检出肿大的淋巴结。

第四节　肝门胆管中分化腺癌

患者 男,64 岁。中上腹闷痛两月余,尿黄一月入院。

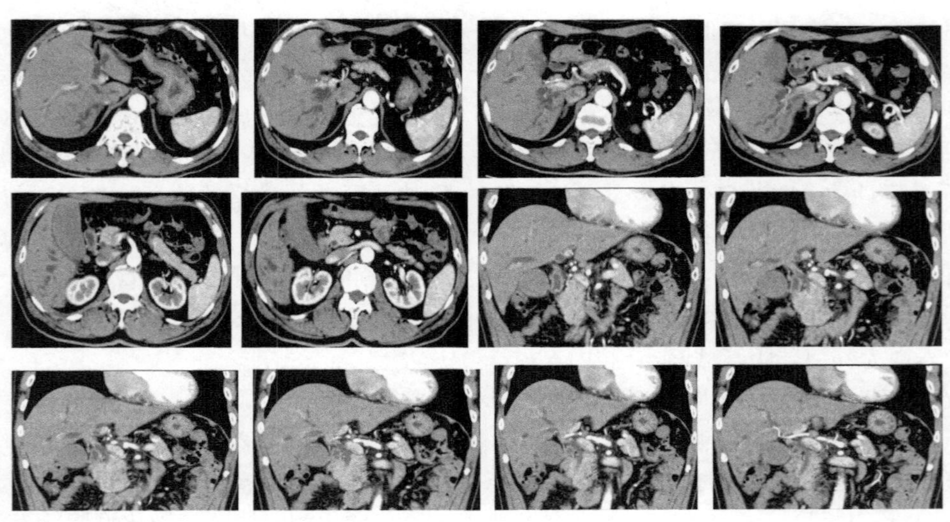

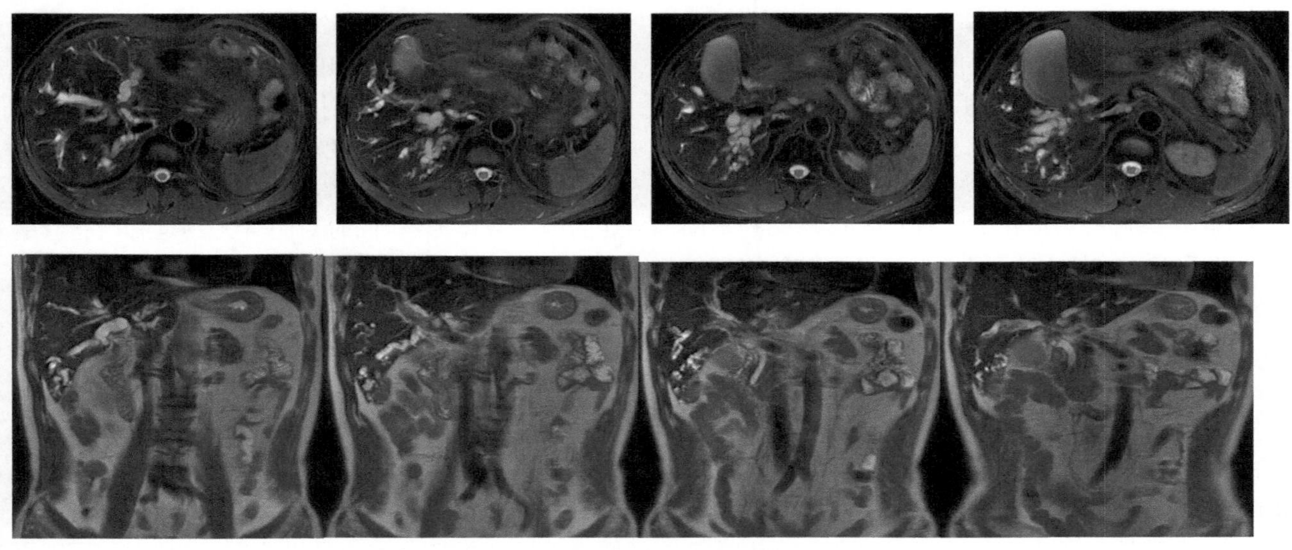

图 16-11-1　肝门部胆管癌与肝门肿大淋巴结

病理检查：肝门部胆管肿物：灰白色组织一块，大小为 4cm × 3 cm × 1.5 cm，切面灰白，质中。常规病理诊断：肝门部胆管肿物切除标本：初步诊断胆管中分化腺癌，待做免疫组化检测进一步证实，并可见癌组织侵及邻近肝组织。免疫组化检测：阳性：CK19，CK18，CEA，CK7，CK8，Villin，CA19-9，CK20（个别+），Ki-67（+，约 60%）；阴性：AFP，Hepatocyte，Vimentin，CD10，CD34。免疫组化诊断：肝门部胆管肿物切除标本：胆管中分化腺癌，可见癌组织侵及邻近肝组织，胆囊未受累及（图 16-11-1、16-11-2）。

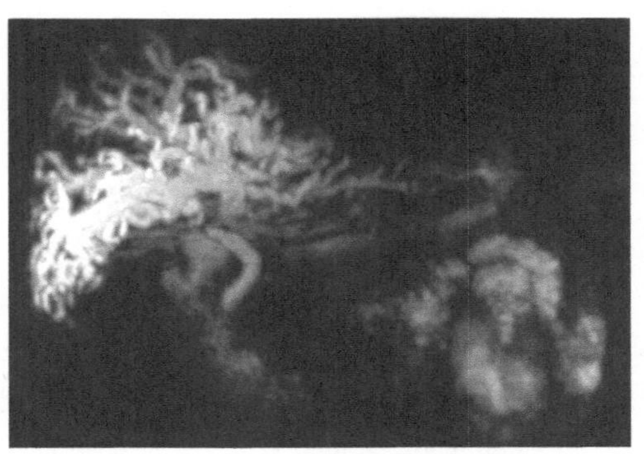

图 16-11-2　肝门胆管中分化腺癌

第五节　肝门胆管癌 MSCT 误诊

肝门胆管癌分型诊断：Bismuth-Corlette 分型用于划分肝门胆管癌的病灶部位，不同类型的肝门胆管癌手术切除率和手术方式均不同。手术一方面要尽可能安全地扩大手术范围，达到断端无残余肿瘤细胞。Ⅰ型及Ⅱ型患者容易确定根治性手术切除的范围；Ⅲ a 型患者一般需要联合肝叶切除，Ⅲ b 型由于左半肝切除影响较小，达到根治性切除的可能性较高，而Ⅲ a 型由于受到剩余肝实质代偿功能的限制，右半肝切除范围有限；Ⅳ型患者由于左右侧肝脏均受累，范围较广，需要结合实际情况判断。

另一方面还必须考虑手术后残余的胆管是否具有足够长度进行胆肠吻合。理论上Ⅰ、Ⅱ、Ⅲ型均属可切除型，而Ⅳ型是否需要行扩大根治术尚有争议。Sakamato 等（1998）报道，自双侧胆管梗阻点沿胆管向肝内侧再延伸 0.5~1.0 cm，作为手术预定切线点，如未超过二级胆管则判断为可以切除。有作者认为，Bismuth-Corlette Ⅰ、Ⅱ、Ⅲ型达到根治性切除的可能性较Ⅳ型高，其中Ⅲ b 型高于Ⅲ a 型，其余病例因侵犯血管、腹腔脏器或转移等情况未能进行肝门胆管癌根治性切除术。不同 Bismuth-Corlette 分型患者行根治性切除术的差异无统计学意义，因此，一方面仍需积累更多病例，另一方面表明 Bismuth-Corlette 分型虽然是判断肝门胆管癌可切除性及手术方式的重要因素，但必须结合分期诊断、患者肝脏储备及全身情况等多种因素综合判断。

大体形态分型：管内结节乳头型及外生肿块型肝门胆管癌因其范围较为局限，在手术中容易确定范围，进行根治性切除，胆管吻合成功率也相对较高;浸润型肝门胆管癌具有沿管壁爬行性生长的特性,容易累及肝内胆管及胆总管,其相应的Bismuth-Corlette分型也往往提示难以进行根治性手术。文献报道,管内结节乳头型与外生肿块型的根治性切除率较高,预后也较好;而浸润型肝门胆管癌手术切除率较低,预后最差。评价大体形态的不同分型及采用的手术方式,同样需要结合其他因素综合判断。

MSCT及重建技术与肝门胆管癌分型诊断:肝门部结构复杂,多套管道系统并行,通过MSCT薄层扫描以及后处理技术,有助于在定性诊断的基础上进一步进行分型诊断。早期的MSCT胆管成像技术采用阳性对比剂进行胆管显影,但对于胆管梗阻患者,尤其是胆管肿瘤患者,应用阳性胆系对比剂可能加重肝脏负担或进一步损伤肝功能,胆系显影的效果也不甚理想。因此,对于胆管梗阻患者,选择MSCT胆系造影法,即用非离子性碘对比剂增强肝实质及其他软组织的密度,使其与胆管腔内的密度差和对比度增大,从而更加清晰地显示胆系。在肝门胆管癌的诊断中,应用较多的MSCT后处理方法主要是多平面重建技术,即应用容积重建数据进行兴趣区的胆管剖面二维重建。一般较多采用的是冠状面或斜冠状面重建,有时可采用多平面重建的特殊形式,即曲面重建显示胆管形态。多平面重建图像更加直观,可以从多个角度显示胆管的纵向剖面结构、腔内外的组织形态以及管壁的情况,同时有助于病灶大体形态的全面显示和准确划分、径线的测量以及CT值测定等。目前MSCT的不足之处在于受射线电离辐射影响以及碘对比剂过敏反应和对肾功能的部分影响。与MR胆胰管造影(MRCP)比较,MSCT的优势在于对胆管内外病变的诊断特异性较强,且对较小的病变漏诊率减少。MRCP尽管可以较为直观地显示胆管树的全貌,但无法判断病灶的准确大体形态,同时对胆管尤其是肝内胆管的受累情况显示尚不满意,必须结合常规MRI检查。此外,MRCP目前扫描时间仍较长,受呼吸和运动伪影影响显著,图像质量常影响诊断。

MSCT肝门胆管癌分型诊断:Bismuth-Corlette分型方面,一组与手术分型的总符合率达86.7%(26/30),较以往文献中提到的准确率高,充分显示了16层以上MSCT对手术的指导价值,但有4例低估了肝内胆管分支的受累范围,误判主要原因可能由于病例均为浸润型,术前未能准确判断肿瘤在肝内胆管管壁中生长的范围,MSCT诊断应注意仔细观察肝内胆管形态及密度的改变,并在重建时尽量选择好的平面,显示肝内胆管的具体受累情况。

大体形态分型方面,该组中MSCT对大体形态分型均与手术中所见相符,符合率较高,可以作为术前大体形态分型的良好手段。肝细胞性肝癌侵犯胆管:有作者曾见一例CT与MRCP均见肝门胆管充盈缺损,肝外胆管如常,肝内胆管蔓藤状扩张,术前诊断为肝门胆管癌,手术发现为一直径约2cm淡黄色结节状包块伴存肝门胆管内癌栓与出血导致肝门胆管梗阻,病理诊断为肝细胞性肝癌。此类病例属于肝细胞性肝癌侵犯胆管导致的误诊。

第十二章　肝门区其他疾病

第一节　肝门部肿瘤 MRI 误诊分析

肝门部肿瘤按其生长形态可分为外生肿块型、浸润型和管内生长型。有研究显示平扫中 T_2WI 对于显示病变及淋巴结肿大、腹水等伴随征象方面敏感性不亚于增强扫描。一组资料单发于肝门区的转移性病变多来自邻近器官（特别是消化系统肿瘤），以直接蔓延方式转移者居多。有作者认为，MRCP 加梗阻部位薄层扫描或增强显示胆管梗阻的准确率高于内镜逆行胆胰管造影（ERCP）和经皮肝穿胆管造影（PTC）。该研究显示 MRCP 对肝门部肿瘤致胆管梗阻水平定位准确率达 93.3%，由于空间分辨力相对低，MRCP 难以区分完全梗阻与高度狭窄，两者均表现为阻塞性改变。动态增强扫描对于肝门部肿瘤鉴别诊断具有重要价值。该组肿块型胆管癌动态增强扫描以延迟期强化为主，体现了癌组织动脉供血不丰富及富含纤维组织、细胞外间隙大的病理组织学基础。

该资料胆管癌组术前定性诊断错误 4 例，其中 2 例于动脉期、门脉期表现为轻度强化，加上并发肝内多发转移灶而误诊为肝门转移性病变，2 例浸润型胆管癌胆管壁增厚、强化而误诊为胆管炎性改变；该组肝细胞性肝癌三期均未见明显强化 2 例而误诊为良性病变，产生病理基础为瘤内血供较少，该作者认为结合患者症状、体征及 AFP 检查非常重要。肝细胞性肝癌动脉期开始强化，门脉期信号仍高于肝组织 2 例，产生原因主要是肿瘤为动脉和门脉双重供血。

肝门转移性病变误诊为胆管癌 3 例、误诊为肝细胞性肝癌 2 例，其中 2 例为富血供性转移性病变。分析这 5 例误诊的主要原因为原发肿瘤病史不详，肿瘤单发且强化方式与肝细胞性肝癌、胆管癌类似所致。

肝门区肿瘤术前评估需了解肿瘤大小、范围、胆管及血管受侵及淋巴结转移情况等。MRCP 整体感强，有利于病变的定位；T_2WI 及增强扫描可以更准确地观察肿瘤边界，3D DCE-MRA 显示的血管改变同血管造影有很高的一致性，3D DCE-MRA 在显示门静脉瘤栓及动静脉瘘方面有独特的优势，但对于血管局部的轻微浸润方面显示欠佳。

该资料胆管癌组术前评估认为可切除的 9 例中。有 3 例分别因术中见病变侵犯 2 级胆管，对侧肝内转移及门静脉浸润而行姑息治疗，术前有 2 例认为病变侵犯 2 级胆管，术中见病变局限肝总管分叉处及左、右肝管予以完全切除，分析这 5 例评估错误的主要原因有：①MRCP 的 MIP 重组图像上扩张的胆管互相重叠，二级分支受累显示欠清，因而影响了病灶范围的判断；②肝门区胆管解剖结构复杂、变异导致对病变是否累及二级分支的定位出现偏差。该组资料中的肝细胞性肝癌组术前评估认为可手术切除、无包膜的肝细胞性肝癌 2 例，因 MRI 术前未显示门静脉左支受侵而行手术，术中见肿块与门静脉左支侧壁有粘连，左肝管与门静脉间部分肿瘤组织未能完全切除，提示肝癌包膜可能是肝门血管受侵的保护性因素。肝门转移性病变术前未能定性而手术探查者不在少数，该组有 4 例术前误诊为胆管癌、肝细胞性肝癌而行手术，术中均未能完全切除。

总之，该研究建议肝门区肿瘤欲行手术者均应行 MRI 平扫联合动态增强扫描、MRCP 及 3D DCE-MRA 等无创性检查，以提供给临床最全面的、较准确的诊断和术前评估信息。

第二节 PTC 检查时肝管汇合处的假性肿瘤

PTC 检查在肝胆疾病的诊断上准确性较高,一般均在 90% 以上。Li 等(1981)报告 4 例梗阻性黄疸病人在 PTC 检查时,对胆管阻塞的原因及部位判断错误,在肝管汇合处表现为肿瘤性梗阻,但实际上 3 例是结石,1 例是胰腺疾病。

导致误诊的原因可能是对比剂和黏稠胆汁难以混合均匀,导致对比剂通过左右肝管汇合处得不到理想的影像。为避免 PTC 时此种假性肿瘤的再现,在注射对比剂前,应当吸取更多的胆管内胆汁,但由于胆系梗阻时胆汁甚为浓稠,这点却难以办到。

造影时病人应当采用直立位,此种体位有利于阻塞部位的确切显示;如果此种体位照片还未得到阻塞部位满意的图像,则宜再用 MRCP 或 ERCP 检查。如果肝门部位确实存在阻塞,肝内胆管一般则出现扩张;如肝内胆管无明确扩张,则说明肝门处多无阻塞。

第三节 假胆管癌征

详见本书 本卷 本篇 第五章 第一节 假胆管癌征。

第十三章　肝外胆管肿块

第一节　肝外胆管细胞癌所致肝实质一过性密度差异

肝实质一过性强化差异是指肝实质血流灌注异常，肝动脉供血增加引起的动脉期肝实质局部强化的现象。影像学上可表现为叶多段性、扇形、多形性及弥漫性等4种形态，最初由Itai等（1982）报道。

诊断标准和分型：一过性肝实质强化差异的诊断标准：CT平扫呈等密度；CT三期动态增强扫描动脉期局部强化呈高密度，门静脉期和平衡期异常强化消退，肝实质密度恢复正常。

测量肝左叶外侧段、肝左叶内侧段、肝右叶前段、肝右叶后段起始部胆管直径。按照测量值将肝内胆系扩张程度分为3级。轻度：肝内胆系扩张直径≤ 5 mm；中度：扩张胆管直径范围6~8 mm；重度：扩张胆管直径≥ 9 mm。为了便于分析将一过性肝实质强化差异形态分为3型。Ⅰ型：沿胆管分布的一过性肝实质强化差异，边界不清，呈柱状或分枝状。Ⅱ型：扇形或不规则片状的一过性肝实质强化差异，边界清楚或不清楚。Ⅲ型：胆囊旁肝实质内弧形片状一过性肝实质强化差异，边界不清。

病理生理学：肝脏血供丰富，由肝门静脉和肝动脉双重供血。肝门静脉是肝的功能血管，将从胃肠吸收的物质输入肝内。门静脉在肝门处分为左右两支，分别进入肝左叶和右叶，继而在肝小叶间反复分支，形成小叶间静脉。小叶间静脉继续分出小支，称终末门微静脉，行于相邻两个肝小叶之间。终末门微静脉的分支与肝血窦相连，将门静脉血输入肝小叶内。

肝动脉血富含氧，是肝的营养血管。肝动脉的分支与门静脉的分支伴行，依次分为小叶间动脉和终末肝微动脉，最后也通入肝血窦。

肝门静脉和肝动脉的血液在肝血窦内混合，肝门静脉和肝动脉供血之间存在代偿，由于正常时肝门静脉压[7 mmHg（1 mmHg=0.133kPa）]明显低于肝动脉压（100 mmHg），所以当肝血窦闭塞或压力增高时，首先发生门静脉供血减少，而肝动脉供血代偿性增多，而较少发生肝动脉供血减少由肝门静脉代偿供血。一过性肝实质强化差异的病理生理学基础是肝动脉供血相对增多，其原因可以为原发性或继发性肝动脉灌注增多。

原发性一过性肝实质强化差异发生时仅存在肝动脉血流增加，肝门静脉内血流无明显减少，常见于富血供的局部病灶、邻近器官的炎症（如胰腺、胆囊等）等，也见于肝迷走动脉，其原因可用“虹吸效应”“窃血”“血池效应”等原理解释。

继发性肝动脉供血增加是指门静脉供血减少时，在神经和体液调节下肝动脉供血相应增加，可由多种原因引起，可见于门静脉或肝静脉栓塞、门静脉受压、长期胆系梗阻等。一过性肝实质强化差异在CT动脉增强扫描时主要表现为动脉期肝实质一过性强化，在CT平扫和CT动态增强的门静脉期及延迟期呈等密度，可表现为各种形态。一项56例研究中，动脉早期发现24例一过性肝实质强化差异，动脉晚期发现32例一过性肝实质强化差异，而且动脉晚期图像显示更清楚，更容易诊断。

Ⅰ型一过性肝实质强化差异

长期胆管梗阻时，胆系扩张，胆管周围血管丛受压，肝窦状隙内压力增加，门静脉血流减少，肝动脉血供代偿性增加，从而形成各种不同形态的一过性肝实质强化差异。长期胆系梗阻所致一过性肝实质强化差异最常见沿胆管分布的一过性肝实质强化差异，呈柱状或分枝状，当断层与胆管走行垂直时显示为环形一过性肝实质强化差异，边界均显示不清（Ⅰ型）。该研究中，中、重度胆系扩张共176段均存在Ⅰ型一过性肝实质强化差异,而46段轻度胆系扩张的肝段仅6段存在Ⅰ型一过性肝实质强化差异,其差异有明显统计学意义。该组认为当长期胆管梗阻、肝内胆管扩张 >5 mm 时常存在Ⅰ型一过性肝实质强化差异。

Ⅱ型一过性肝实质强化差异

该研究中24段Ⅱ型一过性肝实质强化差异分布于重度胆管扩张的肝段,胆管呈柱状或囊状扩张,门静脉显示迂曲、并不同程度受压变窄。

分析Ⅱ型一过性肝实质强化差异主要原因有:扩张胆管压迫门静脉,使得门静脉狭窄,门静脉灌注减少,肝动脉供血代偿性增加;胆管扩张较严重时肝窦阻塞严重,肝静脉窦内压力增大明显,门静脉供血明显减少,肝动脉供血增加明显,这与 Colagrande 等(2004)的研究相一致。另有1段存在Ⅱ型一过性肝实质强化差异的肝段(左叶内侧段)肝内胆管仅中度扩张,但是同一肝叶的左叶外侧段胆管重度扩张,存在明显的Ⅱ型一过性肝实质强化差异,其原因可以用"虹吸效应"解释,即当肝左叶外侧段动脉供血明显增多时,肝左叶供血增加,导致肝左叶内侧段供血也有所增加,进而形成一过性肝实质强化差异。

研究表明肝内胆管重度扩张时,Ⅱ型一过性肝实质强化差异阳性组和阴性组胆管直径的均数存在明显差异。Ⅱ型一过性肝实质强化差异阳性组的95%可信区间下界为9.3 mm。该组认为当胆管内胆管扩张 >9.3mm 时95%患者存在Ⅱ型一过性肝实质强化差异。

Ⅲ型一过性肝实质强化差异

该组56例中22例在胆囊旁肝实质内发现Ⅲ型一过性肝实质强化差异,且胆囊均明显扩张,该研究将测量胆囊的最大横径作为参数。研究结果显示Ⅲ型一过性肝实质强化差异阳性患者的胆囊横径均数明显高于阴性患者,差异具有统计学意义。

Ⅲ型一过性肝实质强化差异阳性组的95%可信区间下限为28.2 mm,该组认为胆囊横径 >28.2 mm 时95%患者存在Ⅲ型一过性肝实质强化差异。其原理与Ⅰ型及Ⅱ型一过性肝实质强化差异的原理相似,即胆囊明显扩张时,压迫肝窦状隙,使得肝门静脉供血减少,肝动脉供血相应增加。影像学表现虽与胆囊炎所致一过性肝实质强化差异相似,但原理不同。后者是由于多种炎性介质作用,使胆囊旁肝实质肝动脉供血原发性增加,同时肝细胞肿胀使得肝门静脉供血减少,肝动脉继发性供血增加所致。

综上所述,肝外胆管细胞癌所致胆系扩张的一过性肝实质强化差异的影像学表现主要有3种方式:Ⅰ型:沿胆管分布的柱状或分枝状一过性肝实质强化差异,边界不清,肝内胆管扩张 >5 mm 时常见;Ⅱ型:扇形或不规则片状一过性肝实质强化差异,边界清楚或不清楚,肝内胆管扩张 >9.3 mm 时常见;Ⅲ型:胆囊旁肝实质内弧形片状一过性肝实质强化差异,边界不清,胆囊横径 >28.2mm 时常见。

鉴别诊断:一过性肝实质强化差异,虽然不是肝内病灶本身的异常强化,但是多种肝内、外许多疾病都可以直接或间接导致肝脏血液灌注的改变,进而形成一过性肝实质强化差异。在肝外胆管细胞癌的诊断过程中,Ⅰ型一过性肝实质强化差异需与癌细胞沿胆管浸润及其他胆管疾病(如硬化性胆管炎等)鉴别;Ⅱ型一过性肝实质强化差异出现时需与肝内转移瘤、肝内其他局部病变等鉴别,以免误诊为肝内转移瘤;而胆囊炎、胆囊转移瘤等疾病均可导致与肝外胆管细胞癌所致的Ⅲ型一过性肝实质强化差异表现相似。因此正确认识肝外胆管细胞癌所致一过性肝实质强化差异,对于肝外胆管细胞癌的诊断和鉴别诊断及其预后评估都具有重要临床意义。

第二节　误诊病例简介:肝外胆管囊腺瘤与胆总管囊肿

胆管囊腺瘤是发生于肝脏的一种囊性肿瘤,常发生在肝内胆管,占80%~85%,被认为是一种少见病,罕见发生于肝外胆管。瘤体一般为多房性,囊壁内层为柱状或立方形黏液上皮细胞,其能分泌大量黏液,上皮细胞下层存在致密的基质细胞层,其能产生卵巢样的间质。胆管囊腺瘤常发生于女性患者,40岁左右为好发年龄,发生在儿童及青少年者罕见,可发生癌变。该病病因尚不明确,一种假说可能与胚胎期胆管发育迷路有关;另一种假说为起源于异位的卵巢或胚胎前肠残余。大体病理表现为囊性肿物,表面光滑,呈苍白或暗褐色。其内可见分隔,有胶状黏液样物质,有时可见乳头状增生。显微镜下有三层结构:第一层由能分泌黏蛋白的柱状或矩状上皮细胞组成;第二层由梭形细胞组成的致密细胞基质;第三层为胶原结缔组织。

临床上以右上腹疼痛不适为最主要表现,占75%,其他如腹部包块、黄疸等少见。囊肿较大时可触及右上腹囊性包块。据相关文献报道,多数患者血清癌胚抗原、CA199 和 CA125 可明显升高,且与疾病进展情况呈正相关。一例患者以上腹部不适为主要症状,与文献报道一致。但该例患者血清癌胚抗原、CA199 和 CA125 均为阴性,与多数文献报道不相同。

目前报道的胆管囊腺瘤影像诊断局限于肝内胆管,胆总管内囊腺瘤影像学报道罕见,有作者查阅文献国内仅有 1 例胆总管囊腺瘤的影像学报道,与该例胆总管囊腺瘤一样,在 CT、MRI 平扫上均表现为胆总管囊状扩张,壁光滑未见增厚及壁结节,囊液密度及信号均匀,囊内未见分隔,肝内胆管轻度扩张。这 2 例影像学表现与肝内胆管囊腺瘤表现的肝内低密度囊性占位伴囊内分隔及壁结节明显不同。CT 多平面重建可直观反映扩张的胆总管与肝内胆管相通的关系。MRCP 可立体显示扩张的胆总管与肝内胆管的关系,与多平面重建比较更具立体感。CT 增强后表现为囊状扩张的胆总管壁持续性轻度强化,与文献报道的强化特点相符。

该例病变在 CT、MRI 上均表现为单纯的胆总管囊状扩张,胆管壁光滑未见壁结节,扩张的胆管呈单囊特征,其内未见分隔,是将其误诊为胆总管囊肿的主要原因。

鉴别诊断:胆总管囊肿表现为肝外囊性占位,密度均匀,边缘光滑,壁薄而均匀,肝内胆管不扩张或轻度扩张,即使扩张的肝内胆管也有其特点,呈球状或梭状,外周胆管几乎不扩张,不同于囊腺瘤引起梗阻性黄疸所致的肝内胆管扩张形式。该例在影像学表现上与胆总管囊肿类似,部分囊壁持续性轻度强化可作为鉴别特征,但最终诊断需病理。

肝囊肿多为单囊,囊液密度均匀,壁薄,增强囊壁无强化。一般没有临床症状,多在体检时发现。

肝脓肿(包括细菌性肝脓肿及阿米巴肝脓肿)可表现为多囊及分隔,但囊壁一般较厚且不规则,边缘大多欠清晰,多为不均匀低密度,增强扫描后出现典型的“环征”,部分脓肿内可见含气影像表现,临床上肝脓肿大多有急性感染症状,如寒战、高热及白细胞计数增高等。

肝包虫病影像学上多表现为单囊或囊中囊,“水上浮莲”是其特征性改变。临床上多有牧区接触史,实验室血清学检查有特异性。

综上所述,该例胆总管囊腺瘤表现不典型,无论是临床特征还是影像学表现均无明显特点,与胆总管囊肿等无法鉴别,是误诊的主要原因。该例报道的意义在于认识不典型胆总管囊腺瘤的影像学表现,在今后临床工作中碰到类似肝外囊性占位时要注意囊腺瘤的可能。

第十四章 胆管结石

第一节 肝外胆管结石 MRCP 的表现

肝外胆管结石，MRCP 表现为胆管腔内圆形或椭圆形无信号或低信号区，MRCP 诊断肝外胆管结石的准确率为 94%~97%。MRCP 适用于诊断肝外胆管结石并可显示小至 2 mm 的结石，这是因为正常胆管结石表现为高信号强度胆汁中的低信号区。大量研究表明：MRCP 对肝外胆管结石诊断的敏感度和特异度分别为 81%~100%；阳性和阴性预测值分别为 82%~100%。

鉴于 MRCP 具有很高的阴性判断价值，对于肝外胆管结石患者，其主要作用不是用于确定肝外胆管结石，而是排除肝外胆管结石。一旦腹痛病人被排除了患有肝外胆管结石，那么就不必进行内镜逆行胆管造影检查，免除了不必要的痛苦。

MRCP 有助于诊断具有复杂症状的胆管结石，如 Mirizzi 综合征。该病表现为肝外胆管被阻塞胆囊管的结石所压迫。MRCP 的多层面扫描可以识别梗阻性结石和长的胆囊管，后者平行于肝外胆管走行，从而使病人易患 Mirizzi 综合征。

一、结石的表现

胆系结石的特征：胆系结石有各种成分，在 MR 影像中几乎都是低信号，在胆总管内呈圆形、卵圆形或多面形的充盈缺损，周围绕以高信号的胆汁，影像如同传统的直接胆管造影。极少数的结石内有混杂的高信号，属色素软结石，易脆裂，更易为内窥镜拉网排石成功，此征象可提供治疗时参考。

嵌顿性结石在最大信号强度投影影像中就能展示，见大块无信号的结石嵌于胆管致梗阻，梗阻端呈弧形、凸面向上的杯口状充盈缺损，在乳头水平呈典型的“新月”征。

胆系结石合并胆管扩张的有 88%。

胆管内结石虽然 MRCP 空间分辨率不如 ERCP，但它有较高的对比分辨率，直径小至 2~3mm 的结石也能发现。在梗阻以上扩张胆管内的小结石，源图像可以显示。多发结石在肝外胆管（肝总管和胆总管）表现为不均匀的信号，周围有很薄的线，两侧面的线呈“轨道”征，有时胆总管勾画很差，要用源图像帮助估价。有的结石胆管扩张很轻，表现为腔内多而无信号的圆形影，至少在 2 个源图像层面上呈现才能诊断为结石。

二、诊断中应注意的几个问题

观察胆管结石用小角度旋转最大信号强度投影影像，以分离重叠于胆管或十二指肠液的结石；斜矢状位（30º~45º）层面对于发现肝外胆管结石最有用，因为此平面平行于胆总管的行程，旋转的最大信号强度投影在展示胆囊管汇入部也是有用的；在结石的诊断中源图像比最大信号强度投影能提供更多的结石信息，在较小结石的诊断中更为突出；在近乳头部胆总管小结石诊断有困难时轴位源图像有帮助。

三、MRCP 对胆系结石的诊断限度

肝外胆管腔内的低信号区并非结石的特征表现，血凝块、肿瘤、空气、流动效应均可表现为低信号。相反，并非所有结石都表现为低信号。一些作者报道 5 例结石内出现高信号成分，认为不同人群中结石结构和成分不同，高信号代表具有较长 T2 值含液多的胆泥成分。

最大信号强度投影像虽能从不同角度展示结石形态，但较小结石的信号缺失区会在重建过程中被周围高信号胆汁所掩盖，且原始图像更利于显示结石的边缘，能比最大信号强度投影像提供更多信息，

因此，原始图像的重要性被多个作者所强调（16-14-1）。

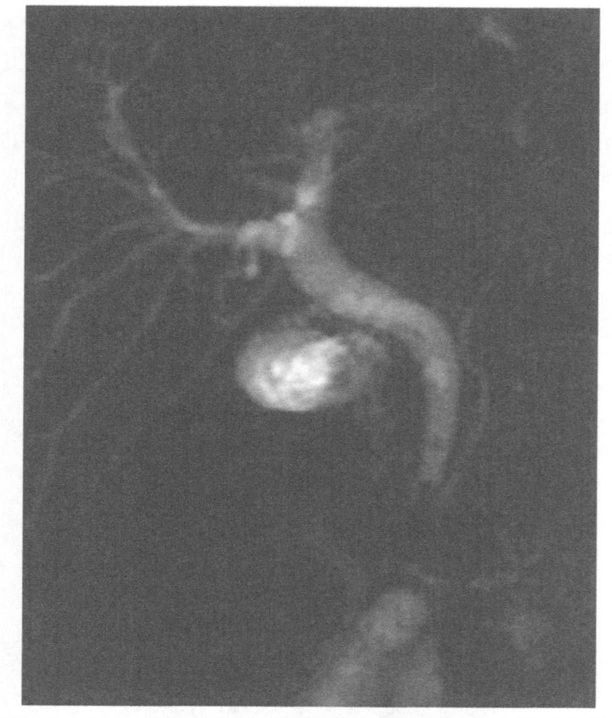

图 16-14-1　MRCP：肝外胆管结石；胆囊管低位左位汇入肝外胆管

许多学者研究表明在诊断肝外胆管结石时，MRCP 的准确度很高，其敏感度为 71%~95%。曾有作者报道潜在假阳性为胆管积气所致，在横断面图像可鉴别肝外胆管结石与胆管积气的气液平面。

需要注意：①与气泡不易辨别，气泡可以来自胆管 - 十二指肠瘘或有括约肌切开术后；②有时结石与实质背景之间会缺乏对比度，导致漏诊，特别是结石紧贴胆管壁者；③肝外胆管下 1/3 腔内由于胆汁流动增加所致的低信号会造成假阳性的诊断。

不少医院已将 MRCP 作为胆囊切除术前的检查常规，以降低各种方式的胆系结石手术中胆管损伤率。由于 ERCP、术中胆管造影等侵袭性检查不再提倡作为术前的检查常规，临床上以诊断为目的的检查已逐步为 MRCP 所替代。应该强调，MRCP 结合 MRI 原始图像的综合观察与分析的重要性，还要了解和熟悉 MRCP 的诊断误区，才能使胆系结石误诊率进一步降低。然而内镜超声在此具有优势。一些作者报道胆胰管的 MR 仿真内镜（MRVE）技术，即在 MRCP 资料作为原始图像的基础上显示胆胰管内腔。MR 仿真内镜或许可协同提高 MRCP 对胆系结石的诊断准确率。

第二节　MRCP 结合 T_2WI 与 MSCT 诊断肝外胆管结石

在比较两种检查方法的优劣时，常用到的指标是灵敏度和特异度，然而有的检查方法灵敏度高但特异性低，而特异度高的检查方法灵敏度又低，这样就不能笼统地说哪一种成像方法最好。ROC 曲线是包含各种临界值时灵敏度与特异度的相互关系的图形，成功地将灵敏度与特异度这 2 个基本指标通过曲线下面积（Az）值直观地表示出来，可以得出灵敏度和特异性相结合的比较，成为综合判断 2 种方法何者为优的较好的统计方法。

一般而言 Az 值越大，该种检查方法的效能越高。Az =0.5 说明实验没有诊断价值；0.5~0.7 说明实验欠准确；0.7~0.9 说明实验中度准确；0.9~1 说明高度准确。在一项研究中，2 种检查方法 Az 值均 >0.9，说明 2 种检查方法对胆管结石均具有高效能。

胆管结石的发病率高，检查方法也很多，由于 ERCP 操作复杂、可引起并发症，而 B 超易受操纵者经验水平和患者肠气的影响，这 2 种方法临床应用的某些缺陷或不足凸显了 MSCT 和 MRCP 在诊断胆管结石方面的优势，因此 MSCT 和 MRCP 应用越来越普及。

随着科学的发展，MSCT 和 MRCP 在技术上也有了很大的改进。受机器质量和扫描技术的影响，许多文献报道 MSCT 和 MRCP 对胆管结石的灵敏度、特异性、准确率均有一定的差异。该项研究采用的是 16 排及 64 排 MSCT 和 1.5T 磁共振扫描仪，同时进行了多平面重建处理以及薄层扫描，因此 MSCT 和 MRCP 对胆管结石的检出率都很高。MRCP 是利用胆汁和胰液含有大量水分、并且 T_2 显著长于周围组织的特点，采用 T_2WI 突出显示前两者的高信号，通过最大信号强度投影（MIP）重建获得类似直接造影的胆胰管图像。

多平面重建是以轴位像为依据，可以在任意切面上对图像进行重建,不仅能直观显示胆管内结石范围以及结石的大小、梗阻位置,还能了解其与周围组织的解剖关系,通过多角度观察,可以直观地显示扩张的胆总管、胰管的全貌。MSCT 薄层扫描结合多平面重建提高了医生的诊断准确率。

除了设备和扫描技术因素外,结石的诊断还受到结石的成分和大小的影响。

胆管结石的主要成分为胆固醇、胆色素及钙盐等,根据成分不同,CT 扫描图像可以表现为高密度、低密度和混杂密度。色素类结石中的主要成分是各种钙盐,在 CT 上表现为高密度影,胆固醇结石的主要成分是胆固醇结晶, CT 上表现为低密度影,如含钙盐结晶和胆固醇 2 种成分,则在 CT 上表现为混杂密度影,结石中含胆固醇成分越多,则 CT 上显示的密度越低。胆管结石以高密度结石和混杂密度结石多见。胆管高密度结石所占比例为 20.0%~29.4%,混杂密度为 41.2%,软组织密度结石为 17.7%,等密度结石为 11.7%。

MSCT 具有较高的密度分辨率,对高密度结石可明确诊断。该组 21 例高密度结石 CT 均做出了正确诊断,确诊率为 100%。但对软组织密度结石和等密度结石及泥沙样结石有时诊断困难,可引起误诊和漏诊。

MRI 扫描 T_1WI,胆系结石由于含钙和胆固醇多少不同,表现为低信号、稍高信号或等信号,但 T_2WI 均为低信号。MRI 既可显示含钙多的结石,也可显示 CT 不能发现的等密度结石,检出率较高。不同的结石在 MRCP 上均表现为低信号,结石的典型表现为圆形充盈缺损,周围包绕高信号的胆汁,常合并梗阻以上胆管轻至中度的扩张,也可表现为高信号管腔内的不规则状、砂粒状低信号。

结石按大小可分为: <5 mm 的微小结石, 5~9 mm 的小结石,10~15 mm 的中结石,>15 mm 的大结石。MRCP 对结石的检出率与结石的大小有关。

一些学者报道 MRCP+ 常规 T_2WI 对 >5 mm 结石的检出率为 100%,而对 <5 mm 的结石的检出率只有 46.88%,结合薄层扫描后可提高到 93.75%。主要原因是 MRCP 空间分辨率有限,且 T_2WI 程度重、层厚较厚引起的部分容积效应,使得小结石易被周围高信号胆汁遮挡而难以显示。

有文献报道 MRCP 难以发现 <3mm 结石,故这时需结合轴位薄层扫描像,可较好地显示结石细节情况,准确率可提高到 94%~97%。该组病例有 3 例微小结石患者, MRCP 原始图像未见结石,轴位 T_2WI 于胆总管下端见点状低信号,后 ERCP 证实为泥沙样结石。

MRCP 难以明确、直观地诊断胆管泥沙样结石,而 MR 常规 T_2WI 上,胆总管泥沙样结石均特征性地显示为胆总管内分层状改变,上层为均匀高信号的胆汁,下层为低信号的泥沙样结石,两者之间存在明确的分界面。MRI 常规 T_2WI 序列图像扫描基线轴面垂直于胆总管长轴方向,可较为直观地显示胆管泥沙样结石的分层状改变(图 16-14-2)。

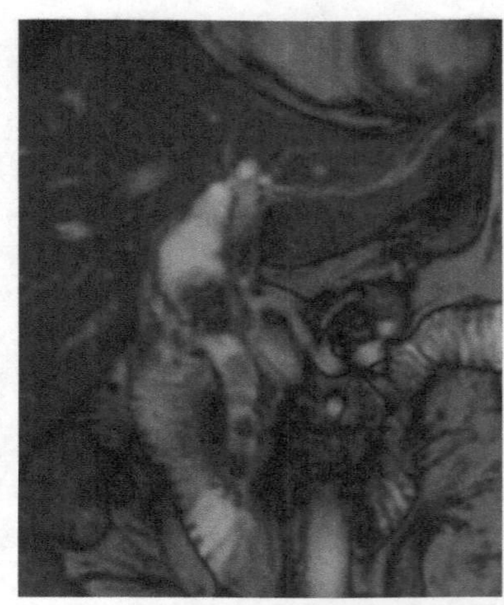

图 16-14-2 MRI 冠状断面图像示肝外胆管多粒结石,肝外胆管扩张

CT 增强扫描对结石的发现与平扫比较并无明显差别,但增强后有利于轻微扩张胆管的显示,且对部分紧贴胆管壁的结石的轮廓勾画更清楚。而且,通过增强,对诊断不明的病变进行观察,基本上能够排除其他病变的可能,胆管结石病变不强化,而胆管炎、肿瘤强化。文献报道胆管结石时,在结石平面或其下方出现局限性同心圆样胆管壁增厚。管壁增厚平均 >2 mm,但常不超过 5 mm,而正常肝外胆管的管壁厚度 <1.5 mm,此征象有助于微小结石的诊断。总之,胆管结石成分不同、大小差异,在影像学上的表现也不一样,因此 MRCP 结合 T_2WI 与 MSCT 两种检查方法对胆总管结石的检出率也存在差异。根据以上研究得出以下结论:两种检查方法的所有 Az 值均 >0.9,说明 MRCP 结合 T_2WI 与 MSCT 诊断准确性均较高,均可作为胆管结石主要的检查方法。MRCP 结合常规 MRI T_2WI 薄层扫描价值比 MSCT 更高。

第三节　胆管内的假结石

在严重的胆管炎，管壁增厚，黏液产生增加和/或上皮脱屑，管壁的游离的漂浮物以及黏液均可在胆系造影中伪似结石而造成解释困难。在胆管探查术及取石术后问题更为复杂，术后T管造影尤其如此。有时，碎屑的征象是特征性的，呈现为不规则形、线形或匐行性透光影。如胆胰管下端括约肌功能正常，这些碎屑可逐渐排出；如引流通畅，胆管炎迅即消退。在探查手术后胆管造影发现可疑充盈缺损时，复习回顾术前造影片对于正确解释常有益处。直接法胆系造影（含PTC、ERCP、术中及术后之引流管造影等）时，胆管中浓稠的胆汁可造成透光区，被称作混淆缺损。

Train等（1987）观察到6例胆管下端长期梗阻的病人，用30%泛影葡胺行胆管造影时，胆囊管和扩张的胆总管交界处有透光影，延迟照片时消失，胆囊管有对比剂充盈，考虑为胆汁和对比剂两种液体的黏稠度、表面张力和密度不同，相互影响的结果，并用简单实验证明此种说法。正常胆汁的黏度大于稀释的对比剂，长期胆管梗阻时，胆汁的黏稠度大为增加。胆汁虽较黏稠，但其密度较低。两种不同黏度的液体开始接触时，即使是可溶性液体，也将互相取代，黏度差别越大，取代越明显。这种物理现象可以说明胆囊管开口处最初对比剂不与胆汁混合的原因。两种液体表面张力的差异促进上述现象的出现。

水溶性对比剂主要成分是水，其表面张力大于油脂或净化剂。胆汁内有胆盐和卵磷脂，其表面张力较低。表面张力高的液体趋于黏附在表面，对比剂开始黏附在胆管壁上，逐渐与胆汁混合，尤似一滴水滴在玻板上形成球形不散的原理相似。

总胆管括约肌段在解剖上与X线表现上常有变异，应用标准的2~3次照片技术，对括约肌段的开关机制及形态变化常可了解。但偶尔可将关闭相的括约肌表现误为下端结石，这种情况曾一度令人烦恼，只在ERCP及MRCP问世后，详细了解了括约肌活动的不同周期形态变化，才对此有了进一步的认识。括约肌收缩不仅使胰腺段远端表现如排笔一样平齐，而且可上凸，造成弧形充盈缺损，酷似结石或其他病变。但多次照片可见该影动态变化则使问题迎刃而解。Mujahed和Evans（1972）报告3例胆管造影时的假结石充盈缺损，这些充盈缺损只出现于总胆管的远端，只有上缘可看见，它凹向上，通常涉及整个胆管腔，而不伸开管腔，也不引起胆汁通过括约肌的梗阻。在特征上它是周期性的，在收缩期它出现于总胆管远端，松弛时它即消失。该作者认为此充盈缺损大概是由于胆胰管十二指肠连接区肌肉结构突出或排列特别所致。

第四节　MSCT胆系三维成像与胆管系统结石

螺旋CT在我国已广泛应用，MSCT也已成为目前应用的趋势。MSCT工作站三维成像功能随着计算机软件、硬件的不断发展也日益丰富和强大起来。用于观察胆系结石的MSCT三维后处理成像方法主要有最大密度投影、表面遮盖显示法和表面透明法，曲面重建是将弯曲的胆管人为地“拉直”在一个平面上观察的二维成像方法，以及用MSCT仿真内镜观察胆管腔内的结石。

一、MSCT胆系三维成像技术特点

最大密度投影清晰显示胆系的细微立体解剖结构及空间分布情况，胆囊内和胆管内的结石表现为充盈缺损区，胆总管内的结石充盈缺损区近端边缘可呈“杯口状”，缺损区密度均匀。表面遮盖显示法图像可以从多方位、多角度观察胆管树形态，立体感较强，对于结石所造成的胆管内对比剂显影中断征象显示清晰，但不能直接显示胆管内的结石，可利用“切割”软件切除部分胆囊壁或胆总管壁，充分暴露结石影。但表面遮盖显示法是通过选取一定的阈值进行滤过，对阈值以下的胆管末梢细节显示不佳（图16-14-3）。

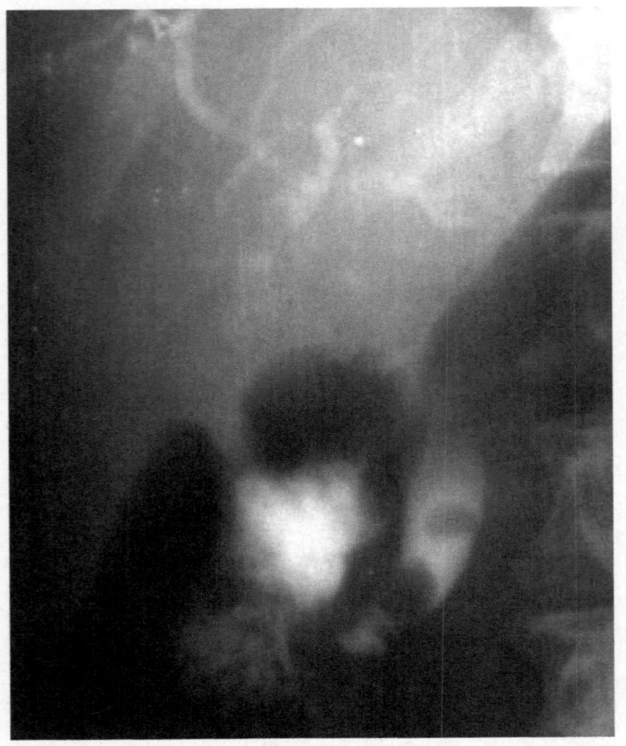

图 16-14-3 ERCP:肝外胆管下段两粒结石,胆总管切迹和括约肌段清楚可见

表面透明法图像显示的胆树为透明状,可以显示胆系结石的轮廓,对周围没有胆管分支重叠的胆总管或胆囊内结石轮廓显示较为清晰。曲面重建可将弯曲走行的胆管人为地“拉直”在一个平面上观察,但有时胆管较细并过于弯曲时,通过矢、冠状面曲面重建出的胆管边缘不光整呈锯齿状。

二、MSCT 胆系三维成像技术的临床应用

临床用于诊断胆管系统结石的无创性检查方法包括 B 超、CT、螺旋 CT 胆系成像、磁共振胆胰成像,特别是近年推出的螺旋 CT 胆系成像、MRCP,都发挥着重要作用。

胆结石 B 超检查前准备工作相对简单,有着便捷、费用相对低廉等优势,但发现结石的能力则依赖于操作者的经验。磁共振胆胰成像是用于针对胆系、胰腺管疾病新的无创性检查方法,并已在临床应用推广, MRCP 可以用于胆系、肝脏多种外科手术前,如腹腔镜胆囊切除术、肝脏切除和部分肝脏移植。经皮肝穿刺胆管造影(PTC)和内镜逆行胆胰管造影(ERCP)的优势在于除了做胆系结石的诊断工作外,还可同时承担进一步的治疗工作,如利用 PTC 做梗阻性黄疸的引流, ERCP 做十二指肠乳头切开、碎石、网篮套取结石等措施。但 PTC/ERCP 是有创的检查手段,可以造成出血、炎症等并发症。

对于胆囊结石患者腹腔镜胆囊切除手术已成为很普通的外科治疗措施,相对于开腹胆囊切除术,腹腔镜也带来了如胆汁渗漏和胆管结扎等胆系损伤的危险,尽管这种危险发生率常常低于 1%,胆管变异是最常见的胆管树发育变异,也是对于胆管外科手术来说最危险的因素之一。

螺旋 CT 胆系三维成像在以上各方面同样发挥着重要作用,尤其对于不适于或禁忌做 MR 的患者。MSCT 胆系三维成像可以立体、直观再现胆树形态,特别是用于了解涉及胆系的各种肝脏肿瘤和胆管肿瘤手术前、经腹腔镜或开腹做胆囊切除术前、做 PTC/ERCP 前正常胆系解剖结构以及常见和不常见的胆管和胆囊管变异,避免对变异的胆管结扎或切开造成胆系损伤显得尤为重要; MSCT 胆系三维成像同样可以用于胆囊切除术后复查的病人。

对于因肝硬化等疾病造成的肝功能异常、胆红素增高和急性胆管梗阻造成胆系分泌功能减退,可造成胆系对比剂充盈不佳,影响螺旋 CT 胆系三维成像结果,则是其不足之处。

第五节 胆管内未怀疑的结石

在手术时,对于那些无胆系结石病史及症状的病人,如其肝外胆管外观正常,一般都不再作总胆管探查术。Fraha 和 Pearson(1976)总结自己病例时指出,进行常规的术中胆系造影发现此类未怀疑结石病人的发生率为 6%,回顾归纳文献资料的发生率为 4%~10%。

Chatterjee 和 Jones(1978)报告为 8.3%。Berei(1981)报告为 5%,他指出,如不常规地进行术中胆系造影,每 100 例总胆管结石病人中至少有 5 例带着漏诊的结石离开手术室。该作者推而广之,假定胆囊切除术病人中有 20% 具总胆管探查指征并行此手术,每年 50 万例胆囊切除术中有 40 万例均不行此探查术,其中 5% 未怀疑结石而漏诊,则为 25 000 例,确为不小的数目。

结石在胆管及胆囊中自发地活动是难以预测的。在总胆管内隐藏一枚结石,在其出现症状之前可潜存数月至数年,如首次手术漏诊,行第二次手术

时可能因为粘连而毗邻关系不清，产生并发症而出现困难，若是老人，则更增危险。如常规施行术中胆系造影，在首次手术即发现直径小到 2~3mm 的结石，对病人确系福音。为寻找小的结石，多次照片（6~12 次）及每次照片只增加少量对比剂是一较好的方法，而对比剂太多太浓则无疑要漏掉小的结石。

第六节　胆管结石的诊断陷阱和误诊

一、诊断陷阱

在多角度重建图像上可清晰地显示多方位的胆、胰管树全貌，对胆系结石的信号、大小、形态、数目、梗阻部位和胆管扩张程度提供了可靠的诊断依据。

胆系结石的一般表现为圆形或卵圆形的充盈缺损，周围围以高信号的胆汁；嵌顿性结石则表现为边缘光滑的杯口状压迹，有时因为成分的不同表现为混杂信号，常合并梗阻以上胆管轻到中度的扩张。诊断中要密切结合源影像及鉴别胆管内气体、血栓、血凝块等形成的充盈缺损的假象。肝外胆管腔内的低信号区并非结石的特征表现，血凝块、肿瘤、空气、流动效应均可表现为低信号。相反，并非所有结石都表现为低信号。Chen 等（1996）报道 5 例结石内出现高信号成分，认为不同人群中结石结构和成分不同，高信号代表具有较长 T2 值含液多的胆泥成分。值得注意的是，胆系小结石有时被高信号的胆汁掩盖而不易显露，对显示小结石，MRCP 的源图像可补充重建图像的不足。因而必须着重强调在诊断胆系结石时，综合观察和分析 MRCP 源图像的重要意义。

有作者指出，需要注意：①与气泡不易辨别，气泡可以来自胆管 - 十二指肠瘘或有括约肌切开术后；②有时结石与实质背景之间会缺乏对比度，导致漏诊，特别是结石紧贴胆管壁者；③肝外胆管下 1/3 腔内由于胆汁流动增加所致的低信号会造成假阳性的诊断。

残余结石在造影诊断中应注意：①造影显示的充盈缺损应与气泡仔细鉴别；②不要满足于肝外胆管显影，应通过体位变化，及增加对比剂的注入量，使两侧肝内胆管都满意充盈后再行照片，否则，势必遗漏肝内胆管的病变；③肝内胆管分支稀少，变细和硬化，都提示该肝内胆管内可能有结石存在。

二、胆总管结石诊断中的误诊

MRCP 诊断胆总管结石相对比较容易，与常规胆管造影的诊断标准一样，结石表现为卵圆形低信号区，周围由高信号胆汁环绕。MRCP 诊断结石的准确性主要取决于对常见误诊原因的认识。最常见的误诊原因：最大信号强度投影重建图像未显示结石；胆总管内多发结石呈弥漫性低信号，类似于胆管狭窄；胆管内气体引起的敏感性伪影；酷似小结石的气泡。

小结石：与最大信号强度投影相关的伪影，并不影响诊断直径大于 10mm 的大结石，即使在最大信号强度投影重建图像上，也很容易分辨出充盈缺损及其周围环绕的高信号胆汁。但对小结石，有必要分析原始图像。在最大信号强度投影图像上包围结石的高信号胆汁可掩盖小结石，出现与 ERCP 相类似的误诊，后者由于胆总管过度充盈对比剂可掩盖小结石。在一组 51 例胆总管结石病人的研究中，56.8% 的结石在最大信号强度投影图像上显示，结石的显示主要依赖于结石大小，但即使比较大的结石（直径范围在 5~10mm）在最大信号强度投影图像上也会漏诊（占 54.2%）。因此，对所有的病例都应该同时观察最大信号强度投影图像和原始图像。

多发结石：多发结石完全充填胆总管时可出现误诊。由于在多发嵌顿的结石之间有很少量胆汁，结石表现为极不均匀低信号，同时伴近端胆管显著扩张，MRCP 看起来像近端胆管双向狭窄，而原始图像可做出正确诊断。

第七节　肝内胆管变异与胆管结石

肝内胆管变异临床常见，变异率可达 37%，其解剖学、胆汁动力学和诊治均有一定特殊性。随着介入放射学、外科学及其他相关学科的发展,对肝内胆管变异的解剖规律和临床相关性的深入研究愈加具有实际意义。一组学者曾对 300 例肝移植供体行术中胆管造影研究,结果显示了 7 种肝内胆管分支类型,最常见的变异类型为右后支胆管直接汇入肝总管或左肝内胆管,约占 11%,其次为右前、右后支胆管在同一位置汇入左肝内胆管,其他变异类型较少见,包括右肝内胆管或副肝内胆管引流至胆囊管等。

一、MRCP 检查技术及其对胆胰管树的显示

MRCP 是临床广泛开展的一种无创性胰胆管成像技术,在不需要对比剂、非侵袭和可重复性方面明显优于 ERCP,特别是对于 ERCP 检查失败的病例,MRCP 是一种首选的替代检查方法。多种脉冲序列均可获得 MRCP 图像,但成像的时间和质量却不尽相同。一组病例中 2D MRCP 采用 SSh-TSE 序列,3DMRCP 采用 3D-HRTSE 序列。

2D SSh-TSE 序列主要优点是扫描速度快、显示管道结构连续性好、一般不出现阶梯样伪影。主要缺点是不能获得薄层原始图像,容易遗漏小病变、对迂曲细小的管道结构显示效果欠佳致。3D-HRTSE 序列配合呼吸门控技术进行三维容积采集,扫描后根据原始图像行最大信号强度投影重建,获得立体的胆管树图像。主要优点在于可获得薄层原始图像,有助于小病变的显示、图像可进行各种后处理。主要缺点是扫描时间相对较长,如患者呼吸不均匀则图像质量很差。

该组资料中 3D-HR TSE 序列激发后采用了半扫描技术获取约半数原始矩阵,填充半数 K 空间,经半傅里叶转换组建图像,这在一定程度上减少了运动伪影,信噪比及空间分辨率也得到相应提高。其中大部分 3D MRCP 重建图像能很好地显示肝内胆管走行汇合情况,但也有部分病例重建图像显示不佳。对这部分病例通过结合 2D MRCP 图像或根据 3D 原始图像追踪其走行,一般均可获得更好的显示。

可见 2DSSh-TSE 序列和 3D-HRTSE 序列在胆管树的显示方面各有优势和不足,临床检查中最好两种方法联合应用,并注意对薄层原始图像的观察,必要时可与常规 MRI 相结合。

二、MRCP 对胆管结石的显示

MRCP 对胆管结石有较高的敏感性(86%~100%)和特异性(85%~100%)。结石表现为胆管内的局限性圆形或线样低信号,部分或完全被高信号的胆汁包绕,嵌顿结石可以被胆汁不完全包绕,类似于狭窄。对于肝内胆管结石,MRCP 较 ERCP 具有更高的敏感性(97% 与 59%)。一般认为薄层序列对于显示结石较好,厚层序列可能会由于部分容积效应使结石显示不清。但是部分研究显示,厚层块半傅立叶单次激发快速自旋回波(HASTE)和弛豫增强快速采集(RARE)序列对于胆管结石与薄层成像具有相似的敏感性。

MRCP 显示胆管结石的不足之处,主要在于伪影造成的假阳性。气泡、血块、息肉、金属、流动相关伪影均可呈现类似于胆管结石的信号。有研究显示对于上述部分伪影的鉴别,借助 T_1WI 可能会有所裨益。考虑到上述影响因素及 MRCP 空间分辨率的限制,该组对最大径 <1.0cm 的管腔内充盈缺损或 3D 重建图像肝内胆管结石表现不典型者,采取结合 3D 原始图像和常规 MRI 的方法以求最大程度地排除假阳性病例。

三、肝内胆管变异与肝内胆管结石间的相关性

肝内感染、胆汁淤滞、胆管蛔虫等因素是原发性胆管结石的主要病因,在肝内胆管变异伴发肝内胆管结石的病例中也存在上述影响因素。此外,肝内胆管变异者发生肝内胆管结石还可能与其解剖特点有关。

研究统计结果表明变异的肝内胆管引流系统较正常型更容易发生肝内胆管结石,而且具有显著统计学差异。分析其结石的易患原因,一般认为走向异常、合并开口异常的叶、段胆管,容易引起胆流异常,继而诱发感染,最终导致结石发生。

有学者研究表明,肝内胆管变异造成胆流异常具体可能包括以下机制:

(1)汇合角度异常:正常左右肝内胆管的汇合角度一般 <110°,如变异胆管与所汇入肝内胆管的交角过大,则 2 支汇合管胆流方向近似相向,导致两侧胆流均呈滞流状态,胆流受阻而诱发结石。一组病例观察,右叶变异胆管与所汇入肝内胆管的交角多数大于此角度,这可能是右叶肝内胆管结石发生

率高的原因之一。

(2)汇合的2支胆管切面积相差过大:正常肝内胆管二级以上分支均呈"Y"型汇合,其汇合角度与两分支胆管切面积、胆汁流量的关系一般均符合Roux定律,符合此定律则胆汁流动所消耗的功率最小,反之则易形成湍流。如果汇合的两分支管切面积相等,则两分支管对称于主管中轴的延长线,其夹角相等。当两分支管切面积相差过大,在胆流作用下细管和粗管间的夹角将逐渐增大趋于直角以致形成湍流,而诱发结石。回顾该组病例,右叶肝内胆管汇入左肝内胆管或肝外胆管等两汇合支切面积相差悬殊的情况的确比较常见。

(3)血管压迫:正常情况下,进入肝内的肝动脉、肝内胆管和门静脉三者由格里森鞘包绕共同走向肝内,当变异肝内胆管越过中线单独走向对侧时,胆管和血管走行相互分离,肝血管可能从其前方或后方越过,而从前方越过纤维鞘者可对胆管形成明显的压迫,造成受压部以上的变异肝内胆管扩张和胆汁滞流,这种横跨型变异在该组病例中同样比较常见。

综上所述,肝内胆管变异可能是其本身和其余肝内胆管结石的重要易患因素。对于存在肝内胆管变异的患者,手术中不仅要遵循胆管手术的一般原则,还应着眼于改善和纠正胆汁流体力学的障碍,以减少肝内胆管结石发生或再发的可能性。

对肝内胆管结石的手术患者,建议术前常规作MRCP检查,注意有无肝内胆管变异并了解其和结石的关系。MRCP检查发现存在肝内胆管变异时,应留意是否合并肝内胆管结石,同样当检出肝内胆管结石时,也应注意是否有肝内胆管变异存在,以降低漏诊率。MRCP在肝内胆管解剖类型的鉴定和肝内胆管结石的检出、定位方面具有很高的应用价值。

第八节 黏胆症

详见本书 本卷 第十五篇 第一章 第五节 黏胆症。

第十五章 肝外胆管其他情况

第一节 胆总管十二指肠瘘

胆总管十二指肠瘘相对少见。其形成的病理变化主要为胆管结石引起的慢性炎症刺激致管壁增厚、糜烂、破溃,与周围组织发生粘连,继而影响到十二指肠而与其形成瘘管。气体可由十二指肠进入肝内外胆管而致胆管积气。CT诊断胆总管十二指肠瘘比较困难,但仔细观察胆总管管壁周围及与十二指肠的关系,可以获得一些有价值的诊断信息。一例胆总管管壁明显增厚,周围脂肪间隙模糊,与肠道分界不清,加上PTC检查早期对比剂即进入肠道,故应考虑到胆总管和肠道间有瘘管形成可能。

第二节 总胆管-十二指肠瘘并十二指肠溃疡

慢性消化性溃疡并发总胆管-十二指肠瘘十分少见,一般说来,此瘘多继发于胆系结石。慢性十二指肠后壁溃疡穿孔偶尔导致总胆管与十二指肠交通。

总胆管-十二指肠瘘主要见于男性病人,临床上无特征性表现,上升性(返流性)胆管炎为此种胆-肠瘘少见的表现,一旦出现返流性胆管炎的症状和体征,可作为诊断的线索。此瘘通常为影像学检查发现。

第三节 肝外胆管的正确识别

Lating 和 Jeffrey(1980)报告2例病人超声检查时,在右腹部的纵断扫描时观察到一扩张的管状充盈液体的结构,位于门静脉的前方,疑为扩张的总胆管;在邻近的矢状旁断面扫描时发现,上述所谓扩张的总胆管实际上是位于门静脉前方的胆囊颈。

我们在ERCP检查时也发现,当胆囊颈管较长或/和胆囊管低位开口而胆囊管又正与总胆管影像重叠投影时,如不注意,则可将扩张的胆囊管误认为总胆管,或是因此诊断总胆管扩张,或是将胆囊管的螺旋瓣影像重叠于胆总管内误认为总胆管内结石影。

有作者指出,超声检查时偶尔肝动脉可类似于扩张的胆管。横断扫描见一扩张的管状结构,位于门静脉的前面,在形态学上它为肝动脉或扩张的胆管;在其他横断图像上见此管状结构起源于腹腔动脉干,实为肝动脉;在更为颅侧的断面上,可见到正常大小的胆管,密切伴随门静脉的前支。

在超声检查时,有时总胆管可类似于门静脉的分支。总胆管在颅侧与门静脉密切接触,随着总胆管的逐渐向尾侧行进,总胆管转向门静脉后方,然后进入十二指肠。矢状面扫描常显示总胆管与门静脉紧靠并列,由于换能器角度变更,此二结构之间的界面可能变得不那么明显,导致总胆管表现如同肠系膜上静脉那样的静脉结构,而出现混淆与误诊。由于总胆管特征性地位于后方,且有向尾侧的成角,使其容易与肠系膜上静脉分辨开来,另外,总胆管更为平行于下腔静脉与主动脉。

我们在 ERCP 检查时，发现一例肝胆管结石病人右肝管前下支明显扩张并含大量结石，其走行向下伸长，加上肝外胆管显影不佳，则可将右前下支肝管误认为明显扩张的肝外胆管。因此，在 ERCP 灌注对比剂时务必密切随时观察，否则容易造成影像混淆和错误诊断。

第四节　肝外胆管测量

传统上，按胆囊管汇入处将肝外胆管分成肝总管和胆总管，但在 CT 横断图像上不容易显示胆囊管的汇入处，因此不能像传统那样分段，为了便于观察，我们将肝外胆管分为胰上段和胰腺段与括约肌段进行分析。所谓胰上段，即指胰腺段以上的肝外胆管，它包括肝总管及胆总管十二指肠上、后段。正常及无胆胰疾病的病人的肝外胆管胰上段普通 CT 显示率低，也难以观察，但是，高分辨率 CT 扫描则使其显示率大大提高。为了更好地观察肝外胆管胰上段，一项研究选择螺旋 CT 增强扫描的样本，其显示率为 52%，较一些文献报道的 66% 低，其原因之一可能为所选择病例均为常规扫描，未进行薄层扫描。除了技术方面的原因外，我们考虑还有一些因素可能影响其显示，如肝门区占位、门静脉海绵样变、肝裂太宽、腹水、胰腺炎、腹膜炎、手术后等。

肝外胆管胰上段表现为圆点状低密度影，增强后不强化，密度与胆汁相似，有时可见胆管壁的强化。正常肝外胆管与肝动脉及门静脉一起位于肝十二指肠韧带内，胰上段肝外胆管位于门静脉的右前方者，位于门静脉左前方者为肝动脉。有作者报告，胆总管位于门静脉右侧者占 55.0%，位于门静脉右前方者占 45.0%。该组位于门静脉右前方者 95 例，占 94.1%，右侧者 4 例。在腹部普通 CT 增强扫描图像上，如何寻找和观察肝外胆管胰上段，该组的体会是：首先在增强扫描门脉期找肝外段门静脉，肝外胆管胰腺段一般位于它的右前方，而肝动脉则位于门静脉左前方；或先找到肝外胆管胰腺段（一般比较容易找到），然后向上寻找，也容易找到；另外，窗技术的运用也很重要。

在活体，胆管内径的测量受检查方法影响甚大。外科法测量的是胆管外径，受管壁厚度的影响，而且外科法不能选择正常人进行测量，因此其正常值不准确。X 线口服胆囊造影肝外胆管内径受胆胰管下端括约肌的张力和胆囊内压的影响，脂餐后，胆囊收缩，下端括约肌松弛，胆管内压下降，处于排泄状态，其管径小于非排泄状态下的管径。静脉法胆系造影和直接法胆系造影测量胆管不是在生理状态下进行的，而且都属损伤性检查，无法在正常人身上测定正常胆管。超声检查是无损伤性检查，可选择健康人进行在完全生理状态下进行，主要观察总肝管，因肠气干扰，对胆总管观察较差。CT 横断图像是在完全生理状态下测量胆管大小，是目前活体研究中较为理想和准确的方法之一。

Sample 等（1978）运用超声进行测量，提出 6mm 为正常值，6~8mm 为可疑患病。以此区别内、外科黄疸，敏感性为 85%~100%，特异性为 75%~100%。Cooperberg 等（1980）以 4mm 作正常标准区别内外科黄疸，其敏感性为 98.8%，特异性为 86.7%；以 5mm 作标准，敏感性降低为 94%，特异性不变。Foley 等（1980）在 CT 图像上测定正常肝外胆管的前后最大径，发现最小者为 2.8mm，一般为 4~6mm。

因为正常的肝内胆管在 CT 扫描上常不能显示，过去认为在 CT 图像上显示出肝内胆管即是胆管扩张和阻塞。然而，随着 CT 技术的发展，现在有高达 40% 的病人可见正常粗细（1~3mm）的肝内胆管，而无胆系疾病。认识上述表现对评价可疑的胆管阻塞非常重要。

在许多病人中，肝外胆管能够分辨。在对无胆管疾病的 100 例病人的研究中，66 例可以看到肝总管，平均直径为 2.8mm；82 例可见到胆总管，平均直径为 3.6 mm（Marincek 等，1986）。尽管胆总管直径 8~10mm 不能明确界定有无胆总管扩张（Baron 等，1997），但是正常胆总管的直径通常小于 4mm。正常肝管自肝门向肝周逐渐变细。

肝外胆管壁厚度正常应小于 1.5mm。胆管壁强化亦可发生在无胆管疾病的病人中，仅有胆管壁的强化并不是胆管病变的指征。

笔者一组 196 例总胆红素正常者其管径大小为 1~4mm，平均 1.6mm，较文献报道的 3~5mm，平均

2.8mm 为低。其中 1~3mm 的占 99%，根据百分位数法计算得出，正常肝外胆管胰上段内径的 95% 参考值上限为 3.47 mm，我们认为，从活体形态学观点分析，肝外胆管胰上段正常标准的上限似应定在 3.5mm，超过此值则多为病理情况。超声、CT 测量结果基本上是一致的，最大径的平均值及范围皆比以往报告的数据为小，以往我们曾将 7mm 作为正常肝外胆管横径平均值，现在看来似欠妥当。

肝外胆管（括约肌段除外）的壁主要由弹性纤维和结缔组织构成，平滑肌纤维稀少，富有弹性，胆管大小可在短期内发生变化。临床上经常可以看到，许多病人经造影检查只发现轻度扩张的胆管，但并没有阻塞性病变，这种扩张是年龄因素引起的，还是胆系疾病引起的，这直接关系到治疗措施的选择。明确胆管直径与年龄的关系，有助于诊断分析。从该项研究 6 个年龄组肝外胆管的显示率看出，随着年龄的增加，显示率有逐渐增大的趋势，这可能与胆管壁随着年龄的增加而有一定弹性降低、张力降低有关。50 岁以上老年组增宽格外明显。

综上所述，我们认为肝外胆管内径只是一个征象，不宜过于强调它的价值，尤其不应孤立静止地看待它。不仅应全面观察肝内外胆管系统，对其毗邻（肝、胰、十二指肠等）亦应详细了解，这样才能更正确地诊断胆系疾病，实事求是地评价胆管内径的价值，从而减少误诊与漏诊。

我们认为，对活体形态测量的具体数值应该辩证地观察和分析，不应该死板地、绝对地看待具体测量数值，因为多种因素都可对它产生影响，例如：各个作者选择测量样本的数量、选择样本群的标准、测量的方法、样本群的年龄、性别、体重、身高、体质、人种与民族、样本群生活的地域……诸多因素均可在一定程度上改变具体的测量数值。

与具体测量某一数值相比较，作为影像诊断的研究，最好是选择一种质的改变，例如，在纵隔内主 - 肺动脉窗平常不见或只见小片的淋巴组织变成结节状了；骨皮质的完整性破坏了；肠黏膜不仅增厚而且不规则强化了……这些征象的价值就比较高，在它们的基础上进行诊断就会有把握得多，诊断的信心也会增强不少。

第五节　肝外胆管胰上段

传统上，按胆囊管汇入处将肝外胆管分成肝总管和胆总管，但在 CT 横断图像上不容易显示胆囊管的汇入处，因此不能像传统那样分段，为了便于观察，我们将肝外胆管分为胰上段和胰腺段与括约肌段进行分析。所谓胰上段，即指胰腺段以上的肝外胆管，它包括肝总管及胆总管十二指肠上、后段。

在上腹部 CT 扫描的图像上，观察分析的重点之一是第一肝门的观察，它也是观察的难点之一。要观察清楚第一肝门的结构，分析其是否呈现异常，很重要的一点就是认真分析第一肝门的各个组成成分的表现，其中肝外胆管及肝内外胆管连接处的表现常常使人难以捉摸。在平扫时，第一肝门的观察经常造成诊断困难，而在增强扫描时，由于肝动脉与门静脉在不同的时相中都直接呈现出来，观察比较容易；而肝门胆管及肝外胆管胰上段则一般不强化，仍难以分析。因此，研究分析肝门胆管及肝外胆管胰上段是十分必要的。

正常及无胆胰疾病的病人的肝外胆管胰上段普通 CT 显示率低，也难以观察，但是，高分辨率 CT 扫描则使其显示率大大提高。为了更好地观察肝外胆管胰上段，我们选择螺旋 CT 增强扫描的样本，其显示率为 52%，较国内外一些文献报道的 66% 低，其原因之一可能为所选择病例均为常规扫描，未进行薄层扫描。除了技术方面的原因外，我们考虑还有一些因素可能影响其显示，如肝门区占位、门静脉海绵样变、肝裂太宽、腹水、胰腺炎、腹膜炎、手术后等。

肝外胆管胰上段表现为圆点状低密度影，增强后不强化，密度与胆汁相似，有时可见胆管壁的强化。正常肝外胆管与肝动脉及门静脉一起位于肝十二指肠韧带内，胰上段肝外胆管位于门静脉的右前方者，位于门静脉左前方者为肝动脉。大多数肝外胆管胰上段位于门静脉的右前方，少数位于其右水平方向及右后方。

在腹部 CT 增强扫描图像上，如何寻找和观察肝外胆管胰上段，我们的体会是：首先在增强扫描门脉期找肝外段门静脉，根据其与肝外胆管在小网膜缘走行密切关系，就能轻松地找到，肝外胆管胰腺段一般位于它的右前方，而肝动脉则位于门静脉左前方；或先找到肝外胆管胰腺段（一般比较容易找到），然后向上寻找，也容易找到；自然，在 PACS 荧屏上合理的窗技术运用也很重要。

第六节　肝外胆管胰腺段

关于分段观察：按照传统的看法，肝外胆管以胆囊管汇入处为界，可分为肝总管和胆总管，但在普通 CT 横断图像上不容易显示胆囊管的汇入处，因此不易区分开二者，为了便于观察，我们将肝外胆管分为胰上段和胰腺段两段进行分析。所谓胰上段，即指胰腺段以上的肝外胆管，它包括解剖学的肝总管及十二指肠上、后段。在一组 CT 图像上，我们又将胰上段分为肝内段（即为肝实质影像包绕的肝总管）和胰上段（即介于肝内段与胰腺段的一段肝外胆管）进行观察与分析。

显示率的问题：正常及无胆胰疾病的人的肝外胆管普通 CT 显示率较低，也难以观察，但是高分辨率的单排螺旋 CT 扫描则使其显示率大大提高，其技术要求包含螺旋扫描、增强技术、薄层扫描、合理的窗技术的运用等。为了更好地观察肝外胆管胰上段，一项课题选择单排螺旋 CT 增强扫描的样本，其显示率为 52%，但较国内外其他一些文献报道的 66% 为低，其原因有待进一步研究。

肝外胆管表现为圆点状低密度影或裂隙状影，增强后不强化，密度与胆囊内胆汁密度相似，有时可见胆管壁的强化，影响肝外胆管显示的因素有：①技术原因，窗宽、窗位的调节对肝外胆管的显示很重要，扫描层厚越薄，显示的可能性越大，口服对比剂，使十二指肠内充盈对比剂，有利干肝外胆管胰腺段的显示；②增强扫描，正常情况下胰腺强化表现为均匀强化，胰头段胆管与胰腺组织的密度差异更为明显，非常有利于观察胰头段胆管，该组即用此法进行观察，效果相当不错。

年龄与显示率的关系：该组病例按年龄段划分，从各组病例的显示率可以看出，随着年龄的增加，显示率有逐渐升高的趋势，可能与胆管壁随着年龄的增加而有一定的弹性降低，张力降低有关。性别差异：该组男女之比为 3：1，男性病例明显多于女性，这可能与就诊病人的性别差异、肝癌病例男性较多有关。

大小、形状与长度：该组病例肝外胆管胰腺段其管径大小为 1mm~4mm，其中 1~3mm 的占 99%，平均 1.6mm，较文献报道的 3mm~5mm，平均 2.8mm 为低。我们认为，从活体形态学观点分析，肝外胆管胰腺段正常标准的上限似应定在≤ 4mm，超过此值则多为病理情况。肝外胆管胰腺段的形态呈圆形或类圆形，圆形占大多数（88/14），钩突段则由圆形变扁至裂隙状逐渐消失。该组肝外胆管全段长 8mm~32mm，其中 8mm、16mm 的占大多数，平均 11.9mm。大多数位于门静脉的右前方，少数位于门静脉的水平方向或右后方。

在正常及非肝胰疾病的 196 例中，有 94 例（47.96%）的病例肝外胆管胰头段与钩突段均未见显示，而有 102 例（52.04%）的病例肝外胆管胰头段与钩突段显示，直径≤ 4mm，也均无肝胰疾病，从而使我们思考一个问题：即当胆汁流经该处时才显示，且直径≤ 4mm；胆汁未流经该处时，肝外胆管胰腺段处于闭合状态，提示肝外胆管与体内其他管道（输尿管、食管等）有相似之处，均具有收缩功能。而且，我们观察到肝外胆管胰腺段在同一层面的不同时期的直径可以不同，从另一方面也提示肝外胆管具有收缩功能。

胆管流经钩突段：以往，人们一直以为肝外胆管胰腺段只流经胰头段，当其在钩突段看见肝外胆管的影像时也不敢认同。通过观察，我们发现在正常及非肝胰疾病组胆管胰腺段内径≤ 4mm 的 102 例中有 68 例在胰头段与钩突段均可见到，这是值得我们注意的问题。随着断面影像的发展，将胰头再分成胰头段与钩突段已取得人们的共识，因此，对于钩突段的影像学表现越来越受到临床医生的重视。

影响肝外胆管胰腺段显示的因素：①技术原因，窗宽、窗位的调节对肝外胆管的显示很重要，扫描层厚越薄，显示的可能性越大，口服对比剂，使十二指肠内充盈对比剂，有利于肝外胆管胰腺段的显示；②增强扫描，正常情况下胰腺强化表现为均匀强化，胰头段胆管与胰腺组织的密度差异更为明显，非常有利于观察胰头段胆管。随着年龄的增加，显示率有逐渐升高的趋势，可能与胆管壁随着年龄的增加而有一定的弹性降低，张力降低有关。我们认为，从活体形态学观点分析,肝外胆管胰腺段正常标准的上限似应定在≤ 4mm,超过此值则多为病理情况。

断面影像上对胆管胰腺段的认识:我们体会到,上下层面的连续观察对于研究断面图像总有益处。在单排螺旋 CT 增强扫描门静脉强化期找门静脉肝外段,它与肝外段胆管及肝动脉同在一纤维鞘中,走行于小网膜缘中,根据门静脉主干外胆管胰腺段的关系,就能轻松地找到;或先在胰头及钩突找到肝外胆管胰腺段的断面图像,然后向上方层面寻找,则容易找到胰上段;当然,窗技术的运用也很重要。此外、当门静脉主干出现时,肝外胆管胰腺段一般位于它的外前方,而肝动脉则位于门静脉左前方,但是常见的毗邻关系也可以发生变化。

第七节　肝外胆管成像中的误诊

肝脏提供的声学窗使超声易于显示肝门部肝外胆管,而胆总管因十二指肠或结肠气体的影响常显示不清。高分辨力 CT 或螺旋 CT 能很好地显示肝外胆管,尤其是扩张的肝外胆管。增强 CT 动脉期和门脉期显示胆囊壁和肝外胆管壁中等程度强化,腔内充盈的胆汁呈低于肝脏和胰腺更低密度,轴面上胆管呈环状,类似于外周有薄层钙化的透 X 线结石。CT 诊断胆管结石,偶尔出现“假性结石缺损”,为胆囊颈部螺旋皱褶、间隔或炎性增厚的胆囊壁所致,后者行增强 CT 扫描时,胆囊黏膜强化,低密度水肿的黏膜下层可被误认为胆囊内液体,从而形成胆囊结石的假像。

右肝内胆管与左肝内胆管在肝门部汇合,形成肝总管。肝总管长约 2~4cm,位于门静脉前方,可作为 CT 或超声辨认肝门结构的参考。约 80%~90% 的病人胆囊管汇入肝总管右侧壁,约 10%~20% 的病人胆囊管环绕肝总管,汇入肝总管的前壁、后壁或内侧壁。

肝总管和胆囊管在更近端或更远端汇合是一常见变异,见于半数的病人。在距离肝门部较低的位置汇合时,二管延长,平行走行数厘米后合并为一短的胆总管,在影像上相贴近的肝总管和胆囊管表现为双管状结构。由于两者被包埋在一个共同的结缔组织鞘内,手术中正确辨别和分离它们均较为困难,可能导致意外情况的发生,如因疏忽而结扎了肝总管导致胆管梗阻,横切胆管造成术后胆漏或将 T 管误置入胆囊管内。为避免医源性并发症,胆囊切除术时,常保留一个长的胆囊管残端,但这一部位常出现胆汁淤滞、炎症和结石。

低位汇合延长的胆囊管内结石发生率高。嵌顿在胆囊颈或胆囊管的结石压迫和阻塞邻近的肝总管,引起梗阻性黄疸,导致 Mirizzi 综合征。正确诊断 Mirizzi 综合征常依靠胆管造影。其 CT 和超声表现包括胆囊管与肝总管连接处的大结石、肝十二指肠韧带局部炎症和胆囊及肝内胆管扩张。

胆总管长约 4~8cm,直径约 6~9mm,分为胰上段、胰内段和共同管段。80%~90% 的胆总管和胰管有一共同的开口,胆胰液通过这一开口向十二指肠大乳头(Vater 乳头)排空，10%~20% 有两个独立的开口。偶尔,胆总管在距共同管段上缘 2~3cm 处与胰管汇合,导致共同管过长,此类胆胰管异常连接可导致胰液反流和胆管壁破坏,引起管腔扩张和胆总管囊肿。胆总管囊肿常在 1 岁内出现症状,但 20%~30% 的病人可推迟到儿童期或成人期。大约 1/3 的病人出现典型的三联征:右上腹疼痛、黄疸、可触及包块。所有的病人至少有其中一个症状。

直接法胆管造影、肝胆闪烁照相、超声、CT 和 MRCP 均能够正确诊断胆总管囊肿。1 型最常见,表现为胆总管一大的囊状或梭形扩张,约占 75%。2 型表现为胆总管大的憩室相突出,约占 2%。该两型薄壁的胆总管囊肿影像学上类似于重复胆囊或胰腺假性囊肿,胆系其余部分则正常。3 型最少见,胆总管囊肿位于胆总管十二指肠壁内段,呈局限性气球样扩张,约占 1%~2%,影像上表现为胰头内或十二指肠壁内的囊性病变,各种胆管造影方法都能很好显示其特征。4 型表现为肝内外胆管多发的动脉瘤样扩张,约占 18%~20%。

一般情况下,腹部超声、CT 或 MRI 很容易显示节段性或弥漫性胆管扩张,重要的是在连续层面上仔细分析受累的远侧胆管,为鉴别先天性胆管扩张如肝内胆管囊肿和胆总管囊肿,还是结石、肿瘤或其他病变导致的胆管扩张,需要采用多种方法。还应记住,某些正常解剖结构可类似于胆结石,如胆囊间隔、强化的胆囊黏膜或胆管壁均可造成结石的假象。

另一方面，多数透X线的结石，其CT值类似于腔内胆汁，在CT上不能显示。超声也可将结石漏诊，原因是螺旋状黏膜皱襞、间隔或相邻的十二指肠或结肠内的气体和回波反射性物质使结石难以辨认。胆囊和胆管常见的发育变异和异常是造成CT和超声误诊的原因之一。

胆系积气：胆系内常出现气体即胆系积气，尤其常见于有胆系手术史者，如胆肠吻合术、括约肌切开术后。胆系积气可引起敏感性伪影，利用某一扫描序列可将伪影降低到最低限度，如这种伪影在快速自旋回波（turbo SE）序列中是稳定的。极少情况下，过量的气体在胆总管内可形成完全不均匀信号，降低了MRCP的诊断价值。在外科分流、括约肌切开术或ERCP后，看到胆管树内气体即胆管积气并非少见，胆管分支类型与胆管系统解剖一致。偶尔，进行胆总管结石排石时在胆管树内可见到气体。一种潜在的诊断误区是气腹延伸到肝门而误认为是肝管积气。另一种潜在诊断误区是胆管积气与门静脉系统积气的鉴别。

门静脉积气的其他原因包括近期外科手术或是留置导管（包括G管）。门静脉积气通常有典型分支形状，可达到肝脏的周边，与胆管积气不同（胆管积气集中在肝脏的中央部位）。

胆系内气体可由多种原因引起，最常见于ERCP、胆管支架、胆肠吻合术后、胆胰下端括约肌开放状态。胆系内气体可误诊为结石，两者在所有序列中均表现为圆形无信号区。两者的鉴别点为：气体位于胆管的远地位置，而结石位于胆管的近地位置；气体可产生磁敏感性伪影，而结石则无伪影。MRCP对磁敏感性伪影不敏感，不易辨认。

气泡：括约肌切开术后病人胆系内常见气泡。与常规胆管造影一样，在MRCP图像上气泡与结石表现相同，需要与小结石鉴别。鉴别小结石与气泡的有效方法是选择一个与胆总管长轴垂直的平面（通常为倾斜轴位平面）进行MRCP成像。这一额外成像可通过三维序列扫描重建横轴位平面的容积数据获得，也可通过二维成像获得，后者可获得另一组图像。横轴位平面显示胆总管结石位于胆总管的下垂部位，而气泡则位于其非下垂部位。

关于增强后的强化：在静脉注射对比剂后，胆管在正常情况下不强化，这样就易与肝内血管区分。接受肝内小胆管胆汁的左、右肝内胆管下行，在肝门处形成肝总管，在胆囊管并入后形成胆总管，胆总管继续下行进入胆胰共同管入十二指肠。

因为正常的肝内胆管在CT扫描上常不能显示，过去认为在CT上显示出肝内胆管即是胆管扩张和阻塞。然而，随着CT技术的发展，现在有高达40%的病人可见正常粗细（1~3mm）的肝内胆管，而无胆管疾病。认识上述表现对评价可疑的胆管阻塞非常重要。

在许多病人中，肝外胆管能够分辨。在对无胆管疾病的100例病人的研究中，66例可以看到肝总管，平均直径2.8mm；82例可见到胆总管，平均直径3.6mm。尽管胆总管直径8~10mm不能明确界定有无胆总管扩张，但是正常胆总管的直径通常小于8mm。正常肝内胆管自肝门向肝周逐渐变细。肝外胆管壁厚度正常应小于1.5mm。胆总管壁强化亦可发生在无胆管疾病的病人中，仅有胆管壁的强化并不是胆管病变的指征。

肝外胆管：在静脉注射对比剂后，胆管在正常情况下不强化，这样就易与肝内血管区分。接受肝内小胆管胆汁的左、右肝管下行，在肝门处形成肝总管，在胆囊管并入后形成胆总管，胆总管继续下行进入胆胰共同管入十二指肠。

因为正常的肝胆管在CT扫描上常不能显示，过去认为在CT上显示出肝胆管即是胆管扩张和阻塞。然而，随着CT技术的发展，现在有高达40%的病人可见正常粗细（1~3mm）的肝胆管，而无胆管疾病。认识上述表现对评价可疑的胆管阻塞非常重要。在许多病人中，肝外胆管能够分辨。在对无胆管疾病的100例病人的研究中，66例可以看到肝总管，平均直径2.8mm；82例可见到胆总管，平均直径3.6mm。尽管有的作者认为胆总管直径4~6mm不能明确界定有无胆总管扩张，但是正常胆总管的直径通常小于4mm。正常肝管自肝门向肝周逐渐变细。肝外胆管壁厚度正常应小于1.5mm。单纯的胆总管壁强化亦可发生在无胆管疾病的病人中，没有其他胆管异常表现，仅有胆管壁的强化并不一定是胆管病变的指征。

超声扫描见到的一些胆管发育变异：在超声检查中，大约有10%的正常人可见肝动脉位于总肝管的前方。偶尔还见门静脉也位于胆管树的前方。Laing和Jeffrey（1980）在研究超声所见的假性扩张的总胆管时，发现胆囊的连接皱襞位于近侧，造成酷似总胆管的影像，实际上，只是胆囊的一个节段性显示。

胆囊切除术后银夹:胆囊切除术留置的银夹与胆管靠得很近时,有时可类似于胆管结石。利用包括横断面成像在内的两个平面的MR胆系造影成像技术,可鉴别银夹与结石。多数情况下,横断面成像可显示银夹的无信号区位于胆管外,并可见来自于银夹的磁敏感性伪影。

第八节 胆钙乳的动态观察

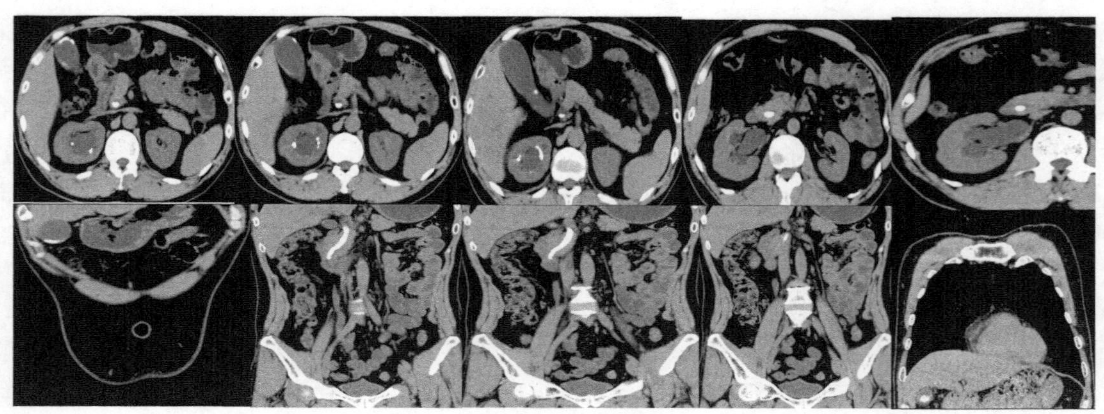

图 16-15-1 胆钙乳的动态观察

患者,男,43岁。

右腰腹部疼痛1月余入院。右肾结石,右侧输尿管结石,胆囊结石,慢性胆囊炎。1月1日CT平扫可见肝外胆管为高密度影充填,且有液平,考虑为胆钙乳。两天后,即1月3日,胸部CT平扫时仍可见胆囊结石,但肝外胆管内的胆钙乳已消失干净。

最初,胆钙乳充满肝外胆管且可见液平。初看酷似引流管内置,但却不见与体外相连;又似胆管蛔虫钙化,但钙化蛔虫体为固体,必导致胆管梗阻,胆管明显扩张,有液平可见,足可否认固体梗阻。胆囊内的胆钙乳与肝外胆管内的胆钙乳一样,也可在短期内消失,在临床上已屡见不鲜,这是值得注意的问题(图16-15-1)。

第十六章　胆管狭窄

第一节　慢性胰腺炎引起的胆管狭窄

85% 的人肝外胆管胰腺段，或被胰腺包绕，或横跨胰腺，因此，胰腺炎或胰腺肿瘤均可侵犯此段引起狭窄。自从 Reiedi（1896）首次报告以来，对于慢性胰腺炎致肝外胆管狭窄渐有了解，但如不注意则可导致误诊。

临床表现：在我们报告慢性胰腺炎并发肝外胆管狭窄 28 例中，有 26 例伴发胆系疾患，表示此症与胆系疾病关系密切。上腹痛和黄疸是本症的主要临床表现，其中黄疸 14 例，占 50%。一组 16 例血清碱性磷酸酶检查中，有 11 例大于正常 2 倍，虽比 Petrozza 等（1984）所报道的低，但是，血清碱性磷酸酶大于正常值 2 倍仍不失为本症的特殊指征，可用于临床病例的筛选。该组作者认为，对于有腹部症状及血清碱性磷酸酶升高的慢性胰腺炎病人，应行 MRCP 或 ERCP 检查，以明确有否肝外胆管狭窄存在。

影像学研究：对于慢性胰腺炎并发肝外胆管狭窄的特征性表现，Desplas（1938）认为，绝大多数表现为梭形僵硬性狭窄。

根据肝外胆管狭窄的表现，可分为如下类型：A 型：肝外胆管胰腺段呈长梭形向心性狭窄，光滑对称，上方有不同程度扩张并移位呈屈膝样，不全性梗阻，括约肌段开闭自如；B 型：肝外胆管括约肌段狭窄，其上肝外胆管呈鸟嘴样扩张；C 型：肝外胆管胰腺段呈沙钟形狭窄；D 型：Da 型，肝外胆管胰腺段现弧形侧方移位，胰腺多伴存假性囊肿；Db 型，肝外胆管胰腺段呈局限性偏心性狭窄；Dc 型，肝外胆管胰腺段表现为管状狭窄伴充盈缺损；E 型：肝外胆管呈现突然杯口状中断，完全性梗阻。

A、C 型为慢性胰腺炎肝外胆管狭窄的特征性表现，Db、Dc 及 E 型仅见于肿瘤。Guien（1971）统计 79 例钙化性胰腺炎中，61% 胆管异常，绝大部分为 A 型改变，C 型占 6%，Da 型仅 4%。正常情况下肝外胆管胰腺段长约 0.8~4.5cm。慢性胰腺炎肝外胆管狭窄的长度随胆管下端进入十二指肠部位不同而变化，一般在 2~3cm 之间。Desplas（1938）首次描述了最常见类型为梭形僵硬性狭窄。Caroli（1953）利用术中胆系造影照片测量将向心性胆管狭窄并胰腺钙化称为 A 型，并强调括约肌的开启。特征性改变为胰腺段或胰后段向心性狭窄，光滑对称，逐渐变细，狭窄长度为 2~3cm，呈进行性不可逆性改变，狭窄上方轻度扩张，移位成角呈屈膝状。据 Sarles（1978）报道，在重症胰腺炎中还有 23% 的病例肝外胆管无异常。对于慢性胰腺炎，应强调早期 ERCP 观察力图在早期无症状时发现肝外胆管狭窄，术前行 ERCP 或 PTC 及术中行胆管造影也不能忽视，以求及时发现和治疗伴随的胆管狭窄。

我们认为，不宜单凭胆管管径缩小不著而否认狭窄，需结合病变处胆管上方的扩张，胆管的移位及成角等表现分析有无狭窄。因为，本症系不全性梗阻，狭窄胆管上方扩张一般较轻；由于狭窄段系胰腺段胆管，其位置较固定，上方扩张胆管压力升高均可导致不同程度的移位和成角；正常胰腺段胆管长约 8~45mm，其长度随胆管下端进入十二指肠部位的不同而变化，因此狭窄段长度多为 10~30mm。

检查程序的选择：由于 ERCP 不仅能较好地显示胆系解剖，还可观察胰管的情况，故可认为 ERCP 是诊断本症的较理想的方法。如果 ERCP 未能满意地作出诊断，还可考虑行 PTC。在慢性胰腺炎手术时，不应放弃术中胆管造影，必要时，宜联合应用上述检查方法，可提高本症的诊断正确率。以往认为超声和 CT 难以显示本症，但 Schulte（1990）等应用增强 CT 观察胆管壁的变化,提出本症可表现为局限性向心性胆管壁增厚大于或等于 2mm,但管壁增厚不大于 5mm。我们在 23 例手术中发现胆管管壁明显增厚 2 例,管壁钙化 1 例,其壁厚为 3~5mm。应用 CT 胆管造影和 MRCP 可提高本症的诊断准确性。

鉴别诊断:在重症胰腺炎患者,慢性胰腺炎的影像学表现伴肝外胆管胰腺段 2~3cm 长的狭窄,其轮廓光滑匀称,为典型的向心性不可逆性改变,诊断并不困难,但有时需与下列疾病鉴别:

(1)胰腺假性囊肿挤压胆管:对于肝外胆管狭窄,应在真性狭窄与外在挤压所致窄小之间进行鉴别,如实在鉴别困难,可行引流及术中胆管造影观察是否有胰腺假性囊肿存在。如果引流后梗阻缓解,黄疸消退,则为假性囊肿压迫所致。

(2)胰腺癌或其他恶性肿瘤侵犯肝外胆管:肿瘤梗阻常为完全性或鼠尾样狭窄;CT 表现为胆管壁局限性或弥漫性偏心性增厚,常厚于 5mm;加之肿瘤本身的表现,颇易区别。区别困难时可行内镜超声检查,它不但可区分胰腺包块的性质,且可确定肿瘤转移情况,以减少不必要的剖腹探查;还可行内镜逆行胰管造影抽吸细胞学检查,它是确定胰腺肿瘤简单、安全、可信、有效的方法。

(3)胆管癌:只侵犯肝外胆管时,狭窄多伴肝内胆管的弥漫性扩张,且多发生于肝门附近,位置较高。肝门以下的肝外胆管胆管癌侵犯胆管壁,多呈现为不规则的团块,胆管壁轮廓不完整,且有不规则明显增厚。大多数学者认为,除非有其他证据,任何局限性肝外胆管梗阻伴胆管扩张都必须考虑为胆管癌,单凭影像学检查难以除外恶性病变的诊断时,需行组织活检确诊。

(4)外伤及医源性狭窄:胆管外伤十分少见。医源性胆管狭窄多位于肝外胆管胰上段,即胆囊管进入肝外胆管处附近,其狭窄段较短,多为局限性环形狭窄,甚至为线状环形狭窄,与本症的表现截然不同。

(5)原发性硬化性胆管炎:多为肝内外胆管同时受累,扩张狭窄交替呈串珠样,局限受累少。

单凭某一影像手段诊断困难者,需联合应用其他手段再行诊断与鉴别诊断。如仍困难,则可考虑经皮细针抽吸,胆管刷洗胆管脱落细胞学检查,ERCP 抽吸细胞学检查及内镜超声检查,必要时可行剖腹探查。

第二节 手术损伤性胆管狭窄

1. 发病机制 手术损伤性胆管狭窄,又称为医源性胆管狭窄,即手术损伤或胆管外伤修复术后的胆管狭窄。在良性胆管狭窄的病因中,大约 90% 是继发于医源性损伤,以胆系手术所占比例为最大,其中又以胆囊切除术为甚,可以这样说,胆囊切除术是导致胆管损伤的主要原因。据我们一组 54 例资料,胆系手术造成的损伤为 53/54 例,其中,绝大多数(48/54)病例都是由于胆囊切除术后,其余病例为胆肠吻合术后,胆系探查术后,胆管损伤修补术后,肝损伤修补术后。黄志强等(1988)总结分析全国以往曾有一次以上胆系手术者 2873 例,发现肝胆管狭窄所占的比例随手术次数增加而依次上升,其中经 1 次手术者狭窄发生率为 29.55%,3 次手术者为 53.22%。

胆系术后引起的肝外胆管扩张的因素中,除因胆囊切除或胆胰管下端括约肌功能失调导致胆管内压力的变化外,残余结石和胆管局限性狭窄等病变引起的胆管梗阻和感染可能是更重要的因素。手术直接损伤,或肝外胆管切口部缝合过紧外,T 管近侧横臂过长,长时间压迫胆管壁造成组织缺血损伤,也可引起总肝管分叉部局限性狭窄。这种狭窄经 T 管造影往往难以发现,待患者出现症状后,通过 ERCP 方才明确诊断。

鉴于此点,有作者提出,一方面应减少胆系术后不必要的 T 管引流,适当地开展胆管切开后一次缝合;另一方面,应重视 T 管放置和缝合的操作技术,选择长度和硬度适宜的 T 管, T 管近侧横臂不宜过长,避免由于位置和长度不当造成 T 管对胆管壁的压迫,避免由于缝合过紧引起总胆管切口部狭窄。

2. 病理学 胆管狭窄处及其附近的周围组织皆显示损伤后的纤维组织增生,瘢痕挛缩。炎性纤维化或纤维组织。胆管狭窄的位置,一般在肝外胆管(即胆总管与肝总管),少数在肝胆管汇合肝外胆管处,以及胆肠吻合口。它们均位于肝外胆管十二指肠上段、后段及其以上部位。由于生长速度较为一致，狭窄段（端）的基本表现是：边缘光滑，整齐，圆钝，两侧对称，管壁柔软，范围局限，未见凹凸不平。在单侧肝管开口狭窄时，早期手术可见到同侧肝脏瘀血肿大，晚期则呈萎缩性改变，体积缩小。

3. 临床表现　反复右上腹痛，发热，黄疸，胆汁外漏。术后出现症状时间长短不一，短者数日，长者数年。研究本症选择病例标准：①均有胆系手术史；②影像学检查清楚显示肝外胆管狭窄；③再次手术证实确实有胆管狭窄。手术史绝大多数为曾做胆囊切除术，其次为胆系探查术，少数为胆肠吻合术、肝破裂修补术、胆管外伤修补术等。实验室检查：血总胆红素增高，直接胆红素增高，碱性磷酸酶增高；甲胎蛋白及乙型肝炎表面抗原试验均为阴性。

4. 影像学研究　基本征象：狭窄位置越高，肝胆管扩张越多，也越明显。扩张的肝胆管一般皆无纡曲，也无枯枝征象。胆囊切除时最易损伤胆囊管汇入肝外胆管附近的肝外胆管，一般位置较高；胆肠吻合术者狭窄最易发生于吻合口处。一次手术引起的狭窄多在胆囊管汇入肝外胆管处附近，而多次手术引起的胆管狭窄的位置则比较分散。

狭窄的形态学特点有四：①杵状狭窄，狭窄端圆钝或略变尖，但无杯口凹陷及凹凸不平，狭窄上方胆管正常或仅轻度扩张，管壁光滑柔软整齐。②局限性环形狭窄，狭窄两端对称光滑，狭窄范围在 3mm 以内，大部分术中胆管被误扎，误缝或横断所致，犹如一个橡胶输液胶管被线横扎。有的病例在狭窄修复术时在狭窄处还可见丝线残迹。③葫芦形狭窄，狭窄上方及下方胆管略有扩张，狭窄处两侧对称向内凹陷，呈中心性狭窄，形如葫芦，系损伤后的胆管壁纤维组织增生，瘢痕形成，管壁均匀增厚，引起管腔狭窄。④悬空形狭窄，狭窄两端对称，但其间悬空不连接，狭窄段长约 20~30mm，中间约有 5mm 长的范围无对比剂显示。

5. 比较影像学　超声与 CT 对显示狭窄以上胆管的扩张情况价值较大，而对狭窄的发现则较差。MRI 及 MRCP 对显示狭窄及周围情况的信息甚为丰富，诊断价值大。

ERCP：大部分病例可以显示狭窄下方的胆管影像，狭窄端表现为杵状，圆钝，光滑或略尖；小部分病例对比剂可显示狭窄情况，并上达狭窄处的上方，显示出狭窄段的整个轮廓，但由于逆行造影注入压力较小，一般仅显示狭窄部位以下的胆管的情况。

PTC：一般能显示狭窄段及肝内外胆管的形态，在狭窄不严重的病例，对比剂能通过狭窄处下流入肠；狭窄严重者，只能显示狭窄上方胆管扩张，无对比剂入肠。PTC 可弥补 ERCP 的不足，PTC 注入对比剂的压力通常大于 ERCP，而且胆管顺行性生理收缩也可能助长这个压力梯度，有助于胆管的显示。术中胆系造影：方便实用，可能了解胆系有无发育变异，避免手术中因解剖异常或辨认不清造成损伤。同时，还可发现其他病变。可对医源性胆管狭窄准确定位。术后 T 管造影：显示肝内外胆管狭窄效果较好。

6. 鉴别诊断　医源性胆管狭窄是因为手术的直接损伤或损伤后的纤维组织增生、瘢痕收缩所致。由于生长速度比较均匀，造影所示狭窄段（端）基本特征是：边缘光滑，整齐且圆钝，两侧对称，管壁柔软，范围局限，未见有凹凸不平及杯口状改变，仔细分析狭窄段（端）的形态，结合病史及症状（手术史，病人年龄一般不大）对鉴别良、恶性病变有重要价值。

在单侧肝胆管开口狭窄时，早期手术可见到同侧肝脏瘀血肿大，晚期则呈萎缩性改变，体积缩小。造影可见对侧肝管虽有扩张，但无纡曲；一般无胆管炎常见的枯树枝征及恶性肿瘤常见的软藤征表现。这与狭窄的程度、位置、时间有关，从症状出现至再次手术时间一般不长，病因明确可有助于鉴别。在胆肠吻合术后，由于胆汁分流，可使残留的肝外胆管变细，此时，应注意与胆管癌鉴别。医源性胆管狭窄尽管胆管变细，但其走行自然，无移位，胆管壁光滑匀称，无僵硬感，再结合手术史容易鉴别。

此外，罕见的胆管憩室如位于肝总管起始部及一侧肝胆管开口上方，可使该侧肝胆管及总肝管局部对称性狭窄，酷似医源性胆管狭窄，可造成混淆。此刻，手术史极为重要。

第三节　胆管狭窄与异位血管压迫

肝门处的异位血管在胆管前横过可致该部胆管发育受阻，久之，管腔相对狭小，在此基础上若有蛔虫钻入,或因胆流不畅而继发感染,便可形成结石,加重梗阻。胆管炎长期反复发作又加重原有狭窄。

若为肝右动脉所致,常可引起总肝管上端狭窄,形成肝内广泛结石,还可有严重的胆汁性肝硬化及门脉高压,这时,由于汇管区纤维组织压迫,门静脉分支稀少,管腔变细,或由于门静脉分支发生短路分流,肝脏门脉血供大为减少,肝动脉血流量则代偿性增加,横跨胆管的肝动脉也随之增粗,又加重了对狭窄部的压迫,造成恶性循环。若走行异常的血管只造成某支肝胆管狭窄,则只有狭窄以上的胆系结石及相应肝叶和肝段纤维化。

异位血管压迫与胆结石所致的狭窄同属于炎性狭窄,二者很难鉴别,诊断常用方法是手术探查。胆系结石引起的炎性狭窄除可发生在胆总管末端外,通常发生在胆总管分支汇合部,而发生在汇合部以下或肝外胆管上的肝外胆管狭窄多为损伤所致。术中发现为后种部位狭窄,若能除外损伤因素,而狭窄部又有异位血管横过并嵌入狭窄环,或将血管游离牵开后,狭窄部上环形凹陷,则狭窄为血管压迫所致。血管走行异常致胆管狭窄,尤其是合并有肝硬化时,既要解除狭窄,又不能损伤血管。交叉换位后,解除狭窄,再作胆管整形及胆肠吻合术,是一种可满足上述要求的较好处理方法。

第四节　胆管狭窄的误诊

诊断胆管狭窄的同时,可能出现胆管狭窄性质和程度的误诊。伪影是由于MRI图像的矩阵较常规MRI图像小或与最大信号强度投影重建有关。仅仅利用MRCP成像来显示狭窄的形态特征不足以做出正确诊断。事实上,矩阵的减少限制了细微结构(如黏膜不规则性)的显示,不注射对比剂,一方面反映了生理状态下的狭窄,另一方面限制了其他特征(如胆管扩张性等)的显示。MRCP是完整腹部成像的一部分,将MRCP和常规成像联合使用,有助于显示狭窄的特征和性质。另一类误诊是对狭窄程度的认识,最大信号强度投影重建图像常过度估计胆管狭窄。在最大信号强度投影图像上,重度狭窄处的少量胆汁不能显示,表现为完全性梗阻的假象。即使很少量的胆汁也能在原始图像上显示,分析原始图像可减少误诊;分析继发征象比如狭窄上方胆管扩张程度,亦可减少误诊。

诊断胆管狭窄的其他问题是不能显示远端萎陷的胆总管,无法确定胆总管狭窄的长度。

肝右动脉横过胆总管可造成胆总管假性狭窄。正常解剖中,肝右动脉行走在近端胆总管的后方,对胆总管可产生一种外压性改变,某些情况下,这种外压性改变可类似于一种轻度狭窄。除了同时分析原始图像和轴面T_2WI外,典型的部位也有助于鉴别真性和假性狭窄。嵌顿于肝段胆管的小结石,周围有极少量的胆汁包围,引起肝段胆管扩张,也可表现为肝内胆管假性狭窄。

第十七章　胆管先天异常和发育变异

第一节　胆管先天性异常

据尸解统计，胆管先天性异常约占2.4%，外科手术统计约占2.8%，术中胆管造影统计约占5%~13%。

迷走肝内胆管：迷走的肝内胆管引流肝实质的某个有限的部分。最常见的，是右叶肝内胆管或是前段支或是后段支引流进入左叶主肝内胆管，而不是右叶主肝内胆管。

迷走的肝内胆管可汇入总肝管、总胆管、胆囊管、或低位汇入右肝内胆管。少见的，迷走的肝内胆管走行经过胆囊床，甚或进入胆囊本身。在后面情况下，在胆囊切除术时它容易发生撕裂，如果未被发现，则可产生术后胆汁瘘。此型迷走肝内胆管直径大于2mm，必须与胚胎残余囊肝管进行区别，囊肝管直径为0.5~1.0mm，甚至当其撕裂时也无重要的临床意义。较少见的迷走肝内胆管是迷走左肝内胆管，汇入总胆管。

肝内胆管的异位汇入：肝内胆管汇入肝外胆管时，有的比正常高，有的又比正常低。当其汇入较正常低时，其临床意义在胆囊手术时，当胆囊管进入右肝内胆管，或右肝内胆管在连接左肝内胆管之前进入胆囊管。

双重胆囊管或双重总胆管：双重胆囊管或双重总胆管十分少见。

囊下胆管：囊下胆管是右叶下部分难见到的小的先天性异常分支，它紧邻胆囊近侧，但它不与胆囊相交通。

先天性气管胆系瘘：先天性气管胆系瘘是罕见的先天性异常，它多伴存呼吸困难，且可咳出带胆汁特征的痰。此瘘通常起始于气管隆突附近，经过横膈，一般交通于左肝内胆管。胆系积气通常见于X线腹部平片上。在以往，此瘘多以支气管造影进行术前的观察。在现在，放射性胆系核素显像可以在术前提供诊断的证据。

第二节　肝间管

胆系的发育变异常见，但真正的副肝内胆管发生率只占1%。Cibney等（1987）报告1例连接左、右肝内胆管之副肝内胆管，并命名为肝间管。左、右胆管系统肝内吻合发生在胆小管之间已为显微镜检证实，然而手术和胆管造影尚未曾发现二者的互通现象。

肝间管的胚胎学发生机制不明，有作者认为肝外残余结构——“迷行管”有时可能位于左、右肝内胆管间，并假定这种“迷行管”代表在肝形成期实质已经萎缩的胚胎肝内胆管。

肝间管也许就是由于胆汁异常地从右肝内胆管引流入胆囊管而致永久遗留下来的迷行管。一般放射科大夫、介入放射学大夫和外科大夫都必须了解这种胆系变异，如不熟悉则可导致解释错误、手术损伤，而造成术后胆漏和狭窄。

第三节 先天性双胆管

先天性双胆管畸形是极为少见的发育异常,有作者认为人类的这种胆管异常与动物(爬虫类,鱼类,鸟类)的两组肝芽相类似。Kodam 等(1980)报告一例,术前经 ERCP 确诊。

在研究胆囊管低位汇合时,我们发现,当胆囊管最低位与肝外胆管汇合时,如果不注意,则可误为此类异常(从图片上看,《中华放射学杂志》1990, 24:288. 报告一例,似乎就是此类情况)

第四节 MRCP 与发育变异

胆囊和胆管的发育变异与胚胎期发育异常密切相关,包括肝内和肝外胆管扩张以及胆总管和胆囊管异常。有作者将胆管扩张分为不同的亚型,包括胆总管憩室和肝内胆管囊状扩张。MRCP 可诊断肝内胆管囊状扩张,在原始图像和最大强度投影重建图像上表现为肝内多发的囊状扩张结构,并互相交通。这种起源于胆管的囊肿由此可与其他病变如多发的单纯肝囊肿和肝脓肿鉴别。临床上特别感兴趣的其他发育变异为副胆管以及胆囊管的异常汇合,尤其是腹腔镜技术应用后更是如此。约 18% 的病人有异常副胆管,多见于右侧胆管系统。引流第 7 肝段或第 8 肝段胆汁的异常胆管,汇入胆总管或胆囊管的变异对手术十分重要,在腹腔镜的操作中,它很容易因疏忽而被切断。

胆囊管与胆总管汇合部的位置变异很大,最常见的汇合部位为胆总管中 1/3 外侧壁,此外还有低位汇合和高位汇合。低位汇合时,胆囊管较长,行走在胆总管内侧,并与之平行,类似于扩张的胆总管。应分析原始图像或斜位最大信号强度投影重建图像,以避免误诊。

第五节 诊断陷阱

有作者注意到,在超声检查中,大约有 10% 的正常人可见肝动脉位于总肝管的前方。偶尔还见门静脉也位于胆管树的前方。Laing 和 Jeffrey(1980)在研究超声所见的假性扩张的总胆管时,发现胆囊的连接皱襞位于近侧,造成酷似总胆管的影像,实际上,只是胆囊的一个节段性显示。

第十八章　原发性硬化性胆管炎

原发性硬化性胆管炎与 IgG4 相关性胆管炎

原发性硬化性胆管炎是一种慢性胆汁淤积性肝病，其特征是肝内外胆管炎症和纤维化，导致多灶性胆管狭窄，最终发展为肝硬化、门静脉高压，因目前尚无有效的治疗药物，故预后不佳。IgG4 相关性胆管炎是近期备受临床关注的一类胆汁淤积性肝病，因其生物化学特点及胆管造影表现与原发性硬化性胆管炎相似，会被认为是原发性硬化性胆管炎的变异形式。但随着对 IgG4 相关硬化性疾病研究的深入，IgG4 相关性胆管炎是否作为这类新的临床疾病实体的独立表现形式也在进一步研究当中。因 IgG4 相关性胆管炎对激素治疗敏感、患者预后良好，掌握原发性硬化性胆管炎与 IgG4 相关性胆管炎间的诊治及鉴别便尤为重要。

（一）原发性硬化性胆管炎

Hoffman（1887）首次报道该病，之后陆续有报道。以前多依据开腹手术病理检查确诊，自 20 世纪 70 年代以来，随着内镜下逆行胆胰管造影（ERCP）和磁共振胆胰成像（MRCP）等检查技术的开展和广泛应用，原发性硬化性胆管炎的发病率和诊断率明显提高。原发性硬化性胆管炎的病因尚不完全明了，研究发现，本病既无胆系结石、外伤、手术史，也无胆系肿瘤存在，而与自身免疫、遗传易感、门静脉及胆系的慢性非特异性感染等因素有关。

其发病可见于任何年龄，但诊断的中位年龄为 40 岁左右，男女比例约为 2：1，约 80% 的患者伴发炎症性肠病，主要为溃疡性结肠炎。因此，“典型”的原发性硬化性胆管炎是一类好发于青壮年、生物化学及临床表现为胆汁淤积性肝病、常伴有炎症性肠病的疾病。

美国胃肠病学会在 2002 年发表了对原发性硬化性胆管炎的诊疗指南，随着更多研究结果的出现，也出现了诸多版本的诊断标准，如 Myens 标准等。欧洲肝病学会（EASL）和美国肝病学会（AASLD）也分别于 2009 年及 2010 年提出了关于胆汁淤积性肝病和原发性硬化性胆管炎的指南。欧洲肝病学会在 2009 年发布的《胆汁淤积性肝病的临床指南》中建议：MRC 显示有典型的原发性硬化性胆管炎改变且排除继发性硬化性胆管炎，无其他可解释的胆汁淤积、生物化学指标升高者可诊断原发性硬化性胆管炎，诊断原发性硬化性胆管炎肝活组织检查是非必需的，但其可评估疾病的活动度和分期。如果高质量的 MRCP 结果正常，诊断小胆管原发性硬化性胆管炎须做肝活组织检查；同样，表现为不对称的血清转氨酶升高和 / 或 IgG 水平升高者，肝活组织检查对判断是否伴发有其他疾病或与其他疾病交替存在有帮助。

美国肝病学会于 2010 年发布的《原发性硬化性胆管炎诊疗指南》中建议：对于有淤胆生物化学表现的患者，应行 MRCP 或 ERCP 检查以明确原发性硬化性胆管炎的诊断；当 MRCP 或 ERCP 发现典型的原发性硬化性胆管炎表现时，不推荐进行肝穿刺；如果 MRCP 和 ERCP 无明显异常发现，建议对患者行肝穿刺活组织检查以明确有无小胆管原发性硬化性胆管炎；如果患者伴有转氨酶异常，建议行肝穿刺活组织检查以明确有无重叠综合征；对于疑诊原发性硬化性胆管炎的患者，建议检测血清 IgG4 以排除自身免疫性胰腺炎。

在上述两个较权威的临床诊疗指南里，对原发性硬化性胆管炎的诊断均是由血清生物化学检测、影像学检查、排除其他淤胆病变及组织学等多方面综合组成，其中 MRCP 和 ERCP 在诊断中尤为重要。Berstad 等（2006）报道 MRCP 与 ERCP 诊断原发性硬化性胆管炎的敏感性分别为 80% 和 89%，特异性分别为 87% 和 80%。Moff 等（2006）对 36 例原发性硬化性胆管炎患者和 5 例对照者进行随机、盲法的研究，结果表明 MRCP 和 ERCP 对诊断原发性硬化性胆管炎及判断是否存在肝内胆管狭窄具有相似的诊断价值，但 ERCP 更有助于判断肝外胆管梗阻及严重程度。

虽然两种检查方法有着近乎相似的诊断准确

性,但 ERCP 有一定的并发症如胰腺炎、败血症等。尽管 ERCP 仍是诊断原发性硬化性胆管炎的金标准,但 MRCP 作为一种无创性检查方法,可以作为怀疑原发性硬化性胆管炎病例的初步检查手段。

(二)IgG4 相关性胆管炎

随着对自身免疫性胰腺炎研究的进展,人们渐渐认识到自身免疫性胰腺炎病变不仅仅局限于胰腺,其胆管病变的表现类似原发性硬化性胆管炎,也能引起梗阻性黄疸。起初这种胆管病变被命名为自身免疫性胰腺炎相关性硬化性胆管炎, Bjornsso 等(2007)建议将之改为 IgG4 相关性胆管炎。

之后,随着对唾液腺、泪腺、腹膜后淋巴结、甲状腺、肾脏等其他受累器官的研究, Kamisawa 等(2004, 2006)提出了 IgG4 相关硬化性疾病这一概念。

IgG4 相关硬化性疾病是以血清 IgG4 水平升高和多部位 IgG4 丰富的淋巴 - 浆细胞浸润为特征的一种综合征,而 IgG4 相关性胆管炎即特指 IgG4 相关硬化性疾病的胆系表现。

IGG4 相关性胆管炎是一类发病机制不明的硬化性胆管炎,以血清 IgG4 水平升高、胆管壁密集浸润 IgG4 阳性的浆细胞为特征。IgG4 相关性胆管炎患者常伴发自身免疫性胰腺炎,且对激素治疗应答良好。早期诊断及治疗对 IgG4 相关性胆管炎患者极为重要,且明确诊断有助于避免过度治疗甚至不必要的手术。

在临床上, IgG4 相关性胆管炎患者的胆系影像学表现与原发性硬化性胆管炎、胰腺癌和胆管癌的表现相近,常易混淆,不能单凭影像学表现来鉴别 IgG4 相关性胆管炎和上述预后不良的疾病。并且,当患者没有伴发自身免疫性胰腺炎表现时,作出 IgG4 相关性胆管炎的诊断也相当困难。因此,需要拟定 IgG4 相关性胆管炎的诊断标准对临床诊治进行指导。

2009 年,欧洲肝病学会在《胆汁淤积性肝病的临床指南》中指出,对 IgG4 相关性胆管炎做出诊断基于患者有典型的硬化性胆管炎的胆系影像学改变,并依据:(1)最近接受胰腺癌 / 胆系外科手术或胰腺活组织检查,发现有自身免疫性胰腺炎 /IgG4 相关性胆管炎特征;或(2)具有典型的自身免疫性胰腺炎影像学改变和 IgG4 升高;或(3)符合下述生物化学、病理学和影像诊断标准中的两项: IgG4 升高,胰腺影像学表现,其他器官的变化包括硬化性腮腺炎、腹膜后纤维化或胃肠道受累和腹部淋巴结肿大及 IgG4 阳性浆细胞浸润,胆管活检每高倍视野中 IgG4 阳性浆细胞 >10;并且予类固醇激素治疗 4 周,胆管支架拆除后,梗阻性胆汁淤积不复发、肝功能试验 <2 倍正常值上限、出现 IgG4 和 CA199 下降,即可诊断为 IgG4 相关性胆管炎。

而日本 IgG4 相关性胆管炎研究委员会、肝胆疾病研究委员会、日本胆系协会等工作组也从 2010 年就开始着手共同制定有关于 IgG4 相关性胆管炎的诊断标准,并在 2012 年推出了基于以下 4 条标准的诊断原则:

(1)特征性胆管影像学表现:肝内和 / 或肝外胆管壁增厚、弥漫或节段性狭窄;

(2)升高的血清 IgG4 水平(≥ 1.35g/L);

(3)同时并存有自身免疫性胰腺炎、IgG4 相关的泪腺、涎腺炎或 IgG4 相关的腹膜后纤维化;

(4)组织病理学特征性表现:①标志性的淋巴或浆细胞的浸润及纤维化;② IgG4 阳性的浆细胞的浸润(每高倍视野中 IgG4 阳性浆细胞 >10 个);③轮辐状纤维化;④闭塞性静脉炎。

需要注意的是,尽管血清 IgG4 升高是 IgG4 相关性胆管炎的特征,但单独血清 IgG4 水平升高不能作出 IgG4 相关性胆管炎的诊断。目前, IgG4 水平诊断 IgG4 相关性胆管炎的敏感性和特异性尚不清楚。总 IgG 水平(≥ 18 g/L)和 IgG4(≥ 1.35 g/L)水平增加显示出相对较高的敏感性。但最近有报道,一些胰腺癌或原发性硬化性胆管炎患者血清 IgG4 水平也升高,并伴有 IgG4 阳性细胞在胰腺和肝脏的显著浸润。

在一些过敏性疾病如寻常型天疱疮和过敏性皮炎等疾病中,血清 IgG4 水平亦升高。

因此,尽管血清 IgG4 是诊断 IgG4 相关性胆管炎的敏感标志,但不是诊断 IgG4 相关性胆管炎的金标准。其他器官的累及是诊断 IgG4 相关性胆管炎的重要线索,如果胆管狭窄患者存在无法解释的胰腺疾病,需提高对 IgG4 相关性胆管炎的怀疑。但是也有些 IgG4 相关性胆管炎患者并没有明显的胰腺疾病的临床或影像学证据,因此,不存在胰腺疾病也不能排除 IgG4 相关性胆管炎的诊断。

虽然 IgG4 相关性胆管炎患者对激素治疗敏感,但对怀疑 IgG4 相关性胆管炎的患者使用激素诊断性治疗仍是危险的,应在激素治疗之前尽量排除恶性肿瘤的可能。在许多患者中,能够得到超声内镜指导下的胰腺活检标本有助于在开始激素治疗之前证实 IgG4 相关性胆管炎的诊断。

综上所述，对 IgG4 相关性胆管炎的诊断是需要结合组织学、影像学、血清学、其他器官累及的表现和对激素治疗的反应等多个方面的特征综合做出。

（三）鉴别诊断

原发性硬化性胆管炎和 IgG4 相关性胆管炎虽皆属于胆汁淤积性肝病，且临床表现和影像学表现等有诸多相似之处，但仍有着各自独特的特点。鉴别二者目的在于，对患者的治疗、并发症处理及预后等存在差异，明确诊断甚至可以避免不必要的手术。

发病年龄上，原发性硬化性胆管炎好发 25~45 的岁青壮年，而 IgG4 相关性胆管炎更多见于老年人（平均年龄 62 岁）。临床表现上，虽然多数原发性硬化性胆管炎和 IgG4 相关性胆管炎患者都会出现黄疸，但原发性硬化性胆管炎患者仍以乏力、瘙痒为主，占到 60% 以上，还可表现为右上腹痛、消瘦等，而 IgG4 相关性胆管炎主要因梗阻性黄疸就诊，大部分患者没有严重的腹痛，其他器官受累时有相应表现如唾液腺肿大等。

在伴发疾病方面，62.5%~90.0% 的原发性硬化性胆管炎患者会合并炎症性肠病，而仅有 0~6% 的 IgG4 相关性胆管炎并发此病，原发性硬化性胆管炎一般不伴有胰腺病变，而 IgG4 相关性胆管炎的患者却常常合并其他 IgG4 相关的疾病，如高达 92% 的 IgG4 相关性胆管炎会有胰腺受累的相应表现，还常并发硬化性泪腺炎、硬化性腮腺炎、腹膜后纤维化等。

病情转归上，约 10%~30% 的原发性硬化性胆管炎患者可能发展为胆管癌，而迄今尚未有 IgG4 相关性胆管炎患者并发胆管癌的病例报道。

血清生物化学检测上，原发性硬化性胆管炎和 IgG4 相关性胆管炎都有胆汁淤积指标（碱性磷酸酶、胆红素）异常的表现，但绝大部分 IgG4 相关性胆管炎患者血清中可检测出高水平的 IgG4，少部分 IgG4 相关性胆管炎患者最初 IgG4 水平尚未升高，但在随访期间 IgG4 水平也逐渐攀升；IgG4 相关性胆管炎患者中 CA199 水平也可升高，但一般不超过 100 IU/ml，而在原发性硬化性胆管炎患者中，CA199 的升高往往预示可能并发胆管癌。对于自身免疫性抗体的检测，抗中性粒细胞胞质抗体是原发性硬化性胆管炎相对特异性的抗体，见于大部分原发性硬化性胆管炎患者，但却在 IgG4 相关性胆管炎患者中罕见。

影像学表现上，有报道节段性狭窄及胆总管低位狭窄在 IgG4 相关性胆管炎比原发性硬化性胆管炎中更常见，相反，带状狭窄和串珠样改变则提示原发性硬化性胆管炎而不是 IgG4 相关性胆管炎。但单纯依靠胆管造影仍难以鉴别，还应结合其他临床表现，如 IgG4 相关性胆管炎患者常有弥漫性腊肠样胰腺水肿伴胰管不规则狭窄的影像学表现，或激素治疗后复查发现狭窄明显改观。

肝组织病理学表现上，原发性硬化性胆管炎典型的肝脏病理学表现为洋葱皮样胆管纤维化，而 IgG4 相关性胆管炎主要为胆管壁的 IgG4 阳性浆细胞大量浸润和轮辐状纤维化；IgG4 免疫染色结果显示 IgG4 相关性胆管炎的 IgG4 阳性细胞 >10 个 / 高倍视野，虽然原发性硬化性胆管炎患者也有门管区胆管和肝外胆管的 IgG4 阳性细胞浸润，但浸润程度明显低于 IgG4 相关性胆管炎患者，IgG4 阳性细胞 <10 个 / 高倍视野；中性粒细胞的浸润常见于原发性硬化性胆管炎，而 IgG4 相关性胆管炎的炎症浸润主要由淋巴细胞、浆细胞和嗜酸性粒细胞组成；部分 IgG4 相关性胆管炎患者活检标本可见以门静脉为基础的纤维化 - 炎症结节，这种结节位于门静脉区，包含淋巴细胞、浆细胞、嗜酸性细胞和成纤维细胞，但在原发性硬化性胆管炎中没有这种结节。

在对治疗的反应及预后方面，IgG4 相关性胆管炎患者对激素治疗敏感，预后相对较好，而原发性硬化性胆管炎对激素和其他免疫抑制剂均疗效欠佳。有症状的原发性硬化性胆管炎患者随访 6 年后，合并肝衰竭、胆管癌等可高达 41%，肝移植是唯一可使患者长期生存的方法。

虽然原发性硬化性胆管炎和 IgG4 相关性胆管炎存在上述诸多不同，但在临床实践中，患者的表现常错综复杂，往往鉴别困难。而且，目前对于两者的确切关系还存在争议。9%~36% 的原发性硬化性胆管炎患者血清 IgG4 水平也会升高，有作者推测这部分患者实际上可能是 IgG4 相关性胆管炎而非原发性硬化性胆管炎。

此外，一些作者发现儿童原发性硬化性胆管炎患者往往激素治疗有效，认为这可能是由于疾病早期胆管壁以炎症反应为主而纤维化轻微的关系。相反，那些对激素治疗无效的 IgG4 相关性胆管炎患者则可能是由于疾病进展,胆管壁炎症轻微而纤维化严重的关系。

有学者认为 IgG4 相关性胆管炎和原发性硬化性胆管炎本质上属于同一疾病谱，IgG4 相关性胆管炎是原发性硬化性胆管炎的早期表现或特殊类型。二者的确切关系仍有待进一步的研究证实。

第十九章　胆系寄生虫病

第一节　胆系蛔虫病

胆系蛔虫病既往是临床上常见的急腹症之一，但是，近年来，由于生活水平日益提高，发病率明显下降。

临床表现：蛔虫是最常见的引起胃肠道寄生性感染的寄生虫之一，典型的成虫长约 15~50 cm，直径约 3~6 mm。蛔虫可在空肠内生活 1~2 年而无任何症状，当蛔虫移行至十二指肠乳头进入胆系内则会导致胆绞痛、胆囊炎、化脓性胆管炎、胰腺炎、肝脓肿甚至败血症等严重并发症，这些因素的刺激可导致胆管癌的发生。胆系蛔虫病多因饮食不卫生不规律、饥饱失常、服用驱虫药量不足等因素，导致胃肠道功能紊乱，蛔虫趁机扰动钻窜入胆系而发病。腹痛常突然发生，典型者表现为剑突下剧烈的阵发性的“钻顶”样绞痛。疼痛发作时病人辗转不安，手捧上腹，弯背屈膝，四肢厥冷，大汗淋漓，疼痛发作后如正常人。常伴有恶心呕吐，发热。查体胆囊区压痛明显。蛔虫死后其崩解的组织碎片和虫卵，可诱发钙盐沉积，促进胆系结石形成，加重对机体组织的损伤。一组 9 例均未见明显胆系结石形成。

影像学研究：B 超检查经济实惠、实时成像，常被列为首选。典型胆系蛔虫表现为不伴声影的管状回声，具有相对低回声的中心和相对高回声的平行双线状壁，实时声像图可显示活体蛔虫的蠕动，但是由于肠气的干扰，会影响胆总管中下段的显示，另外超声诊断的准确性与操作者的经验密切相关。该组有 5 例行超声检查，仅发现胆囊增大，内透声差，但均未发现蛔虫。ERCP 具有诊断和治疗双重作用，可清晰显示胆管内条状充盈缺损，透视下有时可观察到活体蛔虫的蠕动，并可直接取虫。但 ERCP 是一种有创的检查方法，应用时必须权衡操作过程中潜在的并发症。

MRI 为多序列、多方位、多参数成像，胆系蛔虫病具有特异的影像学表现，胆系蛔虫在 T_1WI 上表现为条状稍高信号，在 T_2WI 上表现为条状低信号，活体蛔虫肠道内吞入的液体则表现为低信号中央见线状稍高信号，形成所谓的“三线”征，在横轴位上表现为眼镜征。

该组病例中 8 例 T_1WI 上表现为稍高信号，T_2WI 上表现为低信号，其中 3 例 T_2WI 上条状低信号内见线状稍高信号。由于蛔虫进入胆系前寄生在肠道内，可引起肠道改变，该组病例中 5 例合并肠道积气扩张。

MRCP 利用水成像原理，是唯一非侵入性的显示胆管及胆囊内蛔虫的检查方法，且可同时显示胆管及胰管系统。胆系蛔虫在 MRCP 上表现为条状低信号充盈缺损。该组 9 例在 MRCP 上均可见胆系内条状低信号充盈缺损，且 MRCP 薄层原始图像上显示病变更加清楚直观，可显示常规 MRI 不能显示的病变，不易漏诊，是诊断胆系蛔虫病的首选方法。

鉴别诊断：本病应与胆系结石、沉积物、气体、肿瘤及其他寄生虫等相鉴别。

胆系结石：胆系结石在 T_1WI、T_2WI 及 MRCP 上均表现为低信号，呈圆形或椭圆形。

胆系内的沉积物：多不定形，很少为条状，T_1WI 及 T_2WI 多为稍低信号。

胆系内气体：胆系内气体在 T_1WI、T_2WI 均为极低信号。

胆系肿瘤：胆管癌、胆囊癌显示壁不规则增厚，呈结节状或乳头状，T_1WI 为稍低信号，T_2WI 稍高信号，增强后可有强化。

华支睾吸虫：华支睾吸虫比蛔虫小得多，长

8~15 mm,呈扁平状。

肝片吸虫:肝片吸虫比华支睾吸虫大,但仍比蛔虫细小,长约 8~40 mm。

由于胆系蛔虫病的 MRI 及 MRCP 表现特异,依据临床病史及粪便常规检查多易与其他疾病鉴别。胆系蛔虫病作为一种相对少见的急腹症,早期确诊十分重要,其 MRI 及 MRCP 表现具有特征性,可为临床正确治疗提供充足的依据。

第二节 肝吸虫胆管炎

华支睾吸虫(简称肝吸虫)在我国广东珠江三角洲一带发病率较高,感染率达 4.08%。

进食未煮熟的带肝吸虫的鱼片后,幼虫在十二指肠经肝外胆管、肠黏膜或门静脉寄生于胆管末梢,引起胆管黏膜及周围的慢性炎症,同时破坏胆管的局部免疫防御功能。肝吸虫虫体、黏液团及由肝吸虫引起的泥沙样结石阻塞胆管,细菌从肠道逆行感染引起胆管急性炎症,为吸虫性胆管炎。肝吸虫的肝内胆管扩张程度取决于患者反复感染的程度、病程、体内寄生虫的数量及有无并发症等。

一组 48 例由于临床表现较重,均为急性起病,CT 表现均有肝内胆管不同程度扩张,且肝内胆管扩张多广泛弥漫,部分中重度扩张的胆管自肝门向肝被膜方向均匀扩张。这表明患者反复感染,病程较长较重目并发症较多,同时常伴有多发末梢胆管的小囊状扩张。

该组病例出现末梢胆管小囊状扩张的比例约占 79%(38/48),其原因可能是由于肝吸虫喜在小胆管内寄居生长,其成虫的体宽也与小胆管直径吻合,造成末梢小胆管梗阻扩张及淤胆。由于长期的慢性刺激,胆总管、肝管及十二指肠乳头常表现为胆管壁僵硬,粗细不均匀等慢性炎症引起的管壁增厚及狭窄;另一方面,由于十二指肠乳头及胆总管下端炎性狭窄而开口变小,从上游胆管不断排泄下来的肝吸虫及其代谢产物通过受阻,在胆总管下端形成肝吸虫虫体、虫卵及脱落的上皮与黏液构成的团块,造成阻塞,使梗阻以上胆管、胆总管扩张。肝外胆管的中重度扩张常与肝内胆管的轻度扩张不成比例。

胆囊多表现为炎症改变,胆囊增大,胆囊壁增厚,囊内有时见团状软组织密度影。

当肝吸虫团块造成肝外胆管梗阻时,CT 显示肝外胆管扩张,胆囊增大,可同时伴有肝内胆管扩张,此时如果不重视其肝内胆管扩张的形态,容易与其他胆管阻塞性疾病混淆。

该组 15/48 例肝吸虫术前误诊,其中 8 例显示肝内外胆管不同程度扩张,肝内胆管内或肝外胆管内见高密度影,考虑结石而引起误诊,因为肝吸虫团块中含虫卵多时,虫卵积在一起时密度也较高,同时肝吸虫产物也易形成以其为中心的胆色素性结石,手术证实未见结石形成,其胆管梗阻以虫团梗阻为主。当 CT 表现为肝内外胆管扩张,胆总管壁增厚强化而胰头正常,胆总管下端未见高密度结石时,容易误诊为浸润性肝外胆管癌或壶腹癌,该组有 5 例肝吸虫误诊为胆总管癌及胆胰共同管癌。

该组 2 例 CT 表现为肝内胆管扩张,同时肝实质内见低密度结节状影,边缘相对清楚,增强后病变呈不均匀强化,且延迟强化,病灶有所缩小,CT 误诊为肝吸虫合并肝内周围型胆管癌,但经服吡喹酮治疗后复查,发现肝内低密度灶明显变小,另 1 例基本消失,考虑为肝吸虫病伴炎性肉芽肿形成。此征象可能由于肝吸虫成虫、虫卵的化学毒性作用及机械性刺激引起胆管周围肉芽肿反应。据 Kim(2003)报道,肝吸虫感染所引起的胆管癌在 CT 影像中比普通型胆管癌更易发现,肝内周围胆管可见囊状扩张和纡曲。

总之,肝吸虫性胆管炎及其所引起的胆管梗阻 CT 表现有一定特征性,在鉴别梗阻性黄疸时,肝吸虫团块引起的胆总管梗阻也要重视,特别在肝吸虫疫区,当 CT 显示胆总管梗阻伴有包膜下小胆管呈囊状扩张时,需要考虑肝吸虫团块所致。

第十七篇　胆囊疾病

第一章 胆囊癌

第一节 早期胆囊癌

一、病理学

早期胆囊癌，即癌细胞仅浸润至胆囊黏膜层及固有层内。有作者认为，还应包括浸润至固有肌层的罗-阿窦内，以及浆膜下层罗-阿窦内的癌。早期胆囊癌的肉眼形态，可分为隆起型和表面型。若以早期胃癌的分型为基准，相比其特点表现为：

1型（隆起型）：肿瘤全部或部分呈乳头状或结节状隆起，有的带蒂。

2型（表面型）：无明显隆起。可再分为2a型：为低平的表面隆起性病变；2b型：病变与周围黏膜高度无明显差异。癌组织常于黏膜内水平方向浸润，呈表层扩大型，其范围可达数厘米。据鬼岛宏等（1987）统计，早期胆囊癌中69.4%为2b型及部分具2b型的形态。比早期胃癌、早期结肠癌均高，且为黏膜内水平方向浸润。

3型（陷凹型）：极为少见。

混合型：1型+2a型，2b型+2a型，2b型+1型+2a型，等等。

各型中以表面型为最多见，约占73%，其次为隆起型，约占27%，陷凹型极为少见。

早期胆囊癌合并胆囊结石的发生率相当高，可高达73%左右。隆起型中约有60%合并胆囊结石，表面型中约有79%合并胆囊结石，这是应该十分注意的问题。因此，对胆囊结石患者随时都应提高警惕，考虑是否伴存早期胆囊癌。早期胆囊癌病灶的大小，差别很大。鬼岛宏（1987）统计62个早期胆囊癌病变中，病灶最大径，小者为1mm，大者达120mm，平均为40.9mm，其中直径在10mm以下的小胆囊癌占25.8%；该作者并统计57个早期胆囊癌的面积，最小者为0.1cm^2，最大者为80.5cm^2，平均13.9 cm^2，其中有1/4的病例之癌肿面积占切除胆囊的一半以上。

二、影像学研究

B型超声：超声对胆囊疾病的诊断起着重要的作用：能很好显示胆囊内小的隆起性病变的形态、大小、部位、但可出现假阳性及假阴性；对直径在5~10mm窄基底乳头状病变易于发现，但定性有一定困难；对显示限局性壁肥厚的表面型早期癌与腺肌瘤病等其他胆囊病变的鉴别诊断有一定的价值，表面呈微细或粗大凹凸不平者提示为早期癌，但有一定限度；判断胆囊癌对胆囊壁浸润深度方面有所限制。

超声内镜检查：与一般超声比较，超声内镜检查对胆囊病变影像显示更为清晰，并能因声像图不同而显示出胆囊壁的三层结构，而对胆囊癌浸润深度诊断，早期胆囊癌诊断显示出一定的优越性：①超声内镜检查能清晰地显示胆囊隆起性病变的形态、大小，对良性与恶性病变的鉴别诊断有一定的价值。但对癌存在于腺瘤之中的早期胆囊癌，其癌与腺瘤的界限显示不清；②对胆囊壁结构显示及癌浸润深度的诊断，超声内镜检查能根据声像图的不同，显示出胆囊壁的三层结构，从而可在术前判断胆囊癌对胆囊壁浸润的深度，为早期胆囊癌的诊断提供依据。早期胆囊癌即为癌浸润仅只限于第二层之内，而第三层未受侵犯者；③对2b型早期癌的诊断与慢性胆囊炎的鉴别诊断存在一定的限度。

CT：Thorsen等（1984）报告，在CT图像上，正常胆囊壁厚为1~2mm，超过3.5mm则为异常。胆囊癌约有80%以上的病例为胆囊壁肥厚型及肿瘤形成型。CT对判断胆囊癌的浸润范围有一定的价值，但难以发现早期胆囊癌。对壁肥厚型胆囊癌与胆囊炎的鉴别诊断有一定限度。不规则形的壁肥厚者，癌的可能性大。

直接法胆系造影的薄层法：常规的 ERCP 和 PTC 对早期胆囊癌的诊断价值不大。日本学者户松成等(1986, 1987)将之加以改良，只注入少量的对比剂，利用对比剂与胆汁的比重差，行薄层造影。同时注意不使对比剂与胆汁相混合，变换体位，形成胆汁与对比剂的双对比，从而清晰地显示胆囊黏膜形态以及胆囊内病变的形态。对隆起型及表面型早期胆囊癌的诊断，都有很大的价值。因而，如超声发现胆囊内有小隆起，胆囊壁肥厚，胆囊结石及胆管扩张者，宜行此薄层造影，以发现早期胆囊癌。

X 线血管造影：Folkman 等(1974)报告，胆囊癌直径在 1mm 以下时，无明显血管供应，再生长时，则出现新生肿瘤血管。今野俊光等(1980, 1985)实验研究，胆囊癌直径在 4mm 时，便可见肿瘤新生血管，动脉造影时，从毛细血管期至静脉期可见到肿瘤染色征象；在临床上，肿瘤直径在 15mm 大小时血管造影可清晰显示，从而认为血管造影的诊断价值较大。大川薰等(1987)指出，早期胆囊癌的血管造影主要表现为肿瘤的轻微不规则染色，胆囊动脉无明显异常改变；而浸润至浆膜层以上者，则可见胆囊动脉分支不规则、阻塞及新生血管征象。因此，行胆囊动脉的超选择性造影，若能清楚显示胆囊及其周围动脉形态，则可达到胆囊癌早期诊断的目的。血管造影对胆囊癌的定性诊断及浸润深度的诊断价值，比 B 型超声、CT 及胆系造影都要好。

三、其他检查

经皮经肝胆囊穿刺及细胞学诊断：有作者报告 47 例经手术证实的胆囊癌中，胆囊壁穿刺细胞学的阳性率为 74.3%，胆囊胆汁细胞学阳性率为 77.4%，两者并用的阳性率为 80.9%。对大量胆囊内胆汁进行细胞学检查对诊断早期胆囊癌很有价值，最好对怀疑早期癌的病例，能作胆囊外引流，反复多次地行胆汁细胞学检查，定会提高诊断准确率。

胆囊内胆汁癌胚抗原浓度测定：测定胆囊内胆汁癌胚抗原浓度可作为胆囊良性与恶性疾病鉴别诊断的辅助手段。胆囊癌病例比胆囊内良性病变(胆囊结石、胆囊炎、腺肌瘤病及其他良性隆起性病变)病例的胆囊内的癌胚抗原浓度显示明显增高，这对胆囊内良性与恶性病变的鉴别诊断有很大价值。经皮经肝胆囊穿刺细胞学检查，胆囊内胆汁癌胚抗原浓度测定，及同时并用胆囊造影对胆囊癌的诊断价值很高，而早期胆囊癌在这三项都呈阳性者极少，只根据一项作诊断有时会有假阳性。并且，对充满结石及无明显隆起的早期胆囊癌的诊断，这些检查手段都有很大的限度。

经皮经肝内镜检查：早期胃癌按 X 线检查→内镜检查→活检病理的诊断体系取得了良好效果，因此，有学者提出，早期胆囊癌的诊断也可用 B 型超声作筛选法(简单、易行、且能发现胆囊病变)，对可疑者，即在超声引导下行胆囊内镜检查，并取活检作病理组织学检查，易于发现早期胆囊癌。经皮经肝内镜检查可清楚地观察胆囊黏膜面的形态，直接观察胆囊病变的形态、大小及表面特征，其影像相当清晰，并能放大观察以及取活检行病理组织学检查。因而，有学者提出如下诊断程序：超声检查或 CT 或 MRI(发现胆囊内隆起病变或轻度黏膜增厚)→ ERCP 或超声内镜检查(①不能确诊，但又高度怀疑癌；②确诊癌，尚需了解癌向胆囊管浸润的情况)→经皮经肝直接胆囊内镜检查(①取活检，作病理组织检查；②了解胆囊管有无受侵，确定手术方案)。

第二节　误诊病例简介：直径 0.8cm 胆囊低分化腺癌，侵及浆膜层与胆囊结石

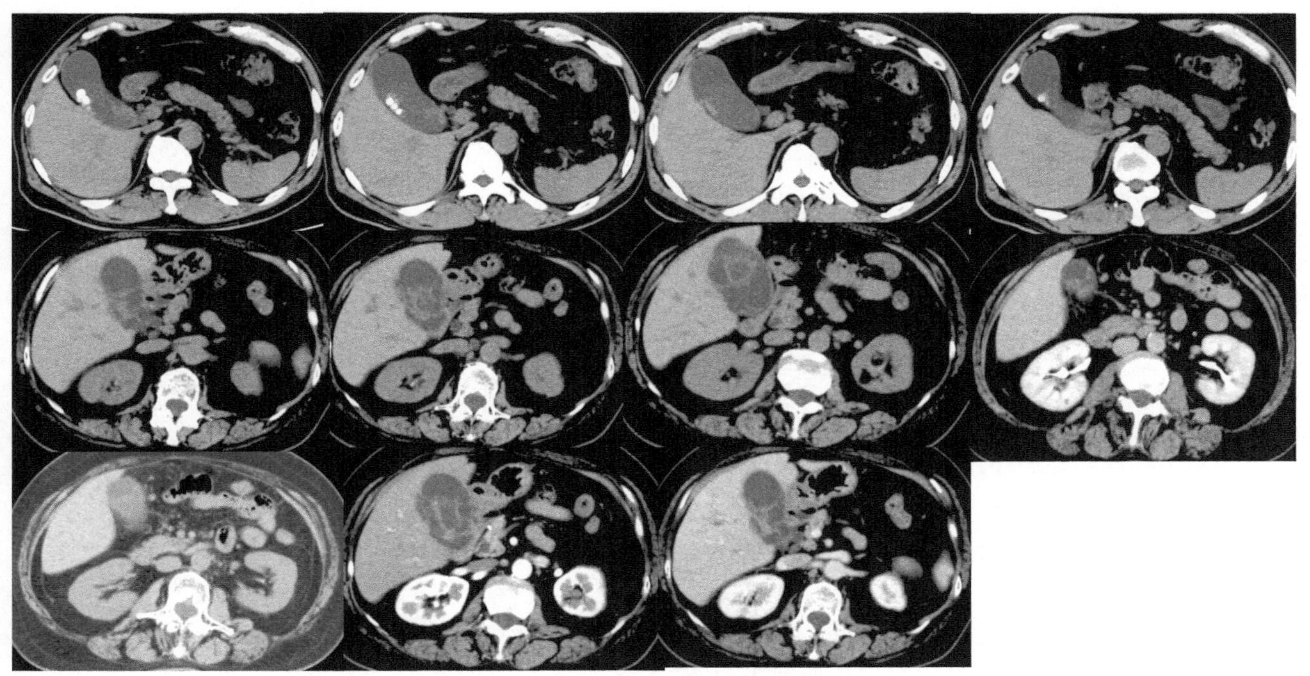

图 17-1-1　直径 0.8cm 胆囊低分化腺癌，侵及浆膜层与胆囊结石

患者，男，58 岁。腹痛 1 月余入院。

CT：胸部 CT 发现胆囊增大，壁增厚，内见多发结节状致密影，考虑胆囊多发结石，慢性胆囊炎。11 天后上腹部 CT 平扫：胆囊增大，约 4.0 cm × 1.0 cm，壁增厚，内见多发结节状致密影，最大约 0.9 cm × 1.0 cm，CT 值 192HU，胆囊管内密度欠均匀。CT 诊断：胆囊多发结石，慢性胆囊炎，与 11 天前 CT 图像比较，胆囊略增大；胆囊管内密度欠均匀。

手术所见：腹盆腔无腹水。胃肠、肝脏未见明显异常。胆囊充血水肿，胆囊增大，大小约 10.5cm × 4.5cm，胆囊壁厚约 0.4cm，大网膜包绕整个胆囊；胆囊床、肝门部未见肿大淋巴结，胆囊三角脂肪堆积较多。术后剖开胆囊见脓性胆汁，胆囊内多枚结石，最大直径约 0.9cm，胆囊颈部及胆囊管可见结石嵌顿。

病理检查：胆囊切除标本：破碎胆囊一具，大小 8cm × 4cm × 2cm，浆膜面光滑，胆囊黏膜面粗糙，局部隆起呈结节状，直径 0.8cm，胆囊壁厚 0.2cm~ 0.4cm。另见黑色结石一堆，总体积 1cm × 1cm × 0.5cm。病理诊断：胆囊切除标本：胆囊慢性炎，局部黏膜面及肌层见不典型腺管，倾向低分化癌，待补充取材及免疫组化进一步确诊。胆囊结石。

免疫组化检测：阳性：CK（L），CK20（局灶 +），Villin，CK8，CK18，CK19，EGFR（++++），VEGF（+++），P-gp（++），TOPO- Ⅱ（++），Tubulin-β（+），5-Fu（+），Ki67（约 70%）；阴性：CK7，CEA，CA19-9，Hepatocyte，Syn，CgA，ERCC-1。免疫组化诊断：胆囊切除标本：胆囊低分化腺癌，侵及浆膜层。

误诊漏诊病例分析体会：回顾 CT 图像，发现当时只看见胆囊结石，却忽略了观察与结石同存的不规则增厚的胆囊壁，在结石处尤其明显，这是一条教训，即观察胆囊结石时不要忘记观察胆囊壁的厚度、轮廓，在增强扫描时观察囊壁的强化更为重要（图 17-1-1）。

第三节　误诊病例简介：胆囊高分化胆管型腺癌

患者，女，60 岁。体检发现胆囊占位一周入院。

入院诊断：胆囊占位；心脏支架置入术后；高血压Ⅲ

级。CT:胆囊窝囊实性占位,胆囊内分隔状软组织影,不规则强化,性质?胆囊淋巴管瘤?不排除恶性肿瘤,建议MRI检查。肝内外胆管扩张。手术所见:腹腔无腹水,肝脏大小形态正常,质软,未扪及明显肿物,胆囊充血、肿胀,质硬,与周围网膜粘连,分离胆囊三角见肝门部淋巴结肿大,质硬,胆囊大小约8cm×3cm,壁厚0.5cm,术后剖视胆囊质硬,胆囊内多个分隔,胆汁浑浊,内充满结石。

病理检查:冰冻病理和常规病理:胆囊加部分肝切除标本:已剖开胆囊一具,大小7cm×5cm×4cm,切面呈囊状,部分囊腔扩张,部分囊腔内含灰黑灰黄色结石,囊壁厚0.2cm;胆囊旁附着肝组织一块,大小4cm×2cm×1.5cm,切面灰黄,质中。冰冻病理诊断:胆囊加部分肝切除标本:结石性急慢性胆囊炎,伴腺肌症形成,并部分腺上皮呈腺瘤样轻至中度异型增生,确诊待常规多块取材。常规病理诊断:胆囊加部分肝切除标本:初步考虑胆囊腺上皮高级别上皮内瘤变伴灶性癌变,累及R-A窦,经多块补取材均未见脉管、神经及周围肝组织累及,待做免疫组化进一步分析。免疫组化检测:阳性:HER-2(+++),CK7,P53(+,约70%),Ep-CAM,CDX2(灶+),Ki-67(+,约60%),SMA(+),CA199,CEA;阴性:CK20。免疫组化诊断:胆囊加部分肝切除标本:结合免疫组化结果,符合胆囊高分化胆管型腺癌。

第四节　厚壁型胆囊癌与慢性胆囊炎鉴别

胆囊癌的病因和发病机制:胆囊癌病因不明,可能与胆囊结石和慢性胆囊炎的长期刺激、胆囊良性肿瘤恶变、胆胰管合流异常、雌激素水平以及致癌物质的长期接触等诸多因素有关。有作者报道胆囊结石发作年龄越小,胆囊癌发病的风险越大。Kumar和Agqurwal(1994)认为部分胆囊癌系胆囊结石及慢性炎症长期刺激,导致上皮细胞化生和异型性增生进而癌变。Nevin等(1976)报道29例胆囊良性肿瘤,其中4例恶变,1例为胆囊息肉恶变,另外3例为胆囊腺瘤恶变。胆胰共同管长度>8 mm,出现胰胆返流,称为胆胰管异常连接。胆胰管异常连接者伴有胆囊黏膜增生、化生等癌前病变概率高于正常人群。

慢性胆囊炎的病因和发病机制:慢性胆囊炎可由反复发作的急性胆囊炎发展而来,且常合并胆囊结石,结石反复嵌顿、刺激胆囊壁引起炎症,炎性渗出物沉积又增加了结石的形成,二者互为因果。由于长期反复发作,造成整个胆囊壁纤维组织增生而增厚甚至钙化,胆囊积液肿大或萎缩。CT表现为胆囊壁增厚较均匀。

值得注意的是慢性胆囊炎的一种特殊类型——黄色肉芽肿性胆囊炎。Yun等(2004)研究发现此病胆囊黏膜表面常有小溃疡形成,胆汁经过溃疡面或破裂的罗-阿窦进入胆囊基质。胆汁降解为不溶性胆固醇及脂质,巨噬细胞在炎症部位吞噬脂肪,形成大而圆的泡沫细胞,由于炎症组织的机化,在胆囊壁内形成黄色肉芽肿。病变较一般慢性胆囊炎严重,多有周围黏连。增厚的胆囊壁内可见大小不一、数目不等的圆形或类圆形低密度灶。增强扫描,胆囊壁内低密度灶(因为其主要由不溶性胆固醇、脂质及巨噬细胞构成)不出现强化,是黄色肉芽肿性胆囊炎特异性CT表现。

影像学研究:大多数学者根据影像学表现将胆囊癌分为三型:①肿块型。胆囊区的软组织肿块,胆囊腔基本闭塞,常伴邻近脏器的直接侵犯;②厚壁型。胆囊壁局限或弥漫性不规则增厚;③腔内型。乳头状肿瘤由胆囊壁凸入胆囊腔内。其中,肿块型最常见,占41%~70%;其次为腔内型,占15%~23%;厚壁型最少见,占13%~25%。

肿块型和腔内型胆囊癌,诊断相对容易,一般不会误诊。而厚壁型胆囊癌为肿瘤局限或弥漫性不规则浸润胆囊壁,引起胆囊壁增厚的一类胆囊癌,与慢性胆囊炎尤其是黄色肉芽肿性胆囊炎,临床与CT表现均有相似之处,故术前误诊率相对较高。该组25例厚壁型胆囊癌患者中,术前6例误诊为慢性胆囊炎,而慢性胆囊炎中也有4例,包括2例黄色肉芽肿性胆囊炎,术前诊断为厚壁型胆囊癌可能性大。

误诊分析:一组通过对25例厚壁型胆囊癌与40例慢性胆囊炎两组病例CT表现的回顾性分析比较,认为造成误诊的原因可能有:①胆囊癌伴有胆囊结石和炎症,放射科医师仅满足于结石性胆囊炎的诊断;②没有仔细观察胆囊壁增厚的形态、特征和胆囊黏膜线是否完整;③对黄色肉芽肿性胆囊炎认识不足;④对二者的鉴别要点缺乏充分的了解。

虽然厚壁型胆囊癌与慢性胆囊炎 CT 表现均为胆囊壁增厚，但以下征象有助于鉴别诊断：

（1）胆囊壁厚度及形态：正常胆囊壁厚度约为 1~2 mm，一般认为胆囊壁厚度 >3 mm 为异常。厚壁型胆囊癌常呈不规则结节状或局限性增厚，最厚：最薄 >2：1，内壁凹凸不平，胆囊壁多僵硬；慢性胆囊炎胆囊壁增厚多呈均匀一致性，最厚：最薄 <2：1，且胆囊壁较柔软。

（2）胆囊轮廓：正常胆囊窝内有一层脂肪组织分隔肝脏与胆囊，CT 表现为胆囊与肝脏间薄层透亮低密度带。厚壁型胆囊癌系恶性病变，易穿透肌层达浆膜层并侵犯胆囊窝内的脂肪组织并向邻近肝脏扩展侵犯，如肝右前叶下段（Ⅴ段）/ 左内叶（Ⅳ段），从而导致胆囊轮廓模糊或与肝脏分界不清。CT 表现为胆囊窝脂肪间隙消失，邻近肝实质内可见异常低密度区，增强后呈不均匀明显强化。而慢性胆囊炎是良性病变，对周围肝脏系慢性炎性浸润，范围较局限，表现为“浸而不连”，肝 - 胆界面常常存在。

（3）胆囊黏膜线的完整性：胆囊内壁（固有层）因含有丰富的毛细血管，在 CT 增强检查图像上，表现为致密、连续光滑的环状线条影，称为胆囊黏膜线。胆囊良性病变，如慢性胆囊炎、胆囊息肉、腺瘤等均不会侵犯、破坏固有层，故 CT 增强检查显示胆囊黏膜线完整存在。少数慢性胆囊炎黏膜线欠完整，是胆囊壁严重纤维化和炎性水肿所致，发生率较低，仅为 10% 左右。而胆囊恶性肿瘤，癌组织侵犯胆囊壁各层，致使固有层内丰富的毛细血管受到侵蚀破坏，CT 增强检查时受到破坏的胆囊黏膜线不再显示，表现为黏膜线中断。

（4）梗阻性黄疸：胆囊癌早期一般不会引起黄疸，如出现黄疸则应考虑：①胆囊内肿瘤已突破胆囊浆膜层直接侵犯肝脏并同时侵犯、压迫肝内胆管，从而引起黄疸；②胆囊癌侵犯胆囊全层后发生肝门部淋巴结转移，压迫肝总管或胆总管，引起黄疸；③位于胆囊颈部的肿瘤早期易经胆囊三角处淋巴结转移，进一步向肝十二指肠韧带内淋巴结转移，压迫胆总管，导致黄疸；④胆囊颈部的肿瘤侵犯浆膜后，可以直接侵犯邻近的肝门肝实质及肝门部胆管，造成肝门部胆管狭窄或阻塞，导致黄疸；⑤门腔间隙 - 胰后组淋巴结肿大并侵犯 / 压迫胆总管，导致低位胆系梗阻；

慢性胆囊炎患者一般不会出现黄疸，一旦出现黄疸，多为结石进入胆总管下段引起胆系低位梗阻或 Mirizzi 综合征引起的高位梗阻。Mirizzi 综合征是胆囊结石少见的并发症，是指胆囊颈管结石嵌顿及局部周围炎引起肝总管狭窄，管壁破坏，造成梗阻性黄疸及肝内胆管炎。

（5）胆囊癌、慢性胆囊炎强化特征与增强扫描价值：虽然二组疾病动脉期、门静脉期和延迟期均呈进行性 / 持续性强化，但增强扫描后可明确有无胆囊黏膜线中断，并可进一步观察有无腹腔脏器转移和淋巴结肿大。

总之，MSCT 能清晰地显示胆囊壁的形态、病变部位、胆囊壁增厚特征及胆囊壁的浸润程度和邻近脏器情况，不仅使胆囊癌在早期得到及时诊断，而且也为与慢性胆囊炎相鉴别提供了较为全面的信息。

第五节　误诊病例简介：高密度胆囊癌与胆囊炎及胆囊结石

胆囊癌是胆系最常见的恶性肿瘤，86% 发生于 50~80 岁，女性多于男性，男女之比为 1:3，一般认为胆囊癌的发生与胆囊结石所伴发的慢性感染造成的长期刺激有关，因为 80% 的病例伴有胆囊结石；半数患者右上腹可触及肿块，转移出现早。

CT 上胆囊癌分为胆囊壁增厚型、腔内型和肿块型：①增厚型，占 15%~22%，表现为壁增厚，大部分为不规则的，少数病例可表现为均匀性增厚，与慢性胆囊炎难以鉴别；②腔内型，占 15%~23%，表现为乳头状、单发或多发腔内肿块，基底部胆囊壁增厚，增强后肿块明显强化；③肿块型，占 41%~70%，表现为胆囊窝内软组织密度肿块，有广泛的邻近肝组织侵犯，常合并胆管梗阻。胆囊癌也常合并胆结石和胆囊炎（占 73%~98%），20% 的患者胆囊壁可见钙化。此例胆囊壁略有强化，胆囊内病灶密度高，强化不明显，很像胆囊结石，而最后通过病理诊断为腺癌，表现为高密度可能与细胞成分密实和钙含量较高有关；回顾性仔细查看 CT 图像后发现，靠近胆囊管颈部局部病变与管壁分界模糊，虽然增强扫描后病变未强化，但是应考虑到病灶与管壁分界的关系，以此来减少对高密度胆囊癌的诊断失误率。

附：具体病例资料：CT 表现：平扫示胆囊较饱满，其体部、颈部及胆管内见多发梭形、椭圆形高密度影,其内密度尚均匀,CT 值约 75 HU,边缘较清。动静脉期增强后病灶强化不明显,CT 值仍保持 75~80 HU,边界尚清,部分胆囊壁略增厚,胆管略扩张。肝、脾及胰腺、双肾等邻近组织未见明显异常,腹膜后未见明显肿大淋巴结影。考虑诊断为胆囊炎伴胆囊结石。手术所见:胆囊约 9.0cm×5.6cm 大小,充血水肿,与周围组织无粘连,胆总管未见明显扩张;切开胆囊标本后在胆囊颈部见一枚直径约 3.0cm 大小肿块。表面呈草莓状改变,未见结石。病理诊断:胆囊中 - 低分化腺癌,部分为黏液腺癌,大小 3.0cm×2.0cm,侵至胆囊壁全层,累及神经,切缘阴性。

第六节　误诊病例简介:胆囊癌误诊为肝脓肿

胆囊癌是胆管系统最常见的恶性肿瘤,分为胆囊壁增厚型、腔内型和肿块型三种类型:①胆囊壁增厚型,CT 表现为胆囊壁增厚,大部分是不规则的,少数病例表现为均匀性增厚,须与慢性胆囊炎鉴别;②腔内型,表现为乳头状、单发或多发腔内肿块,基底部胆囊壁增厚,增强后乳头状肿物明显增强;③肿块型,表现为胆囊窝内软组织密度肿块,几乎所有的病例均有广泛的邻近肝组织侵犯,常合并胆管梗阻,少数肿块型病例难以区分肿块是来自肝脏还是胆囊,肿块型胆囊癌 CT 表现为低或混杂密度,动脉期和门脉期轻度增强,延迟期增强明显;这主要是胆囊癌常常有丰富的间质,CT 对比剂滞留时间长有关。

一例属肿块型胆囊癌,病灶位于肝内,动脉期和门脉期边缘轻度强化,病灶内可见气体密度影,肝内胆管未见扩张,再结合患者发热、寒颤、右上腹疼痛,全身皮肤及巩膜无黄染,白细胞明显增高,很容易误诊为肝脓肿。回顾性分析 CT 片,有一帧图像病灶边缘可见 3 个沉积性小结节稍高密度影,手术证实为结石。术前没有注意到结石的存在,故出现了病灶在肝内的判断错误。

目前胆囊结石与胆囊癌的关系备受人们的关注。胆囊癌合并胆囊结石的发病率为 25%~95%,多数在 50%~70%,而胆囊结石病例中有 1.0%~6.3% 合并胆囊癌。其机制可能为结石长期刺激胆囊黏膜导致慢性炎症和癌变,也可能导致胆囊排空障碍,胆汁淤滞,加上细菌感染等因素,使胆酸转化成有致癌作用的物质。Nerri 等(1988)应用逻辑回归分析法统计出胆囊结石患者胆囊癌发病率比无胆囊结石患者高出 7 倍。因此,病灶内看到结石影,应高度注意胆囊癌的可能性。肿块型胆囊癌与肝内占位鉴别,肿块内结石影具有很大的鉴别诊断价值。

该例误诊为肝脓肿,究其原因主要是没有仔细观察 CT 片,没有发现病灶内的结石影,只停留在病灶内气体影上,仅满足于第一印象而致误诊。病灶内气体提示什么?我们分析研究,可能确实存在胆囊周围炎症或肝脓肿,只是病变主要病灶是胆囊癌,全面诊断应该是胆囊癌合并肝脓肿被误诊为单纯肝脓肿了。这也告诉我们,一些疾病常常是复杂的,不仅是单一的,考虑诊断可适当考虑全面一些,思路开阔一些,切记不要忽略了多因素致病的可能性。

第七节　误诊病例简介:胆囊癌与肝门胆管癌

患者,女,64 岁。腹胀、尿黄 23 天,眼黄 11 天入院。五天前曾在外院住院治疗,外院考虑诊断为肝门部胆管癌,胆囊炎。门诊以肝门部胆管癌收治住院。MRI:MRCP 示肝内胆管、左右肝管明显扩张,最大径约 2.6cm,至肝总管处截然中断,肝门部可见不规则软组织信号影,边界不清,胆总管下段显影无明显扩张,胆囊体积明显增大,壁厚,腔内无明显充盈缺损,胆囊管结构不清;胰腺体积不大,胰管无明显扩张,腹膜后淋巴结肿大,边界不清。MRI 诊断:肝门部占位,考虑胆管细胞癌伴梗阻性肝内外胆管扩张。

手术所见:腹腔少量渗液,胆囊增大约 10cm×4cm,有张力,壁厚水肿。肝脏呈淤胆肝改变。肝十二指肠韧带呈挛缩状态。肿瘤位于胆总管中下段,局部有肿大淋巴结,质硬,不活动。胆总管扩张,直径约 1.5cm,余未见异常。决定行胆管癌根治性切除 + 肝十二指肠韧带骨骼化 + 胆肠吻合术 + 胆囊切除术。

病理检查:胆囊切除标本:胆囊大小 6cm×4.5cm×2cm,浆膜面表面附后少许肝脏组织。沿胆囊颈部切开，可见胆囊内壁弥漫性增厚，切面灰黄，质中，壁厚 1~2.2cm。胆总管中下段切除标本：灰白色组织一块，大小 3.5cm × 2.5cm × 1.5cm，切面灰黄，质中。门静脉前组织；第九组淋巴结；第 12L 淋巴结；第 12P 淋巴结；第八组淋巴结。

常规病理诊断：胆囊切除标本：初步诊断胆囊高中分化腺癌，待做免疫组化检测进一步协助诊断。腺癌组织侵犯胆囊壁全层至浆膜层，但未侵及肝脏组织。胆总管中下段切除标本：胆总管中下段及少量胰腺组织可见腺癌组织累及。门静脉前组织切除标本：可见腺癌组织累及，另检出淋巴结 5 枚未见癌转移。第九组淋巴结切除标本：检出淋巴结 2 枚，其中 1 枚见癌转移。第 12P 淋巴结：检出淋巴结 1 枚，可见癌转移。第八组淋巴结：检出 3 块癌组织结节。第 12L 淋巴结：检出淋巴结 2 枚，均未见癌转移。

免疫组化检测：阳性：CEA，Ck19，CK7，Villin（+），CA125（灶 +），CD34（血管内皮 +），CA19-9（灶 +），Ki-67（+，约 20%）；阴性：AFP，CDX2，Hepatocyte，CD10，CK20，P53。免疫组化诊断：胆囊切除标本：胆囊高中分化肠型腺癌，腺癌组织侵犯胆囊壁全层至浆膜层，并累及胆总管中下段及少量胰腺组织，但未侵及肝脏组织。

误诊病例回顾分析：MRI 检查时注意力完全被肝外胆管的异常表现吸引，忽略仔细观察胆囊的情况，这是一条重要的教训，在 MRI 和 MRCP 检查时务必全面仔细观察胆胰各个部分，该例是误诊，也是漏诊；临床诊断与院外诊断的误导也有一定影响，但属于次要的问题；还有一点教训是胆囊癌侵犯胆囊壁全层后，可向外蔓延，累及其邻近的胆、胰器官及周围组织，出现明显异常的影像学表现，而胆囊癌本身却只是显示胆囊壁增厚，极易被人忽略。

第二章　胆囊神经内分泌癌

原发性肝胆神经内分泌肿瘤

神经内分泌肿瘤是一种起源于肽能神经元和神经内分泌细胞的异质性肿瘤,可发生于全身各器官和组织。近年随着免疫组化技术的进步,其检出率大大增加,但由于其早期诊断缺乏特异性指标常致误诊,胆囊、肝脏是神经内分泌肿瘤发病的罕见部位,诊断更难。

病理学:WHO(2010)对神经内分泌肿瘤修订认为:神经内分泌肿瘤分为神经内分泌瘤,神经内分泌癌(小细胞型和大细胞型),混合性神经内分泌癌和部分特异性神经内分泌肿瘤。

一组6例均属于小细胞型神经内分泌肿瘤,均有淋巴结转移,属于晚期。病理表现为肿瘤细胞高度异型性,体积小或中等,境界欠清楚,坏死明显,可见血管或神经侵犯。

免疫组化对神经内分泌肿瘤诊断有特异性,突触素(Syn)和嗜铬粒素A(CgA)是特异性的指标,分化好的神经内分泌肿瘤强表达Syn和CgA,而NEC则弱表达。另一些多肽激素如胃泌素等在某种特异性肿瘤中表达。该组3例胆囊神经内分泌肿瘤均高表达Syn,其中2例高表达CgA。2例肝神经内分泌肿瘤的Syn染色表达强阳性,2例CgA表达阳性。

(一)原发性胆囊神经内分泌肿瘤

临床表现:胆囊神经内分泌肿瘤非常罕见,近15年仅报道约60例,以中老年为著,女性稍多。该组3例均为老年,其中2例为女性,与文献一致。临床症状有右上腹痛、黄疸、腹部肿块等,而"类癌综合征"少见,表现为腹泻、脸部潮红、高血糖病、心律失常等,可能与神经内分泌细胞分泌的5羟色胺、组胺等有关。该组3例均未见典型类癌综合征。

胆囊神经内分泌肿瘤常伴发胆囊炎、胆囊结石,该组2例均有胆囊结石,有学者认为这与胰多肽分泌增多有关,胰多肽可抑制胆囊的收缩导致胆汁淤积形成胆石。

关于该病起源目前有3种意见:①胆囊多能干细胞的分化;②胆囊颈部残存神经内分泌细胞;③胆囊基底部、体部细胞的肠化生。

影像学研究:原发性胆囊神经内分泌肿瘤从形态学上可分为2型。

(1)厚壁型:胆囊壁局限性增厚,主要位于胆囊颈部和基底部,肿块形态不规则,向腔内外生长,增强后正常胆囊内膜线中断,黏膜强化明显,但结节或肿块强化不明显,肿块向腔外生长时常侵犯肝脏,胆囊窝或肝门部伴或不伴淋巴结肿大。该组1例属厚壁型,肝脏与胆囊分界欠清,增强后肿块轻度强化,与文献报道一致。

(2)肿块型:胆囊正常形态消失,胆囊窝见巨大肿块,密度欠均匀,常出血或囊变坏死,偶见钙化,肿块与肝脏分界不清,有或无肝门、腹膜后淋巴结肿大。增强后肿块不强化或轻度强化,低于或近似正常肝实质,强化形式为环形、分隔样。该组2例均为巨大肿块,1例完全占据胆囊窝,局部向肝缘外突出,呈分叶状,密度欠均匀,见小片状出血及囊变,分析原因可能与瘤细胞的内分泌特性、小细胞肿瘤的高恶性程度有关。该患者随访3月后肿块明显肿大,进一步证实其恶性程度高。另1例偏侧占据胆囊窝,胆囊底部伴多发结石,肿瘤累及十二指肠、胰头,胆总管、肝内胆管、十二指肠降部以上扩张明显,证实该肿瘤恶性程度高。

鉴别诊断:原发性胆囊神经内分泌肿瘤主要与胆囊腺癌鉴别,两者临床表现与发病年龄均相似,若出现类癌综合征,则鉴别较易,另外前者增强后轻度强化,常伴发早期淋巴结或肝转移。

(二)原发性肝脏神经内分泌肿瘤

临床表现:肝脏神经内分泌肿瘤亦罕见,多数由胃肠道和胰腺等转移而来,原发的实属罕见。平均发病年龄45岁,女性稍多,男女比例约1:1.4。该病与肝硬化、肝炎等无明显关系。关于肝神经内分泌肿瘤的起源,Libbrecht和Roskams(2002)认为肝脏祖细胞可以向神经内分泌细胞转化,并分泌CgA;

Roskams(2004)认为胆管上皮细胞可以分泌神经特异化烯醇酶(NSE),证实肝内存在内分泌细胞。

影像学研究:该肿瘤影像学表现主要有2种形式。

(1)单发肿块型:病灶一般较大,直径>5 cm,肿瘤密度欠均匀,中央常有液化坏死,瘤周或瘤内偶见点状或斑片状钙化。增强动脉期肿块强化不明显或明显强化,门脉期减退或逐渐强化,呈肝细胞癌的“快进快出”或胆管细胞癌的“慢进慢出”强化模式。该组2例属于单发肿块型。其中1例瘤内见点状钙化,文献中少见报道,分析原因主要是神经内分泌瘤常形成骨化或钙化,或者瘤内反复出血致钙盐沉积。增强后2例均表现为肝细胞癌“快进快出”的强化模式;强化方式均为环形强化,其中1例行DSA检查表现为“抱球样”灌注,与CT表现吻合。该型常与原发性肝细胞癌、胆管细胞癌混淆。但原发性肝细胞性肝癌常有肝硬化病史,甲胎蛋白明显升高,动脉期强化更明显,与胆管细胞癌鉴别较难,但前者早期一般有淋巴结或肝内转移等征象。

(2)肿块伴子灶型:病灶多发,其中有较大病灶,周边伴多发子灶,肿块密度不均匀,常有囊变坏死、出血、钙化等,早期淋巴结转移常见。增强动脉期呈中度或明显强化,门脉期强化逐渐减退。本型与转移瘤不易鉴别,后者也多发,大小不一,但一般有原发病史,增强后呈环形强化,典型者呈“牛眼征”。该组1例属大肿块子灶型,大肿块中央见片状坏死区,强化明显,呈分隔状、环状强化,影像表现与文献报道一致。

总之,原发性肝胆神经内分泌肿瘤非常罕见,典型的类癌综合征很少出现,诊断较难,若出现以下影像表现时可提示神经内分泌肿瘤:无肝炎、肝硬化背景的患者,肿块巨大,瘤内易出现坏死囊变、出血等征象,尤其是钙化有一定特异性,增强后环形或边缘强化,早期即出现淋巴结转移,排除肝细胞癌、胆管细胞癌后应考虑肝神经内分泌肿瘤;胆囊窝巨大肿块或胆囊壁增厚,中央坏死囊变、出血,增强后轻度环形、分隔样强化,早期淋巴结转移,要想到胆囊神经内分泌肿瘤可能。

第三章 淋巴瘤与淋巴管瘤

第一节 胆囊黏膜相关淋巴组织型淋巴瘤

胆囊恶性肿瘤以上皮来源多见,胆囊黏膜相关淋巴组织型淋巴瘤十分罕见。黏膜相关淋巴组织型淋巴瘤多见于淋巴组织丰富的胃、空回肠、肺等脏器,偶见于甲状腺、唾液腺及肝脏。正常胆囊黏膜层无淋巴滤泡,少量淋巴细胞存在于上皮细胞之间,恶变成淋巴瘤可能与慢性滤泡性胆囊炎或其他理化因素改变导致自身免疫改变有关。发病年龄以中老年为主,临床表现无特异性,胆囊壁明显局限性增厚,易误诊为胆囊癌。

胆囊癌以腺癌多见,分局限型和弥漫型,增厚的胆囊壁多明显强化,易外侵胆囊周围肝组织,实验室检查 CA199 升高较为敏感。

急、慢性胆囊炎多表现为胆囊壁均匀弥漫增厚,囊腔内多可见结石,胆囊壁水肿增厚时表现为分层强化,黏膜层明显强化,临床有急性发作病史。

胆囊腺肌增生症表现为胆囊壁增厚,黏膜层和黏膜下区强化,延迟期胆囊壁强化范围扩大,典型表现可见罗 - 阿窦与胆囊腔相通。

胆囊黏膜相关淋巴组织型淋巴瘤少见,早期病变呈局限性胆囊增厚,中、重度强化,晚期病变也可外侵及淋巴结转移,相关实验室检查无特异性,明确诊断多依靠镜下病理及免疫组织化学检查。胆囊黏膜相关淋巴组织型淋巴瘤与其他淋巴类肿瘤相比,细胞分裂较好,恶性度低,多选择手术治疗,根据术后分期决定是否辅助化疗。

第二节 胆囊淋巴管瘤

淋巴管瘤是一种少见的先天性淋巴系统畸形,约 95% 见于头、颈、腋窝部皮肤和皮下组织,余 5% 见于体部其他部位,如肺、胸膜、心包、食道、胃、空肠、结肠、胰腺、肝、胆囊、肾脏和肠系膜。胆囊淋巴管瘤罕见,仅占腹腔淋巴管瘤的 0.8%~1.0%。

1. 病理学 病理分型:淋巴管瘤分为单纯型、海绵状和囊性 3 个亚型。免疫组织化学 CD31 或Ⅷ因子相关抗原可呈阳性,细胞角蛋白阴性,提示淋巴管瘤起源于集合系统而非原始淋巴组织。14 例中有手术描述的 10 例, 8 例描述病灶起自胆囊体部或颈部浆膜层,胆囊的黏膜面正常。14 例中海绵状 1 例,囊性 8 例,未分型 5 例。单纯型淋巴管瘤由小的薄壁淋巴管构成。海绵状淋巴管瘤由扩张的淋巴管和淋巴样基质构成,且与周围各种正常淋巴系统相通。囊性淋巴管瘤由大小不同的含有平滑肌肌束和胶原束的淋巴系统构成,但是与邻近正常淋巴系统不相通。1 例为海绵状淋巴管瘤,胆囊被多房囊性小泡状病灶包裹呈“蚕茧”样,而胆囊壁完整为特征。

2. 临床表现 胆囊淋巴管瘤大部分无症状,部分表现为右上腹隐痛,可向肩背部放射,进食油腻或辛辣食物后加重。无黄疸和胆绞痛报道,但病灶增大压迫邻近脏器或合并感染、出血、穿孔或撕裂可出现相应症状。1 例表现为突发右上腹痛并胆道感染症状和体征。伴发热、白细胞升高和肝功能轻度异常。其余病例血象、肝功能和电解质正常。另例右上腹疼痛 15 年,以进油腻食物后加重。实验室检查:肿瘤标记物(甲胎蛋白、癌胚抗原、CA199 和

CA125）一般为阴性。

3. 影像学研究　B 超检查 13 例，显示胆囊窝或胆囊周围囊性病灶 7 例，肝下囊性病灶 3 例，胆囊炎 1 例，肝囊肿 1 例，双胆囊 1 例，无一例术前明确诊断。

典型的超声表现为胆囊床单房或多房无回声囊性肿块、内部常有薄壁间隔、胆囊壁完整和黏膜面光滑为特征，合并感染或出血时囊内回声可不均匀。2 例 B 超发现合并胆囊结石。

CT 检查 8 例，6 例表现为胆囊周围、胆囊窝内囊性病灶和多发间隔，1 例表现为胆囊周围积液，1 例误为肝内囊肿。CT 的典型表现为胆囊周围单房或多房水样密度囊性肿块，合并出血或感染囊内密度可增高，1 例显示囊内密度高达 37~60 HU，囊内间隔厚度均匀，囊壁可轻度强化。伴有出血或感染的淋巴管瘤很难与囊性肿瘤鉴别。ERCP 可显示胆囊与肿块的关系，并确定病灶是否与胆囊相通，排除胆系发育畸形和胆汁漏。

1 例血管造影显示病灶血供来自胆囊动脉，提示病灶与胆囊的密切关系。

MRI 检查 6 例，均表现为胆囊窝内多房囊性病灶伴多发细的间隔，胆囊被向下推移 3 例，被包埋 3 例，其中 4 例提示淋巴管瘤诊断。MRI 多平面成像结合 MRCP 有助于全面评价病灶范围及与胆囊的关系。MR 特征为胆囊窝内多房囊性病灶在 T_1 和 T_2 上有不同的信号强度，推测是由于每个囊内的水脂比率不同。而 MRCP 显示胆囊被“淹没”“蚕茧”征为特征。另外，由于病灶起自胆囊体或颈部的肝面浆膜层，因此，胆囊向下推移，病灶与肝组织分界不清亦具特征性。动态 MR 增强扫描显示囊变区在各期都没有强化，但间隔有轻度强化，胆囊壁线性强化，黏膜面完整为特征性表现。

4. 鉴别诊断　由于大多数淋巴管瘤呈多囊、分叶状，位于胆囊一侧或包裹胆囊，与邻近肝内囊性病变、胆系畸形扩张或胆汁漏难以鉴别。若胆囊淋巴管瘤合并出血、感染和撕裂较难与肝血管瘤、囊腺瘤、胆囊周围囊性肿瘤或血管肉瘤鉴别。囊型淋巴管瘤最易误诊为肝囊肿，肝囊肿动态增强不强化。但依据病灶位于胆囊周围，多房囊性和多发间隔，边界清楚但黏附于肝面，胆囊被“淹没”或“蚕茧”征，间隔轻度强化或无强化有助于淋巴管瘤的诊断，B 超或 CT 鉴别较困难，MRI 结合 MRCP 更能显示上述特征。

附：具体研究病例：有作者（2010）共检索到胆囊淋巴管瘤 14 例（中文 5 例、英文 9 例），其中男、女各 7 例，年龄 2 岁半至 66 岁，诊断中位年龄为 36 岁，仅 1 例为儿童，其余均在 25 岁以上。反复发作右上腹隐痛 6 例，时间 2 个月至 10 年，进油腻或辛辣食物后加重 3 例。因其他经 B 超或 CT 检查发现病灶 6 例，无症状 B 超体检发现病灶 2 例，突发右上腹痛 2 天 1 例，该例血常规、肝功能异常，其他 6 例查血常规、肝功能和肿瘤标志物均正常。无明显阳性体征，右上腹轻触痛 3 例，3 例可触及右上腹包块。术中发现合并胆囊结石 2 例，1 例合并胆管泥沙样结石。囊腔内均为淡黄色浆液，2 例伴出血。14 例均成功完整切除胆囊和病灶，其中 5 例腹腔镜，9 例开腹。

第四章 肉芽肿性胆囊炎

第一节 黄色肉芽肿性胆囊炎误诊为胆囊癌

黄色肉芽肿胆囊炎是一种在炎性胆囊内形成瘤样肿块的少见疾病。它是一种良性而有破坏性的胆囊炎性病变,它不同于慢性胆囊炎,其发病机制可能是炎症波及胆囊壁,使罗-阿窦破裂或黏膜形成溃疡,胆汁渗入囊壁间质,在降解中产生的胆固醇和磷脂诱发组织细胞增生,并吞噬胆固醇和脂质形成泡沫细胞;炎症反应又促使慢性炎细胞、嗜酸性粒细胞浸润及成纤维细胞增生,从而产生结节,出现胆囊壁特有的黄色肉芽肿结构。胆汁降解同时胆固醇与黏蛋白释放并能浸润胆囊壁甚至囊壁外其他组织,形成广泛粘连。CT检查常示胆囊壁不规则增厚,并可形成肿块,与邻近肝叶分界不清,而且胆囊癌的发病率高于黄色肉芽肿性胆囊炎,故常容易诊断为胆囊癌局部侵及肝脏。此类病例由于其临床及影像表现的无特征性,常常可造成误诊,因此在诊断胆囊癌的同时,要考虑到黄色肉芽肿性胆囊炎的可能,自然,确诊仍需病理检查。

第二节 肉芽肿性胆囊炎(软斑病)

软斑病是一种少见的炎性肉芽肿性病变,女性多见,发生于泌尿生殖系统多见,发生在胆囊的非常罕见。软斑病术前确诊困难,且发生于胆囊者极少,临床及影像表现缺乏特异性,确诊主要依赖病理。本病需与胆囊癌鉴别。临床表现无特异性,病因及发病机制尚不明确,多认为属慢性感染性疾病,多数学者认为与大肠杆菌慢性感染有关,约40%患者有免疫缺陷性疾病,部分病例伴T淋巴细胞功能降低,巨噬细胞吞噬细菌功能异常。

附具体病例资料:患者,女,56岁,反复右上腹隐痛5年余,2周前出现皮肤巩膜轻度黄染。体检:右上腹部轻压痛,莫非征阳性。实验室检查:总胆红素(TBil)101.6μmol/L(正常参考值:2.0~21.0μmol/L)、直接胆红素(DBil)60.6μmol/L(正常参考值:0.0~8.0μmol/L)、丙氨酸转氨酶(ALT)357 U/L(正常参考值:0~40U/L)、天冬氨酸转氨酶(AST)125 U/L(正常参考值:0~40 U/L)、γ-谷氨酰转移酶(GGT)1403 U/L(正常参考值:8~58 U/L)、碱性磷酸酶(ALP)656U/L(正常参考值:30~125 U/L)。B超示:胆囊底部实质性光团,内见多个强光团,胆囊结石,胆囊炎。CT平扫示:胆囊底部见一3.4cm×3.6cm类圆形软组织密度团块,边缘光整,内见多发小斑点状钙化灶,胆囊颈部及胆总管结石,肝内外胆管、胆总管扩张。CT增强扫描示:胆囊底部病灶明显强化。手术病理所见:胆囊内见多枚结石,底部见一圆形肿物,切面灰白灰褐色,质软。病理见胆囊黏膜破坏,大量炎细胞浸润,以淋巴细胞、浆细胞为主,并见较多组织细胞,多核巨细胞,纤维组织增生,均质变,HE及过碘酸雪夫染色见软化斑小体(Michaelis-Gutman小体),诊断为肉芽肿性胆囊炎(软斑病)。

第三节　黄色肉芽肿性胆囊炎和厚壁型胆囊癌及误诊分析

黄色肉芽肿性胆囊炎临床发病率较低，是一种少见的特殊类型的胆囊慢性炎症，约占所有胆囊炎性病变的 0.7%~13.2%。由于黄色肉芽肿性胆囊炎具有慢性炎性反复过程，刺激胆囊壁增厚纤维化，继而与邻近脏器发生粘连，分界不清，加之临床表现、实验室检查无特异性，术前常误诊为厚壁型胆囊癌，甚至在直视手术中亦难以区分。

一项研究通过分析临床确诊的 22 例黄色肉芽肿性胆囊炎和 25 例厚壁型胆囊癌的临床表现、实验室检查和 CT 表现特征，旨在提高术前对这两种疾病的鉴别诊断能力，降低误诊率。

黄色肉芽肿性胆囊炎是一种以胆囊慢性炎症为基础，同时伴有黄色肉芽肿形成、重度增生性纤维化以及泡沫样细胞为特征的破坏性炎症性病变，由于病史相对较长，慢性反复发作的过程容易引起周围肝脏的粘连形成肿块，往往术前与厚壁型胆囊癌不易区分，鉴别诊断困难，甚至在术中直视下也很难区分，因此，术前正确诊断对于手术方法的选择非常重要，可以避免选择侵袭性的扩大手术。

一、黄色肉芽肿性胆囊炎和厚壁型胆囊癌的临床和发病机制

一项研究结果显示，在黄色肉芽肿性胆囊炎患者中出现右上腹痛慢性反复发作过程、畏寒发热及血白细胞、粒细胞增多的患者较厚壁型胆囊癌增多，而厚壁型胆囊癌中出现黄疸、体重减轻、CA199 增高的患者明显多于黄色肉芽肿性胆囊炎，而其余的临床症状（背部放射痛、恶心、呕吐、食欲不振、CEA 增高）均无明显差异。因此，黄色肉芽肿性胆囊炎和厚壁型胆囊癌的临床表现有很大程度的相似性，在临床实际工作中，单纯根据临床症状很难进行鉴别。文献认为黄色肉芽肿性胆囊炎和厚壁型胆囊癌的发病机制均与胆囊结石和反复性慢性炎症密切相关，Parra 等（2000）认为罗 - 阿窦与黄色肉芽肿性胆囊炎的发生有关，黄色肉芽肿性胆囊炎是急性炎症反应和梗阻的双重结果，胆囊的慢性炎症或结石梗阻造成胆汁淤积，炎性刺激胆囊黏膜面损伤，形成溃疡，渗透入胆囊壁的胆汁产生胆固醇和脂质诱发过敏反应，刺激组织细胞增生，并吞噬胆固醇转化为泡沫细胞和多核巨噬细胞，形成特有的黄色肉芽肿性结节。而厚壁型胆囊癌主要是由于结石、炎症等慢性机械性损伤，刺激胆囊黏膜过度增生，促使胆囊上皮细胞破坏与修复过程交替，继发基因突变形成厚壁型胆囊癌。

该组资料显示，在 22 例黄色肉芽肿性胆囊炎中合并 13 例胆囊或胆管结石，在 25 例厚壁型胆囊癌中合并 8 例胆囊或胆管结石，均说明黄色肉芽肿性胆囊炎和厚壁型胆囊癌的发生与结石密切相关，但是，目前还没有明确证据表明黄色肉芽肿性胆囊炎和厚壁型胆囊癌之间有直接的关联，不能认为黄色肉芽肿性胆囊炎是厚壁型胆囊癌的癌前病变，两者之间没有直接的关系。

二、黄色肉芽肿性胆囊炎和厚壁型胆囊癌的螺旋 CT 表现与鉴别诊断

胆囊壁内低密度结节：胆囊壁内低密度结节是鉴别两者的主要 CT 征象，该组 22 例黄色肉芽肿性胆囊炎中 20 例出现此征象，具有很高的敏感性（90.9%）和准确度（80.9%），而 25 例厚壁型胆囊癌中仅出现 7 例，与文献报道相符。两者的病理基础不同，黄色肉芽肿性胆囊炎中低密度结节是黄色肉芽肿结节，由泡沫细胞、淋巴细胞、浆细胞、核分叶的白细胞、成纤维细胞、脓肿、坏死组织等组成，而厚壁型胆囊癌中出现的低密度结节代表坏死组织和出血灶。

黏膜线的连续与否：黄色肉芽肿性胆囊炎和厚壁型胆囊癌中，胆囊壁多表现为弥漫性增厚，黄色肉芽肿性胆囊炎主要发生在胆囊壁内，肉芽肿将薄层的胆囊肌层连同黏膜层推向胆囊腔，其胆囊腔黏膜面多表现完整，该组 22 例黄色肉芽肿性胆囊炎中 15 例出现连续的胆囊内壁黏膜线，而对照组 25 例厚壁型胆囊癌中仅仅 6 例黏膜线完整，19 例出现胆囊黏膜线的中断、破坏，两者差异有显著性，因此，黏膜线的连续与否这一征象也有助于鉴别，究其原因主要是厚壁型胆囊癌起源于胆囊上皮，恶性肿瘤细胞过度增生从而破坏胆囊黏膜层。

胆管梗阻和淋巴结肿大：黄色肉芽肿性胆囊炎和厚壁型胆囊癌中，胆管梗阻和淋巴结肿大也有差

异性,厚壁型胆囊癌属于恶性肿瘤,更容易侵犯邻近的胆管和肝总管等,或出现淋巴结肿大压迫肝总管,使得肝内胆管出现梗阻征象,与文献报道相符。但是邻近肝脏组织的浸润差异不明显,分别为 14 例和 15 例(P=0.798),黄色肉芽肿性胆囊炎邻近肝脏浸润主要是由于大量炎性细胞浸润,受累肝组织水肿和肝组织纤维增生,而厚壁型胆囊癌主要是癌性浸润,与受侵袭的肝脏形成无分界肿块。

此外,胆囊壁最大厚度,厚壁范围、强化方式、强化程度、邻近肝脏浸润以及周围脂肪间隙清晰征象差异无统计学意义,研究认为黄色肉芽肿性胆囊炎和厚壁型胆囊癌的 CT 表现互相重叠,几乎没有一种征象是某种病变所特有,因此在鉴别诊断上还是有一定困难。

六种阳性征象:该项研究对 22 例黄色肉芽肿性胆囊炎患者的 CT 征象中,六种阳性征象(弥漫性胆囊壁增厚,胆囊壁内低密度结节,连续的黏膜线,增厚的囊壁不均匀强化,邻近肝脏浸润,合并胆囊、胆管结石)的敏感性、特异性、阳性预测值、阴性预测值和准确度进行对照,发现胆囊壁内低密度结节和完整的黏膜线具有很高的敏感性和准确度,因此认为胆囊壁内低密度结节和完整的胆囊内黏膜线在黄色肉芽肿性胆囊炎征象中相对多见,较具特征性,对于诊断黄色肉芽肿性胆囊炎有较大价值,术前需要仔细分析,但最终确诊尚有待于病理诊断。

总之,黄色肉芽肿性胆囊炎和厚壁型胆囊癌在临床和 CT 特征上重叠较多,综合分析其临床表现和影像学特征对于提高黄色肉芽肿性胆囊炎的术前诊断准确率有较高的价值,该项研究认为临床上出现反复的右上腹痛、畏寒发热及血白细胞、粒细胞增多的急性患者,并且 CT 征象上显示胆囊壁内低密度结节、胆囊壁内黏膜线完整常常提示黄色肉芽肿性胆囊炎的诊断,但是若肿瘤标志物 CA199 增高明显,需要考虑厚壁型胆囊癌的可能。

附具体研究资料:收集 10 年期间经手术病理证实的 22 例黄色肉芽肿性胆囊炎资料,其中男 9 例,女 13 例,年龄 34~ 86 岁,中位年龄 60.5 岁,病程 3 个月 ~10 年, 14 例患者病程 >2 年。同时收集该院 5 年期间手术病理或临床综合确诊的 25 例厚壁型胆囊癌资料进行对照,其中男 11 例,女 14 例,年龄 36~79 岁,中位年龄 59 岁,病程 3 个月至 2 年。观察和分析内容包括 8 项:临床症状特点;胆囊增厚情况,并测量增厚的胆囊壁最大厚度和范围,判断局限性增厚(增厚范围 < 胆囊周长 60%)和弥漫性增厚(增厚范围 > 胆囊周长 60%);有无胆囊壁内低密度结节;观察增强后胆囊内壁黏膜线的完整性;胆囊厚壁的强化方式和程度(轻度强化:CT 值增加 <20 HU,高度强化:CT 值增加 > 20 HU);胆管梗阻情况;胆囊和胆管内是否合并结石;周围肝脏是否浸润、周围淋巴结肿大和脂肪间隙是否清晰。

22 例黄色肉芽肿性胆囊炎均行手术胆囊切除并经病理确诊,17 例术前误诊为厚壁型胆囊癌,误诊率为 77.3%,术中发现 12 例与邻近肝脏粘连明显,遂将胆囊连同周围浸润肝脏一并楔形切除。25 例厚壁型胆囊癌, 12 例经手术或活检确诊,余 13 例为临床综合诊断。

第五章 胆囊腺肌增生症

第一节 胆囊腺肌增生症及误诊分析

胆囊腺肌增生症是一种以胆囊黏膜和肌层增生为特点的增生性疾病。胆囊腺肌增生症，又称腺体增生性胆囊炎、胆囊壁憩室症，因其发病率较低，又无典型的临床症状，故容易误诊或漏诊。两组病理学专家分别独立进行的研究提示，本病在国人切除胆囊标本中的发生率为 3.00%~ 3.46%，国外较高。说明胆囊腺肌增生症的实际发生率远较目前影像诊断和临床对其存在的认知为高。

病理学：部分学者研究认为胆胰管汇合畸形、胰液返流刺激与胆囊腺肌增生症的发病有关，还有作者认为胆囊结石及胆囊慢性炎症的长期刺激是导致胆囊腺肌增生症发生的重要因素。病理学主要特点是胆囊壁黏膜层和肌层增生，致使囊壁增厚，且出现多个增生扩大的罗 - 阿窦。在正常胆囊黏膜上偶而能观察到罗 - 阿窦，但是其数量少，体积小（呈小管状结构），并多局限在肌层较浅的部位，且窦隙未扩张成囊状，周围无增生的平滑肌组织环绕及肌层组织结构或排列完好。慢性胆囊炎时，上皮内杯状细胞增多，黏液分泌增多，胆囊内压力增加使肌层互相分离，因胆囊本身无黏膜肌层和黏膜下层，黏膜便可长入肌层并与胆囊腔相通，形成较多较大的罗 - 阿窦。原在黏膜层绒毛之间的罗 - 阿窦由于黏膜上皮增生而数目增多，分支广泛，深入肌层，甚至达浆膜面。有的罗 - 阿窦因其囊内压力增高而明显扩大。罗 - 阿窦在一般染色法的病理切片上其形态酷似腺体，故称为腺体样窦。然而，真正的腺体在胆囊体部是少见的。所谓腺体增生一般是指罗 - 阿窦的增生。若弥漫性分布则可明确为腺肌病，如多数集中在一处形成结节则成为腺肌瘤。

增生扩大的罗 - 阿窦，也称为壁内憩室，其内易淤积胆汁，继发感染，产生窦内结石，即壁内结石。比较局限的腺肌增生，可形成局部结节或“肿块”，一般在胆囊底部；或呈环状分布形成狭窄，在狭窄环远端的囊壁也可被腺肌增生侵犯，胆囊常于狭窄处扭曲、成角。狭窄环远端的囊腔内也易于淤积胆汁，继发感染，产生结石。

显著肌层肥厚是本病胆囊壁增厚的主要原因。胆囊黏膜上皮明显增生，过度增长、突入或穿透黏膜下层和肌层形成壁内憩室、囊肿，或称罗 - 阿窦增生扩大，呈管状、点状、不规则等多种形态，大小各异，其直径多在 0.8cm 以下，2.0cm 以上者少见。罗 - 阿窦的不同形态表现与组织标本的取材切面有一定关系。罗 - 阿窦内充满胆汁或胆泥，或直径 2~3 mm 的结石。腺肌增生症也可合并腺瘤样增生，无蒂，表面光滑，多发或单发。病理组织学检查以黏液腺化生的上皮细胞增生为主，一般无上皮细胞异型性，胆囊底部囊壁呈局限性增厚。

镜下特征主要表现为胆囊壁纤维性增厚，常有淋巴细胞、浆细胞浸润，伴平滑肌细胞的增生肥大，局限性管壁增厚，可达正常时的 3~5 倍。

分型：根据病变范围可分为 4 型。

（1）弥漫型（广泛型），整个胆囊壁呈弥漫性增厚。

（2）节段型（环状型），在胆囊颈部或体部形成节状肥厚，在增厚的胆囊壁中段出现环状狭窄，把胆囊分隔成相互连通的 2 个小腔，以至胆囊形似葫芦。或是发生于体底部广泛性囊壁增厚。狭窄环即为病变处，其远端也可受侵犯。

（3）局限型（基底型），以此型多见，位于胆囊底部，故又名底部型，呈中央凹陷的局限性腔内或腔外圆形隆起性病变。表现为底部结节或“肿块”形成；或如节段型，但狭窄环近底部，使底部形成一小囊腔。

(4)混合型:同一胆囊出现局限型与节段型混合存在的复杂表现,定义病变为2个或2个以上部位起源且彼此间不连续性分布。

在局限型和节段型胆囊腺肌增生症,病变与正常胆囊壁分界明确。

关于癌变:以往多认为胆囊腺肌增生症属良性,近年来报道胆囊腺肌增生症可癌变,在节段型发生癌变的概率要高于其他类型。一些作者报道的节段型发生胆囊癌的概率明显高于非节段型,主张积极手术。罗-阿窦与癌变的关系近年来国内外病理学家们做了一系列的研究工作。一些作者认为个别腺肌增生症可能是癌前期,理由有二:①腺肌瘤病的局限区域覆盖的黏膜含有黏液细胞化生区,表明有癌前期病变的可能;②胆囊结石的患者易罹患胆囊癌,而本病74%~92%病人合并有结石。有作者曾报道1例在节段性腺肌瘤病区域发生非侵袭性癌,肿瘤来源于囊样罗-阿窦的覆盖上皮。另有作者研究表明节段型胆囊腺肌增生症的癌变率较高,尤其见于>60岁的老年患者。

有作者也证实胆囊底部局限型胆囊腺肌增生症即有黏液腺癌并存,在一囊状罗-阿窦内可见癌变细胞侵入乳头状间质内,而胆囊腺肌增生症外胆囊无类似变化,提示胆囊腺肌增生症具有恶性潜能。部分胆囊癌的病理切片中可以在癌灶内或癌灶旁找到罗-阿窦。胆囊结石的患者易罹患胆囊癌,74%~92%胆囊癌患者合并有结石。

临床表现:病人可无症状,或出现上腹部疼痛和不适等主诉,但这些症状缺乏特异性。一组35例报告中,手术及病理组织学检查发现34%病例合并胆结石,83%伴轻度慢性炎症。推测胆囊腺肌增生症患者的临床症状也可能由这些并存疾病引起。

胆囊腺肌增生症病程一般较长,临床症状轻重不一,主要表现为消化不良、食欲减退及上腹胞胀,常有右上腹隐痛,尤以进食脂肪饮食时症状加重或产生胆绞痛,多为合并胆囊结石。如伴有结石,临床症状类似胆囊炎、胆石症;无结石者,起病隐匿,病程缓慢,多无临床症状,但某些病人可有特殊症状,有报道胆囊腺肌增生症病人表现出不明原因的发热。

影像学研究:罗-阿窦首先由口服胆囊造影所发现,随后又被超声、CT和MRI证实。各种影像学检查方法的结果对于胆囊腺肌增生症的诊断和与之紧密相关罗-阿窦征象发现的敏感性、准确性和特异性不尽相同。胆囊腺肌增生症的影像学表现以胆囊壁增厚和罗-阿窦形成为特征。X线胆囊造影、超声、CT和MRI均容易显示胆囊壁增厚,但定性诊断相对困难。所以从影像诊断的角度看,清晰显示罗-阿窦成为诊断本病的重要依据。

X线胆囊造影:本病在未并发严重炎症时,因黏膜增生,胆囊功能往往很好,生理性胆系造影时胆囊显影浓密;又因肌层增生,其收缩功能也很好,一般于脂餐后半小时胆囊已显著缩小,甚至可在一小时内排空。

罗-阿窦显影:正常罗-阿窦不能在胆囊造影相上显示,但是,当其增生扩大时则可表现为胆囊腔周围的壁内憩室,这是本症的直接征象,也是诊断胆囊腺肌增生症的主要依据,一般在胆囊收缩、囊内压力增高时显示尤佳。若窦的颈部有阻塞,窦内有结石和/或胆色素时,对比剂难以进入窦内,罗-阿窦即不能显示。另外,窦腔太小,对比剂的密度不够高、投照条件又不适当,也不能显示。胆囊狭窄部或底部点状透亮阴影:此阴影一般如绿豆至米粒大小,往往于胆囊收缩时显示。在节段型者,此种点状透亮阴影各出现于远、近两囊靠近狭窄环处,胆囊收缩时,两囊进一步分离,两个点状透亮阴影也进一步分离。在底部型者,此种点状透亮阴影出现于胆囊底部。

此征象是诊断本症的可靠征象。一般认为,当部分胆囊被腺肌增生侵犯时,增厚部分与正常的囊壁有突然的分界,当肌层增生部分的囊壁强烈收缩时,该处胆囊壁即形成囊管状,可对正常部分胆囊腔造成局部压迹,形成一小的充盈缺损,即为点状透亮阴影。

在未显示罗-阿窦的病例,当发现此种点状透亮阴影兼有其他一些改变时,诊断基本可以考虑;当胆囊显影原属正常,而胆囊收缩时在底部出现此种透亮阴影,则提示多为本病。

此种点状透亮阴影与阴性结石、炎性息肉、胆固醇息肉、良性肿瘤、息肉样恶性肿瘤等相似,但根据其发生部位、脂餐前后的X线表现容易鉴别。

一处或多处狭窄环(或间隔)及其远端的囊腔:有的节段型仅于胆囊中部显示一处狭窄,形成远、近两个囊(或多个囊),胆囊收缩时两囊(或多囊)互相分离。在底部型者,也可显示狭窄环,环接近底部,其远端形成一小囊腔,狭窄环远端的囊壁一般均受侵犯,胆囊收缩时两囊也互相分离。有时狭窄环及其远端的小囊内腔非常狭窄，甚至闭塞，这时显影的胆囊可表现无异常。胆囊底部出现结节或"肿块"阴影：有的病例胆囊底部出现结节或"肿块"阴影，有的显影胆囊底部显示一边缘模糊的圆形充盈缺损，有的显影的胆囊底部显示一向内的弧形压迹。狭窄环远端囊内结石：在节段型和底部型，皆可出现此征。胆囊持久性扭曲、成角畸形。胆囊外形不规则，但浓缩及收缩功能良好。

要显示上述这些X线征象，适当的投照技术是必要的：①多体位投照，包括俯卧位、仰卧位、直立位、右侧卧位照片。必要时可于电视透视下寻找显示胆囊狭窄与扭曲的最好投照位置。②加压照片，以移去与胆囊重叠的肠气影。③脂餐后胆囊收缩时的照片是相当重要的，往往更能显示罗-阿窦及点状透亮阴影。一般于脂餐后1/2小时照片，但有时需要在脂餐后1小时甚至1个半小时后，待胆囊更明显收缩时再照片。④投照条件必须适当，利用小的照射野是可取的。医生与技师应及时看片，以便决定显示病变最好的时刻及位置。

传统的口服胆囊造影需要罗-阿窦内积存一定量的对比剂，才可被显影。这不仅要求罗-阿窦体积大，且连接胆囊腔和罗-阿窦的管道还应通畅，以使对比剂容易进入。如某些因素导致胆囊不能显影，罗-阿窦就无法显示。

口服胆囊造影表现为：①弥漫型，胆囊壁的边缘不整齐，其周围可见一层环形围绕的多发的小斑点状致密阴影，即"花环征"。②节段型，多发生在胆囊壁的中部呈环形增生狭窄，至胆囊影成葫芦形。③基底型（局限型），位于胆囊底部，呈结节状的充盈缺损，周围见散在的小憩室影。如果罗-阿窦太小而显影不清时，难与胆囊炎和胆囊癌相鉴别，鉴别点主要为后者在口服胆囊造影检查时多可见胆囊腔狭窄及不规则充盈缺损。

MRI：MR多层面、多体位、多序列成像对明确病变程度和类型有独特优势。

在T_2WI，罗-阿窦表现为病变胆囊壁内点状高信号，这主要由罗-阿窦内自由水的含量决定。MRI显示罗-阿窦的能力不仅与脉冲序列参数有关，还与胆汁的浓缩状态有关。随着禁食时间延长，胆汁内自由水含量逐渐减少，T_2WI显示罗-阿窦的敏感性也相应降低。薄层T_2WI显示罗-阿窦明显优于常规T_2WI，可能与该组病例罗-阿窦体积较小，前者有效减小了体积效应有关。在MRCP，罗-阿窦表现为沿高信号胆囊腔边缘分布的局灶性或串珠样点状高信号。MRCP观察胆囊壁增厚虽不理想，但对罗-阿窦整体形态的显示效果是断面影像无法比拟的，尤其在局限型和节段型胆囊腺肌增生症。

与传统的呼吸门控触发三维FSE技术相比，近年出现的SSFSE屏气技术明显缩短了成像时间，提高了图像清晰度，其单层投影技术更成为目前成像速度最快的MRCP方法。虽然Vitellas等（2002）认为单层投影MRCP技术是显示正常胆胰管及其有无狭窄的最佳方法，但该组结果提示，它对罗-阿窦的显示结果并不令人满意。这可能与单层投影MRCP为减小部分体积效应影响而使用较长的有效TE（600ms以上）有关。因为较长的TE使得T2弛豫时间相对较短的浓缩胆汁显示困难，进而造成这些患者的罗-阿窦不能显示或仅部分显示。

有时，胆囊区域虽然存在类似罗-阿窦的点状高信号，但因为胆囊内胆汁浓缩使胆囊轮廓未显示或仅部分显示，故很难判断这些点状高信号是否为可靠的罗-阿窦。

多层连续扫描后通过最大强度投影重建MRCP，虽然扫描时间相对较长，但显示RAS的效果也罗-阿窦较好。没有在同一患者比较这2种MRCP是该研究的不足之处。

在T_1WI，罗-阿窦可表现为低信号、高信号或等信号，这主要与胆汁的浓缩程度有关。虽然T_1WI对罗-阿窦的显示能力明显不如T_2WI和MRCP，但该作者认为，对可疑胆囊腺肌增生症的患者，T_1WI可作为评估胆汁浓缩状况及选择MRCP成像方法的参考。当T_1WI显示胆汁呈现高或等信号时，SSFSE单层投影法MRCP不宜成为唯一选择，此时应降低TE时间，或与多层连续扫描法结合使用，以提高罗-阿窦显示率。

此外，当胆囊内胆汁在T_1WI呈高信号时，对应的T_2WI通常呈等信号，这时在T_1WI判断胆囊壁厚度及病变范围就相对容易。

该组研究还发现，无论在何种序列，罗-阿窦的信号强度可与胆囊内胆汁信号强度相同或不同。在同一病例，不同部位的罗-阿窦信号强度有时也存在较大差别。推测这在一定程度上可能反映了罗-阿窦内胆汁与胆囊内胆汁及不同部位的罗-阿窦内胆汁代谢活动有所不同。在MRCP，罗-阿窦表现为沿高信号胆囊腔边缘分布的局灶性或串珠样点状高信号。胆囊壁局限性或弥漫性变形、增厚,增厚的胆囊壁内多发高信号小囊状憩室,即罗-阿窦增多增大;小囊腔内可伴发相对低信号的结石。MRCP观察胆囊壁增厚虽不理想,但对罗-阿窦整体形态的显示效果是断面影像无法比拟的,尤其在局限型和节段型胆囊腺肌增生症。

由于口服胆囊造影检查准确度和敏感度均不高,目前临床上已不常用。

超声在显示的增厚胆囊壁内的小囊样结构(<5 mm)即罗-阿窦上的平均出现率为90%。然而,CT和MRI显示罗-阿窦的敏感度存在较大差异,研究表明薄层MR-T_2WI 100%、MRCP79%、常规T_2WI 74%、增强T_1WI 68%、常规T_1WI 32%、增强CT 26%、平扫CT为0。一些作者研究证实MRI、螺旋CT和B超对于胆囊腺肌增生症诊断的敏感性分别为93%、65%和43%;特异性分别为93%、85%和89%;准确性分别为93%、75%和66%。

有学者报告一组26例术前影像学诊断和术后病理结果符合率仅为11.5%,经CT术前明确诊断的2例,均因发现罗-阿窦而做出诊断,另外1例由B超发现胆囊底部明显增厚而做出诊断。其余23例均未见罗-阿窦,但术后病理明确证实罗-阿窦存在。考虑可能与以下几点有关:①病变处于早期。该组病例中弥漫型为7例,其中2例胆囊壁增厚<5 mm且均伴有胆囊结石,考虑病变处于早期,B超及CT较难看到罗-阿窦。②技术缺陷。B超较容易受腹部肠气及合并结石的干扰,CT为横断扫描,容易漏诊较小的病变,而且B超与CT的组织分辨率低,不易发现罗-阿窦。③满足于胆囊炎、胆囊结石等诊断,未注意仔细寻找罗-阿窦。

超声检查胆囊壁小囊十分敏感和简便,是目前的首选方法,但由于本病常合并胆囊炎、胆石症、胆汁过分黏稠及积脓等。易造成假阳性,另外附着胆囊壁的胆砂、胆泥或血凝块及胆囊壁血管的强回声均可形成假阳性。有研究表明,超声内镜(EUS)对胆囊腺肌增生症的诊断要优于超声,且超声内镜对胆囊腺肌增生症与胆囊癌的鉴别诊断要优于超声,同时组织谐波显像技术的定位及定性诊断也得到肯定。由于多期动态增强螺旋CT薄层扫描和胆囊CT成像检查对本病的诊断准确度高而得到推广使用。在MRI,半傅里叶采集单次激发快速自旋回波(HASTE)序列MRI技术对本病定性诊断有很高的精准性,并优于CT及超声。

鉴别诊断:胆囊腺肌增生症应与胆囊癌鉴别。后者虽有胆囊壁增厚或肿块表现,但病变部分无罗-阿窦形成,据此诊断特异性可达很高。

此外,如果发现胆囊壁增厚并伴有肝脏浸润或肝内转移,以及区域淋巴结肿大,则应高度怀疑胆囊癌。值得注意的是,节段型胆囊腺肌增生症并存胆囊癌可达6.4%,特别是60岁以上的患者。病理组织学检查时也发现罗-阿窦上皮癌变的个案报道,提示胆囊腺肌增生症有恶性潜能。手术切除病变胆囊是目前治疗本病的有效手段。

鉴于本病的进展、术前性质不明、与恶性病变的鉴别困难且MSCT对判断胆囊腺肌增生症是否恶变缺乏特异性,对那些病程较长且反复发作者或合并胆囊结石者(尤其胆囊壁内结石)、壁不规则增厚而难以排除恶变者以及60岁以上节段型者应尽早行手术切除,术中应行快速冰冻病理切片除外恶变可能。

第二节　胆囊腺肌增生症病例之一

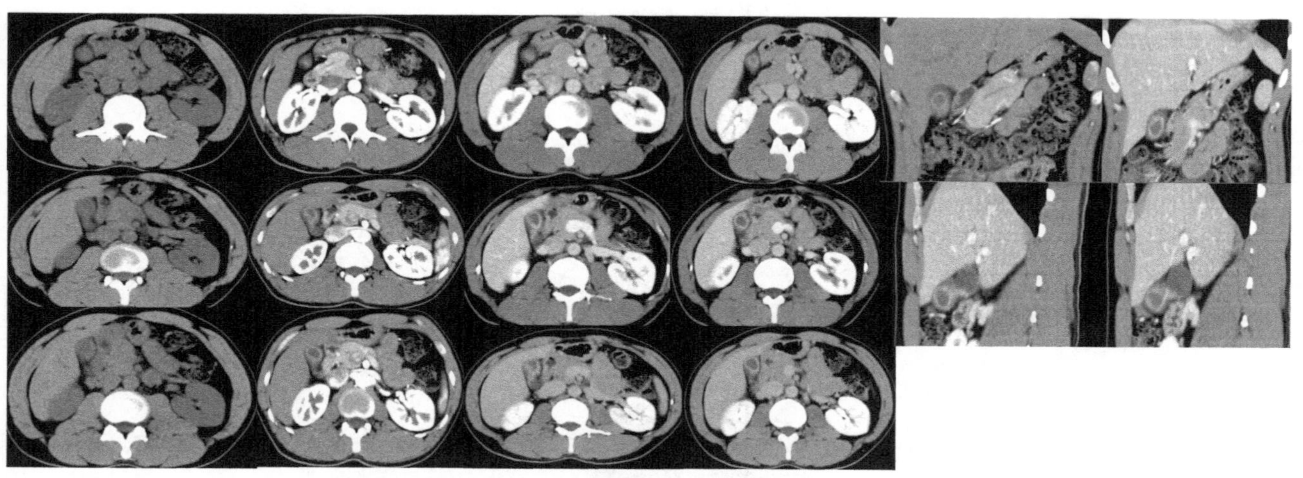

图 17-5-1　胆囊腺肌增生症病例之一

患者，男，30 岁。

手术所见：术中见胆囊无充血、肿胀，胆囊大小约 7cm×3cm，壁约 0.3cm，胆囊底部增厚约 1cm，术后剖视胆囊见胆囊内胆汁浑浊，未见结石及息肉。

病理检查：胆囊一具，大小 7.5cm×4cm× 1.6cm，浆膜面粗糙，黏膜面呈粗网状，壁厚 0.4~1.0cm。病理诊断：慢性胆囊炎伴腺肌症（图 17-5-1）。

第三节　胆囊腺肌增生症病例之二

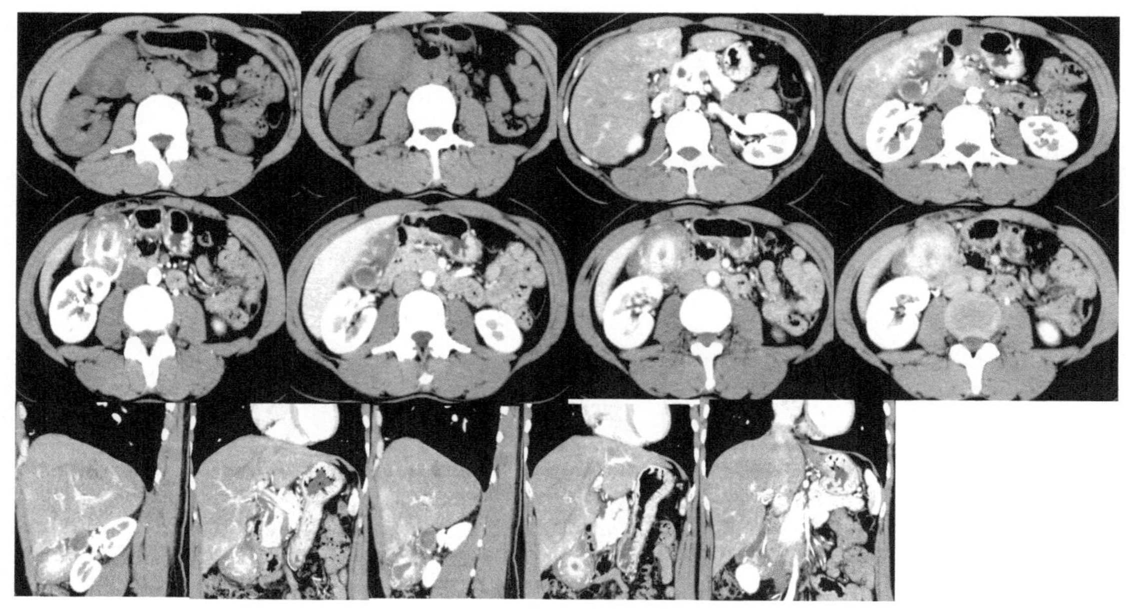

图 17-5-2　胆囊腺肌增生症病例之二

患者,女,43 岁。外院超声提示:胆囊腺肌症?胆囊肿块性质待定?其他病变侵犯胆囊?CT:胆囊壁明显增厚,考虑:胆囊腺肌症,肉芽肿性胆囊炎,胆囊癌不能排除;胆总管略扩张;右肾小结石。腹腔镜胆囊切除术后病理证实:胆囊腺肌增生症(图 17-5-2)。

第四节 慢性胆囊炎伴腺肌病及结石形成

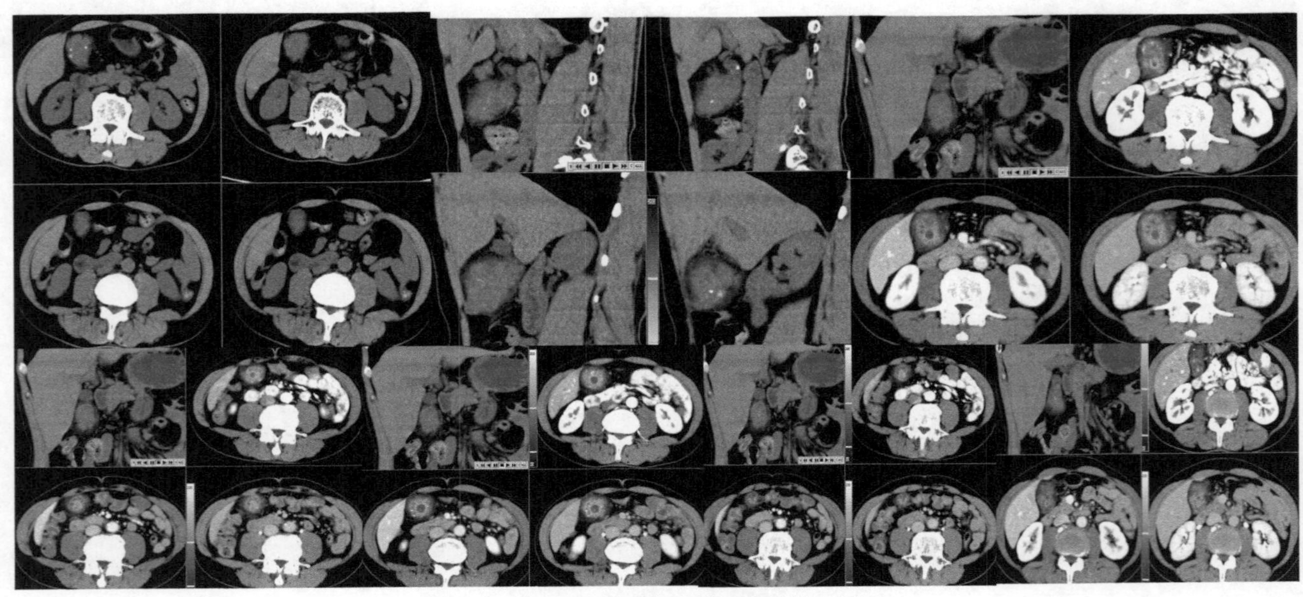

图 17-5-3 慢性胆囊炎伴腺肌病及结石形成

患者,男, 63 岁。因腹痛、腹泻、呕吐伴发热 1 天入院。手术所见:胆囊大小约 8.0 cm × 4cm,胆囊壁厚约 1.5cm,稍毛糙,充血水肿,与肝脏、大网膜稍粘连,胆囊三角脂肪堆积较多。胆囊内可见数枚胆固醇性结石。病理检查:胆囊一具,大小 6.5cm × 4.5cm × 3.8cm,内容物已流失,黏膜面呈细网状,胆囊壁厚 1.15cm。另见淡黄色组织一堆,总体积 4cm × 3.5cm × 1cm。灰黑色结石两枚,总体积 1cm × 0.7cm × 0.4cm。病理诊断:慢性胆囊炎伴腺肌病及结石形成。注:胆囊壁明显增厚,其中见纤维组织增生,部分腺体囊状扩张,淋巴组织增生。另于淡黄色纤维脂肪组织中见扩张管状结构,内衬柱状细胞分化尚好,部分内膜上皮缺失,管壁含平滑肌,伴慢性炎细胞浸润,来源不明,请结合手术部位考虑。(图 17-5-3)

第六章　胆囊其他肿块

第一节　胆囊胆甾醇沉积病

胆囊胆甾醇沉积病，又称草莓胆囊，鱼鳞胆囊。本病较少见，以往多在尸检或标本检查时发现。

病理学：Gluthert（1958）对胆囊胆甾醇沉积病的病理检查研究甚为完整。病变开始于胆囊体部，以后是胆囊颈部，最后是胆囊底部。胆囊胆甾醇沉积病，有 1/3 的病例病变累及整个胆囊，1/3 病例体部或底部受累，1/3 病例病变较为局限。病变可累及胆囊管，但肝外胆管一般不被累及。一些作者根据病变的严重程度将本病分为点状型和息肉型，各型间在临床上症状相同，而 X 线检查的表现却有不同。点状型 X 线检查确诊较难，息肉型 X 线较易诊断。

有学者认为，胆囊胆甾醇沉积病与胆甾醇代谢无关，而与胆囊淋巴液的引流不畅有关。一些学者指出，本病有 5%~10% 的病例与胆囊腺肌瘤病，神经纤维瘤病（一些学者称之为神经类脂质病），或胆囊弹力纤维增多症合并存在。

胆囊黏膜面可见黏膜皱襞普遍增厚，呈淡金黄色并形成网样结构，突出于墨绿色的黏膜上。黏膜皱襞增厚，不规则处则形成粟粒大小（个别可达半米粒大）的息肉样物。

镜检可见黏膜皱襞处顶部上皮脱落，基部上皮有轻度增生。顶部增厚处上皮下黏膜固有层几乎全部被泡沫细胞所占有。其间有少量炎性细胞浸润，还可见管壁肥厚的毛细血管。

临床表现：右上腹疼痛，有时可伴黄疸。进食后可有上腹部饱胀感，尤以进食油腻物后为甚。体检可见右上腹压痛。

影像学研究：在胆囊造影胆囊显影时，可表现为胆囊外形呈不规则的锯齿状。因为，胆囊胆甾醇沉积病是胆甾醇脂及其他类脂物质沉着在黏膜固有层，形成类圆形的颗粒或长线条。这些沉积物多位于黏膜皱襞皱褶部，所以 X 线片上表现为向腔内突出的细锯齿状或毛茸样阴影。胆囊胆甾醇沉积病与胆囊细小结石或泥沙样结石的阴影区别一般不困难，在胆囊结石，胆囊外形光整，在变动体位时有时可见到结石影位置的改变；在限局性胆囊胆甾醇沉积病，表现为固定的边缘整齐的充盈缺损，在切线位上显示较好。胆囊胆甾醇沉积病因胆囊黏膜面的增加而使胆囊吸收增强，因此，在生理性胆系造影时，胆囊内容物可有过度浓缩现象，脂肪餐后可有胆囊过度运动，或胆囊快速排空及早期胆囊排空现象。

第二节　胆囊腺瘤

胆囊息肉样病变，又称胆囊隆起样病变，泛指胆囊壁向腔内呈息肉状生长的所有非结石性病变总称。胆囊息肉样病变主要包括胆囊真性肿瘤性病变，例如胆囊癌、胆囊腺瘤；还包括胆囊非真性肿瘤性病变，例如胆固醇性息肉、炎性息肉、胆囊腺肌增生症等。

胆囊腺瘤多为单发，少数多发，有蒂息肉，直径为 0.5~2.0 cm，甚至可充满整个胆囊，外形可呈乳头状或非乳头状，表面可破溃出血、坏死、感染，是胆囊最常见的良性肿瘤，女性比较多见，男女之比约 2∶7。可发生在胆囊的任何部位，部分病例同时伴有胆囊结石、单纯性胆囊炎等。较多的影像学资料已证实胆囊良性肿瘤具有癌变趋势,被认为是胆囊癌的癌前病变,癌变机会与腺瘤大小呈正相关。很多研究从分子水平也证实了胆囊腺瘤到癌变序贯存在,其癌变经过:腺瘤增生→腺瘤细胞中重度异型增生→癌变,一旦确诊,宜行手术切除。

总体来说,胆囊腺瘤的发病率偏低,虽有癌变的可能性,但对人群构成的威胁并不太大。

临床症状主要有右上腹胀痛不适、纳差等慢性胆囊炎症状,可向右肩背部放射,恶心、消化不良,胆绞痛,发作时伴轻度黄疸,个别病例无明显症状。

胆囊腺瘤诊断主要依赖于影像学检查。目前已公认B超是检查胆囊疾病行之有效的首选方法。B超检查对胆囊腺瘤诊断的敏感性为45%~90%,明显高于MRI和CT检查,B超能直接显示肿瘤大小、部位、形态、肿瘤与胆囊壁关系,有无合并胆囊结石。

胆囊腺瘤在B超上主要表现为胆囊壁向囊腔突起的中等强度回声光团,不伴声影,不随体位改变而移动,有蒂或广基。当发现肿瘤附着处的胆囊壁不规则增厚,提示胆囊腺瘤有癌变的可能。CT平扫诊断价值不大,增强扫描可见囊壁及附壁腺瘤的中等或明显强化,尤其是对腺瘤恶变的诊断有明显的优势,可以提高诊断符合率,而MRI因为多序列成像,信息量丰富,表现为长T1、稍短T2信号影,与囊壁关系紧密,有时与胆囊结石鉴别困难。

该病例进行了上腹部CT平扫和MRI检查,表现较典型,结合B超检查,正确诊断不难。临床检查可将B超结合MRI或CT检查,提高术前诊断符合率,但最后确诊有赖于术后病理检查。

第三节　迷走胰腺

Martinez和Gregg(1973)报告1例手术前口服胆囊造影发现固定的胆囊内的充盈缺损,手术证实为迷走胰腺。与此区别诊断者包括腺肌瘤病、乳头瘤或胆囊癌。迷走胰腺中,大约75%出现于胃、十二指肠与空肠。胆囊内迷走胰腺据该作者意见尚属首例报告,十分罕见。

第四节　胆囊的假肿瘤

Barth等(1981)报告2例小儿,为完全靠肠外给予营养度日而又营养过度者,上腹部皆扪及包块,疑为肿瘤,超声发现为膨胀的胆囊。

正常情况下,胆管和胆囊内胆汁的流动为胆胰十二指肠连接区的括约肌及叶状瓣等结构所控制,在消化间期,括约肌关闭,胆汁进入胆囊贮存、浓缩;进餐时由于神经和激素的作用,引起胆囊排空,即胆囊收缩和括约肌松弛。禁食期间,胆管和胆囊缺乏神经性和激素的刺激,导致胆囊内大量胆汁贮留。在儿童,引起胆囊膨胀的原因还有水肿、结石性胆囊炎、黏膜皮肤淋巴结综合征、家族性地中海热及结节性多动脉炎。

笔者曾见一例右上腹痛急症患者,超声与CT检查均发现胆囊肿大,密度甚高且不匀,CT值75HU,与肝脏密度相近,怀疑胆囊新生物,因系急症不便作更多检查,遂行手术。手术发现胆囊膨胀,其内胆汁约50~60ml,十分浓稠,尤如豆羹状,且混杂小的胆固醇结石;胆囊管增粗,并有两个90º的弯曲;未发现胆囊新生物。类似此类胆汁淤滞导致误诊者,文献也曾见报道,虽属少见,但不能不提高警惕。

第五节　胆囊息肉

Donald(1980)提出超声显像可显示直径小于4mm的胆囊息肉。胆囊息肉应区别于胆囊癌:胆囊息肉,超声显像可见其体积较小,表面光滑,行多方向探查,有时可显示息肉的蒂;胆囊癌则为较大的实质性包块,或呈不规则光团,有时表面呈菜花状,病变基底较宽。

第六节　肝细胞癌侵犯胆囊

肝细胞癌侵犯胆囊罕见。一些作者报道1例38岁男性患者。CT增强扫描见胆囊底部有一肿块，与肝内另一大肿块相连，肝右叶后段示一较小的转移瘤，胆囊无移位，肝内外胆管无扩张。MRI示肝、胆肿块不均质，T2WI为轻度高信号，T1WI为轻度低信号。

增强MRI清晰显示肿瘤为腔内生长。X线选择性肝动脉造影显示肝内肿瘤主要由肝中动脉及肝右动脉供血，界限不清，为富血管性肿瘤。胆囊内肿瘤亦是富血管性肿瘤，由扩张的胆囊动脉供血，胆囊动脉深支已被包绕。病理证实为肝细胞癌侵犯胆囊。

胆囊体部与胆囊窝之间无腹膜被覆，浸润型胆囊癌易穿过该处，常常侵犯肝脏，而肝细胞癌侵犯胆囊却十分少见。肝细胞癌侵入胆囊并形成腔内肿块，极像浸润型胆囊癌。

CT在显示肿瘤位置时表现为肝、胆肿块相连，及X线血管造影显示富血管，皆不易鉴别这两种肿瘤，胆囊动脉分支被包绕有助于浸润型胆囊癌侵犯肝脏的诊断。

在MRI加权图像上，肝细胞癌与浸润型胆囊癌均呈高信号。因胆囊底部附着于肝下方，两个器官之间的肿瘤浸润基本上为垂直方向，冠状面可显示大的肝脏肿瘤向下侵入胆囊，在显示浸润方向上，冠状扫描较横断扫描可获得较多资料。因此，多方向MRI扫描，尤其是冠状扫描，在类似病例，有助于提供一些线索作出正确诊断。

第七节　发生于胆囊的胃肠道外间质瘤

胃肠道间质瘤以往多归为平滑肌肿瘤，近年来随着病理学的发展，尤其是免疫组化及超微结构研究的进展，国内外许多学者提出胃肠道间质瘤实为一组独立的起源于胃肠道原始间叶组织的非定向分化的肿瘤。

胃肠道间质瘤是指从食管一直到直肠的消化道的非上皮淋巴造血组织的呈梭形细胞分化为主的肿瘤，可以发生于胃肠道任何部位，但以胃部最多见。发生在胃肠道的间质瘤在临床上近几年来并非少见，但发生在胃肠道外胆囊的胃肠道间质瘤甚少，病因尚未清楚。

有作者报告一例发生于胆囊的胃肠道外间质瘤。该病例胆囊的恶性病变表现，在CT平扫+增强扫描诊断明确，但间质瘤的影像表现缺乏特异性，难与胆囊癌等肿瘤鉴别，确诊有赖于病理学检查。

第七章 胆囊结石

第一节 单能量成像及能谱曲线与胆囊等密度胆固醇结石

胆囊结石是临床上常见疾病,其主要包括胆色素结石、胆固醇结石,依结石的成分不同,在常规混能CT像上表现为低密度、等密度及高密度,其中,等密度结石极易漏诊,以往只能通过CT胆系造影、超声、MRI及ERCP进行诊断。随着能谱CT应用于临床,使传统的混合能量成像变成单能量成像,并配合物质分离技术、能谱曲线及有效原子序数,使CT诊断等密度结石成为可能。

依结石的成分不同,胆系结石在CT像上可表现为低密度、等密度及高密度,常规CT较容易诊断高密度及低密度结石,但因等密度结石与胆汁密度接近,往往不易被发现。目前,对等密度结石主要依赖CT胆囊造影、超声、MRI及ERCP诊断,但上述几种方法各有其缺点,CT胆囊造影准备时间长,且部分患者对口服造影耐受差;超声诊断率与操作者水平相关,且肥胖患者因腹腔脂肪的干扰影响其诊断率;MRI对结石的诊断率高,但禁忌证较多,费用高且扫描时间长,不适于急诊患者。另外,扫描床重量的限制,使部分肥胖患者不宜行此检查;ERCP属有创性检查,且辐射剂量高,不能作为常规检查。能谱CT的出现为临床提供了一种新的方法。

传统CT设备采用混合能量成像,X线中包含不同能量水平的光子,射线硬化效应导致CT值漂移,从而影响图像质量及病变的诊断。另外,传统CT计算出的CT值是混合能量等效值,即采用平均辐射能的计算方法得到CT值,即:不同的物质可以表现为相同的CT值,这样就影响了一些等密度病灶的检出率。

如何使相同CT值的不同物质分离开来,一直都是放射学家关注、探讨的问题。理论上利用不同能量水平的单能量X线可以得到一系列相应能量水平的CT图像,即能谱成像。每种物质都有其特征X线吸收曲线,在人体中,当X线能量高于40 keV时,作为CT图像重建时体素的衰减曲线为一平滑的曲线,而曲线上的任何两点便决定整个曲线走向,也就是说仅需要两次能量采集即可确定一条特征吸收曲线。

近年来,两款双能量CT已投入临床使用,一种是Simens公司的双源CT,一种是GE公司的宝石能谱。该项研究采用了GE公司的宝石能谱CT。宝石能谱CT采用高(140 kV)、低(80 kV)双能量进行瞬时(<0.5 ms)切换获取两组一致性很好的吸收投影数据,并根据这两组数据确定物质在40~140 keV能量范围内的衰减系数,进而得到101组KeV单能量图像及物质能谱曲线。

有研究证实,结石的CT值与胆固醇含量呈负相关,且绝大多数等密度结石为胆固醇结石。一组中,20例结石经手术及超声证实为胆固醇结石,其在传统混合能量图像上的CT值与胆汁差异不大,肉眼难以分辨,故17例完全的等密度结石全部漏诊。

对结石及胆汁进行单能量成像及能谱曲线分析后,发现所有结石的CT值从40 KeV到140KeV依次上升,其中40 KeV处CT值为负值,相对于胆汁呈低密度,140 KeV处为正值,相对于胆汁呈明显高密度灶,结石的形态及轮廓均显示清晰,而在70 KeV附近结石轮廓及形态均显示不清,统计学分析显示,70 KeV处结石及胆汁的CT值无显著差异,其余各单能量结石及胆汁的CT值均有显著差异,间接说明了在60~70 KeV单能量图像与传统混合能量图像大致相仿。

结石的能谱曲线呈上升型,斜率为正值,其CT

值的变化及曲线类型与腹部脂肪组织的研究结果一致,说明了结石含有脂质成分。

胆汁的曲线 15 例呈轻度下降型，5 例呈平坦型,可能与胆囊内胆泥淤积程度有关。结石及胆汁的曲线在 60~70 KeV 处相交,40KeV 及 140 KeV 处两曲线分离较明显,进一步说明了在 60~70 KeV 处等密度结石无法显示,而在 40 KeV 及 140 KeV 处等密度结石可以清晰显示。

该项研究尚有以下不足:病例较少且未与其他病变进行对比研究,尤其是胆固醇息肉,其 CT 表现与胆固醇结石相似,在临床上易误诊。两者的鉴别诊断尚需进一步研究;该组病例中结石均较大,对等密度小结石的显示能力尚待进一步研究;仅对含脂质等密度结石进行能谱分析,对于极少数不含脂质的等密度结石显示情况及结石具体成分与能谱表现的相关性还需扩大样本量进一步研究。总之,能谱 CT 为临床提供了一种新的诊断胆囊等密度结石的方法,单能量成像及能谱曲线有助于显示常规 CT 不能显示的胆囊等密度结石。

附:具体研究资料:病例入组要求:结石完全呈等密度,常规 CT 平扫不能显示结石;结石呈稍高密度,常规 CT 像上隐约可见,但不能确定其边界与轮廓,不能确诊。

第二节　漂浮结石

在口服胆囊造影时,放射科医生发现漂浮结石这个现象。胆汁的比重(1.01~1.04)一般低于胆囊结石(1.04~1.058),因此,后者趋向于下沉。胆汁通常成层,在顶部为较轻层。口服胆囊造影导致胆汁比重上升,达 1.03~1.085,常引起胆囊结石漂浮在胆汁内,位于接近它们自己的比重层中。虽然超声成像所见的大多数漂浮结石只是在口服胆囊对比剂(如果胆囊有功能的话)给予以后才见到,含气的结石和相当纯度的胆固醇结石在超声成像时也可呈漂浮状,因其比重(1.01~1.035)比较胆汁为低。

漂浮结石,当其非常小时,表现为横贯胆囊腔内的一个中断的水平线状回声。声影可能是模糊的,或者无声影。在直立位再行扫描,将引起结石的再度排列,还可能诱出声影,因为声束对于结石的行列说来,是以平行于行列代替了垂直于行列。较大的漂浮结石可以表现为有声影的线状回声。非常低的比重的结石可以漂浮紧贴胆囊的前壁,从而导致只看见它们的声影。如同上述的技术方面的研究,在口服胆囊对比剂后行超声成像,有时能够解答,由小而无声影的回声层所引起的最初的模棱两可的超声图像。如果这类口服胆囊超声成像未能完成,病人可直接进行口服胆囊造影。

第三节　肺内胆石

详见本书 本卷 第十五篇 第一章 第四节　肺内胆石。

第四节　同一胆囊内各种类型结石

患者,男,89 岁。胆囊多发各种类型结石(图 17-7-1)。

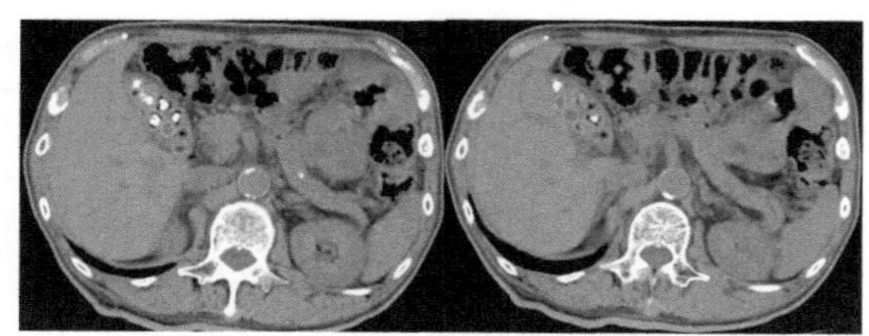

图 17-7-1　同一胆囊内各种类型结石

第五节 CT 对胆石化学性质预测

胆系结石的非手术疗法已成为胆系结石治疗的重要组成部分,特别是高效率胆石溶解剂的产生和胆系介入性放射学的发展,为溶石治疗增添了新的内容。各种溶石剂均只对某种化学类型的结石有效,因此溶石治疗成功的关键在于对某种化学类型胆石患者的选择。

胆囊结石的 CT 表现可分为五种类型:①高密度结石,结石密度显著高于胆汁,其密度均匀或略不均匀, CT 值大于或等于 65HU。从化学成分看,绝大多数为胆色素类结石;②略高密度结石,结石密度略高于胆汁, CT 值为 13~55HU。大多数为胆固醇类结石,少数为混合性结石;③等密度结石,结石密度与胆汁不可区分或不易区分, CT 值小于 10HU。均为胆固醇类结石;④低密度结石,结石密度低于胆汁。皆为胆固醇类结石;⑤环状结石,结石边缘有一高密度或略高密度环状影, CT 值 29~99HU,化学成分为混合性结石;结石中心密度较低, CT 值 -33~-37HU,为胆固醇类结石;两种密度之间界限清楚。

胆囊结石按化学成分分类为:①胆固醇类结石(包括环状结石的核心部分),胆固醇含量为 84.5 ± 8.1%,其 CT 值为 7.9 ± 12.7HU;②胆色素类结石,胆固醇含量 19.04 ± 11.2%, CT 值为 112.86 ± 57.5HU;③混合性结石,胆固醇含量为 57%~66%,CT 值为 50HU 左右。

既往临床以口服胆囊造影时胆囊结石的透光度作为预测胆固醇类结石的标准,但准确性较差。由于 CT 对组织及病变的高度敏感性,密度分辨力高,为胆系结石的定性预测研究提供了有利条件。在胆系结石的 CT 值测定分析中,Moss 等(1980)首先提出结石的含钙量与 CT 值有关。Hickman 等(1986)与 Baron 等(1988)的模型实验结果均表明胆系结石 CT 值与胆固醇含量有明显的负相关,并且提出胆系结石的 CT 值分析有助于预测溶石效果。

一些作者通过体外和体内胆系结石 CT 分析证实了 Hickman 等(1986)的发现,并观察到胆系结石的 CT 值与钙和胆红素含量存在着正相关,这更有利于溶石剂的选择。

胆固醇类结石与胆色素类结石的平均 CT 值有明显差异,使得用 CT 值预测胆系结石化学类型成为可能。该组作者指出,根据该项研究所用的 CT 机(日本岛津 CT-2000T)以 CT 值 40HU 作为区别两类结石的界值,或使预测结果达到较高的符合率。分析胆系结石的 CT 表现可为溶石治疗提供具体指导。对于高密度结石可试用溶胆红素和钙的溶石剂;而对于等密度和低密度结石,应使用溶胆固醇的药物;环状结石则宜先用溶钙药物将外层溶解后,再选用溶胆固醇的溶石剂。

CT 与胆囊结石的定量诊断: CT 对胆囊结石的定量诊断,即结石计数和结石大小的测量,除与 CT 扫描机本身的性能和扫描条件有关外,主要的决定因素是胆囊结石和周围胆汁的密度差异。胆囊胆汁的密度与其浓缩程度有关,而胆汁的浓缩程度则与胆囊的浓缩功能和患者是否禁食有关。一项研究结果表明,胆囊结石的密度,指 CT 值,与其胆固醇含量呈负相关,与其胆红素和钙含量呈正相关,此三种成分以不同构成比形成的胆囊结石,在 CT 图像上可以呈高密度、等密度和低密度影像。等密度结石不能在 CT 图像上被显示。这就是 CT 在诊断胆囊结石时敏感性仅为 70% 和不能反映胆囊结石确切数目的原因。

同一胆囊结石的不同部位的 CT 值也可能不同,形成密度不均匀的结石。如果外周部分和胆汁等密度,或数个结石紧密地堆积在一起,则 CT 图像不能反映胆囊结石的真实大小。

另外,CT 图像层面检查性质,部分容积效应,扫描时病人呼吸的均匀程度,及一切引起 CT 图像产生伪影的因素,也都影响 CT 对胆囊结石的检出、计数和径线的测量。

第六节　胆肠瘘伴结石性肠梗阻

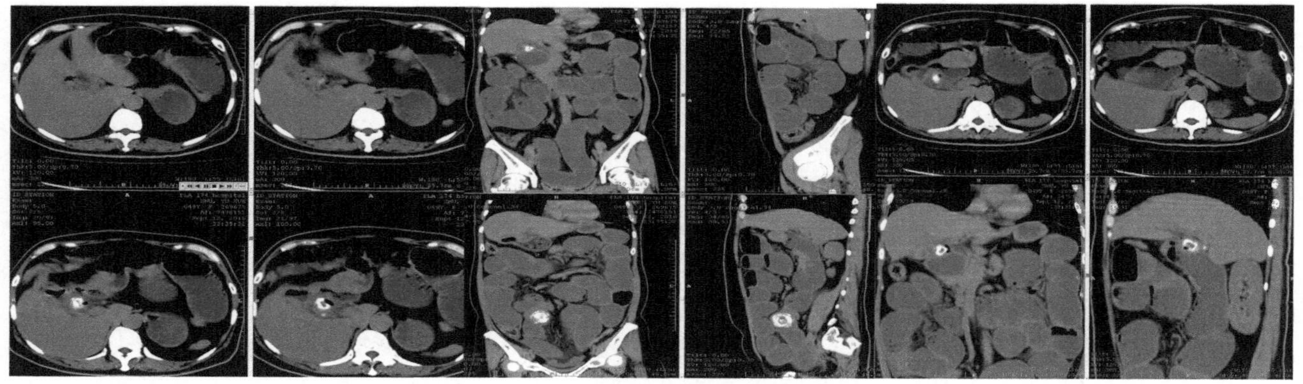

图 17-7-2　胆肠瘘伴结石性肠梗阻

患者，女，49 岁。腹胀伴停止排气、排便半月。患者半月前因进食海鲜等食物后出现腹胀不适，伴恶心、呕吐胃内容物、非喷射性呕吐，腹部胀痛，阵发性发作，无放射痛，进食后加重，并出现肛门停止排气排便，无发热，无畏寒、寒战等，无黑便，无反酸嗳气及呕血等，在外院诊治，未予以特殊治疗，今症状加重，在我院急诊，行 CT 提示：回肠远段混杂密度影，考虑肠结石伴低位小肠梗阻；胆囊结石，慢性胆囊炎急性发作，化脓性胆囊炎待排，请结合临床。予以急诊收住院治疗。起病来，患者精神、睡眠、饮食均差，小便量较少，体重稍有减轻。

入院后予以胃肠减压、制酸护胃、补液及营养支持，患者已排大便后复查 CT 提示，肠梗阻明显好转，回盲瓣肠壁水肿、增厚。临床考虑粪石梗阻后可能，但肠管由于梗阻时间长，肠壁水肿，病人要求出院。

胆肠瘘并继发结石性肠梗阻为胆结石经胆肠瘘或胆胰管下端括约肌进入胃肠道，并发生嵌顿引起机械性肠梗阻，主要包括胆系病变和肠梗阻两方面。该病多见于老年女性患者，患者一般有长期慢性结石性胆囊炎并反复发作的病史，常以持续性中上腹痛、呕吐及肛门停止排气、排便等临床症状就诊。

胆肠瘘伴结石性肠梗阻，由于有特异性的 CT 影像特征，即 Rigler 三联征：①不全性或完全性机械性肠梗阻；②胆系积气；③肠道内异位的结石影。除此外还可见胆囊变形、直接或间接显示胆肠瘘道及其并发症征象；易于与其他原因引起的各类肠梗阻等急腹症相鉴别。因此 CT 检查是胆肠瘘伴结石性肠梗阻最佳及最有价值的检查手段。总之，本病是常发生于老年女性的一种少见病，缺乏特异性，临床上术前诊断较困难。CT（特别是多层螺旋 CT）检查不仅能发现典型肠梗阻征象及梗阻程度，明确梗阻点大致部位，而且能提示胆肠瘘位置，了解胆系有无残余结石，为临床制定治疗方案提供了重要资料（图 17-7-2）。

第七节　胆囊结石化学类型

随着医学技术的发展，胆囊结石非手术疗法发展很快。但是，目前使用的口服或接触性溶石剂大多数只对胆固醇结石有效，因此，非手术治疗前在了解结石特征与胆囊功能状态的同时，确切了解结石的化学类型，是治疗成败的关键。常规 X 线检查经济易行，不仅能了解结石的特征及胆囊功能状态，在预测结石化学类型方面具有较大的发展潜力，因此，重新受到许多学者的重视。

在常规 X 线检查中，胆囊结石的化学类型与多种影像学特征有关，而每一种影像学特征均只是反映了作为某一种类型的结石的倾向性，不能单独作为判断结石化学类型的依据，在实际工作中，必须对每一个因素综合分析，才能较准确地判断结石的化学类型，但这样诊断过程则较为复杂。为简化诊断过程，提高准确率，有必要建立一个统一客观且代表总体概率大小的判别诊断标准。周代全等（1996）

以概率理论为基础,应用计算机通过数学模型推算结石属于某一类别的概率大小来确定结石的类型。该函数式在实际应用中只需将每一例的各变量值代入式中,分别计算出 Y1 和 Y2,比较 Y1 和 Y2 的大小,即可判断出该例结石为胆固醇结石或非胆固醇结石。

利用计算机通过数学模型来推算作为某一类结石的概率,关键要掌握严格统一的赋值标准,不同的赋值方式可以得出不同的判别函数式,而一旦函数式确定,利用该函数式计算的各变量的赋值方式就不能再作变更。该函数式判别结石的正确率为92.7%,错判率为 7.3%,对胆固醇结石的检出率为92.5%,具有较高的实用价值。

该函数式与 Dolgin 等(1981)的判别法比较有下述区别:①结石的化学类型的分类标准不同,Dolgin 等将胆固醇含量大于或等于 50% 者归为胆固醇结石,而该法以大于或等于 70% 为分类标准,其临床实用价值更高;②因素的分类方法不同,Dolgin 等将结石大小按其直径分为小于或等于 6mm 和大于或等于 7mm 两组,将结石的数目分为少于或等于10 粒和多于或等于 11 粒两组,而该法经统计学分析证实,将结石大小按其直径分为小于或等于10mm、介于 11~20mm 之间、大于 20mm 三组,将结石数目分为孤立性、2~10 枚、多于或等于 11 枚三组;①判别分析纳入的因素有差别,Dolgin 等的纳入因素为结石钙化、漂浮、数目、大小、表面特征及人种,该法除未纳入人种外,纳入上述所有因素,另外还增加纳入了具有统计学意义的结石形状、大小均匀性、患者性别、胆囊形态;④ 6 计算方法不同,Dolgin 法须经系数多次计算,而该法采用 Bayes 统计法建立函数式一次运算,计算更为简单。

第八节 X 线检查胆囊结石进入胃壁和胃腔

大的胆囊结石无法通过胆管,常被狭窄的管腔所阻。胆石的压力使已发炎的胆囊局部变薄,变薄处与胃壁周围发生纤维性粘连,其间形成瘘管,结石经瘘管进入胃内。胆囊亦可经类似途径进入十二指肠,然后再逆行入胃。胃内胆石所产生的症状,依结石所在的部位而异。胆石在胃腔内,可以有间歇的不全幽门梗阻的症状,或完全性幽门梗阻的症状;若胆石嵌入胃壁,通常不发生梗阻症状,亦无黄疸。

腹部平片:胆囊 - 胃瘘,或胆囊 - 十二指肠瘘的瘘管内或胆管内常有气体充盈,这些气体都是由胃经瘘管进入胆系的,常可显示胆管的轮廓。如在结石迁移前胆囊管即已闭锁,气体仅可进入瘘管和萎缩的胆囊。如瘘管通畅,以钡剂或有机碘对比剂检查时,瘘管亦可显影;如瘘管因结石或其他原因阻塞,胃内气体未进入胆囊,瘘管与胆管均不会显影。

钡餐检查:胃腔内结石,胃内可见充盈缺损,触诊易于移动。如结石进入幽门时,其 X 线征象类似癌瘤或无蒂息肉。胃壁间的结石可出现一局部肿块,但局部的胃黏膜是完整的,颇类似于胃的良性肿瘤。

第九节 胆石性肠梗阻

胆囊结石进入消化道的途径:胆囊结石可由两种途径自胆系进入消化道:在急性胆囊炎基础上,继发胆囊管的梗阻,使胆囊内压增高,再加胆石的腐蚀作用,造成胆囊 - 肠瘘,导致胆石通过瘘口进入肠腔。此类胆囊 - 肠瘘,大多为胆囊 - 十二指肠瘘,其次为胆囊 - 结肠瘘、胆囊 - 胃瘘,及肝外胆管 - 十二指肠瘘。胆囊结石还可通过扩张的肝外胆管下端的胆胰共同管进入十二指肠,一般认为直径小于 1cm 的胆石较容易经胆胰共同管排至肠道。Review 提到直径小于 2.5cm 的结石可由肠道自行排出。进入肠道的结石直径在 3cm 以上时,则有产生肠梗阻的可能。

临床表现:胆石性肠梗阻常见于 60~70 岁以上的老年肥胖女性。本病需在结石性胆囊炎基础上发病,故患者常有胆系结石的病史,有时甚至在肠梗阻发作中伴有急性胆囊炎的畏寒、发热及放射性疼痛等症状。胆石性肠梗阻的症状和体征与梗阻病变发生部位有关。临床上,常表现为亚急性单纯性机械性肠梗阻，即从发病到手术时间较长。虽梗阻持续较久，经保守治疗并不缓解，但病人一般情况及脱水现象均不太严重，肠腔虽呈中度扩张，但通常无肠壁坏死。

影像学研究：胆石性肠梗阻的X线表现与胆石进入消化道的途径有关。腹部立卧位平片是最基本的X线检查方法，可显示肠梗阻征象，肠内迷走钙化结石及胆系积气征象。结石的发现，对胆石性肠梗阻的诊断固然有助，但必须先除外粪石、输尿管结石、钙化的淋巴结，及位于消化道外的迷走胆石。结石确实在肠内，但无临床及X线肠梗阻证据时，也不能做出本病的诊断。在X线平片上不显影的结石皆为胆红素钙结石。胆系积气，虽可提示有胆系内瘘或胆管下端括约肌松弛，但并无特征性，且显示率也不高。

肠道造影：肠道造影对胆石性肠梗阻的诊断有特殊的价值。经胃十二指肠引流管，作碘水肠道造影，除可证实小肠通道受阻，明确梗阻部位外，还可能显示瘘管，可见肠道内对比剂逆行进入胆系，多呈不规则管状，与腹部平片所示充气胆系影像相符。当此类特征性征象，与肠道积液、积气、扩张等梗阻征象及肠内迷走结石同时存在时，可作为胆石性肠梗阻X线诊断的重要依据。

胆石性肠梗阻少见。诊断依据为肠梗阻征、胆系积气、腹部迷走结石，其中腹部迷走结石是定性诊断的重要依据。但是，除含钙量较高的胆系结石外，腹部平片胆系结石的显示率甚低。胆石进入肠腔后，在移动时可引起不全性肠梗阻。由于肠内容物的沉积，不仅使结石体积增大，而且密度也增高。在积液肠腔衬托下CT能清晰地显示引起梗阻的结石。引起肠梗阻的结石直径一般为3.0~5.0cm，梗阻多发生在管径较小的回肠，一般不易导致肠壁坏死和穿孔。随着结石的移动，发生肠梗阻的部位亦可随之改变。

对高龄女性有小肠亚急性肠梗阻病例，X线检查随访中梗阻并不加剧，腹内有迷走钙化影，或胆系有积气时，应考虑胆石性肠梗阻的可能。对临床拟诊胆石性肠梗阻的患者，可选用合适的肠道造影（碘水造影），以确认瘘管的存在，除外腹内恶性肿瘤病变后，可做出本病的肯定性诊断。

第十节　假性胆囊结石

超声检查胆囊疾病的特异性与敏感性均佳，现已成为胆囊疾病影像诊断的首选方法，但是，文献上报告不少超声检查中的假性胆囊结石，颇值得注意和借鉴。

十二指肠伪似胆囊结石：胆囊常位于十二指肠或横结肠的前面，当十二指肠内含空气而且挤压于胆囊背面时，纵断扫描时则可将十二指肠误为胆囊腔内存有结石。

肠袢伪似胆囊结石：肠袢有中心性回声，肠壁回声较弱，有时可类似胆囊含有结石。但实时超声检查常可观察到肠袢的蠕动，胆囊的正常毗邻关系的进一步分析有助于防止此类混淆。已有几位作者报告肠腔积气可伪似收缩胆囊中的结石。如胆囊未被查见，此类回声区域又邻近于肝，确易造成分辨不清。有时结石与肠气阴影的区别不绝对可靠，如肠气位于左叶的内外段之间裂隙下方，常可误为结石影。如能确定胆囊影位于其右侧，此问题则迎刃而解。

胆囊皱襞类似胆囊结石：常常可见一皱襞沿着胆囊后部行进，接近于胆囊颈，伪似胆囊结石，如其伴存后方的折射阴影，则更易误诊。令病人左侧卧位，在其深吸气时扫描，尽力使胆囊延伸、展开，常可减少这种误解。

胆囊息肉伪似胆囊结石：在有的病人见到一中振幅到高振幅回声出现于胆囊内，可类似结石。熟悉息肉的特征表现有助于鉴别二者。

折射阴影伪似胆囊颈结石：当反射波的临界角遇到或超过二邻近的声的介质（胆囊壁和胆囊内胆汁）之间并伴声波的不同速率时，可出现折射影，如该影邻近胆囊颈，则极易误为该处的结石，需随时警惕之。

胆囊内胆汁淤滞伪似结石：胆汁淤滞形成淤泥，位于胆囊的悬垂部位，可见于住院病人或空腹病人，有时此淤泥在形状上可稍分叶，而伪似胆囊包块或结石。该影后方缺乏声影有助于减少误诊。

第十一节 Mirizzi 综合征

详见本书 本卷 第十八篇 第三章 Mirizzi 综 合征。

第八章　胆囊炎症

第一节　误诊病例简介:胆囊结石并胆囊结核与胆囊癌

胆囊结核主要是结核杆菌通过血液和淋巴循环感染胆囊所致,本病少见。胆囊结核大部分合并有胆囊结石、胆囊炎或胆管梗阻。影像检查无特征性表现,Xu 等(2011)报道,胆囊结核 CT 表现分为 3 种类型:囊壁增厚型,囊壁均匀或非均匀增厚,周围可伴有环形水肿带;小结节型,囊壁结节状或息肉状突入囊腔;肿块型,内可见点状钙化灶及多发低密度区。

一项研究报告一例胆囊结核 CT 表现,胆囊底轻度局限性增厚,增强扫描胆囊壁可见多个分隔,提示脓肿形成。

胆囊结核术前诊断困难,与胆囊癌,慢性胆囊炎等不易鉴别,需结合临床病史、影像检查、实验室检查进行综合分析。以下 4 点支持胆囊结核的诊断:中年患者,伴结核中毒症状;超声及 CT 示胆囊壁增厚、结节或肿块伴钙化,CT 增强扫描胆囊壁强化呈分隔状;胆囊病变伴腹内其他脏器的结核及结核性淋巴结肿大;实验室检查有贫血、红细胞沉降率升高及结核菌相关试验强阳性。

附:具体病例资料:患者,男,73 岁,因右上腹持续性隐痛 2 个月入院。体检:腹软,无压痛及反跳痛,莫菲征阴性。上腹部 CT 见胆囊壁增厚,囊内密度不均匀,与肝脏边界不清;增强扫描胆囊壁不均匀强化,内见分隔状强化影。考虑胆囊癌或炎性病变。手术病理所见:胆囊底部与腹壁粘连,胆囊被大网膜包裹,与胃十二指肠、横结肠广泛粘连,胆囊约 9 cm×5 cm×4 cm,张力高,胆囊壁水肿,内触及多个结石,钳夹胆囊壁破裂后见白色浑浊样脓液流出。病理见大量类上皮样细胞及少量多核巨细胞,外周绕以淋巴细胞浸润。病理诊断:胆囊结核。

第二节　肝局灶性结节增生,慢性胆囊炎伴多发胆固醇息肉

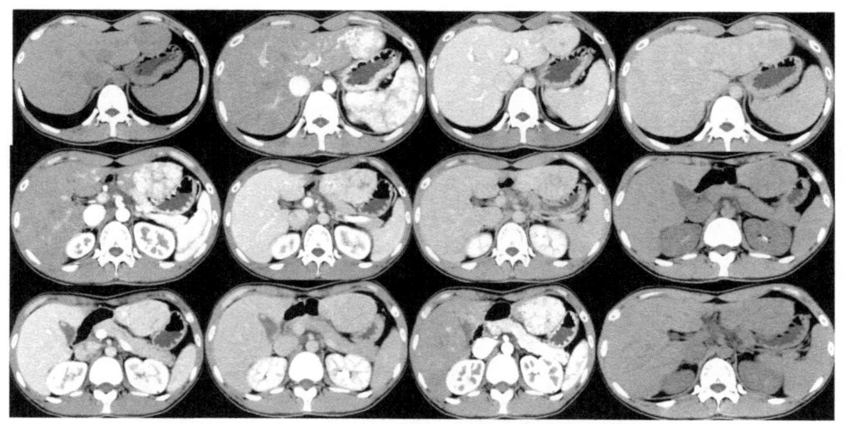

图 17-8-1　肝局灶性结节增生,慢性胆囊炎伴多发胆固醇息肉

患者,男,21岁。

病理检查:肝肿物切除标本:肿物大小为7.5cm×7.5cm×4.5cm,肝被膜完整,表面凹凸不平,切面灰褐,可见瘢痕样纤维间隔,呈分叶状,质中。病理免疫组化诊断:肝局灶性结节增生;慢性胆囊炎伴多发胆固醇息肉(图17-8-1)。

第三节 胆囊结核

发病机制:胆囊结核少见。胆囊结核常继发于体内其他脏器的结核病,甚少为原发性。结核杆菌通过血液传播侵入胆囊,在黏膜层形成干酪样病灶,随后溃破而成为溃疡,病变可沿胆囊壁扩散,或向深部发展,如沿胆管扩散可引起胆管的结核性感染,也可逆流入肝,发生胆系内瘘后可形成结核性肝脓肿,但病变较局限。

病理学:胆囊增大,可触及多个结石,胆囊与胃、横结肠等周围脏器组织紧密粘连,胆囊壁瘢痕肉芽增生明显,胆囊底部穿破入肝实质形成局限性脓肿,脓肿周围亦见瘢痕肉芽组织增生,脓液呈黄白色。胆囊壁增厚达8mm,坚韧,黏膜粗糙不平,并见干酪样坏死物。

影像学研究:各种影像学手段均可见胆囊增大,收缩功能差,胆囊内有多发性结石。结核肉芽肿为实质性病变,特异性甚少,可被误诊为肿瘤或其他病变。

第四节 慢性坏疽性胆囊炎伴结石形成

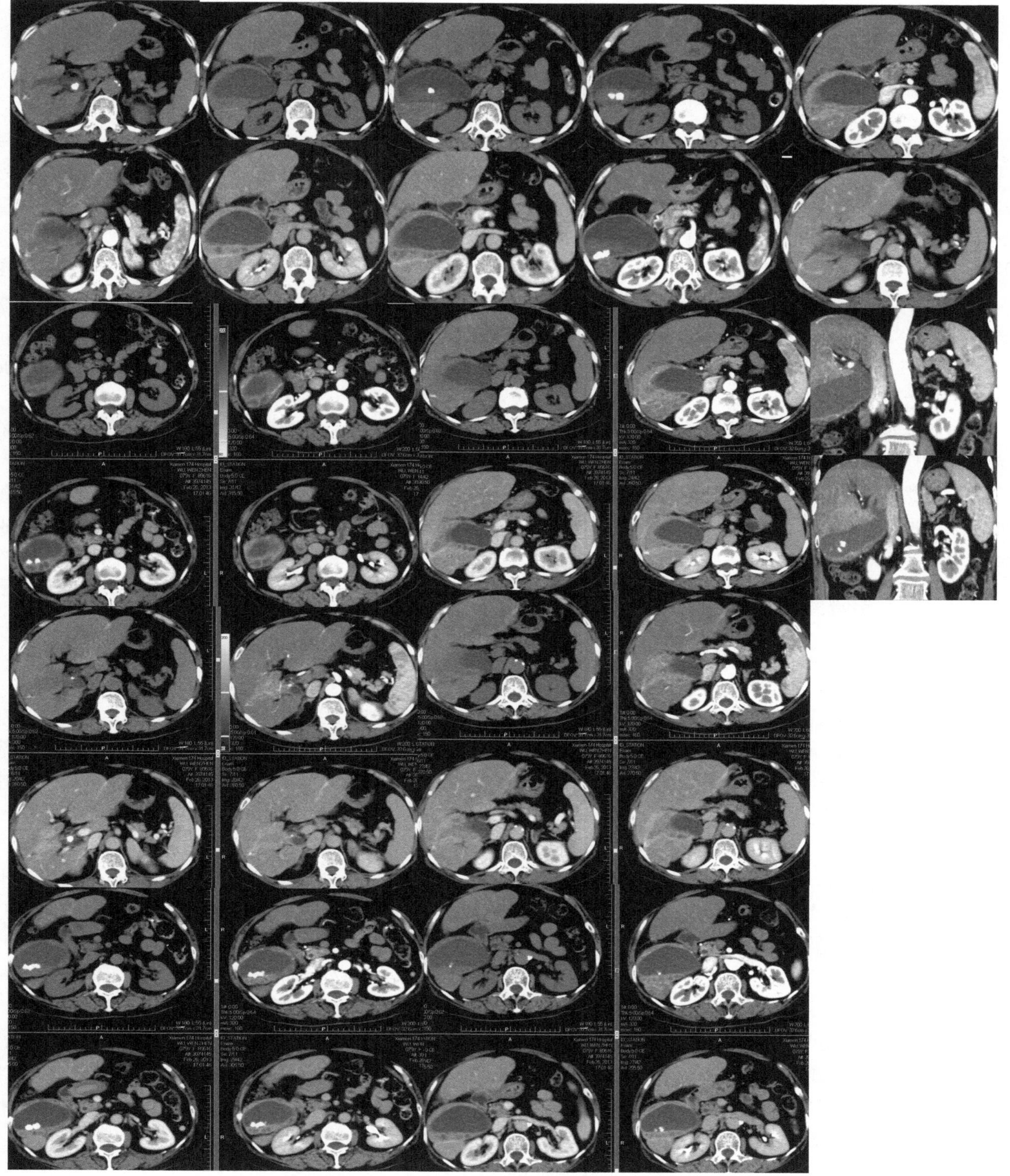

图 17-8-2 慢性坏疽性胆囊炎伴结石形成

病例，女，79 岁。右腹痛 1 月入院。

手术所见：术中见肝脏呈明显小结节性肝硬化表现，呈暗褐色，肝脏萎缩变小，向右侧旋转，胆囊大小约 12 cm × 8cm，壁厚约 1.2cm，胆囊内积脓，胆囊壁部分坏死并慢性穿透，周围被网膜及横结肠和十二指肠包裹，胆囊三角解剖结构不清，胆囊内多个褐色结石，最大者直径约 0.8cm，胆囊颈部结石嵌顿。

病理检查：胆囊组织三块，总体积 8cm × 5cm × 2.5cm，表面充血糜烂，内壁粗糙，呈灰褐色，壁厚 0.5~1.5cm，另见黑褐色结石一堆。病理诊断：慢性坏疽性胆囊炎，伴结石形成（图 17-8-2）。

第五节　钙胆汁（乳状胆汁）

钙胆汁，又名乳状胆汁、石灰胆汁、胆钙乳，是以胆汁内的微粒状物质（碳酸钙、磷酸钙、以及胆红素钙）沉淀于胆囊中，造成半液状或灰泥样物质而形成。

物理学上，钙胆汁的浓度各有不同，从浓稠的液体到油灰样团块，甚或为坚硬固体，均有报告。它的颜色可为白色、黄色、棕色或黑色，颜色深浅皆仰赖于其中胆色素含量的多寡。

与胆囊结石的发病率相比，钙胆汁实属少见，在大多数病例都伴存于胆囊管的结石性梗阻和慢性胆囊炎。一般它发生于部分性或完全性胆囊管梗阻时，此类梗阻常由结石引起。钙胆汁几乎总是伴有胆囊结石。

一、影像学研究

超声成像：十分类似于胆囊结石，出现有回声及声影的物质沉积于胆囊的低坠部分。此特点也可表现介于胆泥与胆结石之间：高回声影的物质蓄积于胆囊腔的低坠部分，形成液 - 液平，且成像光亮的胆汁位于上方。当超声有怀疑时，X 线平片总是可以确诊。

X 线腹部平片：可显示胆囊的弥漫性不透光，有时稍现结节状表现。十分类似于正常功能的胆囊。X 线水平投照可显示钙胆汁的下坠成层表现，从而做出诊断。在口服胆囊造影时，受累的胆囊功能通常降低（它们可浅淡显影），如果在造影前未拍摄平片，则可能出现危险，即将它诊断为正常。一些学者报告 6 例（5 例女性）X 线平片观察本症，以后随访中发现 1 例钙胆汁影完全消逝，另外 5 例钙胆汁量明显减少，皆伴存多发性胆囊结石。5 例为胆囊疾病症状（即上腹和右上腹痛，食入脂肪难以忍受），只有 2 例有黄疸和绞痛。在 X 线平片上，胆囊区钙胆汁显示为不同量的致密碎片影，有时伴存阳性胆囊结石。

钙胆汁影的形状常随病人体位而发生变化。在以往报告的病例中，胆囊造影通常显示功能减退或丧失，但在该作者 3 例胆囊造影中 2 例胆囊适当显影。他们着重指出，钙胆汁的自发流出并不如以前想象的那样难见，它可以出现于有黄疸或无黄疸者，也可见于有胆绞痛或无胆绞痛者，亦能如同胆囊结石自发流逝那样常见。

CT：虽然少有因钙胆汁而行 CT 扫描者，但在因其他疾病进行 CT 检查时，见到钙胆汁表现为胆囊密度明显升高，除非钙胆汁完全充满胆囊（此类情况很少），可见钙胆汁的液平面。MSCT 三维重建更可仔细观察它的表现。

在临床工作中，我们发现，钙胆汁并不像以前认为的那样少见，而是时有遇见。

有时在 CT 平扫时看到钙胆汁，病人并无胆系的症状和体征，只是因为其他疾病进行胸部和腹部常规 CT 平扫，尤其是一些身患非胸腹部的恶性肿瘤进行化疗或 / 和中草药治疗的病人，以及一些没有腹部症状和体征的健康的年青人，一般在随访不久即消失干净，不再见到，间隔时间跨度从几天到十几天。我们推测，胆汁的代谢表现不是一成不变的，时时刻刻都可能有变化，经常随着病人的饮食改变、不同的药物摄入及病人的生理状态的不同而发生一些变化，钙胆汁并不只出现于结石性胆囊炎病人。

鉴别诊断；需要考虑鉴别的情况是：出血性胆囊炎、胆系出血、对比剂摄入而尚未很好混合。钙胆汁的衰减值高于血液，而是否为对比剂则可由病史来排除。

第九章　胆囊壁的其他情况

第一节　胆囊的连接皱襞

Sukov 等(1979)在研究连接皱襞(junctional fold)时,发现此皱襞在超声扫描图像上可表现为一息肉,也可呈现为一包块,同时显示胆囊内的多重反射(混响)伪影。改变角度再扫描,可见此皱襞连接于胆囊壁上。据统计,在人群中正常可见大约 45% 的人出现此连接皱襞。此皱襞还可在超声图像上将胆囊分成两个独立的腔隙,再斜行探查,又可见二腔交通,该皱襞一直可见。突出的连接皱襞还可使胆囊变成僧帽畸形和 / 或 Z 字形,可见该皱襞发自胆囊前部,而假性淤泥能见于胆囊后部,这是由于层面厚度伪影的缘故。Fiske 和 Filly(1982)就此曾行详尽讨论。

第二节　超声和 CT 所见胆囊壁的厚度

在超声和 CT 检查中,经常需要评价胆囊壁的厚度问题。有时,胆囊较小,由于餐后胆囊收缩,囊壁较厚,不应误诊为慢性胆囊炎的小的皱缩胆囊。在蛋白过低症病人,可见胆囊壁增厚,腹水患者的胆囊壁也较厚。

第三节　慢性乙型肝炎患者胆囊壁水肿

胆囊壁水肿:胆囊壁水肿是一种常见的病理现象,可出现在急性胆囊炎、病毒性肝炎、肝功能衰竭及急性链球菌感染后肾小球肾炎等疾病中。胆囊壁水肿的 MRI 表现较具特征性:在 T_2WI 上呈明显分界的两层,与病理对照研究显示外层的高信号对应水肿的浆膜下层,内层的低信号对应完整的肌层和黏膜层。

胆囊多呈梨状,位于肝下胆囊窝内,借结缔组织附着于肝脏,分为底、体、颈三部分,颈部和胆囊管相连:胆囊壁由黏膜、肌层和外膜三层组成。黏膜层包括黏膜上皮和固有层,黏膜上皮为单层柱状,固有层为薄层结缔组织,有较丰富的血管、淋巴管和弹性纤维。肌层较薄,肌纤维排列不甚规则,有环行、斜行、纵行等。外膜较厚,为疏松结缔组织,含血管、淋巴管和神经等,外膜表面大部覆以浆膜。正常的胆囊壁在 MRI 上常无明显的分界,呈均匀厚度的一层结构。胆囊壁增厚水肿在 T_2WI 上呈清楚分界的两层:高信号的外层和低信号的内层;与病理对照研究显示高信号的外层对应水肿的浆膜下层,低信号的内层对应完整的黏膜和肌层。胆囊壁水肿的强化特征:水肿的外膜层无明显强化, T_2WI 表现为低信号的黏膜和肌层强化明显,浆膜可呈线状强化。

多种病因:胆囊壁水肿可见于多种疾病,也是病毒性肝炎的一种常见肝外表现。慢性肝炎、肝硬化时其形成机制可能与下列因素有关:①慢性肝炎、肝硬化时门静脉压力增高使门静脉属支 - 胆囊静脉回流受阻,可导致胆囊收缩下降,胆囊壁增厚水肿;②低蛋白血症导致血浆渗透压下降造成胆囊壁水肿;

③肝、胆淋巴液回流受阻,部分淋巴液可能滞留于胆囊壁内;④肝炎病毒对胆囊壁直接侵蚀;⑤邻近肝实质的炎症、坏死导致胆囊壁充血水肿。

影像学研究:对胆囊壁水肿的正确认识有助于减少误诊,判断肝内病变的严重程度。超声和CT的研究均发现胆囊壁增厚水肿可以提示病毒性肝炎肝内急性炎症的存在。

研究显示慢性乙型肝炎胆囊壁水肿的MRI,特别是脂肪抑制T_2WI能敏感地发现胆囊壁增厚、水肿,其MRI表现为胆囊壁增厚呈分层现象,外膜层的疏松结缔组织明显水肿,T_2WI呈高信号。对于慢性乙型肝炎,从炎症活动度中度开始就出现胆囊壁水肿,其出现与中重度炎症活动度有关,与慢性肝炎纤维化程度无关。胆囊壁水肿的程度与炎症活动度及纤维化程度关系不大。以胆囊壁水肿作为判断慢性肝炎炎症活动中重度存在的标准,具有较高的特异性和阳性预测值,但其敏感性较低。

鉴别诊断:胆囊壁水肿见于多种疾病,如急性胆囊炎、肝炎、肝硬化等,甚至在一些肾脏疾病也会引起胆囊壁的增厚水肿。这些疾病大都有典型的临床症状、体征及实验室指标,与慢性肝炎导致的胆囊壁水肿不难鉴别,如急性胆囊炎时除有腹痛及"墨非征"阳性外,常可见胆囊结石及胆囊腔的扩大积液,与慢性肝炎时胆囊腔的缩小不同。

总之,MRI能够较全面地描述胆囊壁水肿。对于慢性乙型肝炎,胆囊壁水肿的存在与中重度炎症活动度有关,与肝纤维化程度无关。胆囊壁水肿的程度与炎症活动度及纤维化程度均无关。对于慢性乙型肝炎,胆囊壁水肿的MRI征象可以作为判断中重度炎症活动存在的一个指标,具有较高的特异性和阳性预测值,但其敏感性较低。

第四节　误诊病例简介:胆囊穿孔、腹腔包裹性积液误诊肝包虫

由于胆管、胆囊、胆总管结石阻塞,80%胆囊炎可急性发作,严重的炎变可引起胆囊壁化脓。由于胆囊内胆汁不断淤积,排出受阻内压增加和胆囊壁的炎性水肿充血,发生化脓性胆囊炎穿孔,在胆囊窝区形成包裹性积液。一例患者因在20年前做过两次肝包虫摘除手术,胆囊穿孔形成包裹积液呈多发类圆形囊性低密度影有分隔,且位于肝下缘胆囊窝区与肝界分解不清,腹膜炎的典型临床症状不明显,故误诊为肝包虫。

但是,若仔细回顾性分析,可不难诊断,化脓性胆囊炎穿孔形成包裹性积液:有胆囊炎病史,肝内外胆管扩张,胆囊、胆总管结石梗阻,易引起胆囊炎急性发作,治疗不及时会引发胆囊穿孔;腹腔包裹性积液位于胆囊窝内与胆囊分辨不清,似胆囊增大改变;三维重建示胆囊与腹腔包裹囊肿分离中间形成通道。

所以,影像诊断医师在诊断时一定要密切结合临床表现,深入地观察,全面综合分析。

第十章　胆囊发育变异和先天异常

第一节　胆囊形态变异和异常

胆系的胚胎学:胚胎第3周肝胆系统开始发育,于原始前肠腹侧发出一个对裂芽,这一内胚层憩室较大的头侧部分被称作肝部,代表肝实质和肝内胆管始基;较小的尾侧部分被称作囊部,形成胆囊和肝外胆管。胚胎第5~7周,增生的内胚层细胞空泡形成,使这些结构出现了一个开放的腔。第12周,随着肝脏发育成熟,肝内胆管伴随门静脉分支生长,并排泄分泌胆汁。因此,在妊娠的前3个月,遗传因素、环境因素、母体的局部或全身状况都会影响到肝胆系统的正常发育。

胆囊的影像检查:腹部平片通常不能显示胆囊,只有在胆囊腔内含有阳性对比剂、气体、不透X线的结石、钙胆汁或囊壁钙化形成瓷瓶样胆囊时,才得以显示。断面成像能很好显示胆囊,特别是禁食胆囊处于扩张状态时更易显示。胆囊常表现为梨形,附着于肝右叶和方叶下面,突入叶间裂。

诊断胆系疾病,可利用各种影像学技术,以超声最常用,最好使用实时超声和5.0MHz的探头。病人应禁食12h,使胆囊充盈胆汁,以便更好地显示腔内结石、肿块、胆囊壁厚度和黏膜分隔。每一个超声图像仅覆盖一个薄的矢状面或横断面,深度有限,因此,在同一时间内不能观察到整个胆囊结构,易造成误诊,尤其是位于胆囊颈或胆囊管的小结石,常被十二指肠内气体掩盖;胆囊萎缩或异位时,也容易误诊。

CT或MRI断面成像技术上固有的局限性,也影响着胆囊病变的显示。因此,要认真做好每一种检查,并仔细分析研究,确保胆囊和胆管的完全显示,才利于正确诊断结石或观察病理改变。常规腹部成像常见到胆囊位置、形态、数目的发育变异和先天性异常。虽然多数无临床意义,但可能会误诊为胆囊病变,也可能增加胆系手术或介入治疗中损伤的危险性。

胆囊的先天变异和异常:胆囊的先天变异和异常可分为形状、大小、数目与位置的改变四类。胆囊或胆管发育变异和发育异常并不少见,多数经手术或尸检偶然发现,随着被疑有胆系疾病或无相关腹部疾病影像学检查的增多,发现也随之增加。罕见的胆囊和胆管解剖形态给影像科医师的诊断带来了困难,也容易造成术中意外事故和医源性损伤,尤其对于腹腔镜下胆囊切除术,在这种视野有限的情况下更是如此。

从另外角度看,胆囊的先天变异和异常还可分为:形态异常,胆囊憩室,胆囊缺如,胆囊位置异常,肠系膜异常。胆囊常见的先天异常为大小与形状的异常,少见的先天异常有:双重胆囊,胆囊分开,甚至胆囊管也分开;胆囊缺如,少数病例还可见到胆囊管。

胆囊发育不全:胆囊缺如可见于某些动物,如鼠和马。而人类可出现胆囊和胆囊管发育不全,其发生率大约占新生儿的1/6000,女性与男性之比为3:1,具有家族性。

50%的病人同时伴有其他异常,包括先天性心脏病、肛门闭锁、直肠阴道瘘、气管食管瘘、无脾、马蹄肾及其他多种异常。

在报道的200余例胆囊发育不全中,多数是经手术或尸检意外发现的,大约半数的病人出现餐后腹痛或胆绞痛、厌脂肪餐及其他症状,这些临床表现均是因胆道运动障碍或胆总管结石所致。术前的影像检查未显示胆囊,常归因于慢性胆囊炎所致的胆囊萎缩,因而使某些病人去接受不必要的胆囊切除术,术中才惊奇地发现胆囊缺如。因此,超声、CT或胆管造影未显示胆囊和胆囊管时,应考虑到胆囊发育不全。

胆囊发育不全或胆囊退化常见于儿童早期即有胆汁淤滞的病人,其主要原因可能是胆管闭锁、新生儿肝炎或胆管炎和胆囊纤维化。

重复胆囊:人类重复胆囊的发生率约为 1/5000,但在驯养的哺乳动物中却十分常见。真正的重复胆囊(双胆囊畸形)有两套独立的胆囊和胆囊管,后者可汇合后开口于肝外胆管(Y 型),或分别在不同的部位开口于肝外胆管(H 型)。两个胆囊常彼此相邻,位于胆囊窝内。

副胆囊也可位于肝内或其他部位,引流至左或右肝管。单个或两个胆囊病变或结石并不少见。正确认识这一异常,可避免术中意外事故的发生或将来不必要的二次手术。

双腔胆囊(胆囊分隔)是指由一个隔膜将胆囊分割成两个毗邻的腔,与真正的重复胆囊相比,它仅有一个胆囊颈和胆囊管。胆囊先天性大憩室也可出现类似的表现。

MRCP、口服胆囊造影、直接胆管造影或 ERCP 充盈胆囊腔,可正确诊断重复胆囊或双腔胆囊;超声或 CT 也可显示这些异常。需要与胆囊窝内重复胆囊相鉴别的病变包括胆总管囊肿、胆囊憩室、折叠胆囊、局灶性腺肌瘤病、胆囊周围积液或积脓。

诊断陷阱:口服胆囊造影时,胃幽门的轴位像与胆囊影重迭,形似裂隙状胆囊结石。偶尔十二指肠球部气体轴位像出现于上腹部平片上,可伪似气肿性胆囊炎伴胆囊结石。

第二节 胆囊结构变异和异常

由于胆囊解剖、腔内胆汁充盈程度、病变侵犯范围的不同,以及邻近结构的外部压迫,胆囊的大小和形态在影像学检查中可出现很大变化。

胆囊分隔:胆囊形态最常见的变异是所谓的自由帽畸形,发生率约 5%,,它大约出现于 2%~6% 的人群中。此名字的由来是,类似天主教红衣主教的红帽的形状的帽子,被古希腊的奴隶领袖戴上,作为他们解放的象征。其特征是胆囊底部出现一个黏膜间隔或皱襞。横断面 CT 或超声图像上,自由帽畸形,也被称作僧帽畸形或变异,可类似于重复胆囊或双腔胆囊,在分隔的胆囊底部可出现胆汁淤积和结石。

以往,学者们都认为僧帽状胆囊无临床意义,只是胆囊底部纠集或皱折。目前,不少学者指出,当此类底部皱折(事实上,不少已有胆囊内部分隔)不影响胆汁的进出时,它可无临床症状,仅为一无症状的先天变异而已;当其影响胆汁的进出时,常可促使炎症发生与形成结石,多有临床表现,此刻,则不应称作先天变异,事实上已为先天异常了。僧帽状胆囊口服胆囊造影的表现颇具特征性。

类似的皱折可出现于胆囊的更近侧,在此类病例,这征象必须与有时见于腺肌瘤病的增厚的分隔区别。在腺肌瘤病,口服胆囊造影时刺激后检查常可见罗 - 阿窦(R-A 窦)充盈。

不论是在腺肌瘤病的分隔胆囊,还是突出的僧帽状胆囊畸形,在 CT 扫描图像上均可伪似双重胆囊。适当的使用薄层扫描,加上实时超声成像,则可除外双重胆囊。十分少见的情况,多发性薄的分隔出现于胆囊中(先天性多分隔胆囊)。在此类先天异常,胆汁可以停滞于分隔的小囊内,促使结石易于形成。在先天性分隔胆囊与环状腺肌瘤病,胆系核素显像,能显示远侧部分一个或多个延迟充盈,相当于这些部分胆汁有淤滞。外表观察,多分隔胆囊是轻微结节化。组织学上,分隔的壁为表面两层上皮组织夹着一薄层肌肉组织。口服胆囊造影与超声检查可以明确诊断先天性分隔状胆囊。

正常的胆囊管内可见 Heister 螺旋皱襞(胆囊颈螺旋瓣),其功能是根据胆管腔内压力调节胆囊的充盈和排空。有些病人的螺旋襞或黏膜间隔可延伸至胆囊颈,在 CT 图像上类似于结石,超声对螺旋襞之间的小结石可能漏诊。

多隔胆囊:多隔胆囊是一种少见的先天性异常,由多个黏膜间隔将胆囊分隔为多个相互连通的腔,它是由于发育中的胆囊不完全的空泡形成或上皮层过度内折所致。多隔胆囊可具有正常的形态和功能,但易发生结石。口服胆囊造影、CT 或超声能很好地显示其特征性形态,表现为蜂窝状或多囊状胆囊。脱落的胆囊上皮和息肉状胆固醇异常沉积表现可类似于多隔胆囊,需要与之鉴别。

胆囊畸形:一种少见的先天性或后天性胆囊畸

形，影像学上易于混淆。例如，胆囊腔局限性环状狭窄使胆囊呈葫芦状，胆囊的长轴层面可表现为双腔胆囊或分隔状胆囊，但在轴面 CT 层面上，由于容积效应，该狭窄区的表现可类似于胆结石。

胆囊憩室：在 CT 或超声图像上，胆囊表现为变形的多囊结构，而非圆形或梨形，这种少见的形态见于先天性胆囊憩室，或见于腺肌瘤病所致的后天性假性憩室。后者的特征是黏膜增生，突入胆囊壁肥厚的肌层形成罗基坦斯基 - 阿索夫（Rokitansky-Aschoff）窦（简称罗 - 阿窦），可呈局灶性、节段性或弥漫性分布。超声图像上，这些壁内假性憩室表现为增厚的胆囊壁内多个无回声区，可含有产生回声的结石。弥漫性生长的腺肌瘤病的 CT 表现十分有特征，胆囊变形或呈分叶状，周围绕以成簇的囊状结构，并可突入邻近的肝实质。

第三节　胆囊数目的变异和异常

先天性胆囊缺如：胆囊的先天性缺如，在人类是十分少见的情况（在马与鼠则为正常的表现），它的出现，不是归因于胆囊胚芽发育的缺如，就是由于胚胎发育时再管道化的失误。胆囊管可与先天性胆囊缺如一起缺如，也可单独存在。

与先天性胆囊缺如同时伴存的状态包括：胆系闭锁、左侧同质异构（多脾症）、直肠阴道瘘、肛门闭锁、单骨或多骨缺如。但是，病人其他部位也可以完全正常。

在过去，本症都是依靠于对右上腹有症状病人的手术，口服胆囊造影或静脉胆系造影有时胆囊不显影而做出诊断。今天，当怀疑有本症时，可用超声或 CT 合并核素显像进行证实。如果细心的超声检查在通常胆囊的部位未发现胆囊，在 CT 和胆系核素显像腹部未见到胆囊影像时，在不见外科手术瘢痕的情况下，先天性胆囊缺如必须考虑。

双重胆囊与三重胆囊：双重胆囊是极为少见的先天性解剖异常。在确定诊断之前，两个分离的胆囊腔与两条分离的胆囊管必须观察到。两条胆囊管可能在进入肝外胆管之前互相连接。额外的胆囊可能是异常的胆囊，但是，在双重胆囊，一般说来两个胆囊的大小大致相等。

病因学理论包括，胆囊管、肝内胆管或总胆管囊袋化发育的持续，它们在正常情况下应该退化或进行不完全性再管状化。三重胆囊在人类极为罕见。一个分叉的胆囊有两个腔，但只有一条胆囊管。上述胆囊数目上的先天异常，除了它们可能倾向于产生结石和 / 或出现间歇性胆囊管梗阻以外，其临床意义甚小。一个先天性胆囊憩室容易与双重胆囊或分叉胆囊混淆。囊性肝内胆管的持续存在的结果，可以或可能不引起胆汁淤滞和结石的形成。在组织学上，它含有正常胆囊壁的所有各层结构。

第四节 假的双胆囊

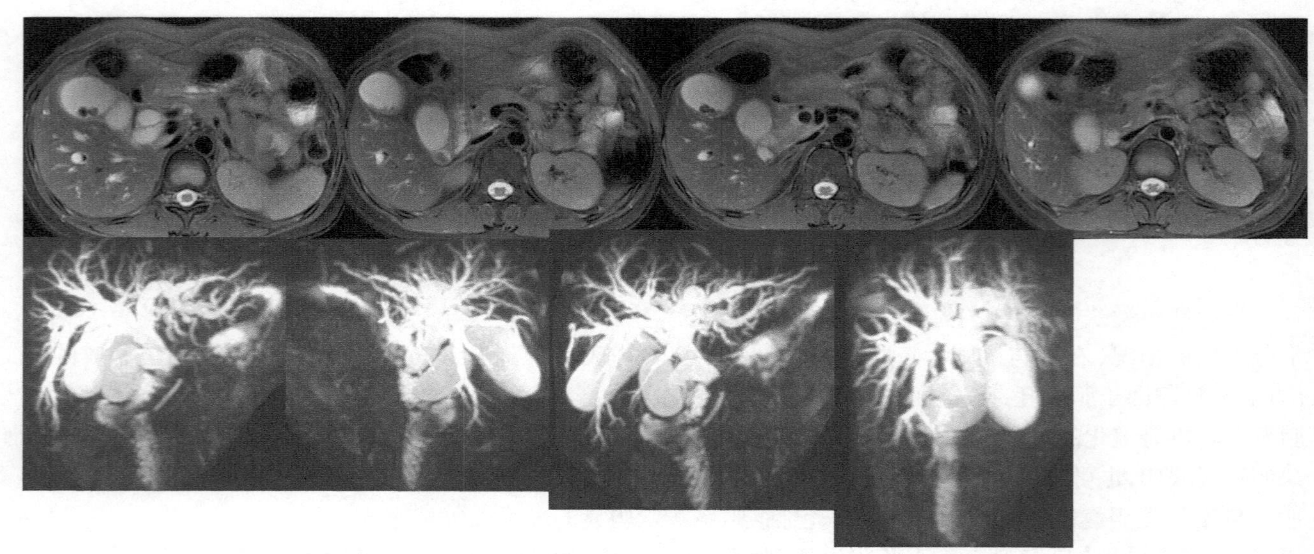

图 17-10-1 假的双胆囊

患者,女,24 岁。患者于 5 年前无明显诱因,渐出现右上腹部疼痛不适,呈持续性胀痛,无放射痛,未随体位、饮食改变而变化,无畏寒、发热、黄疸,疼痛持续约半小时自行缓解,无恶心、呕吐、返酸、嗳气,未予诊治,症状反复发作,今以腹痛待诊住院诊治。

手术所见:可见胆囊结石和肝外胆管结石。术前 MRI 怀疑双胆囊,实际上是一个胆囊,另一个较小的囊状影为扩张的胆囊管造成。

双胆囊发生率为 1/3000~1/4000,系胚胎期形成胆囊及胆囊管的胚芽组织分为 2 个部分,各自发育成独立的胆囊及胆囊管。双胆囊可都在肝右叶,或一右一左,或一下一上,或一大一小,每个胆囊都有自己的胆囊管,且分别汇入胆总管或联合成"Y"形总胆囊管后再汇入胆总管(图 17-10-1)。

第五节 胆囊位置的变异和异常

胆囊位置异常可分为:漂浮胆囊,肝后和肾后胆囊,肝内胆囊,肝上胆囊,左侧胆囊,横位胆囊。其中以后位胆囊最为少见。异位胆囊内不透 X 线的结石可类似于邻近脏器钙化的囊肿或肿瘤。胆囊位置异常可增加手术或介入治疗的难度和医源性损伤。

(1)漂浮胆囊:胆囊异位的一个常见原因是由于肠系膜附着部松弛导致胆囊过度移位,也就是说,最常见的位置异常是漂浮胆囊,也称游离胆囊,它倾向于发生扭转或出现经小网膜孔的疝。漂浮胆囊完全为腹膜包绕,并且以一系膜附着于肝脏。正常情况下,胆囊表面有腹膜覆盖,固定在肝下面。大约 4%~5% 人群的胆囊和部分胆囊管由一个长度不同的肠系膜系带悬吊在肝下面,被称为"游离、游走或悬垂胆囊"。这种可移动性胆囊可远离肝脏而移至中腹部或左侧腹部,或呈管状逐渐延长达盆腔。此类胆囊也可突入网膜孔,发生自发性扭转和缺血性坏死。非疝入的胆囊发生扭转比疝入的胆囊扭转多见,女性与男性之比约为 3:1,此类病人典型者为 60 岁至 80 岁的瘦小老妇。其症状与体征类似于急性胆囊炎。如不治疗,可进展为坏疽,且可出现腹膜炎。影像学表现的特点是非结石性胆囊炎的表现。

胆囊通过小网膜孔发现疝,可以是间断性的和无症状的,也可引起不明确的不适感,或发生绞窄。非绞窄病例的常规的影像学表现包括:显影的胆囊向中线移位靠近十二指肠球部，胆囊似乎悬挂在球部尖端上方，最好的观察方法是口服胆囊造影后再作上消化道钡餐检查。CT 和超声成像的表现可能是非特异性的，只显示一个囊状的结构位于小网膜囊内。如果其内存在着胆囊结石，则可提示正确的诊断。在放射性核素显像时，如果能排除核素示踪剂返流进入胃，与胆系核素显像进行比较，常对诊断有帮助。在已发生了绞窄的病例，为做出诊断，常常必须经皮进行穿刺抽吸。在 CT 或超声图像上，位于一个少见部位的游离胆囊可类似于软组织肿块或囊性病变，但细心观察可发现它与肝门部相连接，在肝下胆囊窝内无胆囊结构。

（2）肝后和肾后胆囊：这两种少见类型的异位胆囊分别位于肝脏或右肾后方。断面成像中，该类型异位胆囊如果不行胆管造影使之充盈对比剂，可能误诊为肾脏、肾上腺或肝囊肿。异位胆囊内不透 X 线的结石可类似于邻近脏器钙化的囊肿或肿瘤。胆囊位置异常可增加手术或介入治疗的难度和医源性损伤。胆囊 99% 位于肝主叶间裂水平的肝下内侧面，肝主叶间裂在 CT 图像上作为左右叶的分界标志，大多数人的胆囊偏下前方。Gross（1936）报告 5 例手术证实的肝后胆囊，Blanton 等（1974）报道 1 例放射性核素检查因肝后区有核素缺损区而疑肝内病变，后经静脉法胆系造影证实为肝后胆囊，首次于手术前诊断了肝后胆囊。Nardi 等（1988）用超声和 CT 诊断 2 例肝后胆囊。

胚胎发育：胚胎发育第四周初，在前肠与卵黄蒂交界处内胚层增厚，向腹侧生长出一囊状突起，即肝憩室，从其头端分出头支和尾支，头支发育成肝脏和肝管，尾支发育成胆囊和胆囊管。在肝憩室的头支尾支分化过程中，胆系原基发生异位或游移，则可形成胆囊异位。

临床表现：肝后胆囊的病人发生胆囊炎时，可产生酷似胸膜病变的胸痛，胸膜反应，肩痛及肾盂肾炎等症状体征，术前明确诊断对外科医生手术处理方法的选择亦有重要的指导意义。Nardi 等（1988）报道的 2 例病人均有严重的肝硬化，1 例为酒精中毒性肝硬化，1 例为肝色素沉着症，他们皆伴有明显的肝右叶萎缩，肝左叶增生。因此，该作者认为，胆囊异位不是由于先天发育异常而是继发性的，是由于明显的形态学紊乱导致胆囊沿着一个轴逆转所造成，但是，该作者同时复习了 150 例肝硬化病人的资料，均未见类似的肝后胆囊征象，于是，他本人对上述提法也未能持肯定态度。国人刘爱莲等（1992）报告 2 例肝后胆囊病例，亦有轻度的肝形态学改变，但都不足以诊断肝硬化，而且，该组作者也复习了 150 例肝硬化病人资料，虽然这些病例皆有不同程度的肝叶比例失调，胆囊移位，胆囊旋转，胆都未形成肝后胆囊，因此，他们认为肝后胆囊是一种先天发育异常，而不是肝硬化所致。

影像学研究：由于肝后胆囊在 CT 扫描时易误诊为肝内病变，提高对肝后胆囊的认识是非常重要的。在 CT 扫描时，正常胆囊窝处未见到胆囊者，不能只考虑为胆囊缺如，胆囊畸形或慢性胆囊炎所致的胆囊萎缩，也应考虑有异位胆囊的可能，应注意在其他部位寻找有无可疑的胆囊影，确诊须进行 CT 胆系造影，此时，可清楚显示与胆管系统同时显影的胆囊而予确诊。除 X 线胆囊造影所见胆囊位置变异可导致漏诊外，Greaves 等（1983）介绍超声检查胆囊时还发现肝后方的胆囊：胆囊位于通常胆囊位置的外侧，纵断观察可见囊状结构，肝的主叶裂也移向右侧。肝肿大还可将胆囊向左侧推移。肝后胆囊亦应注意与局限性肝包膜下积液，右肾上腺病变，右肾上极突出的囊肿或肿瘤相鉴别。

（3）肝前胆囊：显著前位的胆囊位于肝和腹壁之间，超声扫描如不留心，可将之误为一脓肿。

（4）肝内胆囊：肝内胆囊，意指胆囊位于肝内，胆囊部分或全部包埋于肝实质内，它完全被肝实质包围，约占人群的 9%。尽管部分地埋置于肝实质中并不难见，但完全性地位于肝内却十分少见。在超声或 CT 图像上，肝内胆囊表现类似于肝囊肿、脓肿或坏死囊变的转移灶，根据它与肝叶间裂及胆囊管的关系可做出正确诊断。肝内胆囊排空和功能受周围肝实质的影响，易产生结石。急性胆囊炎体检时，由于其位置深，又无腹膜炎征象，临床表现容易与其他病变混淆。此类胆囊患病时，行胆囊切除术非常困难，而且，这可能是由于放射性核素肝 - 脾显像的错误解释所致。如果考虑有肝内胆囊的可能性时，放射性胆系核素显像应避免可能产生的错误。超声成像与 CT 扫描也出现错误，但不如核素硫胶显像那么常见。

肝内胆囊病人无论是开腹胆囊切除术或是经腹腔镜胆囊切除术，均易引起肝脏损伤和出血，增加了手术难度。术后 CT 复查，在切除的胆囊区域常可见到胆汁或血液聚集，类似于术前的胆囊、肝囊肿或脓肿。

(5)肝上胆囊:这一少见的先天性异常与肝右叶前段发育不良和结肠肝区上移有关。肝硬化时右叶萎缩可出现类似的表现。CT 或超声显示右侧膈下异位的胆囊,类似于肝周液体聚集或脓肿。异位胆囊可位于腹膜后间隙、肝内、肝上、镰状韧带和前腹壁等处。肝上胆囊相当少见,考虑其胚胎学关系为肝右叶缺乏正常的生长,留下胆囊"搁浅于"肝上部位,造成结肠肝曲也移向颅侧。肝上胆囊在核素肝胆显像与 X 线口服胆囊造影一般难以发现而造成误诊。

Faintuch 等(1980)报告 3 例肝上胆囊,皆伴肝发育不良和结肠肝曲上移。Regen 等(1965),Anderson 等(1970),Blanton 等(1974)及 Youngwirth 等(1983)相继报道肝上胆囊的个案。他们指出,当核素肝胆显像或 X 线口服胆囊造影未看见胆囊时,应随时想到肝上胆囊的可能。这些检查的观察范围宜包括所有膈下区域。

(6)左侧胆囊:左侧胆囊,既可以是全内脏转位的一个内容,也可以是一个孤立的表现。胆囊还可横亘位于中线(不确定的位置)。胆囊位于左上腹部,当这一典型部位见于全内脏转位的病人时,肝脏、胆囊和其他内脏之间的关系保持正常,但它们是正常关系的镜像。左侧胆囊也见于因肠系膜附着处发育缺陷所致的游离胆囊、中肠旋转不良或单独发生。

在报道的大约 50 例左侧胆囊中,多数胆囊位于肝左叶下方和镰状韧带左侧,胆囊管越过中线汇合至胆总管或左肝管。如果 CT 或超声在正常胆囊窝位置看不到胆囊,应考虑到左侧胆囊的可能性,并仔细观察肝左叶下方区域。左侧胆囊病人可能同时伴有其他先天性异常(如多脾、下腔静脉与半奇静脉连接中断)。Naganuma 等(1998)和 Maetani 等(1998)相继报告了与胆囊异位有关的各种异常的超声和 CT 表现。

(7)其他位置异常:胆囊的其他少见位置异常包括:靠近脊柱的后份、沿着下腔静脉、在镰状韧带内、在横行巨结肠内、甚至在前腹壁内。这些少见位置异常,除可能引起影像学的问题外,一般少有临床意义或无更大的临床意义。胆囊位置上的发育变异很大,偶尔可低于肝下缘,亦可位于结肠肝曲附近。

(8)后天性胆囊异位:肝硬化引起肝萎缩时,胆囊向前移至肝脏与腹壁之间的腹膜腔隙内,影像表现类似于先天性肝上胆囊。后天性胆囊异位也见于肝段切除术后或右肾切除术后,可活动的胆囊易下垂至术后的空虚区域。

第六节 胆囊大小的异常

胆囊发育不全:发育不全的胆囊或发展不健全的胆囊是先天性的异常,但无明确的临床意义。此类体积较小的胆囊有功能,不含有结石,可除外慢性胆囊炎。

关于小胆囊:小胆囊另外的原因,在儿童与青少年,应该除外囊性纤维化。胆囊异常见于囊性纤维化病人中的 1/3~1/2,其典型的征象包括:体积小、功能差、边缘不规则、蹼样的分隔、而且通常无结石。在病理检查时,可见异常的胆囊中含有浓稠的色淡的胆汁,细胞内和黏膜下囊肿内的黏液蓄积。在文献上,胆囊壁增厚的病因学讨论甚多,有作者在有关超声诊断的论著中提到,胆囊收缩是一常见原因,此种真正的胆囊壁增厚只在空腹病人中观察到,此刻,胆囊正居于最强烈的收缩状态中。Vogler Ⅲ 等(1986)指出,在 CT 图像上,由于病人进餐,胆囊收缩可造成胆囊十分缩小,而不应误为慢性胆囊炎的皱缩或挛缩的小胆囊。

第十一章 胆囊创伤与胆囊术后

第一节 腹腔镜胆囊切除术的并发症

详见 本书 本卷 第十五篇 第九章 第二节 腹腔镜胆囊切除术的并发症。

第二节 诊断陷阱：胆囊切除术后银夹

胆囊切除术留置的银夹与胆管靠得很近时，有时可类似于胆管结石。利用包括横断面成像在内的两个平面的 MR 胆管成像技术，可鉴别银夹和结石。多数情况下，横断面成像可显示银夹的无信号区位于胆管外，并可见来自于银夹的磁敏感性伪影。

第三节 误诊病例简介：胆囊切除术后，肝内胆管细胞癌与炎症性纤维增生

患者，女，60 岁。胆囊切除术后 4 年，右上腹闷痛 3 月入院。CT：胰腺轻度萎缩，正常强化，组织密度均匀，未见明显高或低密度影，胰管稍扩张，宽约 0.32cm。腹膜后未见明显肿大淋巴结。胆囊切除术后。肝门结构不清楚，肝门区约 3.0cm × 5.0cm × 3.5cm 软组织块，平扫 CT 值 35~44HU，增强三期逐步强化，CT 值分别为 58、71、83HU，右肝内胆管扩张，内见多个斑片状高密度影，右肝后右下段萎缩，胆总管下端无梗阻。CT 诊断：胰腺轻度萎缩，胰管稍扩张，胆囊切除术后改变；肝门区软组织影逐渐强化，性质？炎症性纤维增生？术后改变？请结合临床。右肝内胆管多发结石、扩张，右肝后叶下段萎缩，胆汁性肝硬化可能。MRI：肝右叶及尾状叶增大变形，左外叶体积明显缩小并见分叶状软组织肿块影，T_1WI 低信号，T_2WI 压脂稍高信号，边缘模糊，内见不规则扩张的肝内胆管影，肝门结构不清，肝门区及腹膜后可见多个肿大淋巴结影，部分融合，边界不清。MRCP 示肝内外胆管扩张，以右后叶下段明管明显且管腔内见多个大小不等的结石影充填，肝总管及胆总管中上段扩张，最大径约 1.2cm，下段逐渐变细，管腔内未见明显异常信号影，胆囊缺如呈术后改变，胰管轻度扩张。MRI 诊断：肝右叶肝内胆管多发结石伴肝内外胆管及胰管扩张；肝左外叶异常信号影，考虑：胆管癌，慢性炎症？伴肝门及腹膜后淋巴结肿大，请结合临床。

手术所见：大网膜与右侧腹壁粘连，松解粘连后暴露肝脏，见胆囊缺如，左肝萎缩变硬，第一肝门粘连严重，胰头区可触及质硬肿物，与周围组织粘连成团，右肝后叶可触及结石，胃肠未见明显异常。切取左肝变硬肿块送冰冻病理检查，检查回报考虑胆管癌。故术中诊断肝门部胆管癌伴腹膜后转移，行肿瘤姑息治疗。病理检查：冰冻病理及常规病理：肝左内叶切除标本：不规则软组织一块，大小 8cm × 4cm × 2cm，切面灰黄灰白，质中偏韧。冰冻病理诊断：肝左内叶切除标本：镜下可见腺癌组织侵犯肝小叶，结合临床病史，初步考虑胆管癌，待做常规石蜡切片及免疫组化检测进一步明确。常规病理诊断：肝左内叶切除标本：中分化肝内胆管细胞癌，癌组织

侵犯周围肝组织。免疫组化诊断:肝左内叶切除标本:中分化肝内胆管细胞癌,癌组织侵犯周围肝

组织。

第十二章　胆囊其他疾病和诊断陷阱

第一节　胆囊的假肿瘤

详见本书 本卷 本篇 第六章 第四节　胆囊的假肿瘤。

第二节　胆囊核素显像的假阴性

Echevarria 等(1980)报告 2 例急性胆囊炎患者,1 例手术证实为急性坏疽性出血性胆囊炎,胆囊腔内有多数小结石,另例临床上为一过性胆囊管阻塞,最后排出结石;但他们的肝胆核素显像都未发现胆囊的异常。急性胆囊炎几乎都是胆囊颈内结石在胆囊管口处嵌塞的结果,胆汁淤积引起胆囊壁的炎性改变;5%~8% 的病人为急性非阻塞性胆囊炎。该作者指出,单纯从胆囊核素显像阴性实不能排除所有的急性胆囊炎。

第三节　超声扫描中的假胆囊

在超声检查时,充盈液体的十二指肠肠袢可被误认为胆囊影像。但仔细观察则可发现此假胆囊的壁不甚清晰,其内容物通常无回声。再横断扫描,可见真正的胆囊与上述假胆囊彼此靠近。纵切真正的胆囊,则见它的壁显示清晰,而其内容物是透声的。另有作者报道,在胆囊切除术后的病人,手术野的血肿和纤维化形成,可在纵切超声图像上显示为假性胆囊。

第四节　胆囊内众多小的回声区

Gooding(1981)在讨论胆囊空肠造口吻合术病人超声扫描时指出,胆囊内返流的食物颗粒可佯似胆石的表现,同样,在胆胰管下端括约肌切开术后食物返流入胆囊,引起众多的小回声区,颇似结石,引起误诊。

第五节　胆囊的影像学检查及诊断陷阱

腹部平片通常不能显示胆囊,只有在胆囊腔内含有阳性对比剂、气体、不透 X 线的结石、钙胆汁或囊壁钙化形成瓷瓶样胆囊时,才得以显示。断面成像能很好显示胆囊,特别是禁食胆囊处于扩张状态时更易显示。胆囊常表现为梨形,附着于肝右叶和方叶下面,突入叶间裂。

在美国,成人胆结石和胆囊炎发病率高,每年手术者几乎达60万,每年的医疗费用超过50亿美元。诊断胆系疾病,可利用各种影像学技术,以超声最常用,最好使用实时超声和5.0MHz的探头。病人应禁食12h,使胆囊充盈胆汁,以便更好地显示腔内结石、肿块、胆囊壁厚度和黏膜分隔。每一个超声图像仅覆盖一个薄的矢状面或横断面,深度有限,因此,在同一时间内不能观察到整个胆囊结构,易造成误诊,尤其是位于胆囊颈或胆囊管的小结石,常被十二指肠内气体掩盖;胆囊萎缩或异位时,也容易误诊。

CT或MRI断面成像技术上固有的局限性,也影响着胆囊病变的显示。因此,要认真做好每一种检查,并仔细分析研究,确保胆囊和胆管的完全显示,才利于正确诊断结石或观察病理改变。常规腹部成像常见到胆囊位置、形态、数目的发育变异和先天性异常。虽然多数无临床意义,但可能会误诊为胆囊病变,也可能增加胆系手术或介入治疗中损伤的危险性。

第十八篇　胆囊管疾病

第一章　胆囊管疾病

第一节　胆囊管发育变异及病变

胆囊管的发育变异及病变在临床上有重要意义，精准的影像学检查能避免胆系手术时损伤胆囊管，对明确胆囊切除术后综合征的病因也能提供参考。一般说来，胆囊管长约35mm，直径约3mm，靠近胆囊段的胆囊管有螺旋形黏膜皱襞，称为Heister瓣形皱襞，近胆总管段较为光滑，结构并不复杂。然而，它在临床上却有着重要意义，若对其发育变异不熟悉，则可能在做内镜及外科手术时产生困惑。

1. 胆囊管的发育变异和先天异常　开口位置的发育变异：有的胆囊管开口较高，在肝门区，因而肝总管短，胆总管长；有的开口很低，接近十二指肠，因而肝总管长，胆总管短。少数胆囊管开口于胆总管的左侧，经胆总管的前或后方，迂回至右侧与胆囊连接，这种胆囊管特别长，可导致引流不畅，并发胆囊炎。

Ichii等(2002)依据走行及开口位置不同，将胆囊管解剖分为6型：右侧开口(Ⅰ)；左侧开口，在胆管前走行(Ⅱ)；左侧开口，在胆管后走行(Ⅲ)；在肝门区开口(Ⅳ)；在胰腺段胆管开口(Ⅴ)；其他类型(Ⅵ)。

Fric等(1990)调查了1 574例行ERCP检查的病人(男706例，女868例)，发现乳头区憩室(PPD)在低位胆囊管(乳头上5mm内)中频繁出现($P<0.001$)，女性乳头区憩室伴低位开口胆囊管者与不伴低位胆囊管开口者有显著性差异($P<0.05$)，原因不能简单归于年龄因素，低位胆囊管开口可能是病因，因为它影响了胆汁的运输，所以低位胆囊管伴乳头区憩室是一种新的综合征。

Gallonay(1984)报道了一例十二指肠组织易位于胆囊管，非常罕见。

Cabajo-Caballero等(1997)指出，胆囊缺如亦罕见，多伴有胆囊管的缺如。

胆囊和胆囊管的先天性异常，其临床意义在于，进行胆系外科手术时，必须要熟悉先天异常，从而避免意外损伤，影像诊断工作者也必须具备这种知识，以便合理解释影像。

2. 胆囊管发育变异的临床研究　近年来，有研究表明胆囊管的变异与结石形成有关。在结石形成过程中胆囊起重要作用，但胆囊管的形态和开口位置的不同也可能影响这个过程。

Caroli等(1997)研究了胆囊管长度和开口位置对胆结石形成的影响。将1992—1994年间270例做了ERCP的病人随机分为无胆石组(113例，男65例，女48例)和有胆石组(157例，男73例，女84例)，对胆囊管长度及其开口位置分别作了详细的记录。结果发现胆囊管汇入左侧肝管是结石形成的易感因素，而胆囊管的长度与结石形成无直接关联。

Castelain等(1993)将168例经ERCP检查胆囊管显影的病例分为3组：第1组57例，无胆结石；第2组27例，有胆囊结石，胆管无结石；第3组34例，胆管结石伴或不伴有胆囊结石。测量胆囊管最宽径及最窄径。最大直径第3组为(7.72 ± 2.29)mm，第2组为(4.59 ± 1.13)mm，第1组为(2.63 ± 0.67)mm，三者之间有显著性差异($P<0.001$)。最小径：第3组为(5.00 ± 0.99)mm，第2组为(3.10 ± 0.62)mm，第1组为(1.83 ± 0.53)mm。

最大径与最小径的不同表明了胆石病不同程度的进展，胆管结石组的胆囊管比其他二组增粗明显，似说明胆管结石伴存的炎症可能累及胆囊管。此外，胆囊管直径的增加可实现碎石术后胆石的排出，也有利于ERCP或腹腔镜胆囊切除术的操作。

通常认为胆囊运动功能减退是胆囊结石形成的

最初原因，但胆囊管开口位置的不同也起重要作用，因开口位置在左侧时，胆汁通过胆囊管的阻力增加，从而使胆囊内容物（如胆固醇结晶）冲洗效应减弱，易于沉积下来。

Uetsuji 等（1993）经术前术中胆系造影及术中肉眼观察胆囊管汇入总肝管的部位，将 468 例胆系疾病病人和 39 例胆囊管低位汇入并且长度增加者编为一组，与 358 例患有胆结石，但胆囊管汇入正常者进行对比研究。低位汇入组胆总管短，发生了严重的并发症：7 例胆石性胰腺炎，7 例 Mirizzi 综合征，3 例胆囊癌，2 例汇合口结石，1 例胆囊管扩张。证明了胆囊管异位汇入可造成胆汁滞留和 / 或胰液返流入胆管，使并发症增多，同时造成胆胰管粘连，导致手术困难。

第二节 胆囊管疾病

胆囊管的病理情况，包括：胆囊管炎症（含急性胆囊炎、慢性胆囊炎、瓷样胆囊、钙胆汁、胆囊积水、胆系内瘘），结石，扩张，狭窄或 / 和梗阻（可为部分性、完全性梗阻，其原因可以是炎症水肿及粘连、结石、肿瘤、Mirizzi 综合征）以及胆囊手术后胆囊管残端过长、假胆囊形成等。常见的胆囊管疾病有结石、Mirizzi 综合征、胆囊管十二指肠瘘、胆管阻塞、胆囊管肿瘤、硬化性胆管炎侵犯胆囊管；另外，胆囊管也可被邻近的恶性肿瘤或炎性疾病侵犯。肝移植或胆囊切除术后，残留的部分胆囊管可发生病变，已知的术后综合征包括残留胆囊管过长、残留胆囊管结石、胆囊管瘘、T 管位置不正。

一、胆囊管结石

胆囊管疾病中以结石最常见，临床上 95% 的急性胆囊炎病例都是由胆囊管结石梗阻引起。直径 <3 mm 的小结石可排出胆囊管。当出现胆囊管结石时，一般都以急性胆囊炎住院治疗，如症状不缓解，通常都是腹腔镜或开腹手术处理，所以，作为影像诊断来说，很少有病人因胆囊管结石来科进行检查，因而影像诊断学的文献上，对胆囊管结石的研究甚为缺乏。然而，由于胆囊切除术后一些病例残留胆囊管过长，而出现胆囊管残留结石，此时才有可能对胆囊管结石进行观察、分析和研究，导致胆囊管结石在临床影像诊断中并不多见的假像。

胆囊管残留结石，可分为两种情况：一是胆囊手术时，手术医生未完全取出胆囊管内的结石而残留下来，在胆囊切除手术后不久复查即可见到残留过长的胆囊管内还残留着较小的少数结石。一是残留胆囊管过度，随着手术后胆囊管炎症的残留和发展，逐渐又产生了新的胆囊结石，这在临床上屡见不鲜，有的残留过长的胆囊管内的结石还相当大，相当多，用手术残留的结石难以解释。

胆囊管与总胆管成像时的重叠及直接胆系造影时胆囊管充盈不全均可造成“结石”的假象，胆囊管结石或胆囊管走行异常可误诊为包块和肿瘤。所以，熟悉胆囊管正常及异常的影像表现以及相关疾病的形成过程，对提高诊断水平及避免误诊很有帮助。

二、胆囊管残端过长与胆囊切除术后综合征

过长的胆囊管残端（长度 >1.5 cm）有可能需行再次胆系手术。腹腔镜胆囊切除术后，可由于金属夹的滑脱引起胆囊管残端瘘。

胆囊切除术后，胆囊管残端究竟留多长？这在临床研究的论文中常有争论，各位学者意见不一，要求严格者提出以 0.5cm 为好，一般认为留下 1.0cm 属于可容忍范围，一些文章中提出小于 1.5cm 为标准，根据我们的临床经验，我们赞成以短于 1.0cm 为标准较好，如能短于 0.5cm 为最好。从多年的临床经验看，胆囊管位于肝总管后面或侧面伴随下行，易被肝总管遮掩或被对比剂影重迭，在手术中正位 X 线照片和手术野均难以发现，只有通过斜位照片才能辨认胆囊管汇入处，这样，就给不了解胆囊管低位汇入的手术医生设下陷阱，常常导致常规胆囊切除术后胆囊管残留过长，不可避免地出现“胆囊切除术后综合征”。自然，现在术前 MRCP 可清楚显示胆囊管的情况，为手术医生帮助不少。

胆囊管残端过长，一直被认为是“胆囊切除术后综合征”的一个重要原因。我们在临床所见到的胆囊管低位汇入者，胆囊管残端长约 40mm 左右，在最低位汇入病例残端更长，长约 54mm 以上，均等于或超过正常胆囊管长度的最大值 40mm，说明此类残端确实太长，不是一个“端”而是一条“管”，不宜

称为胆囊管残端，而应称为残留胆囊管，即一般所说的“残留假胆囊”，它可成为长而大的死腔，或因原有的感染源，或因胆汁反流，极易发生感染，构成术后所谓残留胆囊炎的临床症状。

这些术后病例，皆因术前不了解不认识胆囊管低位汇入，术时由于视野有限或经验不足，很难发现胆囊管的全貌以及低位汇合，自然不可能注意分离或难以分离长度增加的胆囊管全长，而只按常规手术（这在腹腔镜切除胆囊术尤其明显），导致胆囊管残端遗留过长，形成残留胆囊管，成为假胆囊。术前如行 MRCP、ERCP 或 PTC，了解胆囊管低位汇入的位置，对于手术计划的制订及手术程序的安排，均是必要的。

胆囊切除术后有 85% 病人能完全解除术前的症状，但约 5% 的病人术后与术前一样仍有严重的上腹痛，称为胆囊切除术后综合征，原因可能为胆系梗阻、遗留的胆管结石、胆囊管残端过长、胆胰管下端括约肌狭窄或运动障碍。有关胆囊切除术后综合征已有大量报道。近年腹腔镜胆囊切除术普及，但却很少有文献报道它是否能导致胆囊管残端综合征以及能否用来治疗这种综合征。

Rozsos 等（1997）经过对 8 例病人 7 年的随访，发现胆囊残端或胆囊管残端可能是造成这种综合征的直接原因。但关于这点还有争论。

Rogy 等（1991）认为胆囊切除术后综合征可能源于不同的胆系病理改变，他们研究的目的在于评价胆囊管残端综合征的原因。过长的胆囊管残端（>1.5cm）有可能需再次行胆系手术，322 例病人胆囊切除术后 10 年内进行过二次胆系手术，35 例（10.8%）发现有明显长的胆囊管残端，其中 24 例在探查时发现胆囊管有病理改变，14 例为胆总管结石，6 例为胆胰管下端括约肌狭窄，3 例为慢性胰腺炎，1 例是因肝炎造成症状。

余下的 11 例，8 例胆囊管残端有结石，1 例有胆囊管残端十二指肠瘘，1 例是因缝线肉芽肿引起症状，仅有 1 例未发现其他异常，再次手术后 4 年，此病人仍产生了同以前一样的胃肠症状。于是该作者认为，胆囊管残留本身不一定是术后综合征的原因，切除全部胆囊管并不能杜绝术后综合征的出现。

胆囊管残端过长者出现的症状，多半是由于隐匿结石、胆汁淤积、神经性疼痛、慢性炎症及肉芽肿形成所致，也可能为残端囊肿形成、胆囊管断端愈合不佳、异物、瘢痕组织牵拉胆管、胆囊管局限狭窄和纤维化、粘连引起胆囊管狭窄和扭转所致。

Trondsen 等（1997）研究了阻塞小鼠胆囊管的后果。121 只小鼠进行手术，40 只行胆囊管结扎（L 组），41 只结扎后向后侧引流（LE 组），40 只对照（S 组）。

10 只来自胆囊管结扎和胆囊管结扎后向后侧引流组的小鼠分别在 1 周、1 个月、3 个月、6 个月后死亡。14 只发生胆囊扩张，其中 7 只来自胆囊管结扎组，7 只来自胆囊管结扎后向后侧引流组，都发生在 3~6 个月后。其他鼠胆囊均小于手术前体积（P<0.0001）。胆囊周围纤维化和粘连在胆囊管结扎、胆囊管结扎后向后侧引流组很普遍，胆囊管结扎后向后侧引流组更甚。

胆囊管结扎组中有 16 只小鼠发生胆囊壁炎症，胆囊管结扎后向后侧引流组中有 28 只，对照组仅有 2 只，胆囊管结扎后向后侧引流组比胆囊管结扎组明显（P<0.002）。胆囊管结扎后向后侧引流组发生 11 只胆囊积脓，轻微胆管炎在胆囊管结扎后向后侧引流组中比胆囊管结扎组更普遍（P<0.0001）。结论：显微镜下观察到胆囊管阻塞炎症发病率很高。

胆囊切除术后有 85% 病人能完全解除术前症状，但约 5% 的病人术后与术前一样仍有严重的上腹痛，称为胆囊切除术后综合征，原因可能为胆系梗阻、遗留的胆管结石、胆囊管残端过长、胆胰管下端括约肌狭窄或运动障碍等。过长的胆囊管残端（>1.5cm）有可能需行再次胆系手术。腹腔镜胆囊切除术后，可由于金属夹的滑脱引起胆囊管残端瘘。

三、胆囊管残端瘘

Mergener 等（1999）发现，近年随着腹腔镜的广泛应用，胆囊管残端瘘的发生率也随之升高。主要是由金属夹的滑脱引起，有作者在腹腔镜中采用可吸收缝线结扎胆囊管，明显降低了残端瘘的发生。超声及 ERCP 在胆囊管残端瘘早期诊断中起重要作用，ERCP 还可行乳头切开术或放置支架治疗。

一些学者介绍一例胆囊切除术后 20 年出现胆囊管残端 - 十二指肠瘘的病人，此症十分少见，据当时该作者介绍，文献上只报告过三例胆囊管残端内瘘的病案，一为漏至十二指肠，一为胃，一为结肠。所有 4 例皆为胆囊切除术后数年出现。

在无选择的胆囊切除术后病人中，胆囊管残端真正的发生率不详，在经历总胆管探查与胆囊切除术者，有作者统计，明显长的残端遗留占 63%。与此类似,反复胆系探查发现胆囊管残端者,30%有胆结石位于胆囊管残端。在胆囊切除术后,胆绞痛与黄疸消退,症状与体征减轻,通常由于总胆管结石的排出,偶尔,肝外胆管梗阻的解除可源于胆系内瘘的出现。

自发性胆系内瘘的原因一般皆为胆石通过所致,只有10%病例为其他疾病(例如:消化性溃疡、胃肠道新生物等)引起。胆囊已切除者,内瘘源于胆石者十分少见。

过长的胆囊管残端(>1.5 cm)有可能需行再次胆系手术。腹腔镜胆囊切除术后,可由于金属夹的滑脱引起胆囊管残端瘘。

胆囊切除术后,胆囊管残端究竟留多长?这在临床研究的论文中常有争论,各位学者意见不一,要求严格者提出以0.5cm为好,一般认为留下1.0cm属于可容忍范围,一些文章中提出小于1.5cm为标准,根据我们的临床经验,我们赞成以短于1.0cm为标准较好,如能短于0.5cm为最好。

四、胆囊管与肿瘤

Chijiiwa等(1993)统计了1976—1990年间14例经治疗的日本胆囊管癌病人和18例西方国家报道的同类病例,以研究胆囊管癌的临床特征。日本和西方胆囊管癌病人平均年龄均为62岁,男女比例3.5:1。其中8例有胆石存在(西方组6例,日本组2例),明显低于胆囊癌病人,尽管侵犯很深。胆囊管癌预后较好,少有淋巴结及远处转移。

Ohtani等(1994)统计了120例病人的121处原发肝外胆管癌与胆囊管开口位置之间的距离,64例肿瘤(53%)在开口位置5mm内,14例接近开口位置,18例在胆囊管内,32例在胆管末梢,有超过半数的原发性肝外胆管癌在胆囊管开口位置5mm内和下方的胆管内,他认为应进一步研究这一区域是否有特别的致癌因素。

第三节　胆囊管疾病影像学检查

胆囊管可通过不同的影像学方法显影。静脉胆系造影用于胆结石诊断的阴性预测值几乎为100%,但有对比剂过敏的可能,而且不能显示胆系阻塞段以下的部位,现基本已摒弃。

目前常用于胆系疾病诊断的影像学方法有超声、CT、逆行性胆胰管造影(ERCP)、磁共振胆胰管成像(MRCP)。超声、CT对于扩张的胆管可以显示,但是对于在正常范围内的胆管、胆囊管却很难显示。

ERCP已成为胆系成像的参照标准,然而它不能成为一项常规的术前检查方法,因为可能发生并发症或插管失败。常见的并发症是由于胰管过度充盈所致,大约有1/3的病人在ERCP术后发生无症状的血清淀粉酶增高,原因为对比剂剂量较大,注射速率过快,导致胰管过度充盈,引起三级胰管的破裂,X线片上可见胰实质中有对比剂的积聚,临床表现为较长时间的腹痛及背痛,此类病人往往在24小时内发生急性胰腺炎,发生率可达1%左右。

MRCP是近年来迅速发展起来的一种无创性胆胰管成像新技术,能多角度、多方位显示胆系解剖结构,现已广泛应用于胆系疾病的诊断,其临床价值已与有创性ERCP检查相近。MRCP、MSCT三维重建或直接的胆系成像是目前最好的检查方法。

一、MSCT

MSCT进行胆囊管三维重建:当前常用的技术有容积补偿、表面补偿及生理性成像分析。重建过程并没有改变CT像素,它只是将原始图像从另外的角度重新组合,矢状、冠状、斜行是标准的重建方法。其他的重建技术还有最大密度投影、最小密度投影及变量层厚重建,CT灌注不但可以重建胆系影像,还可以通过对比剂排泄时间测定胆系的生理参数。

腹腔镜胆囊切除术前,弄清胆囊管的解剖非常重要,Ichii等(2002)对胆系的三维影像进行了研究,50例病人在胆系造影后行MSCT检查,42例胆囊管显影(84%),其中30例(60%)为Ⅰ型,9例(18%)为Ⅲ型,Ⅱ、Ⅳ、Ⅴ型各1例。同时测量了胆囊管的长度,并发现长度小于或等于2cm的胆囊管显影时间短于长度大于2cm的胆囊管的显影时间,两者之间有显著差异($P<0.01$)。

Kobayashi等(1996)将螺旋CT三维重组胆囊管的影像与ERCP及静脉滴注胆系造影(DIC)进行了比较,主要从胆囊管是否显示及其长度和变异3

方面评价。三维技术显示了 168 例中 157 例的胆囊管(93.5%),而静脉滴注胆系造影中的 89 例有 81 例显示不清晰(91%), 23 例做三维 CT 和 ERCP 的病人中,有 20 例检测胆囊管的效果与 ERCP 相当,2 例优于 ERCP, 1 例比 ERCP 差。CT 三维重建技术有助于在腹腔镜胆囊切除术前明确胆囊管的长度及其变异,可替代 ERCP。

二、MSCT 和 MRCP 比较

MSCT 胆系造影可清楚地显示变异胆管和胆囊管,但是 MRCP 却可能由于十二指肠及肝管的重叠而显影不满意。

Shinichi 等(1999)对 1996 年 11 月至 1998 年 8 月间陆续做腹腔镜胆囊切除术的 120 例病人进行了研究,其中 114 例有胆石症,6 例有胆囊息肉。18 例做了螺旋 CT 胆系造影术后被怀疑有迷走胆管或胆囊管,其中 16 例病人又做了 MRCP。这 16 例又与术中胆系造影做了比较。结果 13 例胆管变异与 3 例胆囊管变异按术中胆系造影被分为 6 种类型,螺旋 CT 胆系造影检出了所有变异,而 MR 胆系成像却有 7 例变异未检出,假阴性的结果主要是由于胆囊管注入胆管的部位被变异的胆管干扰,或变异的胆管被十二指肠干扰。

MRCP: MRCP 技术是一种综合了 PTC 和 CT 优点的新的诊断方法。它主要是采用梯度回波序列和快速自旋回波序列以及二维、三维多平面、多体位(主要是冠状位和斜冠状位)成像,并用最大强度投影重组影像,简便直观,不依赖于对比剂,无电离辐射,无创伤痛苦,检查迅速。它利用 MR T_2WI 使含水结构显影的特点,以增强胆管内液性信号来显示胆管影像。可清楚地显示肝内外胆管和胆囊,准确显示胆管梗阻部位。

它利用磁共振水成像的原理,采用重 T_2 加权成像技术,增强体内胆汁、胰液等近似静止状态的液性结构的信号(呈高信号),而周围的实质器官显示为低信号,从而突出了胆胰管的影像,能多平面、多角度、多方位显示胆囊管、胆管及胰管管腔的形态学状态,以此对胆胰管疾病作出诊断。与 ERCP 和 PTC 相比,它简便直观,不依赖于对比剂,无电离辐射,无创伤痛苦,检查迅速。

MRCP 检查技术: MRI 在腹部成像中起着越来越大的作用,以前多局限于实性器官(肝、肾)异常的检查,现在对胆胰管系统及肠道检查的应用亦日渐广泛。快速 MR 技术利用长 T2(>1.5 秒)探测肝胆的液体信号,无需对比剂就可产生高质量的 2D 或 3D 的 MRCP 影像。

检查前 8h 需禁食,扫描前 15min 肌肉注射 20mg 山莨菪碱以抑制胃肠蠕动,从而减少伪影,提高 MRCP 影像质量。检查前训练病人呼吸,平静呼吸及屏气动度应保持一致,嘱病人最大时间屏气,力求配合,以避免呼吸运动对 MRCP 影像的影响。

检查前口服枸橼酸铁铵可使 MRCP 影像质量明显提高,减少胃肠道液体的干扰,从而提高胆囊管的显示率。因为枸橼酸铁铵是一种顺磁性对比剂,可使 T_1 值明显缩短,因而长期以来枸橼酸铁铵一直是作为一种水溶性阳性对比剂而被研究和使用;同时它缩短 T_2 值,降低其造成的背景高信号干扰,从而使胃、十二指肠腔内液体高信号显著降低或完全消除,使 MRCP 影像质量明显提高,特别是对易被胃窦、十二指肠重叠的胆囊管,胆总管中下段的形态和边缘细节显示更为清晰。

最初曾尝试用稳态序列自由成像,但由于敏感性强,对流动的液体及血管的搏动亦显影。后多用 RARE 和 FSE 成像,由于回波时间长,只有静止的液体空间显影,而其背景因信号丢失显影被抑制, RARE 和半傅里叶 RARE 技术已被广泛用于 MRCP 诊断。

硬件和软件技术的进步使 MRI 大大降低了因肠蠕动和呼吸造成的伪影,从而使解剖细节的成像更加完美,FSE 成像时间也大大缩短,一方面病人容易接受,另一方面也提高了设备的使用效率。呼吸门控三维 MRCP 的节段回波平面成像迅速、可靠,并可从多个方向成像,能有效降低重叠及运动伪影,这对明确胆管正常或异常的解剖颇有临床应用价值。

MRCP 技术已由早期的梯度回波(GRE)技术发展到快速自旋回波(FSE)技术,其中应用最广的是单次激发快速自旋回波序列(SSFSE),其成像速度快,层厚薄,空间分辨力及信噪比高,并可在原始冠状面成像基础上,利用最大信号强度投影技术对原始图像进行重组,同时采用脂肪抑制技术、屏气扫描及多角度放射状扫描,获得与 ERCP 相似的影像。

对于屏气合作欠佳病例,采用呼吸门控 3D MRCP 可同样获得较满意 MRCP 图像。虽然 3D MRCP 扫描时间短,其重建图像可多角度、多方位显示胆系全貌,但是对于小直径的胆囊管及胰管的显示不如 2D MRCP。

3D MRCP 作快速恢复快速自旋回波序列(FRFSE)扫描,加脂肪抑制及呼吸门控技术,3D MRCP(FRFSE)相对于传统 2D MRCP(SSFSE)而言,胰胆管显示率明显提高,可多角度、多方位显示胆囊管、胆管及胰管管腔的形态学状态,可避免成像重叠,具有较高的准确性、特异性和敏感性。MRCP 结合冠状位原始图像及横断位 T_2WI,可了解肝内外胆管、胆囊及胆囊管的解剖结构关系,可观察胆囊管汇入肝外胆管的方式及汇入部位,观察胆囊管长度、内径、走行及与肝外胆管轴线的成角,并可发现胆囊管的各种发育变异。

MRCP 的胆囊管成像:腹腔镜胆囊切除术前常规 MRCP 观察胆囊管的解剖及变异,从而减少医源性胆系损伤,减少胆系术后并发症的发生,对病人的治疗方案、手术步骤及预后有着十分重要意义。不少学者的研究发现,胆囊管的长度、走行及汇入变化较大,MRCP 能清晰显示胆囊管和胆囊管汇合肝外胆管的发育变异。

MRCP 能良好地显示胆囊管的病变。有作者通过 MRCP 与超声的比较发现,对于评价胆囊管结石及其引起的胆囊管梗阻,MRCP 明显优于超声。

一些作者研究发现,MRCP 对诊断因胆囊管结石引起的 Mirizzi 综合征亦具有重要作用,并可发现胆囊管瘘。还有学者报道,MRCP 可显示胆囊切除术后胆囊管残端结石及胆囊管残端的扩张。由此可见,MRCP 不仅能清晰显示胆囊管的解剖和变异,而且对胆囊管疾病的诊断具有重要作用。

MRCP 对胆囊管与其注入肝管部位的评价:在不同技术的对比及呼吸诱导三维多层技术的临床价值研究方面,Tsunoda 等(1998)对 10 例志愿者分别用呼吸门控二维、呼吸诱导二维、呼吸诱导三维单层和多层技术行 MRCP 检查,证实非屏气 MRCP 对胆囊管和非扩张性胆管显影较差,而呼吸诱导三维多层技术是最优的。另有 35 例病人行这项技术检查,对胆囊管及其与肝管结合部的成像进行评价,其中 8 例与 ERCP 比较。用这项技术的 93% 病人和志愿者的显影很充分。同时还评价了胆囊管及其结合部的变异,发生率与以前的报道一致。MRCP 观察到的解剖结构变化与 ERCP 基本接近。

MRCP 对胆囊扭转的术前诊断:这种病的征兆往往很隐蔽,Matsuda 等(2000)报道了一例 78 岁女病人,超声和 CT 均诊断为胆囊炎和结石,静滴法 CT 胆管造影未显示胆囊及肝外胆管的扭曲,胆囊管显示因阻塞而中断。MRCP 显示了肝外胆管由于胆囊管的牵拉形成的 V 型扭曲,胆囊管扭曲且远端变细,胆囊扩大并偏离腹中线,胆囊、肝外胆管、胆囊管的信号存在差别,据此诊为胆囊扭转。这对胆囊切除术时避免损伤胆管很有意义,对有急性胆囊炎或不明原因急性腹痛的老年人,MRCP 可能会做出准确诊断。

MRCP 的优缺点:MRCP 具有无创性、能反复应用和无需对比剂等优点,能较好地反映胆胰管解剖关系和病理变化,获得不亚于 ERCP 的图像质量,结合源图像和常规 MRI 图像,提供比 CT、PTC、ERCP 更多对诊断有价值的资料,有助于制定合理的手术方案,适用于病情轻重不一的各类病例。MRCP 检查不仅可显示梗阻的部位和梗阻的程度,还可以显示梗阻周围软组织的情况。

MRCP 与 ERCP 相比较,胆肠吻合术后、胃毕Ⅱ式吻合术后的患者均能行 MRCP 检查,但不能行 ERCP 检查,急性胰腺炎患者可行 MRCP 检查,但不能行 ERCP 检查,后者可能引起严重并发症,特别是在 ERCP 检查失败的病例,MRCP 是最好的选择,可以作为一种首选的替代检查方法。一组大部分病例采用屏气多角度 2D MRCP 扫描、可显示胆囊管的形态、走行及汇入肝总管的位置,结合常规图像、3D MRCP 原始图像和最大强度投影、遮盖表面显示重组图像进行观察可提高清晰度和明确汇入位置。

MRCP 的局限性在于空间分辨力的限制,难以清楚显示胰管的分支,对轻度狭窄及微小结石不能显示,由于高信号的液体掩盖,对胆总管末段与胰管汇合处分辨不清,胆管狭窄长度往往因十二指肠降段不显影而不能判断。因此,对 3D MRCP 源图像及最大强度投影、遮盖表面显示重组图像的观察十分重要。

MRCP 不能进行活检或介入治疗,对大量腹水和某些体内有金属内置物(如胆管支架、心脏起搏器、血管支架)的患者无法进行检查,这也是 MRCP 的不足之处。

随着 MRCP 技术的进步,用其诊断胆管阻塞的存在及程度已相当准确,然而,其缺陷也日益暴露。包绕在稠密胆汁中的小胆石或息肉样瘤在最大强度投影(MIP)重建时有可能不显示,呼吸控制不好时,可形成胆管变异假象(异常接口、双胆管)。

胆管外因素(腹内金属夹、胃十二指肠内气体)

能导致肝外胆管周围信号缺失，从而造成胆管狭窄或阻塞的假象。肝右动脉、胃十二指肠动脉的搏动也可造成肝外胆管假性阻塞。胆管内因素（气体、出血、碎片、碘对比剂）也可造成假性阻塞或充盈缺损，甚至胆囊胆管不显影。采用合适的 MR 技术（如腹内有银夹时行脂肪抑制技术，不应使用 MRCP）及结合临床仔细分析影像结果对避免这些不足非常重要。

三、肝区闪烁扫描（HBS）和 MRCP 联合检查胆囊术后综合征

核医学检测技术对胆系疾病的诊断和超声、磁共振、X 线检查比较，在动态观察、功能分析、定量测定方面更有其独特之处。此法简便、无创、灵敏度高、安全实用，并可在合乎生理条件下进行，可为胆系疾病的早期诊断和疗效观察提供有价值的信息。

诊断胆系疾病所用显像剂一般多采用 ^{99m}Tc 标记的亚氨基二乙酸（IDA）类药物如 ^{99m}Tc-EHIDA，但此种显像剂在高胆红素血症时摄取较差，影响图像质量，目前对抗高胆红素的吡哆醛氨基酸类衍生物 ^{99m}Tc-PMT 得到了广泛的应用。

它们能被肝多角形细胞快速摄取，继而排至胆汁内，胆汁内浓度高，肝内外胆管显示清晰。显像方法是应用 SPECT（或 γ 相机）在注入显像剂后做连续多次动态显像（必要时做延迟显像），根据显像所见进行形态与功能定性、定量分析。但其影像与其他检查方法比较仍有一定差距，因此更多用于功能检查。

Dimonte 等（1998）研究了肝区核素显像和 MRCP 联合检查胆囊术后综合征的作用。他收集了 1997 年 6 月至 1998 年 2 月间 5 例女病人，3 例行外科手术，2 例行腹腔镜手术。5 例病人均有胆系痛，但无胆汁淤积及肝功改变，MRCP 显示 1 例正常，其他病例显示有胆管树扩张、严重的胆总管狭窄、因残留 1 枚 6mm 结石而扩张的残留胆囊管，胰管正常。肝区核素显像表明所有病人均有胆汁流动延迟（注射 185MBq^{99m}Tc- 甲溴苯宁后 3 小时内排空），3 例残留胆囊管（RCD）未显示，肝区核素显像检测到 3 例早期肝功能不良。

肝区核素显像、MRCP 分别检测胆管树的功能与解剖，对肝功和胰管形态的研究也提供了数据。检出的辅助功能及胆汁输送的改变，如严重的胆胰管下端括约肌痉挛、非开放性扩张的残留胆囊管及残留胆囊管结石，可能是胆囊术后综合征的原因。总之，肝区核素显像、MRCP 联合检查是诊断胆囊切除术后综合征的一种无创、简单、准确的方法，并能筛选出需要进一步行外科手术的病人。

第四节　胆囊管 MRCP

胆系结石是临床上的常见病和多发病，其中以胆囊结石更为多见。腹腔镜技术由于创伤小、腹腔术后粘连概率低及住院时间短等特点，现已成为临床胆囊切除术的首选治疗方法。然而，Taourel 等（1996）统计，腹腔镜胆囊切除术所致胆管损伤发生率为 0.2%~0.3%，比传统剖腹胆囊切除术时的 0.1% 增加了一倍以上。由于胆囊管是连接胆囊和肝外胆管的重要结构，导致胆管损伤与胆囊管的形态学及发育变异有着密切的关系。

胆囊管是连接胆囊和肝外胆管的重要结构，它在胆囊和肝外胆管之间输送胆汁，常呈管状或蜿蜒扭曲状走行，其形态的变化还与胆囊的充盈情况有关。靠近胆囊段的胆囊管内有 5~12 个新月形的皱襞（螺旋瓣），它有助于保持胆囊管开放，并控制胆汁流出。胆囊管汇入点变异很大，范围可从肝门部至胆胰管括约肌水平。

胆囊管发育变异通常没有临床意义。但是，在合并胆系疾病需做胆囊切除术时，术前如果对胆囊管解剖及变异认识不足，易导致疾病误诊，易导致术中胆源性损伤，并可导致术后胆系瘘发生率等并发症增加。

一、影像学研究

目前常用于胆系疾病诊断的影像学方法有 B 超、CT、ERCP、MRCP。B 超、CT 对于扩张的胆管可以显示，但是对于在正常范围内的胆管、胆囊管却很难显示。ERCP 已成为胆系成像的参考标准，它可以清楚显示胆囊管解剖，然而它不能成为一项常规的术前检查方法，因为可能发生严重并发症或插管失败。

MRCP 是一种无创性胰胆管成像技术,具有操作简单、快速成像、无创伤的特点,并能多角度、多方位显示胆系解剖结构,现已广泛应用于胆系疾病的诊断,其临床价值已与有创性 ERCP 检查相近。

近年来,随着软、硬件的迅速发展, MRCP 已由早期的梯度回波技术发展到快速自旋回波技术,其中应用最广的是单次激发快速自旋回波序列,其成像速度快、层厚薄、空间分辨率及信噪比高,并可在原始冠状面成像基础上,利用最大信号强度投影(MIP)技术对原始图像进行三维重建,同时采用脂肪抑制技术,获得与 ERCP 相似图像。

对于屏气合作欠佳病例,采用呼吸门控 3D MRCP 可同样获得较满意 MRCP 图像。虽然 3D MRCP 扫描时间短,其重建图像可多角度、多方位显示胆系全貌,但是对于小直径的胆囊管及胰管的显示不如 2D MRCP。

Taourel 等(1996)对 171 例 MRCP 图像分析发现,胆囊管显示率为 74%, MRCP 可以较好地显示胆囊管。在另项研究 149 例中,胆囊管显示率为 82%,部分病例可以显示胆囊管螺旋瓣。

Taourel 等(1996)发现 MRCP 可观察胆囊管走行形态、汇入位置及方向。

Taourel 等(1996)对 171 例 MRCP 图像分析发现,胆囊管中间汇入占 17%;平行走行占 25%,变异右肝管占 9%。Dusunceli 等(2004)统计了 581 例 MRCP,结果发现长胆囊管占 1.7%,中间汇入占 0.63%,低位汇入占 3.8%,短胆囊管占 0.2%,变异右肝管占 4.8%。有作者对 801 例 MRCP 研究表明,胆囊管变异占 5.9%。

变异胆囊管多伴有胆囊、胆囊管和 / 或胆总管结石及炎症。上述研究结果的差异,可能与:①样本含量大小;②种族差异;③地区分布差异;④研究方法差异等有关。

腹腔镜胆囊切除术前常规 MRCP 可观察胆囊管发育变异,从而减少医源性胆系损伤,减少胆系术后并发症的发生,对患者的治疗方案、手术步骤及预后有着十分重要的意义。

附:具体病例资料:观察项目和标准:胆囊管呈平行走行的诊断标准是胆囊管与胆总管平行距离不少于 20 mm,胆囊管中间汇入是指胆囊管汇入胆总管的左侧,长胆囊管是指其长度 >6 cm。

在 MRCP 图像上多角度、多方位观察胆囊管显示情况,部分病例结合 SSFSE 序列轴位 T2WI 观察胆囊管显示率,观察并测量胆囊管长度及管径,并统计胆囊管走行形态、汇入位置高低、汇入方向及各种发育变异。观察胆囊管发育变异与胆囊管疾病的相互关系。

一项 149 例研究结果显示, MRCP 上胆囊管显示清晰合计 122 例,显示率为 82%(122/149),部分病例可以显示胆囊管的螺旋瓣。胆囊管长度为(20.83 ± 8.92)mm,直径为(2.82 ± 1.04)mm, 70%(85/122)呈管状走行, 30%(37/122)呈扭曲状走行。

66%(80/122)在肝外胆管全长的中 1/3 处汇合入胆总管,上 1/3 占 31%(38/122),下 1/3 占 3%(4/122)。胆囊管汇入肝外胆管右侧占 74%(90/122),左侧(中间位)占 3%(4/122),前和后占 23%(28/122)。73%(89/122)胆囊管呈斜角汇入, 15%(18/122)呈螺旋状, 12%(15/122)平行状走行。

MRCP 可清晰观察胆囊管变异。在 122 例中,胆囊管变异占 20%(24/122),其中呈平行走行 54%(13/24),低位汇入占 17%(4/24),中间汇入占 17%(4/24),长胆囊管占 4%(1/24),胆囊管囊肿 4%(1/24),汇入变异右肝管占 4%(1/24)。其中变异右肝管 1 例伴结石形成,胆囊管囊肿 1 例伴有胆囊炎。

第五节 误诊病例简介:胆囊管与胆钙乳

患者,女, 77 岁。腹痛、恶心呕吐 1 小时急诊入院。急诊 CT 示:胆囊多发结石,慢性胆囊炎;胆总管下段结石伴胆总管中上段扩张。两天后 CT:胆囊多发结石,慢性胆囊炎,胆囊管及胆总管稍高密度影,考虑胆钙乳,请结合临床。七天后 CT:结石性胆囊炎,胆钙乳已消失,胆囊壁局限性增厚明显,怀疑胆囊肿瘤侵犯胆囊周围。

住院两周后行胆囊切除术,术后病理诊断:胆囊切除标本:慢性结石性胆囊炎伴 R-A 窦形成。

临床经验告诉我们,胆囊内的胆钙乳经常出现变化,其中的原因尚不清楚,总的印象是应当动态观察胆钙乳。但在回顾总结该病例时,考虑胆囊管内胆钙乳的变化如此迅速,超过以往的临床观察动态变化的时间,心中总有疑惑,再与临床联系,这才恍然大悟，发现住院两天后CT所发现的胆钙乳实际上不是真正的胆钙乳，而是ERCP注入的对比剂，自然，住院七天后胆钙乳已消失也属误诊。这样看来，紧密结合临床确实是防止误诊的有力措施。

住院第二天急诊ERCP+EST+ENBD手术，术中见胆总管结石伴急性胆管炎，憩室内乳头。造影见肝内胆管、胆总管扩张，胆总管见一大小约0.9cm透光区，行乳头括约肌切开及球囊扩张，见脓性胆汁流出，使用网篮取出黄色结石1枚，球囊清理胆管，复透透光区消失。

在ERCP注入对比剂的病人，经常发生胆囊内充满对比剂，而只有胆囊管内有对比剂这种情况并不多见，确实值得我们警惕。

第二章　胆囊管的发育变异和先天性异常

第一节　胆囊管的发育变异和先天性异常

胆囊和胆囊管的先天性异常：胆囊和胆囊管的先天性异常，其临床意义在于，进行胆系外科手术时，必须要熟悉先天异常，从而避免意外损伤，影像诊断工作者也必须具备这种知识，以便合理解释影像。胆囊管与胆管的变异，胆管的变异通常没有临床意义，然而，靠近胆囊或胆囊管的胆管走行异常，或者呈空虚状汇入胆囊或胆囊管时，胆囊切除术就存在很大风险。异常胆管呈空虚状汇合胆囊管的占1%~2%。胆囊管发育变异通常没有临床意义。但是，在合并胆系疾病需做胆囊切除术时，术前如果对胆囊管解剖及变异认识不足，易导致疾病误诊，易导致术中胆源性损伤，并可导致术后胆系瘘等并发症的发生率增加。

发育变异与胆囊结石及炎症：胆系结石是临床上的常见病和多发病，其中以胆囊结石更为多见。腹腔镜技术由于创伤小、腹腔术后粘连概率低及住院时间短等特点，现已成为临床胆囊切除术的首选治疗方法。然而，Taourel 等（1996）统计，腹腔镜胆囊切除术所致胆管损伤发生率为 0.2%~0.3%，比传统剖腹胆囊切除术时的 0.1% 增加了一倍以上。由于胆囊管是连接胆囊和肝外胆管的重要结构，导致胆管损伤与胆囊管的形态学及发育变异有着密切的关系。变异胆囊管多伴有胆囊、胆囊管和 / 或胆总管结石及炎症。多位作者的多项研究结果报告的差异，可能与：①样本量的大小不一样；②种族差异；③地区分布差异；④研究方法及检查手段的差异以及对变异胆囊管的认识和研究水平有关。

胆囊管的发育变异：胆囊管的发育变异很常见，有作者统计约占 18%~23%。另有学者报告，胆囊管发育变异发生率为 5.0%~22.7%，一组资料胆囊管发育变异发生率 5.9%（53/900）。包括：胆囊管汇合肝外胆管位置变异（低位、最低位、高位、异位、过长与过短、缺如）、汇合形状的变异（螺旋状、平行走行，汇合的角度，迂曲，成角，扭折）以及汇合部位的变异（非肝外胆管：右肝管、左右肝管汇合处、左肝管）。

MRCP 可以较好地显示胆囊管的发育变异。一些学者对 171 例病人的 MRCP 影像分析发现，胆囊管显示率为 74%；胆囊管低位汇合于肝外胆管占 9%，中间汇合肝外胆管占 17%；胆囊管与肝外胆管平行走行占 25%，变异右肝管占 9%。

有作者对 801 例 MRCP 研究表明，胆囊管变异占 5.9%。另有学者统计 581 例 MRCP，发现长胆囊管占 1.7%，异位汇合占 0.63%，低位汇合占 3.8%，短胆囊管占 0.2%，变异右肝管占 4.8%。一项研究发现，胆囊管内侧汇入发生率 17%，汇入右肝管发生率 9%，与肝总管并行发生率 25%。

胆囊管汇合肝外胆管位置的变异：有的胆囊管汇合肝外胆管位置较高，在肝门区，因而肝总管短，胆总管长；有的汇合肝外胆管位置很低，接近十二指肠，因而肝总管长，胆总管短。一般认为，胆囊管通常在肝外胆管全长的中 1/3 处汇合胆总管，如果不将肝外胆管括约肌段包括在内，将其余肝外胆管分作十等分，胆囊管汇合肝外胆管位置常常在肝外胆管上半，大约在 3/10 处及其附近，也即是肝总管与胆总管的比例大约为三七开。一组 MRCP122 例中，66%（80/122）在肝外胆管全长的中 1/3 处汇合肝外胆管，上 1/3 占 31%（38/122），下 1/3 占 3%（4/122）。

一、高位汇合

胆囊管可以汇合于左右肝管汇合处。一组内侧汇入发生率 18.9%，汇入右肝管发生率 18.9%，与肝总管并行发生率 16.9%，该组显示汇入左右肝管汇合处发生率较高，达 39.6%，胆囊管变异容易并发胆囊病变，如结石和炎症，发生率 47%，合并胆系疾病发生率 98%，该组除 1 例肝内多发囊肿外， 52 例均有胆系疾病。

二、低位汇合

我们将胆囊管汇合于肝外胆管全长（括约肌段除外）下半者，称为胆囊管低位汇合。在胆囊管低位汇合中，约有 1/10 的病例胆囊管汇合于肝外胆管胰腺段与括约肌段交界处，即十二指肠壁外处，称之为胆囊管最低位汇合。一些学者认为，胆囊管通常在肝外胆管全长的中 1/3 处汇合胆总管约占 75%，约 10% 汇合入远 1/3。另有作者认为，胆囊管低位为胆囊管汇合于肝外胆管的下半或远 1/3 段（图 18-2-1）。

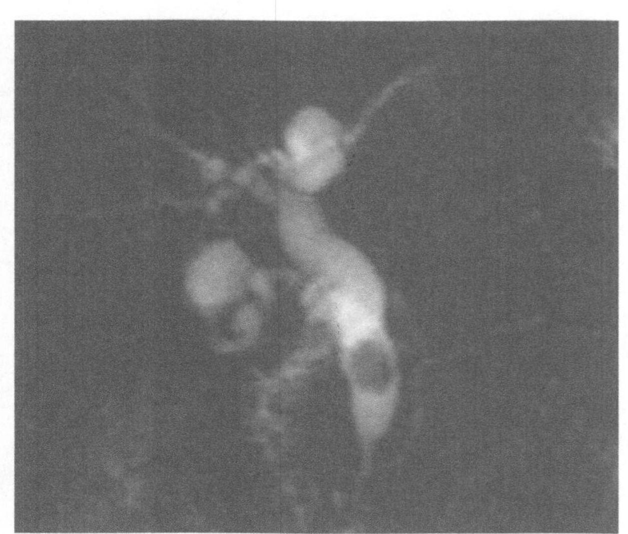

图 18-2-1　MRCP：胆囊管低位异位汇入肝外胆管，肝外胆管结石正位于汇入口下方，括约肌段可见绒毛瓣

胆囊管低位汇合，可至胰腺内、胆胰共同管水平的十二指肠内，胆囊管直接汇合十二指肠内非常罕见，低位汇合变异约占胆管变异的 55%。胆囊管低位汇合势必伴存胆囊管长度的增加。据国内外解剖学者研究，正常成人的胆囊管长度约为 25~40mm。低位汇合的胆囊管平均长度比正常最大值都长许多。一些作者提出，长胆囊管是指其长度 >6 cm。

胆囊管低位汇合伴乳头区憩室：有作者调查了 1 574 例行 ERCP 检查的病人（男 706 例，女 868 例），发现乳头区憩室在低位胆囊管（乳头上 5mm 内）中频繁出现（$P<0.001$），女性乳头区憩室伴低位汇合胆囊管者与不伴低位胆囊管汇合者有显著性差异（$P<0.05$），原因不能简单归于年龄因素，胆囊管低位汇合可能是病因，因为它影响了胆汁的运输，所以低位胆囊管伴乳头区憩室是一种新的综合征。

三、最低位汇合

胆囊管最低位汇合与胆胰管下端括约肌的功能：正常人体解剖学研究发现，肝外胆管越近括约肌段处，肌纤维越多，而使管腔保持一定张力，胆囊管汇合部位越低，括约肌影响胆囊管内容物的进出也就越严重。胆囊管在括约肌段上端汇合总肝管，不仅影响胆囊内胆汁的引流，而且也可能对胆汁从总肝管排泄有所妨碍。汇合部位正居括约肌段上方，很有可能妨碍括约肌段的正常关闭和开放，引起功能紊乱，从而导致总肝管内胆汁排空障碍，同时为肠道感染逆行进入胆系创造某些条件。胆囊管与总肝管交叉与伴行，对总肝管内胆汁排泄也可能造成阻碍。

胆囊管最低位汇合与连接区结构异常：胆囊管最低位汇合括约肌段的上方，直接涉及胆胰管十二指肠连接区的解剖构造。从广义上讲，它也是连接区先天性结构异常的一种表现，而不应只看作先天变异。我们所见 9 例胆囊管最低位汇合的病例，皆伴存胆囊结石、胆囊炎及胆管结石，此类先天性结构异常可能就是这些疾病的解剖学病因因素之一。因此，我们认为，临床上对此类先天异常应给予足够的必要的重视（图 18-2-2）。

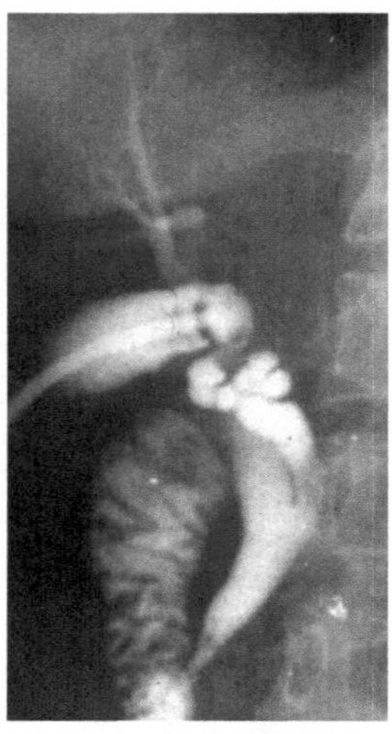

图 18-2-2　引流管造影：扩张的胆囊管从左侧低位汇入扩张的肝外胆管，括约肌段可见小结石

四、在影像诊断时，胆囊管低位汇合可引起的误诊

假性胆囊管低位汇合：在肝外胆管胰腺段因疾病显示不良时，可将胆囊管正常汇合位置误认为低位汇入。此时，注意观察整个肝外胆管的形状、长度和走行，有利于识别真象。

螺旋瓣与假结石：在胆囊管低位汇入时，胆囊管常可与肝外胆管影像重叠，胆囊管内的螺旋瓣影像如不注意可误为肝外胆管内的结石影。

五、胆囊管汇合肝外胆管位置的方位

一些作者依据胆囊管走行及汇合肝外胆管位置不同，将胆囊管分为6型：①右侧汇合；②左侧汇合，在肝外胆管前走行；③左侧汇合，在肝外胆管后走行；④在肝门区汇合；⑤在胰腺段胆管汇合；⑥其他类型。

少数胆囊管汇合肝外胆管壁的的左侧，经肝外胆管的前或后方，迂回至右侧与胆囊连接，这种胆囊管特长，可导致引流不畅，并发胆囊炎。

有作者统计国人296例标本，胆囊管汇合肝外胆管右壁为84.1%，汇合前壁6%，后壁7.4%，左壁2.5%。另有作者统计800例胆囊管汇合处标本，汇合右壁者占89%，汇合左壁8.6%，后壁2.39%。

MRCP可清晰观察胆囊管变异。一组122例MRCP中，胆囊管汇合肝外胆管右侧占74%(90/122)，左位占3%(4/122)，前位和后位占23%(28/122)。

另有作者指出，胆囊管汇合于肝外胆管右侧占49.9%，左侧占18.4%，前或后占31.7%。

少数胆囊管汇合于胆总管的左侧，经胆总管的前或后方，迂回至右侧与胆囊连接，这种胆囊管特长，可导致引流不畅，并发胆囊炎。从胆囊管低位汇合资料看，胆囊管汇合左壁者所占比例甚大。左位汇合势必导致胆囊管围绕总肝管走行，妨碍胆囊内容物的进入与排出。

六、螺旋形汇合

胆囊管汇合可呈前、后螺旋形汇合肝总管。其具体表现，可以是胆囊管旋前于肝总管内侧汇合；也可以是胆囊管旋后于肝总管内侧汇合。在这类的情况下，胆囊管围绕总肝管走行，势必妨碍胆囊内容物的进入与排出。一组122例MRCP中，73%(89/122)胆囊管呈斜角汇合，15%(18/122)呈螺旋状，12%(15/122)平行状走行。一些学者发现，正常情况下，大约73%胆囊管呈斜角汇合肝外胆管，17%胆囊管呈螺旋状围绕肝外胆管。另有作者指出，10%胆囊管在汇合前与肝外胆管呈平行状走行(图18-2-3)。

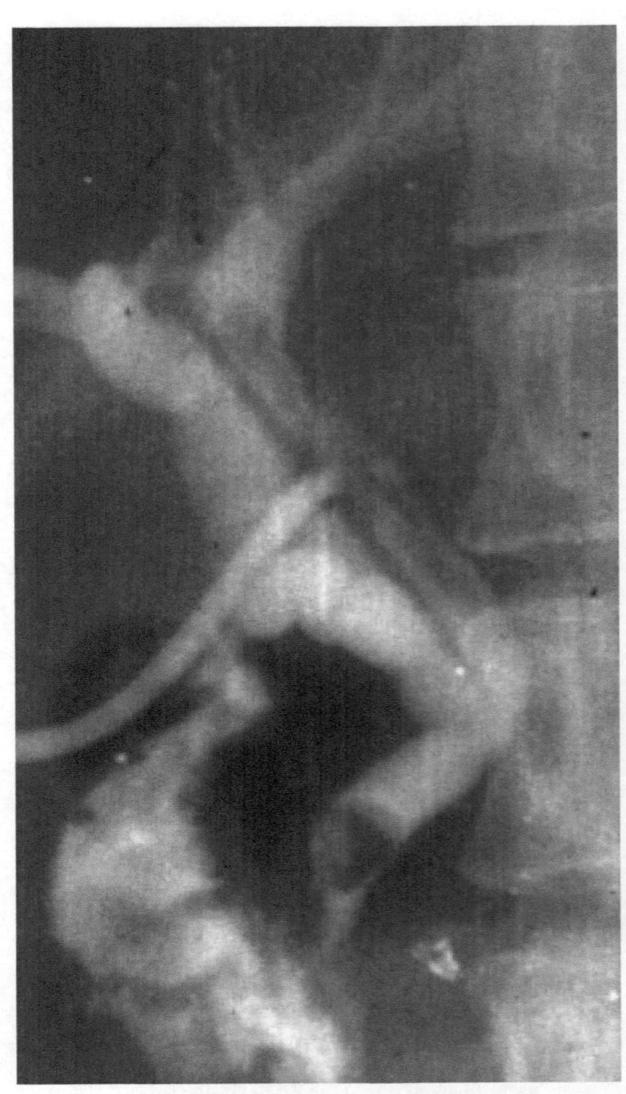

图18-2-3 T管造影：扩张的过长的胆囊管残端低位前位汇入肝外胆管，括约肌段上方可见类圆形结石影

七、平行汇合

一些作者报告，在胆管造影中，胆囊管与肝外胆管呈平行走行占10%，两者伴行距离较长常提示有共同的纤维鞘。另有作者认为，与肝总管并行2cm以上称为并行走行。由于有纤维鞘包绕，胆囊管汇合于肝外胆管就有两个汇合处，一为真正的汇合处，

即在纤维鞘中较低位置二者实际汇合处；一为假汇合处，即为胆囊管从纤维鞘露出与胆囊连接处，在手术时，由于看不见纤维鞘内的实际汇合点，经常将假汇合处误为真汇合处而进行切断，必要的结果是造成胆囊管残留过长。

胆囊管与肝总管并行时，在外科手术或腹腔镜切除胆囊时，有可能将并行肝总管误认为胆囊管而予以钳夹、离断，而急性胆囊炎或慢性胆囊炎急性发作的患者，并行胆囊管与肝总管更不易分离，手术容易导致肝总管损伤。

八、胆囊管汇合肝外胆管的角度

在尸体解剖学文献中，常常可以看到胆囊管汇合肝外胆管的角度的测量，在临床活体的观察研究中则少有观察和分析，据我们观察，这个角度在同一活体常有变化，在不同的个体变化更大。分析原因可能是，除了它们共同被一纤维鞘包裹、胆囊管平行于肝外胆管走行时该角度变化较小以外，在活体这个角度常出现变化：不同的呼吸时相直接影响腹腔内压力的升降，导致该角度的变化；进食与否直接影响胆囊的充盈与排空，常常改变该角度的大小；胃肠的蠕动，尤其是邻近胆囊及胆囊管的十二指肠降段及结肠肝曲收缩与舒张、充盈与排空更是直接对该角度造成影响。

九、胆囊管的其他发育变异和先天异常

胆囊管汇合于非肝外胆管：胆囊管可汇合左肝管、右肝管及左右肝管分叉处，并可呈空虚状汇合肝总管或右肝管；胆囊管汇合于右肝管较汇合于左肝管多见。在一组 122 例 MRCP 中，长胆囊管占 4%（1/24），胆囊管囊肿 4%（1/24），汇合变异右肝管占 4%（1/24）。其中变异右肝管 1 例伴结石形成，胆囊管囊肿 1 例伴有胆囊炎。

胆囊管过短或缺如：胆囊管过短或缺如，长度小于 5mm，胆囊颈部直接汇入肝外胆管；胆囊缺如罕见，多伴有胆囊管的缺如。胆囊管过短时术中牵拉胆囊，胆总管被拉直，易误认胆囊管而伤及胆总管。

胆囊管囊状扩张：在胆囊管囊性扩张者，术中易将胆囊管囊状扩张的囊腔当作胆囊的颈部，而将胆总管当作胆囊管而错误切断。

十二指肠组织易位于胆囊管：曾有作者报道一例十二指肠组织易位于胆囊管，非常罕见。

双胆囊管（可伴有或不伴存双胆囊）：更为少见。

如果术前对胆囊管的上述变异认识不足，可导致胆系瘘发生率增加。

十、胆囊管变异的临床研究

研究表明胆囊管的变异与结石形成有关。在结石形成过程中胆囊起重要作用，但胆囊管的形态和汇合位置的不同也可能影响这个过程。

Deenitchin 等（1998）研究了变异胆囊管和胆结石的关系。1979 至 1993 年间将 500 例做了 ERCP 的病人进行随机分组（表 18-2-1），250 例无胆结石，250 例有胆结石，测量并比较了胆囊管长度、内径、外形及其与胆囊轴线的成角。有结石组胆囊管又长又细（平均长 48mm，内径 4mm），无结石组胆囊管平均长 28 mm，内径 7 mm，两者相比有显著性差异，$P<0.001$。由此得出结论：变异胆囊管多伴胆结石。

表 18-2-1　胆囊管发育变异与胆囊结石的关系

	胆囊管长度（mm）	胆囊管内径（mm）	胆囊管与胆囊夹角（°）	胆囊管畸形发生率（%）
有胆结石组	48	4	84	99
无胆结石组	28	7	119	29

研究表明，胆囊管的变异可导致胆囊管自身疾病，一些作者研究表明变异胆囊管多伴有胆囊及胆囊管结石，并可造成梗阻性黄疸。另有学者发现胆囊管异位汇入可造成胆汁滞留和 / 或胰液返流入胆管，产生胆胰管粘连，可导致梗阻性黄疸，并造成手术困难。胆囊管结石对伴行肝外胆管压迫可引起 Mirizzi 综合征，可造成胆管梗阻。胆囊管与胆总管成像的重叠可造成结石的假象，胆囊管结石或胆囊管走行异常可造成包块和肿瘤的假象。

MRCP 用于显示各种胆管先天畸形。其诊断肝内胆管畸形准确度为 98%，胆囊管发育异常准确度为 95%。当腹腔镜下胆囊切除术开始普及后，术前确定胆管变异已引起注意，因为这些发育变异增加了无意中结扎胆管的危险性。当怀疑胆管结石时，MRCP 可确认胆囊位置并可显示胆管和胰管的异常连接。如果要实施胆囊切除，MRCP 可用来确定包含于胆囊的胆囊管的长度。

胆管发育变异可导致腹腔镜胆囊切除术中胆管损伤的危险性增加，MRCP 能准确诊断胆管变异从

而降低这一危险。Taourel 等(1996)在 171 例 MRCP 检查中发现低位胆囊管汇合 11 例(9%),中间胆囊管汇合 22 例(17%),胆囊管与总胆管平行 31 例(25%)及右肝管走行反常 12 例(9%)。由此可见,胆囊管的发育变异在临床上有重要意义,熟悉胆囊管的发育变异的影像表现以及相关疾病的形成过程,对提高诊断水平及避免误诊很有帮助。

第二节 胆囊管的活体形态学

一、胚胎学与组织学

在胚胎发育过程中,肝憩室的尾支远端膨大形成胆囊,基部变细形成胆囊管,当十二指肠壁发育生长不平衡,导致胆总管转位,当胆总管由腹侧经过外侧和背侧转至十二指肠内侧时,胆囊管也随着胆总管的起始部转向左侧。肝憩室尾支继续延长膨大,使胆囊进入肝下面的胆囊窝内。这样,就可发生胆囊管低位汇合,胆囊管延长及汇合口异位等一系列发育异常。

二、一般表现

胆囊管是连接胆囊和肝外胆管的重要结构,通过它,胆汁在胆囊和肝外胆管之间进出。胆囊管长度 2~4 cm,直径 1~5 mm,常呈管状或蜿蜒扭曲状走行,其形态的变化还与胆囊的充盈情况有关。靠近胆囊端的胆囊管内有 5~12 个新月形的皱襞,呈螺旋形突入管腔形成螺旋瓣,又称为 Heister 瓣形皱襞,它有助于保持胆囊管的开放,并控制胆汁的流出。近肝外胆管端的胆囊管段较为光滑,结构并不复杂。

一项 100 例中国正常成人 ERCP 测量的研究,发现胆囊管汇入口在肝外胆管(含括约肌段)全长的中 1/3 段者最多,占 73%,上 1/3 段占 20%,下 1/3 段占 7%。

一组 122 例 MRCP 中,66%(80/122)在肝外胆管全长的中 1/3 处汇合肝外胆管,上 1/3 占 31%(38/122),下 1/3 占 3%(4/122)。

胆囊管从胆囊颈行向左后下方,多从肝总管右侧汇入肝总管形成胆总管。胆囊管与肝总管相遇后立即进行汇合者较少见,多数胆囊管与肝总管相遇后平行下降一短距离,然后再汇合。胆囊管通常在肝外胆管全长的上 1/3 处汇合入胆总管,然而,胆囊管的汇入点变化很大,范围可从肝门部至胆胰共同管水平。

胆囊管开口在肝门区时,肝总管短,胆总管长;胆囊管开口位置很低时,接近十二指肠,因而肝总管长,胆总管短。

有作者报告一组 149 例 MRCP,其胆囊管显示清晰合计 122 例,显示率为 82%(122/149),部分病例可以显示胆囊管的螺旋瓣。胆囊管长度为(20.83 ± 8.92)mm,直径为(2.82 ± 1.04)mm,70%(85/122)呈管状走行,30%(37/122)呈扭曲状走行。

Dasgupta 等(2005)发现,正常情况下,大约 73% 胆囊管呈斜角汇入胆总管,17% 胆囊管呈螺旋状围绕胆总管,10% 胆囊管在汇合前呈平行状走行。

胆囊管汇入肝外胆管右侧占 49.9%,左侧占 18.4%,前或后占 31.7%。少数胆囊管开口于胆总管的左侧,经胆总管的前或后方,迂回至右侧与胆囊连接,这种胆囊管特长,可导致引流不畅,并发胆囊炎。

三、关于肝外胆管的分段

传统看法是按胆囊管汇入肝外胆管处将肝外胆管分为上下两段,上为总肝管,下为总胆管,胆囊管汇入的位置直接影响总胆管的长度:低位汇入,总胆管变短;最低位汇入,总胆管则不存在。

Hand(1963)从解剖学角度提出,将肝外胆管分为:壁薄腔宽的上段和壁厚腔窄的下段(即传统称呼的括约肌段)。从影像诊断学和活体形态学来看,我们认为这样分段比较好,其理由是:①在临床上活体检查时,括约肌段在影像检查时常呈动态变化,扩张和收缩频繁而且明显,其影像表现甚不固定,变化很大;②在 80% 左右的人群中,事实上,括约肌段主要是包含着胆胰共同管,即胆管与胰管汇合后形成的共同管道,理应隶属胆管和胰管共有,而不应全属胆系;③括约肌段的功能与上段的功能差别甚大,它不只是单纯的胆汁的通道,而且在调节胆汁和胰液的流动(包括:流动量、流动速度、流动方向以及流动闸门的开闭等)方面起着重要的作用;④括约肌段及其内部的叶状瓣的活动及其调节相当复杂。

因此，将括约肌段加上十二指肠乳头统称为胆胰管十二指肠连接区的作法，远比将它只划归于总胆管为佳。鉴于此种考虑，我们在测量肝外胆管及总胆管的长度时，均将括约肌段除外，这样，不仅可比性较强，测量更准确可靠，而且也更为合情合理。

第三节　胆囊管先天异常

一、胆囊管的先天异常

有作者研究手术解剖学时指出，胆囊管的先天异常有：①胆囊管肥大，颇似胆囊管缺如；②汇注到胆囊管的副肝胆管，在行胆囊管切断时要注意保存副肝胆管；③胆囊管替代总胆管，提示胆系手术要十分小心，以保证胆汁通畅；④胆囊后胆囊管，如哈德门袋膨出，匐于胆囊管上方，很像胆囊管缺如，遇此情况时，在分离胆囊颈部时，切勿损伤其深侧面的胆囊管。

二、胆囊管最低位汇入肝外胆管

胆囊管最低位汇入括约肌段上方，直接涉及胆胰管十二指肠连接区的解剖构造。从广义看，它也是连接区先天性结构异常的一种，而不应看作为先天性的发育变异。我们报告一组 9 例最低位汇入者，皆伴存胆囊结石、胆囊炎、胆管结石，此种结构的先天异常可能就是这些疾病的病因学方面的解剖因素之一，准确地说，这类先天异常事实上是先天畸形。因此，我们认为，临床上对此类先天畸形应给予必要的重视（图 18-2-4、18-2-5）。

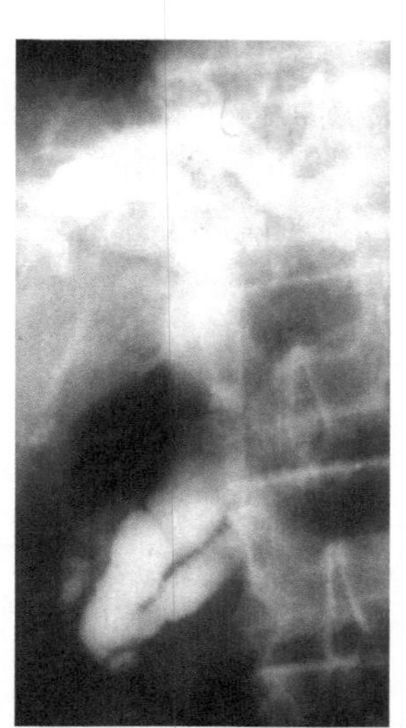

图 18-2-4　ERCP：扩张的胆囊管最低位汇入扩张的肝外胆管，汇合处正位于肝外胆管括约肌段上方，即十二指肠壁浆膜层上。

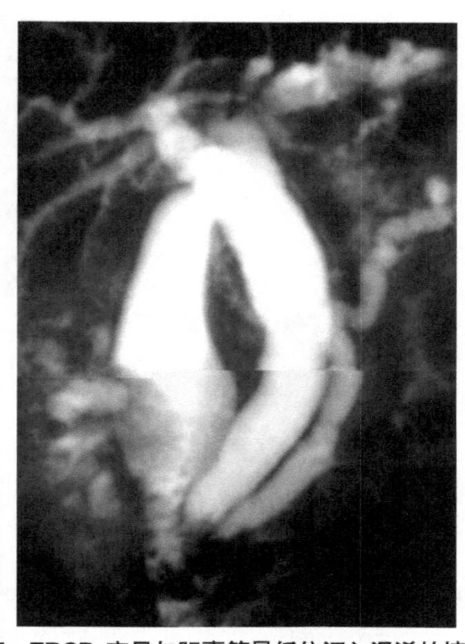

图 18-2-5　ERCP：容易与胆囊管最低位汇入混淆的情况——扩张的肝外胆管与主胰管下端的汇合，此时，胆胰共同管未显示。

总胆管与主胰管开口处形成的隆起，即十二指肠乳头（Vater 乳头）。它一般为 1.0cm × 0.5cm × 0.5cm，大小变异颇大，小者仅 1~2mm 直径，大者可为 1cm 以上，但很少超过 1.5cm。

三、胆囊管与总肝管的连接异常

胆囊管与总肝管连接水平的异常甚多见，从肝门到后下，甚至低至十二指肠上部之下。当连接过低时，此二管在其行程中，以纤维组织紧密相连，很难以分开。胆囊管可走行到总肝管的左后方，或在其前方，在后者的左侧表面与之连接。偶尔，胆囊管可连接于右肝胆管。

肝胆管和胆囊管的长度及其连接的角度变异甚大。胆囊管管径与长度的变异较大。胆囊管一般多在十二指肠上缘以上约 2.5cm 处与总肝管汇合，但也可与总肝管紧密黏着向下行走一段距离，或与总肝管并行至十二指肠或胰腺头部后面再汇合，此时胆囊管与总肝管都比较长（图 18-2-6）。

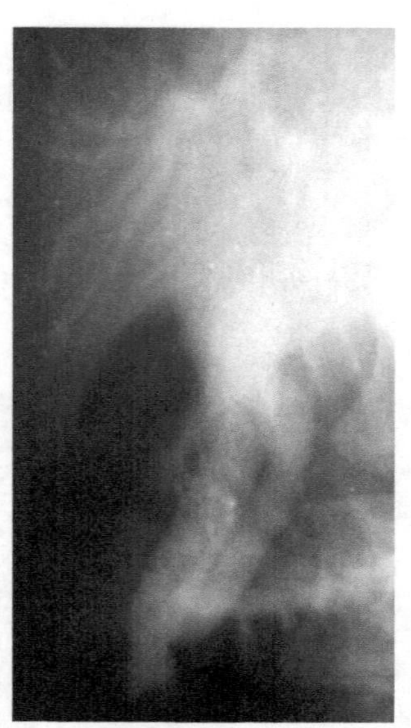

图 18-2-6 ERCP:扩张的胆囊管最低位汇入扩张的肝外胆管,汇合处正位于肝外胆管括约肌段上方,即十二指肠壁浆膜层上。肝外胆管与最低位汇入的胆囊管紧邻平行走行且被包裹在同一纤维鞘膜囊内

第四节 先天性胆囊及胆囊管缺如

先天性胆囊及胆囊管缺如很少见,至 1970 年文献记载仅有 150 余例。但是,先天性胆囊及胆囊管缺如伴发结石者并不罕见, Gerwig 等(1961)复习 55 例,有 20 例伴存结石。

先天性胆囊缺如,常伴存胆囊管缺如,多合并有胆管结石,大都有肝内外胆管扩张,但是,有的胆管也可不扩张。有时,肝外胆管扩张,并无结石发现。

一、临床表现

先天性胆囊及胆囊管缺如的临床发病率为 0.03%~0.065%,在尸检,其发现率则高达 0.155%~0.37%。患者缺乏临床特征,可毫无症状,或有不同程度的胆系疾病症状,并发结石者多有梗阻性黄疸及胆管疾病症状,故临床常诊断为胆囊炎或胆系结石。

二、影像学研究

当病人在口服胆囊造影时,胆囊未见显示,或一再不显影,宜注意是否为先天性胆囊及胆囊管缺如,进一步再行超声显像、CT、MRCP、ERCP 等检查,可有助于诊断。先天性胆囊及胆囊管缺如需与后天性胆囊炎症性萎缩区别,并需探寻有无肝内胆囊及左位胆囊,以及少见的腹壁内胆囊,镰状韧带内胆囊,及腹膜后腔胆囊。术中或术后胆管造影是诊断先天性胆囊及胆囊管缺如更为可靠的方法,并能了解有无胆系的其他先天性畸形。

第五节 胆囊管发育变异

胆石症是临床上的常见、多发疾病,其中以胆囊结石更为多见。目前,腹腔镜胆囊切除术已成为胆囊结石外科治疗的首选治疗方法。然而, Taourel 等(1996)统计,腹腔镜胆囊切除术所致胆管损伤发生率为 0.2%~0.3%,比传统剖腹胆囊切除术所致的发生率(0.1%)增加了 1 倍以上,这与术前对胆囊管的解剖及变异认识不够有着密切的关系,胆囊管发育变异是导致胆囊切除术复杂化的重要因素,也是医源性胆管损伤的主要危险因素。

目前常用于胆系疾病诊断的影像学方法有超声、CT、磁共振胆胰管成像(MRCP)、逆行性胆胰管造影(ERCP)。超声、CT 对于扩张的胆管可以显

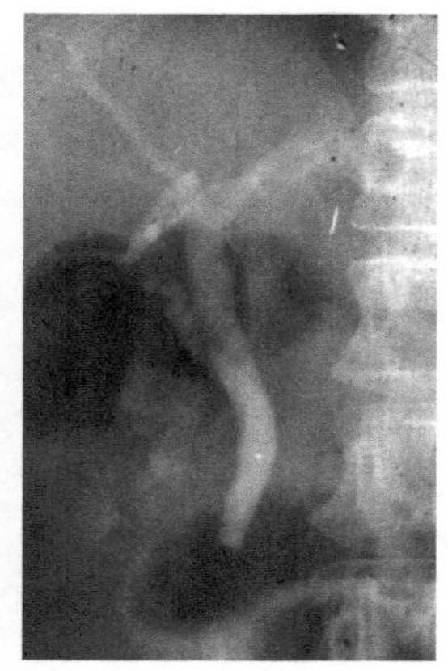

图 18-2-7　胆囊管的发育变异

示，但是对于在正常范围内的胆管、胆囊管却很难显示。

ERCP 已成为胆系成像的参考标准，然而它不能成为一项常规的术前检查方法，因为可能发生严重的并发症或插管失败。MRCP 是近年来迅速发展起来的一种无创性胆胰管成像新技术，能多角度、多方位显示胆道解剖结构，现已广泛应用于胆系疾病的诊断，其临床价值及其优点已超过有创性 ERCP 检查。

一、胆囊管的发育变异

胆囊管的变异很常见，占 18%~23%。包括：胆囊管汇合肝外胆管位置变异（低位、最低位、高位、异位、过长与过短、缺如）、汇合形状的变异（螺旋状、平行走行，汇合的角度，迂曲，成角，扭折）以及汇合部位的变异（非肝外胆管：右肝管、左右肝管汇合处、左肝管）。主要有如下类型：

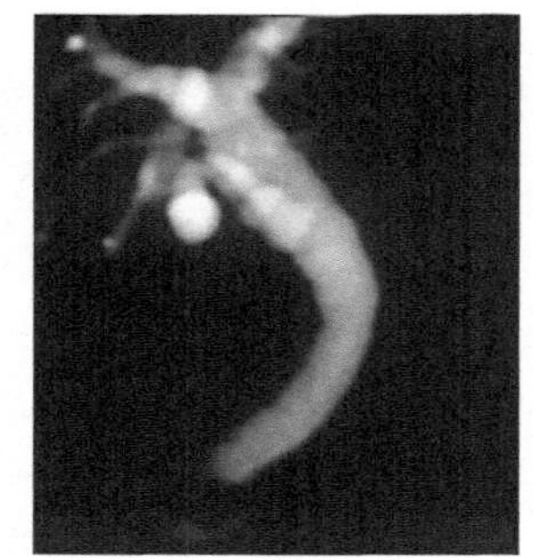

图 18-2-8

（1）胆囊管汇入位置的变异：胆囊管通常在肝外胆管全长的中 1/3 处汇合入肝外胆管约占 75%，约 10% 以上汇入肝外胆管的下半或远 1/3，即为低位汇入。胆囊管低位汇入肝外胆管，可至胰腺内、胆胰共同管水平的十二指肠壁内，但是，胆囊管直接汇入十二指肠内非常罕见，低位汇入变异约占胆管发育变异的 55%；

（2）胆囊管汇合部位的变异：高位汇入，即胆囊管汇入左右肝管汇合处；胆囊管汇入左肝管、右肝管；胆囊管汇入可呈前、后螺旋形汇入肝总管；胆囊管可呈空虚状汇入肝总管或右肝管；

（3）胆囊管汇合形状的变异：胆囊管与肝总管并行 2cm 以上称为并行，约占 10%，如果两者伴行距离较长常提示有共同的纤维鞘，并且胆囊管过长，常常可导致手术时误为胆囊管正常汇入，而造成术后胆囊管残留过长（18-2-7）。

胆囊管与肝总管并行二者并行，可以互相平行，胆囊管可以围绕肝总管螺旋绕行：胆囊管旋前于肝总管左侧汇入或前侧汇入；胆囊管旋后于肝总管左侧汇入或后侧汇入；

（4）其他少见变异包括：胆囊管过短或缺如，长度小于 5mm，胆囊颈部直接汇入肝外胆管；胆囊管过短时术中牵拉胆囊，胆总管被拉直，易误认胆囊管而伤及胆总管。胆囊管囊状扩张，在此种情况，术中易把囊腔当作胆囊的颈部，而将胆总管当作胆囊管而切断。双胆囊管（可有或无双胆囊）。曾有作者报道一例十二指肠组织易位于胆囊管，非常罕见。

二、胆囊管的发育变异的临床意义

研究表明，胆囊管的发育变异可导致胆囊管自身疾病，Caroli-bosc 等（1997）及 Deenitchin 等（1998）研究表明变异胆囊管多伴有胆囊及胆囊管结石，并可造成梗阻性黄疸。

胆囊管的发育变异是一种较常见的发育变异，其临床意义在于，进行胆系外科手术时，必须要熟悉先天异常，从而避免意外损伤，影像诊断工作者也必须具备这种知识，以便合理解释影像。如存在胆系疾病需行手术时，这些发育变异会给手术带来较大风险。随着腹腔镜胆囊切除术在临床上的广泛应用，术前常规了解胆囊管的发育变异就显得相当重要（图 18-2-8）。

胆囊管的发育变异的临床意义还在于，除了上述术后胆囊管残留过长外，还有，在手术时，靠近胆囊或胆囊管的胆管走行异常，或者肝总管呈空虚状汇合胆囊或胆囊管时，胆囊切除时就存在很大风险，可导致手术医生误将肝总管认为是胆囊管进行结扎，造成不应有悲剧性后果。异常胆管呈空虚状汇入胆囊管的占 1%~2%。

如果术前对胆囊管的上述发育变异认识不足，易导致疾病误诊，易导致术中胆源性损伤，并可导致胆系瘘等并发症的发生率增加。

Uetsuji 等（1993）发现胆囊管异位汇入可造成胆汁滞留和 / 或胰液返流入胆管，产生胆胰管粘连，可导致梗阻性黄疸，并造成手术困难。

胆囊管结石对伴行肝外胆管压迫可引起 Mirizzi 综合征，可造成胆管梗阻。胆囊管与肝外胆管成像的重叠可造成结石的假象，胆囊管结石或胆囊管走行异常在影像上可造成包块和肿瘤的假象。

由此可见，胆囊管的发育变异在临床上有重要意义,熟悉胆囊管的发育变异的影像表现以及相关疾病的形成过程,对提高诊断水平及避免误诊很有帮助。

三、MRCP 诊断胆囊管发育变异

MRCP 结合冠状位原始图像及横断位 T_2WI,可了解肝内外胆管、胆囊及胆囊管的解剖结构关系,可观察胆囊管汇入肝外胆管的方式及汇入部位,观察胆囊管长度、内径、走行及与肝外胆管轴线的成角,并可发现胆囊管的各种发育变异。

评价胆囊管的发育变异,应结合 MRI 断面图像和 2D、3D MRCP 原始图像和(最大强度投影、遮盖表面显示)二维重组图像,仔细观察胆囊管形态、胆囊管与肝外胆管汇合处的情况、胆囊管的走行。

胆囊管与肝总管并行时,有可能将并行肝总管误认为胆囊管而予以钳夹、离断,而急性胆囊炎或慢性胆囊炎急性发作的患者,并行胆囊管与肝总管更不易分离,手术容易导致肝总管损伤。胆囊管囊性扩张者,术中易把囊腔当作胆囊的颈部,把胆总管当作胆囊管而切断。胆囊管过短时术中牵拉胆囊,胆总管被拉直,易误认胆囊管而伤及胆总管。

Crist 和 Gadacz(1993)报道常见易引起腹腔镜胆囊切除术术中胆囊管损伤的发育变异有以下几种:①胆囊管与肝总管并行 2cm 以上;②胆囊管汇入异常,通常胆囊管汇入胆总管右侧,变异时胆囊管汇入左侧壁,可旋前汇入及旋后汇入,亦可汇入左右肝管或左右肝管汇合处;③胆囊管粗大;④胆囊管过短或缺如。据文献报道胆囊管发育变异发生率为 5.0%~22.7%,该组资料胆囊管发育变异发生率 5.9%(53/900)。

MRCP 不仅可以显示胆囊管发育变异,而且也可显示胆管树变异和胆系疾病,Taourel 等(1996)对 171 例病人的 MRCP 影像分析发现,MRCP 诊断肝管和胆囊管变异的符合率达 98% 和 95%,敏感度达 71% 和 86%。胆囊管显示率为 74%;胆囊管低位汇入占 9%,肝总管左侧汇入占 17%;胆囊管与肝管平行走行占 25%,变异右肝管占 9%。

一组 53 例研究中,内侧汇入发生率 18.9%,汇入右肝管发生率 18.9%,与肝总管并行发生率 16.9%,该组显示汇入左右肝管汇合处发生率较高,达 39.6%,胆囊管变异容易并发胆囊病变,如结石和炎症,发生率 47%,合并胆系疾病发生率 98%,除 1 例肝内多发囊肿外,52 例均有胆系疾病。

Dusunceli 等(2004)统计了 581 例 MRCP,结果发现长胆囊管占 1.7%,胆囊管汇入肝外胆管非右侧壁占 0.63%,胆囊管低位汇入占 3.8%,短胆囊管占 0.2%,变异右肝管占 4.8%。还有作者对 801 例 MRCP 研究表明,胆囊管变异占 5.9%。

MRCP 也能良好地显示胆囊管的病变。Park 等(1998)通过 MRCP 与超声的比较发现,对于评价胆囊管结石及其引起的胆囊管梗阻, MRCP 明显优于超声。

Choi 等(2000)研究发现,MRCP 对诊断因胆囊管结石引起的 Mirizzi 综合征亦具有重要作用,并可发现胆囊管瘘。Rubini 等(1999)报道, MRCP 可显示胆囊切除术后胆囊管残端结石及胆囊管残端的扩张。由此可见, MRCP 不仅能清晰显示胆囊管的解剖和变异,而且对胆囊管疾病的诊断具有重要作用。

变异胆囊管多伴有胆囊、胆囊管和 / 或胆总管结石及炎症。多位作者的多项研究结果报告出现一定的差异,可能与:①样本量的大小;②种族差异;③地区分布差异;④研究方法及检查手段的差异等有关。

腹腔镜胆囊切除术前常规 MRCP 可观察胆囊管的解剖及变异,从而减少医源性胆系损伤,减少胆系术后并发症的发生,对病人的治疗方案、手术步骤及预后有着十分重要意义。

第六节 胆囊管低位汇入综合征

一般认为,胆囊管汇入肝外胆管处,常位于肝外胆管的上半段,即总胆管的长度与肝外胆管全长之比约为 0.7,换言之,即总肝管与总胆管长度比较,为三七开。我们将胆囊管汇入处在肝外胆管全长(括约肌段除外)下半者,即比值小于 0.5 者,称为胆囊管低位汇入。

在胆囊管低位汇入中,约有 1/10 的病例胆囊管汇入于肝外胆管胰腺段与括约肌段交界处,即十二指肠壁外处,称之为胆囊管最低位汇入。

一些学者认为,胆囊管通常在肝外胆管全长的

中 1/3 处汇合胆总管约占 75%，约 10% 汇合入远 1/3。另有作者认为，胆囊管低位为胆囊管汇合于肝外胆管的下半或远 1/3 段。

胆囊管低位汇合，可至胰腺内、胆胰共同管水平的十二指肠内，胆囊管直接汇合十二指肠内非常罕见，低位汇合变异约占胆管变异的 55%（图 18-2-9）。

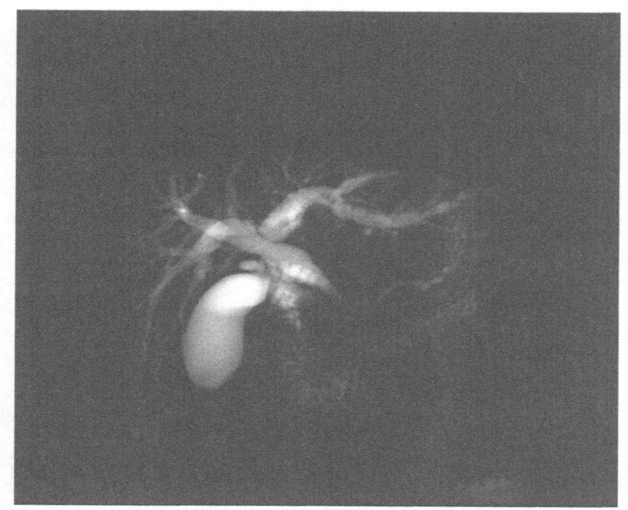

图 18-2-9　MRCP：扩张的有螺旋瓣的胆囊管低位异位汇入扩张的肝外胆管下端，即最低位汇入

一、胆囊管低位汇入的影像学表现

1. 胆囊管长度明显增加　胆囊管低位汇入势必造成胆囊管长度增加。据国内外尸体解剖学研究，正常成人的胆囊管长度约为 25~40mm，低位汇入者的胆囊管平均长度比正常最大值都长许多。一些作者提出，长胆囊管是指其长度 >6 cm。

部分胆囊管低位汇入病例和全部最低位汇入病例的胆囊管，与总肝管并排伴行一段距离后，再汇入总肝管，从影像学观察，只有一个汇入处；而从尸体解剖学和外科手术学看，除该汇合点外还有一假汇合点，即胆囊管与总肝管相遇后，首先共同为结缔组织鞘包绕一起并排下行，从结缔组织鞘外观看似已汇合，实际上为假汇合，如从该处切断和结扎胆囊管，势必导致胆囊管残留部分过长。

2. 胆囊切除术后胆囊管残端过长　从多年的临床经验看，胆囊管位于肝总管后面或侧面伴随下行，易被肝总管遮掩或被对比剂影重迭，在手术中正位 X 线照片和手术野均难以发现，只有通过斜位照片才能辨认胆囊管汇入处，这样，就给不了解胆囊管低位汇入的手术医生设下陷阱，常常导致常规胆囊切除术后胆囊管残留过长，不可避免地出现“胆囊切除术后综合征”。自然，现在术前 MRCP 可清楚显示胆囊管的情况，为手术医生避免误入此类陷阱帮助不少。

胆囊管残端过长，一直被认为是“胆囊切除术后综合征”的一个重要原因。我们在临床所见到的胆囊管低位汇入者，胆囊管残端长约 40mm 左右，在最低位汇入病例残端更长，长约 54mm 以上，均等于或超过正常胆囊管长度的最大值 40mm，说明此类残端确实太长，不是一个“残端”而是一条“残管”，不宜称为胆囊管残端，而应称为残留胆囊管，即一般所说的“残留假胆囊”，它可成为长而大的死腔，或因原有的感染源，或因胆汁反流，极易发生感染，构成术后所谓残留胆囊炎的临床症状。

这些术后病例，皆因术前不了解不认识胆囊管低位汇入，术时由于视野有限或经验不足，很难发现胆囊管的全貌以及低位汇合，自然不可能注意分离或难以分离长度增加的胆囊管全长，而只按常规手术（这在腹腔镜切除胆囊术尤其明显），导致胆囊管残端遗留过长，形成残留胆囊管，成为假胆囊。术前如行 MRCP、ERCP 或 PTC，了解胆囊管低位汇入的位置，对于手术计划的制订及手术程序的安排，均是必要的。

3. 胆囊管的异位汇入　胆囊管一般从肝外胆管右侧壁汇入肝外胆管。但是，少数（尸体解剖学与手术解剖学观察约为 15%）胆囊管可从非右壁汇入，即从左壁、前壁或后壁汇入，我们将之称为胆囊管异位汇入，据我们研究，胆囊管低位汇入者约有 3/4 以上都合并异位汇入。

在一组 54 例胆囊管低位汇入肝外胆管病例中，有 32 例（59.3%）胆囊管从左侧壁汇入，前壁汇入 8 例，后壁 6 例，右壁汇入仅 8 例。在另组 9 例胆囊管最低位汇入肝外胆管的病例中，4 例汇入左壁，4 例从左前方汇入，1 例从前方汇入，皆非从右壁汇入。在 CT 与 MRI 的横断图像上，清楚可见胆管汇入肝外胆管方位，远比以往 ERCP 和 PTC 所获图像更为准确和清楚。

从胆囊管低位汇入资料看，胆囊管汇入左壁、后壁及前壁者所占比例甚大，这样的异位汇入势必导致胆囊管围绕总肝管走行，围绕的严重程度各个病例不尽相同，但它们都妨碍胆囊内容物的进入与排出，从形态学的角度给胆囊及胆管病变的发生创造了条件。

4. 胆囊管扩张　在我们观察到的低位异位汇入的胆囊管病例中,胆囊管大多呈普遍性一致性扩张;少数病例胆囊管的胆囊端较为细窄,与正常胆囊管相差不大,然而其肝外胆管端却明显扩张,遂形成长颈的喇叭状外形。上述两种情况都说明,胆囊管发生了炎症或/和胆囊管胆汁流通出现了梗阻情况,可以解释患者的临床症状。只有个别病例胆囊管无明显扩张,似说明个别胆囊管低位异位发育变异,但当时还未出现病理性改变,还未发生临床症状。

关于胆囊管两端内径的差异,我们观察到在胆囊管低位异位汇入组中,约有 20% 病例的胆囊管两端内径相差较大,即近胆管段较近胆囊段明显扩张,究其原因,考虑有下述三个因素:先天性发育异常;胆囊管近胆管端易受胆管疾病的影响,胆管感染时易逆行侵及该段胆囊管,胆管扩张时,胆囊管汇入处相应扩张,随之近胆管段也扩张;胆囊管近胆管段无螺旋瓣,尤易扩张。

5. 胆囊管的瓣膜减少　与正常组比较,在我们观察到的低位异位汇入的病例,胆囊管的瓣膜明显减少,约有 40% 的病人,胆囊管少瓣或无瓣。

正常成人胆囊管黏膜可有 5~12 个新月形皱襞凸入管腔内,它连续规则地斜行环绕胆囊管,表现为螺旋状黏膜皱襞。在胆囊管低位汇入组中,胆囊管无瓣或少瓣者常多于一般情况,分析其原因,主要是因为胆囊管扩张,使螺旋瓣本身的深度变浅,瓣膜变平,从而影响螺旋瓣的显示,至于是否与先天发育因素有关,则有待进一步观察。

关于螺旋瓣的作用,以往认为它可控制胆汁的出入,使胆囊管不能过度膨大或缩小;目前认为螺旋瓣内有平滑肌,螺旋瓣的作用主要是保持胆囊管的恒定开放,有利于胆汁的流通,在胆囊或肝外胆管内压力变化时,防止胆囊管的扩张或萎陷。

胆囊管低位汇入时,螺旋瓣本身的深度变浅,瓣膜变平,甚至螺旋瓣缺如或数目减少,皆不利于保持胆囊管的恒定开放,可能导致胆汁流通的障碍。同时,胆囊或胆管内压发生变化时,均可涉及胆囊管的内压变化,尤其当胆胰管下端括约肌病变(如痉挛、狭窄或梗阻)时,胆管内压升高,胆汁向上方反流,胆囊与胆囊管等缓冲地带也随之扩张,这是一种病理生理机能代偿的表现。

6. 常伴发胆囊和胆管病变　在胆囊管低位异位伴发胆囊病变的病例中,以胆囊结石为最多。在一组 54 例低位异位汇入中,有 39 例伴发胆囊结石;9 例最低位异位汇入病人,每例都伴存胆囊结石。

在胆囊管低位异位伴发胆管病变的病例中,以肝内外胆管结石为最多。在该组 54 例低位异位汇入中,有 34 例伴存肝内外胆管结石;最低位异位汇入的 9 例病人,全部都伴存肝内外胆管结石。

胆囊管低位异位汇入总肝管,给肠道逆行胆系感染创造了有利条件,汇入部位越低越靠近胆胰管下端,感染越重,胆囊管最低位异位汇入者,胆系感染最为严重。

在最低位异位汇入者, ERCP 检查逆行注入对比剂时,常常都是对比剂首先进入胆囊管,使之显影于总肝管以前。这除了与患者俯卧位右侧抬高(在胆囊管左位或左前位汇入总肝管者,对比剂自然容易进入胆囊管)的体位因素有关外,汇入位置最低也有一定的作用。同理,肠道逆行感染也会更容易累及胆囊。

在该组胆囊管最低位异位汇入的 9 例中,除 1 例外, 8 例均可见总肝管扩张,且为肝胆管结石伴肝胆管炎。在该组,有 8 例均见胆囊管从总肝管右侧与总肝管交叉,再从总肝管前方或后方绕到它的左侧,与总肝管一起并排伴行长段距离,然后再汇入总肝管的下端。另 1 例胆囊管从总肝管右侧逐渐移行到总肝管前方,再汇入总肝管。

在这 9 例中,胆囊管与总肝管均现扩张,但胆囊管明显细于总肝管者有 8 例, 1 例胆囊管与总肝管直径基本相等,皆为 6mm,在总肝管上段二管交叉,然后并排伴行 50mm 后,抵达总肝管下端,汇入总肝管,形成括约肌段。

7. 乳头区憩室　有作者调查了 1 574 例行 ERCP 检查的病人(男 706 例,女 868 例),发现乳头区憩室在低位胆囊管(乳头上 5mm 内)中频繁出现($P<0.001$),女性乳头区憩室伴低位汇合胆囊管者与不伴低位胆囊管汇合者有显著性差异($P<0.05$),原因不能简单归于年龄因素,胆囊管低位汇合可能是病因,因为它影响了胆汁的运输,所以低位胆囊管伴乳头区憩室是一种新的综合征。

二、在 X 线诊断时胆囊管低位汇入可引起的误诊

1. 假性胆囊管低位汇入　在肝外胆管胰腺段因疾病显示不良时,可将胆囊管正常汇入位置误认为低位汇入。此时,注意观察整个肝外胆管的形状,长

度和走行，有利于识别真象。

2. 螺旋瓣与假结石　在胆囊管低位汇入时，胆囊管常可与肝外胆管影像重叠，胆囊管内的螺旋瓣影像如不注意可误为肝外胆管内的结石影。

三、胆囊管最低位汇入与胆胰管下端括约肌的功能

解剖学研究发现，肝外胆管越近括约肌段处，肌纤维越多，而使管腔保持一定张力，胆囊管汇入部位越低，括约肌影响胆囊管内容物的进出也就越严重。胆囊管在括约肌段上端汇入总肝管，不仅影响胆囊内胆汁的进出，而且也可能对胆汁从总肝管排泄有所妨碍。汇入部位正居括约肌段上方，很有可能妨碍括约肌段的正常关闭和开放，引起功能紊乱，从而导致总肝管内胆汁排空障碍，同时为肠道感染逆行进入胆系创造某些条件。胆囊管与总肝管交叉与伴行，对总肝管内胆汁排泄也可能造成阻碍。

四、胆囊管最低位汇入与连接区结构异常

胆囊管最低位汇入括约肌段的上方，直接涉及胆胰管十二指肠连接区的解剖构造。从广义上讲，它也是连接区先天性结构异常的一种表现，而不应只看作先天变异。我们所见 9 例胆囊管最低位汇入的病例，皆伴存胆囊结石，胆囊炎及胆管结石，此类先天性结构异常可能就是这些疾病的解剖学病因因素之一。因此，我们认为，临床上对此类先天异常应给予足够的必要的重视。

五、胆囊管低位汇入综合征

胆囊管低位汇入常伴存汇入异位，低位汇入势必导致胆囊管长度增加，汇入低位加异位多造成胆囊胆汁引流不畅，加上胆囊管螺旋瓣的欠缺等各种因素，均给胆囊内容物的引流造成困难，而且低位汇入（尤其是最低位汇入）给肠道感染逆行累及胆系创造有利条件。因此，胆囊管低位汇入者胆囊疾病发病率甚高。这些情况都说明，上述解剖结构的改变，已成为胆囊疾病的产生和发展的病因学因素。因而，我们认为，胆囊管低位汇入和异位汇入，与其看作是一种先天变异，倒不如看作先天异常更为恰当。综上所述，我们提出“胆囊管低位汇入综合征”这一概念，来概括此类先天异常，力图引起更多的讨论和关注。

胆囊管低位汇入综合征包括内容为：胆囊管低位汇入，胆囊管长度增加；胆囊管异位汇入；出现胆囊疾病的症状和体征；常规胆囊切除术后，胆囊管残留过长，原胆囊疾病的症状体征无明显好转。

第三章 Mirizzi综合征

第一节 Mirizzi综合征之一

Kohr(1905)早就报道胆囊管结石嵌塞和炎症引起肝总管不全性机械性梗阻。Mirizzi称之为功能性肝管综合征,意指胆囊管结石炎症产生的胆汁流梗阻,由于胆管下端括约肌痉挛而加重。因胆囊管或胆囊颈结石嵌顿引起肝总管梗阻称为Mirizzi综合征,又称肝管综合征。它是由术中胆系造影的先驱者,阿根廷外科医生Mirizzi(1948)发现的。

Mirizzi综合征是慢性胆囊炎的一种不常见的并发症,其内涵是结石嵌顿于胆囊管、胆囊颈、胆囊管残端内,导致总肝管梗阻。出现此种梗阻,不仅仅是单纯的结石的机械性因素,还有周围慢性炎症反应的积极参与。

发病机制:Mirizzi综合征更多出现于胆囊管先天异常者,或胆囊管低位汇合肝外胆管的病人。此类情况具有较长的胆囊管,而且与总肝管同被一筋膜鞘包裹。大多数胆囊管都是从肝外胆管右侧壁汇入,而容易患Mirizzi综合征的因素是,胆囊管从左侧壁汇入或胆囊管围绕肝外胆管螺旋状走行。有作者研究120例术中胆系造影,见18%病例胆囊管汇入肝外胆管处位置低下,胆囊管其长轴与肝总管走行一致,认为这种低位的胆囊管汇合及胆囊管和肝总管平行走行易发生Mirizzi综合征。一些学者提出,Mirizzi综合征可由于手术创伤,肝管肿瘤,硬化性胆管炎,增大的胆囊管淋巴结,胆囊管肿瘤结节,急性胆囊炎或胆囊癌等引起。

Lubbers(1983)指出,“Mirizzi括约肌”没有足够的解剖学存在的证据,他还综合有关报道,提出Mirizzi综合征缺乏确切含义。

虽然发病原因各不相同,胆囊病变与肝总管受累情况也互不一致,但其共同特征为一异常的肝总管狭窄。随着胆系影像诊断学的迅速发展,Mirizzi综合征的病例报告日渐增多,对于Mirizzi综合征的认识亦趋深化。

Clemett和Lowman(1965)在观察大量临床病例的基础上,提出Mirizzi综合征病例具有的4个要素:①与肝总管并行的胆囊管发育变异;②胆囊管或胆囊颈结石嵌顿;③因结石本身或结石周围继发局部炎症引起肝总管不全性机械性梗阻与梗阻性黄疸;④胆管炎反复发作及持续黄疸后并向肝硬化发展。

目前,多数学者认为,胆囊颈或胆囊管的嵌顿性结石和伴发的炎症累及并压迫肝总管,引起肝总管狭窄及不完全梗阻,继发胆管炎和黄疸症状者,即为Mirizzi综合征。

Mirizzi综合征并不是一种少见病,其发病率不超过胆系手术的2%,术前诊断比较困难,如果不充分了解及认识此病将导致胆管损伤。

一、Mirizzi综合征分型

两型:McSherry(1982)提出的分类法分两型。Ⅰ型:肝总管被胆囊管或胆囊颈的结石压迫;Ⅱ型:结石侵蚀肝总管,瘘管形成。

四型:Csendes(1989)将其分为四型。Ⅰ型:胆囊管或胆囊颈结石嵌顿并压迫胆总管;Ⅱ型:胆囊管与胆总管之间的侵蚀融合少于胆总管周径的1/3;Ⅲ型:胆囊管与胆总管之间的侵蚀融合为胆总管周径的2/3左右;Ⅳ型:胆囊管与胆总管之间的侵蚀融合累及整个胆总管壁。

四型:Nagakawa(1997)根据诊断与治疗特点提出新的分类方法,Ⅰ型:胆囊管或胆囊颈结石压迫胆总管;Ⅱ型:胆囊管与胆总管之间有融合;Ⅲ型:胆囊管结石压迫右肝管;Ⅳ型:胆囊管内无结石,由于胆囊三角炎症纤维化致胆管狭窄。

二、病理学

Mirizzi 综合征是胆囊管或胆囊颈结石嵌顿或合并炎症引起胆管梗阻，有或无胆瘘形成。其临床病史及体格检查均无特异性，术前诊断很困难，常出现黄疸，多诊为胆管炎，而 Mirizzi 综合征是梗阻性黄疸不常见的病因，若不认识此病，或术前未能正确诊断，则术中很易造成胆管损伤，横断胆总管为常见的错误。所以，了解 Mirizzi 综合征解剖及病理生理知识有助于正确地诊断和成功的处理。

胆囊管低位开口是一个关键的易患因素，有作者统计，在胆系手术病人中胆囊管低位开口约占18%~49%，其结果导致胆囊管与肝总管并行一段，若胆囊颈或管有结石嵌顿，反复发作的急性炎症最初使胆囊扩张，所累及区域的结构发炎及增厚，然后胆囊靠近肝总管或胆总管近端，胆囊壁与胆管壁发生粘贴，并压迫胆管产生梗阻性黄疸，结石引起压迫性坏死和进一步急性炎症，这时胆石可能侵蚀邻近的胆管壁产生胆瘘，大部分患者的胆囊管消失，产生更大的瘘，随着时间推移，结石可慢慢地移至胆管内，产生管壁完全坏死。

Mirizzi 综合征的临床重要性：Mirizzi 综合征术前诊断对治疗方案的选择十分重要，因为随着微创手术治疗胆石症（经腹腔镜胆囊切除或取石）的广泛开展，明确诊断可以帮助临床医生对患者采用开腹手术还是腹腔镜手术有重要指导意义。Mirizzi 综合征伴有炎症和粘连会阻碍腹腔镜手术时对胆囊三角的分离，可能导致腹腔镜手术失败，再选择开腹或损伤胆管产生严重的并发症，增加医疗风险和隐患。

未认识的 Mirizzi 综合征的后果包括：继发于胆囊和肝十二指肠韧带内的炎症反应的肝外胆管的狭窄；结石嵌顿于总肝管并侵蚀，形成胆囊 - 胆瘘，并伴存一个炎症包块所围绕共同腔隙。由于本病缺乏特征性临床表现，临床诊断较为困难，加之其特殊病理基础，局部解剖关系不清，若术前不能确诊又无警惕，而当作一般胆囊结石处置，则术中由于广泛而严重的粘连，使胆囊切除困难，稍不小心则很容易损伤周围脏器。轻率的胆囊剥离，则可损伤胆囊管，甚至可误将胆总管当作长而扩张的胆囊管予以结扎或切断，造成灾难性后果。因此，提高对 Mirizzi 综合征病理基础及 X 线表现的认识，术前确诊并掌握好治疗原则甚为重要。

三、临床表现

黄疸、上升性胆管炎或仅只怀疑为胆囊炎的症状是 Mirizzi 综合征通常的临床表现。如果病人未行治疗，则可能出现复发性胆管炎，以及胆汁性肝硬化。

正确的术前诊断是极为重要的。在胆囊切除术时，逆行分离胆囊底至胆囊颈，以便游离胆囊时，手术医生通常是结扎首先看见的小口径的含胆汁的管道，一般情况下，这就是胆囊管。但是，在 Mirizzi 综合征病人，此管道将不是胆囊管，而是总胆管，因为此结构从近侧梗阻处看相当细小，由于胆囊结石和周围的炎症，胆囊管已不容易识别。上面这情况是在胆囊炎或 / 和胆系结石的不正确术前诊断之后出现的。

由于 Mirizzi 综合征临床表现缺乏特异性，给术前诊断带来困难。一组资料中，23 例患者中就诊时曾经有黄疸病史 12 例，仅占 52%，且即使有黄疸还需要和其他引起黄疸疾病相鉴别，因此，单纯依赖临床表现和体征对 Mirizzi 综合征诊断十分困难，临床往往需要求助于影像学检查。

有作者报告，一例术前错误诊断为癌的患者，且在手术中竟还得到“证实”，实际上，这却是一个围绕着胆囊和肝十二指肠韧带的广泛的炎症粘连的团块，伪似不能手术切除的新生物，不适当的手术则随之而至。此类未确认出的胆系内瘘，可能在术后漏出胆汁；在手术时还可能将嵌顿着的结石遗漏。

四、影像学研究

比较影像学：Mirizzi 综合征的诊断主要依靠影像诊断。在 X 线检查口服胆囊造影时，胆囊多不显影。静脉胆系造影时，胆囊胆管显影浅淡，甚至不显影，确诊率甚低。由于 B 型超声的准确性和可重复性较差，而且所得信息有限，不宜单独作为确诊 Mirizzi 综合征的方法。但是，超声和 CT 对胆管腔外恶性病变的鉴别很有价值，因此，对于 PTC 和 ERCP 检查后某些病例的鉴别诊断，它们都有着重要的作用。以前最可靠的检查方法是直接法胆系造影，现在 MRCP 及 MSCT 的三维重建完全可以胜任本病的诊断。术前主要依靠 PTC、ERCP，至于二者孰优孰劣，谁首选，谁补充，各学者意见不甚一致，这在各地各单位也不尽相同。在早期，通过影像检查诊断 Mirizzi 综合征主要依靠直接法胆系造影。目前，虽然有腹部 B 超、MRCP 和 CT 检查在胆囊和胆管疾病的诊断中已经普遍应用，使胆囊和胆管疾病的诊断水平大为提高，但对 Mirizzi 综合征的术前诊断仍面临较大的挑战。

一组 25 例中，术前仅 24% 的病例被正确诊断，不足总病例数的 1/4。该组术前诊断率较低的原因在于临床医师和影像科医师对本病认识不足。有些病例的影像表现虽然具有特征，但因诊断医师不了解此病而未能做出明确诊断，而是仅仅局限于描述客观征象，或是仅诊断胆囊结石、胆管结石或肝内、外胆管扩张，影像报告中缺乏进一步的综合分析与主观能动性判断。

超声：超声与普通 CT 扫描二种技术通常都是最早进行的检查。不幸，它们所见的征象均非特异，并且诊断困难。如果看见三联征：结石嵌顿于胆囊颈、肝胆管与总肝管扩张、总胆管无异常，则可提示诊断。有时，还能显示总肝管的移位。有作者报告，有的可见邻近于胆囊的一个不规则的腔隙，伴有或不伴有一个结石被逐出的表现。超声在肝外胆管床的位置可见到两条平行的管状结构，再加上胆囊管残端有一结石，也可提示诊断。一个炎症性包块的存在，能支配解释超声或 CT 图像，提示为胆囊癌、胆管癌甚或胰腺癌的程度。一组 15 例患者均行超声检查，14 例提示胆系结石，说明超声对胆系结石的诊断是敏感和准确的，但对 Mirizzi 综合征尚难做出明确的诊断。在梗阻性黄疸的患者超声检查可以对胆系结石进行较好的筛选作用。

一般认为，本病的 B 超声像图可出现如下表现：①胆囊颈或胆囊管有一个固定的结石强回声，结石直径通常 >1.0 cm，直径较小的结石常能自然排出；②胆囊颈部水平以上的胆管扩张，即肝总管和肝内胆管出现不同程度的扩张；③扩张的肝总管或胆总管在结石下方管径突然变为正常；④胆囊肿大与积液，囊腔内显示多发结石，胆囊壁增厚呈现炎症改变。普遍认为，如果胆囊管、肝总管及门静脉的影像呈现“三管征”，即应考虑为本病。

X 线检查：X 线平片可显示一个大的单个钙化的结石，紧邻肝门附近，结合临床表现，可提示诊断。直接法胆系造影典型的表现为：胆管位于胆囊管或胆囊直接对应之处可见较宽的弧形充盈缺损，边缘光滑，经常在侧壁，有时因胆囊管与肝总管之间的关系偶尔也在中间，其上胆管扩张，扩张胆管于结石以下突然变成正常的胆管，胆管多表现为部分梗阻，少数时表现为完全梗阻。

Mirizzi 综合征的典型表现有：①肝总管光滑的弧形外压性变窄。受压方向随胆囊管与胆总管粘连位置不同而异，以外侧多见，内侧及中位受压者较少见；②胆囊多不显影，胆囊管或胆囊显影时，可见紧靠受压的肝总管的透光结石影；③肝胆管常有轻度至中度扩张，伴慢性胆管炎表现；④胆总管在大多数病例均无异常，偶尔可见有继发性结石的阴影；⑤胆系内瘘的表现。

内瘘的发生率相当高，但显示率很低。不显影的胆囊与肝总管之间出现不规则的对比剂充盈，或透视下见胆囊与胆总管同时显影而胆囊管不显影，或胆囊与结肠同时显影，这些征象均提示胆系内瘘可能存在。

但是，应该注意，肝总管外压变窄及胆囊颈或胆囊管结石嵌顿等 X 线征象都是非特异的。急性胆囊炎、胆囊癌、胆囊管癌、胆管癌、原发性硬化性胆管炎，胆管医源性狭窄或良、恶性肝门部淋巴结肿大、胰腺癌等皆可使肝总管受压变窄。因此，在考虑诊断 Mirizzi 综合征的同时，需排除上述疾病才能确诊，此时，应结合临床表现，X 线征象，以及超声与 CT 检查的资料，进行综合性诊断。

直接法胆系造影常能作出正确的诊断。如果考虑恶性病变是超声或 CT 图像的基础，术前常需作直接法胆系造影以了解手术入路地图，或作为胆汁引流的一部分，给予正确术前诊断的机会。主要的征象是胆囊管汇入总肝管区及其附近，总肝管呈现光滑的曲线形节段性狭窄，或出现外侧的外压性压迹。令人遗憾的是，如果结石未出现钙化，而且又存在上述主要征象，鉴别诊断应该有肝门周围淋巴结肿大、胆囊癌或慢性胆囊炎引起的胆囊肿大、肝肿瘤、胰腺肿瘤、胰腺假性囊肿。

在直接法胆系造影时应用延迟照片，对比剂或是途经胆囊 - 胆瘘，或是经不完全梗阻的胆囊管，使任何造成损伤的结石，都可能描绘出梗阻点的轮廓，从而确诊。此外，直接法胆系造影可用于描述总肝管任何狭窄的范围与严重性。如果因为怀疑恶性病变而做血管造影，可能看见在肝动脉外侧出现曲线形的压迹，因其邻近总肝管，故不需惊奇。

从理论上讲，直接法胆系造影应能显示胆系瘘管的形态，但尚未见到明确显示瘘管的报道。因此，对 Mirizzi 综合征的分型，单纯依靠影像表现还不能做出，主要还是根据手术结果方能得出诊断。术中根据不同的分型可采取不同的手术方式，主要有胆囊切开取石造瘘术、单纯胆囊切除术、胆囊切除胆管修补T管引流术及胆囊切除，胆管空肠Roux-Y吻合术，也有用腹腔镜行Mirizzi综合征手术的，对于不能耐受手术的患者，可经内窥镜取石，并结合体外微波碎石，内支架支撑也取得了良好效果。因Mirizzi综合征与肿瘤恶变有某种关联，因此若术中诊为Mirizzi综合征，应行胆囊快速冰冻病理检查，以决定手术方式。

CT：肝内胆管轻中度扩张，肝外胆管胰腺段正常，胰腺段以上水平梗阻，若没有肝门肿块，梗阻点附近又有结石则应考虑为Mirizzi综合征。因直接法胆系造影上肝总管宽的弧形压迹也可以是肝门区转移癌、胆囊癌或其他疾病引起，而CT的应用可弥补直接法胆系造影的不足，不仅可观察胆管周围结构的情况以除外其他病变，同时可明确扩张的胆管和结石；根据病程及有无瘘管形成，CT显示的胆囊可增大、缩小、正常，有时也可以显示不清，但胆囊壁常增厚，胆囊颈附近常可发现不规则的腔及结石，此时可用侧卧位及薄层扫描加以证实；正常人胆囊形状朝向胆囊管应越来越细，若颈部增宽或不规则就应引起注意。腹部CT检查能较好地显示胆囊和胆管中的含钙结石。本病的CT表现包括：①肝内胆管及胰腺上段肝外胆管扩张；②肝门区多囊与多管征，周围的脂肪间隙模糊；③胆囊颈增宽；④胆管中含钙结石；⑤胆囊结石和/或胆囊壁增厚，胆囊周围的脂肪间隙模糊。

单一的CT图像诊断Mirizzi综合征的敏感度、特异度、阳性预测值、阴性预测值和准确度分别为42.0%，98.5%，93.0%，83.5%和85.0%，CT检查与MRCP检查联合应用可以明显提高术前诊断本病的敏感性和准确性，以及观察者之间的一致性。

CT，特别是增强CT，可以显示扩张的肝内胆管及正确判断梗阻水平和梗阻原因。当存在以下征象时应考虑Mirizzi综合征可能：胆囊管与肝总管连接部位结石和肝内胆管和胆囊管扩张，胆囊增大及胆囊炎表现。由于胆系结石可能因含胆固醇不表现为高密度，可能与胆汁或周围软组织呈现等密度，CT仅能显示超声检出结石的79%，因此，CT对Mirizzi综合征诊断仍然存在一定困难。一组资料中，8例接受CT检查患者中，仅4例检出胆囊颈部或胆管结石，也只有3例术前提示Mirizzi综合征可能，因此，对肝内胆管扩张、梗阻水平位于肝总管且缺乏占位性病变征象的患者，应进一步建议MRCP或/和ERCP检查。

MRCP：无创伤性的磁共振胆胰管成像，是一种较好的选择，因为这种技术不需要插管注入对比剂，即可完成且可进行三维立体观察胆系情况，同时也可像CT一样观察胆管周围结构，除外其他疾病。

MR检查，特别是MRCP能无创显示胆系和胰管解剖结构，并能清晰显示结石，而且无辐射，结合MR动态增强还能检出肝内一过性动脉期强化。肝内一过性动脉期强化虽然不是胆管炎特异性征象，可见于富血供肿瘤（血管瘤、局灶结节增生和肝癌）周围，也可见于异常血管供应和动静脉瘘周围，但对胆管炎作为一种辅助征象有一定的提示诊断价值。

在胆管疾病中，肝内一过性动脉期强化的病理基础有以下3种可能：一是扩张胆管周围血管丛受压导致门脉血供降低进而引起动脉血供增加补偿；二是胆管炎时，急性炎症导致血管扩张，特别是肝动脉扩张；三是存在炎症时门脉受压，肝动脉供血的代偿。

一组资料，MRCP于全部18例接受MR检查患者检出胆囊管或胆囊颈部结石及肝内胆管的扩张，但MR报告术前诊断仅11例提示Mirizzi综合征，可能与放射诊断医生对Mirizzi综合征认识不足有关。同时，胆囊管低位汇合是Mirizzi综合征易感因素，一组资料于23例患者中，12例观察到胆囊管低位汇合，正确术前诊断及检出相应发育变异对治疗方案选择和避免术中胆管损伤具有重要临床意义。

MRCP检查具有非侵入性、无需使用对比剂、患者易于接受等优势，其对胆囊胆管疾病的成像和诊断效果接近通过应用碘对比剂后完成的X线胆系造影。如果MRCP再结合常规MRI的横断面T_1WI和T_2WI表现，就不仅可以显示胆系解剖与梗阻性病变，还可以进一步观察胆管周围组织的结构与解剖形态，提高对胆系疾病的诊断水平的档次。

一组19例行MRCP检查，检查报告中术前诊断Mirizzi综合征5例，占检查例数的26%，明显高于同期B超检查结果。但MRCP的这个结果同样不能令人满意，诊断医师对病人的临床表现缺乏足够的了解，可能是该组术前诊断率较低的原因之一。

在目前，由于Mirizzi综合征临床缺乏特异性，术前诊断比较困难，术中易造成胆管损伤，因此应该充分地了解和认识该病，并综合超声、CT 及 MRI、直接法胆系造影（ERCP、PTC）多种影像学表现来做出准确诊断。

CT 和 MR 能检出 Mirizzi 综合征所致肝内胆管扩张、邻近肝总管的胆囊管或胆囊颈部结石及胆管炎，由于 CT 对胆系结石的检出存在一定限制，MR 特别是 MRCP 对 Mirizzi 综合征诊断优于 CT。熟悉 Mirizzi 综合征影像学表现有利于术前正确诊断，为临床治疗方案的选择提供指导，改善患者预后，有重要临床意义。

Mirizzi 综合征实际上是胆囊结石的一种并发症，以病人出现胆系症状、黄疸和外压性肝总管狭窄为特征。了解与认识 Mirizzi 综合征的临床和影像特征是提高术前诊断水平的重要环节。在临床工作中如果发现患者有较长的胆囊结石和间歇性腹痛病史，急性胆囊炎与胆管炎反复发作，近期出现皮肤与巩膜黄染，医师应想到本病可能性。

在综合分析各种影像检查结果的基础上，术前正确诊断本病是能够实现的。影像检查还有助于显示局部解剖细节，明确病变严重程度，指导手术方案选择（如通过 ERCP 置入胆管内支架、经腹腔镜切除胆囊、开腹手术），尽可能避免在手术操作过程中意外损伤胆管。Mirizzi 综合征可以合并胆囊腺肌瘤病和胆囊癌，也应引起注意。

第二节 Mirizzi 综合征之二

因胆囊管或胆囊颈结石嵌顿引起肝总管梗阻称为 Mirizzi 综合征。该病最早由阿根廷外科医生 Mirizzi 于 1948 年描述，Mirizzi 综合征包括以下四点：①胆囊管存在解剖结构上的变异，与肝总管并行。②结石嵌顿于胆囊管或胆囊颈。③结石本身或周围继发感染引起肝总管的机械性梗阻。④反复发作的胆管炎。Mirizzi 综合征并不是一种少见病，其发病率不超过胆系手术的 2%，术前诊断比较困难，如果不充分了解及认识此病将导致胆管损伤。

CT 表现：肝内胆管轻中度扩张，肝外胆管胰腺段正常，胰腺段以上水平梗阻，若没有肝门肿块，梗阻点附近又有结石则应考虑为 Mirizzi 综合征。

因直接法胆系造影上肝总管宽的弧形压迹也可以是肝门区转移癌、胆囊癌或其他疾病引起，而 CT 的应用可弥补直接法胆系造影的不足，不仅可观察胆管周围结构的情况以除外其他病变，同时可明确扩张的胆管和结石；根据病程及有无瘘管形成，CT 显示的胆囊可增大、缩小、正常，有时也可以显示不清，但胆囊壁常增厚，胆囊颈附近常可发现不规则的腔及结石，此时可用侧卧位及薄层扫描加以证实；正常人胆囊形状朝向胆囊管应越来越细，若颈部增宽或不规则就应引起注意。当因患者自身原因或其他因素使直接法胆系造影不能进行或未成功时，无创伤性的 MRCP 即成为一种较好的选择，因为这种技术不需要插管注入对比剂即可完成且可进行三维观察胆系情况，同时也可像 CT 一样观察胆管周围结构，除外其他疾病。

直接法胆系造影表现：胆管位于胆囊管或胆囊直接对应之处可见较宽的弧形充盈缺损，边缘光滑，经常在侧壁，有时因胆囊管与肝总管之间的关系偶尔也在中间，其上胆管扩张，扩张胆管于结石以下突然变成正常的胆管，胆管多表现为部分梗阻，少数时表现为完全梗阻。

综上所述，由于 Mirizzi 综合征临床缺乏特异性，术前诊断困难，术中易造成胆管损伤，因此我们应该充分地了解和认识本病，并综合超声、直接法胆系造影（ERCP、PTC）、CT 及 MRI 多种影像学表现来做出准确诊断。

第四章　关于胆囊管残端

第一节　胆囊管残端-十二指肠瘘

Van Houten 和 Lewicki（1973）介绍一例胆囊切除术后20年出现胆囊管残端-十二指肠瘘的病人，此症十分少见，据当时该作者所知，文献上只报告过三例胆囊管残端内瘘的病案，一为漏至十二指肠，一为胃，一为结肠。所有4例皆为胆囊切除术后数年出现。

在无选择的胆囊切除术后病人中，胆囊管残端真正的发生率不详，在经历总胆管探查与胆囊切除术者，有作者统计，明显长的残端遗留占63%。与此类似，反复胆系探查发现胆囊管残端者，30%有胆结石位于胆囊管残端。在胆囊切除术后，胆绞痛与黄疸消退，症状与体征减轻，通常由于总胆管结石的排出，偶尔，肝外胆管梗阻的解除可源于胆系内瘘的出现。

自发性胆系内瘘的原因一般皆为胆石通过所致，只有10%病例为其他疾病（例如消化性溃疡、胃肠道新生物等）引起。胆囊已切除者，内瘘源于胆石者十分少见。

第二节　再显性胆囊

再显性胆囊，是指胆囊切除术后残存的胆囊管扩张，在影像学检查时呈现类似胆囊的影像，又称为假胆囊、小胆囊。一组作者报告4例，表现为肝外胆管外侧相当于胆囊区有一圆形低密度阴影或回声暗区，其直径分别为2.5cm、2cm、2.3cm、1.8cm，其中2例合并胆囊管结石。残留胆囊管过长的原因是术中结扎胆囊管时距肝外胆管太远，但残留胆囊管扩张的原因尚未明确。一种意见认为是胆囊切除术后，胆胰管下端括约肌有暂时性的痉挛所致，但对这种见解认识尚不一致。

另一种意见认为，残存的胆囊管成为胆汁的贮存所，但因不能收缩而逐渐扩张，造成胆汁的淤积，继之易引起感染、炎症和结石的形成。

胆囊管残留过长的检查方法甚多，包括B型超声、MRCP、CT、PTC、ERCP等。有时，为排除十二指肠球部病变的可能性，可同时进行钡餐检查（图18-4-1）。

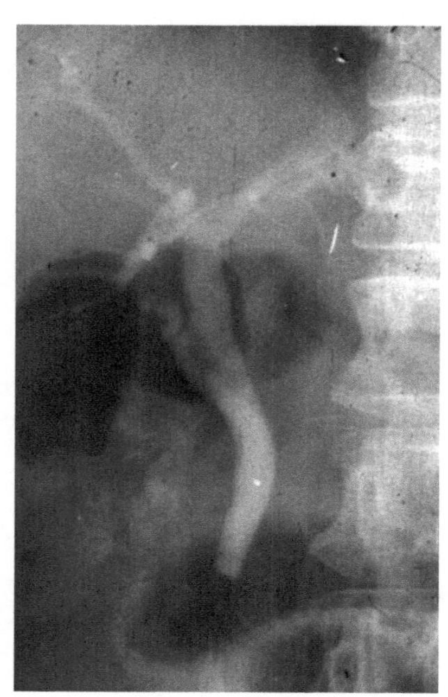

图 18-4-1　ERCP：过长的胆囊管残端低位异位汇入肝外胆管，该例括约肌段处于收缩状，而使肝外胆管下端呈杵状表现

胆囊管残留过长需与非典型十二指肠憩室、肝外胆管囊肿等鉴别。

扩张的残存的胆囊管内产生结石,使其远端穿破而与十二指肠球部或其他脏器形成瘘管,目前报告的有胆囊管残端 - 十二指肠瘘、胆囊管残端 - 结肠瘘、胆囊管残端 - 胃瘘。

第三节 胆囊管残端与胆囊管低位汇入

请详见本书 本卷 本篇 第二章 胆囊管的发育变异和先天性异常 第一节至第六节各节内容。

第十九篇　胆胰管十二指肠连接区疾病

第一章 胆管低位梗阻

第一节 低位梗阻性黄疸的分型

有作者回顾性分析105例低位梗阻性黄疸患者的CT和内窥镜逆行胰胆管造影(ERCP)的影像资料,将胆系扩张分为下列7种类型:Ⅰ型为肝内、外胆管及胆囊均重度扩张;Ⅱ型为肝外胆管、胆囊重度扩张伴肝内胆管轻度扩张;Ⅲ型为肝内、外胆管重度扩张伴胆囊不扩张或轻、中度扩张;Ⅳ型为肝外胆管重度扩张伴肝内胆管和胆囊不扩张或轻、中度扩张;Ⅴ型为肝内胆管重度扩张伴肝外胆管及胆囊不扩张或轻、中度扩张;Ⅵ型胆囊重度扩张伴肝内、外胆管不扩张或轻、中度扩张;Ⅶ型为肝内、外胆管及胆囊均不扩张或轻、中度扩张。

105例低位梗阻性黄疸中33例为肿瘤性病变,72例为非肿瘤性病变。肿瘤性病变中,Ⅰ型16例,Ⅱ型10例,Ⅲ型4例,Ⅳ型1例,Ⅶ型2例。非肿瘤性病变中,Ⅰ型4例,Ⅱ型4例,Ⅲ型9例,Ⅳ型33例,Ⅴ型2例,Ⅵ型11例,Ⅶ型9例。Ⅰ、Ⅱ型扩张和Ⅲ至Ⅶ型扩张在肿瘤和非肿瘤病变中差异有统计学意义。

低位梗阻性黄疸病变性质和肝内、外胆管及胆囊扩张程度密切相关:Ⅰ型和Ⅱ型扩张提示绝大多数为肿瘤性病变,少数为嵌顿性结石。Ⅲ至Ⅶ型扩张常为胆管、胆囊结石及炎症。

胰头部肿块和胆管内的高密度结石是低位梗阻性黄疸的直接征象,对诊断具有定性作用,但低位梗阻性黄疸病变出现典型直接征象仅占30%以下。因此,多数患者诊断的确立依赖于胆系的扩张、胆管下端形态等间接征象。

胆系活体形态学:胆系主要由肝内、外胆管及胆囊共同组成。正常情况下,肝内、外胆管及胆囊其管腔大小可根据生理需求在一定范围内调整。根据一些学者的研究,正常肝外胆管管径为3~11 mm,平均为5~6 mm;肝内胆管左、右支管径在2~9 mm,平均为3~4mm。ERCP对胆囊一般仅能部分显示,其显示率取决于逆行造影时,对比剂注入量和注射压力大小,以及胆囊颈部有无嵌顿性结石等。而CT和超声则无此限制,但需多层面观察。病理情况下,如胆管炎症、结石和肿瘤或先天性异常等均可引起胆汁排泄障碍,从而使胆系发生不同程度的扩张。

胆系扩张表现:该组105例低位梗阻性黄疸中,Ⅰ、Ⅱ型胆系扩张和Ⅲ、Ⅳ、Ⅴ、Ⅵ、Ⅶ型胆系扩张在低位梗阻性黄疸的病变(肿瘤、非肿瘤)中差异有统计学意义($\chi2 = 47.33$, $P<0.001$),表明肿瘤性胆系扩张绝大多数为Ⅰ、Ⅱ型胆系扩张,非肿瘤性胆系扩张绝大多数为Ⅲ、Ⅳ、Ⅴ、Ⅵ、Ⅶ型胆系扩张。

由于Ⅰ、Ⅱ型胆系扩张为全程重度扩张(肝内、外胆管及胆囊重度扩张)和肝外胆系重度扩张(肝外胆管及胆囊重度扩张),说明此2种形式的扩张其梗阻程度重,梗阻发生急,且此梗阻进行性加重,符合胆管下端癌及连接区癌等生长速度快和进行性加重的生物学行为。

一些作者报道肝内、外胆管一致性扩张呈软藤样改变提示为肿瘤可能性大。该组Ⅰ、Ⅱ型胆系扩张患者中,除了肝内、外胆管和胆囊一致性重度扩张外,还含有肝外胆系(肝外胆管和胆囊)同步一致性重度扩张患者。因此,可以认为肝外胆系(肝外胆管和胆囊)同步一致性重度扩张为肿瘤性胆管扩张更合理。

这是由于胆管下端肿瘤梗阻后,导致胆汁通过排泄障碍,而致肝内、外胆管和胆囊内压力均增高;但由于肝内胆管因周围有肝组织的支撑且离梗阻端较远,而肝外胆管及胆囊仅有少量支撑组织且离梗阻端较近,因此,在发生低位胆系肿瘤性梗阻时,肝外胆管及胆囊首先发生重度扩张,而肝内胆管重度扩张则发生较晚或相对较轻。也就是说肿瘤引起的胆系急性梗阻,早期即可引起肝外胆管及胆囊急性扩张,晚期可引起全程胆系扩张。

Ⅲ、Ⅳ、Ⅴ、Ⅵ、Ⅶ型胆系扩张,该组统计学结果显示其梗阻原因主要为胆管(囊)结石或炎症或胰头慢性炎症,极少数为肿瘤。根据流体力学拉普拉斯 Laplaopk 定律和帕斯卡(Pascal)定律(Himal, 2000; Schlosser 等, 2001),胆管内结石绝大多数可在胆管内移动,胆管有一定程度扩张收缩能力,胆汁可排入十二指肠,因此,胆管内结石在一定时间内可无阻塞或仅有胆汁的排泄欠通畅,即无胆系扩张或仅有轻度胆系扩张。

但随着时间延长,胆管内结石在狭长的胆管内移动,而使胆管内壁黏膜损伤,加上胆汁的排泄欠通畅,而使胆管壁发生炎症。久而久之,可使胆管壁毛糙、增厚,胆管的收缩扩张能力下降,而发生相应程度的代偿扩张,即在较晚期时出现肝外胆管扩张。而胆囊和胆管的发病机制虽一样,但其病理过程可不完全同步。因此,胆系结石和炎症引起的低位梗阻的管腔扩张程度轻,其肝外胆管和胆囊的扩张程度常不一致。

同时,胆管结石、胆管炎患者,在 CT、MR 等图像上可显示管壁增厚,增强后可见胆管壁强化;胆管炎严重者,管壁的外层也有炎性渗出、粘连,可使胆管形态变成椭圆形或不规则形,管壁不清,这些征象有益于鉴别诊断。

而对于胆总管下端嵌顿性结石患者,因其结石嵌顿于胆管下段不能运动,而使胆汁通过发生严重障碍,可引起梗阻以上胆系的急性重度扩张,其胆系扩张不符合上述流体定律,管腔扩张程度和形式可完全和肿瘤(胆管下端癌和连接区癌)性胆系扩张呈一样改变。除了胰头部无肿块外,常可见胆总管下端高密度结石的“靶征”,同时可见扩张胆管壁增厚现象;这是由于胆管内大结石在嵌顿之前,常在胆管内存在一相当长时间,大部分已形成慢性胆管炎,增强后可发现增厚扩张的胆管,这些对鉴别诊断有重要参考价值。

胆囊被切除的患者如有肝外胆管重度扩张或肝内、外胆管重度扩张者,因胆囊状况的真实性被掩盖,其胆系扩张类型的划分受到干扰,应采用上述结论作客观分析。

第二节 胆管低位梗阻 CT 诊断标准

肝内、外胆管扩张程度、形态和肝外胆管壁增厚 CT 诊断标准:①按肝内胆管 1~2 级分支的直径将肝内胆管扩张程度分为轻度(<3 mm)、中度(4~5 mm)、重度(>6 mm)。②依肝外胆管扩张最明显处直径将肝外胆管扩张程度分为轻度(5~10 mm)、中度(11~20 mm)、重度(>21 mm),肝总管直径 >4 mm 为扩张,胆囊横径 >45 mm 为增大。③肝内胆管扩张形态可分为:竹节状,分支稀少,呈条状,由近及远逐渐变细;剑鞘状,近端胆管扩张显著,远端突然变细;软藤状,肝内胆管明显迂曲扩张。④肝外胆管梗阻端的形态可分为:漏斗型,扩张肝外胆管在梗阻端呈渐进性狭窄,狭窄范围 >10 mm;截断型,扩张的肝外胆管在 10 mm 以内突然消失。

第三节 低位梗阻性黄疸病因病理

低位梗阻性黄疸临床上很常见,病因复杂,简介如下。

括约肌段的良性狭窄:在大多数病人,炎症和瘢痕性改变是括约肌段狭窄的形态学基础,这是由于胆囊结石疾病细菌感染的小管性或淋巴性播散。括约肌段狭窄的影响是胆胰管压力升高和胆胰液流动减少。在手术时可能发现胆管扩张,余压增加,排出降低,而且,在瘢痕性狭窄探针不能通过。只在炎性狭窄是可逆性的,但是永久性的改变是不确定的。因此,治疗是必须的,首先是用器械扩张到 4~6mm。一组作者在 921 例内镜括约肌切开术中,发现有 110 例(12%)是括约肌段的良性狭窄。其中,96 例为胆囊切除术后,14 例胆囊尚存。

括约肌段狭窄的诊断是以 ERCP 发现胆管扩张

作根据的。但是,这并不是特异性征象,因为在胆囊切除后,在括约肌正常张力情况下,胆管可以变得扩张;同时,胆管扩张是括约肌段狭窄的一个诊断标准,而胆系核素扫描时的异常发现,和胆汁淤滞相符合的实验室同存的征象不能避免。与外科手术相比,内镜括约肌切开术是括约肌段狭窄首选的治疗方法。然而,出现于括约肌段狭窄的内镜括约肌切开术的并发症,比胆管结石(8.8%)为多(13.6%)。出血和胆管炎是并发症过多的原因。

括约肌段炎症:有作者报告14例继发性括约肌炎病人的乳头活检情况,1例为肌束周围与肌束内的中度纤维化,而其他病人为乳头黏膜糜烂伴胆系内容的嵌入;6例为肝的囊尾蚴病,只有3例可见到胆管黏膜下水肿。胆系结石对括约肌段的影响与结石的嵌顿与排出所引起的创伤有关,这是括约肌成形术的适应证。在肝的囊尾蚴病穿孔进入胆系时不出现括约肌疾病,是个信号,只有水肿改变,囊尾蚴病的治疗的效果是可逆的。

有作者报告一例获得性免疫缺陷综合征11月幼儿,由于溃疡性乳头炎引起胆汁淤滞,经内科治疗而好转。对此类病人可以反复地进行内镜复查追踪,以评价是否有继发括约肌段狭窄的危险。一些作者指出,与胆系结石相关的十二指肠乳头炎的病理特点的分析,主要在胆管的扩张、胆系内部压力、乳头炎的组织病理学特点等。其结论是:就其本身而论,胆管扩张的主要原因表现为乳头的病理性改变;乳头炎伴发胆系结石同胆固醇结石,是继发于胆囊排出的胆囊结石;胆红素钙结石主要形成于乳头炎的结果。在某些病例,蛔虫病在他们的过去病史中考虑为乳头炎的病因;这也提示,如乳头炎进展,乳头的功能不全将出现。

“假肿瘤”:有作者报告49例胆胰共同管周围肿瘤的内镜表现,其中38例为肿瘤,11例为炎性非肿瘤性病变(假肿瘤)。只靠内镜观察难以区别二者。除了在肿瘤组胰管趋向于扩张,在假肿瘤组胆囊结石更为常见以外,两组的胆胰管造影表现基本类似。

在34例胆胰共同管肿瘤中,内镜活检做出正确诊断者为28例。11例假性肿瘤中有2例由于内镜活检怀疑为肿瘤而行手术探查。在肿瘤组有19例行胰十二指肠切除术,7例行分流手术,7例内镜括约肌切开术,只有5例因未能成功地进行胆系引流而死亡,一年生存率为44.7%。相反,在假肿瘤组,在内镜括约肌切开术后,平均追踪24个月(范围为12~41个月),只1例89岁老翁因其他不相关的原因死亡外,余皆健存。

胆胰共同管区的良性肿瘤包括:平滑肌纤维瘤、脂肪瘤、神经类肿瘤、血管瘤以及类癌。最常见的良性肿瘤是绒毛状腺瘤。

在临床病史、临床检查、血液学检查以及生化检查资料,在肿瘤组与假肿瘤组之间都互相重叠。对区别诊断有帮助之处是,在假肿瘤组均未扪及胆囊,而在肿瘤组中却有42%的病人可扪及胆囊,即Courvoisiers定律阳性。十二指肠镜检查两组所见类似,它们都有肝外胆管扩张。在肿瘤组胰管扩张较重,但这点帮助只适用于少数病人。11例假肿瘤病人中有6例在ERCP检查时发现胆囊结石,而只有2例结石出现于肝外胆管,另2例以前曾行胆囊切除术。这似乎提示病因学因素,可能与结石通过胆胰共同管期间,造成炎症变化,导致假肿瘤形成。Baggenstoss(1938)报告100例尸解病例有18例腺瘤性增生,他指出,在息肉、腺瘤状增生和十二指肠乳头的低度的乳头状癌之间十分类似。此假说是进步的,因为乳头是一个区域,是乳头黏膜的局灶性(酶和胆盐)刺激的上皮移行区,在息肉状增生的发展中承担重要作用。一般而论,不少作者认为此假说甚为正确。

如果怀疑内镜所见为恶性者,可在内镜括约肌切开术后几天,再进行反复的内镜活检,这样,常常可以增加诊断恶性病变的正确性。胆胰共同管组织周围炎症反应的吸收,再次活检查结果则大不相同。如仍然怀疑恶性,可在作根治术前再行手术活检冰冻切片确诊。

第四节　胆胰管连接区梗阻

胆胰管连接区梗阻的检查方法:胆胰管连接区梗阻是梗阻性黄疸常见的梗阻部位,其梗阻的原因较复杂,CT常规增强扫描常难以明确诊断。诊断困难的原因是多方面的,使病灶充分地显示出来,是准确诊断的关键之一。

低张CT增强扫描的目的是使胃肠道扫描时处于低张状态，使十二指肠充分扩张，同时减少胃肠道蠕动所致的伪影，更好地显示病变。有作者对47例CT平扫拟诊为胆胰管连接区梗阻的患者采用低张CT增强扫描，较好地显示了梗阻部位的改变，提高了梗阻原因诊断的准确性。该研究在扫描前12分钟左右时肌注654-2，扫描前嘱患者尽量多饮水，使胃肠道在扫描时处于低张状态。为了及早显示胆胰管连接区，改变了常规自上向下的扫描方法，采用自下向上的扫描方法，即自十二指肠水平段向肝顶方向扫描。这种方法的优点是可避免遗漏胆胰管连接区，及早发现遗漏，及时更改扫描范围，更好地了解胆胰管连接区的增强情况。同时尽可能缩小扫描的范围，对胆胰管连接区进行动态扫描，更有利于显示胆胰管连接区的增强表现及泥砂样结石。

近年来，屏气磁共振胆胰管造影（MRCP）的临床应用使胆胰管连接区梗阻的检查方法发生了很大的变化，MRCP在显示梗阻端的形态、显示结石的信号等方面有优势，提高了胆胰管连接区梗阻的病因诊断和鉴别诊断能力。有作者认为，MRCP在直接显示病灶，在显示病灶本身的强化等有时尚不如低张CT增强扫描。有作者在实际工作中，对胆胰管连接区梗阻患者应用MRCP检查，但尚不能明确诊断时，后采用CT低张增强才明确诊断的。该作者认为CT，尤其是MSCT低张增强扫描，速度快、层厚薄、胃肠道气体干扰少，可多方位成像及三维重建，显示病灶更直观，仍然在某些方面具有优势，可与MRCP相互补充，相互印证。

胆胰管连接区梗阻的CT征象：胆胰管连接区梗阻因梗阻的时间和程度不同有不同的CT表现，肝内胆管扩张的形态常能提示肝外胆管梗阻的性质。软藤状胆管扩张常提示肝外胆管梗阻时间较短，梗阻程度较重，梗阻原因往往是胆胰管连接区占位病变。软藤状胆管扩张的形成机制主要是正常的胆管（即扩张度好的胆管），因下端梗阻而胆管内压升高所致，末梢的小胆管也扩张，CT表现为扩张的胆管影延伸至肝的边缘部分。

残根状胆管扩张常提示梗阻原因往往是肝外胆管下段结石。残根状胆管扩张的形成机制主要是因为梗阻时间长，梗阻程度较轻，胆管扩张以肝门邻近的肝段胆管为主，同时因为肝脏有不同程度的胆汁性肝硬化及末梢胆管的硬化，因此末梢的胆管不扩张或不能扩张，CT表现为扩张的胆管比较短而直，分支也少，呈残根状。

至于不典型的胆管扩张，其原因与肝脏的背景情况、病程的长短及梗阻的程度等有关。一组研究中连接区癌病例中有些在扩张的十二指肠降段显示了乳头状软组织结节影，并有较明显的强化，为连接区癌的征象；有的病例显示了“半月征”，为起源于管壁的肿瘤向腔内生长，使圆形的水样密度影形成半月形缺损，也是连接区癌的征象；一些病例在环形扩张的十二指肠影内可见环形扩张的胆总管影，即“双环征”。“双环征”的出现，是由于十二指肠处于低张状态，在横断面图像上，降段扩张呈环形，同时又由于肝外胆管梗阻、肝外胆管内胆汁淤积引起肝外胆管扩张且拉长，并向十二指肠内坠降。所以在同一层面上可见2个环形影套在一起，即环形的十二指肠影内套着扩张且下坠的环形肝外胆管影，“双环征”是连接区癌较为特征性的征象。

第五节　十二指肠壁内胆胰共同管内异位胰腺致梗阻性黄疸

异位胰腺，又称迷走胰腺，凡在正常胰腺以外生长的，与正常胰腺组织既无解剖上又无血管联系的孤立的胰腺组织均称为异位胰腺，为一种少见病，异位胰腺导致梗阻性黄疸更为少见。其确切胚胎学机制尚不清。异位胰腺可发生于任何年龄，可见于腹腔的任何部位，以胃及十二指肠最多见，亦有发生于纵隔的报道。

异位胰腺多无临床症状，患者往往以合并疾病而就诊或常在体检时无意中发现。在胆总管周围的异位胰腺，在婴幼儿时期很小，不引起梗阻，随年龄的增长，异位胰腺缓慢增大，到一定年龄后，这种增大就会停止，此时与胆总管为毗邻关系，并不产生压迫，在某些因素作用下，出现异位胰腺的增生、炎症或癌变等，对胆管产生压迫，则引起黄疸。一例出现黄疸考虑为十二指肠壁内异位胰腺对胆总管下端压迫所致。

异位胰腺发生于胃壁时钡餐造影可见典型X线征象为脐样凹陷和导管征，有此征象者多可确诊为异位胰腺，但上述两种征象不常见。

十二指肠壁内异位胰腺 MSCT 扫描平扫示十二指肠胆胰共同管处肠壁局限性增厚，宽基底与肠壁相连并部分呈结节样向腔内突起致肠腔狭窄，其密度与同层面正常胰腺一致；增强扫描动脉期及静脉期异位胰腺强化程度、消退速度与正常胰腺一致。

该例异位胰腺在 CT 上显示其表面较光整，整个平扫及增强过程中均显示异位胰腺与肠壁无分界。MSCT 可准确的发现病灶，但对其定性诊断尚存在困难，且需与各种富血供的肿瘤性病变相鉴别。手术探查和病理检查仍为诊断本病的最为重要的手段。

异位胰腺缺乏特征性的临床表现和有效的检查手段，极易误诊，其并发症较多，且比正常胰腺更易恶变，故一旦发现，无论有无症状，均以早期手术治疗为宜。

第六节　胆管下端高分化胆管型腺癌

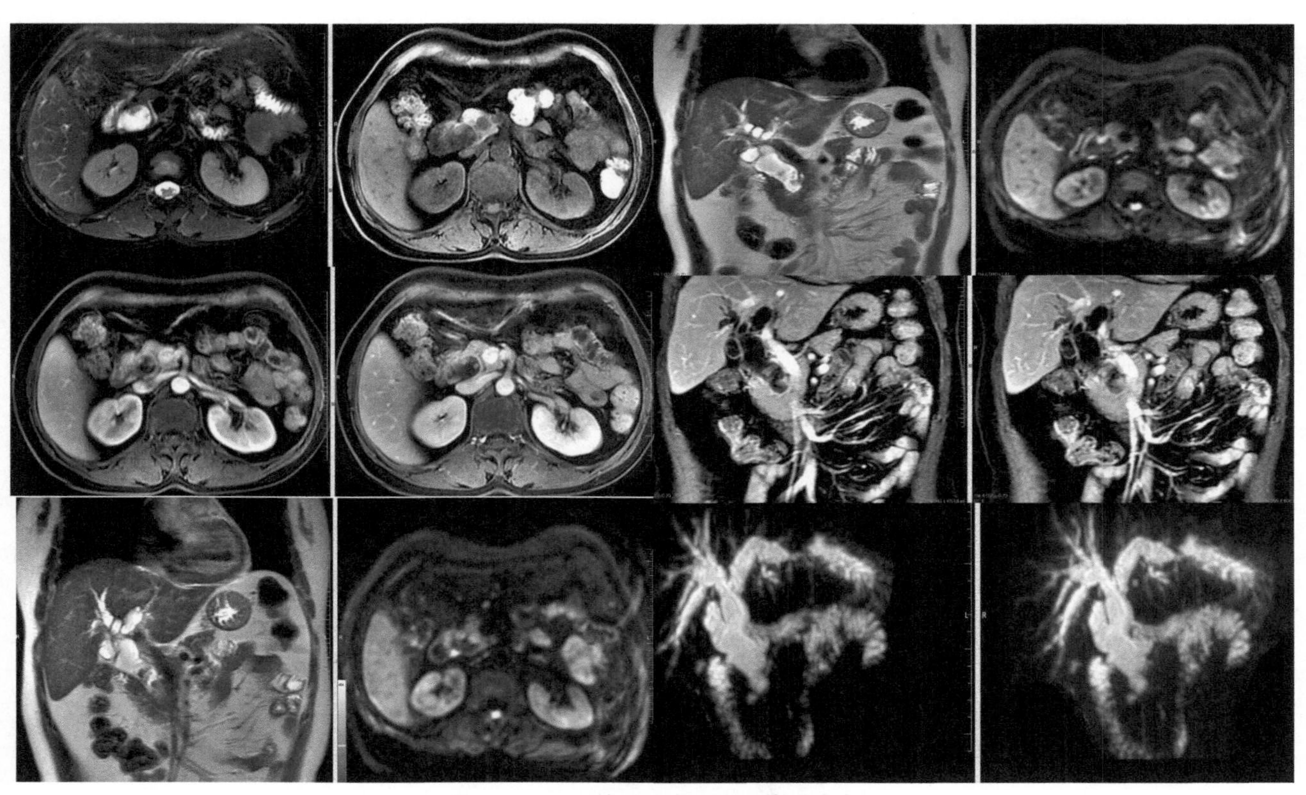

图 19-1-1　胆管下端高分化胆管型腺癌

患者，女，52 岁。反复上腹部闷痛不适 2 月入院。

手术所见：胆囊缺如，胆总管内径约 3cm，术中胆道镜探查示胆总管下段及十二指肠乳头可见两个内生性肿物大小约 1.2cm × 1.1cm × 1.0cm，质中，胰腺质地正常。

病理检查：胆总管下段肿物：管壁样组织一块，大小 2.3cm × 1.5cm × 0.7cm，表面附一乳头状广基肿物，肿物大小 1.5cm × 1.3cm × 0.5cm，切面灰白灰黄，质软，界限尚清。常规病理诊断：胆总管下段肿物：乳头状肿瘤，局部细胞层次增多，轻度异型，但未见明确浸润，肌层尚完好。目前倾向交界性，与高分化腺癌或腺瘤癌变难以鉴别，待充分取材及石蜡切片进一步诊断。病理检查：A“胆道下段肿物”：灰褐色组织一块，大小 1.7cm × 0.7cm × 0.3cm，切面灰白灰褐，质中；B“胰十二指肠”：胰腺，大小 7cm × 4.5cm × 2cm，切面灰褐未触及结节及病灶，十二指肠，长 13cm，直径 1.8cm，肠黏膜未见明显异常；C“上切缘”：灰褐色组织一块，大小 0.9cm × 0.8cm × 0.2cm；D“第 7 组淋巴结”：灰黄色组织一块，大小 1.1cm × 0.5cm × 0.3cm；E“第 8A 淋巴结”：灰黄灰褐色碎组织一堆，总体积 3.5cm × 3.0cm × 0.7cm，检出淋巴结样物 3

枚,直径 0.6~1.8cm,切面灰白质中;F“第 12H 组淋巴结”:灰白色组织一块,大小 1cm × 0.9cm × 0.3cm;G“第 16 组淋巴结”:灰黄灰褐色碎组织一堆,总体积 2.2cm × 2.0cm × 0.5cm;H“第 12B 淋巴结”:灰褐色组织一块,大小 2.6cm × 2cm × 0.6cm,切面灰白,质中;I“第 12L 淋巴结”:灰褐色组织三块,总体积 2.5cm × 1.2cm × 0.8cm × 0.3cm;J“第 9 组淋巴结”:灰黄色组织一块,大小 2cm × 1.6cm × 0.3cm;K“第 14 组淋巴结”:灰褐色组织两块,总体积 0.9cm × 0.8cm × 0.5cm。

免疫组化诊断:①“胆道下段肿物切除标本”:胆管内高分化胆管型腺癌。②“胰及十二指肠切除标本”:均未见肿瘤组织累及。③“上切缘切除标本”:未见肿瘤组织累及。④淋巴结清扫:送检的“第 8A 淋巴结”0/3,“第 16 组淋巴结”0/10,“第 12B 淋巴结”0/1,“第 12L 淋巴结”0/2,“第 9 组淋巴结”0/3,“第 14 组淋巴结”0/1。综上,共检出淋巴结 20 枚,均为阴性。⑤送检的“第 7 组淋巴结”及“第 12H 淋巴结”为纤维脂肪组织,未检出淋巴结(图 19-1-1)。

第七节 MRCP 双管征的讨论

磁共振胆胰管成像(MRCP)提供了胆胰管疾病丰富的形态学诊断信息,可以和经内窥镜逆行胆胰管造影(ERCP)相媲美,现已成为诊断胆胰管异常的重要方法。

胰管和胆管扩张是胆胰管疾病常见而重要的征象,他们可分别独立发生或同时发生。当胰管和胆管同时扩张时称为“双管征”。此征象最初应用在 ERCP 中,MRCP 沿袭使用了“双管征”这一术语。MRCP 显示“双管征”具有重要的临床诊断意义,它高度提示恶性病变可能,尤其是胰头癌,但应排除良性疾病。

MRCP 检查技术:恰当的 MRCP 技术是清楚显示“双管征”的保证。磁共振成像技术的进步,如使用相控阵线圈提高了空间分辨力,缩短了 T1 和 T2,可以一次屏气检查整个上腹部,同时评价胆胰管、胰腺实质、邻近软组织和血管。

MRCP 的扫描脉冲序列有多种,包括 2D 快速自旋回波(FSE)序列、3D FSE 序列、单次激发快速自旋回波(SSFSE)序列、稳态自由进动梯度回波序列以及 3D FSE 和平面回波成像(EPI)相结合的技术。但较常用的是重 T_2WI SSFSE 序列,它有两种不同而互补的扫描方式:单一厚层 SSFSE,和多个薄层 SSFSE,两者各有优缺点。

单一厚层 SSFSE 扫描的层厚一般是 30~50 mm,最大的优点是成像时间短,可在同一胆胰管层面重复扫描以进行动态 MRCP 检查,观察胆胰管下端括约肌功能状态。单层采集的最大缺点是扫描野内其他含有液体的结构或者腹水能形成容积效应,遮盖胆胰管结构。为了克服这一缺点,一般要求病人检查前 4 h 禁水或者在扫描前口服 T2 阴性对比剂,以消除胃肠道液体的高信号。但口服阴性对比剂可能干扰十二指肠和连接区周围癌的观察。

多个薄层 SSFSE 扫描可以避免容积效应,其层厚一般是 4~5 mm,或更薄(2 mm),TE 较单层采集短,分支胰管也能较好显示。当怀疑胆胰管恶性梗阻或者单层采集发现覆盖伪影时可以采用多层采集。多层扫描完成后,可应用 MIP 技术进行各个层面的三维重组,形成立体影像。重组的影像质量优于单层采集的影像质量。

激发促胰液素分泌 MRCP(s-MRCP)是更高级的胆胰管成像技术,可以观察胰腺功能。促胰液素刺激胰腺外分泌腺体分泌胰液和碳酸氢盐,胰管内胰液容量持续性增加。在开始的 5 分钟内,促胰液素能使正常人胆胰管下端括约肌收缩,造成暂时性的胰管压力增高。采用单一厚层 SSFSE 扫描时,若能显示肝外胆管、胰管及十二指肠的结构,则可以动态扫描,观察胰液从胰管流入十二指肠。激发促胰液素分泌 MRCP 能够评估胰腺的外分泌功能,更好地评价括约肌和胰管的解剖,减少了假阳性诊断。缺点是费用高及促胰液素应用受限。

胆胰管解剖及正常 MRCP 表现:通常情况下,胆总管与胰管有 3 种汇合方式:①两管在肠壁内汇合(约占 60%),汇合后的管腔略现扩大,共同开口于十二指肠大乳头;②两管平行走行(约占 38%),呈“双管腔”,共同开口于十二指肠乳头尖部;③两管分别独自开口(约占 2%)。也有极少数胆总管与胰管在进入十二指肠壁前汇合,形成较长的共同管。

胆总管长 4.1~8.0 cm,直径 6~8 mm。可分为十二指肠上段、十二指肠后段、胰头段及十二指肠壁内段4部分。MRCP可显示98%正常人的胆总管,可鉴别95%的正常和异常。

胰管走行变异很大,尤其是在胰颈主胰管和副胰管交界处,可呈弯曲状,突然成角或折曲成襻。正常主胰管直径一般小于3mm,显示率取决于所使用的MRCP序列。采用SSFSE技术,胰头、体、尾主胰管的显示率分别为97%、97%和83%,分支胰管的显示率较低。但MRCP可清楚显示梗阻性病变引起的胆胰管扩张。

"双管征"的鉴别诊断:"双管征"是胆胰管病变的重要征象之一,也是影像学诊断的重要依据,曾被认为是胰头癌的典型征象。但实际上"双管征"并不是一个特异性征象,还可见于其他恶性病变,如连接区癌、胆总管下段癌、十二指肠乳头癌、淋巴瘤和转移瘤,恶性胰腺导管内乳头状黏液性肿瘤;良性病变包括慢性胰腺炎、连接区先天性狭窄、胆胰管下端括约肌纤维化或机能障碍、胆管结石嵌顿;其他罕见的原因有原发性腹膜后纤维化、卡波西肉瘤和寄生虫感染。

常规胆胰管造影检查鉴别良恶性胆胰管梗阻的原则也适用于MRCP。MRCP显示"双管征"时,应全面分析其扩张形态、扩张程度、梗阻部位、梗阻端形态及狭窄段长度等征象,同时结合横断面T_1WI和T_2WI表现做出鉴别诊断。

恶性病变的"双管征"通常表现为胆胰管明显扩张,狭窄段较长,边缘不规则,不对称性阻塞,可伴有垫肩征,胆管突然中断,出现肿块;而良性病变的"双管征"表现为胆胰管扩张程度较轻,狭窄段较短,边缘光滑,对称性狭窄,管腔逐渐变细。

连接区周围癌:连接区周围癌包括连接区癌、胰头癌、胆总管下段癌及十二指肠癌。它们的临床特点和解剖位置、治疗方法类似,但长期预后不同,所以有必要鉴别诊断。

"双管征"是连接区周围癌常见而重要的征象。MRCP是显示"双管征"理想的方法,结合常规横断面T_1WI和T_2W1以及增强扫描,其对诊断连接区周围癌及评价肿瘤侵及范围有重要作用。连接区癌的肿块一般较小,可有胆管增厚或向十二指肠突出。MRCP常显示明显的胆总管扩张和轻到中度的胰管扩张。有作者发现52%的连接区癌病例可见"双管征",十二指肠腔至扩张的胆胰管末端的距离为2~9 mm,平均5 mm。胆胰管末端边缘常不规则,以钝圆及新月状常见,扩张的胆总管末端形态在不同的层面或投照方向是可以变化的,分支胰管扩张少见。

有时连接区癌与其他造成连接区梗阻的疾病(如胆胰管下端括约肌纤维化或机能障碍、胆管结石嵌顿)较难鉴别。在评价连接区梗阻时,应考虑到MRCP的这种限度。

胰头癌引起胰管阻塞,导致远端胰管扩张。肿瘤侵犯胆总管时,引起胆总管扩张,出现"双管征"。一些作者研究发现62%的胰头癌病例可见"双管征",十二指肠腔至扩张的胆胰管末端的距离为14~42 mm,平均25mm。

胰头癌的"双管征"管腔末端突然截断,可见多种形态,包括钝圆状、鸟嘴状及鼠尾状。"双管征"梗阻端可见实质肿块,在动态钆对比剂增强时早期强化不明显。

有时,梗阻近端和远端的两段胰管和胆管表现为4个分离的管腔,即"四节征"。MRCP上,胰头癌胰管改变的主要特征包括:扩张胰管管腔光滑,多呈明显扩张,并常在胰头肿块处截断,分支胰管扩张多见。而其他连接区周围癌的分支胰管扩张少见。

胆总管下段癌累及连接区或胰腺时,可引起梗阻性胆胰管扩张,形成"双管征"。扩张的近端胆管、不扩张的远端胆管和扩张的胰管可形成"三节征"。管腔梗阻端表现为管腔闭塞、管壁增厚或腔内息肉样结节。在T_1WI上,胆管癌一般为低或等信号(相对于肝),在T_2WI上信号表现多样,多呈中度或明显高信号。静脉团注钆对比剂后,肿瘤最初仍为低信号,随后缓慢地进行性强化,且从病灶周边开始,逐渐向病灶中央进展,高峰强化时间为注射对比剂后120 s。

连接区周围十二指肠癌在MRCP表现为肠腔内菜花状或息肉状充盈缺损,部分病例无明显肿块,但可见肠壁环形增厚,肠腔狭窄,伴有胆胰管不同程度扩张而出现"双管征"。

慢性胰腺炎:慢性胰腺炎出现"双管征"较少见。胆管扩张的机制为胰腺肿胀压迫胆总管。在MRCP上,扩张胆总管的特征为由上至下逐渐变细,扩张胰管的特征为粗细不均,且不规则。如果慢性胰腺炎伴有炎性肿块,可类似肿瘤,但这时可见未阻塞的胰管穿过肿块,即"胰管穿过征"。早期分支胰管扩张和钙化是慢性胰腺炎最突出而特异的征象。主胰管和分支胰管的其他改变包括串珠样扩张和狭窄、轮廓不规则,有时可见假囊肿及充盈缺损(结石、黏液栓或碎屑形成)。

胰腺导管内乳头状黏液性肿瘤：胰腺导管内乳头状黏液性肿瘤是一种在胰腺导管内产生黏液的肿瘤，多见于男性及老年人。由于影像检查技术的普及和发展，其发现率有逐渐增高趋势。本病源于胰管上皮的乳头状增生，肿瘤细胞高柱状富含黏液，生长缓慢，但可以癌变。该肿瘤为恶性时，由于黏液过度分泌，导致主胰管和/或主要分支胰管扩张，局限性导管扩张常常形成囊样结构。晚期大量黏液造成胆总管末端及连接区梗阻，引起胆总管扩张，形成“双管征”。

胆管结石：胆管结石一般不会引起“双管征”。但当结石位于连接区时，也可引起胆管和胰管同时轻度扩张而出现“双管征”。在大多数病例中，结石与肿瘤容易鉴别。在MRCP，胆管结石表现为在高信号管腔内出现低信号充盈缺损，且轮廓清楚锐利，周围几乎被高信号胆汁围绕。但有时胆道积气、血块、蛋白栓或肿瘤组织形成的充盈缺损可类似胆总管结石。有作者认为轻度重T2WI或钆对比剂增强扫描有助于鉴别结石与其他病变。

寄生虫感染：Dearden等(2004)报道了1例MRCP显示十二指肠内寄生虫感染引起的“双管征”，胰腺及邻近组织未见肿块。超声提示肝内外胆管扩张，但未见结石。ERCP检查发现十二指肠黏膜水肿，连接区结构模糊不清，无法定位。组织活检证实为十二指肠原位粪类圆线虫感染。粪类圆线虫属土壤传播的肠线虫类寄生虫，流行于热带。此病人经治疗后症状消失，复查MRCP显示扩张的肝外胆管和胰管已完全恢复正常。

MRCP与ERCP的比较：ERCP仍被认为是诊断胆管梗阻性疾病的“金标准”，但它并不完美。MRCP的出现减少了ERCP的使用。MRCP检查的适应证较广，适合于ERCP检查不成功或有ERCP禁忌证的病人，尤其适用于ERCP操作困难、危险或禁忌的病人；但幽闭恐惧症、体内有心脏起搏器及人工耳蜗植入等病人禁忌。与ERCP比较，MRCP无需特殊准备，无需麻醉，无创，费用低，无辐射，不需对比剂，无并发症，操作者依赖性小，梗阻近端胆管显示清楚且可评价管外病变等；但缺点是空间分辨力低，不能活检及治疗，而ERCP兼有诊断和治疗双重作用。因此，两者在临床应用时可互为补充，但不可相互代替。

综上所述，MRCP显示“双管征”具有一定优势。虽然“双管征”不是一个特异性征象，但它更多见于恶性病变。鉴别诊断需综合分析“双管征”的形态、胆胰管扩张程度、梗阻部位、梗阻长度及梗阻端形态等征象，同时需结合横断面T_1WI和T_2WI表现。

第八节 胆胰管括约肌段狭窄

详见本书 本卷 本篇 第七章 第一节 胆胰管括约肌段狭窄。

第九节 胆胰管十二指肠连接区梗阻鉴别诊断

当临床发现梗阻性黄疸时，CT检查可判断梗阻的平面，如梗阻平面位于胆胰管十二指肠连接区时，鉴别诊断应从下述几个方面去考虑。

慢性胰腺炎：慢性胰腺炎局限性胰腺肿大者，常见于胰头部，又称作假肿瘤性胰腺炎。病人有反复发作黄疸及慢性胰腺炎病史，往往有胆系结石、胆系蛔虫、十二指肠憩室等疾患为诱因。其中约一半的病例，由于炎症纤维组织增生而引起肝外胆管胰腺段狭窄，致狭窄上方扩张。此类胰腺炎的CT表现为扩张的肝外胆管外形光滑，自上而下逐渐均匀变细，终止于胰头区，肝外胆管的横断面一直保持圆形。胰头可见均匀密度的局限性肿块，或仅表现为胰头肿大，体尾部无异常，增强扫描见胰头密度较为均匀。如能发现肿大的胰腺与周围粘连，胰腺有不规则钙化影，同时有慢性胰腺炎病史或胰腺炎的其他表现，结合ERCP和超声所见，以及反复发作的病史，则支持慢性胰腺炎的诊断。

胰头肿瘤：胰头癌压迫和侵犯肝外胆管常造成肝外胆管胰腺段突然中断，或从圆形变为不规则形。肝外胆管受侵犯侧可见胰头肿块。尽管如此，CT发现单纯胰头肿块，而不伴有其他良、恶性征象时，仍有部分病例难以明确诊断，可建议进一步作ERCP、内镜胰腺超声等影像学检查，结合临床化验做出判断，或者进行临床随访，或者在影像技术导引下进行穿刺活检，依靠细胞学检查确诊。在此，尤其值得注意的是，在慢性胰腺炎的基础上可并发胰腺癌，如穿刺活检为阴性时，并不能完全排除胰头癌的可能。所以，如仍难鉴别时，只能作剖腹探查，进行细致的组织学检查方能确诊。

胰头癌：胰头不规则肿大，变形，增强扫描见强化的胰头中的小叶结构消失，并可见低密度灶，为癌肿间质纤维化或坏死所致，如发现胰头前方呈毛刺状，则为癌肿侵入胰周脂肪的表现. 老年人胰腺萎缩，小叶间隔宽，脂肪及纤维组织充填呈羽毛状，易发现较小的等密度肿瘤。在胰头癌，有胆管系统和胰管的扩张，其"双管征"的两管之间多有明显的软组织影将两管分隔，扩张的肝外胆管环多数由大圆形突变成小圆形后突然消失，程度较肝外胆管癌和连接区癌轻。

胰腺继发性肿瘤：胰腺周围淋巴结转移或淋巴瘤也可引起胰头增大，甚至胆管下端梗阻，需结合临床及CT其他表现来做出鉴别诊断。

胆胰管十二指肠连接区癌：胆胰管十二指肠连接区癌与胆管下端胆管癌的CT表现常常相近，其主要表现为低位胆管梗阻和肝外胆管的突然中断，部分患者在中断的部位可见腔内软组织肿块，或显示胆管壁不规则增厚，从而提示梗阻是由于腔内肿瘤引起。

一般来说，在CT图像上，胰头与胆胰管下端如未见明确肿块，仅见肝外胆管和/或胰管扩张，则倾向于胆管下端癌和连接区癌。但小的胰头癌实难与它们鉴别。进一步确诊，则需结合临床表现与各种影像学检查（含：MRCP、内镜超声、ERCP、PTC、低张十二指肠造影等）资料进行综合分析。

在晚期病例，胆胰管十二指肠连接区癌、胰头癌和胆管下端癌均可能侵犯周围脏器，形成巨大肿块，使临床和影像诊断鉴别更为困难，甚至病理区分也可发生困难。此时，在临床处理上大同小异，但预后有所不同。胆管全程成比例重度扩张，可见"双管征"（双管影紧靠在一起）和"双环征"，扩张的肝外胆管的环影由大圆形突然消失。

共同管癌：除梗阻性胆管、胆囊扩张外，可在胆管下端发现肿块，在十二指肠乳头部见到对比剂充盈缺损。如肿瘤侵犯胰头，则胰头肿大或见低密度病灶。共同管癌表现为胆管末端软组织肿块，突向十二指肠乳头内侧，在胰头钩突的外侧；增强扫描时该肿块有强化，密度低于正常胰腺，有界线，而增强的胰腺小叶结构正常。

胆胰共同管结石：胆胰共同管结石的鉴别诊断一般不困难，在CT图像上，可见胆胰共同管有高密度或中等密度结石影，或与胆管壁形成晕环征或新月征，则可明确诊断。

有时，胆胰共同管结石排出后，由于扩张的肝外胆管没能及时回缩，或由于肝外胆管壁弹性回缩力降低（年迈或感染因素），导致扩张的肝外胆管仍显扩张状态，但在CT图像上却未见结石影，或其他因素不能轻易肯定梗阻存在，需密切结合临床黄疸消退情况及胆红素水平做出正确判断。如仍有可疑，应加作ERCP或/和PTC，以明确诊断。相反，临床上确有梗阻性黄疸存在，少数病例不能显示胆管扩张，可能因梗阻程度较轻，时间较短，或梗阻呈间歇性，或同时伴有胆管炎存在，对这类病例，都适于进行ERCP或/和PTC检查。

在绝大多数情况下，用CT薄层扫描，可发现胆胰共同管内钙化密度的结石，患者常有反复发作的绞痛及黄疸病史。在个别情况，CT对胆胰共同管胆固醇成分的低密度结石难以确定。对于诊断不明的病例，需要采用薄层高分辨技术，使用不同的体位，有助于病变的发现。值得注意的是，胰头区的高密度影不一定总是胆管结石，胰腺区的淋巴结钙化、胰颈后方增强的门静脉均可被误认为是结石。

下述情况也应注意：胆管结石排出后，肝外胆管壁因弹性减退或消失，难以恢复原状，胆管系统仍呈现扩张状态，可造成胆管梗阻的假象。肝内胆管因为四周都是肝脏实质，梗阻消除后，一般肝内胆管的扩张也消失，从而恢复原状。测定血清胆红素，可有助于判断有无梗阻存在。结石引起的梗阻常为不全性，或为间歇性，胆管扩张的程度有时可以很轻；CT测定肝外胆管的直径多在正常范围（小于或等于6mm）内，或在临界范围（6~8mm）内，但临床上血清胆红素常有升高。

综上所述，有结石病史的病人，肝外胆管扩张不一定总是意味着存在梗阻。相反，轻度结石性梗阻，或短期梗阻的病人，胆管也可不出现明显扩张。对于CT表现的分析，必须随时紧密结合临床情况，方不致于误诊。

胆管下端癌:胆管下端癌表现为胆管下端突然不规则狭窄,管壁增厚或管腔内、外有结节;有强化,但比正常胰腺为低。肿瘤直径小于 0.5cm 的胆管下端癌,往往仅见低位梗阻性胆管扩张,而难以发现肿块。肝外胆管的下端管壁偏环形增厚,胆管系统的扩张较重,无胰管的扩张。低位梗阻性黄疸病因复杂,一般病灶很小就会引起临床症状,因此病人就诊早,而原发病灶较小,不易检出,此时薄层重建显得特别重要;而间接征象一般很明显;通过这些征象的分析,能明显提高病变诊断的准确性,以便对患者及时治疗,提高生存率。

第十节　假胆管癌征

详见本书 本卷 第十六篇 第五章 第一节　假胆管癌征。

第二章　胆胰管十二指肠连接区癌

第一节　胆胰管十二指肠连接区癌

大体病理及其CT表现：连接区癌大体病理形态分为乳头型、共同管内型和混合型，以乳头型最为多见，常呈膨胀性向腔内外生长，并向十二指肠腔内突出，表现为十二指肠壁乳头部的局限性肿块，一组15例均为乳头型连接区癌，也证实该型连接区癌最为普遍。

乳头型易在薄层（层厚≤5mm）扫描图像上见到十二指肠乳头部局限性充盈缺损的肿块影，并且增强扫描可见肿瘤较周边正常十二指肠壁强化更显著，这是诊断乳头型连接区癌最直接的CT征象。至于共同管型连接区癌，肿瘤常向胆总管下端蔓延生长，CT图像上十二指肠腔内乳头部见不到充盈缺损的肿块影；而混合型连接区癌则间于二者之间，CT图像上可在十二指肠腔内乳头部见到充盈缺损的肿块影而得以诊断。事实上，临床实际工作中，混合型常归属于乳头型这一类。

任何肿瘤的生长均依赖一定动脉血的滋养，连接区癌也不例外，故增强动脉期CT扫描，可见肿瘤明显的均匀强化或周边环状强化，更容易与周围正常的十二指肠壁的强化鉴别。门脉期扫描，肿瘤虽仍然强化，但与周围正常十二指肠壁间的强化的差异减小。由于连接区癌肿瘤常较小，肿瘤内坏死不多见，故肿瘤呈均匀强化，尤其门脉期强化更趋均匀一致；肿瘤周边的环状强化，缘于肿瘤周边动脉血供更丰富。如果肿瘤较大，肿瘤中央可出现液化坏死区，该组有2例见此征象。

MSCT扫描速度快、图像清晰，其获得的原始图像可在工作站进行多种图像后处理，而且能进行多期动态增强扫描，在十二指肠乳头癌的诊断中具有较大的优势，而且可确定肿块的部位及周围情况，了解肿块的强化模式。

乳头型连接区癌MSCT平扫表现为十二指肠乳头区圆形、椭圆形软组织肿块，边缘较规则，密度较均匀。多期增强扫描中，动脉期轻度强化，静脉期强化程度增加，延迟期强化程度减退。以静脉期强化最明显。胆总管中重度扩张，梗阻端形态呈截断状突然狭窄，肝内胆管轻中度扩张，与肝外胆管扩张程度一致。部分病例胰管扩张，呈双管征。

多平面重建图像的优势是可任意轴向和角度旋转，多方位观察，多平面重建冠、矢状面影像比标准轴面影像更有助于解剖的理解，能直观反映肿块和肿瘤处肠壁情况。多平面重建可显示十二指肠乳头区软组织肿块突入十二指肠腔内。

乳头型连接区癌浸润生长明显而不形成明显肿块，主要表现为乳头区局部肠壁增厚，胆胰管扩张程度较轻。显示局部肠壁环状增厚，增强扫描见明显强化。

乳头型连接区癌的CT鉴别诊断：胰头癌、胆总管下端癌和连接区癌是胰头及胆胰管十二指肠连接区常见的恶性肿瘤，虽然三者引起的临床症状很类似，同时治疗方法均采用胰十二指肠切除为主要术式。

但是需要指出的是胰头癌的切除率低，仅在5%~25%不等，并且预后差，5年生存率一般在5%左右；而连接区癌和胆总管下端癌的切除率及预后要好得多，切除率达60%~70%，5年生存率可达40%。因此，术前对三者的鉴别诊断，对外科医生手术中具体操作的实施与预后的判断均有极大帮助和指导意义。

临床上，患者均有不同程度的梗阻性黄疸的表现，CT图像上也必然可见到肝内胆管和胆总管不同程度的扩张。至于胆囊的扩大，只要不是慢性胆囊炎所致的胆囊萎缩，胆囊也必然会扩大。根据活体形态学研究，胆总管和胰管共同形成胆胰共同管而开口于十二指肠乳头者，占 75% 左右，故连接区癌者，胰管也常常合并扩张。该组 15 例患者，均见到不同程度的肝内胆管、胆总管和胰管的扩张以及胆囊的增大，也说明这一点。而胆总管下端癌除在胆总管下端区域可见肿块外，常常仅有胆系的扩张，却没有胰管的扩张，这点有助于二者的鉴别。胰头癌因具有围管性浸润的生物学特性，也往往有胆系和胰管的扩张，但胰头癌在动脉期扫描时常呈强化不明显的低密度肿块影而可与连接区癌区别。

该组病例左、右肝内胆管起始段扩张的最大直径小于 1.2cm 者占 80%（12/15），胆总管扩张的平均最大直径为 1.9cm，胰管扩张的平均最大直径为 3.5mm，胰体尾萎缩者仅见 1 例。

有作者曾测量 50 例胰头癌和 10 例胆总管下段癌，左、右肝内胆管起始段扩张的最大直径小于 1.2cm 者仅为 23.5%，明显低于连接区癌者；而胆总管和胰管扩张的程度却差别不大，同时胰头癌伴胰体尾明显萎缩者占绝大多数（88.5%）。故可认为，肝内胆管扩张不显著和胰体尾无萎缩者，有助于连接区癌的诊断。此与连接区癌肿瘤较小，没有完全阻塞连接区有关。

影响乳头型连接区癌 CT 诊断的技术因素：该组平扫仅见 5 例十二指肠腔内乳头部有充盈缺损的肿块影，并且肿瘤均较大（瘤径 >3.0cm），该作者认为主要由于：①连接区癌肿瘤本身均较小（该组有 10 例瘤径≤ 3.0cm）；②未采用薄层扫描；③肿瘤与周围正常肠壁的密度差异小，故应强调薄层增强扫描有利于显示肿瘤的轮廓。该组 15 例在薄层增强扫描 CT 图像上均可显示肿瘤的轮廓、大小以及明显的强化等。这是由于肿瘤血供相对周围正常肠壁的血供丰富，进而增加二者的密度差异，加之采用薄层扫描，故肿瘤显示率高。肿瘤强化明显，动脉期 CT 值达 76.5~81.6HU，门脉期达 60.2~68.2HU，均明显高于周围正常肠壁，通过与 5 例平扫肿瘤 CT 值的测定比较，肿瘤增强 CT 值动脉期提高 36.3HU，门脉期提高 19.7HU。

由于动脉期和门脉期肿瘤的增强程度比较差异不大，并且均能显示肿瘤的轮廓、形态和大小等，好像动脉期扫描似乎无必要。但事实上，梗阻性黄疸的病人作 CT 检查，除明确梗阻平面外，更需进行鉴别诊断，尤其对胰头及胆胰管十二指肠连接区的梗阻性黄疸者，常需与胰头癌鉴别，动脉期增强扫描对显示胰头癌，尤其是小胰头癌为最佳时相，故主张不应放弃动脉期的扫描。何况，动脉期扫描对显示动脉血管，特别是作三维血管成像更有利。

清楚显示连接区癌的肿块，病人检查前的准备十分重要，除需 8 小时禁食外，口服足量的清水更显重要，从而使十二指肠尽量扩张，当然检查前 10 分钟给予一定量的平滑肌松弛药（如盐酸山莨菪碱），更有利于十二指肠充分扩张，从而提高连接区癌肿瘤的显示率。但一般认为只要服水量足，基本能满足诊断的要求。另外，薄层增强扫描更显必要，如果采用 1~3mm 层厚的扫描或进行重建，相信对肿瘤的检出率会更高。随着 MSCT 在临床的应用，对十二指肠乳头状连接区癌的诊断与鉴别诊断水平必将进一步提高。

MRI：MRI 对软组织病变显示敏感，能清楚显示肿瘤的部位、大小，判断肿瘤的浸润范围，MRCP 能显示胆管梗阻的水平，肝内外胆管及胰管扩张形态、程度以及梗阻端的形态，以及充盈良好的十二指肠的管腔形态，且为无射线辐射、创伤的影像学检查，对十二指肠乳头癌的影像学诊断具有独特的优势（图 19-2-1）。

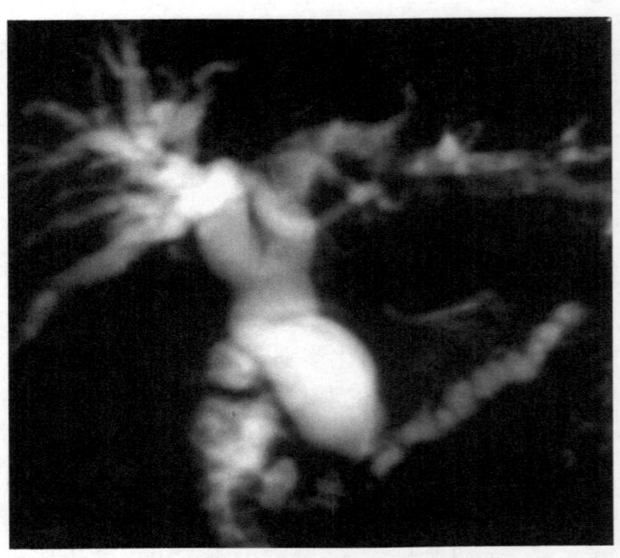

图 19-2-1 MRCP：连接区癌引起的胆胰管扩张

乳头型连接区癌的 MRI 表现：十二指肠乳头区充盈缺损是十二指肠乳头癌的直接征象，由于乳头型连接区癌容易较早侵犯胆胰管括约肌段以及胆胰管下端，造成胆胰管梗阻扩张，临床较早出现黄疸、腹痛等症状，因此乳头型连接区癌患者往往能较早就诊，肿块形态较小。大部分病例表现为乳头区肿块，肿块较小者 MRI 信号往往均匀，病灶 T_1WI 呈略低或中等信号，T_2WI 呈中等或不均匀略高信号。肿块增大后容易出现液化坏死，MRI 信号往往不均匀。增强后病灶强化较明显，小病灶强化较均匀，较大病灶者强化不均匀。

部分乳头型连接区癌浸润生长明显而不形成明显肿块，影像学主要表现为乳头区局部肠壁不规则增厚，可见局限性肠壁僵硬，增强后不规则强化。

乳头型连接区癌的 MRCP 表现：单次激发厚层投射 MRCP 检查，与传统的多层面采集获得原始图像后进行三维重建 MRCP 技术诊断价值相似，且具有成像时间短、图像无需重建、无呼吸伪影等优点，因此该组病例全部采用单次激发厚层投射技术进行 MRCP 检查。

乳头型连接区癌累及胆胰管括约肌段则引起胰胆管梗阻扩张表现，若胰胆管为共同开口受肿瘤侵犯或胰胆管同时受累，可见胰胆管梗阻扩张表现，呈现“双管征”，由于恶性梗阻较完全，因此梗阻扩张胆管往往为重度扩张，常呈“软藤征”改变。少数肿瘤仅累及胆总管下端，则仅表现为胆管扩张，而胰管梗阻表现不明显。

若肿瘤无胆胰管侵犯，则胆胰管无梗阻表现，一些病例仅见胆管轻度扩张，少数病例胆胰管未见扩张。对于梗阻扩张的胆管 MRCP 能很好地显示梗阻端的形态，胆总管下端的梗阻系乳头型连接区癌直接侵犯所致，因此大部分的梗阻端形态为截然中断表现。若肿瘤进一步向管腔内生长，可见梗阻端肝外胆管内的充盈缺损改变，扩张的肝外胆管下端可见小结节状充盈缺损；肿瘤以侵犯胆管壁为主的话，梗阻端形态往往呈“鸟嘴状”狭窄。

部分病例未见明显梗阻者，均为十二指肠局部肠壁增厚，而无明显肿块形成，未见梗阻原因为肿瘤以肠壁侵犯为主，而不累及胆胰管开口。

MRCP 除了能显示胆胰管之外，同时能显示液体充盈良好的十二指肠的形态以及其与胆胰管的关系，十二指肠降部内乳头区可见充盈缺损。利用低张 MRI 结合 MRCP 可以很好地提高十二指肠乳头区结构的显示。如临床诊断胆总管下端梗阻并高度怀疑乳头型连接区癌，应做低张 MRCP 及适当充盈十二指肠，同时做增强扫描以显示十二指肠壁及肿瘤增强情况。

对乳头型连接区癌的诊断，应该强调 MRI 及 MRCP 联合检查，以提高诊断准确性。MRI 可以很好地显示十二指肠乳头部肿瘤的形态特点，结合 MRCP 可以清楚地显示癌肿引起的肝内外胆管扩张形态与程度，尤其是肝外胆管的扩张形态及狭窄端特征性的“鸟嘴状”狭窄和截断改变。MRI 及 MRCP 联合检查是诊断乳头型连接区癌一种敏感且无创伤性的检查方法，具有较高的诊断价值。

胰头癌表现为胰头区软组织肿块，T_1WI 呈稍低信号，T_2WI 呈等或略高混杂信号。胰头癌为少血供肿瘤，动态增强扫描各期信号强度均低于正常胰腺组织。

胆总管下端癌表现为受累胆管壁不均匀增厚，胆管腔内软组织信号结节，动态增强 MRI 动脉期及门静脉期均出现明显强化。MRCP 示受累节段胆管腔狭窄，梗阻平面以上的胆总管及肝内胆管明显扩张。胆总管下端结石在胆总管下端常形成倒杯口状狭窄，也应与鉴别，但结石在 T_1WI 和 T_2WI 上均呈极低信号，往往伴有肝内胆管结石和胆囊结石，并且为多发。

第二节 胆胰共同管周围癌

胆胰管十二指肠连接区癌，即胆胰共同管周围癌，以前也称为“壶腹”周围癌，是指起源于胆胰共同管、胰头部胆总管或胰管上皮以及十二指肠乳头及周围（以乳头开口为中心，直径 2cm 的区域）黏膜的恶性肿瘤的总称。胆胰共同管周围癌占消化道肿瘤的 5%。

胆胰管十二指肠连接区组织结构多样、复杂，胆胰共同管周围癌早期鉴别诊断有一定难度；对于不同起源的肿瘤，其发生率、手术切除率和预后均有差别。胆胰共同管周围肿块和低位胆管梗阻是胆胰共同管周围癌的共同表现，但不同组织学起源的肿瘤各有特点。胆胰管十二指肠连接区周围肿瘤临床三联征是黄疸、疼痛、体重减轻；放射学三联征是胆管扩张、胰管扩张、胆胰共同管周围包块。有此两个三联征可以提示诊断为共同管周围肿瘤。

肿块：肿块是最常见的直接征象。胆胰共同管周围癌大部分呈稍长 T_1、稍长 T_2 信号,肿块大小不一。胰头癌肿块常较大,与周围组织分界不清;中心位于十二指肠腔外,十二指肠常受压变形或移位。增强扫描各期强化低于正常胰腺组织。胆总管下端癌肿块一般较小,呈胆总管腔内结节或管壁增厚,少向肠腔内突出,但胆管梗阻重。增强扫描各期强化明显,并有延迟强化。胆胰共同管癌及十二指肠乳头癌肿块中心位于十二指肠腔内,形成充盈缺损,两者表现相似,增强扫描各期呈均匀或环状中度强化,但十二指肠乳头癌延迟强化明显(图 19-2-2)。

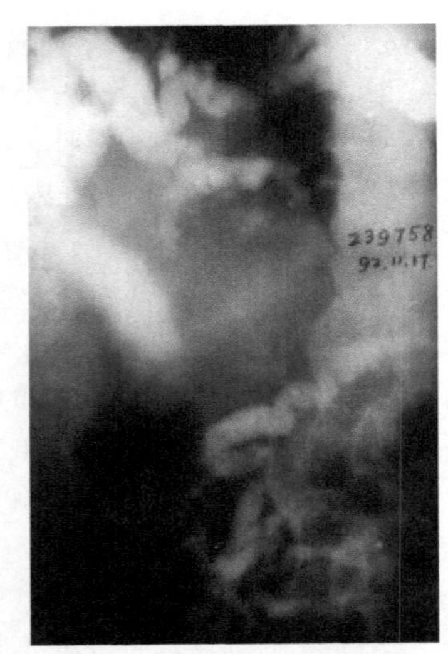

图 19-2-2 ERCP:胆胰管下端恶性梗阻所致肝内胆管软藤状扩张和胰管的迂曲扩张

通过 MRI 平扫和三期增强可将绝大部分胰头癌区别开来,但对鉴别胆胰共同管癌及十二指肠乳头癌仍有困难。

肝内胆管"软藤"状扩张:"软藤"状扩张是胆胰共同管周围癌的一个重要征象。一组中出现胆管"软藤"状扩张 46 例,占 90.2%。胰头癌梗阻水平较高,位于钩突平面以上,胆胰管间有肿块故间距较大(>5mm)。胆总管下端癌胆管梗阻水平位于钩突平面,胆总管下端狭窄或中断;胆总管下端癌胆管"软藤"状扩张的比例最高,该组 8 例,占 100%。胆胰共同管癌及十二指肠乳头癌梗阻水平位于钩突平面以下,扩张胆胰管间距 <5 mm。

"双管征":"双管征"是胆胰共同管周围癌的另一个重要征象。胰头癌出现"双管征"的比率最高,该组 19 例,占 86.4%,因为胰头癌起源于胰管上皮,且具有围管性和嗜神经性生长的生物学特性,所以胆胰管阻塞严重,易形成分离的"双管征"。国内外学者报道"四管征"是胰腺癌的典型特征,"四管征"是指肿块上方扩张的胆总管,肿块远侧扩张的胰管,肿块下方相对正常的胰管及胆总管。该组仅见 4 例。胆总管下端癌出现"双管征"者较少,该组 3 例,文献报道"三管征"是胆总管下端癌的特异征象(指梗阻近、远端胆总管,未扩张的主胰管),该组 2 例见"三管征"。胆胰共同管癌和十二指肠乳头癌呈并行"双管征",早期胆胰管狭窄较轻时可无"双管征",该组胆胰共同管癌 10 例,占 83.3%;乳头癌 8 例,占 88.9%。

血管侵犯、淋巴结转移:周围血管是否侵犯和淋巴结及其他脏器转移是评价肿瘤可切除性的两个重要征象,MRI 三期增强扫描对显示胆胰共同管周围和门静脉系统血管是否受侵犯很重要。该组中 15 例淋巴结转移,3 例周围脏器转移。

ERCP 表现:内镜下胰头癌侵犯肠壁位于乳头上方,通常乳头外观尚正常。造影显示主胰管胰头段不规则狭窄或闭塞,上游胰管明显扩张;同一平面胆总管偏心性狭窄,边缘毛糙,有时还伴有向胰管方向的成角和推移,在胆总管末端往往还有一小段正常的胆管。

胆总管下端癌内镜下乳头表面黏膜一般完好,肿瘤侵犯胆管末梢时可见乳头轻度增大,其形态变化较乳头癌为轻。通常胆管造影仅显示梗阻以下的胆管,借助导丝可显示狭窄段胆管长度,以及梗阻以上扩张胆管,胆管走行方向通常无改变。

胆胰共同管癌和乳头癌的内镜下表现为乳头或胆胰共同管区肿大隆起,常呈不规则结节状,表面完整或溃烂,乳头开口不清。造影表现为胆胰共同管汇合区管腔明显变窄或闭塞,形态不规则,两侧不对称。胆胰共同管癌和乳头癌一般在十二指肠镜检查时,通过肉眼观察即可得到初步诊断,并可进行活检及内镜直视下刷取细胞取得病理证实。

MRCP 与 ERCP 对胆胰共同管周围癌诊断的比较:MRCP 具有安全、无创、适应证广泛等优点,三维成像类似于直接胆胰管造影,可显示整个胆胰系的全貌,是目前诊断恶性梗阻性黄疸最常选择的方法。MRCP 不仅能提供生理状态下胆管树整体图像,并同时显示梗阻上端与下端的情况,结合梗阻端形态及源图像可对梗阻的性质作出判断;尤其是结合 MRI 多种序列及动态增强,可观察管外组织结构的变化,在评价肿瘤范围、阻塞部位和范围、有无肝实质侵犯和远处转移等方面明显优于 ERCP。

MRCP 最大缺点是不能取得病理信息，对于乳头及胆胰共同管周围病变诊断受限。

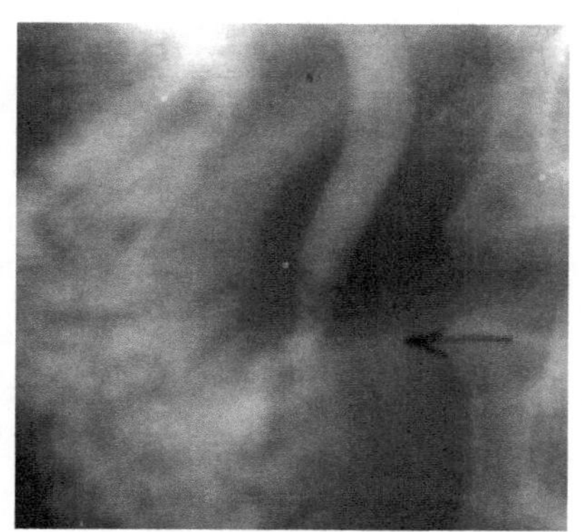

图 19-2-3　ERCP：在肝外胆管括约肌段清楚可见三条横行的绒毛瓣的细线状充盈缺损，呈倒人字形。

ERCP 是早期诊断胆胰共同管周围癌的重要手段，对胆胰共同管微小肿瘤的定位与定性诊断明显优于其他检查，是目前公认的诊断胆胰管疾病的金标准。它能在内镜下对十二指肠乳头区黏膜直接观察和切取活组织病检，并能提供直接清晰的胆胰管影像；部分治疗性 ERCP 技术已达到了外科手术相同的疗效。该组 ERCP 对十二指肠乳头癌确诊率达到 100%（图 19-2-3）。

但 ERCP 也有其局限性，当胆管完全梗阻时，只能显示梗阻以下胆管，对手术治疗有参考价值的病变段范围难以显示；由于对比剂注射压力影响常夸大胆胰管扩张程度；缺乏对肿瘤周围浸润和淋巴结转移的判断，无法评价肿瘤的可切除性。另外，ERCP 属于一种侵入性检查，有发生胰腺炎等并发症的风险。

胆胰共同管周围病变的临床诊断主要依赖于影像学，MRCP 和 ERCP 各有其优势，MRCP 结合常规 MRI 对胰头癌及胆总管下端癌优势明显，对各类胆胰共同管周围癌周围毗邻关系的评估准确。尤其适合于一般情况差、不能耐受 ERCP 检查及已行胃肠改道手术的患者。可作为优先选择的检查方法。ERCP 对胆胰共同管癌及十二指肠乳头癌早期诊断价值突出，同时可以取活检，这是其他检查方法所不能比拟的。结合患者自身情况，综合利用各种影像学方法，争取对不同类型病变选用敏感性最高的方法。胆胰共同管癌表现为肝外胆管下端偏心性狭窄，十二指肠相对应部位的肿块充盈缺损影，胰管全程扩张，与扩张的肝外胆管并行，呈“双管征”，两者走行有聚拢趋势。

上述征象在三维的 MRCP 皆能清楚显示，由于它是三维，并且可多角度观察，远比 ERCP 观察更为全面和准确。MRCP 不仅观察管腔内的改变，而且可观察管腔外乳头及胰头组织的变化，对连接区周围癌范围的确定十分有利。

第三节　“壶腹”周围癌

早期诊断“壶腹”周围癌的临床意义：“壶腹”周围癌主要指胰头癌、“壶腹”癌、胆总管远端癌及十二指肠乳头癌。大量研究显示不同病理类型间的“壶腹”周围癌的术后中位生存率存在较大差异，特别是胰头癌的病变进程、影像学表现、治疗方案的选择与其他“壶腹”周围癌有所不同，其中位生存期明显低于其他病理类型的“壶腹”周围癌。临床常将“壶腹”癌、胆总管远端癌及十二指肠乳头癌统称为“壶腹”部癌，故胰头癌与“壶腹”部癌的早期明确诊断对患者的预后有重要的临床意义。

“壶腹”周围癌的特征性影像学表现：“壶腹”周围癌的特征性影像学表现主要指胰头 -“壶腹”区软组织肿块及病变水平以上胆胰管系统不同程度的扩张。文献报道 MRI、超声对“壶腹”区肿块显示率分别为 100%、81. 08%。一组 79 例“壶腹”周围癌中，胰头 -“壶腹”区肿块 74 例，利用常规 MRI 检查肿块显示率为 93.67%，超声肿块显示率为 83.54%（66/79）。这与 MRI 检查具有较高的组织分辨率，可多方位、多角度、多层面成像，而超声检查因受腹壁脂肪及肠道内气体的干扰对“壶腹”区病变显示欠佳有关。

胰头 -“壶腹”区软组织肿块常导致病变水平胆总管及胰管梗阻，并伴病变水平以上胆胰管不同程度扩张。不同病理类型的“壶腹”周围癌所致胆胰管扩张程度不同。

该组研究显示胰头癌及“壶腹”部癌均以Ⅲ型至Ⅳ型扩张为主，Ⅰ型至Ⅱ型与Ⅲ型至Ⅳ型之间差异有统计学意义（χ^2=7.670，P=0.006），但灵敏度及特异度均不高。若以Ⅲ型～Ⅳ型扩张及胰头无明显增大为标准，诊断“壶腹”部癌的灵敏度为 83.30%，特异度可达 93.90%，对提高“壶腹”周围癌的鉴别诊断，特别是胰头癌与“壶腹”部癌的早期诊断水平，制订适当的治疗方案，延长患者中位生存期有重要的临床意义。MRCP 联合常规 MRI 及超声检查在“壶腹”周围癌诊断中的优势：常规超声检查因无创、简便、高效、经济而成为“壶腹”周围癌首选的检查方法。超声检查对肝内外胆管扩张十分敏感。超声检查中胰头癌主要征象为胰头区低回声肿块，主胰管扩张，肝内外胆管扩张、胆囊增大、“平行管征”等。“壶腹”部癌的超声典型征象为胰头“壶腹”区的低回声结节，边境不清楚，部分浸润到周围组织，胆总管及胰管扩张。由于“壶腹”部体积小，位置深，而易受肠道内气体干扰，因此，利用超声检查“壶腹”部肿块较困难。该研究常规超声检查对“壶腹”周围癌的显示率为 83.54%，低于常规 MRI 检查（93.67%），又因超声诊断依赖于操作者的临床经验和操作技巧，重复性欠佳。目前，超声检查只作为黄疸待查或可疑“壶腹”区病例的初筛检查手段。

常规 MRI 检查对胆总管及十二指肠腔内外病变的信号变化具有较高的灵敏度与特异度，而 MRCP 检查则利用水在重度 T2WI 上极高信号的特点，同时结合脂肪抑制、预饱和、流动补偿、相控阵线圈等技术重建而成，能清晰显示胆胰管的影像。

Adamek 等（2000）研究显示 MRCP 在检测胆胰管扩张和狭窄方面的灵敏度可达 93% 以上。与 ERCP 和经皮肝穿胆管造影（PTC）相比，MRCP 无需对比剂，安全无创，病人无痛苦，检查成功率高，诊断准确性高，对无法耐受 ERCP 或 PTC 检查的患者，MRCP 是较有效的影像学检查手段。但因 MRCP 对胆胰管病变信号变化缺乏特异性而易导致漏诊、误诊及无法显示病变形态学变化、信号特点等缺陷，对梗阻性病变诊断具有一定困难。MRCP 联合常规 MRI 及超声检查技术可以弥补其对微小病变信号分辨差、对管腔内病变信号表现缺乏特异性等缺点，对提高“壶腹”周围癌，特别是胰头癌与“壶腹”部癌的早期鉴别诊断有重要意义，可为临床选择适当治疗方案及是否需要 ERCP 检查提供有效的影像学信息。

第四节　胆胰管十二指肠连接区高中分化腺癌

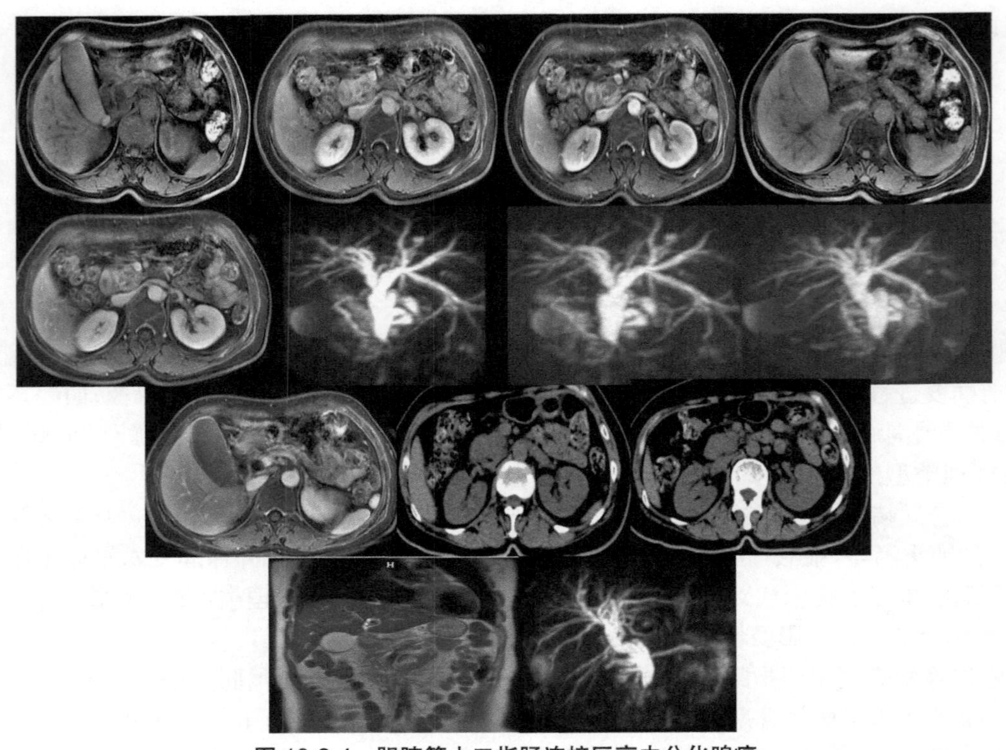

图 19-2-4　胆胰管十二指肠连接区高中分化腺癌

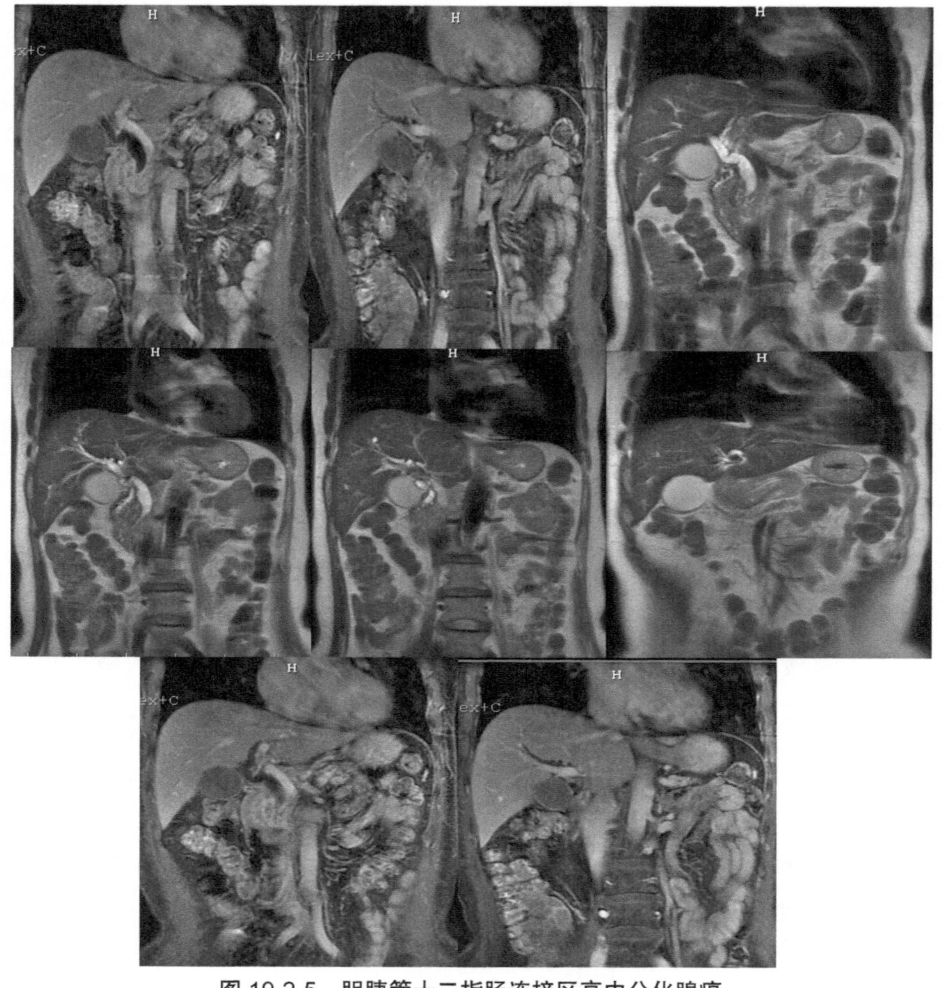

图 19-2-5 胆胰管十二指肠连接区高中分化腺癌

患者，女，57 岁。因发现血糖高 8 年，加重伴消瘦 2 个月余入院。行 CT 检查提示：右肺中下叶微小结节，建议随访；肝外胆管下段可疑占位，伴肝内外胆管扩张，建议 MR 检查。甲胎蛋白：3.44ng/ml、糖类抗原 125：9.10U/ml、糖类抗原 19-9：1982.57U/ml ↑、癌胚抗原：7.34 ng/ml ↑。

病理检查：胆胰共同管肿物，大小 5cm × 3.8 cm × 3.5 cm，肿物切面灰白质中，其余肠黏膜皱襞明显。肠外膜及肠周脂肪组织检出淋巴结样物 4 枚，直径 0.8~1.2 cm。第 8 组淋巴结：灰黄色组织一块，大小 2.5 cm × 2.5 cm × 0.3 cm。常规病理诊断：胆胰共同管肿物切除标本：胆胰共同管高中分化腺癌，侵犯十二指肠壁全层至肠黏膜下层，可见癌组织局部侵犯胰头组织，并见癌组织侵犯间质神经及血管组织，肠管两侧切缘均为阴性，肿瘤细胞耐药及预后检测待免疫组化报告。淋巴结清扫：送检第 8 组淋巴结检出 1/4；自检肠外膜及肠周淋巴结 0/3。以上共检出淋巴结 7 枚，其中 1 枚可见癌转移。

免疫组化检测：阳性 CK7，CA19-9，Villin，CK20（个别 +），VEGF（2+），EGFR（3+），Tubulinβ（+），TOPO Ⅱ（+），Ki-67（+，约 15%）；阴性：5-FU，ERCC1，P-gP。免疫组化诊断：胆胰共同管肿物切除标本：胆胰共同管高中分化腺癌，详见常规组织学报告（图 19-2-4、19-2-5）。

第五节 胆胰管十二指肠连接区癌

胆胰管十二指肠连接区癌少见，发病率为 0.01%~0.04%（Montag 等，1990；Rubin 等，1991）。过去，由于诊断技术水平有限，术前常不能与其他周围癌区别而统称为"壶腹"周围癌。近年来，现代影像技术的进展及在临床的广泛应用表明,胆胰管十二指肠连接区癌与其他周围癌,完全能够,而且也非常必要区分开来。

1. 病因学　目前仍不甚清楚,可能为多因素所致。

良性肿瘤:胆胰管十二指肠连接区良性肿瘤以乳头状腺瘤为多,它和胃肠道乳头状腺瘤一样,都可发生恶变。胆胰管十二指肠连接区癌的病理学检查也见33.5%~52%(Liu等,1983)是乳头状腺癌。家族性息肉病中,除结肠之外,十二指肠是第二个常见的息肉好发部位,且息肉常集中在乳头附近。此病可同时合并腺癌(Jarvinen等,1983),其中胆胰管十二指肠连接区癌约为2.8%(Sener等,1984)。一些学者(Hayes等,1987;Jarvinen等,1983;Kurtz等,1987)认为,腺瘤到腺癌是一个连续的过程,即腺瘤是腺癌发展过程中的一个阶段或先期病变。病理检查所观察到的连接区腺瘤表面有癌灶存在,以及81.2%胆胰管十二指肠连接区癌中有残留的腺瘤组织的报道(Kurtz等,1987)都支持这一观点(图19-2-6)。

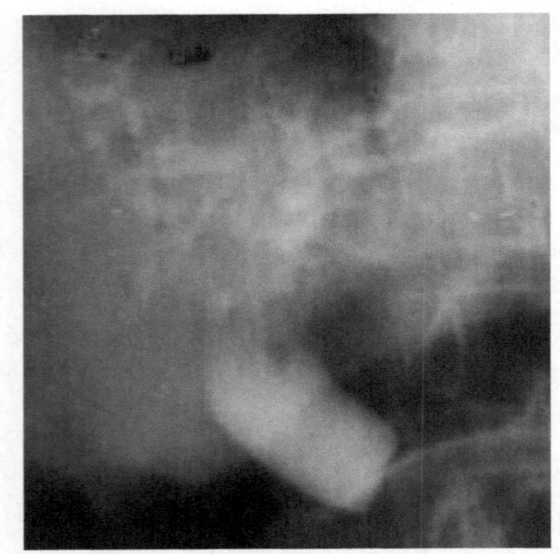

图19-2-6　ERCP:连接区癌导致明显扩张的肝外胆管下端的杵状征

遗传因素:Austin(1988)对2周内先后发现胆胰管十二指肠连接区癌的两同胞兄弟进行研究,并综合分析胆胰管十二指肠连接区癌与Gardner综合征和家族性结肠息肉病的关系,认为遗传因素对发病确有一定的影响。

胆系结石与胆系肿瘤的关系:胆囊癌合并胆囊结石的发生率高达80%,胆胰管十二指肠连接区癌合并胆系结石的发生率为25%~35%,Ryan(1986)通过分析小肠绒毛病变的分布规律,推测胆胰管十二指肠连接区癌与胆汁和胰液中的致癌物质有关。

2. 病理学　胆胰管十二指肠连接区癌,起源于连接区之共同管黏膜上皮,或胆管下端黏膜上皮,或胰管下端黏膜上皮。癌多呈息肉状或结节状,表面凹凸不平,常有糜烂或溃疡。肿瘤大小不等,直径在0.4~15.0cm之间,平均3cm左右。大体形态上可分为十二指肠乳头型,共同管内型和混合型,以乳头型为多见。乳头型表现为十二指肠壁内局限性肿块,呈膨胀性向肠腔内生长;共同管内型癌肿向胆胰管下端蔓延生长,此型与胆管下端癌难以区分。

癌肿呈息肉样或结节状,表面凹凸不平,乳头癌常呈菜花状,其表面多有糜烂或溃疡。肿瘤大小不等,一般位于乳头部的肿瘤较大,最大者直径可达8cm;位于管腔内者一般较小,最小者直径仅0.5cm。组织学类型皆为腺癌,且以腺癌和乳头状腺癌为主,高分化腺癌所占比例较大,黏液癌和未分化癌占极少数。大多数肿瘤恶性程度低,转移时间较晚。

分型:按大体形态可分为管腔内型、乳头型和混合型。以癌的原发和所占据的部位为基础,可将连接区癌分为六型:1型,癌局限于乳头的十二指肠黏膜;2型,癌局限于共同管;3型,癌局限于胆管末端;4型,癌局限于主胰管末端;5型,癌局限于共同管和胆胰管末端;6型,癌肿不仅侵犯共同管和胆胰管末端,而且还侵犯十二指肠黏膜。

3. 临床表现　胆胰管十二指肠连接区癌男性多见,男女之比大于2:1,病人大部分年龄在40岁以上,平均50~55岁。据我们1991年43例报告,男性37例,女性6例,年龄38~69岁,平均52.4岁。最常见症状是黄疸,其次是食欲不振、上腹部闷胀不适和疼痛、消瘦、发热、腹泻、黑便等。病例的主要症状为:黄疸(42/43),上腹胀痛或闷胀不适(33/43),纳差(25/43),体重减轻及乏力(各为24/43)。主要体征为:巩膜皮肤黄染(39/43),肝肿大(28/43),胆囊肿大(26/43)。传统地把黄疸作为早期症状,无痛性进行性黄疸是典型表现。当今概念发生变化:本症的最早期的表现和典型症状并非是黄疸。

上腹部痛、上腹部闷胀不适、纳差、体重减轻、乏力等症状体征,常在黄疸出现前早已存在,这是由于肿瘤组织的阻塞,胰管胆管内压力升高,胰液胆汁分泌排泄不畅所致,在胆管胰管代偿性扩张适应阶段,临床上可不出现黄疸。因此,如能高度重视这些早期症状，并积极地利用现代影像技术检查病人，定会有利于本症的早期发现。

临床观察和实验研究表明，肝外胆管梗阻时，胆管扩张是比黄疸更为敏感的征象。胆管内压正常为0.49~1.47kPa（50~150mm 水柱），肝分泌压为 2.94~3.43kPa（300~350mm 水柱），只有当胆管内压上升超过肝分泌压时，胆红质才会逆流入血而出现黄疸。而在肿瘤缓慢生长和逐渐加重胆管堵塞过程中，胆管系统逐渐扩张和加强排空以克服和减少内压升高引起的损害，尽可能地适应内压升高，胆管内压在一定时期内维持在肝分泌压之下，临床上并不出现黄疸。因此，在连接区癌引起胆管梗阻的早期，常常无黄疸却有胆管的扩张。动物实验也证明，胆管梗阻时，胆管扩张总是先于黄疸出现。有作者报告，在黄疸不是最初症状的胰腺癌病人，黄疸出现距最初症状出现的间隔时间平均为 3 个月，最长可达 22 个月。

此外，注意黄疸和胆囊肿大等体征，血液生化检查中的胆红质和转氨酶的分离现象对本症有诊断和鉴别诊断的意义。胆胰管十二指肠连接区癌可合并慢性胆囊炎、慢性胰腺炎、胆系结石、胃幽门乳头状瘤、异位胰腺等。

4. 影像学研究　B 型超声对胆管扩张的显示率高，并能直接显示胰腺的图像，因此，有作者指出，对40 岁以上不明原因出现消化道症状者，应首选超声检查，一旦发现胆管胰管扩张及胆囊肿大，对提示诊断有重要意义，其主要目的是从中筛选可疑病例，如同时发现胰头区有肿块或低密度区，则更有诊断价值，即使未找到病因亦应高度警惕，进一步作 CT、MRI、MRCP、ERCP、PTC、生化检查、免疫学及病理细胞学等检查，以期得到早期诊断。超声检查的优点是扫描范围宽，提供信息多。它能发现胆囊肿大，胆管和主胰管扩张，从而准确地确定梗阻的部位和范围。同时还能显示胆胰管十二指肠连接区病变与胰腺等邻近组织和器官的关系，了解肝脏、胆囊、胰腺和其他部位胆管的情况，甚至可能提供有关淋巴结情况，对鉴别诊断和制定治疗措施十分有益。有作者指出，鉴于胆管扩张出现于黄疸之前，在临床上，对于不明原因难以解释的上腹部痛或上腹不适者，可用超声检查作为筛选手段。在一个无胆管手术病史的病人，肝外胆管直径超过 8mm 足以证实肝外胆管下端出现梗阻。

声像图表现肝外胆管与胰管均明显扩张，并可在胆胰管汇合处，胰头的右侧或右后侧显示边缘不规整的低回声光团。光团较小，其直径多为20~30mm，与胰头有较为明确的分界。对肝外胆管和胰管均明显扩张而初检时未能显示病变者，除应随诊复查外，尚应进一步行 CT，MRI，MRCP，PTC 或 ERCP 等影像学检查，以免漏掉较小的病变。

超声检查的定性诊断常有一定限度。一是发现病灶有一定的困难：超声检查可受胆系术后和肠道气体等因素影响，而使病变不能显示或显示不清，足以证实肝外胆管下端出现梗阻；临床要求检查部位不明确和检查重点不突出，也给发现病灶带来难处。二是即使发现管腔内病变，有时还需要与胆固醇结石和良性肿瘤等鉴别，尤其是合并结石存在时，定性诊断更为困难。但是如果改进和提高检查技术，有目的有重点地检查胆胰管十二指肠连接区，诊断准确率定会有较大提高。

超声误诊原因分析有三。

（1）定性不准确：①由于该解剖部位较深，胰头癌，胆胰管十二指肠连接区癌和胆管下端癌三者所处部位相似，特别是中晚期癌肿浸润、粘连、转移等造成病灶扩大界限不清，解剖毗邻关系紊乱，因此，从声像图上鉴别困难，不易准确定性；②腺癌组织结构较均匀，透声较好，声像图表现为实质性低回声，特别是坏死、液化时易误诊为囊肿；③癌肿组织坏死，纤维化导致回声增强，同时声能的吸收也可形成后方声衰减而误诊为结石；④胆胰管十二指肠连接区癌影像重叠于胰头中间，胰头肿块较小未超出胰头正常范围者易于漏诊，有时仅提示胆管下端梗阻，而未能提示病因。

（2）干扰因素：腹壁肥厚，消化道气体干扰，图像显示不清晰。

（3）经验不足：未扫查到病变部位，或对异常声像图，特别是早期阶段的表现不能辨认而造成漏诊。

CT 扫描：与超声检查的优点一样，CT 扫描的范围宽，提供信息甚多。它也能发现胆囊肿大，胆管和主胰管扩张，从而准确地确定梗阻的部位。同时，它还能显示连接区病变与胰腺等邻近组织和器官的关系，了解肝脏、胆囊、胰腺和其他部位胆管的情况，甚至可能提供有关淋巴结的情况，对鉴别诊断和制定治疗措施十分有益。

但是，CT 在定性诊断上常有一定的限度。一是难以发现病灶，CT 常因扫描程序选择不当而漏扫，或扫描层面不到位使病变未能显示，或显示不清。

此外,还与临床要求检查部位不明确和检查重点不突出有关。二是即使发现管腔内病变,有时还需要与胆固醇结石及良性肿瘤等相鉴别,尤其是合并胆石时,定性诊断往往有一定困难。但是,如果能够改进和提高检查技术,有目的有重点地检查连接区,诊断的准确率则有较大的上升。例如,CT 检查能够采用左侧卧位时以空气衬托病变,行薄层扫描技术等,都可提高乳头型胆胰管十二指肠连接区癌的显示率。Ricardo 等(1988)认为超声检查连接区肿块的敏感性高于普通 CT。比较二者检查胆胰管十二指肠连接区癌的优缺点来看,超声在某些方面超过普通 CT。

可显示胆管扩张和胆囊扩大,有的病例还可见到乳头肿大、胆管内靶征、胆囊结石。CT 扫描重点不在连接区和扫描技术不当等,是病变显示率低的主要原因。

对乳头型胆胰管十二指肠连接区癌,扫描时易受诸多因素(例如:肠道蠕动,检查前对比剂服用的时间和剂量,扫描层距等)的影响,对乳头大小,轮廓的改变观察不及 X 线十二指肠低张造影。观察乳头本身的大小轮廓及有无溃疡,低张十二指肠造影优于 CT;而观察乳头周围结构有无侵犯及淋巴结转移, CT 优于低张十二指肠造影。因此,两种检查方法必须优势互补,方能提出较为准确的诊断。

X 线十二指肠低张造影:在二十世纪六十年代,此法是诊断胆胰管十二指肠胆胰管十二指肠连接区癌的最佳手段,随着超声、CT 和 ERCP 的出现,此法已逐渐被淘汰。X 线表现可分为直接征象和间接征象:

直接征象:乳头型和混合型可见乳头及其周围的正常形态消失,代之以边缘不规则和密度不均匀的充盈缺损或龛影或钡斑;癌肿较大时可出现反 3 征,连接区的纵行皱襞和包皮及小带破坏,甚至邻近十二指肠的黏膜破坏和消失,肠壁僵硬和不规则性肠腔狭窄。

管腔内常常仅见到大而光整的乳头,或乳头及其周围呈结节状改变。有的病人十二指肠可出现功能障碍,诸如局限性痉挛和激惹,排空延迟等。十二指肠乳头旁憩室可能受压、移位和变形,以及边缘不整等。在十二指肠上部外上缘常可见到扩大的胆囊和总胆管的压迹,此种间接征象在三种类型胆胰管十二指肠连接区癌中均可见到,并且,它的出现可早于黄疸的出现,对早期诊断胆胰管十二指肠连接区癌有着重要意义。胆胰管十二指肠连接区癌可导致胰腺炎,因而有时可见十二指肠痉挛,肠环扩大,肠黏膜增粗和紊乱。

又可将连接区癌分为肿瘤型与溃疡型,肿瘤型:可由肿瘤的形态、大小、所占据的部位及浸润程度、被覆黏膜的状态而呈现不同的 X 线形态。共同特征为乳头及近侧纵行皱襞的正常形态消失,代之以不规则的局限性充盈缺损,正面观可见肿瘤形态。当癌肿侵犯十二指肠黏膜时,可见乳头周围横行皱襞中断和破坏,一般易与良性疾病区别。但在早期癌及黏膜下癌(只侵犯胆胰管下端或 / 和共同管,而十二指肠黏膜未受侵蚀),只见到乳头及近侧纵行皱襞肿大,周围横行皱襞无中断破坏现象,只靠低张造影,则与良性疾病鉴别困难。此时,可进一步作 CT 和 / 或超声、MRI、MRCP、胆胰管造影、内镜、活体组织学及细胞学检查。 溃疡型:在降段乳头部位呈现边缘不整的充盈缺损,其内有不规则的阴影斑(溃疡形成),多有周围皱襞的中断破坏。此型与胰头癌相比更为局限,且腔内的隆起性病变为其特征,一般鉴别不难。鉴别困难者,可进一步采用 CT 和 / 或超声、MRI、MRCP、胆胰管造影,以及内镜检查。

间接征象:于十二指肠上部外上缘常可见扩大的胆囊和总胆管的压迹。胆囊扩大可在十二指肠降段上部的外缘形成较大而浅的弧形压迹,总胆管扩张有两种表现:一是在球后形成一垂直带状压迹;一是在同一部位形成局限性圆弧状压迹。此种征象在三种类型肿瘤中均可见到,并且,它的出现可早于黄疸,对早期诊断胆胰管十二指肠连接区癌有意义。本症可导致胰腺炎,因而有时可见十二指肠痉挛,肠环扩大,肠黏膜增粗和紊乱。低张造影可发现十二指肠降段内侧不规则充盈缺损、球后段总胆管压迹增宽、十二指肠上曲外上方胆囊压迹扩大等征象。此法对乳头型肿瘤的诊断有一定的价值,对管腔内肿瘤则爱莫能助。

直接法胆胰管造影的表现:ERCP 对于诊断胆胰管十二指肠连接区癌比较理想。它具有一定的优点:通过内镜能直接观察到乳头部癌肿及邻近十二指肠情况。十二指肠镜能在近距离观察乳头,而乳头肿瘤时乳头的肿大和表面溃烂,故当内镜接触到乳头时,极易出血。乳头开口又常被肿瘤阻塞以致于插管失败;直视下采取活体组织,经病理检查可于术前即明确诊断。通过逆行胆胰管造影以了解内镜观察不到的共同管及附近管腔内的状况,或为乳头切开进行活检提供资料；了解胆胰管排泄胆汁与胰液的功能，可见全部胰管和/或胆管有不同程度的扩张和对比剂排空延迟；返流或排泄的对比剂可显示乳头肿瘤和十二指肠的轮廓。当年，ERCP 的问世，已使胆胰管十二指肠连接区癌的诊断准确率由以往的 25% 提高到目前的 73%~100%。在内镜直视下，可观察到肿瘤呈菜花状，乳头增大并充血水肿，乳头呈息肉状。如插管造影成功，可见管腔内不规则充盈缺损，其中位于肝外胆管远端者居多，主胰管远端及共同管内者较少，显影之胆胰管常有梗阻和扩张，肝内胆管扩张多呈软藤表现。

其他直接法胆系造影：含 PTC、术中胆管造影、术后 T 管造影。可见肝外胆管远端充盈缺损，肝内胆管扩张迂曲，有时仅见肝内胆管软藤状扩张而不见其下端病变的表现，这常常是因为 PTC 造影技术不当（诸如：未作立位观察，未多轴位观察，注入对比剂过少等导致下端病变未能显示；对肝外胆管的应有的长度不甚了解而未进一步往下方观察；满足于肝内胆管软藤状扩张的发现，加上注入对比剂困难，即中断造影，草率地诊断为下端病变），肝外胆管由于长期梗阻而产生的胶冻状胆汁的占位使对比剂难以充盈。

在各种直接法胆系造影中，胆胰管十二指肠连接区癌可表现为：管腔内型和混合型常为管腔内不规则的充盈缺损或呈杯口状缺损；乳头型表现为共同管或胆胰管末端呈圆钝的 V 字形改变，不规则的偏侧性狭窄。

大多数病例都有不同程度的胆胰管梗阻表现：梗阻较严重者，胆管和胰管普遍扩张和纡曲，状似软藤；部分可见双管征，即胆管胰管均现扩张。

动态观察对比剂排空时，由于排泄阻力增大，可见癌肿未波及的括约肌段胆管有明显的强烈收缩，对比剂呈细线状或滴状排泄。完全梗阻者，尤其是乳头型，ERCP 常常造影失败，但多数经镜下观察到菜花状肿物和活检即可确诊。

胆胰管十二指肠连接区癌直接征象：内镜下见到充血糜烂的菜花状或息肉状肿块；　直接法胆系造影见胆胰管腔内充盈缺损，或不规则性管腔狭窄；低张法十二指肠钡剂造影示十二指肠腔内隆起，或凹陷性病变，或见反 3 征；CT 显示突入十二指肠壁不规则局部增厚，腔内肿块，总胆管靶征突然消失；B 型超声探及十二指肠腔内低回声肿物。

胆胰管十二指肠连接区癌间接征象：内镜见十二指肠乳头充血水肿、糜烂或结节状改变；肝外胆管与主胰管扩张呈双管征，肝内外胆管呈软藤状扩张；对比剂从胆管胰管排空困难；十二指肠的胆囊和肝外胆管压迹明显；低张法十二指肠钡剂造影显示胰腺炎的间接征象。这些间接征象可出现于早期胆胰管十二指肠连接区癌，应给予足够重视（图 19-2-7）。

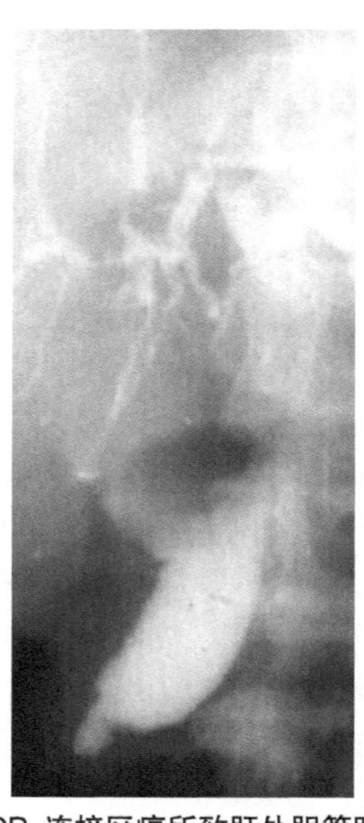

图 19-2-7　ERCP：连接区癌所致肝外胆管明显扩张，其下端呈下凸表现，肝内胆管扩张，括约肌段僵硬且可见充盈缺损

血管造影：腹腔动脉造影和肠系膜上动脉造影时，可能见到胰十二指肠动脉，尤其是胰十二指肠动脉的后上支呈现不规则、增粗、僵直、中断、成角弯曲，以及肿瘤血管。有时可见斑片的肿瘤染色。

胆胰管十二指肠连接区癌的早期诊断：胆胰管十二指肠连接区癌临床分期：1 期，癌瘤局限，无向周围组织浸润和转移；2 期，癌瘤侵犯周围组织和/或有局部淋巴结转移；3 期，癌瘤向远处转移。Nix（1983）认为，癌块直径小于 8mm 者，均未见浸润十二指肠；直径大于 15mm 者，才会侵犯胰腺，或出现胰腺周围淋巴结转移。

胆胰管十二指肠连接区癌的早期诊断，是建立在高度重视和充分认识其早期症状的基础上，在黄疸出现之前而不是之后，即不失时机地进行有效的影像学检查。

超声，上部胃肠道钡餐检查，低张十二指肠造影等是较常用的筛选方法，常常最早发现胆胰管十二指肠连接区癌的早期间接征象。一旦发现总胆管和胆囊扩大的征象,怀疑胆胰管十二指肠连接区癌时,MRCP、ERCP 应是首先选择的影像检查。乳头型和混合型胆胰管十二指肠连接区癌,通过内镜直接观察和有效地活检,即可于术前确诊。

低张十二指肠造影,需要造影质量高,有清楚显示乳头及其周围微细结构的正位象,才可能发现较小的病变。管腔内型和混合型胆胰管十二指肠连接区癌,共同管或胆胰管末端偏侧性不规则狭窄是 MRCP、ERCP 等直接法胆系造影的特征性表现。乳头增大并呈炎性改变,胆胰管内对比剂排空延迟也属于早期征象。

梗阻性黄疸病人行直接法胆系造影检查时,造影的技术是十分关键的环节,要力求显示胆管的全程,有意识地行立位观察和拍摄胆胰管括约肌段的异常情况,对于发现早期胆胰管十二指肠连接区癌颇为有益。

家族性腺瘤性息肉病患者的胆胰管十二指肠连接区癌发病率约为普通人群的 1 000 倍(Alexander 等, 1989),因而,对此类患者进行检查和定期复查,对胆胰管十二指肠连接区癌的早期诊断有意义。

Menzel 等(1997)在 51 例非常小的胆胰管肿瘤病例中对导管内超声、内镜超声、ERCP、CT 等诊断技术进行比较。在 ERCP 检查时,导管内超声的换能器置于胆胰管系统内进行观察,这是迅速简单和可靠的方法,它可提供有价值的管道周围有关的资料。

在胰癌的诊断上,它的敏感性为 85%(6/8),ERCP 为 37%(3/8),内镜超声为 50%(4/8), CT 为 37%(3/8)。在胆管肿瘤,它们的敏感性分别为 89%(8/9),78%(7/9),33%(3/9),33%(1/3)。在 ERCP 检查时,将小的超声导管换能器系统置入胆管或/和胰管,技术简单,而并发症很少,对于小的胆胰管病变的精确诊断,它可给 ERCP 增添有价值的研究资料。

对于胆胰共同管癌, Shirai 等(1997)在研究连续的 39 例胰十二指肠切除术和淋巴结根治术病人,和 1447 个淋巴结切除标本中检查肿瘤的转移。发现 39 例中有 31 例病人 97 个淋巴结有转移,其分布为:胰十二指肠后组 20/21,胰十二指肠下动脉组 12/21,胰十二指肠前组 3/21,肠系膜上动脉干 3/20,肝外胆管周围组 3/21,肝门后组 2/21,主动脉旁组 3/5。在肝动脉、胆囊管、胃周围、右侧腹腔干、中结肠动脉或右腔静脉组淋巴结都未发现转移。该作者指出,胆胰共同管癌的淋巴道转移,主要是转移到胰十二指肠后组,然后到胰十二指肠下动脉组,最终抵达主动脉旁组(图 19-2-8)。

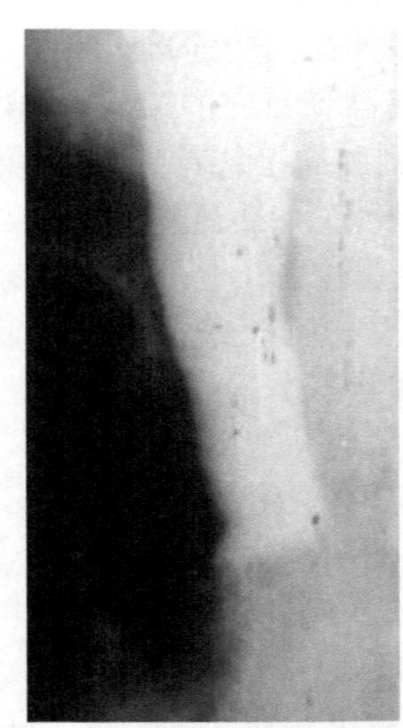

图 19-2-8 ERCP:连接区癌导致明显扩张的肝外胆管下端呈不规则杵状

Low(1997)通过对 514 例逆行胆管造影的回顾性分析,发现有 50 例为恶性胆管狭窄,其中以胰癌(21/50)最为常见。肿瘤侵犯处的胆管造影形态学是非特异性的,包含固有的肩征及逐渐变尖等征象。胰管扩张出现于胰癌组的 80%,具有相对特异性。其他的侵犯胆管的恶性病变包括有:胆管癌、转移、胆胰共同管癌以及胆囊癌。与胰癌一样,病变的形态学表现(即肩征与逐渐变尖、狭窄的长度、近端胆管扩张的严重程度等)对病理的特异性诊断均帮助不大。Williams 等(1997)报告 1 例病人的切除标本中,在胆胰共同管区同时存在有腺癌与类癌两种疾病。

5. 鉴别诊断 连接区良性肿瘤:连接区良性肿瘤常伴十二指肠多发性腺瘤,且体积较小,边缘常光滑,有蒂,多有轻度或无明显的胆胰管梗阻。有的病例,在临床和 X 线表现上酷似胆胰管十二指肠连接区癌而无法进行鉴别。此时则须借助于活检。

胰头癌:胰头癌与胆胰管十二指肠连接区癌的临床表现常常相似,而影像表现则较容易鉴别:在直接法胆系造影,前者表现为总胆管梗阻平面较高,并且常向右上方移位甚至出现成角畸形;后者梗阻平面较低,总胆管无移位表现。超声检查和 CT 扫描常可显示两者肿瘤的大小和部位的差异。

胆系结石:胆系结石在连接区共同管内嵌顿,这在内镜下可以鉴别。低张十二指肠造影多显示乳头增大，但边缘光整，乳头及其周围的正常结构无破坏和消失。此外，病史和临床症状有助于鉴别。

胆胰管十二指肠连接区癌，由于解剖位置特殊，较易早期发现。一般病程较短，病灶较小，转移较晚，手术切除率高，预后较好，5年生存率为32%~62%，10年生存率可达42%（Hayes等，1987）。如能早期诊治，胆胰管十二指肠连接区癌的预后将会更令人满意。

第六节　共同管癌

发生于胆管下端、胰头、共同管或十二指肠乳头部的癌肿，有作者将之统称为共同管周围癌。上述不同起源的肿瘤，虽临床表现及外科手术方法相似，但切除率及预后不同，如共同管癌切除率可达40.0%，术后5年生存率43.2%，而胰头癌手术切除率约9.8%~26.7%，术后5年生存率仅只3.4%。因此，需于手术前加以区别，早期诊断及治疗，对预后极为重要。

1. 影像学研究　胰头癌：胰头不规则肿大，变形，增强扫描见强化的胰头中的小叶结构消失，并可见低密度灶，为癌肿间质纤维化或坏死所致，如发现胰头前方呈毛刺状，则为癌肿侵入胰周脂肪的表现。老年人胰腺萎缩，小叶间隔宽，脂肪及纤维组织充填呈羽毛状，易发现较小的等密度肿瘤。

共同管癌：除梗阻性胆管、胆囊扩张外，可在胆管下端发现肿块，在十二指肠乳头部见到对比剂充盈缺损。如肿瘤侵犯胰头，则胰头肿大或见低密度病灶。

共同管周围癌共有的间接CT表现：肝内外胆管扩张，常为中度以上，扩张的肝外胆管突然中断于胰头以下，胆囊也扩大。双管征系胰头部胰管和胆管均有扩张，说明胆管下端病变引起低位梗阻性胆胰管扩张。

共同管癌，胆管下端癌，如已侵犯胰头，则表现类似于胰头癌。胰头癌如侵犯十二指肠及胆管下端，则呈围管浸润。有些病例术前难以确定肿瘤来源而统称为共同管周围癌。

结合超声、CT、MRI及MRCP检查，必要时需进行ERCP综合诊断，对术前早期诊断共同管癌很有必要。综合诊断共同管周围癌检出率可达93%。CT可为首选检查方法。

快速动态增强加薄层CT扫描：采用此技术可以发现胰头低密度缺血的癌肿，可与增强的胰头组织形成对照；同时可使胰血管显影，明确癌肿有无侵及周围组织，尤其是肠系膜上动脉与静脉，腹腔动脉及门静脉。上述血管被侵以及肝与腹膜后淋巴结转移等为不可切除的表现。而个别直径小于1cm的淋巴结转移，普通CT可能漏诊而仍可切除。直径小于1cm的多发性肝转移为不可切除，但普通CT扫描可以漏诊。

2. 鉴别诊断　胆管下端结石：在绝大多数情况下，用CT薄层扫描，可发现钙化密度的结石，患者常有反复发作的绞痛及黄疸病史。在个别情况，CT对胆管下端胆固醇成分的低密度结石难以确定。

限于胰头的慢性胰腺炎：较少见。病人有反复发作黄疸及慢性胰腺炎病史，往往有胆系结石、胆系蛔虫、十二指肠憩室等疾患为诱因。CT图像上可仅表现为胰头肿大，体尾部无异常。增强扫描见胰头密度较为均匀，如能发现肿大的胰腺与周围粘连，扩张的肝外胆管逐渐变细且光滑等典型变化，结合ERCP和超声所见，以及反复发作的病史，可免误诊。

胰腺继发性肿瘤：胰腺周围淋巴结转移或淋巴瘤也可引起胰头增大，甚至胆管下端梗阻，需结合临床及CT其他表现来作出鉴别诊断。

胰头癌与胆管下端癌或共同管癌的普通CT鉴别诊断：胰头癌表现为胰头变形、增大，增强扫描后胰头结构消失，有不规则形低密度病灶。共同管癌表现为胆管末端软组织肿块，突向十二指肠乳头内侧，在胰头钩突的外侧；增强扫描时该肿块有强化，密度低于正常胰腺，有界限，而增强的胰腺小叶结构正常。胆管下端癌表现为胆管下端突然不规则狭窄，管壁增厚或管腔内、外有结节；有强化，但比正常胰腺为低。肿瘤直径小于0.5cm的胆管下端癌，往往仅见低位梗阻性胆管扩张，而难以发现肿块。

第七节 胆管下端小的高分化胆管型腺癌

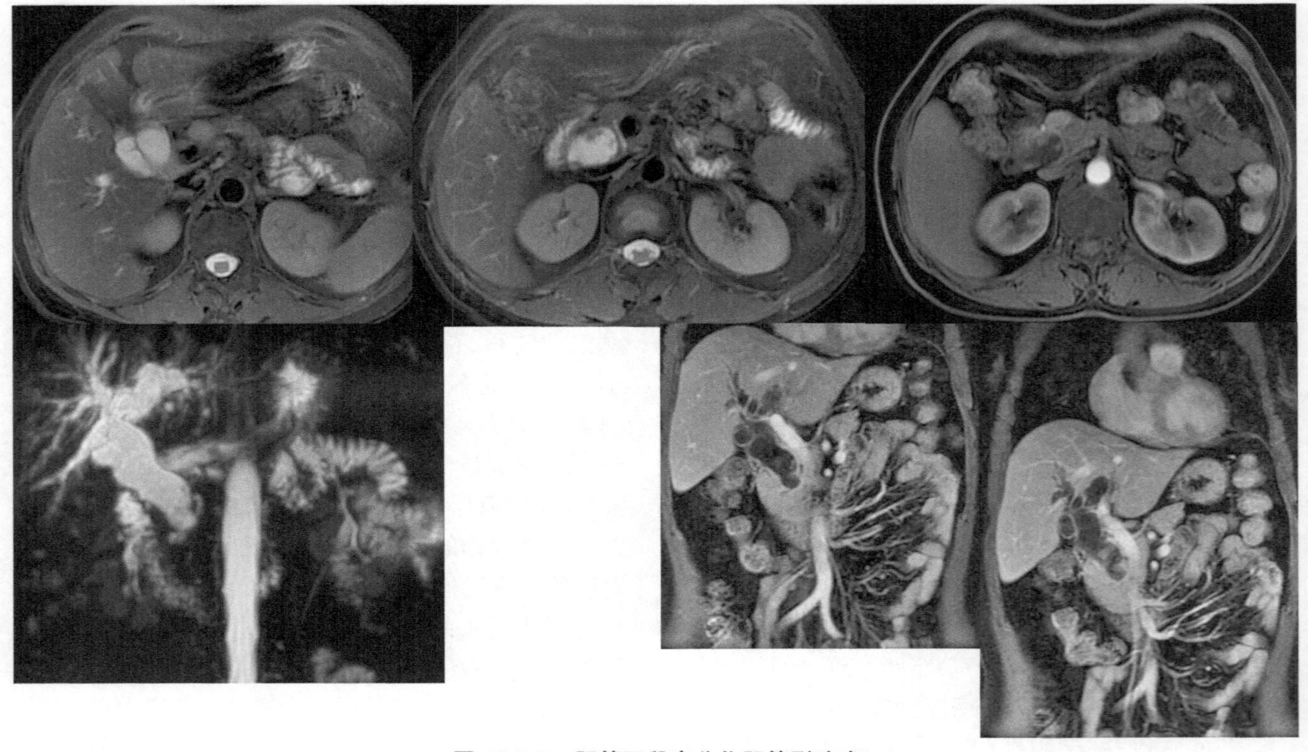

图 19-2-9 胆管下段高分化胆管型腺癌

患者,女, 52 岁。反复上腹部闷痛不适 2 个月入院。外院 CT 提示胆总管扩张。门诊拟胆总管结石收治住院。CT:胆囊管低位异位汇合于肝外胆管,胆囊管残端过长;周围淋巴结未受侵犯。肝内外胆管及胆总管明显扩张,胆总管下段阻断,原因不明,建议 MRI 检查。MRI:胆总管下段实性占位,考虑:腺瘤(恶变可能);胆总管癌,伴胆总管及肝内胆管向心性扩张,请结合临床。

手术所见:胆囊缺如,胆总管内径约 3cm,术中胆道镜探查示胆总管下段及十二指肠乳头可见两个内生性肿物,大小分别为 1.2cm × 1.0cm 和 1.0cm × 1.0cm,质中,胰腺质地正常。

病理检查:胆总管下段肿物:管壁样组织一块,大小 2.3cm × 1.5cm × 0.7cm,表面附一乳头状广基肿物,肿物大小 1.5cm × 1.3cm × 0.5cm。切面灰白灰黄,质软,界限尚清。病理诊断:胆总管下段肿物:乳头状肿瘤,局部细胞层次增多,轻度异型,但未见明确浸润,肌层尚完好。目前倾向交界性,与高分化腺癌或腺瘤癌变难以鉴别,待充分取材及石蜡切片进一步诊断。

病理检查:胆管下段肿物切除标本:灰褐色组织一块,大小 1.7cm × 0.7cm × 0.3cm,切面灰白灰褐,质中。胰十二指肠切除标本:胰腺:大小 7cm × 4.5cm × 2cm,切面灰褐,未触及结节及病灶,十二指肠:长 13cm,直径 1.8cm,肠黏膜未见明显异常。病理诊断:胆管下段肿物切除标本:胆管内高分化胆管型腺癌。胰十二指肠切除标本:均未见肿瘤组织累及。共检出周围淋巴结 20 枚,均未受肿瘤侵犯(图 19-2-9)。

第八节　误诊和漏诊病例简介:胆胰共同管周围高中分化腺癌

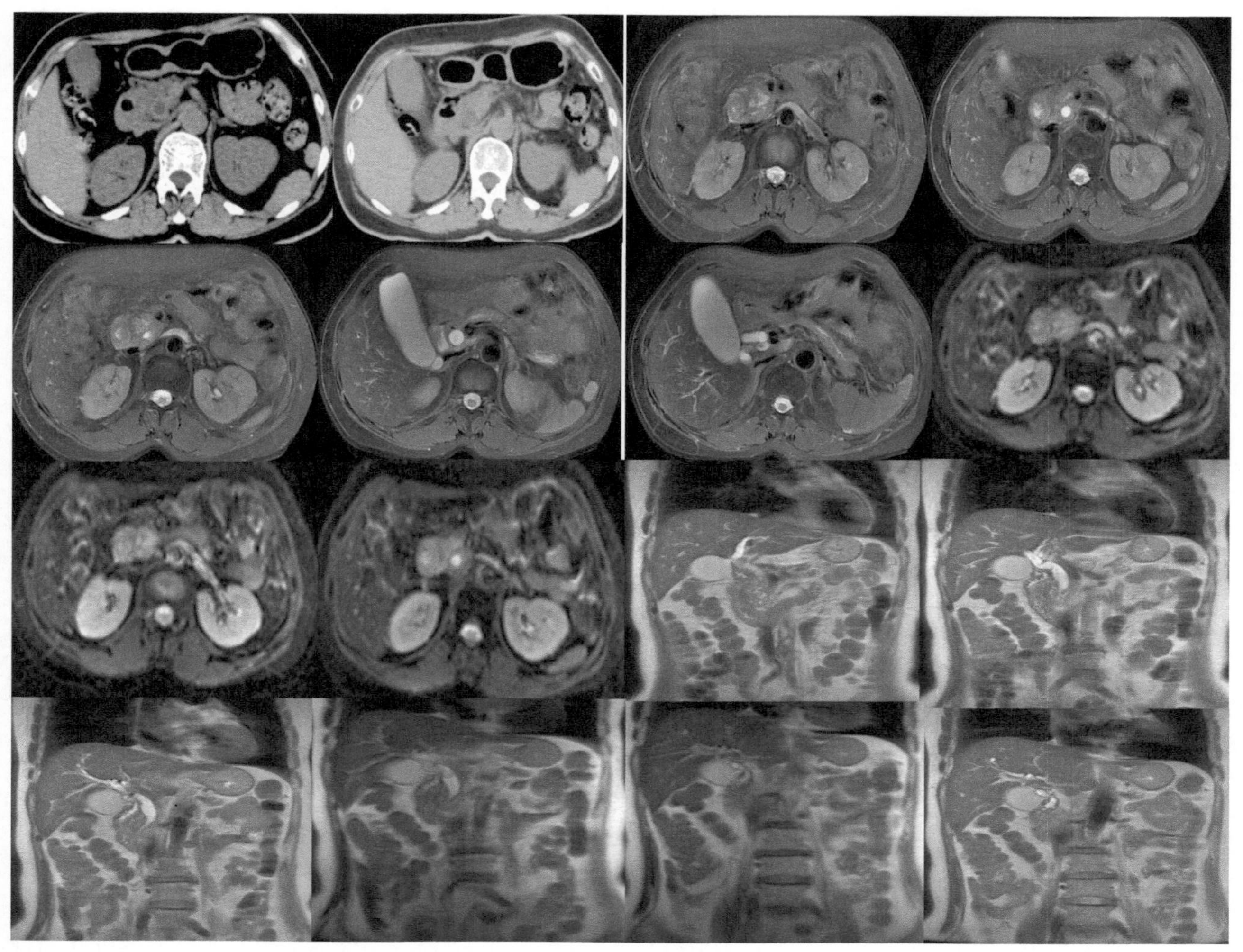

图 19-2-10　胆胰共同管周围高中分化腺癌

患者,女，57 岁。手术后病理检查:胰十二指肠切除标本:胆胰共同管周围肿物 5.0cm× 3.8cm×3.5cm,肿物切面灰白,质中。免疫组化病理诊断:高中分化腺癌,侵犯十二指肠壁全层至肠黏膜下层,局部侵犯胰头组织,侵犯间质神经与血管组织,周围淋巴结 1/7 可见癌转移。

误诊和漏诊病例分析：CT 和 MRI 检查只做平扫,未做增强,导致误诊。平扫观察十分粗糙和欠认真,从图像上可见胆管下端及邻近胰腺与十二指肠壁密度与信号强度都有变化,已呈团块状,但报告的医生却不认识;胆管下段细长,MRI 冠状断面清楚可见,亦视而不见,一点都未考虑有占位存在。这些都是误诊的原因(图 19-2-10)。

第三章 胆胰管十二指肠连接区其他肿瘤

第一节 胆胰共同管的腺瘤及有关问题

胆胰共同管的腺瘤:胆胰共同管的绒毛状腺瘤是不常见的疾病。胆胰共同管是孤立性绒毛状腺瘤最少见的部位之一。一些作者报告6例,平均年龄68岁,4例为女性。3例病人术前内镜诊断中有2例确诊。5例病人经局部切除肿瘤,1例行根治性胰十二指肠切除术。该作者回顾文献上共报告此类肿瘤38例。十二指肠的绒毛状腺瘤十分少见。Molgal等(1987)报告一例75岁老妇十二指肠内有广泛的绒毛状腺瘤,侵犯降段与胆胰共同管。

胆胰共同管区的乳头状小管状腺瘤非常少见,它有潜在的恶性倾向。除非它引起梗阻性黄疸,在手术前诊断总是困难的。偶尔,当病人感到上腹部非特异性不适时,它可被超声检查、CT或ERCP发现。有作者报告一例共同管区的乳头状小管状腺瘤,该病人表现为普遍性搔痒和体重减轻,但无黄疸。

继发于胆胰共同管的活动性腺瘤的间歇性胆系梗阻:目前,胆胰共同管的绒毛状腺瘤的良性性质已成为问题,因为经手术证实,有25%以上的"良性"腺瘤实为恶性病灶。在纤维内镜使用之前,尽管偶尔在低张十二指肠造影或PTC有所怀疑,但术前能够诊断绒毛状腺瘤者极为少见。虽然此类病变通常引起胆系进行性梗阻,但最初的症状可以是间歇性的。

胆胰共同管肿瘤最常见的初期症状是非特异性的上腹不适。但是,随着病变的进行性发展,可以出现梗阻性黄疸和胆绞痛。上部胃肠道出血和十二指肠梗阻是不常见的晚期表现。实验室检查价值有限,最多见是发现胆汁淤滞性黄疸。

一些作者报告一例病人,胆胰共同管内的绒毛状腺瘤脱垂,进出于肝外胆管下端,导致间歇性胆系梗阻。诊断的最初线索是暂时性的体温升高、肝的生化检查异常以及超声发现肝外胆管稍有扩张。最初的ERCP检查观察到胆管内息肉状包块,再做内镜,发现它脱垂于十二指肠中。病人经历黏膜下切除和双重括约肌成形术后,胆胰管梗阻得以解除。

胆胰共同管是孤立性绒毛状腺瘤最少见的部位之一。Rosenberg等(1986)报告6例,平均年龄68岁,4例为女性。3例病人术前内镜诊断中有2例确诊。5例病人经局部切除肿瘤,1例行根治性胰十二指肠切除术。该作者回顾文献上共报告此类肿瘤38例。

胆胰共同管的腺瘤与腺癌:Caruso等(1987)研究胆胰共同管3例腺瘤和5例癌肿的组织学,同时以糖类抗原19-9单克隆抗体确定抗原的诊断意义,发现在腺瘤,某些结构不良的腺体对糖类抗原19-9显示一种弱阳性,而在共同管肿瘤,此抗原存在于腺瘤性的残渣中,以及分化良好的腺癌区域内。此观察指出,内镜检查与大体-镜下观察是评价共同管肿瘤定位的基础。在腺瘤和癌中,糖类抗原19-9的免疫学发现提示它们的组织学关系,但它不用于它们的区别诊断。

非典型性上皮增生与胆胰共同管癌:Kimura等(1988)为了评价非典型性上皮增生与胆胰共同管癌之间的关系,在老年组尸解病例进行组织学、组织化学以及免疫组织化学的观察。

上皮增生的非典型程度在组织学上分为五级,其在576例尸解病例中的发生率分别为:1级为正常上皮增生,占65.8%;2级为轻微非典型与非恶性上皮增生,占30%;3级为中度非典型上皮增生,介于良恶性之间,属边缘性的,占3.1%;4级为严重非典型上皮增生,可能有恶性变化,占0.9%;5级上皮增生为明显的癌肿，占 0.2%。在胆胰共同管处非典型上皮增生的发生率最高。

与癌有关的抗原，即癌胚抗原（CEA）和糖类抗原 19-9（CA19-9）免疫组织化学染色，和黏蛋白高碘酸 -Schiff（PAS）和阿辛兰（AB）的 pH2.5 和 pH1.0 的组织化学染色显露出 1 级上皮增生与 2 级上皮增生的大多数癌胚抗原是阴性，而阿辛兰阳性，pH2.5；3 级上皮增生与 4 级上皮增生癌胚抗原与阿辛兰均为阴性；5 级上皮增生癌胚抗原阳性而阿辛兰阴性（$P<0.01$）。

癌胚抗原结合阿辛兰 pH2.5 染色有助于正常上皮增生到非典型性上皮增生，中度到重度非典型上皮增生，以及癌肿之间的组织学诊断。对于非典型性上皮增生之间的关系的研究显示，某些胆胰共同管癌可发生于非典型上皮增生。

腺瘤与腺癌紧密相关：Yamaguchi 等（1987）将一组 109 例共同管癌与 5 例腺瘤，对每例的肿瘤组织以 5mm 一层切断。按照肿瘤侵犯的范围的镜下所见，胆胰共同管的癌肿分为四级。12 例为 1 级者，其侵犯境界限于括约肌内，显示无淋巴结侵犯，5 年相对生存率为 85%，这样即是共同管的早期癌。除 2 例不便分级的肿瘤外，其余 95 例分别分级为 2、3、4 级，这些，肿瘤均侵犯超过括约肌境界，5 年相对生存率分别为 11%、25%、24%。

在 109 例癌肿中，20 例在肿瘤的边缘有一不容争辨的腺瘤区域，5 例腺瘤，2 例较大的非典型性上皮病灶，提示癌为原位癌。这些征象提示，在胆胰共同管的腺瘤与腺癌之间有着紧密相关。十二指肠乳头腺瘤中的癌极为少见。一些作者报告一例 73 岁老妇，在乳头腺瘤中出现腺癌，内镜诊断为乳头癌合并腺瘤。肿瘤组织学检查见乳头腺瘤中显露有表浅的腺癌。在有的病例，乳头癌可从该区以往存在的腺瘤发展而来。该作者认为，当腺瘤出现于胆胰管十二指肠连接区时，宜进行胰十二指肠切除术。肝外胆管的良性肿瘤十分少见，这些良性肿瘤的局灶性切除后，有较高的再发生率，已为人们熟悉，但个别肿瘤可以恶变则很少引起注意。有作者报告一例良性共同管周围肿瘤局灶性切除后四年复发，发展成为分化良好的乳头状腺癌，然后进行胰十二指肠切除术进行根治。

绒毛状腺瘤：十二指肠的绒毛状腺瘤十分少见。在广泛应用纤维内镜之前，十二指肠和胆胰共同管的息肉状上皮性肿瘤很少能在术前诊断出来。它们的症状是非特异性的。只有高度怀疑它才可能做出早期诊断。如诊断延迟，则可能出现危及生命的并发症，增加恶性变的机会。Celik 等（1986）报告 11 例共同管的绒毛状肿瘤和 2 例发生在十二指肠的新生物。Molgal 等（1987）报告一例 75 岁老妇十二指肠内有广泛的绒毛状腺瘤，侵犯降段与胆胰共同管。

第二节　十二指肠乳头肿瘤样表现的鉴别诊断

从 1985 到 1989 年，Chang（1990）回顾该医院 1 500 例 ERCP 且伴有乳头照片的病例，内镜发现其中有 63 例乳头呈肿瘤样表现。从临床和影像学表现认为所有病例均是共同管周围恶性肿瘤，但无组织学证实。剖腹术发现 14 例为良性病变，31 例为共同管周围恶性肿瘤，2 例病人为乳头的转移性肿瘤，故总数为 47 例。外科病理报告、手术医生的观察以及标本照片都用来确定肿瘤的定位。然而，有 2 例共同管周围恶性肿瘤的起源处难以清楚确定。所有 3 例慢性胰腺炎的诊断都是在剖腹手术时通过活检做出来的（表 19-3-1）。

良性病变者，临床追踪至少 8 个月（范围为 8~45 个月）。病例根据大体观察可分为三组：第 1 组为乳头肿大，但覆盖着正常黏膜；第 2 组为乳头表现外在性生长，伴或不伴溃疡，其区别的特点为外在性病变；第 3 组为乳头表现为溃疡性肿瘤包块，区别特点为肿瘤有溃疡。

良性病变中，8 例病人中的 5 例为“其他”，有胆囊结石 2 例，总胆管结石 2 例，肝内胆管结石 1 例；其他病人早在 18 个月之前因为胆囊结石和肝外胆管结石，经历了胆囊切除术和总胆管取石术。所有 6 例有胆囊结石和胆管结石的病人都分在第 1 组。

该作者指出，该项研究支持十二指肠大乳头非肿瘤性肿大，与胆囊结石或胆管结石存在和 / 或通过该处有关的推测。但也可得出初步结论，在良性和恶性病变的区别中，没有独特的内镜表现，但是，可以这样说，一个溃疡性肿瘤包块多半意味着是恶性肿瘤。

表 19-3-1:内镜所见乳头区的肿瘤样表现的不同原因

原因	乳头肿大伴正常黏膜	向外生长的包块	溃疡性包块(病例数)
原发性恶性肿瘤			
胆胰共同管	2	12	5
胰腺	1	6	1
肝外胆管下端		2	
共同管周围区	2		
转移性恶性肿瘤			
齿龈癌			1
淋巴瘤		1	
良性病变			
慢性胰腺炎	1	2	
共同管腺瘤	1	2	
其他	7	1	
总数	14	26	7

一些作者发现,单纯引起乳头及其近侧纵行皱襞肿大者,多为一些良性疾病,如:胆系结石、胆囊炎、胰腺炎等引起的乳头炎;胆管结石嵌顿在胆胰共同管;胆囊切除术后综合征等。而乳头及其近侧纵行皱襞肿大,同时伴有形态异常者,多为该区恶性肿瘤。

第三节 括约肌区域病变分类

Martin 等(1987)报告 109 例连续尸检,且特别注意括约肌区域的大体和镜下观察。有 24 例患胆系疾病,7 例胰腺疾病。按照以往的组织学描述,选择一组 18 例呈病理性改变的括约肌。在此组中,胆系疾病不是更为常见(28%)比之于正常括约肌组(21%),反之,在胆系疾病组中没有更多的括约肌病变(21%)比之于无胆系疾病组(15%)。慢性胰腺炎更常见伴存于异常的括约肌,但是在这些病例中,另外伴存的病变(酒精中毒、青铜色糖尿病)也能解释胰腺炎的发生。胆胰括约肌的病理性改变是常见的,通常是不易被察觉的。这些表现不是单纯的发育变异,因为有 5 例无疑是病理性的,而且伴存括约肌段明显增厚,和纤维性腺瘤病理表现。此项研究显示硬化性胆胰括约肌炎是存在的,但是相当少见。

第四节 胆胰共同管肿瘤分类

Ponchon 等(1989)报告 52 例胆胰共同管肿瘤,经内镜检查,特别是内镜括约肌切开术和网篮活检后,组织学分类为:腺癌为 26/52 占 50%,腺瘤为 18/52 占 35%,腺瘤与癌为 8 例占 15%。在 37%(19/52)病例中,内镜观察乳头正常,只有在括约肌切开术后才发现肿瘤。用网篮取除、激光治疗,或括约肌切开术后再用上述两手段去除腺瘤做了 11 例。继后活检显示腺瘤组织残存或复发只有 1 例,其他 10 例追踪 39 个月一直良好,示腺瘤已完全去除。浸润性肿瘤能迅速导致十二指肠梗阻。

第五节　胆胰共同管错构瘤

胆胰共同管肿瘤是少见病，但它们中，许多都是恶性病变，良性病变有：腺瘤、腺肌瘤、平滑肌瘤、类癌、神经纤维瘤、粒状细胞胚瘤、错构瘤等。虽然经过广泛手术切除后，恶性肿瘤的预后相当良好，但在良性病变则大可不必进行那样的手术。因此，对此类病人的适当处理，正确的组织学诊断是必要的。MRCP、ERCP 的广泛开展为胆胰共同管区病变的诊断提供了有力的手段。然而，在内镜所见、影像学表现的基础上，有的病例甚至在内镜活检后，在良性与恶性病变的鉴别诊断上仍然有不少的困难。

胆胰共同管错构瘤极为少见，其临床表现和内镜所见可以相当复杂。共同管肿瘤的临床表现变化较大。有的病人可以一直无明显症状，而另外的病人可出现隐蔽性上消化道出血，或更典型的上腹痛与黄疸。胆囊常常肿大。事实上，胆囊疾病与胆胰共同管肿瘤常常可能同存。在这情况下，注意力多集中在胆囊，而导致胆胰共同管肿瘤的漏诊。在一组 12 例胆胰共同管肿瘤病人中有 9 例，在肿瘤确诊以前都曾做过胆囊切除术。

有时，腹痛与变动不定的黄疸可能被解释为胆囊疾病的表现，而导致胆囊切除。而在另一方面，出现胆管扩张，但无胆囊结石，则应当警觉地排除胆胰共同管肿瘤的可能性。

在诊断胆胰共同管肿瘤时，ERCP 检查常规应有相互相关的三步：①乳头的检查；②组织活检；③胆胰管的造影。内镜检查时，乳头常常肿大、不规则，而且分叶。虽然一个向外生长的溃疡性包块伴自发性出血多提示为恶性，其他的内镜表现常为非特异性，可能观察到一些非新生物性的表现，诸如一个总胆管囊肿、嵌顿性共同管结石或乳头炎。乳头可能肿大呈结节状，并存溃疡，这在一般良性肿瘤是较为少见的表现。这样，内镜所见无恶性疾病的特征性表现，组织学的检查是正确诊断所必需的。

然而，使用常规的活检钳所得到组织学标本可能诊断价值较低。使用电烙器网篮进较大颗粒的活检已证明诊断的正确性较高，自然，此法可能加杂明显的出血，但是正确诊断的获得比这更为重要。胆胰共同管肿瘤最常见的放射学表现是胆管扩张或/和胰管扩张。肝外胆管末端的不规则的充盈缺损伴胆管引流延迟，在许多病人都能见到。肝外胆管末端常常较粗大，而不是逐渐变尖。因此，造影时获得良好的胆胰管末端的点片甚为重要。

第四章　十二指肠乳头及乳头区憩室

第一节　MRCP 诊断乳头区憩室综合征

十二指肠乳头区憩室,是起自十二指肠大乳头周围 2~3 cm 的一种外向性囊袋状突起,多见于老年人,是消化系统常见病,大部分无临床症状。由于其解剖位置与胆胰管关系密切,有时也可引起胆胰系统症状,临床上称之为乳头区憩室综合征(Lemmel's syndrome)。

对有胆胰系症状的十二指肠乳头区憩室患者来说,影像学检查的关键不仅仅是要发现有无十二指肠乳头区憩室或胆胰系病变,而且要更进一步判断十二指肠乳头区憩室与胆胰系病变两者间可能的关系,即是否为乳头区憩室综合征,以利于临床医生选择治疗方案。

1. 十二指肠乳头区憩室发生机制　十二指肠憩室绝大部分位于胆胰共同管周围,可能与该部位是胚胎前肠和中肠的愈合部,有胆胰管、血管通过,为一薄弱区有关。文献报道十二指肠乳头区憩室发现率为 2%~22%,多发生在老年人,且随着年龄的增加而增加。

某院在两年半期间内共进行 MRCP 检查 661 例,发现十二指肠乳头区憩室 49 例(占 7.4%),根据十二指肠乳头区憩室与乳头的位置关系把十二指肠乳头区憩室分为 3 型,即憩室开口于十二指肠乳头区肠壁的乳头区型(周围型)、乳头开口于憩室内的憩室内型(憩室内乳头)及乳头开口于憩室颈的边缘型,周围型又可分为乳头上型和乳头下型。这几型中,憩室内乳头型、边缘型及乳头上型易引起胆胰系症状。

2. 十二指肠乳头区憩室与胆胰疾病的关系　十二指肠乳头区憩室与胆胰系病变的关系密切,一般认为十二指肠乳头区憩室与胆石症发生有关,所致的胆石症主要为胆总管结石而非胆囊结石,同时也发现十二指肠乳头区憩室与胆囊切除术后胆总管复发结石有关。十二指肠乳头区憩室与胰腺炎关系密切是由于胆石症的存在,即十二指肠乳头区憩室首先易发生胆总管结石,继之发生胆源性胰腺炎。

十二指肠乳头区憩室易合并胆胰系病变即乳头区憩室综合征的原因目前认为与括约肌功能异常及十二指肠乳头区憩室对胆总管末端的机械性压迫有关。憩室炎症等的长期刺激使括约肌功能受到明显影响,胆管内压也相应改变,继而引起肠液逆流,导致细菌逆行生长繁殖,从而发生胆胰疾病。一些作者研究憩室的形态,发现与胆胰共同管关系密切者能持续地压迫胆胰共同管,导致胆胰管内压力增高,出现胆管梗阻征象。憩室与胆总管关系愈密切,体积越大,则梗阻越明显。该组资料中引起胆总管末端受压的十二指肠乳头区憩室都较大,直径都大于 1.5 cm,且多属于边缘型和乳头上型。

另外,憩室内乳头是一种较特殊的类型,虽没有直接压迫胆总管,但由于憩室内食物残渣的堆积可导致胆汁引流不畅,或细菌增殖引起憩室炎、乳头炎,也会导致胆汁排空不畅。

3. 比较影像学　X 线钡餐造影虽能看见十二指肠乳头区憩室,但不能显示胆胰管的情况。

内窥镜逆行性胰胆管造影在十二指肠乳头区憩室的诊断中起着较重要的作用,它能在内镜下直视乳头区憩室的开口和显示胆胰管的病变,但大多情况下不能显示憩室本身,无法显示十二指肠乳头区憩室与胆胰管远端的解剖关系。

影像上要证实十二指肠乳头区憩室与胆胰疾病的关系,其直接证据是显示胆总管受压梗阻,间接证据是发现胆管扩张、胆管排空差、并除外其他病变。乳头区憩室综合征的诊断不仅仅是要揭示有无十二指肠乳头区憩室及胆胰系病变，更重要的是揭示胆胰管与十二指肠乳头区憩室的解剖关系。MRCP 不需造影剂即可清楚显示胆胰管系统的解剖形态。目前对肝外胆管及主胰管的显示率达 100%，对非扩张的肝内胆管外 1/3 的显示率也超过 90%。胆总管远端与胰管汇合后形成胆胰共同管，此区较短，且周围有胆胰括约肌收缩，管内含液很少，甚至无液体，常规 MRCP 显示该部位往往受限。

Koike 等（2000）和 Cappeliez 等（2000）用脂餐和胰泌素刺激后，进行药物动力学的 MRCP 检查，可清楚显示该部，如动态扫描，还可在一定程度上观察乳头的功能状态。

正常情况下或胰泌素刺激下十二指肠腔内含有一定量的液体，因此 MRCP 除可清楚显示胆胰管系统外，还可显示十二指肠结构，从而帮助分辨共同管，还可判断胆系外病变对胆胰管系统的影响。利用同层动态 MRCP 可很好评价胆胰括约肌功能，提高对共同管及其周围病变的捡出率，是常规 MRCP 形态学研究的重要补充，具有很好的临床应用前景。

MRCP 可以同时显示胆系及胰管，对胆胰管的显示也基本达到了 ERCP 的效果。对胆系病变尤其是对胆系结石的诊断价值已有较多的论述，目前已逐步替代诊断性 ERCP，成为观察胆管形态的最好的可替代性方法。

对胰腺分裂、环胰等先天变异及急慢性胰腺炎、胰腺癌、胰腺黏液性肿瘤等胰腺良、恶性病变也有较高的诊断价值，可替代或部分替代 ERCP、CT 的作用。

MRCP 的另一个潜在的用途是胆囊切除术前显示胆管是否有发育变异以减少术中胆管损伤的危险性。由于十二指肠内液体的存在或于检查前饮水，使 MR 对胆胰管成像的同时，亦使十二指肠显示，达到了类似十二指肠造影的目的。该组资料中有 49 例病人做了 MRCP 检查，除了清晰显示胆胰管系统有无病变外，有 46 例还明确显示了十二指肠乳头区憩室的形态及其与胆总管末端之间的解剖关系，初步显示了 MRCP 对乳头区憩室综合征的诊断价值。Kurihara 等（2000）曾报道 1 例十二指肠乳头区憩室致阻塞性黄疸病例，进食后症状加重，MRCP 检查清晰地显示了憩室对胆总管末端的外在性压迫。

与 ERCP 相比，MRCP 的明显优势是非侵害性，完全摒弃了 ERCP 的危险性，此外还能观察到梗阻近端的胆胰管情况，也不受限于术后解剖结构改变的病人。整个操作简便，成像时间短，成功率高且不依赖于操作者水平。如结合 MR 常规扫描还可判断肝、胆、胰腺、腹膜后隙有无病变及腹腔血管状况，在临床上有着广阔的应用价值。

第二节　乳头区憩室和憩室内乳头

十二指肠憩室是消化道中常见的病变，一般对其临床意义估计不足。在上消化道造影时，其发现率为 2%~5%，仅次于结肠，十二指肠是胃肠道憩室的第二个好发部位。它们是先天抑或后天性的，一直存在争议。憩室最常出现于十二指肠降部的内侧面，属于胆胰管十二指肠连接区，且多系偶然发现。十二指肠憩室大多（约 75%）位于十二指肠降段内侧壁，即胆胰管十二指肠连接区的乳头及其附近，称乳头区憩室。

1. 命名　乳头区憩室以往名称甚多，如：乳头旁憩室、壶腹旁憩室、乳头周围憩室、Vater 乳头区憩室、十二指肠降段内侧憩室、憩室内乳头、胆胰管异位插入乳头以及迷走乳头等。我们认为，这些都反映了对同一事物观察的不同着眼点，为避免名称上的混乱，建议用乳头区憩室这一名称囊括憩室内乳头和乳头周围憩室。乳头区憩室，乃指以乳头为中心，半径 30mm 的圆周内的各种类型的所有憩室。由于其解剖位置与胆胰管关系密切，有时也可引起胆胰系统症状，临床上称之为乳头旁憩室综合征（Lemmel' s syndrome）。

2. 分类和分型　十二指肠憩室的分类是基于憩室起源的推测，根据病变形成可分为先天性和后天性，真性先天性憩室极少，且含有肠壁的各层；获得性憩室又分为原发性和继发性两类。乳头区憩室根据病理腔内有无肌层可分为真性憩室和假性憩室，还可根据憩室突出方向分腔内憩室和腔外憩室，腔内憩室非常罕见，可能出现在正常胎儿发育过程中的重建，多数十二指肠憩室为腔外憩室。有作者将十二指肠乳头区憩室乳头上型、乳头内型憩室归为 A 型，其他乳头旁憩室归为 B 型，发现 A 型十二指肠乳头旁憩室是胆总管结石复发的独立危险因素。

3. 病理学　原发性憩室,是黏膜、黏膜肌或黏膜下组织通过肠壁局限薄弱处凸出。胚胎学研究发现,十二指肠乳头区是前肠和中肠的汇合部,为先天性肠壁薄弱区;同时,此处也是胆胰管共同汇合进入肠道处,缺乏结缔组织支持,为一菱形薄弱区,正如小肠憩室与结肠憩室好发于血管进出处的情况一样;胆胰管下端括约肌收缩牵拉十二指肠壁,对乳头区憩室的发生起了一定的作用;再加上肠腔内压力的增高使该薄弱区的肠壁向外疝出,久之,则形成憩室。这是乳头区最常见的憩室。也有作者报道十二指肠乳头区憩室患者十二指肠较长,其末端高于十二指肠球底部,易导致十二指肠排空延缓,内压增加,所以导致憩室形成。上述解释可以说明为什么乳头区憩室的发现率随着年龄的增高而增加,多见于 50~60 岁年龄段。

有作者认为,由于乳头区肠壁薄弱,加上后天的胆胰管下端括约肌收缩牵拉肠壁,肠腔内压升高,使该薄弱区的肠壁向外疝出,久而久之则形成憩室,故又称它为继发性乳头区憩室,我们认为,从根本上讲,它也应归属于原发性憩室。继发性十二指肠憩室,不变地见于十二指肠第一段,常由消化性溃疡或胆系结石对肠壁的牵拉所致。还有一种比较少见的获得性憩室,发生于人体与体外压力急剧变化时,多发生于潜水员。

4. 临床表现　多数十二指肠憩室是无症状的,仅 5% 的患者因憩室压迫周围组织、出血、感染、穿孔等表现出相应的临床症状。一些作者统计,乳头区憩室伴存胆系胰腺疾病者甚多,为 77/111 例(69%),大部分病例症状较轻。其中十二指肠穿孔被认为是十二指肠乳头区憩室最少见但最为严重的并发症,死亡率高达 20%。

性别和年龄:有作者报告女性多于男性,而在国内多份资料中均称男性多于女性,这有待进一步研究。大多数作者指出,大部分乳头区憩室见于中老年人,年龄为 30~78 岁。我们(1995)报告一组 45 例十二指肠乳头区憩室在 40~65 岁多见,尤以 50~65 岁更多,说明随着年龄增大,憩室的发生率就越高,这一点也符合憩室的发生机制。

5. 影像学研究　憩室的发现:十二指肠憩室是消化道常见疾病之一,其发生率变化不一。乳头区憩室,因无特殊临床症状而常被合并症所掩盖,故临床表现呈多样化,常于某种检查时偶然发现。根据不同的检查方法,憩室的发生率差异甚大。一些作者在 100 万份病例中发现乳头区憩室发生率为 0.11%。归纳文献,见常规单对比钡餐检查对十二指肠乳头区憩室的发现率为 1%~6%,一般为 2% 左右;低张法双对比钡餐检查发现率为 13%~21%,一般为 16% 左右;尸检发现率为 2.2%~22%,一般为 8% 左右;内镜发现率最高,为 5%~23%,一般为 10% 左右;ERCP 发现率低于内镜,其原因是对比剂进入憩室的机会远不如内镜观察。但检出率都大大高于一般 X 线检查。低张十二指肠造影与 ERCP 同时进行,不仅可提高憩室的检出率,而且更有利于研究憩室与胰胆系病变的关系。十二指肠乳头区憩室表现为十二指肠降段内侧与胰头之间的囊袋状影,多数可见气 - 液平,部分病灶内可见内容物残留,导致密度不均匀呈网织样改变,部分憩室可疝入胰头内,其密度与潴留物有关,可为气囊、液囊或液 - 气囊。

对于十二指肠乳头旁憩室的诊断多依赖于消化道造影及十二指肠镜检查,但 Schnueriger 等(2008)报道因憩室炎憩室颈部黏膜水肿,憩室颈部狭窄,致十二指肠镜检容易漏诊。另外,十二指肠憩室颈部狭窄及憩室腔内充满食物残渣时也可致消化道造影出现假阴性结果。

一些作者认为,CT、MRI 对十二指肠憩室检出敏感性低,MSCT 检出率仅为 18.75%,不能检出直径 <1.0 cm 的病灶,十二指肠憩室的检查仍有赖于无创的钡餐造影。而另有作者认为,CT 对十二指肠憩室的检出被低估是对此病的 CT 表现认识不足。

MSCT 可以通过重建了解憩室与十二指肠乳头、胆总管的确切关系,区分憩室类型,还可以通过仿真内窥镜了解憩室腔内情况,可以为临床提供更多有益的信息。

最重要的是,MSCT 在检出憩室的同时可以对肝胆胰脾疾病做出及时的诊断,提示憩室与胆胰系统疾病的相关性,以便更好地帮助临床了解胆胰系统疾病的发生原因,提供致病线索,拓宽临床医生对该病的认识,从而做出正确的诊断与治疗。

一组 22 个十二指肠乳头区憩室均位于十二指肠系膜缘,表现为胰头右后方囊袋状向外突起,其内多为气体密度影,也可出现液 - 气平面及筛板状结构。原始轴位像结合 MSCT 后重建技术可显著提高对十二指肠乳头区憩室的诊断率,明确病变与十二指肠壁及十二指肠乳头的关系。憩室内可见筛板状结构，经多平面重建后均可见狭窄的憩室颈部与十二指肠腔相连。此筛板样结构可能为十二指肠内压增高使肠内容物进入憩室腔，炎症刺激导致憩室颈部狭窄，食物残渣滞留憩室内所致。

十二指肠乳头区憩室内有液 - 气平面，且常伴存明显上腹部症状及肝内、外胆管扩张，憩室内的液 - 气平面可提示憩室炎的发生。但所有患者中仅有部分病例可观察到憩室壁的强化，这可能与十二指肠乳头区憩室的位置有关，周围强化的胰头组织，使部分轻度强化的憩室壁缺乏组织对比。十二指肠乳头旁憩室伴出血患者可见高密度对比剂进入憩室腔。

一些学者认为十二指肠乳头上型及乳头内型憩室与胆管结石形成关系更为密切，利用 MSCT 后处理技术多平面重建可从不同斜面观察憩室、胆总管两者之间的关系，明确憩室与胆总管的位置，可判断憩室是乳头上型及乳头内型憩室、乳头旁型憩室，为临床治疗提供参考。利用 MSCT 的多平面重建在观察十二指肠乳头区憩室全貌、十二指肠乳头区憩室与胆胰管解剖关系有着其他检查方法不可相比的优势，且又能作为鉴别梗阻性黄疸的病因、急慢性胰腺炎诊断的检查手段，既能显示憩室，又能发现胆胰疾病。通过多平面重建发现乳头上型及乳头内型憩室往往可直接压迫胆管及胰管，容易致胆胰疾病的发生。

该组研究提示，十二指肠乳头区憩室与胆胰疾病的形成关系十分密切，也是胆管结石形成的因素之一，憩室直径大小是一个潜在的重要因素。十二指肠乳头旁憩室具有较为典型的 CT 特征，MSCT 能较全面地对十二指肠乳头旁憩室进行评价。

MRCP 检查发现并诊断十二指肠憩室有较多的报道，十二指肠憩室内含液体、气体，MRCP 显示肠外囊袋状影，内含气液平面等特征性表现，显示有较高的诊断准确性。

有作者报告一组 49 例病人 MRCP 检查，除了清晰显示胆胰管系统有无病变外，有 46 例还明确显示了乳头旁憩室的形态及其与胆总管末端之间的解剖关系，初步显示了 MRCP 对乳头旁憩室综合征的诊断价值。Kurihara 等(2000)曾报道 1 例乳头旁憩室致阻塞性黄疸病例，进食后症状加重，MRCP 检查清晰地显示了憩室对胆总管末端的外在性压迫。

Tsitouridis 等(2003)研究的一组病例 MRCP 发现十二指肠憩室的敏感性仅为 34.8%(23/66)，认为发现率取决于憩室的大小及其含水量。但完全含液的十二指肠憩室还可能被误诊为胰头的囊性肿瘤。

6. 十二指肠腔内憩室　十二指肠憩室绝大多数为腔外憩室，腔内憩室非常罕见，文献报道不足 100 例。一般认为，十二指肠腔内憩室的发生与肠壁先天性发育异常有关，肠管局部残留的隔或蹼突向腔内形成腔内憩室，并在肠蠕动的作用下逐渐增大，形成风向袋状结构。

与腔外憩室不同，十二指肠腔内憩室的两面均被覆黏膜层，黏膜层下只有薄的纤维肌层，血供很差，易发生缺血坏死或穿孔。除少数患者憩室与肠壁的全周附着外，大多数情况下其附着点小于肠壁周径的一半，当憩室附着于肠壁全周时，食物只能通过位于憩室中央或周边的小孔进入十二指肠远段。十二指肠腔内憩室可合并其他先天性畸形，如唐氏综合征、肠旋转不良或各种疝、肛门闭锁、胆管畸形、环状胰腺和先天性心脏病等。诊断十二指肠腔内憩室的主要方法为上消化道造影。典型表现为十二指肠腔内充满钡剂的囊袋状结构及其周围的边界光整的线样透亮线，称为风向袋征，线样透亮线代表憩室壁。并发十二指肠梗阻时，梗阻近段十二指肠及胃腔明显扩张。

CT 横断面典型表现为双腔征；十二指肠局部层面见双重管腔，内含液体及肠内容物，有时还能见到内层管壁不连续、局限性断裂，代表憩室的裂孔，同时通过各断面的重建 CT 图像，可以清楚地看到风向袋征。憩室局部增厚时表现为十二指肠腔内肿块。虽然风向袋征是十二指肠腔内憩室的特异性表现，但有时需与十二指肠息肉、十二指肠肿瘤、胆总管囊肿、肠套叠等鉴别，这时内窥镜检查对鉴别诊断有帮助，在十二指肠内壁上可见盲袋状结构。

CT 表现为双腔征时，主要应与肠套叠鉴别。前者 2 层管壁间间隙较宽，间隙内只能观察到液体密度影即肠液，而后者 2 层管壁间间隙窄，间隙内能观察到被套入的肠壁外的脂肪密度影。

乳头区憩室的数目与大小：单憩室 95/111 例(85.6%)，双憩室 16/111 例(14.4%)。憩室最大直径 30mm，多数憩室的直径为 5~10mm。双憩室多位于乳头上方或两侧。乳头旁并憩室下唇开口 10/111 例(9%)。憩室内乳头 18/111 例(16.2%)。憩室的直径越大，伴发胆胰疾病的概率越高。

乳头区憩室的形态；乳头区憩室多为圆形或卵圆形，呈向内突出边缘光滑完整的圆弧形阴影。乳头区的占位病变，肝外胆管扩张，嵌顿性结石或乳头炎性肿大均可压迫憩室使之变形，如有炎症粘连，可见憩室轮廓不规则。

关于憩室内容物：憩室内容物的信号特征决定其MRI表现，通常憩室内含有气体、液体和食物，憩室内形成的气液平面是辨认十二指肠憩室的特征性表现，一组病例中仅占51.7%（30/58）。而相当一部分憩室呈完全液性或气性，造成在MRCP上诊断的困难。该组有5例全含气，厚层MRCP图像不能显示憩室，在MRCP和横断位各序列图像上呈低信号，极易漏诊。无气的憩室全含液体成分，在MRCP图像上较易发现，较多的憩室内因含食物呈不均匀信号，该组中23个无气憩室有15个呈不均匀信号，另外8个呈均匀液性信号，需与胰腺囊性占位相鉴别。Macari等（2003）报道的7例CT、MRI初始描述为胰腺囊性肿块，最终证实为十二指肠憩室，充满液体。其中3例回顾性诊断发现憩室，另4例回顾性诊断也不能与囊性肿块鉴别，鉴别诊断包括胰腺囊性肿瘤、胰腺假性囊肿，胰腺囊性占位形态较固定，内部信号均匀。十二指肠憩室出现憩室炎、憩室出血和憩室穿孔等并发症少见，憩室炎和憩室出血无憩室外征象时，MRI诊断困难，憩室炎有时可见憩室周围T2WI高信号渗出，憩室穿孔时出现憩室周围渗出外，在后腹膜或腹腔内见到游离气体。

7. 乳头区憩室与胆系病变的关系　十二指肠憩室临床报道或研究最多的是乳头旁憩室伴发胆管疾病。Lemmel（1934）首先发现了十二指肠憩室与胆胰疾病的关系，并使用“乳头综合征”来描述这种关系，亦称为Lemmel综合征。伴发的疾病包括胆管炎症、肝外胆管结石、胆囊炎胆囊结石和胰腺炎。

从大量的统计学资料来看，乳头区憩室与胰胆系病变的发生有着密切的联系。根据Landor和Fulkerson（1966）等作者统计，乳头区憩室并发胆系结石者占31%~49%，而十二指肠水平段憩室并发胆系结石者仅有13%；憩室并发胆系疾病更为常见，一般为60%以上，甚至可高达80%以上。反之，从胆系结石并发乳头区憩室的发生率来看，也可说明两者的密切关系。Spuy（1979）报告107例胆系结石中，伴有乳头区憩室者占20.6%，而其他病变伴有憩室者仅为2.5%。有胆系手术史的病例，伴有乳头区憩室者也较多。Spuy（1979）报道29例中有5例，占17.2%，贾雨辰等（1984）86例胆系术后综合征中，伴有憩室者占19.8%，60例憩室中有21例（35%）发生胆系术后综合征。这可能与引起胆系病变的外在因素乳头区憩室未解除，从而导致术后症状不能缓解或容易复发有关。

是否胆系或/和胰腺疾病发病率在原发性乳头区憩室必定增高，目前尚未定言，但是，许多研究认为，在某些情况下，憩室可成为胆胰管梗阻的原因：①由于憩室排空不良致其内部压力升高，或因憩室腔较大致食物残渣大量贮留，机械性地压迫胆管胰管，造成胆汁胰液排泄不畅。②胆胰管下端括约肌功能紊乱，闭锁不全，容易发生逆行感染，细菌过量繁殖引起胆系胰腺感染，从而出现反复发作的胆管炎、黄疸、胰腺炎。Lotveit等（1976）报告，乳头区憩室病例的胆汁细菌培养阳性率很高，细菌属于肠道菌群。当胆汁淤滞或有细菌感染时，游离胆红素与钙结合，可形成胆红素钙结石。③憩室内滞留物的化学刺激和细菌可引起憩室炎及其周围炎，进而发生乳头炎。早期为括约肌痉挛，黏膜水肿充血，后期则形成缩窄性乳头炎。这些都说明乳头区憩室对胆胰疾病的发生存在较大的病理学影响。

有鉴于此，有作者指出，乳头区憩室常常伴存胆系炎症和结石，建议采用“十二指肠乳头区憩室胆系病变综合征”这一更为符合临床实际的名称。

乳头区憩室与胆系结石：不少作者指出，在十二指肠憩室和胆系结石之间有着因果关系，在胆囊切除术后，憩室持续存在，可使胆系结石容易复发，为证实这种理论，Lotveit等（1982）研究101例已行胆囊切除术后二年以上无症状者，现出现症状疑胆胰系疾病再行检查和手术。由于年轻人憩室较少，该组选择病人均在60岁以上。乳头区有憩室组32例，无憩室组69例；101例中有复发结石者50例，憩室组为28/32（87.5%），无憩室组为22/69（31.9%），两组之间差别显著（$P<0.01$），此结果支持乳头区憩室容易患胆系结石的假说。Kennedy等（1988）指出乳头区憩室与胆系结石关系也十分密切。

乳头区憩室与肝外胆管扩张：乳头区憩室并发胆系疾病的病例常显示肝外胆管扩张。据统计，ERCP发现此类病例肝外胆管宽度大于15mm者占58%~71%。中野哲（1974）认为肝外胆管扩张与憩室大小有关，直径在2cm以上的憩室有75%可见到肝外胆管扩张。

乳头区憩室与乳头炎：有作者认为，缩窄性乳头炎90%继发于胆系结石等胆系疾病，而原发性乳头炎可能与乳头区憩室有关。

乳头区憩室与胰腺炎：对乳头区憩室与胰腺病变的关系尚有不同的看法，一般认为无明确的关系，但据中野哲（1974）的研究，尿淀粉酶的升高与憩室的大小有关，大的憩室常常伴有胰腺炎，8%伴存胰癌。贾雨辰等（1984）60例乳头区憩室中有胰腺炎10例，占16.7%，但多为反应性胰淀粉酶升高，有明显胰腺炎征象者仅3例。

乳头区憩室与胰腺癌：对于乳头区憩室与胰腺癌的关系，多数作者持否定态度。但是，Feldman（1957）指出，乳头区憩室常埋藏在胰腺头部实质中，由于这种密切的解剖学关系，乳头区憩室伴发胰头癌的机会要比一般想象的高许多。该作者复习1957年以前的文献，仅有20例乳头区憩室伴发胰腺癌，而贾雨辰等（1984）报告60例乳头区憩室中就有9例，说明其发生率比较高，这是一个值得注意的问题。

8. 憩室内乳头　憩室内乳头，表示胆胰管开口于憩室内，有作者称之为“乳头异位型”，国内文献报告均甚少见，我们（1995）报告11例。我们认为，从广义上讲，这是胆胰管十二指肠连接区异常的一种，属于胆胰管异位开口的一种，对胆胰疾病具有重要的病因学意义。

Costopoulos等（1967）指出，Baldwin（1911）在尸检时发现4例，继后也有作者陆续少数病例报告，都怀疑它与胆胰疾病的发生关系密切。有作者统计，憩室内乳头约占憩室的17%（松川，1977），Nelson（1976）在T管造影中发现有3%的胆总管开口于憩室之内，贾雨辰等（1984）发现2例，占52例内镜检查的3.8%。由于此类畸形的存在，括约肌功能不全，容易发生逆行性胰胆管感染。Vicecoute等（1984）对乳头区憩室病人的胆胰管下端括约肌进行测压研究，并与无憩室组对照，发现主要指标差别十分明显，憩室组压力明显低于对照组（其中，在基础压力、峰值压力对比皆是$P<0.01$，压力波高度$P<0.02$），两组压力波频率无明显差别。

我们（1995）报告45例乳头区憩室中，并发胆胰疾病为：①憩室内乳头11例全部都伴存胆胰疾病；②34例乳头区憩室中，91%并存胆胰疾病。自然，收集到的这些病例，之所以进行ERCP检查都是因为胆胰疾病而来，不能代表普通人群中的发病率。

一组6个憩室内乳头型十二指肠乳头区憩室中，仅1例因行肾上腺肿瘤术前检查时偶然发现；另5例均有明显胆胰管梗阻症状，其中4例并发肝内外胆管扩张；1例并发急性胰腺炎。因此憩室内乳头型十二指肠乳头旁憩室应引起临床的足够重视。

9. 乳头区憩室并发胆胰疾病影响因素　憩室的位置：Eggert等（1982）观察到有菌胆汁胆囊炎和胰腺炎的组织学表现和胆系内结石的发生率，随着憩室与胆胰共同管开口间的距离的缩短而增加。越靠近乳头，胆胰发病就越多，憩室内乳头胆胰疾病发病率最高。乳头上方的憩室比下方者容易引起症状，这可能与胆胰管从后上内方进入十二指肠有关。

胆胰管下端括约肌，作为胆胰系统细菌屏障作用的生理功能，由于乳头区憩室的存在而被破坏，使胆系胰腺感染的机会明显高于无乳头区憩室的患者。Osncs等（1977）在174例ERCP检查中，发现乳头区憩室40例（23%），其中在有胆胰疾病的患者组，乳头区憩室的发现率为35%；而在无胆胰疾病的患者组，其发现率仅为6%。李智华等（1991）在ERCP检查时发现，乳头区憩室患者的胆管生理性蠕动减弱，胆胰管连接区形态可有异常改变，尤其是憩室内乳头患者更为明显。憩室与胆胰共同管开口的距离：贾雨辰等（1984）报告60例憩室中，除1例多发者一处憩室位于第三段外，其余都在距乳头2cm之内。

憩室的大小：憩室越大越易出现症状。随着年龄增加，憩室逐渐变大，数目也可能逐渐增多。有学者发现，尿淀粉酶升高与憩室大小密切相关，大憩室常常伴存胰腺炎。

虽然大的憩室容易压迫胆胰共同管引起胆管扩张或引起胆胰其他疾病，但这仅是因素之一，更重要的是憩室与胆胰管开口之间的距离和憩室的位置。因此，我们在观察乳头区有无憩室时，还应着重观察乳头开口的位置及与憩室之间的关系。当憩室处于舒张状态（即其内充满对比剂）时，容易诊断；若憩室内因食物残渣干扰造影图像或憩室处于收缩状态时，诊断可出现困难。此时，应注意动态观察十二指肠轮廓外有无致密影或黏膜影伸出，以确定是否有憩室存在。

乳头区憩室作为病因学因素，引起胆胰病变的发病机制似可概括如下：①憩室作为“占位病变”，机械地挤压胆胰管下端，导致胆汁、胰液排泄不畅，淤滞，梗阻，有利于胆系结石的形成和感染的发生，尤以憩室内乳头和大憩室病例显著。②憩室内容物滞留感染，出现憩室炎症，进而蔓延至乳头及胆胰管,促使胆胰病变的发生。③胆胰管下端调节胆汁胰液的排空机制包括两部分:一为胆胰管下端括约肌(以往称为 Oddi 括约肌),一为胆胰共同管和/或胆胰管下端丰富的黏膜的叶状皱襞(或称为叶状瓣,绒毛瓣),炎症对它们均极为不利。乳头区憩室之所以重要,盖因乳头的缘故。乳头炎症初期为黏膜水肿、充血、括约肌痉挛,以后黏膜溃烂、叶状瓣减少或消失、逐渐形成瘢痕,纤维化和狭窄,胆胰共同管僵硬,导致闭锁不全,严重影响胆汁和胰液的排空;胆胰管下端括约肌压力降低,功能失调,加之闭锁不全,上可导致胆胰管内压力下降,胆汁胰液排空无力;下可引起十二指肠内容物(自然也包含憩室内容物)向上逆流,进入胆胰管,造成逆行性感染,促进胆系结石形成。

随着年龄增长,憩室的发生率上升,上述诸因素协同作用,且随着机体的抵抗力降低而逐渐加剧,胆胰病变发病率不可避免地逐渐增高。

10. 鉴别诊断　憩室内容物的信号特征决定其 MRI 表现,通常憩室内含有气体、液体和食物,憩室内形成的气液平面是辨认十二指肠憩室的特征性表现,该组病例中仅占 51.7%(30/58)。而相当一部分憩室呈完全液性或气性,造成在 MRCP 上诊断的困难。该组有 5 例全含气,厚层 MRCP 图像不能显示憩室,在 MRCP 和横断位各序列图像上呈低信号,极易漏诊。

无气的憩室全含液体成分,在 MRCP 图像上较易发现,较多的憩室内因含食物呈不均匀信号,该组中 23 个无气憩室有 15 个呈不均匀信号,另外 8 个呈均匀液性信号,需与胰腺囊性占位相鉴别。Macari 等(2003)报道的 7 例 CT、MRI 初始描述为胰腺囊性肿块,最终证实为十二指肠憩室,充满液体。其中 3 例回顾性诊断发现憩室,另 4 例回顾性诊断也不能与囊性肿块鉴别,鉴别诊断包括胰腺囊性肿瘤、胰腺假性囊肿,胰腺囊性占位形态较固定,内部信号均匀。十二指肠憩室出现憩室炎、憩室出血和憩室穿孔等并发症少见,憩室炎和憩室出血无憩室外征象时, MRI 诊断困难,憩室炎有时可见憩室周围 T_2WI 高信号渗出,憩室穿孔时出现憩室周围渗出外,在后腹膜或腹腔内见到游离气体。

Hariri 等(2005)报道 1 例十二指肠乳头区憩室腔内充满液体病例,与胰头部囊性肿瘤难于鉴别。但他们同时提出若能了解十二指肠憩室发生的位置及在憩室内存在少量气体则有助于对十二指肠乳头旁憩室做出正确诊断。

11. 误诊病例简介　有作者指出,十二指肠乳头区憩室往往因十二指肠蠕动排空快,憩室不易充盈而漏诊;另外,钡剂反流入胰胆管又可误为乳头区憩室。十二指肠降段憩室内可生长腺瘤,但憩室内团块状食物残渣也可形成充盈缺损,易误诊为憩室内肿瘤。

从影像学方面讲,乳头区憩室一般说来易于发现和诊断,然而,有关误诊的报告亦不少。Nelson 等(1976)列举不少 X 线诊断误诊和漏诊的病例。

Hasan 等(1988)报告 2 例 PTC 检查时将憩室误诊为壶腹周围肿瘤,同一作者(1991)报告 1 例乳头区憩室伴梗阻性黄疸,超声检查将中等大小的憩室引起的胰头肿块误诊为胰头癌。

Bellamy(1993)指出,当凸出的黏膜皱襞环绕憩室颈部时,直接法胆系造影可呈现为憩室内充盈缺损,而成为壶腹区周围的假肿瘤。

在 CT 图像上,十二指肠憩室可类似脓肿或穿孔的溃疡,发生在十二指肠内侧壁的愈合后的溃疡可能被误诊为憩室,但溃疡和脓肿伴发的炎症反应的不规则外形和急性临床表现则与憩室有着本质的区别。如果仍有疑问,需要借助上消化道造影予以鉴别。

在某些情况下,为液体充盈的十二指肠憩室可被误诊为胰腺的低密度肿块,取卧位使气体进入憩室则可与胰腺肿块区分开。

有作者报告一组 65 例 MRCP 中有 11 例将内含气液平面的十二指肠球部影像误诊为十二指肠憩室,因此在发现十二指肠肠外气液平面时应同时观察不同断面图像,正确认识胃十二指肠走行。该组误诊率较高的主要原因为影像征象认识不足,通过学习和讨论,回顾误诊病例都能得到正确的判读。

十二指肠乳头区憩室诊断的临床意义:十二指肠憩室的 MRI 诊断具有较高的准确性,其临床意义远非憩室诊断本身,其临床意义在于胆系炎症和结石的病因诊断和对 ERCP 及内镜下治疗有指导意义。研究显示乳头区憩室和胆管扩张及结石的相关性,在发现肝外胆管下端狭窄,肝外胆管扩张的病例,仔细观察有无乳头旁憩室的存在,对狭窄的良恶性鉴别诊断有帮助。其次乳头区憩室可造成 ERCP 的检查困难,影响肝外胆管结石内镜下取石操作。研究显示,内镜下发现肝外胆管结石的病例有 40% 合并乳头区憩室,因此明确乳头区憩室的部位、大小对肝外胆管结石和肝外胆管下端狭窄的 ERCP 检查和内镜下治疗计划的制定有指导意义。

12. 有症状与无症状　Fellbaum 等（1987）指出，乳头区憩室在临床上，可表现为有症状的和无症状的两型。它们的切除由于手术的危险性较高而导致苦恼。关于无症状的乳头区憩室是否为手术的适应证问题，学者们意见不尽一致。该作者通过尸解病理研究发现，在无症状的乳头区憩室病例，未见到肝、胰以及胆系的病理性改变，也无憩室炎或憩室周围炎的表现。同时，他们也未发现无症状的乳头区憩室与上腹部器官的病理性改变相关的迹象。因此，手术切除乳头区憩室，似应限制于有症状者。

13. 对十二指肠乳头区憩室应给予必要的重视　在钡餐检查时，十二指肠乳头区憩室是众所周知的，首先用 X 线观察乳头区憩室是在 1913 年，随着时代的前进，钡餐检查经常发现乳头区憩室，但传统看法认为它是无症状的，无害的，所以常常习惯地告诉病人："没有什么关系"，"不是什么大问题"，但是，事实上并非如此。我们认为，应从病因学的高度来评价乳头区憩室的临床意义，改变传统的看法，应把憩室的出现作为胆胰病变的"信号"来看：当病人上腹痛进行钡餐检查时，如果发现乳头区憩室，应给予足够重视，宜建议病人进行胆胰系统的深入检查（包括超声检查、CT 扫描等），如有可能，应行 MRCP 或 / 和 ERCP，观察憩室与乳头的关系，测量憩室与乳头之间的距离，了解是否为憩室内乳头，如果是，是更应重视，然后与临床医生共商治疗措施，力争早诊早治，不让胆胰疾病进一步恶化。

第五章 胆胰管十二指肠连接区结石

第一节 胆胰管十二指肠连接区结石

胆胰管十二指肠连接区结石,又称为共同管结石,胆管下端结石,胆管下段结石,胆总管下段结石。超声显示扩张的肝外胆管内有强回声光团伴后方声影,为肝外胆管结石的主要特征。共同管结石引起胆管扩张程度较共同管癌为轻,且呈不完全性胆管梗阻。而结石嵌顿于共同管上口者,其上游肝外胆管扩张则较为显著。共同管结石也可引起主胰管扩张,但发生率较低。有作者曾报告5例胆管下端结石,其中2例静脉胆系造影显影不良,低张十二指肠造影时,钡剂逆流进入胆管,衬托出胆管下端的阴性结石;另3例静脉胆系造影可见肝外胆管扩张,但未见结石影,然而低张十二指肠造影显示十二指肠乳头增大,呈类圆形充盈缺损改变,提示结石存在,后经手术证实。

胆管下端结石在低张十二指肠造影可有如下表现:

(1)胆管下端结石嵌入胆胰共同管,十二指肠乳头水肿,增大:造影可见其为边缘锐利的多边形或类圆形充盈缺损,直径多大于15mm。它可在降段相当于乳头处,显示形如钝角、直角或锐角的角形充盈缺损,其边缘非常锐利,有的甚至推压邻近的肠黏膜皱襞,但皱襞并无中断或破坏的表现。成角的边长依结石的大小而定。这是由于结石具有多面形的特征所致,它不同于乳头部肿瘤的表现。

(2)钡剂逆流进入共同管:钡剂逆流进入共同管内,深约1.5~2.5cm,居于结石透明阴影周围,可把结石显示出来,其大小,形态及位置均清楚可见。此征出现率虽不高,但有确诊的价值。其反流的发生固然可能与炎症后期引起的括约肌功能不全,结石轮廓不规则从而造成空隙,容许钡剂潜入有关,但低张技术的应用也可能是其原因之一。

(3)十二指肠外压征:充填于肝外胆管下端的结石对紧邻的十二指肠推压,可使相应肠段在低张造影中出现喇叭状、橄榄状、弧形压迹和阻断征等X线表现。这些表现与填塞于总胆管下端内结石的位置、大小、数目和嵌顿情况有关,故具有特征性诊断意义。这些征象中,任何一种均有助于总胆管下端结石的诊断,若出现多种形式的压迹,其诊断意义更大。

俯卧位较仰卧位好,以较清楚地显示这些征象,因在俯卧位时,扩张的总胆管和结石能更紧密地间接地压在相邻的十二指肠壁上,同时,俯卧位起着相当于加用压迫器的作用。

(4)十二指肠球部上缘喇叭状压迹,或球部橄榄状压迹:在充盈钡剂的球部上缘可显示上宽下窄的喇叭状外在压迹,或在球部显示纵行的橄榄状压迹。

(5)十二指肠球后段阻断征:大多数病人球部与降段之间的球后段几乎全无钡剂存在,有的仅隐约显示1~2条被拉直了的横行黏膜皱襞,颇似完全阻断,其压迹边缘常常并不直。此征在俯卧位更为明显显示。

(6)十二指肠降段上部内侧缘弧形压迹:此压迹可深可浅,亦可为单弧或双弧。

(7)十二指肠球部或球后段纵行柱状外在压迹:十二指肠球部后段出现纵行带状透亮影,即笔杆征,为肝外胆管扩张压迫所致。此压迹边缘光滑整齐并较直,压迹区内常可见到数条黏膜皱襞,仰卧位与俯卧位表现常不一致。

(8)十二指肠球后段或降段上部外侧弧形压迹:在十二指肠球后段或降段上部外缘可出现光滑弧形压迹,为增大的胆囊压迫所致,表示胆管下端多有梗阻，胆囊因之扩张。

Neitlich 等（1997）比较未增强扫描的螺旋 CT 与 ERCP 发现总胆管结石的情况，在 13 个月时间内对 51 例（年龄范围 18~94 岁）临床怀疑胆系结石的病例，均在 ERCP 前作螺旋 CT 平扫。螺旋 CT 扫描可评估有无胆管结石、共同管结石、胆囊的情况及胆囊的结石、肝内胆管扩张、肝门处及胰头处胆管的大小。ERCP 评估胆管或共同管结石，以及胆管的扩张情况（图 19-5-1）。

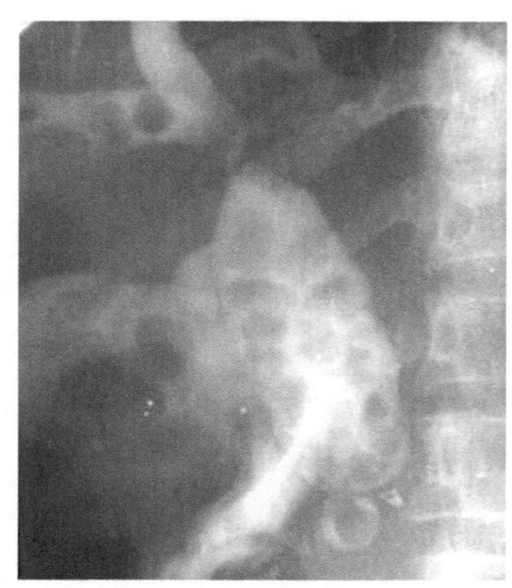

图 19-5-1　PTC 及手术病理证实：肝内外胆管明显扩张，其内含多发性结石，肝外胆管括约肌段结石清楚可见

在螺旋 CT 平扫时，ERCP 所发现有总胆管结石的 17 例中有 15 例为螺旋 CT 所看见。3 例嵌于共同管内的结石全为螺旋 CT 所发现。另外，在螺旋 CT 有一假阳性发现。在总胆管结石中，螺旋 CT 的敏感性为 88%，特异性为 97%，正确率为 94%。结果证实，螺旋 CT 平扫，在怀疑胆系结石时，有助于评估。

总胆管下端结石低张造影所见和临床表现不够典型的病人，常须与胰头癌、共同管癌和总胆管下端癌相区别。

胰头癌：超声、CT 和 MRI 对本病的诊断有确诊的意义。如未行上述三项检查，在 X 线造影时胰头癌可有十二指肠降段中部的不规则充盈缺损，可有倒 3 征、十二指肠环扩大及胃窦部的垫压征，这些征象在结石都难出现。

共同管癌：共同管癌与共同管结石一样，可出现乳头的充盈缺损、球部的柱状征，但缺乏乳头的角形变化。增强扫描时可见肿瘤病变呈现强化的征象。

总胆管下端癌：总胆管下端癌与共同管结石一样，可出现球部上缘喇叭征及降段内壁上部单弧形压迹征，但时与共同管结石不同，当出现这些征象时，都有球后段的不规则的不成比例地外压迫征象同时伴存。这在超声、CT 和 MRI 均可明确显示。

第二节　结石的影像学研究

CT：普通 CT 与 MSCT 检查均可见肝外胆管胰腺段远侧、胆胰共同管部出现稍高密度或高密度结节状影，其上游肝外胆管常有扩张。普通 CT 由于层厚不薄，细小的共同管结石本身常难显示，只能看见其上游肝外胆管扩张而怀疑下端梗阻的原因可能是结石。对于不典型的等密度结石的准确诊断，CT 平扫有一定困难，此时 CT 增强扫描或 / 和 MRI 扫描是必须的。增强扫描：经静脉团注有机碘对比剂后，不同期相扫描后，胰腺实质、周围血管及肝外胆管壁得到明显强化，胆管腔内容物密度不变，两者形成鲜明的对比，极易观察共同管内的结石。如诊断还有困难，则应加做 MRCP 进一步检查。

MRI 及 MRCP：在临床上，专门为了诊断胆胰共同管结石而行这两项检查者甚为少见，一般都是为了寻找肝外胆管下端梗阻的原因，区别肿瘤梗阻与非肿瘤梗阻时才进行此项检查。有关详细内容请参见本书 本卷 本篇 第二章　胆胰管十二指肠连接区癌。

结石的自然消失：Schneider 与 Seitz（1986）报告在 84 例超声检查发现肝外胆管结石的病人中，有 16 例可见结石自发通过乳头。结石的通过，是由超声、ERCP、术中胆管造影以及临床证实的。15/16 经过乳头的结石病人都有右上腹痛，3 例病人有急性胰腺炎发作，5 例有血清淀粉酶过多。胆红素水平下降、碱性磷酸酶的丙种 GT 值小，均提示结石通过胆胰共同管。20 世纪 70 年代英文文献中也曾有作者报告，具有“本茨征”的胆囊结石可能出现崩裂，变成直径小于 10mm 的小结石，从而经胆管下端排到肠道，出现结石自然消失的后果

鉴别诊断：胆胰共同管结石的鉴别诊断一般不困难，在 CT 图像上，可见胆胰共同管有高密度或中等密度结石影，或与胆管壁形成晕环征或新月征，则

可明确诊断。

有时，胆胰共同管结石排出后，由于扩张的肝外胆管没能及时回缩，或由于肝外胆管壁弹性回缩力降低（年迈或感染因素），导致扩张的肝外胆管仍显扩张状态，但在CT图像上却未见结石影，或其他因素不能轻易肯定梗阻存在，需密切结合临床黄疸消退情况及胆红素水平作出正确判断。如仍有可疑，应加作MRCP、ERCP或/和PTC，以明确诊断（图19-5-2）。

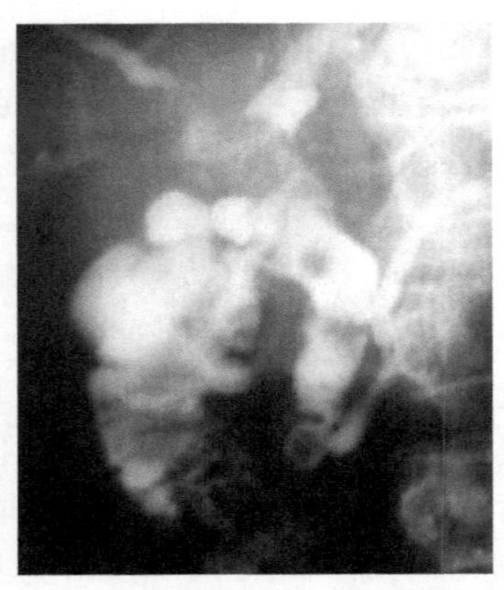

图19-5-2 ERCP：胆胰管扩张，肝内外胆管结石，肝外胆管括约肌段结石，明显扩张的胆囊管低位左位汇入肝外胆管

相反，临床上确有梗阻性黄疸存在，少数病例不能显示胆管扩张，可能因梗阻程度较轻，时间较短，或梗阻呈间歇性，或同时伴有胆管炎存在，对这类病例，都适于进行MRCP、ERCP或/和PTC检查。

在绝大多数情况下，用CT薄层扫描，可发现胆胰共同管内钙化密度的结石，患者常有反复发作的绞痛及黄疸病史。在个别情况，CT对胆胰共同管胆固醇成分的低密度结石难以确定（图19-5-3）。

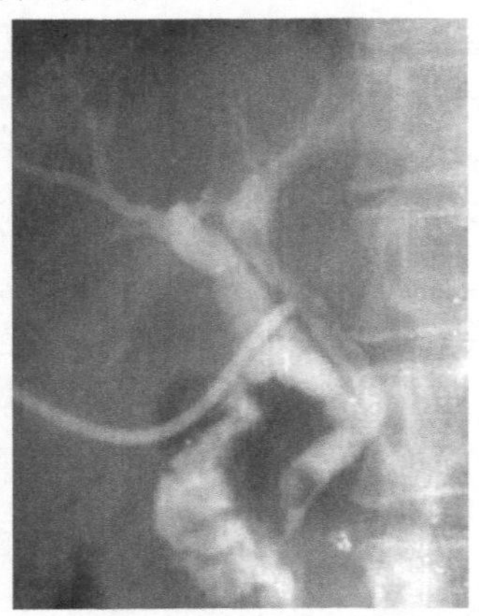

图19-5-3 T管造影：扩张的术后残留的胆囊管低位左位汇入肝外胆管，肝外胆管括约肌段结石位于括约肌段上部导致肝外胆管梗阻

值得注意的是，胰头区的高密度影不一定总是胆管结石，胰腺区的淋巴结钙化、胰颈后方增强的门静脉均可被误认为是结石。下述情况也应注意：

胆管结石排出后，肝外胆管壁因弹性减退或消失，难以恢复原状，胆管系统仍呈现扩张状态，可造成胆管梗阻的假象。肝内胆管因为四周都是肝脏实质，梗阻消除后，一般肝胆管的扩张也消失，从而恢复原状。测定血清胆红素，可有助于判断有无梗阻存在。

结石引起的梗阻常为不全性，或为间歇性，胆管扩张的程度有时可以很轻；CT测定肝外胆管的直径多在正常范围（小于或等于4mm）内，或在临界范围（4~6mm）内，但临床上血清胆红素常有升高。

综上所述，有结石病史的病人，肝外胆管扩张不一定总是意味着存在梗阻。相反，轻度结石性梗阻，或短期梗阻的病人，胆管也可不出现明显扩张。对于CT表现的分析，必须随时紧密结合临床情况，方不致于误诊（图19-5-4）。

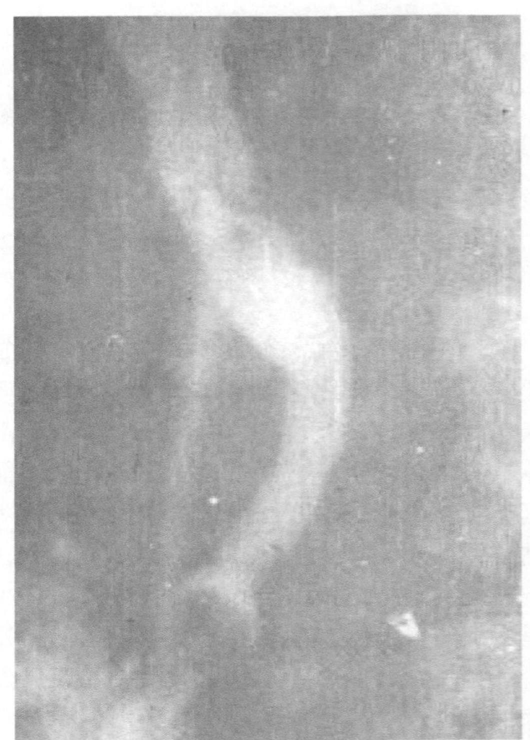

图19-5-4 术后T管造影：肝外胆管扩张，肝外胆管下端典型的杯口征，提示括约肌段结石引起的充盈缺损

第三节　胰头区的高密度影

值得注意的是，胰头区的高密度影不一定总是胆管结石，胰腺区的淋巴结钙化、胰颈后方增强的门静脉均可被误认为是结石。

下述情况也应注意：胆管结石排出后，肝外胆管壁因弹性减退或消失，难以恢复原状，胆管系统仍呈现扩张状态，可造成胆管梗阻的假象。肝内胆管因为四周都是肝脏实质，梗阻消除后，一般肝胆管的扩张也消失，从而恢复原状。测定血清胆红素，可有助于判断有无梗阻存在。结石引起的梗阻常为不全性，或为间歇性，胆管扩张的程度有时可以很轻；CT测定肝外胆管的直径多在正常范围（小于或等于6mm）内，或在临界范围（6~8mm）内，但临床上血清胆红素常有升高。

综上所述，有结石病史的病人，肝外胆管扩张不一定总是意味着存在梗阻。相反，轻度结石性梗阻，或短期梗阻的病人，胆管也可不出现明显扩张。对于CT表现的分析，必须随时紧密结合临床情况，方不致于误诊。

第六章 胆胰管下端括约肌闭锁不全

第一节 新生儿胆胰管下端括约肌闭锁不全

本症十分少见。Frates(1965)报告2例,均伴存十二指肠闭锁和环状胰腺。Kirks和Baden(1973)报告一例唐氏综合征患者,出现完全性远段十二指肠梗阻伴存本症。Rosenblatt(1967)报告2例空气返流入胆系伴十二指肠梗阻。Caffey(1972)也曾举例介绍十二指肠狭窄婴儿钡剂返流入胆系。在X线照片上,肝影内可见线状空气条纹影,在新生儿期,此类表现通常表示空气位于门静脉系统内,在胆管树内者极少。一般说来,在常规腹部X线检查中,对于门静脉系统积气与胆系积气难以区别,在新生儿尤甚,但是,如从影像上能够确定胆外胆管蒂或胆囊的所在,则可排除门静脉积气的可能性。Atkinson等(1977)在讨论本症时指出,十二指肠远端梗阻的病例出现本症,可能源于十二指肠内压高于胆管树处腔内压的升高。有的病例手术发现无确切的胆胰下端共同管,此类解剖结构的变异也为本症的一个原因。

第二节 成人胆胰管下端括约肌闭锁不全

成人胆胰管下端括约肌闭锁不全,常见于中老年女性。病因不明,某些病例的病因可能为先天性。由于括约肌闭锁不全,致使肠道内少量气体逆行进入胆管,在右上腹X线平片上可见到肝外胆管少许积气,但胆管形态大小无异常可言。胆管可能有轻度炎症致使病人感到右上腹不适。本症一般为功能性病变,可归之为良性病变,具有暂时性和可恢复性的特点。

部分病变可为器质性的改变,表现为僵硬的缩窄性闭锁不全,其病理表现为瘢痕形成,原因为括约肌病理性破坏,医源性括约肌切开术后或胆管大结石排出后。

第三节 十二指肠-胆系逆流的少见原因

在没有胆系-十二指肠瘘的情况下,胆总管下端开口异常可引起十二指肠-胆系返流,Chermet等(1975)统计以往法文文献中有13例胆总管开口于十二指肠球后部引起此类返流的报道。

该作者报告一例67岁老人有类似的表现,分析研究系因溃疡周围瘢痕化与收缩,导致胆总管高位开口,并有十二指肠乳头关闭不全,术中胆系造影证实诊断,并清楚见到胆总管远端呈鱼钩状开口进入十二指肠球后部。

第四节　胆胰管下端括约肌闭锁不全鉴别诊断

胆囊及胆管内积气：常表示与胃肠之间有异常通道形成，最常见者有胆系穿孔，并瘘道形成，此外，胰管内亦可见气体；十二指肠球部溃疡穿孔并与胆系交通；消化道癌肿累及胆系，胰腺炎以及胆管与胃肠吻合术等均可见有气体。此外，短期内由胆管排出结石而引起括约肌短时功能失调，亦可有胆管积气；有时胆管内蛔虫亦可短时间内带入少量气体。

如有肝内胆管积气，则须与肝静脉内积气区别，肝静脉与肝内胆管的解剖学分布不同是其鉴别的要点。胆囊积气：一般是因产气细菌引起的胆囊感染所致。胆囊炎：往往有胆囊扩大，钡餐无胆管内钡剂逆流改变。

第七章 胆胰管下端括约肌段狭窄

第一节 胆胰管括约肌段狭窄

胆胰管下端括约肌紊乱所引起的症状类似于各种原因所致的胆胰管梗阻。不论它是由于括约肌段的纤维化，还是生理功能的障碍，它的临床表现都是括约肌段受累。典型地，括约肌段狭窄可能难与胆系结石区别，因为它可伴存反复的右上腹痛或上腹痛，有胆汁淤滞或胰腺炎或二者兼有的实验室资料，而且在影像学检查时可见到胆管和/或胰管的扩张。

1. 病因学 原发性括约肌段狭窄可以是括约肌段先天性异常的结果。括约肌段的急性和慢性炎症可引起狭窄。内膜组织异位，类似于前列腺增生所见那样，也可引起流出道狭窄。继发性括约肌段狭窄可出现于胆系结石或/和胆管结石，直接的机械性损伤下端括约肌，或胆系的连续刺激导致括约肌段反射性痉挛。括约肌段狭窄的90%是来自于这些原因。以往的外科手术处理是较为少见的原因。良性和恶性括约肌段周围的新生物必须除外。

有趣的是，括约肌段的功能性狭窄可与胰腺分裂同时伴存。已发现后者出现于3.3%慢性腹痛经ERCP检查者，而在以往有胰腺炎历史者它更为常见(占12%)。继发性括约肌段狭窄：由于胆管结石及手术器械创伤括约肌段黏膜，形成炎症，纤维化；慢性胰腺炎合并胆系疾病时，可致括约肌段狭窄。

原发性括约肌段狭窄：指原发性括约肌段功能不全，造成胆汁引流不畅，形成慢性炎症，导致纤维化。

2. 临床表现 括约肌段狭窄可出现右上腹痛，伴存胆汁淤滞或胰腺炎或两者的实验室表现，这主要仰赖于受侵犯的括约肌段的范围。胆管括约肌的单独狭窄可以出现，而只侵犯胰管括约肌者则甚为少见。胆胰管下端括约肌最常受到侵犯，使其与胆管结石难以区别。

3. 临床诊断标准 临床上有反复发作右上腹痛、右上腹不适，可伴有发热、黄疸，若再加上下述情况一项者，即可确定为括约肌段狭窄：测定胆管内压超过150mm水柱，可提示此段不全性梗阻；手术探查胆管4号探针或12号导尿管不能通过肝外胆管下端进入十二指肠，或用力通过时有明显阻力；ERCP插管时见十二指肠括约肌段部炎症、缩窄；ERCP造影时发现有肝外胆管扩张，对比剂由肝外胆管内排出延缓，括约肌段压力升高；经内镜括约肌切开术(EST)后，随访见临床症状明显改善或消失。

纤维性括约肌段狭窄：胆管造影通常可显示一定程度的胆管扩张，伴胆管下端一长段光滑的狭窄或鸟嘴状狭窄。可见到括约肌段上方的狭窄前扩张。对比剂的引流延迟也支持这诊断(有作者报告，静脉胆系造影时，在正常情况下，胆囊切除术后，在仰卧位，胆管排空时间为45分钟)。在胰管造影片上，可观察到主胰管有轻微的扩张。尽管完全性梗阻通常提示为恶性梗阻，但是，在良性狭窄和恶性狭窄之间进行区别仍然是困难的。胰高血糖素可松弛括约肌，有利于插管，以及区别痉挛与解剖学的狭窄。有作者报告，在括约肌段狭窄病人，ERCP的成功率只有82%，因此，有时还需PTC进行补充。在外科学文献上，括约肌段狭窄者，从肝外胆管到十二指肠，不容易通过3号Bakes扩张器。

功能性括约肌段狭窄：在ERCP时，进行括约肌的内镜测压，可以显示在括约肌的收缩相，压力异常高且伴逆行性收缩，和矛盾的胆囊收缩素八肽反应。测压可以帮助单纯的功能性括约肌段狭窄与其他原因的胆囊切除术后疼痛进行区别。在功能性狭窄与纤维性狭窄之间的压力差别很小。功能性狭窄显示

非线性压力 - 直径相关，当探针直径增加时可随之扩张。而纤维性狭窄不能为探针扩张或只能轻微地被探针扩张。

4. 并发症　胆管炎：括约肌段狭窄使胆汁排出不畅，淤积，导致胆管炎。胰腺炎：胆胰管括约肌段有胆胰共同管者约占 80%，当共同管发生狭窄时，引起胆汁反流与混流，故常常引起或并发慢性胰腺炎。

5. 影像学研究　括约肌段正常 X 线表现：括约肌段上宽下窄，呈漏斗状。从括约肌段的宽度、长度、形状、轮廓以及其宽度与胰腺段远端宽度的比值等项的动态观察清楚地表明：括约肌段收缩与扩张是经常性的，其宽度，长度、形状、轮廓及比值等随时都在变化，并不是静止不动的。了解正常括约肌段的 X 线表现后，方能判断括约肌段是否狭窄。

括约肌段狭窄的影像学表现：确定括约肌段是否有狭窄存在，应注意观察括约肌段形态及宽度的变化。当有狭窄时，在直接法胆系造影（多次照片及录像）观察，可见括约肌段变窄，无扩张的表现，而且呈现僵硬，其宽度及形状前后一致不变，并可见括约肌段以上胆管扩张。

肝外胆管下端及括约肌段形态改变，可呈杵状、鸟嘴状、杯口状及囊状。通过手术结果结合照片观察发现：肝外胆管下端呈杵状或杯口状，大多为括约肌段全段有较严重的狭窄（一般通过 8F 导尿管较困难）或合并有胆管下端结石；肝外胆管下端呈浅杯口状，还见于僵硬括约肌段向上端胆管胰腺段逆行顶入；括约肌段呈鸟嘴状，为括约肌段有一段较长狭窄，狭窄可以较轻，一般不伴有结石；肝外胆管括约肌段呈囊状，多为胆胰共同管狭窄，胆管括约肌段尚可部分扩张；肝外胆管下端狭窄伴变形、移位，常提示合并有慢性胰腺炎

括约肌段狭窄，肝外胆管一般都有不同程度的扩张。狭窄越重，时间越长，胆管扩张的程度也就越显著。肝外胆管因长期扩张，导致管壁弹力减低，甚至可继发肝外胆管囊柱状扩张。肝外胆管扩张是诊断括约肌段狭窄的重要征象。

括约肌段狭窄的患者，肝外胆管也可不扩张。这见于下述情况：肝外胆管经（胆囊造瘘、T 管、PTCD 等）引流后，虽括约肌段狭窄，但因胆汁已被引流，胆系内压力降低，肝外胆管扩张减轻以至于不扩张；非扩张性胆管梗阻，与括约肌段狭窄有关的因素有梗阻病程的长短、肝外胆管壁长期慢性炎症及管壁增厚、硬化，以至于肝外胆管下端虽显著狭窄，病人也有黄疸出现，但肝外胆管却并不扩张；合并有肝总管狭窄及结石性梗阻的黄疸病人，肝外胆管可以不扩张。此时不能忽视括约肌段狭窄的存在。

上述三种情况肝外胆管非扩张型括约肌段狭窄的病人，超声和 CT 往往漏诊，PTC 和 ERCP 对此类病人诊断比 CT 和超声要优越。因此，肝外胆管不扩张，并不能完全否认括约肌段狭窄的存在。在直接法胆系造影时，括约肌段狭窄还可根据由胆管排出至十二指肠内的对比剂较少，或无对比剂排出，以此推测肝外胆管下端可能有梗阻。但是，十二指肠内的对比剂不少并不能除外括约肌段狭窄，这需结合当时摄片时注药的压力、剂量、速度，以及照片的时间等多种因素综合考虑。在静脉法胆系造影胆管显影时，可见胆管延迟显影及持续显影，肝外胆管胰腺段下端呈杵状，其上段扩张，括约肌段不易显示。

6. 鉴别诊断　肝外胆管下端假性梗阻：此症与括约肌段暂时痉挛，及当时胆管内注入对比剂的量，及其推注药时的压力有关。X 线片上，可见肝外胆管括约肌段呈鼠尾状变细，或胰腺段下端呈杯口状或杵状改变，其肝外胆管亦可稍现扩张。但是，如行动态观察，或多次反复透视照片，这些表现并不恒定，在临床上病人也无胆管梗阻的症状和体征。

对于胆系术后，直接法胆系造影显示肝外胆管直径大于 1.0cm 以上者，如在复查照片见肝外胆管直径逐渐增宽，而临床上又有症状者，方可考虑可能有括约肌段狭窄。

肝外胆管下端恶性梗阻：胆管下端癌及胆胰管十二指肠连接区癌，病程较短，且为持续性无痛性黄疸。直接法胆系造影可见胆管下端呈向心性不规则狭窄，多为较完全性梗阻，边缘毛糙不整，肝胆管扩张纡曲，多呈软藤征。而括约肌段狭窄一般病程较长，梗阻为不全性，边缘较规则光滑。ERCP 对鉴别尤其有用。

第二节　括约肌段狭窄的影像诊断

超声检查:括约肌段狭窄可出现胆管扩张,有时出现胰管扩张。有作者用超声研究胰管与肝外胆管的直径,在静脉注射肠促胰酶后,发现括约肌段狭窄且有症状的病人,有 83% 胰管的直径增粗。在外科括约肌切断术后成功率(疼痛解除)的 90% 有阳性结果。

核素检查:肝胆核素显像有诊断价值,放射性核素从胆到肠的时间延长,超过 45 分钟,提示为括约肌段狭窄。ERCP 常可证实放射性核素检查所见。99mTc-IDA 肝胆核素显像,在功能性和解剖学的括约肌段狭窄的非损伤性筛选工作中,承担着主要角色。在一组括约肌段狭窄病人的研究中,有异常表现的病人的基础括约肌压为 38.5mmHg(比较于正常的 15 ± 4mmHg)。显像异常的标准包括:胆 - 肠时间延长(超过 1 小时),异常时间 - 活性动态(管道的放射活性为 2 小时,等于或大于 1 小时),梗阻(肠无放射活性),以及明显的管道扩张。核素显像还用来客观地了解治疗的反应。在另一组报告,以 ERCP 作为金指标,肝胆核素显像发现了 10 例括约肌段狭窄中的 9 例。在可见的胆胰管道中保持放射活性 2 小时,考虑为异常引流的最好的指征。

CT:当超声检查显示解剖结构不是很理想时,CT 的用处只在于显示没有包块性病变(尽管这并不能完全除外新生物的存在)。

ERCP:对于括约肌段狭窄,以前最有用的检查方法是 ERCP。它可直接观察括约肌段的情况。括约肌段及其周围十二指肠的肿瘤可以确定,还可以用钳夹或网圈进行乳头的活检,以支持诊断。为得到组织学标本有时还须行内镜下括约肌切断术。此外,分泌物的抽吸、细胞学检查、括约肌的测压以及为了 X 线摄片行造影剂的灌注,皆可同时进行。

第三节　括约肌段的良性狭窄

在大多数病人,炎症和瘢痕性改变是括约肌段狭窄的形态学基础,这是由于胆囊结石疾病细菌感染的小管性或淋巴性播散。括约肌段狭窄的影响是胆胰管压力升高和胆胰液流动减少。在手术时可能发现胆管扩张,排出降低,而且,在瘢痕性狭窄探针不能通过。只在炎性狭窄是可逆性的,但是永久性的改变是不确定的。因此,治疗是必须的,首先且器械扩张到 4~6mm。Tulassay 等(1987)在 921 例内镜括约肌切开术中,发现有 110 例(12%)是括约肌段的良性狭窄。其中,96 例为胆囊切除术后,14 例胆囊尚存。括约肌段狭窄的诊断是以 ERCP 发现胆管扩张作根据的。但是,这并不是特异性征象,因为在胆囊切除后,在括约肌正常张力情况下,胆管可以变得扩张;同时,胆管扩张是括约肌段狭窄的一个诊断标准,而胆系核素扫描时的异常发现,和胆汁淤滞相符合的实验室同存的征象不能避免。与外科手术相比,内镜括约肌切开术是括约肌段狭窄首选的治疗方法。然而,出现于括约肌段狭窄的内镜括约肌切开术的并发症,比胆管结石(8.8%)为多(13.6%)。出血和胆管炎是并发症过多的原因。

第四节　胆胰共同管假性肿瘤

详见本书 本卷 本篇 第八章 第三节 胆胰共同管假性肿瘤。

第八章　胆胰共同管及其周围疾病

第一节　胆胰共同管周围病变

胆胰共同管周围区是指胆胰共同管周围 2 cm 之内的区域，其结构包括胰腺头部、钩突部及胰管末端、胆胰共同管、十二指肠乳头和胆总管下段。胆胰共同管由胆胰共同管和十二指肠主乳头组成，周围环绕胆胰管下端括约肌。

胆胰共同管病变的种类可分为肿瘤及肿瘤样病变、炎症、先天性变异等（表 19-8-1）。由于该区域解剖复杂，组织结构多以及各结构紧密相邻，其临床症状及影像表现有很多相似之处，但不同病变的临床预后截然不同。因此，正确诊断及鉴别诊断对治疗及预后非常重要。

表 19-8-1　胆胰共同管周围病变的起源及种类

病变起源	病变种类
胰腺	胰头癌、神经内分泌肿瘤、囊腺瘤、实性假乳头状瘤、淋巴瘤、胰母细胞瘤、急性胰腺炎、慢性胰腺炎、胰腺囊肿
胆胰共同管及十二指肠	胆胰共同管癌、十二指肠乳头癌、腺瘤、间质瘤、淋巴瘤、十二指肠乳头炎、十二指肠乳头区憩室
胆总管下段	胆总管下段癌、囊腺瘤 / 癌、胆总管结石、胆管炎、先天性胆管扩张
其他	胰腺导管内乳头状黏液性肿瘤、环状胰腺

影像检查方法：胆胰共同管周围病变的影像学检查方法有 CT、MRI、超声、经皮经肝穿刺胆管造影（PTC）、经内镜逆行胆胰管造影（ERCP）、磁共振胆胰管成像（MRCP）及正电子发射体层摄影术（PET/CT）等。其中 CT 特别是多层螺旋 CT（MSCT）对胆管及胆胰系病变显示较清晰，能显示病变的直接或间接征象，成为胆胰共同管周围病变的首选检查方法；超声因其有操作简便、无创伤、可重复检查等优点，可用于胆胰共同管周围病变的筛查，但其易受肠腔气体的干扰，并与操作者的临床经验密切相关；

MRCP 是观察胆胰管系统解剖和病理形态的方法，不需要使用对比剂即可进行多平面成像，可从多角度全面显示胆系的结构，明确梗阻的部位、范围；PTC 及 ERCP 由于其具有介入治疗作用，加之 ERCP 对病变的活检定性作用，依然为诊断胆胰系疾病的“金标准”，但因其为有创检查，且随着 CT 及 MRI 新技术的推广和应用，其临床应用已日趋减少。

PET/CT 技术是融合同位素和 CT 断层扫描两种技术而成的新技术，主要用于检测全身及骨的转移。

一、胆胰共同管周围区各种病变的影像学研究

（一）起源于胰腺的病变

1. 胰头癌　胰头癌是胰腺最常见的肿瘤，约占胰腺癌的 60%~70%。CT 表现为胰头部低或等密度实质性肿块，增强扫描瘤体强化程度大多低于正常胰腺实质。若胰头内胆总管、胰管同时扩张，形成所谓“双管征”；有时，梗阻近端和远端的两段胰管和胆管表现为 4 个分离的管腔，即“四管征”，为诊断胰头癌的特异征象。胰头癌在 MRI 上表现多样，多数呈低、等 T_1 和等 T_2 信号。MRCP 征象为胆总管胰头段及主胰管胰头段被癌瘤组织破坏中断，二者之残留近段均有扩张及信号增高，并且扩张的两管不能相交，一些作者称该种征象为“不相交征”，认为是胰头癌的特异征象。典型早期胰腺癌的 PET 表现为胰腺癌瘤体局限性摄取增高灶，其标准摄取最大值（SUVmax）>2.5；晚期胰腺癌还可伴有胰腺周围、腹膜后和其他脏器代谢增高灶（转移灶）。

2. 胰腺内分泌肿瘤　胰腺内分泌肿瘤仅占胰腺

肿瘤的1%~2%。根据是否分泌激素分为功能性和无功能性。功能性胰腺内分泌肿瘤体积较小,CT平扫一般呈等密度,部分可见到细小的线状或结节状钙化。MRI上肿瘤一般呈长T_1、长T_2信号,含胶原和纤维较多的肿瘤T_2WI可呈低信号,脂肪抑制T_1WI显示病灶更清晰。胰腺内分泌肿瘤属富血供肿瘤,增强后明显强化,瘤体周边环形薄壁高密度强化环为胰腺内分泌肿瘤特有征象。无功能胰腺内分泌肿瘤多有包膜,体积较大,瘤体内囊变、出血、钙化多见。

3. 胰腺囊腺瘤　胰腺囊腺瘤包括浆液性囊腺瘤和黏液性囊腺瘤。浆液性囊腺瘤为良性,几乎无恶变倾向。胰头浆液性囊腺瘤CT表现为胰头单腔或多腔的囊性病变,壁厚薄不均,病灶中心出现钙化,尤其是"星芒"状瘢痕伴钙化,对浆液性囊腺瘤的诊断有特征性意义。MR平扫T_1WI为低信号,T_2WI为"蜂窝"状的高信号,囊壁光滑,内壁可见壁结节。增强后囊隔和囊壁不同程度强化,呈"蜂窝"状,中心瘢痕可延迟强化。

黏液性囊腺瘤CT表现为多房水样低密度病变,囊壁厚薄不均,T_1WI上呈高低混杂信号,T_2WI呈高信号,增强后壁、分隔和实体部分均较明显强化。黏液性囊腺瘤若囊壁不规则增厚,出现壁结节则具有高度潜在恶性,瘤体越大,癌的可能性也越大。若囊内见"岛"状实质性肿物、囊壁钙化、囊肿周围有浸润征象等都高度提示囊腺癌的可能。

4. 胰腺实性假乳头状瘤　胰腺实性假乳头状瘤仅占胰腺肿瘤的1%~2%,年轻女性发生率较高。CT表现一般为边界清楚的类圆形、低或等密度混杂肿块,多有完整包膜,内部可有出血、坏死和钙化,一般不伴有胆总管或主胰管的扩张。MR表现为T_1WI上呈低信号,T_2WI上呈不均匀高信号或混合性信号的病灶,如肿瘤内出血可出现T_1WI呈不均匀高信号,增强扫描实性部分明显强化。

5. 胰腺淋巴瘤　胰腺淋巴瘤罕见,绝大多数为全身淋巴瘤对胰腺的浸润,主要病理类型是B细胞非霍奇金淋巴瘤。CT表现为胰头及体部体积增大,弥漫分布低密度肿块,密度较均匀,体积较大,一般病例报告直径常>7 cm,增强扫描肿块可呈环状或结节状轻度强化。常伴有胰头旁、后腹膜、肝门等部位淋巴结肿大。MRI表现为弥漫性或局限性胰腺肿大,呈等T_1、等T_2信号。

6. 胰母细胞瘤　又称儿童型胰腺癌,是一种少见的恶性肿瘤,常见于1~8岁儿童,平均年龄4.1岁,好发于胰头或胰尾。CT表现为低密度实性肿块,多呈分叶状,肿瘤有完整或不完整包膜,增强后轻度强化,常伴有区域性钙化、出血、坏死及囊变。MRI表现为等长T_1、长T_2信号,胰腺实性肿块伴钙化及坏死且有包膜,是该瘤的影像特点。

7. 急性胰腺炎　胰头部胰腺炎常继发于胆总管结石和ERCP检查。CT表现为胰头体积增大,轮廓不规则,密度稍减低,边缘模糊不清。坏死灶呈更低密度,如伴出血可见点片状高密度影夹杂其中。MRI平扫表现为胰腺局部或广泛增大,边缘模糊,呈混杂样信号,胰头旁可有大量渗出、假性囊肿、周围包裹积液的形成,增强扫描病变组织呈"渐进式"强化。

8. 慢性胰腺炎　慢性胰腺炎根据不同的发病机制,可分为3种。

(1)自身免疫性胰腺炎:是由自身免疫炎症介导、以胰腺肿大和胰管不规则狭窄为特征的一种特殊类型慢性胰腺炎,约占慢性胰腺炎发病率的5%~6%。典型的自身免疫性胰腺炎特点:胰腺弥漫性受累,胰腺实质密度(信号)减低,以胰头为主,边缘光滑,密度较均匀,DWI上呈分散或沿胰腺长轴分布的高信号,大部分病灶增强后延迟强化;主胰管狭窄及胰腺段胆总管狭窄合并近端胆管扩张;胰腺钙化或囊肿较少见。激素治疗后肿块明显缩小,可能遗留胰腺萎缩。ERCP显示主胰管弥漫性不规则狭窄,累及胆管时表现为节段性胆管狭窄。

(2)肿块型胰腺炎:好发于胰头,约占慢性胰腺炎的10%~36%。一般表现为形态不规则、边界不清晰的低密度肿块,增强后轻度强化,等或低于胰腺实质密度。肿块内部可伴有囊状低密度,周边厚环状强化,主胰管及其分支呈不规则扩张并穿过肿块,即"胰管贯穿征",约20%可见"双管征"。

(3)沟部胰腺炎:沟部是十二指肠和胆总管间胰头的一部分。其特点为胰头与十二指肠间纤维瘢痕的形成。影像学表现为胰头和十二指肠之间的薄片状肿块且伴有十二指肠壁增厚,肿块呈低回声(密度),T_1WI呈低信号,T_2WI呈等或轻度高信号,增强后延迟强化。MRCP显示胰头段胆总管狭窄。有文献报道约15%~30%的病例会发生恶变。

9. 胰腺假性囊肿　胰腺假性囊肿是最常见的胰腺囊性病变。一般继发于急、慢性胰腺炎或胰腺创伤。胰头部的假性囊肿CT表现为胰头内大小不等的圆形或类圆形水样密度，增强后可轻度强化。MRI 表现为 T_1WI 呈均匀低信号，T_2WI 为均匀高信号。如囊内伴有蛋白成分、坏死组织碎片和出血使 T_1WI 上信号不同程度增加，T_2WI 上信号不同程度减低。

（二）起源于胆胰共同管及十二指肠的病变

1. 胆胰共同管癌　胆胰共同管癌，又称共同管型胆胰管十二指肠连接区癌，以乳头状腺癌和管状腺癌多见，占胆胰共同管周围癌的 10% 左右。其超声、CT、MRI 表现为：胰头前方、胆管下端软组织肿块，增强扫描呈轻至中度均匀或不均匀强化，可呈延迟强化；部分癌肿较小不能明确显示，但胆总管远端与胰管近端的间距缩小，一般认为扩张的双管靠近（扩张的胆胰管末端间距≤ 5 mm）常见于胆胰共同管癌，如扩张的双管分离（扩张的胆胰管末端间距 >5 mm）常见于胰头癌。MRCP 表现为扩张的胆总管于胆胰共同管部截断，胆总管下端呈不规则或"鼠尾"状突然变尖狭窄与十二指肠相对应部位的充盈缺损（图 19-8-1）。

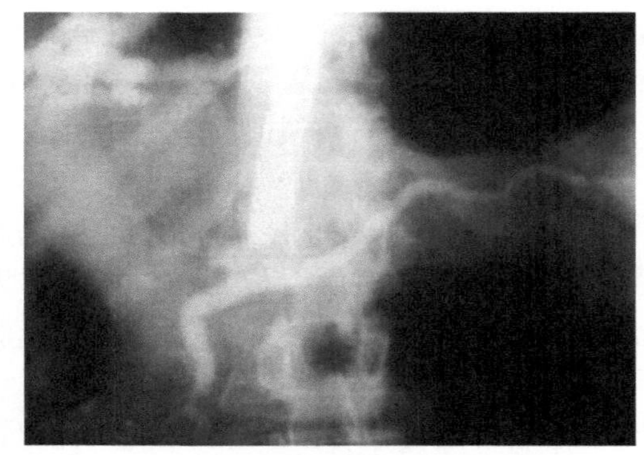

图 19-8-1　ERCP：胆胰管下端恶性梗阻引起的双管征，肝外胆管扩张明显，但其内对比剂浓度远比主胰管低，导致影像浅淡

2. 十二指肠乳头癌　即乳头型胆胰管十二指肠连接区癌，十二指肠乳头癌分为肠型和胆胰管型。CT、MRI 表现：胰腺钩突底部、十二指肠降段内侧乳头区软组织肿块，密度（信号）多均匀，边缘多清楚；胰头一般不大，相邻肠壁不规则增厚，肠腔狭窄。肿块长轴常与十二指肠长轴一致，与十二指肠肠腔断面呈"双环征"且内环相切。增强扫描呈轻至中度均匀或不均匀强化。病变穿透浆膜时，可累及胰头。肝内外胆管呈软藤状扩张，扩张胆管于胆胰共同管区突然截断或呈"鸟嘴"状狭窄，可有主胰管的扩张呈"双管征"。低张十二指肠造影主要征象为腔内不规则充盈缺损及恶性龛影、黏膜破坏、管壁僵硬、蠕动消失、管腔环形或不规则狭窄等。

3. 十二指肠腺瘤　十二指肠腺瘤是由腺上皮发生的良性肿瘤，多呈息肉状。约占十二指肠良性肿瘤的 69%，肿瘤常单发。CT 表现为局部肠腔内软组织肿块，平扫密度均匀，边缘光滑，可伴有胆胰管扩张、胆囊增大，增强后呈轻至中度均匀强化。低张十二指肠造影表现为十二指肠腔内圆形或椭圆形轮廓光滑的充盈缺损；有糜烂或溃疡形成时可显示钡斑与龛影，肿瘤区域黏膜皱襞可消失但黏膜正常。多发性腺瘤呈多个小圆形充盈缺损，类似"蜂窝"状；带蒂腺瘤可引起肠梗阻或套叠，加压可显示蒂部，且有移位为其特点。

4. 十二指肠间质瘤　胃肠道间质瘤是由 Mazur 等（1983）提出的，发生在十二指肠者极少见，多位于十二指肠降段和水平段。典型的 CT 表现包括良性者体积较小，密度均匀，轮廓清晰，边缘光滑锐利，无或浅分叶，与管壁有蒂相连突向肠腔内生长，邻近肠黏膜结构清晰，呈中度至明显均匀增厚。恶性者体积较大，呈明显分叶状或不规则形，密度不均匀，病灶内常有坏死或囊变，常呈外生型生长，轻中度不均匀强化，坏死或囊变区不强化。MRI 上胃肠道间质瘤信号不均匀，T_1WI 以等信号多见，T_2WI 呈高信号为主的混杂信号。

5. 十二指肠淋巴瘤　十二指肠恶性淋巴瘤很少见，占小肠恶性淋巴瘤的 10%~15%，绝大多数是 B 细胞型非霍奇金淋巴瘤。可分为五型，即：浸润型、肠腔动脉瘤样扩张型、息肉肿块型、肠系膜型和混合型。根据分型不同，CT 表现呈多样性。主要表现为多发节段性肠管管壁增厚伴肠系膜淋巴结肿大，肠腔内分叶状息肉样软组织肿块，但病变肠管的黏膜多连续，肠管形态仍能保持一定的扩张度和柔软度，常无梗阻现象，增强后呈轻至中度强化。

6. 十二指肠乳头炎　十二指肠乳头炎是指累及覆盖乳头黏膜的炎症性改变。影像表现为乳头增大，直径≥ 10mm，十二指肠内充盈缺损，边缘光滑，增强后明显强化。胆管梗阻程度及其继发性改变也较轻，并与乳头部肿块大小不相称。治疗后可明显好转或消失。

7. 十二指肠乳头区憩室　又称胆胰共同管周围憩室，是起自十二指肠大乳头周围 2~3 cm 的一种外向性囊袋状突起。因其解剖位置与胆胰管的关系密切，可引起胆胰系统并发症，临床上称之为 Lem-

mel's 综合征。典型的 CT、MRI 表现为十二指肠环内侧与胰头间类圆形的囊袋状气体或液体密度(信号)影,与十二指肠关系密切或与肠腔直接沟通,其内可见气-液平面,如憩室内容物残留,则密度不均匀(信号混杂),腔内呈"网织"状或"筛板"状结构。

(三)起源于胆总管下段的病变

1. 胆总管下段癌 胆总管下段癌是指发生于胆总管胰头段的恶性肿瘤,多为分化较好的腺癌。依据肿瘤的生长特性分为肿块型、管壁浸润型及内生型,其中浸润型最多见。内生型 CT、MRI 见胆总管腔内或乳头处结节状软组织肿块;浸润型或结节型则表现为胆管壁局限性或弥漫性增厚,管腔"圆锥"状、"鼠尾"状逐渐变窄或突然截断。增强扫描肿瘤呈明显强化和管壁不规则的环形强化,且具有延迟强化的特点。当累及胆胰共同管或胰腺时,可引起胰管扩张。MRCP 可显示梗阻下方正常胆总管而表现为"三管征"(指梗阻近、远端胆总管、主胰管),一般认为"三管征"是胆总管下段癌较特征性的影像学表现 (19-8-2)。

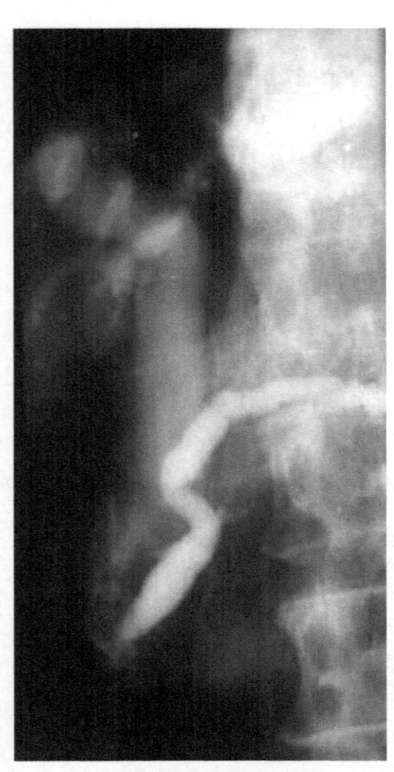

图 19-8-2 ERCP:胆胰管下端恶性梗阻引起的双管征

2. 胆总管下段囊腺瘤/癌 胆管囊腺类肿瘤是少见的肝内外胆管的肿瘤,多发生于肝内,中年女性好发。囊腺瘤发生于胆总管下段时 CT 主要表现为胆总管下段囊性肿块,边界清晰,囊液密度均匀。囊腺瘤多为多房,囊壁及囊内分隔厚薄一致,囊腺癌多为单房,可见乳头状结节突起,增强扫描囊壁、分隔、壁结节呈明显强化。部分囊腺癌内可见钙化,囊壁结节及不规则钙化被认为是囊腺癌区别于囊腺瘤的特征性表现。MRI 表现为囊液呈长 T_1、长 T_2 信号,但各腔内的信号多不一致。其信号强度主要取决于囊液的黏稠度、蛋白含量、含铁血黄素等。

3. 胆总管下段结石 胆总管结石的声像图表现为胆管腔内出现强回声光团,后方伴有声影,其形态恒定不变,结石阻塞近端的胆总管扩张,结石回声与胆总管管壁之间分界清楚。CT 平扫结石可分为高密度、等密度、低密度 3 种类型,以高密度结石常见,表现为梗阻以上胆管扩张,结石部位层面扩张的胆管突然消失,于充满低密度胆汁的扩张胆管中央或后部可见高密度结石影,形成所谓的"靶征"和"新月征"。MRI 表现为 T_1WI 上为高信号或低信号,T_2WI 上呈低信号或无信号,以及近端胆总管扩张。MRCP 表现为扩张的胆总管下端呈倒"杯口"状充盈缺损,为胆总管结石的典型征象。

4. 化脓性胆管炎 化脓性胆管炎,又称复发性化脓性胆管炎。CT 表现:常伴有肝内外胆管高度扩张、管壁增厚及胆汁密度增高,胆总管直径常大于 20 mm,扩张的胆管内有时可见结石影,十二指肠乳头增大且呈明显不均匀强化。

5. 胆总管下段囊肿 胆管囊肿为先天性胆管壁发育不良所致的胆管扩张,发病年龄在 10 岁以下者占 52%~81%。根据发生的部位不同分为五型:Ⅰ型,胆总管呈囊性扩张;Ⅱ型,胆总管局部呈憩室样扩张;Ⅲ型,胆总管囊肿突人十二指肠壁内;Ⅳ型,肝内外胆管的多发囊肿;Ⅴ型,局限于肝内胆管的囊肿,即 Calori 病。

典型 CT、MRI 表现:胆总管下段囊状、柱状或憩室状扩张,边缘光滑,壁薄而均匀。肝内胆管可无扩张或呈梭状扩张;增强扫描无强化,部分可见点状强化。若囊肿内出现壁结节及囊壁不规则增厚,增强扫描呈明显强化提示恶变(图 19-8-3)。

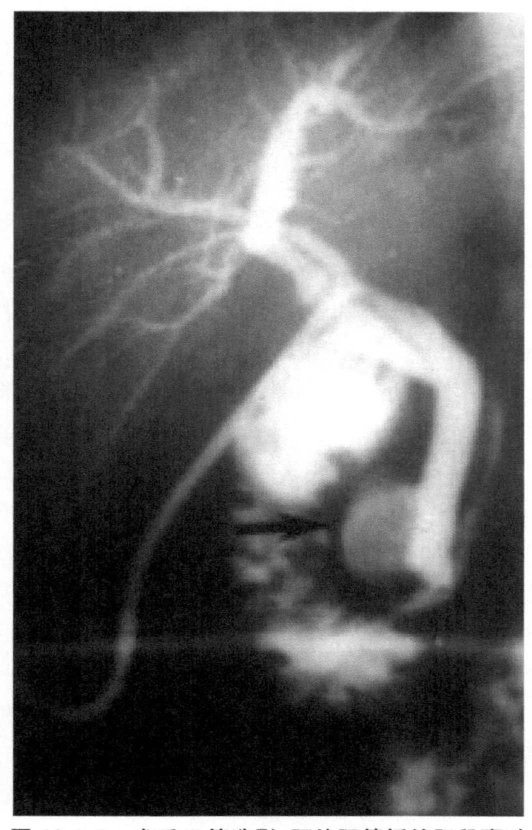

图 19-8-3 术后 T 管造影：肝外胆管括约肌段囊肿

除部分胆总管结石表现为高密度，十二指肠乳头憩室可见气 - 液平外，其他各种病变在 CT、MRI 上表现具有许多相似之处，故平扫鉴别困难（图 19-8-4）。

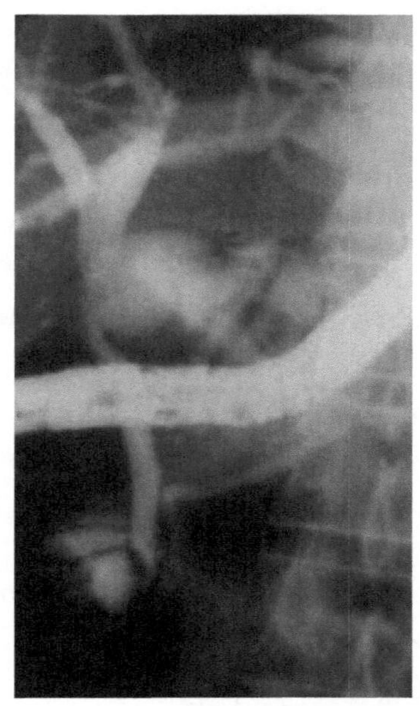

图 19-8-4 ERCP：轮廓不甚规则的肝外胆管括约肌段囊肿

（四）其他

1. 胰腺导管内乳头状黏液性肿瘤　导管内乳头状黏液性肿瘤罕见，好发于老年男性。按发生的部位可分为主胰管型、侧支胰管型和混合型。主胰管型主要表现为主胰管弥漫和 / 或节段扩张，伴有壁结节，常合并胰腺实质的萎缩，可伴分支胰管的扩张，当肿瘤位于胰头时可见肿瘤上段胆管扩张。分支型可见于胰腺各个部位，主要见于胰头和钩突，表现为和主胰管相交通的单房或多房囊性肿瘤，常伴有分隔和壁结节。ERCP 表现为扩张的胰管内可因伴有浓缩的黏液或肿瘤结节所致充盈缺损。

2. 胰腺分裂　是指胰腺发育过程中，两胰芽融合失败形成。伴有胰腺炎发生时表现为胰头腹侧或背侧局限性密度（信号）异常，增强扫描呈明显的延迟强化，偶可见到多房状表现，炎症吸收后可遗留不均匀脂肪沉积。

二、各种征象对胆胰共同管周围区病变的诊断价值

胆胰共同管周围区病变的主要影像表现可概述为直接征象和间接征象，其直接征象为胰头胆胰共同管部类圆形或伴分叶不规则软组织肿块，平扫时，

增强扫描时，肿块强化程度可表现为 3 种：不强化，主要见于胰头部假性囊肿、十二指肠乳头憩室、胆总管下段囊肿等；轻中度强化，主要见于胰腺黏液性囊腺瘤、胆胰共同管癌、十二指肠乳头癌、十二指肠间质瘤、胆管囊腺癌等；明显强化，主要见于胰腺内分泌肿瘤、十二指肠乳头炎、胆总管下段癌。

间接征象较多，概述为胰管、胆管的扩张常见扩张形式有“双管征”，最常见于胰头癌（扩张的双管分离）和胆胰共同管癌（扩张的双管靠近）。“三管征”是胆总管下段癌的特征性表现。“四管征”见于胰头癌。“胰管贯穿征”常见于胰腺炎性肿块。

胆总管下端及胰管形态改变：“靶征”“新月征”“杯口征”见于胆总管下段结石。“鼠尾状狭窄”可见于胆管癌及部分胆胰共同管癌。“截断征”常见于胰头癌、胆总管下段癌，其扩张的胰管或 / 和胆管末端突然截断，断端可呈“虫蚀”状、“鸟嘴”状及“鼠尾”状等形态，常伴有近端管腔扩张。“串珠样”改变常见于慢性炎症，同时多伴肿块处胰管渐行性、穿通性狭窄。胰腺周围渗出、肾周筋膜增厚可见于急、慢性胰腺炎。假性囊肿常见于胰腺炎，偶见于胰腺癌。钙化常见于慢性胰腺炎，也可见于胰管结石、

囊腺瘤等。

胰腺头部增大伴胰腺尾部萎缩，常见于胰头癌。

第二节 胆胰共同管假性肿瘤

Leese 等（1986）报告 49 例胆胰共同管周围肿瘤的内镜表现，其中 38 例为肿瘤，11 例为炎性非肿瘤性病变（假肿瘤）。只靠内镜观察难以区别二者。除了在肿瘤组胰管趋向于扩张，在假肿瘤组胆囊结石更为常见以外，两组的胆胰管造影表现基本类似。

在 34 例胆胰共同管肿瘤中，内镜活检做出正确诊断者为 28 例。11 例假性肿瘤中有 2 例由于内镜活检怀疑为肿瘤而行手术探查。在肿瘤组有 19 例行胰十二指肠切除术，7 例行分流手术，7 例内镜括约肌切开术，只有 5 例因未能成功地进行胆系引流而死亡，一年生存率为 44.7%。相反，在假肿瘤组，在内镜括约肌切开术后，平均追踪 24 个月（范围为 12~41 个月），只 1 例 89 岁老翁因其他不相关的原因死亡外，余皆健存。

胆胰共同管区的良性肿瘤包括：平滑肌纤维瘤、脂肪瘤、神经类肿瘤、血管瘤以及类癌。最常见的良性肿瘤是绒毛状腺瘤。

在临床病史、临床检查、血液学检查以及生化检查资料，在肿瘤组与假肿瘤组之间都互相重叠。对区别诊断有帮助之处是，在假肿瘤组均未扪及胆囊，而在肿瘤组中却有 42% 的病人可扪及胆囊，即 Courvoisiers 定律阳性。十二指肠镜检查两组所见类似，它们都有肝外胆管扩张。在肿瘤组胰管扩张较重，但这点帮助只适用于少数病人。11 例假肿瘤病人中有 6 例在 ERCP 检查时发现胆囊结石，而只有 2 例结石出现于肝外胆管，另 2 例以前曾行胆囊切除术。这似乎提示病因学因素，可能与结石通过胆胰共同管期间，造成炎症变化，导致假肿瘤形成。Baggenstoss（1938）报告 100 例尸解病例有 18 例腺瘤性增生，他指出，在息肉、腺瘤状增生和十二指肠乳头的低度的乳头状癌之间十分类似。此假说是进步的，因为乳头是一个区域，是乳头黏膜的局灶性（酶和胆盐）刺激的上皮移行区，在息肉状增生的发展中承担重要作用。Leese 等（1986）报告病例称此假说甚为正确。

如果怀疑内镜所见为恶性者，可在内镜括约肌切开术后几天，再进行反复的内镜活检，这样，常常可以增加诊断恶性病变的正确性。胆胰共同管组织周围炎症反应的吸收，再次活检查结果则大不相同。如仍然怀疑恶性，可在作根治术前再行手术活检冰冻切片确诊。

第三节 PTCD 术中对比剂胰管逆流与共同管的关系探讨

胆胰下端括约肌功能、结构正常时，胆汁与胰液通过共同管或各自进入十二指肠，不会相互返流到胰管和胆管，否则可造成急慢性胰腺炎、胆管结石、慢性胆管炎、胆囊炎甚至胰腺、胆管、胆囊癌变。近年不少研究表明胆胰管异常合流与上述疾病关系密切。

有作者通过观察 134 例梗阻性黄疸患者的经皮肝穿胆管造影（PTC）片，选出有胰管逆流的 39 例，并测量其共同管的长度，进行分析。目的是通过对合并胰管返流的胆管病变患者，观察其与共同管的关系，验证以往文献的推测。

一些作者统计 50 例成年国人离体标本，把胆总管、胰管的汇合方式分为 4 型：Ⅰ型，两管完全分开，分别开口于十二指肠的不同部位，较罕见；Ⅱ型，两管并行进入十二指肠壁并在同一十二指肠乳头部分别开口，较少见；Ⅲ型，两管通过胆胰共同管进入十二指肠，此型以是否长于 12 mm 又分 2 种亚型，ⅢA（长共同管型），共同管长度 >12 mm，和ⅢB（短共同管型）。Ⅲ型的胆总管和胰管汇合成胆胰共同管，斜行穿过十二指肠壁，终止于十二指肠乳头口。胆胰共同管的平均长度，文献中无公认的数据，根据部分学者对 23 例成年国人新鲜标本解剖测量发现，随着共同管延长，胆、胰管汇合角增大。

胆总管胰管汇合部，由四部分括约肌共同构成胆胰管下端括约肌，调节胆囊充盈，控制胆汁胰液的排出，维持胆管系统和胰管系统的正常压力。胆总管括约肌为发达的平滑肌组织，位于胆总管与胰管汇合之前；胰管括约肌为一薄层环行肌；共同管括约肌环绕在共同管周围；纵肌束为一薄的扇形肌膜组织，位于胆总管和胰管之间作为共同管壁，研究发现此结构作用十分关键（图 19-8-5）。

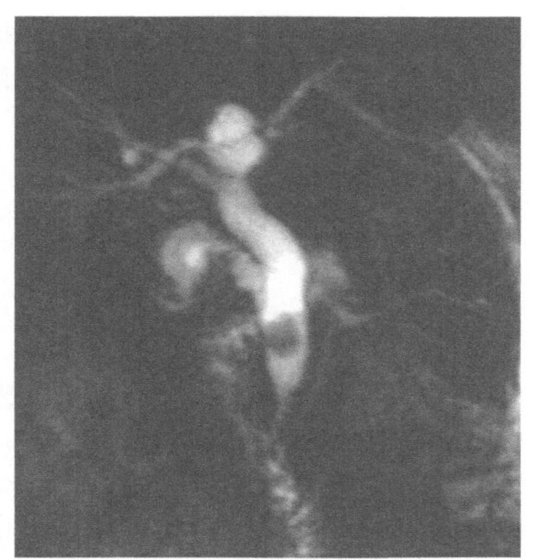

图 19-8-5　MRCP：肝外胆管扩张，肝外胆管结石，正常的括约肌段清楚可见横行的三条绒毛瓣引起的细线状充盈缺损，导致括约肌段呈现锯齿状外形

一般认为对比剂胰管返流与两种因素有关：纵肌束缺如；胆胰管下端括约肌功能障碍。

共同管较短的病例，其胆总管、胰管汇合前走行近似平行，胆胰管汇合的角度较小，因而纵肌束形成一层薄而长的薄膜，起到活瓣的作用；而共同管较长的病例因其胰胆管汇合位置高，角度大，汇合前缺乏平行走行阶段，使纵肌束汇合后部分短而宽，造成胰管出口闭合不全，活瓣功能丧失，结果胰液在较高的压力下较易向胆管逆流。

胆胰括约肌功能障碍也是导致胆胰逆流的主要原因（Hakamada，1997）。胆胰下端括约肌功能异常见于两种情况：胆胰下端括约肌狭窄，由于慢性炎症和／或胆总管纤维化导致部分或完全括约肌狭窄；胆胰下端括约肌功能障碍，即括约肌高压带间歇性功能性阻塞，由括约肌痉挛、肥厚、去神经所致。

胆胰下端括约肌功能异常的动力学改变包括：由于胆总管末端、胰管纤维化或痉挛导致基础压升高，此改变是诊断胆胰括约肌功能障碍的金标准；逆行性收缩波增加；周期性收缩频率增加。

括约肌功能障碍病因十分复杂，由于受神经 - 体液调节，有研究证实胆总管周围分布的神经对胆胰下端括约肌有明显的抑制作用，并与胆管的压力关系密切。

以上研究可以提示，胆总管、胰管高位汇合，汇合角较大，减弱了纵肌束的调节作用，胰液返流入胆管，导致胆管的慢性炎症或纤维化，进而引起胆胰下端括约肌功能障碍，胆总管、胰管压力升高，而胆胰管压力升高促进神经 - 体液的正反馈调节，进一步加重了胆胰括约肌功能障碍。

纵肌束缺如及胆胰括约肌功能障碍使胰液和胆汁相互返流成为可能，并导致多种胆管、胰管疾病，胆汁和胰液相互混合后，被胆汁激活的胰淀粉酶及胆汁内由卵磷脂氧化后生成的脱磷酸卵磷脂，具有强烈的细胞毒作用。

胆管壁及胰管壁在胆胰混合液的长期刺激下发生慢性炎症、增生，及肠上皮化生，并促进胆结石形成，胆结石和胆管慢性炎症也可相互促进，加速疾病的进展。Hakamada 等（1997）总结的大宗病例显示，经长期随访（15 个月至 20 年，平均 18 年），在慢性炎症长期刺激下，胆管发生癌变的概率约 7.4%。

根据该组病例共同管的长度分析，可以认为，由于胆管疾病导致梗阻性黄疸有多种病因，但与共同管的长度关系密切，其机制即由于共同管较长导致纵肌束构造不完全，胆、胰管汇合角度大，部分胆汁、胰液异位返流，使胆胰括约肌功能障碍进行性加重，最终可导致严重后果。该组病例共同管的平均长度大于正常人；胆管原发病变组与继发及外压性胆管病变组相比，共同管差异有显著性，说明胆管疾病与共同管长度关系密切。该研究更证实以前的研究，即共同管异常可导致多种胆胰管疾病（图 19-8-6）。

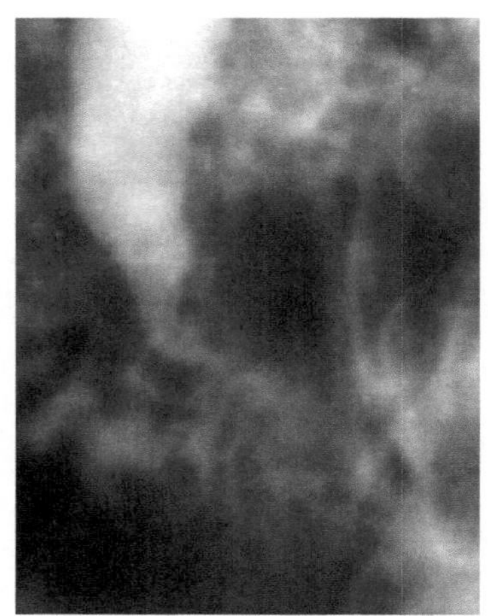

图 19-8-6　ERCP：肝外胆管扩张，肝外胆管括约肌段外形呈不规则锯齿状，提示存在绒毛瓣。

第四节 共同管的暂时性水肿或痉挛

Thompson 等(1987)报告,在 53 例前瞻性连续性肝外胆管探查术病人的探查后胆管造影中,有 12 例无对比剂进入十二指肠,其中 11 例进行胆管镜检查,观察胆管的解剖情况与胆胰共同管来评价病人。发现 10 例病人共同管并未扩张,共同管的暂时性水肿或痉挛继发于手术性创伤、结石的去除、或其他疾病,皆为内镜做出诊断,每例病人均行手术和术后胆管造影证实。这些病人术后行胆管造影随访,均观察到共同管开放,胆汁自由流入十二指肠,无狭窄或结石。上述资料说明,手术胆管镜可以观察和评价胆系及胆胰共同管的解剖或病理情况。

第五节 共同管区的误诊

胆总管远端解剖结构细小,含胆汁量少,产生的信号弱, MRCP 显示共同管区十分困难。为提高该区域的显示,一种有效的方法是检查前口服冷开水,以充盈和扩张十二指肠,这样,乳头部炎症所致的小突起能被很好地显示出来。

分析常规 T_1WI 有助于排除共同管和共同管周围肿块性病变。

然而,鉴别共同管小肿瘤与炎症所致的乳头部狭窄在所有病例都难以作到。

其他误诊与嵌顿于乳头内的小结石有关(若结石周围无液体包围,则显示结石非常困难),也与胆总管远端不典型的形态结构有关,它可类似于嵌顿的结石。对于这两种情况,有必要分析原始图像,以提高诊断正确率。

第六节 十二指肠壁内胆胰共同管内异位胰腺致梗阻性黄疸

详见本书 本卷 本篇 第一章 第五节 十二指肠壁内胆胰共同管内异位胰腺致梗阻性黄疸。

第九章　连接区的检查技术

第一节　MRCP 与低位梗阻定位、定性

病变的定位：在低位胆系梗阻定位诊断中，整个胰管均扩张则提示病变多位于胆胰共同管；整个胰管未显影或显影但不扩张，则提示病变可能居胆胰共同管之上方，未侵及或不全侵及胆胰共同管；胰头段胰管未显影而体尾段扩张，则多提示为胰头病变；少数病例的胰头段主胰管扩张而体尾段不扩张，乃因主副胰管相通，开口于十二指肠副乳头所致。

定性分析应注意之处：MRCP 定性诊断准确率在 64%~98% 之间。其中对低信号结石诊断具有特异性，但应注意：①结石好多发，一组 23 例胆系结石中 18 例并存胆囊结石，11 例见有左、右肝管及总肝管结石，7 例胆总管内结石呈串珠状；②图像重建后，胆汁高信号往往掩盖细小结石的低信号，以至见不到结石影，该组 7 例经三维最大强度投影重建后结石未显影，经 5~7mm 层厚选择性最大强度投影重建后见到结石影，而源图像显示小结石更加明显，因此必须结合源图像诊断；③腔内血块、小乳头状瘤、息肉等病变在重 T_2WI 上亦呈低信号，与结石信号类似，给鉴别诊断带来困难。

胆胰管十二指肠连接区癌可在胆管梗阻端或高信号的十二指肠腔内见到低信号肿瘤影，反向摄片病变显示更佳，源图像上更清晰易辨，如伴胰管明显扩张，定位定性诊断具一定特异性。一组 5 例胆胰管十二指肠连接区癌源图像上见到明显低信号病变影，故诊断正确，1 例十二指肠乳头部腺瘤呈混杂低信号，误诊为胆胰管十二指肠连接区癌。

MRCP 对胰腺段胆管癌、胰头癌、转移癌的鉴别比较困难，该组 2 例胆管癌均诊断错误。此外，对低位炎性梗阻性病变，因多伴有结石或胰腺炎，虽居胆胰共同管处，但其影像表现复杂，诊断也较困难。该组 2 例胆胰管十二指肠连接区炎性病变 MRCP 未能作出定性诊断，经十二指肠电子内镜及病理活检诊断为炎症。MRCP 诊断胆胰管十二指肠连接区炎性病变应在明确除外其他病变，特别是除外腔内小的胆胰共同管癌后，方可考虑，必要时应进行随访，在此，ERCP 较 MRCP 优越。

MRCP 诊断低位梗阻的优势和限制：无创性 MRCP 开始用于临床即显示出其优越性，虽然在治疗上不能取代 ERCP 和经皮经肝胆管造影（PTC），但在诊断上它基本可替代作为纯诊断手段的 ERCP，或作为内镜及介入治疗前的初步检查，使其更具目的性；在 ERCP 存在技术困难和解剖因素影响不能进行插管时，MRCP 检查非常有效；MRCP 较 ERCP 和 PTC 具有明显的优势，它可获得相关的肝脏和胰腺的 MR 断面图像，能直接观察到管腔内外病变情况，因此 MRCP 诊断低位胆系梗阻性疾病潜力巨大。

MRCP 尚存在的一些不足：重建后图像容易掩盖小病变，必须结合源图像诊断；对胆管内病变信号表现缺乏特异性，易导致误、漏诊；对恶性梗阻性疾病定性诊断尚存在一定困难，有待深入总结；对炎性病变诊断特异性差；不能如同 ERCP 那样进行活检或治疗。

就像普通胆管造影，胆胰共同管成像目前还不可能区分嵌入的结石与胆胰共同管内在的病变。但是，MRCP 仍不失为一种无创性诊断低位胆系梗阻性疾病的有效技术。

第二节 脂餐和胰泌素刺激后的MRCP

MRCP不需对比剂即可清楚显示胆胰管系统的解剖形态。目前对肝外胆管及主胰管的显示率达100%,对非扩张的肝内胆管外1/3的显示率也超过90%。胆总管远端与胰管汇合后形成胆胰共同管,此区较短,且周围有胆胰括约肌收缩,管内含液很少,甚至无液体,常规MRCP显示该部位往往受限。

Koike等(2000)和Cappeliez等(2000)用脂餐和胰泌素刺激后,进行药物动力学的MRCP检查,可清楚显示该部,如动态扫描,还可在一定程度上观察乳头的功能状态。

正常情况下或胰泌素刺激下十二指肠腔内含有一定量的液体,因此MRCP除可清楚显示胆胰管系统外,还可显示十二指肠结构,从而帮助分辨共同管,还可判断胆系外病变对胆胰管系统的影响。利用同层动态MRCP可很好评价胆胰括约肌功能,提高对共同管及其周围病变的检出率,是常规MRCP形态学研究的重要补充,具有很好的临床应用前景。

MRCP可以同时显示胆系及胰管,对胆胰管的显示也基本达到了ERCP的效果。对胆系病变尤其是对胆系结石的诊断价值已有较多的论述,目前已基本替代诊断性ERCP,成为观察胆管形态的最好的方法。

对胰腺分裂、环状胰腺等先天异常及急性胰腺炎、慢性胰腺炎、胰腺癌、胰腺黏液性肿瘤等胰腺良、恶性病变也有较高的诊断价值,可替代或部分替代ERCP、CT的作用。

MRCP的另一个潜在的用途是胆囊切除术前显示胆管是否有发育变异以减少术中胆管损伤的危险性。由于十二指肠内液体的存在或于检查前饮水,使MR对胆胰管成像的同时,亦使十二指肠显示,达到了类似十二指肠造影的目的。

第十章　胆胰管异常连接

第一节　胆胰管异常连接与 MRCP

胆胰管异常连接系日本学者 Kozumi（1916）首次提出，是指胰管和胆管在十二指肠壁外合流的先天性异常，常形成过长的共同管，十二指肠乳头部括约肌不能作用于胆胰管合流部而导致胰液与胆汁相互混合而逆流入胆管，导致胆系及胰腺的一系列病理变化。

研究表明胆胰管异常连接与许多胆、胰腺疾病和肝脏损伤（如先天性胆总管囊肿、胆石症、胆囊炎、胆囊癌、胰腺炎、胰腺癌、肝硬化等）密切相关。因此诊断胆胰管异常连接对预防相关疾病的发生至关重要。自胆胰管异常连接被提出以来，其诊断标准一直未能统一。共同管的长度是关键性指标，但判定共同管长度的标准也不尽一致。多数研究者认为成人共同管长度≥ 15 mm，小儿≥ 5 mm，即可诊断为胆胰管异常连接。此外，胆胰管异常连接的诊断还应将共同管的长度与胰、胆管汇合部是否位于狭窄部近端来结合判断。

在诊断胆胰管异常连接疾病的检查方法中，主要有内镜逆行胆胰管造影（ERCP）和磁共振胆胰管成像（MRCP）；ERCP 是诊断胆胰管异常连接的金标准，但为有创性检查，且易导致相关并发症。MRCP 是发展最快的影像学检查技术之一，目前广泛应用于临床。由于 MRCP 的无创性，且可多方位清楚显示胆胰管解剖结构，在诊断胆胰管异常连接及相关疾病中的价值获得了临床的认可，并已成为诊断胆胰管异常连接的首选检查方法。

一、胆胰管异常连接的分型与 MRCP 表现

目前胆胰管异常连接有多种不同的分型标准。Yamauchi 等（1987）根据胰及胆管汇合方式的主次分为：胆 - 胰型（B-P 型），即胆总管汇入主胰管形成共同管，此型多合并有胆管扩张；胰 - 胆型（P-B 型），即主胰管汇入胆总管，多合并有胆系结石。

Todeni 等（1984）根据胆胰管的汇合角度将胆胰管异常连接分为 4 型：①直角汇入型（符合 B-P 型）；②锐角汇入型（符合 B-P 型）；③复杂汇入型；④正常角度型。

Komi 等（1984）将胆胰管异常连接分为：A 型，胆管汇入胰管；B 型，胰管汇入胆管；C 型，副胰管同时显影。

随后，Komi 等（1992）根据共同管有无扩张及胆胰管汇合角度，将胆胰管异常连接分为 3 型：即Ⅰ型（B-P 型）、Ⅱ型（P-B 型）及Ⅲ型（复杂型）。Ⅰ型指胆总管与胰管成直角相汇，根据共同管是否扩张进一步分为Ⅰ A 型（不合并扩张）和Ⅰ B 型（合并扩张）。Ⅱ型指胆总管与胰管成锐角相汇，根据共同管是否扩张进一步分为Ⅱ A 型（不合并扩张）和Ⅱ B 型（合并扩张）。Ⅲ型指副胰管显影，有或无复杂的管网连接。根据共同管有无扩张、主副胰管是否相通等进一步分为 3 种亚型：Ⅲ A 型（胰腺分裂合并胆管扩张），Ⅲ B 型（主胰管缺如）和Ⅲ C 型。Ⅲ C 型又分为Ⅲ C1 型（主胰管和副胰管之间有细小的交通分支）、Ⅲ C2 型（共同管、主胰管和副胰管三者管径相通）和Ⅲ C3 型（管道系统部分或全部扩张）。

虽然目前胆胰管异常连接的分型各异，但总体分类标准一致，影像学上多采用 B-P 型、P-B 型、复杂型的分型方法。

有作者认为 B-P 型在 MRCP 上主要表现为胆管呈囊状或梭形扩张，扩张下方的胆管末端常有明显狭窄段，且以近似直角或钝角与主胰管汇合。P-B 型在 MRCP 亦表现为胆管扩张呈球囊状或梭形，但扩张程度较轻，近连接处之末端胆管可有轻度或无

明确狭窄段,胰管与胆总管多呈锐角汇合。复杂型较少见,尚未见相关MRCP表现的报道(图19-10-1)。

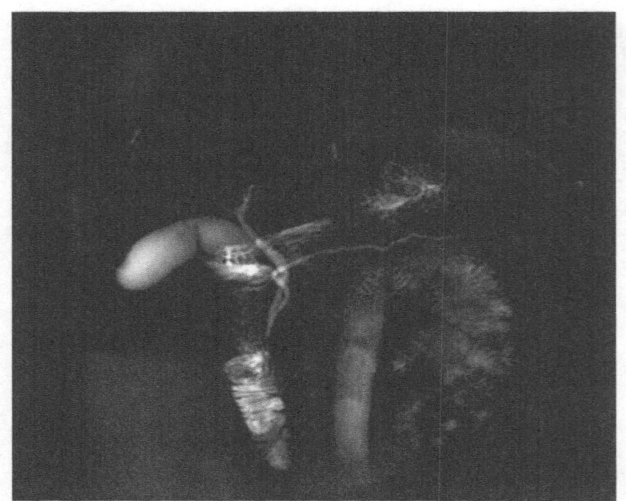

图19-10-1 MRCP:胆胰管异常连接:胆胰共同管长度远超过8mm

MRCP在胆胰管异常连接及其相关疾病中的应用

MRCP在胆胰管异常连接的应用:Park等(2005)通过分析MRCP和ERCP对胆胰管异常连接的诊断价值,发现MRCP的敏感性和特异性均很高。MRCP可显示90%的胆胰管异常连接共同管长度、合流形式及胆管扩张情况,对胆管扩张型胆胰管异常连接及相关疾病的显示效果与ERCP相近或优于ERCP,是诊断胆胰管异常连接的可靠方法。对超声检查提示胆管扩张、不明原因的胰腺炎或上腹痛病人(尤其年轻病人),应首选MRCP筛查。但MRCP仍有局限性,如共同管相对稍短的胆胰管异常连接诊断困难,胰管分支和胆管外周分支显示空间分辨力稍低,不能清楚显示婴幼儿的肝内胆管和胰管结构。

此外,由于MRCP是屏气扫描,共同管长度易随胆胰管下端括约肌周期性变化而变化,测出的共同管长度要比ERCP短。但MRCP局限性随3D MRCP新技术而得到改善,必将对胆胰管异常连接的诊断提供帮助。

MRCP在先天性胆总管扩张症的应用:MRCP是一种无创、便捷、有效的检查方法,能清楚地显示胆胰管解剖结构,并对胆管囊肿做出准确的诊断、分型及定位,其定位准确率可达100%,并能清楚显示胆管囊肿的合并症。先天性胆管扩张症在MRCP上有特征性表现,即扩张的胆管与胆管相通,胆管扩张的形态、位置也有其特点,但有时需与肝囊肿、胰腺囊肿等其他上腹部囊性病变相鉴别。目前对MRCP能否取代ERCP诊断先天性胆总管扩张症仍有争议,部分研究者认为MRCP可完全取代ERCP诊断先天性胆总管扩张症,但也有研究者认为MRCP对胰管及胆胰管汇合处的解剖结构显示模糊,且MRCP有过度评价胆管的狭窄程度。胃肠道内的气体、血管搏动伪影等均可导致胆管的假性狭窄。对婴幼儿囊肿型胆管扩张症,MRCP显示胆胰管异常连接欠佳。

MRCP在胆囊炎和胆石症的应用:目前,超声被公认为临床筛选胆系结石的首选方法,但对于胆总管结石,MRCP明显优于B超。MRCP诊断胆总管结石的敏感度为100%,特异度为91%。MRCP可以判断胆系结石的部位、数目、大小及形态,同时可以判断梗阻部位及胆总管的扩张情况,还可清楚显示增厚水肿的胆囊壁及胆囊周围的积液,从而有助于正确诊断急性胆囊炎及其并发症,鉴别并发黄疸的原因。MRCP具有无创性、安全性及较高的诊断准确性,在胆总管结石的诊断方面具有明显优势。但MRCP也有一定的局限性,如胆管内血块及气泡均表现为低信号,与结石鉴别困难,同时还对结石的诊断容易出现较高的假阴性,应注意随访。

MRCP在胆系肿瘤的应用:MRCP能清楚显示病变部位及胆胰管扩张或狭窄程度,同时还可显示病变部位远近端及周围的情况,尤其在显示胆胰管走行、肝内外胆管树及管腔方面具有直观性。在3D MRCP成像上还可清晰显示肿块浸润的范围及梗阻上下两端的胆道状况,对确定分型和诊断有较多的帮助。Manfredi等(2001)研究表明MRCP对肝门部胆管癌术前分型准确率达91.3%。MRCP的缺陷在于空间分辨率不如ERCP。当胆管内有支架或胆系积气、出血和腹水时易导致MRCP诊断误差。因此,在诊断胆系肿瘤时,MRCP应结合MRI其他序列检查以提高诊断率。

MRCP在胰腺炎的应用:MRCP诊断胰腺炎的准确率较高,可较好地显示胰腺炎胰管的状态及假性囊肿,胰腺炎MRCP特征表现为“胰管穿透征”,即主胰管完整并连续地穿过炎性肿块而无中断。此外,MRCP还能明确主胰管与胆总管的汇合分型,清晰显示胆胰管树的形态。但MRCP空间分辨力较低,对胰管的轻微狭窄或扩张难以清楚显示。

MRCP 在胰腺癌的应用：MRCP 诊断胆胰系恶性占位的敏感度达 100%，特异度和准确度达 99%，明显优于超声及 CT。MRCP 不仅能够显示胰腺病变部位、主胰管的狭窄或扩张程度、囊状肿瘤形态及肿瘤内部结构，还可清楚地显示肿瘤侵犯范围及与周围结构的关系，有助于肿瘤的分期和定性诊断。但 MRCP 对总胆管下段、胆胰管连接区和胰头部恶性肿瘤准确定位性差，MRCP 必须结合 MRI 其他序列检查才能做出综合判断。同时，MRCP 也是鉴别胰腺癌和胰腺炎的重要方法。胰头癌在 MRCP 上的典型表现为胰管和胆总管呈连续性扩张，并在肿块处截断，肝内外胆管均扩张呈“软藤征”。

胆胰管异常连接及相关疾病的检出率的增加，对提高胆胰管异常连接的诊断和预防治疗相关疾病具有重大的临床意义。但胆胰管异常连接的分型及 MRCP 的诊断标准尚未统一，胆胰管异常连接相关疾病的致病机制有待明确，这需要研究者对胆胰管异常连接的临床特点、实验室检查、影像学检查等方面做进一步的研究，以便制定统一的标准，有利于胆胰管异常连接及相关疾病的早期发现、及时正确的治疗。近年来随着 MRCP 技术的不断发展与成熟，主胰管和胆总管的位置关系、共同管长度、结构以及是否合并胆管扩张已能清晰显示。MRCP 作为一种无创性的检查方法，已逐渐取代 ERCP，有望成为胆胰管异常连接及相关疾病诊断的首选检查方法。

第二节　关于胆胰管异常连接的形成

胰腺起源于中肠的肝憩室，由腹侧和背侧胰原基共同发育而成。腹胰由左侧腹胰原基和右侧腹胰原基融合形成。在早期，这两个原基均有各自的原基管汇入肝憩室。腹胰形成后，左侧腹胰管逐渐消失；约于胚胎第 6~7 周，腹胰绕肠轴旋转与背胰融合。在此过程中，若腹胰或肝憩室发育不良，就有可能形成胆胰管异常连接。例如，左侧腹胰原基和右侧腹胰原基融合后，若前者的原基管不消失，或同时存在肝外胆管下端闭塞，则肝外胆管通过左侧腹胰管与胰管系统交通，形成胆胰管异常连接和先天性胆管囊肿等（大井至，1982）。

Wong 和 Lister（1981）对 32 例 6~22 周龄人胚的胆胰管部作连续切片证实，在胚胎第 8 周前，胆总管和主胰管在十二指肠外衔接；此后，胆胰管连接部逐渐移入十二指肠腔。至出生后，此种移动仍在进行。若因某种原因使此种正常内移中止，即形成胆胰管异常连接。此时，影像学上可见肝外胆管和主胰管在十二指肠壁外汇合，共同管过长，胆胰管连接角较钝（图 19-10-2）。

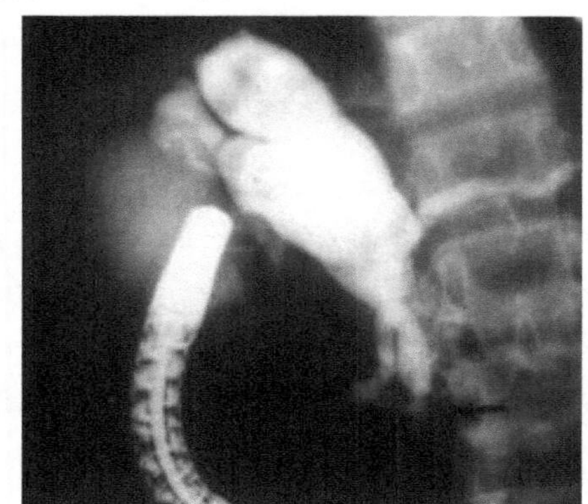

图 19-10-2　ERCP：复杂型胆胰管异常连接，肝外胆管囊状扩张明显，主胰管显著扩张

第三节　胆胰管异常连接

胆胰管异常连接是指主胰管和肝外胆管在十二指肠壁外汇合，胆胰管下端功能失调，引起胆汁和胰液混流，继而导致一系列胆胰疾病，这是一种先天性异常。

十二指肠乳头开口位置代表胚胎早期肝憩室的发生部位，因乳头位置定位于胚胎 22 天，而胆胰管汇合发生于胚胎 5~6 周的腹胰背胰融合阶段。由此推测胚胎早期肝憩室发生异位可能是胆胰管异常连接的致病因素之一；异位使腹胰与背胰间距增大，在二者融合过程中，胆胰管汇合形成的共同管和胆总管受到牵拉，导致共同管过长。

Arima 和 Akita（1979）将胆胰管异常连接与异

常长的共同管分开讨论。我们认为,事实上,从解剖学观点看,两者相互依存,不可分割。因为,十二指肠乳头范围有限,若胆胰管在十二指肠壁外汇合,势必引起共同管伸长,反之亦然。

自 Babbitt 报道先天性胆管囊肿合并胆胰管异常连接,提出新的病因学观点以来,这一异常连接及其与胆胰系疾病的病因学联系愈益得到重视。现在已认识到,胆胰管异常连接不仅可合并先天性胆管囊肿,而且与胆囊癌、胆管癌、胆系结石及胰腺炎等之间也有很大的相关性。并且先天性胆管囊肿又是一公认的影响胆系癌发生的重要因素。

胆胰管异常连接的分类:确定胆胰管的连接异常以后,需进一步对胆胰管异常连接进行分类诊断。胆胰管异常连接的分类方法不统一。

古味等(1977)将胆胰管异常连接分为四类,并统计 183 例 ERCP 资料,此四类在成人和儿童分别占的比例如下:①胆总管汇入胰管;成人 64%, 儿童 65%;②胰管汇入胆总管;成人 27%, 儿童 7%;③胰管分为二支,分别开口于十二指肠,而胆总管汇入其中一支胰管;成人 2%, 儿童 17%;④复杂连接;成人 7%, 儿童 11%。

Kimura 等(1981)把胆胰管异常连接分为:A 型:P → B(胰→胆连接,主胰管注入肝外胆管)型,和 B 型:B → P(胆→胰连接,肝外胆管注入主胰管)型。但此两种类型往往不能包含全部胆胰管异常连接。有些病例很难划归某一类型,如总胆管注入主胰管钩突支,总胆管注入主胰管而副胰管流入正常的十二指肠乳头等。这些病例的病理关系比较复杂,巫北海与吕维富(1993)将之划作胆胰管异常连接的复杂型。

Kimura 等(1985)报告 65 例胆胰管异常连接,其中 P → B 型和 B → P 型分别为 42 例(64.6%)和 23 例(35.4%)。巫北海与吕维富(1993)报告 59 例胆胰管异常连接, P → B 型和 B → P 型分别为 34 例(57.6%)和 18 例(30.5%),复杂型 7 例(11.9%)。

古味(1991)在其旧的分类法基础上进一步提出新的分类。1 型:1a,胆总管汇入主胰管;1b,在 1a 基础上有共同管扩张。2 型:2a,主胰管汇入胆总管;2b:在 2a 基础上有共同管扩张。3 型:3a,副胰管直接汇入十二指肠,主胰管汇入胆总管;3b,主胰管汇入胆总管后,二者又分别开口于十二指肠;3c1,胆总管分支汇入主胰管,胆总管和主胰管分别开口于十二指肠;3c2,主胰管呈弓形分支,分别开口于十二指肠,胆总管汇入其中一侧支上;3c3,在 3c2 基础上有主胰管弓形分支扩张。

X 线直接法胆胰造影及诊断标准:直接法胆胰造影包括 ERCP、PTC 及术中与术后胆胰管造影等。胆胰管异常连接的诊断,需肯定胰管和胆管在十二指肠壁外汇合,合并其他胆胰系病变的存在,同时除外该区及邻近的肿瘤、结石、炎症,及十二指肠乳头区憩室等因素所致胆胰管连接区后天性形态学的改变。环状胰腺及胆胰管双开口者一般不属于本症之列。

Nagata 等(1985)诊断胆胰管异常连接的标准是:① X 线直接法胆胰管造影片上见胰管和胆管在胆胰管下端括约肌形成的切迹以上汇合;②胆胰管共同管长度大于或等于 15mm;③胆汁内胰淀粉酶水平大于或等于 10 000IU。

胆胰管汇合之共同管长度的异常判断标准不尽一致:Misra(1990)认为共同管长度大于或等于 8mm 即属异常长共同管;而 Kimura 和 Ono 等的标准分别为大于 15mm 和大于 6mm。日本胆胰管异常连接研究会认为,成人共同管长于 10mm,小儿共同管长于 4mm 诊断为异常长共同管比较确切。共同管进入十二指肠壁的角度也可以影响测量的结果。

有学者对 100 具成人尸体检查结果显示,正常共同管的长度平均为 4.4 mm。多数学者测量后认为,成人共同管长度 >5 mm 即可诊断为胆胰管异常连接。有作者报道胆胰管下端括约肌长度平均为 6 mm,超出此范围共同管将失去该括约肌的控制。

我们认为,在成人,共同管长于和等于 6mm 划作异常较为妥当,同时,共同管长度的评价还须综合考虑胆胰管连接的形态、年龄、体质、检查体位、摄片时呼吸时相、投影学与摄片当时情况,及放大率等诸多有关因素。

目前诊断标准为:①胆胰管在十二指肠壁外高位汇合,十二指肠降段切线位摄影时共同管长度 ≥ 6mm;②肝外胆管与主胰管汇合角度增大(>45°),胆汁内胰淀粉酶含量高(>1000U/L);③肝外胆管与主胰管之间存在未退化的背侧胰管等异常交通,导致胆汁和胰液逆流。具备其中一条即可诊断。

胆胰管异常连接与胆管扩张的关系:Arnolds(1906)首先报道先天性胆管扩张与胆胰管异常连接间的联系。自 Babbitt(1969)报告先天性胆管扩张合并胆胰管异常连接提出新的病因学观点以来,胆胰管异常连接与胆胰系病变的病因学联系愈益受到重视。

此后，许多作者相继作了报道。Jona、Ono、Sameshima 报道先天性胆管囊肿合并胆胰管异常连接分别占 100%、68% 和 47%。Kimura 等（1976）认为胆管注入胰管类型的胆胰管异常连接者更倾向于合并先天性胆管囊肿。奥平（1990）指出此类胆管囊肿的胆管壁上可合并胆管癌或同时合并胆系结石。Okada（1990）调查 100 例胆胰管异常连接合并先天性胆管囊肿病人，其中圆柱状扩张和囊状扩张分别占 23 例和 77 例（图 19-10-3）。

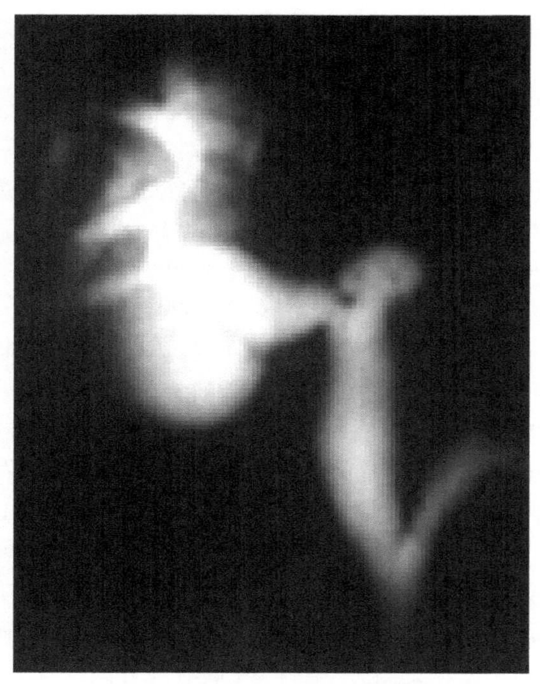

图 19-10-3 PTC：动物（狗）试验：人为手术造成胆胰管异常连接后，导致肝内外胆管明显扩张

胆胰管异常连接合并先天性胆管囊肿的发生机制研究甚多。Babbitt 等认为，可能系异常长共同管的胆胰管括约肌发育不良致肝外胆管和主胰管的压力梯度逆转，使胰液流入肝外胆管，诱发胆管炎反复发作，管壁增厚和狭窄，最终导致扩张。Oguchi（1988）研究胆管壁的病理学结构，发现多数胆胰管异常连接合并胆管囊肿者，均有胆管上皮增生，替代单层柱状上皮细胞，且有小圆细胞浸润及管壁纤维化。Fujii（1990）应用肝胆管核素显像证实此类患者胆汁在肝外胆管中滞留的时间显著延长，胆汁流过十二指肠大乳头的时间也显著延迟。Kimura 等（1985）和 Misra（1990）等推测，可能系高位汇合的胆胰管失去胆胰管下端括约肌的调控，导致出现胆管扩张等一系列胆胰疾病。

胆胰管异常连接与胆系癌：Kimura 等（1976）认为，胆→胰型连接者更倾向于合并先天性胆总管囊状扩张，之后又发现在胆管癌合并胆胰管异常连接的病例中，胆总管囊状扩张最为多见；而在胆囊癌的病例中，胆总管多不扩张，且胆胰管连接形式多为胰→胆型（92.9%）。

Aoki 等（1987）的 569 例胆胰管异常连接中，大多数有肝外胆管扩张（囊状 44%，梭状 23%，圆锥状 17%），131 例（23%）有胆系癌，其中胆囊癌、胆管癌和肿瘤来源不明者分别为 93 例、31 例和 7 例，253 例胆管囊状扩张病人中只有 30 例（12%）与胆系癌（胆囊癌 9 例，胆管癌 21 例）有关，但 80 例无胆管扩张的病人中 49 例（61%）有胆系癌（胆囊癌 44 例，胆管癌 4 例，肿瘤来源不清 1 例）。Yamauchi 等（1987）对 24 例胆胰管异常连接研究的结果与 Aoki 等的结果接近。Tanaka 等（1993）将这种高的癌肿发生率解释为：胰液返流入胆囊，引起慢性胆囊炎伴小肠上皮化生，形成癌前病变，进而发展为分化癌；胆囊内胆汁的浓缩机制也可以促进癌的转化。青木春夫（1990）统计 569 例胆胰管异常连接中的 131 例胆系癌，其中胆管癌、胆囊癌和癌肿原发部位不清者分别占 54%、16.3% 及 12%。Ono 和 Kato 分别报道，在胆系癌中以胆囊癌多见（占 57%~77%）。在胆管癌合并胆胰管异常连接的病例中，肝外胆管以囊状扩张最为多见；而在胆囊癌病例中，肝外胆管多不扩张，且胆胰管异常连接的类型多为胰管注入胆管型（占 92.9%）。

Shimada（1991）用氨基丙基键洗脱药桶及液相色谱分析仪提取和分离胆汁中的磷脂，胆胰管异常连接病例胆汁中溶血卵磷脂的浓度和比例以及磷脂酶 A_2，淀粉酶活性等均显著增高。该作者认为，返流胰液中的磷脂酶 A_2 可使卵磷脂转化为溶血性卵磷脂，后者具有细胞毒性作用，损害细胞，引起胆系黏膜增生及化生，最终导致出现胆系癌。Chijiiwa 等（1993）研究 1586 例 ERCP 资料，胆胰管异常连接占 1.56%，75% 的胆胰管异常连接患者合并胆总管囊肿，而无胆总管囊肿的胆胰管异常连接患者中 67% 患有胆囊癌。胆胰管异常连接与先天性胆总管囊肿密切相关（92%），而有胆总管囊肿的患者中 9% 伴有胆囊癌或胆管癌（图 19-10-4）。

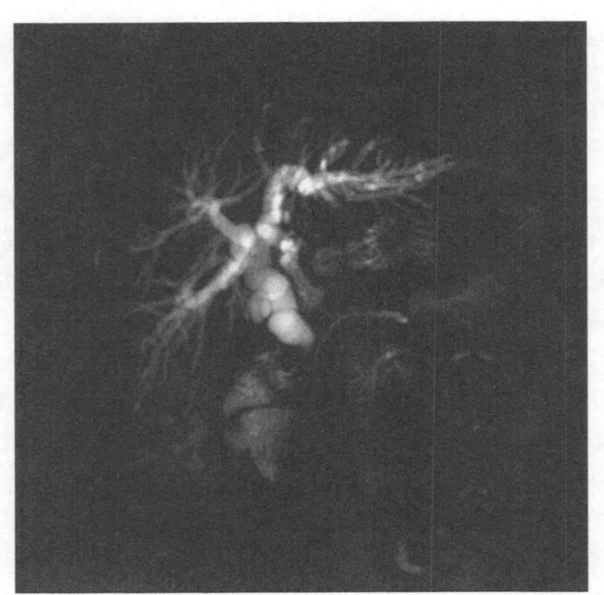

图 19-10-4 MRCP：肝内外胆管扩张，胆囊已切除，残留胆囊管低位异位汇入肝外胆管，肝外胆管括约肌段过长，为胆胰管异常连接的一种

既往不少文献中，胆系结石在胆囊癌患者中的发生率为 60%~70%，认为是胆囊癌的主要发病原因，且有病理学研究支持。Chijiiwa 等（1993）发现，胆系结石在无胆胰管异常连接的胆囊癌患者中出现率为 54%，而伴胆胰管异常连接的胆囊癌患者中无一例发生胆系结石，表明在伴胆胰管异常连接的胆囊癌患者中，胆系结石并不是主要病因学因素。这些病人的胆囊黏膜，通常出现与癌前病变有关的过度增生或化生，在胰液持续流入胆囊的动物模型中，已复制出此类黏膜改变。

尽管胆胰管异常连接与胆囊癌密切相关，但胆胰管异常连接在原发性胆囊癌中的频度知之甚少。Chijiiwa 等（1993）考察 53 例原发性胆囊癌，ERCP 显示良好的 37 例中 4 例（11%）与胆胰管异常连接有关，与普通人群胆胰管异常连接发生率（1.56%）相关非常显著（$P<0.001$）。

胆总管和胆囊双癌的情况少见。Ikoma 等（1992）统计 1992 年 5 月以前的此类报道共 32 例，其中 37.5% 合并胆胰管异常连接，与胆胰管异常连接的连接类型无明显关系。胆总管癌多局限于黏膜层，在发生上和胆囊癌有无直接联系尚无定论。

胆胰管异常连接与胆系结石：宫野（1985）认为胆胰管异常连接与胆系结石联系密切。但 Misra（1990）回顾性分析 95 例胆系结石的胆胰管汇合情况，发现 67/95 例（70%）主胰管和肝外胆管为双开口，而正常对照组及胆囊癌组中胆胰管双开口者仅分别占 37% 和 33%，并且 95 例胆系结石中只有 1 例共同管过长。该作者推测，这种在胆系结石病例中主胰管与肝外胆管双开口显著增多的原因有二：①此类患者胆胰管下端括约肌功能紊乱，使胆汁在胆管和胆囊中淤积时间过久，形成结石；②在有共同管的人群中，胰液中的糖原和水解蛋白可溶解而成为胆石核心的黏蛋白。

胆胰管异常连接与胆囊炎：宫野等（1985）认为，胆胰管异常连接与胆囊炎联系密切，且这类病例胆汁中淀粉酶浓度增高。Yamamoto 等（1991）研究 39 例胆胰管异常连接胆囊黏膜的组织学结构，认为胆囊上皮的增生多与胆胰管异常连接的胰液返流有关；而上皮的化生则多与胆石长期慢性刺激有关。巫北海与吕维富（1993）分析胆囊炎和胆囊结石在胆胰管异常连接和正常胆胰管连接两组的发病率无明显差异，该作者推测其原因，可能系胆囊经胆囊管汇入肝外胆管位置离胆胰管下端有一定距离，虽有胰液返流肝外胆管，常有下游总胆管尤其是扩张总胆管的“缓冲”，故可能较少受到直接侵害。

胆胰管异常连接与胆管炎：巫北海与吕维富（1993）通过对照分析发现，胆胰管异常连接组胆管炎的发生率明显增高。Neiderhiser 等（1973）将 0.5mmol/L 或 1.0mmol/L 溶血性卵磷脂分别注入豚鼠胆管内，6 小时后出现严重的炎性反应。Shimada 等（1991）应用氨基丙基键洗脱药桶及液相色谱分析仪对胆管中胆汁的磷脂进行分离和提取，成功地证实胆胰管异常连接患者胆汁中溶血卵磷脂的浓度及磷脂酶 A_2，淀粉酶活性等，均显著升高。Shimada 等的研究证实，在胆胰管异常连接的患者，胆管内胆汁的溶血性卵磷脂浓度可高达 4.44mmol/L。推测此种溶血性卵磷脂对胆管上皮可能产生毒性作用，使其溶解，脱落及炎性细胞浸润。

胆胰管异常连接与胰腺炎：Opic（1901）在胰腺炎患者的胆胰管共同管内发现嵌入性胆石，推断胰腺炎可能与胆汁返流有关，从而提出了著名的共同管理论。Kato（1983）报告 77.8% 的胆胰管异常连接患者合并胰腺炎，与之对照的正常胆胰管连接仅 36.9% 合并胰腺炎。

Armstrong（1986）前瞻性研究胰腺炎患者的胰管返流的情况，其中 62.3% 的病例有胆汁的胰管返流，与对照组（14.6%）有显著差异。此结论与 Kelly（1976，1980）等的统计结果一致。直接法胆管造影可见此类病例的胆囊管，肝外胆管和共同管均显著增宽；胆胰管的汇合角增大。胰管往往呈蛇行样扩张，不规则，可在共同管内见到结石。术中胆系造影可见对比剂自肝外胆管返流入主胰管。宫野（1985）认为，在肝外胆管纺锤形扩张的胆胰管异常连接病例，合并胰腺炎的频率尤其高。这些病例往往有共同管十二指肠壁内段功能性或器质性狭窄（包括胆囊-胆胰管下端括约肌反射功能失调，结石或蛋白栓梗阻等），共同管十二指肠壁外段多扩张。共同管内压升高，使胆汁向胰管内返流，激活胰酶，引起胰腺炎。目前，普遍认为，胆胰管异常连接合并胰腺炎实为胆源性胰腺炎。

Yamashiro（1984）的实验动物模型成功地复制出胰腺炎。须田对胆胰管异常连接病例的胰腺组织行病理切片，见胰管上皮变性，剥脱。在小叶间，尤其是胰管周围出现纤维化及杆菌的集落。该作者推测，胰管内的细菌可能产生多糖分解酶，破坏胰管的保护屏障，加之胆汁的返流等因素，最终引起胰腺炎。

巫北海与吕维富（1993）在两组对照中，胆胰管异常连接组胰腺炎的发生率显著高于对照组（$P<0.05$），该组的肝外胆管宽度，胰头段胰管宽度及胆胰管夹角也大于对照组（分别为 $P<0.05$，$P<0.001$，$P<0.05$）。该作者观察发现：在胆胰管异常连接合并胰腺炎的病例，胰管的影像学变化较为显著，尤以胰头部明显，胰管内常见有蛋白栓，总胆管胰腺段多无缩窄，手术探查时胰头形态及质地多无异常。而在正常胆胰管连接组，胰管的改变较少，总胆管胰腺段多有缩窄，与上方正常或扩张的胆管形成截然分界，手术探查时多有胰头肿大或缩小，质地多较硬。产生上述差别的病理及病因学机制尚待进一步考察。

胆胰管异常连接与先天性胆管闭锁：胆胰管异常连接常与先天性胆管闭锁同时存在。尸检证实，先天性胆管闭锁的患儿 50%~70% 合并胆胰管异常连接。Chiba（1990）统计 28 例先天性胆管闭锁，共同管显示清晰的 18 例中有 16 例共同管长度在 4~10mm 间，依日本胆胰管异常连接研究会之诊断标准，此 16 例应属胆胰管异常连接之列。其中，有 14 例胆胰管连接方式为主胰管注入肝外胆管（87.5%）。

胆胰管异常连接合并胰管环状重复畸形：胰管环状畸形属对称性重复，此种畸形可导致胰腺局部肿大和胰管引流不畅。胆胰管异常连接合并这种畸形，不仅使胰液排空缓慢，而且更加重胆汁向胰管的反流，导致胰腺疾病的发生率增高。

胆胰管异常连接合并胰腺融合畸形：胆胰管异常连接合并胰腺分裂胰腺分裂，是指胰腺胚胎发育在第 8 周左右，背侧与腹侧胰管系统未能融合，这是胰管先天性异常最常见的一种。公认的观点是，胰腺分裂若合并副乳头狭窄，则可致胰液引流障碍，从而诱发胰腺炎。当胆胰管异常连接合并胰腺分裂时，可反复发生梗阻性黄疸及胆管炎，可能系胰液反流至胆管所引起。

胆胰管异常连接合并腹背胰融合异常：在胚胎发育融合时，背胰管远侧构成主胰管体尾部，腹胰管构成主胰管的胰头段及钩突支。肝外胆管再与主胰管汇合成胆胰共同管。腹背胰融合异常，可致钩突支明显增粗、扭曲，在与主胰管汇合处形成局限性扩张，而胆管下端狭窄且又汇入钩突支，从而形成过长的胆胰共同管。

胆管异常汇入副胰管时，不仅形成过长的共同管，而且胆汁需经副乳头引流。

第四节　胆胰管异常连接合并胆管扩张

胆胰管异常连接是由于胆管和胰管在十二指肠壁外提前汇合，胆胰管共同管过长，致使胆胰括约肌不能调节、控制胆胰管连接区而引起胆胰管连接区流体力学异常。

胆胰管异常连接患者若延误治疗，可以导致胆系结石、慢性胆管炎症、胰腺炎甚至胆系肿瘤的发生，因此采取合理和影像检查，对于患者的早期诊治十分重要。

胆胰管异常连接是一种少见病，可发生于任何年龄，10 岁以下女性儿童多见，尤其是婴幼儿发病率最高。

患者主要临床表现为腹痛、黄疸和腹部肿块 3 大症状，但部分患者表现为呕吐和发热，部分患者合并胰腺炎、胆总管结石和胆囊炎。

<1 岁的患者,主要临床表现为黄疸、陶土样大便,部分患者发生哭闹等症状; >1 岁的儿童,主要临床表现以腹痛、呕吐、发热等症状为主。

大部分胆管扩张首先由超声发现,一组 3 例患者于产前行超声检查,即发现先天性总胆管扩张症。该组有 16 例患者术前行超声检查,结果显示超声均能准确地诊断总胆管扩张症,而且能精确测量胆总管囊性扩张(又称胆总管囊肿)的直径,与此同时,超声可以观察胆囊炎症、胆囊和胆总管内蛋白栓形成情况。

该组中 11 例患者出现胆囊壁增厚,系胆胰管异常连接患者合并胆囊慢性炎症所致,该结果与文献报道相类似,提示该征象为胆胰管异常连接的诊断依据之一。但超声不能很好地显示胆胰管异常连接共同管,对于胰液和胆汁反流的诊断无能为力。

该组有 18 例行腹部 CT 检查,与术中胆系造影及术后病理分型对比显示,CT 可以显示肝内外胆管扩张情况、胆系阳性结石、胰腺炎及其程度;利用增强 CT 检查,可以很好地观察胰管的扩张情况,该组有 3 例患者 CT 发现胰管和胆管汇合于十二指肠外并确诊为胆胰管异常连接。

然而 CT 显示胆胰管共同管率较低、不能测量共同管长度,因此 CT 在胆胰管异常连接中的诊断率较低。Watanabe 等(1997)应用滴注胆管造影螺旋 CT 诊断胆胰管异常连接,此方法不仅从形态上显示胆胰管异常连接,而且从功能上证实胰液胆汁的相互反流,但由于对比剂的昂贵,患者需要接受大剂量的辐射而在我国儿童患者中尚未广泛开展。

MRCP 是利用胆汁胰液的自然对比,可以显示胆胰管的三维结构以及胰管、胆系的细微差别。该组病例有 17 例行 MRCP 检查,与术中胆系造影和术后病理对照,结果发现 MRCP 不仅清楚显示总胆管扩张症,还可以清楚地显示胆胰管共同管及胆胰管异常连接。但儿童胰管细小,肠道内液体信号的干扰,胰管分支显影率较低。

一些作者采用口服稀释 5 倍 Gd-DTPA 液后行 MRCP 检查,研究结果提示该法能有效地降低胃肠道液体高信号强度、改善 MRCP 图像的质量和胰管的显示率。

有学者通过注射促胰液素刺激胰腺外分泌后行动态 MRCP,观察胆胰管异常连接患者胆管及胆囊的注射药物前后的动态变化,如果胆管提前显影,则提示有胰液向胆管反流,且可以很好地显示胆胰管异常连接共同管,同时可以评价胰腺外分泌功能。

Tiscornia 等(1988)报道,口服柠檬橙汁能强烈刺激胰腺外分泌功能。随后 Chu 等(2010)将柠檬橙汁液口服后行动态 MRCP,研究结果表明胰管显示率明显提高,使得胆胰管异常连接诊断率进一步提高。由于其为非侵入性检查方式,并有取代 ERCP 的趋势,由此认为 MRCP 为儿童胆胰管异常连接首选诊断和术后随访的方法。

胆胰管异常连接合并胆管扩张症手术治疗中,广泛采用术中胆系造影,观察胆总管囊肿形态、胆胰管共同管、胆管的通畅情况、胆胰管括约肌的功能情况,同时观察肝门及肝内胆管形态。

该组病例术中胆系造影成功率为 98.2%,胰管显示率为 61.3%,对于胆总管囊肿巨大、

十二指肠向前移位者,共同管显示欠佳,使得胆胰管异常连接诊断率受限。但术中胆系造影除了用于观察胆胰管合流、胆胰管括约肌的功能情况,更重要的是该法能很好地显示胰管,以免术中损伤胰管。

总之,超声、CT、术中胆系造影和 MRCP 均对胆胰管异常连接患儿胆管扩张及其并发症的显示具有一定价值。CT 对胆胰管合流于十二指肠外显示率较低,但 CT 能对胆胰管周围组织结构显示清晰;而超声不能直接观察胆胰管异常连接共同管,但能很好地观察胆囊增厚及胆结石情况; MRCP 不仅能显示总胆管扩张症,而且可以明确显示胆胰管共同管,应为儿童胆胰管异常连接诊断首选的方法。

第五节 胆胰管异常连接与胆囊管最低位汇入总肝管

胆胰管异常连接,又称作异常胆胰管连接,是指主胰管和肝外胆管在十二指肠壁外汇合,胆胰管下端功能失调,引起胆汁和胰液混流,继而导致一系列胆胰系疾病,这是胆胰管十二指肠连接区的一种先天性异常。

据近年国内外研究发现,胆胰管异常连接是一种病因学因素,在它的基础上,胆系胰腺疾病的发病率都有不同程度的增高,按照发病率增高的程度,以

胆管囊肿的发病率增高最为明显，然后，依次为胆囊炎、胆囊结石、胆管炎、胰腺炎、胆囊癌、胆管癌、胰腺癌等。

与胆胰管异常连接十分类似的情况是胆囊管最低位汇入总肝管，在临床表现与病理学上二者颇为相似，仅解剖学上略有不同，我们认为，它们都是属于胆胰管十二指肠连接区的先天性异常。对于胆胰管异常连接和胆囊管最低位汇入总肝管，影像诊断方法主要是MRCP、CT三维重建、ERCP、PTC、术中胆管造影、术后胆管引流管造影等。

病理学：Wong和Lister（1981）对32例6~22周龄人胚的胆胰管连接部作连续切片观察证实，在胚胎第8周前，胆总管和主胰管在十二指肠壁外衔接。此后，连接部逐渐移入十二指肠壁。至出生后，此种移动仍在进行，如某种病因使此种正常内移中止，即形成胆胰管异常连接。

Kimura等（1985）把胆胰管异常连接分为P→B（主胰管注入肝外胆管）型，和B→P（肝外胆管注入主胰管）型。该组作者报告65例胆胰管异常连接，其中P→B型和B→P型分别为42例（64.6%）和23例（35.4%）。

但此两种类型往往不能包含全部胆胰管异常连接。有些病例很难划归某一类型，如胆总管注入主胰管钩突支，胆总管注入主胰管而副胰管流入正常的十二指肠乳头等。这些病例的病理关系比较复杂，我们（1993）将之划作胆胰管异常连接的复杂型。在我们当时报告的59例胆胰管异常连接中，P→B型和B→P型分别为34例（57.6%）和18例（30.5%，复杂型7例（11.9%）。

Arima和Akita（1979）将胆胰管异常连接与异常长的共同管分开讨论。我们认为，事实上，从解剖学观点看，两者相互依存，不可分割。因为，十二指肠壁内段胆胰管长度有限，若胰管与胆管在十二指肠壁外汇合，势必引起共同管伸长，反之亦然。有作者指出，胆胰共同管长度超过6mm者即应划归胆胰管异常连接。

自Babbitt（1969）报道先天性胆管囊肿合并胆胰管异常连接，提出新的病因学观点以来，这一异常连接及其与胆胰系疾病的病因学联系愈益得到重视。现在已认识到，胆胰管异常连接不仅可合并先天性胆管囊肿，而且与胆囊炎、胆囊癌、胆管癌、胆系结石及胰腺炎等之间也有很大的相关性。

临床表现：在临床上，胆胰管异常连接病人常有胆胰疾病的症状与体征，但一般都根据其伴存的疾病的表现，诊断为胆囊炎、胆囊结石、胆管结石、胆管囊肿、胰腺炎、胆囊癌等，当临床根据其诊断进行手术（诸如：胆囊切除术、胆管探查术、胆管取石术、胆管囊肿切除术等）治疗后，病人的症状与体征通常改变不明显，而常被称作胆囊切除术后综合征，或胆系手术后遗症。此时，如作MRCP、ERCP或PTC检查，方发现病人实为胆胰管异常连接。再针对此症手术后，临床症状与体征常常可以得到缓解或逐渐消失。

影像学研究：胆胰管异常连接主要依靠MRCP、CT胆系三维成像及X线直接法胆管胰管造影进行诊断。胆胰管异常连接的诊断，需肯定胰管和胆管在十二指肠壁外汇合，合并其他胆胰系病变的存在，同时应除外该区及邻近的肿瘤、结石、炎症、及十二指肠乳头区憩室等因素所致胆胰管连接区后天性形态学的改变。环状胰腺及胆胰管分别开口者一般不属于本症之列。

胆胰管汇合之共同管长度的异常判断标准不尽一致：Misra（1990）认为共同管长度大于或等于8mm即属异常长共同管；而Kimura和Ono等的标准分别为大于15mm和大于6mm。日本胆胰管异常连接研究会认为，成人共同管长于10mm，小儿共同管长于4mm诊断为异常长共同管比较确切（户谷拓二，1987）。

我们认为，在成人，共同管长于和等于8mm划作异常较为妥当。同时，在进行胆胰共同管长度的评价时，还须综合考虑胆胰管连接的形态、年龄、体格、检查体位、呼吸时相、投影学与摄片当时情况，及放大率等诸多因素。

胆囊管最低位汇入总肝管：胆囊管低位和异位汇合于总肝管，在临床上并不少见，但最低位汇合则所见不多，我们曾报告9例。最低位汇合，即胆囊管汇于肝外胆管的最低部位，即汇入十二指肠外壁处，也即是汇入壁内段（括约肌段）的上方。此时，一般所谓的胆总管已不存在，肝外胆管只有总肝管和括约肌段两段，总肝管甚长，它不仅位于十二指肠上方，而且位于十二指肠后方及胰腺后方，直达十二指肠降段中部的肠壁，接受胆囊管的汇入，进入肠壁，形成括约肌段。

胆囊管低位汇入总肝管势必影响胆囊内胆汁的引流。胆囊管低位必定带来胆囊管变长，胆囊管最低位汇入，必使胆囊管变得最长。我们一组胆囊未切除的4例胆囊管平均长度为79.50mm,远比一般人长许多。胆囊已切除的5例胆囊管残端平均长度为54.02mm,也比胆囊管解剖学正常平均值(40mm)长。

胆囊管与总肝管交叉伴行,左位(异位)汇入也有碍胆汁引流。胆囊管最低位汇入总肝管给肠道逆行胆系感染创造有利条件。该组病例逆行注入对比剂时,常常对比剂都是首先进入胆囊管,使之显影于总肝管之前,这除了与患者俯卧右侧抬高(胆囊管左位或左前位汇入总肝管)体位因素有关外,汇合位置最低也可能起到一定作用。同理,肠道逆行胆系感染累及胆囊也会更容易。

从解剖学知道,肝外胆管越近括约肌段处,肌纤维越多,而使管腔保持一定张力,这对此类胆囊管最低位汇入的胆囊内胆汁的引流,可能也有妨碍。该组所有病例皆有胆囊结石与胆囊炎,盖与上述诸因素有一定关系。

胆囊管在括约肌段上端汇入总肝管,不仅影响胆囊内胆汁的引流,而且也可能对肝胆汁从总肝管排泄有所妨碍。因为汇入部位正居括约肌段上方,很有可能妨碍括约肌段的正常关闭与开启,引起功能紊乱,从而导致总肝管内胆汁排空障碍,同时为肠道感染逆行进入胆系创造某些条件。

胆囊管与总肝管交叉伴行对总肝管胆汁排泄也可能有妨碍。该组9例均有总肝管结石与炎症,其中6例伴存肝胆管结石,我们考虑也可能与上述因素有一定的关系。

胆囊管最低位汇入壁内段(括约肌段)上方,即正好在十二指肠壁外部分,直接涉及胆胰管十二指肠连接区的解剖构造,从广义看,它与胆胰管异常连接一样,也是胆胰管十二指肠连接区先天性结构异常的一种,而绝不仅只是一种先天变异。

因为,从该组9例小范围看,它常伴存胆囊结石、胆囊炎、总肝管结石与肝管结石,此种结构的先天异常可能就是这些疾病的病因学方面的解剖因素之一。因此,我们认为,临床上对此类先天异常应给予必要的重视。

第六节 十二指肠乳头异位与胆胰管异常连接

胆胰管走行曲度较大时,分别沿汇合处胆总管、胰管内侧管壁作切线,其夹角即胆胰管汇合角度。若胆胰管走行较平直,则直接作两管的长轴线,其夹角认为是二者汇合角度。

十二指肠乳头是由胆总管与主胰管汇合斜行穿入十二指肠降段内侧壁,局部肠黏膜皱襞向肠腔内突起形成的乳头状结构,其开口多位于十二指肠降段中1/3部(约占66%),27%在降段下1/3部,约3%在降段的上1/3部,位于十二指肠水平段附近者仅有4%。尸检报告乳头位于十二指肠降部中1/3位置约占67%,余位于降部上1/3或以远部位。解剖学认为乳头开口于十二指肠降部中段为正常,开口于降部中段以远者为十二指肠乳头开口异位。

PTC诊断十二指肠乳头开口异位及其临床意义:一项课题的研究对象均为因阻塞性黄疸行PTC介入治疗的患者,PTC通过顺行性胆管造影可动态观察介入术后胆管通畅、胆胰管汇合形态等情况,较CT和MRCP对胆管内腔形态的显示更为准确和直观,定性诊断率高。

实践表明,PTC在显示胆胰管汇合状态的同时,借助胆胰管和十二指肠显影可准确反映十二指肠乳头的位置分布、是否存在十二指肠乳头开口异位、胆胰管异常连接等情况。一些作者通过PTC影像学方法对十二指肠乳头开口异位、胆胰管异常连接及二者关系进行分析,以期提高传统X线十二指肠造影和十二指肠镜或ERCP检查时对十二指肠乳头开口异位、胆胰管异常连接的认识,达到早期诊断胆胰管异常连接的目的。

十二指肠乳头开口异位与胆胰管异常连接的临床相关性分析:该研究中,PTCD术中共确诊胆胰管异常连接患者31例,其中乳头位于十二指肠降部中1/3者占38.71%(12/31),余61.29%(19/31)位于降部中1/3以远部位,接近文献报道的67.8%~71.1%。

进一步统计结果显示乳头异位位置越远,胆胰管异常连接共同管越长($P<0.05$),但对胆胰管汇合角度无显著影响;胆胰管异常连接患者中十二指肠乳头开口异位发生率较高,与文献报道一致。

国内学者报道在伴有胆胰管异常连接的先天性胆管扩张症患儿及其他成人胆胰疾病患者中,十二指肠乳头开口异位发生率显著高于不伴胆胰管异常连接的患者，且乳头异位越远，共同管越长，越易发生胆胰逆流。病理证实多继发一系列胆管或胰腺病理改变，如胆管癌和胰腺癌。这种异位间接提示胆胰管异常连接、先天性胆管扩张症的胚胎学成因。

乳头开口位置代表胚胎早期肝憩室的发生部位，因乳头位置定位于胚胎22天，而胆胰管汇合发生于胚胎5~6周的腹胰背胰融合阶段。由此推测胚胎早期肝憩室发生异位可能是胆胰管异常连接的致病因素之一；异位使腹胰与背胰间距增大，在二者融合过程中，胆胰管汇合形成的共同管和胆总管受到牵拉，导致共同管过长。

十二指肠乳头开口异位与胆胰管异常连接共同管长度密切相关，而共同管长度异常是诊断胆胰管异常连接的关键指标。这为常规X线上消化道造影预测胆胰管异常连接提供了可能，即通过判断显影的十二指肠乳头位置，预测是否存在胆胰管异常连接。造影时若发现乳头位置向远端异位，应注意想到是否伴存有胆胰管异常连接；而胆胰管异常连接与诸多胆胰疾病有重要的病理联系，尤其是与胆系癌相关。

在十二指肠乳头开口异位患者中，胆胰疾病发病率增加，乳头周围黏膜病变也增多，此类疾病缺乏特征性的临床表现，易误诊为胃肠道病变，或首先进行X线上消化道造影或胃十二指肠镜检查以诊断或排除胃肠道疾病。提高对十二指肠乳头开口异位的认识，重视十二指肠乳头开口异位与胆胰管异常连接的密切关系，将有利于以传统的上消化道造影技术早期诊断胆胰管异常连接，尽早施以干预治疗；或进一步明确胆胰管异常连接合并的胆胰疾病尤其恶性肿瘤，以早期诊断，改善此类疾病的预后。

我们认为，乳头与十二指肠降段关系，在活体与非活体肯定有差异。用消化道检查去间接推论有无胆胰管异常连接是否符合事实，值得研究。目前，异常连接的定义尚无定论，更何况如此？共同管长度的标准也有争论，都是我们应该深入研究的问题。

第七节　PTCD术中对比剂胰管逆流与共同管的关系探讨

详见本书 本卷 本篇 第八章 第四节　PTCD术中对比剂胰管逆流与共同管的关系探讨。

第八节　胆胰管异常连接合并胰腺融合畸形

胆胰管异常连接合并胰腺分裂：胰腺分裂，是指胰腺胚胎发育在第8周左右，背侧与腹侧胰管系统未能融合，这是胰管先天性异常最常见的一种。公认的观点是，胰腺分裂若合并副乳头狭窄，则可致胰液引流障碍，从而诱发胰腺炎。当胆胰管异常连接合并胰腺分裂时，可反复发生梗阻性黄疸及胆管炎，可能系胰液反流至胆管所引起。

胆胰管异常连接合并腹背胰融合异常：在胚胎发育融合时，背胰管远侧构成主胰管体尾部，腹胰管构成主胰管的胰头段及钩突支。肝外胆管再与主胰管汇合成胆胰共同管。腹背胰融合异常，可致钩突支明显增粗，扭曲，在与主胰管汇合处形成局限性扩张，而胆管下端狭窄且又汇入钩突支，从而形成过长的胆胰共同管。胆管异常汇入副胰管时，不仅形成过长的共同管，而且胆汁需经副乳头引流。

第九节　胆胰管异常连接合并胰管环状重复畸形

胰管环状畸形属对称性重复，此种畸形可导致胰腺局部肿大和胰管引流不畅。胆胰管异常连接合并这种畸形，不仅使胰液排空缓慢，而且更加重胆汁向胰管的反流，导致胰腺疾病的发生率增高。

第十节　胆胰管汇合情况与急性胰腺炎发病关系的研究

急性胰腺炎发病因素多，发病机制复杂，胆管疾病，如结石或肿瘤梗阻，是引起急性胰腺炎的重要病因。但除此之外的其他诱因，诸如酗酒、高脂血症、暴饮暴食等，少数人患病究其原因可能解剖上存在着某种差异。部分学者对此已有关注，并进行相关研究，但多采取非活体解剖的方式，病例数较少，且非生理状态，故而有所限制。

以往，有学者从胰管的形态学方面推测，以下情况可能易患急性胰腺炎：胆胰管汇合角度较大；胰管较粗，腔内压降低；存在共同通道并较长；胆胰共同管嵴膜不明显，"瓣膜"作用小；胆、胰管末端括约肌欠发达；除结石外的其他因素致胆胰共同管梗阻。但由于当时检查设备受限，检查例数或尸检例数较少，而且缺乏无创、生理状态下、可以整体直观显示胰胆管的检查手段，一直没有确切的结论。MRCP的出现使得这些问题得以解决。

胆胰管汇合类型是否为明显共同管型与急性胰腺炎发病关系：由于急性胰腺炎的发病有"共同通道或共同管"学说，而三种胆胰管汇合类型中只有明显共同管型有共同通道，所以该组首先观察明显共同管型汇合与急性胰腺炎发病关系。结果为 $\chi^2=0.455$（$P>0.05$），说明是否为明显共同管型汇合与急性胰腺炎的发病没有必然联系。

有无胰管变异与急性胰腺炎发病关系：该组数据中 OR=8.34，$\chi^2=18.935$（$P<0.01$），证实胰管变异与急性胰腺炎的发病有密切关系，而且胰管变异是急性胰腺炎发病的一个高危因素。这可能与"存在十二指肠乳头功能不全和胰液流量增加，二者相互作用可以使背侧胰管的压力增加"有关，但具体原因有待进一步证实。在该组病例的观察中同时发现，同样有胰管变异时，胰腺炎的发生概率也是不同的，例如胰头处副胰管多而杂或是胰腺分裂时更容易合并有胰腺炎，但是由于该组胰管变异的病例数较少，无法进行详细的分类及统计学分析，所以有待进一步的研究。

共同管长度与急性胰腺炎发病关系：随着共同通道的增长，OR 及 χ^2 值也随之增长，且 P 值均 <0.05，表明共同通道长度越长，患急性胰腺炎的危险性越大。一些学者从解剖学的角度证实了这一点：共同通道越长，"使两管之间的隔膜短而宽，这一缺陷使其不能遮盖胰管口，'活瓣'功能不全而抗胆汁返流能力下降"，从而更易发生急性胰腺炎，当共同通道长度 >15 mm 时，称之为胆胰管异常连接。

胆胰管汇合角度与急性胰腺炎发病关系：该组中胆胰管汇合角度在 50° 以下时病例组与对照组并无统计学差异；而 >50° 时则有显著的统计学差异（$P<0.01$）。说明胆胰管汇合角度在一定范围内时对急性胰腺炎的发病并无影响，而随着汇合角度的增大，大于一定限值时，急性胰腺炎的发病率明显增加。这也可能与汇合角度过大时胆汁返流的概率也随之增加有关。

综上所述，急性胰腺炎的发病在解剖上与胆胰管的汇合情况有一定关系，如有胰管变异、共同通道较长、胆胰管汇合角度过大都是急性胰腺炎发病的危险因素，但由于该组病例数较少，仅仅是一个初步的探讨，结论尚需进一步完善，并有待于更大样本数的研究。

第二十篇　胰腺疾病

第一章　关于胰腺肿瘤

第一节　诊断陷阱：酷似原发性胰腺肿瘤的胰腺及胰周疾病

发育变异和先天异常：正常的十二指肠：有的病人 CT 扫描提示胰腺头部增大，但在口服阳性对比剂后，再重复 CT 扫描，却显示正常的胰腺头部，及含对比剂的正常十二指肠和胆囊，事实上是充盈液体的十二指肠呈现低密度，与胰头紧邻而被误认为胰腺头部肿大。

慢性胰腺炎行 Puestow 术后：在慢性胰腺炎行 Puestow 术后，CT 扫描显示与空肠吻合的胰管明显扩张，酷似胰腺囊性肿块，如不了解手术情况则容易误诊。

环状胰腺：在环状胰腺，CT 扫描显示胰腺组织环绕十二指肠；在 ERCP 图像上，还可显示主胰管缠绕十二指肠内的内窥镜，并且环状胰腺使胆总管狭窄，其近端扩张。

十二指肠旁索带：十二指肠旁索带结构有时可被液体充盈，此时，CT 扫描则可能显示液体充盈的十二指肠旁索带围绕在十二指肠周围，在横断图像上容易被误作胰腺肿块；但在冠状多平面重建则可显示出十二指肠旁索带全貌，从而避免误诊。

胰腺组织内的迷走脾：在胰腺组织内的迷走脾，轴位增强 T_1WI 可显示胰腺内一个与脾脏等信号强度病灶；冠状 T_1WI 图像显示胰腺包绕着这个异常信号灶。

先天性胆总管囊肿：CT 常规横断扫描可显示扩大的冗余的胆总管胰腺段，酷似胰头内囊性病灶，但在 ERCP 检查时，则可显示对比剂进入囊肿内。

一、胰腺炎症或感染性病变

胰腺炎并发症：CT 平扫时，可显示出血型胰腺炎伪似胰腺不均匀性肿块。在一些有胰腺炎病史的老年病例，CT 平扫和增强时可显示整个胰腺多发厚壁囊性病变，术前可误诊为导管黏液蛋白乳头状瘤，术后病理证实为多发假性囊肿。

自身免疫性胰腺炎：自身免疫性胰腺炎可表现为胰头肿大，密度不均匀，有时血管周围炎形成不均匀的团块，容易和肿瘤血管受侵相混淆。有的罹患本病的腹痛患者，MRI T_2WI 和 MRCP 显示肝外胆管胰腺段长段均匀狭窄，但却没有信号异常的广泛胰头增大。轴位 MRI T1WI 可显示胰尾增大，周围有低信号边。

胰周淋巴结肿大或淋巴瘤：在腹腔淋巴瘤的病人，有时胰腺体部附近淋巴结肿大，易和胰体肿块混淆。

胰腺转移性肿瘤：在临床上，胰腺转移性肿瘤很少见，有作者报告，乳腺癌转移到胰腺可产生胰腺整体弥漫性肿大，其密度不均匀，增强时强化也不均匀；平扫时与弥漫性胰腺炎症性水肿类似，但其强化表现则完全不一样。有的肾细胞癌转移转移到胰腺，表现为与肾肿块一样的强化特点，这为诊断肾细胞癌转移提供一定帮助。

二、胰腺邻近结构病变

纤维组织细胞瘤：有的纤维组织细胞瘤病人，表现为胰腺区多个大小不等的低密度病灶，增强扫描时也呈略低密度，尤如黏液的表现，在临床上，最初被误诊为胰腺黏蛋白腺癌，手术后病理确诊为腹膜后纤维组织细胞瘤。

肠系膜类癌：肠系膜类癌可在 CT 平扫上显示肠系膜根部胰头附近一不均匀性肿块，其内可见钙化，如不注意，可被误诊为胰腺头部肿瘤。

肠系膜硬纤维瘤：肠系膜硬纤维瘤 CT 显示腹腔巨大卵圆形肿块，胰腺背侧受压，容易误诊为胰腺来源的肿块。

胃间质瘤累及胰腺：有的胃间质瘤侵犯胰腺，与胰腺分界不清,此时,多平面重建可以帮助了解肿瘤的起源。

十二指肠淋巴瘤:十二指肠淋巴瘤可以侵犯胰腺,与胰腺分界不清,但是胃肠检查可以显示十二指肠本身的病变及黏膜的变化。

十二指肠腺癌:十二指肠腺癌常常侵犯胰腺,也表现为低密度肿块影,但其强化特点与胰腺癌不一样。

脾血管瘤:脾血管瘤可大可小,小者一般与胰腺无关,大者则可侵犯胰腺尾部,导致诊断混淆。

左侧肾上腺外副神经节瘤:有的左侧肾上腺外副神经节瘤可向前挤压胰腺体尾部,有的时候在横断图像上二者分界不清,则可与胰腺肿物混淆。

三、血管性病变

肠系膜上动脉瘤:在有的肠系膜上动脉动脉瘤病人,增强 CT 显示胰头区被附壁血栓包绕的强化的动脉内腔,若没有动脉期内腔强化的影像,很可能被误认为是胰头病变中囊腺瘤,被附壁血栓包绕的动脉内腔缩成一团,尤如囊腺瘤中的壁结节。

门静脉栓塞:门静脉栓塞时,增强扫描一直呈现为胰腺内的低密度病灶,容易被误诊为胰腺肿块。

第二节 浸润性胰腺导管腺癌,高分化

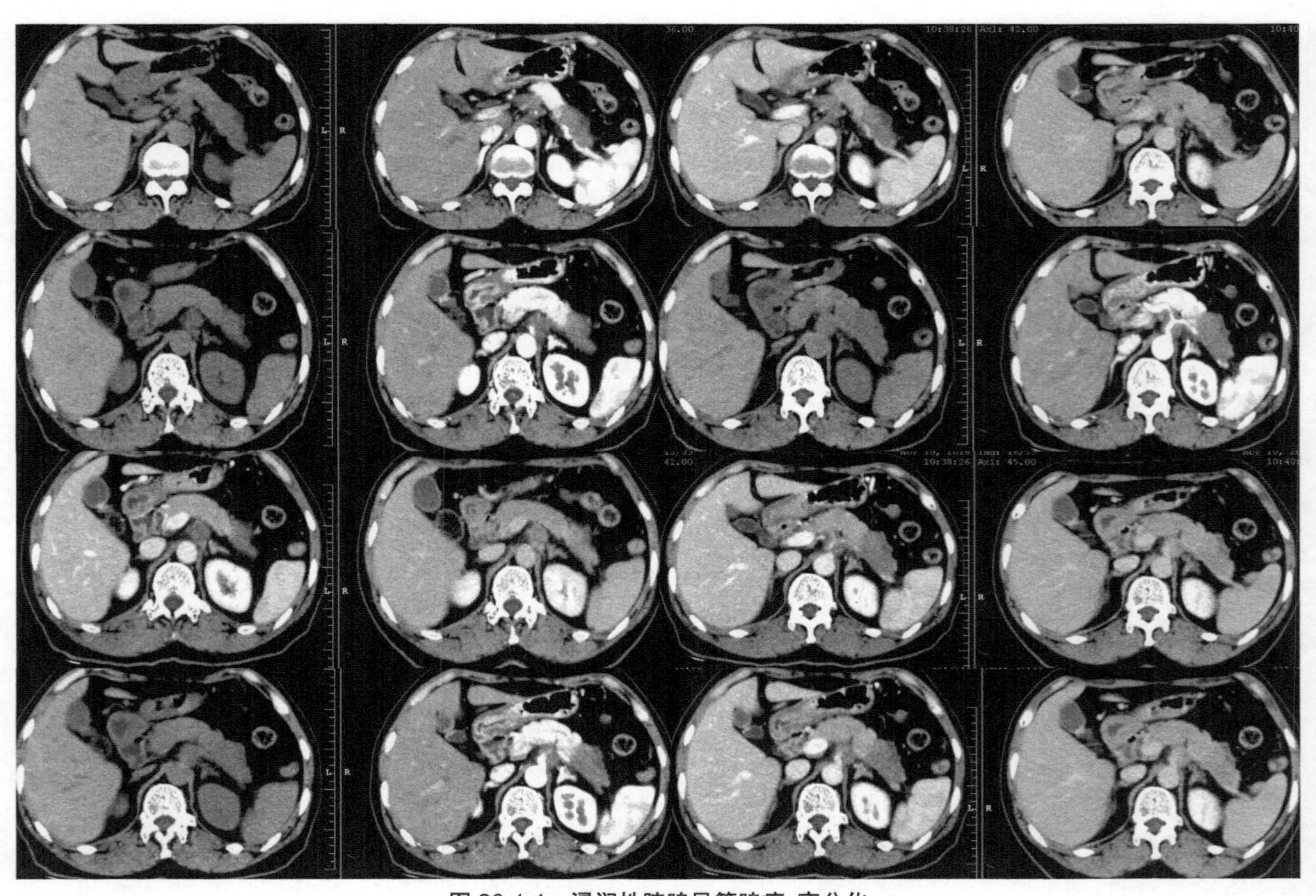

图 20-1-1 浸润性胰腺导管腺癌,高分化

患者,女,60 岁。

手术所见:腹腔无腹水,无种植转移,肝脏未及转移灶,胃肠未见异常,肿瘤位于胰体尾部交界处,大小约 5 cm×4 cm,质硬,活动度差,肿瘤累及腹腔干及分叉部血管,质硬,包裹。

病理检查:胰体尾肿物:胰腺肿物一块,大小 7 cm×4.5 cm×2.5 cm,切面灰白灰黄,质中偏硬。常规病理诊断:胰腺肿物切除标本:浸润性腺癌,大小 7 cm ×4.5 cm ×2.5 cm,侵

及周边纤维脂肪组织及淋巴结，局部可见侵及神经组织。切缘可见少量癌组织。

免疫组化检测：阳性：AAT，AACT，CK19，CA19-9，CK7，CK20，Villin，CK8，CK18，EGFR（3+），PgP（3+），Topo Ⅱ（+），ERCC-1（3+），VEGF（3+），Tubulinβ（+），Ki-67（+，约50%）；阴性：CD10，Mncin-2，CgA，5-Fu，CDX-2，Vimentin。免疫组化诊断：胰腺肿物切除标本：浸润性胰腺导管腺癌，高分化，大小 7 cm × 4.5 cm × 2.5 cm，侵及周边纤维脂肪组织及淋巴结，局部可见侵及神经组织（图 20-1-1）。

第三节　胰腺肿瘤的分类

见表 20-1-1。

表 20-1-1　胰腺恶性肿瘤根据细胞起源的分类

导管细胞起源	结缔组织起源	腺泡细胞起源	不确定组织来源的
导管腺癌	平滑肌肉瘤	腺泡细胞癌	胰腺母细胞瘤
黏蛋白过度分泌性癌	恶性纤维组织细胞瘤	腺泡细胞囊腺癌	
黏蛋白巨细胞肿瘤	恶性血管周围细胞瘤		
巨细胞癌	骨源性肉瘤		
腺鳞癌	横纹肌肉瘤		
黏蛋白胶样癌	恶性神经鞘瘤		
实性乳头状上皮性肿瘤	脂肪肉瘤		

源自 Gore RM 和 Livine MS.eds.Textbook of Gastrointestinal Radiology，2000，WB Saunders Company PA，USA.

第四节　易与原发性胰腺肿瘤混淆的胰和胰周疾病

CT、MRI 以及超声对诊断胰腺和胰周疾病有了明显的进步，但是，上腹部（腹腔内及腹膜后）复杂的解剖结构给诊断带来了一定的困难，多种良、恶性病变与原发性胰腺肿瘤相似，在临床诊断工作中常常造成混淆。

CT：虽然胰腺肿瘤可以选用多种检查手段，但是 CT 检查具有最明显的优势，其次是 MRI。MSCT 可薄层扫描，多时相采集（动脉期、胰腺实质期和门静脉期），用多种后处理技术显示胰腺，比如多平面重建和容积再现等。其突出的优点是可以获得高质量的非轴面扫描图像，这对于评价周围血管是非常有帮助的。曲面重建除了可以整体显示胰腺和肝外胆管以外，还可以用单纯的二维图像显示多个不同斜面的结构。患者检查前禁食 3 h，扫描前口服 1 000ml 水，其他约 300ml 水在采集数据前即时喝下，对比剂用高压注射器以 3~4 ml/s 的流率团注，使用对比剂跟踪模式。注射后约 70 s 获得胰腺实质期薄层容积数据，随后得到门静脉期数据，真正的动脉期扫描是用来评价血管性病灶（例如胰岛细胞瘤）和胰腺癌的强化表现。三维图像可在后处理工作站上处理。

MRI：快速成像明显扩大了 MR 在评价胰腺病变方面的作用，高性能的 1.5T 和 3.0T 扫描仪以及呼吸门控技术使磁共振具有强大的组织对比能力，还具有提供高分辨力的各向同性体素的能力。其独特作用在于胰腺肿瘤 CT 难以明确诊断时可以作为辅助检查，例如病灶较小，还没有引起组织变形的胰管腺癌和胰岛细胞癌。还可以诊断肝外胆管结石，胰管结石，胆管癌，也可以进一步评价胰腺增大的病例（例如，早期自身免疫性胰腺炎）。

MR 是无创性评价胰管以及肝外胆管之间关系的常用方法，MRCP 可以迅速完成，快速二维及三维成像序列可以提供肝外胆管和胰管的高分辨力图像。MR 成像一般采用相位阵列线圈。常规轴面及冠状面 2D 和 3D 梯度回波 T_1WI 完成后，采用同相位和反相位 T_1WI 以及脂肪饱和 T_1WI 获得腹部和薄层胰腺的扫描（层厚为 2~3 mm）。T_2WI 包括轴面和冠状面半傅立叶驰豫强化快速采集和单脉冲快速自旋回波 T_2WI 序列，连同脂肪饱和呼吸门控快速自旋回波 T_2WI 序列。根据试验性注射或对比剂跟踪算法，动态 2D 和 3D 梯度回波 T_1WI 用薄层采集胰腺图像。虽然会产生一些“噪声”，但是，通过良好的后处理，可以显示主要血管之间的精确关系。薄的与较厚的 2D 与 3D 图像或者半傅里叶低转换角的 MRCP 可以很容易地完成并评价胆胰管的解剖。

超声：常规腹部超声评价胰腺疾病时是有局限性的，主要用于腹痛患者的筛选，评价胆囊和胆管以及囊性病变，近来，超声设备的进展，例如：彩色多普勒序列和声学以及合成图像等，大大改善了患者胰头和胰体的显示；内镜超声可以提供胰腺囊性肿瘤高分辨力的图像，明显提高了小肿瘤的显示率，并且可以取样活检。但是，超声检查与操作者有很大关系，并且和医院特色也有一定的关系。

PET 和 PET/CT：表现疑似胰腺癌时，PET 是有益的补充，可以探测出远处转移灶，评价肿瘤的活性，检测肿瘤对治疗的反应，尤其是非黏液性肿瘤。一项胰腺病变结合 PET/CT 检查的试验显示，在胰腺良、恶性病变的鉴别方面，敏感性显著提高而特异性无显著性差异。

一、发育变异及可能混淆的病变

发育变异和先天异常：正常的解剖结构和前肠道的异常可疑似原发性胰腺肿瘤。正常十二指肠第四部分或邻近胰尾的近段空肠，密度较高的邻近的肠管或冗长的、扩张不全的胃底可以与肿块类似，CT 扫描时口服阳性对比剂或 MR 成像时喝水就很容易区分。胰头或胰颈部侧面轮廓的改变也是很常见的，它也可能类似胰腺肿块，典型的病例在 CT 增强时，该小叶与邻近实质等密度，在动脉期和门静脉期显示出正常的胰腺强化。

胰腺分裂：胰腺分裂起源于胚胎期背侧和腹侧胰管的异常融合，是最常见的先天性发育变异，一般人群中患病率接近 10%，它和临床的关系经常在复发性胰腺炎时讨论到，虽然很少，但它可以导致胰头的扩大并被误认为肿块。

环状胰腺：环状胰腺是第二常见的先天性变异，导致胰腺组织部分或全部环绕着十二指肠降部，如果钡餐检查发现十二指肠乳头水平的狭窄，就需要考虑环状胰腺的可能，ERCP 或者无创性的 MRCP 可以显示环绕十二指肠的胰管。

十二指肠重复畸形和十二指肠憩室：十二指肠重复畸形和十二指肠憩室，在 CT 和 MRI 上也可能误当成胰腺的肿块，尤其是它们的内容物是纯液体的时候。虽然胃肠道中重复畸形很少见，但发生在胃十二指肠区域的约占 12%。他们通常不相通，在十二指肠降部和水平部的肠系膜侧最常见，患者典型的表现是梗阻症状，但是也可以发展为胆系梗阻和胰腺炎。在钡餐检查中，十二指肠通常表现为被“C”形环内的肿块压迫，十二指肠重复畸形表现为位于或邻近十二指肠壁的圆形光滑的囊，囊内充满液体。十二指肠憩室常在上消化道钡餐检查中发现，检出率可达 14.5%，它可以是先天性管腔内的，但通常是后天向外受压形成，许多腔内的憩室位于十二指肠降部，在钡餐检查中表现为典型的“风向袋”畸形，充满对比剂的憩室突出到真正的管腔外。但是，如果憩室完全充满液体或其他物质而没有充满钡剂的话，就和囊性的胰腺肿瘤很相似。在磁共振 T_2 像上，十二指肠憩室可以同时包含高信号和低信号的区域，分别对应于液体和气体。另外，MSCT 和冠状面容积再现法可以更好的显示薄的、腔内憩室的囊壁以及十二指肠和胰腺之间界面的分割。

脾脏的变异：脾脏的变异，例如副脾或者脾组织植入也可以和胰腺肿块相似，副脾在人群中的发生率大约 10%，^{99m}Tc 硫胶、放射性标记的热破坏红细胞及 ^{111} 铟标记的自体血小板可以用来区分胰腺组织或是脾脏。

先天性胆总管囊肿：先天性胆总管囊肿是少见的先天胆管畸形，常在婴儿期和少年期发病，表现为肝外胆管囊性或梭形扩张，和胰头部的囊性肿块相似。^{99m}Tc 标记的肝内胆管核素显像可以有助于证实是否分泌到胆总管囊肿中，另外 ERCP、经皮肝穿刺胆系造影以及术中胆管造影可以确诊。MRCP 也能够确诊并且可以无创性的显示该解剖结构，胆系增强 CT 或 MRI 也有助于达到这一目的。

二、胰腺炎性或感染性疾病

胰腺炎在影像诊断和临床上，由于病理状况和临床表现与胰腺恶性肿瘤类似，因此常会进行外科切除手术。

慢性胰腺炎：慢性胰腺炎常常合并一定范围内的胰腺解剖的异常，包括胰腺的萎缩和增大，胰管的扩张。慢性感染导致的胰腺实质局部增大有时仅根据形态学特征或 CT 和 MRI 增强检查还是很难和胰腺癌进行鉴别。一方面，慢性胰腺炎的炎症性改变可以导致局部淋巴结的肿大和血管受累，更容易怀疑是恶性病变；另一方面，胰腺癌经常由慢性胰腺炎发展而来，这两种状况可以共存。有作者认为在胰腺感染性病变和肿瘤的鉴别方面，MRCP 优于 MR 和 CT 成像，研究还认为 MRI 使用锰福地吡增强，可以提高检出率和更好显示局部胰腺病变的特点。

沟形胰腺炎：沟形胰腺炎一种少见的节段性慢性胰腺炎，也可以和胰头癌很相似，这种病变局限在胰头、十二指肠和肝外胆管之间的凹槽内，磁共振 T_1WI 可以发现位于胰头和增厚的十二指肠壁之间低信号薄片状病变，动态 CT 可以显示强化不明显的似纤维样病变的病灶扩散在胰头和十二指肠之间。

急性胰腺炎：急性胰腺炎的合并症，例如出血、假性囊肿形成及胰周脂肪坏死也可以类似胰腺肿瘤。

自身免疫性胰腺炎：自身免疫性胰腺炎典型的征象是弥漫性的胰腺肿大，但是，局灶性的也可以表现为胰头部清晰的肿块，CT 提示自身免疫性胰腺炎的特征包括轻度的胰周感染，没有钙化，没有血管包埋在内；在 ERCP 和 MRCP 图像上，多处胆管的狭窄和主胰管弥漫性不规则狭窄是另外的特征表现。在合并同时存在自身免疫性疾病的情况下，例如原发性硬化性胆管炎、溃疡性结肠炎等，确定该诊断就可以避免不必要的外科手术。

寄生虫囊肿：寄生虫囊肿虽然在胰腺中非常少见，但也偶有报道，例如胰腺棘球绦虫，它可以是单房或多房，也可以是混合囊，由于仅根据影像学表现来把它们和其他的囊性肿块加以区分非常困难，所以，诊断这一疾病时应该考虑地区的流行性疾病情况。

胰周淋巴结肿大：肿瘤新生物、炎症或感染性病变等所致的淋巴结肿大，可以混淆为胰腺的病灶。这些淋巴结在门腔静脉周围、肝门附近、胰周以及腹腔周围。

淋巴瘤：非霍奇金 B 细胞类型的淋巴瘤所致的巨大淋巴结，可以类似胰腺癌，通常，肾静脉平面以下有肿大淋巴结时，要考虑淋巴瘤可能，而不支持胰腺癌的诊断。

转移性肿瘤：来源于食管、胃、结肠、乳腺、肾上腺和肾脏的恶性肿瘤的转移灶，也可以表现为该区域淋巴结的受累，找到原发灶可以明确诊断。

伴有淋巴结增大的炎性病变：伴有淋巴结增大的炎性病变，包括肉芽肿性病变（例如结节病）和血管增殖性病变（例如巨大淋巴结增生症）也可以表现为该区域淋巴结的增大，虽然结节病的表现非特异性，但是如果肝脏或脾脏有伴随表现，以及典型的肺门周围和气管旁淋巴结病变或肺实质性的改变存在，结节病还是可以诊断。

巨淋巴结增生症：巨淋巴结增生症的表现是不固定的，但是有明显增强的腺病。

淋巴结结核：胰腺和胰周的淋巴结结核，虽然少见，但是也可以和胰头癌混淆。肺部结核还没有明显表现时，系膜、网膜和胰周的淋巴结常已经受累，增强 CT 可以显示增大的、多房的淋巴结，有时候中心强化不明显而周围环状强化。

当不支持肉芽肿性感染而表现为低密度淋巴结时，可能需要考虑为肠脂肪肉芽肿症。最后，移植患者术后表现为巨大的淋巴结肿大时，需要考虑淋巴增生性障碍。在淋巴结和胰腺之间有完整的脂肪层，或者胰腺受压前移，有助于区分是胰周淋巴结肿大，还是胰腺肿瘤。

血管性病变：胰腺血供虽然来自前肠道，但还是有部分是肠系膜上动脉和腹腔动脉的侧支血管供血，异常状况时，例如变异的血管，或者继发于胰腺炎并发的假性动脉瘤，或者外科血管的吻合在常规图像上可和肿块类似，尤其是管腔内完全栓塞，CT 上没有强化的时候。

急性胰腺炎患者中，10% 的病例合并有假性动脉瘤，最常受影响的是脾动脉。光谱多普勒超声可以在假性动脉瘤内显示紊乱的动静脉组合血流，彩色血流多普勒超声可以在无回声的肿块中显示双向血流（“流出和流入信号”）以及“旋涡”血流模式。

由于三维 MSCT 血管造影使诊断的特异性得到明显的改善。也可以行超选择性的常规血管造影检查。静脉也可以被误认为胰腺肿块。例如，在动脉期没有强化的门静脉，在门静脉或下腔静脉栓塞时强化不明显的侧支血管。在鉴别门静脉系统还是胰腺实质性病变时,主张使用钆对比剂的三维磁共振血管造影成像。

三、胰腺周围结构的疾病

周围结构的多种病变,尤其是大的或者浸润性病变可以被误认为原发性胰腺肿瘤。他们可以起源于后腹膜、肠系膜、胃肠道、肾脏、肾上腺或者神经系统。

腹膜后病变,例如血肿、纤维化或者肿瘤新生物可以类似胰腺肿块。

有些肠系膜病变(例如萎缩性肠系膜炎)或肿块(例如良性肿瘤,纤维瘤,硬化性肠系膜炎),除非它和胰腺之间的界面得到确认,否则,可能诊断困难。

相关的胃的肿块包括胃底或胃后壁的肿瘤,巨大的胃淋巴瘤和巨大的外生性胃肠道间质瘤(胃平滑肌瘤,平滑肌肉瘤等),可以形成一个坏死中心并被误认为囊性胰腺癌。

胃的假性肿瘤包括胃的憩室等,三维 CT 或 MRI 可以很好地显示这些肿块的特征并确定它们的起源。

许多十二指肠病变可能与胰腺疾病混淆。肿瘤性病变,例如淋巴瘤、腺癌、平滑肌肉瘤、十二指肠梭形细胞肉瘤、布氏腺瘤及十二指肠转移性肿瘤等,可以和原发性胰腺肿块相似;良性病灶包括充满液体或碎屑的憩室、血肿、穿孔的包裹,重复性囊肿,平滑肌瘤。

邻近的空肠曲,尤其是密度较高时,可以和胰尾部分叶状或者卵圆形肿块类似。小肠的腺癌和多种小肠的肿瘤可以和胰腺疾病相似,但是,使用足够的口服对比剂并且多平面观察可以做出鉴别。

薄层 CT 冠状面或非轴面三维重建有助于检测出细小的十二指肠腺癌。肿瘤经常表现为偏心性或者环形肠壁增厚累及一小段肠管,致"苹果核"的外观,和钡餐检查中的所见相似。CT 肠镜检查也是有一定用处的。

脾脏组织有时候和胰尾紧密相连,像原发的富血管的胰腺肿块。其他的脾脏肿块,例如淋巴瘤,如果是弥漫性的,也可能累及胰尾。脾脏疾病,包括囊肿,转移和血管瘤也可以表现为起源于胰腺。

巨大的肾脏肿块,尤其是累及肾脏上极(左肾最明显)也可以和原发的胰腺肿块相混淆。这些肿块可以是实质性肿瘤、囊肿或是血肿。肾脏的淋巴瘤也可能累及胰腺。

肾上腺疾病也可以像胰腺疾病,右侧肾上腺巨大的病变在这种情况下常常诊断困难,尤其是巨大的肾上腺嗜铬细胞瘤可能表现为胰腺起源。

最后,肾上腺以外的神经组织的肿瘤,比如肾上腺外的嗜铬细胞瘤(神经节细胞瘤)和神经鞘瘤也需要考虑。

四、胰腺转移性肿瘤

在晚期恶性肿瘤患者尸体解剖过程中,有 3%~12% 的患者胰腺发现有转移性病灶,并且,有胰腺转移病灶的患者绝大多数也有胰腺外的转移,通常转移到胰腺的原发性肿瘤可能来源于肺、胃、十二指肠、乳腺、肾脏、黑色素瘤、淋巴瘤和骨肉瘤。

转移灶对于转移到胰腺特定部位没有特异性,CT 表现包括单个的局限性肿块,多灶性结节,以及腺体弥漫性的浸润。大多数转移性病灶表现为边界清晰的单个巨大的肿块,但是,来源于卵巢囊腺癌和黑色素瘤的转移灶的特点是囊性病灶。转移性病灶增强方式是多种多样的,经常类似于原发性肿瘤的强化特点。超声或者 CT 引导下的细针穿刺活检对于影像学像原发性囊性胰腺肿瘤的病灶可以得到较好的确诊,从而避免开放性胰腺活检。

在所有转移到胰腺的肿瘤中,淋巴瘤、肾癌、黑色素瘤和原发性胰腺肿瘤的鉴别最困难,因为它们的转移灶有单发趋势,经常没有确定的其他部位的转移。这种单个的胰腺转移灶在 CT 扫描时和胰腺原发件肿瘤难以区别。一般而言,倾向转移性病灶的图像特点包括病灶的多发、富血管供应和图像特点与特定的原发性肿瘤相一致,例如,由于顺磁性的黑色素物质、黑色素瘤在磁共振 T_1WI 相上是高信号的。已知的原发性恶性肿瘤的临床病史可以有助于鉴别诊断。

五、其他的胰腺疾病

和胰腺原发性肿瘤相似的另外一组疾病是对于药物和毒素非常敏感的代谢性疾病。发病个体是中老年人,在相对很少累及的区域产生假肿瘤,有代表性的是位于胰腺钩突与胰背之间。手术导致的解剖改变,包括肾切除术、Wipple 手术和 Puestow 手术,由于密度较高的输入肠袢或胰腺的移位都可以显得像胰腺肿块一样。

胰腺的脂肪替代可以出现在纤维囊泡症、肥胖、糖尿病、库欣综合征以及 Shwachman-Diamond 综合征(一种少见的与胰腺外分泌功能不全有关的先天性疾病)患者身上。

局灶性脂肪替代的区域或替代不足有时候可以类似肿块。结合脂肪饱和序列的化学位移 T_1WI 磁共振成像可以用来区分这一改变。含脂肪的区域相对于周围实质在同相梯度回波 T_1WI 图像上显示为等信号甚至高信号,反相梯度回波可以典型显示为低信号,由此来确定脂肪的存在。

认识上述这些可以混淆成胰腺肿瘤的变异和疾病,以及知道各种成像方法的优劣,对于选择检查方法和处理是非常重要的。一个不确定的病灶,影像学表现可能是胰腺来源时,需要考虑较多的鉴别诊断,根据临床病史和理想的 CT 和 MRI 图像特征,鉴别诊断的范围可以大大缩小。CT 和 MRI 成像技术的进展可以大大改善胰腺恶性肿瘤的鉴别能力。

第五节　胰腺实性假乳头状肿瘤(SPN)

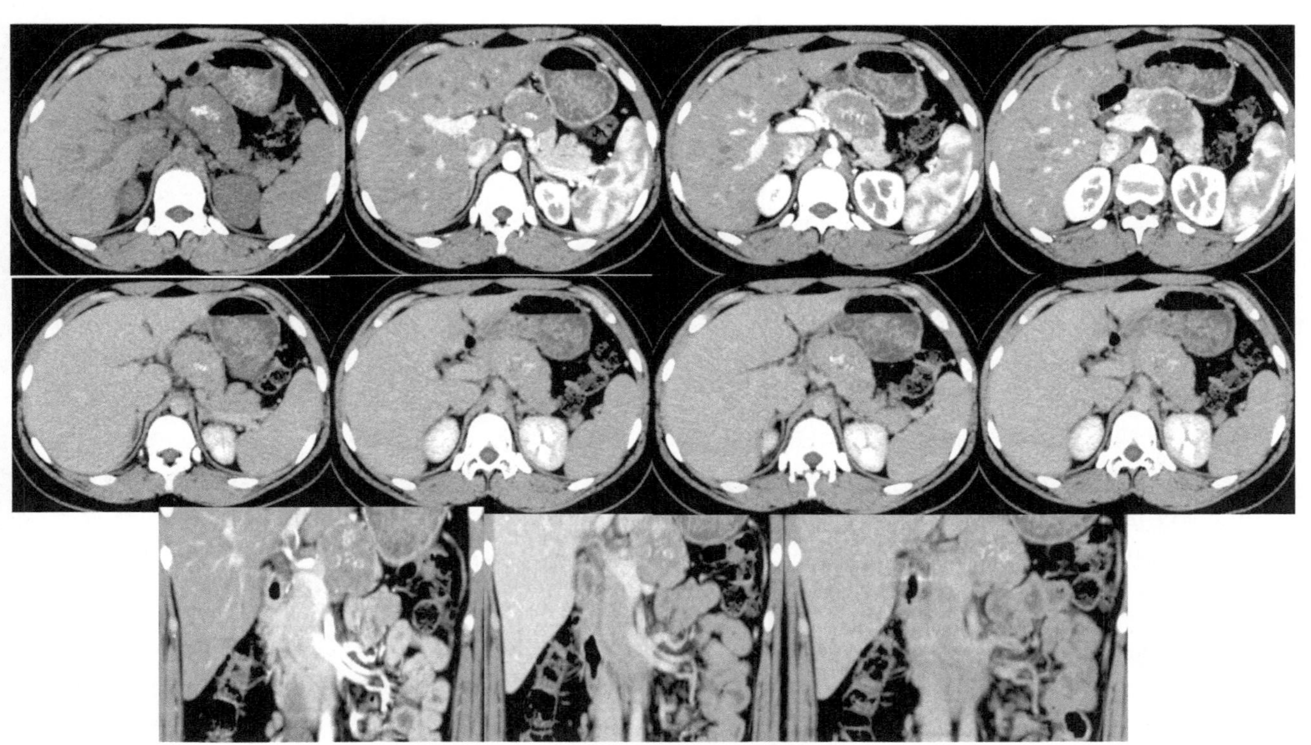

图 20-1-2　胰腺实性假乳头状肿瘤(SPN)

患者,女,15 岁。该病例年轻,胰腺病灶少血供,有钙化,渐进性强化,边界欠清。

病理检查:胰腺肿物切除标本:肿物大小为 5cm × 4.5cm × 4.5cm,肿瘤未见包膜,肿瘤细胞胞浆丰富,轻度核异型,倾向低度恶性肿瘤。免疫组化诊断:胰腺实性假乳头状肿瘤(SPN)(图 20-1-2)。

第二章　早期胰癌与小胰癌

第一节　关于早期胰癌与小胰癌

需要指出的是,小胰癌并不等于早期胰癌。Moossa 提出临床病理上早期胰癌的标准是:①肿瘤最大直径≤ 2cm;②胰周包膜无浸润;③没有远处转移;④切除标本上无淋巴结转移。

尽管小胰癌体积较小,远处器官转移及淋巴结转移并不少见,不能仅仅因为原发肿块较小、无浸润征象,就认为可以切除。

第二节　早期胰腺癌

早期胰腺癌一直是影像诊断的难点,现代医学影像技术的发展,使早期胰腺癌诊断成为可能。近年来,胰腺癌的发病率及死亡率均有逐渐升高的趋势,虽然诊断胰腺癌的方法很多,但在临床确诊时多属晚期,仅 10%~15% 可手术治疗。早期发现并手术切除肿瘤是治愈胰腺癌从而提高生存率的关键。现代医学影像技术的发展使早期胰腺癌的诊断成为可能。

一、早期胰腺癌的概念

目前对早期胰腺癌的界定尚存有异议。Moossa 等根据临床病理将早期胰腺癌定义为肿块最大径≤ 2.0cm,胰周被膜无浸润,无远处淋巴结转移,切除标本上无淋巴结转移。

美国癌症联合会将肿瘤局限于胰腺内,最大径≤ 2.0cm,无淋巴结转移,无血管侵犯的 T1aN0M0 作为早期胰腺癌的诊断标准。临床工作中通常将肿块最大径在 2.0cm 以下的小胰腺癌称为早期胰腺癌。与≥ 2.0cm 胰腺癌相比,早期胰腺癌手术切除机会大,其术后 5 年生存率也有明显提高,约在 30% 以上(Yamaguchi 等,1999)。然而,随着对早期胰腺癌临床病理研究的深入,发现早期胰腺癌淋巴浸润和胰周神经侵犯的发生率很高(Yamaguchi 等,1999)。研究还表明,早期胰腺癌术后长期存活者,其肿瘤最大径一般不超过 1.5cm。因此有学者认为,作为早期胰腺癌的诊断标准肿瘤最大径应比 2.0cm 更小。

Tsunoda 等(1998)通过对 347 例肿瘤最大径≤ 2.0cm 的胰腺癌资料进行研究,发现肿瘤≤ 2.0cm 者中仅 41.7% 属 T1 期,其 5 年生存率不到 50%。而肿瘤最大径≤ 1.0cm 的 33 例早期胰腺癌和 12 例原位癌, 5 年生存率达 100%。因此认为应将肿瘤最大径≤ 1.0cm 作为划分早期胰腺癌的诊断标准,原位癌或有微小浸润的管内癌,不论其大小,也列入早期胰腺癌的范畴。Ariyama 等(1998)也认为将局限于胰管上皮最大径≤ 1.0cm 的肿瘤作为早期胰腺癌比较合适,他对 77 例此类早期胰腺癌进行随访,5 年生存率达 100%。

二、早期胰腺癌的影像研究

CT:CT 自临床应用以来,以其密度分辨力高、重复性好而成为胰腺肿瘤最重要的影像检查手段。由于胰腺癌大多属少血供肿瘤,CT 平扫时早期胰腺癌多呈等密度改变,再者因肿瘤体积小,很少引起胰腺形态和轮廓的改变,致使 CT 平扫时早期胰腺癌极易漏诊。

CT 薄层动态增强扫描，使早期胰腺癌的低密度得到一定的显示，早期胰腺癌的检出率明显提高，可达 80%，被认为是当时最佳的影像诊断技术。但由于常规 CT 扫描速度的限制，常规动态增强扫描很难在动脉期内完成全胰腺的扫描，而且，对早期胰腺癌低密度的显示还不够满意，早期胰腺癌的检出仍存在一定的难度。螺旋 CT 极大地提高了扫描速度，使在胰腺动脉期和肝门脉期内分别完成全胰腺扫描成为现实。

很多学者对胰腺螺旋 CT 双期扫描的扫描时相，对比剂的注射量及速率进行了详尽的研究，综合文献报道，胰腺螺旋 CT 双期扫描的主要参数通常为动脉期延迟时间为 35~40 秒，门脉期为 65~70 秒，对比剂用量约 90~150ml，注射速率 3ml/ 秒。研究发现在胰腺动脉期，正常胰腺实质明显强化而肿瘤强化不明显，两者密度差异增大，因此非常有利于早期胰腺癌的检出（Lu 等，1996）。

Furukawa 等（1996）对 22 例≤ 2.0cm 的早期胰腺癌进行了螺旋 CT 双期扫描，有 21 例（95%）肿瘤在动脉期明确显示。Choi 等（1997）比较了螺旋 CT 动脉期和延迟期对早期胰腺癌的显示差异，动脉期肿瘤检出率为 90%，而延迟期仅 50%，且在动脉期 80% 的病灶显示优于延迟期。因此，Choi 认为由于螺旋 CT 扫描速度快，使全胰腺在强化最显著时完成，因而肿瘤 - 胰腺对比强烈，小病灶易于检出。目前，MSCT 双期薄层扫描已成为发现早期胰腺癌的最佳扫描方法。早期胰腺癌除了显示为低密度肿块的直接征象外，其间接征象的显示对诊断也有重要价值。间接征象主要包括肝内外胆管及胰管扩张，胰腺体、尾部萎缩，胰腺形态或轮廓改变。由于肿瘤具有围管性浸润生长的特性，常压迫胆总管或阻塞主胰管而导致其远侧扩张，胰体、尾部萎缩。有时可因阻塞形成潴留性囊肿，并可诱发急性胰腺炎。然而，受肿瘤大小及所处部位的影响，或因肿瘤突出胰腺轮廓向外发展，可无肝内外胆管扩张，或仅显示轻微的胰管扩张。

Yamaguchi 等（1999）对 8 例≤ 2.0cm 的早期胰腺癌进行研究，发现 3 例无或仅有轻微浸润的早期胰腺癌的唯一 CT 征象是主胰管或分支胰管的扩张。Tsuchiya 等（1999）分析了 36 例 1.0cm 的早期胰腺癌的 CT 表现，9 例（26%）显示了肿块，20 例（57%）在 CT 上仅表现为胰管扩张。Yamaguchi 等（1997）还报道了 2 例原位胰腺癌，CT 无胰管扩张表现，胰尾部却发现囊性病变。据此推测，囊性病变可能是早期胰腺癌的前期征象。

由此可见，主胰管或分支胰管的扩张在影像诊断胰腺癌时具有非常重要的意义，它可能是早期胰腺癌的唯一 CT 征象。对高度怀疑早期胰腺癌的病例，即使是微小的异常影像表现，都应进行全面而细致的胰腺检查，以便发现早期胰腺癌。

MRI：由于呼吸运动、肠蠕动的影响，MRI 应用于胰腺检查的初期效果并不理想，随着 MR 成像速度加快，图像信噪比提高，快速回波、呼吸抑制、抑脂技术等的应用，胰腺癌的检出率明显提高。胰腺癌在 MRI T_1WI 上呈低信号肿块，可与正常胰腺组织区分，但边界欠清。T_2WI 上肿瘤呈高信号。联合应用脂肪抑制（FS）的平扫 T_1WI，不管使用 SE 序列还是梯度回波序列，均可使胰腺组织的信号强度明显提高，与周围组织和低信号的肿瘤对比更佳，有利于检出胰腺肿瘤和显示胰腺的毗邻关系。

近年，研究显示，多数作者更倾向于采用快扫的脂肪抑制梯度回波作 T_1WI，如扰相梯度回波成像（SPGR）和快速小角度激发成像（FLASH）等，可在一次屏气间完成整个胰腺扫描，伪影少，且可用于多时相动态增强扫描，以观察胰腺及肿瘤的血流动力学变化。

平扫的 T_2WI 多采用脂肪抑制的 FSE 序列，但伪影较多，有时可采用单次激发 SE 代替 FSE 序列完成 T_2WI 来降低运动伪影，但同时降低了信噪比。脂肪抑制的 T_2WI 主要用于显示肿瘤局部浸润情况，亦可较好地显示肿瘤内部的液化坏死。

目前，动态增强 MRI 在胰腺肿瘤诊断中的应用越来越受到重视，与平扫 MRI 相比，动态增强 MRI 有较多优势：①由于使用对比剂，提高了胰腺 - 肿瘤的信号强度差异，有利于小胰腺癌的检出，更有利于发现 1cm 以内的早期胰腺癌；②清晰显示胰周血管，结合多平面重建和血管三维重建，可对胰周血管情况做出评价；③有利于显示肝内小转移灶。

然而，由于胰腺血流动力学特点不同于肝脏，因此，动态增强扫描应综合考虑数据采集的时间、对比剂的用量及注射速率、个体循环差异等诸多因素，才能获得较好的动态增强 MRI 效果。早期动态增强 MRI 研究多采用手推对比剂后即行屏气扫描，无精确的扫描时间窗。Kanematsu 等（2000）应用高压注射器作小剂量试验，测定对比剂到达腹主动脉的精确时间，研究不同延迟扫描时间胰腺及其周围血管的信号强度变化。结果显示,当对比剂使用量为0.1mmol/kg,速率为3.0ml/秒时,分别延迟15秒和45秒作两次屏气梯度回波序列扫描,能较佳地显示胰腺实质和胰周血管。关于对比剂用量,Coche等(1999)认为应采用标准剂量(0.1mmol/kg)进行MRI动态增强扫描,但亦有作者认为使用双倍剂量的动态增强扫描有利于提高薄层扫描的信噪比(Ichikawa等,1997)。注射速率一般认为2~3ml/秒较为合适。

Ichikawa等(1997)对21例胰腺癌进行了螺旋CT和动态MRI的对比研究,其中6例肿瘤最大径小于2.0cm,CT发现病灶3例,MRI发现5例。认为动态增强MRI在早期胰腺癌检测方面优于CT。Irie等(1997)对8例直径2.0cm的早期胰腺癌进行CT、MRI比较研究,结果显示,CT发现5例,MRI发现7例,其中1例由于血供相对丰富而为CT和动态MRI所遗漏,却被MRI T_1抑脂序列清晰显示出来。此研究中,MRI发现早期胰腺癌的最小肿瘤直径为0.8cm。该学者认为,MRI特别是MRI T_1抑脂序列为检测早期胰腺癌的首选方法。

磁共振胆胰管成像(MRCP)成像原理为利用重T_2,使慢流或静态的液体在重T_2WI上呈明显高信号,突出胆胰管的影像以达到成像的效果。MRCP成像多采用2D或3D FSE序列。随着一些成像序列如单次激发半傅里叶采集重T_2WI技术的不断开发应用,胆胰管成像日趋完美。MRCP对正常主胰管的显示率可达81%~96%,3D MRCP还可较好地显示主胰管的全长。MRCP可明确显示胰腺癌所致的主胰管异常,如不规则狭窄、中断及ERCP所不能显示的肿瘤远侧端胰管扩张。作为无创性的胆胰管成像技术,MRCP是ERCP检查失败或不能行ERCP检查者的最佳替代方法,同时MRCP还可提供比ERCP更多的有关胰管周围组织的相关信息。

在技术更新方面,运用脂肪抑制技术,减少了胆管周围脂肪组织的信号强度,有利于胆管的显示;而流动补偿技术及呼吸抑制技术的应用,提高了图像质量。应用新技术所获得的MRCP图像可与ERCP相媲美,并在一定程度上取代了ERCP。

Diehl等(1999)对胰腺癌MRCP与ERCP进行了比较,发现MRCP与ERCP的诊断准确率分别为80%、85%,阳性预测值分别为85%、88%,而MRCP结合MRI原始图像后的诊断准确率和阳性预测值可达到88%、91%。

Reinhold等(1996)认为,MRCP可显示91%~100%的胆管梗阻及85%~100%梗阻水平的情况,其敏感度为86%,特异度为95%,准确度为97%。由此可以看出,MRCP结合MRI图像对胰腺癌的诊断准确率已达到或超过ERCP。MRCP和MRI原始图像的相互补充更有利于显示早期胰腺癌的直接或间接征象,因而更有利于早期胰腺癌的检出。

MRI内镜技术,采用快速扰相梯度回波技术,将射频线圈置于十二指肠降段,对胰腺进行平扫或增强扫描,可获得更为清晰的胰腺图像。Inui等(1998)对22例行MRI内镜检查,13例被证实为胰腺癌,肿瘤及扩张的胰管清晰可辨。因此,MRI内镜新技术可对胰腺肿瘤提供更精确的诊断,可用于早期胰腺癌的检测。

CT、MRI导引下细针穿刺活检(FNAB):对怀疑为胰腺癌的病人行术前影像导引下细针穿刺活检有利于疾病确诊,从而减少术前待诊时间。文献报道,术前影像导引下穿刺活检的诊断准确度为69%~76%。Graham等(1994)对83例可疑病人行CT导引下细针穿刺活检,结果63例证实为胰腺癌,其中4例为二次穿刺活检确诊,总准确度为76%。他认为影响细针穿刺活检的主要因素有5类,即临床病史,穿刺途径,CT所示肿瘤大小、部位、有无坏死。其中以肿瘤大小对细针穿刺活检影响最大。随着肿瘤直径减小,细针穿刺活检诊断准确度下降。因此对于高度怀疑早期胰腺癌的病例,应重复细针穿刺活检以提高诊断准确度。但也有学者对此提出异议,认为穿刺活检可造成针道种植等问题,穿刺后短时间内手术切除肿瘤是避免上述问题的有效途径。

MRI导引下经皮细针穿刺活检为MRI介入新技术,由于早期胰腺癌病灶小,平扫时CT常呈等密度,给CT导引下穿刺活检带来了困难。MRI具有优越的软组织分辨力,可显示CT平扫时呈等密度的微小病灶,且可清晰显示病变位置与相邻器官及血管的空间结构关系。文献报道,MRI导引下穿刺定位精确度可局限在2~3mm直径范围内,结合对早期病灶有较好显示的MRI T_1抑脂序列,将非常有利于早期肿瘤的术前定性诊断。目前此项技术尚处于初步应用阶段,相信随着此项技术的进一步完善,定会提高早期胰腺癌的术前诊断水平。

综上所述,虽然早期胰腺癌的CT、MRI诊断技术有一定进展,但仍存在不少问题:① CT、MRI对早期胰腺癌的诊断还须积累更多的资料与经验；②两者的比较影像学研究应在不断技术更新的基础上进行；③对正常大小的隐匿性转移淋巴结的鉴别和胰周淋巴及神经浸润的影像诊断将是影像学面临的难题。诸多问题表明早期胰腺癌诊断仍较困难，但可以预见，CT 和 MRI 在诊断早期胰腺癌方面将会起到越来越重要的作用。

第三节　关于小胰癌

胰腺癌的影像诊断主要依赖对肿瘤直接及间接征象的把握，小胰癌由于病灶较小，很少引起胰腺形态轮廓的变化，因此，胰腺 MRI 信号的变化显得尤为重要。

正常胰腺组织富含水样蛋白，而胰腺癌含量很低，因此，在脂肪抑制 T_1WI 序列上正常胰腺组织呈高信号，而胰腺癌则呈低信号，该序列由于降低了图像的背景噪声，胰腺癌病灶呈明显低信号，与正常胰腺组织形成鲜明对比，研究显示，脂肪抑制 T_1WI 上胰腺癌与正常胰腺组织的信号对比度最大，有利于小胰癌的检出，可以发现直径 <1.0cm 的肿瘤。该组病例于脂肪抑制 T_1WI 呈低信号者 18 例，等信号 3 例，其中 1 例病灶直径约 7 mm。

胰腺血供丰富，而胰腺癌属于少血供肿瘤，在增强的动脉期信号多低于正常胰腺，使胰腺 - 肿瘤的对比明显提高，更有利于显示在脂肪抑制 T_1WI 像上呈等信号的小肿瘤；随着增强时间的延迟，门静脉期时，对比剂积聚于胰腺癌间质内，肿瘤呈逐渐强化趋势，故对癌灶的显示不如动脉期，但门静脉期有利于判断胰腺癌周围血管侵犯情况及有无淋巴结肿大、肝脏有无转移等，对胰腺癌的术前分期及评估具有重要意义。

Ichikawa 等（1997）对 21 例胰腺癌的对比研究取示，增强 MRI 在早期胰腺癌的检出上优于螺旋 CT。薄层扫描序列的应用，减少了扫描的容积效应，更有利于小病灶的显示。该组病例均行 MRI 脂肪抑制 T_1WI 序列增强薄层扫描，动脉期肿瘤病灶均呈明显低信号，肿瘤与正常胰腺对比明显，因此，对怀疑胰腺癌的患者，应在注射对比剂后逐期行薄层扫描，获得胰腺各期图像，注意观察胰腺信号变化，以便检出小胰癌。

MRCP 利用重 T_2WI 技术来直接显示胆、胰管形态和结构，可了解有无梗阻或变异，在诊断方面大多可替代逆行胆胰管造影（ERCP）。Adamek 等（2000）对 124 例临床高度怀疑胰腺癌的患者分别实施 MRCP 和 ERCP，发现 MRCP 与 ERCP 诊断胰腺癌的敏感性相似。与 ERCP 比较而言，MRCP 具有无创、简便、多方位成像的优势，可清晰显示胰、胆管梗阻性病变的梗阻平面，对于主胰管被肿瘤浸润而阻塞者，MRCP 还可显示其远侧端扩张的胰管，有利于对病灶做出准确诊断。根据胰、胆管扩张的形态特点可以对病变性质做出较为准确的判断，有利于胰腺炎和胰腺肿瘤的鉴别。

Ichikawa 等（2001）报道的一组 66 个病灶的研究显示，MRCP 显示主胰管穿过炎性肿块呈光滑的狭窄性改变或无异常，并称之为“胰管穿透征”，而恶性肿块则表现为病灶区主胰管的阻塞中断，伴有远端胰管的连续性扩张，单用 MRCP 的“胰管穿透征”鉴别两者的敏感性、特异性和准确性分别高达 85%、93% 和 92%。从该组病例分析，MRCP 可准确显示肿瘤导致的胆胰管中断和扩张，对确定肿瘤部位及其大小有重要参考价值。

小胰癌多发生于胰头和钩突部，该组 21 例中就有 14 例肿瘤位于胰头和钩突部，由于肿瘤具有围管性浸润生长的特性，易压迫胆总管下端引起梗阻性胆管扩张，或阻塞胰管引起远侧段胰管扩张。因此，小胰癌早期就可表现出显著的间接征象，而 MRCP 在显示胆胰管扩张方面具有明显优势。该组 21 例中有 13 例表现为肝内、外胆管不同程度扩张，21 例主胰管出现不同程度扩张，MRCP 均清晰显示了胆胰管的形态和结构，根据胰管中断的发生情况，可以初步确定病灶的部位及大小，指导下一步的操作，以获得有利于诊断的影像证据。T_1WI 脂肪抑制序列，MRCP 及脂肪抑制 T_1WI 薄层增强扫描序列是检出胰腺肿瘤的最佳组合，特别是对小胰癌的检出。

早期发现小胰癌，还必须重视其早期临床表现，可以认为应对 40 岁以上出现黄疸，上腹部不适，腰背部痛，体重减轻等早期可疑症状予以重视。对于血胰淀粉酶升高的患者，切勿因得出胰腺炎的诊断而忽视了小胰癌的存在，小胰癌阻塞胰管可诱发胰腺炎,该组 1 例患者因急性胰腺炎入院治疗,血胰淀粉酶每逢进食后升高,经 MRCP 和 MRI 增强扫描,发现直径 7 mm 小肿瘤阻塞主胰管,后经手术病理证实。

MRI 具有较高的软组织分辨率,多参数、多方位成像的优势,对胰腺癌可疑患者可行多期相薄层增强扫描,而 MRCP 在显示胆、胰管结构方面又具有独特的价值, MRCP 结合 MRI 图像,对小胰癌的诊断更具重要临床价值。

第四节 有关钩突的病变

钩突下方为十二指肠水平部。钩突一般与左肾静脉同一层面。当钩突形态变圆,边缘变凸时,应提示有肿瘤的可能。

有作者报告 14 例胆总管下端癌中,手术所见和病理检查均有胆管、胰腺及其外围受累者 5 例,其中 4 例 CT 检查评价准确,均表现为钩突内侧的不规则低密度肿块影,并与肠系膜上动、静脉关系密切。有 2 例肿块影完全包绕肠系膜上动脉或腹腔干,增强扫描见这些腹膜后的肿块影显示轻度强化。尽管病理证实胆总管癌周围的胰腺组织有侵及,但 CT 显示胰腺内的病灶远不如腹膜后病灶清楚明显。

当肿瘤向钩突内侧侵及,尤其是包绕门静脉和肠系膜上动、静脉时,神经丛的受侵往往越加明显。在无胰腺外肿瘤浸润的 5 例中,有 3 例为胰腺内神经受侵, CT 显示了位于胰腺内的肿瘤病灶,病理检查也证实在神经周围间隙内有癌细胞浸润。虽然有 1 例胰腺内神经受侵者 CT 未见明确的肿瘤病灶,但术后 6 个月即发现包绕在腹腔干和肠系膜动脉周围的复发肿块影。

在 2 例肝门胆管癌病例中,均有肝十二指肠韧带内的神经丛受侵,增强检查时出现胆总管壁的强化,病理证实强化的管壁为富含肿瘤血管的肿瘤组织浸润所致;同时 CT 还可见胆总管和肝固有动脉之间的脂肪间隙密度略增高,病理证实为受侵的神经周围纤维性变所致。尽管在 10 例中有 6 例淋巴结转移,但在肠系膜上动脉、腹腔干及肝固有动脉周围的淋巴结却没有转移。该作者认为,只要在 CT 图像上发现有不规则的软组织肿块影从胰腺钩突的内侧向肠系膜上动、静脉和 / 或腹腔干等蔓延时,即应考虑腹膜后神经丛的受侵。

胰位于脾静脉之前,胰体位于肠系膜上动脉与静脉之前。钩突位于肠系膜血管之后,比较于整个十二指肠水平段,它有一短的横行范围。由于它的后面关系着肠系膜上血管,一个来自于胰头钩突的包块可误为十二指肠肿块,反之亦然。

胰腺癌病灶处胰腺肿大并形成肿块。在 CT 图像上,表现为病灶处前后径增大与限局性凸出,超出邻近正常胰腺轮廓 3mm 以上的隆起,占 90% 以上的病例。癌肿多发生于胰头区。

有作者指出,胰腺前后径增大的标准为:胰头 >29.3mm,胰体 >23.6mm,胰尾 >21.2mm,胰头钩突 >10mm。肿块的形态近似圆形、椭圆形或不规则形;边缘多不光整,与正常胰腺分界不清,此为恶性肿瘤不规则性生长与向周边浸润的结果。胰癌病变区除胰腺肿大外,胰腺还可能显示为正常大小,约占 7% 左右。

另有作者报道 12 例直径在 20mm 以下小胰癌,超声直接显示肿块影 10 例,胆胰管均扩张者有 9 例,可见超声检查不仅可用于胰癌的筛选,而且对小胰癌的诊断也很有用。超声对伴存胰管胆管扩张的小胰癌的单独确诊率达 73%,应该注意的是这些表现并无特异性,尤其是超声对轻度的血管和后腹膜的浸润不能确定,而且直径在 10mm 左右又无胆胰管扩张的钩突部癌及弥漫性癌,则很难发现。

ERCP 可出现假阴性,在两个因素可影响其对癌的诊断。第一是照片的质量,第二是胰癌或合并胰腺炎等其他病变的形态学分析。当 ERCP 因种种原因(胆胰管下端肿瘤浸润、主胰管内结石梗阻或胰腺钩突部肿块引起胰管梗阻等)而不能显示胰管的影像时,可通过超声导向经皮胰管穿刺造影获得胰管的图像。

胰头钩突癌的诊断,可根据钩突前后径 >10mm,其轮廓变圆隆或呈分叶状,钩突与肠系膜上动脉及肠系膜上静脉间的脂肪消失,胰胆管扩张等征象确立诊断,一般不易漏诊。

第三章　胰腺癌的术前分期与手术切除性评价

第一节　不可切除的主要原因

Warshaw 将血管侵犯、肝转移、腹膜转移作为胰腺癌无法切除的三个原因。Diehl 又增添了淋巴结转移和胰周侵犯（十二指肠除外）两个因素。因此，准确及时地发现这些 CT 征象非常重要。

血管侵犯：胰周血管侵犯为不可切除的最常见原因。Freeny 报道约 84% 的胰腺癌患者出现血管侵犯，血管受累的概率依次为肠系膜上动脉、肠系膜上静脉、下腔静脉、肝外门静脉、腹腔动脉、主动脉。Steven 研究了 86 例手术证实的胰头癌病人，发现除主要大血管外，胰周小静脉（胃结肠干、胰十二指肠前上静脉、胰十二指肠后上静脉的浸润也是胰腺癌扩散的可靠征象。若将此加入胰头癌可切除性的标准，则将估计肿瘤可被切除的准确率由 22% 提高至 29%，而估计肿瘤无法切除的准确率由 73% 提高至 80%。

血管侵犯按程度分六种类型：A 型，脂肪分隔邻近血管和肿瘤和 / 或正常胰腺实质；B 型，正常胰腺分隔邻近血管与低密度肿瘤；C 型，低密度肿瘤与邻近血管无法分隔且凸向血管；D 型，低密度肿瘤与邻近血管无法分隔，进入管腔内或部分包绕血管；E 型，低密度肿瘤包绕邻近血管，其间无脂肪存在；F 型，肿瘤使血管闭塞。A、B 型被认为是可切除病变，E、F 型无法切除，C、D 型应考虑是否同时行血管切除术。

早期研究中，发现血管侵犯的敏感度自 36% 至 67% 不等，运用螺旋 CT 双期扫描后将敏感度提高至 88%。Diehl 认为原因有二，一是在动脉期对病变区进行了薄层（层厚 3mm）扫描，二是大剂量团注及于主动脉强化峰值开始螺旋扫描有利于胰周血管的最佳强化。

螺旋 CT 可显示所有主要胰周血管（脾动脉、脾静脉，腹腔干，肠系膜上动脉、肠系膜上静脉，胃十二指肠动脉），但对小动脉显示稍差（前胰十二指肠动脉显示率 100%，后胰十二指肠动脉 39%，后下胰十二指肠动脉 14%）。这主要是由于胰腺动脉期增强，与小动脉缺乏对比，正常胰腺表面小结节也掩盖了胰周小动脉。与此同时，胰周小静脉在螺旋 CT 双期扫描中显示较好。

Suresh 等对正常胰腺行螺旋 CT 胰腺期、肝期双期增强薄层扫描结果显示，胰周小静脉（后上胰十二指肠静脉、前上胰十二指肠静脉、胃结肠静脉干）在胰腺期的显示率较高（分别为 88%、93%、98%），明显优于肝期。

血管造影曾被认为是判断胰腺癌侵犯血管的最可靠的方法，Kancko（1997）对比了螺旋 CT 和血管造影两种方法，认为螺旋 CT 在以下四个方面优于血管造影：①螺旋 CT 为无创伤性检查方法；②螺旋 CT 能显示肿瘤与胰周动脉的真实关系；③螺旋 CT 能显示血管周围外膜的改变；④螺旋 CT 可显示主要血管的三维立体结构及其毗邻关系。

有无转移：无法正确术前分期的最常见原因是没有发现肝转移。约 40% 螺旋 CT 认为可以切除的胰腺癌患者术中由于发现肝转移而无法切除。这种转移瘤多较小，直径约 2~10mm，CT 不易发现，但术中穿刺及触摸很明显，薄层扫描（3~5 mm 层厚）可提高其检出率。另外，肝内直径不大于 15mm 的小病灶中，约 50% 为良性病变，故当发现肝内小病灶时应注意鉴别其良、恶性。

第二节　胰头癌周围淋巴结转移

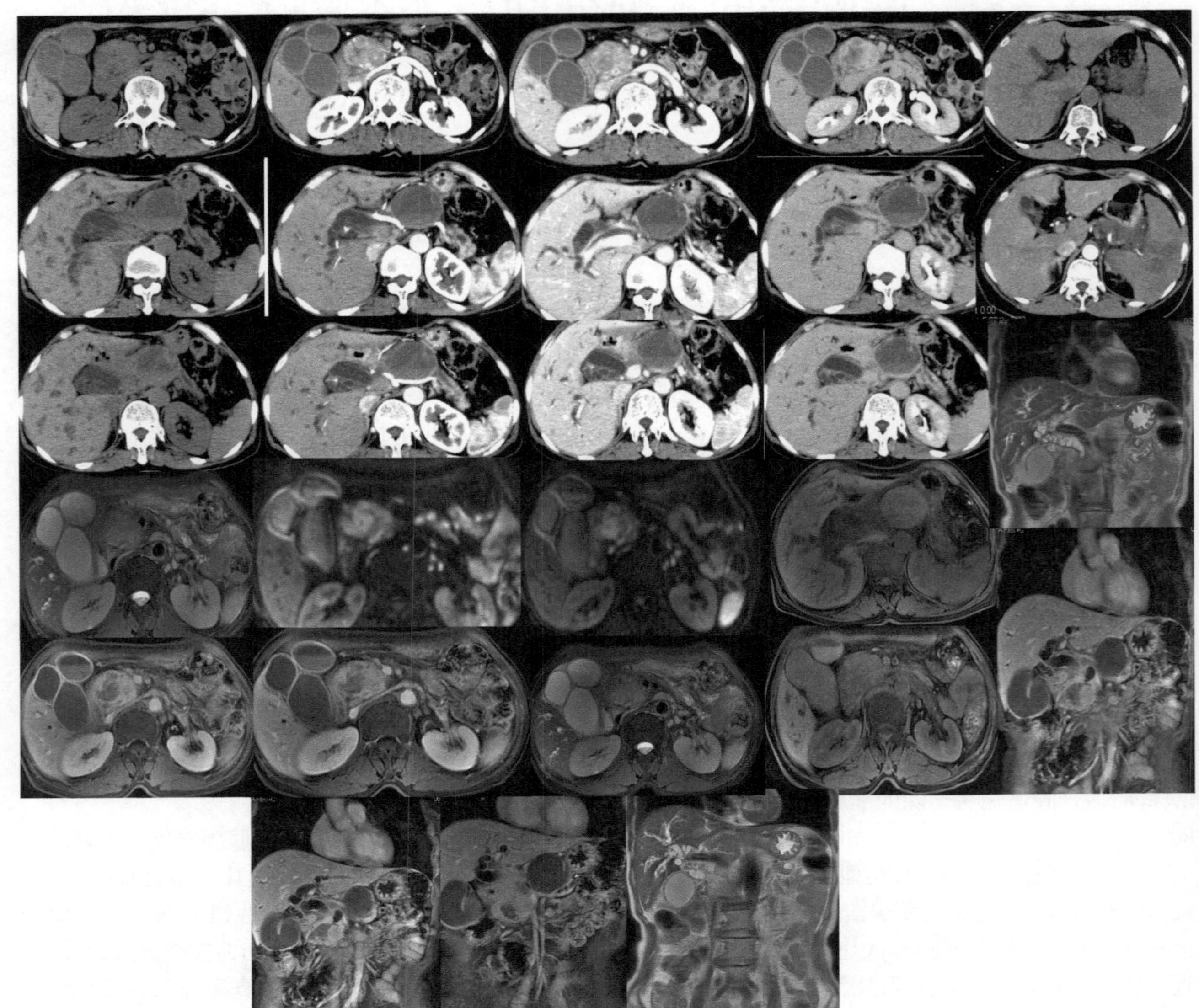

图 20-3-1　胰头癌周围淋巴结转移

患者,女, 60 岁。因上腹胀痛,黄疸入院。有“慢性胰腺炎,胰腺假性囊肿史”。

病理检查:十二指肠淋巴结切除标本:灰黄色组织一块,大小 1.8cm × 1.2cm × 0.7cm,切面灰黄、质软。常规病理诊断:十二指肠淋巴结切除标本:淋巴组织中可见转移性腺癌病灶,待作免疫组化检测进一步探讨其来源。免疫组化检测:阳性: CA19-9;阴性: CEA, CK7, CK19, CK20, Villin, CA125, ER, PR, AFP, Hepatocyte。免疫组化诊断:十二指肠淋巴结切除标本:淋巴组织中可见转移性腺癌病灶,结合临床病史,符合来源于胰腺癌转移(图 20-3-1)。

第三节　远处转移灶

远处转移灶也是造成胰腺癌切除失败的主要原因。胰腺癌的远处转移主要包括肝脏及腹膜的转移。螺旋CT在门静脉相可很好显示大于8~10mm的肝内转移灶，肝内转移灶的显示率为75%。但普通螺旋CT对肝内微小转移灶及腹膜转移灶的检出率较低。

第四节　术前分期

国际抗癌协会根据胰腺癌原发肿瘤、局部淋巴结、远处转移三方面的情况制定了TNM分期法。该种分期方法较为复杂，于是制定了一种较为实用的简单分期方法将胰腺癌分为四期：Ⅰ期，胰腺肿大，无周围血管和脏器侵犯；Ⅱ期，胰腺癌侵犯周围组织；Ⅲ期，局部淋巴结转移；Ⅳ期，肝或其他脏器转移。该法认为Ⅰ期为手术切除指征，Ⅲ、Ⅳ期为无法手术切除的指征，Ⅱ期能否切除尚有争论。

第五节　胰腺低分化癌伴坏死，侵犯脾脏

患者，女，67岁。左上腹痛1月余入院。

手术所见：胰体尾与脾门、横结肠脾曲、左肾上腺及后腹膜组织粘连紧密，呈一大小约15×10cm肿物，边界不清，质硬，脾动脉脾静脉与胰尾粘连紧密，无法游离。肠系膜上动脉及腹主动脉旁可触及多发肿大淋巴结。用超声刀游离胰颈部与周围组织的粘连，从胰腺下缘分离出肠系膜上动脉及肠系膜上静脉，清扫肠系膜上动脉旁及腹主动脉旁肿大淋巴结；在胰腺的上缘，分离出脾动脉，见脾动脉部分被淋巴结包绕，清扫淋巴结后切断脾动脉，断端双重结扎；在胰腺的背面，分离出脾静脉，切断脾静脉，近端断面缝扎，远端则予以结扎。使用切割闭合器切断胰尾，无损伤线U字缝合胰腺断端以防止胰瘘。将胰腺断端托起，向后继续分离胰腺断端与后腹膜组织粘连。分离胃脾韧带，脾结肠韧带及脾脏与后腹膜粘连，最终将胰体尾、脾脏与肿物整块切除。

病理检查：胰腺体尾部及脾脏切除标本：胰腺低分化癌伴坏死，侵犯脾脏，可见脉管内癌栓，胰体断端切缘为阴性。左肾上腺切除标本：肾上腺组织未见癌组织累及，内可见血肿形成，周围脂肪组织中检出疑似节细胞神经瘤一枚。淋巴结清扫：肿瘤周围组织中，共检出淋巴结23枚，其中17枚可见癌转移（图20-3-2）。

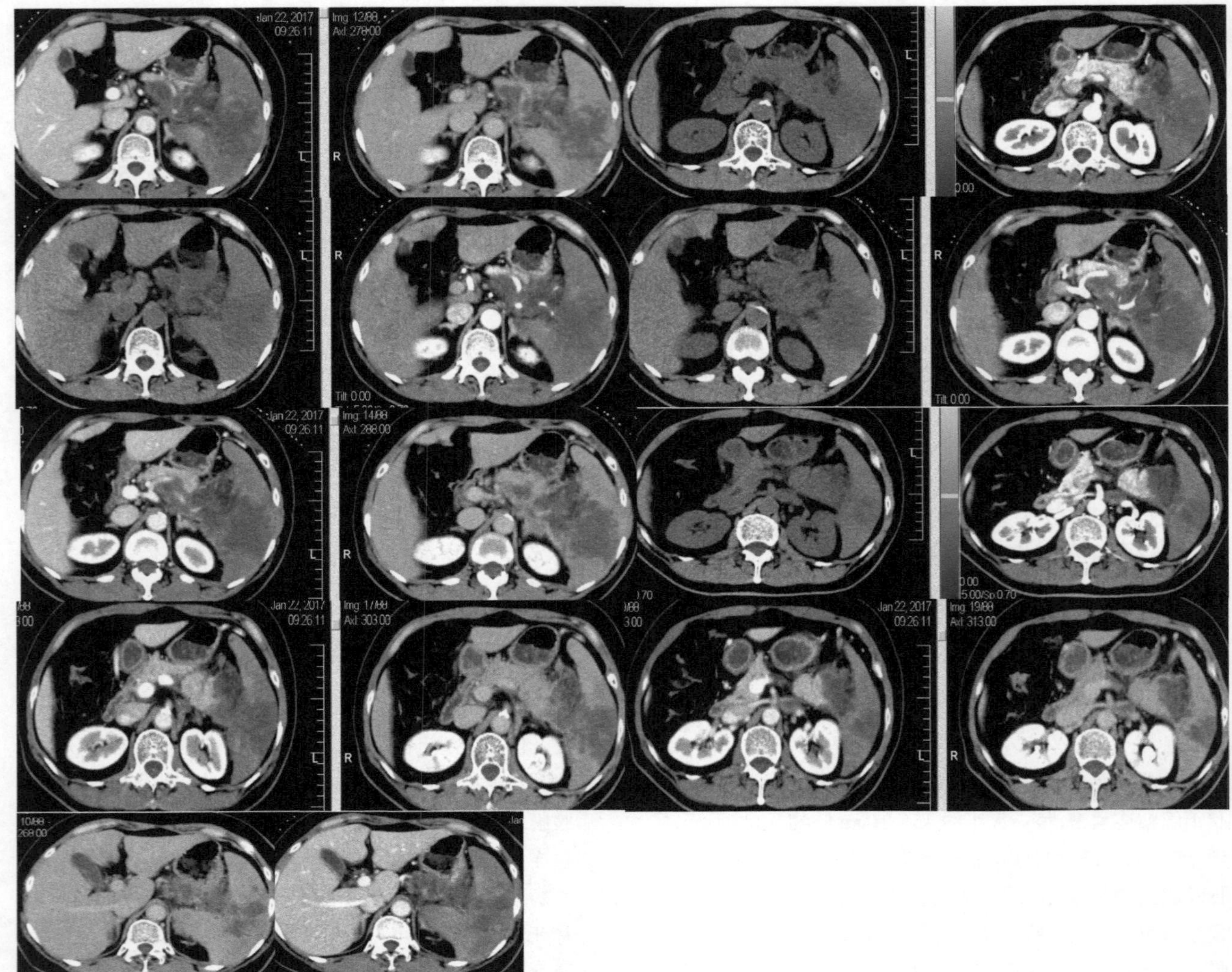

图 20-3-2 胰腺低分化癌伴坏死,侵犯脾脏

第四章　胰腺癌

第一节　误诊病例简介：胰腺中低分化囊性腺癌与间质瘤

患者，男，58 岁。体检发现胰腺占位 1 个月入院。CT 诊断：十二指肠降段及胰头不规则等低密度占位，性质待定：间质瘤？神经鞘瘤？胰头癌？建议 MRI 检查；胰腺明显萎缩，呈线样，胰体部囊肿。

MRI：胰头及十二指肠间隙内可见分叶状异常信号影，大小约 6.4cm × 4.1cm × 6.7cm，T1WI 略低信号，T2WI 不均匀高信号，囊性部分信号更高，DWI 呈较高信号，边界清楚，胰头受压结构不清，胰体尾体积缩小；MRCP 示肝内外胆管及胰管形态如常。MRI 诊断：胰头及十二指肠间隙内占位，考虑间质瘤，淋巴瘤？建议增强扫描。

手术所见：腹腔内无明显腹水，盆腔、肝脏、大网膜及腹主动脉旁未扪及明显转移灶；胆囊约 7cm × 3cm，无明显充血水肿，内未扪及结石；肝十二指肠韧带未触及明显肿大淋巴结，胆总管直径 0.8cm，管壁未见明显水肿增厚；切开十二指肠侧腹膜探查胰头部可见一成人拳头大小肿物，界限不清，移动性差，术中切取 1.5cm × 1.5cm 大小肿物送检，切开组织呈鱼肉状，冰冻病理示上皮性肿瘤（具体性质及类型不明确）。

病理检查：胰十二指肠切除标本：紧靠一侧切缘的肠管外侧可见一多房囊性肿物，送检前已剖开，大小 5.5cm × 4.0cm × 1.2cm，表现附着少量碎组织。另见灰褐色碎组织一堆，总体积 5.0cm × 5.0cm × 4.0cm。常规病理诊断：胰十二指肠切除标本：初步诊断胰腺中低分化囊性癌，待做免疫组化检测进一步协助诊断。癌组织侵犯十二指肠黏膜下层，十二指肠两切缘均为阴性，肠外膜及肠周自检出淋巴结一枚未见癌转移。

免疫组化检测：阳性：CA19-9，CK7，CK19，Villin（散在 +），CEA（小灶 +），P16（灶 +），CD117（小灶 +），CD34（血管内皮 +），PAS 染色，AB 染色，P53（+，<5%），Ki-67（+，<10%）；阴性：CA125，AFP，CK20，CgA，SyN，CD56，NSE。免疫组化诊断：胰十二指肠切除标本：免疫组化检测结果支持胰腺中低分化囊性腺癌，侵及十二指肠黏膜下层。

第二节 胰腺导管腺癌,Ⅱ级

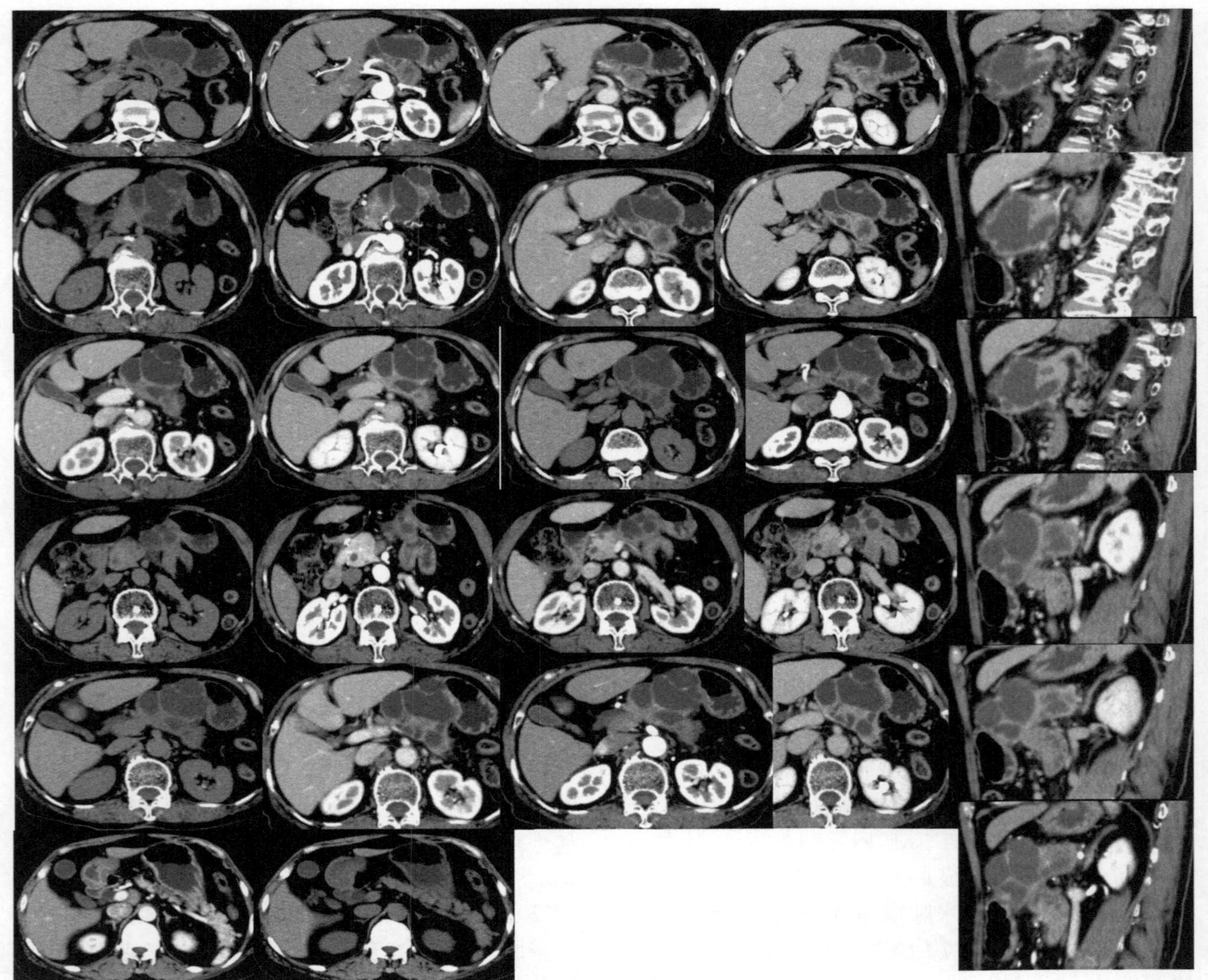

图 20-4-1 胰腺导管腺癌,Ⅱ级

患者,女,77 岁。反复腰背部痛 1 周入院。

病理检查:胰腺肿物切除标本:灰白色组织一块,大小 10cm × 6cm × 4cm,表面附脂肪,切面灰白质韧,与周围边界不清。脾脏切除标本:脾组织一个,大小 9.5cm × 7cm × 5cm,切面灰红质软,表面见一结节,直径 0.5cm。病理诊断:胰腺导管腺癌,Ⅱ级,大小 10cm × 6cm × 4cm,伴灶性坏死,浸润至边缘纤维脂肪组织,累及少数神经。胰腺旁淋巴结(-),0/5。脾脏充血出血,伴小动脉硬化,未见癌侵犯(图 20-4-1)。

第三节　中低分化胰腺导管腺癌，侵及十二指肠黏膜下层

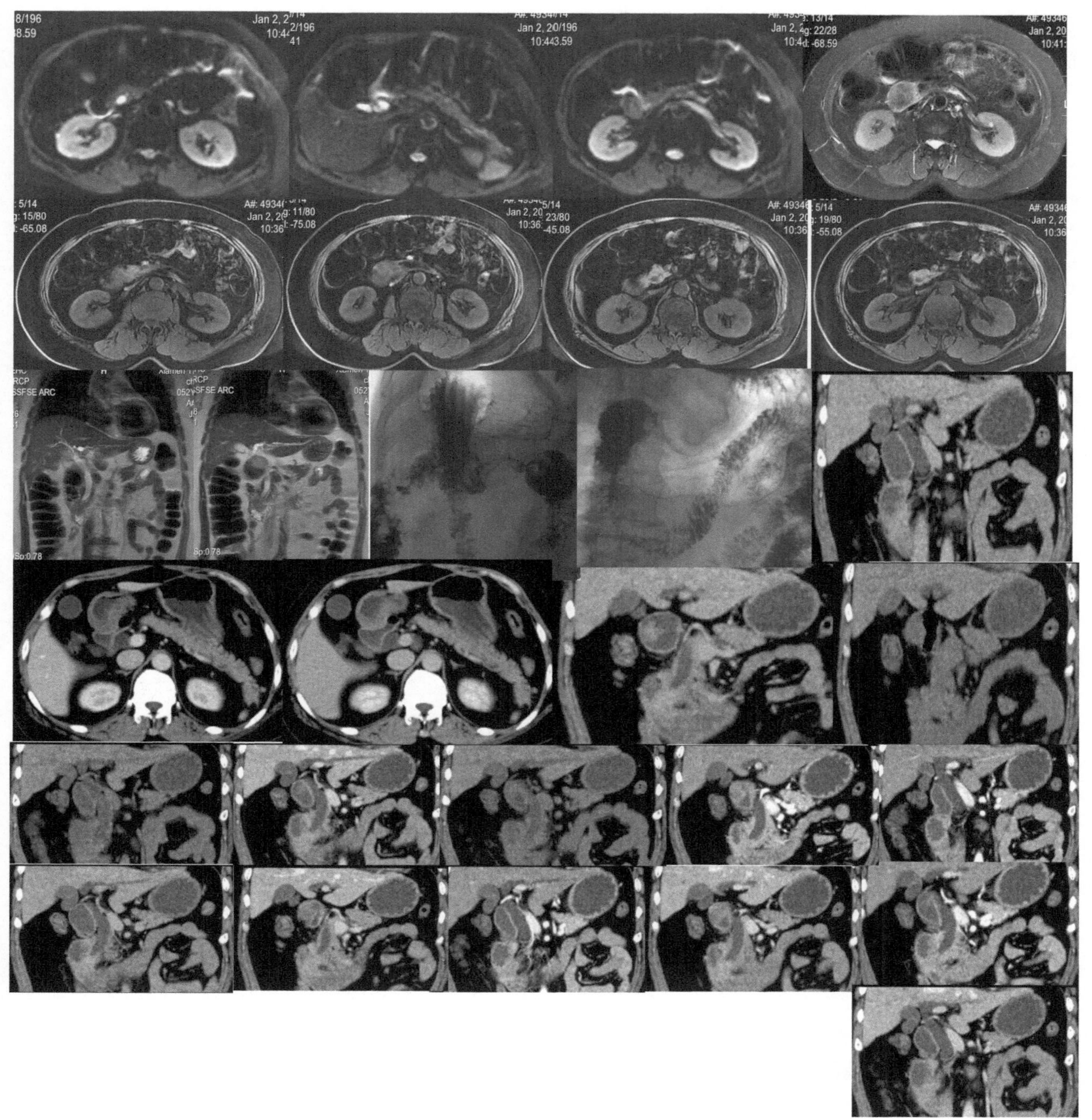

图 20-4-2　中低分化胰腺导管腺癌，侵及十二指肠黏膜下层

患者，女，52 岁。3 天前出现无明显诱因出现左腹部闷痛，外院 CT 示：十二指肠降部管壁稍增厚。昨日胃镜提示十二指肠球部及降部未见明显异常。浅表性胃炎。今天胃镜提示十二指肠水平部改变，考虑肿瘤可能。CT 检查考虑十二指肠壁病变侵犯乳头。双对比胃肠造影提示十二指肠水平段见约 3cm 局限性管腔变窄，十二指肠水平段占位？

病理检查：胰、十二指肠及胆囊切除标本：标本为切除的部分胃、十二指肠及胆囊。其中十二指肠一段，长27cm，管径2cm，于十二指肠乳头处见一肿物，大小2.5cm × 2cm × 0.6cm，切面灰白，质硬，与周围组织界限不清。附部分胰腺组织，大小6.5cm × 2cm × 0.5cm，十二指肠周围检出淋巴结样物4枚，直径0.5~1cm。常规病理诊断：胰、十二指肠及胆囊切除标本：初步诊断中低分化胰腺导管腺癌，侵及十二指肠黏膜下层，待做免疫组化进一步确定。十二指肠切缘及胃吻合口切缘均为阴性，胃壁及胆囊组织均未受癌组织累及。免疫组化检测：阳性：CA19-9，CK7，CK20（散在+），Villin，EGFR（3+），VEGF（2+），P-gP（2+），Tubulinβ（+），TOPO Ⅱ（+），CD34（血管内皮+），Ki-67（+，约20%）；阴性：ERCC1，5-FU。免疫组化诊断：胰、十二指肠及胆囊切除标本：中低分化胰腺导管腺癌，侵及十二指肠黏膜下层（图20-4-2）。

第四节　胰腺间变细胞癌

胰腺间变细胞癌是一种罕见的胰腺外分泌肿瘤，多见于60~80岁老年男性，该病影像表现无特异性，定性诊断困难。有作者认为胰腺间变细胞癌与胰腺导管腺癌影像表现有区别，常规CT表现为胰腺形态不规则、体积相对较大的外生性或分叶状肿块，实质内可见中心坏死区，类似黏液囊腺瘤或囊实性肿块，增强后肿块表现为不均一、中等程度的强化。

动态增强CT动脉期周围实性部分强化，中心可见片状低密度区。门静脉期肿瘤周边实性部分强化范围较动脉期有扩大，强化程度略增高，强化壁厚薄不一，中心坏死区无强化，与邻近胰腺实质对比明显，延迟期周围实质为略高密度影，强化范围无明显变化，可能与该例延迟强化时间较短有关，增加延迟时间瘤体内对比剂退出会有差异（图20-4-3）。

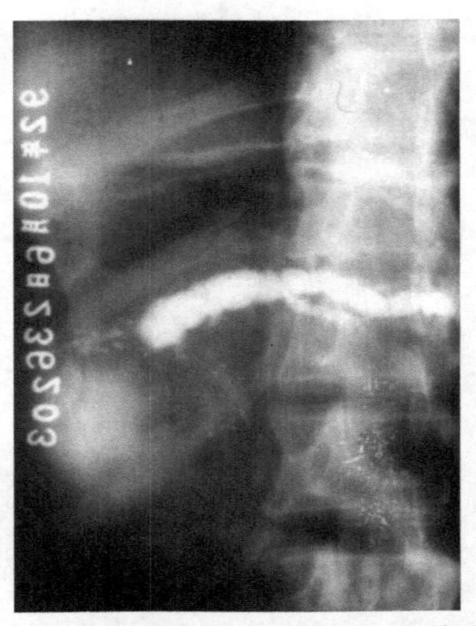

图20-4-3　ERCP：可见胰头癌引起的主胰管明显扩张迂曲，胰头部类圆形包块被细小胰腺导管包裹，包块内有部分对比剂，手术病理证实该包块正是胰头癌

胰腺间变细胞癌极易向胰腺周软组织、胃壁、脾、腹膜等周围结构侵袭蔓延，一例CT未见有明确肝转移征象，病变主要累及前方的胃后壁、周围软组织及肠系膜血管等。

胰腺间变细胞癌的淋巴结转移早，且范围广，可出现在胰腺远隔淋巴结和胸腔内淋巴结，该例未见有明确肿大的区域淋巴结。由于有囊变坏死区，MRI以混杂信号为主，对肿瘤定性帮助不大，但其定位及显示软组织较CT敏感。螺旋CT、MRI等多平面、多期成像方法，可充分认识肿瘤本身血供以及周围累及情况，与常见胰腺导管腺癌有区别，对提示诊断、术前直观判断肿瘤的可切除性很有帮助。

第五节　表现为囊性肿块的胰腺癌

胰腺癌表现为囊性肿块者不多，诊断时易误诊为胰腺炎，假性囊肿形成。

要注意囊肿的下游的实性肿块，囊壁增厚及壁结节的出现。壁厚而不均匀，发现壁结节提示囊腺癌可能性较大。同时，要结合周围结构的间接改变及转移征象，特别是胰腺肿物后方肠系膜上动脉的受侵，常是胰腺癌的重要特征。

有作者报告 10 例此类病人中，有 8 例出现此征，其病理基础与肿瘤浸润血管周围的淋巴管，及反应性结缔组织增生有关。

一组作者报告 120 例胰腺癌中有 10 例（占 8.3%）表现以囊性为主，其中胰腺癌合并上游潴留性囊肿 4 例，表现为边缘光滑的类圆形囊肿，壁薄，囊内 CT 值类似水，特征为在囊肿的下游或胰头方向有实性肿块；胰腺癌中央坏死 2 例，CT 图像上癌肿近乎全部呈一低密度厚壁囊性肿物，边界不规则，囊内密度较均匀，肿块后方与肠系膜上动脉粘连；1 例还有肝转移，病理见肿瘤坏死未完全液化而呈鱼肉状，镜下为微囊性改变；另有囊腺癌 3 例，胰腺黏液细胞腺癌 1 例。

第六节　胰颈中高分化腺癌伴大量坏死

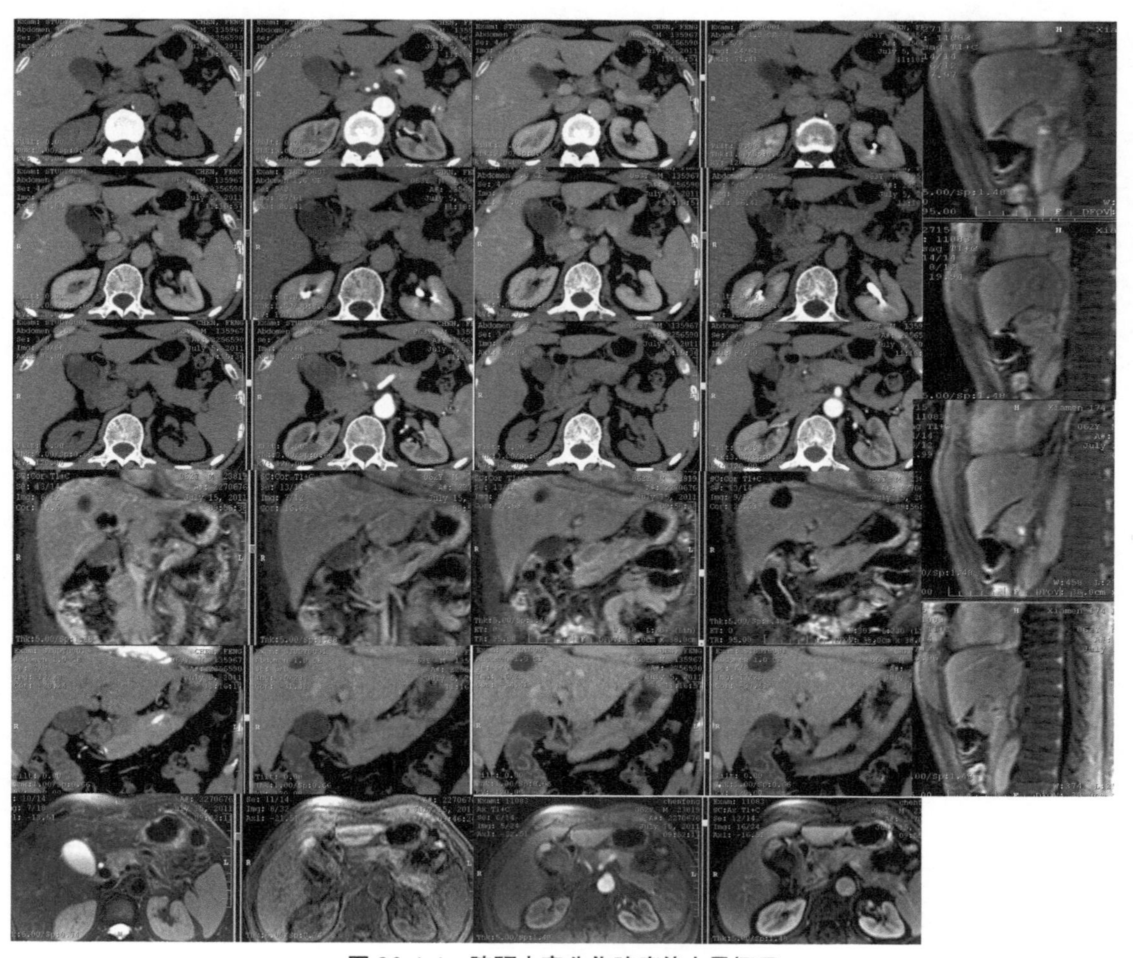

图 20-4-4　胰颈中高分化腺癌伴大量坏死

患者,男,62 岁。发现胆囊结石 1 月,突发右上腹疼痛 1 天入院。

手术所见:胰头颈部上缘可及一质地坚硬肿物,大小 2cm × 3cm,右侧壁向十二指肠浸润生长并侵犯十二指肠浆肌层,后下壁侵犯肝动脉并与其紧密粘连,局部有淋巴结肿大,腹腔无明显腹水。胆囊约 9.5cm × 3.5cm,内有大量结石,胆总管直径约 1.5cm,肝脏呈轻度肝硬化表现,表面未见明显肿物。腹腔盆腔及大网膜未见明显肿瘤种植和转移,切除胰头肿物术中送病理检查,结果回报示胰腺癌,决定行胰十二指肠根治性切除。

病理检查:部分胃 + 十二指肠 + 胰腺切除标本:胃体积 8.5cm × 4cm × 3cm,胰腺体积 6cm × 3.5cm × 2.5cm,十二指肠长 13cm,远切端直径 1.5cm,肠管部分剖开,胃黏膜皱襞消失,十二指肠未见明显异常,胰腺剖开可见一灰白结节,体积 2cm × 2cm × 2cm,切面灰白,质中,其余未见明显异常。胆囊切除标本:胆囊一条,体积 13cm × 4cm × 3.5cm,剖开胆囊内可见大量的黑色结石,最大体积 3cm × 2.5cm × 2cm,胆囊壁厚 0.2~0.3cm。常规病理诊断:胰头(腺癌)及十二指肠切除标本:胰头导管腺癌,Ⅱ级,胰腺十二指肠交界处有癌侵犯至十二指肠深部肌层及浆膜。胃壁、胃切缘、十二指肠壁和切缘均阴性。胆囊切除标本:胰腺癌侵犯胆囊(从黏膜到肌层)。慢性结石性胆囊炎。淋巴结清扫:第 8 组淋巴结 0/2,但较大淋巴结旁的软组织有转移癌。第 12 组实为纤维脂肪组织未见转移灶。

免疫组化诊断:胰颈旁肿物切除标本:中高分化腺癌伴大量坏死(图 20-4-4)。

第七节 胰头腺癌

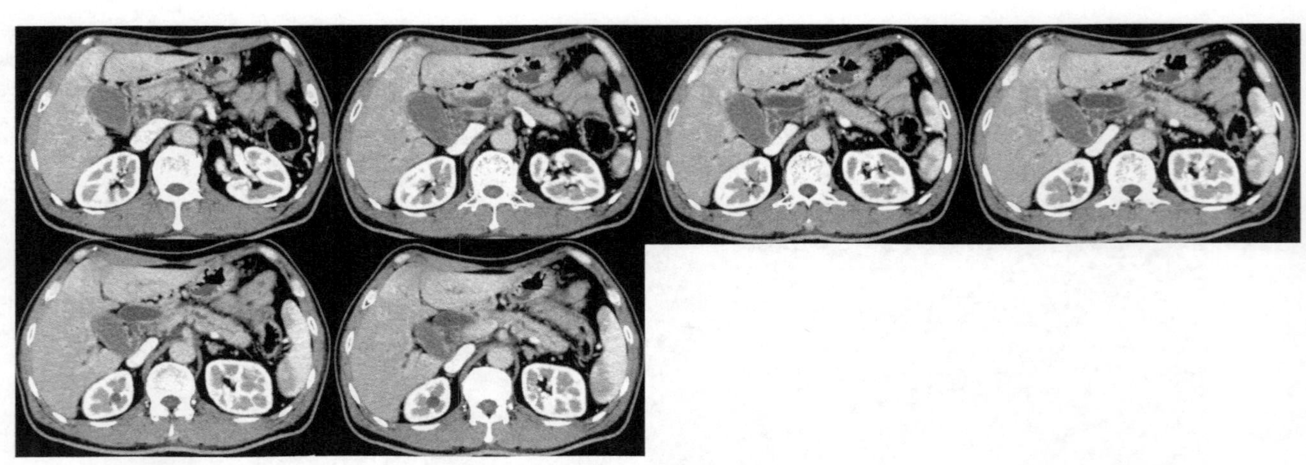

图 20-4-5 胰头腺癌

患者,男,64 岁。CT:胰头占位性病变。扩张的胆囊管低位汇入肝外胆管,肝外胆管明显扩张,主胰管明显扩张。术后病理诊断:胰头腺癌。肿瘤大小为 4cm × 3cm × 2cm(图 20-4-5)。

第五章　胰腺的部分影像学检查

第一节　逆行胰管造影术中的充盈缺损原因

伪影：最常见的管内充盈缺损是注入的气泡。这些气泡通常呈圆形，或近椭圆形，易于识别，且同时可勾画出胰管的形态。气泡常是多发、连续的。透视下很容易看到气泡随着少量对比剂的注射而移动，或者可显示出气泡从导管口被注入。气泡也可吸回到导管中。当病人的位置改变时，胰管内的气泡将升到胰管最高处。一个大的气柱影可造成干扰，使主胰管显示不清。当较多的对比剂被注射到充气段时，胰腺影会发生腺泡化改变。胰管内气体的存在也能与狭窄胰管混淆，或被误认为胰管梗阻。注射时对比剂的外渗可能误诊为扩张且扭曲的胰管内不规则肿块，当注射前确定胰管内导管口的位置困难时，或插管时无意中插入胰管的一侧分支后，注射对比剂常可发生对比剂外渗。

炎症：胰腺的炎症可导致多种不同类型的胰管内充盈缺损，最常见的是胰管内结石。蛋白质性的栓子与胰腺的慢性炎症有关。这些蛋白质栓子的磷酸钙不断增多，最终生成管腔内钙化的结石，可在慢性钙化性胰腺炎较晚期发现。在ERCP，这些结石在不同的发展阶段可显示或不显示出钙化。注射对比剂前的X线片对显示这些结石的钙化有帮助，而这些结石可被随后注入的对比剂所遮盖。CT对确定胰腺内的细微钙化有较高敏感性。角形的边缘，多发和可移动性等特点，可将结石与其他的充盈缺损区分开。当腹痛是由于胰管内结石引起时，外科或内镜介入治疗可适当缓解胰管的梗阻。

胰腺慢性炎性病变中一种不常见的发现是在主胰管内存在胶状管型。罕见情况下，在急性胰腺炎病人的主胰管中可看到为数众多的小的充盈缺损。虽然ERCP在胰腺炎的急性期是禁忌的，但当胆总管结石为胰腺炎病因之一而拟使胆总管显影时，胰管可以被无意中注入对比剂而显影。这些充盈缺损被认为与胰腺自身溶解的碎片有关。

当胰腺炎伴有假性囊肿形成时，后者在ERCP检查中充盈对比剂的概率约为70%。

新生物：由胰腺新生物造成的胰管内充盈缺损并不多见。这些胰管内的病灶与肿瘤本身或凝胶管型的分泌物有关。良性胰管内肿块罕见，其中以胰管内乳头状瘤最常见，它可单发或多发，和黏蛋白分泌过多有关。

最常见的胰腺恶性肿瘤——胰管腺癌，通常与胰管狭窄或切断术有关。有时类似胰管内充盈缺损或息肉状肿块，与胰管内乳头状瘤非常相似，或者像一个增大而又不规则扩张的主胰管。腺癌很少发生黏蛋白分泌过多形成的斑块或息肉状病变。

胰管被黏蛋白充盈最常发生于胰腺的黏蛋白囊性肿物。过多的凝胶物质可以引起主胰管的扩张并伴有向下端括约肌段的扩展，甚至扩展到胆胰管汇合的远端。

黏蛋白性囊性肿物的一种变异是管性黏蛋白性囊腺瘤或囊腺癌。在ERCP图像上，最常表现为钩突支的扩张，其内被黏蛋白管型所充填。一些小的充盈缺损也许和小的乳头状肿瘤有关。这些扩张的胰管由增生的乳头状上皮排列而成，这些增生上皮可以是非典型性的或是明显恶性的。

第二节　胰腺疾病中不熟悉的 X 线征象

有作者著文讨论胰腺疾病的不熟悉或未应用的 X 线征象。

在上消化道钡餐检查时,胆囊或肝外胆管扩张,它压迫充盈钡剂的十二指肠而出现不同类型的切迹,此切迹由于区别诊断甚为广泛,故难以简单地评价。十二指肠空肠曲的挤压移位也评估困难,因其正常位置变化甚大。钡剂反流进入总胆管是胰十二指肠疾病可靠指征。

局部十二指肠痉挛,大概源于局灶性神经肌肉刺激,低张十二指肠钡餐检查观察此征最佳,十二指肠外部常被侵犯。

第三节　胰腺超声检查的误诊

与肝脏相比,胰腺超声表现通常呈等或稍高回声。胰腺超声虽然在多数病人可见到胰头和胰体,但胰尾的显示则需要胃充满水后检查,以避免气体重叠产生伪影。正常胰管 80% 表现为被回声壁勾画出的窄带状低回声线影,宽径为 2mm。胰头或胰体附近的肠管可类似胰腺低回声肿块,为排除肿瘤有必要行 CT 检查。另外,扩张的远端胆总管可被怀疑为胰头的无回声肿块,为避免这种误诊,同样有必要行 CT 检查。

超声扫描中其他类似胰腺或胰腺病变的结构包括肝左叶外侧段的后部(第 2 肝段),这是因为血管周围脂肪造成的声波衰减,导致肝左叶外侧段后部回声较前部(第 3 肝段)减弱所形成。肝尾叶的乳头状突起和肿大的门腔静脉淋巴结也可误认为胰腺。

马蹄肾和腹膜后纤维化,当超声上表现为一腹膜后中线声谱带时,也类似于胰腺肿块。

胰腺超声检查中有三个正常结构可被误认为胰管扩张:第一个是分隔胰腺后缘和脾静脉的脂肪层;第二个是脾动脉或静脉,特别当血管迂曲且与胰腺存在容积效应时;最后一个是包裹在肝左叶和胰腺之间塌陷的胃窦。

第六章　MRI、CT 与胰腺癌

第一节　3.0 T MR 不同扩散加权成像与胰腺癌

MR DWI 具有成像速度快，图像后处理简单、实用性强等优点。为突出上腹部病灶的对比度，通常要结合一定的脂肪抑制技术。为了增加 DWI 的稳定性和提高其对肝内病灶定量及定性的诊断率，除常规应用较多的憋气 DWI 外，呼吸门控 DWI、呼吸门控脂肪抑制 DWI、自由呼吸脂肪抑制 DWI 都在探索性研究中。

3.0 T 主磁场强度使得图像信噪比理论上比 1.5 T 提升 2 倍，从而成为高空间分辨率及缩短腹部成像时间的基石。然而，与 1.5 T MR 比较，3.0 T MR 所带来的更大的能量沉积、磁敏感伪影、呼吸运动以及胰腺周围肠道和血管运动的敏感性使得胰腺 DWI 更具有挑战性。

为了突出病灶与胰腺组织的对比度，提高检出率，大多胰腺 DWI 扫描技术均结合各种脂肪抑制技术，包括频率选择饱和脉冲、频率选择反转恢复脉冲及反转恢复脉冲，一项研究应用反转恢复脉冲脂肪抑制技术。

另外，与 1.5 T MR 比较，3.0 T MR DWI 序列会导致上腹部脏器更多的伪影，从而影响图像观察，甚至 ADC 值测量。保持较高的对比噪声比及对比度是应用不同序列提高病灶检出率的前提条件。该项研究中，呼吸门控反转恢复脂肪抑制 DWI 的对比噪声比及对比度均相对高于其他序列，证明其有助于胰腺癌病灶的检出。因该序列经过 220 ms 的反转后，正常胰腺中沉积的高信号脂肪组织被抑制，因此病灶组织与正常胰腺组织的对比增加，而无反转恢复技术的序列，胰腺组织的信号高低不均，致使胰腺癌的高信号被正常组织掩盖，因而其对比噪声比及对比度下降，不利于病灶的检出。自由呼吸反转恢复脂肪抑制 DWI 由于呼吸运动的影响，导致对比噪声比略有下降，且病灶的轮廓模糊，不利于病灶的观察。

组织 ADC 值的大小与细胞密度、纤维含量、血供、生理运动及伪影程度有关。通常情况下，细胞密度越大、纤维含量越大、血供越少，组织的 ADC 值越小。

影响 ADC 值的生理运动包括呼吸运动、心脏血管搏动、肠管及其内容物蠕动等，这些生理运动可夸大水分子运动，导致组织 ADC 值的增加，或者运动导致伪影致使 ADC 值的增加或减少。

该项研究中，邻近胰腺指的是胰腺癌近段无癌胰腺区，远端炎症区指的是由于胰管扩张而导致癌灶远端胰腺发生炎性病变。

胰腺癌的典型组织病理学特征为恶性细胞伴大量促结缔组织增生的间质成分混杂侵袭性生长，组织内水分子的扩散受限程度理论上要高于正常胰腺组织，因此其 ADC 值应低于邻近正常胰腺组织。

该项研究 X、Y、Z 轴扩散梯度憋气 DWI 和 Z 轴扩散梯度憋气 DWI 序列的胰腺癌、邻近胰腺及远端炎症 ADC 值无统计学差异，说明 3.0 T MR 憋气扩散序列所导致的胰腺信号不均致使 ADC 值不稳定，而呼吸门控 DWI、呼吸门控反转恢复脂肪抑制 DWI 和自由呼吸反转恢复脂肪抑制 DWI 显示的胰腺癌、邻近胰腺及远端炎症 ADC 值统计学有差异，且胰腺癌的 ADC 值统计学上均低于邻近胰腺及远端炎症 ADC 值。

由胰管阻塞而引起的远端胰腺炎性病变，其 ADC 值随炎性进展的状态不同而不同，急性炎症由于炎性细胞的渗出和血管通透性增加导致的水肿致使自由水分子增多，扩散受限程度不等，ADC 值增加或者会轻度降低；而慢性炎症由于炎性肉芽肿及纤维成分的增加,水分子的扩散受限更加明显,ADC 值降低更为明显,该项研究中入选病例的远端炎症有急性渗出性表现,也有纤维增生的慢性炎性病理状态,因而各序列 ADC 值与正常胰腺及胰腺癌的大小相比变化较多。

总之,呼吸门控 DWI、呼吸门控反转恢复脂肪抑制 DWI 及自由呼吸反转恢复脂肪抑制 DWI 上所测量的 ADC 值比 X、Y、Z 轴扩散梯度憋气 DWI 和 Z 轴扩散梯度憋气 DWI 能够更好地反映胰腺癌、邻近胰腺及远端炎症的组织病理状态,而呼吸门控反转恢复脂肪抑制 DWI 既能突出胰腺癌与胰腺的对比度,又能更清晰地观察胰腺及病灶的大小与范围,在临床上有助于胰腺癌的筛查与诊断。

第二节 误诊病例简介:胰腺癌与实性假乳头状瘤

患者,女, 35 岁。体检发现胰腺占位 10 天入院。外院 CT 平扫提示胰腺体部占位,建议增强扫描。门诊 CT 直接增强扫描:胰腺体部可见类圆形软组织密度块影,大小约 3.1cm × 2.6cm,增强三期 CT 值分别是: 64~73HU, 63~78HU, 71~85HU,内可见斑片状无强化区,胰管无明显扩张,胰腺轮廓清楚,腹膜后未见明显肿大淋巴结。CT 诊断:胰腺体部占位,考虑实性假乳头状瘤,神经鞘瘤? 建议 MRI 进一步检查。

手术所见:腹腔无腹水,胰体部可见一大小约 5 cm × 4 cm 实性肿物,边界清楚,脾动脉脾静脉与胰体肿瘤粘连紧密,无法游离。肝、脾、肠未见明显异常。行胰体尾切除 + 脾切除术。

病理检查:胰体尾肿物 + 脾切除标本:胰腺大小 10.0 cm × 4.5 cm × 3.0 cm,胰体部见一结节,大小 3.0 cm × 3.0 cm,结节切面灰红,质软,与周围界限尚清,其余切面灰红,质软。脾大小 10.0 cm × 4.7 cm × 3.5 cm,切面暗红,质软,未见明显异常。病理诊断:胰体尾肿物 + 脾切除标本:镜下可见形态较一致的肿瘤细胞呈实性排列,初步考虑为胰腺癌,肿瘤分类待做免疫组化检测进一步证实。脾脏未见癌组织累及。

误诊病例回顾分析:该病例年龄是胰腺实性假乳头状瘤的好发年龄,加之体检发现,无临床症状,三期增强扫描影像学表现与胰腺癌典型表现有一定差异,导致误诊。回顾分析发现,胰腺癌的发病率远高于实性假乳头状瘤,其影像学表现多种多样,不典型者不在少数,因此,在胰腺占位性病变的鉴别诊断中,首先还是应该想到胰腺癌,这就是经验之谈。回顾仔细观察影像,发现病灶中已出现坏死,呈现为斑片状无强化区,病灶侵犯血管,但这些表现却均被诊断医生忽略,是导致误诊的重要原因。

第三节　误诊病例简介：胰腺中低分化囊性腺癌，侵及十二指肠黏膜下层

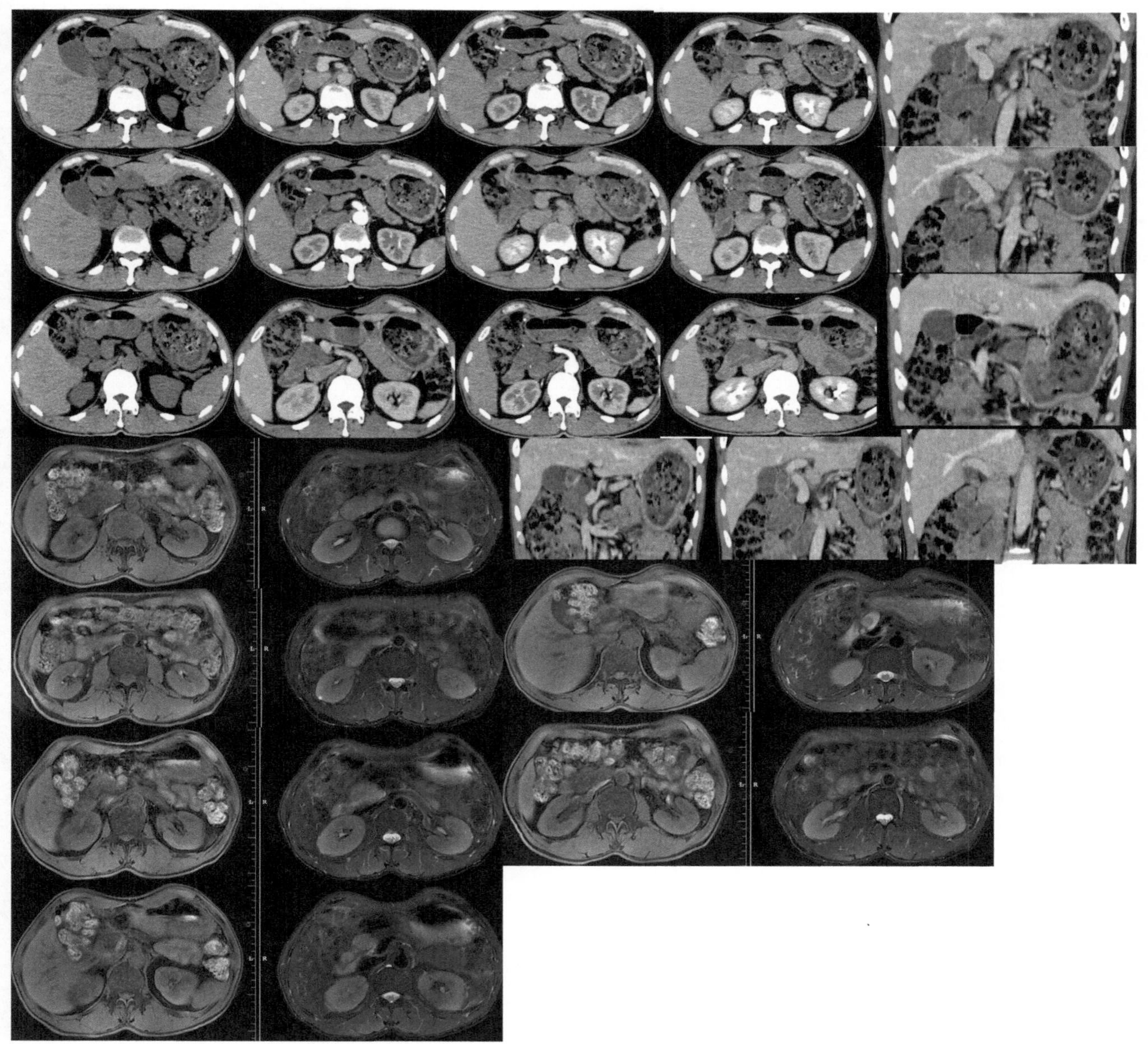

图 20-6-1　胰腺中低分化囊性腺癌，侵及十二指肠黏膜下层

病例，男，58 岁。CT 拟诊：十二指肠降段及胰头不规则等低密度占位，性质难定，①间质瘤？②神经鞘瘤？③胰头癌？ MRI 拟诊：胰头及十二指肠间隙内占位，考虑间质瘤，淋巴瘤？

病理检查：胰十二指肠切除标本：肠管一段，长 13cm，直径 2cm，皱襞明显，紧靠一侧切缘的肠管外侧壁可见一多房囊性肿物，送检前已剖开，大小 5.5cm × 4cm × 1.2cm，表面附着少量碎组织。另见灰褐色碎组织一堆，总体积 5cm × 5cm × 4cm。胆囊切除标本：大小 7cm × 4.5cm × 4cm，囊腔内充满墨绿色胆汁，黏膜面光滑，壁厚 0.1cm，未见结石、息肉及占位。第 12R 淋巴结：灰白色组织一块，大小 1cm × 0.4cm × 0.3cm。第 12L 淋巴结：灰褐色组织一块，大小 1cm × 0.7cm × 0.4cm。第 9 组淋巴结：灰褐色组织三块，总体积 2.5cm × 1.8cm × 0.5cm。

常规病理诊断:①胰十二指肠切除标本:初步诊断胰腺中低分化囊性癌,待做免疫组化检测进一步协助诊断。癌组织侵及十二指肠黏膜下层,十二指肠两侧切缘均为阴性,肠外膜及肠周自检出淋巴结1枚未见癌转移。②胆囊切除标本:胆囊组织未受癌组织累及,呈慢性炎,黏膜上皮大部缺失。③送检“第12L淋巴结切除标本”检出淋巴结0/2,“第9组淋巴结切除标本”检出淋巴结0/7,“第12R淋巴结切除标本”为纤维脂肪组织,未检出淋巴结及癌转移结节。以上共检出淋巴结10枚,均未见癌转移。

免疫组化检测:阳性:CA19-9,CK7,CK19,Villin(散在+),CEA(小灶+),P16(灶+),CD117(小灶+),CD34(血管内皮+),PAS染色,AB染色,P53(+,<5%),Ki-67(+,<10%);阴性:CA125,AFP,CK20,CgA,SyN,CD56,NSE。免疫组化诊断:胰十二指肠切除标本:免疫组化检测结果支持胰腺中低分化囊性腺癌,侵及十二指肠黏膜下层。

误诊分析:胰腺囊性腺癌,病变较少见,并侵及十二指肠黏膜下层,境界不清,对于肿瘤来源于胰头还是来源于十二指肠黏膜难于分辨(图20-6-1)。

第七章　CT、MRI 以外的其他影像学检查

胰腺癌超声检查

直接征象：大多数为胰腺局限性肿大，少数为弥漫性肿大，小的胰腺癌不引起胰腺大小和形态的变化；在胰头癌，胰头呈局限性增大或隆起；癌肿内部回声呈低回声型（约占一半病例）、强回声型（20%左右）、混合型（11%左右）、等回声型（2%左右）、无回声型（3%左右）。较小的癌肿（直径20~40mm）以低回声型多见（占84%左右），而较大的癌肿因肿瘤内出血、坏死，可有多种回声表现。有的胰头癌内部光点粗大不均匀，边缘不规则，呈分叶状，向外突起或向周围浸润，肿瘤后方回声衰减（占21%左右）或回声增强（3%）。

继发征象：胰管扩张（约占 1/3 病例）。显示胰管缩短和扩张，是胰头癌与胆胰共同管癌鉴别的重要特征；胆管扩张（约占 3/4 病例）；胰腺周围血管受压，移位和浸润（约占 6%）。当胰头癌压迫相邻的下腔静脉及其他血管时，可使其变形或移位。有作者报告 10 例有下腔静脉受压表现者，其中 8 例最后确诊为胰头癌，另 2 例为胆胰共同管癌。肝和腹腔淋巴结转移（约占 6%）。

鉴别诊断如下：

根据典型的声像图可以提示胰腺癌的诊断，但声像图无特异性，应注意与其他疾病鉴别。

胰岛细胞瘤：一般能与胰腺癌区别，若瘤体大，特别是无功能性胰岛细胞瘤常表现为混合型回声，鉴别较难，依靠血管造影显示胰岛细胞瘤富血管的变化，可与表现为少血管的胰腺癌鉴别。

胆胰共同管癌：共同管癌较胰腺癌更易引起胰管和胆管的扩张，其阻塞肝外胆管的水平更低，一般不引起胰头外形和大小的变化，可作鉴别的参考，进一步应结合 MRCP、CT、ERCP 诊断。

慢性胰腺炎：慢性胰腺炎所致的局限性胰腺肿块与胰腺癌极难区别。有作者指出，胰腺炎胰管扩张的程度较胰腺癌为轻，表现粗细不均匀，管壁不规则，而胰腺癌胰管呈串珠状，管壁较光滑，并有胰管中断现象。但是，只凭胰管的超声征象鉴别两者是很不可靠的，胰腺的穿刺活检有且于确诊。

有学者认为，超声诊断胰腺癌并不逊于 CT，声像图的阳性发现，提供了进一步的诊断线索，特别是超声判断胆管的扩张十分准确。有的病人血清胆红素无异常，临床尚未出现黄疸，超声却早期发现了胆管扩张，因此，应用超声发现临床黄疸前胆管扩张，有可能检出早期胰腺癌。

第八章　胰腺癌的综合诊断

第一节　胰腺癌的综合诊断

尽管诊断技术突飞猛进的发展,但胰腺癌病人在确诊后很多都已难手术切除,手术切除后的5年生存率也很低,在5%以下。因此,不少作者提出,疑存胰腺癌的病人影像学评估应有四个主要的目标:

首先,对检查的小部分病人提供迅速而准确的诊断,同时费用最少,尽可能降低胰腺癌的发病率;其次,确定疾病的范围,决定肿瘤是否能手术切除;第三,以非手术性经皮胰腺活检证实临床和放射学诊断;第四,对于不能手术切除的胰腺癌病人提供非手术性缓解性治疗,包括经皮胆系引流和内脏神经阻滞等。

胰腺癌的诊断,可以利用综合的方式或计算手段来最有效地实现。此处所讨论的计算手段只是部分作者的意见,不一定是最好的,也不是唯一的评估疑存胰腺癌的病人的方法。此类计算手段,应涉及到每个单位,而且反映关注胰腺癌的诊断和治疗的影像诊断医生、内科医生、外科医生的观点。

检查程序的选择,部分由放射科的设备的有效利用和影像诊断专家的见解来决定,部分与内科医生与外科医生设计的治疗措施需要的就人而论的特殊知识有关。对怀疑胰腺癌者进行评估所使用的检查程序的不同,仰赖于病人有无黄疸出现。

对非黄疸病人,CT常常作为首选手段,可能有4种诊断:胰腺无异常发现;孤立的胰腺包块;胰腺包块伴存转移,即是,CT征象提示胰腺外的肿瘤扩展,诸如肝转移或淋巴结转移,邻近器官受侵或胰周血管受犯;胰腺包块伴辅助征象(如胰管内钙化或假性囊肿),提示有炎症性疾病。

胰腺无异常发现:对于发现胰腺癌,普通CT的敏感性约为92%,漏诊约为8%。虽然如此,因为敏感性低于100%,CT所示正常并不能完全摒除存在异常的可能性,它们或是胰腺癌,或是伪似胰腺癌症状的其他疾病。这样,如果临床高度怀疑胰腺疾病,而CT却未发现异常,病人则宜再做MRCP、ERCP。一般说来,对于排除胰腺疾病,MRCP、ERCP最为敏感,极少有胰腺癌在CT、MRCP和ERCP均未发现异常者。

尽管MRCP、ERCP发现胰腺癌高度敏感,但它难以确定胰腺癌的范围和可切除性。另外,炎症和肿瘤的胰腺造影表现在某些病人实难区分。为此,MRI、血管造影可作为进一步评估的手段。

胰腺包块:局灶性或弥漫性胰腺肿大是一非特异性征象,炎症和肿瘤均可产生。如果只是一个孤立的胰腺包块,即是缺乏附加的允许区别炎症和肿瘤的CT辅助征象时,MRCP、血管造影可作出特异性诊断。起初,有的作者在CT发现孤立胰腺包块时加作MRCP、ERCP,然而,发现不少胰腺包块病人临床都强烈怀疑为肿瘤,MRCP、ERCP也可见到肿瘤的征象,最后还需血管造影确定切除的可能性。这样,病人需接受三项费用较贵的检查进行评估。因此考虑ERCP可以免除,只用MRI、MRCP、血管造影作为孤立性胰腺包块的进一步评估,因为,它既可提供特异性诊断,又可确定肿瘤切除的可能性。

在某些难以解释胰腺轻微的轮廓不规则的病例,高分辨CT扫描可能了解到胰腺实际的解剖学情况。在可疑的病例,MRI、MRCP、血管造影或ERCP都能帮助做出正确诊断。

胰腺包块伴存转移:如果一个胰腺包块和伴存的胰外肿瘤的侵犯征象已被确定,做出不可切除胰腺癌的CT诊断是能够令人信赖的。在此类病人,诊断可为经皮活检证实。CT导引下内脏神经阻滞可用来减轻疼痛。Freeny 和 Lawson（1982）的病例中，CT 诊断为不可切除的胰腺癌而不需另加影像学检查者超过 80%，胰腺外的肿瘤侵犯、肝转移以及区域性淋巴结受累，分别占病人的 62%、47% 与 25%（图 20-8-1）。

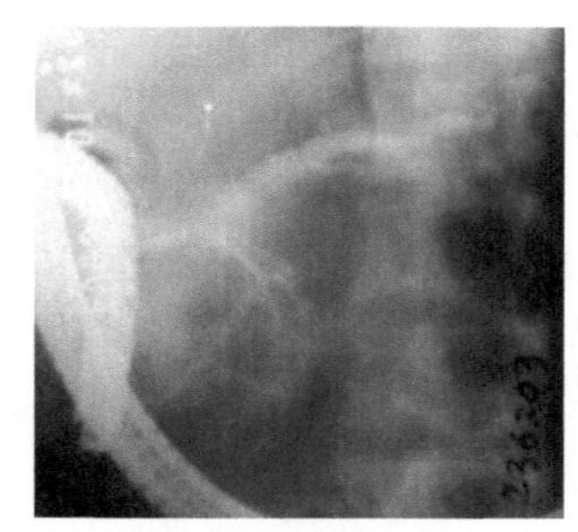

图 20-8-1　ERCP：手术病理证实胰头癌。主胰管明显扩张纡曲，胰头癌导致主胰管梗阻且扩张的胰管小分支包裹肿瘤，肿瘤内对比剂呈絮团状显示

胰腺炎性包块：在某些怀疑胰腺肿瘤的病人，CT 图像上的表现可能更为适合于炎性疾病（急性或慢性胰腺炎）。反之亦然。这样，为了正确诊断，必须仰赖于临床和实验室发现附加的诊断学检查（诸如 ERCP 或血管造影）。

有黄疸的病人的影像学评估：梗阻性黄疸，可为炎性病变和肿瘤病变引起，包含：胰腺炎、胰腺癌、转移性肿瘤以及胆系的原发性疾病（诸如：胆系结石、硬化性胆管炎等）。由于这些疾病临床鉴别常有许多困难，CT 所提供的广泛的诊断信息，使其成为评估梗阻性黄疸病人的首选检查方法。

尽管超声发现梗阻性扩张的胆管十分准确，但它常难以明确梗阻的病因。另外，胰腺癌的许多辅助征象（含区域性淋巴结受累或血管受犯等）超声成像发现较少。然而，CT 通常可确定梗阻的水平和病因疾病的范围以及梗阻的肿瘤的切除可能性。

患胰腺癌但不能切除的黄疸病人，可能用非手术的缓解性经皮胆系引流进行治疗。诊断的组织学证实依赖于经皮活检，其导引手段或是超声，或是 CT。

有梗阻性黄疸的胰腺癌病人，缺乏肿瘤不可切除的 CT 征象者，在胰腺手术之前宜行血管造影。动脉造影给手术医生提供血管走行的图示，在某些病例，还可能显示出肿瘤不可切除的征象，手术则可避免进行。除非对胆管梗阻平面有疑问，或准备进行胆肠吻合术，直接法胆系造影通常都不一定再做。

胰腺轮廓异常，在 CT 扫描容易发现，但再作 MRI、血管造影（动脉相和静脉相）和 ERCP 都未发现胰腺轮廓异常部位出现异常时，多说明临床症状不一定是由胰腺所致。

CT 扫描对于胰腺内较为深在的小胰腺癌难以发现，而 MRI、MRCP、ERCP 和血管造影对之则较为敏感，这是此类检查的优点所在。

第二节　MR 多种成像技术综合诊断

MR 多种成像技术（包括动态增强断面 MR 扫描、MRCP 和 MRA）对胰腺癌的术前诊断与分期及其手术切除性评价的总的准确度可达 94%。Catalano 等（1998）报道 MR 综合诊断 23 例胰腺癌，结果肿瘤均被检出并获准确分期。Trede 等（1997）对 58 例胰腺肿瘤进行了 MR 综合诊断，并与超声、CT、ERCP 和传统血管造影作对照研究，结果显示，MR 综合检查对胰腺癌局部蔓延、淋巴结转移、血管浸润和肝脏转移的诊断准确性均高于其他检查方法（分别为 95.7%、80.4%、89.1% 和 93.5%），虽然尚无统计学上的显著性差异，但采用 MR 多种成像技术一项检查即可同时了解肿瘤、胰胆管和血管等多方面情况，进行胰腺癌的术前诊断、分期及手术切除性评价，起到 CT、ERCP 和血管造影等多项检查的诊断效果。

MR 动态增强成像对于胰腺癌的诊断和术前分期有较为重要的意义，T_1WI 脂肪抑制图像胰腺癌呈低信号肿块而正常胰腺组织呈高信号，但是胰腺癌合并慢性胰腺炎可以导致这种对比差异的降低，这种情况并非少见。T_2WI 图像显示胰腺癌的价值有限。由于大多数胰腺癌为乏血供，其在动态增强扫描时动脉期呈现明显的低信号，由于肿瘤与正常组织间存有较大的信号差异，有助于检出尚未引起形态改变的小病灶。在延迟扫描时肿瘤呈等信号或稍高信号，边缘模糊。

胰头癌常引起胆总管和胰管的狭窄和阻塞，在 MRCP 上可表现为“双管征”及胰管和胆总管下端的截断表现，这种表现通常为胰头癌或胆胰连接区癌所致某些癌肿在检查时可仅表现为胰管和胆总管的扩张和截断,而无明显的异常信号病灶出现。

由于胰腺有丰富的淋巴回流、没有纤维包膜,胰腺癌易早期发生局部淋巴结和邻近组织的浸润和转移。肿瘤浸润在 T_1WI 脂肪抑制图像呈现为邻近后腹膜脂肪内条状高信号改变。脂肪抑制的动态增强 MRA 三维成像可以很好地显示血管包绕或阻塞以及局部的血管解剖改变。动态增强 MR 血管成像通过注射对比剂,采用快速序列屏气扫描,克服了以往时间飞跃法和相位对比法的缺陷,综合观察原始图像和重建图像可清楚显示病灶与血管的关系。

MR 检查在其他胰腺良性肿瘤的检测方面也有相当的作用,如富血供的胰岛素瘤在 MR T_1WI 图像呈低信号, T_2WI 图像呈相对高信号,动态增强呈均匀强化或环状强化,表现较为特殊,可帮助检出较小的肿瘤。

MR 综合诊断还具有无创伤性、安全、简便、病人易于接受等优点。

综上所述,脂肪抑制 T_1WI 和动态增强扫描是胰腺癌诊断与鉴别诊断的最佳 MR 检查技术。断面 MRI 与 MRCP、MRA 技术的综合应用,可进行准确的胰腺癌术前分期和手术切除性评价,提供超声、CT、ERCP 和血管造影等多项检查的信息。可以预计,随着 MR 成像技术的不断发展与完善,胰腺癌的分期诊断和手术切除性评价将越来越准确、简便。

第九章　胰腺癌的鉴别诊断

第一节　假肿瘤性慢性胰腺炎

慢性胰腺炎偶尔可呈现一局灶性的非钙化包块，颇似肿瘤，难与癌肿区别。Lammer 等（1985）报告此类病人 21 例，其中大多数病人均经 2 种或更多的影像检查方法研究，因其影像诊断（16 例考虑为癌，5 例考虑胰岛细胞瘤）为可切除的胰腺肿瘤，有 17 例做了剖腹手术（9 例部分胰腺切除术，8 例手术取多处活检），4 例未手术而行穿刺活检。全部病人组织学诊断皆为慢性复发性胰腺炎。包块位于胰头者 12 例，胰体 4 例，胰尾 5 例。17 例行 CT 检查，均见胰内小包块，平均 CT 值与其余胰腺组织相等，增强扫描时 6 例包块有小的低密度中心，等密度 10 例，高密度 1 例。每例胰的轮廓均清楚，其中 5 例在包块之后可见扩张的胰管，3 例胰尾组织萎缩。超声检查 10 例皆见边界清楚且有分叶的包块，回声增加 2 例。回声降低 8 例。感染征象，诸如胰周纤维化，格氏筋膜增厚或钙化，CT 与超声均未见到。

18 例做 ERCP，10 例可见主胰管有单一长的狭窄，因为狭窄段的侧支不能充盈及狭窄近侧分支正常而考虑为癌，3 例有主胰管的完全梗阻；2 例可见小腔，其内表面不规则；5 例总胆管胰腺段狭窄伴狭窄前扩张。11 例行血管造影，7 例见富血管性包块；5 例临床怀疑胰岛细胞瘤；4 例为胰外分泌性肿瘤，其胰头部血管减少；1 例有肠系膜上静脉的胰内闭塞。

17 例行剖腹术，每例均见硬块；2 例胰尾及包块有轻微感染性水肿；3 例虽然 X 线检查上只见 1 个包块，手术见为 2 或 3 个包块；3 例见胰周围肿大炎症性淋巴结；手术大夫不能排除新生物者 15 例，8 例行多次手术活检而避免做部分胰切除术，余 2 例病因为穿透性胃溃疡。

Sarles 等（1965）将慢性胰腺炎分为原发性钙化性胰腺炎、梗阻性胰腺炎（原有良性或恶性的胰管或胆管梗阻）和不明原因的胰腺炎。按照他们的观察，原发性钙化性胰腺炎开始为一小病灶或者少数不规则分布的病灶。只要胰管不受侵犯，此疾病保持局灶性。该作者认为假肿瘤性胰腺炎不能作为慢性胰腺炎的一个特殊亚型，它似乎是慢性胰腺炎的一个早期阶段，为一不常见的大的原发性病灶。这相当于慢性胰腺炎较早期阶段 CT 观察所见到的局灶性肿大，在 69%~75% 的病例以后变成弥漫性肿大。

慢性胰腺炎的一个特征性表现是钙化，但它要 1~3 年才变得在 X 线检查时看得见。早期慢性胰腺炎也可在 CT 检查时呈现为一局灶的非钙化性肿块，如果实验室发现是非特异性，又是在慢性胰腺炎进展阶段，CT 未见胰周纤维化，实不能排除一个早期胰腺癌。甚至，一个还能切除的胰癌的特征性 CT 表现——轮廓清楚的包块，常常为小的低密度区，伴存主胰管胰尾段扩张，有时周围实质萎缩——可见于假肿瘤性胰腺炎一半以上的病例。胰癌超声检查特征性地显示一局灶性包块与回声降低、紊乱，这些最常见于假肿瘤性胰腺炎，而不显示通常见于慢性胰腺炎的那类表现：弥漫性肿大伴回声增强或混杂，以及钙化。

因此，如果超声发现一回声降低的胰块，而无胰腺炎的临床表现，就不得不用另外的方法去排除一小胰癌。对于区别胰腺疾病的良、恶性，MRCP 与 ERCP 最为恰当，然而胰腺炎可伪似任何类型肿瘤的导管变化。在长而孤立的不规则的狭窄和不伴有其余胰腺的炎症的梗阻之间做出恰当的区别有时确实很难做到，乃因假肿瘤性胰腺炎构成一种不常见的大的局灶性胰腺炎，其余胰腺组织无炎症改变。

假肿瘤性胰腺炎血管造影不是表现为一无血管包块，就是显示为局灶性多血管性包块。小的多血管的包块总必须怀疑为早期胰腺癌或胰岛细胞肿瘤。Herlinger和Finlay(1978)指出较小的癌可比大肿瘤的异常血管为多，因后者血管的包裹与闭塞减少血液供应。直接邻近于癌的局灶性胰腺炎可表现为局灶性多血管，或在CT表现为一包块。如果临床症状和实验室发现提示有胰岛细胞瘤存在，因为胰岛的数目和大小相对地增加，不仅在X线表现上，而且有时在组织学上，与局灶性胰腺炎的区别诊断都变得很困难。

在少见的情况，增生的胰岛细胞能直接接触于神经纤维，甚或进入神经周围间隙，造成一早期侵袭性癌的印象。在血管造影或CT显示的炎症性包块也可为穿通性胃或十二指肠溃疡引起。

第二节 误诊病例简介

胰癌大多数为局部侵犯胰头或体尾部，少数为弥漫性浸润。癌的晚期如局部较明显增大，一般不难确诊，但是如果仍然保持正常外形，则难免误诊。

有作者报告二例误诊病人，在事后回顾性观察，1例胰尾后缘较僵硬，前缘轻微隆起，对于75岁老人，应考虑外形普遍增大，此例尸解发现较广泛的间质增生和明显纤维化，考虑可能是胰腺虽有癌细胞弥漫性浸润而体积不大的原因；另1例胰头稍大。

该作者分析导致误诊的另一原因是胰癌转移的征象明显，1例肝转移的表现很像肝硬化及在其基础上发展起来的肝癌，另1例有明显的十二指肠受侵犯。

文献报告胰癌引起十二指肠受侵犯并不少见，可高达20%以上，主要侵犯降部，但亦有少数可侵犯球部。未密切结合临床及化验改变也是误诊原因之一，二例均有血糖高及血淀粉酶高。Nardi指出，老年人，尤其男性，如近期发生糖尿病并伴腹部症状，应疑及胰癌。

第三节 慢性胰腺炎误诊为胰腺癌

胰腺炎是临床常见病、多发病，按照病程可分为急性和慢性胰腺炎。急性胰腺炎一般分为急性水肿型(轻型)胰腺炎和急性出血坏死型(重型)胰腺炎2种。急性胰腺炎发病急，症状严重，通常表现为腹、背痛，有些有明确诱因，如暴饮暴食、胆囊结石及胆管结石等；其血尿淀粉酶的明显升高、CT扫描下胰周的广泛渗出和肾周筋膜增厚对于诊断此病有重要意义。

慢性胰腺炎的误诊：慢性胰腺炎的发病率在我国有明显上升趋势，已成为消化系疾病中的常见病，诊断易出现漏诊和误诊。究其原因，主要是由于慢性胰腺炎临床症状不典型，临床医师对该病的认识欠缺，而目前的诊断手段(CT，超声)存在一定不足。

有作者报道了213例慢性胰腺炎患者，有72例长期诊断为慢性胃炎或萎缩性胃炎，65例诊断为慢性腹泻、肠炎或慢性结肠炎，24例诊断为胆系结石或胆囊术后综合征等，诊断为胰腺新生物或胰腺癌8例，临床症状极不典型。该组患者的临床病程均为慢性，有1例甚至没有任何症状，在查体时发现病灶。

2005年南京慢性胰腺炎诊治指南在排除胰腺癌的基础上，建议将下述4项作为慢性胰腺炎的重要诊断依据：①典型的临床表现(腹痛)；②病理学检查；③影像学上有慢性胰腺炎的胰胆改变征象；④实验室检查有胰腺外分泌功能不全依据。①为诊断所需，②阳性可确诊，①+③可基本确诊，①+④为疑似患者。虽然影像学检查方法对于确诊慢性胰腺炎很重要，但目前CT和超声检查并不能让临床满意，超声引导下细针穿刺或手术成为不可避免的最后手段。有作者报道了12例肿块型慢性胰腺炎患者，术前仅有4例影像学检查给出了正确诊断。

一组回顾性分析了16例误诊的慢性胰腺炎病例，发现有一些征象具有明确的指导诊断的意义。共有4例患者胰头内可见腹腔干及其分支“穿行”，这种穿行并不是真正的穿过胰腺，征象的成因可能是胰头炎性水肿、渗出和坏死物增多，体积增大进而包绕动脉造成“穿行”假象。而肿瘤的生长对动脉的影响往往是侵犯和推挤（淋巴瘤除外），这一点是共识。因此，这种“伪动脉穿行征”可以作为胰腺肿瘤与炎症的重要鉴别点。

7 例患者胰腺病变呈囊实性病灶，囊壁较厚而密度均匀、形状规则，增强扫描动脉期呈“靶征”，延迟后囊壁持续强化，病灶范围缩小。这种强化方式符合一般脓肿的典型表现，原因是脓肿的多层构成结构，外层为纤维肉芽组织，强化效应较明显，内层为炎症、坏死组织，没有强化，有别于胰腺癌常见的强化方式，即不强化或轻度强化。

有的患者的胰腺病灶内可以见到纤维分隔，这种结构在胰腺癌，特别是囊腺癌中经常可以见到，使病灶呈多囊改变，不作为鉴别要点。其他一些患者的胰腺病灶完全呈囊性，没有强化和渗出，其位置在胰腺头部内，和胰腺假囊肿一般位于胰腺边缘不同；要和胰腺真性囊肿和胆总管囊肿相鉴别，但是正确诊断的概率不大。

而肝门部及腹主动脉旁可以见到钙化的淋巴结，对于慢性胰腺炎的诊断具有重要意义。

双管征是胰腺癌常见、重要征象，在该组 16 例患者中有 2 例发现，虽然出现概率较低，但提示慢性胰腺炎双管征存在的可能性。

CT 增强三期扫描对于慢性胰腺炎诊断非常必要。Hollett 等（1995）研究了 120 例正常胰腺的螺旋 CT 双期扫描结果，指出动脉期胰腺 CT 值比实质期平均高 20 HU，有利于胰腺病灶的检出。Hattori 等（2009）测量了 23 例胰腺癌患者肿瘤三期的 CT 值，分别为（61 ± 13）HU、（80 ± 13）HU、（86 ± 11）HU，虽然胰腺癌大部分为乏血供肿瘤，但是具有动脉期 - 静脉期 - 延迟期肿瘤 CT 值的递增，动静脉期 CT 值差值超过 20 HU。该组测量了 13 例患者三期扫描的慢性胰腺炎病灶实质部分的 CT 值，虽然呈递增趋势，但是动静脉期强化的绝对值均不超过 10 HU；由于样本量小，不具有统计学意义，但是值得深入研究，对于慢性胰腺炎诊断有提示性作用。

慢性胰腺炎的 CT 分型：由于存在误诊因素，诊断容易进入误区，依据慢性胰腺炎的 CT 表现可以分为 4 型：①实性肿块型；②囊肿型（包括单囊和多囊）；③混合型（囊实性）；④经典型（有急性胰腺炎反复发作病史及 CT 表现出现胰腺钙化、胰周渗出及肾前筋膜增厚）。慢性胰腺炎临床表现一般比较有特点，结合病史及 CT、超声检查诊断相对简单，但仍有例外。

误诊分析：腹腔无渗出，血、尿淀粉酶水平不高，缺乏典型的 CT 表现是慢性胰腺炎误诊的主要原因。病灶周边延迟强化环可能系炎性肉芽组织，表现类似于假包膜，相对具有特异性，可作为鉴别诊断的依据。伪动脉血管穿行征则提示病灶对周边组织缺乏压迫，是胰腺炎与胰腺癌的生长方式不同所致，可以作为鉴别的重要 CT 征象。

而肿大淋巴结和双管征不能作为胰腺癌的特异性征象，但是具有提示作用。

所以慢性胰腺炎的诊断需要结合临床、实验室及影像学辅助检查等多种手段，综合判断，才能把误诊概率降到最低。

第四节　误诊病例简介:胃与十二指肠交界处慢性炎性增生团块与胰头癌

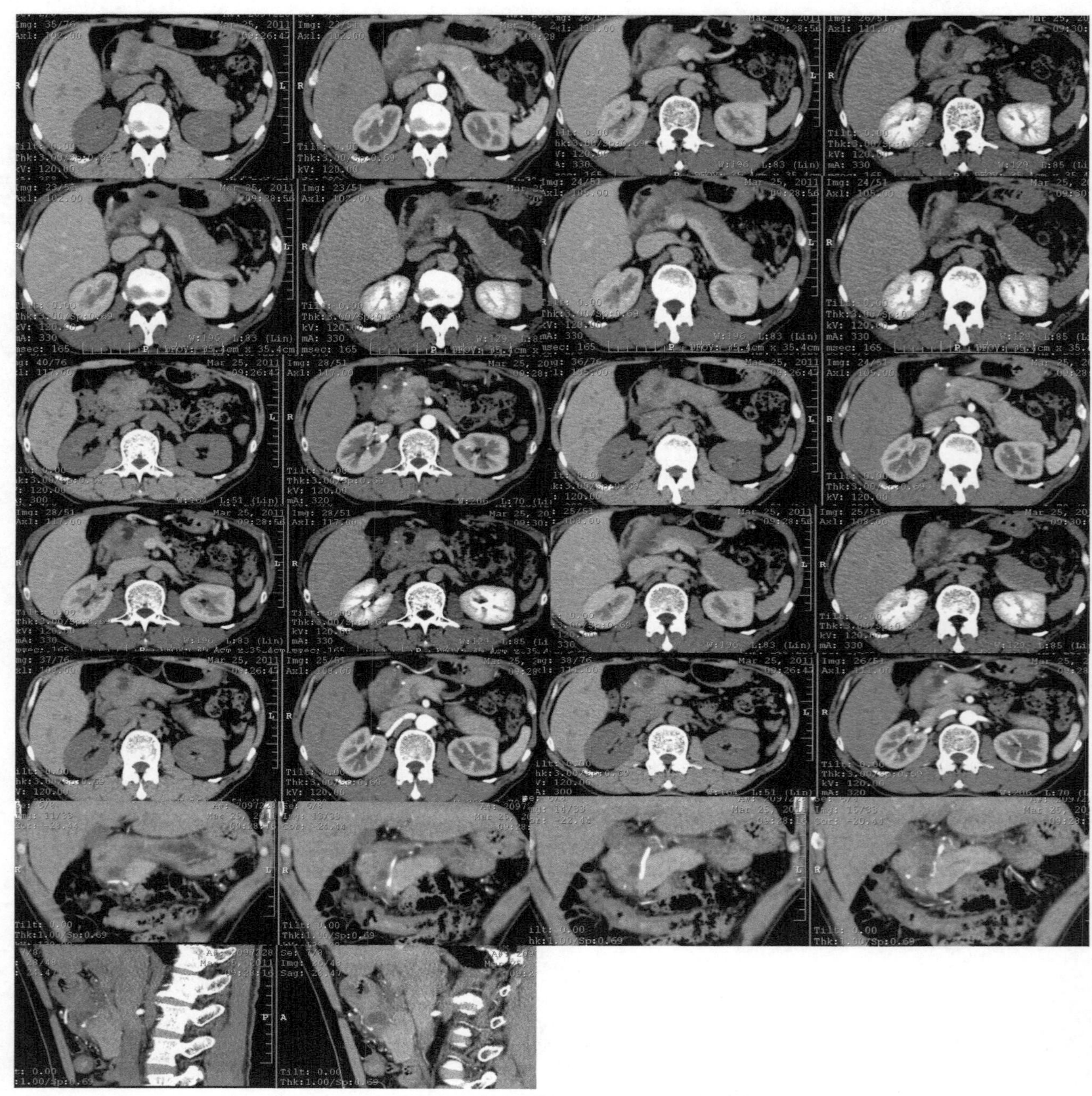

图 20-9-1　胃与十二指肠交界处慢性炎性增生团块与胰头癌

患者,男,50 岁。

CT 诊断:胰头占位,考虑胰腺癌可能,与胃窦粘连,前方腹腔内多发小淋巴结。胰管稍扩张。肝右后叶膈顶低密度灶,转移? 肝左外叶上段血管瘤。

手术所见:胰头部可见一肿物,大小约 5cm× 3cm,质较硬,边界不清,与十二指肠及胃窦部粘连紧密。

病理检查:胰头肿物、胆囊、及远端胃、部分十二指肠切除标本:总体积 30cm×8cm×6cm,沿胃壁及肠壁剪开,在距胃切端 11cm，距十二指肠切端 12cm 的胃与十二指肠交界处见一椭圆形肿物，该肿物临床已切开，肿物位于十二指肠浆膜外，将肠壁拱起并推向肠腔，总体积 7cm × 5cm × 4.5cm，切面灰白淡黄，质中，包膜完整。肿的周边检出淋巴结数枚。胆囊一具。

病理诊断：胰头肿物、胆囊及远端胃、部分十二指肠切除标本：胰腺小叶存在，其内可见胰岛，小叶内细胞排列呈腺泡状，有的呈梁状；小叶间成纤维细胞增生，淋巴细胞及浆细胞灶性浸润，灶区中性粒细胞大片浸润并伴间质水肿及片块状炎性坏死。切除的部分肠黏膜及胃黏膜呈轻度慢性炎症改变。慢性胆囊炎伴 R-A 窦形成。讨论：本例胰腺组织结构完好，间质慢性与急性炎症并存，灶区坏死，肌成纤维细胞小片状增生，但界限不清，与组织混杂，未形成真正的炎性肌成纤维细胞性肿瘤。整个病变呈慢性炎性增生的病理学形态改变（图 20-9-1）。

第五节　胰腺癌和炎性胰腺肿块鉴别

胰腺癌和肿块型胰腺炎均好发于胰腺头部，其 CT 表现非常相似，因此其鉴别诊断较困难，是临床手术前诊断的难题。一项课题发现胰腺癌的漏诊率为 7.6%，误诊率为 4.5%，而肿块型胰腺炎的误诊率则高达 52.6%，正确认识胰腺癌和肿块型胰腺炎的各种 CT 征象对该 2 种病变的诊断和鉴别诊断具有重要意义。

肿块的密度、强化程度：肿块本身的 CT 值对胰腺癌和肿块型胰腺炎的鉴别价值不大，而胰腺癌和肿块型胰腺炎肿块相对于正常组织的强化程度的高低对鉴别诊断有价值，前者强化明显（值得注意的是，二者相对而论，尽管胰腺癌一般少血供，但其强化程度竟高于肿块型胰腺炎），提示胰腺癌的可能性大；后者强化中等，提示肿块型胰腺炎的可能性大。

胰头肿块伴腺体尾部萎缩：多数学者认为此征象支持胰腺癌的诊断，该组资料亦提示胰头肿块伴腺体尾部萎缩这一 CT 征象支持胰腺癌的诊断。

胰头肿块伴体尾肿大：该组发生在胰腺癌中为 10.61%（7/66），出现在肿块型胰腺炎中为 84.21%（16/19），两者差异有统计学意义，表明胰头肿块合并胰腺体尾肿大对肿块型胰腺炎的诊断有重要价值。由于肿块型胰腺炎是胰腺反复炎症，通常整个胰腺都有炎性改变，因此患者胰头部肿块常合并胰体尾部慢性炎症，胰腺体尾部常有纤维组织增生和炎性细胞渗出，而致胰腺体尾部肥大。Neff 等（1984）报道，15%~30% 的慢性胰腺炎可形成肿块型胰腺炎，虽然炎性肿块大多数发生在胰头区，病变不局限在胰头肿块区，非肿块区（胰腺体尾）也常受累，只不过未在胰腺体尾部形成明显肿块，但可见胰腺体尾通常肿大。

胰胆管扩张：由于胰腺癌常具有围管性生长的特点，常压迫胆总管和 / 或阻塞主胰管而导致胆管和胰腺管及其分支胰腺管的扩张，所引起的胰胆管扩张早期为轻度，晚期常为重度扩张，为进行性加重。但在肿块型胰腺炎中，这是由于胰腺纤维化压迫、牵拉胰腺管而导致不规则扩张，同时胰腺头部的假性炎性肿块压迫胆总管下端而至胆管下端炎症及扩张，这一过程相对较漫长，因此肿块型胰腺炎也可引起胰胆管扩张，常为轻、中度扩张。

该组胰胆管扩张在胰腺癌和肿块型胰腺炎间差异不明显，可能与该研究分类不细有关。由于胰胆管扩张较复杂，从扩张的程度上可分为轻、中和重度；从扩张形式上可分为单纯胰管扩张、单纯胆管扩张和胰胆管同时扩张，另外还有一些特殊类型的扩张，如“双管征”、“三管征”和“四管征”等。

扩张的胰管穿过胰腺肿块：扩张的胰管穿过胰腺肿块，又称“胰管贯穿征”，对肿块型胰腺炎的诊断具有一定价值。因此，对于胰腺肿块合并胰腺管扩张患者的 CT 扫描，扩张胰管全程的显示能提高鉴别诊断的能力。由于胰管全程 CT 显示较困难，应行 MR 胆胰管成像（MRCP）或内镜逆行胰胆管造影（ERCP）等检查，有益于胰腺肿块病变性质的鉴别。

胰腺钙化：多数学者认为此征象是慢性胰腺炎的较特征性表现，但 Lesniak 等（2002）报道，胰腺钙化可出现在胰腺假性囊肿、囊腺瘤、非功能胰岛细胞瘤、胰腺癌、胰母细胞瘤以及正常脾动脉和脾静脉等，但发生率较慢性胰腺炎低。该研究结果显示胰腺钙化这一征象对肿块型胰腺炎具有诊断价值。

肾前筋膜增厚和胰周渗出：肾前筋膜增厚出现在胰腺癌和肿块型胰腺炎中的发生率差异有统计学

意义,说明该征象的出现提示肿块型胰腺炎的可能性大。胰周渗出在胰腺癌和肿块型胰腺炎中的发生率差异无统计学意义,说明该征象对胰腺癌和肿块型胰腺炎的鉴别价值不大。由于通常认为胰周渗出为胰腺炎症所致,但胰腺癌患者向胰腺周围侵犯时所造成的CT表现和胰周渗出相似,鉴别诊断时应慎重。

胰腺肿块合并胆管炎、胆结石:肿块型胰腺炎的病因常为胆源性,常合并胆系炎症如胆管炎、胆总管结石、慢性胆囊炎。该组资料显示此征象出现在胰腺癌和肿块型胰腺炎中的发生率差异有统计学意义,因此,胆总管结石和胆管炎的存在是诊断肿块型胰腺炎的一个有价值的证据。

肿块内小囊状低密度区:胰腺癌和肿块型胰腺炎均可见小囊状低密度区,前者是由于肿瘤生长迅速而致的瘤体坏死,后者是由于炎性坏死和小脓肿等。该组资料显示该征象对两者的鉴别意义不大。

综上所述,正确认识胰腺癌和肿块型胰腺炎的各种CT征象对该2种病变的诊断具有重要意义。

我们认为,在临床上分析研究时,切记不要将胰腺癌与炎性胰腺肿块置于对立的位置,非你即我,非此即彼,它们可以合并在一起,只不过以谁为主要成分而已。这在人体各部位都可找到类似的情况,诸如肺结核与肺癌,即可在肺结核的基础上出现肺癌,或合并肺癌;胆囊炎和胆囊癌,即可在胆囊炎基础上出现胆囊癌,二者都可合并存在,并非两者一定对立。

第六节　胰腺癌与慢性胰腺炎鉴别诊断

胰腺癌和慢性胰腺炎的临床表现缺乏特征,影像学检查在发现病变和定性诊断方面起重要作用。胰腺癌以导管腺癌最常见,约90%来源于导管上皮,少数发生于腺泡细胞。慢性胰腺炎是由多种病因引起的胰腺腺泡破坏及萎缩、间质纤维化、结缔组织增生等病变,以病程渐进及反复为特点。两者均含有胰腺实质萎缩及纤维化、导管上皮细胞增生或化生引起的继发性改变,如囊变、导管狭窄及扩张、假性囊肿、钙化等,影像表现存在诸多相似之处。常规CT和MRI等检查存在一定局限性,鉴别诊断困难。

MRCP技术:3.0T MRCP能清晰显示信号强度相对较弱的主胰管及其扩张分支胰管、胆囊管及复杂肝内细小胆管形态结构,为慢性胰腺炎和胰腺癌的诊断和鉴别诊断提供了丰富的信息。文献报道2D和3D MRCP各有优缺点:2D屏气扫描图像,受呼吸运动影响小,图像背景抑制较好,分辨率高,但细节显示较差;3D呼吸门控触发扫描图像,能多方位、多角度MIP重组,观察细微病变,同时原始图像层厚较薄,病灶组织分辨率较高。2D和3D结合应用可以提高MRCP显示胰胆管病变的能力。MRI常规T_1WI和T_2WI可从整体上反映胰腺病变的信号、形态及邻近解剖关系,所以MRCP结合常规MRI检查更具诊断价值。一组病例均进行2D和3D MRCP,并辅以横断面T_1WI和T_2WI扫描。

MRCP对分支胰管形态学的价值:胰腺导管系统由主(副)导管、各级小叶间导管、小叶内导管等构成,从胰头至胰尾有15~20对小叶间分支导管与主(副)导管延续,形成胰腺导管树状结构。正常胰腺导管的二级分支主要包括钩突支、头上(下)支、体上(下)支、尾上(下)支。与ERCP注射对比剂后的压力作用成像不同,MRCP多在生理状态下成像,不易观察正常的胰管分支。在超高场MRCP上正常分支胰管极少显示,即二级分支胰管有时呈发丝样浅淡显示(使用促胰液素刺激胰腺分泌后MRCP上能较好显示分支胰管,但多应用于胰腺外分泌功能检查)。因此,在自然状态下MRCP上如果清楚显示分支胰管,并且分支胰管形态异常即可视为分支胰管扩张。

目前影像学对分支胰管扩张的研究多见于胰管内黏液乳头状瘤,其分支胰管型和混合型分支胰管扩张有一定的影像学特征,表现为分支胰管或主胰管扩张,呈单囊或多囊状,囊内有附壁结节、黏液栓子或分隔,病灶与主胰管相通,主胰管不同程度扩张,十二指肠乳头膨大。该组资料表明,慢性胰腺炎和胰腺癌均可引起不同程度的胰腺导管系统局部狭窄或梗阻,造成主胰管和分支胰管扩张,但以往这方面的影像学研究报道不多。

慢性胰腺炎和胰腺癌分支胰管扩张的机制和意义:该组资料显示,小囊状分支胰管扩张在慢性胰腺炎（42.2%）较胰腺癌（20%）多见，且部分主胰管轻度扩张的慢性胰腺炎病例亦能见到小囊状扩张的分支胰管。慢性胰腺炎可能因胰腺纤维化、导管上皮增生、胰管内胰石及蛋白栓等改变引起主胰管及其分支局部狭窄、梗阻，导致分支胰管小囊状扩张，或形成小潴留性囊肿。随主胰管全程分支胰管扩张者在慢性胰腺炎（77.8%）较胰腺癌（56.7%）多见，而仅胰腺远段（体尾）分支胰管扩张慢性胰腺炎（22.2%）少于胰腺癌（40%），但慢性胰腺炎分支状分支胰管数目和扩张程度较胰腺癌明显。可能的原因是慢性胰腺炎的胰腺纤维化程度较胰腺癌广泛，且慢性胰腺炎有腺泡萎缩、导管壁局限性增厚等改变，引起导管系统的各级胰管局部狭窄及其远端扩张；而胰腺癌近端狭窄或梗阻后首先影响主胰管，随主胰管压力逐级升高，远段分支胰管顺应性扩张。

慢性胰腺炎引起胰管内压升高，可达 30~50 厘米水柱（正常时低于 20 厘米水柱），同时引起胰腺组织压升高。该组 1 例胰头癌仅见肿块附近 1 支分支胰管分支状扩张，但主胰管扩张不明显，其远侧分支胰管也未显示，可能与肿块累及邻近分支胰管，而主胰管尚未受累有关。此外，与胰腺癌比较，该组慢性胰腺炎分支状分支胰管的外形更不规则，也可能与两者的纤维化程度差异有关。总之，慢性胰腺炎和胰腺癌的分支胰管扩张在形态、发生部位和扩张程度方面存在一定差异。了解分支胰管扩张的 MRCP 表现有助于正确理解所见异常影像及提高对其鉴别诊断能力。

第七节　胰头部肿块型慢性胰腺炎

胰头部肿块型慢性胰腺炎是节段性慢性胰腺炎的一种特殊类型，临床表现为梗阻性黄疸和胰头肿块，与胰头癌十分相似。

一、病因及临床特点

肿块型慢性胰腺炎为节段性慢性胰腺炎的一种特殊类型，又称为假肿瘤性胰腺炎，93% 的炎性肿块位于胰头部，可能与此处胰管解剖特点有关。胰头上部是由副胰管（Santorini 管）引流的，该管开口于十二指肠小乳头，66% 的正常胰腺小乳头关闭，胰液逆流至与 Santorini 管以锐角相连的主胰管（Wirsung 管），当管内蛋白质沉淀物增多，胰液黏稠度增加，分泌量增多时，胰液引流受阻，首先满溢至 Santorini 管引流区域的胰头部实质内。肿块型胰腺炎的病因，国外以慢性酒精中毒为主要原因，国内以胆源性为主，其他原因还包括高脂血症、遗传性和自身免疫异常等。一组 30 例中，25 例伴有不同程度胆系炎症。临床上，慢性胰腺炎患者平均年龄为 48 岁，比胰腺癌患者平均发病率值小，且以男性多见，患者一般情况良好，常表现为反复发作性上腹部隐痛，部分患者伴有轻度间歇性黄疸。

二、病理机制与影像学研究

胰头部肿块：该组病例的判断标准是胰头部局限性增大，前后径 >2.93cm，同时胰头与 胰体部直径的比值 >1.32。根据该组胰头部慢性肿块型胰腺炎的 CT 表现特点，该组将其划分为 4 型，即单纯肿块型、肿块内伴假囊肿型、肿块内伴钙化型和混合型。

单纯肿块型，该组占 23.3%，多呈类圆形，直径为 3~4cm，边缘较规则，肿块大于 4cm 时边缘多不规则。病理机制为炎症迁延不愈反复发作，胰腺组织变性坏死，腺泡萎缩，胰腺小叶间或胰管周围纤维组织增生和慢性炎性细胞浸润而形成炎性肿块。CT 平扫示胰头部软组织肿块，呈等密度或略低密度，密度均匀，边界多不清晰，无明显分叶。

肿块伴假囊肿型，该组占 20%。假性囊肿的形成是慢性胰腺炎的特征性表现。CT 平扫示胰头肿块内密度不均，可见多个或一个囊状低密度影，囊内密度较高，CT 值平均为 25 HU，囊内壁光滑无结节。肿块内伴钙化型，该组占 46.7%。钙化为慢性胰腺炎的特征性表现，形成原因为胰液的蛋白质慢性沉淀并阻塞胰管导致钙质沉积。此型最多见，CT 表现为胰头肿块内砂粒样或斑点状钙化。混合型，该组占 10%。该型较为少见，钙化位于上方中心部位，假囊肿分布于钙化周围，囊肿大小不等，形状不规则，其形成机制与上述两型相同，仔细观察其分布特点，推测胰头内钙化阻塞胰腺导管的开口，从而导致胰液的聚积，这一点有待进一步证实。

增强后 75% 炎性肿块于动脉期轻度强化，静脉期及延迟期呈现逐渐强化，CT 值增加 20~40HU。

假囊肿增强后囊壁及囊内容物无强化,周围的胰腺组织均匀渐进性强化,与不强化的囊肿形成密度差,有一定特征性。15% 肿块于动脉期明显强化,密度高于体尾部,除可能由于炎性肿块血供较丰富外,还可能由于慢性胰腺炎急性发作时,血管活性物质释放引起血管扩张,毛细血管通透性增加。10% 炎性肿块无明显强化,这可解释为慢性胰腺炎晚期,动脉内膜下或中层纤维化,管壁增厚,另外肿块内纤维组织增生较明显致使炎性肿块血供减少也是无强化的重要原因。MSCT 能够进行薄层动态多期增强扫描,清晰显示炎性肿块的血流灌注情况,对该病的诊断及鉴别诊断具有重要意义。

胰管扩张:胰头部炎性肿块处胰管多正常或狭窄、贯通病灶,远端胰管多呈串珠状扩张,主胰管管径平均为 5mm,同时多数伴有胰管内钙化。沿主胰管走行的钙化是诊断胰头部肿块型胰腺炎的可靠征象。其病理基础为胰腺纤维化改变,使胰腺增大变硬,后期发生萎缩,导致胰管不规则扩张,而胰液的蛋白质沉淀可能是胰石形成的基础。该组 10 例可见主胰管穿过炎性肿块呈光滑的狭窄性改变或无异常,即胰管穿透征。MSCT 局部放大、薄层扫描技术能够良好地显示胰管形态学的改变,另外还可以利用曲面重建成像将胰管的全长显示在同一层面上,能直观显示胰管有无扩张、管壁有无增厚及腔内结石情况。

胆管扩张:因胰头肿块纤维化压迫及炎性浸润远端胆总管引起管壁纤维变性导致不全性胆管梗阻,狭窄段位于胰内胆管段,多在 2 cm 以上, CT 表现为胆总管轻中度不规则扩张,直径平均为 9.2mm,壁厚 2~3 mm,无突然中断、变形,下端逐渐狭窄呈“尖嘴状”改变。多平面重建能够清晰显示此征象,肝内胆管扩张少见。增强后管壁呈环形强化。

胰周血管的改变:慢性肿块型胰腺炎由于反复发作及胰液的渗出,胰周血管间隙内脂肪间隙模糊。炎性肿块可压迫胰周血管移位,该组 23 例肠系膜上动脉、肠系膜上静脉、腹腔干及其分支和门静脉等血管周围脂肪间隙欠清晰,但未消失。3 例表现为肿块与肠系膜上静脉紧贴,管腔无明显变形。所有病例均无血管包埋侵犯现象。另外胰腺炎时肠系膜上静脉扩张,肠系膜上动、静脉的比值小于 1。这可能由于血管活性物质改变了胰腺的血流情况。相反在胰腺癌时,肠系膜上动脉直径增大。MSCT 能在极短的时间完成胰腺多期增强扫描,使胰周血管在最佳灌注期内得到清晰显示,结合精细的容积扫描及不同方位多平面重建图像重组可获得清晰的血管图像,了解血管与炎性肿块之间的关系。

肾前筋膜或肾周筋膜增厚:是提示胰头慢性炎症的重要征象,这是由于胰腺发生炎症时,胰组织充血水肿,胰液渗出,使胰腺组织坏死出血,由于胰周缺乏完整包膜,炎性渗出物及坏死物向胰周及肾旁间隙内扩散,累及肾前或肾周筋膜使其增厚。

三、胰头部肿块型慢性胰腺炎与胰头癌的鉴别

胰头部肿块型慢性胰腺炎与胰头癌鉴别较难,即使根据病史、体征及影像特征,甚至术中所见也难以和胰头癌相鉴别,而且临床上多数胰腺癌常合并慢性阻塞性胰腺炎。

以下五方面可以作为与胰头癌相鉴别的要点:①癌肿内一般不会见到钙化,炎性肿块内钙化相对多见;②胰头癌为少血供肿瘤,各期强化均不明显,炎性肿块大多为延迟强化,至平衡期与胰体尾呈等密度;③胰头癌的胆总管及胰管至肿块处呈突然中断,即双管征,慢性肿块型胰腺炎胆总管下段呈逐渐变细的尖嘴状改变,主胰管呈串珠状扩张同时伴有胰管内结石和 / 或钙化,胰管扩张的比例高于胆总管扩张的比例,用胰管穿透征鉴别两者的特异性高达 93%;④炎性肿块可压迫胰周血管移位,血管周围脂肪间隙模糊,胰头癌时肿瘤多包埋血管,胰周动静脉受累不仅是诊断胰腺癌的确切标准,同时还是癌肿不可切除的可靠征象;⑤炎性肿块多伴有肾前筋膜增厚,癌肿一般很少引起肾周筋膜增厚。

第八节　胰十二指肠沟区病变的鉴别诊断

胰十二指肠沟:胰十二指肠沟是胰腺和十二指肠之间的一个潜在间隙,其内侧是胰腺头部;外侧是十二指肠降段的浆膜面;胰十二指肠沟的后界是十二指肠第三段或下腔静脉,由于总胆管远端常位于胰腺头内或其后部附近,所以总胆管远端常横贯于胰十二指肠沟的后部;胰十二指肠沟的前界与十二

指肠球部和胃窦邻接。该部的形态学能清晰地显示在 CT 和 MRI 上，正常情况下，胰十二指肠沟内有少数小的淋巴结，一般不易在影像上显示。正常情况下，有时 CT 平扫不易区别胰头和十二指肠的界限，可误诊为胰头增大。

胰十二指肠沟区的病变：起源于该区的病变大致可分为五类，即：胰腺、十二指肠、淋巴系统、胆胰管连接区和血管疾病，了解该区的形态学表现，能精确地判断病变的起源和性质。在诊断时还要考虑与门腔静脉间隙和附近大血管病变的鉴别。

发育变异：胰腺局部膨隆为发育变异。环形胰腺：为先天性发育异常，胰腺组织部分或全部包绕十二指肠降段肠腔。影像可见十二指肠狭窄、下端胆管狭窄和其上段胰、胆管和胃扩张。

一、胰腺病变

（一）沟部胰腺炎

沟部胰腺炎是节段性慢性胰腺炎的一种特殊类型，亦称沟槽状胰腺炎，病变涉及十二指肠、胰腺头和总胆管下段的胰十二指肠沟区域，可分为两种类型：纯沟型为病变仅限于胰十二指肠沟内；节段型病变侵犯胰腺头部并有沟部瘢痕组织形成，这是该病的病理组织学特点。致病原因还不太清楚，可能与胃溃疡、胃手术后、胆系病变、胰头囊肿、十二指肠壁内真性憩室和十二指肠壁内胰腺异位等病变有关。临床症状可能有腹痛、复发性呕吐、黄疸和体重减轻等。不少病例因误诊为胰腺癌，而行手术切除。因此，应加强对该病的认识。该病由 Becker（1973）首先提出，过去认为很少见，但一些作者报告 123 例经手术病理证实的慢性胰腺炎中，有 30 例属于沟部胰腺炎。以往发现较少，可能是因为认识不足。该病和一般慢性胰腺炎一样，没有年龄和性别上的差异。

有作者报告 6 例，因疑为胰头癌而行胰十二指肠切除，术后病理证实为沟槽状胰腺炎。该组 6 例患者中，临床表现包括波动性黄疸，上腹部隐痛不适、呕吐、体质量减轻，术前诊断为胰头癌；手术后，除 1 例死于术后并发症，1 例失访外，余 4 例至今存活。该组作者认为沟槽状胰腺炎的临床表现和影像学检查均无特异性，超声内镜检查有助于诊断；诊断时，应注意与胰头癌相鉴别。

影像学研究：CT 的检查包括 CT 平扫、动态 CT 和大剂量增强扫描。平扫可见胰头和十二指肠区实质性块影；动态 CT 对病变的范围显示的更清楚；大剂量 CT 增强扫描显示病变为非均质性强化，或可见到十二指肠壁内囊腔、胰十二指肠沟和十二指肠壁增厚以及肠腔狭窄。有时可见胆胰管扩张、胰头萎缩和钙化。该病在 MRI 上的表现是，病变呈薄片状块影，在 T_1WI 上呈稍低信号，在 T_2WI 呈等或稍高信号，增强扫描于十二指肠和胰头之间可见延迟强化。在鉴别诊断方面，需要考虑胰头癌、十二指肠癌、总胆管癌和急性胰腺炎伴发蜂窝织炎。胰头癌常有密度减低区，增强扫描仔细观察强化的变化，有助于胰头癌和胰十二指肠沟炎的鉴别，癌肿侵犯的范围较广，常波及胰周组织和十二指肠。上消化道钡餐检查，有利于观察十二指肠肿瘤的定位和定性；MRCP 可鉴别总胆管癌和胰十二指肠沟炎，后者表现为长段光滑性狭窄。

（二）胰腺炎

急性胰腺炎可伴发胰腺周围间隙，包括胰十二指肠沟的液体潴留，但不同于胰十二指肠沟炎，急性胰腺炎的积液和炎症反应，变化较快，短期复查可以吸收，或有假性囊肿形成。在 CT 上表现为胰腺密度轻度下降，胰腺轮廓模糊。在 MRI T_1WI 上呈低信号，T_2WI 上呈高信号，增强扫描胰腺呈均质高信号，胰腺周围的炎性反应，在 T_2WI 上也呈高信号。

慢性胰头炎性肿块以纤维化改变为主，在 T_1WI 和 T_2WI 上均呈低信号，动脉增强扫描在各期，纤维化区无强化或强化程度与正常部位的胰腺一致。而胰头癌在动脉期表现为低信号，没有强化表现，或仅有肿块边缘轻度强化，且肿块边缘较清楚。

自身免疫性胰腺炎，又称为硬化性胰腺炎、非酒精性导管破坏性慢性胰腺炎，为胰腺炎的一种特殊类型。本病具有如下特点：无胰腺炎急性发作史；无酒精滥用史；血清 γ- 球蛋白或 IgG 含量增高；自身抗体存在；CT 等影像检查可见胰腺弥漫增大，包膜增厚；MRCP 显示胆胰管不规则狭窄或肝内外胆管狭窄伴扩张；激素治疗效果良好，治愈后甚少复发；可并发或不并发其他自身免疫性疾病，如原发性硬化性胆管炎、慢性特发性肠道炎症、干燥综合征、系统性红斑狼疮以及特发性腹膜后纤维化等。

（三）胰头癌

腺癌是胰腺导管细胞腺癌的简称，占胰腺恶性肿瘤的 95%，近 2/3 的胰腺癌发生在胰头部。因为早期出现梗阻性黄疸，发现时肿瘤一般体积较小。小于 2cm 在 CT 平扫上往往呈等密度不易发现，但可引起胆胰管扩张。MRI：肿瘤细胞在 T_1WI 低信号、T_2WI 高信号。对于局限于胰腺轮廓内的小肿瘤，MRI 优于 CT。外生性胰小管腺癌是胰头部的胰管腺癌向外生长形似胰十二指肠沟的肿瘤。

（四）胰腺腺鳞癌

胰腺腺鳞癌在临床上比较罕见，文献上又称腺棘癌（adenoacantuoma）、黏膜表皮样癌（mucoepidermoid carcinoma）等，组织学特点是腺癌细胞群中混杂有不同数量的鳞癌细胞。国外文献报道仅 140 余例，国内偶有报道。影像学特征与胰腺导管癌无明显差异。如果 CT 或 B 超发现呈浸润性生长且瘤体较大的胰腺肿块有中央坏死，提示有腺鳞癌的可能。

（五）胃泌素瘤

胃泌素瘤由 Zollinger 和 Ellison（1955）首先报告，又称为卓 - 艾综合征（Zollinger-Ellison syndrome，ZES）。90% 以上的胃泌素瘤发生在称之为"胃泌素瘤三角区（gastrinoma triangle）"，三角区的尖顶起自胆囊管和胆总管的汇合部，下至十二指肠第二、三段连接处，内至胰腺颈、体交界处这一解剖区域。瘤体一般较胰岛素瘤为大，平均 4cm（0.2cm~20cm），50% 以上是多发的，大约 1/2~2/3 的胃泌素瘤是恶性的。临床主要表现有消化性溃疡、腹泻、脂肪泻。

影像学研究：CT 的敏感性较高，平扫呈等或低密度，质地均匀，边界清楚；CT 增强扫描动脉早期显示较清晰，实质期瘤体密度较淡。对 CT 可疑的病例进行 MR 检查，能进一步明确病灶，脂肪抑制 T_1WI 呈低信号，T_2WI 上呈高信号，增强扫描呈均质或环形强化。胃泌素瘤在 CT 上除能看到肿瘤本身外，时间久者，尚可显示胃、十二指肠黏膜肥厚等异常征象。

（六）胰腺脂肪瘤

脂肪瘤是常见的间叶性肿瘤，多见于结肠，而胰腺脂肪瘤甚为少见，Katz 等（1999）报告 4 例。复习文献以往仅有 5 例报道。无临床症状，多为中年男性，多为作腹部 CT 检查时偶然发现，表现为胰实质内边缘清楚的脂肪性肿块，大小在 1.4cm × 2.0cm~4.5cm × 5.3cm 之间，但有大至 30 cm × 20 cm 者。老年人或肥胖者胰腺内脂肪浸润，偶见于胰腺头部，其形态呈斑点状或索条状，易误诊为肿瘤。

（七）胰腺肉瘤

胰腺肉瘤非常罕见，仅占胰腺恶性肿瘤的 0.6%，胰腺癌与肉瘤的比例约为 184：1。原发于胰腺的肉瘤有未分化肉瘤、纤维肉瘤、恶性纤维组织细胞瘤、卡波西肉瘤、平滑肌肉瘤、恶性神经鞘瘤、横纹肌肉瘤等。实际上，大多数胰腺肉瘤是未分化癌的肉瘤样分化，或者是腹膜后肉瘤侵犯胰腺。本病好发于青年和婴幼儿。临床常有腹部不适，食欲不振，腰背酸痛，偶尔可见黄疸。肿瘤大者，可触及包块，质硬，有压痛。平滑肌肉瘤可能起源于胰管或血管，胰腺肉瘤恶性程度很高，常为多血管性的，易有早期肝转移。CT 表现可为较均匀的实质性肿块，或为高度不均质强化的肿块，肿瘤内有坏死区。影像学上不能与腺癌区别。

（八）囊性肿瘤

浆液性囊腺瘤，又称小囊性腺瘤，以胰体尾多见，是胰腺囊性肿瘤中最常见的良性肿瘤。MRI 表现为境界清楚的 T_1WI 低信号、T_2WI 蜂窝状高信号病变，肿瘤内小囊多而密集，小囊直径一般小于 2cm；在 T_2WI 上小囊和间隔清晰可见，壁光滑，囊内壁可见壁结节，不侵犯周围脏器，增强后囊壁、囊内分隔及壁结节有轻至中度强化，中心瘢痕可延迟强化。

二、十二指肠病变

（一）十二指肠壁囊性营养不良

十二指肠壁囊性营养不良是一个少见病种，Potet 和 Duclert（1970）首先报道，其后主要在欧洲文献研讨。本病可以单独存在，但常常与慢性胰腺炎特别是胰沟部胰腺炎并发。以往有些文献可能把本病误诊为十二指肠囊性重复畸形。本病的主要病理变化特点是增厚的十二指肠壁内出现小囊肿，小囊多位于十二指肠内侧壁，极少数发生在外侧壁，囊肿位于黏膜下或肌层，其内面覆盖以类似胰腺管的立方上皮，小囊腔为纤维组织包埋，病变部位可能原有异位的胰腺组织和慢性胰腺炎。根据囊腔大小，病变常表现为大于 1cm 的囊状外观，有时囊腔较小，类似实质性病变的表现。

影像学研究：在影像诊断学，囊腔容易在超声和 CT 上发现。在超声图像上，于增厚的十二指肠壁中有椭圆形单房或双腔低回声区。胰头往往增大伴有慢性胰腺炎表现，如主胰管扩张、钙化和假性囊肿。在 CT 上典型表现为十二指肠内壁增厚，平扫与胰腺对比呈等密度，增强早期呈低密度，螺旋 CT 动脉期呈更低密度，门脉期十二指肠壁的纤维层又与胰腺呈等密度。增厚的肠壁中常有小囊腔。一些作者报道 10 例，对该症在超声和 CT 的表现作了详细的描述，CT 上 9/10 例显示十二指肠壁增厚，7/10 例有小囊腔，肠壁增厚和小囊同时存在的占 6 例，1 例仅有小囊而没有肠壁增厚，3 例仅有十二指肠壁增厚呈实质性，小囊不明显，易误诊为胰腺癌。有时病变发展缓慢，开始囊腔不清楚，数月后变为明显囊肿。

（二）十二指肠憩室

典型的十二指肠憩室发生于乳头周围，十二指肠降段的内侧，或位于第三段十二指肠沟内，常有气体存留。十二指肠憩室易误诊为肿瘤、脓肿或囊肿等。憩室内潴留食物残渣，可导致胰十二指肠炎。口服钡餐检查，有钡剂或气体进入囊腔内，有助于憩室的正确诊断。有时，憩室内无气体存留，不易与胰腺肿瘤鉴别，再次复查会有气体进入。

（三）外生性十二指肠腺癌

外生性十二指肠腺癌往往是十二指肠乳头周围的腺癌向外侵犯，瘤体常呈息肉状向胰十二指肠沟内突出。消化道检查可见十二指肠黏膜破坏，肠梗阻或胆管阻塞征象。

（四）十二指肠淋巴瘤

十二指肠淋巴瘤甚为少见，不易与癌肿鉴别。

三、淋巴系统病变

胰十二指肠沟内的淋巴结，特别是肝脏和胆系的淋巴管沿肝十二指肠韧带引流，肝十二指肠韧带就在胰十二指肠沟内，或其邻近，因此肝、胆、胰和十二指肠的病变均可引起胰十二指肠沟的淋巴结肿大。要区别单个肿大的淋巴结与胰腺肿瘤是比较困难的，一般来说，胰腺肿瘤常向内侵犯，容易引起胆胰管阻塞。常见的淋巴系统病变是转移瘤和淋巴瘤。

（一）转移性肿瘤

随着 CT 的普及应用，胰腺转移瘤的发现逐渐增多，胰腺的转移多见于肿瘤的晚期，常伴有全身广泛转移。在原发病灶中，肾癌最常见。初次发现原发灶到胰腺转移的时间，在数月到数年之间。值得特别提出的是，有肾细胞癌的患者，5~10 年后可有胰腺孤立性转移。

胰腺的转移瘤无特殊的好发部位，大多数转移灶呈大的孤立结节，边缘清晰，也可能为多发病灶，少数为弥漫性浸润，1/3 的转移灶可见胰管扩张，阻塞胆管的较少见。增强后的 CT 表现有多种多样，常与原发灶相似，肿瘤较大时，显示为非均质性，转移瘤由多血性原发灶而来的，特别是肾细胞癌与其原发灶的强化特点相同。腹膜后和腹腔神经丛附近转移瘤，介入治疗有较好的疗效。能使 35% 的淋巴结消失，止痛疗效 80% 以上。

（二）淋巴瘤

淋巴瘤分为霍奇金淋巴瘤和非霍奇金淋巴瘤两大类。胰腺淋巴瘤又有原发性和继发性之分。原发性淋巴瘤可表现为孤立性肿块、多发性结节和弥散性病变三种类型，以单发肿块为主，约 16% 为弥散型，无包膜，边缘清楚。继发性淋巴肉瘤常为多发或弥漫性分布。

在 CT 上有 2 种表现，局限性单个或多发肿块或由于肿瘤浸润胰腺呈弥漫性增大。在 CT 图像上很像急性胰腺炎，但临床无急性胰腺炎征象，血清胰蛋白酶不升高。尽管有肿块包绕胰周血管，但胰管扩张的极其少见，这点有别于胰腺癌。在肾静脉平面以下出现淋巴结肿大也有利于淋巴瘤的诊断，可排除胰腺癌的可能。一旦影像诊断怀疑淋巴瘤，应进行穿刺活检进一步明确诊断，避免不必要的手术治疗。有作者提出瘤内出现钙化和坏死可排除非霍奇金淋巴瘤的可能。

（三）淋巴管瘤

淋巴管瘤是淋巴系统的良性肿瘤，好发于儿童的颈部（75%）和腋窝部（20%），腹部病变多见于腹膜后和肠系膜。胰腺的淋巴管瘤十分罕见，仅有数例报道。占全身淋巴管瘤的 1% 以下。可长很大才出现症状。肿瘤呈多囊性肿块，可大至 10 cm，外围有薄的纤维性包膜，囊内含有血性、浆液性或淋巴性液体。可能为先天性淋巴管发育畸形，由于淋巴管引流受阻，引起淋巴管扩张，显示为不同大小扩张的淋巴管，其中有薄的间隔。可在胰腺内生长，也可有蒂与胰相连。病理上分两种类型，简单型（毛细血管型）和海绵状型（囊状水瘤）。淋巴管瘤 CT 表现为单房或多囊性肿块，薄的间隔有强化，囊壁薄偶有钙化。螺旋 CT 多层面重建可显示瘤蒂。这些病变不易与假性囊肿、包虫囊肿和囊腺癌等病变鉴别。

（四）巨淋巴结增生症

巨淋巴结增生症比较少见，多发性更为罕见，有作者报告一例，同时有纵隔和腹部病变。巨淋巴结增生症是一种非肿瘤性免疫增生性疾病，病因不明，可能与疱疹病毒 8（HHV-8）感染有关。该病首先由 Castleman 等（1954）报道，此后命名为 Castleman 病，以往文献报告有许多同义名，如良性淋巴瘤、巨大淋巴组织增生症、淋巴结错构瘤、血管性淋巴组织错构瘤等。该病可发生于淋巴结存在的任何部位,一些作者统计400例,以胸部纵隔最为常见(70%),其次为颈部(40%)、腹部(12%)、腋部(4%)。多发性病变,以肺内和纵隔同时发病为多见,少数为胸、腹部同时发病,腹膜后也不少见。

巨淋巴结增生症的主要病理改变是淋巴组织和小血管的肿瘤样增生,组织学上分为三型:第一型是透明血管型或血管滤泡型,约占80%~90%,肿块大小不等,直径在3~10 cm之间,大多为单发肿块,一般无临床症状;第二型为浆细胞型,约占10%~20%,肿块一般以多结节型为主,常有发热、贫血、血沉加快;第三型为中间型或混合型。

影像学表现

一些作者报告10例,其中局限性9例,弥漫性1例。局限型9例病理诊断均为透明血管型,表现为单发肿块6例,单个较大肿块周围伴有小的子灶3例。CT平扫与肌肉相比呈等密度;动态增强多数病变(5/7例)在动脉期和延迟扫描均持续高度强化,强化程度接近大动脉。MRI平扫与肌肉相比T_1WI表现为低信号或等信号,T_2WI呈高信号,动态增强扫描病灶的强化方式与CT一致。4例肿块(直径>5 cm)增强扫描内部见裂隙状和放射状的CT低密度区和MRI低信号区,病理证实为较多纤维成分。弥漫型1例为浆细胞型,表现为腹膜后多个软组织结节,轮廓光整,明显强化。该作者认为,腹部巨淋巴结增生症的影像学表现与病理类型密切相关。局限透明血管型巨大淋巴结增生症的特点是单发肿块或单发较大肿块周围伴有小的子灶,强化密度与信号接近大动脉,较大肿块内部增强后可出现裂隙状或放射状CT低密度和MRI低信号区发生于肝门部的巨淋巴结增生症,在影像学上酷似肝内肿瘤。

CT:与肿块的细胞类型有关。局限型,平扫大多显示病灶边缘清楚而均匀的低密度区,少数中间可见点状钙化或较低密度区,动态增强扫描动脉早期显示迅速均匀强化,其程度与主动脉相仿;少数病灶平扫呈均匀低密度区,增强扫描动脉期呈高密度,门脉期和延迟期逐渐变为等密度,部分可见早期强化和延迟强化。肾上腺区和腹膜后亦为好发部位,偶尔可见钙化。罕见于胰腺,文献报告仅7例。

MRI表现:T_1WI病灶呈均匀中低信号,T_2WI病灶显示为明显高信号。动态增强扫描 动脉期病灶表现迅速均匀强化,呈明显高信号,有时可见星状低信号瘢痕;门脉期和延迟期持续强化。

四、胆胰管连接区周围肿瘤

胆胰管连接区周围肿瘤,旧称壶腹周围肿瘤,系指胆胰管连接区、胆总管下端、胰管开口处、十二指肠乳头及其附近的十二指肠黏膜等处的癌肿。这些来源不同的肿瘤,由于其所在的特殊解剖部位,有着相同的临床表现,手术时也难以将其截然分开,故常作为一个类型,统称为胆胰管连接区周围癌。胆总管远段癌形似胰十二指肠沟的肿瘤,其主要表现是肿瘤部胆管突然中断和近侧胆管扩张,但阻塞部位于胆胰管连接区,则不能确定其原发部位,即使组织学上鉴别肿瘤原发于胆管、胰腺还是十二指肠也不可能。一例胆胰管连接区周围癌,CT增强扫描显示肝外胆管下端低密度肿块位于胰头和十二指肠之间;MRCP显示肿块位于肝外胆管、主胰管和十二指肠之间。

五、血管内癌栓和血管瘤

在鉴别胰十二指肠沟区病变时,还需想到肝癌等所引起的血管内癌栓,癌栓好发于门静脉,向肝外发展的癌栓可侵犯肠系膜上静脉和脾静脉。

肠系膜上静脉内癌栓的影像学表现是,CT增强扫描的门静脉期可显示肠系膜上静脉内圆形或类圆形充盈缺损。

脾静脉内癌栓表现为CT增强扫描门静脉期脾静脉内圆形充盈缺损;还可表现为CT增强扫描门静脉期门静脉内圆形充盈缺损及其周围广泛侧支循环形成,即门脉海绵样变。

除上述门静脉和肠系膜上静脉癌栓外,尚可见到门静脉瘤和肠系膜上动脉的动脉瘤。门静脉瘤可能与先天性畸形有关。门静脉瘤在CT上显示瘤体逐渐为对比剂所充盈,门静脉血管造影能更好地显示瘤体与附近血管的关系。

肝外门静脉瘤的影像学表现:CT增强扫描肝外门静脉呈现囊状扩张,有对比剂充盈;门静脉血管造影显示瘤体为对比剂均匀填充。

肠系膜上动脉动脉瘤的影像学表现:CT增强扫描显示胰头区被附壁血栓包绕的强化的肠系膜上动脉的内腔;若没有动脉期肠系膜上动脉内腔强化的影像,很可能被误认为是胰头病变。

第十章　胰腺囊性病变

第一节　胰腺囊性肿瘤 CT 诊断与处理对策

胰腺囊性肿瘤是一种少见的肿瘤，占整个胰腺肿瘤的 1% 左右，占胰腺囊性病变的 10%~15%，但随着体检普及和断面影像诊断技术（超声、CT、MRI）广泛使用，近年其检出率或发病率有增加趋势。

简要分类：临床上常见和普遍所指胰腺囊性肿瘤主要包括：浆液性囊腺瘤、黏液性囊性肿瘤和导管内乳头状黏液性肿瘤，几乎占整个胰腺囊性肿瘤的 90% 左右。胰腺囊性肿瘤根据良、恶性可分为囊腺瘤和囊腺癌；依据肿瘤囊性成分又可分为浆液性囊腺瘤和黏液性肿瘤，黏液性肿瘤包括黏液性囊性肿瘤和导管内乳头状黏液性肿瘤。其次，还包括胰腺原发实质性肿瘤囊性变，如最常见实质性假乳头状肿瘤、非功能性胰岛细胞肿瘤、腺泡细胞囊腺癌、腺鳞癌巨细胞肿瘤和成熟囊性畸胎瘤等；胰腺转移性肿瘤的囊性变，最常见为胃癌、肾癌和黑色素瘤的胰腺转移。

鉴别诊断原则：胰腺囊性肿瘤间鉴别以及与胰腺囊性病变、胰腺肿瘤的囊性变的鉴别存在难点，CT 表现或征象有一定的重叠。Sahani 等依据 CT 特征，分为 4 型。Ⅰ型者，病变包括最多见的假性囊肿，其次为真性囊肿、大囊型浆液性囊腺瘤，极少部分黏液性囊腺瘤和分支型导管内乳头状黏液性肿瘤，Hippel-Lindau 综合征者，胰腺也呈多个囊样病变。结合曾有胰腺炎病史，则提示为假性囊肿。如多平面重建或 MRCP 显示胰腺主胰管与囊性病变相通，则为分支型导管内乳头状黏液性肿瘤机会显著提高。Ⅱ型者，只见于良性小囊型浆液性囊腺瘤，有典型 CT 征象。Ⅲ型者，大囊型浆液性囊腺瘤和黏液性囊腺瘤（癌）均可相似表现，难以鉴别。Ⅳ型者，包括黏液性囊腺癌、实质性假乳头状肿瘤、非功能性胰腺神经内分泌肿瘤、腺泡细胞囊腺癌和主胰管型 / 混合型导管内乳头状黏液性肿瘤。它们 CT 鉴别有一定的难度，确诊依赖病理。

临床处理对策：总之，囊性病变直径 <3cm 者，90%~95% 为良性，临床可随访。如临床患者有明显肿瘤压迫不适，也可采取手术治疗。对于Ⅰ型者，根据临床和 CT 难以鉴别时，其发生恶变倾向的概率为 1/3，即黏液性囊腺瘤和分支型导管内乳头状黏液性肿瘤具有恶变倾向，如果暂时不手术，必须密切随访；Ⅱ型 CT 表现者，属良性肿瘤，肿瘤较大，临床征状明显者，可手术切除；至于Ⅲ型 CT 表现者，建议临床积极手术，因发生恶性的概率为 1/2；Ⅳ型者，均为恶性或恶变倾向肿瘤，临床手术为首选。

第二节　胰腺囊性病变钙化

详见本书 本卷 本篇 第二十五章 第五节　胰腺囊性病变钙化。

第三节 关于胰腺囊性病变

胰腺的囊性病变,约 80%~90% 为胰腺假性囊肿,而大约 10%~20% 为囊性肿瘤。胰腺囊性病变大多为黏液性囊性肿瘤、浆液性囊性肿瘤和导管内乳头状瘤,其他囊性病变所占比例不足 10%,因此,胰腺囊性病变的鉴别主要集中在胰腺假性囊肿、黏液性囊性肿瘤、浆液性囊性肿瘤和导管内乳头状瘤这几种病。

胰腺肿瘤和胰腺假性囊肿是两类性质截然不同的胰腺囊性病变,治疗方法完全不同,精准医学,影像先行,影像的鉴别诊断更显意义重大。

胰腺囊性病变影像诊断思维主要包括四步骤。第一步,确定是否有胰腺炎病史;第二步,胰腺囊性病变分为大囊型、微囊型、寡囊型和其他(即小于 10% 部分),分析病例影像所见囊性病灶进行分类:第三步,临床血清肿瘤标记物水平为基准结合常见胰腺囊性病变的影像各自特点进行分析;第四步,影像结论并决定临床的治疗方案。

胰腺囊性病变影像诊断思维三部分中,最重要的无疑是胰腺囊性病变病灶本身的特点,传统意义的影像学习和分析方法是把需要诊断的病变的影像特征与疾病对号入座,优点是典型的可以做出明确诊断,不典型的就会不知所措。

进一步而言,这样也不符合影像逻辑的思维方式,比如对胰腺囊性病变病灶而言,首先看到的是胰腺上的囊性肿块,影像的思维方式是对常见囊的特点进行分类概括,形成思维流程导图,如胰腺囊性病变分为大囊、微囊和寡囊型,再对每种囊的影像细节特有之处分析,再结合特定的临床资料做出进一步的诊断和处理。

针对一例胰腺囊性病变而言,合理的影像诊断思维包括四步骤:第一步,明确是否有胰腺炎病史,该例没有胰腺炎病史,无法做出明确的胰腺假囊肿的诊断。这里需要强调的是,如果有可以做出明确胰腺假囊肿的诊断,但是如果没有明确的胰腺炎病史,很少一部分患者也可能是胰腺假囊肿。第二步,该例为胰腺病变为大囊型。第三步,血清学肿瘤标记物 CA19-9 明显升高,提示胰腺恶性肿瘤,因而黏液性囊性肿瘤和局限性导管内乳头状黏液瘤均符合。囊性肿块细节特点观察,发现其与胰管不通,导管内乳头状黏液瘤被排除,黏液性囊性肿瘤符合,进一步观察囊壁及细节,发现其内有分隔、囊壁结节,黏液性囊性肿瘤伴浸润性癌诊断成立。第四步,影像评估为临床高风险恶性肿瘤,影像提供了手术的依据。

总之,胰腺囊性病变影像表现有一定的特征性及规律性,影像学的诊断对良、恶性的鉴别及后续治疗方案的选择而言具有重要的价值,掌握胰腺囊性病变的影像学特征并作出正确的诊断依赖于科学的影像诊断思维,其在胰腺囊性病变临床实践中具有重要意义。

第四节 误诊病例简介:胰腺癌被误诊为胰腺囊腺癌

患者,女, 77 岁。反复腰背痛 1 周,外院诊断胰腺囊肿入院。CT 平扫和增强扫描提示:胰腺体积明显增大,占据小网膜囊,胰体尾部密度下降且不均匀,可见多发性囊状低密度影,囊腔大小不等,囊壁厚薄不均匀且部分轮廓欠清,胰腺边缘不光整,与胃后壁分界不清;增强后胰腺病灶呈不均匀强化,囊状低密度影强化程度不一,部分囊壁可见强化,边缘欠光整,胰腺内动脉分支轮廓不规则;肝外胆管扩张;腹腔及腹膜后淋巴结肿大。诊断意见:胰腺体尾部囊实性肿块性质待定,考虑囊腺癌可能性大,不除外囊腺瘤。怀疑腹部淋巴结转移。肝外胆管扩张原因待查。

病理检查:①胰腺肿物,灰白色组织一块,大小 10cm × 6cm × 4cm,表面附脂肪,切面灰白质韧,与周围边界不清。病理诊断:胰腺导管腺癌,Ⅱ级,10cm × 6cm × 4cm,伴灶性坏死,浸润至边缘纤维脂肪组织,累及少数神经。②胰腺囊肿壁:囊壁一块,病理诊断:胰体尾部囊壁组织切除标本:囊壁被覆单层立方上皮,囊壁间质大量淋巴细胞和一些中性粒细胞浸润并有平滑肌组织,符合囊肿伴感染。

回顾性误诊分析发现；病灶区增强后强化程度远低于胰头区，说明病灶区为少血供，理应倾向考虑为胰腺癌；CT 所见低密度区大小不等，大者相当大，但不膨大，说明其内张力不高，实质上并不都是囊肿，许多实为坏死区；临床诊断为胰腺囊肿对影像诊断有一定的误导；体尾部囊肿表现吸引观察的注意力，对该区实质部分观察不仔细；胰腺导管腺癌伴灶性坏死呈现低密度，与囊肿的表现混为一谈，导致误诊。

第十一章　胰腺囊腺瘤与囊腺癌

第一节　CT能谱成像鉴别胰腺寡囊型浆液性囊腺瘤与黏液性囊性肿瘤

胰腺囊性病变包括肿瘤性和非肿瘤性病变，其中肿瘤性病变常见的有胰腺浆液性肿瘤、黏液性囊性肿瘤及囊实性的胰腺实体假乳头肿瘤；非肿瘤性的病变主要有假性囊肿和真性囊肿。胰腺浆液性肿瘤根据大体和组织学表现的不同分为浆液性微囊腺瘤、寡囊型浆液性囊腺瘤及其他少见类型。术前明确胰腺囊性肿瘤的性质对于制定临床处理方案非常重要。

寡囊型浆液性囊腺瘤(大囊型浆液性囊腺瘤)在大体形态及影像表现上与黏液性囊性肿瘤较为类似，术前往往不容易区分。对于寡囊型浆液性囊腺瘤与黏液性囊性肿瘤的术前鉴别诊断研究前期较多集中于临床及影像学描述性形态特征方面，其敏感度与特异度各研究之间差异较大。对于囊液的生化及肿瘤指标分析和囊壁的细胞学检查，需在内窥镜超声引导下穿刺吸取囊液，为有创性检查且技术难度较高，广泛应用存在一定局限。

CT能谱成像是在双能量扫描条件下实现的CT功能成像技术，不但能够获得基物质密度值及其分布图像，还能获得不同千电子伏(keV)水平的单能量图像。该组选择碘-水和钙-水作为2对基物质。CT能谱成像可以显示不同病变和人体组织随着X线能量水平(keV)的变化而变化的X线衰减系数(HU)，从而产生反映不同病变和人体组织对于X线的特征性能谱曲线，同时根据所得的能谱曲线能够计算出该病变或组织的有效原子序数。由此可见，CT能谱成像是具有多参数、定量分析的新成像模式。

一般特征：与黏液性囊性肿瘤相比，浆液性囊腺瘤恶变的可能性较小，所以对于一些不适于手术的患者可进行临床随访观察，但是寡囊型浆液性囊腺瘤在术前不易与黏液性囊性肿瘤相鉴别。根据文献报道，病灶多位于胰头部、呈多囊状和分叶状、囊壁不强化是寡囊型浆液性囊腺瘤区别于黏液性囊性肿瘤的特征，黏液性囊性肿瘤较寡囊型浆液性囊腺瘤更易发生于女性患者。一项该研究中没有观察到病灶位置和性别构成的差异，可能是病例数较少的原因，由于该研究主要是针对CT能谱成像的定量指标，故未对文献中提及的常规影像形态特征进行统计分析。该研究结果显示，寡囊型浆液性囊腺瘤病灶较黏液性囊性肿瘤小，与文献报道结果一致，该组病例显示黏液性囊性肿瘤的患者年龄一般较寡囊型浆液性囊腺瘤患者大，且多数因相关临床症状而就诊。

CT能谱特征参数：以往研究结果显示，寡囊型浆液性囊腺瘤的囊液与黏液性囊性肿瘤的囊液在化学成分和物理特性方面存在明显差异，黏液性囊性肿瘤的囊液黏稠、蛋白较多(包含部分肿瘤标记物)游离水分较少，并有文献报道黏液性囊性肿瘤的囊液黏稠度高于浆液性囊腺瘤的囊液。该研究结果显示，寡囊型浆液性囊腺瘤与黏液性囊性肿瘤的囊性成分在CT能谱成像特征上有明显差异，主要表现在低能量水平的CT值、有效原子序数及基物质浓度方面。常规CT所采用的混合能量X线所产生的衰减平均效应会降低组织的低对比分辨率，而CT能谱成像提供的单能量图像可以弥补这方面的不足。

寡囊型浆液性囊腺瘤与黏液性囊性肿瘤的囊液密度较低，用常规CT值进行测量时是难以区分的，两者在70~80keV(相当于常规CT的120~140 kVp)附近能谱曲线是非常接近和/或相交的；而在低能量水平(40~50 keV)时两者具有明显的差异。

虽然常规 CT 的 CT 值难以区分浆液与黏液，但有效原子序数和高密度基物质(碘、钙)浓度的差异反映了黏液性囊性肿瘤的囊液质量高于寡囊型浆液性囊腺瘤的囊液。

多参数联合诊断：以往研究结果显示，鉴别寡囊型浆液性囊腺瘤与黏液性囊性肿瘤缺乏单一的特异性指标，联合多个相关指标才能提高诊断效果。与常规 CT 相比，CT 能谱成像提供了更多的定量指标和分析工具。众多指标在日常临床诊断工作中的综合评估较为困难，该研究把传统的临床指标与 CT 能谱成像定量指标相结合，判别分析结果显示样本回代符合率高(100%)，所得判别函数具有很高的判别能力。该研究也存在一些明显的局限性：病例数较少；对于胰腺黏液性囊性肿瘤未作进一步的分类；缺乏手术标本离体测量与分析结果和回顾性分析。这些不足之处需要在今后的研究工作中通过扩大样本量、增加体外实验和前瞻性研究来完善。

第二节　浆液性囊腺瘤

浆液性囊腺瘤较黏液性囊腺性肿瘤少见，在胰腺囊性肿物约占 1/3，女性明显多于男性，男性与女性之别约为 1∶4.5。发病平均年龄为 62 岁。

浆液性囊腺瘤大体病理见肿瘤多发生在胰头，直径 1~25cm，平均 7cm，剖面见许多直径为 2~15mm 的小囊，呈蜂窝状，故又称微囊型囊腺瘤。肿瘤表面可有多分叶，中央可有星状纤维瘢痕，瘢痕内尚可有钙化。Kabayashi 等报道浆液性囊腺瘤也可呈一个大囊，或仅有数个小囊。细胞富含糖原，又称富含糖原的囊腺瘤。一般认为本病无恶变的可能，如果影像表现典型，患者年老、无症状，可以不必手术切除。

CT 增强扫描呈轮廓清楚的分叶状肿物，血供丰富，分隔内有广泛的毛细血管网，肿瘤可明显强化而呈蜂窝状肿物，可见中央的星状瘢痕及其钙化。有时由于小囊过于细小，CT 上可表现为实性肿瘤。

MRI 可见分叶状肿物，T_1WI 上为低信号，轮廓光整，不侵犯周围脏器；T_2WI 上呈蜂窝状的高信号，其内多个小囊肿和间隔清晰可见，偶可见壁结节。增强扫描示瘤壁、间隔有轻到中度的强化，肿瘤呈细小分隔及微小或多房囊性改变，蜂窝状，中央可见星状瘢痕及钙化，多房囊内容物无强化。由于 MRI 较 CT 能更好地显示肿瘤囊性成分的形态和大小，MRI 有利于确定肿瘤的囊性性质，MRI 更容易鉴别浆液性和黏液性囊腺瘤。

第三节　胰体浆液性囊腺瘤

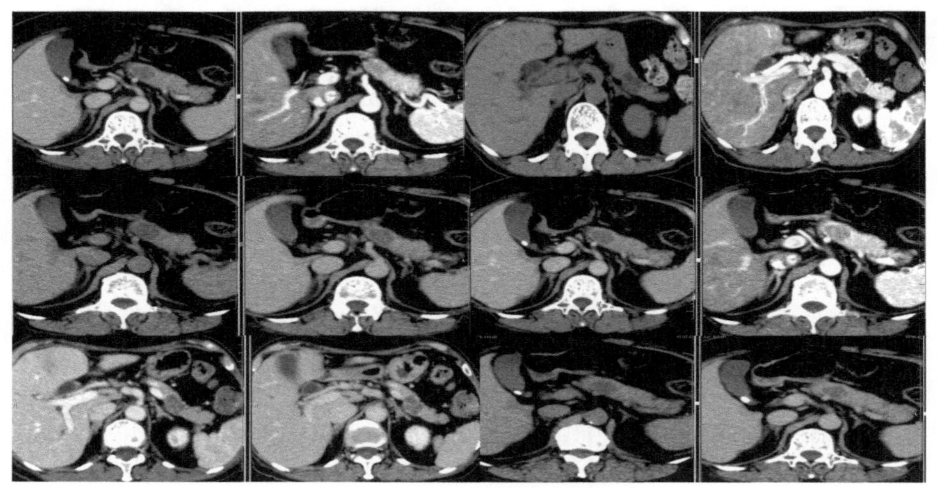

图 20-11-1　胰体浆液性囊腺瘤

患者,女,63 岁。反复右上腹闷痛 4 个月余入院。

病理检查:胰腺肿物切除标本:胰腺一段,大小 7.5cm×3cm×2.5cm,一端可见一灰白色结节,结节大小 2cm×2.2cm×2cm,切面灰白,质中,偏脆,与周围界限欠清。常规病理诊断:胰腺肿物切除标本:符合浆液性囊腺瘤,待免疫组化进一步确诊。免疫组化及组织特染检测:阳性:CK(P),CK(L),CK8,CK18,CK19,CK7,CK(H)(局灶),EMA(局灶),Ki-67(2%),AB,PAS;阴性:CK20,CEA,ER,PR,CD31,CD34,D2-40。免疫组化诊断:胰腺肿物切除标本:浆液性囊腺瘤(图 20-11-1)。

第四节　小囊性囊腺瘤,大囊性囊腺瘤或腺癌

小囊性囊腺瘤是良性肿瘤,多见于老人,以多发性小囊为特征。CT 图像上,该肿瘤中央常有瘢痕;在 MRI 增强 FLASH 图像上可见瘢痕延迟强化。

大囊性囊腺瘤或腺癌是含有黏蛋白的恶性或潜在恶性的肿瘤,中年女性较多见。肿瘤较大(平均直径 10cm),为多房状,有包膜,大的不规则的囊性腔隙被厚的间隔分开。最常见的位置是胰体和胰尾,易向邻近组织和器官侵犯。原发肿瘤和转移瘤产生的黏蛋白偶使其在 T_1WI 和 T_2WI 上呈高信号。

第五节　胰体尾浆液性微囊性腺瘤

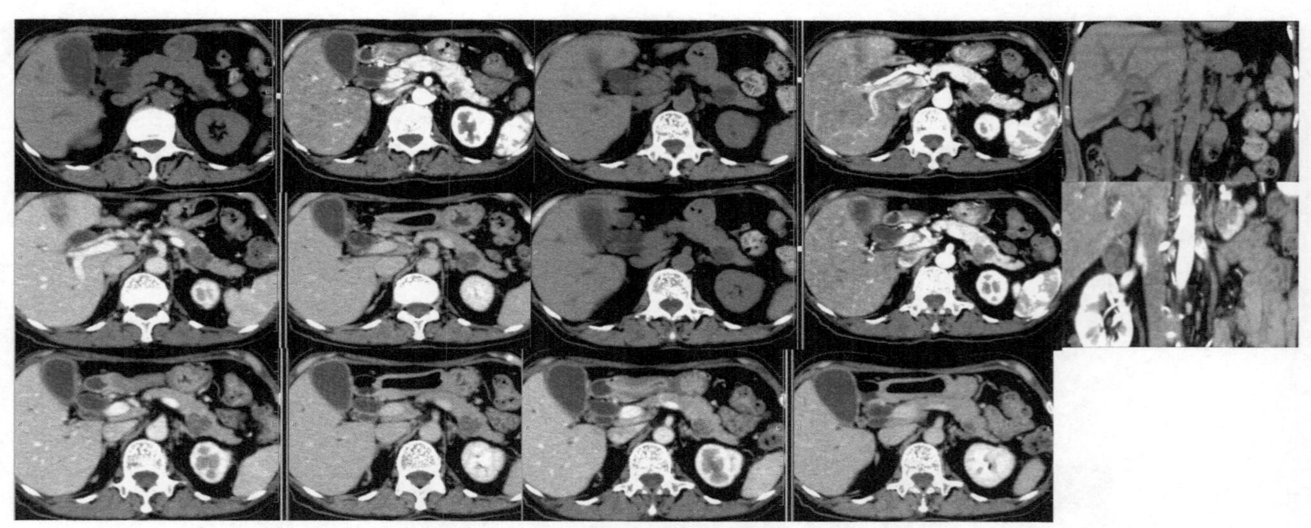

图 20-11-2　胰体尾浆液性微囊性腺瘤

患者,女,78 岁。因反复右上腹痛 5 个月余,再发 19 小时入院。病理检查:脾、胰体尾肿物切除标本:大小 8.5cm×4cm×2.5cm,胰体尾切面可见一灰白色结节,面积 2.5cm×1.5cm,结节呈多囊性,囊腔的直径约 0.2~0.4cm,结节与周围边界较清,胰腺周边带有脂肪。脾脏大小 8cm×6cm×3.5cm,切面紫红,未触及结节及质硬区。常规病理诊断:胰体尾肿物切除标本:初步诊断浆液性微囊性腺瘤,待免疫组化检测进一步证实。脾脏切除标本:红髓白髓界限清楚,未见异常。免疫组化检测:阳性:CK7,CK8,CK18,CK19,EMA,NSE,CA19-9(局灶),Ki-67(<5%);阴性:Vim,CEA,CgA,Syn,CD34。免疫组化诊断:胰体尾肿物切除标本:免疫组化支持浆液性微囊性腺瘤(图 20-11-2)。

第六节 胰腺先天性囊肿

胰腺先天性囊肿为胰导管的内皮细胞发育异常，临床上少见，约占全部胰腺囊肿的 10%~15%。多见于小儿，尤其女婴，常为多发性，一般较小，多数无症状，也有文献报道发病时表现为胰腺炎的成年患者。直径自几毫米到 3~5 cm，也有文献报道直径达 15 cm 者。内壁光滑，被覆扁平或低柱状上皮，有时上皮完全萎缩，囊内含有浆液、黏液或者感染出血而形成的混浊液体。囊肿内不含实性组织成分、间隔或类似肿瘤的赘生物。紧贴囊旁的胰腺组织没有炎症，不粘连。大多数先天性囊肿为偶然发现，囊肿的特征为不与胰管的分支交通。

CT 显示胰腺内水样密度肿物，CT 值一般为 0~20 HU，壁薄光滑，囊内无间隔及软组织结节。静脉注射对比剂后无强化，胰腺其余部分正常。

MRI 上符合单纯囊肿的表现，为长 T_1、长 T_2 信号，囊壁薄而光整。

一例为成年女性，与本病好发年龄不一致，影像检查偶然发现胰腺病变，虽病变大小在先天性囊肿常见范围内，MRI 检查基本符合囊肿的表现，且周围胰腺组织无病变，但囊壁上的一个小的壁结节与先天性囊肿囊内无软组织结节的特点不符，故误诊为囊腺瘤。

胰腺先天性囊肿患者一般情况良好，血液生化检查多正常，影像表现上较难与囊腺瘤鉴别，术前诊断多较困难，文献报道者多为术后通过病理组织学检查才最终确诊。

第七节 胰管黏液囊性瘤的导管淤积变型

详见本书 本卷 本篇 第二十章 第六节 胰管黏液囊性瘤的导管淤积变型。

第八节 胰腺浆液性囊腺瘤病例

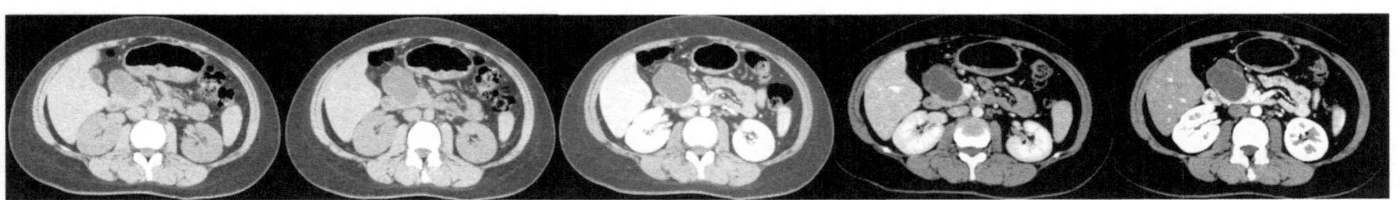

图 20-11-3 胰腺浆液性囊腺瘤病例

患者，女，26 岁。

手术病理证实：胰腺浆液性囊腺瘤（图 20-11-3）。

第九节 浆液性囊腺瘤与黏液性囊性肿瘤的鉴别

浆液性囊腺瘤与黏液性囊性肿瘤的鉴别至关重要，前者只有大于 40mm 病例才建议处理，后者则需手术处理。

下列征像有助于两者的鉴别：①前者发病年龄略高于后者，胰头多见，后者胰体尾部多见；②前者由多个小囊组成，为小囊性病变，子囊囊腔直径多 <10.0 mm，切面呈蜂窝状，囊大小相对较一致、外周囊相对稍大；后者为单个或多个较大囊腔，为大囊性病变，子囊一般少于 6 个，囊大小无一致性，且囊腔直径多 >20 mm；③前者切面中央有放射状钙化，后者囊壁或囊内分隔有钙化;④前者囊内信号均匀,后者 T_1WI 信号稍高,多信号不均匀;⑤前者多囊肿块间隔较厚,可呈囊实混杂病灶,后者不出现混杂病灶。约 30% 浆液性囊腺瘤为单囊性病变,囊内均匀水样信号有助于鉴别。

有研究认为对于浆液性与黏液性囊腺瘤的鉴别诊断主要依靠病变位置和是否出现钙化。病变位于胰腺头颈部和存在中心钙化,提示为浆液性囊腺瘤;而肿瘤位于胰腺体尾部和病变无钙化则更支持黏液性囊腺瘤/癌的诊断。

Curry 等(2000)报道 22 例胰腺浆液性囊腺瘤中无 1 例有边缘钙化, 4 例有中心钙化,而 28 例胰腺黏液性囊腺瘤/癌中 7 例有边缘钙化、1 例有中心钙化。有研究认为病灶中心的星状瘢痕及瘢痕钙化是浆液性囊腺瘤的特异性表现,但很少见到。

研究显示囊的数目和大小对于浆液性囊腺瘤和黏液性囊腺瘤的鉴别诊断有一定意义。浆液性囊腺瘤囊直径多小于等于 2cm,数目大于 6 个,而黏液性囊腺瘤单房直径多大于 2cm,囊的数目小于等于 6 个。

但 Lewandrowski 等(1992)提出大囊型胰腺浆液性囊腺瘤的概念,以区别于经典的微囊型胰腺浆液性囊腺瘤,此类型病变的囊壁上皮细胞与典型的微囊型浆液性囊腺瘤并无区别,但病变由单囊或少数大囊构成,囊腔直径 >2cm,二者在影像上难以区分,常会被误诊为黏液性囊腺瘤/癌。

根据病变轮廓、囊的数目和最大囊直径、发生部位、钙化情况、囊壁特征及囊壁乳头对于浆液性囊腺瘤与黏液性囊腺瘤/癌具有较高的鉴别诊断价值。但两者在 CT 表现特征上存在重叠,对于这些不典型病例的诊断,应结合多种影像学检查方法如 MR、超声内镜、细针穿刺囊液细胞学检查及囊液肿瘤标记物检测等诊断技术来提高胰腺囊腺瘤的正确诊断率。

有研究报道 MSCT 显示为单房病变或实性病变的浆液性囊腺瘤,在 MR 检查中 T2WI 像上显示为典型的高信号多房性囊肿,并可分辨 CT 图像未能显示的分隔信号,表明 MR 具有一定的鉴别诊断价值。多种诊断技术的联合应用,如细针穿刺囊液细胞学检查及囊液的生化分析及肿瘤标记物的测定,有可能提高对非典型病变的诊断准确性。

第十节 胰腺浆液性囊腺瘤

患者,女, 75 岁。反复左上腹闷痛 10 余年,加重半年入院。

手术所见:腹腔无腹水,胰体尾部与脾门及后腹膜组织粘连紧密,可触及一大小约 7cm×6cm 囊实性肿物,边界不清,质中,脾动静脉与胰尾粘连紧密,无法游离。肝脏、脾脏、肠管未见明显异常。

病理检查:胰体尾肿物及脾脏:部分胰腺组织一块,大小 8cm×5cm×3cm,切面呈多房囊性,囊腔直径 0.5~1.5cm,腔内含透明样液,囊壁光滑,壁厚 0.1cm,胰尾部表面连接脾脏,脾脏大小 8.5cm×5cm×2cm,切面红褐质中。常规病理诊断:胰体尾肿物及脾脏肿物切除标本:初步诊断胰腺浆液性囊腺瘤,待免疫组化进一步明确诊断;淤血性脾脏肿大。免疫组化检测:阳性: EMA,CK7,CK8,CK18,CK19,CK(P),CK(L),Vimentin,Ki-67(+,约 1%);阴性: CEA,Syn,CgA,F8,D2-40,CD34,Actin,S-100,Desmin,CD31。免疫组化诊断:胰体尾肿物及脾脏肿物切除标本:胰腺浆液性囊腺瘤(图 20-11-4)。

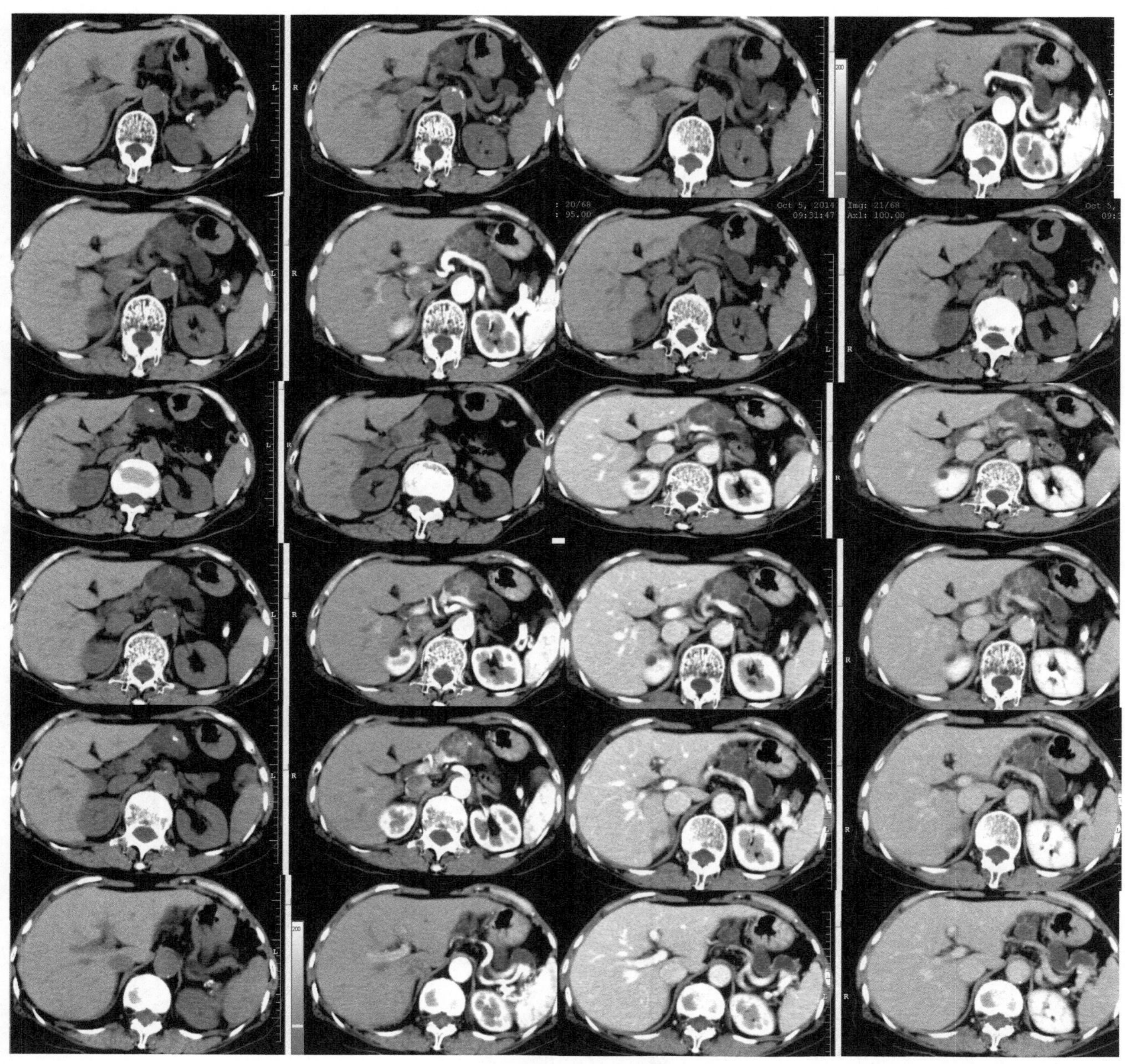

图 20-11-4 胰腺浆液性囊腺瘤

第十一节 胰腺黏液性囊腺瘤

患者，女，43 岁。两年前无意中发现上腹包块，质地稍硬。偶有腹胀，伴里急后重，大便 2~3 次 / 日，量少，成型。患者未重视，两年来腹部包块逐渐增大。

手术所见：进腹后，吸尽腹盆腔积液。首先分离其上覆盖大网膜，用超声刀游离，注意保护胃网膜左、右血管，将大网膜与肿瘤分开并切除部分大网膜，继续沿肿块边缘游离，将肿瘤与横结肠、十二指肠、空肠、回肠分开，直至胰腺上缘，继续仔细分离，证实肿瘤来源于胰尾处，距肿瘤 3cm 处用闭合器闭合部分胰尾，移除标本。

病理检查：腹膜后肿瘤切除标本：分叶状囊肿两个，大者大小 20cm × 15cm × 6 cm，小者大小 15cm × 14cm × 5cm，切面呈多房状，内含胶冻状黏液，局部见少量灰黄油脂样物，未见毛发。大者表面附少量大网膜样物质，大小 11cm × 8cm × 2cm，小者表现附少量灰黄组织，似胰腺，大小

4.5cm × 3cm × 1cm。另见大网膜一块，大小 20cm × 11cm × 2.5cm，未触及结节。常规病理诊断：腹膜后肿瘤切除标本：考虑胰腺黏液性囊腺瘤，大小 20cm × 15cm × 6 cm~15cm × 14cm × 5cm。注：请结合手术所见，排除卵巢来源；肿瘤外侧分别附少量胰腺组织和大网膜组织，局部附少量实体形细胞团，待免疫组化协助定性。

免疫组化检测：阳性：CK7，CH-L，CK-L；阴性：CK20，CK-H，CgA，Vimentin。免疫组化诊断：腹膜后肿瘤切除标本：腹膜后黏液性囊腺瘤，肿瘤外侧局部附少量实体性细胞团，免疫组化提示其兼有神经内分泌及腺上皮分化，性质不明。请注意随访（图 20-11-5）。

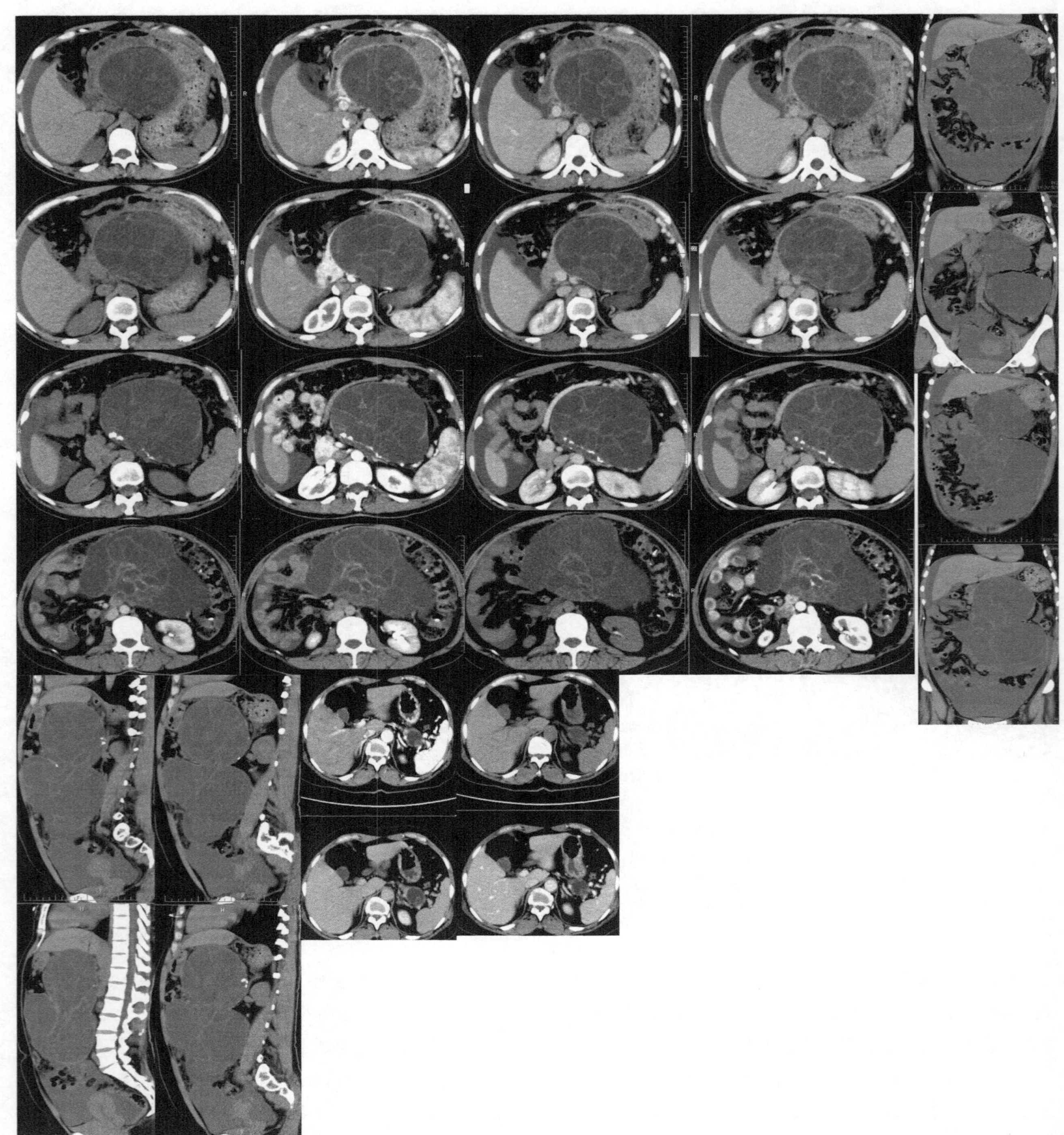

图 20-11-5 胰腺黏液性囊腺瘤

第十二节　误诊病例简介：胰腺浆液性囊腺瘤与扩张的主胰管

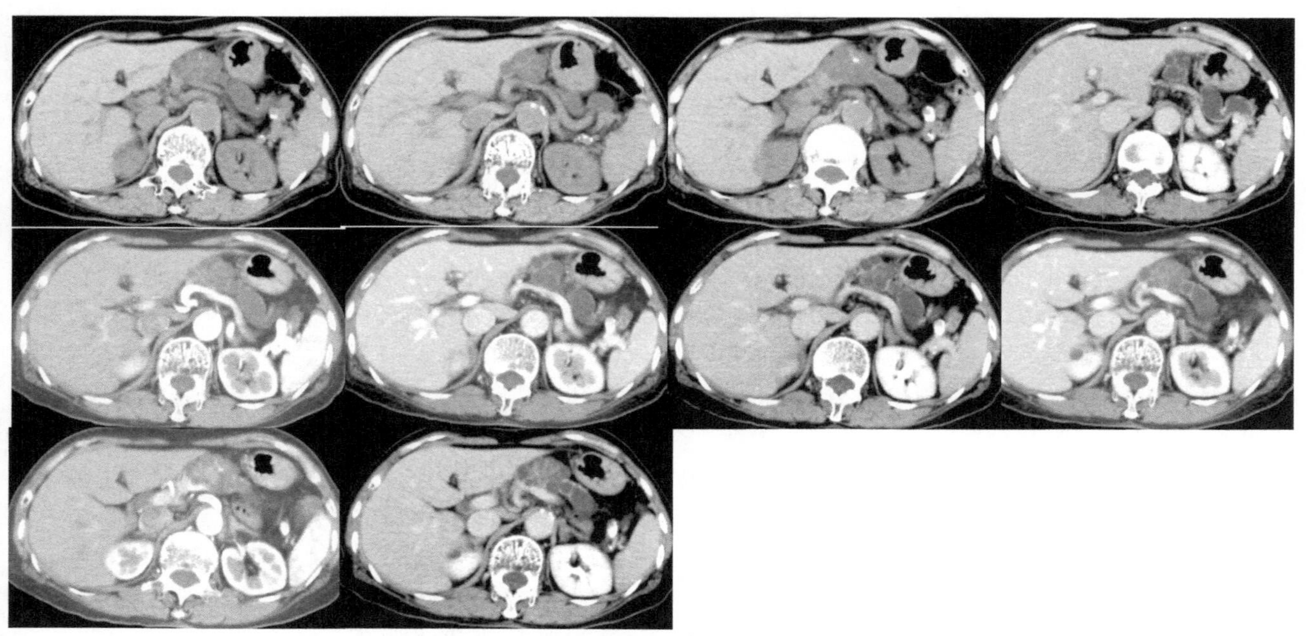

图 20-11-6　胰腺浆液性囊腺瘤与扩张的主胰管

患者，女，75 岁。

病理学检查：胰腺组织一块，肿瘤大小为 8cm × 5cm × 3cm，切面呈多房囊性，囊腔直径 0.5cm~ 1.5cm，腔内含透明样液，囊壁光滑，壁厚 0.1cm。免疫组化诊断：胰腺浆液性囊腺瘤。

CT 增强扫描诊断时，误将胰尾囊腔认作扩张的主胰管（图 20-11-6）。

第十二章 胰腺假性囊肿

第一节 位于纵隔的胰腺假性囊肿

胰腺假性囊肿出现于纵隔十分少见，Kirchner(1977)报告2例并回顾英语文献上已报告的14例且加以讨论。出现于纵隔的胰腺假性囊肿大多位于后纵隔，一般是途经主动脉裂孔和食管裂孔穿过横膈进入纵隔。临床症状有胸痛、腹痛和呼吸困难。

胰腺假性囊肿是胰腺分泌物、血和坏死物的包裹，常为胰外伤或胰腺炎症所致。虽然它通常位于腹部小网膜囊，但它常可沿着阻力最小的方向进行扩展，进入纵隔即为其例。

Kirchner分析16例，男女发病相等，年龄为10个月至73岁，仅3例为小儿。主诉皆只涉及胸部，但在大多数病例的病史常提示曾患胰腺炎或淀粉酶阳性，只2例扪及腹部包块。在成人，酒精中毒是常见病因，而在小儿，外伤则更为常见。此外，在儿童还应考虑滥用药物的因素。纵隔的胰腺假性囊肿可引起食管和胃向左下移位，胸腔积液，肺基底部浸润或肺不张，纵隔感染或脓肿以及少有的胰腺钙化。Edell等(1979)报告3例纵隔胰腺假性囊肿，产生吞咽因难。患者有慢性酒精中毒，经常发生腹痛和呕吐，偶尔有胰腺炎症状发作。X线胸片显露一纵隔包块，上部胃肠道钡餐检查示胃后包块，食管远端有光滑的壁外的压迫。超声检查发现胰尾巨大的假性囊肿扩展进入纵隔，从而明确诊断。Shah等(1980)报告1例纵隔胰腺假性囊肿压迫心脏，引起超声图像改变，假性囊肿引流后，异常的超声图像消失。

第二节 胰腺假性囊肿表现类似肾囊肿或肾周囊肿及脓肿

Lilienfeld等(1976)报告3例排泄性尿系造影时断层摄片容易误诊为厚壁肾囊肿或肾周囊肿的胰腺假性囊肿，并详细分析了产生此种现象的各方面原因。而且该作者还提示，在滴注法排泄性尿系造影断层摄片时见到厚壁囊性空腔，除考虑坏死性肾上腺类瘤、感染性肾囊肿、肾痈及肾周围脓肿外，还应考虑到胰腺假性囊肿。Heckman等(1975)著文报告了胰腺假性囊肿表现类似于肾周围脓肿。

第三节 胰腺假性囊肿对肾脏的犯及

胰腺假性囊肿可以直接侵犯肾脏及输尿管，产生症状及X线表现，宛如原发性尿系病变一样。在肾的不典型的非血管性病变及腹部包块伴存肾疾患征象的区别诊断中应考虑胰腺假性囊肿的可能性。Atkinson等(1973)报告4例病人，有3例为胰腺假性囊肿侵犯肾脏，排泄性尿系造影表现为肾内病变，其中2例肾动脉造影也认为属肾脏病变；1例为胰腺假性囊肿引起输尿管移位，而类似巨大的腹膜后包块。

Rosenquist(1973)报告胰腺假性囊肿的不寻常的表现，其中1例表现为影响左肾下极的腹内包块，1例呈现为骶前包块。此外，Gorder和Stargarder

(1969)还报告了胰腺假性囊肿X线表现酷似肾内包块的病例。

第四节　胰腺假性囊肿的自发性内引流

胰腺假性囊肿的自发性破裂是常见的并发症，大约出现于5%的病人，其中一半引流直接进入腹腔，立刻发生休克与腹膜炎，死亡率甚高，文献报告约为50%~70%。但如能迅速诊断，进行急症手术，大部分病人可因此获救。另外一半病人破裂引流进入胃肠道，导致症状和体征的暂时或持久的缓解。

Cosio和Onstad(1972)统计以往报告指出，胰腺假性囊肿的发生率大约为住院病人的1/22 000，而仅有47例胰腺假性囊肿破裂的报告。该作者报告1例极其少见的分别内引流到十二指肠和结肠的病例，女性54岁，因呕吐与腹泻入院，发现大的感染性胰腺假性囊肿，手术前钡灌肠不仅充盈结肠，还途经瘘道抵假性囊肿，又到达小肠。手术见巨大假性囊肿充满腹膜后间隙、胰区及小网膜囊，并延伸向下抵达盆腔，二瘘管分别位于中段降结肠、十二指肠与假性囊肿之间，胃及空回肠如常。

Guyer和Amin等(1970)报告2例胰腺假性囊肿自发破裂入胃者，Leopold等(1972)报告假性囊肿引流入十二指肠病例。Clements等(1976)报告自发性内引流6例均经X线检查证实，皆有胰腺炎的病史，3例在X线检查前未疑及假性囊肿，其他3例在内引流前2~26日扪到腹部包块。1例引流到胃，3例到十二指肠，1例到食管，1例引流到左半结肠。该作者认为，胰腺假性囊肿自发内引流到胃肠道起初是有益的，但常可合并胃肠道出血，感染也可随自发引流扩散至结肠，则对病人不利。

Sugawa等(1977)报告经ERCP发现的4例胰腺假性囊肿内引流到胃的病例。通过内窥镜向主胰管注射对比剂时清楚显示囊肿与胃的交通，从而有助于手术途经的设计。胰腺假性囊肿自发内引流入胃肠道可能导致囊肿消退，但并不意味着手术可以避免，因为它只是暂时性的缓解。

第五节　胰腺假性囊肿

患者，女，53岁。

病理检查：胰腺囊肿壁手术送检标本：胰腺囊肿壁为粉红色组织2枚，总体积0.3cm×0.3cm×0.2cm。病理诊断：胰腺囊肿壁手术送检标本：为纤维组织构成的囊壁样组织，局部区小血管增生，并有淋巴细胞及中性粒细胞浸润，符合囊壁组织。胰腺囊肿壁切除标本：灰褐色不规则组织2块，总体积2.5cm×2cm×0.4cm，切面灰褐质中。符合胰腺假性囊肿。注：另见少量小肠组织(图20-12-1)。

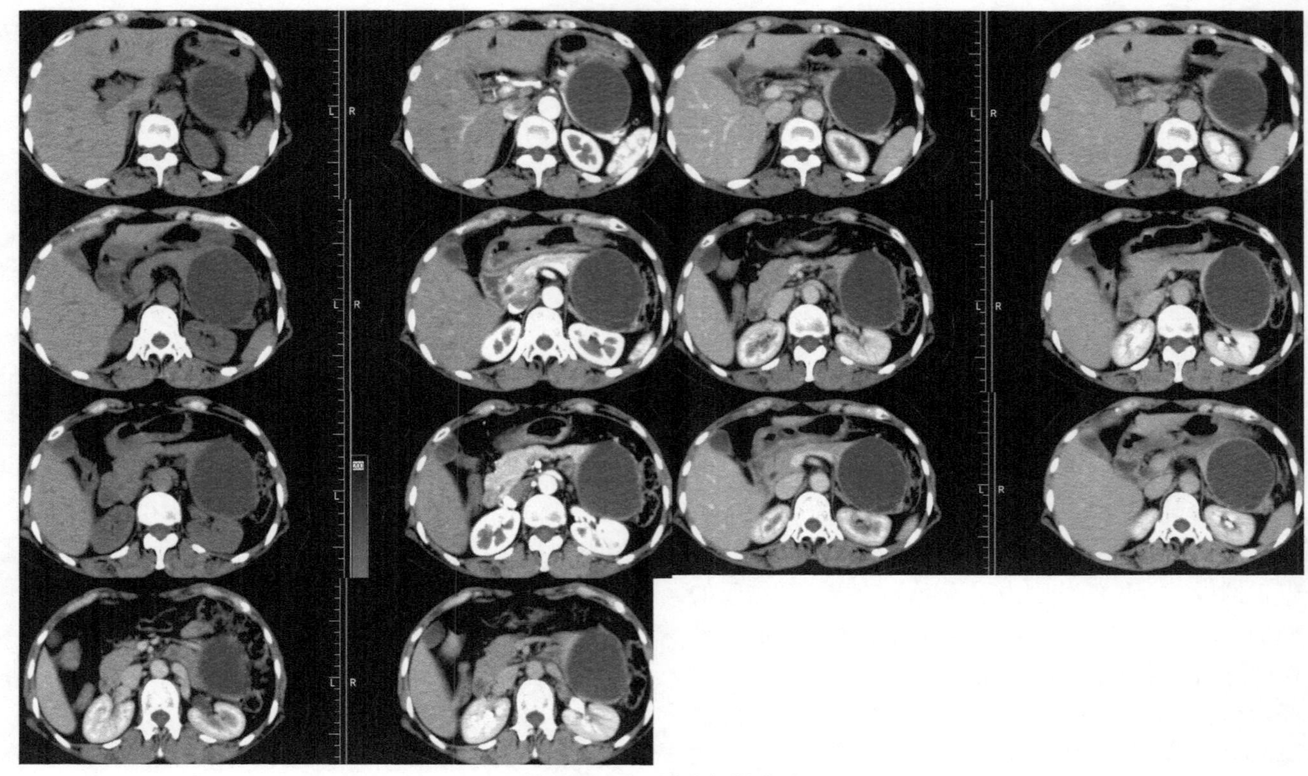

图 20-12-1 胰腺假性囊肿

第六节 其他少见部位的胰腺假性囊肿

Bellon 等(1979)报告十二指肠壁内的胰腺假性囊肿。这些假性囊肿可能是壁内、壁外的压迫性病变，它可有多发性的部位，甚至遍及胃肠道。在严重的胃肠道的外在性压迫或壁内病变区别诊断时，需要考虑此类假性囊肿。胃肠道它处的壁内的胰腺假性囊肿报告甚少，Shockman 和 Marasco (1967)指出它可出现于结肠，Radke 和 Bell(1966)报告 1 例胃壁内的假性囊肿。侵犯十二指肠者，最常见于第二段肠壁外侧或后外侧，内后侧较少。

Warchaw 等(1972)与 Rmaer 等(1974)分别撰文讨论位于脾内的胰腺假性囊肿，且指出它可以成为脾肿大的一个原因。

第七节 胰腺假性囊肿的并发症

一支动脉为假性囊肿侵蚀是少见而危险的并发症，血管造影发现者更少。如果胰腺假性囊肿与胰管相交通，则有可能有相当的出血进入胃肠道。L'Hermine 等(1971)报告 8 例病人，一个特征性的征象是胰腺内坏死空腔内的对比剂池，且与动脉交通，一般见于腹腔动脉注射对比剂后 2 秒或 3 秒的照片。其中 6 例有 2 例犯及胃十二指肠动脉，4 例犯及脾动脉，仅见 1 例为主要动脉分支显影中断。

胰腺假性囊肿和假性动脉瘤的紧急出血是胰腺炎之最迅速致命的并发症。Stabile 等(1983)报告 8 例，皆为急性胃肠道出血，2 例伴存腹腔内出血。术前内脏的血管造影准确地确定了出血的部位，大大有利于手术计划的设计。急症剖腹与动脉结扎施行于 7 例，1 例血管栓塞处理成功。此组死亡率为 12.5%，比文献报告 123 例一组的 37% 要低。

第八节　胰腺假性囊肿与左肾

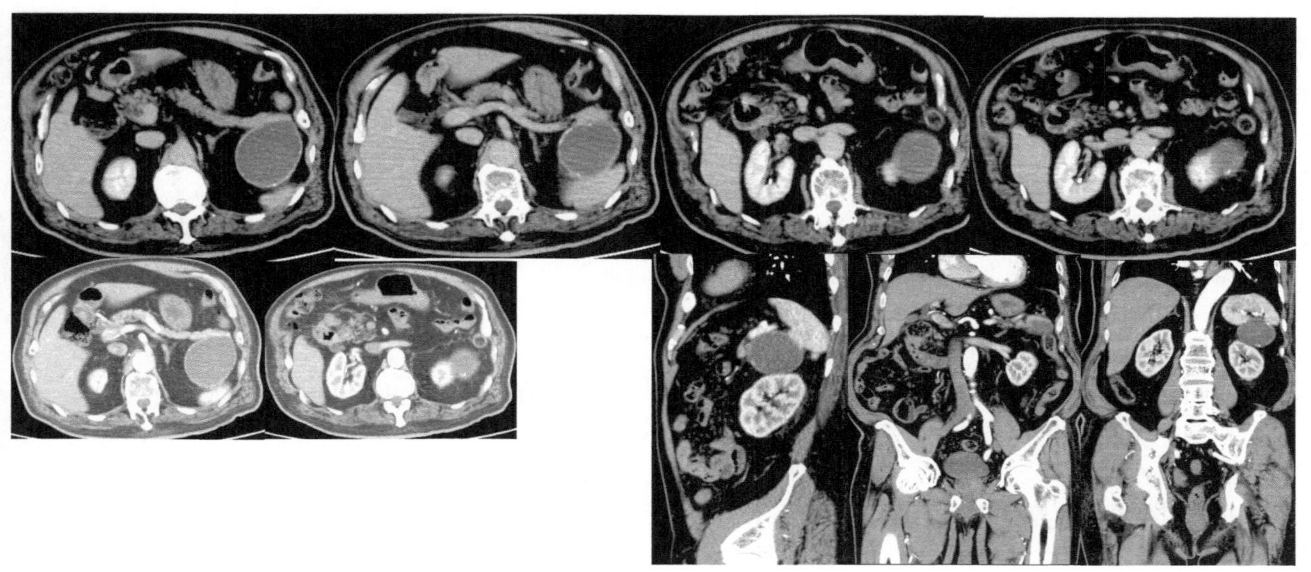

图 20-12-2　胰腺假性囊肿与左肾

患者，男，74 岁。

手术病理证实：胰腺假性囊肿。横断图像与肾分不开，冠状面和矢状面重建图像见其与左肾可以分开，可能只累及左肾筋膜。手术证实这个判断（图 20-12-2）。

第九节　胰腺假性囊肿蛋壳状钙化

我们曾发现 1 例中腹部钙化，X 线检查腹部正位片上，见此完整的蛋壳状钙化重叠于第 2 腰椎体左侧缘，侧位片见其位于脊柱前方，手术病理见其为一完整的薄壳鸡蛋状团块，适位于胰腺体部内，为胰腺假性囊肿蛋壳状钙化。

第十节　不典型部位胰腺假性囊肿与 CT

胰腺假性囊肿为胰腺炎的并发症，发生于急性胰腺炎者占 2%~3%，发生于慢性胰腺炎者达 30%，胰腺假性囊肿内为封闭的含淀粉酶和脂肪酶的液体，并非由上皮包被，而是由一纤维囊包裹。

胰腺假性囊肿无自发回复倾向，总保持与胰管的交通。假性囊肿常发生于胰内或胰腺周围，重症胰腺炎者，假性囊肿还可由腹膜后蔓延至盆腔及肠系膜根部或结肠系膜，非典型部位胰腺假性囊肿（如发生在纵隔、脾脏等处）较少见。

可将假性囊肿的部位分为四类：胰腺内，胰腺周围紧邻器官内，胰腺内和胰腺周围混合型，非典型部位（肝内、纵隔内等）。

对假性囊肿，可测量其横径及前后径，定出大小，选择兴趣区测量其密度。有作者在 236 例胰腺炎病人中，CT 发现 85 例有假性囊肿，占 36%，其中 87 例急性胰腺炎内有 18 例（21%），149 例慢性胰腺炎中有 67 例（45%）。85 例假性囊肿中，孤立性囊肿 34 例（40%），多发性囊肿 51 例（60%）。

19 例假性囊肿发生在不寻常部位，即非典型假性囊肿，位于肝、脾、胃壁及纵隔内。在肠系膜根部或结肠系膜处的假性囊肿未计入非典型组。

非典型假性囊肿出现于一处者有 14 例，出现在多处者有 5 例，16 例病人除了非典型部位假性囊肿外，同时还有胰内或胰周假性囊肿。非典型部位假性囊肿平均 CT 值为 16.4HU（±12.6），其余 66 例胰内和胰周假性囊肿的 CT 值为 14.7HU（±10.9），密度无明显差异。19 例非典型部位假性囊肿中，男性 16 例，女性 3 例。所有非典型部位假性囊肿通过囊液的穿刺抽吸，放置引流管或手术采样证实。

Luetmer 等的 56 例慢性胰腺炎病人中发现有 30%（17 例）患假性囊肿，值得注意的是为数较多的假性囊肿（21%）发生于急性胰腺炎者，而文献中报道急性胰腺炎发生假性囊肿的仅有 2%~3%

按假性囊肿的大小、部位，可发生疼痛、出血、破裂、脓肿等并发症。

根据对炎性胰液蔓延并最终形成假性囊肿的引流途径的分析，对非典型部位假性囊肿的诊断较为容易。

上腹部韧带是重要的引流途径，首先是胃肝韧带和肝十二指肠韧带，其次是脾肾韧带和胃脾韧带。这些韧带是腹膜后组织的皱折，并包含动脉，静脉，淋巴管和脂肪组织。胰腺炎的炎性液体可流入韧带的夹层中，并经此途径抵达腹膜被覆的某一器官。

肝十二指肠韧带和胃肝韧带与肝脏相联系，经此韧带假性囊肿会扩散至肝包膜下；胃肝韧带与腹膜后相连并连接胃小弯与肝脏，向上通往静脉韧带裂隙，向下通往肝门，胃肝韧带的腹膜下组织紧密连接于肝脏的格氏鞘中；肝十二指肠韧带位于胃肝韧带的下缘，并将胰腺和肝门广泛连接起来。

在 8 例患肝包膜下假性囊肿的病例中，还发现有 6 例分布于胃肝韧带和肝十二指肠韧带不同大小的假性囊肿。

脾肾韧带将胰尾和脾门连接起来，并与肾动脉远端联系，胰尾脾门相连关系解释了假性囊肿发生于脾脏的问题。胃大弯与脾之间进一步的联系是靠胃脾韧带，此韧带与脾肾韧带的连续性使胰胃相连，故假性囊肿通过此引流途径可以蔓延至胃大弯。

在胃脾韧带的假性囊肿偶尔会被误诊为发生于网膜囊的胰周假性囊肿。当炎性胰液于腹膜后向上，或经食管裂孔、主动脉裂孔，或经横膈的椎前肌间隙扩散至纵隔时，即产生纵隔假性囊肿。

非典型部位胰腺假性囊肿的鉴别诊断，包括包裹性腹腔积液、脓肿、棘球蚴囊、坏死的转移肿瘤和淋巴瘤、胆管囊肿。在纵隔部位需与支气管源性囊肿区别。

第十一节　误诊为胰腺假性囊肿的一些情况

1. 超声诊断胰腺假性囊肿的陷阱　超声检查是一种公认的诊断胰腺假性囊肿的手段。Miller 等（1978）讨论了在超声诊断中容易与胰腺假性囊肿混淆的病变，包括：胆囊破裂胆汁漏出，肝包虫囊肿、胰腺脓肿、霉菌性动脉瘤、胰腺囊腺瘤、脾囊肿、平滑肌肉瘤和胃底液体等。

2. 胰管囊状扩张误为假性囊肿　Kuligowska 等（1981）指出，在超声检查时发现整个胰腺有多发性囊状区，考虑为多发性分散的假性囊肿。再作 ERCP，却发现实际上是胰管的广泛的囊状扩张。

3. 左肾静脉曲张伪似胰腺假性囊肿　超声检查左肾前出现一低回声包块时，有几种常见病因应予考虑：肾和胰的低回声新生物、胰尾的假性囊肿、肾上腺包块、胃肠内液体；另外的可能性包括：胰周围淋巴结、小网膜囊或腹膜后脓肿及血肿、贮尿囊肿、局限性腹腔内液体积聚或脾动脉的动脉瘤。静脉结构的异常通常不考虑在区别诊断中。

Spira 等（1982）报告 1 例门静脉高压病人血液分流，导致左肾静脉血流增加及静脉曲张，呈现为低回声包块，伪似胰腺假性褒肿。

第十二节　胰腺假性囊肿

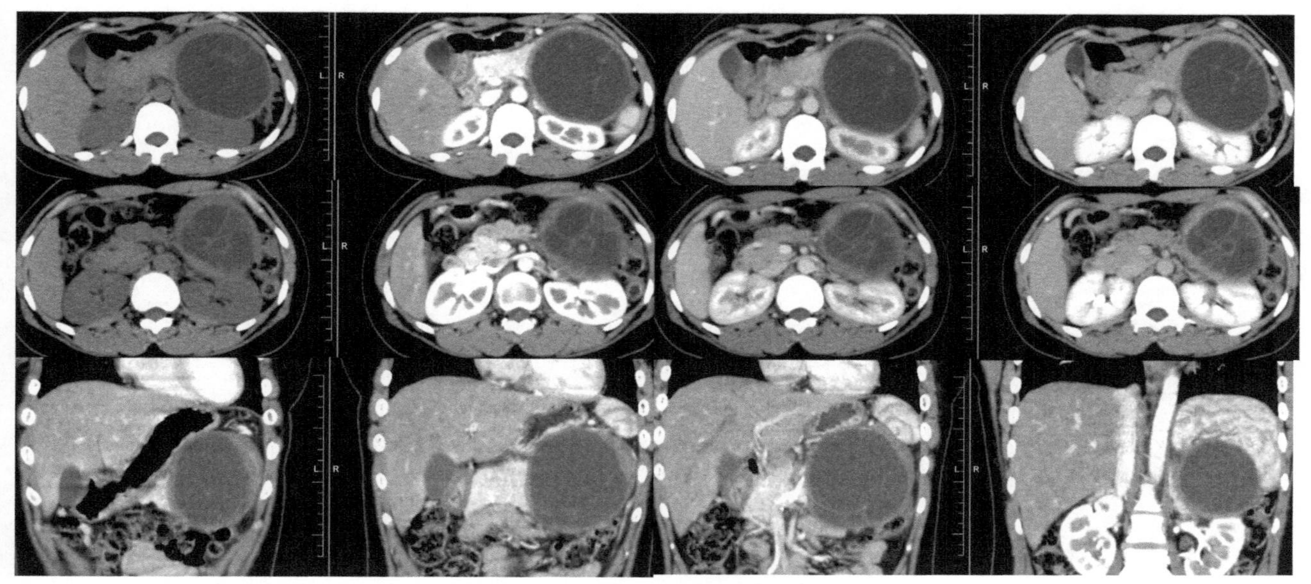

图 20-12-3　胰腺假性囊肿

患者,女,22 岁。

病理检查:冰冻病理:胰腺囊肿壁切除标本:鲜红色不规则组织一块,体积 1.5cm × 1cm × 0.5cm,切面灰白,质中。冰冻病理诊断:(胰腺囊肿壁)经冰冻标本深切,纤维及胶原组织中局灶区见少量胰腺腺体组织伴间质慢性炎细胞浸润,符合良性(囊壁)病变。

常规病理:胰腺囊肿壁切除标本:灰褐色不规则组织一块,体积 2cm × 1.5cm × 0.6cm,切面灰白,质中。常规病理诊断:胰腺囊肿壁切除标本:胰腺囊肿壁内纤维组织增生,其中散在少量腺泡和导管,少量慢性炎细胞浸润,囊壁无上皮衬覆,结合临床,符合胰腺假性囊肿(图 20-12-3)。

第十三节　胰腺假性囊肿的动态变化

在研究影像诊断的误诊时,经常都应想到病情的动态学变化,病变与病情一样,绝非一成不变,而是每时每刻都在变化,用超声观察胰腺假性囊肿就是生动例证。

Sarti(1977)报告三例胰腺假性囊肿,采用超声连续追踪观察,发现超过以往一般人认为的动态性变化:一个大的假性囊肿竟在 6 天内形成,而另外二例假性囊肿在观察期间均自发性消退干净。此发现启示人们,对胰腺假性囊肿是否需手术干预,以及手术的时间皆需重新考虑。

第十三章　胰腺导管内乳头状黏液性肿瘤

第一节　MSCT及MRI对胰腺导管内乳头状黏液性肿瘤的诊断

胰腺导管内乳头状黏液性肿瘤，是一种好发于老年男性的胰腺囊性肿瘤，表现为低侵袭性、淋巴结转移率小和复发率低等特点，临床预后良好，因其外科治疗方法与胰腺癌明显不同，故导管内乳头状黏液性肿瘤的正确诊断对临床手术术式的选择具有重要意义。

导管内乳头状黏液性肿瘤是一种发生在主胰管及大的分支胰管内乳头状生长的黏液样肿瘤，大约占胰腺外分泌性肿瘤的1%~2%，胰腺囊性肿瘤的12%。

Ohhashi等(1982)首次报道了4例胰腺产黏液腺癌。随后陆续有一些报道，该肿瘤曾有不同的命名，如产黏液癌、高分泌黏液癌、导管内乳头状肿瘤、导管高分泌黏液肿瘤、导管内癌、导管产黏液肿瘤、导管扩张型黏液性囊腺瘤和囊腺癌、胰腺导管内乳头状黏液性肿瘤。

WHO(1996)将具有向性索基质分化倾向伴有卵巢样间质的囊性肿瘤定义为黏液性囊性肿瘤，具有向胃和肠上皮分化倾向由黏液产生性上皮乳头状增殖形成的肿瘤定义为胰管内乳头状黏液性肿瘤。

病理学：根据WHO(2000)有关导管内乳头状黏液性肿瘤分类标准，将其分为腺瘤、交界性肿瘤、原位癌及腺癌4种病理类型，并将原位癌和腺癌归为恶性。

组织学上导管内乳头状黏液性肿瘤是扩张的导管衬覆高柱状黏液性上皮，部分区域由立方或柱状上皮细胞围绕一纤维血管轴心形成乳头结构。肿瘤内的不同区域细胞均呈异型性。一组11例中，腺瘤6例，交界性肿瘤4例，腺癌1例。

临床表现：该肿瘤好发于老年男性，男女比例为1.4∶1。发病年龄60~70岁，平均63~66岁。该组11例中，男性多于女性(9∶2)，平均年龄71.8岁，与文献相比，该组患者男明显多于女，可能为样本量少所致。

导管内乳头状黏液性肿瘤具有生长缓慢、低度恶性、淋巴结转移率小和复发率低及极少侵犯周围组织的特点。具有较高的手术切除性，临床预后较好。其临床症状和体征取决于导管扩张的程度和产生黏液的量。临床表现多为腹痛，体重下降，部分患者表现为呕吐及腹泻、黄疸等，部分无明显症状。

该组1例主胰管型导管内乳头状黏液性肿瘤患者，胰管扩张明显，症状相对较明显，临床出现胰腺炎症状。6例出现上腹部不适，食欲下降特征，4例患者为体检或偶然发现。

影像学研究：影像学分型：根据肿瘤的起源及影像学表现不同，通常把导管内乳头状黏液性肿瘤分为3种类型：主胰管型，主胰管扩张，而肿瘤主要存在于主胰管；分支胰管型，分支胰管扩张而肿瘤不存在于主胰管；混合型，肿瘤既存在于主胰管又存在于分支胰管。

MSCT常规横轴位可显示囊性病变及胰管扩张程度。高分辨率薄层图像可观察胰腺导管扩张、胰腺囊性病变关系和腔内壁结节等细微的病理改变，并清楚显示肿瘤的范围且准确判断其大小，CT检查还可显示十二指肠乳头有无增大，也可观察并发胰腺炎时所导致胰周围脂肪间隙模糊。图像后处理技术中曲面重建可以将胰管全程显示在1帧图像中，可清晰展示胰管情况及囊性病变与主胰管间的交通，几乎可与MRCP相媲美，因此曲面重建对导管内乳头状黏液性肿瘤诊断及分型具有重要帮助。增强扫描可显示囊性病变、壁结节、软组织肿块强化程度及邻近关系。该组9例采用MSCT扫描，曲面重建可清晰显示胰管扩张程度、范围、囊性病变和主胰管关系，以及腔内壁结节。该组中2例发生在胰头部的分支胰管型导管内乳头状黏液性肿瘤表现为胰头多房囊性病变，内分隔厚薄不均，主胰管扩张不明显，显示与主胰管关系不明确，术前误诊为胰腺囊腺瘤。

MSCT对于判断导管内乳头状黏液性肿瘤良、恶性方面，文献报道当病灶直径>3 cm、扩张胰管的附壁结节较多或大、主胰管扩张>10 mm、胆总管扩张、胰周淋巴结肿大和邻近血管受侵犯，以及患者出现胆系梗阻表现，提示恶变，因此导管内乳头状黏液性肿瘤术前正确诊断及判断良、恶性对临床具有重要意义。该组1例主胰管弥漫性串珠样扩张，直径约1.8 cm，内伴壁结节，术后病理诊断为腺癌。

MRI具有较高的软组织分辨率，可清晰显示囊性病变形态、内部成分及壁结节，对细小分隔及囊性病变的显示优于CT。

MRCP能更好地显示导管内乳头状黏液性肿瘤的发病部位、主胰管及分支胰管迂曲扩张程度及数量、囊性肿瘤内部结构（如分隔和壁结节的存在），该组作者认为与曲面重建相比，MRCP还可清晰显示主胰管和囊性病灶的沟通，通过三维旋转，可多角度观察胰管扩张程度及囊性病变之间的关系，更有利于导管内乳头状黏液性肿瘤的诊断。

另外，MRCP相对ERCP快速、简便、无创、可重复性好，因不受导管内稠厚黏液的影响，MRCP显示囊状扩张的分支胰管的数目可明显多于ERCP，测量扩张管腔的大小也更真实可靠。对胰管远端的显示明显优于ERCP。

鉴别诊断：胰腺囊腺瘤：胰腺囊腺瘤好发于老年女性，表现胰腺单发或多发的囊性病变，囊性病变可单房或多房，也可伴壁结节，并有强化，但囊性病变不与胰管相通，不伴胰管扩张。

胰腺假性囊肿：胰腺假性囊肿常为胰腺炎或胰腺外伤后所致，表现为单房囊性病变，内密度均匀或不均匀（伴有出血或坏死时），内壁光滑，壁可略增厚，常伴周围脂肪间隙模糊，结合病史不难诊断。

实性假乳头状瘤：实性假乳头状瘤好发于年轻女性，单发或多发囊实性肿块，边缘清楚，包膜完整，增强后呈渐进性强化，临床症状不明显。

慢性胰腺炎：在慢性胰腺炎，主胰管扩张一般较局限，常见于年轻患者，可见到胰管结石或钙化和假性囊肿的形成，胰腺周围脂肪间隙模糊，部分导管内乳头状黏液性肿瘤患者可同时合并慢性胰腺炎，但观察到十二指肠乳头有黏液流出及主胰管内肿瘤组织后可基本排除胰腺炎。

第二节　胰腺导管内良、恶性黏蛋白性肿瘤的MRCP鉴别诊断

胰腺导管内黏蛋白性肿瘤的特点为胰管及胰腺间质内大量黏蛋白形成并潴留，黏蛋白液流动致十二指肠乳头扩张。病理学包括良性、恶性多种改变。影像学鉴别其良恶性对选择适当的治疗方式尤为重要。

回顾MRCP表现，对主胰管型肿瘤，观察主胰管扩张最大径值、部位、扩张范围、管腔内充盈缺损。对胰管分支型肿瘤，分析其囊性病变的最大直径、部位、囊腔内充盈缺损、相应的主胰管扩张情况。主胰管直径大于5mm为扩张。并就MRCP充盈缺损与病理所见对照研究。该项研究结果显示，主胰管型中4例良性肿瘤主胰管最大直径10~12mm，平均11mm，6例恶性肿瘤主胰管最大直径15~30mm，平均20mm，有统计学差异（P<0.05）。良性肿瘤组主胰管扩张最大直径位于胰头2例，胰体、尾各1例，恶性肿瘤组位于胰头、体各3例，良恶性之间无差异。所有病例主胰管扩张最大径值部位与肿瘤主体部位一致。良性肿瘤组主胰管扩张为1~2节段性扩张，恶性肿瘤组为弥漫性扩张。1例良性肿瘤MRCP未见充盈缺损；而显微镜检查示主胰管腔内小壁结节，直径3mm（假阴性1例）。恶性肿瘤组3例充盈缺损直径大于10mm，并经手术病理证实；1例充盈缺损小于5mm，而切除标本的显微镜检查未见主胰管腔内壁结节（假阳性1例），恶性组无假阴性病例。

胰管分支型中良性肿瘤（17个），囊性病变最大径值10~45mm，平均24mm；恶性肿瘤组（7个）最大径值20~55mm，平均35mm，二者之间有统计学差异，但数值交叉较多。良性肿瘤组位于胰头11例，胰体5例，胰尾1例，恶性肿瘤组胰头5例，胰体2例，良恶性之间无差异。良性肿瘤组MRCP未见充盈缺损，与切除标本显微镜检查结果一致，恶性肿

瘤组 3 例可见 MRCP 上的充盈缺损,病理标本上可见壁结节。良性肿瘤均无主胰管扩张,恶性肿瘤中除 1 例外均有相应主胰管轻度扩张,5~10mm 不等。

Irie 等(2000)认为，MRCP 是鉴别胰管内黏蛋白性肿瘤良恶性的有效手段，MRCP 见到主胰管腔内或囊内充盈缺损提示恶性可能,主胰管型肿瘤如主胰管弥漫性扩张或直径超过 15mm,胰管分支型肿瘤伴有主胰管扩张,多为恶性肿瘤表现。

第十四章　胰腺实性假乳头状瘤和胰腺实性假乳头状癌

第一节　胰腺实性假乳头状瘤肝转移

胰腺实性假乳头状瘤约占胰腺原发肿瘤的0.17%~2.50%，年轻女性多见。WHO(2004)肿瘤组织学分类将其统一命名为实性假乳头状瘤，定义为由形态比较一致的细胞形成的实性巢状和假乳头结构的上皮性肿瘤，常伴出血及囊性变，通常为良性，偶尔可为恶性。

免疫组化研究发现实性假乳头状瘤在胰腺内、外分泌和局灶性上皮均有表达，提示实性假乳头状瘤可能起源于胰腺胚胎多能干细胞。实性假乳头状瘤病理成分不同，影像学表现亦不同。肿瘤由实性区、假乳头区及二者的过渡区组成。

实性区由较为一致的瘤细胞构成，呈片块状或巢状排列，影像学表现为相对均匀的实性成分，实性区亦可因退变、坏死出现微囊，表现为实性成分中的小囊变灶；假乳头区肿瘤细胞排列成片状、索条状或围绕血管及坏死区呈放射状、假乳头状排列，为实性假乳头状瘤的重要病理学特征，影像学表现为不均匀的囊实性区；二者间的过渡区细胞成分相对较少，肿瘤组织围绕血管形成假菊形团，同时离血管较远的区域易发生坏死，表现为完全的囊性区。

实性假乳头状瘤具有延迟强化的特点，即实性成分于动脉期、门脉期、延迟期逐渐强化，这是因为实性区与假乳头区之间的过渡区形成假菊形团，相对较少的肿瘤细胞呈网状排列并形成血窦，因此影像学上表现出类似海绵状血管瘤延迟强化的特点，但三期强化程度均低于正常胰腺实质，囊性成分始终无强化。病灶内间隔的强化也体现出延迟强化的特点，且强化程度多高于肿瘤实性部分，仅在动脉期强化程度低于胰腺实质。一例肝脏转移病灶因与实性假乳头状瘤的组织同源，故在影像上与胰腺原发病灶表现一致。

实性假乳头状瘤是一种具有低度恶性倾向的肿瘤，其生物学行为相对良好，复发和转移不常见。文献报道约15%的患者出现肝转移和腹膜转移，总体5年生存率约95%，发生转移的患者行转移灶切除及术后复发患者再次行手术切除均可取得较好的效果。

附：具体病例资料：患者，女，14岁，右上腹不适半年，B超示肝右叶多发囊实性混合回声病灶，提示肝脏占位病变；血常规、肝、肾功能、电解质、肿瘤标记物甲胎蛋白、癌胚抗原、CA19-9均未见异常。

CT检查：CT平扫示肝右叶多发囊实性占位病灶，边界光滑，实性成分沿囊壁呈壁结节状散在分布，囊内可见纤细分隔；增强扫描动脉期、门脉期、延迟期示囊壁、实性壁结节及纤细分隔呈持续不均匀强化。CT检查后补充询问病史，患者4年前曾行胰腺体尾部实性假乳头状瘤切除术，考虑为转移性病灶。遂行右半肝切除术，术中所见：肝脏表面光滑，肝右叶可见2个巨大囊性占位，大小约10cm×10cm，内囊液为暗红色，囊壁上有水泡样突起，左肝未见异常。病理肉眼及光镜所见：右半肝切面呈囊实性，可见坏死，瘤组织呈巢团状排列，浸润性生长，细胞形态较一致。病理诊断：(右半肝)恶性肿瘤。免疫组化诊断：(右肝)胰腺实性假乳头状肿瘤肝转移。

第二节　胰腺实性假乳头状瘤

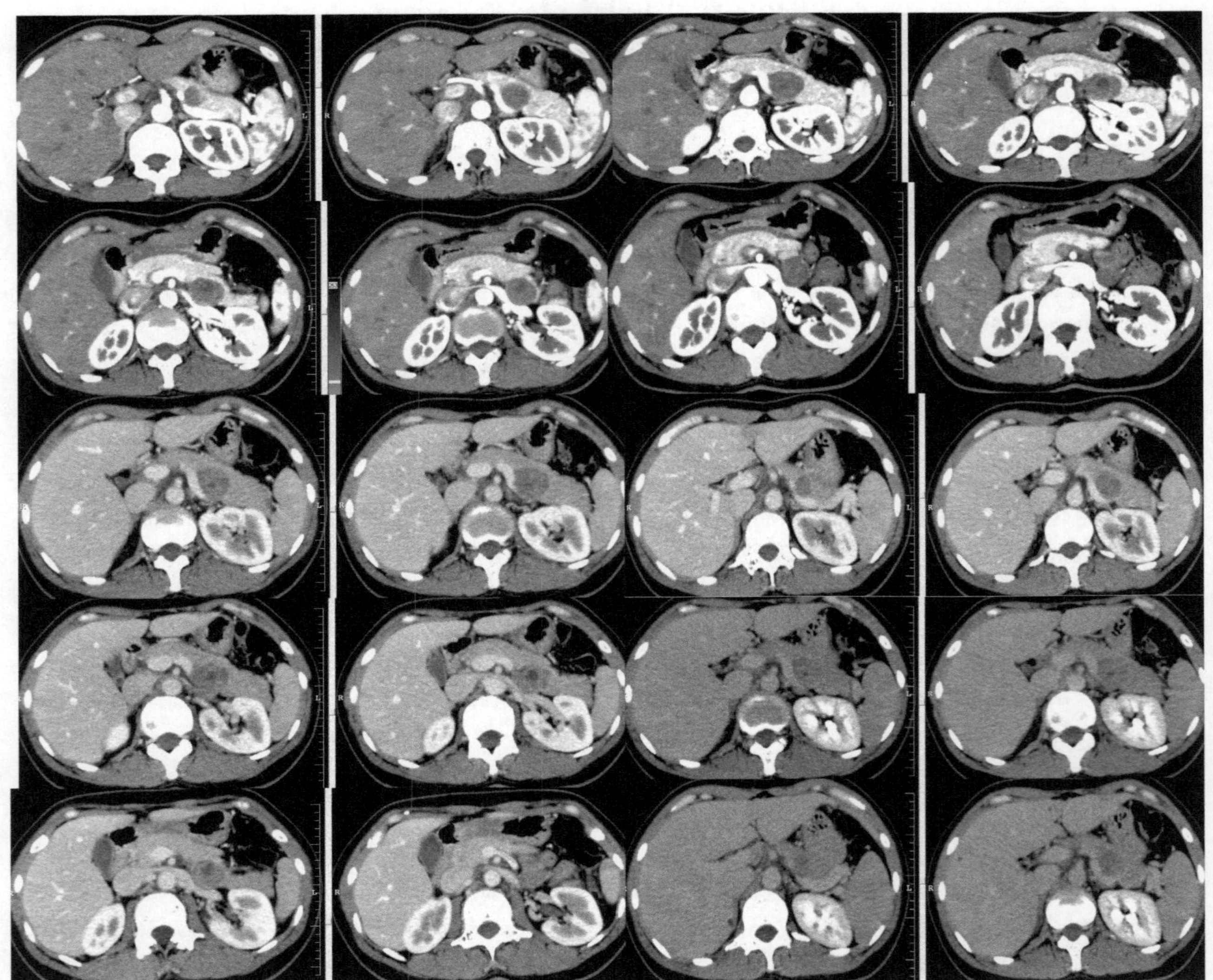

图 20-14-1　胰腺实性假乳头状瘤

患者,女,36 岁。体检发现胰腺占位 10 天入院。

手术所病理检查:胰体尾肿物与脾切除标本:切除胰腺大小 10cm×4.5cm×3cm,胰体部见一结节,大小 3cm×3cm,结节切面灰红,质软,与周围界限尚清,其余切面灰红,质软。脾大小 10cm× 4.7cm×3.5cm,切面暗红,质软,未见明显异常。常规病理诊断:胰体尾肿物与脾切除标本:镜下可见形态较一致的肿瘤细胞呈实性排列,初步考虑为胰腺癌,肿瘤分类待做免疫组化检测进一步证实。脾脏未见癌组织累及。免疫组化诊断:胰体尾肿物与脾切除标本:胰腺实性假乳头状瘤,切缘阴性,脾脏未累及(图 20-14-1)。

第三节　误诊病例简介:胰腺乳头状囊性肿瘤

详见本书 本卷 本篇 第二十章 第二节 误诊病例简介:胰腺乳头状囊性肿瘤。

第四节　胰腺实性假乳头状肿瘤

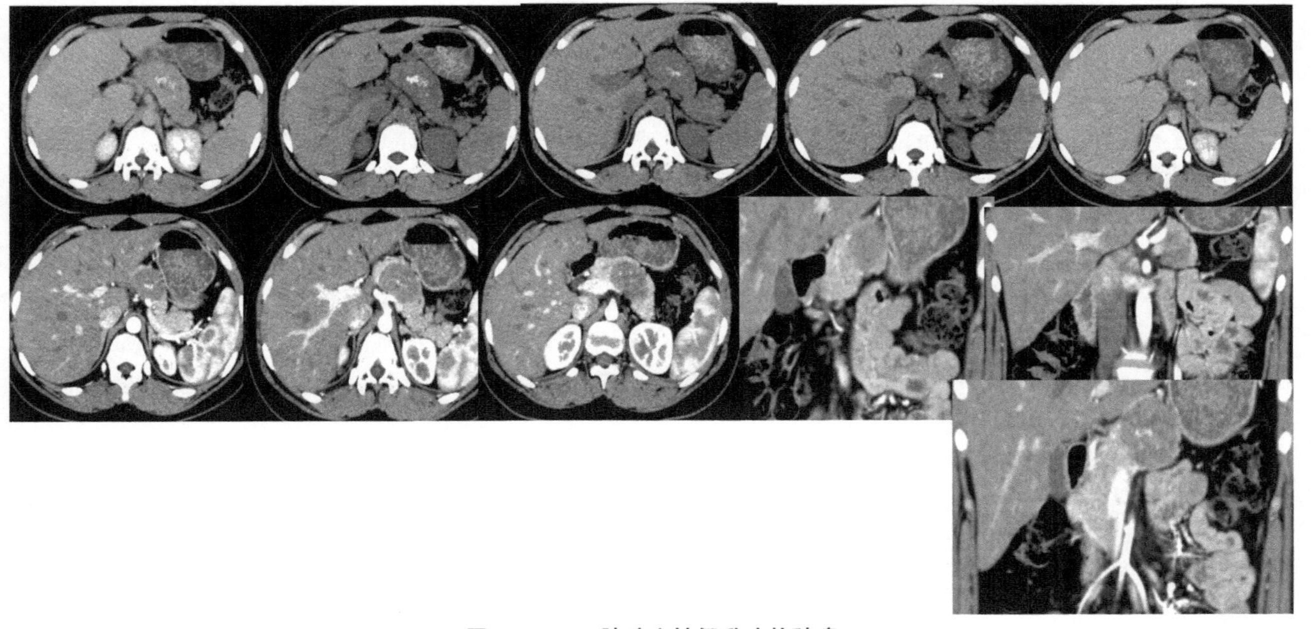

图 20-14-2　胰腺实性假乳头状肿瘤

患者，女，15 岁，因体检发现胰腺占位 20 天入院。

病理检查：冰冻病理诊断：胰腺肿物及脾脏切除标本：肿物大小为 5cm × 4.5cm × 4.5cm，肿瘤未见包膜，肿瘤细胞胞浆丰富，形态较温和，伴轻度核异型，倾向低度恶性肿瘤（如实性假乳头状肿瘤或神经内分泌肿瘤），确诊待常规及免疫组化。胰腺切缘、胰尾及脾脏均未见肿瘤累及。免疫组化诊断：胰腺肿物及脾脏切除标本：结合免疫组化检测结果，符合胰腺实性假乳头状肿瘤（SPN）（图 20-14-2）。

第五节　胰腺实性假乳头状瘤误诊分析

胰腺实性假乳头状瘤是一类少见、组织发生未定、具有低度恶性潜能的胰腺肿瘤，发病率约占胰腺肿瘤的 1%~3%。由 Frantz（1959）首先报道，曾有多种名称，诸如：实性乳头状肿瘤、乳头状囊腺瘤、实性囊性乳头状上皮肿瘤、Frantz 瘤等，WHO（2000）国际肿瘤组织学分类最终将其统一命名为胰腺实性假乳头状瘤，分类为生物行为未定或交界性恶性潜能肿瘤。该病术前诊断准确率不足 50%。

组织起源及发病机制：胰腺实性假乳头状瘤的组织起源及发病机制目前尚不清楚。WHO（2000）胰腺肿瘤分类中将其列为胰腺外分泌肿瘤，但免疫组织化学及超微结构显示，该肿瘤有胰腺外分泌、内分泌及上皮表达的多向分化表型，提示肿瘤可能起源于多潜能干细胞，其多向分化的表现可能是多潜能干细胞沿不同方向或不同阶段分化的结果。

胰腺实性假乳头状瘤好发于年轻女性，10 岁以下儿童及 50 岁以上发病者较为少见，一组 8 例患者均为女性，平均年龄 29.8 岁，与国内外文献报道基本一致。国内 1 组 293 例胰腺实性假乳头状瘤的研究报道该病男女发病比例为 1∶8.2，表明本病具有明显的性别分布趋势，但该组研究 ER 表达阳性率仅为 25%（2/8），并未发现雌激素受体与肿瘤发生密切有关。

根据国内外文献报道，雌激素可分为Ⅰ型和Ⅱ型，相应受体亦分为 α、β 亚型。Carbone 等（1989）发现 ER 表达阴性可能与免疫组化染色针对 ERα

有关。Morales 等(2003)对 7 例胰腺实性假乳头状瘤患者行 ERα、ERβ 免疫组化染色,结果显示阳性例数分别 2 例和 6 例,从而解释了胰腺实性假乳头状瘤明显女性多发,但 ER 表达多为阴性的现象。

该组病例的 CT、MRI 表现显示胰腺实性假乳头状瘤具有一定的影像学特征。胰腺实性假乳头状瘤多为单发,肿瘤体积较大,好发部位无明显特异性。该组 8 例病变均为单发肿块,胰头、胰体、胰尾均有,病变直径平均值约 6.3 cm,且最大层面主体均位于胰腺轮廓之外,这点与胰腺其他肿瘤,如胰腺癌、胰腺内分泌肿瘤的表现差异较大,是一个较为重要的鉴别点。但也正因为病变主体位于胰腺之外,该组病例术前有 2 例误诊为起源于胰腺组织之外的肿瘤,1 例诊断为异位嗜铬细胞瘤,1 例诊断为血管肉瘤。因此,术前诊断该病时,一定要仔细分析病变与胰腺的定位关系,减少误诊。

该组病例 6 例 CT 表现边界清晰,2 例因部分肿瘤细胞增生活跃,呈浸润性生长,边界欠清晰;3 例 MRI 均显示低信号包膜影,与病理对照 8 例病变均有完整或不完整的包膜。CT 虽显示病变边界清楚,但不能清晰显示包膜结构,而 MRI 显示病变的包膜明显优于 CT 检查,这对鉴别诊断胰腺肿瘤具有重要的意义。

该组 2 例病例包膜不完整,术后病理证实病变伴有周围组织浸润,因此结合文献报道,推测可以将包膜完整与否作为判断肿瘤侵袭性的一个重要依据。

胰腺实性假乳头状瘤通常由不同比例的囊实性成分组成,完全囊性或完全实性罕见,该组病例以囊实性相间例数最多,占 62. 5%(5/8),其次为囊性为主者 37. 5%(3/8),未见完全实性病变。病理上肿瘤内部常常会发生出血、坏死、囊性变、泡沫细胞聚集和胆固醇性肉芽肿形成等,从而造成病变内部成分复杂,CT 及 MRI 表现病变密度或信号不均匀。

囊性部分多靠近肿瘤的中心区域,在 CT 上呈低密度区,病理上为瘤体内充满黄色液体的囊变区或陈旧性出血。但 CT 仅能发现新鲜出血,表现为高于软组织密度、低于钙化密度的高密度区,而陈旧性出血在 CT 上不能与实性成分的软组织密度明显区分,而因为肿瘤内部出血多为慢性出血,CT 较难明确显示。

该组中 1 例病例 CT 显示病变为不均匀低密度,而 MRI 明确显示了肿瘤内部慢性出血改变,同时,MRI 在胆固醇性肉芽肿的显示亦明显优于 CT。许多学者认为肿瘤内出血亦为胰腺实性假乳头状瘤区别于其他胰腺肿瘤的重要特征之一,出血系远离血管周围的肿瘤细胞发生退变所致。胰腺实性假乳头状瘤内尚可见钙化,该组 3 例肿瘤内可见条状或斑点状钙化影。

增强扫描胰腺实性假乳头状瘤呈现“渐进性强化”的特点,实性区血供相对比较丰富,动脉期呈周边或不均匀强化,静脉期和平衡期强化程度逐渐增加,但强化程度低于正常胰腺组织的强化程度。文献报道胰腺实性假乳头状瘤具有延迟强化的特点,即实性成分动脉期、门静脉期、延迟期逐渐强化,这是因为实性与假乳头之间的过渡区形成假菊形团,相对较少的肿瘤细胞呈网状排列,之间形成血窦,因此影像学上表现出延迟强化的特点。一些学者认为该强化方式与海绵状血管瘤相似。

胰腺实性假乳头状瘤的临床表现并无特异性,往往因腹部隐痛不适或体检时发现腹腔肿物而就诊。且由于胰腺实性假乳头状瘤瘤体质地较软,生长缓慢,即使肿瘤位于胰头部,也很少引起胆总管或胰管的扩张,较少出现黄疸症状,这也是该肿瘤的特征性表现之一。该组病例中 3 例肿瘤位于胰头部,仅 1 例伴有胰管轻度扩张,均无胆总管扩张。此特点与胰腺癌截然不同,可作为胰腺实性假乳头状瘤的诊断依据之一。

该组病例中所有患者的血、尿淀粉酶、血糖及肿瘤标记物(CEA、CA19-9、CA125)均在正常范围内,这与一些学者的 293 例胰腺实性假乳头状瘤临床荟萃分析中的研究结果基本一致,除极少数病例血清总胆红素轻度升高外,肝肾功能、血糖、电解质、淀粉酶以及肿瘤标记物(AFP、CEA、CA19-9、CA125、CA242 等)水平均未见明显异常,此特点亦是与胰腺其他肿瘤鉴别诊断的依据之一。

虽然胰腺实性假乳头状瘤的影像学表现具有一定特征,但术前诊断仍有一定难度,误诊率较高,本病误诊主要与以下因素有关:本病是胰腺的少见肿瘤,对其认识不足;胰腺实性假乳头状瘤瘤体偏小且以实性结构为主,囊性表现不明显时,尤其是 CT 对囊实性成分显示不如 MRI,在影像学上易误诊为胰腺癌或其他胰腺无功能性神经内分泌瘤;当肿瘤较大时,可在腹膜后形成巨大占位,致使在影像学上定位困难,较难判断其组织来源;当肿瘤以囊性成分为主时,胰腺实性假乳头状瘤需与胰腺囊腺瘤、胰腺假性囊肿等进行鉴别，仅从影像表现较难鉴别，需要密切结合临床及实验室检查。

该组病例术前误诊率为37.5%，较文献报道的误诊率已有降低，误诊率降低与近年影像技术快速发展和临床上对该病的认识增加有关。

总之，胰腺实性假乳头状瘤是一种好发于年轻女性的低度恶性或具恶性潜能的肿瘤，肿瘤细胞以纤维血管为轴心形成分支状的假乳头结构是其组织病理学特征性改变。本病临床症状较轻，无特异性表现，CT和MRI表现具有一定的特征性，MRI对病变包膜、内部出血、胆固醇结晶等成分的显示优于CT检查。

胰腺实性假乳头状瘤多为良性过程，但具有侵袭性，可局部复发，手术切除是本病的首选治疗，即使复发或转移，手术后患者的生存时间仍较长。

第六节　误诊病例简介：胰头实性假乳头状肿瘤与胰腺假性囊肿

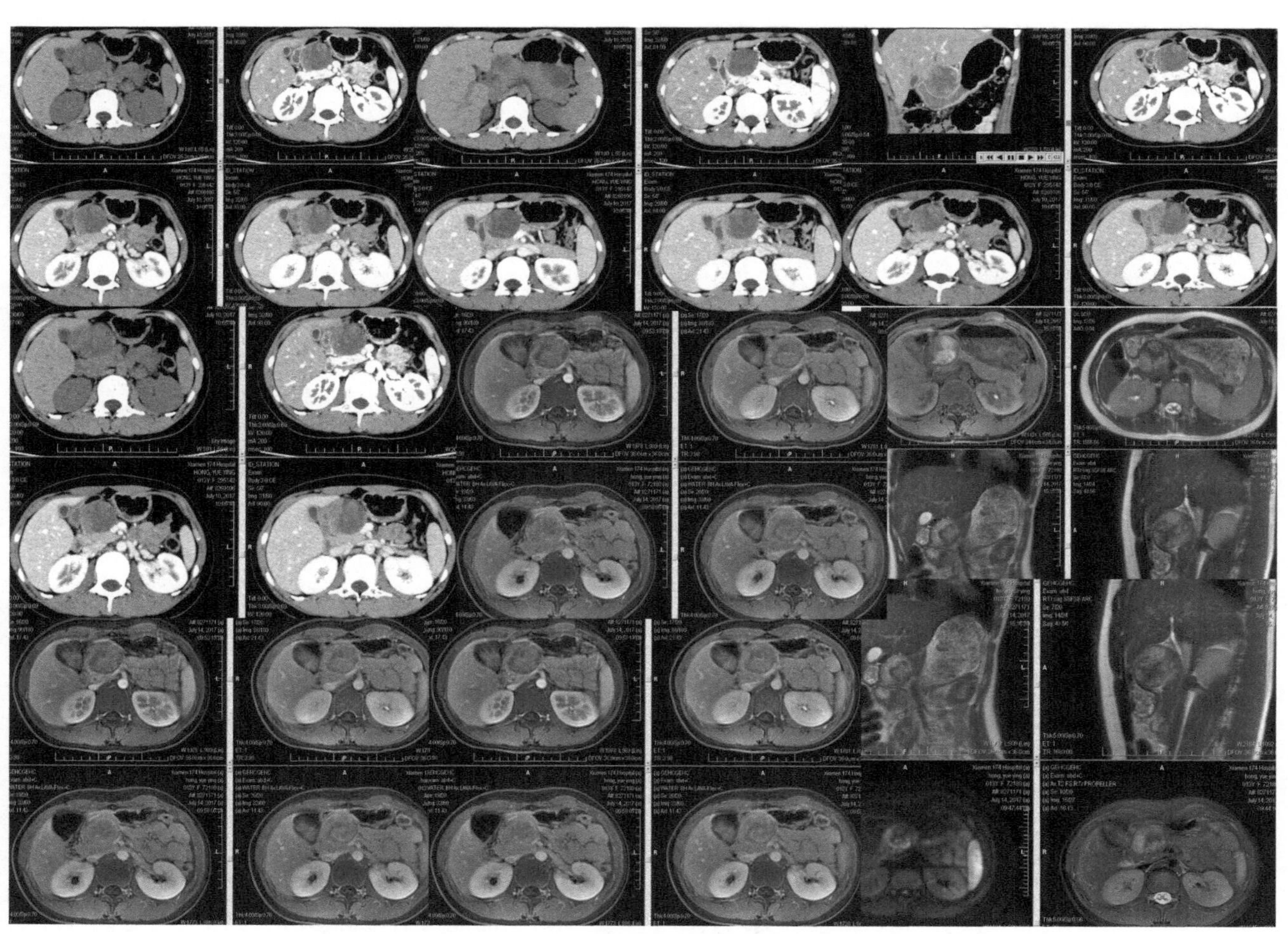

图20-14-3　胰头实性假乳头状肿瘤与胰腺假性囊肿

患者，女，16岁。缘于1个月前因腹部外伤后出现上腹部疼痛，呈闷痛性质。外院CT提示：胰头颈部囊实性占位，考虑：肿瘤性病变可能性大，血肿待排，建议进一步检查。今来院，门诊拟"胰腺假囊肿"收住入院。病理检查：胰腺肿瘤切除标本：灰红色不规则组织一块，大小约5cm×4cm×2.7cm，送检前已剖开，切面灰红灰褐，质中；于切面可见一囊腔，最大径约2.5cm，囊内充满砖红色物质，囊内壁尚光滑；肿物似有包膜。常规病理诊断：胰腺肿瘤切除标本：考虑胰腺实性假乳头状肿瘤，待做免疫组化检测进一步证实。免疫组化检测：阳性：β-catenin（核+），Vimentin，AAT，AACT，

CD56,CD10(灶+),Syn(灶+),CK18,CK8(灶+),P53(+,约30%),Ki-67(+,<5%),CK(P),CD34(血管内皮+),PAS染色;阴性:CK19,CK7,Villin,CK20,CgA,CA19-9。免疫组化诊断:胰腺肿瘤切除标本示胰腺实性假乳头状肿瘤(图20-14-3)。

第七节 胰腺实性假乳头状瘤与恶性胰腺实性假乳头状瘤

胰腺实性假乳头状瘤是一种少见的胰腺肿瘤,最早由Frantz(1959)报道,曾被称为实性和乳头状肿瘤、乳头状囊性肿瘤、实性-囊性肿瘤、实性乳头状上皮肿瘤、乳头状上皮肿瘤等。WHO(1996)正式将其命名"实性假乳头状瘤",而恶性者称为实性假乳头状癌。胰腺实性假乳头状瘤发病率仅占胰腺所有肿瘤的0.13%~2.70%,占胰腺囊性肿瘤的6%~12%。胰腺实性假乳头状瘤多呈良性或低度恶性,但肿瘤发生转移的发生率可达15%。

胰腺实性假乳头状瘤多发生于20~30岁女性,Papavramidis等(2005)总结了718例胰腺实性假乳头状瘤,男女发病比例约1:9.78,平均发病年龄为21.97岁。一组39例男女发病比例约1:2.9,平均年龄33.2岁,与文献报道略不同,考虑与病例数相对较少有关。

胰腺实性假乳头状瘤的临床表现无明显特异性,包括腹部不适或腹痛,少数可触及上腹部肿块。文献报道约70%~90%的病人可表现出临床症状。无临床症状的患者是由于其他原因行腹部超声或CT检查时意外发现。该组中有8例即为体检时发现。

胰腺实性假乳头状瘤预后良好,其5年生存率高达95%~100%,多数患者病灶切除后可长期生存,因此早期诊断对于指导临床治疗及预后的判断具有重要价值。

影像学研究:胰腺实性假乳头状瘤一般瘤体较大,肿瘤可有包膜及假包膜形成,一般边界清晰。包膜增强后可显示明显的延迟强化。该组病例均为单发,肿瘤长径2~17 cm,平均7.5 cm,大小与良、恶性无关,该组2例恶性大小仅3~4 cm。胰腺实性假乳头状瘤可发生于胰腺的任何部位,最常见于胰腺尾部或头部。该组20例位于胰腺头颈部,其中5例位于钩突部,19例位于胰腺体尾部。

病理上胰腺实性假乳头状瘤由实性片状、假乳头状区及两者的过渡区构成,假乳头状结构的黏液变性、出血、坏死,构成肿瘤囊实性成分相间改变的基础。

CT表现取决于肿瘤实性和囊性结构的比例和分布,按实性和囊性结构的比例不同,可将CT表现分为3种类型:以囊性结构为主;以实性结构为主;囊实混合性结构为主。该组中21例胰腺实性假乳头状瘤以实性结构为主;11例以囊实性混合结构为主;7例以囊性结构为主。胰腺实性假乳头状瘤在CT上的表现与其囊实性成分的比例及分布密切相关。CT平扫表现为胰腺内的囊实性肿块,实性结构呈等或略低密度,增强扫描动脉期呈轻度强化,门静脉期及延迟期呈明显强化,即呈现渐进性强化,且囊实性成分的分界于静脉期显示更为清楚。瘤内可以出现坏死、液化及囊性变,共同组成肿瘤的囊性区,一般呈低密度,增强扫描无强化。双期和三期增强扫描能明确体现肿瘤渐进性延迟强化的特点。

钙化和分隔是胰腺实性假乳头状瘤的特征,文献报道约30%病例可发生钙化,该组16例发生钙化,占41%,钙化多位于实性区及包膜内,以小结节状多见,提示肿瘤生长缓慢和生长时间较长。无论胰腺实性假乳头状瘤位于胰腺的任何部位,均较少引起胆总管和胰管扩张。即使胰管扩张,其程度也较轻,与胰头区肿瘤的大小不成正比。胰管扩张与肿瘤压迫、浸润胰管及胰腺慢性炎症等诸多因素有关。该组资料表明,增强MSCT能显示肿瘤与周围血管及组织结构的关系,多平面重建显示效果更好。CTA能够较好显示肿瘤与动脉的关系,CTV则能够显示肿瘤与静脉的关系。但MSCT评价瘤周组织受侵情况的能力有限,确切的恶性证据需待病理证实。胰腺实性假乳头状瘤对动脉和静脉,都以推移为主而不是侵犯,与胰腺癌侵犯血管的表现不一样,可以作为鉴别诊断的依据。

胰腺实性假乳头状瘤是一种有恶性潜能或低度恶性的肿瘤。据WHO分类标准,恶性胰腺实性假乳头状瘤有明确的诊断标准:明确的神经周围侵犯、血管侵犯或侵犯深入至周围组织。有下列征象者可考虑为恶性胰腺实性假乳头状瘤：肿瘤明显突破包膜并浸润胰腺实质；直接侵犯门静脉、肠系膜上静脉等邻近大血管和/或浸润邻近脏器；胰周淋巴结转移性肿大；出现远处脏器转移，如肝脏、腹膜、卵巢等。

然而，胰腺实性假乳头状瘤生物学行为特殊，即使良性胰腺实性假乳头状瘤也具有恶性潜能，缺少以上恶性表现时也有发生转移的可能。即使出观包膜及周围胰腺浸润，预后亦较好。包膜完整与否是判断肿瘤性质为良性或低度恶性的重要依据。

鉴别诊断：胰腺实性假乳头状瘤比较少见，因此常常误诊为胰腺其他良性肿瘤或胰腺癌，而一旦肿瘤巨大即被诊断为胰腺癌，往往采用化疗及放疗，对患者造成更大损伤。因此，鉴别诊断对确定治疗方案十分重要，无论胰腺实性假乳头状瘤是否为恶性，首选治疗方式均为手术切除。

有一些要注意。

（1）囊腺瘤：囊腺瘤分为浆液性囊腺瘤和黏液性囊腺瘤。病灶也呈囊实性，边界清楚，可伴胰管扩张，但囊腺瘤好发于中老年女性，壁结节及分隔与胰腺实性假乳头状瘤渐进性中度强化的实性成分不同，且病灶中心星状瘢痕伴钙化是浆液性囊腺瘤的特征性表现，而黏液性囊腺瘤可见壳状、条状钙化。当边界不清晰，囊内间隔、囊壁欠规则、邻近器官受累或远处转移时，应考虑囊腺癌。

（2）胰腺癌：胰腺癌一般发病年龄明显高于胰腺实性假乳头状瘤，常有CA19-9的明显增高，无明显边界及包膜，可因缺血、坏死而发生囊变，多在瘤体中央区，形态不规则，与实性部分分界不清，囊壁不完整，厚而不规则，或无明确囊壁显示。增强扫描实性部分呈轻度强化。胰腺癌多数发生在胰头，常向后侵犯周围血管神经，出现胆胰管明显扩张，淋巴结肿大及远处转移的概率远高于胰腺实性假乳头状瘤，且胰腺癌具有累及周围血管的特性。

胰腺假性囊肿：胰腺假性囊肿者常有胰腺炎或外伤史，病灶以囊性为主，囊内极少有间隔，囊壁一般较薄、多不光整，无壁结节，囊腔多与胰管相通，其出血所致的高密度灶不会出现逐渐强化；部分可伴有慢性胰腺炎的胰腺改变，如胰腺萎缩、胰实质或胰管的钙化、胰管不规则扩张等。

此外，胰腺实性假乳头状瘤还需与胰岛细胞瘤囊变、胰管内黏液乳头状瘤以及胰周肿瘤性病变等相鉴别。

总之，胰腺实性假乳头状瘤好发于年轻女性，临床上没有特异性症状，CT表现为囊实性肿块，常较巨大，边界清晰，实性部分和包膜渐进性强化，部分肿瘤可见钙化，多数不伴有胰管或胆管的扩张，具有一定的特征性，结合临床和MSCT特征可以做出准确诊断。

第八节　胰腺囊实性乳头状瘤误诊分析

详见本书 本卷 本篇 第二十章 第一节　胰腺囊实性乳头状瘤误诊分析。

第九节　胰腺实性假乳头状肿瘤（SPN）

男，52岁。

术后病理免疫组化诊断：胰腺实性假乳头状肿瘤（SPN），为低度恶性胰腺外分泌部上皮性肿瘤。4.5cm × 4cm × 4cm，切面灰黄质中，境界尚清（图20-14-4）。

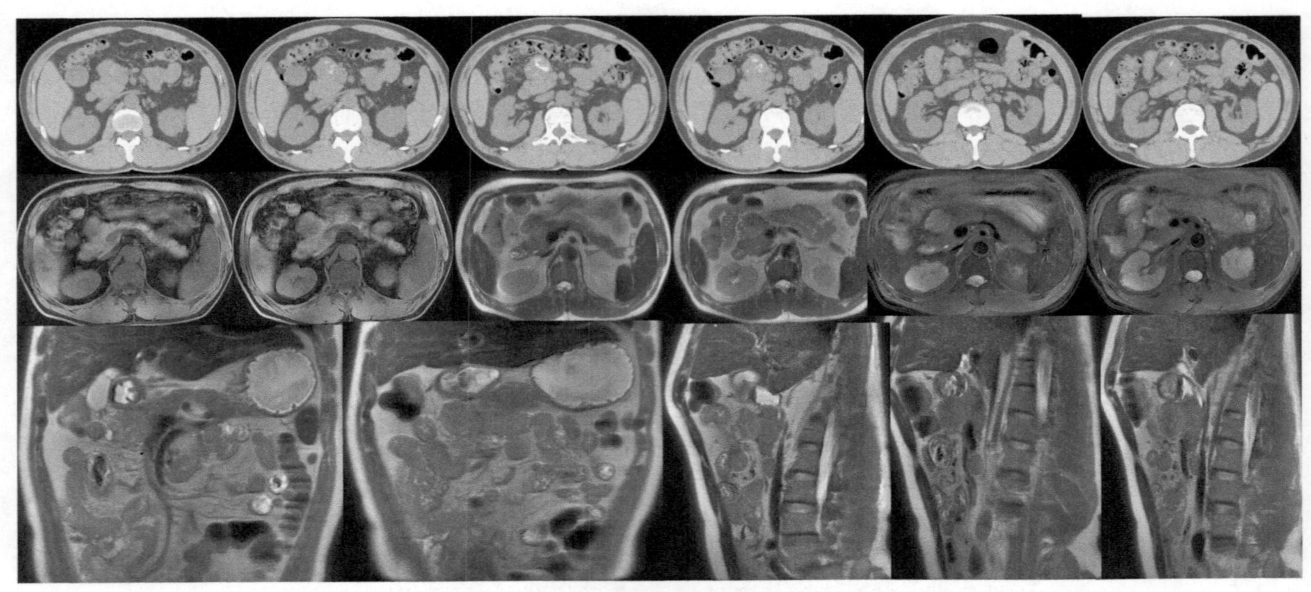

图 20-14-4 胰腺实性假乳头状肿瘤

第十节 胰腺实性假乳头状瘤典型与不典型表现

胰腺实性假乳头状瘤是一种少见、独特的胰腺良性或低度恶性的肿瘤。主要发生于青年女性，以往临床及影像学对其认识较少，容易误诊为胰腺无功能腺瘤、囊腺瘤或腹膜后肿瘤。胰腺实性假乳头状瘤约占胰腺外分泌肿瘤的 0.13%~2.7%，因其发病率低及术前误诊，使得发病率难以准确计算。Frantz(1959)首次报道，病变好发于 20~40 岁育龄期女性，偶发老年女性和男性。女性发病率约占 87.5%~91.7%，一组 7 例均为女性，平均年龄 29 岁，未见男性患者，可能与病例样本量小有关。

临床上曾命名为实性乳头状上皮瘤、实性 - 囊性肿瘤、乳头状囊性肿瘤、实性囊性乳头状腺泡细胞瘤和 Frantz 瘤等，但这些命名均不能准确从镜下及肉眼水平表达该肿瘤特征。

WHO(2004)肿瘤组织学分类中将其统一命名为实性假乳头状瘤，定义为由形态比较一致的细胞形成实性巢状和假乳头结构的上皮性肿瘤，常有出血及囊性变，此瘤通常为良性，偶尔可为恶性。其中 14.7% 有复发及转移等恶性倾向。

一组 7 例中，有 1 例手术提示肿瘤突破包膜，且与脾血管分离困难，病理报告低度恶性潜能。胰腺实性假乳头状瘤组织起源仍不明确，有学者认为可能源于胰腺的多潜能干细胞，表现为导管、腺泡和内分泌以及血管瘤样分化。

影像学研究：胰腺实性假乳头状瘤的 CT 表现与病理基础密切相关，其病理学检查见肿瘤实质均由实性区、假乳头区及二者的过渡区以不同比例混合组成。实性区肿瘤细胞排列成巢状或片块状，假乳头区肿瘤细胞以纤细的纤维血管为轴心形成分支状假乳头，假乳头表面细胞呈复层排列囊性结构。远离血管周围的肿瘤细胞产生退行性变表现为同程度的坏死、液化、囊性变及陈旧性出血。

根据囊实性结构比例不同分为：囊性成分为主型、囊实成分相近型及实性成分为主型。其 MSCT 表现取决于肿瘤实性结构和囊性结构的比例和分布。

该组术中及大体标本显示 4 例包膜完整，边界清楚，其中 1 例侵及包膜，且与脾血管粘连，病理报告肿瘤有潜在恶性倾向，而术前 MSCT 示肿块边缘光滑清晰，与周围组织界限清楚，未见脾血管受侵征象，因此认为 MSCT 尚不能准确评价肿瘤包膜完整性及血管受侵情况。

30% 的胰腺实性假乳头状瘤可见细条状或斑点状钙化，且以边缘区多见。该组 2 例伴钙化，发生率占 28.57%。MSCT 对钙化显示明显优于 MRI。

该组囊性为主型 2 例，囊实性相近型 1 例，

MSCT表现为有覆壁结节的囊性肿块及囊实相间的肿块。实性为主型4例，MSCT表现为实性肿块内囊性部分呈裂隙样及斑片状低密度影，其手术病理为肿瘤细胞的坏死、液化、囊性变及陈旧性出血，对陈旧性出血的MSCT诊断不及MRI。

增强扫描囊性成分不强化；而实性成分因假乳头区肿瘤以纤细的纤维血管为轴心形成假乳头结构，表现为明显强化，且呈渐进性强化特点。

因胰腺实性假乳头状瘤质地较软，生长缓慢，即使位于胰头部，也很少会引起胆管或胰管扩张，常常向腹腔及腹膜后相对空虚部位生长。

肿瘤较大时可压迫引起周围结构如胃、十二指肠、血管移位，由于胰腺与脾静脉的特殊解剖关系（脾静脉紧贴胰腺后方走行），因此当胰腺实性假乳头状瘤瘤体较大时，压迫脾静脉，致脾静脉回流受阻，大量静脉血可通过胃网膜静脉-胃结肠干-肠系膜上静脉回流至门静脉系，形成典型“发夹样”改变，造成门静脉循环压力增高而门静脉压力正常即出现胰源性门静脉高压。该组胰尾部1例胰腺实性假乳头状瘤伴有该征象，同时伴脾淤血肿大。

MSCT常规轴位可显示肿瘤大小、形态、位置及强化特点。其图像后处理技术，如：多平面重建可以多方位显示除肿瘤本身特征之外，同时可多角度观察邻近脏器受压及侵及情况，最大密度投影、容积再现可清晰显示邻近血管受推压改变，特别是当脾静脉受压导致胰源性门静脉高压时，可观察其侧支循环，有助于判断侧支血管的走行、位置及曲张程度。容积再现显示立体感及周围解剖结构清楚，利于临床医生观察。

典型与不典型表现：胰腺实性假乳头状瘤的MSCT典型影像学征象：发生于胰腺任何部位，胰头及胰尾多见，而非胰腺实质内，常突出胰腺轮廓之外，常向腹腔及腹膜后空虚处生长；肿瘤呈圆形、类圆形囊实性肿块，囊实性成分不等，肿瘤形态规整，边界清楚，可见包膜；增强后实性成分动脉期轻度强化，静脉期强化程度进一步加强，而囊性部分始终不强化；肿瘤与邻近组织分界清楚，可造成邻近器官及血管推压移位。长期压迫脾静脉可造成胰源性门静脉高压。位于胰头部病变，少有胆管及胰管扩张；腹腔及腹膜后无肿大淋巴结影像。

不典型表现：肝转移；胆管梗阻征象；肿瘤突破囊壁，侵及胰腺实质；与非功能胰岛细胞瘤类似表现；高密度钙化；男性患者。

总之，胰腺实性假乳头状瘤是一种预后较好的肿瘤，临床及MSCT表现有一定特征性，对于发生于年轻女性胰头或胰尾的囊实性肿块，边缘清楚，包膜完整，且临床症状不明显，应考虑到本病可能。手术切除是胰腺实性假乳头状瘤唯一根治方法，即使伴有转移病灶，完全切除并可获得长期生存期，治疗不充分或未经治疗，可明显恶变并发生转移。MSCT对其正确诊断、制订手术方案及评价预后有重要意义。

第十一节　胰腺实性假乳头状瘤误诊讨论

胰腺实性假乳头状瘤是一种少见的良性或低度恶性的胰腺肿瘤，近年来逐渐被临床、影像和病理所关注。胰腺实性假乳头状瘤约占胰腺外分泌肿瘤的1%~2%，WHO（1996）正式将其统一命名为胰腺实性假乳头状瘤，将其新分类为生物学行为未定或交界性恶性潜能的肿瘤。胰腺实性假乳头状瘤好发于30岁左右的女性，胰尾部最多见，约占56%~77%，其次为胰头部约占34%。胰腺实性假乳头状瘤临床症状无特异性，患者多无意中或体检时经超声发现腹部包块，可伴有腹部隐痛、腹胀等。

胰腺实性假乳头状瘤的诊断需密切结合临床病史及影像学表现，一组8例中仅4例术前做出正确诊断，2例误诊为胰腺癌，2例误诊为胰腺囊腺瘤，可能与该病的发病率相对较低，对此病的认识不足有关。螺旋CT双期增强可清楚地显示胰腺实性假乳头状瘤瘤体、胰腺组织和胰周血管的增强变化和特征，故应重视该检查对胰腺实性假乳头状瘤的诊断价值。

胰腺实性假乳头状瘤瘤体形态规则，多呈圆形或卵圆形，位于胰腺的边缘处，体积较大，常突出于胰腺轮廓之外。胰腺局部增粗，与肿瘤交界处呈杯口状改变。肿瘤多有较厚且完整的包膜，与周围组织分界清晰。瘤细胞围绕纤维血管排列形成假乳头状结构是胰腺实性假乳头状瘤的特征性组织学改变。

螺旋CT凭借极高的密度分辨率能够清晰地显

示该特征，特别是增强检查在周围未强化的囊性部分的衬托下，明显强化的乳头状结构显示更为清晰。该组 4 例增强后可以明确的见到自囊壁向腔内突出的假乳头状结构，该征象为诊断胰腺实性假乳头状瘤的可靠征象。

CT 平扫胰腺实性假乳头状瘤实性部分呈等密度或略高密度，CT 值为（41.09 ± 6.38）HU，囊性部分呈低密度。增强后动脉期瘤体实性部分的 CT 值为（43.82 ± 10.35）HU，实质期 CT 值明显增加为（48.91 ± 9.93）HU，但仍低于正常胰腺组织的强化。囊性部分各期未见强化。

肿瘤强化在实质期明显高于动脉期（P = 0.005），强化曲线为逐渐上升型，与肿瘤具有类似于海绵状血管瘤的血窦有关。渐进性强化可能是诊断胰腺实性假乳头状瘤的比较特征性的表现。胰腺实性假乳头状瘤由于生长缓慢且质地较软，生物学特性为不易侵犯胰周血管、胰管及胆管。瘤体较大时，周围的脏器血管受挤压而移位，但脂肪间隙往往存在。双期增强可使胰周血管在最佳灌注期内得到清晰显示，从而能够更好地辨别血管与肿瘤之间的关系。

胰腺实性假乳头状瘤即使位于胰头部，也很少引起胰管及胆管扩张，这与胰头癌的围管性浸润生长明显不同。该组 1 例位于胰头者符合此特征，没有胰管及胆管与胰周血管的侵犯，但术前缺乏认识，误诊为胰头癌。综上所述，胰腺实性假乳头状瘤的诊断要点为：临床多见于年轻女性，无明显症状；肿瘤呈圆形或类圆形多位于胰腺的边缘处，有完整的包膜，与胰腺交界处呈杯口状改变；肿瘤内可见假乳头状结构，为本病的特征性表现；肿瘤囊实性相间，呈“浮云征”；双期增强特点，肿瘤实质期强化明显高于动脉期；临近脏器血管受推压移位，但很少有受侵征象；不伴有胰管及胆管的扩张。

胰腺实性假乳头状瘤的 CT 表现需与其他胰腺病变相鉴别。

囊腺瘤（癌）：分为浆液性囊腺瘤（癌）和黏液性囊腺瘤（癌），多发生于 40~60 岁女性，囊内分隔粗细不均，多有壁结节。肿瘤内有无假乳头状结构为囊腺瘤与胰腺实性假乳头状瘤的重要鉴别点。

胰腺癌囊变：多发生在胰头部，囊变位于中央区呈不规则形，与实性部分分界不清，肿瘤易导致胰管及胆管扩张与血管的侵犯。肿瘤在各期均无明显强化。

胰腺假囊肿：常有胰腺炎或外伤手术史，囊壁较薄而均匀，无壁结节或乳头状突起。

总之，胰腺实性假乳头状瘤是一种很少见的良性或低度恶性肿瘤，螺旋 CT 双期增强能够显示胰腺实性假乳头状瘤的血供特点及生物学行为，结合临床病史大部分肿瘤可以在术前做出明确诊断，为临床手术方式的选择及预后评估提供重要的资料依据。

第十五章　胰腺内分泌肿瘤

第一节　胰岛素瘤 MRI 漏诊

胰岛素瘤是一种少见的内分泌肿瘤，发病率约10万分之一，是较常见的功能内分泌肿瘤，90% 胰岛素瘤为良性，手术切除是唯一可以治愈的方法，而胰岛素瘤一般体积非常小，定位相对困难，且影像学表现多样。因此术前明确肿瘤的部位、大小和毗邻关系非常重要。

病理学：肿瘤大体呈圆形或类圆形，肿瘤有包膜，与周围正常组织界限清楚或较清，瘤细胞排列呈梁索样、腺泡样或巢片样分布，瘤细胞形态一致或相对一致，胞浆丰富红染，可见嗜酸性颗粒，瘤细胞核圆形或卵圆形。

临床表现：本症具有经典的 Whipple 三联征，包括空腹时低血糖发作，空腹或发作时血糖 <2.8 mmol/l（50 mg/dl），进食或静脉推注葡萄糖可迅速缓解症状。一组 43 例术前均有 Whipple 三联征。7 例曾被误诊为癫痫。10 例合并肝内胆管结石、胆囊结石、脂肪肝，2 例为合并垂体腺瘤。2 例异位胰腺，分别位于十二指肠水平部上方和左肾门水平脊柱旁，因此为减少漏诊，胰腺动态扫描时范围应该大一些，最好按腹部的范围扫描。

影像学研究：该组 43 例胰岛素瘤良性单发 40 例（93%），多发 3 例（7%）；2 例合并甲状腺腺瘤、垂体微腺瘤、胸腺瘤。胰岛素瘤约 90% 以上是单发良性肿瘤，少数为多发性肿瘤或恶性胰岛素瘤。

Falchetti 等（2008）报道胰岛素瘤中约有 10% 为多发肿瘤，而且此类肿瘤多合并多发性内分泌肿瘤综合征，在多发性内分泌肿瘤综合征中最常见的内分泌肿瘤主要是甲状旁腺瘤、胰腺内分泌瘤和垂体腺瘤，而以胰岛素瘤为首发临床症状的多发性内分泌肿瘤综合征 -1 型约占 10%~30%。该组中 3 例是多发，在胰腺分别有 3、5、7 个病灶，其中 2 例合并垂体腺瘤、甲状腺腺瘤，临床上被诊断为多发性内分泌肿瘤综合征 -1 型。该组 40 例均呈明显强化，均在动脉期与周围组织对比最佳。6 例动脉期呈等信号，静脉期明显强化。

胰岛素瘤和其他功能性胰岛细胞瘤同为富血供肿瘤，极少数肿瘤为乏血供的胰岛细胞瘤，绝大部分肿瘤增强后明显强化，尤其在动脉期上显示最佳。胰岛素瘤 T_1WI 呈低、稍低或等信号，T_2WI 呈稍高信号，T_2WI 抑脂呈高信号，DWI 呈高或稍高信号。

该组中 31 例呈高或稍高信号，12 例阴性，分析原因可能为层厚 6~8 mm 太厚，而病灶较小，最小者直径仅 3.7 mm；此外，部分患者呼吸伪影较大，影响图像质量。因此，薄层扫描和患者良好的配合很重要。

由于胰岛素瘤含有丰富的血窦，因此在 T2WI 抑脂序列上信号较正常的胰腺实质高，从而清楚显示瘤灶。正常的胰腺实质内含有丰富的含水蛋白，而胰岛素瘤内没有含水蛋白，因此在 T1WI 上胰岛素瘤的信号较周围正常胰腺实质信号低，从而清楚显示瘤灶。

DWI 上，胰岛素瘤信号较周围正常胰腺实质高，推测其原因可能是胰岛素瘤内部结构排列较致密，并且血窦分割较多，瘤灶内水分子受限程度较明显。

该组 22 例病灶发生在胰体尾部，占 51. 2%，与文献报道胰岛素瘤多发生在胰体尾部基本相一致，绝大多数学者认为是胰体尾部胰腺的 β 型胰岛细胞较多的缘故。

90% 的功能性胰岛细胞瘤直径 <2.0 cm。该组 43 例手术证实 55 个病灶，长径 0.37~2.6 cm，平均 1.0cm，其中 48 个 <2.0 cm，占 82.8%，与文献报道大

致相符。3 例恶性胰岛素瘤中,1 例胰腺病灶及转移灶多期增强扫描无明显强化,另 2 例动脉期显示病灶最佳,且病灶较大,长径 >3 cm。

鉴别诊断:胰岛素瘤的诊断主要依靠临床表现,饥饿试验和生化指标,影像学诊断主要为临床提供术前定位。由于其通常合并 Whipple 三联征,诊断并不困难。仍需与胰腺癌、胰岛细胞增生症、胰腺副脾等鉴别。

胰腺癌:胰腺癌通常为乏血供肿瘤,增强扫描强化不明显,不容易导致低血糖,而胰岛素瘤通常为富血供肿瘤,增强扫描强化明显,且常合并低血糖。

一些学者报道 1 例胰腺混合性导管内分泌癌误诊为胰岛素瘤,因其具备典型的 Whipple 三联征,CT 表现为胰尾部占位,增强扫描明显强化,动脉期病灶显影最佳,临床和影像学诊断为胰岛素瘤,病理为混合性导管内分泌癌。

混合性导管内分泌癌为胰腺导管腺癌的一种亚型,进展较快,其特征为在原发肿瘤及其转移灶中可见导管细胞和内分泌细胞,其中内分泌成分占 1/3~1/2,内分泌表现为神经内分泌标记和 / 或激素产物,如胰岛激素、胰岛淀粉样肽等。

胰岛细胞增生症:胰岛细胞增生症为非胰岛素瘤源性低血糖综合征的主要原因,该病极其罕见,多发生于小儿,成人少见。增生的胰岛细胞呈弥漫性分布,可以引起胰腺局部轮廓突起,但其边界与正常胰腺组织分界不清,影像学上无特征性表现,其临床诊断标准内容繁多,病理上与胰岛素瘤亦难以鉴别。该院曾有 1 例病理诊断胰岛细胞增生症,但临床诊断为胰岛素瘤,并且影像学表现动脉期显示最佳。

胰腺副脾:胰腺副脾以胰尾较为多见,且体积较小,动脉期呈明显强化,易误诊为胰腺富血供肿瘤,但副脾动脉期呈花斑样强化,且无 Whipple 三联征。

MRI 漏诊原因:该组 MRI 漏诊 7 例,1 例位于胰头前缘极小病灶,MRI 平扫及 LAVA 动态增强均未见显示,而经宝石 CT 能谱处理后,动脉期可见异常强化灶,手术及病理证实为胰岛素瘤;3 例在 MRI 平扫时类圆形异常信号,T_1WI 抑脂及正反相位呈低信号,DWI 和 T_2WI 抑脂序列,其中 1 例 MRI 平扫时胰尾部较小外生性类圆形异常信号,LAVA 增强扫描各期未见显示;另 1 例病灶位于胰颈肠系膜上静脉旁,误认为是肠系膜上动 / 静脉,胰岛素瘤体积较小。

分析原因:T_2WI 抑脂序列对病灶敏感;少数胰岛素瘤乏血供,增强后不强化。充分认识胰岛素瘤的影像学表现和胰腺毗邻的血管解剖有利于减少漏诊。

另有 3 例良性多发,15 个病灶;其中 1 例病史 40 年,手术及病理证实共有 3 个大小分别为 0. 7cm、0.4cm 和 1.2cm 的胰岛素瘤,MRI(层厚 5mm)上仅看到 1.2cm 的病灶,但 CT(层厚 2.5mm)双期增强上看到 3 处病灶;另外 2 例多发胰岛素瘤亦出现类似情况,CT 增强扫描能显示全部病灶;这与 MRI 层厚较大而 CT 层厚和间隔较小(2. 5mm)有关。故建议加做胰腺动态 CT 薄层扫描多发胰岛素瘤以防止漏诊。

总之,MRI 检查是胰岛素瘤术前诊断重要的影像学方法之一。针对临床怀疑为胰岛素瘤的病例应尽量减小扫描层厚和间隔,3.0~5.0mm 为宜;应将 MRI 多期增强与平扫 MRI 各序列相结合,因后者较前者可以提供更多的诊断和鉴别诊断信息,特别是对乏血供胰岛素瘤更具有诊断意义,可以避免多期增强未强化的肿瘤被漏诊的可能。DWI 和平扫 MRI 压脂序列相结合能提高诊断胰岛素瘤的敏感性。

第二节 胰腺小功能性腺瘤的检出:MR 成像序列选择

胰岛素瘤作为最常见的胰岛细胞肿瘤通常直径小于 2cm,因此胰腺功能性肿瘤的定位对于放射学家是个挑战。而可靠的术前定位方法有助于制定准确的治疗方案并可避免探查性剖腹手术。Thoeni 等(2000)连续对 28 例病人进行前瞻性研究以确定:MRI 检出 $\leqslant$ 2cm 胰岛细胞瘤的敏感性与特异性、最佳的 MR 成像序列以及要达到正确和有效诊断所需的最少序列。

28 例中,包括女 17 例、男 11 例,平均年龄 48 岁(18~82 岁)。28 例中 19 例行胰腺腺瘤手术切除,病理学检查 17 例为胰岛素瘤、2 例为胃泌素瘤。

仔细对照手术、病理与 MRI 所见的肿瘤大小和部位。MRI 检查前 4 小时患者禁食,检查前将导管置于肘前静脉内,用于检查中滴注 0.9% 生理盐水

250ml。检查使用 1.5T MR 仪与体线圈。所用自旋回波(SE)序列均加预饱和及高频相位编码的呼吸抑制技术。毁损梯度回波(SPGRE)成像用于屏气扫描与流动补偿。SE T_1WI 扫描时先无脂肪抑制、后应用频率选择性脂肪抑制技术,接着作有与无脂肪抑制的 T_2WI 扫描,最后 10 例也同时作 FSE T_2WI 扫描。前 12 例作快速 SPGRE 屏气的平扫与注射 Gd 剂的增强扫描,后 16 例作快速多层面 SPGRE 平扫与增强扫描。

阅片医生解释与分析图像时不知道患者的手术与临床检查结果。将 MRI 的结果与手术、病理和/或临床随访结果对照,确定所有 MRI 序列的敏感性、特异性以及阳性与阴性预测值。用对比噪声比(CNR)将病灶显示的程度量化。

20 例 MRI 检查确定 17 例有胰腺肿瘤,另 3 例有功能性胰岛细胞瘤的临床表现,而 MRI 未发现肿瘤。阅读所有图像,其阳性预测值为 100%,特异度为 100%,阴性预测值为 73%。20 例中 15 例脂肪抑制 T_1WI 与 SPGRE 平扫发现证实为胰岛细胞瘤的病灶(75%),增强 SPGRE 发现 12 例肿瘤(60%),17 例无脂肪抑制 SE T_2WI 扫描中 11 例显示了肿瘤(65%),脂肪抑制 T_2WI 13 例显示病灶(65%),10 例 FSE T_2WI 中 7 例发现病灶(70%)。

2 例病人的病灶在所有序列上(包括增强扫描)均漏诊,其病灶与正常的胰腺等信号,其中 1 例位于胰腺头部,未引起外形的改变;另 1 漏诊的瘤灶不能与十二指肠壁区分。

与周围正常的胰腺组织相比,腺瘤为较低或较高信号。注射钆剂后显示肿瘤的 12 例中,胰岛细胞瘤 4 例表现为边缘环状强化,中央为低信号,1 例瘤灶中央强化,周围为低信号,绕以正常强化的胰腺;另外 7 例瘤灶为均匀强化。

该组 MRI 检出 2cm 及以下的胰岛功能性肿瘤的敏感度为 85%,与有创性检查手段相似,而优于大多数 MRI 文献报道的结果。该研究结果较好,缘于改良的序列设计、较好的梯度场与线圈,使之可进行快速扫描、具较高信噪比以及钆剂增强早期相图像质量优良。该研究与其他作者的结果一致,即脂肪抑制下 SE T_1WI 是检出小的胰岛肿瘤最好的序列,但该研究中 SPGRE 平扫可检出同样多的病灶,而数据采集时间较短。只有当 T_1WI 与 T_2WI 均未显示病灶或二者不足以确诊,而临床上高度怀疑胰岛细胞肿瘤时才需要行增强扫描。

MRI 漏诊胰岛细胞肿瘤的原因包括:患者肥胖、呼吸不规则致图像质量不良、患者不合作、病灶极小、病灶内广泛纤维化以及肿瘤异位,如位于十二指肠壁内。该作者推荐使用脂肪抑制 SPGRE T_1WI 与 FSE T_2WI 扫描 MR 成像技术作为检查小胰岛细胞肿瘤的手段。

第十六章　胰腺神经内分泌肿瘤

第一节　胰腺神经内分泌肿瘤的良、恶性

病理学：病理上，胰腺神经内分泌肿瘤多数带有部分或完整的包膜，胰腺神经内分泌肿瘤通常较大，瘤内常有坏死和囊性变，部分肿瘤有间质内不规则团块状钙化或微小钙化小球(砂砾体)。电镜下多数胰腺神经内分泌肿瘤可找到神经分泌颗粒，免疫组织化学染色显示 CgA、NSE 及 Syn 等阳性。

临床表现：胰腺神经内分泌肿瘤是起源于胰腺导管上皮多能干细胞的一类少见肿瘤，发病率低于十万分之一。胰腺神经内分泌肿瘤早期常无症状，当肿瘤生长至一定大小、压迫或浸润邻近脏器和结构时，方产生相应的临床症状和体征，如上腹部不适和疼痛、梗阻性黄疸、黑便等。

关于恶性胰腺神经内分泌肿瘤的认识：目前，对恶性胰腺神经内分泌肿瘤的诊断尚缺乏统一的标准，有学者认为，虽然恶性胰腺神经内分泌肿瘤具有体积较大、出血坏死、瘤细胞异型性与核分裂象较多、局部浸润或侵犯血管及神经周围淋巴间隙等恶性肿瘤的一般特点，但单从病理改变判断胰腺神经内分泌肿瘤的良、恶性存在一定的限度，只有当发生其他脏器和淋巴结转移时才是诊断恶性的可靠依据。另有学者认为，除转移外，周围组织浸润和血管侵犯应该作为恶性胰腺神经内分泌肿瘤的诊断指标，甚至有学者提出，因胰腺神经内分泌肿瘤大多是恶性的，即使缺乏血管或神经周围的浸润，也不能排除潜在恶性行为。

一组 12 例诊断为恶性的胰腺神经内分泌肿瘤中，1 例仅病理见侵及包膜，无包膜外侵犯，其余向包膜外浸润，累及十二指肠 9 例，累及胆总管 4 例、胰管 1 例，累及血管 4 例，侵犯腹膜后神经及肠系膜根部和大网膜各 1 例，而淋巴结转移仅有 4 例，无一例出现脏器转移。因此，可以认同某些学者观点，若把有无转移作为判断恶性胰腺神经内分泌肿瘤的唯一标准，将延误部分潜在或低度恶性胰腺神经内分泌肿瘤患者的彻底治疗，故应将病理形态学改变，肿瘤侵犯包膜、血管，局部组织浸润，淋巴结及脏器转移等，均纳入诊断恶性胰腺神经内分泌肿瘤的标准。

影像学研究：功能性胰腺神经内分泌肿瘤由于早期即有临床内分泌症状，影像发现时平均直径 <2 cm，而非功能性胰腺神经内分泌肿瘤通常较大，直径 >5 cm，该组功能性胰腺神经内分泌肿瘤平均直径约 1.5 cm，非功能性胰腺神经内分泌肿瘤平均直径约 6cm。

功能性胰腺神经内分泌肿瘤平扫时密度均匀，常呈等密度或稍低密度，在 MRI 上多呈长 T_1、长 T_2 信号，FS T_1WI 及 FMPSPGR 平扫序列多为低信号，且显示病灶较常规 SE T_1WI 更清晰，胰腺轮廓一般无改变或改变不明显。

增强扫描时由于功能性胰腺神经内分泌肿瘤血供丰富，动脉期肿瘤明显均匀强化，部分可近似于血管强化。结合典型临床表现和实验室检查指标，功能性胰腺神经内分泌肿瘤诊断不难，影像学检查的目的主要是术前定位，以便手术治疗。该组 10 例功能性胰腺神经内分泌肿瘤中，8 例呈上述改变，仅 2 例出现囊变坏死和环形强化。

胰腺神经内分泌肿瘤待临床发现时，体积较大，平扫时密度较胰腺实质稍低或呈等密度，其内常可见更低密度坏死或囊变区，其信号亦呈不均匀长 T_1、长 T_2 改变。虽然胰腺神经内分泌肿瘤也富血供，肿瘤坏死和囊变不明显者，呈明显均匀的强化；肿瘤伴有坏死、囊变时，强化不均匀或呈环状强化。

该组 16 例胰腺神经内分泌肿瘤有 13 例出现不同程度的囊变坏死，呈不均匀或环状强化，约占

81%，但 87%（14/16）仍以中度到明显强化为主，显示其富血供特征。

另外，在增强扫描中，有 15 例肿瘤出现瘤体周边环形薄壁明显强化，强化程度高于正常胰腺及瘤体内部，这与病理所见肿瘤有完整包膜且包膜血窦丰富一致，此征象在胰腺其他肿瘤中很少见，故可以认为瘤体周边环形薄壁（包膜）明显强化为胰腺神经内分泌肿瘤另一特征性的影像表现。

有学者认为，肿瘤内发现钙化有助于胰腺神经内分泌肿瘤的诊断，该组 26 例胰腺神经内分泌肿瘤中 4 例肿瘤内出现钙化。

胰腺神经内分泌肿瘤良、恶性的判断：识别恶性征象、评价良、恶性是胰腺神经内分泌肿瘤术前影像学检查的一项重要内容，能够为临床进行术式选择及切除范围提供参考依据。

胰腺神经内分泌肿瘤大部分有完整或部分的包膜，这也是胰腺神经内分泌肿瘤多境界清楚、非浸润性生长的病理基础。但恶性胰腺神经内分泌肿瘤常侵及包膜或向包膜外侵犯，导致肿瘤与周围组织局部粘连、肿瘤的局部浸润、侵犯血管，甚至出现淋巴结和脏器的转移。这些征象均应纳入诊断恶性胰腺神经内分泌肿瘤的标准。

该组 26 个病灶中 20 个有完整或不完整的包膜。14 例良性胰腺神经内分泌肿瘤中 12 例有完整且光滑的包膜，影像上表现为边界锐利清楚的圆形或类圆形肿块，肿块多为胰腺内生长，少数较大者呈外生性生长，邻近组织结构为受压推移改变；

12 例恶性胰腺神经内分泌肿瘤中，8 例有完整或部分包膜，其中 7 例出现包膜外侵犯，CT 或 MRI 上可见肿瘤局部边缘毛糙，与邻近血管或十二指肠分界不清，累及胆总管时则有低位胆管梗阻的表现，但以胆总管扩张为主，另外 4 例无明显包膜存在，肿瘤向周围广泛浸润性生长，除有邻近血管、十二指肠或胆胰管的侵犯外，还出现腹膜后神经或肠系膜、大网膜的浸润。增强扫描时由于胰腺神经内分泌肿瘤多强化明显，与周围结构的关系显示得更加清楚，如果有脏器的转移（常常是肝脏首先受累），还可以显示富血供的转移灶，该组除 4 例有腹膜后淋巴结转移外，无一例出现脏器转移。

鉴别诊断：当胰腺神经内分泌肿瘤出现上述恶性征象时，应注意与胰腺癌的鉴别。胰腺癌多为乏血供，强化程度低于正常胰腺实质，且有明显围管性浸润和嗜神经生长的特点，侵犯胰管和胆总管（指胰头癌）引起的胰管和/或胆总管扩张、胰腺萎缩较胰腺神经内分泌肿瘤更常见且明显，胰腺癌因有嗜神经生长的特征，临床上患者经常有顽固性腹痛。

当胰腺神经内分泌肿瘤发生明显囊变时，需与胰腺囊腺瘤或癌鉴别。囊腺癌多为大单囊，少数呈多囊，囊壁厚薄不一，囊内可有粗细不均的分隔，并可见壁结节，增强后囊壁、分隔及壁结节可轻度强化，而胰腺神经内分泌肿瘤的囊壁及实性成分多为中到明显的强化。

第二节　胰腺神经内分泌肿瘤,肝脏转移性胰腺神经内分泌肿瘤

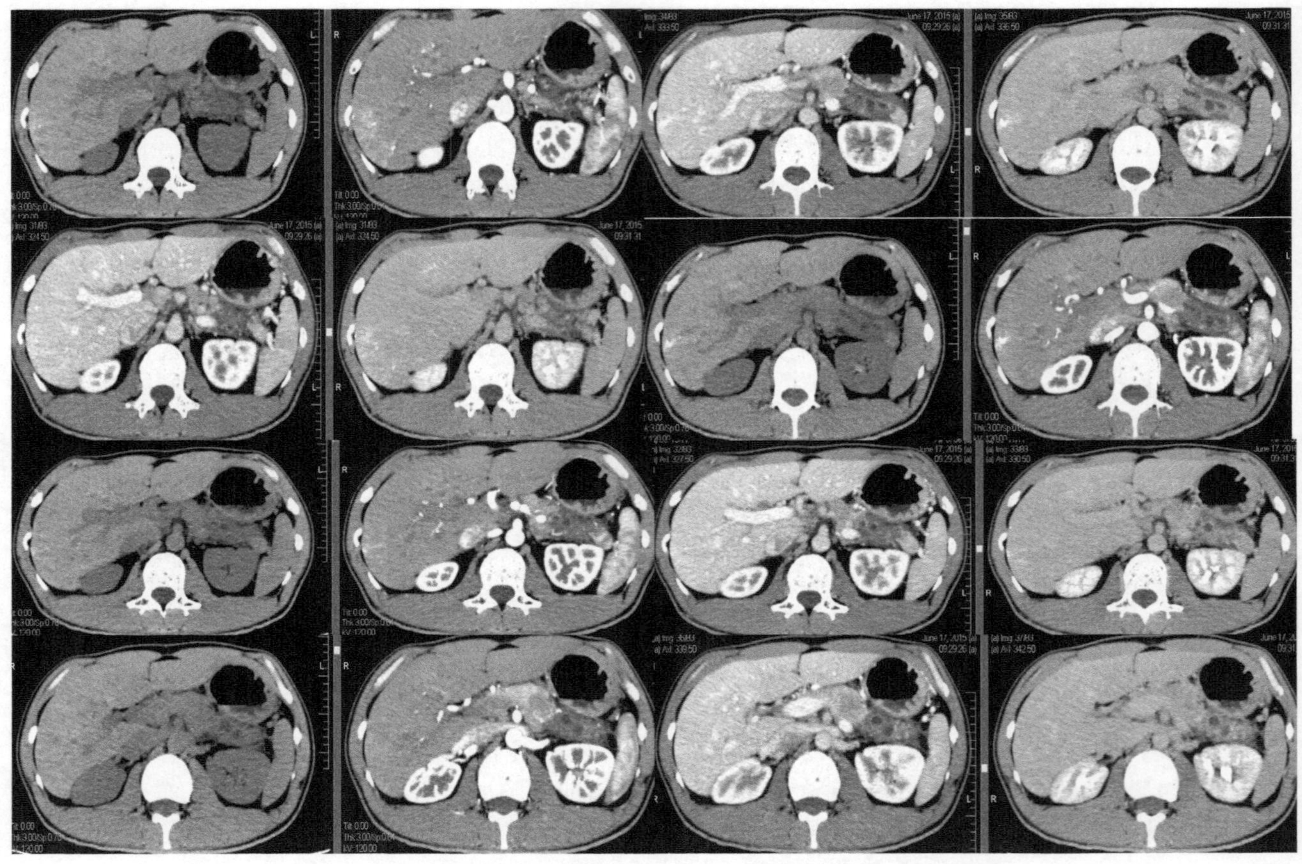

图 20-16-1　胰腺神经内分泌肿瘤,肝脏转移性胰腺神经内分泌肿瘤

患者,男,35 岁。

手术所见:胰腺体尾部可探及一大小约 6.5cm × 4.5cm × 2.5cm 质硬组织,活动性差,瘤体与脾动脉起始部关系密切,肝脏表面可见多发白色小结节,大小约 1~8mm,最大结节位于胆囊床旁,约 8mm。腹腔内未见腹水,大网膜、肝十二指肠韧带、胃、十二指肠、小肠及结肠及其系膜未见转移癌结节。遂行胰体尾切除 + 脾切除 + 肝组织活检及肝脏肿瘤烧灼术。病理检查、免疫组化诊断示胰腺神经内分泌肿瘤、肝脏转移性胰腺神经内分泌肿瘤(图 20-16-1)。

第三节　胰腺类癌

类癌,又名嗜银细胞癌,是一种少见的生长缓慢且低度恶性的神经内分泌肿瘤。85%~90% 的类癌发生在胃肠道,以阑尾、回肠、直肠、胃多见, 10% 的类癌发生于支气管,其余则发生于胸腺、卵巢等部位,胰腺类癌极少见。在临床上,根据 Modlin 等(2003)统计,胰腺类癌仅占所有类癌的 0.58%(79/13715)。

病理学:病理形态及免疫组织化学检查是胰腺类癌确诊的关键,通常表现为体积较大的肿块,边缘光滑,有包膜,出血、坏死多见。癌细胞多由小圆形细胞组成,细胞排列呈实性巢状、小梁状、腺泡状、片状、弥漫状,间质血管丰富。

由于类癌能合成和分泌较多的5-羟色胺，后者经降解，形成5-羟吲哚乙酸经肾排出，因此测定血中5-羟色胺、尿中的5-羟吲哚乙酸浓度具有诊断意义。免疫组织化学染色NSE、Syn、CgA及5-羟色胺可为阳性，尤其5-羟色胺有高表达率。

临床表现：类癌起源于胚胎原始肠道黏膜的Kulschitzsky细胞或嗜铬细胞，该类细胞具有嗜铬亲银特性，能产生小分子多肽类或肽类激素，如5-羟色胺、缓激肽、组胺、儿茶酚胺等，此类物质作用于心血管、呼吸道及胃肠道，表现为面色潮红、周围性水肿、哮喘及腹痛、腹泻，该症状群临床称之为类癌综合征。

胰腺类癌起源于胰导管黏膜的肠嗜铬细胞（EC），是一种低度恶性、生长缓慢的恶性肿瘤。由于癌组织可以分泌5-羟色胺或5-羟色氨酸（5-HTP），部分患者在临床上可出现类癌综合征，类癌综合征的发生率约为23.3%~34%，且其中多数患者伴有肝脏转移。

胰腺类癌的男女比例为1∶1.1，平均年龄为48.9岁，约44.9%的肿瘤发生于胰头，其次为胰尾占21%，由于肿瘤血供丰富，66.7%的病例继发肝脏转移，因此5年生存率仅为28.9%。

影像学研究：胰腺类癌的影像诊断文献报道较少，有作者报道1例位于胰颈体部，CT、MRI均表现为轮廓光整、密度与信号均匀、与周围正常胰腺分界较清晰的肿块，CT双期增强扫描，肿块均较平扫明显强化。Kim等（2005）报道1例胰腺类癌呈圆形肿块，邻近的主胰管扩张，肿块与周围结构境界清楚。

胰腺类癌具有以下CT表现：肿块好发于胰头、胰体部。肿块较大但边缘光整。Soga（2005）统计156例胰腺类癌，测得其平均直径约6.86cm。上述表现与胰腺类癌的生物学特征有关，由于属于低度恶性肿瘤，生长缓慢、侵袭性低，患者带瘤时间长，因此就诊时肿瘤通常较大。

平扫时肿瘤密度不均，易发生囊变坏死。此与病理上所观察到肿瘤易于出血坏死相吻合。增强后肿瘤明显强化，尤以动脉期明显。胰腺类癌属于富血供肿瘤，病理通常可见间质血管丰富，且易出血、坏死，但病理只能观察到类癌组织的一部分，而CT则能反映整个病灶的不均匀强化程度，因此，CT能更为全面地评价类癌组织的血供情况。

肿瘤血供丰富，其发生肝转移的概率相对较高，且转移瘤亦均表现富血供的特点。

比较影像学：超声、CT、MRI及内镜超声对胰腺类癌的诊断都有帮助，^{99m}Tc或^{111}In标记的生长抑素单光子发射计算机体层成像（SPECT）扫描可对80%类癌病灶定位。Perez-Fidalgo等（2006）认为^{18}氟代脱氧葡萄糖（^{18}F-FDG）PET评价胰腺类癌不如^{111}In-奥曲肽SPECT扫描。Orlefors等（2005）的研究表明，^{11}C-5-HTP PET检测神经内分泌肿瘤较敏感，尤其检测小病灶比SPECT、CT多，可见正电子核素标记的胺前体显像剂有望在胰腺类癌的诊断中发挥重要作用。

鉴别诊断：胰腺癌：胰腺癌多发生在胰头，肿块多呈等、低混合密度，境界不清，可出现“双管征”，由于绝大多数胰腺癌属于乏血供肿瘤，增强后强化程度通常低于正常胰实质，这些特点与胰腺类癌不同，再结合相关实验室检查可鉴别之；

囊腺瘤和囊腺癌：囊腺瘤和囊腺癌均以囊性成分为主，单囊或多囊，可见壁结节，囊腺癌实质部分较多时与类癌在平扫时不易鉴别，但其强化程度低于胰腺类癌，可区分。

胰腺实性假乳头状瘤：胰腺实性假乳头状瘤好发于胰腺体尾部，多为体积较大的囊实性肿块，有完整包膜，与胰腺类癌相似，但其钙化较常见，发生率约30%，且增强后动脉期通常仅轻度强化，门静脉期或延迟期强化更为明显，但仍低于正常胰实质强化程度，可作鉴别诊断。

无功能性胰岛细胞瘤：无功能性胰岛细胞瘤通常体积较大，境界清楚，密度不均匀，易囊变、坏死，增强后实质部分强化显著，胰腺类癌与其鉴别困难，需结合临床症状及相关血液学检查。

腹膜后脂肪肉瘤：腹膜后脂肪肉瘤CT表现为密度不均匀，边缘不清楚，呈浸润性生长的肿块，若病灶内见到脂肪密度可与本病鉴别。

第四节　胰腺神经内分泌肿瘤转移至肝脏和周围淋巴结

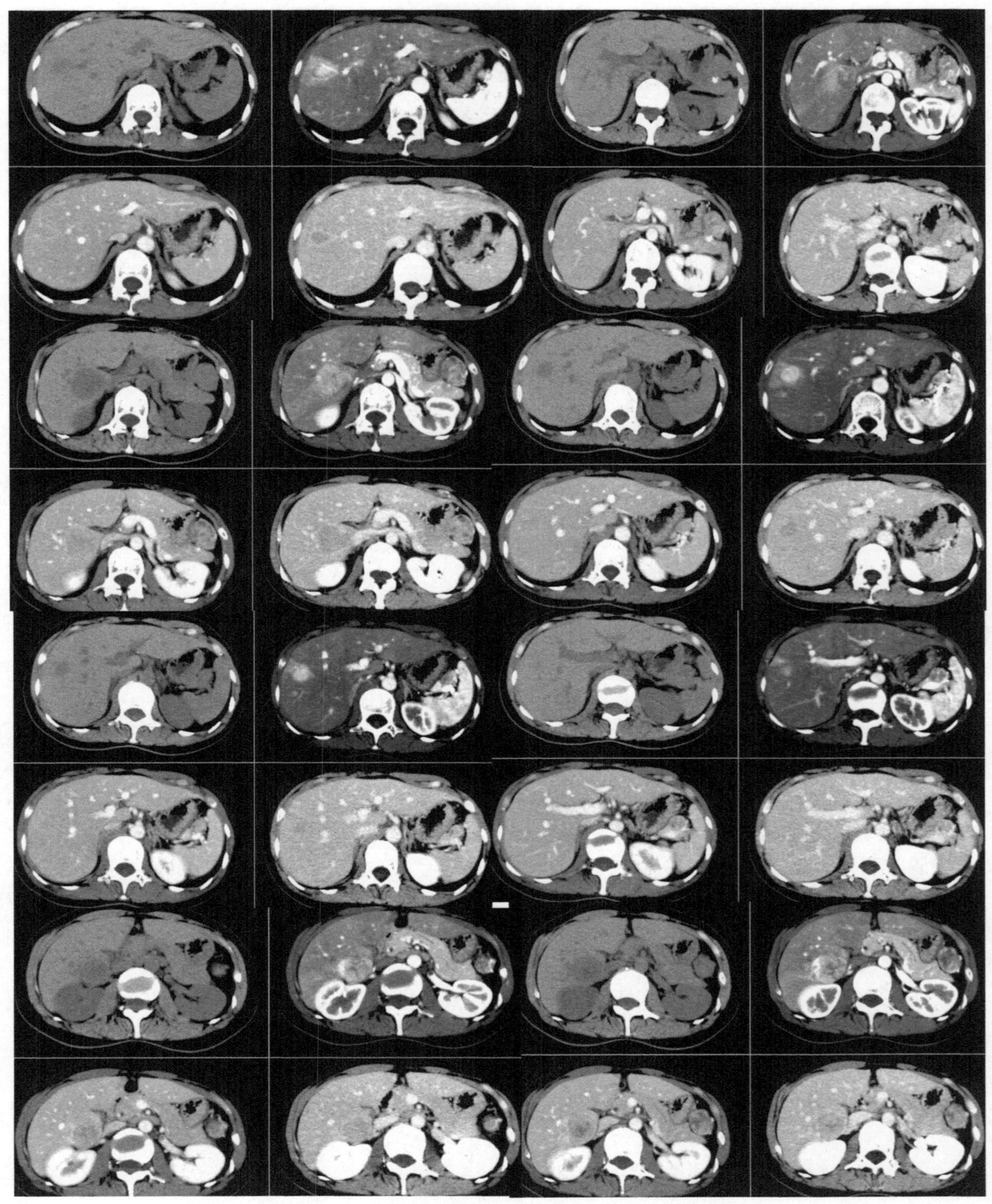

图 20-16-2　胰腺神经内分泌肿瘤转移至肝脏和周围淋巴结

患者，女，47 岁。体检发现肝占位 1 天入院。

手术所见：腹腔无腹水，胰体尾部及脾门可见 4 cm × 3 cm × 3 cm 结节状肿物，边界尚清，质中，脾动脉静脉与胰尾粘连紧密，无法游离。右肝近脏面可见一大小 4 cm × 3 cm 肿物，边界清楚，局部向外突出，术中彩超定位下可见肝右叶多个占位，脾脏及肠管未见异常。

手术名称：剖腹探查 + 胰尾肿物切除 + 脾切除 + 肝脏肿物活检 + 肝肿物射频消融手术。

病理检查：冰冻病理及常规病理：胰尾肿物及脾脏：切除标本一具，胰腺组织大小 6cm × 4cm × 2.7cm，切面见一结节样肿物，大小约 4cm × 2.5cm × 2.5cm，切面灰白灰褐伴出血，质中，肉眼观未侵及脾脏；脾脏大小 7.5cm × 5cm × 3cm，切面红褐，质中，未触及肿物；胰腺周围附有少量脂肪组织，检出淋巴结样物一枚，大小 1.8cm × 1.4cm × 0.7cm，切面灰褐，质中。冰冻病理诊断：胰尾肿物及脾脏切除标本：初步考虑胰腺内分泌肿瘤，其肿瘤性质、分类及分级待做常规石蜡切片及免疫组化检测进一步协助诊断，脾脏未见肿瘤组织累及。常规病理诊断：胰尾肿物及脾脏切除标本形态学符合神经内分泌肿瘤（G2 级）或肝细胞癌，待免疫组化进一步确诊；脾脏未见肿瘤累及；胰腺周围脂肪组织中检出淋巴结 1 枚，可见肿瘤转移（图 20-16-2）。

免疫组化检测：阳性：CK（P），Syn，CD56（大部分 +），CgA（散在 +），NSE，CK18，CK8，S-100，AACT（小灶 +），CK19（部分 +），CA19-9（散在 +），CD99（小灶 +），Ki-67（+，约 3%）；阴性：AAT，Vimentin，Hepatocyte，CD10，CD34，AFP，PAS 染色。免疫组化诊断：胰尾肿物及脾脏切除标本：胰腺神经内分泌肿瘤（NET，G2 级。核分裂数约 2~3/10HPF，增值指数约 3%），切缘阴性。肿瘤转移至肝脏和周围淋巴结，脉管内未见癌栓，神经未见累及。

胰腺神经内分泌肿瘤的 G 分类：1 级（grade 1，G1）肿瘤细胞增殖率低，是典型的分化良好的肿瘤；3 级（grade 3，G 3）肿瘤细胞增殖率高，是典型的分化差的癌。2 级（grade 2，G2）肿瘤的临床和预后方面有两面性：在没有恶性依据的肿瘤，G2 可能提示复发风险增加，需要密切随访；在恶性肿瘤，G2 可能提示生物学行为更具侵袭性，需要更激进的治疗方案。所有胰腺神经内分泌肿瘤均具潜在恶性，但区别在于侵袭性行为或转移的可能性不同，且胰腺神经内分泌肿瘤的 G 分类与患者生存期密切相关（图 20-16-2）。

第十七章 胰腺其他恶性肿瘤

第一节 胰腺单发转移瘤与胰腺癌的CT鉴别诊断

胰腺转移性肿瘤在临床上少见,其CT表现形式主要有三种:单发结节型、多结节型及胰腺弥漫增大型,其中以单结节型最为多见,术前最易误诊为原发胰腺癌。

胰腺单发转移瘤与原发胰腺癌的影像学表现存在差异,仔细分析其影像特征大多可作出正确诊断。

胰腺单发转移瘤与原发胰腺癌的影像学表现有较多相似之处,也有各自的特征性。一般认为以下几方面可作为胰腺单发转移瘤与原发胰腺癌的CT鉴别诊断要点:

(1)好发部位:胰腺单发转移瘤可发生于胰腺的任何部位,无明显好发倾向;胰腺癌60%~70%发生于头部,其次为体部、尾部或者头体部。

(2)病灶边缘是否清晰:胰腺单发转移瘤多为圆形、类圆形,部分为不规则形,绝大部分边缘清晰规则;胰腺癌多以浸润性生长方式向周围扩展使其形态多不规则,边界不清。

(3)周围血管有否侵犯:胰腺癌常常侵犯周围血管,而胰腺转移瘤周围血管侵犯非常少见,一组13例胰腺单发转移瘤无一例周围血管侵犯。Klein等(1998)报道胰腺转移瘤66例,仅2例见周围血管脂肪侵犯,且原发肿瘤均为乳腺癌。

(4)胆胰管有否扩张:该组13例胰腺转移瘤中,仅有3例合并胰管及胆管轻度扩张,而其余10例未见此征象,与原发胰腺癌的CT表现有明显差异。这可能是癌组织起源及病灶部位不同所致。

(5)胰腺癌大多起源于胰腺导管上皮细胞,具有围管性浸润的重要生物学特征,因而容易阻塞胰管,使胰管扩张;胰头癌常侵及胆总管的胰内段,使梗阻近端的胆总管、胆管及胆囊扩张。而转移瘤是原发癌细胞脱落后通过血行或淋巴道转移至胰腺,并非起源胰管,其肿瘤组织虽可侵犯胰腺导管上皮,但其发生率较低。

(6)胰腺萎缩:胰腺癌肿瘤组织侵犯胰腺及胰管后,肿瘤远端由于血供和排泄受阻导致胰体、胰尾萎缩;而胰腺转移瘤组,因胰管及血管累及少,胰腺体尾部萎缩比率小。

(7)密度与强化方式:胰腺癌与转移瘤都可导致胰腺外形变化,胰腺内肿块多表现为低或等密度,也可为高密度,两者无明显差异。增强扫描胰腺单发转移瘤因原发肿瘤不同有多种不同强化方式。相对具有特征性的是肾癌转移,因其为富血供肿瘤而强化明显。胰腺癌均呈低密度表现,部分病灶边缘为规则或不规则强化,反之正常胰腺强化明显且密度均匀,致使肿瘤轮廓、形态显示更清楚。

(8)胰腺单发转移瘤虽具有一定影像特征,但仍有部分与原发胰腺癌表现相仿,影像鉴别困难,此时结合临床非常重要。

患者若有原发肿瘤病史,则高度提示转移瘤诊断。发生胰腺转移的常见肿瘤有肺癌、结肠癌、乳腺癌、肾癌及胃癌等。有关原发肿瘤发病率的报道并不一致,Klein等(1998)报道按发病率高低依次为肾癌、肺癌、乳腺癌。Merkle等(1998)报道依次为肺癌、乳腺癌和肾癌,但也有文献报道胃癌和肺癌最多见。肺癌中又以小细胞肺癌最多。

在原发胰腺癌中,肿瘤标志物CA19-9阳性率达80%~90%,而转移性胰腺癌中,CA199多在正常范围内。因此,检测CA19-9对于鉴别胰腺转移和原发肿瘤具有一定的意义。

总之,胰腺单发转移瘤具有一定的影像学特征,综合分析病灶形态边缘、有无周围血管侵犯及有无胰管、胆管扩张等继发征象有助于与原发胰腺癌鉴别。而临床肿瘤病史及生化检查对两者鉴别诊断具有重要提示意义，但最终确诊仍需穿刺活检或手术病理检查。

第二节　误诊病例简介：肾癌胰腺转移瘤

胰腺转移瘤少见，原发肿瘤主要来源于肺、胃肠道、肾脏、乳腺和皮肤（黑色素瘤）。有关原发肿瘤中各种类型肿瘤发病率报道并不一致。一些报道肾癌发生胰腺转移的较多。

胰腺转移瘤患者可以出现消化道出血，腹部疼痛、阻塞性黄疸、体重下降、胰腺内分泌功能异常等症状，但肾癌的胰腺转移瘤患者约 50% 无症状，诊断很困难。肾癌手术切除后到发现胰腺转移的时间很长，有报道间隔时间在 10 年或 10 年以上。

不同组织来源肿瘤的胰腺转移瘤 CT 表现不尽相同。肾癌的胰腺转移肿块常表现为富血供，均匀强化或边缘强化，这种强化方式反映了肾癌的多血供特点，与少血供、不强化的胰腺癌肿块容易鉴别。

肾癌胰腺转移瘤与无功能胰岛细胞瘤较难鉴别，两者都可以单发或多发，它们的增强特点相同，都是富血供，当肿瘤长大到一定程度时，中心易发生坏死或囊变。

该例病灶多发，CT 增强动脉期显示 4 枚结节直径 1cm 左右，境界清，3 枚均匀强化，1 枚呈环形强化，从 CT 图像上很难鉴别转移瘤与胰岛细胞瘤，此时病史很重要，患者既往有肾癌手术史，术前应该首先考虑转移，但是，由于病灶多发，术前诊断为多发性胰腺神经内分泌肿瘤。

总之，有肾癌病史、动脉期胰腺内多发明显强化结节影者宜首先考虑肾癌胰腺转移。

第三节　胰腺巨大非霍奇金 B 细胞淋巴瘤，倾向 Burkitt 淋巴瘤

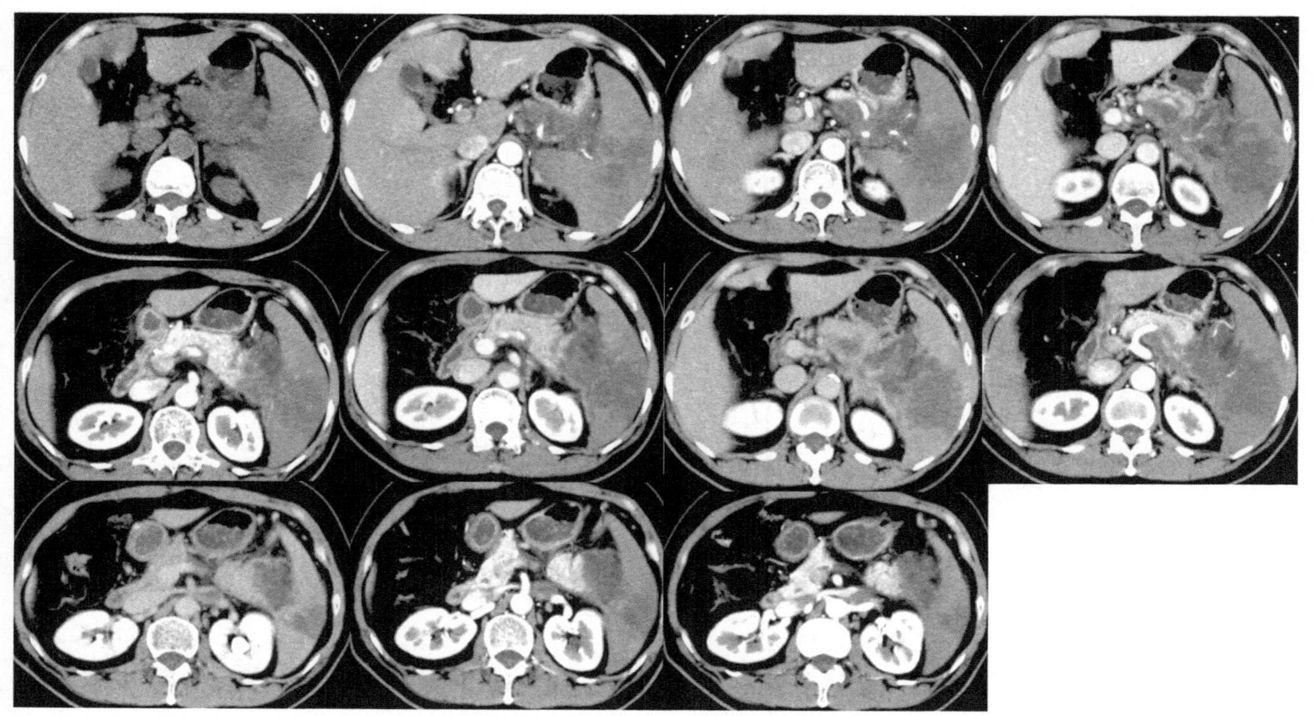

图 20-17-1　胰腺巨大非霍奇金 B 细胞淋巴瘤，倾向 Burkitt 淋巴瘤

患者,女,67岁。术后病理免疫组化诊断:胰腺巨大非霍奇金B细胞淋巴瘤,倾向Burkitt淋巴瘤,可见坏死及脉管内瘤栓,肿瘤侵及脾脏。

从发病率来看,脾脏淋巴瘤似乎远比胰腺原发性淋巴瘤多见,该病例可能是脾脏淋巴瘤侵犯胰腺,多为胰腺继发性淋巴瘤(图20-17-1)。

第四节 胰腺转移瘤

胰腺转移瘤较少见。近年来由于MSCT技术的发展,胰腺转移瘤的检出率较前有大幅度的提高;而放化疗的进展,使晚期患者的生存时间相对延长,亦使胰腺转移的发生较前增多。因此,提高胰腺转移瘤诊断的准确性对治疗和预后有着重要意义。

恶性肿瘤患者尸检发现1.6%~11.0%伴有胰腺转移;而胰腺恶性占位性病变中2%~5%为胰腺转移瘤。发生胰腺转移的常见肿瘤为肾细胞癌、肺癌、胃癌、乳腺癌和结直肠癌,其次为恶性黑色素瘤和平滑肌肉瘤。

一组56例资料显示,最常见的原发肿瘤为肺癌和胃癌。在肺癌中,又以小细胞肺癌居多(78.6%),这可能是因为小细胞肺癌恶性程度较高,易通过血行转移播散的原因。胃癌发生胰腺转移的概率高可能与位置毗邻有关。

胰腺转移瘤可以侵犯导管上皮细胞而被误诊为胰腺癌,也可造成急性胰腺炎,导致患者症状各异且不典型,如腹痛、背痛、恶心、黄疸、黑便、上消化道出血及体重下降等。但也有部分患者无症状。该项研究中,反复上腹痛或上腹不适者最多见(55.4%),背痛和黄疸各占7. 1%。在部分临床表现为腹痛、恶心的患者中,可见胰头部转移灶及显著扩张的胰管。

胰腺转移瘤可发生于胰腺任何部位,在胰头、体、尾部的分布无显著差异。其形态主要有3种表现:最常见者为局限性单发结节灶,实性居多,边界清晰;其次是多发结节;第三是弥漫性病变。Klein等(1998)发现3种形态所占比例分别为78.8%、16.7%和4.5%,该项研究结果与此接近,分别为67.9%、21. 4%和3.5%。

除以上3种类型外,该项研究结果显示部分胰腺转移瘤为囊性病灶,即囊性转移。表现为囊变的4例胰腺转移瘤中,3例原发灶为肺鳞癌,1例为卵巢囊腺癌,提示囊性胰腺转移的发生与原发肿瘤的囊性成分和肿瘤易坏死有关。

该项研究中,仅有8例(14.3%)合并胰管扩张,且病灶大部分位于胰头部,这可能与肿瘤的位置及邻近转移淋巴结压迫胰管所致。胰腺癌起源于胰腺导管上皮细胞,很容易引发胰腺导管中梗阻、扩张。而转移瘤是原发肿瘤通过血行或淋巴道转移至胰腺,其肿瘤细胞并非起源于胰管上皮,一般不造成胰管扩张,除非转移瘤浸润到胰导管上皮细胞或位于胰头的病灶压迫胆总管可引起胰管扩张。

胰腺癌多伴外侵,周围脂肪密度增高,可见条索影,并常累及周围血管;胰腺转移瘤大部分边界清晰,周围脂肪间隙存在,很少侵犯包膜外。该项研究中56例仅有2例侵犯胰腺周围血管,因此是否侵犯周围血管是两者重要的鉴别点之一。少数胰腺转移瘤伴外侵,周围脂肪间隙模糊,可伴有脾梗死,与胰腺癌鉴别困难。

来源于胃或结肠黏液腺癌的胰腺转移瘤可伴有钙化,可能与原发灶病理类型有关。

该项研究为三期扫描,发现在增强早期(25 s左右)病灶显示最清楚,门静脉期或延迟期部分病灶略呈等密度,因此多期扫描对于诊断胰腺转移瘤有重要价值。胰腺转移瘤的强化表现可为囊变(无强化)、轻度强化、环形强化或显著强化,其强化方式主要与原发肿瘤类型及血供有关,如表现为显著强化的4例均来源于肾癌。

胰腺转移瘤的强化方式与大小有关,直径<2 cm者以轻度均匀强化为主,而>2 cm的病灶以环形强化为主,可能是随病灶体积增大,血供不足致肿瘤坏死所致。该项有12例为环形强化,其中8例直径>2cm。如有原发肿瘤病史,病变无显著强化,应高度怀疑胰腺转移瘤。如增强扫描病变显著强化,同时有肾癌病史,应高度怀疑为胰腺转移瘤,但同时需排除胰岛神经内分泌肿瘤、胰内副脾、动静脉瘘、脾动脉的微动脉瘤等富血供病变。在诊断困难的情况下,经皮穿刺活检往往是有意义的检查方法。

不同种类的原发肿瘤发生胰腺转移的间隔时间差别很大,肺癌多为同时发现转移灶;而肾癌发生胰腺转移的间隔时间最长,有文献报道其中位间隔时间为9.1年。该组中间隔时间最长者为1例肾透明细胞癌患者（术后 8 年）发生胰腺转移瘤。

胰腺转移瘤多发生于肿瘤患者的晚期，该组资料显示，发生胰腺转移瘤时，85.7%（48/56）已发生其他部位或多部位转移，仅有 14.3%（8/56）未发现其他部位转移。一旦发现胰腺转移瘤，常提示已处于晚期，预后较差。但对极少数患者，手术切除可以取得良好的效果。

总之，胰腺转移瘤 MSCT 表现有一定的特征性：常表现为胰腺单发或多发结节，为圆形或椭圆形，边缘较清晰，少有胰腺实质外侵犯和胰周血管受累，增强扫描常为乏血供，肺鳞癌和卵巢癌可表现为囊性转移，肾癌胰腺转移为富血供。

结合病史，大多数可与胰腺癌鉴别，对临床治疗方案的选择有重要意义。

第五节　误诊病例简介：起源于胰腺的孤立性纤维瘤

孤立性纤维瘤属于成纤维细胞 / 肌成纤维细胞来源的中间型肿瘤（偶尔有转移），是一种罕见的软组织肿瘤。孤立性纤维瘤最初曾被认为仅起源于脏层胸膜的间皮细胞，目前普遍性的观点认为孤立性纤维瘤是一种可以发生于全身任何部位的肿瘤，除胸膜腔以外，好发于头颈部、纵隔、腹腔后、盆腔、腹腔等，其他如脑膜、肝脏也有报道，源于胰腺的孤立性纤维瘤少见报道。

孤立性纤维瘤组织学表现为无异型的梭形细胞肿瘤无定向排列，细胞密度分布不均，细胞密集区及疏松区（后者含丰富的胶原纤维）间隔分布，并可见灶性分布的血管外皮瘤样结构，但目前发现其他许多良恶性肿瘤包括孤立性纤维瘤都具有“鹿角状”分支血管这种组织学构象。免疫表型显示肿瘤细胞 CD34、Vimentin 弥漫性阳性，CD99、bcl-2 也可显示阳性。

血管外皮瘤肿瘤细胞呈梭形，经典的血管外皮瘤血管丰富，具有特征性不规则分支状血管 - 鹿角状血管，免疫表型：Vimentin 阳性，CD34 阴性、局灶性阳性或仅表现为血管阳性，血管外皮瘤 / 孤立性纤维瘤均属于成纤维细胞 / 肌成纤维细胞来源肿瘤的中间性肿瘤，两者在病理及组织学方面重叠表现很多。WHO（2002）软组织肿瘤中两者并列提出视为同一起源的肿瘤。有部分学者认为处于免疫表型极端的肿瘤可做出定性诊断（即 CD34 弥漫性阳性、血管外皮瘤样结构灶性分布为孤立性纤维瘤，血管外皮瘤样结构弥漫分布、CD34 灶性、阴性或仅血管阳性为血管外皮瘤）。

鉴别诊断：起源于胰腺的孤立性纤维瘤罕见报道，该例主要与胰腺癌鉴别。胰腺癌 90% 以上 CA19-9 含量明显升高，因其含有较多纤维间质以及周围供血小动脉内膜增生导致其血管腔变窄，上述原因可能导致胰腺癌为乏血供的病理学基础。该例增强扫描动脉期即可见肿瘤内结节明显强化，强化幅度与周围正常胰腺实质强化幅度相似，并有延迟强化的趋势，而胰腺癌因其乏血供的特征，动脉期强化幅度明显低于胰腺实质，此点有助于两者的鉴别，但此为个案尚无统计学意义。

因胰腺癌及孤立性纤维瘤实质内均可含有较丰富的纤维间质而影响对比剂的廓清，均可出现延迟强化。推测延迟强化征象只可减小胰腺肿瘤的鉴别诊断范围，对肿瘤定性价值有限。

总之，原发于胰腺的孤立性纤维瘤极其罕见，如胰腺发现肿瘤，实验室检查 CA19-9 不高，增强扫描肿瘤实质于动脉期明显强化且有延迟强化的特点，应想到本病的可能，确诊仍依赖于病理及免疫组化。

第十八章 胰腺其他包块

第一节 误诊病例简介:胰腺结核与胰腺癌

胰腺结核十分少见。临床表现及影像学征象不具有特征性,常误诊为胰腺肿瘤、慢性胰腺炎等疾病,其原因可能是胰酶影响结核分枝杆菌在胰腺着床,然而当结核杆菌突破了这道防线,就可以引起感染。腹部结核常累及脾、肝脏和结肠等器官,很少单独侵及胰腺, Bhansali(1977)报道在300例腹部结核中未发现一例, Auerbach(1994)报道297例死于播散性结核尸检结果,胰腺受累率为4.7%, Paraf等(1969)在一组526例播散性结核的尸检中,发现胰腺或胰周受累仅有11例。近年来有关胰腺结核的报道有所增加,与结核菌耐药性和各种免疫缺陷人群(如获得性免疫缺陷综合征和器官移植患者)的增多有关。一组2例均无其他脏器结核的临床表现。

临床表现:胰腺结核起病缓慢而隐匿,病程大多较长,临床症状和体征均无特异性,该组例1有腹痛、恶心、呕吐、消瘦、乏力症状,同时因为病灶阻塞胰管,胰管扩张,血、尿淀粉酶升高,临床有伴发急性胰腺炎的表现。例2因病灶阻塞胆管,引起间接胆红素升高,出现黄疸。实验室检查无特异性。

影像学研究:CT主要表现为胰腺本身病灶及胰外病变两个方面。

胰腺病灶的表现:胰腺结核好发于胰头部,体尾部也可发生,亦可累及整个胰腺,其影像表现与病理相对应,可表现为胰腺局灶性肿块、多发结节病灶、胰腺弥漫性增大。局灶性病变表现为位于胰腺的低密度肿块(干酪型或增殖病灶),当部分液化时则表现为囊实性肿块,完全液化时为囊性病变,常有多数分隔,坏死、液化区无强化,增殖病灶可有轻度强化,一般低于周围正常胰腺实质及病灶周边强化。

该组2例均发生在胰头,为局灶性病变,仅例1行CT检查,胰头部病灶为增殖性病灶,动脉期扫描无强化,门静脉期有轻度强化,但低于周围正常胰腺组织。

胰外表现最常见的是淋巴结肿大。可发生在胰周、肠系膜、肝门部、脾门等部位,可部分融合成团达数厘米。CT平扫为低密度结节灶,增强扫描为均匀的环状强化,伴有中央轻度强化或无强化为其特征, Pombo等(1998)报道6例中有5例为环状强化。

肿大淋巴结表现为轻度强化的结节可能为增殖性病灶,部分患者淋巴结可出现钙化,特别是病程长或经过抗结核治疗者。该组例1动脉期表现为淋巴结环状强化,门静脉期病灶内强化不均匀,与文献报道相同。2例均无腹部其他脏器结核的表现。

胰腺结核的MRI表现,也有胰腺本身和胰外结核两种表现,胰腺本身结核多发生于胰头部,属于慢性炎症,有作者报道应用磁共振VIBE序列鉴别胰腺癌与肿块型胰腺炎,肿块性胰腺炎的磁共振VIBE序列表现:边界不清、散在分布、信号混杂不均,容易出现T_2WI高信号、T_1WI低信号,可出现胰管穿通征,不容易侵犯周围血管。

该组例1患者, MR平扫为胰头部等低混杂T_1WI信号、等高混杂T_2WI信号的病灶,边界不清,增强扫描无明显强化,未累及周围血管。VIBE序列三期扫描,动脉早晚期,肿块强化不明显,其内信号不均。门静脉期病灶不均匀强化,可见胰管穿通征,与肠系膜上静脉之间的细小脂肪间隙存在。病理报道以增殖性病灶为主,并少许干酪样坏死,MRI表现与病理结果一致。

例2患者, MR平扫为胰头部长T_1、长T_2信号的病灶,边界不清,增强扫描无明显强化,未累及周围血管。VIBE序列三期扫描,动脉早期,肿块强化不明显。动脉晚期：肿块边缘轻度强化，其内信号不均匀，并可见细小分隔。门静脉期：肿块内细小分隔及边缘轻度强化，肠系膜上静脉之间的细小脂肪间隙存在。病理见干酪样坏死，周围包绕上皮肉芽组织，其中见郎格汉斯巨细胞。MRI 表现与病理吻合。

胰外表现主要为门腔间隙的淋巴结增大，MRI 的表现平扫为等低混杂信号，增强为环状强化，其内信号不均，与 CT 增强相似，但 VIBE 更能显示其内结构和成分，可以鉴别淋巴结内有无干酪样坏死。

有文献报道，运用 PET/CT 对 FDG 的吸收来评价胰腺的肿瘤，但是，FDG 并不是肿瘤的特异吸收试剂，肺结核患者对 FDG 的吸收也很敏感。PET/CT 被用于区别胰腺的结核和肿瘤，敏感性和特异性分别为 88%~94% 和 83%~88%，但对该组例 1 患者是失败的。该组仅例 1 行 PET/CT 检查，例 1 PET 显像见上腹部正中偏右局限性摄取 FDG 明显异常增高灶，呈团块状，最大 SUV 值为 14.9，同时 CT 定位于胰头后份软组织区占位，形态不规则，大小约 4.5 cm × 3.1 cm × 6.0cm。与胰体间似有包膜分隔，2 h 后延迟显像，见该病灶摄取 FDG 增加，最大 SUV 值为 15.9。PET/CT 融合图像考虑恶性肿瘤可能性大。

诊断评价及限度：胰腺结核鉴别诊断困难，主要由于临床表现与放射学检查均缺乏特异性，而且往往容易被 B 超和 CT 误诊为胰腺癌。该组 2 例均误诊为胰腺癌，可能的原因是：临床表现和实验室检查均无特异性。CT、MR 及 PET/CT 均高度怀疑胰腺恶性肿瘤，缺乏胰腺结核的影像学特异性。胰腺结核合并胰腺外结核较少，造成诊断困难。

但是从 MR 的 VIBE 序列三期扫描的表现与病理对照仍然有一定联系，可作为鉴别诊断的参考：病灶分界不清，强化不均匀；病灶很大时仍然很少累及血管；胰管穿通征；病灶内有分隔，边缘与分隔可同时强化；腹腔内有淋巴结增大，增强有明显环状强化。

具有以上征象，提示胰腺慢性感染可能性大。同时结合年龄，可以除外胰腺癌可能，该组例 1 患者为男性，18 岁。有报道胰腺癌极少发病在 40 岁以前。

但是，结核的不同时期，病理表现不同，鉴别仍然有一定的限度，对于不能确诊者，而且合并有胰管或胆管梗阻者，应及时行手术治疗，并做病理检查。对明确诊断者，正规抗结核治疗 6 个月以上可有明显的疗效。

第二节　假肿瘤性慢性胰腺炎

详见本书 本卷 本篇 第九章 第一节 假肿瘤性慢性胰腺炎。

第三节　误诊病例简介:胰头神经鞘瘤与胰头癌

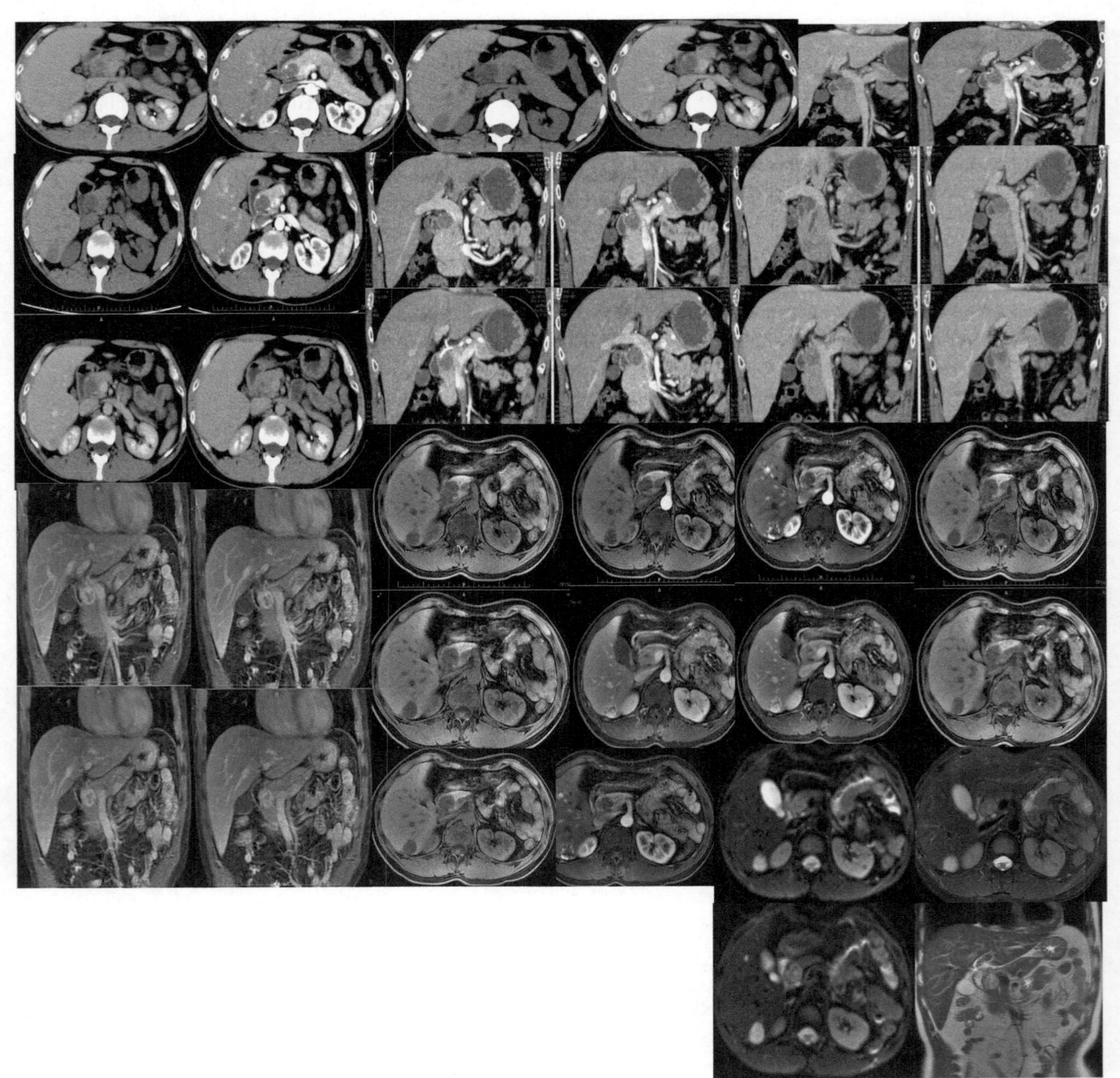

图 20-18-1　胰头神经鞘瘤与胰头癌

病例,男, 43 岁。患者于 1 个月前在外院体检时发现胰头占位性病变,无腹痛、腹胀,无黄疸等不适,近 10 天反复出现脐周闷胀不适,无腹痛,大便正常。近日在我院再次行肝胆胰脾 CT 平扫 + 增强检查示:右肝多发血管瘤;双肾多发错构瘤;胰头区占位。今门诊以"胰腺瘤"收住入院。CT 诊断:右肝多发血管瘤;双肾多发错构瘤;胰头区占位,性质待定,建议 MRI 平扫 + 增强扫描。MRI:诊断:胰头占位,考虑胰腺癌;肝右叶多发血管瘤;左肾多发错构瘤。

手术所见:决定行胰头肿物切除术 + 胆囊切除术。病理检查:胰头肿物切除标本:结节样肿物一个,大小 2.5cm × 2cm × 1.5cm，切面灰黄，质中，包膜完整。胆总管旁淋巴结：灰红色组织一块，大小 3cm × 1.5cm × 0.4cm，切面灰白，质中。常规病理诊断：胰头肿物切除标本：初步诊断良性梭形细胞肿瘤，考虑为神经鞘瘤。胆总管旁淋巴结切除标本：检出淋巴结 3 枚，镜下见淋巴细胞呈反应性增生，待做免疫组化检测进一步证实。免疫组化检测：阳性：CD3（T 细胞 +），CD45RO（T 细胞 +），CD5（T 细胞 +），CD20（B 细胞 +），CD79α（B 细胞 +），Kappa 链（散在 +），Lambda 链（散在 +），CD35（树突细胞网 +），CD21（树突细胞网 +），CyclinD1（个别 +），Bcl-2，Ki-67（+，约 10%，主要集中于滤泡生发中心）阴性：CK（P）。免疫组化诊断：胰头肿物切除标本：胰头神经鞘瘤。胆总管旁淋巴结切除标本：慢性淋巴结炎，淋巴细胞呈反应性增生。

误诊分析：腹部的神经鞘瘤以腹膜后发生者居多，发生于内脏者罕见，其中较常见的部位是胃肠道，而胰腺则是这种肿瘤的一个特别少见的发生部位；恶性神经鞘瘤不能与常见的胰腺癌鉴别。本例肿瘤位于胰头，其轮廓规则、包膜完整，主胰管和胆总管均无扩张表现。平扫 MRI 虽不具特征性表现，但 T_1WI 动态增强晚期不均匀增强，因此应当考虑为乏血供性的神经源性肿瘤（图 20-18-1）。

第四节　误诊病例简介：胰腺内异位副脾

副脾是胚胎第 5 周时位于胃背系膜中的脾芽融合失败所致，为位于正常脾脏之外，与正常脾脏结构相似、功能相同的组织，其发生率约为 10%~30%，其中约 16.8% 位于胰尾部。

但胰腺内异位副脾的影像学报道较少，且易误诊为其他胰腺肿瘤而进行不必要的活检或手术。因此，认识胰腺内异位副脾的影像学特征非常重要。

病理学：大体标本上胰腺内异位副脾一般呈暗红色，周围有纤维组织构成的包膜与邻近的胰腺组织相隔。在组织学上胰腺内异位副脾与正常脾脏结构相似，也含有红髓及白髓，红髓由脾索和脾血窦组成，动脉周围淋巴鞘、淋巴小结和边缘区构成白髓。

与正常脾脏相比，胰腺内异位副脾的间质成分较为丰富，内含一些胰腺腺泡、胰岛及细小导管；某些区域胰腺内异位副脾与邻近胰腺组织的界限较薄或模糊，部分与胰腺组织混合，甚至在胰腺内异位副脾中心可见胰腺组织。

临床表现：据报道男性中胰腺内异位副脾较女性为多，约为后者的 2.7 倍；患者的平均年龄约 40.8 岁；一般无明显临床症状，多因体检发现或其他疾病检查时发现。实验室检查多在正常范围，部分胰腺内副脾表皮样囊肿患者的血清糖链抗原 CA19-9 升高。

影像学研究：胰腺内异位副脾一般为圆形、卵圆形的单发的实质性肿块，边界清晰，其直径一般为 1~2.5 cm 之间，亦有 >4 cm 的报道。当有血液系统疾病或其他疾病时如白血病、淋巴瘤、血小板减少等，脾脏体积会相应增大，而胰腺内异位副脾的大小也会有相应改变。

胰腺内异位副脾中，副脾基本均位于或非常接近胰腺尾部尖端处，一般距胰腺尾部尖端 3cm 之内。多数情况下，胰腺内异位副脾一部分被周围胰腺组织包绕，一部分位于胰腺表面，被胰周脂肪组织包绕，且多凸向胰腺背侧生长。而较小的胰腺内异位副脾则可能完全被胰腺包绕，但这些小胰腺内异位副脾在影像学上容易漏诊。

CT 扫描表现：胰腺内异位副脾多表现为胰尾部类圆形软组织肿块影，其 CT 平扫密度与脾脏相似。在动态增强 CT 扫描各期，胰腺内异位副脾的强化程度与强化方式均与脾脏相似，且密度均高于胰腺。动脉期胰腺内异位副脾多表现为不均匀强化，这可能是因为红白髓内的血流速度不一致所致，这与脾脏的“花斑样”强化表现相似。胰腺内异位副脾也可表现为均匀强化，特别是当胰腺内异位副脾体积较小时。门静脉期胰腺内异位副脾表现为均匀强化，且与脾脏强化程度一致。

Miyayama 等（2003）学者对 3 例患者行 CT 动脉造影（CTA）时发现 CT 增强扫描过程中表现为均匀强化的胰腺内异位副脾，在 CTA 上早期亦可表现为不均匀强化（注入对比剂后 13s 左右），而在后期则表现为均匀强化（注入对比剂后 24s 左右）；另外还发现在胰腺内异位副脾与其周围的胰腺组织间存在一裂隙样结构，提示病变来自胰外。

误诊分析：该组两名患者均为男性，年龄均高于文献报道的平均年龄，其中 1 例因体检发现，另 1 例因贫血入院检查时发现，均未出现与胰腺内异位副脾相关的临床症状；二者的肿瘤标志物均在正常范围。该组两例胰腺内异位副脾均位于胰尾部，例 1

距胰腺尾部尖端约 0.5 cm,例 2 位于胰腺尾部尖端,均为边界清楚的单发实质性肿块,且凸向胰尾背侧生长,与文献报道一致,但所见胰腺内异位副脾体积均较大,其中第 2 例可能与脾脏切除后副脾代偿性功能亢进有关。

病例 1 中胰腺内异位副脾的 CT 表现非常典型,动脉期为不均匀强化,门静脉期均匀强化,强化程度与强化方式均与脾脏一致,且密度高于邻近胰腺;但仍误诊为胰尾部肿瘤性病变,这可能是因为对胰腺内异位副脾的典型 CT 表现认识不足所致。

而病例 2 中胰腺内异位副脾在动脉期表现为轻度均匀强化,密度低于胰腺,这与 CT 典型表现不一致;且国内外文献较少见胰腺内异位副脾增强 CT 扫描时密度低于邻近胰腺的报道,仅见 1 例相关报道,该组作者认为这可能与肝硬化致脾脏增强延迟有关;另外,患者年龄较大且病情复杂,以贫血为突出表现,故虽然患者肿瘤标志物正常范围而仍误诊为胰尾部肿瘤而行手术治疗。

因此,当胰尾部出现圆形或卵圆形、单发、边界清晰的实质性肿块,位于胰腺尾部尖端或非常接近胰腺尾部尖端处,在 CT 增强扫描各期其强化程度与强化方式均与脾脏相似时,需考虑胰腺内异位副脾这一诊断。

若诊断存在疑问,可进一步行其他影像学检查,如超顺磁性氧化铁(SPIO)增强 MRI 扫描。SPIO 进入体内后易被网状内皮细胞识别并吞噬,而肝窦及脾脏均富含网状内皮细胞,故 SPIO 易聚集于肝、脾内,致肝、脾的 T_2 弛豫时间显著缩短和信号丢失,T_2WI 上信号明显下降,且胰腺内异位副脾的信号下降程度与脾脏相似;^{99m}Tc- 热变性红细胞显像(^{99m}Tc-HDRBC 显像):脾组织,包括胰腺内异位副脾可选择性自循环系统清除衰老、变性的红细胞,对 ^{99m}Tc-HDRBC 的摄取率可达 90%,可达到选择性脾显像的目的;这几种检查方法均有助于确诊。

胰腺内异位副脾常没有明显的临床症状且不需要手术等特殊处理,因此,需正确认识其影像学表现而避免不必要的活检甚至手术。位于胰腺尾部尖端或非常接近胰腺尾部尖端处的单发的圆形或卵圆形、边界清晰的实质性肿块,在 CT 增强扫描各期其强化程度与强化方式均与脾脏相似,增强扫描早期表现为不均匀强化等特征均有助于胰腺内异位副脾的诊断。若诊断存在疑问时可行 SPIO-MRI 增强扫描或 ^{99m}Tc-HDRBC 显像确诊。

第五节 胰腺的假性肿瘤

肠袢伪似胰腺肿瘤:Churchill 等(1978)指出,在 CT 图像上,未为造影剂充盈的小肠肠袢可伪似胰腺包块,此类肠袢可表现为胰体或胰尾区域的边缘不清楚的软组织密度块影。经口服造影剂使该肠袢充盈后再行 CT 扫描,则可证实该假包块实为肠袢引起。在胰腺疾病的影像诊断方法中,超声作用巨大,然而,对于胰尾的病变的诊断却因为左半结肠脾曲的关系而变得复杂起来。Berger 等(1977)报告 3 例超声诊断的胰尾明显肿块,以后证实均为充满粪便的结肠所造成,它们正好位于左肾及胰尾的前面。

扩张而充满液体的胃类似左上腹包块:胃排空障碍的病人,或在超声检查前病人曾饮入大量液态食物,可造成胃充盈而又扩大,超声检查时可伪似左上腹的囊性包块。但是,细心观察可以发现,此结构有蠕动可见,而识别出是胃。有时还必须再吞服一杯水,以显示胃内的微小气泡的旋涡,这是一种区别扩张装满液体的胃与胰腺假性囊肿的较好方法。

第六节　误诊病例简介：脾脏破裂伴出血，胰体尾部及胃后壁之间侵袭性纤维瘤病

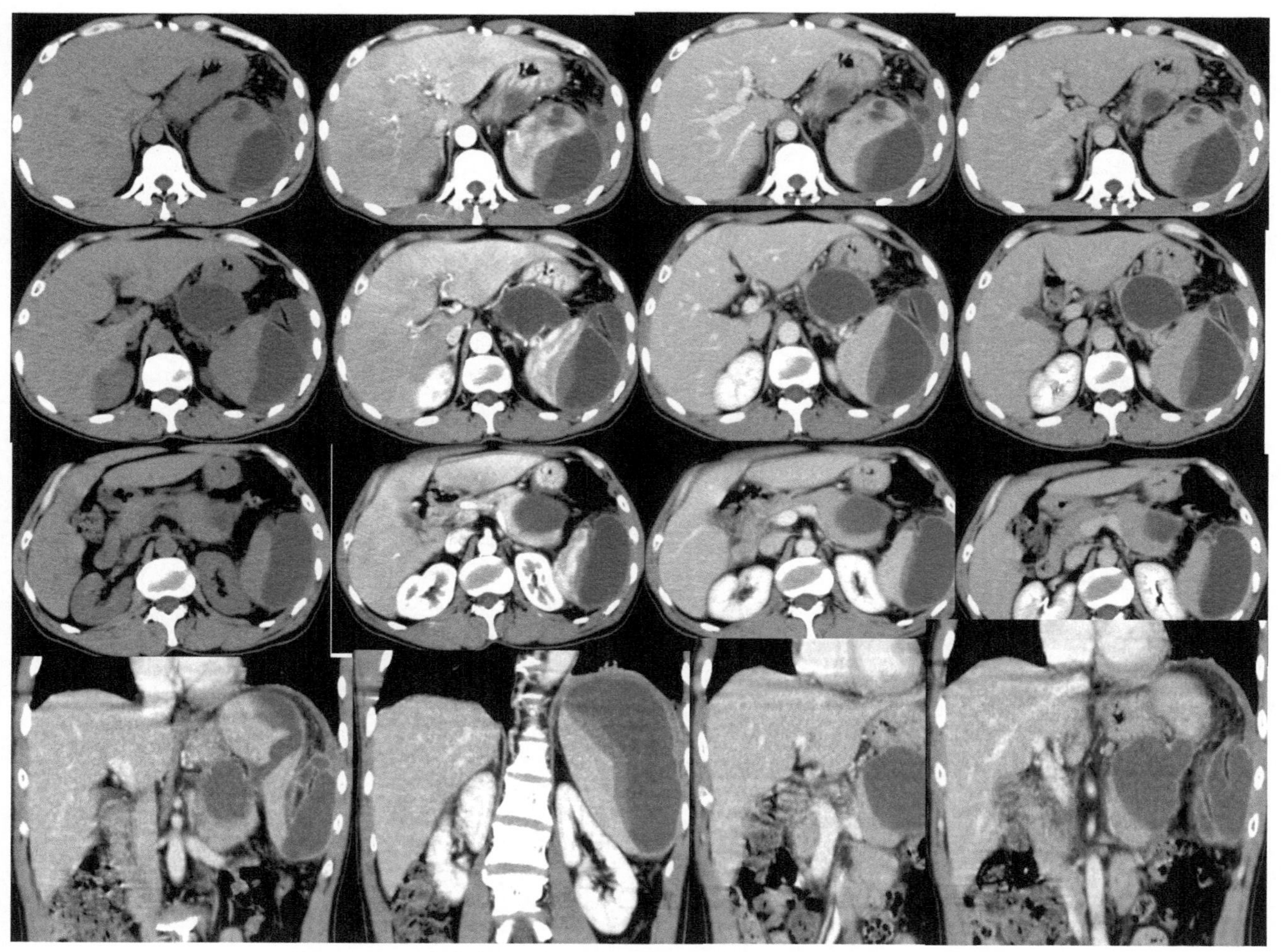

图 20-18-2　脾脏破裂伴出血，胰体尾部及胃后壁之间侵袭性纤维瘤病

患者，男，46 岁。无明显诱因出现左腹疼痛一年。

CT 诊断：胰尾部及脾脏囊性占位，胰腺假性囊肿及脾包膜下积液可能性大，病理检查：脾脏切除标本：体积 11.5cm × 8cm × 3cm，脾脏表面被膜破裂，凹凸不平，可见两个缺损区，面积分别为 2.5cm × 1.5cm，4.5cm × 2cm，切面紫红，呈实性，未见囊腔，缺损区可见明显出血，被膜下有明显出血带。胰体尾部及胃后壁之间肿物切除标本：肿物大小 9.5cm × 6.5cm × 5cm，伴出血、坏死、囊性变，有包膜，与胰腺分界清楚。

常规病理诊断：送检脾脏 11.5cm × 8cm × 3cm，表面及切面均见缺损及出血，被膜下亦出血带。镜下除充血出血外，未见特殊改变，考虑为脾破裂伴出血，或继发于血肿的脾假性囊肿。胰体尾部及胃后壁之间肿物切除标本：胰体尾部及胃后壁之间梭形细胞肿瘤，9.5cm × 6.5cm × 5cm，伴出血、坏死、囊性变，未见胰腺组织，具体类型待免疫组化协助诊断。

免疫组化检测：阳性：Vim（++），Actin（++），SMA（+++），β-catenin（+++），CD99（++）；阴性：CD117，DOG1，Nestin，S-100，CD34，Bcl-2。免疫组化诊断：腹腔内（胰体尾部及胃后壁之间）韧带样型纤维瘤病，伴出血坏死、囊性变，局部细胞增生较活跃。注：本病又称侵袭性纤维瘤病，属于中间型肿瘤，由成纤维细胞和肌成纤维细胞构成，有复发倾向，请注意复查（图 20-18-2）。

第十九章 胰腺先天异常和发育变异

第一节 胰腺分裂与诊断陷阱

胰腺分裂是一常见的先天异常,是胰腺发育过程中腹侧和背侧胰腺始基融合失败形成。因此,有两个分离的引流管进入十二指肠:胰头和钩突经主胰管引流入主乳头,胰体和胰尾经副胰管引流入副乳头。这种异常在尸检中占4%~11%,在ERCP检查中占3%~4%。

在CT图像上,一些胰腺分裂病人中可见到胰头和胰颈外形异常。Zeman等(1988)报道的12例胰腺分裂病人中有5例胰头增大。当在薄层CT扫描中见到明显分离的两部分胰腺或未融合的导管系统时,C T偶尔能作出胰腺分裂的诊断。

两部分胰腺会引起胰头扩大,或被脂肪裂分离。有时背侧胰腺的脂肪浸润可与腹侧胰腺分开。这使得胰头内部超声表现有所差别。由腹侧胰芽形成的腹侧胰腺回声较背侧胰腺弱,这可能是因为脂肪的相对含量不同所致。由于胰腺脂肪沉积随年龄而增加,因此,这一情况在老年人更明显,不应与病理情况混淆。

当胰体、胰尾发生萎缩或发生胰腺炎时CT和超声检查可把未累及的胰头疑为一假肿瘤。酒精中毒者偶尔会观察到孤立的腹侧胰腺炎,可能是回流入腹侧胰腺的胆汁和酒精的协同作用所致。因为胰腺分离,背侧胰腺不出现这种回流。虽然ERCP是确诊胰腺分离的传统方法,但MRCP有替代ERCP的趋势。

第二节 成人完全性环状胰腺并急性胰腺炎

环状胰腺是一种少见的先天性发育畸形,其发病机制目前尚无定论。

临床上将环状胰腺分为成人型和儿童型,又根据包绕程度分为完全性环状胰腺和不完全性环状胰腺,以后者较常见,即环状胰腺仅部分包绕十二指肠,约占十二指肠全周的2/3~4/5。

本病多见于男性,临床表现根据十二指肠的狭窄程度和伴随的其他病理改变而不同。新生儿多在出生后1周内发病,表现为急性完全性十二指肠梗阻,常伴有其他先天性疾病。成人型多见于20~40岁,多表现为十二指肠慢性不完全性梗阻,如反复发作的上腹部疼痛和呕吐,呈阵发性,进食后加重。有的患者可并发消化性溃疡、急性胰腺炎、胆管梗阻等。

环状胰腺的影像学检查主要有上消化道钡餐、CT、MRCP与ERCP等。

上消化道钡餐能显示十二指肠降部的狭窄,近段肠腔扩张;MRCP与ERCP可显示环状胰腺的副胰管;CT不仅能显示十二指肠肠腔狭窄和扩张,还能直接显示环绕十二指肠的环状胰腺组织,与胰腺体尾部相连,且密度一致,增强扫描,与正常胰腺组织同步强化。据此可以诊断。

特别是MSCT的多平面重建功能,可以从冠状位和矢状位观察,清晰显示环状胰腺与十二指肠的关系。部分患者还可以发现环状胰腺内的副胰管,对临床诊断和治疗具有重要意义。

成人型环状胰腺主要应与胰头癌、胰腺炎及十二指肠肿瘤等鉴别。检查前口服阳性对比剂,使十二指肠得到良好的充盈,是观察胰腺和十二指肠关系的关键。增强扫描,根据环状胰腺与正常胰腺组织同步均匀强化的特征,鉴别一般不难。

第三节　环状胰腺和半环状胰腺

在环状胰腺和半环状胰腺这种先天异常中,环状胰腺常表现为扁带状胰腺组织完全或部分环绕十二指肠第二段。这种先天异常在近半数病人新生儿期即出现临床表现,另一半成年后才有症状。CT 表现常不具特征性,可显示为胰头增大,增大胰头的中心有一液性低密度区,代表狭窄的十二指肠腔内的液体。如果口服阳性对比剂,中心区将呈高密度。如果十二指肠充盈水或钡剂不佳,那么只能看到胰头增大。因此,环状胰腺可与肿瘤混淆,特别在有十二指肠梗阻症状的成年人。

第四节　误诊病例简介:异位胰腺与胃肠间质瘤

异位胰腺是正常胰腺解剖部位以外的孤立胰腺组织,与正常胰腺无解剖学联系。异位胰腺在临床上较少见,可引起消化道出血、溃疡、梗阻、炎症等并发症;异位胰腺的常见部位是上消化道,以胃最多见,其次是十二指肠和空肠。一例发生于回肠末端,病变位置深,是胃镜、结肠镜诊断的盲区;病变小,常规 CT 较难发现,动态容积 320 排 CT 发现了该病变,但术前误诊为间质瘤。异位胰腺外观形态与正常相似,但无被膜,其中央稍凹陷,常有胰管开口。镜下所见为正常胰腺组织,有腺泡、导管等小叶结构,约 1/3 的病例可见胰岛,具有分泌功能。一些学者指出,小的异位胰腺常无分泌功能,具有分泌功能的异位胰腺可形成囊性病变。

异位胰腺根据其病理学成分分为 3 种类型,Ⅰ型是以腺泡为主要成分的腺泡型;Ⅱ型是以导管为主要成分的导管型;Ⅲ型是腺泡、导管混合型。异位胰腺组织的强化方式必然与组织的构成有密切关系。与正常胰腺相比较,Ⅰ型,异位胰腺显著强化,明显高于正常胰腺;Ⅱ型,以导管为主要成分的异位胰腺强化程度明显弱于正常胰腺、甚至弱于背部肌肉组织;Ⅲ型,其强化方式及程度接近于正常胰腺。

该病例异位的胰腺组织以腺泡成分为主,属于Ⅰ型,增强后病灶显著强化,且明显强于正常胰腺。异位胰腺的其他特征性影像学表现有:发生于上消化道腔内隆起的异位胰腺可表现为宽基底的圆形充盈缺损,加压后出现“脐样征”,如伴有胰腺导管开口于上消化道,表现为细蒂状致密影,称“中央导管征”;异位胰腺发生囊变后,CT 平扫呈低密度,增强后呈环状强化。

异位胰腺病理成分多样,其影像学表现亦千变万化,增加了术前诊断的难度,临床上发生于消化道的异位胰腺,常被误诊为胃肠道间质瘤,影像学表现两者相似,鉴别困难,当 CT 平扫和增强表现与正常胰腺组织接近时,可提示该诊断。

第五节　误诊病例简介:胃异位胰腺囊腺癌

胃异位胰腺并不少见,由此可发生胃异位胰腺肿瘤。Claudon 等(1988)报道 2 例异位胰腺囊肿的 CT 及超声征象。有作者报告 1 例,为男性 51 岁,不明原因低热 20 余天,体检发现左上腹包块,质较软,能移动,大小约儿拳。CT 示左上腹囊性占位,卵圆形,大小约 6.0cm×9.0cm,囊壁厚度在 0.5cm~2.0cm 之间,囊肿与胃大弯紧密依附。CT 增强扫描示囊壁有强化,囊内呈液性密度,其 CT 值为 -3.2HU。胰腺大小、轮廓无异常。CT 提示源自胃壁的囊性占位。

手术发现囊肿在胃大弯肌层下,切除囊肿内含淡黄色液体,囊壁有形状不规则的附壁结节。病理光镜和电镜示上皮起源的囊性乳头状瘤,有嗜酸性变,囊肿来源于异位的胰腺导管。病理诊断为胃异位胰腺囊腺癌,术后 18 个月随访,患者健在。本病术前 CT 确诊困难,需与胃壁血肿、胃平滑肌肉瘤坏死鉴别,定性诊断有赖于手术和病理检查。

第六节 误诊病例简介:胃体小弯异位胰腺与固有肌层间质瘤

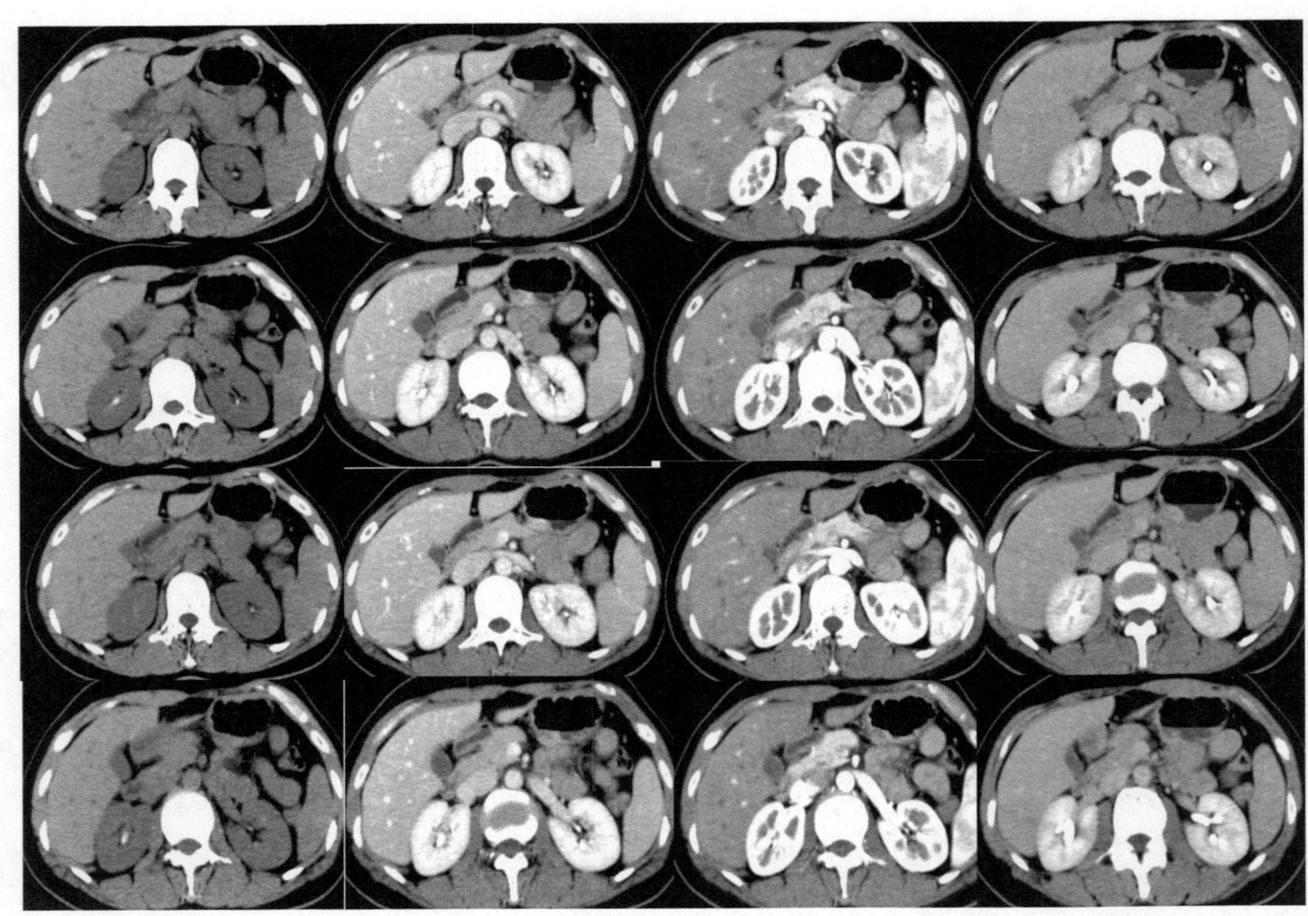

图 20-19-1 胃异位胰腺囊腺癌

患者,女,29 岁。反复上腹痛 1 年余入院。于 4 日前就诊我院门诊行胃镜检查示:胃体下部后壁近胃角处见一约 1.5cm 黏膜隆起,表面光滑;于昨日于我院行超声内镜检查示:胃体黏膜下肿物(固有肌层间质瘤可能,内部血管?坏死?),今为行肿物切除,再诊我院,门诊拟“胃占位性病变”收住入院。

CT:胃充盈良好,胃体小弯侧局部可见类圆形软组织影,大小约 1.5cm × 0.6cm,平扫 CT 值约 53HU,边界清楚,增强扫描病灶明显强化,三期 CT 值分别为 105HU、121HU、107HU,周围脂肪间隙清楚。腹腔及腹膜后未见明显肿大淋巴结。

手术所见:肿瘤位于胃体小弯侧,大小约 4cm × 2cm,边界稍清楚,未突破浆膜层,与周围组织无粘连。

病理检查:胃部肿物切除标本,胃组织一块,大小 6.5cm × 4.3cm × 1cm,胃黏膜中央见一溃疡,大小 3.5cm × 1.5cm,溃疡部切面灰黄,质中,其余胃黏膜未见明显异常。病理诊断:镜下见胃固有肌层内有胰腺腺泡、导管及胰岛,并见导管扩张,符合异位胰腺。轻度慢性浅表性胃炎伴异位胰腺处被覆胃黏膜脱落。四周切缘均为阴性(图 20-19-1)。

第七节　背侧胰腺发育不全和假性发育不全

Gold(1993)报告一例背侧胰腺发育不全和一例假性发育不全。

前者为一 70 岁老妇,大量进食后上腹疼痛,无恶心呕吐和腹泻;伴存成年性糖尿病、

高血压和冠状动脉心脏病;肝肾和胰腺功能未见异常。

超声示肝组织回声轻度不匀,胆囊和胆管未见异常,近胰头处有一直径 20mm 肿块,考虑为胰腺脂肪性变。CT 显示胰腺体和尾部缺失,20mm 肿块与胰头相连,钩突部分脂肪性变,胆总管未见异常。

随后,ERCP 显示位于脊柱右侧的主胰管短而扭曲,近胆胰共同管处略有扩张,在相当超声和 CT 所示肿块区,ERCP 片上显示胰头部周围有正常胰腺腺泡显影,说明该肿块是由于背侧胰腺发育不全而致的腹侧胰腺代偿性肥大。

后者为一 55 岁男性,表现为首次腹痛发作。物理检查除血清淀粉酶 3 500U/L,WBC 23 000/ml 外,均无异常。超声显示胆囊内许多小结石,胆总管无异常。CT 显示胰腺水肿,胰腺周围无积液。诊断为胆囊结石诱发胰腺炎,行保守治疗。

2 周后,病人上腹痛加重,血清淀粉酶 66U/L,WBC 17 000/ml,复查 CT 示 24cm × 16cm × 10cm 大小范围的液体占据了整个胰颈体尾和胰头的大部分。在 CT 导向下,穿刺引流了 1 300ml 无感染的混浊黄褐色液体。因患者继续低热,WBC 计数仍高,遂行手术。术中清除了 900ml 浓稠脓性液体,发现仅有小部分胰腺为出血性坏死性胰腺炎。

胆管造影显示对比剂反流到胰头正常胰管内,并进入坏死的胰腺床和小网膜囊内。引流清除了胰体尾,保留胰头。随后病人体温下降,病情好转。

6 月后 CT 随访,胰头及钩突无异常,无炎症和积液。该病例伴有胰腺肥大,加上免遭萎缩的胰腺钩突,其表现类似于胰背侧发育不全,同时在临床上又无胰腺外分泌功能障碍。

胰腺背侧的原基发育不全是一种非常少见的先天性畸形。自然,急性胰腺炎后出现胰腺萎缩也是非常少见的情况。

第八节　消化道异位胰腺

异位胰腺是一种先天性发育畸形,可发生于任何年龄,以 40~60 岁常见,可能与胚胎时期胰腺组织的异常迁移有关,其确切胚胎学机制尚不清楚,异位胰腺可发生于腹腔的任何部位,以十二指肠最多见(约占 27.7%),其次是胃和空肠,少数发生在胆囊、胆管、脾等消化道以外的部位。有作者报告一组 6 例(胃 2 例,十二指肠 2 例,空肠 2 例)。胃部异位胰腺多发生在胃窦部大弯侧或小弯侧等典型部位,最常见的部位是位于距幽门 1~6 cm 的胃窦大弯侧,其余的位于胃体部和底部等不典型部位,直径一般 1~3 cm。该组 2 例均位于胃小弯侧,其中 1 例为胃体小弯侧,1 例为胃窦小弯侧,胃部病灶最长径约为 2 cm,与文献报道类似。

影像学研究:十二指肠异位胰腺主要位于十二指肠乳头以上,尤以十二指肠球部较多见,该组 1 例位于球部。Wei 等(2011)报道胃部异位胰腺结节的长径 / 短径(LD/SD)(1.81 ± 0.23)明显大于十二指肠异位胰腺结节(1.32 ± 0.18);十二指肠异位胰腺结节因其肠壁紧张性较胃壁低,蠕动较频繁,使得其较胃部异位胰腺结节更小、更圆。该组胃部 2 例,长径 / 短径分别为 1.46、1.41,十二指肠 2 例长径 / 短径分别为 1.14、1.15。该组胃部异位胰腺结节的长径 / 短径大于十二指肠者,与该文献类似。小肠异位胰腺多见于近端空肠。该组 2 例均位于空肠。有文献报道空肠异位胰腺多呈梗阻性,病灶直径 >3 cm 可发生肠套叠,发生肠套叠的肿块内有系膜脂肪伴有局部急性和慢性的炎症和纤维化;也可呈憩室性,异位胰腺生长在憩室内,有憩室炎的症状,CT 显示含空气和坏死物质的厚壁囊腔。该组 1 例可见肠套叠,但直径约为 2 cm。小肠异位胰腺可伴有急性胰腺炎和假性囊肿形成。

胃、空肠和回肠的异位胰腺结节大小对症状产

生有差异性，症状的产生主要与异位胰腺的解剖位置和并发症有关，与结节的功能状况和病变发展程度亦有一定的关系。消化道异位胰腺 CT 平扫多表现为圆形或卵圆形，密度多均匀，边界清楚，与胃肠道壁呈广基底连接，向腔内生长多见，若显示"中心脐凹征"，则可以诊断异位胰腺。该组患者未见明显"中心脐凹征"。

口服泛影葡胺阳性对比剂 CT 呈圆形或卵圆形，边缘清楚，与胃肠道呈广基底的充盈缺损，突向腔内，该组 2 例均可见。CT 增强扫描的强化方式与异位胰腺病理组成相关，腺泡为主要成分者强化显著，高于正常胰腺，门静脉期强化减退亦快于正常胰腺；导管为主要成分者，强化明显弱于正常胰腺，甚至弱于背部肌肉组织；腺泡导管混合型其强化近于正常胰腺。

Cho 等（2000）认为 CT 增强能提高异位胰腺检测率，其中门静脉期能较好显示黏膜下型的异位胰腺覆盖有完整黏膜。该组 6 例，强化均近于正常胰腺，其中 3 例门静脉期可见病灶内侧面黏膜完整，黏膜强化明显；2 例因口服阳性对比剂难以显示黏膜强化情况。

消化道异位胰腺可发生囊性变，CT 平扫呈低密度，增强后囊变区不强化，边缘强化。囊性变可能是因为异位胰腺发生慢性胰腺炎，合并假性囊肿；也可能是起源于导管上皮的囊肿，内衬有分泌功能的上皮；或胰腺导管异常囊形扩张，扩张的导管破裂，周围伴有轻度炎症，而并非真正意义上的囊肿。该组 2 例可见小囊变区。

比较影像学：消化道异位胰腺临床上较为少见，缺乏特异性症状，对该病认识不足，易误诊。尽管 CT 表现难以对消化道异位胰腺作出明确诊断，但其发生部位具有特征性，胃部异位胰腺多发生在胃窦部大弯侧或小弯侧等部位，十二指肠异位胰腺多见于十二指肠乳头以上，以十二指肠球部居多，小肠异位胰腺多见于近端空肠；不同强化方式与其病理组成相关；内层黏膜强化明显；特征性的"中心脐凹征"；腔内生长的方式等，对本病确诊有一定帮助。

MRI 对该病的诊断有重要价值，与正常胰腺的信号是一致的。随着影像技术水平的提高，消化道异位胰腺会越来越多的能在术前作出诊断。

鉴别诊断：消化道异位胰腺需与间质瘤、神经内分泌肿瘤等鉴别。有文献报道 86% 的消化道异位胰腺向腔内生长（该组 6 例均为腔内生长方式），可有助于与其他肿瘤鉴别，其中间质瘤腔外生长多见。此外，增强扫描间质瘤强化程度较异位胰腺明显，神经内分泌肿瘤强化则更为明显。十二指肠异位胰腺还需与十二指肠布氏腺腺瘤鉴别，后者多呈息肉样突起，可有蒂，MRI 上 T_1WI 呈高信号具有一定的特征，T_2WI 呈等信号，增强后呈中等强化。

附：具体研究资料：6 例异位胰腺均为单发病灶，其中发生在胃部 2 例，均位于胃小弯侧；十二指肠 2 例，其中球部 1 例，降部 1 例；小肠 2 例，均位于空肠。6 例术前均诊断不明确或误诊。CT 测量病灶大小为 1.2 cm × 1.3 cm~2.0 cm × 2.0 cm。其中胃部病灶最长径为 2.0 cm；十二指肠病灶最长径为 1.5 cm；小肠病灶最长径为 2.0 cm。3 例病灶呈卵圆形，2 例呈圆形，1 例为分叶状，CT 平扫病灶大多密度均匀，边界清楚，与胃肠道壁呈广基底连接，向腔内生长多见，2 例可见小囊变区。2 例口服 2% 泛影葡胺患者的病灶呈圆形充盈缺损 1 例，卵圆形充盈缺损 1 例，边缘均光整。CT 增强扫描，6 例均呈明显强化，强化方式类似于正常胰腺，其中 4 例均匀强化，2 例小囊变区未强化。

第九节　迷走胰腺或副胰及误诊漏诊分析

迷走胰腺或副胰，亦称异位胰腺，凡在胰腺本身以外生长的、与正常胰腺组织既无解剖上的联系又无血管联系的孤立的胰腺组织。最常发生在十二指肠、近段空肠和胃等部位，消化道异位胰腺多无症状，常在其他疾病术中或偶然发现；消化道异位胰腺 CT 表现多样，易与消化道其他肿瘤相混淆，而导致不必要的手术。

病理学：异位胰腺是一种常见的先天性发育畸形，其发病机制尚不清楚，绝大多数认为可能是胚胎时期背侧和腹侧胰腺始基随着原肠上段旋转过程中，1 个或几个始基保留在原肠壁内，随原肠纵行生长而将胰腺始基带走而形成异位胰腺。异位胰腺的尸检发生率为 0.55%~13.7%，30~50 岁常见，以男性居多；胃、十二指肠、空肠、回肠、食管、麦克尔憩室、结肠、胆囊、脐、输卵管、纵隔、脾脏及肝脏均可发生异位胰腺，而 70% 发生于胃、十二指肠及空肠，尤其是十二指肠乳头周围区。异位胰腺可以发生于黏膜下层（73%）、肌层（17%）及浆膜层（10%）。一组22例中分别为30%、40%、15%，另可见15%（3例）位于浆膜外，并且有孔与消化道相通。

临床表现：多数异位胰腺患者多无症状，>1.5 cm时可能会引起症状，常合并其他病变在术中发现。而异位胰腺所引起的症状主要是由其所在的部位决定，异位胰腺可以引起同正常胰腺一样病理变化，包括急性及慢性胰腺炎、假性囊肿、消化道出血、卓艾综合征、甚至癌变，在胃肠道时可以引起梗阻及肠套叠。Park等（2000）报道无论内分泌型及外分泌型均可引起急性或慢性胰腺炎。该组22例病人中2例表现为肠梗阻：1例为男性，3岁，表现为急性腹痛6h，术中表现为回肠末端异位胰腺合并麦克尔憩室；另1例为男性，53岁，反复腹痛腹胀1个月余，术中见十二指肠异位胰腺合并十二指肠溃疡，可能与异位胰腺的分泌导致十二指肠溃疡、水肿而发生肠梗阻。12例表现为餐后上腹部胀痛，最长1例表现为反复发作20年，其中7例合并其他疾病，而剩余5例中2例血液生化提示慢性胰腺炎改变，而正常部位胰腺未见异常改变。因此，病程较长，正常部位胰腺未见异常改变，而生化系列异常或临床表现为慢性胰腺炎时，对异位胰腺有较大的提示作用。

异位胰腺的影像表现及其病理相关性：Gaspar-Fuentes（1973）按异位胰腺构成比例将Heinrich（1909）提出的3型异位胰腺修改分为4型：Ⅰ型，由类似正常的胰腺组织，即腺泡、胰管和胰岛细胞组成而出现非正常部位；Ⅱ型，仅由胰管构成；Ⅲ型，由腺泡组织构成（外分泌型）；Ⅳ型，由胰岛细胞构成（内分泌型）。腺泡、胰管和胰岛细胞的密度与强化程度并不一样，由不同比例的腺泡、胰管及胰岛细胞构成的异位胰腺其密度及强化方式亦不相同，因此异位胰腺的强化方式与异位胰腺的病理组成密切相关。

实际异位胰腺并不是由哪一种单一细胞组织构成，Park等（2000）按其临床表现将其分成完全型和不完全型2类，并认为几乎所有完全型（Ⅰ型）异位胰腺增强后表现接近于正常胰腺的强化，而不完全型（Ⅱ～Ⅳ型）表现为中等或弱强化。

该组资料中13例增强后6例呈明显强化，类似正常胰腺强化，强化后的衰减均匀或不均匀，5例呈分叶状；1例行CT重建后可见异位胰腺由肠系膜上动脉供血，而其他异位胰腺未见明显的供血血管，文献亦未见相关报道，6例中4例显示中央脐凹征，深约3~5 mm；病理提示正常胰腺腺泡组织为主，中央可见扩张的胰管。3例呈中等强化，延迟后密度降低不明显，病理提示以胰管和少量的腺泡组成。3例强化不明显，低于肌肉密度，病理显示以胰腺导管及增生平滑肌为主；1例成囊样改变，呈边缘中等强化。病理示以大量的胰岛细胞为主，可能与胰岛细胞分泌的胰液无法排出有关。

异位胰腺的漏诊及误诊分析：消化道异位胰腺术前诊断较难，其漏诊原因常见于：胰腺炎及梗阻症状急性发病病人，消化道准备欠佳时，常常易漏诊；发现等密度病灶，误以为消化道食物而漏诊；病灶较小时，局部增厚，考虑为胃肠蠕动局部增厚而漏诊；合并其他疾病时，以单一疾病考虑，该组病例中9/22例因合并其他疾病漏诊。

异位胰腺易与胃肠道其他肿瘤混淆，最常见于胃肠道间质瘤、息肉、淋巴瘤、类癌、淋巴结及胃癌。文献报道关于异位胰腺的诊断方法较多，但均为提示性作用。上消化道造影显示黏膜突起伴有脐凹征其灵敏度及特异度分别为87.5%、71.4%。该组中1例行上消化道造影，但异位胰腺较小而漏诊。CT增强后，异位胰腺内可见线样脐凹征或线样低密度影（胰管）为异位胰腺的特点之一。CT增强后行多平面重建及CT仿真内镜对显示胰管也较有优势，同时仿真内镜对观察肠道黏膜破坏有一定的提示作用。Hazzan等（2002）认为中央有脐凹征为异位胰腺的特点，但这种特点很难在<1.5 cm的病灶中发现。

异位胰腺诊断主要集中在术后病理诊断，而在术前诊断较少，术前诊断异位胰腺可以决定手术的方式，减少病人不必要的痛苦和经济损失；异位胰腺因腺泡、胰管和胰岛细胞组成比例不同而表现出不同的影像特点。

以下征象对诊断具有提示作用：①发病时间较长，多在餐后症状加重；②浆膜层或浆膜外显示等密度或囊性结节时，结节周缘可见渗出性改变，血液生化检查提示胰腺炎改变，而免疫组化检查肿瘤系列未见异常时，应该考虑异位胰腺可能；③CT检查胃肠道实性结节，呈广基底，分叶状，尤其病灶位于十二指肠，增强后强化方式及延迟扫描与胰腺相似，最大密度投影及仿真内镜可见脐凹征时，对异位胰腺的诊断可以更加肯定。同时，无论胃肠道内外发现可疑结节需要增强时,都应在肠道充分准备的情况下进行,必要时可以清洁肠道行仿真内镜检查。

附:具体研究资料:收集经临床及病理证实的异位胰腺22例,男14例,女8例,年龄3~72岁,平均(44±16)岁。12例表现短期内腹部疼痛,6例表现为超过1年的反复腹胀及餐后钝痛,1例表现为腹部包块,3例无症状。14例行胃镜检查,5例行超声内镜检查,1例行上消化道钡剂造影,2例因肠梗阻无内镜检查。

异位胰腺的外观及分布:22例中,16例表现为广基底呈线条样改变,5例表现为团状呈浅分叶,1例表现为囊样改变。胃大弯2例,胃小弯4例,胃窦9例,十二指肠3例,空肠2例,回肠2例,病变均为单发,最小直径1.2 cm,最大直径6 cm,平均最大径(2.6±1.1)cm。22例异位胰腺中,黏膜下层8例,肌层8例,浆膜层3例,浆膜外3例。异位胰腺的CT征象及强化表现:22例异位胰腺均行CT检查,13例行CT增强检查,平扫9例中2例CT密度基本接近胰腺,增强后13例中6例呈明显强化,类似正常胰腺强化,强化后均匀或不均匀,5例呈分叶状;6例中5例显示中央脐凹征,深约3~5 mm;3例呈中等强化,延迟后衰减不明显;3例强化不明显,低于肌肉密度;1例成囊样改变,呈边缘中等强化,病理示由大量的胰岛细胞及少量胰管构成;13例增强病例中2例诊断为异位胰腺,6例诊断为间质瘤,1例诊断为囊肿,1例考虑为胃癌,2例诊断为淋巴结。9例因合并其他疾病而漏诊。

第十节 异位胰腺肿瘤

异位胰腺是指正常胰腺位置以外的胰腺组织。与正常胰腺组织一样,异位胰腺组织也可发生肿瘤样病变,即异位胰腺肿瘤。对于异位胰腺肿瘤的影像学表现,报道并不多见,但异位胰腺肿瘤的发生率并不少见。

定义与发生机制:异位胰腺,又称为迷走胰腺,其定义为正常胰腺位置以外的胰腺组织,两者之间没有解剖上的联系,拥有独立的血液供应和神经支配。Klob(1859)首次从病理学上证实本病的存在。异位胰腺是一种先天性异常,其发生机制尚未完全清楚,多数学者认为是由于胚胎时期胰腺原基与原肠粘连或穿透原肠壁,并随原肠纵向生长及旋转而被异常移植;也有人认为是由异常部位的内胚层细胞异向分化或化生而来。

异位胰腺组织可具有正常胰腺组织的任何组织成分,但往往由导管和周围产生黏蛋白的腺体组成。正常部位胰腺的任何疾病均可发生于异位胰腺,如急慢性胰腺炎和囊肿等,当然,肿瘤性病变也可在异位胰腺组织中发生。异位胰腺并不少见,文献报道尸检中的发现率为0.6%~13.7%。上腹部手术时,每500例中可发现1例(De Castro Barbosa,1946)。异位胰腺组织发生的肿瘤亦不少见,有几十例个案报道。有报道异位胰腺组织比正常胰腺组织更易发生恶变(Cho,2000)。虽然发病率不高,但可对病人的健康产生严重危害。

临床表现:异位胰腺肿瘤根据肿瘤有无内分泌功能,临床表现差异较大。无内分泌功能的肿瘤可无任何临床症状,偶为腹部手术或尸解发现;但肿瘤较大时可产生压迫症状,如发生于胃窦部的肿瘤可引起幽门梗阻;发生恶变后常有上腹部疼痛、不适等症状。胃肠道出血有时可为发生于胃肠道的异位胰腺肿瘤的唯一症状。Souilamas等(1993)报道了1例引起直肠出血的异位胰腺组织发生的囊腺癌。而有内分泌功能的异位胰腺肿瘤可出现相关的内分泌症状,如异位的胰岛素瘤会引起低血糖等。

影像学研究:有作者认为,对于异位胰腺肿瘤,影像学表现除定位作用外并无特异性。但有研究发现发生于异位胰腺组织的肿瘤仍有一定的影像学特点。

肿块的发生部位:异位胰腺肿瘤多发生于胃肠道,包括胃、十二指肠、空肠、Meckel憩室、胆囊和食管等处,尤其好发于胃窦部(Yamagiwa,1977),少数也可发生于结肠系膜和脾脏。发生于空腔脏器壁内者的一个显著特点是位于黏膜下层和肌层,很少累及黏膜和浆膜,这与发生于空腔脏器的常见肿瘤(如胃癌、肠癌等)显著不同。在胃肠道造影检查时表现为外压性充盈缺损,而往往没有黏膜皱襞的破坏,但常会形成溃疡,开口于黏膜表面;在CT检查中直接表现为黏膜下层或肌层的占位性病变。如Halkic等(2001)报道的1例发生于食管胃连接处的异位胰腺癌,其胃肠道造影中的表现即为外压性充盈缺损,而无黏膜的破坏。

肿块的形态和边界:病灶均表现为圆形或卵圆形肿块,良性者多边界光滑,恶性者边缘呈锯齿状与周围组织分界欠清。肿瘤直径多为数厘米,有内分泌功能者体积较小。肿瘤生长较慢,但恶性者的生长速度较快。Ura 等(1998)报道了 1 例异位胰腺恶变的病例,恶变前随访病灶大小无明显改变,恶变后 1 年内大小由 1.8 cm × 1.3cm 增大到 3.3cm × 3.0 cm。

肿块的密度:术后病理证实,绝大多数病灶不论良恶性,除了肿瘤的实质性成分之外有囊样的区域,主要由扩张的胰腺导管构成。病灶囊壁厚,其内有实性分隔。CT 检查病灶实性成分平扫多呈等密度,囊性成分呈液体密度。肿瘤内可有钙化,多见于良性肿瘤。增强后囊性成分无强化,实性成分可明显或不明显强化。Nisar 等(2002)报道了 1 例发生于脾脏的异位胰腺癌,病灶呈囊实混合性,实性成分增强后强化不明显,呈相对低密度灶。而 Tolentino 等(2004)报道 1 例发生于十二指肠的异位胰岛细胞瘤,增强后呈明显高密度。多数作者认为,异位胰腺组织和肿瘤组织中的实性成分的强化方式与以下几种因素有关:

病灶的组织构成:Park 等(2000)认为未恶变的异位胰腺组织有以下 3 种强化方式:①均匀明显强化,与正常位置胰腺的表现相似,这是因为病灶主要由与正常胰腺组织一样的腺泡组成;②强化不明显,病灶主要由导管和增生肥大的肌肉组织组成,而胰腺腺泡成分很少;③病灶呈囊性,无强化,这是因为病变主要为假性囊肿,大部分由扩张的导管构成,只有很少量的腺泡成分。而起源于异位胰腺组织的肿瘤,其强化方式必然也与组织的构成有密切关系。

肿瘤是否具有内分泌功能:与起源于正常部位的胰腺肿瘤一样,起源于异位胰腺组织的胰腺肿瘤,如不具有内分泌功能的恶性者,由于其生长迅速,血液供应不足,将表现为少血供的肿瘤,在 CT 增强扫描后强化不明显呈低密度病灶。但如果异位胰腺肿瘤具有内分泌功能,由于其代谢旺盛,如同正常部位的内分泌肿瘤一般,增强后会有明显强化,呈富血供肿瘤表现。

肿块占位或压迫征象:起源于幽门处的异位胰腺肿瘤,幽门梗阻可能为唯一放射学征象,起源于肠管管壁的异位胰腺肿瘤,会导致管腔狭窄,严重者可能会发生梗阻。发生于胆胰管十二指肠连接区或胰头附近的异位胰腺肿瘤,可引起胆道系统的梗阻扩张,这些表现在 CT 或 MR 影像上均可清晰显示。

转移:恶性的异位胰腺肿瘤,往往发生转移。如发生于胃的异位胰腺癌,往往会有胃周淋巴结的转移,部分病例还可有肝脏等其他脏器的转移。

其他:一些异位胰腺发生的病变在异位胰腺肿瘤中亦有可能见到,如位于十二指肠的异位胰腺,由于炎症反应,往往会有十二指肠肠壁的增厚,这一表现可与肿瘤性病变并存。

正常位置的胰腺组织无异常病变。

诊断:尽管有上述改变,但许多异位胰腺肿瘤影像学表现不典型,确诊有赖于活检或手术、病理结果,多数文献报道在术前均未能做出正确诊断,有时甚至组织学方法确定肿瘤来源于异位胰腺也有困难。对于异位胰腺肿瘤的良恶性鉴别,Guillou 等(1994)曾提出诊断异位胰腺恶性肿瘤的 3 个标准:①肿瘤必须在异位胰腺组织内或其附近;②必须能观察到从胰腺结构到癌组织之间有直接的跃迁;③非肿瘤的胰腺组织至少要包括发育完全的腺泡和导管结构。

影像学上如具有以下 4 点征象可提示为恶性的异位胰腺肿瘤:①肿瘤向周围组织侵犯。位于空腔脏器壁内的肿瘤,侵犯黏膜或浆膜;位于胸腹腔间隙内的肿瘤,侵犯周围血管、神经等组织。②肿瘤内部密度不均匀。虽然不论良恶性异位胰腺肿瘤多有囊性区域,但恶性者其内密度更不均匀,囊、实成分相间分布,混杂不规则。③出现淋巴结转移或远处其他脏器的转移。④肿瘤短期内生长迅速。

异位胰腺肿瘤一般需与下列疾病进行鉴别:

(1)胰腺肿瘤:CT 检查发现正常部位的胰腺组织没有异常改变即可排除胰腺肿瘤。但当异位胰腺肿瘤病灶与正常的胰腺组织非常邻近时,有时会难以区别。经 CT 薄层扫描并行多平面重组,或 MRI 多方位扫描后,可进行鉴别。

(2)胃肠道肿瘤:良性的异位胰腺肿瘤需与胃肠道良性肿瘤如平滑肌瘤鉴别,异位胰腺肿瘤往往会形成溃疡,开口于黏膜表面,行胃肠道造影检查时可表现为“线样征”,而平滑肌瘤等无此表现。且异位胰腺肿瘤多为囊实性,与平滑肌瘤等实质性病灶不同。

恶性的异位胰腺肿瘤需与胃肠道恶性肿瘤进行鉴别,胃肠道恶性肿瘤起源于黏膜层,首先破坏黏膜组织,造成黏膜皱襞的中断、破坏;而异位胰腺肿瘤起源于黏膜下层或肌层,即使侵犯黏膜层造成黏膜破坏,其病灶中心仍位于黏膜下层或肌层内。

(3)淋巴瘤与淋巴结转移:淋巴瘤或转移淋巴结在 CT 平扫时多为密度均匀的软组织肿块,增强后轻度强化,与异位胰腺肿瘤为囊实混合性密度、增强后不强化或明显强化不同;且淋巴瘤或转移淋巴结常为多发肿块,与异位胰腺肿瘤为单发病灶不同。

(4)异位嗜铬细胞瘤:嗜铬细胞瘤的CT影像特点为明显强化和有囊性变,与有内分泌功能的异位胰腺肿瘤表现相似,但病人多有典型的临床症状,可利于鉴别。

(5)神经源性肿瘤:包括神经鞘瘤、神经纤维瘤和神经节细胞瘤。大多为均匀低密度病灶,与异位胰腺肿瘤的囊实混合性密度不同。

总之,无论通过临床症状还是影像学检查,在活检或手术之前确诊异位胰腺肿瘤是困难的。异位胰腺肿瘤的影像学表现多不典型,但仍具有一定的特点,当出现以下表现时应考虑到异位胰腺肿瘤的可能:病灶位于空腔脏器黏膜下或胸、腹腔的间隙内,较少侵及黏膜层;CT检查时病灶密度不均匀,为囊实混合性密度;增强后,如肿瘤无内分泌分化,表现为相对低密度区;如肿瘤有内分泌分化时,强化非常明显;正常位置的胰腺未见异常。如果病灶密度异常不均匀,短期内明显增大,侵犯周围组织,出现附近淋巴结或远处脏器的转移,则高度提示为恶性病变。

第十一节　背胰发育变异

胰腺的发育变异并不少见,许多观点源自有限的尸体解剖,与活体所见出入不小。相对腹胰变异类型而言,背胰变异相对简单,多为形态异常,不伴有胰腺炎等合并症。

背胰局部突起:为最常见的背胰变异类型,多位于胰颈,少数位于胰体,表现为胰腺局部突起。所有病例均突向胰腺腹侧或腹外侧,无1例突向胰腺背侧。由于缺乏认识,常被误诊为胰腺或胰旁病变。

胰尾增宽:关于胰尾增宽,复习文献未见专门定义,结合传统解剖概念,认为以下3点可作为"胰尾增宽"诊断标准:横断面图像上,胰尾最大宽径超过2.5 cm为"可疑增宽",超过3.0 cm为"胰尾增宽";平扫及增强图像上,其质地与其他胰腺组织同步,未见到异常密度/信号灶;增宽的胰尾内,胰管结构、粗细、走行正常。胰尾属腹腔内位,容易发生旋转,其增宽的形态多样,由于缺乏认识,临床上时有将"胰尾增宽"当做"胰腺肿块"而进行手术治疗。

背胰缺如、背胰发育不全:"背胰发育不全"少见,常合并其他异常。一组9例中,有5例合并腹胰缺如和多脾综合征。诊断时,应与慢性胰腺炎导致的胰腺体尾部萎缩(假性发育不全)鉴别,胰腺炎病史和影像学特点是其鉴别点。背胰完全缺如则极其罕见,CT、MRI图像上只见到代偿性增大的胰头。

胰腺脂肪裂:胰腺脂肪裂罕见,常位于胰体胰尾交界处或腹胰-背胰交界处,呈横行的脂肪密度裂隙,与胰腺断裂不同,胰腺脂肪裂没有外伤史、胰周渗出、出血、胰腺病变等外伤相关的影像表现。多平面重建图像提示该裂隙为胰腺周围脂肪组织嵌入。

胰腺分叉:胰腺分叉有2种表现形式,一种为增宽的胰腺内有脾静脉穿过,有学者将其作为独立的变异类型,另有作者通过连续薄层图像分析,认为这种"胰腺分叉"其实是脾静脉与胰尾增宽的组合表现,不应作为孤立变异类型看待;另一种"胰尾分叉"为胰腺实质分叉,没有脾静脉穿过,应看作是重复胰腺的一种类型。

背胰变异并不少见,多为形态异常,常为其他原因腹部检查中偶然发现,相对腹胰变异而言,几乎没有胰腺炎等并发症。CT、MRI图像上,变异的背胰组织质地、密度/信号与正常胰腺相仿,多平面重建、MRCP能准确显示胰腺毗邻关系和胰管结构,对判断背胰变异意义重大。只要提高认识,扫描规范,背胰变异不难诊断。

第十二节　误诊病例简介:小肠脂肪瘤伴异位胰腺致小肠套叠

详见本书 本卷 第二十五篇 第七章 第一节　误诊病例简介:小肠脂肪瘤伴异位胰腺致小肠套叠。

第二十章　胰腺其他囊性疾病

第一节　胰腺囊实性乳头状瘤误诊分析

胰腺囊实性乳头状瘤属少见病。胰腺囊实性乳头状瘤以往报道较少，近期由于对本病认识提高，报道渐多。本病命名较多，包括：胰腺实性－假乳头状瘤、胰腺乳头状囊性及实性瘤、胰腺乳头状囊性肿瘤、胰腺乳头状上皮瘤、乳头状囊性瘤、乳头状囊性癌及胰腺囊实性腺泡细胞瘤。亦有将此瘤首先提出者 Frantz 名字命名本病。由于本病罕见，文献中大组病例甚少，多以个案或小组病例报道。Lam 等（1999）复习文献，收集报道仅 452 例。Papavramidis 等（2005）收集英文报道为 718 例，并统计该瘤为胰腺肿瘤的 2.5%。Casadei 等（2006）收集胰腺肿瘤 772 例，其中胰腺囊实性乳头状瘤 4 例（占 0.5%），为同组胰腺囊性肿瘤的 5.5%（4/73）。

病理学：病理上，胰腺囊实性乳头状瘤常显示完整包膜，瘤体内易发生坏死、出血和钙化，一组 8 例均见不同程度坏死，其中 6 例坏死区内液体呈褐色，提示陈旧性出血。

临床表现：胰腺囊实性乳头状瘤好发于年轻女性，该组 8 例中占 6 例（75%），女性平均年龄仅 25 岁。2 例男性患者发病年龄相对较大。本病临床症状多不明显，常仅表现为上腹部疼痛，部分可无明显自觉不适，部分患者常由于体检或因其他疾病检查偶然发现。

影像学研究：胰腺囊实性乳头状瘤可位于胰腺各部。

CT 表现肿瘤界限清楚，常可显示清楚包膜，肿瘤内易出现坏死或／和出血，表现为密度不均，部分肿瘤表现为明显囊性结构，囊壁显示乳头样隆起，肿瘤边缘及瘤体内常见钙化，表现为瘤体内结节状及边缘厚薄不均壳状钙化，该组 5 例（63%）显示此征象。增强扫描，肿瘤组织动脉期多为轻度强化，实质期则多为中度或明显强化，囊变及坏死区无强化征象。

MRI 表现：肿瘤与正常胰腺组织界限清楚，T_1WI 肿瘤实质常为低信号，坏死及囊变区显示更低信号，肿瘤内亚急性出血可表现为高信号，该组 3 例 MRI 扫描中，1 例表现此征象。T_2WI 肿瘤呈不均匀高、低混杂信号。MR 增强扫描胰腺囊实性乳头状瘤常显示轻～中度不均匀强化，肿瘤界限清楚，常可更清楚显示包膜结构。

误诊分析：因胰腺囊实性乳头状瘤属罕见病变，文献报道胰腺囊实性乳头状瘤影像诊断术前误诊率多较高，Panieri 等（1998）报道 12 例，术前仅 4 例（33.3%）诊断正确。Casadei 等（2006）4 例报道，术前正确诊断 1 例（23%）。该组 8 例，术前根据影像学表现，仅 1 例提出该病诊断。影像学上常误诊疾病包括：胰腺癌、胰腺囊腺癌、胰腺囊性肿瘤（浆液性或黏液性囊腺瘤）、胰岛细胞瘤、假性囊肿等。分析相关肿瘤，胰腺癌及胰腺囊腺癌除发病多为高龄老年患者外，肿瘤常无包膜，向外侵袭性生长，易突破胰腺被膜侵犯周围组织，如血管结构等。胰腺周围淋巴结及肝内转移常见，胰管扩张多明显。增强扫描多轻度强化。

胰腺浆液性或黏液性囊腺瘤亦好发于老年患者，前者肿瘤内常表现为多发小囊状低密度结构及间隔；后者常显示多发大囊性结构及间隔，增强扫描期间隔结构显示更为清楚。胰腺浆液性或黏液性囊腺瘤均可出现钙化，但其钙化率较低，且很少显示多发较大结节样及肿瘤边缘较厚不规则壳样钙化。

功能性胰岛细胞瘤多较小，且增强扫描早期强化明显，无功能性胰岛细胞瘤可较大，但瘤体明显囊肿坏死，肿瘤内显示乳头状结构及明显钙化少见。

胰腺假性囊肿多可追溯胰腺炎或胰腺外伤史,囊壁较规则,无乳头样结构以及周围筋膜增厚等间接征象,往往诊断本病不难。该组8例胰腺囊实性乳头状瘤术前影像学诊断中,3例提示占位,2例误为囊腺瘤,1例可疑胰腺癌,1例考虑无功能性胰岛细胞瘤,1例因肿瘤钙化较多而倾向结核。但仅表现为胰腺结核而无周围淋巴结结核性表现,似难用结核解释胰腺病变性质,况且胰腺结核少有以明显肿块形式表现。胰腺囊实性乳头状瘤生物学行为多属于良性过程,肿瘤生长缓慢,一般不引起胆管扩张,少数可引起胰管轻度扩张。胰管扩张原因认为主要与肿瘤生长部位有关,肿瘤位于胰头部可引起胰管扩张,由于胰腺囊实性乳头状瘤生长缓慢,引起胰管扩张多不明显。该组1例肿瘤位于胰头部,显示胰管扩张征象。该组7例位于胰体及尾部胰腺囊实性乳头状瘤无1例引起胰管扩张。

胰腺囊实性乳头状瘤可自发性破裂,该组见1例。而该组1例患者同时发现胰腺囊实性乳头状瘤、腹主动脉旁嗜铬细胞瘤及肾透明细胞癌,更属罕见。胰腺囊实性乳头状瘤虽属少见肿瘤,但正确认识胰腺囊实性乳头状瘤影像学表现,结合该肿瘤好发于年轻女性,临床表现多轻微或无明显症状等特点,多数胰腺囊实性乳头状瘤是可以正确诊断的。

第二节　误诊病例简介:胰腺乳头状囊性肿瘤

乳头状囊性肿瘤是一种相当少见及组织起源尚有争议的肿瘤,又称乳头状囊性上皮肿瘤、实性乳头状肿瘤等,常见于年轻女性,平均年龄21.8~23.9岁,老年妇女和男性罕见。

乳头状囊性肿瘤可发生于胰腺任何部位,多位于胰头或胰尾部,胰腺之外亦可发病。临床上可无症状或仅有上腹部不适感,因此术前常被误诊。CT上乳头状囊性肿瘤多表现为囊实性圆形肿块,边界清晰,其内无分隔,增强后实质部分可有强化。

一例为胰体尾部类圆形肿块,平扫其密度均匀,增强后呈不均匀明显强化,内有小囊状不强化区,与胰腺非功能内分泌肿瘤及血管瘤鉴别困难。且该例患者为男性,而乳头状囊性肿瘤女性易发病,进一步增加了定性诊断的难度。多数乳头状囊性肿瘤能被完整切除,预后较好,少数患者术后可复发或远处转移,因此对乳头状囊性肿瘤行手术后的患者有必要进行定期影像学复查,以便及时做出相应的处理。乳头状囊性肿瘤的确诊需依靠手术和病理诊断。

第三节　胰腺囊性畸胎瘤

胰腺囊性畸胎瘤是先天性肿瘤,因畸胎瘤内含内、中、外三个胚层成分,故可有钙化、骨化及脂肪结构,一般病史甚长,临床症状轻微,Mester(1990)报告一例,当时他追溯文献共有9例报告。在国内,有作者报告1例,该例为中年妇女,左上腹摸到约鸡蛋大小包块7年,质硬,有轻触痛,CT扫描示胰尾囊性占位,呈分叶状,大小约6.0cm×8.3cm,囊壁完全钙化,其厚度约1.2~2.5cm,此类钙化可谓既厚实又完整,囊内液性密度区CT值为-12.6HU,在囊肿的内后方可见局限性脂肪密度区,手术示胰尾肿瘤,囊壁坚实钙化,囊内有毛发和黄色液体,病理诊断为胰腺囊性畸胎瘤。

第四节　其他胰腺恶性或潜在恶性囊性肿瘤

其他胰腺恶性或潜在恶性囊性肿瘤,包括囊性胰岛细胞瘤、淋巴瘤、未分化癌和囊性转移瘤等。胰岛细胞肿瘤中的胰岛素瘤、胰高血糖素瘤、胃泌素瘤及非功能性神经内分泌肿瘤在罕见的情况下可能出现囊样表现,文献中仅有散在个案报道,诊断主要依赖临床表现及内分泌学检查。胰腺的原发淋巴瘤极为罕见,多数系胰周病灶侵入胰腺。超声上病灶可显示均匀低回声而近似囊肿表现。CT上出现囊性成分系肿瘤坏死所致。

未分化癌、巨细胞肿瘤及肉瘤等原发于胰腺者极罕见，通常是起自胰周而继发累及胰腺。巨细胞肿瘤在组织学上分 2 型：多形型及破骨细胞型。前者高度恶性，预后差；后者与骨巨细胞瘤的组织学相同，预后较好。肿瘤的囊性改变乃系中心坏死所致。

肉瘤中最常见的是平滑肌肉瘤，至 2002 年仅有 21 例报道。病人年龄 14~80 岁，男性好发，肿瘤大小为 2.0~25 cm，CT 上呈均匀实性或不均匀密度，囊性表现与肿瘤坏死有关。强化扫描肿瘤有不均匀或边缘强化。MR T_1WI 上呈不均匀低信号，T_2WI 上呈不均匀高信号。

胰腺转移瘤少见，一组 2 587 例连续尸检中，261 例（10%）有胰腺转移。原发灶多来自乳腺、肾、肺、黑色素瘤或胃肠道。呈囊性表现的转移瘤多系中心坏死或囊性变所致。

第五节 胰腺囊性病变钙化

多种胰腺囊性病变可出现囊壁或囊内钙化。

囊内钙化：一组可见 2 例，分别为囊腺瘤和囊腺癌各一例。在 CT 图像上钙化为斑片状，良性囊腺瘤钙化密度高，量较多，散见于整个囊腔内；囊腺癌钙化量较少，为小斑点状，密度低而边界模糊。

囊壁钙化：最厚者达到 2cm。依 CT 图像可分为：连贯性环形囊壁钙化：多为外伤性假性囊肿和良性囊腺瘤。表现为连贯不间断环状钙化，钙化厚而光滑，密度高，在 CT 图像上为完整的环状，在 X 线平片上表现为蛋壳状，手术标本见亦为禽蛋样，大小及形状不一。断续不连的环形钙化：多为囊腺癌，囊壁为软组织密度，其间混杂有条状、斑状钙化，钙化密度低，可间断地包绕整个囊壁。局限性囊壁钙化：多见于胰腺假性囊肿。钙化厚薄不均，密度高，常局限于囊壁的某一侧。

胰腺囊性病变钙化不常见，可见于胰腺假性囊肿、胰腺囊腺瘤、胰腺囊腺癌、胰腺神经鞘瘤、胰腺囊性畸胎瘤、胰母细胞瘤等。Hertzanu 等（1989）认为，胰腺囊性病变钙化在 CT 图像上无特征性，难以依据钙化来做出定性诊断。

事实上，胰腺囊性病变钙化率不高，环形钙化更少见，应考虑到钙化实际上是各类组织退变的共同病理转归，只凭 X 线照片或 / 和 CT 图像上显示的钙化去作定性诊断确有一定困难。但是，通过钙化这一征象结合其他情况进行分析，常可对定性诊断提示一些有价值的信息。

厚壁连贯性环状囊壁钙化的病理基础，是囊壁组织因慢性炎症，出血或囊液酸碱度的改变而造成纤维退变，导致钙盐沉积，提示为病程较长，发展较慢的病变。胰腺囊腺癌钙化发生机制尚不明确，其囊壁钙化可表现为密度低，钙化斑条断续不连，胰母细胞瘤钙化也有如此表现。胰腺假性囊肿钙化常为偏侧性条状，其厚度约为 0.5~1.5cm，患者多有反复发作的胰腺炎病史，结合病史及囊肿的部位和形态进行分析，多可做出正确的定性诊断。

第六节 胰管黏液囊性瘤的导管淤积变型

胰腺囊性肿瘤少见，报道只占胰囊性病灶的 12.8%，其中又分为浆液性和黏液囊性瘤，后者常是恶性或恶性前期表现。Ohta（1992）报道 7 例胰腺黏液囊性瘤的导管淤积变型影像学（含 ERP、CT 及血管造影）表现并与巨囊型黏液囊性瘤比较。

黏液囊性瘤导管淤积变型的 X 线和病理特征为：胰腺囊肿，其大小直径约 3~4cm，有弥漫的导管淤积形状，为多房性囊肿，并与主胰管相通；组织学上囊肿为多房性，其上皮由产生黏液的高柱状上皮组成，伴存变形，为单层或复层，与巨囊性黏液囊性瘤难以区别。

黏液囊性瘤的导管淤积变型与巨囊性黏液囊性瘤的区别在于：前者发病年龄较大，男性较多，85% 有腹痛无腹块，后者 40% 有腹痛及腹块；前者 70% 有淀粉酶升高，而后者无；后者有主胰管移位或梗阻，而未见前者表现的胰管扩张或由黏液引起的充盈缺损。

该作者指出，如胰腺囊肿有弥漫的导管淤积形状,并在胰腺造影中与主胰管相通,应高度疑及胰管黏液囊性瘤的导管淤积变型。

第七节 胰腺先天性囊性病变

大多数先天性胰腺囊肿为多发性,罕见孤立性。它们多属常染色体显性疾病,除多囊肾外,肾外囊肿可累及肝、胰、脾、子宫内膜、卵巢、精囊、附睾及甲状腺。Nicolau 等(2000)在 213 例常染色体显性多囊肾的腹部超声检查中发现,67% 有肝囊肿,5% 有胰腺囊肿,胰腺囊肿的大小从镜下至数厘米。胰腺真性囊肿多见于婴儿,系胰导管异常发育所致。囊肿大小从镜下至数厘米,单房或多房,有一上皮内衬,内含浆液。淋巴上皮性囊肿罕见,至 2002 年仅见 40 例报道。常见于中老年,囊肿大小为 1~17 cm,内含角化物质。

第八节 胰腺囊性和囊实性病例误诊分析

日常工作中,因一些因素的干扰,部分胰腺囊性和囊实性病例会出现误诊,一些作者根据一组病例的误诊情况,分析了如下几种易于造成误诊的原因,并加以讨论。

"影像表现不典型"与对病变认识的不足:通过该组病例研究,该组作者认识到所谓"病变表现不典型",其实往往伴随着诊断医师对病变认识上的某些不足,从而造成误诊。如实性假乳头状瘤一般好发于年轻女性(平均 24 岁),有报道 30 岁以下患者占 90%,该组病例中 83.3%(5/6 例)为女性,66.7%(4/6 例)在 30 岁以下。

一般来说,年轻女性仅有轻微症状的境界清楚的胰腺肿块,且胰管一般不扩张时才应当考虑实性假乳头状瘤的可能,而该组误诊病例表现为胰头区肿块伴胰体尾萎缩、主胰管扩张,且年龄偏大(42 岁),并不符合以上临床和影像的典型征象;另一方面,实性假乳头状瘤的血供比胰腺癌更丰富、较大的胰腺癌对邻近脾静脉及其他大血管的侵犯概率很高等方面认识上的不足也是造成误诊的因素之一。

再如,胰腺假性囊肿多呈水样密度影,囊壁薄而光滑,常由纤维组织构成,不同时段检查可见病变有所变化。而该组误诊的假性囊肿呈囊实性,囊壁及实性部分轻度强化,且 6 个月后复查病变无变化,故误诊为囊腺瘤。分析其原因有可能是病变含有蛋白质及坏死物质等使部分囊内成分密度增高,且囊壁部分粘连造成不典型的强化表现。

想要克服该类原因误诊,影像诊断医师应当在掌握各病种典型表现的同时,对其不典型表现也应有充分的认识,并通过长期的临床经验积累、大量文献的阅读、扩大知识面和不断更新自己的知识储备来完成。

结合临床不够:胰腺假性囊肿常表现为薄壁囊性病变,其内少有分隔及壁结节,增强后囊壁光滑锐利,伴慢性胰腺炎时常可见到胰腺萎缩、钙化,胰管扩张,扩张的胰管内可有钙化,因其单纯影像表现极易与胰腺囊性肿瘤相混淆,因此胰腺炎病史的临床信息就尤为重要;同时还应注意到当假性囊肿伴胰管扩张,又不伴有钙化及明确胰腺炎病史时与导管内乳头状黏液性肿瘤鉴别较困难,该组病例中尚未发现这种情况。另外,误诊为胰腺囊性病变的实性假乳头状瘤,虽然一都分误诊原因是其囊性成分较多,但未注意到患者是 24 岁女性这一典型临床特征也是造成误诊的重要原因。通过该组资料的分析,充分表明了临床资料对于影像诊断的重要性,应引起诊断医师的足够重视。

检查方法的局限性:如较常见的分支胰管型导管内乳头状黏液性肿瘤,多表现为位于胰头或钩突区的囊实性肿块,其内可有强化的分隔和壁结节,主胰管和 / 或分支胰管扩张,其与囊腺瘤的主要鉴别为邻近扩张的胰管与病变相通,利用 MR 和 MRCP 检查可以有助于显示该结构,提高导管内乳头状黏液性肿瘤的诊断正确率。该组 CT 误诊的导管内乳头状黏液性肿瘤病例正是由于随后进行的 MR 及 MRCP 检查清楚显示病变与增宽的主胰管相通才得以纠正。又如浆液性囊腺瘤常表现为多发微囊,中央部可见延迟强化的放射状纤维瘢痕为其典型表现。其微囊结构单凭 CT 图像往往很难清晰显示，而 T_2WI 在这方面则有明显优势，该组误诊病例即是因缺乏 MR 图像而不能清楚显示微囊结构导致的误诊。再如黏液性囊腺瘤常位于胰体尾处，呈多房水样密度，可有钙化、分隔或壁结节，其囊内分隔有时只能在 MR 图像上显示，特别是在 T_2WI 和抑脂的 T_1WI 增强图像上（分隔在 T_2WI 像上呈相对低信号，T_1WI 强化后呈中等度强化），而 CT 在这方面则显示欠佳。

正如该组误诊病例 CT 表现为大单囊，因其没能显示囊内分隔这一典型表现加之囊壁又无钙化，而误诊为胰腺囊肿。由此可见，MR 检查在某些胰腺囊性病变的诊断中是不可或缺的重要检查手段，有时只有完善 MR 检查，才能帮助提高诊断准确率。

图像细节观察不仔细：这类误诊的出现往往伴随医师经验的不足和工作态度的不严谨，如该组中胰腺癌伴囊变误诊为囊腺癌的病例。虽然胰腺癌囊变后，有时表现极像胰腺囊性肿瘤，但仔细观察胰腺癌本身的特点，如病变远端胰管扩张，局部脾静脉受累等，均提示胰腺癌的可能性。另外，胰腺癌的囊变常位于肿块的偏中心部分，囊变区内无分隔，囊变区壁厚不均匀，这些也可借以与其他病变相鉴别，诊断不困难。细节观察不仔细往往会造成不必要的误诊情况，因此要求诊断医师一定要养成认真观察细节以及病变周围征象的良好习惯以及严谨踏实的工作作风。总之，充分提高对胰腺囊性和囊实性病变不典型表现的认识水平，注重影像表现的细节观察，密切结合临床，并正确选择影像检查方法是提高诊断准确率，避免误诊的保证。

第二十一章　重症急性胰腺炎

第一节　重症急性胰腺炎的影像分类

重症急性胰腺炎：重症急性胰腺炎常引起胰腺实质及胰周组织的损坏，并伴有休克、弥漫性血管内凝血、严重代谢紊乱及多脏器衰竭，还可出现胰腺坏死、脓肿、假性囊肿、瘘管及假性动脉瘤等局部并发症。增强 CT 及 MRI 在区别正常胰腺与胰腺坏死、判断胰周炎性病变及液体聚积作用方面相似。MRI 的多平面成像，可判断液体聚积、假性囊肿与上腹部结构的关系。MRI 发现出血、瘘管、周围脏器炎症较 CT 敏感，而发现气泡、钙化、假性动脉瘤 CT 优于 MRI。

急性胰腺炎临床症状及体征多变，而重症急性胰腺炎常伴有多脏器衰竭及脓毒血症。急性胰腺炎的病因有暴饮、暴食、胆石症、手术及 ERCP 检查后、胰腺癌，少见病因则有环形胰腺、异常胆胰管连接、胆管囊肿。

当伴有休克、肺功能不全、肾衰、胃肠道出血、弥漫性血管内凝血、严重代谢紊乱等脏器衰竭和 / 或胰腺坏死、脓肿、假性囊肿等局部并发症时，称为重症急性胰腺炎。

下列因素对急性胰腺炎的早期诊断判断其严重程度：确定临床病程、估计预后有很大关系：①胰腺坏死的程度；②出现胰外脂肪组织的坏死；③胰源性腹水中血管活性物质及毒性物质的数量及其生物性质；④胰腺坏死的感染。急性胰腺炎的早期诊断及其严重程度的判断，对于及时治疗、密切监视重症病人、加强护理极其重要。临床依据多种参数记分对急性胰腺炎进行分类。比如 Ranson、Imrie、APACHE Ⅱ、SAP 等，但其复杂性限制了它们在临床实践中的应用。20 世纪 80 年代，CECT（增强 CT 扫描）用于早期发现胰腺坏死，确定胰腺及胰周炎性改变。现在，它已成为确定胰腺炎严重程度及其预后的基本方法。MRI 在确定胰腺坏死及其范围、液体聚积（积液）方面与 CT 同样有效。

急性胰腺炎的增强 CT 分类：通过对胰腺及继发性胰外征象的分析，可以初步判断急性胰腺炎的严重程度。非增强 CT 可以确定胰腺水肿，常伴有肠系膜和肾周脂肪水肿、胸腔积液、肠麻痹等胰外征象。增强 CT 检查可以确定胰腺坏死的范围。在胰腺动脉灌注高峰，大剂量注射含碘对比剂（400mg I/kg 体重），可以显示重症急性胰腺炎的胰腺 CT 值明显减低。伴有大量灶性坏死区的出血坏死性胰腺炎在增强后不能清晰地显示坏死区，但其强化密度较正常胰腺及水肿性胰腺炎明显减低。

静脉团注对比剂的第 1 分钟，胰腺的强化较为明显，此为区分重症胰腺炎及水肿性胰腺炎的有效方法，重症胰腺炎胰腺强化值低于 30HU。通过评估胰腺及胰周感染和积液的出现及其程度，加上增强 CT 时出现胰腺坏死，可以进行急性胰腺炎分类。另外，胰腺的强化可分为密度均匀及不均匀，后者的未强化部分大约占全部胰腺的 30%、30%~50%、50% 以上。形态和坏死两种诊断指标的结合，形成急性胰腺炎的另一个诊断指标——CT 严重性指数（CTSI）。它能更精确地反映急性胰腺炎的病变严重程度。

急性胰腺炎的增强 MRI 分类：增强后 MRI 在区别正常胰腺及坏死胰腺、判断胰周炎性改变及液体聚积的作用方面与 CT 相似。T_1WI 脂肪抑制像上，正常胰腺信号高于肝脏。这是因为胰腺腺泡中的水性蛋白及脂肪抑制技术时图像信号强度再分级的缘故。

轻度急性胰腺炎时，胰腺保持正常形态和信号特征。病情加重，显示胰腺肿大及低信号。但其对胰周水肿不敏感，它与周围脂肪信号相等。采用4s回波非增强 T_1WI FLASH 能够区别胰周水肿和腹膜后脂肪。T_1WI 未抑脂像对胰周感染非常敏感，表现为胰腺边缘模糊。病情进一步加重，液体可在胰周组织、次级小叶及其他部位聚积，在 T_2WI 更易发现。

非增强 MRI，坏死的信号强度与发炎的腺体无明显差异。

重症急性胰腺炎时，胰腺实质的强化更加不均匀，而且很快减弱。在发现胰腺坏死方面 MRI 优于 CT。强化后重症急性胰腺炎的信号强度明显低于轻度急性胰腺炎。高磁场梯度强度的 MRI 在鉴别轻、重度急性胰腺炎方面优于低磁场梯度强度的 MRI。

MRI 的多平面成像能力对于评价液体聚积或假性囊肿与上腹部结构的关系很有用。无并发症的假性囊肿 T_1WI 为低信号，T_2WI 为高信号，注射钆剂无强化。血性液体聚积在 T_1WI、T_2WI 均为高信号。出血或蛋白碎片在混合性假性囊肿内形成独立的低信号层。

T_2WI 脂肪抑制像脉冲序列因其可以区别复合液体聚积内的液体及固体成分而曾被作为介入治疗前的主要影像检查方法。CT 图像上的气体在 MRI 质子密度图像上表现为稀疏的点状低信号。但是，MRI 发现气泡和钙化的能力较 CT 低。梯度回波图像对气体引起的伪影的敏感性有助于气泡的识别。MRI 可以比 CT 更清晰地显示出血、十二指肠炎及十二指肠狭窄。

第二节　胰管中断综合征

胰管中断综合征（DPDS）是指多种原因所致的胰腺的主胰管与消化道（十二指肠）的连接性中断，从而使断端远侧部分胰腺组织分泌的胰液不能正常排入消化道，继而引发胰瘘、胰周脂肪坏死、胰腺包裹性坏死（WON）、慢性胰腺炎、胰源性腹腔积液、胰源性门脉高压等一系列严重并发症的综合征。

胰管中断综合征的病因，包括急性坏死性胰腺炎、慢性胰腺炎、胰腺手术、恶性肿瘤、腹部外伤等，其中以急性坏死性胰腺炎的发生率最高。

关于胰管中断的诊断普遍认为 ERCP 是金标准，但 ERCP 为侵入性检查且因其无法对断裂另一端的胰管显影，故 ERCP 对主胰管中断的评价是不完全的。而 MRI 联合 MRCP 为无创性检查，既能显示胰腺及胰周改变，又能对断裂主胰管的近端和远端情况进行分析，故对急性坏死性胰腺炎所致的主胰管中断综合征的评估更有优势。

目前有一些文献报道用胰泌素刺激 MRCP 评价主胰管中断、胰瘘等，但尚未系统阐述急性坏死性胰腺炎致主胰管中断综合征的相关 MRI 表现，有作者收集一组经手术证实的急性坏死性胰腺炎后胰管中断综合征病例。

临床上引起胰管中断综合征的原因很多，譬如腹部外伤致胰腺撕裂伤，胰腺外科术后致主胰管损伤破裂，慢性胰腺炎致主胰管不均匀性狭窄、中断破裂继发假性囊肿，但最常见的病因为急性坏死性胰腺炎。

要确诊“主胰管中断”需要同时满足3个特征：①胰腺坏死的厚度超过2 cm；②胰腺坏死部位的上游（即胰尾侧）可见胰腺组织残存；③胰管造影术中注射入主胰管的对比剂出现外溢。要达到第3个条件，只能靠 ERCP 术（传统意义上 ERCP 是诊断胆胰管疾病的金标准），不过 ERCP 属有创性检查，该检查本身不适合急性胰腺炎（尤其是重症），且 ERCP 无法观察胰腺本身及离断胰腺上游组织的情况，因此 MRI 结合 MRCP 是很好的影像学检查手段。

传统的影像学检查技术对急性坏死性胰腺炎的诊断为增强 CT 检查，不过对于存在局部并发症的急性坏死性胰腺炎患者，后期若需要多次复查，则 MRI 检查可以避免过多辐射剂量的问题。相比较 CT 而言，对于并发胰管中断的急性坏死性胰腺炎 MRI 检查的优势和特点有：无辐射问题；MRI 软组织分辨率高，结合多个序列对胰腺及胰周病理状态细节的显示更丰富；压脂 T_2WI 和 MRCP 对主胰管的解剖特征显示更佳。

该组纳入的26例胰管中断综合征患者临床上按新亚特兰大分类为中度重症/重症急性胰腺炎，患者发病后首次 MRI 检查均为急性坏死性胰腺炎，其 MRSI 评分平均8.9分，影像学上为重症急性胰腺炎，与临床相符。该组急性坏死性胰腺炎坏死类型皆为胰腺和胰周坏死型,即胰腺实质内坏死和胰周组织(主要是脂肪)同时存在坏死,这一分型在病理学上最为常见。

急性坏死性胰腺炎的胰管中断:该组病例胰腺实质内坏死厚度平均 2.4cm,大部分(65.4%)表现为透壁性胰腺坏死、小部分(34.6%)呈厚层性胰腺坏死,这与上述提到的主胰管中断诊断的必备条件之一,胰腺坏死的厚度超过 2 cm 相符合;正因为坏死的深度已突破胰腺实质本身厚度的二分之一(厚层性)至全层(透壁性),故主胰管受累亦出现坏死,继而破裂中断,使得胰液持续性外瘘导致后期局部并发症的出现。

同时,就胰腺实质坏死范围而言,该组多数为大面积坏死(>50%),少数为中等面积坏死(30%~50%),这一现象可解释两方面的结果,一是相应的 MRSI 评分较高,故对应重症急性胰腺炎;二是坏死的范围越大,累及主胰管的长度就更长,这也构成主胰管坏死、中断的原因。Tann 等(2003)回顾性分析经外科证实的 26 例主胰管中断病例的 CT 和 ERCP 表现,发现 ERCP 显示所有病例主胰管在胰内液性积聚处梗阻,且 54% 的病例见对比剂外溢征象:在 CT 上沿着主胰管走行可见一孤立的、平均面积达 27 cm^2 的胰内液性积聚且合并上游残存的胰腺实质显示。这也说明坏死程度对于主胰管中断的影响。就胰腺坏死的部位而言,该组常见的在胰颈体和胰体区,所以后期主胰管在胰体部中断者最多。

主胰管中断综合征的直接征象:该组病例从急性胰腺炎发病随访平均 35 天后,复查 MRI 的特征为大多数(73.1%)在 MRI 的不同序列上可观察到主胰管中断的影像学表现,就胰管中断的位置而言,最常见的是在胰体部中断(57.9%),其次是胰体尾交界区中断(26.3%)和胰颈部中断(15.8%),部分患者 MRI 上未见上述直接征象,可能与扫描层面、层厚及主胰管被累及较重使其与坏死灶分界模糊而显示不清、胰体尾区坏死范围广使得残存的一点胰尾组织内的主胰管难以显示等有关。

此外,该组在 MRI 的不同序列上发现多数患者上游(胰尾侧)残存胰腺组织内的主胰管如“苹果柄”状走行至胰内 / 胰内外包裹性坏死处“截断”且近似直角汇入病变并相通,即“主胰管中断综合征”的出现,这可以解释部分患者腹部包块逐渐增大、腹胀加重的临床表现,原因是残存胰腺组织持续的胰液分泌从中断破裂的主胰管处外瘘至胰腺包裹性坏死内,使其逐渐增大,此时需要外科手术处理。

主胰管中断综合征的间接征象:即局部并发症胰腺包裹性坏死形成,正如该组病例在急性胰腺炎的后期均见这一局部并发症。这里需要说明的是,“主胰管中断综合征”的患者因主胰管破裂中断胰液不断外瘘从而在胰内外缓慢形成由纤维囊壁包裹的液性积聚影,既往称胰腺假性囊肿形成,但在亚特兰大分类里,将其更名为胰腺包裹性坏死形成,原因是这类患者均为急性坏死性胰腺炎,对应胰腺及胰周存在不同程度的坏死,后期(通常为 4~6 周)在胰腺内部或胰腺外周形成囊壁成熟的包裹性液性积聚,但此种积液内部并非单纯的囊液,它还含有或多或少的非液性物质影(实性或半实性的坏死碎片物)。

该组急性坏死性胰腺炎在病程后期发现的 37 个包裹性坏死病灶以单发居多,少数系多发包裹性坏死,病灶最大径 4~24.5 cm 不等,按包裹性坏死病灶分布以胰内和胰周同时受累最常见,这与首次 MRI 上胰腺坏死类型以胰腺和胰周均有坏死的病理特征相一致。该项研究的局限性是病例组未行 ERCP 检查,缺乏相关的影像学对照。

综上所述,若急性坏死性胰腺炎胰腺实质坏死表现为厚层性胰腺坏死或透壁性胰腺坏死时,患者会继发主胰管坏死中断,在这类患者的病程后期(通常 >4 周)可见胰腺内或胰腺内外同时受累的胰腺包裹性坏死形成,上游残存胰腺内主胰管如“苹果柄”状近似直角汇入胰腺包裹性坏死内并相通。该组作者认为可将这一序贯性表现称之“厚层性 / 透壁性胰腺坏死 - 胰管中断 - 胰腺包裹性坏死”三部曲。在 MRI 上,充分认识主胰管中断综合征的这一系列征象,有助于指导临床治疗方案的选择。

第二十二章　急性胰腺炎

第一节　胆胰管汇合与急性胰腺炎

急性胰腺炎发病因素多，发病机制复杂，胆管疾病，如结石或肿瘤梗阻，是引起急性胰腺炎的重要病因。但除此之外的其他诱因，诸如酗酒、高脂血症、暴饮暴食等，少数人患病究其原因可能解剖上存在着某种差异。部分学者对此已有关注，并进行相关研究，但多采取非活体解剖的方式，病例数较少，且非生理状态，故而有所限制。以往，有学者从胰管的形态学方面推测，以下情况可能易患急性胰腺炎：胰胆管汇合角度较大；胰管较粗，腔内压降低；存在共同通道并较长；胆胰共同管嵴膜不明显，“瓣膜”作用小；胰、胆管末端括约肌欠发达；除结石外的其他因素致胆胰共同管梗阻。但由于当时检查设备受限，检查例数或尸检例数较少，而且缺乏无创、生理状态下、可以整体直观显示胰胆管的检查手段，一直没有确切的结论。MRCP 的出现使得这些问题得以解决。

胆胰管汇合类型是否为“Y”型与急性胰腺炎发病关系：由于急性胰腺炎的发病有“共同通道”学说，而三种胆胰管汇合类型中只有“Y”型有共同通道，所以一组首先观察“Y”型汇合与急性胰腺炎发病关系。结果为 χ^2=0.455（P>0.05），说明是否为“Y”型汇合与急性胰腺炎的发病没有必然联系。

有无胰管变异与急性胰腺炎发病关系：该组数据中 OR=8.34，χ^2=18.935（P<0.01），证实胰管变异与急性胰腺炎的发病有密切关系，而且胰管变异是急性胰腺炎发病的一个高危因素。这可能与“存在十二指肠乳头功能不全和胰液流量增加，二者相互作用可以使背侧胰管的压力增加”有关，但具体原因有待进一步证实。在该组病例的观察中同时发现，同样有胰管变异时，胰腺炎的发生概率也是不同的，例如胰头处副胰管多而杂或是胰腺分裂时更容易合并有胰腺炎，但是由于该组胰管变异的病例数较少，无法进行详细的分类及统计学分析，所以有待进一步的研究。

共同通道长度与急性胰腺炎发病关系：随着共同通道的增长，OR 及 χ^2 值也随之增长，且 P 值均 <0.05，表明共同通道长度越长，患急性胰腺炎的危险性越大。一些学者从解剖学的角度证实了这一点：共同通道越长，“使两管之间的隔膜短而宽，这一缺陷使其不能遮盖胰管口，‘活瓣’功能不全而抗胆汁返流能力下降”，从而更易发生急性胰腺炎，当共同通道长度 >15 mm 时，称之为胆胰合流异常（AJPB），即胆胰管异常连接。

胆胰管汇合角度与急性胰腺炎发病关系：该组中胆胰管汇合角度在 50° 以下时病例组与对照组并无统计学差异；而在 50° 以上时则有显著的统计学差异（P<0.01）。说明胆胰管汇合角度在一定范围内时对急性胰腺炎的发病并无影响，而随着汇合角度的增大，大于一定限值时，急性胰腺炎的发病率明显增加。这也可能与汇合角度过大时胆汁返流的概率也随之增加有关。

综上，急性胰腺炎的发病在解剖上与胆胰管的汇合情况有一定关系，如有胰管变异、共同通道较长、胆胰管汇合角度过大都是急性胰腺炎发病的危险因素，但由于该组病例数较少，仅仅是一个初步的探讨，结论尚需进一步完善，并有待于更大样本数的研究。

第二节　急性胰腺炎对肝脏损害的CT观察

详见本书 本卷 第十二篇 第一章 第六节　急性　　胰腺炎对肝脏损害的CT观察。

第二十三章　自身免疫性胰腺炎

第一节　IgG4 相关自身免疫性胰腺炎误诊为胰腺癌

IgG4 相关性疾病是一种与自身免疫有关的系统性炎症纤维化疾病，具有独特的临床、影像及病理学特征，常累及胰腺、肝脏、胆管等多个器官，部分可多器官同时或相继受累。IgG4 相关自身免疫性胰腺炎（autoimmune pancreatitis，AIP）分为两种亚型：淋巴浆细胞硬化性胰腺炎（LPSP）和特发性导管中心性慢性胰腺炎（IDCP）。有学者研究报道亚洲的 IgG4 相关自身免疫性胰腺炎病人几乎均为淋巴浆细胞硬化性胰腺炎，欧美国家的病人两种亚型都存在，目前地域性差异的机制尚不清楚。

IgG4 相关自身免疫性胰腺炎起病较为隐匿，若病变位于胰头患者，多数以无痛性梗阻性黄疸为首发症状，黄疸有时呈波动性。部分患者表现为上腹部轻度压痛、血糖增高、乏力、脂肪泻、体重减轻、新发或加重的糖尿病等症状。另外，IgG4 相关自身免疫性胰腺炎常伴有硬化性胆管炎、硬化性涎腺炎、腹膜后淋巴结肿大、腹膜后纤维化及间质性肾炎等。IgG4 相关自身免疫性胰腺炎的影像学表现随着病变类型、纤维化及浸润程度的不同而表现出很大差异。CT 和 MRI 常见的影像表现是：胰腺局灶性或弥漫性增大，常伴胰腺小叶结构的缺失而呈腊肠样肿胀外观；动态增强扫描见胰腺实质均匀延迟强化，密度高于正常密度；胰周低密度囊状边缘（胰腺周围纤维化所致）；不规则主胰管和 / 或胆总管狭窄；主胰管上段扩张不超过 5mm。

此外，胰腺重度纤维化可导致胆总管胰腺段狭窄及近端扩张；20%~79% 的 IgG4 相关自身免疫性胰腺炎患者可见近段胆管及肝内胆管呈不规则狭窄，类似于原发性硬化胆管炎，前者狭窄范围广且狭窄近端胆管扩张明显，后者多为囊样、串珠样及枯枝样狭窄。

IgG4 相关自身免疫性胰腺炎最常见且最严重的误诊是位于胆胰管十二指肠连接区与胆囊管之间的胰腺癌及胆管癌（以胰腺癌居多）；而二者的治疗和预后完全不同，IgG4 相关自身免疫性胰腺炎只需要激素治疗，而胰腺癌、胆管癌常需根治性治疗。两者有着相似的临床表现，发病于中老年伴无痛性梗阻性黄疸、轻度腹部疼痛、体重下降等。由于胰腺体积增大（特别是胰头部局部增大），胰管、胆管同时受阻塞，在 CT 曲面重建、MRCP 表现为“双管征”，同时可伴有胆总管中上段扩张、胆囊肿大，因此极易误诊。

由于 IgG4 相关自身免疫性胰腺炎发病率低于胰腺癌，因此要诊断该疾病必须排除胰腺癌：IgG4 相关自身免疫性胰腺炎是 IgG4 相关性疾病的一部分，常伴有胰腺外损害，如硬化性胆管炎、泪腺肿大等；胰腺弥漫性肿大、延迟强化、囊状边缘在 IgG4 相关自身免疫性胰腺炎患者常见，而胰腺癌患者少见且胰腺癌边缘不光整、部分伴有胰腺萎缩；IgG4 相关自身免疫性胰腺炎患者 CAIgG4 明显增高且高于正常上限 2 倍以上，胰腺癌患者不升高或轻度升高；IgG4 相关自身免疫性胰腺炎患者血清 19-9 轻度增高，而胰腺癌患者常明显增高。在 CT 灌注成像方面，自身免疫性胰腺炎患者由于其内大量炎性细胞浸润，所以其组织灌注量较正常胰腺组织明显减低，但其强化的方式与正常胰腺组织仍相似；而胰腺癌由于肿瘤纤维化、肿瘤组织邻近由小动脉内膜增生所致的血管硬化以及肿瘤侵犯血管引起血流减少，肿瘤组织坏死使肿瘤局部灌注明显减低，也有助于胰腺癌鉴别。但这些鉴别方法均不是特异的，临床上有较多 IgG4 相关自身免疫性胰腺炎被误诊为胰腺癌的报道，因此，影像学表现不典型者，应考虑

CT、超声引导下穿刺活检进行进一步鉴别。

误诊原因分析:该例为老年男性患者,有与胰腺癌有着相似的临床表现(腹痛、黄疸为主),超声与MRI显示胰头部肿块形成伴胆总管下段闭塞、肝内外胆管扩张,血CA19-9升高,这些是该例术前考虑胰腺癌的主要原因。

第二节 IgG4相关疾病的影像学表现

IgG4相关疾病(IgG4-RD)作为一组新近认识并于2010年宣布的系统性炎症纤维化疾病,已引起国内外学者的广泛关注。影像检查对于诊断IgG4相关疾病具有重要价值,放射科医师有必要熟悉和深入了解此类病变。

IgG4相关疾病的定义:IgG4相关疾病是IgG4阳性浆细胞浸润不同组织或器官,导致该组织或器官肿大的硬化性病变。其特征为患者血清IgG4升高,激素治疗有良好疗效。

对IgG4相关疾病的认识过程:Yoshida等(1995)首次提出了自身免疫性胰腺炎(AIP)的命名。Kamisawa等(2003)报道AIP与Riedel甲状腺炎、腮腺和泪腺Mikulicz病及颌下腺Kuttner瘤均由IgG4阳性的浆细胞浸润造成,由其导致不同器官的硬化性疾病。Takahashi等(2010)报道IgG4相关疾病为一新的综合征,并得到国际上的认可。2011年10月,相关专家在美国波士顿召开了国际座谈会,确定此类疾病统一命名为IgG4相关疾病,各器官疾病的命名均以"IgG4相关"开头(表20-23-1)。

表20-23-1 各受损器官IgG4相关疾病的推荐命名

受损组织器官	推荐命名	受损组织器官	推荐命名
胰腺	IgG4相关性胰腺炎(Ⅰ型自身免疫性胰腺炎)	腹膜后	IgG4相关腹膜后纤维化
眼	IgG4相关眼病	肠系膜	IgG4相关肠系膜炎
泪腺	IgG4相关泪腺炎	皮肤	IgG4相关皮肤病
眼眶软组织	IgG4相关眼眶炎性假瘤	淋巴结	IgG4相关淋巴结病变
眼外肌	IgG4相关眼肌炎	胆系	IgG4相关硬化性胆管炎
眼眶	IgG4相关眼眶炎(包括泪腺炎、眼外肌受累及其他眶内合并症)	胆囊	IgG4相关胆囊炎
涎腺	IgG4相关涎腺炎(IgG4相关腮腺炎、IgG4相关颌下腺炎)	肝脏	IgG4相关肝病
硬脑膜	IgG4相关硬脑膜炎	肺部	IgG4相关肺病
脑垂体	IgG4相关脑垂体炎	胸膜	IgG4相关胸膜炎
甲状腺	IgG4相关甲状腺炎	心包	IgG4相关心包炎
		肾脏	IgG4相关肾病(IgG4相关肾小管间质性肾炎、IgG4相关膜性肾小球肾炎、IgG4相关肾盂炎)
主动脉	IgG4相关主动脉炎和/或主动脉周围炎		
动脉	IgG4相关周围动脉炎	乳腺	IgG4相关乳腺炎
纵隔	IgG4相关纵隔炎	前列腺	IgG4相关前列腺炎

IgG4相关疾病概况:IgG4相关疾病是一类原因不明的慢性进行性自身免疫疾病。患者血清IgG4升高,受累组织和器官由于大量淋巴细胞和IgG4阳性浆细胞浸润,同时伴组织纤维化而发生肿大或结节性(增生性)病变。IgG4相关疾病可多器官同时或相继受累,也可只累及某一器官。受累器官广泛,几乎可累及全身各个器官。

IgG4相关疾病好发于老年人,尤以男性多见。无特异性临床症状,根据发病部位不同表现为相应的症状。单个或多个器官或组织呈弥漫性或局限性肿胀增大，形成类似肿瘤的肿块。实验室检查：球蛋白增高，抗核抗体、类风湿因子等自身抗体阳性，血清 IgG4>1.35 g/L。组织学检查：病变部位大量淋巴细胞和浆细胞浸润伴纤维化，其中有大量 IgG4 阳性的浆细胞。

IgG4 相关疾病中，最早被研究的是 IgG4 相关性胰腺炎（Ⅰ型自身免疫性胰腺炎）。IgG4 相关性胰腺炎是最常见的 IgG4 相关疾病病变，可同时累及胰腺外多个器官。自身免疫性胰腺炎占慢性胰腺炎的 2%~11%，男性患病率高于女性至少 2 倍，患者年龄多大于 40 岁，平均年龄为 60 岁。

IgG4 相关性胰腺炎的临床症状较轻微，表现为部位模糊的上腹部疼痛、波动的梗阻性黄疸、体质量减轻和脂肪泻。合并 2 型糖尿病的患病率为 43%~68%。上述症状经皮质醇治疗后均可好转。Fujita 等（2012）报道，3%~9% 的 IgG4 相关性胰腺炎因误诊为胰腺癌而手术。

本病常用的有 2 个诊断标准，影像检查在本病的诊断中具有重要作用。

美国 Mayo 诊所标准（2006）：即 HISORt 标准，其中 H 为组织学，I 为影像学，S 为血清学（IgG4>1.4 g/L），O 为其他器官受累：胆管、腮腺和 / 或泪腺、纵隔淋巴结、腹膜后和肾，Rt 为对激素治疗有良好反应。符合以下 3 条标准中的 1 条或以上即可诊断：①组织学检查符合自身免疫性胰腺炎；②具有特征性的影像表现伴有 IgG4 升高；③具有特征性的影像表现并对激素治疗有良好反应。

Ⅰ型自身免疫性胰腺炎诊断标准共识：由国际胰腺病协会于 2010 年制定（表 20-23-2）。符合下列之一者可确诊为Ⅰ型自身免疫性胰腺炎：①组织学诊断 1 级标准（H1）；②影像学胰腺 1 级（P1）+ 任意一项非影像学标准；③影像学胰腺 2 级（P2）+ 任意 2 项以上其他的 1 级标准（包括胰管 2 级标准）；④影像学胰腺 2 级（P2）+ 血清（S）或其他器官受累（OOI）1 级标准 + 激素治疗反应（Rt），或 + 胰管 1 级标准（D1）+S 或 OOI 或 H2 级标准 +Rt。以下情况考虑可能为Ⅰ型自身免疫性胰腺炎：影像学胰腺 2 级（P2）+S 或 OOI 或 H2 级标准 +Rt。

表 20-23-2　Ⅰ型自身免疫性胰腺炎的诊断标准

标准	1 级	2 级
P：胰腺影像	典型：弥漫性肿大伴延迟强化（常伴有低密度晕征）	不典型：节段性和 / 或局限性肿大，伴延迟强化
D：胰管表现	长（>1/3 主胰管长度）或多处狭窄，无远端胰管扩张	节段性和 / 或局限陛狭窄，无远端胰管扩张（导管直径 <5 mm）
S：血清学检查	IgG4 大于正常上限 2 倍以上	IgG4 大于正常上限 1~2 倍
OOI：其他脏器受累	A 或 B	A 或 B
	A：胰腺外器官组织学检查（下列任意 3 项）	A：胰腺外器官组织学检查（下列 2 项）
	显著的淋巴浆细胞浸润并伴纤维化，无粒细胞浸润	显著的淋巴浆细胞浸润，无粒细胞浸润
	席纹状纤维化	大量（>10 个 / 高倍视野）IgG4 阳性浆细胞
	闭塞性静脉炎	
	大量（>10 个 / 高倍视野）IgG4 阳性浆细胞	
	B：典型的影像学证据（至少 1 项）	B：体检或影像学证据（至少 1 项）
	近端（肝内或肝门部）或近远端胆管多发节段狭窄	涎腺或泪腺对称肿大
	后腹膜纤维化	肾脏受累的影像表现
H：胰腺组织学	下列至少 3 项	下列任意 2 项
	导管周围淋巴浆细胞浸润、无粒细胞浸润	导管周围淋巴浆细胞浸润、无粒细胞浸润
	闭塞性静脉炎	闭塞性静脉炎
	席纹状纤维化	席纹状纤维化
	大量的（>10 个 / 高倍视野）IgG4 阳性浆细胞	大量的（>10 个 / 高倍视野）IgG4 阳性浆细胞
Rt：激素治疗	2 周内胰腺、胰腺外器官影像表现迅速好转	2 周内胰腺、胰腺外器官影像表现迅速好转

根据胰腺受累的范围，IgG4 相关性胰腺炎可分为弥漫型和局限型。影像表现包括：胰腺弥漫或节

段性肿大。胰管不规则狭窄，但其后方胰管扩张不明显。胰腺病变区 CT 平扫呈低密度。MR T_1WI 呈低信号、T_2WI 呈轻度高信号。CT 和 MRI 增强病变区早期强化较弱，延迟期出现不均匀雪花状强化。

胰腺周围出现包壳状低密度或晕征，为炎症所致胰周渗液、蜂窝织炎或纤维化组织；如果为纤维化组织，长时间延迟可有对比剂充盈。低密度包壳或晕征是本病特征性的表现，56% 的患者可有此表现。低密度晕征出现在病程的某一阶段，有些患者第 1 次检查可仅见胰体尾局限性肿大，无低密度晕征，且胰腺穿刺活检无肿瘤证据，而后继续复查出现典型的低密度晕征。如果为胰头部病变，胰头内胆总管段受累狭窄。

IgG4 相关性胰腺炎合并胰腺外其他器官 IgG4 相关疾病：88% 患者合并 IgG4 相关硬化性胆管炎；33% 患者合并肾脏 Ig4 硬化性病变；10%~20% 的患者出现后腹膜纤维化；33% 患者合并硬化性肠系膜炎；6%~17% 患者同时出现炎症性肠病；31%~54% 患者有血管壁受累。IgG4 相关的淋巴结肿大表现为 IgG4 阳性的浆细胞弥漫浸润淋巴结。淋巴结长径可达 2 cm，可表现为腹部（后腹膜、胰腺周围、肠系膜）、纵隔、肺门、颈部淋巴结肿大，其中胰腺周围、纵隔淋巴结肿大最常见。淋巴结肿大对激素治疗有效，肿大淋巴结的组织类型包括多中心巨淋巴结增生症样、滤泡增生、滤泡间扩大、生发中心样进行性变和结节性炎性假肿瘤样 5 种改变。

亚型：分为 2 个亚型，分别为淋巴浆细胞性硬化性胰腺炎（Ⅰ型自身免疫性胰腺炎、IgG4 相关的胰腺炎）以及特发性导管破坏性胰腺炎（Ⅱ型自身免疫性胰腺炎）。Ⅱ型自身免疫性胰腺炎的病理表现为中性粒细胞浸润导管上皮及腺泡，造成导管破坏，一般无或有很少（<10 个 / 高倍视野）IgG4 阳性浆细胞，血清 IgG4 正常，除了约 30% 患者可伴有炎症性肠病（如溃疡性结肠炎外），一般不伴有其他器官的病变。Ⅱ型自身免疫性胰腺炎患者年龄较Ⅰ型患者低约 10 岁，性别无差异。

胰腺外 IgG4 相关疾病可单独存在，头颈部是 IgG4 相关疾病的好发部位。涎腺：淋巴细胞性泪腺涎腺慢性肿大（Mikulicz 病）、慢性涎腺炎（Küttner 病）。眼眶：淋巴细胞性泪腺涎腺慢性肿大（Mikulicz 病）、慢性泪腺炎、眼眶炎性假瘤、眼眶淋巴增生和三叉神经炎。甲状腺：桥本甲状腺炎、慢性纤维性甲状腺炎。其他部位：包括副鼻窦炎、脑垂体炎、喉部黏膜下病变、头颈部淋巴结肿大等。

IgG4 相关疾病是一种好发于中老年男性、原因不明的自身免疫性病变。IgG4 相关疾病可以累及全身各器官，包括Ⅰ型自身免疫性胰腺炎、IgG4 相关硬化性胆管炎、Mikulicz 病（淋巴细胞性泪腺、涎腺慢性肿大）、Küttner 瘤（硬化性涎腺炎）、眼眶炎性假瘤、慢性硬化性泪腺炎、特发性后腹膜纤维化、慢性硬化性主动脉炎和主动脉周围炎、板状甲状腺炎和桥本甲状腺炎、IgG4 相关间质性肺炎和肺炎性假瘤、IgG4 相关的肾小管间质性肾炎等。这些病变可以单独发生，也可同时发生在同一患者。皮质醇对 IgG4 相关疾病有良好的疗效。

Ⅰ型自身免疫性胰腺炎是 IgG4 相关疾病中最常见的病变。对于不伴有胰管扩张的胰腺弥漫性或局限性肿胀，要警惕自身免疫性胰腺炎的可能性。影像上有自身免疫性胰腺炎的典型表现，则应建议作血清 IgG4 测定或激素试验性治疗，必要时行穿刺活检明确诊断。放射科医师认识自身免疫性胰腺炎非常重要，及时正确诊断可避免患者进行不必要的手术。

第二十四章　胆源性胰腺炎

急性胰腺炎病因最常见的是胆源（石）性和酒精（酗酒）性，两者占 90% 以上。另有 10%~30% 的急性胰腺炎因无法确定病因而被定为特发性（不明原因）胰腺炎。近年来，随着多种物理影像诊断技术的应用，能使胆系疾病，尤其是胆管内小结石、微结石、胆泥和胆汁结晶体等得以显示，2/3 的“特发性胰腺炎”病人获得胆源性胰腺炎的正确诊断，使胆石成为急性胰腺炎的主要致病因素。胆源性胰腺炎是胆系结石诱发的胰腺炎。一般认为，30%~74% 的胰腺炎病人有胆系结石，Cole（1938）推断 60% 的胰腺炎病人有胆系疾病。

病因病理学：Bernard（1856）首次发现胆汁和胰腺炎的关系。目前，对胆源性胰腺炎的病因病理学有三种解释。

共同管学说：Opie（1901）首次观察到胰腺炎患者胆胰共同管有结石嵌塞，创立了共同管学说。直到 Acosta、Ledsesma 和 Kelly（1975）分别证实胆源性胰腺炎是由于胆胰共同管被一个移动的结石短暂地嵌塞后，这个理论才被接受。即当一块胆石经肝外胆管排出后，嵌塞在胆胰共同管，使之梗阻，胆汁经共同管返入胰管，而引起胰腺炎。结石一般较小、轻，表面不平整，其直径比共同管的长度小。当结石阻塞共同管时，共同管内还有空隙使胆汁存留并返流入胰管。使共同管阻塞的原因，除结石经共同管排出以外，还可以是结石通过共同管时引起长期的慢性刺激，造成胆胰管下端括约肌产生刺激性炎症、水肿和纤维化，或共同管的先天性异常，或后天性括约肌纤维化和 / 或癌肿。胆管下端结石间接压迫胰管也可导致胰管阻塞。Hand 认为 80% 的人群有胆胰下端共同管，Sterling 指出共同管进入十二指肠的最小长度是 5mm，是胆汁生理性返入胰管所必须的。有功能的共同管，不仅易形成返流，还可使结石排出。一个足够小的结石和一个足够长的共同管，是共同管被结石阻塞后胆胰管间返流的先决条件。在早期发现一个嵌塞结石，和以后将结石排入大便中的关系，强烈提示胆源性胰腺炎的病因，涉及胆石从胆管排入十二指肠造成共同管暂时性阻塞，因此产生返流性胰腺炎，这与胆胰共同管这个功能性的共同管道密切相关。

共同管阻塞形成暂时性的共同通道闭塞，胆汁在非生理性高压下逆流入胰管，使胰管系统渗透压增加，出现间质性水肿。并且，胆源性胰腺炎病人胆汁常被感染，化学成分也不正常，在生理压力下经共同管逆流入胰管时，也可引起胰腺炎。

十二指肠液返流学说：当结石排出时，可造成胆胰管下端括约肌功能失调，或其他原因使共同管部分阻塞，导致十二指肠内容物返流，引起胰腺炎。但是，Acosta（1982）认为，结石排出时，括约肌段是开放的，暂时允许十二指肠液返入胰管，从而引起胰腺炎。

Neoptolemos（1989）认为，移动的结石可造成胆胰共同管出现裂口，导致活化的十二指肠酶返入胰管。十二指肠液返流学说能解释酶的快速活化和继发的病理学和生物化学变化的所有过程。在动物实验中用此法可诱出典型的胰腺炎。

不流动学说：Neoptolemos（1989）认为，当一个大结石存留在胆管下端时，可间接地压迫胰管造成阻塞。最靠近短暂阻塞部位的胰腺腺泡细胞膜和小胰管破坏，导致活化的胰酶逸出进入到周围组织，引起胰腺炎症、水肿和局部缺血，同时，肝外胆管受阻，造成急性逆行性胆管炎，肝外胆管扩张。

Neoptolemos（1989）将本症病程分为两期：第一期结石移动引起症状发作。一般是轻度发作，多为胆汁返流入胰管所致，但也应考虑结石排出可造成胆胰管下端括约肌功能障碍，使十二指肠液返流入胰管。第二期是胆管下端存留的大结石所致。此处靠近胰管，大结石间接地压迫胰管，造成阻塞，不仅可造成重症胰腺炎的发作，而且可引起急性胆管炎。这种分期法将上述三个学说综合到一起，可以较满意地解释胆源性胰腺炎的病因病理学。

我们赞成大多数学者的观点,可以认为,是综合因素引起胆源性胰腺炎。

尽管急性胰腺炎的发病机制并不完全明了,但已有实验证明当胰腺管被暂时或持久阻塞,胰管内压力升高达 60cm 水柱(正常值不超过 12cm 水柱)时,可引起胰腺腺泡膜的破裂,使胰酶释放入胰腺间质组织而引发胰腺炎。

在胆源性胰腺炎中,结石嵌塞不同程度地阻塞胆总管、胰管后,胰管内压力升高,胰液渗溢到胰腺间质内,激活蛋白水解酶,引发胰腺的组织自溶,产生无菌性急性胰腺炎;返流入胰管的胆盐同时激活胰脂肪酶,导致脂肪坏死。

然而临床上并不是所有的胆系结石(包括胆总管结石)病人,都会引发急性胰腺炎。Arendt 等(2000)认为正常时胰管压力要高于胆管内压力。由一块结石引起的单纯胆管十二脂肠连接区梗阻,并不会引起胆 - 胰返流。为此,该作者设想有两块结石同时迁移、嵌塞在胆胰共同管的上下,在胆总管内产生有毒的胆 - 胰液,使压力梯度发生逆转,有毒的胆汁进入胰管从而引发胰腺炎。

Kim 等(2000)的研究也证实了由结石继发急性胰腺炎与结石的多少(多于 20 颗)、大小(含有直径 <5mm 的结石)相关,而与结石的色素成分无关。Schleicher 等(2001)的研究发现人工封闭网状内皮系统能促使轻度胆源性胰腺炎进展为严重坏死型胰腺炎。由此证实胆管阻塞引起的肝网状内皮系统机能障碍,在胆源性胰腺炎的病理过程中可能是一个协同因素。

Chebli 等(2001)发现胆汁结晶体(胆汁沉淀物中出现的胆固醇单水化合物和 / 或胆红素钙微结晶)不但是引发胆源性胰腺炎的病因之一,且在对复发性胰腺炎病人做胆汁结晶体的针对性治疗后,胰腺炎的复发次数明显减少。这都说明了胆系结石所造成的阻塞是急性胰腺炎发病、进展、恶化、复发的关键因素。及时发现和去除胆系结石,对胆源性胰腺炎的防治至关重要。

第二十五章　胰腺结石和胰腺钙化

第一节　胰腺结石

胰腺结石和胰腺钙化：胰腺结石，又称慢性钙化性胰腺炎，习惯被称为胰腺钙化，在慢性胰腺炎中发生率较高，约占40%，此症首先由De Graaf(1667)报道。胰腺结石是由黏蛋白组成的蛋白栓沉着，并阻塞胰管，继以钙质沉积并与脱落上皮及碎屑共同构成的一种复合物。胰腺钙化，习惯上已将它与胰腺结石等同起来，事实上，胰腺内高密度影应当分为两类：一为胰腺结石，即胰管结石，它居于胰管的各级分枝中，其大小不等，形状各异，可在胰管内移动，容易用手术方法取出；一为假性结石，即名符其实的胰实质钙化，钙质弥漫性地(广泛或局限)沉淀于胰腺实质腺泡内，实质钙化体积小如针尖，呈比较均匀的弥漫分布，与胰管关系不明确，单纯手术难以取出。

病因学和病理学：近年来，随着酒精的摄入量的增加，胰腺结石有不断增多的趋势，而且，由于影像学检查技术的进展及普及，此病的发现率越来越多。

胰腺结石的病因存在地区性差异。在美国、南非及巴西，最常见的病因是慢性酒精中毒，而在印度尼西亚、乌干达等热带国家的胰腺结石，则被认为与蛋白质-热卡营养不良有关。遗传性慢性胰腺炎也常引起胰腺钙化。

甲状旁腺功能亢进、胰腺癌、胆系结石，甚至一些药物的使用也能导致胰腺钙化。如Dastur等报道一例60岁的胰腺黏液腺癌病人，用阿霉素、5-Fu和CCNu(doxorubicin Cycleothyl)化疗三周后CT检查发现胰头钙化，而化疗前CT扫描却没有这种表现。

尸解发现胰腺结石甚少，Stobble在一组27 787例尸解中仅发现43例胰腺结石。

关于慢性酒精中毒引起胰腺结石的机制研究较多。Howard认为，酒精中毒平均9年发生胰腺炎，其后6年发生胰腺钙化。甚至在停止饮酒后，病变还继续发展。长期慢性酒精刺激，使胰管出现明显的黏液样变，胰管上皮失去冲洗作用和润滑作用，胰管内胰液淤积形成结石；也可因胰管上皮吸收增加，固体物质浓缩产生淤积；并且胰管壁无平滑肌纤维，不能通过肌肉收缩蠕动来消除淤积，客观上为结石形成创造了条件。

Nakamura等通过13例胰管三维结构重建，在投射显微镜下观察，发现慢性酒精中毒性钙化性胰腺炎病人的胰管内常见蛋白栓，有时含有黏蛋白，其表面钙质沉淀就逐渐形成结石。这提示胰液的蛋白质沉淀是胰腺结石形成的最初表现。Sarles认为，胰液中的蛋白质浓度升高，碳酸氢盐降低，也可导致蛋白质沉淀。

关于胰腺钙化与胰腺外分泌功能不全的关系，Lankisch等的研究指出，随着胰腺外分泌功能不全严重程度的增加，胰腺钙化更为常见。但是，定性分析证实，胰腺钙化并不完全代表胰腺严重外分泌功能不全(50%假阳性)；重度外分泌功能不全也不一定有胰腺钙化。

胰腺结石由93%的碳酸钙，少量可溶性盐及大约7%的有机物组成。它造成胰管梗阻，致使胰腺实质破坏、萎缩、不规则纤维化和脂肪浸润。多数病人的胰管及其分枝出现各种不同程度的狭窄和扩张，这些变化一般发生于梗阻处的远端，梗阻处近侧存留正常胰腺组织。Banks认为，胰腺结石的长期刺激可导致胰管上皮不典型增生，甚至癌变。

临床表现：我们收集24例胰腺钙化中，17例位于胰头区，其中11例手术病理证实为胰腺结石。17例中有7例为满布胰腺的钙化，7例中有2例因糖尿病而不宜手术,余 5 例手术中有 3 例手术病理证实为胰腺癌。

X 线腹部平片:胰腺结石,由 93% 的碳酸钙、7% 的有机物及少许可溶性盐组成,故大多数胰腺结石能在 X 线腹部平片上显示。胰腺结石多位于第 12 胸椎至第 3 腰椎之间,一般居中线偏右,常为多发性结石,多数为 5~10 枚,单发少见。它以胰头部最多,向胰尾逐渐减少。当胰腺结石散布于整个胰腺或连续分布于主胰管中时,它的排列与胰腺走行甚为符合,即:从右下前走向左上后。如摄侧位照片,可见结石位于腰椎前 1/5 与其前方 2.5cm 范围内,比一般泌尿系结石稍微靠前。胰腺结石可随呼吸相不同而上下移位 1~2 个椎体高度。当胰腺结石的密度较低时,容易被腰椎椎体附件影及肠内容物所掩蔽而造成漏诊,必要时应行斜位摄片(特别是右前斜位),并注意做好清洁肠道的准备。阅片时,注意分析胰腺结石的形态,有助于正确诊断。胰腺结石常为斑点状、圆形及多角形,最具特征性的是沿胰腺走行的铸形结石及串珠状结石。有的胰腺结石中央密度较低,可能代表胰腺结石蛋白等有机物组成的结石核心。

胰腺结石大小不等,形态各异,遗传性慢性胰腺炎的胰腺结石一般比较大。我们所见的最大的胰腺结石为 2cm × 3cm × 5cm,呈多角形, CT 值为 330~500HU,中间密度明显减低。另见一例胰头部多发结石,呈分叉状,分叉的两支可能分别表示主胰管和副胰管被结石充填。

Glinsky 等认为,腹部平片发现胰腺钙化仍然是诊断慢性钙化性胰腺炎最简便最可靠的指征。在平片检查时,应注意和腹腔其他钙化(如:胆系结石、淋巴结钙化、结核性腹膜炎等)鉴别,有时还要与消化道憩室内的残存钡剂鉴别。Glinsky 等按重度、中度、轻度钙化和无钙化把胰腺各区钙化密度分为 3、2、1、和 0 级,由胰头向胰尾逐渐降低。根据胰腺结石的大小可分为大(直径大于 5mm)和小(直径小于 5mm)两类结石。尽管胰腺结石在腹部平片上表现较为特殊,但是,由于 X 线照片的密度分辨力甚低,它决定了这些征象只能在疾病的晚期才能发现,而且轻度病变颇易于漏诊,因此,在腹部平片检查时应特别仔细。

超声:慢性胰腺炎的特异性形态学变化,包括结石、胰管扩张及囊肿,超声均能作出准确诊断。由于慢性炎症,胰腺可出现弥漫性或局限性病变。Sandral 认为,如果有纤维化或钙化,胰腺的边缘可以不规则,实质回声增强。胰管可狭窄、不规则或扩张,梗阻最常见的部位是胆胰管十二指肠连接区。胰腺结石的特异表现是胰腺内强回声光团,如果结石特别大时,其后方可伴存声影。认为超声对结石的敏感性高于 X 线检查的说法不甚恰当。Alpern 报道 25 例腹部平片或 ERCP 证实有胰腺结石者,超声只证实 19 例局部有不均匀的高密度回声,超声检查也发现不了小的钙化。该作者认为,胰腺实质的高密度回声与 X 线照片上的钙化没有直接联系,这可能是由于伴有重度纤维化的胰腺炎及胰腺结石与周围结构的声阻抗缺乏差别的缘故。有时,超声对胰腺结石的发现率较低,可能与肠道气体干扰及检查者的操作技巧欠佳有关。

现代高分辨力实时超声能精确地观察胰腺实质和胰管,慢性胰腺炎的形态学变化,胰腺结石、胰管扩张及囊肿,超声均能确诊。胰腺结石病例 74% 可获得结石的回声, 30% 可见到胰管扩张的部位。当 X 线腹部平片疑存胰腺结石者,可首先选用超声检查进一步诊断。

钡剂胃肠检查:胰腺结石与胆囊阳性结石及肾铸形结石一样,在钡剂胃肠检查时,如仔细观察,可偶然被发现。在胰腺结石病例,如胃的张力较高,胰腺结石多位于胃窦的下方;如胃的张力较低,胰腺结石则位于胃窦的上方,立位观察时,胰腺结石位于胃角的上方。了解这些特点,有助于钡餐检查时发现胰腺结石。

CT:CT 的密度分辨力约高于 X 线检查 10 倍以上,一些细小的胰腺结石,即使是轻微的一点钙化,也能被 CT 发现。了解胰腺实质的各种病理变化,判断胰管梗阻是源于结石还是源于肿瘤,CT 在目前也优于其他影像学检查。对胰腺结石诊断不能肯定,或诊断困难,或鉴别诊断有问题者,应行 CT 扫描。Haaga 等曾见 1 例主胰管内有一枚结石,由于长期梗阻,整个胰腺自溶,仅剩下扩张的胰管,周围有脂肪浸润。

ERCP:ERCP 的应用,使人们不用手术就能使胰管显影,清楚地观察胰腺结石及胰管的继发性改变。尽管 ERCP 可出现并发症,再加上超声、CT 等扫描技术的提高,使得人们重新评价它的价值,但是,没有胰管异常的直接证据,外科医生们常常不愿手术。我们不能只满足于发现胰腺结石,还应进一步了解它所引起的胰管的继发性改变,在这方面,

MRCP 和 ERCP 有其独到之处。Gilinsky(1984)报道 69 例胰腺结石的胰管造影，32 例有大胰腺结石者，30 例发现胰管梗阻，其中 18 例由胰腺结石引起，另 12 例由胰管狭窄所致；37 例小胰腺结石者，仅 1 例显示胰管有梗阻。这说明，胰管的梗阻率与胰腺结石的大小成正相关，胰头的结石更易阻塞胰管。该作者回顾性分析发现，3、2、1 和 0 级胰腺钙化者，胰管显示梗阻分别为 66%、19%、10% 和 0%。Bornman 认为，如果副胰管相当通畅，则主副胰管汇合处近侧的狭窄或梗阻不一定引起胰液排出障碍，这种情况出现率约为 20%，应引起注意。胰管扩张明显时，大的胰腺结石在充盈良好的胰管中为相对低密度影；而胰管中度扩张，对比剂较淡时，胰管内大的胰腺结石则显示为相对高密度影，此时，小的胰腺结石则极易被掩蔽。有时，在胰腺结石周围有一毛糙的透亮环，这可能与其外周附着有机物有关。

胰腺结石需与下列疾病鉴别：胆系结石，右侧肾脏和右侧上段输尿管结石，腹腔淋巴结钙化。

第二节　胰腺结石与胰腺癌

自 Opitz(1901)首次报告胰腺结石并发胰腺癌以来，其发生率各作者报道不一。Netto(1960)报道为 25%；Howard 与 Jordan(1963) 报 道 为 9.4%；Johnson(1963)复习 1925—1962 年世界文献报道的 653 例胰腺结石，其中 24 例合并胰腺癌，发生率为 3.7%；石井(1979)报告为 8%；我们 11 例手术与病理证实的胰腺结石中，发现 3 例胰腺癌；如从弥漫性胰腺结石分析，我们 7 例弥漫性胰腺钙化中，2 例因糖尿病不宜手术，余 5 例手术，发现 3 例皆伴存胰腺癌。

病理学：胰腺结石与胰腺癌的关系，目前尚不清楚。Stable(1970)认为胰腺的钙化沉积物通过长期慢性刺激或引起胰腺癌。化学分析证明：胰腺结石的前驱物——蛋白栓，由浓缩的胰酶蛋白组成，与其接触的胰管上皮可发生糜烂、脱落、增生和鳞状化生，胰腺结石本身的长期机械刺激也可致胰管上皮不典型增生、化生以至癌变。

但是，Stable 又认为，胰腺癌也可能发生于胰腺结石出现之前，它似乎也可以是胰管梗阻、胰液淤积，及胰腺结石形成的原因之一。而 Friedman 指出，胰腺结石很可能不在胰腺癌之前发生，而家族性胰腺炎则可以发生在胰腺癌之前。我们认为，胰腺结石与胰腺癌两者确有因果关系，但是，孰因孰果，则须仔细分析具体病例来确定。

临床表现：单纯胰腺结石与胰腺结石并发胰腺癌，两者临床表现相似，均有腹痛、腹部不适、食欲不振、消瘦无力、腹泻、黄疸等，前者黄疸一般较轻，后者黄疸明显且呈进行性加重。便血是胰腺癌的又一症状，有时还可在腹部能扪及包块。

我们所见 3 例胰腺结石并发胰腺癌，术前均诊断为慢性胰腺炎与胰腺结石，手术与病理确诊为胰腺癌伴转移。其中 1 例首次手术时诊断为胰腺结石，并在术中清除结石，半年后症状复发且加重，再手术时方发现胰腺肿块，病理确诊为胰腺癌。

腹部 X 线平片：可见胰腺弥漫性钙化，遍及整个胰腺，且以胰头部为最密集。我们 3 例在平片上均见到胰腺弥漫性钙化，手术证实皆为胰腺结石，其中 2 例是在胃肠钡餐发现胰腺结石后才补摄平片。

胃肠钡餐检查：许多患者均是在钡餐检查时首先发现胰腺结石。Netto(1960)报告 6 例全是如此，我们 3 例中有 2 例也是这样。钡餐检查除检查胃肠外，观察胰区、胆区有无钙化，也应作为检查内容的一部分，尤其在胃肠道无异常发现时更应如此，因为胃肠疾病的症状体征与胆胰疾病的症状体征常常混淆不清。

超声检查与 CT：当钡餐或平片发现胰腺结石时，宜再行 B 型超声或 / 和 CT 扫描，以观察胰腺实质的情况，这是早期发现胰腺结石伴胰腺癌的有力措施。

Frick(1984)报道利用 ERCP 技术，向周围胰管注入少量对比剂，使胰腺实质密度增加，CT 扫描可发现胰腺癌的充盈缺损，这种被称为 CT-ERCP 的方法，对胰腺癌的实际范围的显示优于单纯 CT 和单纯 ERCP，对早期诊断有一定价值。但是，大多数学者对 CT-ERCP 都持反对意见，其原因是此种方法对胰腺实质损伤较重，对比剂引起的胰腺炎对病人的伤害，远较发现不甚确切的充盈缺损给病人带来的益处为大。

ERCP：此项检查能否发现并发的胰腺癌，取决于肿瘤的大小和位置。肿瘤大，位于胰管内或胰管附近，则容易发现，反之则难。绝大多数胰腺的腺癌与胰管上皮癌，胰管可出现不规则梗阻、中断，狭窄段胰管周围及胰尾段有不规则斑点状影，胰管内偏心性充盈缺损，主胰管及总胆管突然中断。当ERCP发现胰腺结石后，不应只想到慢性胰腺炎，把一切异常征象均用慢性胰腺炎解释，而应想到也可能有胰腺癌伴存，应行进一步检查与分析。胰腺的腺泡上皮癌表现为主胰管受压移位，肿瘤包绕可使病变区胰管侧支僵硬。胰腺的黏液癌可引起胰管不规则囊状憩室状扩张。Itai 等(1987)报道 6 例黏蛋白高分泌性胰癌，过多的黏蛋白和肿瘤亦可引起主胰管扩张变形，或出现明确的充盈缺损。

胰腺血管造影：在 CT、超声问世之前，胰腺血管造影被认为是诊断胰腺癌的最精确的首选方法，它可显示肿瘤引起的血管受压、侵蚀、狭窄、移位或中断，以及肿瘤所在部位的充盈缺损，并可判断胰腺周围有无肿瘤浸润和转移，以估计病变能否手术切除。目前，血管造影一般皆结合介入放射学进行。

第三节 胰腺结石并发胰癌

胰腺结石并发胰癌首先由 Opitz(1901)报道。此后一些学者对本病时有总结，但其发病率各说不一。Johnson(1963)复习了 1925—1962 年世界文献报道的 653 例胰腺结石，其中 24 例合并胰癌，占 3.7%。张万强与巫北海(1991)在 20 例胰腺结石中发现 3 例合并胰癌。胰腺结石与胰癌的关系目前还不太清楚。人所共知胆囊结石与胆囊癌有明显联系，Stabble 等(1970)认为，像慢性胆囊炎胆系结石会引起胆囊癌一样，胰腺钙化沉积物通过长期慢性刺激也可引起胰癌。

Banks(1979)报道，化学分析证明胰腺结石的前驱物——蛋白栓，由浓缩的胰酶蛋白组成，它可使胰管上皮糜烂、脱落、增生和鳞状化生。胰腺结石本身长期机械刺激也可致胰管上皮不典型增生、化生，以至癌变。因此，Johnson(1963)指出，慢性胰腺炎病人胰癌的发生率高于普通人群，慢性胰腺炎伴结石者胰癌的发生率高于无钙化的慢性胰腺炎病人。Ammann 等(1980)报道的 246 例胰腺炎中，仅 1 例非钙化性胰腺炎并发胰癌。

胰腺结石合并胰癌的影像学表现，除了有胰腺结石的表现外，其他影像学征象与单纯胰癌相仿。但是，胰腺结石合并胰癌的患者发病年龄比较年轻，较一般癌龄提前，近期病情明显加重，腹部平片均发现弥漫性胰腺结石。

Netto(1960)报道了经 X 线、手术或尸解证实的 24 例胰腺结石中，有 6 例合并胰癌，其腹部平片皆可见弥漫性胰腺结石。因此，对弥漫性胰腺结石患者，如果其病情呈进行性加重，用慢性胰腺炎，胰腺结石难以解释时，即使比较年轻，也要高度怀疑合并胰癌。须选用超声、CT、MRI、胰腺动脉造影等先进的影像学检查，必要时及早手术探查、活检，这对早期诊治有着一定的价值。

第四节 胰腺钙化的区别诊断

随着影像诊断手段的发展和机器设备的更新，在临床上胰腺钙化发现率越来越高，由于 CT 扫描的密度分辨率高于传统 X 线检查大约 10~100 倍，因此 CT 检查发现胰腺钙化率更高。

据 Ring 等(1979)分析，在欧美城市居民中，大约 90% 病人的胰腺钙化出现于酒精性胰腺炎。而据我们有限资料及国内有关材料分析，在我国，胰腺钙化大多见于慢性胰腺炎患者，这与国外差别甚大。

遗传性胰腺炎在 X 线检查时可以怀疑，它常有大而圆的胰腺钙化，此类病人的阳性家族史是重要的诊断因素。当胰腺钙化伴发肾结石时，应怀疑甲状旁腺功能亢进，宜再行生物化学检查。少数病人有渐进性囊性纤维化和真性糖尿病者也可见胰腺钙化。

在不发达国家，胰腺钙化常伴存于蛋白质营养缺乏。

在美国，大约有 2%~4% 的胰腺钙化病人同时存在胰腺癌，他们常有酒精中毒和慢性胰腺炎，可能是胰腺恶性病变发展的促进因系。当钙化与胰腺癌一起出现时，通常表示以往即有胰腺炎；偶尔，胰腺钙化只见于肿瘤近侧，导致胰腺管闭塞，则以前多未患胰腺炎。肿瘤性胰腺钙化可见于囊腺瘤和囊腺癌，这类钙化有时颇为特殊，呈现放射辐射状，常可提示诊断。海绵状淋巴瘤的钙化也具特征表现。

胰腺钙化除胰腺腺体组织内钙化外，还有胰腺导管内的致密影，即胰腺结石，它可伴存于慢性胰腺炎，它也可不出现胰腺疾病的临床症状，但却常常有非特异性胰腺管狭窄伴狭窄梗阻上游的钙质存积或结石形成。

胰腺假性囊肿蛋壳状钙化：我们曾发现 1 例中腹部钙化，正位片此完整的蛋壳状钙化重叠于第 2 腰椎体左侧缘，侧位片见其位于脊柱前方，手术病理见为一完整的薄壳鸡蛋状团块，位于胰腺体部，为胰腺假性囊肿蛋壳状钙化。

第五节　胰腺囊性病变钙化

详见本书 本卷 本篇 第二十章 第五节　胰腺囊性病变钙化。

第二十六章 胰腺结核

第一节 误诊病例简介:胰腺结核与胰腺癌

详见本书本卷本篇第十八章第一节 误诊病例简介:胰腺结核与胰腺癌。

第二节 极易误诊的胰腺结核

胰腺结核非常少见,极易误诊。胰腺结核的影像表现主要表现在胰腺病灶本身和胰外病变两方面。

1. 胰腺病灶表现 胰腺结核好发于胰头,体尾部亦可发生,也可累及整个胰腺;可表现为胰腺局灶性肿块、胰腺内多发结节病灶、胰腺弥漫性肿大。

(1)胰腺局灶性肿块:局灶性结核多位于头颈部,大小不等,其直径从数厘米至10厘米。

主要表现为位于胰腺的低密度肿块(干酪型或增殖病灶),当部分液化时,则表现为囊实性肿块;完全液化时为囊性病变,常有多数分隔。增强扫描见肿块周边明显强化及分隔强化,坏死、液化区无强化,增殖病灶可有轻度强化,一般低于周围胰实质及病灶周边强化。病程长者可出现钙化,但其发生率并不高。

(2)胰腺内多发结节病灶:胰腺内多发结节病灶表现为整个胰腺不规则结节样肿大,其内见多个灶性低密度区。增强扫描见结节状病灶周边强化,结节本身无强化或轻度强化。此型可能为血行播散感染表现。

(3)胰腺弥漫性肿大:胰腺弥漫性肿大表现为胰腺密度普遍性降低,周边模糊,与胰腺炎类似,增强扫描胰实质不均匀强化。常伴有胰周淋巴结增大、融合,增强扫描呈花环状强化。可能为粟粒型胰腺结核或反应性胰腺炎,因病灶太小难以显示,仅表现为胰腺弥漫性肿大和不均匀强化,结合胰周淋巴结表现有助于胰腺结核的诊断。

2. 胰外表现 (1)淋巴结:胰腺结核最常见的胰外表现是腹腔淋巴结肿大。可发生在胰周、肠系膜、肝门部、脾门等部位,大小不等,部分融合成团,其直径可达数厘米。CT平扫表现为低密度结节灶,增强扫描为均匀的环状强化,伴有中央轻度强化或无强化为其特征。肿大淋巴结表现为轻度强化之结节可能是结核增殖病灶,部分患者淋巴结可出现钙化,尤其是病程长者和经抗结核治疗者。

(2)腹腔实质脏器:肝、脾、肾等腹部实质器官也是血行播散型结核的好发部位。胰腺结核可伴有肝、脾肿大,包括反应性肝脾肿大和结核浸润,前者更多见。粟粒型肝、脾结核常不能被影像学检查发现,而仅表现为肝、脾肿大,术中可见肝、脾表面的粟粒结节,伴发肝、脾之局灶性病灶则罕见,但免疫机能低下者,如获得性免疫缺陷综合征患者,则易于见到。

3. 鉴别诊断 (1)局部肿块型胰腺结核:局部肿块型胰腺结核术前常误诊为胰腺癌,特别是胰头癌,误诊原因有以下三个方面:胰腺结核发病率很低,临床医师警惕性不足,而胰腺癌为常见病;二者临床表现和影像学征象相似,都好发于胰头部,临床表现为腹痛、腹块并可伴有梗阻性黄疸,CT上常表现为局部软组织肿块,并可伴有肿块内不同程度坏死、胆胰管扩张、胰体尾部萎缩以及邻近淋巴结肿大等;对胰腺结核的影像学特征认识不够。

局部肿块型胰腺结核与胰腺癌的鉴别要点：①临床表现不同，胰腺结核可见于较年轻者，有较长时间的低热、盗汗等症状，结核菌素试验阳性及胰外结核的临床表现；而胰头癌常见于40岁以上患者，有进行性黄疸、消瘦、恶液质等症状、体征。②胰腺结核可出现较为特征或与胰腺癌有鉴别价值的CT表现：胰内多发结节灶；肿块内斑点状钙化灶；干酪样坏死可很明显，而呈单房或多房囊样肿块；呈蜂窝状强化的软组织肿块，偶尔肿块内有气体；可伴有胰外结核，特别是特征性淋巴结结核。而胰腺癌肿块内罕见钙化，坏死程度一般较轻且不规则，肿块内无气体，增强后呈不均匀强化而无蜂窝状强化，早期即有胰管破坏，胆胰管扩张更常见。少数鉴别困难者应及时穿刺活检或剖腹探查，以免延误治疗时机。

（2）囊性胰腺结核：囊性胰腺结核与胰腺囊性肿瘤鉴别困难，但后者多为中年以上妇女，囊壁上可有壁结节。另外穿刺抽取囊液有助于鉴别诊断，结核性脓肿多为坏死物或乳白色物质，囊腺癌多为黏液或无色透明液体。囊性胰腺结核尚需与胰腺脓肿、假性囊肿鉴别，胰腺脓肿多数病例有胰腺炎病史而淋巴结常无明显肿大，假性囊肿以单房多见，胰腺脓肿胰周围渗出明显，抗生素治疗有效。

（3）多发结节型胰腺结核：多发结节型胰腺结核还需与淋巴瘤和转移瘤鉴别，综合分析临床病史、实验室检查及影像学表现对作出正确诊断必不可少。

第三节　胰腺结核的诊断思维

由于胰腺结核通常表现为环形强化的肿块伴有中央坏死的出现，因此需与胰腺肿瘤伴囊变坏死、胰腺囊实性肿瘤等鉴别。胰腺囊实性肿瘤种类繁多，临床特征常不明显，影像学表现又具有交叉性，诊断较为困难。

根据影像学表现，多发微囊型肿块多考虑为浆液性囊腺瘤，患者多无症状出现，建议随访观察：若出现腹痛或黄疸等表现，需考虑手术切除。

影像学上表现为较大单发囊性病灶时，特别是女性患者，且病灶位于体尾部者，首先考虑黏液性囊性肿瘤，但寡囊型浆液性囊腺瘤与黏液性囊性肿瘤表现类似，浆液性囊腺瘤囊液的CEA水平一般低于5 ng/ml，鉴别困难时需进行内镜超声引导下的穿刺活检。

约1/3的黏液性囊性肿瘤为恶性，一般可见结节或者直径大于4cm。对于体积较小的病灶，以前推荐终身随访，由于患者年纪较轻，且病灶多位于胰腺体尾部，较易手术，为免除长期随访，故现多建议手术切除，除具有侵犯性的恶性肿瘤，一般不需术后随访。

影像学上表现为较大多发囊性病灶时，特别是出现与胰管交通时，首先考虑导管内乳头状黏液性肿瘤。当肿块累及主胰管或同时累及主胰管和分支胰管时，须手术切除，因此观察病灶是否累及主胰管对诊断尤为重要。

对于分支胰管型导管内乳头状黏液性肿瘤，恶变率约1%，当出现黄疸、主胰管扩张及强化的实性肿块时，应考虑恶变的可能。其他征象，如直径大于3 cm，但无壁结节时，可考虑随访。反之，若出现壁结节者，即使病灶体积小于3 cm，都需考虑恶变可能。另外，胰腺炎、生长迅速、主胰管直径快速变化及胰腺萎缩等特征，虽然尚未明确，但值得警惕。

与黏液性囊性肿瘤术后无需长期随访不同，即使是非侵犯性导管内乳头状黏液性肿瘤，仍具有多发性（21%~40%）、进展性的特征，故术后需密切随访。

当影像上表现出边界清楚、密度不均匀的囊实性肿块，特别是年轻女性患者时，应考虑到实性假乳头状肿瘤，虽然该肿瘤为良性表现，但仍有不到20%的病灶侵犯血管、周围神经，可有淋巴结、肝转移等表现。

当影像学上出现囊性病灶，伴环形强化，并内部分隔或实性成分者，应考虑胰腺神经内分泌肿瘤，其中囊性者约占17%，且大多为无意中发现、无功能型，但影像学上囊性神经内分泌肿瘤难以与黏液性囊性肿瘤鉴别，需要通过内镜引导下穿刺活检。神经内分泌肿瘤囊液的CEA水平一般低于5 ng/ml，且细针穿刺活检细胞学检测含量较高。由于仅从大体形态及活检，一般难以确定胰腺内分泌肿瘤的良、恶性，因此对于怀疑此病者均应考虑手术切除。

原发局灶性胰腺结核与胰腺癌表现类似，特别是在出现梗阻性黄疸或伴有胆总管、胰管扩张时，两者鉴别存在困难。胰腺癌通常出现坏死,类似胰腺结核的干酪样坏死,但很少囊变,一般出现囊变者体积较大(平均 7 cm)。此时要高度注意临床指标,胰腺结核患者年龄相对较轻,通常没有肿瘤指标的升高:而胰腺癌常见于老年人,往往出现肿瘤指标的升高。

影像学上,超声、CT 和 MRI 都能发现胰腺的病灶,增强 CT 扫描可见病灶及其周围肿大淋巴结具有延迟环形强化的特点、胆胰管的扩张程度与胰腺肿块不成比例、压迫血管和胆管而非侵犯等特征有助于胰腺结核的诊断。

MSCT 血管成像不管是动脉还是静脉都只是受压而非侵犯,这与胰腺癌不同,但也有文献报道胰腺结核可见血管受累的表现。鉴别困难时,首先通过影像学检查如 CT 对病灶可切除性进行评估,如果病灶无法切除,则需采用内镜超声引导下细针穿刺活检、超声或 CT 引导下的活检等方法获取组织进行病理或微生物检查。

胰腺结核伴有广泛腹膜后、肝门淋巴结肿大时,需要与淋巴瘤相鉴别。两者在临床上都可以出现发热、消瘦、腹痛等症状,在影像学上都表现为局灶性的胰腺病灶伴有淋巴结肿大,都少有胆管梗阻的表现或肿块与胆管扩张不成比例,且淋巴瘤亦可表现为弥漫性累及。淋巴瘤好发于 50 岁左右的中年人,胰腺病灶和肿大淋巴结在 CT 上均表现为密度均匀的实质性,增强扫描有轻度均匀强化,伴有胰管狭窄或轻度扩张的表现,肿大的淋巴结往往融合成团块状,且具有包绕血管的特性;而胰腺结核多见于 30~40 岁中青年人,胰腺病灶和肿大淋巴结都具有环形强化的典型表现,淋巴结较少融合,且很少侵犯血管,与淋巴瘤包绕血管的特点不同。胰腺结核有时类似急慢性胰腺炎的表现,出现冷脓肿时则需要与胰腺脓肿或假性囊肿相鉴别。此时需要密切关注临床病史和表现,而影像学的价值在于明确胰腺病灶及其范围。

总之,对于胰腺肿物而言,临床上有结核病史而没有肿瘤指标的升高、影像学上胰腺病灶具有典型环形强化、肿块虽大却没有梗阻性黄疸或肿块与胆管扩张程度不成比例的中青年人,要想到胰腺结核的可能性,鉴别诊断困难时则需要活检以获得最终诊断,尽量避免延误诊治或不必要的手术。

第四节　胰腺结核

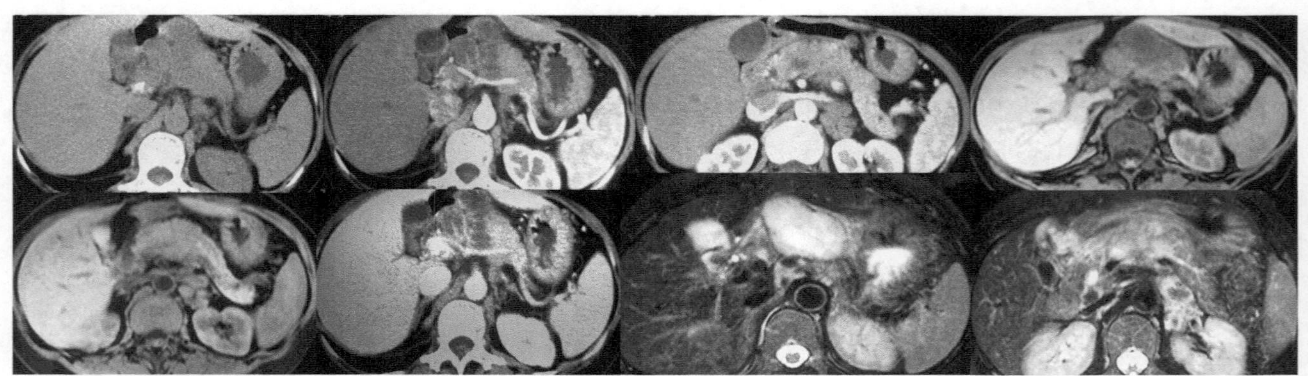

图 20-26-1　胰腺结核

患者,女性, 50 岁。中上腹隐痛 3 个月余入院。 3 个月前无明显诱因出现中上腹隐痛不适,向腰背部放射,进食后加重。皮肤、巩膜无黄染。无寒战、发热;恶心、呕吐;腹泻、便秘。

病理诊断:胰腺结核(图 20-26-1)。

第二十七章　慢性胰腺炎

第一节　三种慢性胰腺炎

慢性胰腺炎侵犯胰腺两个部位以上，经影像学检查和手术证实无实质性硬性包块者，称为慢性弥漫型胰腺炎。

Alpern（1985）和 Luetmer（1989）称慢性胰腺炎累及局部者为慢性局灶性胰腺炎。

慢性胰腺炎也可因小叶间或胰管周围纤维组织增生和慢性炎性细胞浸润形成炎性肿块（即称肿块型胰腺炎），因它极难与肿瘤鉴别，亦称为假肿瘤性胰腺炎（Lammer，1985）。

以上三种慢性胰腺炎之临床症状相似，但手术和影像学检查发现有所不同，观察了解病变的范围和能否查明胰腺炎性肿块是鉴别的关键。

第二节　有关慢性胰腺炎的诊断标准

一些作者提出有关慢性胰腺炎的诊断标准如下：手术或其他方法得到组织病理学诊断； 有胆系疾病史，术中探察见胰腺呈慢性胰腺炎形态改变，但未扪及硬性胰腺肿块和附近淋巴结肿大；胰腺结石或胰腺钙化伴一种影像学检查见到胰腺炎症表现；胰腺外分泌功能试验相当长时间内呈现异常；典型临床症状，体征持续一年以上，同时上述五项中有疑诊，治疗好转者。

如病变已累及胰腺体积一半以上，同时无实质性胰腺肿块，方能诊断为慢性弥漫型胰腺炎。

第三节　CT 检查中胰管扩张的意义

在 CT 横断扫描时，正常大小的胰管并非总可见到。正常人的主胰管平均直径的范围，从 30~50 岁年龄组的 3.3mm 到 70~90 岁组的 4.6mm。

然而，扩张的胰管却容易在正常胰实质影像中以低密度的线状结构显现出来，尤以胰腺中心部位更为明显。Haunz 和 Bag-genstoss（1950）在尸解胰腺癌病人时发现继发于胰癌的胰管扩张，直径平均为 2.5cm，至少比正常值大三倍以上。在 CT 图像上，低密度的胰腺假性囊肿、脓肿有时可与扩张的胰管混淆。

Seidelmam 等（1977）指出，分隔正常胰腺与脾静脉的脂肪层可误为扩大的胰管。胰管扩张可出现于胰新生物与胰腺炎，“双管征”有助于确定梗阻的平面（位于胆管与胰管下端共同管之下方），但无助于病因学的诊断（含新生物、结石、狭窄等）。

第四节　假肿瘤性慢性胰腺炎

详见本书 本卷 本篇 第九章 第一节　假肿瘤性　　慢性胰腺炎。

第五节　误诊病例简介：慢性胰腺炎所致的良性病变与恶性肿瘤

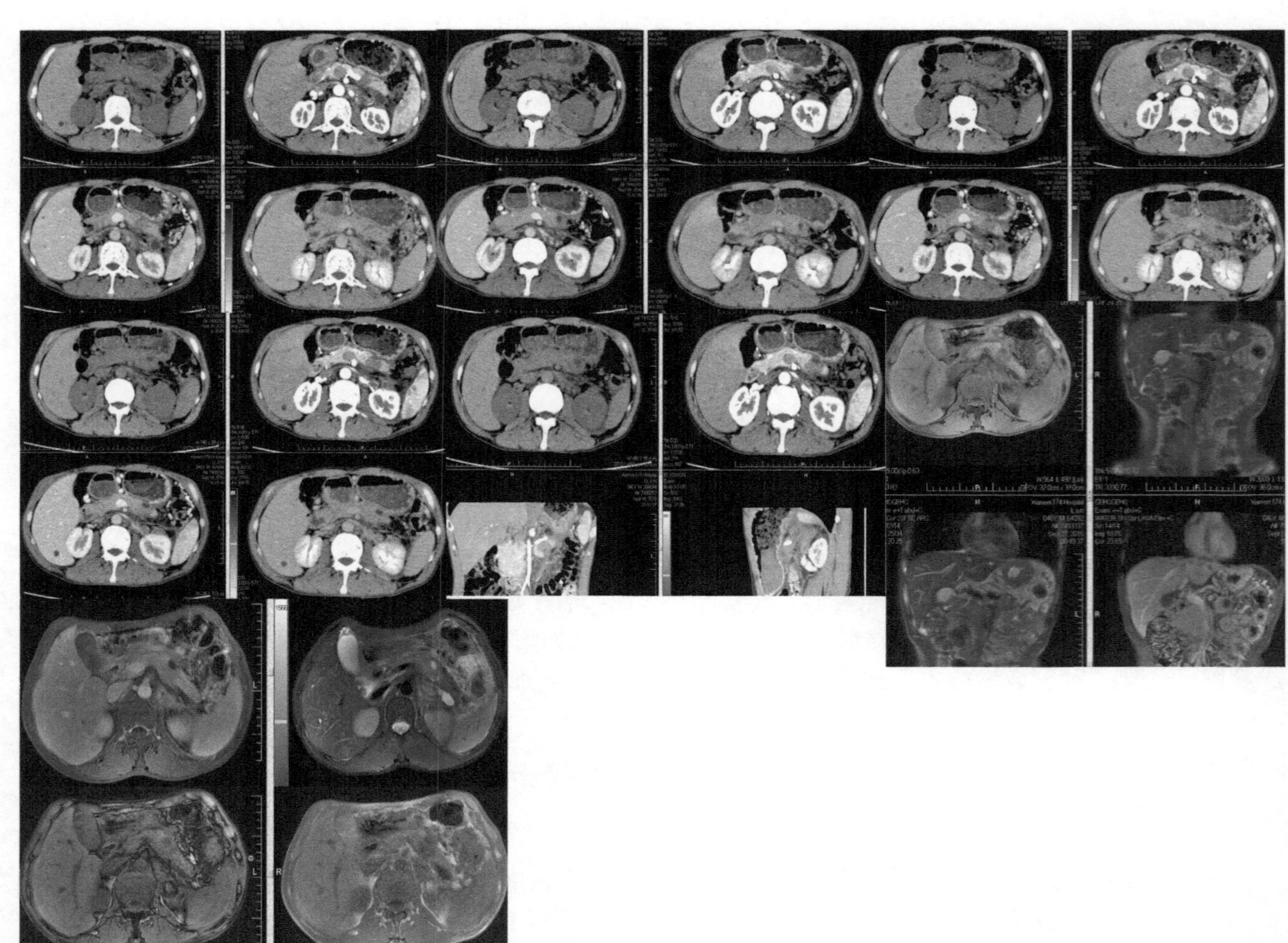

图 20-27-1　慢性胰腺炎所致的良性病变与恶性肿瘤

患者，男，46 岁。反复左腰腹部疼痛不适 1 个月余入院。术前诊断：胰腺恶性肿瘤。

手术所见：见胰体尾与脾门、胃大弯、横结肠脾区及后腹膜组织粘连紧密，无法完全分离，考虑肿物质地硬，术前肿瘤指标升高，故术中决定行肿块整块切除，切除范围包括胰体尾、脾、部分胃壁、横结肠脾区。

病理检查：胰、脾、胃大弯及横结肠：胰腺组织大小 8 cm ×4.5 cm ×4.5 cm，切面见一灰白区，面积约 4 cm ×4 cm，质韧，与周边组织界限欠清；胰腺周围附有脾脏、胃及肠管组织，其中脾脏大小 11 cm ×10 cm ×4 cm，重约 80g，切面呈红褐色，质中；胃大小 8.5 cm ×3.5 cm ×3 cm，胃黏膜呈灰红色，未见明显异常；肠管长 15 cm，两侧切缘直径均为 1.7 cm，肠黏膜呈灰褐色，皱襞明显。冰冻病理诊断：胰、脾、胃大弯及横结肠，切除标本：胰腺体尾部区域软组织结节，镜下见纤维脂肪组织坏死伴成纤维细胞增生及小导管（疑似胰腺小导管）增生，导管上皮未见明确恶性征象，考虑为慢性胰腺炎所致的良性病变，确诊待常规多块取材。常规病理诊断：胰、脾、胃大弯及横结肠切除标本：镜下见纤维脂肪组织坏死伴成纤维细胞增生及胰腺小导管增生，导管上皮未见明确恶性征象，考虑为慢性胰腺炎所致的良性病变，待做免疫组化进一步分析；炎性病变波及脾门、胃大弯及横结肠外膜纤维脂肪组织（图 20-27-1）。

第六节　自身免疫性胰腺炎

详见本书 本卷 本篇 第二十三章　自身免疫性胰腺炎。

第七节　误诊病例简介：胰体尾部慢性胰腺炎与胰体尾部肿瘤

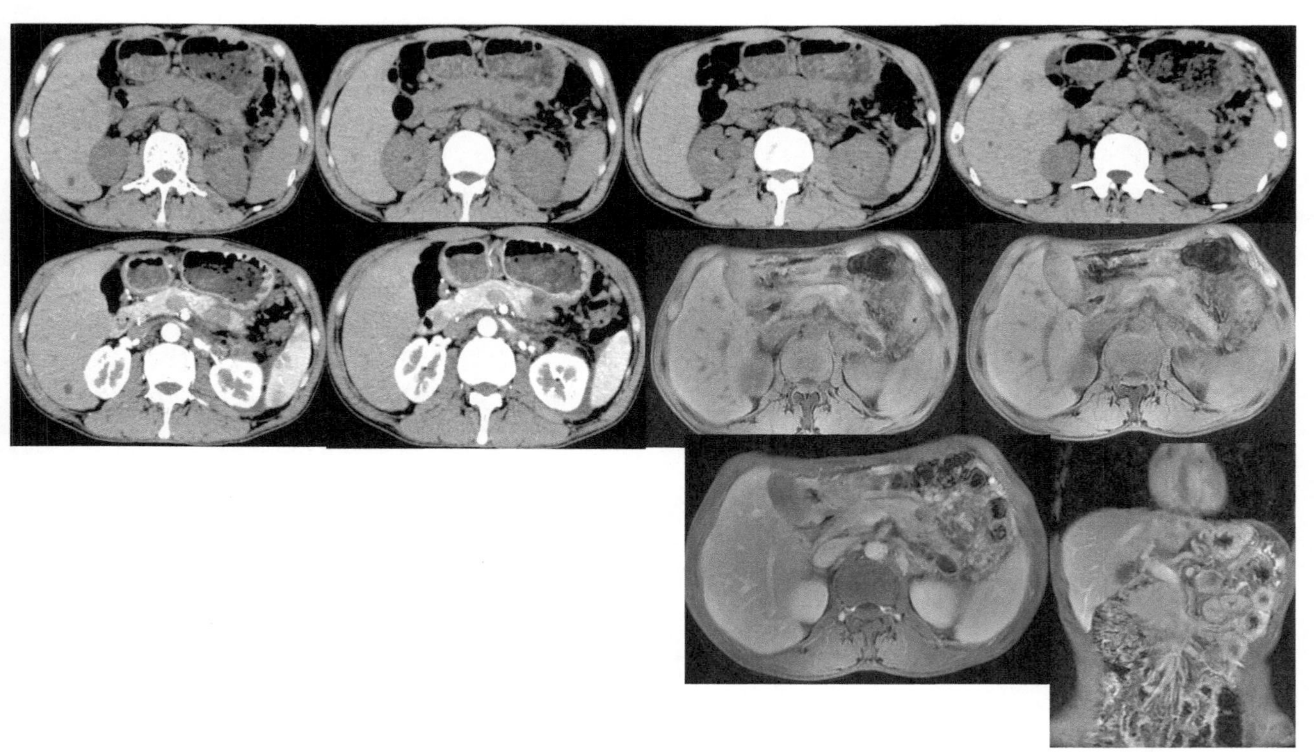

图 20-27-2　胰体尾部慢性胰腺炎与胰体尾部肿瘤

患者，男，46 岁。超声与 CT 平扫发现胰体尾部肿大，实验室检查提示 CA19-9 升高，考虑胰体尾部肿瘤，术后病理免疫组化诊断为慢性炎症。

术后病理免疫组化诊断：胰体尾部慢性胰腺炎伴纤维脂肪组织坏死及纤维组织显著增生，并胰腺导管增生。炎性病变累及脾门、胃大弯及横结肠外膜纤维脂肪组织。（图 20-27-2）

第二十八章 关于糖尿病

第一节 糖尿病胰腺的密度、轮廓和厚度

Gilbeau(1992)用CT扫描分析57例糖尿病患者的胰腺密度、轮廓和厚度。病人分为三组:胰岛素依赖型20例,未用胰岛素治疗也非胰岛素依赖型者25例,用胰岛素治疗但非胰岛素依赖型者12例,并且与对照组的相应结果作了比较(对照组57例非糖尿病者年龄与糖尿病组相近)。研究结果发现:对照组与糖尿病组不同组织之间的胰腺密度无统计学差异。在对照组中,40岁以上胰腺分叶的出现率高于40岁以下者,41~60岁和61~90岁的糖尿病病人,其胰腺分叶的出现率明显高于相应的对照组;与对照组相比,未用胰岛素治疗糖尿病病人的胰体明显缩小,而胰头与胰尾缩小不显著;胰岛素治疗的病人与对照组相比,胰腺各部分均变小。各组病人的胰尾大小均与病程长短有明显关系,胰体大小与年龄密切相关。对照组中年龄与胰腺大小无关。胰岛素依赖型病人的基础血清C肽水平明显低于非胰岛素依赖型且未用胰岛素治疗的病人,和非胰岛素依赖型经胰岛素治疗的病人。

该作者指出:糖尿病患者的胰腺小于对照组,这与以前的尸检发现相符。胰岛素治疗病人的胰腺较未用胰岛素治疗的缩小明显,这一发现和C肽测定结果提示胰岛素治疗的病人有胰岛素分泌降低;胰体似乎是受侵很严重的部分;非依赖型病人需胰岛素治疗似乎与胰头缩小有关,在这些病人,胰腺的萎缩是一种进展过程的表现,首先累及体部,然后是整个胰腺,而头部最后受累。因此,胰腺CT检查可以帮助发现那些有患糖尿病危险的病人(胰腺萎缩)以及非胰岛素依赖型糖尿病病人和那些不久需胰岛素治疗的病人。

第二节 脂肪萎缩性糖尿病

脂肪萎缩性糖尿病是一种少见的胰岛素抵抗性糖尿病,病因不明,由Ziegler(1928)首先报道。影像学表现包括软组织和骨骼异常,软组织异常主要是脂肪含量明显减少或消失,无确切的皮下脂肪层。Garg(2000)用MR检查脂肪分布发现,在某一特定的部位尚有脂肪残存,即在眼眶、手掌、足、头皮、会阴、关节周围及脊柱椎间孔内尚存有脂肪。乳腺、舌、颊部等亦残留少量脂肪。骨骼异常表现为关节周围骨质内出现透亮区或局灶性硬化,也可出现溶骨性病灶,在MRI上表现为液-液平面,增强后表现为环行强化。骨干皮质增厚、骨髓过度生长,增强后骨髓腔表现为弥漫性强化。外周骨骼缺乏脂肪,在T_1WI上表现为低信号,T_2WI短反转恢复序列表现为高信号。一例显示躯干骨形态、密度未见异常。胸腰椎MRI表现为T_1WI高信号,脂肪抑制像信号减低,提示骨髓腔内存在脂肪,但信号欠均匀,可能有脂肪减少,需要定量检查才能进一步明确。

脂肪萎缩性糖尿病需与以下疾病鉴别:

(1)神经性厌食症:神经性厌食症骨髓MRI表现与脂肪萎缩性糖尿病类似,均出现体部软组织脂肪减少,但神经性厌食症的X线平片不会出现液-液平面。

(2)局限性脂肪萎缩:局限性脂肪萎缩体部脂肪丧失常常以上肢为主,而脂肪萎缩性糖尿病表现

为弥漫性。

（3）畸形性骨炎：两者均可见颅骨和长骨骨干皮质增厚，但畸形性骨炎导致骨小梁增厚紊乱，好发于老年人，脂肪萎缩性糖尿病以青年女性多见。

（4）纤维结构不良：在纤维结构不良，其透亮区常有斑点状钙化，表现为磨玻璃样。

（5）骨坏死：骨坏死范围局限，病灶周边有边缘清晰的环状钙化，这和脂肪萎缩性糖尿病不同。

第二十九章　关于胰腺周围血管

胰头周围门静脉-肠系膜静脉系统的解剖及变异

关于胰头周围动脉系统的发育变异已有较多文献报道,但有关此区域门静脉肠系膜静脉系统的发育变异鲜有文献报道。随着 CT 技术迅猛发展,其空间分辨力可达亚毫米(0.4 mm)水平,使得增强 CT 三维血管成像的准确性极大提高,对门静脉-肠系膜静脉系统解剖和变异的在体研究也更深入。一组作者通过复习相关文献,对胰头周围门静脉-肠系膜静脉系统的解剖及变异进行讨论,旨在为外科医师进行胰-十二指肠区域手术获得更准确的静脉血管解剖信息、降低并发症和提高恶性肿瘤手术切除率(切缘阴性)等提供一定的指导和帮助,推动外科手术技术的进一步发展。

一般情况下,门静脉由肠系膜上静脉和脾静脉在下腔静脉前方和胰颈上部的后方于 T12 至 L2 水平汇合而成,汇合部多位于相应平面椎体右缘,部分位于椎体中部略左,少数可位于脊柱左缘或右缘数厘米处;其斜向右上方入肝十二指肠韧带,在肝固有动脉和胆总管后方上行至肝门,分为左右两支入肝。门静脉收集腹盆部消化道(包含食管腹段,除外齿状线以下肛管)、脾、胰腺和胆囊的静脉血。

肠系膜上静脉:肠系膜上静脉是门静脉最大的属支,起自右髂窝的盲肠、阑尾和回肠末端静脉,依次经右输尿管、下腔静脉、十二指肠水平部、胰头钩突前方上行,至胰颈部后方与脾静脉几乎成直角汇合成门静脉。

一般位于肠系膜上动脉右侧,也可位于其左侧或前方。肠系膜上静脉主要收集空肠、回肠、盲肠、阑尾、升结肠、横结肠右半部和胰腺等脏器的静脉血流。

Sakaguchi 等(2010)将肠系膜上静脉分为单支主干型(Ⅰ型)和双支主干型(Ⅱ型),由于肠系膜上静脉与肠系膜上动脉的相对位置在胰十二指肠区域手术中十分重要,故据此又将其分别分为多种亚型。Ⅰ型:具有单一总主干,占绝大多数(约占 76.5%),其以第一空肠静脉走行于肠系膜上动脉的腹侧或背侧分为两个亚型。

Ⅱ型:不形成单一总主干,而由左、右两主干构成,根据左主干的汇入位置将其分为Ⅱ m 和Ⅱ p 两个亚型。Ⅱ m 型(约占 16.5%)两主干同时于脾门静脉汇合处汇入,左主干可走行于肠系膜上动脉的腹侧或是背侧;Ⅱ p 型(约占 7%)左主干汇入脾静脉,此型中左主干均走行于肠系膜上动脉的腹侧。Katz 等(2008)将左右主干分别称为空肠干和回肠干。

第一空肠干:Kim 等(2007)提出了第一空肠干的概念,即引流近端空肠血流入肠系膜上静脉的第一条分支主干,是一根由第一空肠静脉和许多引流近端空肠循环的小分支组成的主干。依据其分支走行可分为 3 型:Ⅰ型,第一空肠干经肠系膜上动脉背侧走行至左腹部(约占 64%);Ⅱ型,第一空肠干横跨肠系膜上动脉背侧后突然全部(Ⅱ a 型)或者部分(Ⅱ b 型)转向右腹部(约占 17%);Ⅲ型,第一空肠干经肠系膜上动脉腹侧走行至左腹部(约占 19%)。其中Ⅰ型最为常见,Ⅲ型则常与多种发育变异合并存在,包括非单支主干型肠系膜上静脉、肠系膜下静脉直接汇入第一空肠干等。对此发育变异的正确认识在胰十二指肠切除术中极为关键。同时其还指出,Ⅱ型变异与肠旋转不良、肠扭转致肠缺血等表现并无一定相关性。

根据肠系膜上静脉与第一空肠干的不同形态表现及位置关系又可作如下分类:即肠系膜上静脉主要属支和较大或较小的第一空肠干汇成肠系膜上静脉单一总主干后汇入脾静脉;肠系膜上静脉主要属支和较大或较小的第一空肠干直接共同汇合入脾静脉而不形成单一总主干。这与前述单支主干型和双支主干型肠系膜上静脉分类描述类似。其中较大的第一空肠干指直径与肠系膜上静脉主要属支直径相仿者。

胃结肠静脉干:胃结肠静脉干,又称作亨利氏干,最早由德国学者 Henle(1868)提出,存在于约

70% 的人群中，主要由胃网膜右静脉和右半结肠引流静脉（包括右结肠静脉、上右结肠静脉、中结肠静脉）、胰十二指肠静脉属支（包括胰十二指肠前上静脉、胰十二指肠前下静脉）中的一条或数条汇合而成，走行于胰头前方并常于脾门静脉汇合处下方约 3 cm 处汇入肠系膜上静脉总干或其右主干。

胃结肠静脉干横径约 3~10 mm，长度往往小于 25 mm，其绝大部分开口于肠系膜上静脉的右外侧或是右前方，少部分可开口于其前方或左前方。Sakaguchi 等（2010）指出，胃网膜右静脉和上右结肠静脉共同汇合形成胃结肠静脉干是其中最常见的类型。Hongo 等（2010）和 Ibukuro 等（2001）认为胃结肠静脉干主要由胃网膜右静脉、胰十二指肠前上静脉以及上右结肠静脉或右结肠静脉共同组成，于胰腺钩突水平汇入肠系膜上静脉。认清胃结肠静脉干及其组成发育变异，可以很大程度上避免胰 - 十二指肠区域手术中因相关血管撕裂损伤引起的出血。

结肠静脉：右结肠静脉常可缺如且均为单支，其可参与构成胃结肠静脉干，也可于胃结肠静脉干 - 肠系膜上静脉汇合处附近直接汇入肠系膜上静脉。

上右结肠静脉又称作副右结肠静脉，存在于大于 90% 的人群中，引流结肠肝区的血流，一般无伴行动脉，最常见为参与构成胃结肠静脉干后汇入肠系膜上静脉，也可直接汇入肠系膜上静脉。

中结肠静脉大部分为单支，也可为多支构成，主要于胃结肠静脉干 - 肠系膜上静脉汇合处头端、同平面或是尾端，脾门静脉汇合处下方约 4 cm 处汇入肠系膜上静脉，也可汇入胃结肠静脉干、肠系膜下静脉甚至是脾静脉或右结肠静脉。

另外，约 70% 人群同时存在副中结肠静脉，其可汇入肠系膜上静脉、胃结肠静脉干亦或是脾静脉、肠系膜下静脉。

脾静脉：脾静脉较粗大，但不如脾动脉那样弯曲，其起自脾门，于胰腺后方右行，横跨左肾前上方，经腹腔干和肠系膜上动脉之间至腹主动脉前方终于胰颈后方汇入脾静脉。常有胃网膜左静脉和数条引流胰腺小分支静脉汇入。脾静脉从脾门至脾门静脉汇合处总长约 15 cm，不同文献报道略有差异。脾静脉主要位于脾动脉的后方，也可位于其旁侧或极少数情况下位于其前方。Shah 等（2005）曾报道 1 例走行于胰体尾前方的脾静脉，可能与早期胚胎发育异常有关。

肠系膜下静脉：肠系膜下静脉起自直肠上静脉，主要引流降结肠、乙状结肠及直肠的血流，其主要由 3 条属支即左结肠静脉、乙状结肠静脉和痔上静脉组成，后两者常合为一总干后与左结肠静脉汇合。肠系膜下静脉的分型和比例各文献报道略有差异。Sakaguchi 等（2010）根据肠系膜下静脉汇入点的不同将其主要分为 4 型，按发生率由高到低分别为汇入脾静脉（SP 型，约占 68.5%）、肠系膜上静脉（SM 型，约占 18.5%）、脾门静脉汇合处（C 型，约占 7.6%）以及肠系膜上静脉左主干（L 型，约占 5.4%）。

每一型中，根据肠系膜下静脉与肠系膜上动脉的相对位置又可以分成多种亚型：SP 型中肠系膜下静脉可走行于肠系膜上动脉的左侧或头侧，SM 型和 C 型中肠系膜下静脉可走行于肠系膜上动脉的腹侧或头侧，L 型中肠系膜下静脉可走行于肠系膜上动脉的腹侧或左侧。

Kim 等（2007）指出，肠系膜下静脉可分别汇入脾静脉（约占 53%）、肠系膜上静脉（约占 31%）、脾门静脉汇合处（约占 12%）以及第一空肠干（约占 4%），而后者第一空肠干均走行于肠系膜上动脉腹侧。

胃左静脉：胃左静脉起于胃小弯的上部，沿胃小弯在小网膜中自左向右下行，其分型为汇入脾静脉（SP 型，约占 46%）、门静脉（P 型，约占 39%）以及脾门静脉汇合处（C 型，约占 15%）。

SP 型中胃左静脉可走行于脾动脉的腹侧及背侧、腹腔干的腹侧、肝总动脉的腹侧及背侧，P 型中胃左静脉可走行于肝总动脉的背侧或肝固有动脉的腹侧，C 型中胃左静脉可走行于肝总动脉的背侧、腹侧以及脾动脉的腹侧。在进行胰 - 十二指肠切除术合并部分门静脉切除的患者中，胃充血、胃排空延迟等时有发生，因此术前需要清楚了解肠系膜下静脉和胃左静脉的解剖走行，选择恰当的手术方式，以更好地保护或是重建这些血管，减少手术并发症。

胰十二指肠静脉系：胰头血供主要由两条静脉弓，即胰十二指肠后上静脉与胰十二指肠后下静脉吻合形成的后弓与胰十二指肠前上静脉和胰十二指肠前下静脉吻合形成的前弓共同引流。胰十二指肠后上静脉是胰头最大的引流静脉，主要引流胰头及十二指肠后部的血流，其经胆总管和十二指肠降部之间上行，可走行于胆总管的前方，也可以走行于其后方，小部分可有双支分别走行于胆总管前、后方，极少部分者与钩突静脉汇合为一支,其主要于脾门静脉汇合处上方 1.5~3.0 cm 处汇入脾静脉后外侧壁或是直接引流入肝内。

胰头及十二指肠的前部主要由胰十二指肠前上静脉(胰十二指肠前上静脉)引流,其横行于胰头的前表面,主要通过共同构成胃结肠静脉干于脾门静脉交汇处下方 1.5~3.5 cm 处汇入肠系膜上静脉,或是直接汇入肠系膜上静脉;部分人存在双支胰十二指肠前上静脉,小支往往于主支下方走行且直接汇入肠系膜上静脉。

胰十二指肠前下静脉横行于钩突和十二指肠水平段之间,胰十二指肠后下静脉则横行于胰头的后部,两者常汇合成胰十二指肠下静脉后或不合并而分别汇入第一空肠干,亦可汇合后共同汇入肠系膜上静脉或是分别汇入第一空肠干与肠系膜上静脉。

以上静脉有时因发育不良而并非存在于所有人群中。

正常情况下,相比胰十二指肠后上静脉和胰十二指肠前上静脉,胰十二指肠后下静脉和胰十二指肠前下静脉常因管径细小或是被周围结构掩盖而较难分辨出,但当肿瘤累及使得肠系膜上静脉在第一空肠干平面以上闭塞时,胰十二指肠下静脉会相应扩张,起到侧支旁路作用,此点一定程度上也可以作为肿瘤累及此区域门静脉肠系膜上静脉的标志;而当其他胰周静脉包括第一空肠干、胃结肠静脉干、胰十二指肠后上静脉和胰十二指肠前上静脉等扩张而胰十二指肠前下静脉、胰十二指肠后下静脉、胰十二指肠下静脉受累阻塞未见时提示肿瘤可能已累及十二指肠水平部;由于相关解剖结构的邻近性,胰十二指肠下静脉受累常提示胰腺外第二部分神经丛(肠系膜上动脉至钩突中界区域)受肿瘤侵犯;胰十二指肠下静脉和第一空肠干受累则提示肠系膜根部肠系膜上动脉已被肿瘤累及。

清楚认识以上静脉发育变异,可以指导外科医生术前尽早发现异常、确定肿瘤累及情况、明确分期以制定最佳的手术方案。

胰头周围还存在许多细小静脉,如直接横行汇入脾静脉或是肠系膜上静脉的胰头部小静脉,主要走行于胰头内侧并汇入脾静脉后壁的钩突静脉,由一条或数条横穿胰腺下部的静脉汇合而成并最终于胰颈水平汇入脾静脉、肠系膜上静脉或是肠系膜下静脉的胰中下静脉,垂直穿行于胰颈背部并汇入脾静脉、肠系膜上静脉的胰背静脉等。它们往往十分细小、变异繁多而较难分辨,需要我们进行更深入的探查和更仔细的操作。

胰头周围门静脉 - 肠系膜静脉系统的发育变异复杂,各文献报道略有差异;不同地区、不同人种间发育变异的发生及比例也有待进一步研究。在临床上,我们需要熟悉此类变异的存在,进行具体分析,以求更准确地进行术前评估,减少手术并发症的发生。

如今影像医学发展日新月异,尤其三维增强 CT 血管成像技术等广泛应用,使得门静脉 - 肠系膜静脉系统解剖及变异的影像越来越多地应用于胰十二指肠区域的术前评估中。随着科学技术的不断发展和完善,学科间合作日趋紧密,胰十二指肠区域手术的可行性、准确性及安全性必将得到进一步的提高,更先进的手术技术也将应运而生,为更多的患者带来福音。

第三十章　MRCP 与胆胰疾病

磁共振胆胰管成像与胰管扩张

磁共振胆胰管成像（MRCP）可清晰地显示胆胰管解剖，已成为观察胆胰管形态及诊断胆胰管异常的重要方法。胰管扩张是胆胰系统疾病的常见征象。由于病理改变不同，各种疾病在胰管扩张的部位、程度及外形等方面存在差异。此处仅就 MRCP 检查对于胰管扩张的病因学诊断进行讨论。

胰管的发育：胰腺由腹侧胰芽、背侧胰芽发育而成。两个胚芽及引流管道在胚胎第 7 周相互融合，引流背侧胰腺胰液的 Santorini 管并入引流腹侧胰腺胰液的 Wirsung 管，形成完整主胰管。主胰管沿胰腺长轴走行，沿途收集 20~35 支分支胰管，最后在十二指肠降部壁内与肝外胆管汇合成胆胰共同管，开口于十二指肠大乳头。正常主胰管自胰头到胰尾逐渐变细，边缘光滑，长约 110 mm，管径 2~3mm。文献测量数据显示胰腺头、体、尾部主胰管直径分别为（2.36 ± 0.60）mm、（2.05 ± 0.72）mm、（1.67 ± 0.86） mm。一般认为主胰管直径 >3.5 mm 为胰管扩张。正常分支胰管在常规的 MRCP 中极少显示。因此自然状态下，若在 MRCP 上观察到结构清晰且形态异常的分支胰管，即可视为分支胰管扩张。

胰管扩张的病因学诊断　胰管扩张是胆胰管病变的重要征象之一，但并不是一个特异性征象。多种疾病可引起胰管扩张，但是由于病理改变不同，不同疾病所致胰管扩张的 MRCP 表现特征存在差异。

1. 恶性病变

（1）胰腺癌：是胰腺最常见的恶性肿瘤。90% 以上来源于胰管上皮细胞，少数来源于腺泡细胞，胰腺癌中约 62% 为胰头癌。胰头部胰管狭窄或梗阻后可引起胰管扩张。MRCP 上表现为胰头部胰管不显示，近端主胰管明显扩张，管腔边缘光滑，在胰头肿块处截断。随主胰管扩张，分支胰管出现顺应性扩张。当胰头癌肿块、胰头区肿大淋巴结压迫胆总管或肿瘤直接侵犯胆总管时，可出现胆总管扩张，即“双管征”，且胆胰管呈分离状态，汇合角大。

扩张的胆总管在肿块处截断或管径突然减小。有时梗阻近端扩张明显的胆胰管和末端扩张程度较小的胆胰管表现为 4 个分离的管腔，呈现“四节征”。胰体癌可导致近端胰腺萎缩和胰管扩张，但扩张程度及长度不及胰头癌，胰尾癌较少引起胰管扩张。

（2）十二指肠乳头癌：肿瘤阻塞胆胰管共同开口，使胰管及胆总管内压力增高而扩张。MRCP 中显示十二指肠肠腔至胆胰管梗阻端间距较小，梗阻端呈鸟嘴样、倒杯口状狭窄或突然截断。常见“双管征”，且由于病变发生在胆胰管交汇处，“双管征”呈聚拢趋势，胆胰汇合角小。胰管平滑扩张，程度轻，分支胰管扩张少见，胆管多扩张明显，呈“软藤样”改变。肠腔内可见息肉状肿物形成的充盈缺损，或表现为肠壁增厚与肠腔狭窄。

（3）胆总管下端癌：MRCP 显示管腔内软组织肿块或胆管壁增厚，管腔狭窄或截断，近端胆管扩张。胆管阻塞显著时，肝内胆管扩张呈软藤样，有时达包膜下。当肿瘤浸润胆胰共同管或胰腺组织时，MRCP 显示“双管征”，提示出现胰管扩张。如果胆总管被腔内肿块截断，MRCP 有时显示“三节征”，即扩张的近侧胆管、不扩张的远侧胆管及扩张的胰管。

（4）胆胰共同管癌：胆胰共同管癌是一种少见的起源于胆胰共同管腺上皮的恶性肿瘤，表现为肿块或管壁增厚。MRCP 上肿块显示为高信号胆胰共同管内的低信号充盈缺损，可突入十二指肠腔内。管壁增厚者可仅显示管腔局部狭窄，胆胰管远端呈圆钝状。胆胰共同管癌阻塞胰胆管，出现“双管征”，胰胆管末端至十二指肠乳头间距离短，胆胰汇合角小。扩张的胆胰管末端边缘不规则，呈钝圆及新月状中断，胰管为轻中度扩张，分支胰管扩张少见。

2. 良性病变

（1）胰腺导管内乳头状黏液性肿瘤：胰腺导管内乳头状黏液性肿瘤来源于胰管上皮，生长缓慢，呈乳头状突起并分泌大量黏蛋白,导致胰管囊状扩张,较少伴有胆管扩张。导管内乳头状黏液性肿瘤分为主胰管型、分支胰管型及混合型。分支胰管型导管内乳头状黏液性肿瘤常位于胰头及钩突部,MRCP上显示为单房或多房的囊性肿瘤,呈葡萄串样改变。主胰管型导管内乳头状黏液性肿瘤在MRCP中显示为主胰管弥漫性或节段性扩张、膨大,伴有分隔及壁结节存在,壁结节呈结节状或扁平状,胰腺实质常萎缩,亦可见分支胰管扩张。混合型导管内乳头状黏液性肿瘤同时表现单房或多房的囊性肿瘤及主胰管弥漫扩张。

导管内乳头状黏液性肿瘤晚期大量黏液造成胆总管末端及胆胰共同管梗阻,形成"双管征"。导管内乳头状黏液性肿瘤可发生癌变,病灶大小、主胰管直径、壁结节的存在和大小与恶性程度呈正相关。s-MRCP显示胰腺外分泌功能明显减低。

(2)慢性胰腺炎:慢性胰腺炎是由多种因素引起的胰腺组织炎症,胰腺功能进行性损害,最终导致胰腺内分泌及外分泌功能不可逆性破坏及胰腺、胰管形态的不可逆性改变。

约66%的慢性胰腺炎存在主胰管及分支胰管扩张。MRCP中显示主胰管轮廓不规则,粗细不均,可见多发狭窄及扩张,贯穿整个病变区,呈串珠样改变。分支胰管扩张明显时,形成"湖泊链"样改变。胰管内常可见结石和黏蛋白碎片引起的充盈缺损。在胰腺炎中晚期,胰管明显扩张,往往同时出现胆管扩张。

慢性胰腺炎若伴有局灶炎性肿块形成。MRCP可显示无局部阻塞的胰管穿过肿块,此即"胰管贯穿征"。胆总管受压,出现局部狭窄及近端扩张,扩张程度轻,轮廓光滑,远端逐渐变细,呈锥形狭窄或正常。s-MRCP显示胰腺外分泌功能在重症慢性胰腺炎时明显减低。

(3)急性胰腺炎:急性胰腺炎是胰腺及周围组织被胰腺消化酶自身消化的化学性炎症。急性胰腺炎一般不会引起胰管扩张,甚至有时水肿增大的胰腺压迫胰管,使胰管在MRCP中显示不清或表现为狭窄。但当存在结石、蛋白栓、假性囊肿时,胰管引流不畅,亦可见胰管扩张、连续,边缘光滑。

(4)自身免疫性胰腺炎:自身免疫性胰腺炎是一种特别的胰腺炎症,由自身免疫性因素引起,影像表现为弥漫性胰腺肿大。MRCP中大部分自身免疫性胰腺炎胰管表现为弥漫性不规则狭窄,病变长度常大于3 cm,呈跳跃性分布,在主胰管狭窄区可见分支胰管扩张。部分自身免疫性胰腺炎表现为局部主胰管狭窄伴近端胰管扩张,扩张的胰管直径一般小于5 mm。

自身免疫性胰腺炎对激素治疗敏感,主胰管管径恢复情况与治疗效果呈正相关。当病变累及胆总管下段时可引起胆管狭窄,边缘光滑。

(5)胰腺假性囊肿:在急性胰腺炎和慢性胰腺炎时,可伴有胰管破裂、胰液外渗并形成包裹性积液,此即胰腺假性囊肿,其表面通常覆以完整的非上皮性包膜。假性囊肿可位于胰腺外及胰腺内,后者可与主胰管相通,MRCP有助于显示胰腺内假性囊肿与主胰管的交通情况。胰管周围的假性囊肿可压迫胰管,导致主胰管及分支胰管扩张。

(6)胆胰管下端括约肌功能障碍:胆胰管下端括约肌功能障碍与胆胰管下端括约肌的收缩功能异常有关,可导致胆管及胰管的阻塞性改变。胆胰管下端括约肌功能障碍可分为3型,其中Ⅰ型可见胰管扩张,主要表现为胰头部胰管直径 >6 mm,体部胰管直径 >5 mm,且胰管排空延迟 >9min。

3. 先天性发育异常

(1)胰腺分裂:胰腺分裂是最常见的胰管先天性变异。两胰腺胚芽及引流管道在发育过程中未能融合,使Wirsung管与Santorini管终身保持分离状态。完全性胰腺分裂时,背侧胰管引流大部分胰腺实质的胰液,开口于十二指肠小乳头,腹侧胰管引流胰头部胰液,与胆总管合并开口于十二指肠大乳头。背侧胰管引流区域大,管径粗,但流出道相对狭窄,胰液引流不畅造成胰管功能性扩张。MRCP可见背侧胰管跨过胆总管下端汇入十二指肠,背侧胰管扩张,边缘光滑,部分病例在背侧胰管开口处呈囊状扩张。腹侧胰管常表现为短且极度狭窄。

(2)环形胰腺:环形胰腺为一种少见的先天异常,表现为胰腺完全或不完全环绕十二指肠,通常为降部中段。当环形胰腺较严重时,胰腺组织压迫胆胰共同管,造成胰管开口不畅,胆汁和胰腺分泌受阻,出现胰管扩张,MRCP可显示主胰管迂曲至胆总管外侧环绕十二指肠,远端胰管轻度扩张,常伴有十二指肠狭窄。

(3)胰管损伤及胰腺术后:胰管损伤主要由穿通伤或钝器伤引起,也可由于外科手术引起。MRCP可以显示胰管损伤急性期的胰管断裂及液体积聚。若急性期的胰管断裂未及时进行修复,可形成断裂处胰管狭窄及狭窄近端的胰管扩张，正常胰管与近端扩张胰管之间可见到明显分界。某些胰腺手术后，如胰十二指肠切除术、胆胰吻合术等，经常发生吻合口狭窄，引起胰管扩张改变。

4. 其他少见原因

（1）胰腺结核：胰腺结核较少见，常发生于血供丰富的胰头及钩突部。Rana 等（2011）报道了 1 例伴有胰管及胆总管扩张的胰腺结核病例，影像学可见胰管及胆总管明显扩张，呈现“双管征”，并且可在胰头部及胆总管内见到团块影。

（2）腹主动脉瘤：Fukui 等（2012）报道了 1 例腹主动脉瘤引起胰管扩张的病例，病人以腹部不适就诊，影像学检查发现腹主动脉瘤，并压迫十二指肠、胆总管远端及胰头部，引起近端胆总管、体尾部胰管扩张。

（3）寄生虫感染：Dearden 等（2004）报道了 1 例十二指肠内寄生虫感染引起胰管扩张的病例。MRCP 显示胆管及胰管同时扩张的“双管征”，胰腺及邻近组织未见明显肿块。ERCP 检查见十二指肠黏膜水肿，乳头及胆胰共同管结构模糊。组织活检证实系十二指肠原位粪类圆线虫感染。该病人经抗寄生虫药物治疗后症状消失，复查 MRCP 显示肝外胆管和胰管无扩张。

总之，MRCP 检查在评价胰管扩张方面具有一定优势。虽然胰管扩张不是一个特异性征象，但是在不同疾病可有不同的 MRCP 表现。综合分析扩张胰管的形态、范围、程度、远端有无狭窄或梗阻及狭窄段长度、梗阻端表现等影像特征，一般可以对胰管扩张的病因做出初步判断。结合常规横断面 T_1WI 和 T_2WI 以及动态增强 MRI 表现，往往可以提高对胰管外胰腺实质性病变的诊断准确性。

第三十一章　胰腺创伤及手术后

第一节　胰腺断裂

有作者报告一例上腹部被他人用膝部顶撞伤后16小时,因腹痛、恶心、呕吐行CT扫描,见胰腺体部断裂分离,两断端之间被一纵行带状低密度液体影将之分开,胰腺周围脂肪层增厚模糊,胰体前方及肝脾外侧缘均见低密度液体聚积。手术见胰腺体部完全断裂分离,腹腔内有大量咖啡色液体。

胰腺断裂十分少见,多为脊柱前的外力撞击所致。CT检查能明确显示胰腺断裂的部位和周围组织的情况,为手术提供可靠的依据。

第二节　假性胰腺折断

在胰腺区域,未为对比剂充盈的密集肠袢,在CT图像上,可伪似胰腺的折断。

Jeffrey等(1983)在一怀疑腹部钝伤的病人CT图像上,看见一前后方向走行的不规则低密度线条影,恰邻近胰头区,伪似胰腺的折断,经认真仔细观察和分析,可见极少量高密度对比剂紧邻该影,方考虑其为肠袢,如不留心,此肠袢还可类似胰尾,造成误诊。

第三节　胰十二指肠切除术后改变

胰十二指肠切除术适用于十二指肠肿瘤,肝外胆管胰腺段癌,胆胰管十二指肠连接区癌及胰头癌等,主要有胰十二指肠切除术(Whipple术)、保留胃和幽门的胰十二指肠切除术(PPPD术)以及扩大的胰十二指肠切除术。胰十二指肠切除术切除范围一般包括远端部分胃、十二指肠、胰头部及胆总管下端;保留胃和幽门的胰十二指肠切除术保留了胃的正常生理功能,肠胃反流受到部分阻止,改善了营养状况,不必行胃部分切除,十二指肠空肠吻合较简单,缩短了手术时间。

胰十二指肠切除术后小肠与胰头吻合,小肠可以向胰头部聚集,有时小肠聚集成团,不要误认为肿瘤,可以行增强扫描,并向下逐层观察,可见与小肠相延续,并可以看到小肠黏膜结构。

第三十二章　与胰腺有关的周围组织疾病及全身性疾病

第一节　周围病变累及胰头与胰头 - 连接区癌累及周围结构的CT鉴别诊断

随着CT的普及和检查方法的不断完善，CT已成为胰腺病变的重要检查方法；近年对小胰腺癌的CT诊断研究较多，但由于认识不足及经济条件的限制，在临床工作中，常遇到胰头区较大肿块与周围结构分界不清，是胰头 - 连接区癌累及周围结构还是周围病变累及胰头，对临床治疗方案及评价预后有重要意义。

一些作者回顾性分析36例经临床病理证实的周围病变累及胰头病例的CT表现，并与36例病理证实的胰头 - 连接区癌累及周围结构的病例进行对比分析。

胰腺癌大多来自导管上皮，少数来自腺泡上皮。连接区癌是指连接区总胆管上皮或十二指肠乳头黏膜上皮或主胰管上皮以及它们所属的腺体所发生的癌，胰头癌和连接区癌（特别是发展到晚期）常难区分，因此，把他们并为一组。

周围病变累及胰头组病例，多数是因为胰头周围淋巴结肿大累及胰头所致，该组占75%（27/36），其中转移淋巴结18例，淋巴瘤5例；淋巴结核4例，询问病史或找寻原发病灶有助于诊断转移淋巴结累及胰头；淋巴瘤常常合并有其他部位淋巴结肿大；淋巴结核常有肺部结核灶，且CT征象有一定的特点，表现为平扫时可见环状或弧形钙化，增强扫描时淋巴结环状强化，内缘光滑，中央干酪、液化区无强化。

以下几点可供胰头 - 连接区癌累及周围结构与周围病变累及胰头的CT鉴别诊断：

（1）胰头是否移位，形态是否完整，密度是否均匀，边缘是否光整：胰头 - 连接区癌浸润性生长，进展迅速，体积增大，常有坏死，平扫一般与正常组织呈等密度或等低密度，由于肿瘤多为少血供，增强早期病灶无明显强化，或较晚轻度强化，与正常胰腺组织明显强化形成鲜明对比，特别是胰头 - 连接区癌累及周围结构时，肿块已较大，胰头失去完整的正常形态，密度不均匀，边缘不清，该组36/36均有此种表现，而胰头移位不明显。

周围病变累及胰头时，周围肿块推移或浸润胰头，平扫时肿块与胰头常常不易区分，表现为胰头区密度不均匀肿块，但增强时正常胰腺与肿块强化幅度和时间的区别，使胰头正常组织与肿块区分开来，病变性质不同，表现不同，转移瘤表现为不均匀环状强化，淋巴瘤表现为轻度均匀强化，结核表现为薄壁环状强化；胰头有浸润时，靠近肿块边缘的胰腺密度减低，该组占36%（13/36）；胰头无浸润时，胰头密度无改变，胰头可被推移或被肿块包绕。

（2）胰管、胆管扩张：胰头 - 连接区癌组织学起源于胰管上皮、胆总管上皮、十二指肠黏膜上皮或腺泡细胞，除腺泡细胞癌外，胰头 - 连接区癌具有围管性浸润的重要生物学特征，因此胰头癌常常出现总胆管、肝内外胆管扩张、胆囊增大以及胰管扩张。该组占89%（32/36），出现比例很高，可能与该组病例均为胰头癌晚期有关；而周围病变累及胰头时，由于胰管有胰腺组织的保护，病灶不易累及胰管、出现扩张，该组胰管扩张仅占11%；肝外胆管进入胰腺前因为没有实质脏器的保护，周围淋巴结肿大或肿块压迫、浸润容易引起胆管扩张和胆囊增大，该组占50%（18/36），与胰头 - 连接区癌组比较，胆管扩张程度较轻，伴有胆囊扩大的比例小，胰头 - 连接区癌组78%（28/36）胆囊扩大，而周围病变累及胰头组仅36%（13/36）胆囊扩大。这可能与胆囊管下端梗阻的程度有关。

（3）胰腺体尾部萎缩：胰头 - 连接区发生癌变

时,癌组织侵犯胰管后造成胰管狭窄或堵塞,远端胰管扩张,远端胰腺组织萎缩和纤维化,该组出现率58%(21/36);而周围病变累及胰头时,胰管不易被累及,胰腺体尾部萎缩比率小,该组仅占5%(2/36)。因此,当胰头区肿块伴胰腺体尾部萎缩时,胰头-连接区癌累及周围结构的可能性大,而周围病变累及胰头的可能性较小。

腹水:胰头-连接区癌晚期容易发生腹膜腔转移和累及门脉导致腹腔积液。

胰周脂肪间隙减少或消失:胰头-连接区癌较易侵犯周围脂肪,引起胰周脂肪间隙减少或消失,该组占72%(26/36);周围病变累及胰头组出现率较小,仅占36%(13/36),可能与淋巴结病变占较大比例有关。

胰头周围淋巴结肿大:由于胰头-连接区癌容易发生周围淋巴结转移。

周围病变累及胰头的病变大部分为淋巴结病变,且胰头周围其他癌性病变亦易发生淋巴结转移,因此,胰头周围淋巴结肿大对两者鉴别诊断价值有限。

第二节 位于纵隔的胰腺假性囊肿

详见本书 本卷 本篇 第十二章 第一节 位于纵隔的胰腺假性囊肿。

第三节 坏死性脂膜炎

曹庆选等(1995)报告一例62岁男性病人,全身皮肤结节2月,疼痛伴发热。

皮肤组织活检病理诊断为坏死性脂膜炎,符合胰腺病性脂肪坏死。

随后CT扫描见胰腺体部巨大椭圆形肿块,最大截面15cm×12cm,边缘清楚,有轻度分叶,密度不均;增强扫描见病灶呈不均匀强化,中心有低密度坏死。手术见肿块呈暗红色,表面不规则,质硬,病理诊断为胰腺癌。

该作者指出,结节性脂肪坏死是一种合并胰腺疾患的脂肪坏死性炎症。此病例特点为:从无胰腺及消化道疾病症状,以皮肤病变为主诉;皮肤结节活检提示胰腺病性脂膜炎后方进行胰腺CT检查;胰腺肿块较大,表明病变早已存在,提示胰腺病变可以皮肤病变为首发症状,而脂膜炎可能是继发性表现,此种脂膜炎对诊断有特征性辅助诊断价值。

第四节 胰十二指肠沟区疾病及其鉴别诊断

详见本书 本卷 本篇 第九章 第十一节 胰十二指肠沟区病变的鉴别诊断。

第三十三章　胰腺疾病的一些诊断陷阱

第一节　胰腺脂肪浸润

如果胰腺实质完全被脂肪代替，因胰腺与腹膜后脂肪密度相等，CT 图像上可能见不到胰腺，这种现象偶尔能够在胰腺的其中一段见到，超声上可造成胰腺回声增强。

胰腺脂肪浸润更常发生在老年人和肥胖病人，总是伴有胰腺整体体积减小。当其与肥胖有关时，脂肪浸润可以逆转。

Matsumoto（1995）复习 80 例胰腺不均匀脂肪替代 CT 影像的特点。研究复习 1 000 例 CT 照片，不均匀胰腺脂肪替代的发生率为 3.2%，以 50~69 岁组占绝大多数。该组病例胰头前部均有脂肪替代，提示此部脂肪替代可能早于胰腺的其他部位。

胰腺不均匀脂肪替代可分成两型：

Ⅰ型：胰头的后部不发生明显的脂肪替代。Ⅰa 型：胰腺体尾部无明显的脂肪替代 28 例（35%），平均 CT 值 -10.1HU。在此型，胰头前部的脂肪替代的 CT 值，明显低于胰头后部和胰体尾部。胰头的前后部之间 CT 值差异范围为 20~122HU（平均 77HU）。Ⅰb 型：胰腺体尾部有明显的脂肪替代 29 例（36%），平均 CT 值 -35.5HU。在此型，胰头前部平均 CT 值明显低于胰头后部，胰头前部 CT 值与胰体尾部 CT 值无显著性差异。

Ⅱ型：肝外胆管周围局灶区域不发生脂肪替代。Ⅱa 型：胰腺体尾部无明显的脂肪替代 9 例（11%），平均 CT 值 -27.5HU。在此型，钩突 CT 值均值为 -11.5HU。Ⅱb 型：胰腺体尾部有明显的脂肪替代 14 例（18%），平均 CT 值 -40.3HU。在此型，钩突 CT 值均值为 -27.5HU。胰头后部肝外胆管周围区域 CT 值（平均 15.7HU）明显高于胰腺其他部位的 CT 值，示其密度甚高。

肉眼能分辨的脂肪替代区与非替代区最小 CT 值差别至少为 20HU。

所有重度脂肪替代的胰头前后径，均明显大于对照组。

在Ⅰ型，胰头脂肪替代区前后径与非替代区胰头前后径的比率，和脂肪替代程度有轻度相关（r=0.62），换句话说，非替代区的前后径倾向于较小和在形态上较扁平。

胰腺脂肪浸润还可能与糖尿病、酒精中毒、囊性纤维化、慢性胰腺炎、慢性类固醇摄入及儿童 Schwachman 综合征有关。无论是局部脂肪替代区，或是局部非脂肪替代区，在 CT 图像上均可表现为假肿瘤征象，需要与囊腺瘤、小胰癌及胰岛细胞癌鉴别。

脂肪浸润时，残留的正常胰腺组织在 CT 图像上表现为稍高密度肿块样结构，其与肿瘤鉴别困难。这种情况多发生在胰头，为排除肿瘤，施行 MRI、MRCP 或内窥镜逆行性胆胰管造影（ERCP）检查十分必要。脂肪浸润还可以改变胰腺正常形态。

第二节　胰腺脂肪裂和胰腺假性破裂

胰周脂肪可侵入胰腺，产生类似胰腺裂隙的表现。在外伤病人，这种情况可与胰腺破裂混淆。但是，胰腺脂肪裂病人血清胰酶正常，胰周脂肪保持清晰。

第三节 胰腺超声检查的误诊

与肝脏相比,胰腺超声表现通常呈等或稍高回声。胰腺超声虽然在多数病人可见到胰头和胰体,但胰尾的显示则需要胃充满水后检查,以避免气体重叠产生伪影。正常胰管 80% 表现为被回声壁勾画出的窄带状低回声线影,宽径为 2mm。

胰头或胰体附近的肠管可类似胰腺低回声肿块,为排除肿瘤有必要行 CT 检查。另外,扩张的远端胆总管可被怀疑为胰头的无回声肿块,为避免这种误诊,同样有必要行 CT 检查。

超声扫描中其他类似胰腺或胰腺病变的结构包括肝左叶外侧段的后部(第 2 肝段),这是因为血管周围脂肪造成的声波衰减,导致肝左叶外侧段后部回声较前部(第 3 肝段)减弱所形成。肝尾叶的乳头状突起和肿大的门腔静脉淋巴结也可误认为胰腺。马蹄肾和腹膜后纤维化,当超声上表现为一腹膜后中线声谱带时,也类似于胰腺肿块。

胰腺超声检查中有三个正常结构可被误认为胰管扩张:第一个是分隔胰腺后缘和脾静脉的脂肪层;第二个是脾动脉或静脉,特别当血管迂曲且与胰腺存在容积效应时;最后一个是包裹在肝左叶和胰腺之间塌陷的胃窦。

第四节 CT 部分诊断陷阱

常规腹部 CT 扫描时胰腺的 CT 值类似于肌肉和充液肠管,因此,口服对比剂对区分胰腺肿块与低密度肠曲非常重要。钙化而迂曲的脾动脉在常规腹部 CT 上偶尔可被误认为胰腺钙化,但是薄层 CT 扫描一般能揭示血管钙化的管状形态特点。另外,迂曲强化的脾动脉不应当误认为胰腺小血管瘤。胆胰共同管周围充盈有对比剂的十二指肠憩室可类似远端胆总管结石或胰腺钙化。含有碎屑的十二指肠憩室也可类似胰腺肿块或胰腺脓肿。

第五节 假性胰腺折断

详见本书 本卷 本篇 第三十一章 第二节 假性胰腺折断。

第六节 假胰管

胃壁伪似胰管:超声检查上腹部横断扫描偶尔可观察到一无回声管状结构,位于胰区内,在肠系膜上血管的前方,酷似胰管,实际上却是胃窦部后面的肌壁。而在邻近的横断层面扫描时,在脾静脉的前方可清楚地看见真正的胰管。

脾动脉伪似扩张的胰管:超声检查偶尔在胰腺区横断扫描时,可见一管状结构位于脾静脉前方,极类似扩张的胰尾内的胰管。实际上此管状结构发自于腹腔动脉干,在胰的实质内发现了真正的胰管,从而证实该结构实为脾动脉,而并非胰管扩张。

小网膜囊积液类似扩大的胰管:偶尔,超声检查时小网膜囊内的液体与胰管混淆。认识此类液体位于胰的前面,而不位于胰腺的实质中,从而可作出正确诊断。

脂肪层酷似扩张的胰管:Seidelmann 等(1977)指出,在 CT 横断图像上,正常存在于脾静脉与胰腺之间的脂肪层可十分类似于扩张的胰管。认真观察脾静脉可与胰腺分离开,至少占一半的病例;25% 的病例部分地或不能观察到脾静脉。

CT 图像上熟悉此种正常关系是必要的,如果未正确认识此脂肪层，脾静脉的宽度加上重叠，就会弄错胰大小的测量；认识错误，则可能误认为脾静脉扩张，胰体积增大。

第七节 易与原发胰腺肿瘤混淆的胰和胰周疾病

详见本书 本卷 本篇 第一章 第四节 易与原发胰腺肿瘤混淆的胰和胰周疾病。

第八节 诊断陷阱：酷似原发性胰腺肿瘤一些影像学表现

1. 发育变异和先天异常

（1）正常的十二指肠：有的病人 CT 扫描提示胰腺头部增大，但在口服阳性对比剂后，再重复 CT 扫描，却显示正常的胰腺头部，及含对比剂的正常十二指肠和胆囊，事实上是充盈液体的十二指肠呈现低密度，与胰头紧邻而被误认为胰腺头部肿大。

（2）环行胰腺：在环行胰腺，CT 扫描显示胰腺组织环绕十二指肠；在 ERCP 图像上，还可显示主胰管缠绕十二指肠内的内窥镜，并且环行胰腺使胆总管狭窄，其近端扩张。

（3）十二指肠旁索带：十二指肠旁索带结构有时可被液体充盈，此时，CT 扫描则可能显示液体充盈的十二指肠旁索带围绕在十二指肠周围，在横断图像上容易被误作胰腺肿块；但在冠状多平面重建则可显示出十二指肠旁索带全貌，从而避免误诊。

（4）胰腺组织内的迷走脾：在胰腺组织内的迷走脾，轴位增强 T_1WI 可显示胰腺内一个与脾脏等信号强度病灶；冠状 T_1WI 图像显示胰腺包绕着这个异常信号灶。

（5）先天性胆总管囊肿：CT 常规横断扫描可显示扩大的冗余的胆总管胰腺段，酷似胰头内囊性病灶，但在 ERCP 检查时，则可显示对比剂进入囊肿内。

2. 炎症或感染性病变

（1）胰腺炎并发症：CT 平扫时，可显示出血型胰腺炎伪似胰腺不均匀性肿块。在一些有胰腺炎病史老年病例，CT 平扫和增强时可显示整个胰腺多发厚壁囊性病变，术前可误诊为导管黏液蛋白乳头状瘤，术后病理证实为多发假性囊肿。

（2）自身免疫性胰腺炎：自身免疫性胰腺炎可表现为胰头肿大，密度不均匀，有时血管周围炎形成不均匀的团块，容易和肿瘤血管受侵相混淆。罹患本病的有的腹痛患者，MRI T_2WI 和 MRCP 显示肝外胆管胰腺段长段均匀狭窄，但却没有信号异常的广泛胰头增大。轴位 MRI T_1WI 可显示胰尾增大，周围有低信号边。

3. 胰腺其他肿瘤

（1）胰腺转移性肿瘤：在临床上，胰腺转移性肿瘤很少见，有作者报告，乳腺癌转移到胰腺可产生胰腺整体弥漫性肿大，其密度不均匀，增强时强化也不均匀；平扫时与弥漫性胰腺炎症性水肿类似，但其强化表现则完全不一样。有的肾细胞癌转移转移到胰腺，表现为也肾肿块一样的强化特点，这为诊断肾细胞癌转移提供一定帮助。

（2）胰周淋巴结肿大或淋巴瘤：在腹腔淋巴瘤的病人，有时胰腺体部附近淋巴结肿大，易和胰体肿块混淆。

4. 血管性病变

（1）肠系膜上动脉瘤：在有的肠系膜上动脉的动脉瘤病人，增强 CT 显示胰头区被附壁血栓包绕的强化的动脉内腔，若没有动脉期内腔强化的影像，很可能被误认为是胰头病变中囊腺瘤，被附壁血栓包绕的动脉内腔缩成一团，尤如囊腺瘤中的壁结节。

（2）门静脉栓塞：门静脉栓塞时，增强扫描一直呈现为胰腺内的低密度病灶，容易被误诊为胰腺肿块。

5. 胰腺邻近结构病变

（1）纤维组织细胞瘤：有的纤维组织细胞瘤病人，表现为胰腺区多个大小不等的低密度病灶，增强扫描时也呈略低密度，尤如黏液的表现，在临床上，最初被误诊为胰腺黏蛋白腺癌，手术后病理确诊为腹膜后纤维组织细胞瘤

（2）肠系膜类癌：肠系膜类癌可在 CT 平扫上显

示肠系膜根部胰头附近一不均匀性肿块，其内可见钙化，如不注意，可被误诊为胰腺头部肿瘤。

（3）肠系膜硬纤维瘤：肠系膜硬纤维瘤 CT 显示腹腔巨大，卵圆形肿块，胰腺背侧受压，容易误诊为胰腺来源的肿块。

（4）胃间质瘤：有的胃间质瘤侵犯胰腺，与胰腺分界不清，此时，多平面重建可以帮助了解肿瘤的起源。

（5）十二指肠淋巴瘤：十二指肠淋巴瘤可以侵犯胰腺，与胰腺分界不清，但是胃肠检查可以显示十二指肠本身的病变及黏膜的变化。

（6）十二指肠腺癌：十二指肠腺癌常常侵犯胰腺，也表现为低密度肿块影，但其强化特点与胰腺癌不一样。

（7）脾血管瘤：脾血管瘤可大可小，小者一般与胰腺无关，大者则可侵犯胰腺尾部，导致诊断混淆。

（8）左侧肾上腺外副神经节瘤：有的左侧肾上腺外副神经节瘤向前挤压胰腺体尾部，有时，横断图像上二者分界不清，则可与胰腺肿物混淆。

6. 手术后　慢性胰腺炎行 Puestow 术后：在慢性胰腺炎行 Puestow 术后，CT 扫描显示与空肠吻合的胰管明显扩张，酷似胰腺囊性肿块，如不了解手术情况则容易误诊。

第九节　胰腺移植可能造成的诊断陷阱

胰岛素依赖型糖尿病病人在发病 20 年内，超过 50% 的病人合并有肾脏、视网膜或神经系统疾病。为预防、控制或逆转这类并发症，外科医生选择性地对此类病人行胰腺移植手术。手术过程是：从尸体取出整个或部分胰腺组织，移植到病人盆腔，移植胰腺的胰液引流入小肠或膀胱。外科医生一般偏向全胰腺移植术，因其理论上血栓形成发生率低，而且可以获得更多的 β 细胞岛。在盆腔或腹部 CT 图像上，移植的胰腺表现为一个软组织肿块影，若没有相应的完整的临床资料，就可能造成误诊。

第三十四章 胰腺活体形态学研究

第一节 胰腺大小和形状

胰头的正常前后径约 3cm，胰颈和胰体至多为 2.5cm，胰尾约 2cm。正常情况下从胰头到胰尾逐渐变细，而不是骤然变化。但是，众所周知，胰腺的大小和形态是可变的，偶尔见不到逐渐变细的情况。在这些个体中，胰体和胰尾几乎等厚，个别情况下，胰尾比胰体还厚。

胰腺的大小一般与年龄有关。胰腺随年龄的增长逐渐缩小，因而，在评估胰腺小肿块时，腺体整体观（包括匀称性、密度和轮廓）较绝对测量更重要。

一些个体中，胰腺可弥漫性膨凸而非病理改变。此时，正常胰腺实质的小叶结构、CT 密度和 MRI 信号强度保持正常，胰周脂肪无改变，胰管不扩张。这些特点和表现能将正常膨凸的胰腺与胰腺炎区分开来。

胰头和胰颈的外形异常在胰腺分裂中已有详细描述，但实际上腹侧和背侧胰腺始基有多种融合方式。这将造成胰头部正常胰腺小叶分离，其常可在胃十二指肠动脉外侧或胰十二指肠前上动脉外侧见到。

第二节 老年人的胰腺

胰腺的年龄变化颇为明显，应予注意，以减少误诊。随年龄增长，胰管渐粗，而胰腺实质的脂肪性退变则逐渐明显。但胰腺之轮廓、大小变化不大，CT 图像清楚可见胰腺的脂肪性变。脾静脉邻近于胰腺的后面，伴一细长的脂肪性界面，将胰腺与脾静脉分开。

第二十一篇　脾脏疾病

第一章　脾脏占位性病变与脾脏肿瘤

第一节　脾脏肿瘤及误诊病例

脾脏肿瘤少见,有作者认为与脾脏特有的免疫功能有关。据尸检统计,脾脏良性肿瘤的发生率约为 0.14%,脾脏恶性肿瘤不超过全部恶性肿瘤的 0.64%。良性肿瘤以脾囊肿及血管瘤多见,其他包括淋巴管瘤、错构瘤等;恶性肿瘤以转移瘤、恶性淋巴瘤、血管内皮肉瘤多见,其他极为少见。

脾肿瘤临床表现缺乏特异性,诊断主要取决于影像学检查。尽管超声对发现病灶很敏感,但定性方面较差,因此 CT、MRI 检查是目前诊断脾肿瘤最有价值的影像检查方法,能明确显示肿瘤的部位、形态、大小、血供特点及与周围脏器和血管的关系,其诊断符合率较高,可作为脾肿瘤的首选而有效的检查方法。但目前仍不能在术前很有效地鉴别脾脏肿瘤的良、恶性,最后的确诊取决于病理诊断。

1. 脾良性肿瘤

(1)脾血管瘤:血管瘤是最常见的脾良性肿瘤,是由毛细血管或海绵样扩张血管组合而成,可单发或多发。大多数病例具有类似肝脏海绵状血管瘤的典型 CT 表现,CT 平扫多表现为脾内边界清楚的低密度灶,肿瘤中心或边缘可发生钙化,部分可发生囊变;动脉期扫描病灶周边明显结节状强化,部分可呈全瘤性明显强化;延迟期扫描大多数病灶能完全充填,呈等密度。一组 3 例脾血管瘤 MRI 表现与肝海绵状血管瘤的典型表现类似,典型病例诊断较易。

(2)脾囊肿:可分为寄生虫和非寄生虫性囊肿,前者以包虫性囊肿多见,后者分为真性及假性囊肿。真性囊肿囊壁内含有上皮细胞层,而假性囊肿则无。多单发,也可多发。

CT 表现为大小不一界清的均匀圆形液性低密度灶,CT 值 10 HU 左右,囊壁菲薄,少数囊壁可见弧状钙化,增强扫描病灶内部及壁无增强,边界显示更清。外伤性囊肿内由于出血和机化,囊内可见混合性密度。该组 8 例由于表现典型,术前定性诊断准确,但需与类似单纯囊肿的淋巴管瘤、囊性转移灶等相鉴别。

(3)淋巴管瘤:淋巴管瘤,又称为囊性淋巴管瘤,由囊性扩张的淋巴管构成,病理上可以表现为毛细血管状、海绵状和囊状。CT 扫描可见脾脏增大,内见单个或多个液性低密度灶,囊状区边缘可清或不清,病灶内可见粗大的间隔, CT 值 10~30 HU,增强扫描病灶周边及内部多有粗大间隔且可见轻度强化。该组 2 例均为伴间隔的多囊状改变,平扫边界清,囊内 CT 值 8~15 HU,增强扫描可见囊内间隔轻度强化,此点有助于与其他脾囊肿鉴别。

2. 脾恶性肿瘤　脾淋巴瘤:脾淋巴瘤可分为脾原发性恶性淋巴瘤和全身恶性淋巴瘤脾浸润。脾原发淋巴瘤罕见,大体分 4 型:①均匀弥漫型;②粟粒结节型;③巨块型;④多肿块型。

脾淋巴瘤 CT 表现为脾弥漫性肿大或局限性隆起,脾内多发或单发低密度肿块或结节,部分病灶可发生明显坏死液化,增强扫描脾脏明显强化,而多数病灶强化不明显,呈低密度,部分患者有脾门及腹膜后淋巴结肿大。脾脏原发性恶性淋巴瘤均匀弥漫型和粟粒结节型在 CT 上与全身恶性淋巴瘤脾浸润相似,鉴别主要靠病史。恶性淋巴瘤晚期可累及脾脏,30%~40% 的霍奇金病患者脾受累及。单纯依靠脾大来确定有无淋巴瘤侵犯是不准确的,因为有 1/3 患者脾大而病理上无脾受侵,另有 1/3 患者脾不大但在病理上有脾受侵。

3. 转移瘤　脾血管丰富,但转移瘤却少见,其中以血行转移多见。多见于肺癌、乳腺癌、前列腺癌等患者。脾转移瘤的 CT 表现呈多样化,缺乏特异性,脾轻度增大或不大,脾内单发或多发边缘清楚或不清楚圆形或结节状低密度灶,平扫 CT 值平均为 25 HU,有轻中度不均匀强化,但低于正常脾脏强化;部分可呈囊性或囊实性改变,或者呈等密度,增强扫描有利于发现等密度的病灶。从病史及临床表现大多可鉴别脾多发性转移灶和脾淋巴瘤;而脾囊性转移灶需与脾囊肿鉴别,前者囊壁往往较厚,且有强化,并可见壁结节,典型者呈牛眼征或靶心征。该组 1 例平扫未见异常,增强见多发转移性低密度灶。

4. 误诊病例 脾髓外浆细胞瘤:髓外浆细胞瘤发病率较低,发生脾脏者更为罕见,该组仅 1 例。MRI 平扫脾内见一类圆形病灶,边界尚清楚,大小约为 6.4 cm × 7.2 cm,T_1WI 呈不均匀性低信号区,T_2WI 呈不均匀性略高信号区,动态增强扫描早期病灶呈结节状不均匀性强化,随时间推移,病灶仍呈不均匀高信号区,误诊为纤维血管瘤。分析原因,首先本病罕见,对其认识不足,其次影像检查无特征性表现,所以影像学检查在其定性诊断方面往往比较困难,最终确诊主要是靠病理,这方面经验有待进一步积累病例。综上所述,CT、MRI 平扫及动态增强检查能准确评价各种脾脏肿瘤发病部位、血供特点及与邻近结构的关系,不仅有助于病变的定位、定性,而且在临床术前分期及术后疗效判断等方面有着重要的作用。但对不典型病例,必须结合临床,采用多种影像学检查,综合分析,可大大提高诊断符合率,必要时做穿刺活检以明确诊断。

第二节 误诊病例简介:脾脏上皮样血管内皮瘤合并肝和肾上腺囊肿

血管内皮瘤是一种罕见的血管源性肿瘤,传统病理学分类包括:上皮样血管内皮瘤、梭形细胞型血管内皮瘤、网状型血管内皮瘤、淋巴结多形性血管内皮瘤、卡波西(Kaposi)型血管内皮瘤、血管内乳突状血管内皮瘤及复合型血管内皮瘤。

上皮样血管内皮瘤于 1982 年首次详细报道,近几年国内陆续报道多例发生于软组织、肺、肝、骨、肾脏、腹膜、脑等部位患者,肿瘤位于脾脏者极为罕见。

上皮样血管内皮瘤的病因至今不详,一例患者合并肝及肾上腺囊肿,肝囊肿多以先天性为主,由小胆管扩张演变而成;肾上腺囊肿临床少见,其病因可能为肾上腺淋巴管阻塞、肾上腺组织发育异常或错构、寄生虫感染等,该例为上皮性囊肿。该例肝、肾上腺囊肿均与发育异常有关,因此其脾脏病变可能与先天性组织结构发育异常也有关。

脾脏上皮样血管内皮瘤临床及影像不具有特征性,临床上可以表现为左上腹部包块、发热、上腹不适、腹痛及贫血、体重下降或消耗性凝血功能障碍等。CT 平扫多表现为稍低密度结节或肿块,根据病变大小、生长时间、出血与否及细胞分化程度等不同,可能会出现不同的组织密度、增强方式及强化程度,目前临床病例较少,影像资料匮乏,尚无法形成统一认识。脾脏上皮样血管内皮瘤需要与脾脏血管瘤、淋巴瘤、转移瘤及感染等相鉴别,确诊有赖于病理检查。上皮样血管内皮瘤生物学行为具有潜在恶性倾向,对术后患者应长期随访。

第三节 误诊病例简介:脾脏纤维瘤病

纤维瘤病是(肌)纤维细胞异常增生并具有局部侵袭性但不发生转移的交界性病变,腹腔内纤维瘤病远较腹壁及肢体软组织少,容易误诊。纤维瘤病发病机制不明,可能与手术史、放射性损伤、妊娠、结缔组织基因缺陷和 Gardner 综合征有关,也有研究认为可能与成纤维细胞增生活跃、合成及降解功能紊乱,以致过量胶原沉积有关。

本病组织学上含有分化好的胶原和纤维组织,无变性、坏死、异型等表现,属于良性,但常呈浸润性生长,虽未见转移,但常于术后复发。本病可见于任何年龄,但以 30~40 岁之间多见,腹部纤维瘤病很少见于 20 岁以下的患者,女性比男性更常发病,10% 的患者可有多处病灶。

磁共振可明确病变的范围,其较常见的特征有:浸润性的边界,在所有脉冲序列呈低或中等信号强度,而在细胞成分较多胶原成分较少的病变 T_2WI 可呈高信号。有研究发现在所有不规则边界的肿瘤中有 1 个低信号条带状影,提示为侵袭性纤维瘤病产生的纤维性组织。如果肌腱或筋膜与此低信号条带状影相连,则考虑存在被侵犯的可能。

CT 表现文献报道主要为腹壁肿瘤,平扫时呈等密度,注射对比剂后强化;肿瘤较大时,病灶呈略高或等肌肉密度中有小梁状、条状或呈偏心的较大圆形低密度改变分散其间。

本病比较罕见,发生于脾脏更为罕见,影像学表现为肿块较大,不均匀强化,仅根据患者既往有小肠纤维瘤手术史来诊断很不可靠,与脾脏血管瘤或血管肉瘤在影像学上鉴别困难,主要依靠临床无消瘦、贫血及血小板减少等表现来鉴别。本病术前诊断如何?该作者文中未行介绍。

第二章 脾脏错构瘤

第一节 脾脏错构瘤

脾脏错构瘤是一种罕见的脾脏血管性肿瘤样病变,由各种正常脾脏组织混杂而成。因患者常无特异性症状,多在体检或手术中偶然发现。由于发病率低,易与脾脏海绵状血管瘤及恶性肿瘤混淆。脾脏错构瘤由 Rokitansky(1861)首先提出,系脾脏胚基早期发育异常,使脾正常构成成分的组合比例发生混乱。本病发生部位差异无显著性,可发生于脾脏各个部位,无性别差异,发病年龄以中年居多,绝大多数无特异性临床症状,但女性患者更容易产生症状。少数脾脏错构瘤与血液系统病变有关,偶伴消化不良。曾有报道脾脏错构瘤合并肾脏疾病或身体其他部位的错构瘤。本病单发病灶多见,少数可见多发病灶,边界清楚,但无完整包膜。

1. 影像学研究 脾错构瘤 CT 平扫时往往示肿块呈等或稍低密度,位于脾内或包膜下。当脾内病灶呈等密度时易漏诊,病灶位于脾包膜下者有时仅表现为脾脏轮廓的改变。部分病灶密度混杂,提示有多种成分组成。脾脏错构瘤较少发生囊变坏死,仅极少数以囊性变为主。

当肿块伴有钙化和/或脂肪时被视为 CT 特征性表现。该组 4 例(4/9)脾脏错构瘤发生钙化,钙化可能是因为肿块长期存在,局部缺血等原因,病灶营养不良性钙盐沉着。钙化可位于肿瘤边缘或内部,形态多样,呈点状、粗颗粒样或弧形,亦可呈爆米花样钙化,后者与肺错构瘤表现相似,有一定特点。与肾脏等其他脏器的错构瘤多含有脂肪不同,脾脏错构瘤内含脂肪少见,该组 9 例均未见含脂肪成分,这可能也是导致脾脏错构瘤常被误诊的原因之一。

多期动态增强扫描后,动脉期病灶与脾脏分界清楚,该期强化类型有 3 种:大多数表现为弥漫性不均匀轻度强化及病灶周围斑片状强化;少数表现为动脉期即明显均匀强化,主要见于小病灶,这种强化与脾脏血管瘤非常相似。门脉期,上述 3 种均呈渐进性延迟性强化,病灶密度趋于均匀。延迟期,大多数密度接近或稍高于脾实质,仅少数低于脾实质。极少数以囊性或钙化为主的病灶可无明显强化。

该组 1 例多发病灶中有 1 个病灶以囊性为主,仅边缘强化。1 例“爆米花”样钙化者各期增强均未见强化。Komah 等 和 Gombas(1976)报道 1 例明显钙化伴部分囊变的脾脏错构瘤,腹腔动脉造影病灶几乎无血管。

2. 鉴别诊断 脾血管瘤:脾血管瘤是最常见的良性脉管性肿瘤,以海绵状血管瘤多见,平扫多为低密度,增强早期呈边缘结节状明显强化或均匀强化,而不呈弥漫性均匀或斑块状强化可资鉴别。

脾囊肿:脾囊肿在 CT 上多表现为形态规则,边界清楚,水样密度,增强后不强化。包虫病的脾囊肿常位于脾下极的被膜下,肿块周围可见环形较规则钙化影。

脾脏恶性肿瘤:血管肉瘤常呈分叶状轮廓,侵袭性生长,可突破脾脏包膜侵犯周围结构,有时可见远处转移灶。

淋巴瘤、转移瘤:脾内多发病灶且增强扫描延迟期强化程度低于脾实质时,需与淋巴瘤、转移瘤鉴别。脾脏转移往往有原发病史,且多数已有其他部位(如肝脏)转移。脾脏淋巴瘤多为继发性,常伴浅表淋巴结肿大,钙化少见,增强延迟期淋巴瘤强化较周围脾实质低。

综上所述,脾脏错构瘤的 CT 表现有一定特征性,当 CT 平扫显示脾内等或稍低密度实性肿块,伴或不伴钙化,多期增强扫描动脉期病灶呈弥漫性不均匀轻度强化或周围斑片状强化并随时间延迟呈渐进性强化，延迟期密度接近或稍高于脾实质时有助于脾脏错构瘤的诊断。当脾脏错构瘤的CT表现不典型时，需联合其他影像技术进行综合诊断，最终确诊仍有赖于病理。

第二节　误诊病例简介：脾脏错构瘤与血管瘤

脾脏错构瘤是一种罕见的良性肿瘤，尸检系列的回顾显示其发生率为0.024%~0.13%，脾错构瘤可发生于任何年龄，无性别偏向。脾脏错构瘤由多种正常脾组织异常混合而成，常为孤立性病灶，少数可为多发，其中单发病灶多见。该例术前诊断为血管瘤。

有4种病理类型，即红髓型、白髓型、混合型和纤维型。红髓型含血窦和类似红髓的组织结构，白髓型主要为淋巴组织，同时具有两种类型者为混合型，当病灶内纤维组织占优势时为纤维型，其中红髓型占大多数。

影像表现上病灶呈圆形或不规则形，没有包膜，可压迫周围正常脾组织，境界清楚，偶尔有含铁血黄素沉着和钙化。增强扫描早期呈明显不均质弥漫性强化，延迟后扫描病灶信号可趋向均匀，早期弥漫性不均质强化可以与脾脏血管瘤相鉴别。

第三章 脾脏炎性假瘤

第一节 脾脏炎性假瘤

炎性假瘤是一种特发的非特异性慢性增殖性炎症,多发生于呼吸系统、中枢神经系统及胃肠道,发生于脾脏者罕见,Cotelingam 和 Jaffet(1984)首次报道脾脏炎性假瘤。

1. 病理学 炎性假瘤发病原因及发病机制目前尚不明确,可能与病毒感染、局部贫血、损伤及自身免疫等因素有关,也有学者认为本病是由一种内源性或外源性过敏原引起的变态反应。肿块大多单发,边界清楚或局部呈浸润性,可压迫周围脾脏组织形成假包膜。镜下可见不同数量的淋巴细胞、浆细胞、嗜酸性粒细胞和梭形细胞混合存在,常见中心凝固性坏死,免疫组织化学分析炎症细胞,发现主要为 T 细胞。

2. 临床表现 脾脏炎性假瘤可以发生于任何年龄,常无明显临床症状,多数于体检时发现。

3. 影像学研究 本病的影像表现可能与肿块内纤维组织和炎性肉芽组织的含量多少有关,超声或 CT 可于脾脏内发现单个(极少数为多个)低回声或低密度影,呈圆形或类圆形,边界多较规则,部分可有钙化。CT 增强扫描以病变延迟强化为特点,中央可见纤维成分形成的低密度区。MRI 表现为脾内边界清晰的肿物,内可见砂粒样及片状钙化,提示其为良性病变;有完整包膜,信号以及增强后表现与正常脾实质接近,提示包膜是由于肿瘤压迫正常脾实质所致;肿块于 MR T_1WI 和 T_2WI 多呈等信号,内部可见片状低信号区,提示主要为纤维成分,而病灶内部的凝固性坏死由于无血供则不出现强化。

4. 鉴别诊断 脾脏血管瘤:脾脏血管瘤为脾脏最常见的原发性良性肿瘤,约占脾原发性肿瘤的50%,瘤体常与正常脾实质界限欠清,其影像表现与肝血管瘤类似,增强扫描具有从病灶边缘强化并向中心逐渐充盈的特征性表现。

脾脏错构瘤:脾脏错构瘤是正常脾组织异常混合排列组成,与正常脾组织分界清楚、无包膜,富含血管成分, CT 表现为密度均匀的低密度区,增强扫描明显强化,常有钙化或脂肪成分。

脾脏恶性淋巴瘤:脾脏恶性淋巴瘤 CT 常表现为脾内单发或多发不规则低密度病灶,边界不清,增强扫描呈不规则强化。MRI 常表现为单发或多发大小不等的类圆形肿块,边界欠清, T_1WI 和 T_2WI 表现为不均匀性混杂信号,增强扫描呈不均质强化,脾脏恶性淋巴瘤常伴有脾脏弥漫性肿大,脾门及腹膜后淋巴结肿大和全身淋巴瘤的表现。

脾脏血管肉瘤:脾脏血管肉瘤属原发性非网织细胞性恶性肿瘤,临床症状多有腹痛、发热、贫血及血小板减少等,CT 或 MRI 表现为脾脏肿大,并可见单发或多发大小不等、边界不清的结节灶,有时可见出血征象,增强扫描病灶强化较明显。

脾脏转移瘤:脾脏转移瘤患者年龄常较大,多有明确的原发肿瘤病史, CT 或 MRI 表现为脾脏单发或多发类圆形、不规则形病灶,强化扫描呈轻到中度不均质强化,可见“牛眼征”或“靶心征”,常伴肝脏或其他脏器转移。

当脾脏内出现边界相对清晰的单发肿块时,应仔细分析其影像改变及临床表现,要考虑到炎性假瘤的可能,为临床诊断及制定治疗方案提供一定的帮助。

第二节　脾原发性炎性肌成纤维细胞瘤

病理学：炎性肌成纤维细胞瘤是一种罕见的肿瘤，WHO 软组织肿瘤国际组织学分类专家组将其定义为由分化的肌成纤维细胞性梭形细胞组成、常伴有大量浆细胞和 / 或淋巴细胞的一种肿瘤，既往又称为炎性假瘤。炎性肌成纤维细胞瘤病理表现多为良性，但有些病例可表现为局部浸润生长、复发和远处转移，故可定为交界性生物学特征。

临床表现：炎性肌成纤维细胞瘤临床少见，多发生于肺部，也可见于身体的任何部位，如皮肤下、心脏等，而原发于脾脏的则更少见。脾脏炎性肌成纤维细胞瘤的发病年龄范围较广，多见于中年人，男女无明显差异。一般无明显症状或出现非特异性症状，主要表现为左上腹不适。部分患者可出现发热、乏力、便秘、血尿、体重减轻、贫血和血沉加快等症状。腹部超声、CT 扫描体检时发现脾内占位，常被误诊为恶性肿瘤。

脾脏炎性肌成纤维细胞瘤至今病因和发病机制不明，文献报道其可能与下列因素有关：自身免疫反应；一种内源性或外源性过敏原引起的变态反应；可能发生于手术及外伤后，感染、贫血等因素引起的反应性改变；可能与 EB 病毒感染有关。

在 CT 诊断上本病应与以下疾病相鉴别：①脾淋巴管瘤，CT 显示脾脏常呈弥漫性增大，脾内成单个或多发类圆形低密度灶，密度不均，其内见纤维间隔形成，常以多房性病变存在，增强扫描纤维间隔及边缘区不均匀强化。②脾血管瘤，增强后病灶均匀强化，且随时间延迟逐步充填变为等密度。③脾转移瘤，多数肿瘤边界不清，增强扫描轻、中度强化，可有典型“牛眼征”表现，如有肿瘤史则鉴别不难。

第四章　脾恶性肿瘤

第一节　脾淋巴瘤

淋巴瘤累及脾脏，作为全身淋巴瘤的一种表现相当常见，而原发性脾淋巴瘤则相对少见。

在大体病理检查，脾淋巴瘤有下述四种表现：无肿块均匀肿大；粟粒状肿块；直径 2~10cm 的肿块；单个大肿块。但是，在大体病理检查中，脾也可表现正常，仅在镜下才可见到瘤细胞。根据组织学检查所见，脾淋巴瘤分为两类，即霍奇金淋巴瘤和非霍奇金淋巴瘤。淋巴瘤是脾恶性肿瘤中最常见者，它可产生弥漫性和结节性的脾浸润。在霍奇金淋巴瘤患者，脾脏往往是首先和唯一受累的器官，脾淋巴瘤的影像学检查对其分期和处理有着重要的意义。

核素扫描：淋巴瘤侵及脾脏，在核素扫描时易于形成灶性放射活性减低区。

超声：脾淋巴瘤浸润可表现为弥漫性或局灶性弱回声病变，其边界光滑或不规则，无弱回声晕圈。可伴存脾肿大或不伴脾肿大。弥漫性浸润表现为脾脏内有直径小于 1cm 的斑样不均匀病变，可累及整个脾脏或其一部分。在恶性淋巴瘤患者出现弱回声的脾脏病变，实质上可以肯定是肿瘤形成。脾脏内强回声的淋巴瘤少见。

CT：一些作者认为，CT 不是诊断脾淋巴瘤的一种准确方法，因其 CT 表现各异，而且，已有瘤细胞的脾也可表现完全无异常。本症 CT 表现一般为相对低密度区。CT 是确定脾脏大小的一种可靠方法，但脾肿大不是淋巴瘤累及的可靠体征。尽管多数非霍奇金淋巴瘤病人的脾肿大表明脾脏受累，但多达 1/3 脾肿大病人组织学检查中无脾淋巴瘤的证据。此外，有多达 1/3 各种淋巴瘤病人有组织学上脾受累而无脾脏肿大。一般说来，在非霍奇金淋巴瘤病例，若见脾呈结节状增大，则脾淋巴瘤浸润的可能性极大。

CT 图像上，淋巴瘤累及脾脏有 4 种表现：脾脏均匀肿大；出现直径 1~5mm 的粟粒状病变；可见直径为 2~5cm 的多发性团块；大的孤立性团块。CT 对直径 1cm 或更大的结节检查是可靠的，但对更小的病灶则可靠性较低。

证实脾门淋巴结受累，或局限性脾缺损以及脾肿大，可相当准确地诊断脾淋巴瘤。增强 CT 扫描可显示密度减低，大小不等，单个或多个不均一病变。

选择性增强肝脾实质密度的碘化脂溶性对比剂有助于对细小的淋巴瘤结节的显示，能提高诊断呈局限性缺损表现脾淋巴瘤的准确性，然而，微小的浸润灶仍可能不被 CT 发现。但是，这种对比剂因有一定副反应而尚未广泛用于临床。注入水溶性对比剂后，正常脾脏可显示出很不均匀的强化，与血管造影显示的斑驳状表现相一致。CT 的不均匀增强在淋巴瘤累及脾脏方面的价值有限。

包括 CT 在内的绝大多数影像学手段对脾淋巴瘤的诊断敏感性低，其原因可能是三分之二的病例虽然组织学上见有脾淋巴瘤浸润，但其结节直径均在 10mm 以下，难以检出。

MRI：MRI 在脾淋巴瘤分期方面不如 CT 常用。脾淋巴瘤浸润结节一般在 T_1WI 呈低信号。脾内的非霍奇金淋巴瘤局灶性浸润在 T_2WI 时比脾实质信号强度高，在 T_1WI 上病灶信号强度与脾实质相近。在近期内大量输入液体者，导致脾实质 T_2WI 上信号减低，使非霍奇金淋巴瘤易于显示。注入超顺磁氧化粒子，能大大提高脾淋巴瘤的检出。

血管造影：脾内较大的淋巴瘤结节显示为单个或多个无血管性肿块，边界模糊，可产生动脉包裹征象，细小的肿瘤血管和静脉阻塞等征象。但血管造影对霍奇金淋巴瘤浸润脾的诊断不甚可靠，只有83%的霍奇金淋巴瘤累及脾脏者表现为脾内不均匀的影像，而也有66%组织学正常的脾产生不均匀的影像。

脾肿大对淋巴瘤累及脾的诊断是有限度的。在非霍奇金淋巴瘤患者发现肿块状脾肿大，淋巴瘤的脾浸润的可能性极大。但是，单独出现脾肿大不是霍奇金淋巴瘤的可靠征象，其中1/3无病理性的脾受累。另外，有1/3的霍奇金淋巴瘤和非霍奇金淋巴瘤侵及脾脏，而脾脏体积无异常。脾内淋巴瘤瘤灶的大小在分类上有意义，高度恶性非霍奇金淋巴瘤的局灶性病变直径大于3cm，低度恶性的非霍奇金淋巴瘤和霍奇金淋巴瘤出现局灶性和弥漫性浸润，病灶直径一般小于3cm。

第二节　脾血管肉瘤

脾血管肉瘤属脾原发性非网状细胞性恶性肿瘤，其病因尚不明确，多发生于成年人。临床表现无特征性，大多有上腹不适、腹痛、纳差、厌食、体重减轻、贫血及脾肿大等，其中以贫血最常见。脾血管肉瘤的预后极差，就诊时常已有全身转移，其中以肝转移最为多见，本病的半年生存率仅为20%。

超声检查可明确脾血管肉瘤为实质性肿瘤，Wafula等（1985）指出，无回声区代表着肿瘤内扩大的血管腔，可能为脾血管肉瘤的特征性表现。

脾血管肉瘤CT表现为肿大的脾脏内有多发大小不等的结节状肿块，密度较低且均匀，边界清楚。有时见到出血征象，当肿块内有钙化或含铁血黄素沉着时，其CT值可达100HU以上。在病理上，脾血管肉瘤极富含血管，但脾血管肉瘤在CT增强扫描时却缺乏强化，其机制尚不明；同样，脾血管肉瘤的肝内低密度灶也不强化，故术前常被误认为是肝囊肿。

脾脏X线血管造影可帮助明确肿瘤的富血管性，但它不能鉴别脾血管肉瘤与脾脏海绵状血管瘤。脾血管肉瘤术前诊断非常困难。当临床具有贫血、腹痛、脾脏肿大，B型超声或CT提示脾脏占位的病例，除考虑脾恶性淋巴瘤，脾转移性肿瘤外，还应将脾血管肉瘤列入鉴别诊断的范围。

第三节　脾非霍奇金B细胞淋巴瘤

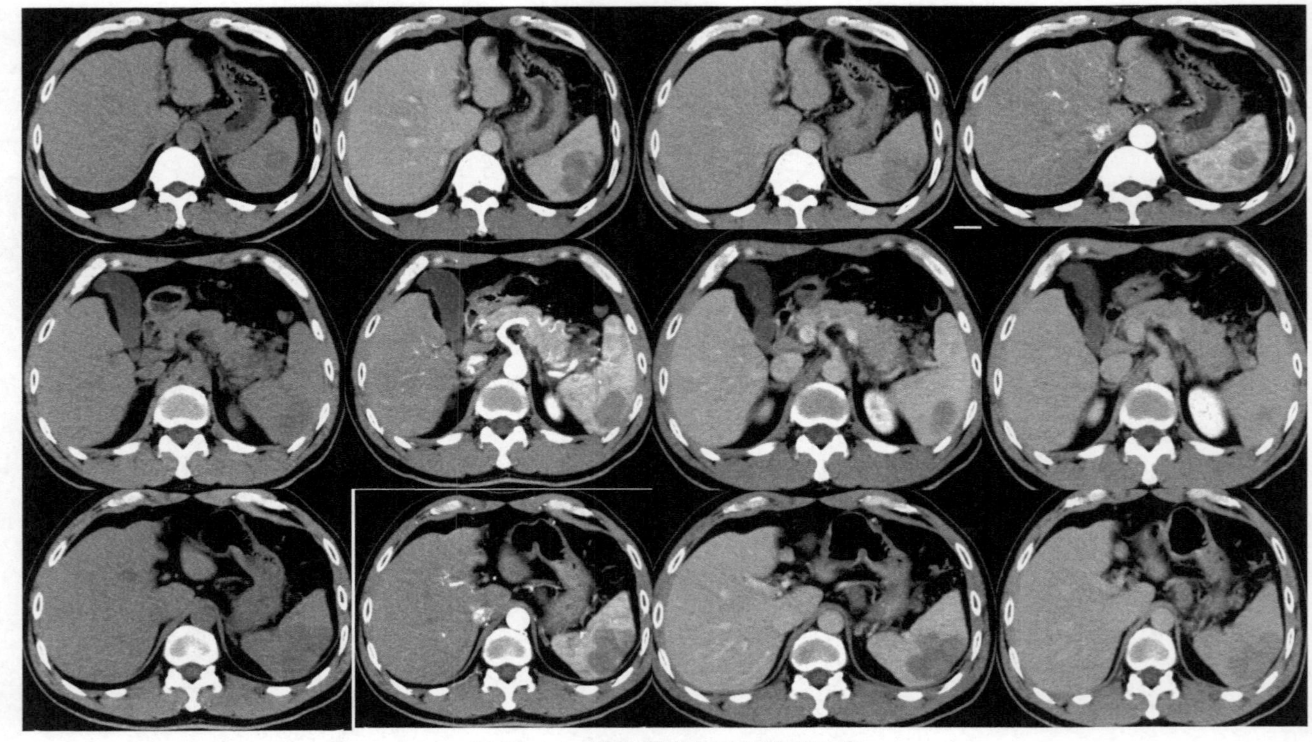

图 21-4-1　脾非霍奇金 B 细胞淋巴瘤

病例,男,40 岁。左上腹痛 9 天入院。

病理检查:脾及胰尾组织:送检不规则组织,总体积约 10cm × 9cm × 5cm,其中见脾门及胰尾组织,大小 7cm × 7cm × 4cm,附着结节状肿物,大小约 6cm × 5cm × 4cm,切面呈灰白及灰褐色,质中,与周围界限不清。肝组织:灰白色组织一块,大小 0.6cm × 0.3cm × 0.2cm,切面灰白,质中。腹腔淋巴结:结节样肿物一个,大小 2.8 cm × 1.8 cm × 1.7 cm,切面灰白,质中。病理诊断:脾及胰尾组织切除标本:初步考虑淋巴瘤,可见瘤组织侵犯脾脏组织。肝组织活检标本:镜下可见正常肝小叶及汇管区结构消失,代之以大小不等、形态各一的假小叶结构,假小叶内肝索排列紊乱,中央静脉缺如,肝细胞浊肿,局灶呈脂肪变性,假小叶间隔有少量慢性炎细胞浸润,符合结节性肝硬化形成的病理学表现。腹腔淋巴结切除标本:初步考虑非霍奇金 B 细胞淋巴瘤(图 21-4-1)。

第四节　脾脏恶性纤维组织细胞瘤

肌成纤维细胞瘤,属恶性纤维组织细胞瘤的一种,起源于具有潜在分化为纤维细胞和组织细胞倾向的未分化间叶细胞。好发于下肢及上肢的深部软组织及腹膜后等处,也可发生于腹腔脏器、心脏、眼眶、喉、肺、脑膜、鼻窦等处,但极其少见。

脾脏恶性纤维组织细胞瘤少见,影像上亦无特征性的征象,且难与炎性假瘤、脾脏脓肿、淋巴瘤、转移瘤及血管瘤鉴别。

但依靠其肿瘤细胞组成及恶性程度,下面几点可提示本病:脾脏形态多不规则,病灶可多发,肿瘤膨胀性生长,可见不完整的假包膜,病灶呈囊实性,低密度病灶内有更低密度坏死区;病灶内部或边缘偶可见点状或条状钙化灶;囊性病灶的囊壁厚薄不均,且边缘不清,可见突向囊内的壁结节;强化呈

"快进慢出"，可见纤维分隔强化，门脉期及延迟期壁结节强化更加明显。

第五节　恶性组织细胞病

恶性组织细胞病是组织细胞及其前体细胞呈系统性、进行性浸润的恶性疾病，较为罕见，而病情进展迅速，常常在6个月内导致病人死亡。主要临床表现有发热、乏力、肝脾及淋巴结肿大。病理上主要表现为肝、脾增大，肝、脾淋巴结、骨髓等造血组织及一些非造血器官和组织中有分化不同阶段的异常组织细胞呈灶性或弥漫性浸润。

脾脏、淋巴结和肝脏是最易累及的器官。受累组织可以部分或全部被破坏，浸润也可以出现粟粒样和小的肉芽肿，但形成巨大肿块的少见。

脾脏的病变也可由于主要脾动脉或其分支动脉阻塞所致，脾脏动脉是终末供血动脉，所以病变通常发生在脾脏的周围部分，在CT检查中通常表现为脾脏周围的低密度病灶。

本病CT表现缺乏特异性征象，与常见的脾淋巴瘤等恶性肿瘤很难鉴别，确诊要靠病理学检查，但CT检查能确定病灶大小，了解病变的范围、周围脏器受累的情况和有无远处转移，为治疗提供重要信息。

第六节　脾转移瘤

尽管脾内有大量淋巴组织，并大量滤过体循环血液，却是肿瘤转移的相对少见部位，脾转移瘤的平均发病率约为3.0%~7.1%。脾转移瘤大多为癌性转移，转移可来自黑色素瘤，卵巢、胰腺、结肠、乳腺及子宫内膜癌，软骨肉瘤和胃淋巴瘤等，脾转移常为恶性肿瘤全身播散的一部分。以往文献认为卵巢癌及黑色素瘤最易发生脾转移，有作者研究发现恶性淋巴瘤最常侵犯脾脏，其中霍奇金病（HD）中30%~40%，非霍奇金淋巴瘤中10%~40%有脾转移。

目前多认为脾转移性肿瘤是指起源于上皮系统的恶性肿瘤，不包括起源于造血系统的恶性肿瘤。脾转移瘤大多数系癌转移，主要经血液途径转移，仅少数经淋巴途径，亦可由邻近器官直接侵犯。脾脏的转移性癌灶肉眼观常表现为多个或单个结节，亦可表现为多数微小结节和弥漫性浸润。

一组病例肠癌、肺癌及胃癌发病率相对较高。发生脾转移的患者多为癌症晚期，并已伴有脾外多器官的转移。脾转移瘤临床表现无特异性，或仅表现为原发肿瘤或全身转移的相应症状。病灶多呈孤立性、多发性或弥漫性浸润。大者肉眼可见界限清楚的圆形结节，位于包膜或脾实质内；小者仅见镜下窦性浸润或微小结节。其形态学特征与原发灶相同，但分化常较原发灶低。血行转移者，瘤组织呈灶性、弥漫性或局限性散在于红髓中，淋巴道转移瘤多位于脾包膜或小梁淋巴管中。

影像学研究：脾脏转移性肿瘤的影像学诊断目前主要依赖于B超和CT扫描，MRI检查的应用也日趋广泛，MRI检查相对于B超和CT扫描有较高的空间分辨率，组织对比度强，结合特定的磁共振对比剂具有定性诊断的优势。

超声：无回声和低回声病变，肿瘤组织界面少，转移灶内部无回声；高回声病变，肿瘤组织界面多，形态多呈不规则状，回声较高，强弱不一，分布不均匀；"靶征"，肿瘤周围水肿或有较多血管者，可出现低回声晕环，较肝癌的声晕宽，中间则是圆形较高回声区，如病灶中央出现坏死、液化则表现为更低的液性低回声。超声诊断脾肿瘤容易，但对肿瘤的良、恶性鉴别比较困难。

CT：CT平扫表现为单发或多发的类圆形低密度结节影，多数境界清楚；弥漫性浸润的肿瘤病灶多为低密度，范围多较广，边界不规则，脾明显肿大。增强后病灶显示更加清楚，部分病灶可以出现环形或不均匀强化，但强化程度不及脾实质。CT扫描对钙化比较敏感，空间分辨率高，在脾疾病尤其是脾外伤，病情稳定者，可作为首选。

MRI：在T_1WI为低信号，出血则为高信号，T_2WI为中等信号，也可为混杂信号；注射Gd-DTPA后呈不均匀强化或"牛眼"状强化，注射超顺磁性氧化铁(SPIO)增强后脾实质为低信号,病灶为高信号。MRI 扫描 SE T_2WI 是脾占位性病变检出的关键序列,对其诊断和鉴别诊断十分重要。经典的 SE T_2WI 有良好的信噪比和组织对比度,在临床应用中价值非常肯定。结合 MR 对比剂能更进一步提高 MRI 检出微小病灶的能力,同时反映靶器官的组织变化。MR 对比剂一直以来是国内外影像学研究的热点。SPIO 是网状内皮系统特异性的纳米级 MR 对比剂,在检测脾脏病变上 SPIO 增强 MRI 明显优于螺旋 CT 扫描,尤其是对脾脏微小病灶(直径 <1 cm)的检测有较高的敏感性和特异性,有助于脾脏肿瘤的诊断与鉴别诊断。Weissleder 等(1987)研究显示 SPIO 增强 MRI 对脾脏的微小病灶(直径约为 0.5 cm)的检测有较高的敏感性和准确性。

鉴别诊断:①多发的囊性脾转移瘤应与脾淋巴瘤鉴别,前者有明确的肿瘤病史,后者临床多有长期发热、浅表淋巴结肿大以及骨髓浸润等征象,且影像学表现具有一定特点。②脾脓肿多数为血行感染所致,特别是免疫功能低下者,常伴有全身感染而发生,常为多发病灶,少数为单发。典型的脓肿可见不规则厚薄不均的脓肿壁,部分病灶脓腔内可见到气体或气 - 液平面,结合脓肿的寒战、高热病史,一般可较好区分。另外,还要与一些脾脏少见的原发性肿瘤相鉴别,如脾脏原发性血管肉瘤等。

尽管脾转移瘤非常少见,但分析和掌握其影像学特点具有重要意义。通过了解脾脏较常见的良、恶性占位性病变的基本特征,结合临床病史可以诊断和鉴别诊断脾转移瘤。为临床的预后和进一步提高患者的生存质量提供重要帮助。

第七节 脾脏 B 细胞淋巴瘤,累及胰腺和肾上腺

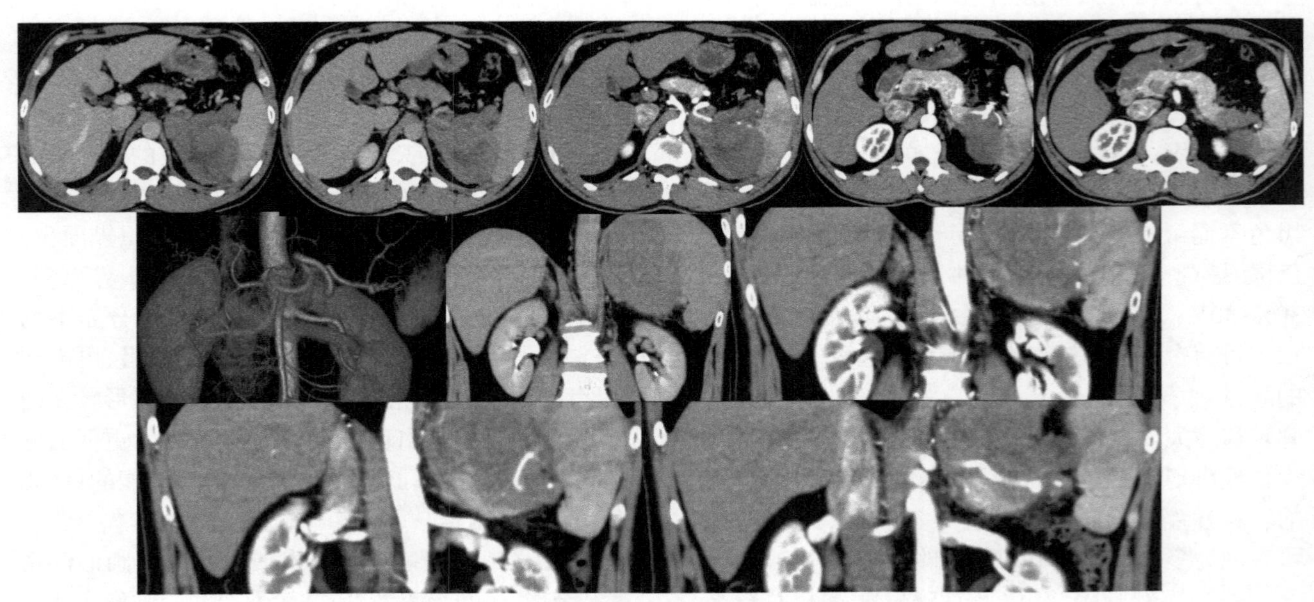

图 21-4-2 脾脏 B 细胞淋巴瘤,累及胰腺和肾上腺

病例,男,50 岁。体检发患者,男,45 岁。

手术所见:脾中下极隆起 2 枚直径约 6cm 肿物,质地硬,浸润胰体尾及左肾上腺并固定。肿瘤广泛粘连,浸润脾动静脉,未浸润胃体,肝内无扪及肿块,腹主动脉旁无肿大之淋巴结,盆腔无扪及种植病灶,术中出血量较多。

病理检查:脾脏及部分胰切除标本:脾脏大小 15.5cm × 9.5cm × 7.5cm,脾脏一端呈隆起状,隆起大小 10.5cm × 10cm × 7cm,切面灰白,质中偏脆,可见坏死灶;部分胰腺组织大小 8.5cm × 5cm × 2.5cm,胰腺组织一端与脾脏及肿物相连,切面灰白,质中,偏脆,肉眼观肿物似胰腺组织;另见部分网膜组织,大小 23cm × 9cm × 3cm,肾上腺皮髓质消失,切面灰白,质中,偏脆。常规病理诊断:脾脏恶性淋巴瘤, 10.5cm × 10cm × 7cm,伴坏死,累及胰腺、肾上腺。网膜组织(-)。淋巴瘤具体类型待免疫组化协助诊断。

免疫组化检测：阳性：CD20，CD79α，MUM1，PAX-5；阴性：CD3，CD45RO，CD23，CD10，CD5，CD56，CD15，CD30，CD7，CD21，GranzymeB，CyclinD1，TIA-1，TdT。免疫组化诊断：脾脏B细胞淋巴瘤，累及胰腺和肾上腺。注：肿瘤由小淋巴细胞构成，弥漫浸润，表达B细胞免疫表型，请注意检查血象中淋巴细胞数量及形态（图21-4-2）。

第五章 脾脏淋巴管瘤

第一节 不常见CT增强表现的脾脏海绵状淋巴管瘤

淋巴管瘤由于淋巴管沿血管神经轴分布,因而全身各部位均可发生,但以头颈部最为常见。发生于脾脏者少见,其发病机制目前认为系淋巴管先天性发育异常,原始淋巴囊不能向中央静脉引流,正常分化良好的淋巴结构异常或未能与正常引流通道建立联系而隔离淋巴管或淋巴囊异常增生扩大所致。本病好发于年幼者,可单发或多发,有时可弥漫累及整个脾脏。脾脏淋巴管瘤一般无临床症状,是否出现症状取决于囊肿的大小和数量。脾脏的淋巴管瘤CT表现文献描述基本一致,即CT平扫示位于脾脏实质或包膜下单发或多发低密度灶,囊壁规则,多无钙化、囊内分隔多见,可纤细或粗大,呈簇状;CT增强后分隔强化明显,囊内容物无强化。

一例CT平扫、增强表现与上述表现有不同之处:平扫低密度病灶中央有不规则形更低密度区域,增强扫描后病灶仅见偏侧性粗大的分隔且呈渐进性持续性强化的特点,但分隔以外的瘤体亦见强化,此点为该例最特殊之处。

为便于观察该组作者采用同一层面近肾脏侧且无明显分隔的区域(3mm^2 的范围)对不同期相的CT值进行测量,动脉期、静脉期及延迟期分别为注射对比剂后35 s、84 s和202 s,测量区域简称“低密度区”。同时测量瘤体中心区域更低密度区域CT值(下简称“更低区”),其测量结果如下:平扫、动脉期、静脉期及延迟期低密度区CT值分别为12.73 HU、61.00 HU、77.10 HU和87.05 HU,更低区分别为31.04 HU、38.06 HU、41.40 HU和45.83 HU,上述两处区域在不同期相下测得CT值可以发现,病灶强化程度随时间推移逐步增强,这种强化方式与文献中所阐述的分隔强化而囊内容物不强化的特点有所不同。

结合该例病理表现,瘤体内更低密度区域的组织成分与其他低密度区一致,只是伴有不同程度的坏死囊变,故强化较弱或强化不明显;肉眼所见非分隔区域的强化较明显,系肉眼难以观察到的弥漫分布的细小的网状分隔强化所致,同时由于脾脏属于血供丰富的器官,故瘤体的血供随之充足,故出现上述较不典型的增强表现。

第二节 脾脏海绵状淋巴管瘤的不典型影像学表现

脾脏海绵状淋巴管瘤是一种少见的脾脏良性肿瘤,由Goldberg(1939)首次报道。检索国内外文献发现相关影像学报道少见,且多以个案形式出现。

1. 发病机制 脾脏海绵状淋巴管瘤是脾脏淋巴管瘤的一种,多被认为是一种错构瘤,而非真性肿瘤。病因有先天和后天因素之说,先天因素认为胚胎发育时部分淋巴管未能与淋巴系统沟通而形成的囊性改变;后天因素认为感染、外伤或其他获得性因素导致的淋巴管引流不畅或阻塞,继而致淋巴管不同程度的扩张。多数认为海绵状淋巴管瘤主要是由先天因素造成。

2. 病理学 脾脏大体上多有肿大改变,临近脾门或被膜下。该组3例脾脏不同程度肿大。2例邻近脾门,1例远离脾门位于脾下极,均突出于脾被膜下,与脾被膜下淋巴管丰富有关。根据脾脏淋巴管扩张程度不同,脾脏淋巴管瘤大体病理分为3型:囊性、实性和蜂窝状。该组 3 例均表现为大小不等的蜂窝状结节，灰红色，质软。组织学上也将其分为 3 型：海绵状淋巴管瘤、囊状淋巴管瘤及混合型淋巴管瘤。该组 3 例病变组织学归为海绵状淋巴管瘤，是由无数大小不等的、扩张的淋巴管组成，管壁厚薄不均，覆以单层扁平内皮细胞，管内充盈着伊红淡染的淋巴液。文献报道 CD9 和 D2-40 是对淋巴管内皮具有相对特异性的脉管标记，一些作者免疫表型检测结果显示 CD9 对脾脏淋巴管瘤具有极高的敏感性。

3. 临床表现　该病好发于儿童，且女多于男。一组 3 例发现时均为成年患者，可能与既往没有体检有关。3 例均为女性，符合女性发病率高的特点。该病多无明显临床症状，少数人表现为左上腹部不适或疼痛、贫血、出血症状。该组 3 例有 2 例是体检发现，1 例表现为左上腹部不适，在外院一直当作胃病治疗，来该院行超声检查后发现病变。

脾脏淋巴管瘤可发生于全身各部位，海绵状淋巴管瘤多见于上肢和腋部，脾脏少见。

4. 影像学研究　（1）超声：该组 3 例均表现为稍强回声光团，形态欠规则，其内可见大小不等液性暗区，病灶周围可见彩流。有 2 例邻近脾门区，与胰腺尾部分界欠清，1 例位于脾下极远离脾门，与胰腺分界清晰。从该组 3 例超声表现分析，超声能够发现病灶所在部位，但是对于邻近脾门的病变不能确定其准确来源，以致对病变进行定性更加困难。

（2）CT：常见 CT 影像学表现基本如下：脾门或脾被膜下单发或多发囊性占位性病变；囊壁边界规则或不规则，与脾实质分界清或不清；囊内部可有网格状、簇状，纤细或粗大分隔，其内可伴有更低密度液性坏死区，钙化罕见；肿瘤 CT 值多位于 30~40 HU 之间；CT 增强后囊壁轻度强化，囊内分隔、间隔或网格呈持续性强化，囊内容物不强化。

该组 3 例 CT 表现部分同上述影像学表现相似，不同点在于增强表现与文献报道不完全相符，除动脉期至静脉期囊壁及其间隔持续性强化外，延迟期囊内容物也发生强化，与一项研究报道的 1 例类似。该组作者分析可能与以下两点有关：其一，脾脏海绵状淋巴管瘤是间叶组织来源，间叶组织在增强时有持续性强化特点；其二，囊内容物内弥漫分布肉眼不可见细小网状间隔。该组 1 例在延迟 30 min 后扫描仍发生强化，且囊内密度更加均匀，CT 值达到 70 HU，比常规延迟期 CT 值 63 HU 还要高，此强化方式在脾脏肿瘤中罕见，该病是否都有此特点须作进一步研究。

（3）DSA：该组 1 例脾动脉造影动脉期表现脾脏下极乏血管区，延迟造影原乏血管区轻度染色，较脾脏实质染色明显减低。DSA-3D 功能成像清晰显示肿瘤供血血管来源于脾动脉分支，供血动脉无明显增粗，环绕肿瘤分布，呈“抱球征”改变，肿瘤内部血管稀少。DSA-3DCT 可显示肿瘤与脾脏的空间关系。DSA 联合 DSA-3D、DSA-3DCT 功能成像可多层面多角度显示肿瘤的血管情况及空间结构关系，有利于脾脏肿瘤的鉴别诊断以及判断是否可行介入治疗。

5. 鉴别诊断　脾脏海绵状血管瘤：本病影像学表现与脾脏海绵状血管瘤极为相似，影像诊断最易混淆，但后者增强后立即强化，瘤周呈“树上挂果”样改变，而前者仅表现为囊壁成间隔强化可作为鉴别；两者在 DSA 表现上也不一样，前者表现为乏血管区，动脉期染色不明显，延迟期轻度染色，后者表现为动脉期就有明显染色。

血管淋巴管瘤（脉管瘤）：其次与血管淋巴管瘤（脉管瘤）鉴别，后者也是起源于间胚叶组织的一种良性肿瘤，组织病理学为脾脏血管组织和淋巴管组织的胚胎发育异常，故而两者影像学表现基本相似，均呈“蜂窝状”改变，增强后间隔持续强化，确诊有赖病理。

除此之外，本病还需与以下 8 种疾病鉴别：①脾囊肿：多为单一囊状结构，少有分隔，囊壁、间隔无强化。②脾包虫病：特征表现为大囊套子囊，囊内间隔及囊壁无强化，可合并肝包虫囊肿。③脾脓肿：临床有寒战、高热症状，实验室检查有白细胞增高，脓肿壁有明显强化及壁外水肿。④脾囊性淋巴管瘤：颈部多见，瘤囊常为圆形或类圆形，边界清楚，囊内密度均匀且与水接近，囊壁轻度强化。⑤脾囊性转移瘤：为囊性或囊实性病灶，壁常不规则增厚，可有壁结节，典型表现为“牛眼征”，可合并其他脏器转移。⑥脾结核：多有肺结核病史，表现为低密度肿块或低密度病变，形态多为圆形或类圆形，少数可有环形强化，可伴有其他脏器的结核浸润，陈旧性脾结核表现为多发针尖样钙化。⑦脾梗死：典型表现脾三角形低密度区，基底部位于脾脏外缘，尖端指向脾门。⑧脾错构瘤：CT 平扫为低密度占位性病变，少数为囊实混合性肿块，边缘清晰，少数可有钙化，内含脂肪时具有特征，CT 增强扫描实性部分呈渐进性均匀强化。

第三节　误诊病例分析:脾血管淋巴管瘤与淋巴瘤或转移性肿瘤

脾血管淋巴管瘤临床少见,临床容易误诊为淋巴瘤或转移性肿瘤。脾血管淋巴管瘤发病率不高,有关影像学报道少见,临床易误诊。一组9例术前CT均未考虑良性病变,其中5例误诊为淋巴瘤,4例误诊为转移性肿瘤。分析其CT表现有助于指导临床诊治。

脾血管淋巴管瘤是由血管和淋巴管胚胎发育异常形成。女性较常见,该组男女比例为1:3.5。脾血管淋巴管瘤与血管瘤或淋巴管瘤类似,可以单发、多发或弥漫性累及整个脾,病变较大,可以引起脾肿大。其病理学基础为血管瘤和淋巴管瘤混合而成,既可以见到含红细胞的异常血管团,也可以见到由内皮细胞组成的含蛋白液囊腔,其间有纤维间隔或脾组织。

脾血管瘤:脾血管瘤可以表现为囊性或实性肿块,但多数表现为含有囊变区的实体肿块。毛细血管型血管瘤平扫为低密度或等密度,增强扫描多为均匀明显强化、边界清楚的结节;而海绵状血管瘤多表现为囊实性肿块,实体部分为等密度或低密度,增强扫描多为花斑样强化,与肝脏血管瘤典型充填式强化不同。条状或结节状钙化可见于血管瘤内部或边缘。

脾淋巴管瘤:脾淋巴管瘤CT表现多为单发或多发边界清楚的薄壁低密度肿块,多位于包膜下,通常无明显强化,增强扫描可以清楚显示其间隔。Pistoia和Markowitz(1988)提出囊壁曲线样钙化有助于淋巴管瘤的诊断。

脾血管淋巴管瘤:脾血管淋巴管瘤CT表现不同于血管瘤和淋巴管瘤,也不是两者CT表现的简单组合。血管淋巴管瘤多表现为囊实性肿块,其实性部分增强扫描多为轻度强化,强化程度低于毛细血管瘤,部分瘤灶的三期增强随时间延长其强化程度渐强,有助于解释其含有异常血管团的成分。间隔可以呈"网格"样强化,该特点类似于淋巴管瘤,但间隔中间成分可以强化,而且平扫密度也较高,又区别于淋巴管瘤。病灶边缘可见粗大血管影,提示病变有较大的供血血管或引流血管。该组有5个无明显强化的瘤灶,均分布在包膜下,符合淋巴管瘤表现,说明此5个瘤灶以淋巴管瘤为主。该组1个瘤灶囊壁有点状钙化,符合脉管来源肿瘤的表现。

鉴别诊断:脾血管淋巴管瘤除需与血管瘤和淋巴管瘤鉴别外,临床还需与淋巴瘤、转移性肿瘤和血管肉瘤等鉴别。淋巴瘤:脾原发性淋巴瘤是最常见的脾脏恶性肿瘤,其CT平扫多表现为低密度结节,增强扫描呈延迟的轻、中度强化,可见"血管漂浮征";未治疗前很少有囊变、坏死或钙化。而脾血管淋巴管瘤粗大血管影多位于瘤灶边缘,且其含有的未强化囊变区多位于脾包膜下,可以与淋巴瘤的坏死区鉴别。血管肉瘤:血管肉瘤是脾脉管来源恶性肿瘤,但临床罕见,其年发病率为0.14~0.25/百万。60%以上患者在就诊时已经存在远处转移,常见部位为肝脏、肺、骨、脑、淋巴结等。其CT表现为脾内均匀或不均匀强化肿块,伴或不伴有巨脾,肿瘤内可有钙化或出血,多数病例有远处转移表现。Thompson等(2005)报道12例,其中9例有坏死,2例表现为血供丰富结节并肝脏转移,肿瘤坏死与远处转移的征象有助于与脾血管淋巴管瘤鉴别。脾转移性肿瘤:脾转移性肿瘤临床非常少见,恶性黑色素瘤、乳腺癌、胃癌、大肠癌等为常见原发灶。脾转移性肿瘤可呈孤立性结节或弥漫性结节。其影像学表现缺乏特征性,临床存在原发灶有助于诊断。

综上所述,脾血管淋巴管瘤女性多见,可以单发,也可以多发。其CT表现与淋巴管瘤和血管瘤有部分重叠,强化方式与其中的血管成分所占比例有关。提高对其CT表现的认识,可以避免部分不必要的脾切除。

第六章　关于脾脏病变

第一节　脾脏病变

脾脏组织学上主要为血窦和淋巴组织，所以脾脏的病变主要为血管瘤和淋巴瘤，其影像鉴别尤为重要。理论上，血管瘤呈现由边缘结节性强化向中心推进的渐进性强化为特点，但实际工作中，脾血管瘤并不具有早期边缘结节状强化的特征，且因时间关系，往往只限于常规的动静脉期及平衡期 2 min 内扫描。而 2 min 内脾血管瘤的强化可不明显或仅轻度强化，因此常常误诊。该组病例中，有 1/3 因未延时扫描而误诊为淋巴瘤、囊肿或淋巴管瘤。究其原因为脾血管瘤的灌注速度较慢，其强化程度和速度均不如肝血管瘤。

由于脾血管瘤的强化速度慢，且 CT 平扫常在病灶的检出及数量上易漏诊和误诊，因此 CT 增强和足够的延时扫描非常重要。一般而论，延时 5~10min 扫描可明确血管瘤的诊断，据该组病例观察，延迟时间可根据病灶大小调整，小病灶 3 min 即可，大部分病灶 5~6 min 可基本充填。

另外 MRI 对血管瘤的诊断帮助很大，通常只需平扫，在 CT 增强不典型或平扫发现脾占位行 MRI 均能明确血管瘤的定性定量诊断，其典型表现为 T_1 呈稍低信号， Trufi 序列呈类似肝内血管 T_2 较高信号，而 Haste 序列呈明显高信号“灯泡征”，病灶边缘清楚。

淋巴瘤分为弥漫增大型、粟粒结节型、肿块型和巨块型。弥漫增大型和粟粒结节型影像表现常仅见脾脏增大。肿块和巨块型 CT 平扫呈稍低密度，增强静脉期病灶显示更清楚，部分边缘不清，肿块呈软组织密度轻度筛孔样强化。

脾脏囊肿常单发，壁钙化为假性囊肿的特征，淋巴管瘤的分叶或花瓣样多房分隔囊性病灶为其特点。发现脾脏囊肿时需注意有无胰腺炎、外伤史、感染或脾梗死等继发所致，否则无壁的囊肿应考虑真性囊肿。

血管瘤与囊、实性肿块（特别是淋巴瘤）的鉴别如下。CT 增强上，淋巴瘤的软组织密度轻度筛孔样强化与血管瘤的液性密度及延时强化不同，而囊肿及淋巴管瘤延迟仍无强化。理论上只要延迟足够的时间，是可以准确鉴别的。但实际工作中，因没有延时而鉴别困难的情况很多，此时采用 MRI 平扫非常有用，淋巴瘤 MRI T_2 序列仅呈稍高信号，低于囊肿和血管瘤信号，且 T_2Trufi 序列上囊肿呈水样高信号，高于此序列血管瘤信号，容易鉴别。

脾脏窦岸细胞血管瘤据文献报道，其延时强化和 T_2 低信号为影像特征，该组仅 1 例符合此特征。错构瘤常含有肿块中心斑块状钙化，不含钙化的脾脏错构瘤易误诊为血管瘤或淋巴瘤，其内密度不均，渐进性延时强化是重要特征。

脾脏的恶性病变除了淋巴瘤外，常见的为转移瘤和血管来源的肉瘤。转移瘤的原发灶常见为消化道肿瘤、黑色素瘤、肺癌、卵巢癌和乳腺癌等，该组的脾转移瘤病例具有此原发灶特点。脾脏的转移瘤常边缘轻度强化或不均匀强化，典型的牛眼征可明确诊断。但转移瘤强化不明显时常难与淋巴瘤鉴别，此时，积极寻找原发灶及肝转移是重要依据，且淋巴瘤发病年龄较轻，常有发热和脾明显肿大可与转移瘤鉴别。

血管来源的肉瘤既具有血管性病变的明显强化特征，又具有恶性病灶的坏死征象，因而病灶常呈现类圆形肿块内实性成分明显强化，坏死区不强化的特点，且具有恶性病灶的易转移特征，常可见肝转移。病灶短期变化大。

脾脏的感染性病变常见脓肿及结核，脓肿的壁常厚薄不均,边缘模糊,较明显强化,可出现脾包膜下脓肿或积液,其发热、腹痛及白细胞升高是重要依据。该组所有脾脓肿患者均具有此病史和体征。

脾结核的诊断较难,因其症状隐匿,临床缺乏特异性,根据病理有4型之分:粟粒型、结节型、脓肿型和纤维钙化型。钙化型易诊断,另外的3型与其他病变的分型有重叠之处,且结节或脓肿病灶常有或无明确强化,与淋巴瘤、转移瘤等难以鉴别,此时,脾外结核的表现为重要依据。

脾脏的梗死常见,常具有典型的楔形,诊断较易。需注意的是感染性病变,如炎症和结核亦可破坏血管壁引起脾梗死,亦可合并肾脏梗死。

脾脏的破裂为急症,出现脾内血肿或包膜下血肿诊断容易,需注意的是迟发性脾破裂和自发性脾破裂应提高警惕。

副脾常见,常有大的主脾和小的副脾,副脾常沿脾血管或脾韧带分布,应注意寻找,其影像特征与主脾一致,主脾术后副脾往往会代偿性增大,有时需一并切除。

种植脾常为脾脏切除或外伤时部分脾组织离开脾窝而异位种植于腹膜后或腹腔内,渐增大为肿块样表现,常误诊为肿瘤性病变。

多脾为多发大小相仿的脾脏,少见,常合并其他器官发育异常。

无脾非常罕见,该组未见此病例。

少见病例,该组3例,影像表现均不典型,常误诊,需依靠病理。

总之,脾脏病变的鉴别常需依赖CT增强,特别是延时约5~6 min扫描即可鉴别血管瘤,或可加扫MRI平扫,其血管瘤、囊性病变及肿瘤性病变T2信号明显不同,有助于鉴别,对转移瘤、脓肿、结核等常见病,需密切结合病史。

其实,脾脏的每一种病变均具有一定的特征性,只有掌握了其影像特征及鉴别的手段,才能对病变的定性有更好的把握。

第二节　脾多灶性病变及误诊分析

一、脾多灶性病变的常见病因

1. 肿瘤性病变　恶性肿瘤:以淋巴瘤和转移瘤多见。脾恶性淋巴瘤多见于继发性脾淋巴瘤,原发性脾淋巴瘤少见。继发性脾淋巴瘤为全身淋巴瘤脾受累,霍奇金淋巴瘤中30%~40%和非霍奇金淋巴瘤中10%~40%侵犯脾。CT表现为脾弥漫增大,内见灶性低密度区,边缘不清,增强不均匀强化,常合并脾外淋巴结肿大,后者对诊断有重要作用。

脾转移瘤的平均发病率约为3.0%~7.1%,多灶性病变占23.3%。CT表现为脾不同程度肿大,内见大小不等低密度区,可囊变,增强扫描示环形强化或不强化,典型者呈"牛眼征",有明确原发灶者易诊断,脾转移瘤的原发肿瘤中,发病率较高的主要有肠癌、肺癌和胃癌。

恶性组织细胞病、白血病脾浸润的CT表现与淋巴瘤、转移瘤类似,诊断主要依靠临床资料、病理学检查,但CT能确定病灶大小,了解病变的范围、周围脏器受累的情况和有无远处转移。

良性肿瘤:血管瘤是脾最常见的良性肿瘤,可为囊性或实性,大小一般为1~3 cm,可单发、多发甚至呈弥漫性病变。

脾多发性血管瘤也称脾血管瘤病。CT平扫为低或等密度区,偶可囊变,增强扫描类似肝脏血管瘤,早期肿瘤边缘结节样强化,延迟扫描逐渐向中心强化,该表现具有特征性意义。

淋巴管瘤少见,CT平扫示脾内多个囊状低密度病灶,CT值常高于一般囊肿,病灶内可见分隔,增强扫描时病灶周围及其内分隔轻度强化,囊内不强化。有学者认为多房、分隔,分叶状轮廓对脾淋巴管瘤有重要价值;囊液CT值为脂肪密度是淋巴管瘤的特征性改变;增强扫描囊壁及间隔轻、中度强化具有鉴别意义。

神经纤维瘤罕见。有学者通过对其他部位神经纤维瘤的研究总结其特点为:属于良性肿瘤,偶有恶变;临床病程长,症状轻缓;肿块常>10 cm,常挤压、推移、粘连周围器官,引起功能障碍,但无侵袭性;CT增强示边缘清楚,多数轻、中度强化,病灶内未强化的低密度区代表坏死、液化或肿瘤黏液样变性。

2. 非肿瘤性病变　主要包括多发脾囊肿、脾结核、脾梗死、多发脓肿等,其中以多发囊肿常见,约占非肿瘤性病变的50%。CT表现为多发性圆形或卵圆形、边界锐利的水样密度区，增强扫描无强化。

脾结核少见，大部分发生于艾滋病或 / 和血行播散性结核患者，CT 表现为多发低密度结节，增强扫描轻度强化，可见散在点状及分叶状钙化灶。

脾梗死是由于脾动脉的分支阻塞，造成局部脾组织的缺血坏死，CT 表现为脾楔形或三角形低密度区，边缘不清，基底位于脾外缘，尖端指向脾门，增强扫描无强化，少数脾梗死伴有包膜下积液，大的梗死灶中央可伴有囊性变，陈旧性梗死灶因纤维收缩，脾可缩小，轮廓呈分叶状。

脾多发脓肿少见，通常合并体内其他器官的脓肿，最常见的原因为血行播散，如感染性心内膜炎，CT 表现为脾多个低密度灶，边缘清或不清，增强扫描呈环状强化，周围见低密度水肿带，典型者脓肿内可见小气泡或液 - 气平面。

二、误诊原因分析

该组脾多灶性病变 CT 误诊 6 例，未做出诊断 3 例。

回顾分析其 CT 资料，1 例转移瘤误诊为恶性淋巴瘤，CT 示脾多发片状低密度区，边缘不清楚，轻度不均匀强化，伴脾门、腹膜后淋巴结肿大，由于当时未查出原发肿瘤，且病变多呈片状，而非结节状，增强扫描也未见明显环状强化。

误诊为转移瘤或恶性淋巴瘤的 1 例恶性组织细胞病和 1 例白血病脾浸润，CT 表现类似，缺乏特征性，诊断主要依靠临床资料。

1 例血管瘤误诊为转移瘤主要由于 CT 增强延迟扫描时间不够，根据多数文献报道，对怀疑脾血管瘤者以注射对比剂后 4~6 min 扫描为宜；其次该患者有支气管肺癌病史，所以首先就做出了转移瘤的诊断，而忽略了对其他征象的分析。

1 例淋巴管瘤误诊为脾囊肿，回顾性阅片发现囊内 CT 值较一般囊肿高，达 26HU，而且囊壁也不如一般囊肿薄、均匀，并有轻度强化，调整窗宽可见部分囊腔有细小分隔。

1 例脾脓肿误诊为转移瘤或恶性淋巴瘤，CT 表现无特征性，因出现脾门淋巴结增大而误诊，回顾分析该例系亚急性细菌性心内膜炎患者，高热，白细胞计数明显升高，脾门淋巴结肿大应是炎症反应的结果，结合临床资料，可做出脾多发脓肿的诊断。

该组恶性淋巴瘤、结核和神经纤维瘤各 1 例未明确诊断。

其中淋巴瘤为脾原发性恶性淋巴瘤，脾外其他脏器未发现异常，CT 检查对此类病例诊断困难。脾结核 CT 检查未发现钙化，在后续检查中发现该患者有肺结核。对怀疑脾结核者可行 CT 薄层扫描，观察是否有钙化灶，同时检查其他脏器，尤其是肺。重视脾外脏器的改变、特别是肺部病变，有利于提高脾结核诊断的正确率。发生于脾的神经纤维瘤，CT 表现缺乏特征性，诊断困难，确诊主要依靠病理学检查。

CT 对脾多灶性病变的诊断价值：脾多灶性病变临床表现缺乏特异性，诊断主要取决于影像学检查。尽管超声检查方便，发现病灶也敏感，但定性诊断较差，而 MRI 对脾钙化灶的显示远不及 CT 敏感。CT 能清楚显示病变的部位、大小、数量、形态、密度以及与周围脏器的关系，对脾多发病变的发现和诊断有重要作用。但对不典型病例，必须结合临床资料，综合分析，必要时做穿刺活检以明确诊断。

第七章　脾窦岸细胞血管瘤

第一节　脾窦岸细胞血管瘤

良性血管源性肿瘤是脾脏肿瘤中最常见的病变,脾窦岸细胞血管瘤属于脾脏血管瘤的一个亚型,又称脾衬细胞瘤,极为少见,病因不明,由 Falk 等(1991)根据免疫组织化学的病理特点提出。

1. 病理学　脾窦岸细胞血管瘤为罕见的良性肿瘤,至今国内外文献报道不足 200 例,涉及影像表现内容的文献则更少,而且主要为个案报道。肿瘤起源于脾脏特有的红髓窦内的上皮细胞(窦岸细胞),故而本病仅发生于脾脏,且常伴有脾脏增大。肿瘤细胞具有内皮细胞和巨噬细胞的特点,同时表达内皮细胞和组织细胞抗原。组织学上,脾脏脾窦岸细胞血管瘤是由脾脏红髓相连的血管性腔道构成,通常它以多发结节的方式累及整个脾脏。

2. 临床表现　脾窦岸细胞血管瘤可以发生于任何年龄,多见于 30~50 岁,无明显性别差异。一项 10 例的研究中患者年龄平均达 56 岁,患病无明显性别差异,与文献报道基本相符。临床上患者多有脾肿大,还可出现脾功能亢进所致的血小板减少和贫血,其他症状无特异性。

3. 影像学研究　有关脾脏脾窦岸细胞血管瘤影像表现的报道多为个案报道。CT 及 MR 平扫表现与血管瘤相仿,CT 表现为等或稍低密度;MR T_1WI 为等或稍低信号的多发结节状,但边界欠清楚;T_2WI 上多呈高信号,少部分因病灶内陈旧出血而呈等或长 T_1、短 T_2 信号。

增强扫描肿瘤表现为类似于脾脏血管瘤及脾脏错构瘤的渐进性增强方式;强化早期,脾脏呈花斑样强化,脾窦岸细胞血管瘤病灶边缘强化被掩盖,故而病灶显示不佳,且边界不清。而静脉期或延迟期呈点状、分隔状或花斑状强化,呈逐渐向内充盈趋势,最终和周围正常脾脏组织相比为高或等密度(信号)病灶;脾窦岸细胞血管瘤病灶内可见陈旧出血,因此在延迟期强化,病灶少数仍呈低密度(信号)。

近年来 DWI 在腹部的应用越来越广,该项研究中的 4 例行 DWI 显示脾窦岸细胞血管瘤病灶大部分为高信号,尤其较大病灶均为高信号。

脾窦岸细胞血管瘤虽然是由类似脾脏血窦的相互吻合的血管腔组成,但其腔隙内可见假乳头样结构突入到腔隙内,乳头样结构内为不等量的纤维结构及内皮样细胞,因此病变为实质性病灶,因而肿瘤内水分子运动明显受限,在 DWI 上显示为高信号。

而脾脏海绵状血管瘤与正常脾脏组织相比无扩散受限改变,故而脾窦岸细胞血管瘤与脾脏海绵状血管瘤在 DWI 有明显差异。

4. 鉴别诊断　海绵状血管瘤:作为血管源性肿瘤不同亚型的脾窦岸细胞血管瘤影像表现,与其他亚型即海绵状血管瘤及脾脏错构瘤有许多相似处。有学者提出,海绵状血管瘤在 T_1WI 信号更低,T_2WI 信号更高,肿瘤的边界清晰,而且内部结构不均,可作为本病的鉴别点。

脾脏错构瘤:脾脏错构瘤由红髓为主的正常脾脏成分混合构成,CT 平扫表现为边界清晰的低密度或等密度肿块,MR T_2WI 上肿瘤因在脾脏正常成分基础上间杂较多纤维组织,因而常呈等、稍低信号,强化表现为早期均匀强化并呈持续延迟强化,且错构瘤常常以单发病灶为主,体积较大。以上特点可与脾窦岸细胞血管瘤鉴别。由于其组织结构与正常脾脏相仿,故而 DWI 无扩散受限改变。综合该项研究发现及复习文献,归纳以下 4 点脾窦岸细胞血管瘤在 CT 及 MRI 上的共同特点:脾脏体积增大;病灶多为多发,且病灶体积较小;病灶增强扫描明显强化,强化方式为向心性;平扫及延迟期病灶不易显示，观察瘤灶数目最佳时期是对比增强扫描的门静脉期。MRI 的特征性表现为 DWI 显示病灶扩散受限，表现为高信号。

第二节　脾硬化性血管瘤样结节性转化

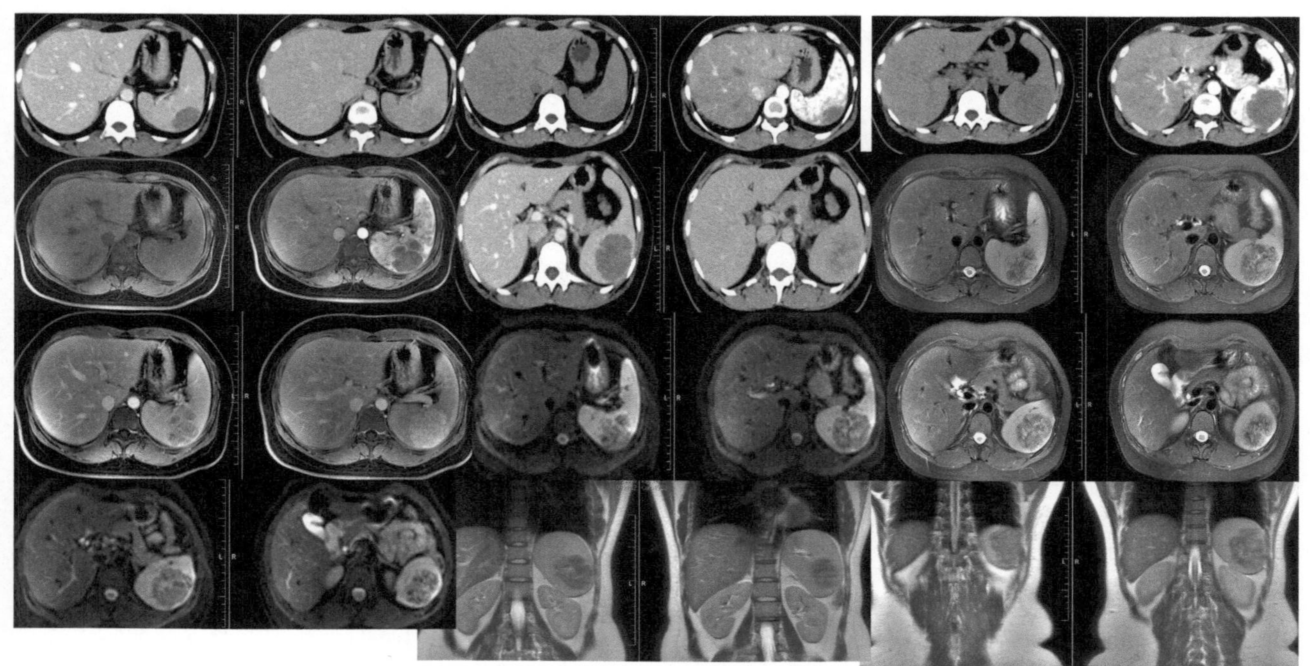

图 21-7-1　脾硬化性血管瘤样结节性转化

患者，女，28 岁。1 周前体检行彩超检查示脾低回声区（大小约为 6.2 cm × 4.8cm），无任何不适；3 天前我院行 CT 检查示肝小囊肿、脾脏后部占位；今日我院行 MR 检查示脾脏后部占位。

手术所见：术中见脾下缘一大小约 5 cm × 5.5 cm × 4cm 瘤体。

病理检查：脾脏及肿物切除标本：灰白灰褐色破碎组织一堆，总体积 12.5cm × 11cm × 4.3cm，其中部分组织似模糊结节状，切面灰白、黄褐相间，大小约 5cm × 4.5cm × 3.5cm，质中偏硬，其余组织为破碎的脾组织，总体积约 7.5cm × 6.5cm × 3cm，切面暗褐色，质偏软。常规病理诊断：脾脏及肿物切除标本：镜下可见在纤维硬化间质中分布着许多血管瘤样结节，部分结节玻璃样变，间质散在淋巴细胞、浆细胞等慢性炎细胞浸润，初步考虑脾硬化性血管瘤样结节性转化，待做免疫组化及原位杂交检测进一步证实。

免疫组化检测：阳性：CD34，CD31，CD8，Vimentin，F8，EMA（散在 +），ALK（散在 +），Actin（小血管壁平滑肌 +），H-caldesmon（小血管壁平滑肌 +），Calponin（小血管壁平滑肌 +），CK（P）（散在 +），Bcl-2（散在 +），Ki-67（+，约 5%），P53（+，<5%）；阴性：CD35，CD21，CD117，DOG1，CD99，Desmin，EBV，Catenin-β。免疫组化诊断：脾脏及肿物切除标本：结合免疫组化及原位杂交检测结果，诊断为脾硬化性血管瘤样结节性转化（SANT），建议术后复查。

脾硬化性血管瘤样结节性转化（SANT）是一种罕见的良性脾脏反应性血管瘤样增生的病变。由 Krishnan 等（1993）报道，称脾索状毛细血管瘤，后来多位学者曾经报道该病例，但颇有争议，Maretl 等（2004）总结 25 例病变，根据其组织学特征、免疫表型正式命名为脾脏硬化性血管瘤样结节性转化。（图 21-7-1）

第八章　脾硬化性血管瘤样结节性转化

第一节　误诊病例介绍:脾脏硬化性血管瘤样结节性转化

脾脏硬化性血管瘤样结节性转化是一种少见的脾脏非肿瘤性血管增生性病变,由 Martel 等(2004)首先提出。硬化性血管瘤样结节性转化发病机制尚不明确,对其命名主要是通过病理学特征定义的描述性诊断:多发的血管瘤样结节分布在纤维硬化的脾脏间质内。该病无特异性临床表现,误诊率极高,应引起重视。各种影像学检查尤其是 CT 及 MRI 检查对其诊断发挥着重要作用。然而到目前为止,关于硬化性血管瘤样结节性转化的文献报道大多集中在病理学特征方面,关于硬化性血管瘤样结节性转化影像表现及特征的文献较少,且大多为个案报道。原发于脾脏的肿瘤性病变相对继发性肿瘤少见,其中最常见的是起源于脾脏红髓的脉管性肿瘤,包括血管瘤、淋巴管瘤、血管肉瘤、错构瘤等,其他比较少见的是血管内皮瘤及窦岸细胞血管瘤等。

1. 病理学　脾脏的硬化性血管瘤样结节性转化是近年来 Martel 等(2004)通过其组织形态学特征和免疫组化表型提出的一种描述性诊断。硬化性血管瘤样结节性转化为非肿瘤性血管增生性病变,其主要特征为多发的血管瘤样结节,常被描述为“结节中结节”。硬化性血管瘤样结节性转化发病机制尚不明确,Martel 等(2004)认为部分硬化性血管瘤样结节性转化病例与血管瘤关系密切。在 2004 年之前,硬化性血管瘤样结节性转化曾经被描述为其他肿瘤性病变,包括错构瘤的变型、多结节性血管瘤及血管内皮瘤等。

2. 临床表现　硬化性血管瘤样结节性转化多见于女性,文献报道男女比例为 1：2;平均年龄为 50 岁(22~74 岁);肿块大小在 3~17 cm 之间;大多无临床表现或因其他病变偶然发现脾脏占位。在一组 4 例中,女 3 例,男 1 例;年龄在 25~62 岁之间,平均 42 岁;病灶均为单发,肿块大小在 2.5~4.4 cm 之间;2 例无任何临床表现而常规体检时发现,1 例因胆囊炎,1 例因门脾静脉血栓偶然发现。这些流行病学特征与以往文献报道的基本相符。

3. 影像学研究　大多数关于硬化性血管瘤样结节性转化的文献报道为对其病理学特征进行描述,关于其影像学表现,尤其是多期相增强扫描 CT 及 MRI 的影像表现的文献报道较少。Li 等(2005)首先对硬化性血管瘤样结节性转化的 CT 表现进行描述,表现为脾内低密度病灶,中央可见钙化点,增强扫描后动脉期及门脉期表现为低密度影而随后周边渐进性强化,延时期中央见无强化区,病灶与周边脾组织分界清楚。随后陆续有学者进行相似的报道,但与之不同的是病灶中央大多无钙化点。该组 3 例 CT 平扫及增强扫描的影像表现与以往文献大致相仿,平扫为低密度影,强化方式为渐进性强化。

Karaosmanoglu 等(2008)首先对硬化性血管瘤样结节性转化的 MRI 表现进行了描述,表现为 T_1WI 及增强扫描后特征性的“辐条轮”征。然而随后有学者的报道提示并非所有的病例均有此特征性表现。在该组 1 例行磁共振检查的患者中病灶表现为 T_1WI 为等信号或稍低信号影;T_2WI 为周边稍高信号中央点状低信号,边界清楚,DWI 示病灶为等信号,增强扫描后呈现与 CT 相似的强化方式:周边渐进性强化,周边强化程度与周围脾组织相似或稍高。T_2WI 图像中内斑点状及短条状低信号,增强扫描后表现为斑点状无强化区。

影像学表现反映了其病理组织学特征。在该组 4 例硬化性血管瘤样结节性转化中,病理学上均显示硬化性血管瘤样结节性转化为脾内孤立的无包膜实性肿块,4 例肿块组织与周围脾组织分界清楚,周边均可见纤维组织层,这正与 CT 及 MRI 平扫及增强时肿块与周围正常脾组织分界清楚相符。需要说明的是,该组 1 例病灶在平扫及增强扫描后各期与周围脾组织分界均不清,推测其原因可能是该患者同时存在脾静脉及门静脉血栓形成,脾脏呈淤血状态,从而使增强扫描后病灶与周边脾组织分界不清。

肿块内多发结节性血管瘤样结节,大小不一,每个结节周围有向心性分布的致密或较致密的胶原纤维组织包绕,由于周围胶原纤维组织的存在,肿块在 MRI T_2WI 仅表现为稍高信号影而非明显高信号。肿块中央绝大部分由致密的梭形细胞构成而血管瘤样结节较少,影像表现为 CT 及 MRI 增强扫描后肿块中央的无强化区和 MRI T_2WI 图像中央低信号。

病理学上裂隙样或不规则的血管腔隙是肿块在 CT 及 MRI 图像上表现为渐进性强化的原因,对比剂通过血管腔隙逐渐向中央的血管瘤结节渗透。

4. 鉴别诊断　硬化性血管瘤样结节性转化需与其他发生于脾脏的良性及恶性的脉管性肿瘤进行鉴别,尤其是与强化方式相似的肿瘤相鉴别。

血管瘤:血管瘤强化模式呈渐进性强化,但在 MRI T_2WI 图像上为明显高信号将有助于鉴别,但仅有 CT 检查或血管瘤不典型时两者鉴别有一定的难度。

窦岸细胞血管瘤:窦岸细胞血管瘤常为多发,体积较小,在影像表现上有助于鉴别。

错构瘤:错构瘤部分可见钙化及脂肪密度,当错构瘤缺少钙化及脂肪成分时,其强化方式亦可为渐进性强化,这时单纯利用影像学对两者进行鉴别比较困难,但错构瘤的临床病史有一定特征,患者可有贫血、血小板减少或全血细胞减少等表现,结合临床病史有助鉴别。

淋巴瘤及转移瘤:硬化性血管瘤样结节性转化还需与淋巴瘤及转移瘤等非脉管性肿瘤鉴别,需结合临床病史,当这些基础病变存在时首先考虑为淋巴瘤或转移瘤,然而可能会造成硬化性血管瘤样结节性转化误诊为淋巴瘤或转移瘤。

总之,硬化性血管瘤样结节性转化的影像学表现具有一定特征,尤其是在 CT 及 MRI 动态增强扫描后的强化方式,然而单纯依靠影像学表现做出初步诊断仍然比较困难。对于大多数放射科医生来说,更重要的是当影像学表现出现上述特征时需要考虑到此病的可能。最终大多数患者确诊还需术后的病理学明确。

第二节　误诊病例介绍:脾脏硬化性血管瘤样结节性转化与血管肉瘤、淋巴瘤

患者,女, 28 岁。体检发现脾脏占位 12 天入院。彩色超声发现脾低回声区,大小 6.2cm × 4.8cm。CT:脾脏后部见类圆形稍低密度影,边界欠清,约 4.7cm × 5.4cm, CT 值 46HU,增强后逐渐强化, CT 值 55~79HU。CT 诊断:脾脏后部占位,淋巴瘤? 建议 MRI 检查。

MRI:脾脏后部可见类圆形异常信号影, T_1WI 等信号, T_2WI 压脂不均匀稍高信号,内可见条片状稍长 T_1 长 T_2 坏死区, DWI 信号不高,大小约 5.9cm × 4.7cm,边界清,边缘呈分叶状;动态增强扫描:动脉期可见结节状强化,静脉期及延迟期逐渐填充,坏死区不强化呈低信号,其内可见裂隙状坏死。脾脏体积无明显增大,包膜光滑。MRI 诊断:脾脏后部占位,血管肉瘤? 请结合临床。

手术所见:腹腔镜下脾脏切除术:术中见脾下缘有一大小约 5.0cm × 5.5cm × 4.0cm 瘤体。将脾脏装入取物袋中,脾脏捣碎的取出。

病理检查:脾脏切除标本:灰白灰褐色碎组织一堆,总体积 12.5cm × 11.0cm × 4.3cm,其中部分组织似模糊结节状,切面灰白,黄褐相间,大小约 5.0 cm × 4.5 cm × 3.5 cm,质中偏硬,其余组织为破碎的脾组织,总体积约 7.5 cm × 6.5 cm × 3.0 cm,切面暗褐色,质偏软。常规病理诊断:脾脏切除标本:镜下可见在纤维硬化间质中分布着许多血管瘤样结节,部分结节玻璃样变,间质散在淋巴细胞、浆细胞等慢性炎细胞浸润,初步考虑脾硬化性血管瘤样结节性转化,待做免疫组化及原位杂交检测进一步证实。

免疫组化检测:阳性: CD34, CD31, CD8, Vimentin,F8,EMA(散在+),ALK(散在+),Actin(小血管壁平滑肌+), H-caldesmon(小血管壁平滑肌+), Calponin(小血管壁平滑肌+), CK(P)(散在+), Bcl-2(散在+), Ki-67(+,约 5%), P53(+,

<5%);阴性: CD35, CD21, CD117, DOG1, CD99, Desmin, FBV, Cateninβ。免疫组化诊断:脾脏切除标本:结合免疫组化及原位杂交检测结果,诊断为脾硬化性血管瘤样结节性转化(SANT),建议术后复查。

第九章　其他脾血管性疾病

第一节　脾动脉瘤与胃出血

内脏动脉动脉瘤的最常见位置是脾动脉，但脾动脉瘤破入胃内却十分少见，当它出现时，幸存者更少。Beeckman 等（1973）报告一例脾动脉瘤破裂成为反复胃出血的原因，该病案 14 天内因突然大呕血两次住院。选择性血管造影见脾动脉瘤，钡餐检查示胃的后内上壁有外在性压迫，手术见一硬块位于胃的后侧，与胰紧密相连，切开包块为血凝块，遂行包块切除，结扎供血动脉，病理证实为脾动脉瘤。术后再做血管造影，见脾动脉受阻，伴存密集的侧支动脉网。

第二节　Klippel-Trenaunay 综合征伴脾血管瘤

Klippel-Trenaunay 综合征，包括皮肤红葡萄酒色血管瘤，静脉曲张，和一个肢体软组织和骨肥大。Klippel-Trenaunay 综合征病变范围广泛，但多累及一侧肢体，常伴发脾血管瘤和 / 或内脏淋巴管瘤。临床如果发现 Klippel-Trenaunay 综合征时，应注意检查内脏，尤其要检查脾脏是否伴有血管瘤和 / 或淋巴管瘤。

CT 平扫可见脾轻度肿大至明显肿大，或脾不肿大，脾内单发或多发低密度肿块，可有斑点状，雪花状钙化；增强扫描大多数病灶强化与脾呈等密度，少数病灶延迟扫描仍不见强化。

脾血管瘤增强表现与肝血管瘤的结节状高密度强化不完全相同，这可能与各自的背景不同有关。脾血管瘤可以恶变为血管肉瘤，表现为密度不均肿块，增强扫描呈不均匀强化，可伴发脾破裂及肿瘤转移等。脾血管瘤须与脾淋巴管瘤鉴别，尤其是 Klippel-Trenaunay 综合征病例，脾淋巴管瘤亦是此综合征常伴发的肿瘤，其 CT 平扫密度较低，CT 值近于水，增强扫描无强化，从而可与脾血管瘤鉴别。

第三节　治疗性脾动脉栓塞与腹腔内游离气体

治疗血液性疾病有时需行脾切除术，但手术常有一定危险性，因而，用导管进行动脉栓塞的介入放射学治疗常被采用。

Allison 等（1981）报告 2 例脾动脉栓塞治疗病案，一例为自体免疫性溶血性贫血，一例为感染后嗜中性白细胞减少。一例栓塞后两周出现发热与脓肿形成，另例栓塞 24 小时后腹痛。两例 X 线检查均见腹腔内游离气体，一例还需手术引流。

虽然临床表现并非在栓塞术后立即发生，但栓塞术后几小时 X 线照片均示脾内游离气体。该作者指出治疗性脾动脉栓塞是腹腔内游离气体的一个新原因，同时，介入放射学者亦应了解这个问题。

第十章 脾囊性病变

第一节 脾脏表皮样囊肿

脾脏囊肿可分为原发性和继发性 2 型,原发性者可分为有上皮被覆的囊肿和寄生虫性囊肿,它们均有境界清楚的囊壁。继发性者则是由外伤引起的假性囊肿,大体标本和镜检均无上皮被覆。脾脏表皮样囊肿属于前者,常为单发性单腔真性囊肿,属于良性病变。

脾脏表皮样囊肿相当少见,仅占所有脾脏囊肿性病变的 2.5%,而有关其影像学表现的报道则更少。文献报道该囊肿最大径可达 18 cm,有作者报告一例达到 29cm,几乎占据整个中上腹部,极其少见。该病变多见于儿童及青年,尤其是年轻女性。一般无临床症状,当病变巨大时则产生相应的压迫症状。

病理上,大体标本显示囊内壁较光整,也可见明显的小梁结构。腔内为清亮液体或含有胆固醇及血液的混浊液体。囊壁由结缔组织构成,多数被覆鳞状上皮,部分被覆柱状、立方或扁平上皮。该例囊壁被覆复层扁平上皮,较少见。囊壁可以钙化,囊肿亦可继发出血、破裂或感染,甚至有该类囊肿恶变的报道。

脾脏表皮样囊肿的组织发生不明,已提出有来自邻近结构的上皮细胞胚胎性包涵物和脾被膜的间皮内陷化生,亦可能为外胚层、内胚层甚至中肾组织的内陷,免疫组织化学的结果与畸胎瘤来源或起源于胎儿鳞状上皮较一致,而不太支持鳞状间皮增生或成熟鳞状上皮的包涵物。

该类囊肿的 CT 表现,一般认为平扫常呈低密度的囊性病变,囊壁可钙化,囊内可见出血的略高密度区,增强检查病灶本身不强化,如有分隔,则显示轻中度强化,周围正常脾组织强化明显。该囊肿需要与脾脏寄生虫性囊肿及假性囊肿相鉴别,仅从影像学表现鉴别诊断较困难,但假性囊肿常有外伤史;而寄生虫性囊肿主要由棘球蚴虫引起,实验室检查对诊断很有帮助。

第二节 多发脾假性囊肿伴钙化

脾囊肿少见,可分为寄生虫性和非寄生虫性,后者又根据囊内壁有无上皮细胞被覆分为真性与假性两大类。一般认为真性囊肿系先天发育异常或组织迷入所致。假性囊肿多与外伤有关。脾假性囊肿多见于中青年,主要以单发囊肿多见。一例为 64 岁老年女性,无明显外伤史,囊肿为多发性,且伴囊壁钙化,甚为少见。

脾囊肿无特征性临床表现,囊肿较大时可出现周围脏器的压迫症状,其术前诊断需依赖影像学检查。B 超表现为脾内边界清楚液性无回声或低回声区。CT 表现为圆形、椭圆形均匀水样密度囊性病变,边缘光整,囊壁较薄,增强无强化;MRI 表现为边缘锐利的囊状均匀长 T_1、长 T_2 水样信号,扩散加权成像(DWI)呈低信号。

该组作者认为该例为脾多发假性囊肿,囊壁有钙化,需与以下疾病鉴别:

多子囊型包虫囊肿:包虫囊肿多有牧区生活史,子囊位于母囊内,CT 或 MRI 扫描可见子囊密度(信号)总是低于母囊密度(信号),母囊壁较厚且钙化多见,增强扫描可见囊壁轻度强化。

脾多发脓肿：脾多发脓肿有高热、寒战病史，囊液密度明显高于水，MRI 表现为 T_1WI 信号介于脑脊液和脾实质之间，DWI 呈高信号，少数可见特征性囊内气体或液 - 气平面，囊壁厚，周围脾实质可见水肿，增强扫描呈明显环状强化。

脾淋巴管瘤：脾淋巴管瘤囊内有粗细不等间隔，囊壁可伴钙化，增强扫描间隔及囊壁不均匀强化。

多发囊性脾转移瘤：脾转移瘤有原发肿瘤史，囊壁较厚，可见附壁结节，牛眼或靶心征为典型表现，增强扫描囊壁呈不同程度强化。

鉴别诊断时还应考虑其他病变，诸如脓肿型脾结核、多囊肾、胰尾假囊肿等。

我们认为，由于该例为多发性囊性病变，并且未提供病理检查结果，是否能够肯定它就是假性囊肿？似乎有一些证据不足，仅供读者参考。

第三节　脾脏内的胰腺假性囊肿

Ramer(1974)介绍一例脾脏内的胰腺假性囊肿，影像诊断显示为脾肿大，其内有充盈缺损，临床症状与体征怀疑胰腺炎和巨脾。该作者强调，脾脏是胰腺假性囊肿的少见部位之一，诚如 Warchaw 等(1972)所述，脾脏内的胰腺假性囊肿是引起脾脏显著肿大的一个病因。

第四节　先天性脾囊肿

脾囊肿可为先天性、外伤性或寄生虫性囊肿。真正的脾囊肿称为表皮样囊肿、上皮囊肿或先天性囊肿，内衬上皮。多数作者认为真正的脾囊肿是由腹膜上皮折叠而成或由陷入脾沟的间质细胞堆积而成。脾囊肿可伴有其他正常脾变异，比如游走脾伴脾囊肿等。

第五节　出血性脾假性囊肿

脾囊肿可分真性囊肿与假性囊肿两种，真性囊肿有分泌性细胞，常见有皮样囊肿、淋巴囊肿和棘球囊肿等；假性囊肿无分泌功能，见于脾血肿、炎症、脾梗死，且常有钙化。

Paris 等(1978)报告 14 例胰腺炎病人的出血性脾假性囊肿，这是胰腺炎少见的加杂症。脾脏肿大可挤压邻近结构，造成移位，甚至导致结肠脾曲的外压性梗阻。

第十一章　脾脏创伤

第一节　CT 图像上的假性脾破裂

CT 诊断脾破裂一般均较准确,极少假阳性。但 Savit(1987)报告一例 CT 误诊为脾破裂者,患者为青年男性,车祸后腹、背及左胁腹痛,排泄性尿系造影已见膀胱破裂伴腹膜外尿外渗,CT 平扫发现脾脏 CT 值低,误为脾床内血肿;同时将其周围含有对比剂高密度的尿液误为急性出血。推测脾脏低密度的原因是由于排泄性尿系造影时患者血压较低,脾内对比剂甚少。

Jeffrey 等(1981)复习 50 例腹部创伤后,经 CT 扫描诊断为脾损伤的 22 例中, 21 例正确, 1 例假阳性,为一 4 岁女孩,假阳性原因为脾脏小、脾周脂肪缺乏和肋骨伪影。其他可能的误诊因素包括运动、条纹状伪影和脾裂隙。

脾裂隙可与脾破裂区别,因其沿脾脏的内侧面,且呈一细的线状影,而包膜下血肿和撕裂几乎总是累及脾脏的外侧面,且伴存游走的腹腔积血。Cholankeril 等(1984)有 3 例患者的肝左叶很像脾周血肿,但如能仔细追踪与肝左叶连接的脾周的密度,则可避免此类误诊。况且也缺乏其他脾撕裂的征象。

Berland 等(1985)报告 3 例创伤后脾呈现低密度, CT 检查前皆现低血压, 1 例误为脾动脉损伤的假阳性。CT 平扫,脾正常密度略低于肝,而在动态扫描及对比剂注射时间延长时,此类关系出现暂时颠倒。Beland 的病例,脾增强扫描时,其密度值至少低于同一层面肝脏 20 HU,他们的病例类似脾梗死。但缺乏脾梗死常见的征象,即增强组织的边缘保持、脾大、局灶性或楔形的缺损以及血管栓塞。他们认为脾强化减少的原因是灌注减少,源于创伤导致的交感神经的刺激。同时发生的低血压也必然减少脾的灌注。另一方面,肝的血流在创伤后大概改变不明显,乃因肝的双重血液供应,以及对肝脏的交感神经性刺激作用较小。

Chamberlain 和 Sherwood(1966)以及 Becker 等(1968)已显示肝正常通过胆系排泄注入对比剂碘量 1%~2%,如未注意肝的密度增高,则可将脾的密度稍低误为病变。Phillips 等(1985)指出在注入 58.4g 碘后 4 小时,肝密度平均增加 22HU。

此外, Jeffrey 等(1981)还报告脾周脓肿可伪似包膜下血肿。积脓常位于内侧的特点,及感染的继发征象均有助于正确诊断。

第二节　误诊病例简介:脾脏破裂伴出血,胰体尾部及胃后壁之间侵袭性纤维瘤病

详见本书 本卷 第二十篇 第十八章 第六节　误诊病例简介:脾脏破裂伴出血,胰体尾部及胃后壁之间侵袭性纤维瘤病。

第三节　外伤性膈疝和脾的疝入

外伤性膈疝并不少见，但是，由于认识不足，发生漏诊误诊者屡见不鲜。

应将下胸上腹部的穿透伤（刺伤、弹伤及牛角穿入伤等），胸腹腰背撞击挤压伤及坠伤等，列为最有可能引起膈肌破裂及膈疝的情况，从而做包括膈肌的胸部的正侧位摄影，常能提示有无膈疝的存在，这是做出正确诊断的最重要的因素。

一旦发生膈肌破裂，自然愈合是不可能的。因腹压有利于腹内容物向上运动进入胸腔，使裂口保持开放，并可引起膈疝。但是，发生膈破裂者，不一定都会发生或立即发生膈疝。Fataar 和 Schulman（1979）报告 47 例膈肌破裂，仅 25 例发生膈疝。发生膈疝的时间可在膈破裂当时，也可在膈破裂后几小时，几天，几月，甚至数年。所以，凡有胸腹损伤病史者，即便初次检查阴性，仍有可能发生膈疝，必要时应予复查。

在不同时间，不同体位检查时，疝影可时大时小，甚至时有时无，其形态可变。

若在胸内出现积气胃肠阴影时，即可确诊。但因疝入内容既有空腔脏器，又有实质脏器，因而可误诊为膈膨升、横膈或肺底肿瘤、胸腔积液、气胸、液气胸、肺挫伤、肺萎陷、肺部感染、肺梗死、先天性肺囊肿、支气管扩张、心包积液等。遇有疑问者，应进一步进行检查。

按疝入内容发生频率排列为：结肠、胃、网膜、小肠、脾、肝等。脾与肝的疝入较为少见，但在一些作者报告 4 例膈疝中，有 3 例见到脾的疝入，1 例见到肝左叶的疝入。

分析其原因，这与膈肌撕裂的部位及撕裂的方向有关：外伤性膈疝膈肌撕裂部位，多见于膈肌顶部后外侧，呈横行或斜行，而该组作者报告病例中，2 例膈肌撕裂均在左侧，呈纵行撕裂，另 1 例从膈后左三角韧带心包处撕裂，达左前方，可能便于脾与肝的疝入。

第四节　自发性脾破裂

Lambert（1992）报道 2 例与溶栓治疗和伴用肝素抗凝有关的自发性脾破裂。

该作者指出，早期诊断至关重要，因此，在作溶栓和 / 或抗凝治疗的患者，或在溶栓期间，如出现不可解释的腹部症状，或低血压，或失血，应考虑此类并发症，宜作 CT 检查。

在决定治疗前，应询问所有病人有关的腹外伤或脾疾患的既往史，以提高对这种可危及生命的并发症的警惕。

第五节　脾外伤诊断的一次教训

脾外伤的直接血管造影征象包括对比剂外渗、动静脉瘘、毛细血管期中脾的不规则显影、随后的无血管的脾髓或血肿形成。间接征象是邻近结构的移位，或脾本身从腹壁和横膈的位移，以及脾内血管束伸直等。

Tuttle（1971）报告 1 例 18 岁青年，选择性腹腔动脉造影示脾内动脉伸直达脾上极，伴对比剂外渗围绕脾上极，考虑为脾上极内大的包膜下血肿，手术却未见包膜下血肿。

再回顾造影片总结教训，发现胃内充盈液体，胃底膨胀挤压脾上极，造成脾内血管与围绕胃底的胃短动脉伸直，术前将胃短动脉误认为脾内血管，且又将扩张的胃黏膜血管延迟照片上的表现混淆为对比剂外渗，故而造成误诊。

第十二章　脾的发育变异和先天异常

第一节　副脾与诊断陷阱

副脾常常是血管造影误诊的源泉,它理应在胰腺肿瘤、肾上腺肿瘤及腹膜后肿瘤区别诊断时予以考虑。特征性的血管造影表现有助于发现和诊断副脾,当它直径大于2cm以上,且其位置不甚典型时,核素显像常有助于诊断。副脾常见。在大宗尸体解剖材料中约占10%(Halpert和Gyorkey,1959),大约80%的病例,它们特征性邻近于脾门,约20%位于胰尾,偶可位于脾动脉沿途或腹腔其他地方,包括空肠壁、盲肠或睾丸;其中10%副脾为多个。副脾的血液供应来自于脾动脉或脾门中脾动脉的分支。血管造影毛细血管期可见其蓄积对比剂均匀,呈类圆形或肾形;如副脾足够大,可见到副脾静脉。当副脾位于脾门中,它的形状特征与血液供应有利于识别。

脾切除术后,副脾增生可类似一大的腹膜后肿瘤;当一个团块发现于脾切除术后,应当考虑副脾的诊断。在先天性溶血性贫血与特发性血小板减少性紫癜症的病人,在其起初颇有作用的脾切除后可出现症状的复发,乃因脾组织或副脾在术后发生了增生。

副脾如位于胰尾区,可为任何支胰的动脉供应,类似于胰的内分泌性肿瘤,如胰岛细胞瘤。在高血压病人主动脉造影片上出现副脾,常使诊断进退两难。当副脾位于肾周间隙,颇难诊断,其血管造影表现可类似于副肾上腺,嗜铬细胞瘤或肾上腺其他肿瘤。

副脾在临床上可类似一些病变,Bass等(1967)报告盲肠处的副脾破裂和蒂扭转时,可伪似急性阑尾炎。Das Gupta和Busch(1960)指出副脾组织产生胃底的凹陷而类似于胃的新生物,在胃肠钡餐检查时造成误诊。Beahrs等(1980)及Glazer(1981)等相继报道在脾的创伤性撕裂后进行脾切除术者,术后两年出现副脾组织的代偿性肥大,CT图像为圆形或边界稍不规则的类圆形等密度阴影,与肝的密度相近。

第二节　脾活体位置与体型关系

人的体型可分为三种:矮壮(胖)体型的脾接近膈肌,位于左侧膈穹之下,有时呈横位,其长径与胸腔垂直,下极平第12胸椎至第1腰椎。瘦高(长)体型的脾贴近胸腹壁,呈垂直位,下极可达第3~4腰椎高度。一般(适中)体型的脾,斜位于膈下左侧的后外方,下极平第2腰椎平面。

活体在影像检查时观察,脾下极可随呼吸而上下移动,平静呼吸时,移动幅度为1~3cm,深吸气时为7~8cm。因此,做各类影像检查时,应尽量让受检查者维持一致的体位及呼吸状态,这是十分必要的。正常脾下极,距髂嵴最高点平面,男性5~8cm,女性7~10cm,一般不低于肋弓下缘;或与肝右叶下缘平齐;另外脾前端不超过腋中线。

第三节　病理误诊病例简介：副脾伴大量钙化与淋巴瘤

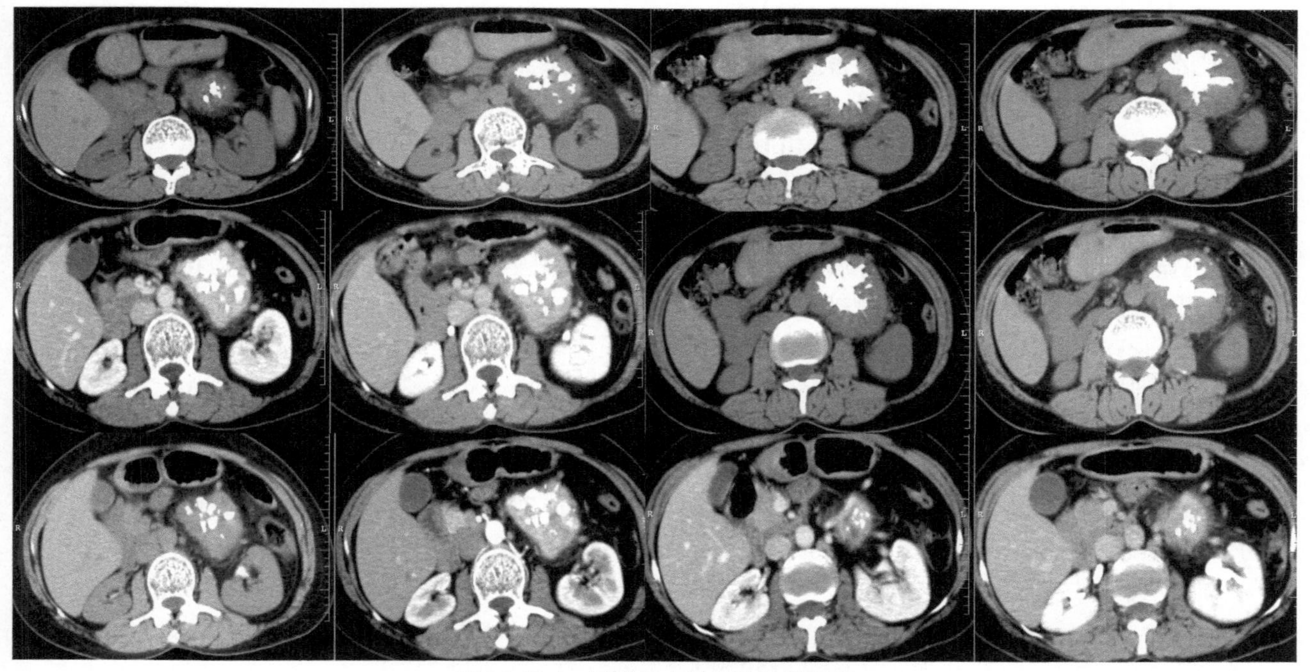

图 21-12-1　副脾伴大量钙化与淋巴瘤

患者，女，44 岁。不规则阴道出血 1 个月，近日阴道出血较前加重，就诊于外院，宫颈活检提示"鳞状细胞癌（高 - 中分化）"。

手术所见：脾脏增大，表面见质硬钙化灶，左侧腹膜后 L1~L5 水平突出一实性肿块，约 12 cm × 10 cm × 8 cm 大小，表面与十二指肠粘连。沿肿瘤右侧缘切开后腹膜，逐层分离肿瘤表面脂肪组织，显露出肿瘤，见其血供丰富，从腹主动脉右侧包绕腹主动脉，固定于腹主动脉及椎体左侧，与周围组织致密粘连。完全切除腹膜后肿瘤，肿瘤质硬，送快速病理检查，回报为淋巴瘤可能。

病理检查：冰冻病理：腹膜后肿物切除标本：灰红色不规则肿物一块，大小 9cm × 9cm × 5.5cm，肿物中央质硬、周边质软，切面灰红灰白。冰冻病理诊断：腹膜后肿物切除标本：钙化或骨化的软组织内见大量淋巴细胞弥漫性浸润，淋巴造血系统疾病可能性大，确诊待常规多块取材及免疫组化。常规病理诊断：腹膜后肿物切除标本示钙化的软组织内见大量淋巴细胞弥漫性浸润，局部血管丰富伴玻璃样变，副脾脏可能性大，确诊待免疫组化。

免疫组化检测：阳性：CD3，CD45RO，CD20，CD79α，CD5，CD23（FCD+），CD21（FCD+），CD35（FCD+），CD10（生发中心），Bcl-2，CD68，CD163，CD31，CD34，F8，κ 链，λ 链，Ki-67（+，约 30%）；阴性：CyclinD1，TdT，D2-40，CD15。免疫组化诊断：腹膜后肿物切除标本，结合免疫组化及组织学图像，符合副脾脏组织伴大片钙化（图 21-12-1）。

第四节　胰腺内副脾

临床和病理：副脾为一种先天性异位脾组织，可能是由于背侧胃系膜内胚胎脾芽的某部分融合失败所致。副脾的发生率为 10%~30%，其最常位于脾门附近，胰尾为第二好发部位，约占副脾的 20%，在临床上仍非常少见。胰腺内副脾患者一般无临床症状，常因体检发现，因其为良性病变，不需要手术切除，但临床上它易与胰腺实质性肿瘤相混淆。因此，如术前能明确诊断，临床只需随访观察，避免不必要的手术治疗。

影像学研究：大小和形态：胰腺内副脾常较小，一般大小为 1~2 cm，Kim 等（2006）报道 7 例，平均大小为（1.5 ± 0.5）cm，病灶呈类圆形，边界清晰，均为单发。

CT 和 MRI 平扫表现：胰腺内副脾表现为胰尾区类圆形软组织肿块影，CT 平扫其密度与脾脏相似。与胰腺实质相比，胰腺内副脾于 T_1WI 上呈低信号，T_2WI 上呈高信号，信号特点与脾脏相似，这主要因为副脾的组织结构与正常脾脏相似。

增强扫描：胰腺内副脾在 CT 和 MRI 增强扫描时均呈明显均匀强化，强化程度与脾脏一致。这可能是由于胰腺内副脾供血动脉来自脾动脉分支。

伴随表现：脾门周围常见其他副脾，该组 3/3 例均见脾门周围副脾。

鉴别诊断：胰腺内副脾少见，认识其影像学表现主要应与胰腺肿瘤鉴别：胰腺内分泌肿瘤：胰腺内分泌肿瘤功能性常见的为胰岛素瘤，其肿瘤亦较小，常早期强化，但患者有明显激素分泌异常的相关临床表现。而非功能性内分泌肿瘤常较大，一般伴有囊变坏死。

胰腺实性假乳头状瘤：胰腺实性假乳头状瘤亦常发生于胰尾，肿瘤常较大，平均约 9 cm，肿瘤一般存在不同程度的坏死或囊变。

胰腺腺癌：胰腺腺癌好发于胰头，肿瘤为乏血供肿瘤，结合增强扫描一般易鉴别。

胰腺转移瘤：胰腺转移瘤少见，一般均为肿瘤晚期，易与本病鉴别，富血供胰腺转移瘤常见于肾癌转移。

比较影像学：目前文献报道的胰腺内副脾大部分经手术证实，事实上，一旦确诊胰腺内副脾无需手术切除，因此术前正确诊断非常重要。目前常见的诊断方法有 CT、MRI 动态增强、超声增强、核素扫描和超顺磁性氧化铁增强 MRI 等。一般来说，CT、MRI 发现胰尾较小肿块（<2.5 cm），密度、信号及强化方式与脾脏相似，则应考虑胰腺异位副脾可能。超声增强检查亦有助于诊断，其强化原理与 CT 和 MRI 相似。据文献报道核素扫描特异性很高，如 ^{99}锝胶体硫，但其分辨力低，不能清楚显示解剖结构，常遗漏小的异位脾。

超顺磁性氧化铁增强 MRI 有望提高诊断的准确性。SPIO 进入人体内后极易被网状内皮系统的细胞识别而被吞噬，由于肝窦和脾脏内富有网状内皮细胞（枯否细胞），其颗粒被吞噬而聚集在肝、脾内，导致肝组织的 T_2 弛豫时间显著缩短和信号丢失，在 T_2WI 上信号明显下降，呈特征性表现。总之，胰腺内副脾的主要影像学表现为发生于胰尾，肿瘤较小，CT 和 MRI 上密度、信号及强化方式与正常脾脏相似，同时常伴有脾门周围副脾。

第五节 副脾有关误诊分析

副脾的发生：副脾为先天性异位脾组织，其发生原因可能是由于背侧胃系膜内胚胎脾芽的某部分融合失败所致，或部分脾组织脱离主脾发育而成。年龄越小副脾发生率越高，成人约 11%，副脾 2 个以上者仅占 3%，通常不超过 6 个。副脾具有脾组织的结构，其血流来自脾血管，单独行走呈蒂状。副脾大多数位于脾门、脾蒂或胰尾部位，少数出现于脾胃、脾结肠韧带内或大网膜、输尿管、卵巢及盆腔内，甚至胰腺、胸腔、腹膜后、阴囊等处。发现与确证副脾的存在可协助脾脏切除方案的制定。

临床表现：副脾一般无明显临床症状，多在查体或因其他病变检查时而偶然发现。当副脾较大时可出现压迫症状、牵拉胃肠道症状。副脾本身的一些病变如：副脾蒂扭转、坏死、梗死或外伤出血等均可出现相应的临床表现。一组 23 例中 1 例脾胃韧带间副脾梗死病例，术前半月即有左上腹疼痛持续近 1 小时，然后自行缓解的临床症状。

影像学研究及误诊原因分析：副脾的 CT 表现特征与主脾相同，主要表现为平扫呈大小不等的软组织结节，圆形或椭圆形，边缘光滑锐利，直径数毫米至十余厘米不等，CT 值均在 40HU 以上。增强后明显均匀强化，强化程度均较平扫提高 50 个 HU 单位。其增强前后 CT 值及增强的方式与主脾相似，因此典型常见部位的副脾诊断多不困难。

副脾主要误诊为左侧肾上腺病变，因副脾紧邻左侧肾上腺，CT 横断面不易分辨来源，但回顾 CT 横断面及相应的多平面重建图像后。病灶显示与肾上腺具有明显的分离征象，提高了病灶的定位诊断；

副脾平扫表现为边界清晰、密度均匀的软组织肿块。增强后均匀强化，类似肾上腺腺瘤；而腺瘤平扫一般低于肌肉密度，增强后通常 CT 值增高小于 60 HU 等；功能性腺瘤还通常使正常肾上腺部分显示纤细等，对上述问题重视不够，是该组 2 例副脾误诊为肾上腺腺瘤的主要原因。

肾上腺嗜铬细胞瘤可表现实质显著强化，但临床有高血压表现和尿儿茶酚胺及其代谢产物的增高。该组 3 例虽均见血压升高，但 CT 诊断时尚没有生化检验资料的支持，此为误诊的另外一个重要原因。因此，在紧邻左肾上腺的占位，要考虑副脾的存在，结合各项生化指标，重视局部薄层扫描与多平面重建等技术的应用，可提高病灶与肾上腺占位的辨别。

此外，由于副脾的 T_1、T_2 信号特点和强化方式与主脾常一致，术前 MRI 检查亦可避免误诊。在副脾的诊断过程中，还应注意其与邻近脏器病变的鉴别诊断：如胃底外生性肿瘤、胰尾胰岛素瘤、脾门转移性淋巴结肿大或淋巴瘤侵犯等。

对位于不典型部位、脾切除后或副脾伴发其他病变（如梗死）等副脾的误诊，更容易发生，更需熟悉副脾可能出现的少见解剖部位、副脾各种病变的临床症状、影像表现，重视超声、MRI 甚至核素扫描等综合考虑，以减少误诊的发生和提高术前的正确诊断率。

第六节　倒置的脾

一般说来，当脾较小且为强壮型体型的人，脾趋向于横位；当脾肿大且为无力型体型的人，脾趋向于垂直；大多数人居于此二型之间，即脾门面向下内、胃底与胃体上部。倒转的脾脏是一种变异，脾门向上指向内侧，或其外侧。

Westcott 和 Krufky（1972）报告 2 例脾的方向异常——倒置，脾门面向上方对着横膈，而脾的隆凸的圆表面却面向下方。脾的最大的面是胃膈面，脏侧通常内凹，被脾门分成至少两个面，前部毗邻于胃，后部毗邻到左肾与肾上腺；下外侧部分常有一压迹，毗邻于结肠的脾曲。手术时，脾常可自由活动，靠邻近器官的压力和悬吊韧带支持。膈结肠韧带从结肠脾曲到膈，大概是最重要的支持韧带，实际上，它构成一支架或吊索，支持脾的下极。

脾的韧带或脾蒂的腹膜有两个反折：前层形成胃脾韧带，后层形成膈脾韧带，脾动脉、脾静脉与胰尾被包含于后份或膈脾韧带两层之中。某些人在脾与结肠之间、脾与后腹壁之间可有粘连，对脾附加以支持。

在一些少见的情况，支持韧带可先天缺如，或变松弛（如妊娠以后及体重突然减少），脾可变得自由活动，只以伸长的胃脾和膈脾韧带附着于胃，它可漂浮或游走进入中腹、下腹、甚或入盆，脾的伸长的蒂如发生扭转，可造成脾的动脉供应与静脉引流障碍。

脾的动脉造影有助于倒置的脾与更严重的情况的区别，脾动脉的横行方向、圆的下缘、边缘光滑、上方的脾门的 V 形轮廓等征像，均有助于此种脾的方向变异与肿块、创伤、以及脾梗死的区别。

第七节　CT 图像上的假性脾破裂

详见本书 本卷 本篇 第十一章 第一节　CT 图像上的假性脾破裂。

第八节　脾组织的分叶和切迹

脾组织的分叶：正常脾脏的大小，形状和位置均可有很大变异。脾组织可膨出或分叶，自脾的脏面向内伸延，位于左肾上极的前方，排泄性尿系造影时可类似左肾或肾上腺肿块的表现，但 CT 扫描不难识别。分叶之间的裂隙很光滑，偶尔可深达 2~3cm。应用脂溶性对比剂有助于鉴别肾脏与脾脏。偶尔脾脏的一个分叶可部分位于左肾之后，将左肾向前推移。

三叶脾：Piekarski 等（1980）讨论脾的 CT 检查时，介绍了三叶脾，该脾颅侧分为三叶，其 CT 横断图像可见三叶完全分开，不相连续，三叶之间的界面为脂肪组织充填的宽窄不等的缝隙，最内侧叶还有钙化，该脾尾侧（即脾体）CT 图像则未再见到分叶，此亦为发育变异。

脾的切迹：脾的形状与轮廓变异不大，脾通常在一定范围内呈现切迹。此切迹大概是由于脾从众多的间质细胞分离的集团结合形成的缘故，这些细胞团的融合与限局化的程度可有不同，融合缺乏则形成一个或多个副脾；融合不全则形成大小不同的脾切迹；十分少见的情况，脾可完全分离成两部分。Kikkawa（1966）指出，在 80%~100% 的脾，切迹出现于上部；在 30%~60% 的脾，下部出现切迹；前面呈现切迹者占 3%~15%；后面及膈面出现切迹甚少。如不了解这些切迹，影像诊断中也可导致误诊。

脾的先天性裂隙导致的误诊：Smidt（1977）报告 1 例腹部闭合伤，核素显像发现脾脏上缘有一裂隙，术前诊断为脾脏血肿，术后方知为先天裂隙。放射性核素显像对腹部外伤的肝、脾检查颇有用处；特别对重危病人早期确定肝、脾的占位性缺损或破裂更是如此；在腹部外伤后体征和症状都不明显，以及肝、脾破裂的潜伏期，核素显像作用甚大。

脾的核素显像异常特异性很少，引起核素显像缺损的疾病包括脾梗死、囊肿、原发或转移性肿瘤。在青少年腹部创伤后，一个充盈缺损通常解释为脾血肿。脾的切迹多沿着上缘，很少沿着下缘，可表现为分叶状脾。Michels（1942）对 50 例脾脏的解剖和脾动脉进行研究，发现脾脏上缘有切迹者占 85%，切迹的数目为 1~6 个，其深度范围是 0.1~4.0cm。

脾脏形态变异：间质细胞团可全部融合形成单一脾脏，但也可能仅部分融合，从而导致脾脏分叶、切迹或裂隙。脾脏分叶多位于脾下极或脾内前方，可由单独一支脾动脉供血，且可压迫胃壁引起胃压迹。脾裂隙可表现为深入脾实质 2~3cm、边缘锐利的裂隙状影像。脾裂隙也可多发。被裂隙分开的脾脏部分可仅由一狭窄组织桥相连，不应与脾破裂混淆。

脾分叶是脾裂隙的一种更轻微的变异，伸入脾实质的裂隙较短。脾分叶在多平面图像上可能更明显。在脾门，间质细胞团也可融合形成一正常脾组织的残留物，称为脾舌。脾舌与胰尾鉴别困难。脾舌也能伸向胃，形成胃的外在性压迫。

第九节　活体脾的大小和重量的变异

在活体，脾的大小和重量可有很大的个体变异。

同一个人，因功能状态不同，脾的大小和构造均可出现变化：血压升高和进食之后，脾均增大；死亡、剧烈运动或饥饿（白髓缩小）之后，脾皆缩小。

同一个人，脾的形状与其周围脏器的功能状态的改变有关：胃腔充满、结肠扩张时，脾略呈四面体形；在结肠空虚时，脾的结肠面则显消逝。

有作者在尸体脾实验超声测量的基础上，提出了在腋后线冠状和前倾冠状扫查测量脾厚和长径的实时超声扫查技术，对 305 例平均 36 岁的正常研究对像（男 148 例，女 157 例），和 160 例脾肿大进行研究和比较，指出这些径线有助于判断脾肿大。但是这些径线值与非活体的解剖学测量不尽相同。脾厚径与解剖学数据接近，而最大长径较实际测量为小，与非活体的解剖学数据有显著差别，应进一步探讨。

第十节　脾形状发育变异引起的混淆

正常脾脏是一卵圆形结构，通常位于左上腹之后外部分，脾的长轴方向、形状及位置可出现不少的变异，Spencer 等（1977）指出，出生时脾长径约为 5cm，其生长与年龄增长呈正比，在成人脾长度的范围为 7~13cm。正常脾长轴指向前下方，然而脾长轴可在任何方向旋转。在核素显像中，颠倒的脾是一难见的变异，可伪似一包块；正常脾的分叶或脾的切迹可能难与梗死、撕裂或其他病理情况区别。创伤或手术可造成脾组织的种植，从而出现脾功能的亢进。

脾的形状和假脾：Gooding（1978）报告难得见到的脾向内后方延伸，超声纵断示脾和一明显包块介于脾和肾之间，实际为脾的下段和内段；超声侧位扫描可见脾与该包块连续；CT 横断图像示脾呈一钩形，外凸内凹，形状颇为奇特。Crade 和 Rosenfield（1979）讨论超声检查脾切除术后病人的假脾，在左侧卧位扫描，脾脏原来位置处有一机化的血肿，而超声所示颇类似脾脏的图像。

脾的发育变异误为肾上腺的包块：Noon 等（1981）报告 CT 扫描将脾的发育变异误为肾上腺的包块，该作者指出，在快速注射对比剂后，通过动态 CT，应用时间 - 密度曲线有可能对此类假性肿瘤做出正确诊断。

第十一节 脾脏位置变异

脾脏的位置与脾肾韧带的长度有关。脾肾韧带一般仅几厘米长，由背侧胃系膜和后腹壁壁层腹膜融合形成。即使脾肾韧带长度正常，脾脏也有一定的活动度，因此，在仰卧位和俯卧位时脾脏的位置稍有不同。在制定治疗方案时要考虑这些因素。如果背侧胃系膜和后腹壁壁层腹膜的融合过早，该韧带消失，在脾脏表面即产生裸区，以致脾脏的一个面不在腹膜内，这可使脾脏与肾脏直接接触。在此种情况下，腹腔积液即不能进入脾的裸区，而只进入脾的腹膜腔内部分。部分脾脏也可直接位于肾脏背侧。

若发生不完全融合，脾肾韧带延长，可导致游走脾。在这种情况下，脾脏位置不断变化，可位于正常位置即左上腹部，也可降至下腹部或盆腔。游走脾可因扭转而产生症状，症状可以是间歇性，也可造成脾梗死。偶尔游走脾无症状，直至成年后才发现。

脾的位置和形状的改变：脾脏的结构柔软，左上腹肿块或器官的增大均可引起明显移位和形状的改变。若附近脏器切除后，脾脏的位置会发生改变，尤其是在左肾切除后，脾脏即占据左肾窝内。偶尔由于脾脏所附着的韧带松弛，脾脏可移至腹内较空虚的部位。

游走脾或游离脾：游走脾是因正常脾脏无固定韧带附着而在腹腔内出现位置变化。游走脾可因不能解释的腹部肿块或脾扭转后的急性腹痛而引起临床注意。CT 或 / 和核素扫描可协助准确诊断。游离脾是另一先天性变异。有时会引起诊断上的困难。此系由于脾脏的悬挂韧带松弛。使脾脏在腹内移动，类似在下腹部出现肿块。此时在脾脏的正常位置看不到脾脏。同时，游离的脾脏有其特殊的外形，注射对比剂后，脾脏的密度明显增高可做出诊断。

游走脾的旋转：游走脾的旋转是一种少见的急腹症的原因，在术前很少做出诊断。Abell（1933）报告 2 例游走脾发生扭转，并回顾文献另外 95 例，其中 88 例为女性，年龄范围 6~80 岁，多数在 20~40 岁之间，最常见症状是扪得腹块，游走的脾可位于腹腔的任何部分，包括盆腔，该组中只有 7 例脾实际位于左上腹。Isikoff 等（1977）报告 1 例游走脾，造影征象诊断误为恶性腹部肿块，患者为女性 22 岁，腹部不适 2 个月，发现左中腹包块，钡剂灌肠提示降结肠近端壁内肿瘤，考虑可能源于间歇性套迭，因临床与 X 线表现不一致而作肝脾 ^{99m}Tc 硫胶扫描，发现肝无异常，左下腹可见中等肿大的脾脏影，手术证实脾游走于左下腹，约为正常脾大小的 4 倍，且被一长蒂悬吊伴存扭转，遂行脾切除。

大多数作者认为，造成此种现象的病因是由于胚胎期背侧胃间膜发育缺陷，导致脾蒂变长，造成脾游走，然后出现扭转。

第十三章 游走脾及其疾病

第一节 游走脾与腹部包块

游走脾的旋转是一种少见的急腹症原因,在术前很少作出诊断。

Abell(1933)报告2例游走脾发生扭转,并回顾文献另外95例,其中88例为女性,年龄范围6~80岁,多数在20~40岁之间,最常见症状是扪得腹块,游走的脾可位于腹腔的任何部分,包括盆腔,该组中只有7例脾实际位于左上腹。

Isikoff等(1977)报告1例游走脾造影征象诊断误为恶性腹部肿块,患者为女性22岁,腹部不适2个月,发现左中腹包块,钡剂灌肠提示降结肠近端壁内肿瘤,考虑可能源于间歇性套叠,因临床与X线表现不一而作肝脾 ^{99m}Tc 硫胶扫描,发现肝无异常,左下腹可见中等肿大的脾脏影,手术证实脾游走于左下腹,约为正常脾大小的4倍,且被一长蒂悬吊伴存扭转,遂行脾切除。大多数作者认为,造成此种现象的病因是由于胚胎期背侧胃间膜发育缺陷导致脾蒂变长,造成脾游走,然后出现扭转。

第二节 游走脾合并脾扭转

临床上游走脾合并脾扭转罕见,多见于20~40岁女性,曾有年龄最小者为2天的报道。

脾扭转的临床症状依脾蒂扭转程度的不同而异。轻度扭转表现为与脾充血有关的慢性腹痛,中度扭转表现为间断旋转引起的间断性腹痛,重度扭转表现为急性扭转导致的脾梗死和脾肿大、累及邻近器官所致的急性腹痛。一例患者表现为慢性经过,临床症状不典型,容易误诊。游走脾主要靠影像学检查确诊。CT不仅可以显示游走的脾,还可了解扭转后脾的血运情况,是术前诊断较理想的方法。该例CT表现脾位于下腹及盆腔,未按正常脾强化模式强化,提示脾缺血;上方可见旋涡状结构,为扭转的脾蒂,可能是实质脏器扭转的特异表现。另外,该例门静脉期肝右叶出现片状低密度灌注异常区。肝灌注异常反映了肝脏血流动力学的改变,见于多种疾病。

该例在排除肝脏自身病变和肠系膜上静脉异常后,应考虑脾静脉血来源不足,这对脾蒂急性扭转的早期诊断有一定提示作用,其临床意义还有待进一步探讨。

游走脾并扭转属于绞窄性急腹症,需要及时诊断和急诊手术治疗。由于脾对机体免疫功能的重要性,对脾倾向于保留手术。这取决于脾的病变程度。对扭转复位后,脾色泽恢复正常,无明显坏疽改变者,可行脾原位固定术。对脾坏死改变者,行脾切除术。

该例患者手术后发现有脾肿大、淤血、坏死,结合临床,考虑为慢性扭转并加重所致,故未能保留脾。

第三节　游走脾与脾梗死

脾位于正常位置以外的腹内其他部位时称异位脾,异位脾脏可复位至脾床称为游走脾。游走脾在临床上少见,多表现为腹部游走包块,临床症状缺乏特异性,约 20% 游走脾可伴脾蒂扭转。此病多见于儿童及 20~40 岁的中青年女性,成年人中多为中年经产妇,可能与妊娠、腹壁薄弱或激素紊乱、手术等所致脾脏系膜及韧带松弛有关。少数脾蒂扭转可伴发邻近部位的胰尾扭转,而发生胰腺坏死,出现胰腺炎症状。一例患者出现腹部游离包块 4 年,但未出现腹痛等症状,故未引起重视,直至出现脾蒂扭转导致腹痛,已出现脾脏梗死,CT 示胰尾部卷曲,胰腺密度尚正常,未见明显异常强化。

影像检查对于游走脾的早期诊断非常重要。

超声:正常脾脏解剖位置探测不到脾脏,而在腹腔其他位置探测到类脾脏声像图,并能显示脾门切迹及脾门血管。

CT:左膈下脾床处正常脾脏影消失,腹盆腔其他位置发现脾脏影像,边缘光滑,密度均匀;增强扫描动脉期及门静脉期呈典型花瓣状强化,平衡期呈均匀强化。当脾门转位而不再朝向内下方时即提示伴发脾蒂扭转,脾门方向的异常及脾蒂“旋涡状”表现是判断脾蒂扭转的重要征象。

脾蒂扭转可分为完全性和不完全性扭转,不完全性脾蒂扭转时,静脉回流受阻,脾静脉迂曲扩张,而脾动脉血供正常,脾脏淤血,可伴脾脏肿大,CT 值减低,脾脏密度均匀,增强扫描显示花斑脾及对比剂消退期延长;完全性脾蒂扭转时,因脾动脉及其分支阻断,可引起脾脏部分性或完全性梗死,CT 表现为脾脏外形肿大,急性期可无明显肿大,边缘均匀光滑,脾脏可见楔形及片状低密度灶,增强扫描无强化。

完全性脾梗死时脾脏密度弥漫性减低,增强扫描三期均未见明显强化。该例脾脏即为完全性脾蒂扭转、脾梗死。

综上所述,CT 检查对游走脾合并脾蒂扭转的诊断有帮助。临床医师根据上述症状、体征,结合腹部 CT 及超声检查明确诊断游走脾、脾蒂扭转及脾梗死后有助于制定治疗方案。脾切除术仅适用于脾梗死的患者,对游走并脾蒂扭转无脾坏死者应选择脾固定术。对无症状性游走脾亦应选择脾固定术,避免脾扭转的发生。

第四节　游走脾影像学检查

游走脾是一种少见的先天性变异,是脾悬韧带过度松弛所致,脾脏可在腹腔游走,类似于腹腔或盆腔肿块,常发生于女性。

CT 表现为脾脏在正常位置缺如,而在其他部位发现具有脾脏外形和强化特征的肿块。

由于肠道气体重叠,超声很难发现异位脾,如果诊断不明,^{99m}Tc- 硫胶体(^{99m}Tc-SC)显像可诊断游走脾。游走脾在临床上没有重要意义,但可能发生扭转。

第十四章 脾脏感染性疾病

第一节 脾脏结核

病理学:本病的致病菌结核杆菌是革兰氏阳性抗酸杆菌。结核杆菌入脾的途径主要有3种:大多数由血行播散引起;经淋巴系统途径转移入脾;邻近器官结核直接累及脾脏。

病理改变:结核菌感染早期产生渗出性病变,在脾内形成结核性肉芽肿,几个结核结节融合成较大结节,病变进一步发展可发生干酪样坏死,当机体抵抗力增强或者有效的抗结核治疗后,干酪样病灶中的结核杆菌代谢低下,繁殖能力被削弱,病灶失去水分而干燥,碳酸钙和磷酸钙沉着形成钙化,少数病人因抵抗力低下或治疗不及时,干酪病灶发生软化或液化,形成半流体或液体物质而形成结核性脓肿。

临床表现:脾结核临床罕见,多见于青壮年,一组10例中位年龄30岁。脾脏结核一般由肺结核通过血液循环播散到脾脏引起,多数为多脏器累及,临床表现常缺乏特异性,主要症状为低热、盗汗、乏力、消瘦、OT试验阳性及血沉增快。少数病人可有脾功能亢进。

体检可发现肝、脾增大,左上腹触痛。Rosengast把脾脏肿大、多血症、发绀症候群称之为"脾结核三主征",但在临床实际中以贫血为多见。

影像学研究:脾结核按CT表现可分为3型,即粟粒型、结节型、脓肿型。粟粒型:常为全身结核的血行播散而感染。CT扫描见脾内弥漫性小结节状低密度灶,增强后病灶无强化。病灶直径<5 mm者,CT检查大多难以发现,仅可见脾肿大,脾脏密度普遍减低。结节型:CT多表现为单发或多发结节状低密度灶或混杂密度灶,边缘清楚或模糊,病灶中心常伴有粉末状、斑点状钙化,增强后可有轻度边缘强化,脾脏可弥漫性肿大。脓肿型:结核结节相互融合或单发病灶发展增大并液化,直径常大于20mm,CT值常在20 HU以下或近似于水密度,增强扫描后病灶中央无强化,边界清楚,呈坏死表现特征,边缘环形强化。有作者将脾结核钙化型单独列出,另有作者将其归入结节型脾结核中一并叙述。

该组中5例脾脏结核伴有后腹膜、肝脾门区多发淋巴结肿大、钙化,3例伴有纵隔内多发淋巴结肿大、钙化,提示结核杆菌经淋巴途径转移入脾,增强后肿大淋巴结呈典型环形强化,有助于该病的诊断。

鉴别诊断:①淋巴瘤是最常见的脾脏肿瘤,病灶偏大,增强后病灶轻度强化,肿大淋巴结呈普遍均匀性强化,结合临床表现、骨髓象、血象等可做出诊断,脾穿刺活检可确诊。②转移瘤:转移瘤多有明确的原发肿瘤,常伴有周围多脏器转移,患者年龄偏大,表现为脾内单发或多发低密度灶,少有弥漫性,病灶相对较大,可出现"牛眼征",无钙化,淋巴结多无环状强化。③脾脓肿:临床表现为寒战、高热、恶心、呕吐、白细胞计数升高,CT表现为单发或多发性较大低密度灶,内壁光整,壁外可见水肿带等。脓肿区内小气泡、气-液面或液-液面,CT增强见脓肿中心有高密度"靶征"、边缘及分隔强化明显等。④脾血管瘤:脾血管瘤多无临床症状,增强病灶呈由边缘向中心扩展持续强化,延迟扫描与脾脏呈等密度。⑤脾囊肿:脾囊肿病灶边缘光滑整齐,增强无强化。

归纳脾结核的诊断要点主要有:①脾结核好发于中青年;②有脾外器官结核病灶或结核病史;③出现急性、亚急性或慢性结核中毒症状及体征;④贫血,血沉加快,中性粒细胞及淋巴细胞数目升高;⑤CT表现为肝脾肿大,脾内单发、多发或弥漫性无强化的低密度病灶,肝门、胰腺周围、脾门、下腔静脉旁淋巴结肿大伴有环形及花环状强化,淋巴结、脾脏等部位的钙化灶;⑥行淋巴结穿刺活检、腹腔镜检及脾穿刺活检病理为结核,浆膜腔液检查发现结核杆菌者;⑦抗结核治疗有效可考虑或诊断为脾结核。

由于脾结核临床缺乏特异性,而脾脏结核 CT 平扫与增强扫描具有一定特征,因此对脾脏结核的确诊具有重要价值。脾脏结核较罕见,影像学经验缺乏,临床资料缺乏,致 CT 误诊率较高,因此有必要加强对本病影像学表现的认识,在日常工作中应重视实验室检查和临床资料,对高度怀疑脾结核的患者,尽早建议临床给予实验性抗结核治疗后复查,同时 CT 或 B 超引导下针吸活检有重要意义,是提高定性诊断,减少误诊的重要措施。

附:具体研究资料:一组 10 例脾脏结核中 7 例误诊:3 例误诊为淋巴瘤,2 例误诊为转移瘤,1 例误诊为脾脓肿,1 例误诊为脾囊肿;仅 3 例正确诊断为脾结核。

第二节　胃内金属异物穿破胃刺入脾引发脾脓肿

脾脓肿较少见,尸检发现率为 0.2%~0.7%,通常是全身感染的一部分。70% 脾脓肿经血行播散引起,15% 由于脾损伤,10% 由于脾梗死,很少由于邻近器官感染的直接侵犯。一般是由于细菌感染,免疫力低下患者则常由于霉菌感染。脾脓肿一般为多发,少数为单发。

一例患者为男性,38 岁,临床上以发热 10 天,咽喉部不适,左上腹痛收治入院。无明显胃穿孔临床症状,考虑为慢性长期磨损和本人特殊体质综合所致。胃内金属异物为一长约 9 厘米的金属丝,穿破胃刺入脾,引发脾脓肿。该例病人不愿意提供既往史。

第三节　胰腺炎的脾实质并发症

Fishman(1995)研究胰腺炎累及脾的 CT 表现时,发现胰腺炎累及脾病变较为少见(发生率 1%~5%),但这些复合病变可危及生命。为避免不良的临床后果,应用 CT 监测病变的范围和发展是很必要的。胰腺炎累及脾病变,主要包括:假性囊肿、脓肿、出血、梗死、破裂和血管损伤。

脾假性囊肿:由于解剖学关系,胰腺假性囊肿可导致脾脏假性囊肿。大多数病人有胰腺炎反复发作史。这些囊肿由于缺少上皮衬壁而被称为假性囊肿。早期,CT 扫描可显示胰尾的假性囊肿,2~6 个月以后的追踪观察发现扩展到脾。多数病例脾假性囊肿是自发的;有些则最终会导致脾出血或脾破裂。假性囊肿所致的脾破裂,是由再发的急性胰腺炎后的脾周围粘连所引起。

脾脓肿:脾脓肿由多种原因所致,而在缺乏脾基本病变或全身疾病时却较少发生。脾假性囊肿也可继发感染产生脾脓肿。其 CT 图像上可见空气气泡,并以持续性发热和进行性加剧的腹痛为其特征。可同时合并出血。脾脓肿还可通过抽出脓液确诊。此外,Jeffey 等(1981)还报告脾周脓肿可伪似包膜下血肿。积脓常位于内侧的特点,及感染的继发征象均有助于正确诊断。

脾出血、血肿及破裂:进入脾的胰酶分解物可腐蚀脾小血管,其结果为脾出血。血液可进入脾假性囊肿内或脾包膜下。如果出血量过大,或可发生真正的脾破裂。若不能及时、准确地诊断,病人血压会迅速下降而进入休克状态。胰腺假性囊肿累及脾或再发的急性胰腺炎常可引发脾破裂。脾假性囊肿病人有脾破裂倾向,甚至很小的损伤都可引起脾破裂。经皮引流可引起腹腔内出血而常被禁忌。

脾血管炎及假性动脉瘤:急性胰腺炎常引起胰腺周围组织炎症,能越过胰腺本身的组织解剖境界,并且包裹或包围邻近的器官和血管结构,因而,胰腺炎可累及小肠系膜,出现炎症改变和水肿,并且蔓延到肠系膜上动脉和静脉周围。此外,脾血管也会受炎症过程的影响。

以上这些改变,在使用动态螺旋 CT 快速血管强化,并且在达到高峰时扫描可充分显示。由于胰酶的毒性作用侵蚀小动脉分支,可导致出血并流入胰液或假性囊肿内。

脾假性动脉瘤可由血管壁受侵而引起。如果不使用动态注射对比法和可靠的数据监测技术,假性动脉瘤容易被漏诊。炎症也可压迫脾静脉或引起血栓形成。在这些病例中,可见到侧支静脉。

脾梗死:局灶性或散发性脾梗死可发生在胰腺炎伴有炎症累及血管的病例中。典型病例有大量的脾血管周围炎症,而炎症压迫被认为是梗死原因。

脾梗死非对比剂增强扫描时,表现为低密度楔形病灶,在强化对比 CT 扫描时的典型表现为一个尖端指向脾门,基底接近脾包膜的无强化的楔形病灶。脾梗死还可发生包膜下血肿。

包膜下积液:CT 表现为透明的液体聚集,使脾实质造成压迹或变平,可按照病灶垂直于器官表面的最大厚度进行量化,分为小于 1cm, 1~3cm,大于 3cm。

另有作者回顾 16 例由 CT 检查胰腺炎时偶然发现的脾实质并发症的临床和放射学结果(以脾动、静脉侵犯为主和脾外假性囊肿脾周蔓延者除外)。12 例为慢性胰腺炎急性发作, 4 例为急性胰腺炎。将 CT 结果与病人的症状、治疗的选择、最终的结果作了相关研究,最后结果显示患者症状呈非特异性, 13 例症状单纯由胰腺炎所致。所有病人均有上腹部疼痛, 2 例有发热。这些患者中脾病变由 CT 检查胰腺炎时或内镜术中偶然发现, 3 例患者出现急性低血压及腹膜刺激征。

14 例(88%)CT 可见脾梗死,其中 6 例为单发小病灶,7 例为多发小病灶,1 例病灶巨大,未见球形梗死灶。11 例(69%)发现脾包膜下积液, 1 例病灶最大厚度小于 1cm, 4 例病灶 1~3cm,大于 3cm 者 6 例。9 例脾梗死和包膜下积液同时存在,其中 3 例有血腹, 2 例血腹巨大并且急性发病,另 1 例血腹位于脾周围。1 例诊为脾内及包膜下脓肿并因急性复发性胰腺炎而并发结肠脾瘘。该作者认为,胰腺炎的脾并发症的急症手术、延迟脾切除术和非手术治疗的选择,主要依据临床表现而不是 CT 结果,但 CT 对发现及随访无症状的并发症有用。

第四节　肝脾结核

肝脾结核常表现为微结节(粟粒性)或大结节(结核瘤)两型。微结节型常发生在粟粒性肺结核病人中,CT 显示无数细小的低密度病灶。大结节型少见, CT 表现为弥漫增大的、直径 1~3cm 大小的低密度病灶或单发的肿块。MR 显示在 T_1WI 上呈低强度和轻度强化的蜂窝样改变。在 T_2WI 上病灶呈高信号,有一个较周围肝实质略低信号的环。微结节型需与转移瘤、真菌感染、结节病和淋巴瘤鉴别。大结节型可误诊为转移瘤、原发恶性肿瘤及脓肿。

第十五章　脾脏增大(脾肿大)

第一节　脾肿大与急性胰腺炎

脾肿大虽不是急性胰腺炎的特有征象,但一项研究显示脾肿大的程度与病情严重程度及临床分级诊断相关。能更精确评价脾大小的指标是脾容积,正常值为(219±76)cm^3,变化范围为4%~8%。有作者采用鼠标手工面积累加法计算研究对象的脾容积。17例急性胰腺炎患者发病4~30天CT扫描复查脾容积为(309.91±209.58)cm^3,其中14例(82.4%)脾容积较发病初增加超过10%。说明脾肿大是急性胰腺炎的一个常见征象。

而脾容积增加显著(≥50%)的5例患者,4例临床诊断为重症急性胰腺炎;Bahhazar急性胰腺炎CT严重度指数(CTSI)评分较高,平均为7分;尿胰酶水平显著增高;住院时间亦明显较长。并发胰腺假囊肿形成的3例患者脾容积均显著增加,其中1例继发感染,发展为胰腺脓肿,1例患者死亡。

急性胰腺炎导致脾肿大的可能原因(Tsushima等,1999)有以下3点:胰腺尾部行经脾肾韧带的两层腹膜之间,脾肾韧带内有脾血管、淋巴、神经走行,而且胰尾部在靠近脾门处有一小部分与脾相接触,当胰尾部及周围发生炎症,会直接或通过脾肾韧带波及脾。胰腺炎还会造成胰床血管(包括脾动脉、胃十二指肠动脉或肝动脉)受压、血栓形成及侧支循环建立,主要累及脾动脉,造成脾充血肿大,而且胰腺病变是脾静脉血栓形成的最常见原因。急性胰腺炎继发脓毒血症,可引发急性脾炎,导致脾肿大。

总之,脾肿大是急性胰腺炎的一个较常见征象,其发生率远高于其他脾并发症。而脾肿大显著病例,常为重症急性胰腺炎且伴严重并发症,预后不良。因此,急性胰腺炎患者早期CT扫描发现脾显著增大,常提示病情恶化可能,临床应密切关注,积极防治重症急性胰腺炎,提高患者治愈率、存活率。

第二节　脾结节病

结节病为系统性疾病,主要累及肺门及纵隔淋巴结,累及腹部者少见,当腹部受累时,全身其他部位往往已表现出结节病的征象。结节病单独发生在脾者更为少见。

脾结节病病例约60%有脾脏肿大,33%表现为脾脏的局灶性病变。超声检查时,可见脾内有非特异性弥漫性回声增强或混杂回声。CT平扫时,表现为不规则的低密度区,增强扫描呈不均匀强化,其间有不规则低密度区。MRI,T_2WI及梯度回波图像表现为弥漫性片状不均匀低信号区,代表慢性纤维化。

一般说来,仅单独发生于脾脏的结节病的影像学表现,无特异性,需与脾脏肿瘤进行鉴别。针吸活检和剖腹探查是确诊的主要方法。

第三节 饮水以后脾体积的变化

在饮水以后,脾体积增大,以往假说认为是由于门静脉血流和压力的增加。Parker 和 Bennett (1971)用 ^{99m}Tc 硫胶行脾显像检查 9 例正常男性青年,发现脾体积变化出现于饮水 5 分钟之后,这些变化主要是由于脾位置改变所致,而门脉血流及压力增加的影响甚小。

脾位置与形状的改变大概是由于饮水后,邻近的胃体积增大,压力增加,将脾向外侧和脚侧推挤。脾位置与形状的这种改变,造成脾体积增大的误解。饮水 30 分钟以后,脾的位置和形状基本上恢复到饮水前的状态。

第四节 脾肿大指数

正常脾大约为 12cm × 8cm × 3cm。脾长径达到或超过 13cm 即可认为有脾肿大。

但在某些病例脾长径的敏感性较低,故 Lackner 提出了"脾肿大指数"的概念,它是指脾脏三个方向上最大径线之乘积,即:脾肿大指数(SI)= 长径(L)× 宽径(W)× 前后径(AP)

脾肿大指数达到或超过 480 表示脾肿大。

将脾肿大指数乘以常数 0.55,还可估计脾的重量(克),正常脾重小于 265 克。

此外,若脾下极低于肝右叶下极水平,或者脾前后径大小超过腹部前后径的 2/3 均可考虑脾肿大。需注意的是,如果肝体积明显缩小,正常脾亦可低于肝右叶下极水平。

第五节 脾肿大的其他重要原因

门脉高压:门脉高压是脾脏肿大的一个常见原因, CT 表现肝尾叶明显的分叶,腹腔积液和侧支血管扩张。用动态 CT 扫描能很好地证实胃、食管静脉曲张和脾周侧支血管曲张。

白血病:白血病病人可有明显脾肿大,但脾常仍有正常均一的 CT 值。可发生自发性白血病性脾破裂。

类肉瘤病:脾肿大作为类肉瘤病的一种表现相对常见。增强前图像表现均一脾肿大,团注对比剂后呈非均一增强。脾类肉瘤病也可表现坏死性肿块伴局限性钙化。

淀粉样变性:实质性脾淀粉样变性有两种表现:累及淋巴样滤泡的结节型和侵犯红髓的弥漫型。CT 表现肿大脾内分散的低密度肿块和无增强的弥漫性低密度脾。脾肿大与受累程度关系不大。

胶质二氧化钍变:胶质二氧化钍颗粒被肝、脾和骨髓的网织内皮细胞吞噬并缓慢再分布至淋巴管。脾胶质二氧化钍变在 CT 图像上表现均匀或点状密度增高。脾髓质纤维化致脾脏变小,密度更高。

髓外造血:它主要与骨髓增生性疾病有关。影像学检查表现为累及肝和脾的局限性占位,可类似肿瘤。

第十六章 脾种植

第一节 腹部脾组织植入

异位脾组织可分为先天性的副脾和获得性的脾组织植入 2 种类型。

副脾在尸检中发生率达 10%~44%。脾组织植入相对少见，它通常是脾脏创伤行脾切除术后脾组织细胞种植于腹膜的结果，其发生机制尚不完全清楚。继发于脾脏创伤的脾组织植入并不少见，在创伤后行脾切除术的患者中，其发生率可达 26%~67%。

异位脾组织可发生于脾组织碎片可以到达的任何部位，它最常发生于腹腔，特别是小肠和大肠的浆膜面、壁层腹膜、肠系膜以及膈肌的腹侧面。脾髓作为静脉栓子，随血行播散，被认为是脾组织植入到这些部位的一种可能的发生机制。从发生脾创伤到诊断脾组织植入的间隔时间自 5 个月至 32 年不等，平均需要 10 年时间。一组 9 例脾脏切除时间平均 17 年。

影像学研究：所见结节形态多数呈圆形、卵圆形，少数表现为扁圆形、半圆形或条片状，其形态与是否受周围解剖结构限制有关，当其生长空间不受限制时，往往呈圆形或卵圆形；当被腹壁等阻挡时，表现为新月形或条片状。植入脾组织的大小可自数毫米至 12cm 不等。该组仅 2 个长圆形结节最大径达 5.0 cm，其余结节直径均在 3.5 cm 以下，据此该作者认为多数脾组织植入结节的直径在 3.5 cm 以下，超过 5.0cm 者不多见。有学者认为，因为脾组织植入结节无单独血供，所以通常不会长得很大。植入脾组织的数目，以多发为特征，其数量可从 1 个到数百个不等，甚至可能数不胜数。该组中，凡继发于脾脏创伤的脾组织植入均为多发结节，即使影像检查仅发现单个结节者，剖腹探查术中均发现腹腔内另有为数众多、米粒至黄豆大小的暗红色无蒂结节散布于腹膜各处，而继发于非外伤性脾切除者腹内仅有单个结节，因病例数尚少，这一现象有待进一步观察证实。

植入脾组织的 CT、MR 平扫表现和在动态检查时的增强类型与正常脾脏完全相同。

CT 平扫表现为境界清楚的均匀偏低密度软组织肿块（与肝脏相比较），注射对比剂后动脉期呈明显均匀或不均匀强化，门静脉期持续均匀强化。MR 平扫在 T_1WI 呈低信号而在 T_2WI 呈高信号（与肝脏相比较），注射对比剂后在动脉期呈现明显均匀或不均匀强化，门静脉期和延迟期变为均匀强化。其独特的不均匀强化一般仅出现在动脉早期，是由于脾组织的红髓和白髓内血流速度不同所致。

该组病例的 CT、MRI 所见基本符合上述表现，但该组大部分结节在门静脉期的强化程度高于动脉期，小部分结节在动脉期的强化程度高于静脉期，推测这可能与该组设置动脉期扫描时间（25 s）过早及不同个体间的血流动力学差异有关。此外，该组所有结节在 CT 扫描动脉期都表现为均匀一致的强化，可能是由于结节较小，红髓和白髓内血流速度的差别相对不大，因而难以在影像上反映出来。

对于既往有脾脏创伤或脾切除术史的患者，一旦发现腹内肿块，特别是脾窝区肿块时应首先想到脾组织植入的可能，其典型的 CT、MR 表现可提示诊断，但确诊有赖于以下几种检查方法：核素扫描是目前公认能够对植入脾组织作出特异性诊断而又无创的检查方法，因为 99mTc- 硫胶体和 99mTc - 标记热变性自体红细胞能够被网状内皮细胞吸收，从而可被用来识别脾组织，后者被证实对脾组织植入诊断具有更高的敏感度和特异度，因而成为目前主要的诊断工具。

应用肝脾特异性对比剂(Ferumoxide)行增强扫描,被认为可以对植入脾组织作出特异性诊断。Ferumoxide是超顺磁性氧化铁(SPIO),能被网状内皮细胞优先摄取,结果使信号强度快速减低,这在SE脉冲序列T_2WI更为确实。因为肝脏和脾脏的肿瘤及其他性质的病变缺乏网状内皮系统的枯否细胞,它们不能吞噬SPIO,因此与脾组织比较它们仍维持原来的高信号,而植入脾组织在应用SPIO后表现为低信号,表明其内存在网状内皮细胞,其确切诊断价值有待临床进一步研究评估。当缺乏上述检查条件时,超声或CT引导下细针穿刺活检是另一种可行的手段,该组有3例即据此获得确诊,但由于脾组织植入结节的包膜菲薄,该法有并发内出血风险,应注意防范。

鉴别诊断:脾组织植入容易与其他很多病变发生混淆,包括副脾、子宫内膜异位、血管瘤、转移癌、腹膜间皮瘤、淋巴结肿大或淋巴瘤等。当脾组织植入结节与肝、肾等脏器关系紧密时更易误诊为相关脏器的实质性病变。仔细分析上述相关病变各自的影像特征,特别是结合是否存在脾创伤及脾切除的病史,对鉴别诊断有极大帮助。

第二节　误诊病例简介:胸壁异位种植脾

异位脾,指脾不在正常的解剖位置而位于体腔其他部位,包括游走脾、副脾、脾弥散(即脾种植)。游走脾多为脾蒂和韧带松弛、过长、或缺失,脾沿左腹向下移动可至脐下或盆腔。

副脾为先天性发育异常而多出的脾。通常为单个,体积较大且位于脾胰韧带附近;有一个脾门和厚的包膜并由脾动脉的分支供血;外观卵圆形,轮廓光整,与邻近结构分界清楚。

脾种植是因脾外伤或切除术引起的自体种植,没有清晰的门样结构,而且通常较小,常为多发,结节形态不规则,小者仅针帽大小,大者数厘米,直径一般不超过3cm,它直接从植入部位获得血供,新生血管穿过菲薄的假包膜进入结节;结节形态多样,由于紧密黏附与植入部位边界相对欠清;此外,与副脾不同,脾种植几乎都有外伤或手术史。

异位种植脾多种植于体腔间隙任何部位或实质脏器:如肝脏、盆腔、胸腔、心包及皮下,最常种植于腹腔,临床常无症状,也有脾种植于特殊部位而引起临床症状,如肠道种植可引起消化道出血。胸腔脾种植较少见,多有胸腹联合外伤史及脾切除史,种植结节均发生于左侧胸腔,常位于脏层或壁层胸膜表面,呈红棕色,临床多无症状,少数有轻微胸痛、轻咳。

胸片及CT无特征性改变,CT平扫常为左侧胸腔单发或多发结节灶,境界清楚,边缘光滑,密度均匀,增强后均匀强化,与胸膜及胸壁肿瘤鉴别极困难,需密切结合病史及胸腔穿刺活检才能在术前明确诊断。

该例术后病理为胸腔异位脾,因患者有胸腹联合外伤及脾切除史,应考虑为异位种植脾。术前误诊的主要原因是对异位种植脾的认识不足,未能密切结合患者外伤、手术史。而且异位种植脾影像学无特征性改变。因此患者若有胸腹联合外伤及脾切除史并伴胸腔结节或肿块,应想到存在胸腔异位种植脾的可能。

第三节　大网膜内部分脾自体移植术后观察

患者,男,36岁。外伤后脾破裂行脾切除及自体脾移植术后。

第一次：10 月 3 日 CT 平扫图像（图 21-16-1）↓

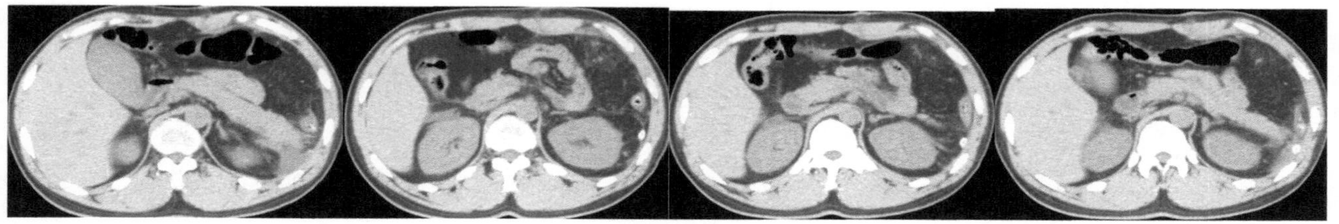

图 21-16-1

第二次：次年 1 月 7 日 CT 平扫图像，前次 CT 扫描后 2 个月复查，大网膜内部分脾自体移植术后，移植脾组织较前明显增大。如不了解病史，只看图像的变化，则可导致不应该出现的误诊（图 21-16-2）。↓

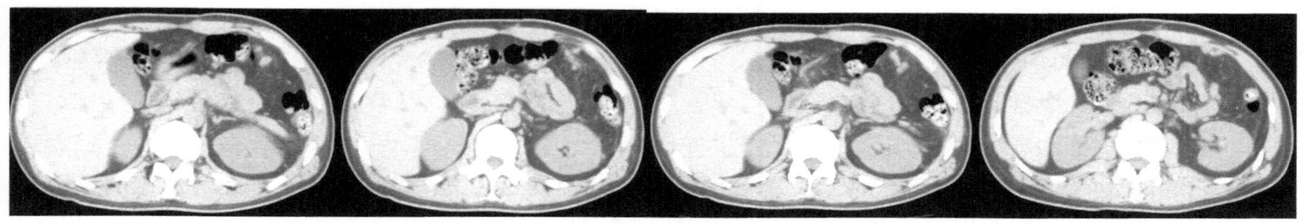

图 21-16-2

关于自体脾移植：脾脏除了具有造血、滤血、破血和储血等功能外，尚具有抗感染、抗肿瘤及生成第八凝血因子（抗血友病球蛋白 AHG）等功能。脾脏释放多种淋巴因子，如趋化因子、移动抑制因子、巨噬细胞激活因子、干扰素、调理素、备解素等。脾切除术后可以造成血液系统、免疫系统紊乱及急性暴发性感染。研究发现，脾脏的确具有不可忽视的抗感染、抗癌等免疫功能。从而导致保脾手术逐渐兴起，其中包括脾脏自体移植。目前自体脾移植主要适用于脾外伤，也有的用于治疗血液病（图 21-16-3）。

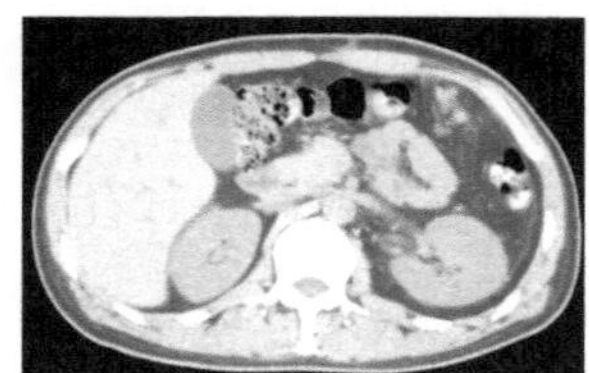

图 21-16-3

根据目前的研究，移植脾组织片主要放在大网膜囊中，这样再生脾的静脉回流与正常脾一样汇入门静脉，这很重要，其理由是肝脏与脾脏在处理抗原上有协作关系。另外，大网膜血运丰富，它可以通过扩散方式在新生血管形成前为移植物提供营养。并且，移植到网膜囊内者生长最好，成活率高，脾功能恢复早。许多证据表明，自体脾移植后再生脾可使滤过机能恢复，血小板可恢复至正常。脾切除术后 IgM 量减少，有再生脾者这种免疫球蛋白恢复正常（图 21-16-4）。

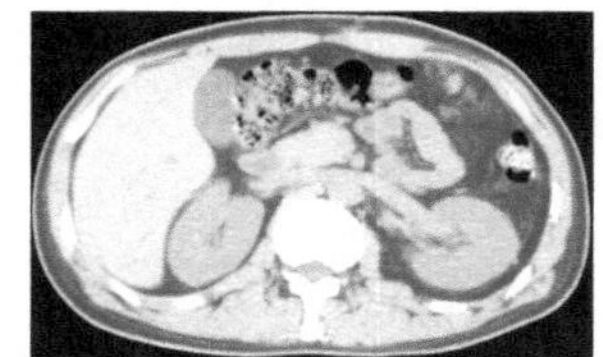

图 21-16-4

第十七章　脾脏其他疾病

第一节　胸内脾功能亢进

脾功能亢进起初均源于腹膜腔内多数脾结节的发展，通常皆起自脾的创伤性破裂。

如果在损伤时脾组织种植于胸腔，则也可出现胸腔内脾功能亢进，但极为少见，截至1971年世界文献仅5例报告，其中含Dalton等(1971)所报告1例。该例系呈现2个小的周围性肺结节，见于腹部枪伤迫使脾切除术后12年时，子弹穿过腹部造成脾破裂；又反跳进入左半胸，显而易见将脾组织种植入胸内。剖胸术见结节直径0.5~2cm，类似小脾，附着于壁层胸膜而不附着于肺内，大者为2.5cm×1.5cm大小。经验告诉我们，如果脾破裂伴有横膈伤，胸腔内脾功能亢进则可能出现。

第二节　脾假性囊肿与脾的钙化

脾囊肿可分真性囊肿与假性囊肿两种，真性囊肿有分泌性细胞，常见有皮样囊肿、淋巴囊肿和棘球囊肿等；假性囊肿无分泌功能，见于脾血肿、炎症、脾梗死，且常有钙化。Paris等(1978)报告14例胰腺炎病人的出血性脾假性囊肿，这是胰腺炎少见的加杂症。脾脏肿大可挤压邻近结构，造成移位，甚至导致结肠脾曲的外压性梗阻。

识别脾内钙化有助于脾疾病的鉴别诊断：引起脾内钙化的病因较多，但肉芽肿是其中最主要的原因。脾肉芽肿钙化呈点状，可伴有肝或肺内钙化。脾附近或脾内静脉石见于血管性异常，如血管瘤病。脾周边部环形钙化见于陈旧性血肿或动脉瘤。脾动脉或动脉瘤的钙化可呈曲线状，常见于脾门部，钙化的动脉瘤较未钙化者不易破裂。脾包虫囊肿仅在明确囊内容物(如：子囊)时方可诊断。卡氏肺囊虫感染后引起的脾钙化最近亦有报道，除脾外，肾及淋巴结亦见钙化。脾梗死后钙化可发生在镰状细胞性贫血病人，但不常见。Magid等(1984)报告1例镰状细胞疾病病人自身梗死，而出现整个脾的钙化。

第三节　脾妊娠

腹腔妊娠是指位于输卵管、卵巢及阔韧带以外腹腔内的异位妊娠，发生率约为1：15 000次分娩，常因临床表现不典型而误诊。脾妊娠是腹腔妊娠的一种，更为罕见。一例表现为脾内侧类圆形低密度灶，CT值9HU，大小约3cm×2cm，边界清晰、锐利，周围为环形软组织略低密度影。近年来，由于对异位妊娠的诊断与治疗技术的提高，尤其是高敏感性的放射免疫β-HCG测定，使异位妊娠患者的死亡率明显降低。异位妊娠患者多因急腹症而就诊，X线平片及透视常无异常。CT扫描一侧附件区或其他部位显示软组织肿块，密度不均，边缘模糊；陈旧性宫外孕为不均匀密度的“囊性”结构，CT值为35~40 HU的滋养层，血运丰富。异位妊娠要紧密结合B超检查及临床，以提高诊断的准确性。

第十八章　脾影像诊断的一些陷阱

第一节　不均匀强化

在CT增强的动脉期，脾脏表现为不均匀强化，不要误认为病变。注射速度越快，这种表现就越明显。可导致脾脏不均匀强化的其他情况包括心输出量降低或通过时间延长，后者见于脾静脉血栓形成、门静脉栓塞或门静脉高压。

造成脾脏不均匀强化的可能机制为血液在通过脾脏的不同组织成分时其血流速度不同。终末动脉输送血液进入脾实质，首先进入白髓，然后进入相对较大容积的红髓。红髓由脾窦和脾索组成。在进入脾静脉窦前，一部分血液从脾窦移出并经脾索缓慢灌注，称为开放性循环。但也有一部分血液绕过脾索，从脾窦直接进入衬有内皮的静脉窦，这条更直接快速的通道叫做闭合性循环。

通过闭合性循环的相对快速灌注可解释为什么灌注早期正常脾脏呈不均匀强化：脾脏中心部分为均匀强化，更靠外周的红髓区域强化较轻且呈不均匀或花斑状。脾脏不均匀强化类型可呈蛇状、索条状、花斑状或条带状，“斑马脾”这一术语也有应用。注药后2min，正常脾脏呈均匀强化。

第二节　正常的脾门脂肪伪似脾内病变

超声检查时，沿着脾的内侧部分的纵行扫描可显示此回声增强区，位于脾实质内。横断扫描时可显示此回声增强区的真实部位，即位于脾脏外、脾门内，实为脾门内的脂肪或脾门附近的肠曲，如不留心，则可误为脾内病变或钙化。

第三节　脾切除术后真、假性包块的超声诊断

脾切除术后，常出现发烧等并发症，它们可能继发于邻近器官（如胰腺）的感染、出血或创伤；术后超声检查所见包块包括膈下脓肿、胰腺炎、胰腺假性囊肿。然而，由于脾的摘除，胃与肠袢可向脾窝移位而类似真性肿块性病变。超声检查时，可以通过对患者进行不同体位（仰、俯卧及侧卧）的扫描来鉴别真、假性肿块。Lee等（1980）报告12例此类病人，认为超声对于评价术后并发症颇为有用，对脾切除术后尤其如此。

了解假性肿块对于避免把胃肠道因病理情况而重新排列误诊为病变十分必要。无论什么时候，充满液体的肠道如果成为混淆的因素，多体位的扫描都是有用的。如用实时超声，只要肠袢有蠕动，证明是肠袢十分简单。

第四节　CT 扫描及一些诊断陷阱

螺旋 CT 一次屏气即可完全扫描整个脾脏，清除了呼吸运动伪影及病变遗漏。当与肝脏一起扫描时，螺旋 CT 快速扫描的能力不仅保障了动脉期和再分配期的扫描，还能进行脾脏灌注计算以及随后的延迟扫描，有助于血管性病变的定性，常规腹部 CT 扫描，一次增强扫描即可满足诊断要求，但分别进行平扫和增强扫描更有助于显示钙化和确定增强程度。

平扫 CT 上脾脏密度均匀，CT 值约 40~60HU，稍低于正常肝脏。脾周的网膜和肠系膜脂肪使脾被膜和脾血管显示清晰。由于脾动脉迂曲走行，在任何扫描层面上均可表现为弯曲索条状、圆形或椭圆形影像。

增强 CT 扫描适用于评价脾实质性病变，能更好确定病变来自脾脏或肾上腺抑或胰腺；团注增强 CT 扫描能使脾脏和脾门血管高密度强化。常规腹部 CT 通常适合于发现肝脏病变，因此常使用的技术指标为：注射速度 2~3ml/s，延迟时间 60~70s。增强 CT 扫描开始时脾脏不均匀强化，但随时间延长而呈均匀强化，最终强化的脾实质密度较肝脏密度低 5~10HU。

脾形态有多种变异，一般的测量值对评价脾的大小并无用处。确定脾体积更精确的方法是脾指数，即脾的长、宽、厚的乘积。长等于可见脾的连续层面数的和；宽是横断图像上脾的最长径；厚为脾门水平测得的脾内外缘的间距。正常脾指数为 120~480cm^3。

脾外侧面有一光滑常呈分叶的外凸缘，它紧邻腹壁和左半横膈。脾门缘常内凹。左肾常在脾后内形成一个凹，在其前内方可见一个不太连续的胃底凹。偶尔可见一个很明显裂隙横穿脾脏，颇似脾撕裂，缺乏脾周血肿可帮助识别这种正常变异。

在平扫 CT 图像上，脾呈均一密度，其 CT 值稍低于肝。数分钟内缓慢注射对比剂时，脾实质 CT 值均匀增加；但是，快速静脉注射时，多数病人脾 CT 值先呈非均匀增加，1 分钟后变均一，说明脾内不同部位有不同血流。切勿将早期注射后的脾密度非均一误认为局限性病变。

脾脏与邻近器官的鉴别：冗长的肝左叶可伸向并紧靠脾脏，产生脾大、脾肿块或脾破裂的假象。这在腹膜腔脂肪少的消瘦病人或儿童中更易发生，导致超声和 CT 诊断困难。

脾下极接近左肾，可产生肾肿块的假象，冠状面重建图像有利于区别这两个器官。

第五节　经动脉门静脉血管造影 CT(CTAP)的脾灌注缺损

经动脉门静脉血管造影 CT 中观察到的脾灌注缺损，与外周注药 CT 增强动脉早期强化的缺损相仿。一组 46 例病人 CTAP 延时 4~6h 以及以后随诊 CT、MRI 研究发现，16 例(30%)显示有脾灌注缺损。这些缺损通常呈楔形，但少部分呈圆形，常位于脾周围。此 16 例病人中除 1 例其他检查证明有脾梗死外，剖腹探查显示所有病人脾脏均正常。这些均被认定为与灌注有关的缺损。因此，在 CTAP 检查中出现的脾灌注缺损时，不要误诊为脾脏占位性病变。

第六节　脾的假性病变

肝伪似脾包膜下血肿：超声检查时，在左上腹纵行扫描可显露正常的脾，在脾上方有时可见一低回声的新月形区域，位于左膈顶下方，酷似脾包膜下血肿或膈下液体积聚；横断扫描时，此低回声区可见来自于肝左叶的外侧缘，且弯向脾的前面。

肝左叶明显增大造成脾的假性缺损：有作者报告核素检查时，10 例肝左叶明显增大的病人，后前位 ^{99m}Tc 硫胶扫描，显示脾脏缺损，而在直立后前位扫描时,这些缺损均不复存在。故除非用其他方法证实,不宜只根据俯卧位扫描所见情况做出诊断。在 CT, Kollins(1978)曾报告肝左叶外段伸展横过身体中线,走向后方而邻近于脾,可伪似脾的撕裂。

在超声检查中,偶尔胃内的气体和液体可伪似脾内或左膈下病变。在吞服水入胃后,则见胃区内有小气泡,从而将胃内容物与脾内或左膈下包块区分开。

第七节　诊断陷阱:脾肺固定术后

布 - 加综合征患者做脾肺固定术后,有的在左下肺出现类圆形致密包块影。X 线正侧位胸片上都可显示。在正位片上可见左膈稍升高。包块经左侧膈顶中心部凸入下肺野。其上缘呈半圆形。光滑规整。高约 3~5cm。左右宽约 4~6cm;下部与膈肌相连。两侧缘与膈肌成钝角。密度高于肺部而低于腹部。侧位胸片显示包块位于后纵隔。与脊柱相重叠。前后缘稍现模糊。在透视下。深呼吸时左侧膈肌与包块同时上下移动。但较右侧膈肌动度弱。

脾肺固定术是外科治疗布 - 加综合征所选用的多种术式的一种。其目的是通过脾肺间毛细血管的产生。建立起侧支循环回流。为使脾肺接触。术中要在左膈顶开窗。并将脾脏上极的包膜切开。然后再将脾上极与肺底部磨擦后互相吻合。使再生毛细血管形成新的侧支循环。术后脾脏仍位于膈下。当膈顶开窗过大或腹腔压力增加时,脾上极可向膈上移位,造成脾疝。在左下肺野显示出包块样影。此包块内毛细血管丰富。血液经增粗的肺静脉回流。包块下部也有致密的血管网络。一般认为,出现此包块是一种正常的术后 X 线表现,对手术效果无不良影响。X 线检查时易将此包块误为占位性病变。此刻,需要熟悉布 - 加综合征的发病史和治疗方法。并注意以下几点:询问有否布 - 加综合征病史及手术史;胸透时嘱患者深吸气,见包块与膈肌分不开而且有同步运动。左侧膈肌活动度减弱或有胸膜粘连改变;较高电压(85~90kV)胸部透视。显示左膈下有与包块紧密相连的密度增高影(此为手术后正常上移的脾下极)。正常胃泡向内侧推移或消失;随访检查,包块无增大或缩小变化。

第八节　MRI 的一些诊断陷阱

MRI 技术:脾脏的 MRI 检查至少要包括 T_1WI 和 T_2WI。自旋回波(SE)、损毁梯度回波(spoiled gradient echo,SGE)和反转恢复序列是产生 T_1WI 的常用序列。SE 序列和快速 SE 序列(如 FSE 或 turbo SE)常用于产生 T_2WI。短 T_1 反转恢复序列(STIR)可用于产生 T_2WI,可选择性地抑制脂肪,提高组织的信号强度,消除化学位移伪影,并减少相位对比伪影。

增强扫描已经成为 MRI 脾脏检查的常规。最常用的方法就是应用非特异性细胞含钆对比剂(如 Gd-DTPA)后行损毁梯度回波序列(如 FMPSPGR 和 FLASH 序列)扫描。理想的 MRI 检查应当为全部脾脏在一次屏气即可全部成像。第一次增强扫描图像应在团注 Gd-DTPA 后 30s 内完成,脂肪抑制序列往往有助于提高损毁梯度回波序列成像图像质量。

屏气 MRI 技术和静脉注射钆对比剂 MRI 增强扫描提高了脾脏的 MRI 评估水平,脾脏的 T_1 和 T_2 弛豫时间与肾脏相似,但长于肝脏。脾脏的质子密度与肝脏相仿。

诊断陷阱:脾脏在传统 SE 序列 MRI 图像上信号均匀,在钆剂增强 MRI 图像上也可呈均匀信号。但在屏气脾脏增强扫描中,脾脏往往呈现独特的增强方式,如在脾脏外围区呈弓形、花斑状的不均匀强化,此种表现与 CT 动态增强表现一致。这可能与血液通过红髓开放和闭合性循环时流动速度的不同有关,另一可能的原因是红髓强化快而白髓强化慢。正常脾脏的延迟 MRI 图像在 2min 内将呈均匀强化。

流动伪影很普遍,并且在相位编码方向上最显著。因此,行横断面成像时,当相位编码方向为水平方向,在主动脉旁或下腔静脉外侧可见到类似脾病变的流动伪影。这些伪影可通过改变相位或频率编码方向消除,但在主动脉或下腔静脉前后方向上仍可留有伪影。

脾脏 MRI 成像也可发生磁敏感伪影,快速梯度回波成像技术常用于脾脏检查,但此 MRI 扫描序列对磁敏感性伪影特别敏感,这能造成手术银夹或其他金属异物区大范围的无信号区。通过降低 TE 和增加接受器带宽,能够减少这些伪影。

另外, MRI 电影技术经常用于评价肝脏。当对肝进行增强对比电影成像时,脾脏根据使用的扫描序列不同而呈弥漫性高信号或低信号,严重限制了脾脏的评估。假如用于脾脏评价,要调整图像窗宽和窗位确保对脾脏的评价满意。

第二十二篇　腹盆部多器官多系统疾病

第一章　免疫缺陷疾病

腹部获得性免疫缺陷综合征

获得性免疫缺陷综合征（AIDS）是由人免疫缺陷病毒（HIV）引起的一种全身性传染病。由于免疫功能受到损害，并发的机会性感染和恶性肿瘤严重危及患者的生命，影像学检查是发现获得性免疫缺陷综合征合并症的重要方法。获得性免疫缺陷综合征合并症可累及人体的多个系统和部位，涉及影像学的多个领域。

消化系统是获得性免疫缺陷综合征的好发部位，发病率仅次于胸部。由于获得性免疫缺陷综合征病人的T淋巴细胞受到人类免疫缺陷病毒的破坏，使机体免疫机能损伤，易发生机会性感染和恶性肿瘤。消化系统获得性免疫缺陷综合征可累及消化道、肠系膜、肝脏、胆系和胰腺，并可累及腹膜和腹膜后淋巴结。主要临床表现包括腹痛、腹胀、腹泻、发热、体重减轻、腹部包块、黄疸和胃肠道出血等，由于症状和体征的非特异性和实验室检查方法的限度，影像学检查对诊断、治疗和随访等起重要作用。

影像学研究：获得性免疫缺陷综合征腹部合并症的病种繁多，表现各异，由于患者免疫力低下，往往合并多重感染，选择合适的影像检查技术有助于疾病的发现和鉴别。超声检查广泛应用于腹部疾病的诊断，对于获得性免疫缺陷综合征这样一个可以累及多个脏器，出现多种表现的综合征，超声检查非常经济、实用、方便，可作为普查的手段，超声携带方便，便于重复检查的特点，可用于观察疗效，为随访患者提供一种安全、廉价的方法。超声引导下活检可缩短确诊时间。与超声相比，CT和MRI在获得性免疫缺陷综合征腹部合并症的检查中，发挥越来越大的作用。首先，可以帮助评价获得性免疫缺陷综合征患者的腹部症状，虽然有时影像所见没有特异性，文献报道只有12%的病例通过CT确定诊断，但对治疗仍有帮助，如对机会性感染进行分期。某些CT征象结合CD4+T细胞计数，可以提示可能的诊断，尽早开始试验性治疗。其次，可以用来观察疗效和评价预后，有些CT征象提示重度免疫抑制，患者预后不佳，这些征象包括肝脏肿块，大量肿大淋巴结及腹水。最后，发现治疗过程中出现的并发症，包括治疗中出现的免疫重建炎性综合征及医源性并发症，有利于及时调整治疗方案。需要强调的是影像引导下穿刺活检对获得性免疫缺陷综合征腹部合并症的诊断和治疗有着非常重要的意义，多数合并症，都要依靠活检来确定诊断。

机会性感染：已经发现任何一种机会性感染的风险都与CD4+T细胞计数有关。大多数细菌感染包括分枝杆菌感染发生在免疫损害的早期CD4+T细胞计数在200~750/μl之间时。原虫和真菌感染如隐孢子虫病和卡氏肺囊虫发生在CD4+T细胞计数低于200/μl以下时，鸟胞内分枝杆菌复合体和巨细胞病毒感染几乎总发生在重度免疫抑制的状态。

1. 获得性免疫缺陷综合征合并腹部结核　免疫功能正常的患者合并结核常表现为肺结核，肺外结核少见，而获得性免疫缺陷综合征患者由于免疫功能低下，发生肺外结核的机会明显上升，腹部是肺外结核最常发生的部位。当CD4细胞数低于（350~400）× 10^6/L时，获得性免疫缺陷综合征患者的结核感染率明显增加，在一般的结核患者中，肺外结核的发生率仅为10%~15%，而获得性免疫缺陷综合征合并结核患者出现肺外结核高达50%以上、肠系膜淋巴结、腹膜、肝脏、胰腺和胃肠道都可能受累。获得性免疫缺陷综合征合并结核感染易于播散，常合并肺结核。获得性免疫缺陷综合征患者合并腹部结核的影像表现通常与非获得性免疫缺陷综合征结核患者不能区分，获得性免疫缺陷综合征结核患者瘘管多见，并可发生在消化道的任何部位。一些作者曾报道获得性免疫缺陷综合征患者合并腹部结核后并发胆管-十二指肠瘘的病例。

人类免疫缺陷病毒感染早期，合并结核影像表现与免疫正常患者结核表现相似，多只累及肺部；获得性免疫缺陷综合征晚期，细胞免疫功能严重受损，结核播散性感染发生率较高，腹部各实质性器官、肠道、淋巴结及腹膜极易受累。

病理上病灶内缺乏上皮样细胞及朗格汉斯巨细胞,巨细胞及淋巴细胞极少,无肉芽肿形成而呈化脓性及凝固性坏死,结核分枝杆菌大量增殖。

获得性免疫缺陷综合征合并腹部结核病例发生于获得性免疫缺陷综合征的各期,有作者报告一组33例血CD4+细胞计数为3×10^6/L~537×10^6/L,平均值为29×10^6/L,CD4+/CD8+比值平均0.084(0.01~0.75),69.7%(23/33)患者CD4+细胞计数≤50×10^6/L,结果显示CD4+细胞计数越低,腹部结核发病率越高,结核病灶的无反应坏死越严重,在CT影像上液化更彻底。在非人免疫缺陷病毒感染的结核患者中只有10%~15%发生肺外结核,而在获得性免疫缺陷综合征合并结核感染患者中则约有50%发生肺外结核,获得性免疫缺陷综合征合并腹部结核常同时累及腹部多器官及组织。

该组33例患者胸部CT扫描均可见肺内不同程度的渗出性或增殖性病灶,其中15例(45.5%,15/33)可见双肺弥漫粟粒样小结节,提示本病感染途径可能是血行播散,腹部结核可能是全身血行播散的一部分。

该类病例腹部CT主要表现有:(1)腹部淋巴结肿大,为最常见表现。在消化系统获得性免疫缺陷综合征很常见,在腹部结核患者占2/3以上。常累及多个淋巴结,以肠系膜和胰腺周围的淋巴结结核常见。受累淋巴结不规则增大,可相互融合,大小为20~50mm。平扫时可见中心低密度坏死,增强扫描淋巴结有环形强化,约40%~70%的病人出现。多数病人具有其他部位的结核。在非免疫缺陷患者中,非典型分枝杆菌感染很少见到,但在获得性免疫缺陷综合征患者中常见,主要是鸟胞内分枝杆菌。Monill等(2001)报道8例由日内瓦分枝杆菌引起的获得性免疫缺陷综合征患者感染,认为CD4+T细胞计数低于100/μl时易出现这种感染,并认为通过穿刺活检可以帮助确立诊断。非典型分枝杆菌感染影像表现为肠壁增厚,肝、脾肿大伴有肝、脾内局部病灶,肠系膜及腹膜后大量肿大淋巴结,融合成团块。非典型分枝杆菌引起小肠感染影像及病理表现与Whipple病相似,常描述为“假Whipple病”,钡餐和CT上表现为轻度肠扩张和广泛、不规则的皱襞增厚。肠系膜及腹膜后经常可见肿大淋巴结,小肠袢因而分离、移位。

(2)肝脏结核:结核菌经血行播散、门静脉途径、淋巴途径和直接蔓延等途径感染肝脏。

病理分型为结核性肝浆膜炎(结核性腹膜炎的一部分)、粟粒型或微小结节型、结核瘤型、肝内胆管型和脓肿型等。临床表现缺乏特异性,有结核中毒征象、肝脾肿大和黄疸。

影像检查:肝、脾低密度结节,脾脏相对容易受累且多表现为粟粒状小结节,增强扫描病灶显示率较高,而平扫有时未能显示病灶;肝、脾结核脓肿,多发生于肝脏,CT表现与细菌性肝脓肿相似,前者多伴肺部、腹腔淋巴结或肠道病变;

CT表现为肝内单发及多发结节病变。粟粒型表现为肝脏和脾脏肿大,有弥漫粟粒结节病灶。结核瘤型表现为单发或多发结节病灶,圆形或类圆形,边界较清楚,病变多位于肝脏边缘部位。CT平扫病灶一般为低密度,增强扫描有的可见边缘强化、病程较长者平扫可为较高密度或有钙化。多合并有其他部位结核,如肺、腹部淋巴结、脾脏等。

影像检查难以作出诊断,须结合肝外结核表现、抗结核治疗复查或行肝穿刺活检。

(3)胰腺:胰腺结核主要来自血行播散性结核和邻近淋巴结核的直接浸润。胰腺结核可发生在胰腺的任何部位。CT平扫见胰腺肿大,可局限在胰头部。CT平扫为低密度灶,增强扫描无强化,或病灶周围有轻微强化。多伴有邻近的淋巴结增大。常有胰腺之外的结核表现。经抗结核治疗病变逐渐缩小及恢复正常。胰腺结核的影像表现缺乏特异性,与局灶性胰腺炎和胰腺癌相似。鉴别诊断应结合其他影像表现,如腹部淋巴结结核的边缘强化、腹水、肠壁增厚,以及肺结核空洞和播散病灶等。

(4)肠道结核,好发于回肠末段及盲升结肠,影像表现为肠壁不规则增厚或肿块形成,邻近大网膜及肠系膜增厚,伴肠系膜淋巴结肿大。

(5)腹膜结核,表现为腹膜广泛增厚,以大网膜增厚明显,呈饼状,可见腹膜多发结节形成及腹腔积液。

(6)其他经血行播散病变,如椎体结核及腰大肌脓肿,前者累及相邻两椎体及椎间盘,椎旁脓肿常见。

获得性免疫缺陷综合征合并腹部结核CT征象的病理基础:①结核脓肿。有作者报告1例CT表现为肝脓肿,肝穿刺脓肿液涂片及培养为结核,而血CD4+细胞计数为7×10^6/L,其病理基础是肝组织大面积的干酪样坏死而缺乏结核结节,免疫正常者中罕见；②淋巴结环状强化，病理基础为淋巴结中央的干酪样坏死，而外围血供存在，重者呈巨大液化坏死灶；③肝脾实质粟粒结节，为结核分枝杆菌血行播散，在实质器官形成弥漫小结核结节，多个结核结节融合形成 CT 所见小低密度灶；④肠壁不规则增厚及肠腔狭窄，为结核菌侵入肠壁淋巴组织而形成溃疡型或增生型肠结核所致；⑤结核性腹膜炎，一般为结核分枝杆菌血行播散所致，亦可能为肠结核及腹部淋巴结结核向腹膜蔓延所致。

国内文献对非获得性免疫缺陷综合征腹部结核的报道以腹腔及腹膜后淋巴结结核为主，感染途径以肠道途径为主，少数为血行播散，腹部淋巴结结核有一定优势解剖分布，实质器官的感染较少。

相对于免疫正常腹部结核患者，获得性免疫缺陷综合征合并腹部结核有如下一定的特点：①感染途径以血行播散途径为主，常合并肺部血行播散性肺结核或全身淋巴结结核病灶，该组 15 例（45.5%，15/33）可见双肺弥漫粟粒样小结节；②获得性免疫缺陷综合征患者腹部结核病灶更倾向于结核脓肿的形成，肿大淋巴结中央液化坏死更广泛、更彻底，病灶中央甚至呈水样密度，增强扫描环状强化；③常多器官受累，以腹腔淋巴结、肝脾、腹膜及回盲部肠道受累为主，相对于非获得性免疫缺陷综合征腹部结核，本病肝脾等实质器官受累较前者多见，肿大淋巴结较广泛，该研究中 16 例（48.5%，16/33）腹部各部广泛淋巴结肿大。上述特点对本病有一定的诊断及鉴别诊断意义。

鉴别诊断：在我国南方及东南亚地区，本病需与获得性免疫缺陷综合征合并马尔尼菲青霉菌病相鉴别，两者 CT 影像相似，本病腹部淋巴结肿大更倾向于累及肝门部及腹膜后淋巴结，脾脏病变更多地表现为弥漫粟粒样小结节；后者腹部淋巴结肿大更倾向于累及肠系膜淋巴结，肝脏病变相对广泛。以上所述肿大淋巴结优势分布及实质器官受累程度不同，可能与两病病原感染途径有关，有助于对两病的影像鉴别诊断，确诊需结合临床体征及病原培养结果。与获得性免疫缺陷综合征合并腹部非结核分枝杆菌（NTM）感染鉴别，非结核分枝杆菌感染主要由鸟 - 细胞内分枝杆菌复合体（MAC）所致，国外文献报道其腹部肿大淋巴结特征性表现为均匀软组织密度，增强扫描无环状强化，且腹部肿大淋巴结发生率（42%）相对较低，而获得性免疫缺陷综合征合并腹部结核肿大淋巴结发生率（69.7%）较高，且表现为中央较低密度的不均匀软组织密度，这对两者鉴别有帮助，但需通过菌种鉴定确诊，结核分枝杆菌只是抗酸杆菌的一种，很多医院特别是基层医院在结核病原检测及培养只局限于抗酸杆菌的检出而未行进一步的菌种鉴定，目前获得性免疫缺陷综合征合并非结核分枝杆菌感染逐渐增多，这提醒影像诊断医师在获得性免疫缺陷综合征腹部 CT 有上述非特异征象时，及在抗酸杆菌阳性患者抗结核治疗无效时应想到非结核分枝杆菌感染可能。

2. 真菌感染　马尔尼菲青霉病：马尔尼菲青霉病是由马尔尼菲青霉菌引起。本病目前已被列为获得性免疫缺陷综合征的指征性疾病，首例人免疫缺陷病毒感染者合并马尔尼菲青霉菌感染于 1988 年在美国报导。东南亚是马尔尼菲青霉菌的流行区。真菌感染是香港获得性免疫缺陷综合征病人死亡的第 6 位原因。在真菌感染中，马尔尼菲青霉菌为第 2 位，仅次于隐球菌感染。病理改变为肉芽肿及坏死。肉芽肿因网状上皮系统感染而形成，常见于免疫正常的患者。坏死见于免疫损害患者。受累器官包括肺、肝、脾、皮肤、血液、骨髓、淋巴结等。

临床表现为发热、体重减轻和贫血。可有头疼、干咳、全身淋巴结增大、肝脾肿大。皮肤病变是本病的特点之一。患者还可并发其他机会性感染，如沙门菌、卡氏肺囊虫、隐球菌等，使诊断增加困难。

腹部 CT 检查表现肠管增宽，肠壁模糊，肠管界限不清，有肠管集中表现，肠系膜增厚和后腹膜多发淋巴结肿大，可同时浸及胸部，肺内有多发结节、单个或多发空洞，支气管血管束增粗、片状实变、肺门淋巴结肿大以及胸腔积液等影像。

食管念珠菌病：食管念珠菌病是胃肠道最常见的机遇性感染。易累及食管下段。临床表现为胸骨后疼痛及吞咽痛，影像上表现为黏膜斑和黏膜皱襞增厚，偶尔由于黏膜下水肿呈“鹅卵石”样表现，进一步发展由于钡剂存留于斑片及假膜间，以及深溃疡和黏膜脱落，食管造影呈明显的不规则的毛糙外观。

3. 其他感染　胃肠道受累在人免疫缺陷病毒感染和获得性免疫缺陷综合征患者中非常常见，获得性免疫缺陷综合征患者中最常见的消化道症状包括腹泻、吞咽困难、腹痛、黄疸、直肠肛管症状和出血。在获得性免疫缺陷综合征感染的初期，食管内镜和食管造影都可在食管下段发现一个大的、浅表溃疡，边缘环绕水肿带，被命名为获得性免疫缺陷综合征相关的特发性食管溃疡,诊断时应进行其他检查除外感染,特别是巨细胞病毒感染。

人免疫缺陷病毒还可以引起低位小肠特发性肠病,表现为慢性腹泻,钡餐和CT上表现为非特异性小肠壁增厚。

疱疹性食管炎在食管双对比造影上显示最好,表现为小的、散在分布的浅溃疡,被正常的黏膜分隔。

巨细胞病毒可在食管黏膜间引起小的、边缘清楚的溃疡。这种浅表的溃疡位于食管中、下段,大于2 cm,溃疡口部可见水肿造成的晕环,与疱疹性食管炎不好鉴别,但可与念珠菌性食管炎区分,也必须通过活检与获得性免疫缺陷综合征相关特发性食管溃疡鉴别。巨细胞病毒还可以引起胃炎和肠炎。胃炎常见于胃窦部,表现为胃壁结节样增厚和管腔狭窄;肠炎表现为受累肠段管壁增厚。

获得性免疫缺陷综合征的其他感染性疾病还包括非结核性分枝杆菌、卡氏肺囊虫和组织胞浆菌感染等,这些疾病不仅累及腹部脏器、胆系和肠腔黏膜,还往往呈现播散性,造成全身多部位感染,如肺内、骨骼和颅内感染等。

4. 实质脏器感染　鸟胞内分枝杆菌复合体是最常见的病源菌,多发生在获得性免疫缺陷综合征晚期,以全身播散的方式出现。CT上有时表现为器官内多发低密度病灶,但更多的只表现为肝、脾肿大,约14%的患者可见中心坏死的肿大淋巴结。腹部器官内结核感染表现为多发低密度病灶,常伴有肠系膜和腹膜后淋巴结肿大。

此外,获得性免疫缺陷综合征患者腹部脏器可并发多种病毒感染,包括乙型和丙型肝炎病毒复合感染、巨细胞病毒、单纯疱疹病毒及EB病毒感染。

CT表现为肝脏肿大,边缘水肿,胆囊壁增厚,肝门部淋巴结肿大,肝炎病毒感染最终可导致坏死后肝硬化。

立克次体感染后肝内可出现杆菌性紫癜,病理表现为肝内多发血窦,没有上皮细胞被覆,在影像上没有特异性表现,小的血窦影像上无法显示,大的血窦在注射对比剂后可表现为低密度灶。Sandrasegaran等(2005)报道杆菌性紫癜增强后的低密度血窦边缘可有均质或结节样强化,但不具特异性。

肝脏还是最易出现卡氏肺囊虫肺外感染的部位,可见于38%的患者,可伴有腹部多脏器受累。影像表现为脏器内低密度及钙化,肺内有卡氏肺囊虫感染的病史可提示诊断。钙化开始被认为是卡氏肺囊虫的特征性表现,近来发现也可见于鸟胞内分枝杆菌复合体和巨细胞病毒感染。

静脉内药物依赖史的获得性免疫缺陷综合征患者易合并肝、脾内脓肿,最常见的是金黄色葡萄球菌,念珠菌感染时可出现肝、脾内微小脓肿。

5. 获得性免疫缺陷综合征相关胆系病变　与获得性免疫缺陷综合征相关的胆系病变包括非结石性胆囊炎和获得性免疫缺陷综合征相关胆管病。非结石性胆囊炎影像表现为胆囊壁水肿增厚,胆囊周围积液,黏膜溃疡,这些表现多见于不能进食、上腹有压痛的患者。获得性免疫缺陷综合征相关胆管病多见于感染获得性免疫缺陷综合征1年后的中年男性,临床表现为碱性磷酸酶、转氨酶及胆红素升高。组织学见胆管黏膜下巨细胞病毒(占21%)和/或隐球菌感染(占32%)。

影像表现为乳头部狭窄、硬化性胆管炎、乳头部狭窄和/或肝内、外硬化性胆管炎及肝外大范围的胆管狭窄。造影显示胆总管变尖、黏膜串珠样改变、肝外胆管不规则扩张,左肝管扭曲、局部不规则囊状扩张。有作者报告一组5例伴肝内胆管轻度扩张,考虑原因为肝门区肿大淋巴结压迫胆管所致。

6. 腹膜后感染　获得性免疫缺陷综合征可引起胰腺、双肾、双侧肾上腺及淋巴结等多个腹膜后脏器的感染。

与获得性免疫缺陷综合征有关的胰腺疾病生前往往难以诊断,多在尸检时发现。ERCP检查在没有机会性感染患者可见胰管分支改变、多发狭窄及广泛的胰管扩张。胰腺结核可继发于胰周淋巴结核。表现为腺体肿大、低密度结节及非特异的团块,由各种机会性感染造成的胰腺炎及胰腺脓肿与非人免疫缺陷病毒感染患者表现类似。

与获得性免疫缺陷综合征有关的肾脏疾病可以出现多种影像表现,包括肾脏肿大、肾内脓肿及肿块,肾实质内钙化及肾盂积水等。各种感染性病变均可引起肾脏脓肿,肾实质内钙化由肺外卡氏肺囊虫感染引起。获得性免疫缺陷综合征肾病可有肾功能不全和蛋白尿,通常在超声上出现回声改变及肾肿大。

腹膜后淋巴结肿大是获得性免疫缺陷综合征患者的常见表现,观察时应注意分析淋巴结的大小、分布及强化形式。由淋巴结反应造成的非感染性淋巴结病变,称为获得性免疫缺陷综合征相关淋巴结病,与 CD4+T 细胞计数有关，通常大于 300/μl，病变淋巴结广泛分布于腹膜后、盆侧壁及小肠系膜，大小均一。

7. 恶性肿瘤　消化系统获得性免疫缺陷综合征相关的肿瘤中以卡波西肉瘤和淋巴瘤多见。

卡波西（Kaposi）肉瘤：卡波西肉瘤源于网状内皮细胞。在获得性免疫缺陷综合征患者中常见，有报道在同性恋或双性恋的获得性免疫缺陷综合征患者中发生率达 50%，可累及皮肤、淋巴结、胃肠道、肺、肝脏及脾脏等部位，主要累及皮肤和呼吸道、其次是消化道和胸腹腔淋巴结。胃肠道各部位均可受累，十二指肠最常发生。典型表现为紫蓝色斑或结节，早期影像检查难以发现，多通过内镜检查确诊。

卡波西瘤灶融合增大，影像表现为黏膜下结节，可伴有脐样凹陷。可见到"靶征"或"牛眼征"。病变扩展到肠壁，则表现为息肉样肿块和皱襞不规则增厚，CT 显示小肠卡波西肉瘤表现为结节状肠壁增厚。肝、脾内卡波西肉瘤表现为肝、脾肿大及增强后小的低密度灶，需要与感染鉴别。典型 CT 表现是肿瘤结节沿血管分布，如在肺内增粗的支气管血管束和肝内门静脉周围。受累淋巴结肿大，肝脏和脾脏增大。MRI 检查可显示肝内血管周围的肿瘤病灶和腹部肿大淋巴结。超声检查在肝内可探及多个沿血管分布的大小不等的强回声结节，增大的淋巴结多位于肝门部和腹腔干旁。

淋巴瘤：获得性免疫缺陷综合征患者发生非霍奇金淋巴瘤的可能性远高于普通人群。消化道是获得性免疫缺陷综合征患者发生结外淋巴瘤的最常见部位，可发生食管狭窄、胃部病变、肠梗阻、肝脏肿块和多组淋巴结增大等。获得性免疫缺陷综合征相关性淋巴瘤不如卡波西肉瘤多见，多为非霍奇金淋巴瘤，发生于非常见的结外部位，如颅内、骨髓和腹腔脏器。

胃肠道是获得性免疫缺陷综合征相关性淋巴瘤在腹部最易累及的部位，有报道发生率可达 54%。主要侵犯胃和末段回肠。钡剂造影消化道淋巴瘤表现为黏膜皱襞不规则增厚，CT 可显示淋巴瘤的肠外病变。肝、脾、胰腺的淋巴瘤 CT 表现为单或多发、结节状等或低密度肿块，腹膜后或肠系膜巨大淋巴结团块也是淋巴瘤的常见表现。

转移瘤：原发灶可能不明确。获得性免疫缺陷综合征患者由于免疫功能下降，肿瘤患者的生存期缩短，肿瘤的侵袭性相对更强，使治疗更为困难。

当获得性免疫缺陷综合征患者出现淋巴结增大、发热、腹痛、腹泻和腹部肿块时，应当考虑到有消化系统的并发症。影像学检查能提供相应的诊断信息，有助于患者得到及时的治疗，可减少有创性检查和感染扩散的可能，也用于判断治疗效果和随访。

总之，影像检查在获得性免疫缺陷综合征诊治，尤其是并发症的诊治过程中发挥越来越重要的作用，对早期发现并发症、及时治疗、指导活检有着重要意义。近来，影像检查在治疗与获得性免疫缺陷综合征相关的急腹症中的作用也逐渐受到人们的重视。

第二章　自身免疫性疾病

详见本书 本卷 第二十篇 第二十三章 第二节　IgG4 相关疾病的影像学表现。

第三章　腹部淋巴瘤

第一节　原发性胃肠道淋巴瘤及误诊分析

原发性胃肠道淋巴瘤是一组起源于胃肠道黏膜下层淋巴组织的恶性肿瘤，是成人较少见的恶性肿瘤，约 60% 的病例只通过 CT 表现就可对肿瘤的组织学类型进行预测。

发病机制：胃肠道淋巴组织是结外淋巴瘤最常见的部位，其病因尚不明确。目前多认为与幽门螺杆菌和 EB 病毒感染、继发性免疫功能异常等有关。按其细胞组成可分为霍奇金淋巴瘤和非霍奇金淋巴瘤，成人以弥漫性大 B 细胞淋巴瘤最常见。

原发性胃肠道淋巴瘤的病变大体表现为胃肠腔内外的肿块，病变与正常组织间常无明确分界，常伴有肠系膜淋巴结的肿大，以上改变是影像学异常的病理基础。

临床表现：一组 24 例中，弥漫大 B 细胞淋巴瘤 18 例，占 75%（18/24），也说明弥漫大 B 细胞淋巴瘤是原发性胃肠道淋巴瘤主要组织来源。该组作者统计文献报道 726 例，发病年龄 4~87 岁，平均 45.8 岁。该组平均 46 岁，与文献报道相近。临床表现无特异性，且具有很大的异质性，不同发病部位的临床表现类似，腹痛为最常见的症状，其次为食欲下降、体重减轻、呕吐、盗汗、消化道出血等。该组病例以上腹部疼痛、恶心、呕吐等消化道症状为主，其中小肠病变以腹痛和黑便为主，结肠病变以腹痛、便血、大便次数改变为主。4 例患者出现不全肠梗阻症状。2 例出现上消化道出血，病程长短不一。

影像学研究：复习文献和分析该组病例发现原发性胃肠道淋巴瘤具有以下主要 X 线特征：①肿块型改变，病变单发或多发，单发时可表现为巨大充盈缺损，边缘欠光整，好发于胃体及胃底部；②溃疡型改变，呈腔内巨大溃疡且深浅不一，同周围正常胃壁界限不清。

CT：原发性胃肠道淋巴瘤的 CT 表现大体为 4 类。弥漫浸润型：主要表现为胃肠道壁的局限或弥漫性均匀增厚，常多个节段受累，其间可间隔正常肠管。节段型：该型多见于肠淋巴瘤，是相对于弥漫浸润型而言的。结节型或息肉型：为单发或多发向腔内生长的肿块，可以是窄基底或宽基底。溃疡型：全部由其他 3 种类型转化而来，其病理基础是肿块本身的缺血坏死，溃疡严重时可诱发胃肠道穿孔；病变增强后呈轻、中度强化，对应肠管大多无明显狭窄反而有轻度扩张。其发生原因是由于肿瘤取代了肠壁的固有肌层并破坏了自主神经丛，从而导致肠壁肌张力的下降，引起管腔扩张，称之为“空气征”。病变段周围轮廓较光整，脂肪层清晰，如脂肪层密度增高且模糊不清，提示淋巴瘤向邻近器官侵犯。

误诊分析：原发性胃肠道淋巴瘤的 CT 表现有一定的特征，但其影像学表现很容易与黏膜来源的癌相混淆。不典型胃淋巴瘤与胃癌相似，不易鉴别。该组病例中有 10 例误诊为癌，其中 4 例胃淋巴瘤导致胃腔狭窄，胃周淋巴结肿大，这些表现与胃癌的某些表现相重叠，而胃癌的发病率明显高于胃淋巴瘤，这可能是造成误诊的最主要原因；另 2 例胃淋巴瘤胃壁弥漫性增厚，误诊为胃癌，可能因为对本病的认识不足导致。

肠道淋巴瘤中以 T 细胞性淋巴瘤相对多见，肠病型 T 细胞淋巴瘤最多，临床上有发热、腹泻、消化道出血，严重时可出现肠穿孔，常误诊为克罗恩病或肠结核，该组有 1 例小肠淋巴瘤误诊为克罗恩病。本病也常引起肠壁的增厚，一般为多节段狭窄，范围较广泛，且有肠系膜侧肠壁为重的偏心性特点，系膜周围淋巴结增生一般较小，当引起瘘道或线样溃疡时,可形成炎性包块,容易形成肠梗阻。

1例误诊为小肠腺癌,因病变侵及周围组织。此外影像科医生对本病的认识相对不足,缺乏对本病的警惕性,诊断时未能考虑。该组中有2例结肠淋巴瘤误诊为癌, CT表现主要有肠壁的弥漫性增厚,肠腔狭窄,但这些表现不具有特异性。

淋巴瘤的特征表现是病变段小肠或结肠出现特征性的管腔扩张,该组中正确诊断6例小肠淋巴瘤和6例结肠淋巴瘤均有此表现。

综上所述,虽然X线、CT影像无法确诊胃肠道恶性淋巴瘤,但可通过影像学表现提示恶性淋巴瘤,结合内镜及手术病理,能够为原发性胃肠道淋巴瘤的诊断提供有力证据,尽早治疗,从而取得较满意的临床疗效。

第二节 胃肠道假性淋巴瘤

详见本书 本卷 本篇 第七章 第五节 胃肠道假性淋巴瘤。

第三节 黏膜相关性淋巴样组织淋巴瘤

黏膜相关性淋巴样组织淋巴瘤,为胃淋巴样增生进一步发展和恶变所造成,胃双对比造影也可显示为胃内多发结节,但其大小甚不均匀,大者常超过3 mm;此外,还可显示黏膜相关性淋巴样组织淋巴瘤的其他表现,包括结节融合、恶性溃疡和胃黏膜皱襞增粗等;胃小区增大所形成的网格状影中,其相对透光区常为>3 mm的多边形。故黏膜相关性淋巴样组织淋巴瘤鉴别不难。克罗恩病的鹅口疮溃疡和胃糜烂灶应与胃淋巴样增生结节表面的脐状凹陷相鉴别,前者的结节状影常较大、较少和散在;而后者的结节小而密集,大小较均匀,且不是每个结节上都有脐状凹陷的表现。至于白血病等恶性肿瘤播散和息肉病。其表现多样,往往应与黏膜相关性淋巴样组织淋巴瘤鉴别。误为淋巴增生样的机会不大。

第四节 弥漫性大B细胞淋巴瘤侵犯肠道、肾上腺、腹膜及腹膜后

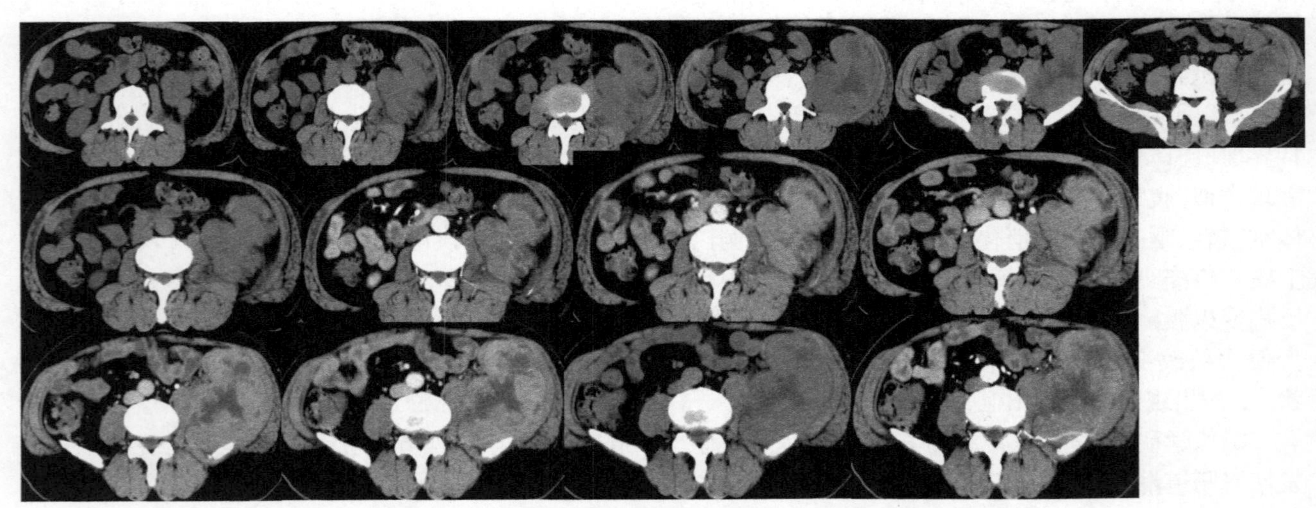

图22-3-1 弥漫性大B细胞淋巴瘤侵犯肠道、肾上腺、腹膜及腹膜后

患者,男,65岁。发现左下腹肿块伴疼痛一个月余入院。

手术所见:腹腔内无明显腹水,左下腹见一大小约

15cm×15cm 肿物，质硬，固定，侵犯隆结肠，与左下腹壁及腰大肌、左盆壁粘连严重，界限不清，肿瘤上缘贴近脾脏下极；左肾上腺可扪及一大小约 3cm×3cm 肿物，质硬，边界尚清楚。

病理检查：左肾上腺及腹膜后肿物切除标本：灰红色软组织一堆，总体积 20.0cm×20.0cm× 13.0cm，其中可见一肠管，长 12.0cm，肠管外侧壁与结节状肿物相连，肠管外可见一结节状肿物，肿物直径 12.5cm，切面灰白，质中，偏脆；另见肾上腺组织一块，大小 5.0cm×3.5cm×2.0cm。病理诊断：左肾上腺及腹膜后肿物切除标本：初步诊断小细胞恶性肿瘤，肿瘤组织累及结肠外膜。另送的游离的肾上腺实质皮髓质结构消失，可见组织学图像类似于腹膜后肿物的异型性小细胞呈弥漫性浸润，待做常规石腊切片及免疫组化检测进一步协助确定肿瘤类型。

免疫组化诊断：腹腔巨大肿瘤根治标本（无法明确原发部位）：非霍奇金淋巴瘤，弥漫大 B 细胞淋巴瘤，生发中心型，肿瘤累及肠壁、肾上腺、腹膜及腹膜后（图 22-3-1）。

第四章 胃肠道间叶组织肿瘤

第一节 胃肠道间质瘤的误诊和漏诊

胃肠道间质瘤是最常见的胃肠道间叶源性肿瘤。随着研究的深入以及靶向药物甲磺酸伊马替尼的使用，MSCT在诊断、治疗随访中的应用，许多不典型病例常常误诊。

病理学：胃肠道间质瘤由Mazur等（1983）根据肿瘤的分化特征而提出。胃肠道间质瘤是一类特殊的、通常CD117免疫表型阳性的胃肠道最常见的恶性间叶源性肿瘤。组织学上有梭形细胞、上皮样细胞、偶见多形性细胞排列呈束状或弥漫状，免疫表型上表达c-kit基因蛋白产物KIT由突变的c-kit或血小板源生长因子受体（PDGFRA）基因驱动。目前免疫组织化学和电镜观察是确诊胃肠道间质瘤的主要病理手段。

临床表现：胃肠道间质瘤好发于中老年人，平均年龄50~60岁，男女发病无明显差异，胃肠道间质瘤可发生于胃肠道的任何部位，其好发部位依次为胃、空肠、回肠、十二指肠、直肠、结肠等，少数可发生于胃肠道外，包括网膜、肠系膜及腹膜等。一组79例中，50岁以上者占76.0%，男女比例为1.47:1。

临床表现无特殊，多与发病部位有关，部分病例为体检时偶然发现。Toshirou和Seishi（2003）认为胃肠道间质瘤的临床表现与肿瘤大小有关，肿瘤直径>3 cm或出现坏死溃疡时，才会出现临床症状。该组间质瘤发生于胃者占62.03%，其次依次为小肠20.25%，结直肠8.86%，腹腔肠系膜6.33%，食管2.53%。通过血行和种植转移，肝和腹膜是其主要转移部位，该组有13例出现转移灶，84.6%转移至肝，38.5%转移至腹膜，腹腔积液罕见，腹膜转移者仅1例出现少量腹腔积液，7.7%转移至肺，未发现其他部位转移灶。

CT诊断及误、漏诊分析：依据肿瘤与胃肠道壁的关系将胃肠道间质瘤分为内生型、外生型、内外生混合型和胃肠外型。结合轴位CT及多平面重建图像，多方位寻找肿块与消化道管壁的关系有助于定位；检查前禁食8 h，扫描前充分充盈胃肠腔，通过多平面重建及多方位重建，对内生型及内外生混合型间质瘤多能准确定位。

该组中发生于食管、结直肠及胃的间质瘤，CT定位准确率较高，而外生型具有在腹腔潜在腔隙发展的特性。由于肿块易坏死，形成溃疡后坏死物质经肠管排除，往往似“假肠腔”，如无法判定肿块因溃疡与肠管相通而形成的假肠腔还是真肠腔，多易误诊。

该组中3例小肠间质瘤和1例胃前壁外生型巨大间质瘤，均因未见肯定肿块与胃肠腔相通而在术前定位错误，而3例胃肠外间质瘤由于与腹腔肠管关系显示不清，误为肠壁来源。其中胃壁前方腹腔巨大肿块与胃前壁、肝左叶之间关系密切，邻近胃黏膜光整连续，无溃疡，误诊为肝左叶外生型恶性肿瘤，术后回顾CTA显示肿块主要由增粗的胃网膜左动脉供血，提示肿块起源于胃。

小肠间质瘤也可见类似的相应肠段血管（动脉和/或静脉）增粗征象；而胃肠外间质瘤，相应肠段血管增粗的征象不明显。结合轴位双期或多期增强扫描和多方位重建图像，并仔细观察肿块与小肠壁及肿块供血血管的关系，有助于定位诊断。

CT上见到与胃肠道管壁关系密切，向腔内、跨腔内外或腔外生长的类圆形、分叶状或不规则软组织肿块，肿块与周围组织境界多较清楚，有不同程度的坏死、囊变，实性部分增强扫描呈富血供肿瘤特点，瘤体早期强化，实质期肿瘤强化更显著，应考虑间质瘤可能。

伴发肿瘤：该组中有 10 例（12.66%）伴发其他肿瘤，其中 6 例间质瘤和 1 例伴发肿瘤术前诊断中漏诊。该组随访的病例中有 4 例术前 CT 未发现胃肠道间质瘤病灶，而在其他伴发肿瘤手术中发现，但复阅 CT 仍未见肿块，因此未纳入该研究。由此可见间质瘤伴发其他肿瘤的比例可能还要高。

间质瘤伴发肿瘤大致可分为：①上皮性肿瘤；②神经纤维瘤病，Yantiss 等（2005）的研究显示神经纤维瘤病患者发生胃肠道间质瘤的部位与 Auerbachs 肠肌层神经丛密切相关，而且瘤细胞的超微结构具有 Auerbachs 神经丛细胞的特点，提示胃肠道间质瘤与神经纤维瘤病在发病机制上存在相关性；③ Carney 三联征。此外，家族性胃肠道间质瘤也值得关注。

在该组中伴发肿瘤多为邻近或原发器官的恶性上皮性肿瘤，伴发肿瘤为上皮性恶性肿瘤（8 例），1 例胃间质瘤，伴发结肠纤维瘤病，1 例伴发子宫肌瘤。术后复习图像分析漏诊原因，一方面是对间质瘤伴发肿瘤的认识不足，影像观察分析不仔细；另一方面是由于呼吸伪影、扫描层面太厚等原因所致图像质量欠佳。

鉴别诊断：除与胃肠道上皮来源的恶性肿瘤鉴别外，还需与以下疾病鉴别：

（1）平滑肌瘤及平滑肌肉瘤：平滑肌瘤起源于食管、胃、小肠肠系膜肌层，膨胀性生长，多有完整包膜，肿瘤外形多较规则，密度较均匀，呈低至中度强化，影像上有时与恶性潜能较低的间质瘤不易鉴别；发生于食管者，平滑肌瘤较多；发生于胃者，间质瘤较多见。平滑肌肉瘤少见，常有出血、坏死、钙化，影像上难与恶性间质瘤鉴别。最终诊断有赖于免疫组织化学及电镜结果。

（2）淋巴瘤：结外非霍奇金淋巴瘤最常见的原发部位中，胃最常见，小肠、直肠、盲肠次之；也可继发于肠系膜、腹膜后非霍奇金淋巴瘤等处淋巴结直接蔓延侵犯肠壁。发生于胃肠道者，胃肠壁多广泛增厚，其程度多较一致，较少形成软组织肿块，管壁多柔软，坏死少见，增强呈中度强化，在肠道者则多段肠道受累，往往伴有多发肿大淋巴结；间质瘤多形成明显肿块，肿块坏死、囊变、溃疡常见，淋巴结肿大罕见；此外，淋巴瘤肠腔是真肠腔，而间质瘤的肠腔是假肠腔。

（3）纤维瘤：纤维瘤是腹膜、肠系膜常见的原发良性肿瘤，好发生于小肠系膜纤维组织。

（4）腹腔黏液瘤：腹腔黏液瘤为阑尾黏液囊肿或卵巢黏液性囊腺瘤 / 癌破裂后，黏液组织及富黏液的柱状上皮细胞散布腹腔，即黏着于腹膜、大网膜、肠壁浆膜，包裹而形成大小不一的肿块。囊壁多薄，不规则，无强化，囊液密度均匀高于水。较大的胃肠道间质瘤瘤体内密度由于瘤内组织坏死液化或黏液变而密度多不均匀，瘤内可见“蜂窝”状小片状低密度或单个或多个大片低密度，坏死区域多不规则；黏液样变是胃肠道间质瘤一个重要的病理特点。

（5）腹膜间皮瘤：腹膜间皮瘤均为恶性，肿瘤沿腹膜表面生长，大网膜增厚成块形成“网膜饼征”，局限性者形成不规则肿块，腹膜、网膜、肠系膜弥漫性增厚，多伴有不同程度的腹腔积液，可沿腹股沟蔓延，伴胸膜受累和淋巴结转移，增强扫描肠系膜血管僵硬呈“星芒”状为其特征性的 CT 表现。胃肠外间质瘤或胃肠间质瘤腹腔种植转移，也表现为腹腔多发大小不一类圆形实性肿块，肿块可伴坏死，无腹膜、网膜、肠系膜增厚，腹腔积液、淋巴结转移少见。总之，胃肠道间质瘤具有一定的影像特点，CT 作为其主要影像评价手段，检查前做好充分地准备，制定合理的检查方案，结合对疾病的全面认识和影像学特点多能做出准确诊断。

第二节　胃肠道间质瘤误诊及漏诊病例简介

胃肠道间质瘤与消化道其他良性肿瘤，尤其是与平滑肌瘤，神经源性肿瘤及息肉在影像学很难鉴别，确诊只有依赖病理组织学检查。

一组 11 例胃肠道间质瘤术前影像学诊断全部误诊，回顾性分析并究其原因主要为对本病的病理、临床、尤其影像学表现认识不足所致。

有作者报告胃部 2 例胃肠道间质瘤肿块定位错误中 1 例发生于浆膜下向胃腔外突出，有一细蒂和胃相连，术前误诊为小肠病变；1 例因肿瘤巨大，瘤内有气体，上消化道钡餐造影可见瘤体坏死腔有一窦道和胃腔相通，术前误诊为胃穿孔、局部包裹性肉芽肿形成。

2 例小肠胃肠道间质瘤定位错误中 1 例系空肠近段病变,误诊为胃病变;1 例回肠下段病变误诊为右侧卵巢肿瘤。另有 1 例曾考虑为升结肠肿瘤,后经 MSCT 三维重建诊断为回肠远段病变。术前通过对肿瘤大小、形态、瘤体密度、强化特征及邻近关系综合分析能初步判断胃肠道间质瘤良恶性,一组 13 例良性胃肠道间质瘤中只有 1 例食管病变因最大径 8.2 cm 沿食管环形生长,术前误诊为恶性。10 例恶性胃肠道间质瘤有 1 例误诊为胃穿孔。由于潜在恶性是病理学分类,影像表现并无特异性, CT 难以鉴别恶性与潜在恶性。

由于肿块易坏死,形成溃疡后坏死物质经肠管排除,往往似“假肠腔”,如无法判定肿块因溃疡与肠管相通而形成的假肠腔还是真肠腔,多易误诊。

第三节　空肠胃肠道间质瘤

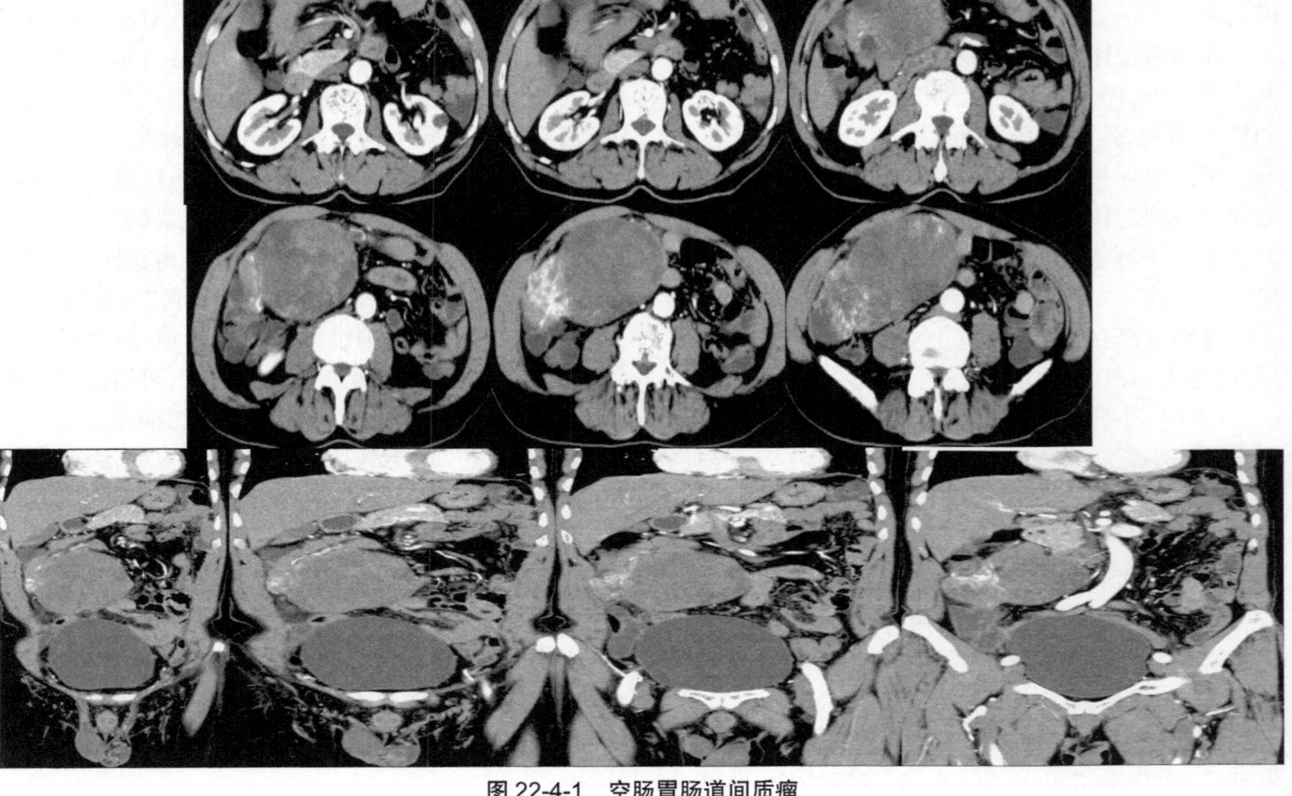

图 22-4-1　空肠胃肠道间质瘤

患者,男,68 岁。术后病理免疫组化诊断:空肠肿瘤切除标本:胃肠道间质瘤,高危险度,瘤细胞较丰富。为灰褐色结节状肿物,14.5cm × 9cm × 6.5cm,切面灰白暗褐色,伴出血及大片坏死,质中偏软,肿物周围大部分区域有包膜,肿物与肠壁局部分不开,肠黏膜皱襞存在。在影像学图像上,清楚可见肠系膜上动脉分支供应肿瘤(图 22-4-1)。

第四节　十二指肠球部远端胃肠道间质瘤(极低危险度)

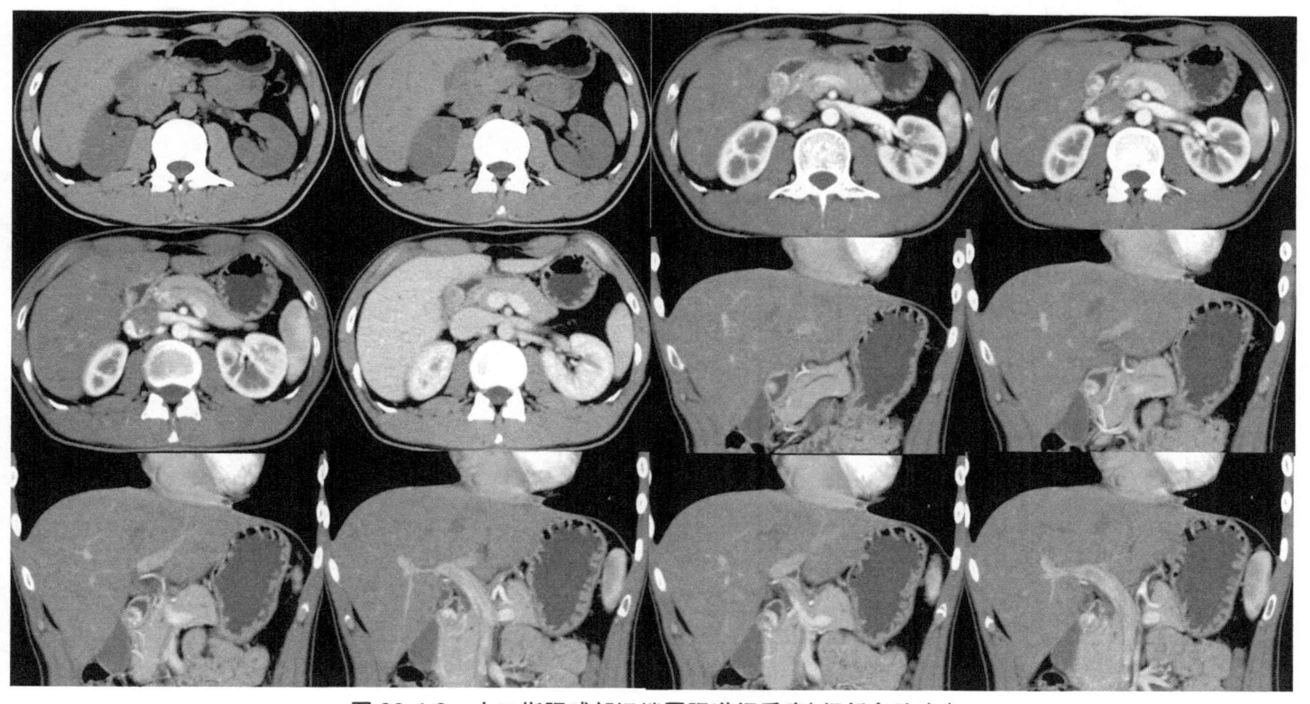

图 22-4-2　十二指肠球部远端胃肠道间质瘤(极低危险度)

病例,男,29 岁。

内镜超声:均质低回声团块,切面大小约 15.6mm×16.3mm,后方浆膜结构清楚。上述图像中,清楚可见充气的十二指肠球部远端一个富血管的强化不均匀的类圆形包块。术后病理诊断:十二指肠球部远端胃肠道间质瘤(极低危险度),瘤细胞较丰富。(图 22-4-2)

第五章 腹部其他恶性肿瘤

误诊病例简介:肝门部囊实性肿块——腹部类癌与胆管囊腺瘤

类癌是一种少见的高分化神经内分泌肿瘤,可见于任何含有神经内分泌细胞的组织,好发于消化道,其次为支气管。中老年人多见,女性占2/3。肿瘤大多数较小,生长缓慢,侵袭性小,但具有恶变倾向,直径<2 cm病变转移很少,>2 cm大多数转移。胃肠道类癌患者临床多表现为腹痛,恶心、呕吐或黑便,酷似癌或溃疡,瘤体较大时引起肠腔狭窄、套叠而致不全梗阻。一例肝门部囊实性肿块术前影像诊断为胆管囊腺瘤。

阑尾类癌多以阑尾炎为首发症状。而腹部胃肠道外类癌多表现为邻近脏器受压(一例符合此种表现)。类癌少数表现为类癌综合征(颜面部皮肤潮红、腹泻、支气管哮喘等),血中也少有激素类物质增高。腹部类癌缺乏特殊影像征象,一些作者归纳如下:肿瘤多单发,表现为不规则软组织团块,密度欠均匀,易发生坏死囊变,增强扫描实性成分强化较明显(该例符合此种表现)。不典型类癌呈不均匀轻中度强化或不强化,肿瘤实性部分动脉期开始强化,至静脉期持续强化。

MRI形态与CT类似,肿瘤信号不均匀,实性成分呈稍长T_1、长T_2信号,强化特点与CT相似,扩散加权成像(DWI)上肿瘤呈高信号。肿瘤血供丰富,多数肿瘤周围或肿瘤内可见流空血管。肿瘤一般与腹腔脏器分界较清,瘤周脏器受压,不同于其他恶性肿瘤直接导致邻近脏器壁弥漫性增厚或肿块,符合低度恶性肿瘤的特点。

鉴别诊断:胆管囊腺瘤:胆管囊腺瘤多数较大,中年女性多见,表现为多囊状,壁厚薄不均,增强扫描动脉期、静脉期、平衡期持续强化,但肝外胆管少见。

神经源性肿瘤:神经源性肿瘤多位于脊柱两侧,倾向于膨胀性缓慢生长,CT表现为类圆形或不规则软组织肿块,边界较清,其内密度不均,部分可伴钙化,增强扫描不均匀强化。

间质瘤:间质瘤腹膜后少见,多与胃肠道关系密切,CT表现为软组织肿块,多数瘤体较大,内可伴液化坏死囊变,增强扫描实性成分强化,肿瘤血供丰富,影像上不易鉴别,需结合临床及实验室检查。

胰腺假性囊肿/脓肿:胰腺假性囊肿/脓肿有胰腺炎或外伤病史。

腹部类癌生长缓慢,病程较长,影像学表现无特异性,但影像学对病灶的发现及诊断提示方面具有重要价值,结合其他临床检查,包括实验室检查等有助于本病的早期诊断。确诊仍依靠病理学检查。

第六章　腹盆部其他肿瘤

第一节　上皮内瘤样病变

上皮内瘤样病变是一种以形态学改变为特征的上皮性病变，包括组织结构和细胞形态学改变，伴随细胞增殖动力学和细胞分化的异常。结构异常指上皮排列紊乱和正常细胞极性丧失；细胞异常指细胞核不规则，深染，核质比例增高和核分裂活性增加。

一组对胃黏膜上皮异型增生随访 6 个月至 8.3 年的研究结果显示：异型增生消退者占 70.9%，加重和癌变占 18.0%，提示胃黏膜上皮异型增生（主要是轻度）是一可逆的过程，经过临床适当的治疗，大部分可消退，仅少数加重或癌变，所以早期诊断具有重要的意义。

MSCT 对胃癌分期的判断具有极大的优越性，其对胃癌的检出率为 80%~88%，然而，目前应用 CT 对胃肠道上皮内瘤样病变进行研究的报道少见。64 排 MSCT 具有卓越的空间分辨率及密度分辨力，易于显示消化道壁增厚及其强化特征，从而有助于提高病变的检出及早期诊断。

根据国际消化系统肿瘤研讨会公布的研究结果，消化系统恶性肿瘤约占所有肿瘤发病的 60%~70%，位居第一，在死亡率“排行榜”上也是“名列前茅”，且呈年轻化趋势。2000 年，国际癌症研究机构首次将上皮内瘤样病变的概念引入胃肠道上皮癌前病变的诊断，以取代以往使用的“异型增生、不典型增生、原位癌”概念。上皮内瘤样病变与癌的关系密切，普遍认为是癌的前期病变，并且提示上皮内瘤样病变部位黏膜发生癌的风险增加，但由于缺乏特异症状，早期难以发现。黏膜活检和内镜黏膜切除术并行病理组织学检查对明确诊断最为重要，但在病理诊断前早期发现尤为重要。

CT 是目前临床应用最为广泛的胃肠道肿瘤影像诊断手段，MSCT 的发展为胃肠道肿瘤诊断提供了更为方便、准确的方法，动态增强或螺旋多期扫描可以观察病变的早期强化和 / 或门脉期、平衡期的延迟强化，有助于早期发现病变。

虽然能谱 CT 在胃的癌前病变及早期胃癌诊断中可以提供定量分析，CT 仿真内镜成像技术对消化道肿瘤的诊断具有一定的应用价值，但特异性和准确性有待进一步提高。

一项研究应用 MSCT 增强扫描的方法对胃肠道上皮内瘤样病变进行血供模式分析，旨在探讨病变的血流动力学改变，从而反映病变的生物学行为及其病理生理学特征，为胃肠道上皮内瘤样病变的诊断、分级及其与胃肠道早期癌的鉴别诊断提供依据。

关于肿瘤强化的基础，不同的作者针对不同的肿瘤都得出类似结论，即肿瘤强化特征主要与对比剂在瘤内微血管的充盈及不成熟的管壁结构有关。

该组资料显示，胃上皮内瘤样病变组与正常对照组间门脉期及平衡期 ΔCT 值比较差异均有统计学意义，结直肠上皮内瘤样病变组与正常对照组间动脉期 ΔCT 值比较差异有统计学意义，表明上皮内瘤样病变已存在微血管改变及不成熟的管壁结构，但胃上皮内瘤样病变组与结直肠上皮内瘤样病变组强化峰值期相不尽相同，可能与病理类型和病变中血管的成熟程度不同有关，确切原因有待进一步研究。

病理研究表明，结直肠高级别上皮内瘤样病变多已经合并癌变。该研究结果显示，结直肠低级别上皮内瘤样病变组与高级别上皮内瘤样病变组之间门脉期 ΔCT 值比较差异有统计学意义，且结直肠低级别上皮内瘤样病变与早期癌之间门脉期 ΔCT 值比较差异有统计学意义，高级别上皮内瘤样病变组门脉期强化程度最高，这一结果与胃肠道癌 CT 增强扫描表现相似，与一些作者的研究结果类似。

该研究由于胃上皮内瘤样病变病例数较少，没有对胃低级别上皮内瘤样病变与高级别上皮内瘤样病变组间进行统计学分析。

该组资料低级别上皮内瘤样病变与高级别上皮内瘤样病变 2 组黏膜厚度差异无统计学意义，可能与上皮内瘤样病变主要为上皮内改变有关，故黏膜厚度对低级别与高级别上皮内瘤样病变不具有鉴别意义。

该研究表明，胃肠道上皮内瘤样病变主要表现为局部黏膜层增厚并有不同程度的强化，胃黏膜局部增厚并有门脉期及平衡期 CT 值均明显增高（ΔCT 值分别为 50 HU、30 HU）、结直肠黏膜局部增厚并有动脉期明显强化（ΔCT 值 30HU），有助于上皮内瘤样病变的诊断及鉴别诊断，但目前尚不能单纯根据 ΔCT 值鉴别上皮内瘤样病变与早期癌。

CT 检查具有快速、薄层、大范围扫描等优点，并能对原始数据进行薄层重建，提高了图像的空间分辨率和时间分辨率，能准确显示胃肠道壁的强化方式及黏膜层增厚的程度，为上皮内瘤样病变的诊断提供依据。

但该研究也存在一定的局限性，由于上皮内瘤样病变概念较新，相关的影像研究的参考文献较少，病例收集数量也较少；此外，胃肠道充盈后整体壁较薄，病变区 CT 值和黏膜层厚度的测量可能存在一定偏差，该研究通过放大原始图像进行测量，以尽可能减少测量误差对研究结果的影响。

第二节　表现较为特殊的腹内侵袭性纤维瘤病

腹腔内侵袭性纤维瘤病相对少见，主要发生于肠系膜或盆腔，很少发生于腹膜后。肠系膜和盆腔病变可有明显的细胞外间质黏液样改变。细胞形态呈良性，无核异型及深染，核分裂象少见。

影像学研究：腹内病变发现时多数较大，呈类圆形或分叶状肿块，某些位于肠系膜根部的病变可较小且形态不规则。相对于其他部位的病变，腹内肿瘤倾向于密度更低且不均匀，增强扫描肿瘤内可见斑片状不强化的低密度区，可能与肿瘤内间质黏液样改变有关。

一组作者报告 2 例腹内病变表现较为特殊：1 例为左上腹腔内病灶，肿瘤侵犯邻近胃壁、结肠、胰腺、脾，并与胃肠道相通形成内瘘，肿瘤内部可见大片液化坏死及气液平面。因其明显的侵袭性生长方式术前误诊为恶性肿瘤。另 1 例发生于胰腺的病变呈明显的囊实性，且病灶形态光整，边界清晰，术前误诊为胰腺囊腺瘤。

胰腺侵袭性纤维瘤病罕见。Amiot 等（2008）回顾既往文献的个案报道仅 9 例，其中大部分肿瘤位于胰腺体尾部，以实性肿块居多，发生囊变者更少见（2/9），术前诊断较难。肠系膜侵袭性纤维瘤病是常见的原发性肠系膜肿瘤之一，患者可伴有 Gardner 综合征。

一些肠系膜或盆腔病变可见明显的间质黏液样改变，表现为 CT 上不均质、不强化的低密度区，并可与胶原成分交互形成“条纹”状或“旋涡”状。目前 MSCT 具有更高的空间分辨率及任一角度多平面重建的优点，对腹内病变及与邻近结构关系的显示具有优势。

鉴别诊断：腹内病变较少见，因累及不同的脏器结构而表现多样。发生在腹腔内的侵袭性纤维瘤病需与胃肠道间质瘤、孤立性纤维瘤、淋巴瘤、软组织肉瘤以及转移瘤等进行鉴别，诊断相对较难。胃肠道间质瘤常发生出血、坏死，密度不均匀。转移瘤有原发病灶。

影像检查可显示病灶的部位、形态和范围，做出定位诊断，在定性诊断方面有一定的困难，一些病例术前曾诊断为纤维瘤、平滑肌瘤、转移瘤（有肝癌切除史患者）等。某些罕见部位如胰腺病变诊断更难，最终需要病理确诊。单靠 CT 表现进行诊断常有一定的难度。

第三节　腹部不典型神经鞘瘤

神经鞘瘤，又称施万细胞瘤，或称雪旺细胞瘤，由 Virchow（1908）首次描述，起源于外周运动神经、感觉神经和脑神经的鞘膜（嗅神经和视神经除外），有完整包膜，常呈孤立肿块，与其所发生的神经粘连在一起，呈偏心性生长，其长轴与神经干方向一致。典型的神经鞘瘤 CT 诊断并不难，不典型神经鞘瘤极易误诊。

腹部不典型神经鞘瘤可以出现以下 CT 征象：

（1）腹部神经鞘瘤以腹膜后最常见，而对于腹部一些少见的发病部位如胃、胰腺、肾上腺等部位的神经鞘瘤的影像表现总结较少。一组总结了 5 例少见部位神经鞘瘤的特点。腹部少见部位神经鞘瘤的大小与发生部位有关，但多 <5 cm。肿瘤多呈圆形或椭圆形；肿瘤境界清楚，边缘光滑，均有完整的包膜；具有典型神经鞘瘤的特征即易囊变，因此肿瘤平扫以囊实性为主；动态增强后实性部分呈进行性中度强化，囊性部分不强化。

（2）肿瘤多发：神经鞘瘤单发多见，多发少见。对于多发神经鞘瘤 1973 年有学者提出神经鞘瘤病这一概念，Michael 等（2006）提出多发神经鞘瘤病的诊断标准：患者年龄 >30 岁且有两个或两个以上非皮内神经鞘瘤，无听神经瘤，无 NF-2 基因突变。神经鞘瘤病一般在 30 岁以上发生，一组 16 例中，有 2 例年龄均 >30 岁，结合影像表现考虑诊断神经鞘瘤病。

（3）完全囊变：完全囊变是神经鞘瘤比较少见的 CT 征象。瘤体完全囊变，呈“纯囊肿”样，囊壁薄且均匀（壁厚约为 3~5mm），囊内外壁均光整，平扫囊内为液性密度；动态增强呈现出薄壁规则环形强化，囊性部分不强化。

（4）厚壁囊变：厚壁囊变和 / 或伴有壁结节，平扫呈厚壁（壁厚 >5 mm）稍低密度灶，囊壁厚薄不均匀，囊内外壁尚光整；增强扫描厚壁、壁结节强化呈“厚壁假囊肿样”改变，囊内低密度区无强化或仅有轻度强化。

（5）钙化：钙化在腹膜后神经鞘瘤内出现的概率并不高，文献报道发生率 < 10%。肿瘤内钙化多呈细点状和肿块边缘的线样钙化，良性神经鞘瘤钙化清楚，钙化出现的比例低，恶性肿瘤钙化常见，部分钙化灶边缘模糊。该组 2 例肿瘤内见钙化，呈点状或环状分布于肿瘤内。

（6）肿瘤供血血管强化：3 例肿瘤平扫密度不均匀，中心囊变呈不规则低密度区；增强扫描动脉期肿瘤周边呈不规则状强化，内部可见肿瘤血管强化或线条状强化，静脉期及延迟期肿瘤周边及内部斑片状强化进一步持续并略增强。

（7）恶性神经鞘瘤的转移：腹部恶性神经鞘瘤以腹膜后多见，肿瘤体积较大，形态不规则，对邻近组织器官压迫、推移、侵犯，可包绕、侵及腹膜后淋巴结、血管，少数肿瘤也可发生肝、肺转移。

神经鞘瘤影像表现与病理关系：神经鞘瘤的影像表现与病理特征相关。神经鞘瘤在病理上是由 Antoni A 区和 Antoni B 区组成，Antoni A 区由密集的梭形细胞构成，细胞核排列为栅栏或旋涡状，境界不清；Antoni B 区瘤细胞稀疏，排列呈网状，基质含水量高。

肿瘤平扫的密度与肿瘤内 Antoni A 区和 Antoni B 区比例、分布密切相关。肿瘤以 Antoni A 区为主时，CT 密度较高；若以 Antoni B 区为主时，CT 为水样低密度，密度低于周围软组织。Antoni A 区和 Antoni B 区多并存于一个肿瘤中，两种结构交织存在，Antoni A 多分布于肿瘤的周边，Antoni B 多位于肿瘤的中心。

由于 Antoni A 区细胞丰富，生长活跃，对 Antoni B 区血液供应产生虹吸效应，容易引起 Antoni B 区的坏死囊变，同时由于 Antoni B 区的组织结构易囊变，从而形成从肿瘤的中心向肿瘤边缘囊变，当肿瘤出现不同程度囊变或黏液样变时，会出现完全囊变、厚壁囊变等不典型征象。

增强扫描强化程度主要与肿瘤内 Antoni A 区的比例、分布密切相关，肿瘤以 Antoni A 区为主时，细胞丰富，一般为富血供区，增强扫描呈中等程度以上强化。少数肿瘤在 Antoni A 区内见到肿瘤的供血血管，增强扫描出现条状强化的血管影。若以 Antoni B 区为主时，CT 为水样低密度，密度低于周围软组织，增强扫描多无强化。

肿瘤生长过程中，肿瘤本身的组织结构、血供的不均匀易造成肿瘤内部组织变性（主要是黏液变或囊变）的多样性，使肿瘤密度变化多样，增强后强化方式不典型。

另外，Hughes 等（2005）发现肿瘤内都未出现明显囊变区，但平扫密度较低，这主要与神经鞘瘤细胞排列有关，细胞排列疏松，施万细胞黏液基质水分含量高及肿瘤内纤维含量多有关。总之，对于不典型神经鞘瘤的影像学诊断较难。该研究之不足在于病例数少，还需要收集更多的病例资料进一步对腹部不典型神经鞘瘤的影像特点进行总结探讨。

第七章　胃肠道疾病

第一节　误诊病例简介：血友病患者之胃肠壁内病变与胃窦癌及胃壁血肿

Wright 和 Matthews（1971）报告 2 例血友病病人胃壁内出血引起诊断困难，1 例考虑为胃窦癌，1 例包块比较大，易扪及，考虑为腹壁血肿。

目前已经认识到，胃肠壁内出血是一种出血性素质和抗凝血治疗的合并症。

Khilnani 等（1964）指出这些病人常常可观察到特征性的 X 线表现，它与胃肠道的其他散在性病变的区别十分重要，因为它不需要手术，经内科治疗即可消散。

一个孤立性血肿可以其密度的增加或以小肠、大肠肠袢的移位而显露。如出血限于肠壁，则可见不同程度的麻痹性肠梗阻、肠腔狭窄或局限的充盈缺损，平片或造影检查时，还可能见到栅栏状缺损。胃壁内出血较少。

Grossman 等（1965）报告 1 例 8 岁血友病患儿的大的胃壁血肿。Rothstein 等（1968）报告 2 例胃底血肿，无出血素质，1 例可能由于酒精中毒后出血，1 例可能继发于手术的压迫性损伤。Wright 和 Matthews（1971）报告之例 1 为胃壁的巨大血肿造成胃的梗阻，例 2 表现为胃底大弯侧巨大充盈缺损，颇类似新生物，2 个月以后好转，6 个月以后即消失。此 2 例均经抗血友病治疗而好转。

第二节　胃肠道的假性病变

有的正常结构可类似病变，胃肠蠕动或病变又可产生人工伪影，胃肠道某段狭窄既可能为一病变或痉挛所致，又可为人工伪影造成。假性病变最重要特点是影像不恒定。真正病变总是存在，可见于每个图像上，而且容易重复显现或复制；然而假性病变则相反，它是暂时出现的，不能见于每个图像上，而且难以重复显现或复制。

第三节　钡剂被覆不良或胃肠扩张不佳

在双对比钡剂检查胃肠道时，如钡剂或液体过量，钡剂被覆黏膜则较差。有作者指出，当钡剂被覆不理想时，实在不行则应改作单对比检查，不然，勉强地作双对比，常可导致漏诊病变。胃肠扩张不佳结果更坏，它可遮蔽大的病变。我们应记住，双对比检查技术失败或空气对比不佳所造成的后果，远比不作该检查的结果还要差。

第四节 胃弥漫浸润型低分化腺癌

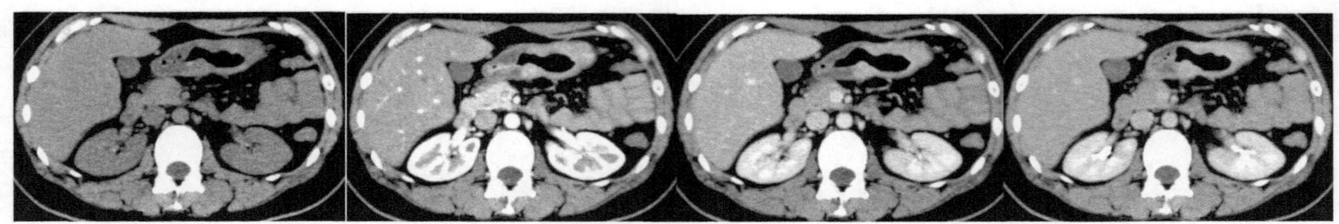

图 22-7-1 胃弥漫浸润型低分化腺癌

患者,女,29 岁。

术后病理免疫组化诊断:胃弥漫浸润型低分化腺癌(大小 6cm × 5.5cm × 1.3cm),部分为印戒细胞癌,侵及浆膜纤维脂肪组织(图 22-7-1)。

第五节 胃肠道假性淋巴瘤

假性淋巴瘤,即淋巴网状细胞增生,为良性非特异性病变,为一种淋巴组织的良性浸润,其特点是淋巴滤泡的大小和数目的增加。本症可发生于多种器官,胃肠道为其好发部位之一。

本症又称作慢性淋巴瘤样胃炎、滤泡性胃炎、反应性淋巴网状(细胞)增生、胃肠道假性白血病、良性淋巴增生、良性淋巴性多发性息肉、淋巴增生、淋巴滤泡局限增生以及良性淋巴样息肉病等。有作者指出,在临床上,内窥镜检、X 线检查和病理上都不易与恶性淋巴瘤或癌肿鉴别,在组织学检查还易被误诊为淋巴肉瘤。

一些作者提示,只有组织学检查才能将真正恶性淋巴瘤与本症区分开,本症组织学表现特点为:真正胚胎中心形成;有多形性炎性浸润;缺乏真正淋巴瘤所引起的淋巴结受累。

本症病因众说纷纭,大多数认为是与溃疡或局限性肠炎有关的炎症过程,有作者认为属错构瘤性病变,也有学者指出胃溃疡经久不愈,由于慢性刺激引起多形性炎症反应,而在溃疡周围形成肿块。病理表现因淋巴组织浸润、增生的程度和范围不同而各异,大体可分:表浅浸润型、黏膜肥大型、弥漫浸润型、局部肿块型和结节息肉型。

本症好发于 40 岁以上,文献上报告最年轻者为 17 岁,可表现为腹痛、黑便、体重减轻、呕血及腹部包块等。在 X 线检查时,胃假性淋巴瘤表现为肿块、胃黏膜皱襞增粗、良性溃疡、胃窦狭窄变形、胃体或胃窦大块充盈缺损并巨大溃疡等。

当其出现于结肠和 / 或直肠时,增生常呈现典型脐样小结节或息肉状;出现于胃时,则表现为一溃疡性包块、浸润性病变、溃疡龛影或肿大的皱襞而类似于恶性肿瘤。有作者报告 2 例胃淋巴增生,X 线与胃镜均见其呈现少见的脐样息肉状改变。肠道假性淋巴瘤好发于回盲部,X 线表现类似真性淋巴瘤,而临床病史却符合局限性肠炎。

第六节 胃肠淋巴增生呈现少见的脐样息肉病变

胃肠道淋巴增生是一良性非特异性病变,特点是淋巴滤泡的大小和数目的增加,名称甚多,诸如:胃肠假性白血病、良性淋巴增生、良性淋巴性多发性息肉、淋巴增生以及淋巴滤泡局限增生等。当其出现于结肠和 / 或直肠时,增生常呈现典型脐样小结节或息肉状;出现于胃时,则表现为一溃疡性包块、浸润性病变、溃疡龛影或肿大的皱襞而类似于恶性肿瘤(Perez 和 Derfman, 1966)。Rahk 等(1971)报告 2 例胃淋巴增生，X 线与胃镜均见其呈现少见的脐样息肉状改变。

胃肠道淋巴增生早在 1838 年即已知晓，Conheim(1865)称之为假性白血病。组织学特点为黏膜下层内淋巴滤泡的大小和 / 或数目单纯的增加，无恶性淋巴瘤病灶那种浸润毁坏的表现。Franken (1970)甚至认为此种增生改变不一定是病理性的。

许多病人结肠受犯出现直肠出血、反复腹泻与腹痛，但其因果关系究竟如何，不少作者认为是个重要问题。本病的少见脐状息肉样改变容易与胃多发性息肉、皱襞的息肉状增厚或多发性迷走胰腺组织相混淆，应予注意。

第七节　诊断陷阱:CT 图像上一些情况类似胃肠病变

Pupole 和 Ruzicka(1984)指出，在 CT 图像上食管裂孔疝可伪似增厚的食管壁或胃食管连接区含气脓肿。偶尔，大的小网膜囊及胰腺假性囊肿伴似扩张且充盈液体的胃，而真正的胃却萎陷缩小位于假性囊肿前方。在肝静脉韧带层面，正常的胃食管连接区可类似一胃的假性肿块，Kaye 等(1980)，Marks 等(1981)及 Balk 等(1984)均作过此类病例的介绍。

胃溃疡穿孔入小网膜囊，造成口服对比剂外渗，充满对比剂的小网膜囊在 CT 图像上酷似充盈对比剂的肠袢，同时可见腹腔气体液体积聚类似充气扩张的结肠肠袢。

有作者指出，弯曲的直肠乙状结肠的体积平均效应，可导致出现直肠内肛管位于肠腔之外的印象，从而可误诊为直肠穿孔。Jeffrey 等(1981)见一手术残留海绵产生一脓肿，海绵为高密度，极类似肠内的对比剂影像。

在 CT 横断扫描图像上，正常胃食管连接区可佯似左上腹包块，此刻可口服对比剂行俯卧或仰卧扫描证实该影实为胃食管连接区。

在结肠肝曲上部充有不规则对比剂，并紧贴肝穹隆外上方，曾被误为钙化的肝肿块。

肠袢类似肿块，肠袢类似肿瘤复发，无对比剂的肠袢形成假肿瘤等在文献上均有不少报告，常用口服对比剂后再重复扫描，一般可澄清问题的真相。

有作者报告幼儿出现腹痛和包块，拟诊为肠套叠(回盲套叠)，本应首先做钡剂灌肠进行诊断，但却先做 CT 扫描，CT 提示为一孤立的腹腔内或腹膜后包块，造成诊断混淆。

CT 图像上，鼻胃管可伪装成几种不同的结构，在广泛腹水病人鼻管可在胃中扭折，向颅侧或足侧再扫描可见鼻胃管的含水银的尖端，水银可引起条纹伪影。

Marks 等(1980)注意到腹水使肠袢移向中线，呈现为粘连于左腹壁的有包裹的气体积聚，颇似脓肿，再尾侧扫描却见腔内有空气及对比剂，证实为降结肠肠袢。

有时在肝肾隐窝内见到不规则气体积聚，考虑为腹内脓肿，再向尾侧扫描却见此脓肿实为肠袢，同时见到邻近的假性增厚(为收缩引起)的胆囊壁。

Newmark 等(1980)曾见到肝左叶外段前方有气体积聚，结合邻近层面分析证实为肠袢，而不应只看一个层面误诊为脓肿或肠腔外气体积聚。

第八节　吻壁现象

双对比检查方法本身可产生一些陷阱，吻壁现象即为其一。在钡剂被覆胃肠道黏膜，气体扩张肠曲时，应努力寻找另外的线形影和新月形影，有时，相对胃肠壁可互相粘贴，尤如接吻，产生假的线影或其他阴影。此类吻壁现象常常是使用压迫后产生的暂时现象，松压后，此现象即刻消逝。如还有怀疑，可设法使该段胃肠壁再行扩张，此现象一般都应该立即消失，如还不消失，则多为真性病变所致。

第九节　不同检查方法的误诊教训

X线腹部平片:在仰卧位片上,有时可见一个圆形的、边缘清楚的软组织块影出现于右上腹部,位于上段腰椎的右侧,重叠于右肾上极。此块影最常见于横型胃和一下垂的胃窦部,此刻,胃居高位,横行于上腹,胃体靠前,胃底胃窦靠后,胃内液体积沉于下垂的部分。

十二指肠球部位于充盈的窦部的后面,全部或部分为胃窦所遮掩,它一般为三角形(斜位及侧位观察尤其如此)或圆形,但比胃窦影为小。因此,当出现上述软组织块影时,首先宜考虑为液体充盈的胃窦,其次才考虑为肿瘤或为液体充盈的十二指肠球部。

有时,在仰卧位平片左膈下左上腹部可见见圆形软组织密度包块影,亦为假性肿瘤,常为胃底积聚液体所致。为排除此类假性肿瘤,可再俯卧位进行检查,块影消失则证明确系假性肿瘤影。自然,钡餐检查及CT扫描则更有助于确诊。

X线检查与CT、MR:腹部假肿瘤性脂肪过多症,为软组织内正常的脂肪组织呈局灶性增殖的结果。一些作者报告2例单纯肥胖病人的假肿瘤性脂肪过多症,在胃肠钡剂检查和淋巴造影时有推挤移位的表现而酷似肠系膜与腹膜后肿瘤。此类表现的良性脂肪性质应用CT及MR检查即一目了然,不需进行手术探查。

关于十二指肠低张造影:十二指肠低张检查对于十二指肠疾病及十二指肠旁区病变的诊断有着重要作用,一般诊断正确率超过常规钡餐检查,特别是小的充盈缺损常规检查常常漏诊,而低张检查却显示较为满意。但是,低张检查使十二指肠环扩张,可能不平衡地增强一个壁内或十二指肠旁病变的表现的考虑;还可能表现十二指肠肠曲内外侧扩张不相称,从而被错误地夸张为异常情况,一些作者报告2例手术证实的正常误诊为异常即为此种情况。

所以,对低张检查与常规检查的比较应一分为二,全面衡量,认真分析研究。

悬挂小滴或钟乳石现象:此现象常可成为溃疡型息肉错误诊断的一个原因,事实上此现象只是暂时的表现,复查或随访常可澄清问题。

第八章　胃肠道炎症

第一节　嗜酸细胞性胃肠炎

嗜酸细胞性胃肠炎，又被译作嗜酸性粒细胞性胃肠炎，系指胃壁和/或肠壁以嗜酸性粒细胞浸润为特征，伴有外周血嗜酸性粒细胞增多及胃肠道症状为主的少见疾病。病变可局限，可弥漫，亦可累及全胃肠道壁各层，影像表现多样，无特异性，容易发生误诊和误治。

病理学：嗜酸细胞性胃肠炎是一种变态反应性疾病，病因至今不明，有人认为嗜酸性粒细胞在胃肠黏膜表面的聚集引发Ⅰ型变态反应是组织损伤的主要机制。本病分4种类型：黏膜病变型，肌层病变型，浆膜病变型及混合型，其中又以黏膜病变型最多见。以上述病理学改变为基础的胃肠钡餐造影表现为胃十二指肠及空回肠黏膜弥漫增粗，或假性息肉样充盈缺损，动力可减弱，管腔狭窄及龛影罕见。累及浆膜者可表现为腹水。一般认为，嗜酸细胞性胃肠炎是一种自限性变态反应性疾病，部分不经治疗而痊愈，但可复发。临床以保守治疗为主，应剔除过敏食物，对激素有特效。

临床表现：嗜酸细胞性胃肠炎由Kaijser（1937）首先报道，迄今世界文献报道约400余例。所有种族、所有年龄段（从新生儿到成人）均有发病，20~60岁为高发年龄，以男性发病为多，男性发病率约为女性的2倍。嗜酸细胞性胃肠炎以胃肠道组织中嗜酸粒细胞异常浸润为特征。嗜酸细胞性胃肠炎的病因尚不明确，一般认为是对外源性或内源性过敏原的变态反应所致。嗜酸细胞性胃肠炎与某些外源性或内源性物质引起的机体过敏有关，有遗传学背景。

嗜酸细胞性胃肠炎诊断标准为：①进食特殊食物后出现胃肠道症状，但要除外寄生虫感染和胃肠道外嗜酸性粒细胞增多的疾病；②外周血嗜性粒细胞增多；③组织学证明胃肠道有1个或1个以上部位的嗜酸性粒细胞浸润。

影像学研究：胃肠双对比造影特点：在造影之前可先行腹部X线平片或进行腹部透视检查，虽表现无特异性但如果发现肠梗阻，可以帮助确定病变主要部位。

嗜酸细胞性胃肠炎可累及全消化道，最常累及胃、十二指肠及空肠，还可以累及结肠、食管甚至肝胆系统等。特征性表现包括黏膜弥漫颗粒样改变、疣状糜烂及溃疡。糜烂和溃疡常多发，好发于胃窦与小肠。还可表现为胃肠蠕动功能差，胃腔内有食物存留，幽门孔黏膜肿胀明显，对比剂通过球部困难等。食管往往有食管贲门裂孔疝和反流性炎症改变。小肠及结肠造影表现有回肠、结肠及盲肠黏膜僵硬、糜烂、肠痉挛、肠腔狭窄。胃肠道双对比造影可清楚显示黏膜皱襞增粗、管腔狭窄的表现，但均无特异性。由于该方法无创伤、直观，可以全方位、大视野确定病变范围和类型，成为诊断本病不可缺少的重要检查手段。

CT表现：与本病的病理改变即嗜酸性粒细胞胃肠壁浸润的深度与广度密切相关，CT检查无特异性，但可以显示肠壁及胃肠道外的病变情况，且CT检查有助于鉴别诊断防止误诊。CT可见胃肠壁增厚，分层状胃肠壁增厚，胃肠腔狭窄，黏膜皱襞粗大，胃肠分泌增多，小肠梗阻等；增强扫描时可见胃肠壁均质性强化，或中度强化，或环形强化，以及肠系膜多发性小结节。

鉴别诊断：本病应注意与其他原因引起腹水嗜酸细胞增多的疾病相鉴别。

伴有胃肠道浸润的高嗜酸性粒细胞综合征：诊断依据主要包括外周血高嗜酸性粒细胞计数增高（$>1.5\times10^9/L$），并至少持续6个月；除外其他引起嗜酸性粒细胞增高的疾病,如寄生虫病或过敏性疾病;必须有器官损伤的证据。最常见的器官损伤为心脏、神经系统、皮肤和肺。单一的消化道受侵犯者罕见,可有染色体畸变。

嗜酸性肉芽肿:主要发生于胃和小肠,呈局限性肿块。病理有嗜酸性肉芽肿混于结缔组织基质中。过敏史少见,周围血中白细胞数及嗜酸性粒细胞常不增加。

寄生虫感染和胃肠道肿瘤:这些疾病中,通常除了胃肠道症状和外周血嗜酸细胞增加,还有其他的临床表现,因此鉴别并不困难。

单纯侵犯食管又称为嗜酸性粒细胞性食管炎,诊断时除须符合以上标准外,还应除外反流性食管炎。

综上所述,X线平片可以发现肠梗阻;胃肠双对比造影优势在于清晰观察黏膜表面,肠壁及外压性病变,虽无特异性,但由于无创伤、直观,可以全方位、大视野确定病变范围和类型,成为诊断本病不可缺少的重要检查手段。CT则能更清楚观察肠壁及肠外病变。而综合观察胃肠壁黏膜皱襞粗大、分层状增厚、肉芽肿等影像特征性,结合外周血嗜酸性细胞增多及过敏史等可有助于确诊本病。

第二节 胃肠道结核

回盲部结核占腹部结核病人的80%~90%,回肠末端瓣膜缘增厚或瓣口狭窄是结核的特征。在早期病例的钡灌肠中可见肠道痉挛、分泌增加和回盲部能动性加大。在钡气双重对比造影上可见线状或星状伴边缘隆起的浅表溃疡。结核性溃疡比克罗恩病的溃疡大,倾向于卵圆形而不是圆形。但结核的肠壁增厚更明显,瘘管和窦道少见。

随着病程进展,出现特征性的变形,包括对称性环状“餐巾环”狭窄和梗阻、收缩、变短和囊袋形成。典型的病人,盲肠可形成截断。这种截断也可见于阿米巴病中,但后者很少如结核那样侵及小肠。肠道的局部狭窄和截断状也可与癌混淆。但盲肠癌很少超过回盲瓣以外。半数胃肠结核病人的CT显示回肠末端和盲肠环形增厚、回盲瓣增大及肠系膜淋巴结肿大。但其他一些表现如回盲瓣的不对称、盲肠内壁增厚、末端回肠病灶向外蔓延和淋巴结肿块都更支持结核病的诊断。

第三节　嗜酸性粒细胞性胃肠炎

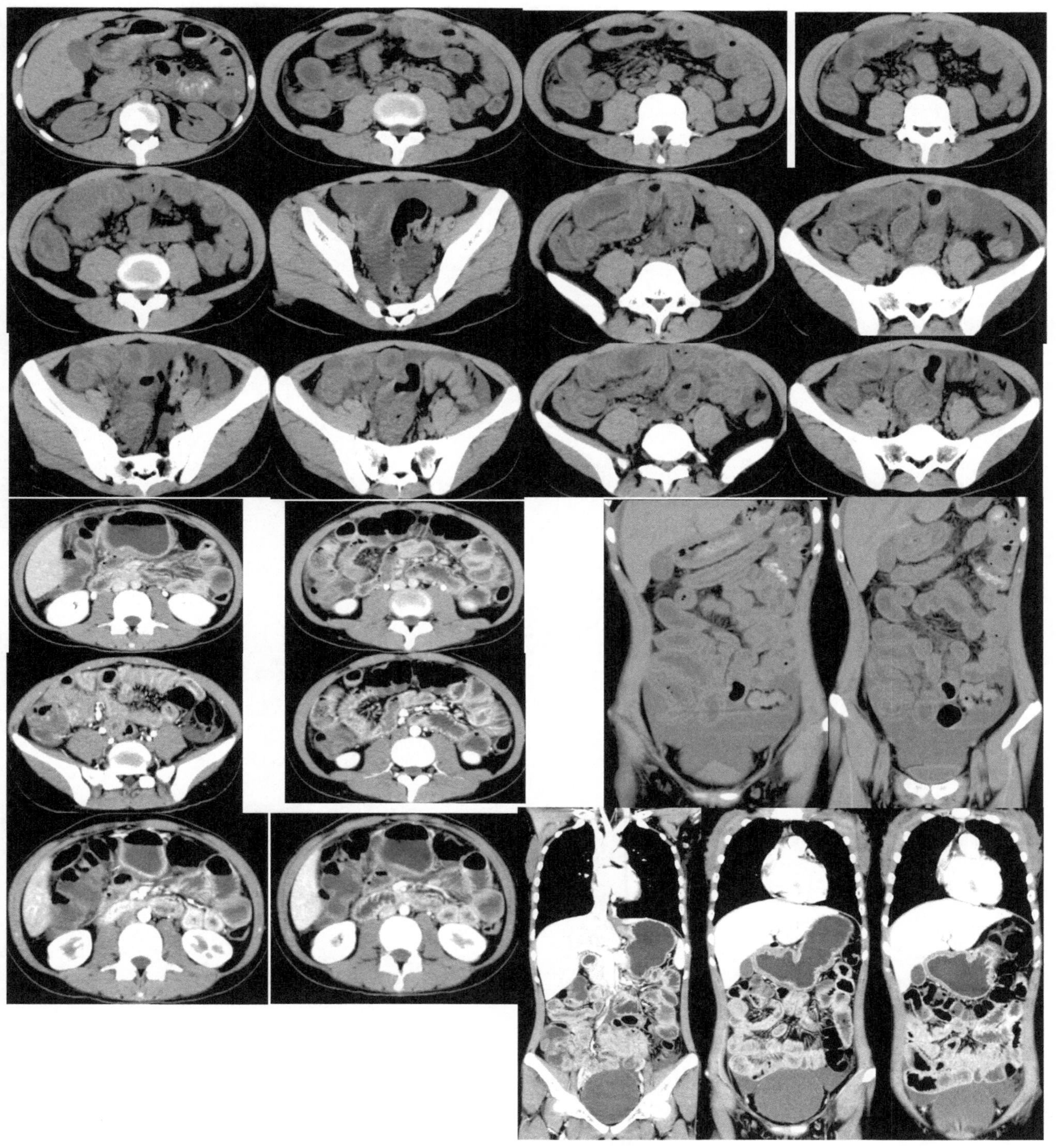

图 22-8-1　嗜酸性粒细胞性胃肠炎

病例,女，16 岁。患者缘于两周前无明显诱因出现脐周疼痛,呈阵发性闷痛,进食后加重,伴偶有大便次数增多，1~4

次 / 日，大便次数多时呈黄色糊状样，便后腹痛缓解，未予重视及治疗。于 1 周前因进食冷饮后出现腹痛加重，以脐周明显，呈阵发性绞痛，排便后可缓解，伴腹泻，7~10 次 / 天，为黄色稀水样便，偶呈黑色，无黏液脓血便，伴呕吐，进食即吐，为非喷射性非咖啡样胃内容物，伴乏力，偶有胸闷，无发热、黄疸，无便血、黑便，无尿频、尿急、尿痛。

实验室检查：嗜酸细胞 6.14×10^9/L、嗜酸细胞 49.1%（明显升高，正常参考值 0.02~0.52 × 10^9/L、5%），白细胞计数 12.52×10^9/L（升高）。免疫球蛋白（IgG.A.M）、自身抗体谱及过敏原检查未见异常。

病理检查：胃窦黏膜活检标本，呈慢性轻度非萎缩性胃炎，未见嗜酸性粒细胞，请结合临床；十二指肠降部黏膜活检标本，呈黏膜慢性炎，建议活检后复查；回肠末段黏膜活检标本，呈黏膜慢性炎，黏膜间质内见散在嗜酸性粒细胞；升结肠黏膜活检标本，呈黏膜慢性炎，黏膜间质内可见少量嗜酸性粒细胞浸润，请结合临床；直肠黏膜活检标本，呈黏膜慢性炎，未见嗜酸性粒细胞。出院诊断：嗜酸细胞性胃肠炎，低钾血症，腹腔积液，盆腔积液，肝功能异常，凝血功能障碍，嗜酸性细胞增多症（继发性？）（图 22-8-1）。

第九章　克罗恩病

一、克罗恩病 MSCT 小肠造影

克罗恩病是一种肉芽肿性炎性病变，其特征是肠壁节段性受累和透壁性炎症。可以累及消化道的任何部分，但以末端回肠和近段结肠最易受累。70% 的病变位于小肠，其中 30% 位于末端回肠。早期主要表现为黏膜或黏膜下层水肿，黏膜面溃疡形成，进而病变累及肠壁全层，导致肠壁纤维化、穿孔，甚至瘘管、窦道形成，造成肠周脂肪、肠系膜以及邻近组织、器官受累。病变肠管呈节段性改变，故又称其为节段性肠炎。

临床上诊断克罗恩病主要依靠消化道造影和肠镜检查，但最终确诊依赖病理。随着 MSCT 技术的迅速发展，以其极高的空间分辨率和时间分辨率和真正意义上的各向同性扫描，使得运用 CT 来诊断肠道疾病成为可能，MSCT 小肠造影的应用日益完善。

MSCT 小肠造影检查方法：检查前准备：准备的关键是取得良好的肠道对比并减少肠蠕动伪影。目前临床上使用较多的肠道对比剂包括水、甲基纤维素和稀释的混悬钡等。一些学者常采用分 4 次口服低密度对比剂 1 500ml，取得了较好的效果。为了减少肠管的蠕动，扫描前 10min 可以静脉注射山莨菪碱（654-2）或胰高血糖素等降低肠道运动的药物。

部分作者采用检查前 1 天进食少渣食物，晚 8 点服 50% 硫酸镁 40ml，酚酞 2 片；检查当日早晨肛门用开塞露 1 支，使小肠和结肠处于空虚状态；检查前，间隔 15~20min 分 3 次服完 1 000~1 500 ml 自制 2.5% 等渗甘露醇溶液（有肠梗阻表现者可酌减），静脉注射 654-2 20mg 后 5~10min 行 CT 扫描，亦取得了很好的效果。

CT 增强扫描及图像后处理：一般静脉注射非离子型对比剂 150 ml，扫描延迟时间对于显示病变肠壁强化程度有重要的作用。有学者通过实验得出：正常的肠壁强化峰值在静脉注射对比剂后平均 50 s 时，即在动脉强化峰值后大约 14 s。观察肠壁的强化程度在诊断早期小肠克罗恩病时非常重要。

扫描范围包括整个腹部（从膈顶至耻骨联合上缘），分别行平扫、动脉期、静脉期和平衡期扫描。将所得原始数据经 0.625 mm 重建后传至工作站，运用多平面重建、曲面重建等后处理技术进行后处理显示肠管；运用最大密度投影显示肠系膜血管及其远端细小分支。

正常小肠的 MSCT 小肠造影表现：十二指肠、空肠、回肠肠管扩展良好的情况下，小肠壁的厚度应 <3 mm，且厚薄均匀。空肠、回肠、末端回肠直径分别为 3 cm、2.5cm 和 2cm，如用低张小肠造影时部分患者空肠直径可达 3.5 cm。正常情况下，十二指肠和空肠的血供较回肠丰富，因此在增强 MSCT 小肠造影时肠壁强化程度明显高于回肠，肠管与周围组织结构之间分界清晰，肠周脂肪密度均匀。

肠系膜血管：正常情况下肠系膜及肠壁血管走行自然，管腔通畅，主干及其分支显示清晰。在增强 MSCT 小肠造影中，可以清晰地显示系膜及肠壁血管的走行、密度、形态，特别是多平面重建和最大密度投影，可同时显示肠系膜动脉和静脉。

肠系膜淋巴结：肠系膜淋巴结沿着系膜血管旁分布，呈圆形或椭圆形的软组织密度影，正常情况下直径不超过 10mm，在肠周脂肪的映衬下显得非常清晰。常规 CT 常难以清晰地显示淋巴结情况。MSCT 多平面重建及最大密度投影能清晰地显示 <5mm 的淋巴结。

小肠克罗恩病的 MSCT 小肠造影表现及其诊断价值：肠壁的厚度和强化特征：克罗恩病是一种透壁性的炎性病变，早期表现为黏膜或者黏膜下水肿、肠壁增厚，而这些改变 MSCT 小肠造影上可以敏感地反映出来。肠壁增厚主要是由于肠壁水肿、淋巴管扩张、胶原纤维增生以及黏膜下层增厚所致，急性期以水肿为主，慢性期表现为纤维组织增生。

严重的肠壁增厚可以导致肠腔狭窄，甚至梗阻发生。正常小肠壁厚度在扩展良好的状态下应<3mm，4mm 就认为是肠壁增厚，增厚一般在 5~10 mm 之间，最厚可达 20 mm。在小肠克罗恩病中，肠壁增厚约占 82%。肠壁厚度在 10mm 以下时常只表现为肠系膜侧增厚而对侧厚度正常，病变肠管肠系膜侧僵硬、缩短，而对侧肠壁呈假憩室样改变。

厚度 >10 mm 时常表现为整个病变肠壁增厚且病变最易出现在末端回肠，病变常呈节段性分布。MSCT 小肠造影通过多平面重建能显示整个肠壁的厚度以及良好地层示病变的节段性特点。但是肠壁的增厚在诊断克罗恩病时不具有特异性。

肠壁的快速强化和肠壁增厚是敏感性最高的征象。典型的肠壁强化是肠壁呈分层状强化，其原因为水肿的黏膜下层在增强扫描时不强化，而浆膜层和肌层强化明显，肠管的轴位像表现为“靶征”。病变早期，肠壁水肿渗出较轻时，肠壁厚度可以正常，但在增强 MSCT 小肠造影上肠壁就可强化。因此，增强 MSCT 小肠造影能够更加敏感地发现厚度正常的炎性肠壁，从而为准确地诊断克罗恩病提供依据。

肠壁强化最为明显的扫描期相是静脉期，一般为动脉期相后 14 s(45~50 s)时最为明显。肠壁的快速强化在诊断小肠克罗恩病时的敏感性为 80%。肠壁的分层和强化增加意味着透壁性纤维化没有出现，即预示着病变处于活动期。

有关正常的肠壁和病变肠壁强化的程度，Booya 等(2006)研究得出：空肠由于黏膜皱襞较多，血供丰富，强化程度明显高于回肠。正常扩张的空肠强化的峰值 CT 值为(113 ± 26)HU，回肠为(72 ± 13)HU；而在回肠克罗恩病时肠壁强化程度明显增加(CT 值高达 119HU)，正常末端回肠 CT 值为 96HU。另外，肠管塌陷时强化程度略高于正常肠壁强化程度。因此，充分的肠道准备和良好的肠腔扩张在 MSCT 小肠造影检查中尤为重要。

肠周脂肪密度和肠系膜血管的改变：肠周脂肪层的变化：由于病变对肠周脂肪的浸润而导致肠周脂肪密度升高(CT 值如水样密度)，边缘模糊，与肠壁之间的脂肪间隙消失，增强时有不同程度的强化。这种病变常出现在系膜侧，并被认为是需要手术治疗的特征性表现。它的出现是炎症浸润的结果，并在事实上代表了病变的活动期，可以促进炎症的进展。而在肠周脂肪出现纤维化时，则强化不明显，提示病变处于静止期，对病情的判定有重要意义。

病变周围肠系膜血管的改变：病变周围的直小血管明显增多、增粗、扭曲，小的直小血管明显突出，提示 C 反应蛋白增高，加之肠周脂肪增生性堆积使得增多的血管呈梳状排列，即“梳状征”。“梳状征”的出现提示病变处于急性炎症期或较为严重的临床阶段。MSCT 小肠造影在诊断小肠克罗恩病时，“梳状征”和肠周脂肪 CT 值的增高特异性最高。

但是，“梳状征”的出现并不是绝对的特异性征象，在 87% 的系统性红斑狼疮和缺血性肠病患者中也可以出现，但是两者都有急性腹痛病史。此外，在血管炎、绞窄性梗阻、肠系膜血管栓塞以及溃疡中也可出现，必须结合病史进行鉴别诊断。

克罗恩病并发症和肠外病变的 MSCT 小肠造影表现及其诊断价值：克罗恩病的并发症包括肠管周围蜂窝织炎、炎性肿块、脓肿、瘘管、窦道和肠梗阻。与传统的 X 线钡剂造影检查相比，MSCT 小肠造影有着更多的优势。克罗恩病是一种透壁性炎性病变，其溃疡和炎症极易穿透肠壁而形成肠管周围蜂窝织炎和脓肿。如肠壁穿孔，邻近肠管可以形成瘘管，或者病变肠管相互粘连造成肠梗阻。MSCT 小肠造影在发现脓肿、肠管的纠集、跳跃性病变及淋巴结的情况方面准确性极高，优于传统的肠道造影检查，且这些征象通常是外科手术的指征。

蜂窝织炎：70% 的克罗恩病有黏膜或透壁性炎症。由于炎性渗出导致病变肠管周围组织炎性充血而血管增多、增粗，系膜脂肪增生、堆积，形成典型的“梳状征”。肠周脂肪密度增加，增强后有不同程度的强化，邻近肠管受压移位甚至梗阻。多平面重建可以清楚地显示炎症累及的范围。

炎性肿块和脓肿：局限性的蜂窝织炎伴大量的非干酪性肉芽肿形成以及纤维组织增生，可以形成炎性肿块。脓肿常出现在系膜或后腹膜，常与病变肠管相连。MSCT 小肠造影上表现为明显强化的软组织肿块影，边界清晰，周围肠管分离移位。若病程较长，肿块中心坏死明显时则增强后边缘强化明显，中心坏死区不强化。如局部病变较为严重，炎症和溃疡已经穿透肠壁侵犯周围大片蜂窝组织时，病变往往以肿块为主要表现。有作者研究发现，46% 的克罗恩病患者有明显的炎性肿块形成。在炎性肿块明显的病例中常伴有腹膜后淋巴结增大。

瘘管：当炎症穿透邻近的肠管、体表皮肤、膀胱以及阴道等结构时可以形成瘘管。MSCT 小肠造影多平面重建可以较为清晰地显示瘘管的存在。但是肠管之间的内瘘 MSCT 小肠造影常难以发现。当病变肠管与周围组织相互粘连、扭曲，形成大片状蜂窝织炎和炎性肿块时需考虑有瘘管形成的可能性。

当与体表有瘘管形成时，MSCT 小肠造影可以见到与体表之间相连的明显强化的条索状影，如与膀胱、阴道等形成瘘管时则可见膀胱或阴道内有对比剂或气体存在。瘘管的出现提示瘘管周围病变处于活动期，但是肛周脓肿则提示慢性过程。

肠梗阻：40% 的克罗恩病患者可以出现肠管的狭窄或者梗阻，甚至以其为主要或为首发的临床症状。急性期或活动期可因肠壁的明显水肿、痉挛所致，而慢性期则由于纤维组织增生所致。MSCT 小肠造影对梗阻的敏感性和特异性分别为 89% 和 100%。多平面重建能明确梗阻的部位、原因，表现为梗阻上段肠管明显积气、扩张且可见气 - 液平面，梗阻点肠壁明显增厚，强化增加，肠腔明显狭窄。

其他：28% 的病例可以出现全身症状，如肝脏脂肪浸润、胆石症、肾石症、骶髂关节炎、肾积水等。由于 MSCT 小肠造影扫描范围包括整个腹部（膈顶至耻骨联合上缘），因此可方便地观察克罗恩病的这些肠外病变是否存在，为全面了解病情提供依据。

二、MSCT 小肠造影在评价克罗恩病病变的活动性以及临床疗效中的价值

肠壁明显水肿、增厚，强化增加且明显呈分层状改变；明显的蜂窝织炎和炎性肿块、瘘管或窦道形成；“梳状征”的出现；肠周脂肪密度的升高等都预示着病变处于急性期或活动期。当增厚的肠壁明显变薄，强化程度降低，肠周脂肪密度下降，瘘管缩小甚至消失则表示临床治疗取得了较好的效果。

MSCT 小肠造影与其他检查方法比较：常规的消化道造影检查，不能观察肠壁的情况，且图像重叠较多容易遗漏某些病变。小肠镜虽然能取得组织学检查，但是在妊娠、肠腔狭窄、梗阻以及有重要的吞咽困难时禁用，并且检查时操作复杂，检查费用较为昂贵，患者耐受性差。近年来发展较快的胶囊肠镜以患者耐受性较好，其敏感性较高已经越来越多地受到了临床关注，但是其检查费用更为昂贵，发现病变不够清晰且梗阻和狭窄仍然是其禁忌证，肠壁的情况，肠周脂肪层的改变，肠外病变情况在上述检查方法中都是盲区。总之，MSCT 小肠造影检查在小肠克罗恩病的诊断、病情严重情况的判断和临床疗效的评价方面有着重要的临床应用价值。

第十章 胃肠道息肉

第一节 胃肠道息肉病综合征

胃肠道息肉病综合征是一组少见病,分为家族性和非家族性。许多病例有恶变的危险。

一些作者报告 MR 检查 6 例胃肠道息肉病综合征病人中,包含家族性腺瘤性息肉病 3 例,Peutz-Jeghers 综合征 1 例,Gardner 综合征 1 例和神经纤维瘤病 1 例。男 2 例,女 4 例,年龄 37~71 岁,所有病人都进行了胃十二指肠镜、乙状结肠镜或结肠镜检查,2 例病人作了 CT 和钡餐检查,最后诊断均经病理组织学检查所证实。

MR 检查应用 1.5T MR 机,选用以下序列:增强前半傅里叶采集单次激发 RARE,增强前扰相梯度回波(SGE),增强前脂肪抑制扰相梯度回波,增强后立即和 2 分钟后脂肪抑制扰相梯度回波。钆对比剂以 0.1mmol/kg 的剂量快速手推团注。2 例病人(Gardner 综合征和神经纤维瘤病各 1 例)只进行上腹部成像。其余 4 例病人进行上腹、下腹和盆腔成像,其中上腹部仅行增强后立即成像,下腹部只进行增强后延迟成像。所有病人在作 MR 前禁食 6 小时。

研究结果显示,息肉呈局灶性、圆形、基底起于黏膜病变,在增强前 T_1WI 和 T_2WI 上,息肉与肠壁信号强度相等,在增强后立即扫描图像上与肠壁增强程度相同,在增强后 2 分钟脂肪抑制扰相梯度回波图像上信号强度从相等到轻度增高。直径大于 2cm 的息肉在增强后 2 分钟图像上显示轻度不均匀增强。MRI 显示的息肉要比在病理组织学上发现的少。直径小于 1cm 的息肉在 MR 上不一定能见到。胃肠道的其他发现还有,在 Peutz-Jeghers 综合征的病人显示继发于息肉的回肠 - 回肠套叠。

胃肠道外的表现包括:在 1 例家族性腺瘤性息肉病病人发现一个 2.5cm 的肾上腺腺瘤,在神经纤维瘤病病人的右肾上腺发现 1 个 1.5cm 的嗜铬细胞瘤,在 Gardner 综合征病人的

肝脏发现有许多肝转移瘤,直径小于 1cm,在 Peutz-Jeghers 综合征病人发现有继发于右肺非小细胞癌的肝转移和骨转移瘤。在该项研究中,直径 >2.0cm 的息肉一般均能发现,而对于直径 <1.0cm 的息肉则效果差,因而尚不能用 MRI 来发现或排除息肉。该作者观察到的一个重要特征是在钆对比剂增强后的图像上息肉与肠壁有同等程度或稍高的强化,能将息肉与不增强的肠内容相区别。

单次激发 T_2WI 序列可以忽略运动造成的伪影并因此能有效地描述肠壁,息肉在脂肪抑制增强扰相梯度回波图像上呈强化的肠壁肿块,这两种方法相结合增强了显示息肉的能力。

第二节 胃肠道假性息肉

Nelson 等(1975)报告 7 例十二指肠的假性息肉,追踪随访 6 月到 15 年,均未发现十二指肠异常。这些假息肉位于十二指肠上曲凹陷部,一直持续存在,可能是上曲内侧面冗长疏松黏膜的堆积所致。

Bockus(1963)指出,在食管胃连接处狭窄病变的近侧可有食管溃疡性病变,在胃出口梗阻的近侧可有胃的溃疡性病变。Eisenberg 等(1977)报告空肠部分梗阻近侧也可有溃疡性病变,但这与以前已

报告过的食管、胃、回肠及结肠不同，这些溃疡性病变呈显著的结节状，术前 X 线诊断常误为新生物，故称之为溃疡性假息肉，鉴别诊断应包括淋巴瘤、癌和类癌。

结肠的假性息肉出现于克罗恩病，在以往 X 线诊断文献中已引起一些注意，但在一段时间中，并未考虑此征是该病的一个征象。

Wolf 和 Marshak(1962)强调克罗恩病的卵石状黏膜和有蒂的假性息肉之间的差别，考虑真正假性息肉少见于克罗恩病。二大组溃疡性结肠炎与克罗恩结肠炎比较，Stanley 等(1971)发现克罗恩病 32 例中无假性息肉，而 Margulis 等(1971)称在 60 例肉芽肿性结肠炎中 9 例有假性息肉，Welin 和 Welin(1976)在其双对比钡灌肠论著中对溃疡性结肠炎中假息肉的表现详加讨论，但未谈论它们在克罗恩病的表现。Freeman 等(1978)报告 8 例克罗恩病的假性息肉，可分为：局限性多发性假性息肉、局限性大的假性息肉、广泛的假性息肉和长指状假性息肉。其中局限性大的假性息肉可伪装成有绒毛的肿瘤，引起肠梗阻，并导致误诊。事实上，克罗恩病的假性息肉不是少见的征象。Keating 和 Mindell (1976)报告一例溃疡性结肠炎，除钡灌肠可见占位效应外，尚有两点使人疑及肿瘤：扪诊上腹有一包块；逆行灌钡时有部分性肠梗阻征象。仔细观察可见包块处包含许多不规则的条纹状钡剂聚集，似绒毛状腺瘤。事实证明该包块是本症的局限性巨大假性息肉。

第十一章 腹部手术后改变

第一节 Billroth Ⅰ式术后改变

详见本书 本卷 第二十三篇 第十八章 第一节 Billroth Ⅰ式术后改变。

第二节 Billroth Ⅱ式术后改变

详见本书 本卷 第二十三篇 第十八章 第二节 Billroth Ⅱ式术后改变。

第三节 贲门胃底切除术后改变

详见本书 本卷 第二十三篇 第十八章 第三节 贲门胃底切除术后改变。

第四节 全胃切除术后改变

详见本书 本卷 第二十三篇 第十八章 第四节 全胃切除术后改变。

第五节 胰十二指肠切除术后改变

胰十二指肠切除术适用于十二指肠肿瘤，肝外胆管胰腺段癌，胆胰管十二指肠连接区癌及胰头癌等，主要有胰十二指肠切除术（Whipple 术）、保留胃和幽门的胰十二指肠切除术（PPPD 术）以及扩大的胰十二指肠切除术。Whipple 术切除范围一般包括远端部分胃、十二指肠、胰头部及胆总管下端，PPPD 术保留了胃的正常生理功能，肠胃反流受到部分阻止，改善了营养状况，不必行胃部分切除，十二指肠空肠吻合较简单，缩短了手术时间。

Whipple 术后小肠与胰头吻合，小肠可以向胰头部聚集，有时小肠聚集成团，不要误认为肿瘤，可以行增强扫描，并向下逐层观察，可见与小肠相延续，并可以看到小肠黏膜结构。

第六节 术后缺损或术后假肿瘤

术后缺损或术后假肿瘤亦可引起误诊。影像诊断医师应熟悉区别活动性十二指肠溃疡与幽门成形术后外凸。最常见的术后假肿瘤是 Nissen 胃底摺叠术后在胃底形成的，该手术是将胃底环绕包围食管末端，以作为对抗胃食管反流的措施，在 X 线平片上则显示为胃底一软块，不应混淆于胃底的平滑肌瘤、胃后壁增厚或含气的脓肿。与此相似，术后盲肠腔中内弯的阑尾残端，勿误为盲肠息肉，该残端特征性地位于回盲瓣下方和盲肠内侧壁。如手术后感染，导管或引流管留置，可造成局限性凸出或线结区，类似于胃肠道感染或溃疡，这在胃造瘘术后最为常见。

第七节 近期造口、吻合术等造成的误诊

外科手术如胃十二指肠吻合术（Biliroth Ⅰ）、胃空肠吻合术（Biliroth Ⅱ）、回结肠吻合术以及包括胆管系统在内的其他类型吻合术，一般不会造成误诊。但在 Biliroth Ⅱ式手术的病人，十二指肠如未充填对比剂，则会与胰头肿块相混淆。空肠和结肠造口术 CT 上很易识别，尤其是静脉注射或口服对比剂时。但在回肠造口术后或回肠膀胱吻合术后，如肠管未充填对比剂，则可被误诊为脓肿或积液。

第十二章　腹部淋巴结及肿瘤转移

第一节　淋巴结转移是胃癌转移的主要方式

淋巴结转移是胃癌转移的主要方式。一项研究以淋巴结直径 >5 mm 作为诊断标准,主要在于淋巴结标准设定过大会造成小的转移淋巴结的漏诊,而过小则造成非转移淋巴结的高估及淋巴结检出困难。文献报道直径 5 mm 以下淋巴结的检出率仅 1.1%,且转移率极低(5.1%);5 mm 以上淋巴结检出率在 45.1% 以上,且转移率在 69% 以上。该组作者对直径 5 mm 以上的淋巴结重点观察,同时结合淋巴结的强化、形态作为诊断标准。该组 CT 对淋巴结转移的诊断准确性为 78.9%,与病理分期一致性良好(P<0.05)。20 例 N0 中 CT 准确诊断 15 例,5 例 CT 示胃周孤立淋巴结,直径约 5~8 mm 且有强化,CT 误诊为有淋巴结转移而高估为 N1,术后病理为非转移淋巴结,其中 4 例为中分化腺癌,1 例低分化腺癌。

11 例 N1 中 6 例 CT 诊断正确,2 例 CT 未发现肿大淋巴结而低估为 N0,但术后病理显示胃周有转移淋巴结;1 例转移淋巴结与肿块融合,CT 误诊为肿块的一部分而低估为 N0;2 例血管旁淋巴结直径 8~12 mm 且轻度强化,CT 误诊为淋巴结转移而高估为 N2,但术后病理证实为非淋巴结转移。26 例 N2 中 CT 正确诊断 24 例,2 例术后病理证实血管旁多发小淋巴结转移,术前 CT 仅检出 1~2 个淋巴结,且认为其直径 <5 mm 而判断非转移淋巴结,该病例为低分化腺癌。

该组病例分析显示:血管周围的淋巴结对比显示明显、检出率较高,而病灶旁淋巴结往往与肿块融合不易分辨,该组 1 例淋巴结误诊为是肿块的一部分而漏诊,因此诊断时一定要注意肿块邻近有无可疑淋巴结。

另外,消瘦患者腹部脂肪少,淋巴结对比显示不明显,扫描时多改变患者体位有助于提高淋巴结的检出率。一些伴有长期胃炎的胃癌患者可出现淋巴结炎性肿大,一般炎性肿大淋巴结无强化或轻度强化,但个别病例出现明显强化时,与转移淋巴结鉴别困难,该组 7 例炎性淋巴结误诊为转移淋巴结。

一般认为,转移淋巴结多肿大明显且有强化,淋巴结短 / 长径之比≥ 0.7,或呈蚕蚀状、囊状、花斑状、串珠状、团状,或侵犯包绕血管;然而早期癌浸润的淋巴结或强化不明显的孤立小淋巴结,CT 鉴别仍很困难。

第二节　淋巴结和淋巴滤泡的发育变异

一组作者发现,在腹股沟、髂外、髂总、主动脉旁及下腔静脉旁淋巴结等处的正常淋巴结的大小,变异很大,一般很少大于 3cm,多呈卵圆形,长径与身体长轴平行,边缘锐利,内部结构呈细颗粒状,但在腹股沟及远端的髂外组淋巴结常由于慢性炎症呈现不规则充盈缺损,淋巴门处亦可因脂肪沉积造成充盈缺损,不应误为异常。

另有学者报告一例成人结肠淋巴滤泡的内窥镜所见。这些淋巴滤泡通常不为内窥镜看见,然而,在结肠黑变病,它们则可异乎寻常地突出,表现为细小白色结节,直径约 1 mm。这考虑为发育变异。此种表现偶尔可在成人结肠双对比钡剂检查时看见。

第十三章 腹盆部其他疾病

第一节 消化道出血的常见病因及其DSA诊断

消化道出血的发病率为(17~144)/10万人，消化道疾病及全身性疾病均可引起。

大量出血者，除有呕血、血便外，同时伴有因血容量减少而导致的周围循环衰竭而危及生命。临床常见的病因有消化性溃疡、食管贲门黏膜撕裂综合征、Dieulafoy病、血管畸形、憩室、息肉、肿瘤、弥漫性溃疡性结肠炎、外伤、重症急性胰腺炎以及医源性损伤等。

胃肠钡餐、内镜、放射性核素扫描及胶囊内镜在不同时期、不同方面对动脉性消化道出血的诊断均起到了重要作用。消化道钡餐检查能较好显示腔内占位性或明显外压性病变，但不能显示黏膜下的血管病变，并要求在出血静止期检查，限制了其在处理急症患者时的应用。纤维内镜检查最直观，其阳性检查结果对引导选择性血管造影检查及介入治疗有积极的意义，但当出血量比较大时，肠腔内充满血液，内镜的使用就受到限制。

ECT核素扫描在定性诊断方面最敏感，出血量在0.05~0.12 ml/min时即可测出，并且由于^{99m}Tc在血液循环中滞留的时间长，检查时间跨度长，故适用于一些间隙性或少量消化道出血的患者，其最大缺点是不能精确定位，对下一步治疗的指导意义有限。

血管造影检查通过显示对比剂外溢及肠腔内的对比剂异常集聚等消化道出血的直接征象，或通过判断导致出血的基础病变的供血动脉来源进行定位诊断，是对消化道出血进行定位的最直观的检查方法。

Nussbaum等(1963)经动物实验表明，当出血量达到0.5 ml/min以上，选择性血管造影即能显示对比剂外溢征象而明确出血部位。同时，血管造影还能显示基础病变异常血管的形态、分布、大小、范围及其与周围血管及器官的关系等间接征象，借此推测病变的性质，进行定性诊断。更重要的是，在血管造影检查发现了出血灶之后，在无相关禁忌证的情况下能够立即实行介入治疗止血，迅速改善失血症状。

与常规血管造影方法相比较，DSA对显示血管结构具有独到的优势。它利用同一部位造影前后2次成像相减原理，避免了非血管组织的重叠，单独显示血管结构，也可清晰显示一些常规造影不易发现的小病灶，更有利于介入栓塞治疗时的定位。

同时，每秒时间内多幅采集技术使对比剂在血管内呈一个动态显影过程，充分地显示动脉、毛细血管及回流静脉，对血管内对比剂外溢、静脉早显等异常征象的实时观察特别有利。连续的血管造影图像，可清晰显示肿瘤的供血动脉及引流静脉，肿瘤血管，肿瘤染色，肿块与邻近血管及脏器的关系，从而进行可能的定性诊断。

由于肿瘤性病变最终需要外科手术根治，在介入处理过程中，还可以在靶血管放置弹簧圈或其他标志物，为外科医师手术提供可靠的导向信息。

对于血管畸形，DSA能够清晰显示出异常血管团的形态特征和病变范围，明确有无静脉早显。动脉瘤血管造影表现一般比较典型，可使荷瘤血管呈卵圆形扩张，或者囊袋状偏于动脉壁一侧。更重要的是，多角度的DSA检查能够全面了解动脉瘤与荷瘤动脉的关系，清晰显示瘤蒂，以指导治疗方案的制订。

DSA对肿瘤性疾病和血管性疾病等异常血管的检出率较高，而对消化道炎性病变、憩室及息肉等检出率相对偏低，导致定性诊断困难。

为提高动脉性消化道出血的血管造影检出率，

应综合分析临床症状和在血管造影检查前进行的其他检查,针对最有可能出血的血管进行超选择插管造影。通过导管对靶血管灌注扩血管药物,行药物性血管造影也有助于异常血管的发现。另外,在出血活动期进行血管造影检查,尽量避免临床止血药物的干预,亦能提高出血的检出率。

第二节 胃肠出血的部分原因

主动脉 - 肠瘘极为少见,主要出现于腹主动脉的动脉瘤,多继发于腹主动脉手术后。

在大量胃肠出血的鉴别诊断中,此瘘应考虑为原因之一。此瘘的病因学讨论包括动脉硬化、霉菌性动脉瘤、梅毒性动脉瘤和创伤后动脉瘤,腹腔内或腹膜后新生物,偶尔为非特异性感染或直接创伤所致。手术后出现的瘘已报告见于主动脉手术后或腹部血管手术后感染。

大多数瘘都出现于动脉瘤与十二指肠之间,Ammann 等(1973)报告 4 例,其中 1 例曾行胃切除术,1 例瘘位于动脉瘤与乙状结肠之间,此症预后不良。

新生儿上消化道出血较少见,大约有一半病儿无器质性改变或凝血障碍。一般说来,食管炎、胃炎、食管溃疡或应激性溃疡、及出血性素质已知为上消化道出血的常见原因。

Cairo 等(1981)首例报告了胃畸胎瘤引起的反复上消化道出血。随后又出现胃排空障碍。腹部 X 线平片示一大钙化性包块使充气胃轮廓外移,触诊为硬而固定无触痛包块。钙化块中有一下颌骨伴存牙结构。超声见平段波混杂密集波,手术切除证实为 10cm × 15cm × 10cm 大的良性畸胎瘤。畸胎瘤常见出现在骨盆、纵隔、腹膜后和颈部,约有 1/3~1/2 具有钙化。

胃的畸胎瘤占小儿畸胎瘤不到 1%,几乎总是良性,它常位于大弯,且男孩多于女孩。该例颇为少见,因其引起上消化道出血,且部位又在小弯,而又是新生女婴。

胃静脉曲张的诊断常有困难,上消化道钡餐检查,甚至内镜都可将胃黏膜皱襞的突起或恶性病变误诊为静脉曲张。Marshall 等(1978)在胃底发现有黏膜皱襞突起或肿块 3 例,其中 2 例皆为钡餐和胃镜误诊,而通过 X 线血管造影及脾门静脉造影确诊。食管静脉曲张的存在,提示可疑及胃静脉曲张。

第三节 胃肠和肠系膜的创伤

在经手术的腹部钝伤病人中,小肠和肠系膜损伤者约占 50%。腔内血管破裂可引起致命的出血,可因为小肠破裂引起腹膜炎。CT 对于小肠和肠系膜损伤的检测很准确。

腹膜内或腹膜后肠腔外气体的显示被认为是小肠破裂的特殊征象,但是比较少见。

小肠破裂的特殊 CT 征象是口服阳性对比剂的外漏。肠壁增厚、中断和肠系膜血肿是小肠损伤的可靠征象。其他 CT 征象包括异常小肠壁增厚和静脉注入对比剂后 CT 值的升高。CT 图像上肠系膜损伤可显示肠系膜的褶间积液(即小肠系膜间积液)。小肠和系膜损伤均可见褶间积液。

胃破裂常发生于饱餐后胃的钝性创伤。常见于儿童。胃前壁最易破裂,其次是胃大弯、胃小弯,最不易破裂的是胃后壁。许多病人创伤位于左侧,最常见于累及脾的创伤。从鼻胃管中可以引流出浓稠的血液。气腹、口服对比剂和胃内容物的外漏均可在 CT 上显示。

十二指肠的钝性创伤通常累及第 2 或第 3 段,十二指肠穿孔和十二指肠血肿的鉴别诊断在临床上非常重要。因为十二指肠穿孔需行急诊手术。而血肿常保守治疗。

十二指肠破裂腔外积气或对比剂外溢见于腹膜后肾周间隙的右前方,并常向腹膜后的其他地方散开。当穿孔靠近屈氏(Treitz)韧带时,在腹腔内也可以见口服对比剂或气体。

十二指肠血肿病人 CT 扫描显示十二指肠壁内块影(血肿),并压向十二指肠腔内。十二指肠血肿的临床表现也很有帮助,因为这些病人由于十二指肠腔阻塞而引起呕吐。十二指肠损伤常伴发胰腺损伤，必须仔细地检查胰腺。

固定点处或固定点附近的空肠和回肠常受伤，如屈氏韧带或回盲瓣。破裂时可见口服对比剂外渗，十二指肠壁增厚、水肿以及在脂肪密度的肠袋之间轨道样积血。破裂多见于肠系膜缘。结肠损伤往往由上腹部挤压伤所致。最常见的损伤位置是横结肠、乙状结肠和盲肠。横结肠的损伤可以引起肌间血肿和没有肠内容物外渗的浆膜撕裂。结肠撕裂伤可发生结肠肠系膜和血管损伤，这些会影响该部分结肠的血运。发生于侧方或是背侧的损伤要进行腹部 CT 三维显示以显示直肠至大肠。病情稳定的腹膜后刺伤病人如果没有结肠穿透伤，可保守治疗。一旦显示结肠穿孔，则需手术治疗。

腹部创伤病人的腹腔肠外积气征象常由于小肠破裂引起，X 线片上显示游离气体是紧急剖腹术的指征之一。然而，在许多钝性创伤病人，CT 虽显示有腔外游离气体但并没有小肠破裂。有研究报道 18 例钝性创伤的 CT 扫描结果，只有 4 例（约占 22%）被证明有小肠破裂。另有研究报道 118 例钝性创伤的腹部 CT 扫描，7 例见到游离的腔外积气，但均无小肠穿透伤。在这两项研究中所有气腹的病人几乎都有胸部创伤，有气胸或机械通气。这意味着空气可能由胸腔进入了腹腔。

口服对比剂对于小肠损伤的 CT 诊断尤为重要，能证明小肠破裂，可更好地显示小肠壁增厚，并能鉴别小肠褶间的液体。小肠对比剂对于胰腺创伤的诊断也有帮助，可衬托胰周水肿或出血。

绝大多数放射科医生都认为常规使用口服对比剂是非常安全的。有研究报道 506 例使用口服和静脉对比剂的腹部创伤 CT 扫描，均未对 CT 扫描产生影响。

腹部钝性创伤可形成肠系膜撕裂伤，继而引起严重的出血和血容量减少。CT 扫描在血腹的病人可以显示肠系膜的血肿形成。

静脉注射对比剂的外漏征可以显示活动性出血的位置。撕裂能影响一段肠的血供而产生局部缺血，严重时可发生肠坏死和腹膜炎。血行阻断的小肠在 CT 上显示为水肿，此时动脉供血完好而肠系膜引流静脉回流受阻。

肠系膜的小撕裂伤起初也许没有临床征象，但不久会有局部小肠梗阻的表现。微小的肠系膜损伤在 CT 上可能仅表现为肠系膜的线征或模糊样改变，代表肠系膜的小血肿或出血。

第四节　胃肠道内异物

胃肠道内的异物，在胃肠双对比造影检查时最易见到是未消化的食物，胃内小块食物粘附胃壁上，其影像与胃息肉难以区分。

未消化的食物，诸如豆芽、豌豆等可见于肠道远端，引起混淆。国外一作者曾报导一例胃肠双对比检查病人，检查前曾食中国菜，检查见回盲部出现多个丝状充盈缺损，误为感染性肠病的息肉（亦为纤维状、丝状充盈缺损），事后证实为食入豆芽所致。

在结肠内粘连的粪便必须与息肉及肿瘤鉴别，前已述及，我们即曾见过将盲肠内粘附的粪结误为盲肠癌施行手术的病例。

熟悉无柄性息肉的特征性表现“投球手帽”征，对于区别息肉与粪便大有帮助。

偶尔，肠内的气泡与黏液条也可引起医师的疑虑，如不注意，则导致误诊。

第五节　误诊病例简介:肠系膜、网膜及淋巴结结核与小肠间质瘤

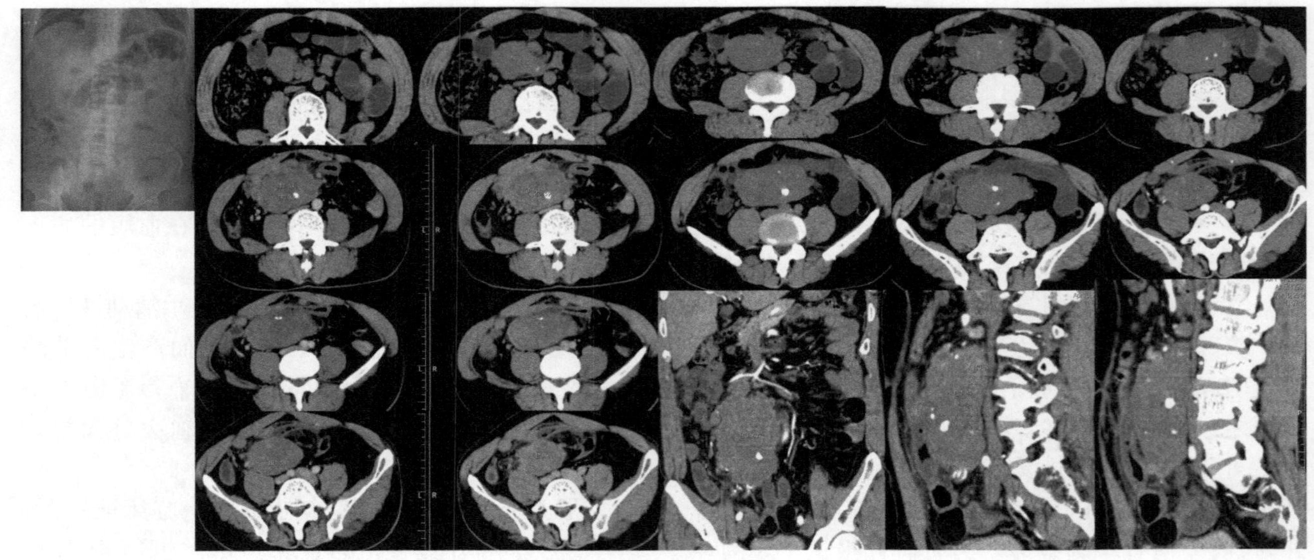

图 22-13-1　肠系膜、网膜及淋巴结结核与小肠间质瘤

患者,男, 57 岁。因腹痛伴肛门停止排气、排便 1 天入院。

手术所见:腹腔少量腹水。肿块位于小肠系膜,距回盲部 15cm,侵犯至浆膜外,与周围肠管粘连缠绕,其中一处肠管与腹壁粘连,游离后,可见直径 1cm × 2cm 灰绿色穿孔灶,考虑穿孔后与腹壁粘连,大网膜及腹膜可见多发白色质硬结节,考虑转移灶。遂行肠系膜肿块切除术和胆囊切除术。

免疫组化检测:阳性: PAS 染色(散在 +),抗酸染色(散在 +),CD68(组织细胞 +),CD163(组织细胞 +),SMA(间质纤维 +), Actin(间质纤维 +), Ki-67(+,约 10%);阴性:CD34,CD117,DOG1,Desmin,S-100,H-caldesmon。免疫组化诊断:腹腔肠系膜肿物及大网膜切除标本:结合免疫组化、组织化学染色检测结果及 HE 组织学图像,符合肠系膜、网膜及淋巴结结核,建议临床完善结核杆菌相关检测以进一步佐证(图 22-13-1)。

第六节　胃肠道充盈缺损较难见到的原因

生殖器官的转移肿瘤:在十二指肠,出现其他器官的转移肿瘤实为罕见,Ngan(1970)报告 4 例十二指肠梗阻均为生殖器官的转移肿瘤所致, 3 例为淋巴播散犯及主动脉旁淋把结,从而产生梗阻的 X 线征象, 1 例为十二指肠第一段的孤立性包块,后者虽然不能排除横结肠播散,但该作者指出,这似为卵巢肿瘤血性转移最好的例证。

感染性纤维性息肉:感染性纤维性息肉,又称嗜伊红肉芽肿,原发于胃者少见,偶见于小肠,侵犯大肠者罕见,后者常伪似结肠癌,在 X 线检查和手术诊断上多令人左右为难。胃肠道的感染性纤维性息肉的病因学尚未明确,这些新生物考虑与弥漫性嗜伊红细胞浸润不一样,它们与肠的嗜伊红肉芽肿无关,也不伴随骨的嗜伊红肉芽肿。Morson 和 Dauson(1979)喜欢感染性纤维性息肉这个名字,因为嗜伊红肉芽肿另外含意是组织细胞病 X 的一部分。

自从 Vanek(1949)报告 6 例本症犯及胃者以来,息肉犯及胃与小肠者已有少量个案介绍,大肠受累者太少,X 线诊断文献上仅几例报告。 Matsuzaki 等(1979)和 Zimmerman(1977)各报告 1 例,一为

升结肠，一为横结肠，X 线照片表现皆酷似结肠新生物。Ferin 和 Skucas(1983)报告 1 例，尽管病人甚为年轻，根据气钡双对比结肠检查仍考虑为结肠腺癌，它为一浸润性病变，位于近侧横结肠，伴存较大的腔内赘生物，组织学证实为本症。息肉小时无蒂，逐渐长大时出现蒂，息肉起于黏膜下，可发生溃疡和出血，其结缔组织基质为嗜伊红细胞与浆细胞浸润，而小动脉为幼稚的成成纤维细胞环绕。

乙状结肠巨大囊肿：乙状结肠巨大囊肿极为少见，尽管它常交通于肠道，在活体仍难以观察和确诊。多数囊肿发现于伴有憩室病者，位于乙状结肠曲的反系膜缘。囊肿通常为孤立的，不与周围其他结构(如膀胱)交通。临床体征与症状无特异性。在组织学上，囊肿为浆膜和一个致密的外层，血管胶原组织覆盖。未见报告有上皮被覆者，但能发现某些平滑肌纤维。病因学不明，肠重复不像是原因，因为病变最常见于 60 岁以上；局部脓肿形成伴随后的慢性囊肿出现可能是其病因。Barratt(1971)讨论了此类病例。

人工全髋置换术所使用的结合剂：Switzer 等(1974)报告一例乙状结肠暂时性腔外的充盈缺损，乃为人工全髋置换术所使用的结合剂造成的。此缺损在手术后即刻出现，当手术野水肿与出血时，缺损则更为明显。如有不透 X 线的物质附加于结合剂上，病因诊断则更明确。

回盲瓣黏膜皱襞过多：当回盲瓣黏膜皱襞过多而形成一唇状突起时，可造成回盲瓣的逆行性脱垂。此突起的瓣在盲肠内产生一充盈缺损。用于扪压或 / 和依靠钡柱的静水压力，凸出的回盲瓣逆行脱垂，造成回肠末端逐渐变尖。瓣装置的这些变化能伴装为病理情况，然而细心地观察可辨别此类变异。

回盲瓣逆行脱垂首先由 Rigler 和 Lasser(1951)报告，钡灌肠检查时，在盲肠内可见一光滑的圆形充盈缺损，此缺损颇为柔软，扪压能改变其形状，用手扪压或 / 和钡柱的静水压，减轻盲肠内的充盈缺损，造成末端回肠的环状缺损。这些征象容易复制，空气造影时更为明显。结肠镜检查有助诊断，手术证实诊断。此症为良性，唇状突起处可见溃疡，为胃肠出血的一个原因。

鉴别诊断有淋巴瘤可产生套迭进入盲肠：回盲瓣的原发性腺癌甚少见，但也可出现类似套迭；回盲瓣类癌慢性套迭也有个案介绍。瓣的逆行脱垂性质柔软，容易脱垂于末端回肠内或外，瓣连接处无肠梗阻。回盲瓣脂肪过多在盲肠内产生一个巨大的压迫，然而真性脂肪过多很少出现逆行脱垂，脂肪过多者瓣的脂肪沉着远远多于本症。

第七节　胃肠淋巴增生呈现少见的脐样息肉病变

详见本书 本卷 本篇 第七章 第六节 胃肠淋巴增生呈现少见的脐样息肉病变。

第二十三篇　胃的疾病

第一章　胃癌术前分期

第一节　MSCT 对胃癌分期误诊病例分析简介(过度分期与分期不足)

一组 41 例的影像分析结果显示，2 位医生判定结果相当一致，医生甲对 80%(33 例)的胃癌浸润情况进行了正确评价，医生乙为 85%(35 例)。前者通过 MSCT 判定胃癌浆膜浸润的敏感度、特异度和准确度分别为 90%、95% 和 93%，后者分别为 80%、97% 和 93%。全部病例中，医生甲做出假阴性诊断 1 例，医生乙 2 例。

11 例病人未被正确分期，其中 6 例过度分期，5 例分期不足(均为硬癌)。

对于 T_1 期肿瘤，医生甲正确分期 13 例，医生乙正确分期 15 例。17 例组织学诊断为 T_1 期肿瘤中，2 例因 CT 表现为突出肿块，伴整个胃壁增厚或浆膜面不规则，强化明显，而由 2 位医生均判定为 T_2 或 T_3 期肿瘤；2 例因肿块与胃大弯侧巨大黏膜皱襞混淆被医生甲过度分期为 T_2 期肿瘤。

T_2 期肿瘤，14 例中 12 例被正确分期，其中 1 例因条带样影自胃外表面延伸至周围脂肪间隙而过度分为 T_3 期。1 例虽胃壁显示清楚但强化不明显而分期不足。

T_3 期肿瘤，8 例中 6 例被正确分期，1 例因位于胃窦后壁，与胰体边界不清而被医生甲过度分期，另 1 例因胃壁外表面显示光滑而被 2 位医生分期不足。

T_4 期肿瘤，2 例均被正确分期。

该项课题作者指出，MSCT 对胃癌的术前分期是一种非常有价值的方法，特别是在对胃癌浆膜浸润程度的评价中具有很高的准确度。

第二节　国际抗癌联盟及美国癌症联合会胃癌 TNM 分期系统(第 8 版)影像相关更新解读

国际抗癌联盟及美国癌症联合会(UICC/AJCC)胃癌 TNM 分期是国际通用的胃癌分期系统，是临床制定胃癌治疗方案、评估预后的重要依据和参考标准，根据临床诊疗进展间隔 4~6 年更新一次。

2016 年 10 月，第 8 版新分期系统发布，其中胃癌的最大变化是在前版单一病理分期(pTNM)的基础上，划分出了临床分期(cTNM)和新辅助治疗后分期(ypTNM)2 个新系统，并对其应用范围和规范进行了初步界定，构建出 3 个分期系统并存的新格局。其目的在于更好地适应肿瘤临床个体化精准医疗的需求以及多学科诊疗协作组(multidisciplinary team，MDT)的推广。

在临床实际操作过程中，当患者确诊胃癌(通常通过内镜活检病理)后，下一步不可避免地要借助临床分期手段判断肿瘤发展程度，指导初始治疗决策；由于缺乏高级别的文献证据及官方分期标准，在第 7 版及以前的胃癌分期系统中，临床医师只能将病理分期(pStage)套用于临床分期(cStage)。

但这种“套用”的问题在于：将显微镜下离体标本的病理特征，直接套用到成像原理不同、分辨率不在一个量级的活体影像学临床分期，缺乏相关依据，使得二者的准确对应成为长久困扰胃癌影像学的难题。

此外，两种分期手段间隔的时滞效应，也会导致 pStage 应用的误差(如接受术前治疗的患者或评估与治疗间隙出现转移的患者等）。简单将病理分期套用于临床分期可能导致分期错误，继而导致后续治疗决策的偏差。鉴于此，结合美国国家癌症数据库和日本静冈癌症中心的 4 091 例胃癌患者数据，第 8 版分期根据胃癌综合治疗特点，划分出了 cTNM 和 ypTNM 2 个新系统，并对其应用范围和规范进行了概述，其中涉及较多的是影像学部分。此处对第 8 版胃癌分期涉及影像学的相关内容更新进行解读。

应用手段选择：胃癌分期依赖的手段包括物理检查、实验室检查、影像学检查、内镜（包括超声内镜（EUS）及细针穿刺）及活检、诊断性腹腔镜探查（包括腹腔灌洗细胞学检查）等。EUS 和 CT（胸部 + 腹部 + 盆腔、口服对比剂、增强扫描）应作为 cTNM 分期的初始影像学手段，PET/CT 和 MRI 可作为进一步精确分期应用的补充手段。

cT 分期：尽管新版分期系统划分出了独立的 cT 分期，但具体分期规定仍沿用病理分期的浸润深度标准。目前影像学诸手段受到分辨率的限制，尚无法准确区分胃壁的 5 层结构（黏膜层、黏膜下层、肌层、浆膜下层、浆膜层），也就难以准确判断癌肿浸润的深度，尤其是菲薄的浆膜层基本无法显示，导致 T_3 和 T_4a 鉴别困难。

第 8 版分期中提到 EUS 有较高的 cT 分期符合率，并在分期应用中作为重点推荐，但根据之前的 Meta 分析结果，EUS 与 CT 的 T 分期准确率差别并不大。2012 年一项 Meta 分析结果显示，CT 胃癌 T 分期准确率为 75%~85%；同期一项关于 EUS 胃癌分期的 Meta 分析显示，EUS 胃癌 T 分期准确率为 75%。在临床实践中，CT 以其简便快捷、经济无创的优势成为胃癌治疗前 T 分期的主要手段。我国在相当一段时期内，CT 可能仍是较多医院唯一可依靠的胃癌治疗前 cT 分期的手段。

第 8 版分期的亮点之一是首次规定了各影像学手段（主要是 EUS 和 CT）在胃癌 cT 分期的操作流程和分期规范。EUS 应用配备多频环扫探头（5.0 MHz、7.5 MHz、10.0 MHz、12.0 MHz）的机型，并简要介绍了操作顺序流程、正常胃壁各层的信号特征及各 cT 分期的征象特点。

所提及的 CT 操作规范包括：①保证胃腔的充分充盈和胃壁扩张；②口服阴性对比剂；③静注注射对比剂多期增强；④多平面重建（MPR）。其中前 3 项是关于前处置和扫描的，旨在得到形态稳定、对比鲜明的胃癌断层图像；最后 1 项则是诊断相关的，因胃癌可沿胃壁 360° 环周生长，仅仅观察轴面图像可能遗漏重要分期征象，故多平面观察在胃癌的诊断和分期中意义重大。

一般认为胃癌 CT 至少需要观察轴面、冠面和矢状面三平面图像，以消除部分容积效应干扰，利于对癌肿浸润胃壁深度的全面、准确观察，及对胃癌侵犯周围脏器的客观评判（如结合矢状面评价胰腺及横结肠侵犯，结合冠状面评价膈肌及肝门侵犯）。

目前国内胃癌 CT 检查提供给临床 MPR 图像的较少，第 8 版分期明确提出 MPR 在胃癌分期的重要性，对于今后的规范化推广具有指南意义。

在分期征象方面，第 8 版分期明确规定了从 cT_1 到 cT_4 各分期的 EUS 征象，但对 CT 征象却只字未提，说明目前胃癌 CT 分期征象尚无统一标准，影像科医师今后在具体操作中仍会面临无指南标准可用的尴尬与挑战，但同时也带来了开展临床研究的新机遇。

近年来围绕胃癌侵出浆膜的判断（cT_3 和 cT_4a）就出现一些分量较高的征象研究，如浆膜侧高强化亮线征用和断层表盘分区法等，胃癌的 CT 分期征象不断完善。第 8 版分期的另一重大变化是将 cT_4b 划分到了Ⅳ A 期，而 pT_4b 仍为Ⅲ期。

结合影像学特征分析，确诊为 cT_4b 的患者多属晚期，侵犯胰腺等周围脏器的同时往往也伴有肝胃韧带、横结肠系膜等周围系膜、韧带、腹膜等结构的浸润和播散，相当部分实际已为Ⅳ期，无法切除。

另一方面，基于 cT_4b 的分期提升，影像学 cT_4b 的判断应该更加严格，对于部分小面积接触或仅是脂肪间隙消失者，多数实际并无侵犯，为避免过度分为Ⅳ期，不宜再作为 cT_4b 考虑。

cN 分期：在解剖描述部分，第 8 版分期明确将远隔（非局域）淋巴结的转移定义为远处转移（M1）而不属于 N 分期，包括胰后、胰十二指肠、胰周、肠系膜上、中结肠、腹主动脉旁及腹膜后淋巴结。影像评估时应注意区分判断。

第 8 版分期规定影像医师应报告伴有恶性征象的肿大淋巴结的数目，同时提出需经 MDT 的复核。本版分期明确提出淋巴结短径 >10 mm 作为可疑转移考虑，对之前不同研究采纳指标（长径或短径）及标准（8~12 mm）的不同进行了统一。

既往 Meta 分析结果显示，EUS 和 CT 判断胃癌 cN 分期的准确率均在 65% 左右的较低水平。第 8

版分期中也提到目前缺乏高证据级别的 cN 分期研究文献，故在 cN 分期时需联合大小、形态和数目 3 个指标进行综合评判，但未给出可供临床操作参考的阈值标准。受到分辨率的限制，目前 CT 难以准确评价直径 5 mm 以下小淋巴结的转移情况，而这部分淋巴结又占据了胃癌转移淋巴结的 1/2 以上。因此，无论联合数目、形态、强化情况等多种指标，或应用能谱 CT 等功能影像学手段，抑或联合各种生物学行为指标建立人工智能模型进行评价，目前均难以解决 cN 分期水平不高的临床现状。

cM 分期：除了上述提及将远隔（非局域）淋巴结转移定为 M_1，胃癌最常见的远处转移位置是腹膜和肝脏。EUS 对远处转移的判断能力有限，仅可观察胃周围器官的病变情况。胸、腹、盆部 CT 是 cM 分期的常用手段，MRI 次之。PET/CT 能够提高 CT 漏检病灶的检出，可应用于 CT 及 MRI 定性困难的病灶。腹腔镜探查联合腹腔灌洗细胞学检查是诊断胃癌腹膜转移的相对可靠手段，可用于确认影像检查未发现的隐匿性转移病灶，第 8 版分期推荐用于 cT_3 以上分期胃癌患者，以及 CT 或 PET 可疑腹膜结节的患者。

综上所述，第 8 版分期划分出 cTNM 和 ypTNM 两个新分期系统，介绍了相关影像学操作流程和规范，提出了规范化前处置、扫描及多平面重建的意义，对相关分期指标和标准进行了初步规定，并对临床 cT_4b 进行了不同于病理 pT_4b 的分期划分。

尽管该版本仍未对影像学尤其 CT 分期征象作出指南规定，无法直接指导临床分期，但作为个体化精准医疗和 MDT 时代背景下的过渡版本，其纲领指向意义高于实用价值，从官方角度为胃癌影像学的临床实践和未来研究方向提供了框架和指引。

第 8 版分期的新变化对影像医师提出了新的挑战，同时也为胃癌影像学带来新的发展机遇；有实力的胃癌研究中心可借助新分期改版提供的机遇，通过大样本及多中心影像学分期研究，推出真正适合临床的 cTNM 分期系统，在胃癌个体化精准医疗中发挥更大作用。

第二章 胃癌分型

胃癌的 Borrmann 分型

胃癌的 Borrmann 分型是由德国病理学家 Borrmann（1926）提出的一种分型方法，主要根据肿瘤在黏膜面的形态特征、外生性和内生性的比例将胃癌分为 4 型：Ⅰ型（结节型），肿瘤向腔内生长，呈息肉状，基底较宽，境界较清楚，溃疡少见，但可有小的糜烂，此型最少见；Ⅱ型（溃疡局限型），肿瘤有较大的溃疡形成，边缘隆起明显，境界较清楚，向周围浸润不明显；Ⅲ型（浸润溃疡型），肿瘤有明显的溃疡形成，边缘部分隆起，部分被浸润破坏，境界不清，向周围浸润较明显，癌组织在黏膜下浸润的范围超过肉眼所见的肿瘤边界，是最为多见的类型；Ⅳ型（弥漫浸润型），呈弥漫性浸润生长，难以确定肿瘤边界，由于癌细胞弥漫浸润及纤维组织增生，致胃壁增厚、僵硬，称“皮革胃”。

Borrmann 分型是胃癌经典的分型方法。1999 年日本胃癌学会（JGCA）制定了新的分类规范，将胃癌分类体系扩大至 6 型，其中将浅表型胃癌定义为 0 型，而将难以分类的胃癌归入 5 型范畴，并在表达进展期胃癌时略去 Borrmann 前缀。2003 年巴黎浅表胃肠肿瘤国际会议亦推荐了该分型标准。

溃疡型胃癌Ⅱ型与Ⅲ型：溃疡型胃癌Ⅱ型与Ⅲ型的 MSCT 表现均可见胃壁增厚，肿块中形成大小、深浅不一的凹陷，多见于胃体和胃窦部，凹陷边缘明显隆起呈堤状。Ⅱ型癌病变范围较局限，胃壁增厚明显，平均 1.5 cm，Ⅲ型胃癌增厚胃壁常呈山坡样起伏，平均厚度约 1cm。Ⅱ型癌边界清楚，呈盘状，常有大而深的溃疡，一组Ⅱ型病例溃疡深度平均 1.3 cm，Ⅲ型癌溃疡平均深度 0.8 cm，可见Ⅱ型癌胃壁增厚较Ⅲ型癌明显，溃疡更深。

增强后增厚胃壁内层呈线状明显强化，门脉期强化区域逐渐扩大直至完全强化，这是进展期胃癌强化的特点，结节状环堤呈不规则团块状强化。

堤壁角：堤壁角是指环堤与胃壁的夹角，它取决于癌周浸润，癌周如无浸润则呈直角或锐角，堤壁角 ≤ 90º，癌周明显浸润则呈斜坡状，堤壁角 >90º，这也是 Borrmann Ⅱ型与Ⅲ型的鉴别要点。

有作者认为环堤完整，有清晰锐利环堤外缘线是 Borrmann Ⅱ型特征性影像征象，可作为与 Borrmann Ⅲ型鉴别的可靠依据。

但是溃疡周围环堤与胃壁相交呈堤状或坡状的判定有时较为困难，这与阅片医生的诊断标准、与病变的发生部位等有关。

Borrmann Ⅱ型癌以团生为主，其环堤境外缘基本反映癌实际浸润范围。Borrmann Ⅲ型癌以弥漫浸润为主，水平浸润范围广泛，肉眼难以准确判定癌实际浸润范围。Borrmann Ⅲ型癌从影像征象判断其浸润范围往往较实际癌浸润范围要小。溃疡型胃癌中以 Borrmann Ⅲ型癌较多见，该组 33 例中 Borrmann Ⅲ型癌 21 例，比例达 64%，与文献报道相符。

胃镜下判断 Borrmann Ⅱ型与Ⅲ型有一定的困难，随着 MSCT 技术的发展，后处理功能的应用，MSCT 对于溃疡型胃癌的诊断及分期，尤其是对于 Borrmann Ⅱ型与Ⅲ型的鉴别诊断其敏感性及准确性将越来越高，这也必然给临床在治疗方案的选择及预后判断方面提供更多的支持和帮助。

第三章　关于进展期胃癌

第一节　进展期胃癌手术可根治性的CT评估

以往认为，Ⅰ、Ⅱ期胃癌可彻底切除，达到根治目的。Ⅲ、Ⅳ期不能彻底切除，应以化疗、放疗、免疫疗法等综合治疗。

近年来，对胃癌生物学行为的研究表明：胃癌分为局限性（膨胀型）与弥漫型（浸润型）2大类，其生物学行为有所不同。前者肿瘤可以巨大，但脏器内浸润范围小，淋巴结转移率低，转移距离近，多为大结节或肿块型，虽然貌似严重，实际上是良好的手术适应证，不可轻易放弃；后者肿瘤在胃壁内浸润范围广，淋巴结转移率高，转移距离远，多为小结节孤立型，对这类患者不能掉以轻心，应切除足够的受累脏器及广泛清扫淋巴结。

随着腹部外科手术领域的不断探索，外科手术水平的不断提高，胃癌术式日益改进，部分Ⅲ期胃癌亦能实行根治术，大大扩大了胃癌手术治疗范围，CT特别是螺旋CT的应用为胃癌的术前诊断、评估提供了强有力的依据。

CT高估和低估原因：CT对腹腔种植性结节显示率较低而导致低估。一组手术发现腹腔转移结节13例中，CT仅报告5例，主要原因有：腹腔转移瘤经常很小，与腹壁、肠壁之间缺乏对比，常难以发现；腹腔范围大，若扫描范围不够充分，常易漏诊；腹腔转移瘤经常发生在伴有腹水或肠梗阻的情况下会增加寻找结节的困难。

消瘦、恶液质病人脂肪间隙消失，对判断周围脏器侵犯带来较大困难。有的病例分别侵犯前腹壁、胰头、肠系膜血管而未报告而导致低估，另有病例报告分别侵犯脾静脉、肠系膜血管而手术未见侵犯而导致高估。单纯只做平扫是导致低估的一个重要原因。因各种原因未能增强扫描者，常有低估和高估的病例。对淋巴结转移的判定目前仅依据淋巴结大小，大小标准不同，其敏感性和特异性亦有较大差异。一组采用8 mm为标准，但仍有部分病例假阳性和假阴性，其原因是CT难以区别炎性反应性增生及癌性转移性病变，因此，单纯依据淋巴结大小判断其有无转移准确率不高。

其他因素：CT诊断医师诊断经验的主观原因、患者检查前准备工作的好坏以及CT机的快速、薄层、大范围扫描能力等机器性能均对CT术前估价产生重要影响。

检查方法对CT术前估价的重要性：患者在检查前禁食12 h，扫描前15 min饮水500 ml，上机时再饮水300 ml，这样能充分充盈胃、十二指肠及空肠，对比度好，伪影很少。少数病例因体质因素不能足量饮水不能强求，胃肠道内气体较多，伪影干扰大，影响了对邻近脏器观察及腹腔种植小结节的检出率。

检查体位：该组部分病例改变了传统的单纯仰卧位扫描，采用双体位扫描模式，即先采用常规仰卧位扫描，发现病变后按不同部位加扫不同的扫描体位。胃窦、幽门部病变加扫右侧卧位，胃底贲门部病变加扫头低足高位，胃体部病变加扫俯卧位。

胃钡餐造影中的体位技术在胃的CT检查得到了创造性的运用。这种扫描模式对判断邻近脏器侵犯及程度起到了举足轻重的作用。采用此方法常可明确诊断，起到了事半功倍的奇妙效果，应受到足够的重视。建议在胃肠道CT检查中多采用这一方法。

增强扫描：在此基础上进行CT双期增强扫描，对浆膜外浸润及邻近器官受侵程度的判断尤其是对附近血管的侵犯情况更加精确，对胃癌分期及术前可切除性估价的正确性得到了大幅度的提高。建议进展期胃癌术前应常规CT增强扫描,这对可否手术和术式选择具有重要指导意义。对胃癌CT诊断的很多研究表明肿瘤的CT分期与手术结果有较高的一致性,不少作者认为有必要将CT疗前分期列为胃肠肿瘤治疗前的常规检查。

总之,术前行CT检查对进展期胃癌治疗方案的制订有着十分重要的指导作用,胃癌病例中若有2个以上周围脏器受侵犯和/或已发生远处转移就不宜行手术治疗。一般CT判断准确率约为93.0%,但对腹腔转移结节的检出尚有一定的困难,有待进一步深入研究探讨。随着螺旋CT、多层螺旋CT的逐渐应用,检查方法的不断改进,对胃癌诊断认识的进一步加深,CT对胃癌的术前指导作用必将越来越重要,是胃癌术前评价的首选检查方法。

第二节 进展期胃癌与胃淋巴瘤鉴别

两组对比观察内容有八项,分列如下:

1. 发病部位及壁厚 胃窦部:胃癌8例,胃淋巴瘤4例;胃体部:胃癌5例,胃淋巴瘤4例;胃窦-胃体部:胃癌8例,胃淋巴瘤5例,其中1例淋巴瘤累及十二指肠球部;胃体-胃底-胃窦部:胃癌1例,胃底部:胃淋巴瘤2例。

胃癌组:受累胃壁厚度0.7~3.7cm,平均1.8 cm。淋巴瘤组:受累胃壁厚度1.0~4.3 cm,平均2.0cm。两组病例在病变胃壁厚度方面差异无统计学意义(2 = 2.49,$P>0.05$)。

2. 强化程度及方式 胃淋巴瘤组:表现为胃壁弥漫性增厚,强化较均匀,强化程度明显低于周围胃黏膜,与肌肉强化程度相仿,黏膜线连续或间断显示。

胃癌组:表现为胃壁不规则增厚,呈条状、板状强化,相应胃壁黏膜消失,病变强化程度高于或与黏膜强化程度相仿,胃壁肌层浑浊或强化程度增高。1例黏液腺癌强化程度与胃淋巴瘤组相仿,但正常黏膜线状强化消失;另1例印戒细胞癌伴黏液腺癌,病变局部强化程度与淋巴瘤相似,其余胃壁与胃癌强化程度一致。

胃癌组(2例黏液腺癌除外)动脉期病变的CT值较平扫平均提高约20 HU,静脉期平均提高约40HU;淋巴瘤组动脉期病变的CT值较平扫平均提高约10HU,静脉期平均提高约20 HU。两组在动脉期和静脉期病变强化程度的差异有显著性意义($P<0.05$),相应期相上胃癌组胃壁强化程度明显高于淋巴瘤组。

3. 病变胃腔内形态及胃浆膜面表现 浸润溃疡型胃癌是进展期胃癌中最常见的表现形式,占该组的77%(17/22),故胃腔内常表现为凹凸不平征象,边缘结节状增厚;而胃淋巴瘤常表现为多发表浅性凹陷,加之胃腔对比剂充盈不佳,常表现为胃腔内较光整,占该组的67%(10/15)。进展期胃癌侵犯胃壁浆膜面常表现为浆膜面凹凸不平、周围脂肪间隙模糊,可见条絮状及结节状软组织密度影,该组占82%(18/22)。

淋巴瘤:浆膜面模糊而周围结节状软组织密度影相对少见,浆膜面结节状突出征象在该组中未见。

4. 胃壁环周浸润 胃癌及胃淋巴瘤中晚期均形成环周浸润,该组病例中胃癌3例,淋巴瘤3例。

5. 腹腔淋巴结 直径超过2 cm淋巴结病例中,胃癌组4例(占18%),淋巴瘤组1例(6%);直径为1~2 cm者胃癌4例(18%),淋巴瘤2例(13%);余14例胃癌及12例淋巴瘤腹腔淋巴结均小于1.0cm或未见。两组病例淋巴结分布无明显特异性,好发部位均为胃小弯上下、幽门上下、胰头周围及腹主动脉周围,均可发生淋巴结融合及坏死征象。

6. 胃腔狭窄征象 22例胃癌病例中15例发生不同程度胃腔狭窄;15例淋巴瘤中8例发生狭窄,其中2例为狭窄与不规则坏死腔并存,形成狭窄后扩张征象,而该组胃癌中未见此征。

7. 远处浸润或转移 22例胃癌患者中有4例发生肝脏多发转移,其中1例并发左侧肾上腺转移,而15例淋巴瘤患者中未出现肝脏浸润征象。

8. 腹水 22例胃癌中3例出现大量腹腔积液,2例少量腹腔积液,而胃淋巴瘤组中仅2例出现少量腹腔积液。

9. 进展期胃癌及胃淋巴瘤发病机制及生物学行为的差异 进展期胃癌起源于胃黏膜上皮或腺体上皮,向周围浸润破坏正常胃黏膜的同时,向下浸润超过黏膜下层,胃癌血供丰富,表现为增强后正常胃壁黏膜线状强化消失,呈条状及板状强化,厚度明显超过胃黏膜,动、静脉期较平扫分别高出15~20 HU及

40~45 HU。

胃淋巴瘤多发生于黏膜下层，因增殖进展使胃壁增厚或皱壁增厚，早期胃黏膜多连续，中晚期出现多发间断胃黏膜线中断。胃淋巴瘤细胞密集，血管较少，动、静脉期分别较平扫 CT 值高出约 8~15 HU 和 15~25 HU。

胃黏液腺癌及胃胶样癌因含黏液及胶样物质而表现为平扫密度较正常胃壁及肌肉低，属胃癌中乏血供肿瘤，强化程度明显低于腺癌及印戒细胞癌等，而与胃淋巴瘤相仿，故两者鉴别存在一定困难，平扫胃壁与肌肉 CT 值比较有一定帮助。

10. 大体形态与增强扫描时强化表现　进展期胃癌及胃淋巴瘤大体形态基本相仿，均可以表现为蕈伞型、溃疡型、弥漫浸润型、局限性增厚、弥漫性增厚，同时由于部分病例胃部病变造成胃腔对比较充盈不佳，对胃壁厚度价值的评估造成一定的偏差，从而失去统计学意义。

胃癌（除外黏液腺癌及胶样癌）富血供，肿瘤生长到一定程度即出现肿瘤局部血供不足而发生坏死，形成溃疡，周围隆起，CT 上表现为凹陷征象。而淋巴瘤血供较差及不同部位淋巴瘤生长速度不一致，常表现为多发的浅表凹陷及隆起，CT 表现胃腔内边缘光整或浅波浪状。进展期胃癌浆膜面浸润常表现为浆膜面凹凸不平、脂肪间隙模糊及内见条状、结节状软组织密度影；淋巴瘤浆膜面浸润相对瘤体本身而表现较轻，浆膜面仍较光整。

11. 周围淋巴结表现　该组 4 例胃癌及 1 例淋巴瘤病例腹腔内淋巴结大于 2.0cm，均表现为胃小弯、胃大弯、幽门上、幽门下、胰头周围、腹主动脉周围广泛淋巴结肿大，均可见融合征象，单纯从肿大淋巴结分布情况很难鉴别两者，但以下淋巴结表现有助于诊断胃癌：胃部病变较小而胃周及腹膜后广泛淋巴结肿大、融合；淋巴结肿大伴淋巴结内细沙状钙化；淋巴结肿大伴周围脏器转移；多发小淋巴结伴腹腔大量积液；对于小于 1.0 cm 淋巴结，出现在远离病变部位，并且多发，往往提示胃癌可能大，而病变周围的小淋巴结对两者的鉴别诊断无明显统计学差异。

12. 胃腔狭窄与柔韧性　进展期胃癌与胃淋巴瘤均可出现胃腔狭窄征象，胃癌常伴有结缔组织反应增生，胃壁僵直，而胃淋巴瘤为淋巴组织在黏膜及黏膜下层浸润增殖，不伴有结缔组织反应性增生，故柔韧性较好。平扫、动脉期、静脉期狭窄胃腔变化较明显，提示胃柔韧性较好，胃淋巴瘤可能大。胃腔假性扩张，CT 上观察到的病变部位胃腔与近端胃腔相仿，常提示淋巴瘤诊断，该组淋巴瘤病例中出现 2 例。

总之，CT 可以通过对胃部病变强化程度、强化方式、病变腔内形态及病变与淋巴结分布、形态、密度相关性进行分析，对鉴别进展期胃癌与胃淋巴瘤有重要意义。

第三节　胃弥漫浸润型低分化腺癌

患者，女，29 岁。反复上腹部疼痛不适 2 个月入院。

免疫组化诊断：①全胃切除标本：弥漫浸润型低分化腺癌（大小 6cm × 5.5cm × 1.3cm），部分为印戒细胞癌，侵及浆膜纤维脂肪组织，可见脉管内癌栓；上切缘及下切缘均为阴性；大网膜可见癌结节。②淋巴结清扫：小弯侧淋巴结 7/19，大弯侧淋巴结 2/3，送检的“12p 组淋巴结” 0/4，“12b 组淋巴结” 0/1。注：肿瘤细胞预后及耐药检测供临床参考。

胃癌是我国最常见的恶性肿瘤之一，好发年龄为 40~60 岁，可发生在胃的任何部位，但以胃窦、小弯及贲门区常见。胃癌起源于胃黏膜上皮，沿黏膜及黏膜下浸润、生长，造成黏膜破坏，局部形成软组织密度肿块，常发生淋巴转移。胃印戒细胞癌的临床特征是弥漫浸润性生长，早期即可发生远处转移，最常见为卵巢或子宫颈（图 23-3-1）。

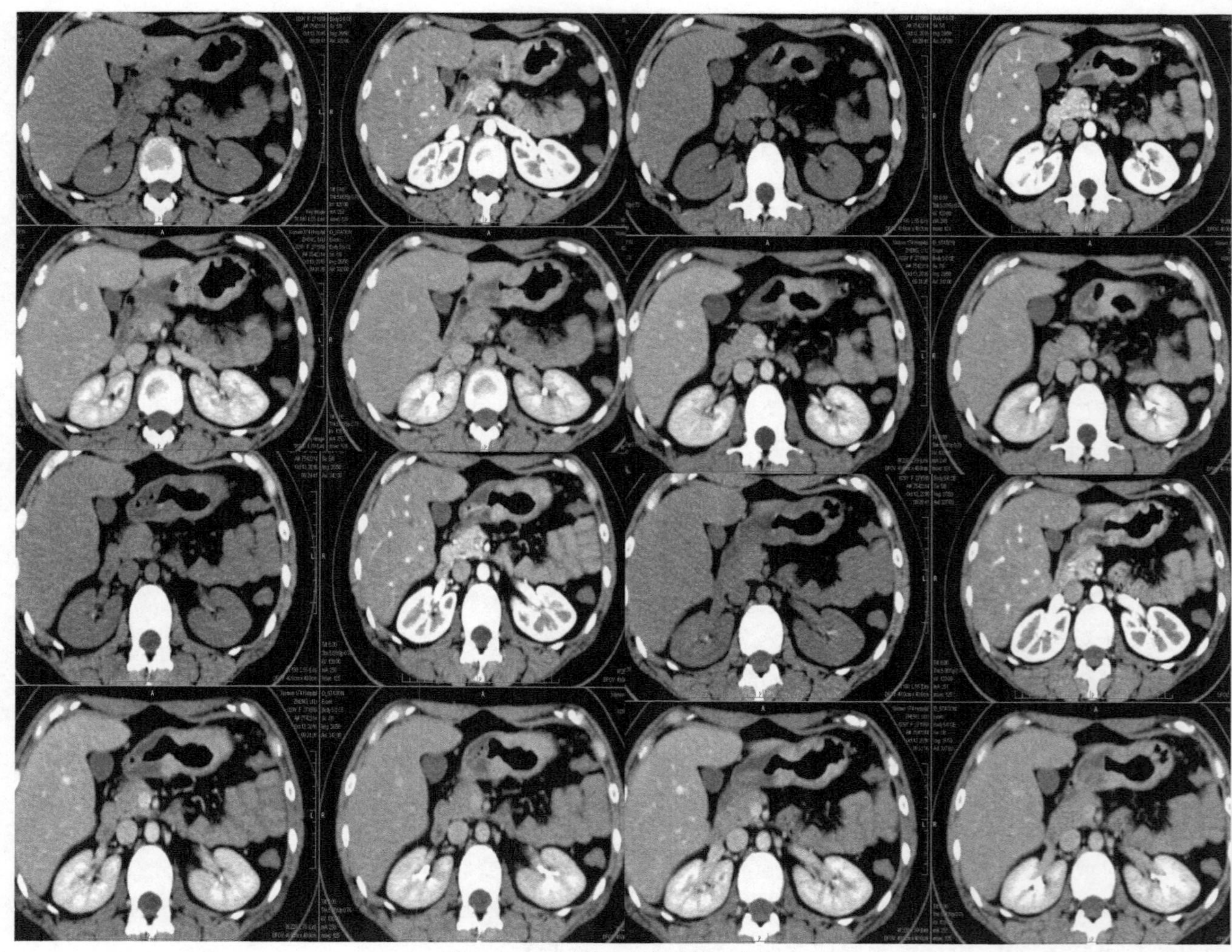

图 23-3-1　胃弥漫浸润型低分化腺癌

第四章　早期胃癌和肿瘤血管生成

第一节　早期胃癌影像学诊断

在世界范围内,胃癌的死亡率高居榜首。早期胃癌根治术后5年生存率为85%~100%,其中始发阶段小胃癌及微小胃癌的10年生存率可达100%,而进展期胃癌只有20%~30%。由于早期胃癌有相当高的治愈率,在临床诊治中具有十分重要的意义,特别是胃癌术前准确的分期对于有效的治疗方案的制订相当重要。

双对比钡餐检查:双对比钡餐检查目前仍为早期胃癌检测的首选方法。优质的双对比像已能发现各型早期胃癌,包括癌灶最大径 <l cm 甚至 0.5 cm 的小胃癌和微小胃癌。

可以提示诊断的重要特征,包括龛影口部和表面的结节状改变,周围不规则的黏膜纠集,胃壁毛糙、僵直、凹陷、双边、边缘毛刺征,黏膜细节的破坏和粗糙、小的充盈缺损。

双对比造影检查对早期胃癌的检出率,国内学者报道最低者为50%,也有高达91%的报道,多数作者的结果介于两者之间。西方学者的研究也有相似的结论。目前的共识是双对比造影检查结合胃镜+活检,这样可以最大程度地提高早期胃癌的检出率,可达95.4%。

目前早期胃癌的临床和病理分型仍然沿用日本内镜协会所制定的标准,熟练掌握不同类型胃癌的表现是诊断的基础。

Ⅰ型和Ⅱ a型:Ⅱ a型约占早期胃癌的9.5%,充盈压迫像轮廓显示为大小不等、粗糙结节状充盈缺损,周围黏膜破坏,粗细不均,紊乱交叉;周围的胃小区增大,胃小沟增粗。隆起的表面有糜烂征象。如果隆起的高度超过4 cm以上或带有蒂的,表面光滑,无分叶现象者不应考虑早期胃癌。

Ⅱ型:形态呈不规则的圆形或椭圆形,边缘清晰,胃壁僵硬。病灶内有的可见颗粒状小隆起(Ⅱ+Ⅱ a)或浅凹陷(Ⅲ+Ⅱ c)。早期胃癌以Ⅱ c型多见,约占全部早期胃癌的40.5%~76.2%。

Ⅱ c型主要表现为黏膜面糜烂,胃小区破坏消失,胃小沟中断紊乱,边缘不规则呈蚕蚀状,无明显边界,黏膜皱襞集中、破坏呈笔尖状、杵状和V字形。病灶较大时可见浅凹陷内伴有小颗粒状隆起(Ⅱ c+Ⅱ a)。高分化腺癌龛影边界一般不明确,造影像呈现淡薄不规则、模糊钡斑,低分化或未分化腺癌则均有明确边界,造影像龛影呈椭圆形、颗粒状及星芒状。黏膜癌龛影表面多较平坦,黏膜下癌表面凹凸不平,切线位龛影口部均可见单发或多发小结节影,此征可区别良性溃疡,对定性诊断有重要意义。

Ⅱ b型多为黏膜癌,如发现胃小区大小不等、破坏、扩大或模糊、消失,病变区的胃小区小沟扭曲断裂,形成不规则的颗粒状或轻度凹凸变化;黏膜皱襞展平和浅淡的染钡区,病变周围呈移行性改变时提示诊断,应行胃镜检查。

黏膜癌胃壁粗糙、趋僵、舒张性较差;黏膜下癌胃壁则明确僵直、凹陷,并可呈现双边,但不论黏膜癌或黏膜下癌,充盈像大多显示有微小边缘毛刺征,此征是诊断早期胃癌极有价值的X线征象。

若龛影周围黏膜全部或部分纠集,终端呈杵状增粗、突然变细、中断改变,说明癌组织侵犯胃壁已深达黏膜下层。

贲门部早期胃癌特征有局限性浅钡斑,龛影以及可透光病灶。所有前壁、小弯和后壁的病灶在半立位、俯卧位、右前位和斜位上均可显示。所有后壁及小弯侧的病灶在半立位、仰卧位、左前位和斜位上均可显示。

早期胃癌龛影周围黏膜改变无一定规律，确诊需结合其他征象，全面观察胃壁及其微皱襞和病灶的特点。除常规摄片外还应仔细分辨有否小的钡剂聚集区、小钡池、局限性大小不等的增生结节、胃壁局限性僵硬、胃壁局部不完整、轻度增厚等，发现疑点及时摄片。

早期胃癌的鉴别诊断十分困难，如表浅型胃癌很容易被误诊为浅表性胃炎，而凹陷型胃癌则可能误诊为良性胃溃疡。此外，胃窦部分Ⅱc及Ⅱc混合型胃癌所致胃窦变形与胃窦进展癌的鉴别也是影像学应该认真探讨的问题。

CT：CT是胃癌术前分期最实用和可靠的方法。CT检测早期胃癌的准确率，各家报道相当悬殊。Lee等（2000）的结果为57%（28/49），而Nishimata等（2003）的研究则显示MSCT（虚拟内镜和多排重建）对胃癌的总体检测率为94%（63/67），其中早期胃癌的检测率为96.7%（30/31）。Lee等（2000）初步评估了包括胃黏膜期在内的双期螺旋CT对早期胃癌检测的有效性，早期胃癌可能出现典型高衰减增强和非典型非高衰减增强方式。

典型高衰减早期胃癌为Ⅰ型增强方式，即出现内侧高衰减层的局部增厚，此种类型双期螺旋CT的检测率为18%（9/49）。

Ⅱ型增强方式，即内侧高衰减黏膜层的中断，而未出现黏膜期外侧低衰减层的增强，此种类型的检出率为30%（15/49）。

Ⅲ型增强方式为高衰减内层局灶性息肉样突出，而在黏膜期没有增厚的低衰减外层正常强化。病灶在延迟扫描中不甚清晰。

早期胃癌在动脉期及门静脉期明显强化，在平衡期强化程度明显下降。另有作者报道部分早期胃癌胃壁呈单层结构，表现为胃壁局限性增厚，动脉期及门静脉期均显示病灶明显强化，平衡期强化程度略有下降；部分患者胃壁呈3层结构，内层于门静脉期强化最显著。

螺旋CT三期增强扫描对胃癌术前分期的诊断价值由于CT设备和检查方法等因素的不同，在CT对胃癌分期的准确性方面意见分歧很大。

胃癌的T分期是影响切除率的主要因素。根据胃癌的CT诊断标准，当胃壁呈多层结构时，早期胃癌（T_1）表现为局部胃壁内层明显强化增厚，中层和外层结构正常，如果胃壁的中层结构中断消失则被认为是进展期胃癌。因此，胃壁多层结构的显示有利于早期胃癌（T_1）和进展期胃癌（T_2~T_4）的鉴别。如果胃壁显示为单层，区分T_1和T_2是困难的，有文献报道早期胃癌可因胃壁呈单层被过估为T_2。

Nishimata等（2003）的工作较为细致，他们的研究表明对于术前T分期，内镜超声和MSCT的总体准确率、敏感性和特异性分别为87.5%、82.4%和96%；及83.3%、69.1%和94.4%。淋巴结转移是胃癌的主要转移途径，工藤明敏等（1991）应用CT对胃癌转移淋巴结进行研究后发现，转移淋巴结多呈囊状、花斑状或串珠状，相对高密度或周边高密度、中心低密度或压迫血管。螺旋CT三期增强扫描对N分期的准确性为85.7%，由于门静脉期脏器强化率及血管显示率最高，因此门静脉期对血管旁淋巴结转移的检出率较高。Nishimata等（2003）的实验也证实了上述的结论，对于术前N分期，内镜超声和MSCT的总体准确率、敏感性和特异性分别为79.1%、57%和9.5%；75%、57.4%和89.3%。

磁共振成像（MRI）：由于MRI扫描时间长，且各种运动伪影的影响较明显，使胃肠道病变的显示能力和清晰度下降，应用受限。现代MRI机采用快速自旋回波技术和呼吸补偿方法，病人可在屏气状态下进行扫描，运动伪影可最大程度得以克服，图像质量明显提高。目前有关MRI检测早期胃癌的报道甚少。Yamada等（2001）通过胃壁所表现出的信号特征来验证早期胃癌评估的正确性。共有15例怀疑早期胃癌患者的手术标本入组研究，MR的图像和组织病理学的结果相比较。在T_1WI和T_2WI上，可以清楚地勾勒出正常胃壁4~6层结构，和组织学分层非常吻合。15例胃癌患者中的14例（93%），其MR上所显示的侵入胃壁的深度和组织病理学分期吻合。有1例患者（7%）MRI上的分期低于组织病理学分期。MR图像上还可以显示出肿瘤的大体特征、溃疡的存在和邻近淋巴结的肿胀。故该组作者认为高分辨率MR对于体外早期胃癌的胃壁侵入的评估有非常高的准确率，因此能够行术前组织病理学的分期。

比较影像学：胃癌影像的作用是尽可能早地诊断出病变并且判断出哪些肿瘤是可以根治的。目前，内镜是胃癌诊断的一种选择方法。如果遇到小的肿瘤必须判断肿瘤浸润的深度（是早期胃癌还是进展期胃癌）时，超声内镜是有优势的，因为它可以获得有关胃壁的高分辨的图像。胃腔外生长的巨大肿瘤的分期最好由注水法CT完成，因为CT可以最为准确地观察周围脏器/结构的浸润,从而有助于制订手术方案。目前MRI尚不适合于胃部影像学的研究。如肿瘤较小及肿瘤合并炎症改变,则MR很难检测。但是假如在1次检查中需要同时获得胃壁的高分辨的图像和识别出胃癌的转移,那么MRI便具有根本上提高胃癌分期的最大潜在优势。

第二节　误诊病例简介:胃小弯印戒细胞癌与胃窦壁稍增厚

病例,男,59岁。上腹部饱胀不适两年加重一个月入院。CT:胃窦壁稍增厚,约0.9cm,增强扫描时呈中度强化,周围脂肪间隙清楚。扫描区内腹腔及腹膜后未见明显肿大淋巴结。CT诊断:胃窦壁稍增厚,请结合内镜检查。

手术所见:胃小弯靠近胃窦部可见一大小1.2cm×1.0cm溃疡病灶,浸润至浆膜外与周边脂肪垂粘连,胃旁淋巴结无明显肿大,肝脏、肠管及盆腔未见明显癌转移结节。

病理检查:胃癌根治标本:胃切除标本大小16.0 cm×4.5 cm×2.5 cm。距幽门6cm处胃小弯侧黏膜平坦,质稍硬,大小3.0 cm×2.5 cm×0.6 cm,其余黏膜皱襞明显。常规病理诊断:胃癌根治标本胃小弯小细胞肿瘤,大小3.0 cm×2.5 cm,位于黏膜层,局部达黏膜下层,肿瘤细胞类型、预后及耐药性免疫组化待报。幽门黏膜慢性炎,重度,较多淋巴滤泡形成。胃体黏膜慢性浅表性胃炎,轻度,伴灶性肠上皮化生。吻合口切缘及幽门口切缘均为阴性。自检胃小弯侧淋巴结8枚,个别可疑有癌转移,待免疫组化证实。自检胃大弯侧淋巴结(-),0/6,大网膜组织未检出癌结节。送检的第8组淋巴结(-),0/4。

免疫组化检测:阳性:CK(L),CK8,CK18,AB,PAS,EGFR(+++),VEGF(+++),Topo-Ⅱ(+++),G-Fu(++),Ki-67(+,80%),Tubulin-β(+);阴性:CK(H),Syn,CgA,CD56,CD117,DOG1,H-caldesmon,Calponin,P-gp,ERCC-1,CD68,CD163,CK45,CD34。免疫组化诊断:胃癌根治标本,胃小弯印戒细胞癌,大小3.0 cm×2.5 cm,侵及深肌层,详见常规病理报告。自检胃小弯侧淋巴结8枚,其中2枚可见癌转移。

误诊漏诊分析体会:回顾性再次认真观察CT图像,发现术前观察太粗糙,欠认真,对胃壁的几层观察欠仔细,对黏膜观察尤其欠妥,这就是教训。众所周知,胃的癌肿都最早起源于黏膜,对黏膜的观察尤其重要,在增强扫描时,务必观察强化黏膜的完整性、均匀性及其各期相表现的动态变化,这对于诊断早期胃癌是必不可少的。

第五章 胃癌的转移

第一节 胃癌的淋巴结转移

详见本书 本卷 第二十二篇 第十二章 第一节 淋巴结转移是胃癌转移的主要方式。

第二节 淋巴结转移是胃癌的主要转移途径

淋巴结转移是胃癌的主要转移途径,工藤明敏等(1991)应用CT对胃癌转移淋巴结进行研究后发现,转移淋巴结多呈囊状、花斑状或串珠状,相对高密度或周边高密度、中心低密度或压迫血管。

关于胃癌的CT分期评价:文献报道对于胃癌的CT分期评价不一,以往的报道较为乐观,但晚近的大部分报道较悲观。对于这些文献的评价很难形成定论,主要是由于在如何衡量病变淋巴结的大小、形态等方面标准不一。CT的局限性在于确定胃壁的浸润深度及检出在正常大小淋巴结上发生的病理改变。CT分期过低,主要是由于对正常大小的淋巴结已发生癌转移,或腹膜及肝脏内小转移灶不能检出。CT分期过高,主要是由于尚未穿透胃全层的癌肿,其周围脂肪层消失,另外,将反应性增生或炎性淋巴结的肿大判为转移。如贴近胃壁的病变淋巴结与胃癌病灶本身有时也难以鉴别,也导致分期不准。

转移淋巴结的大小的讨论:淋巴结大小、形态及强化程度:CT诊断淋巴结转移主要依据淋巴结大小、形态及强化程度:淋巴结<10 mm伴有中度/明显强化,或>10 mm,或周边高密度中心低密度,淋巴结短/长径之比≥0.7,淋巴结呈蚕蚀状、囊状、花斑状或串珠状,压迫和包绕血管或融合成团块状,为淋巴结转移阳性。该CT标准可较准确反映胃癌淋巴结转移,但部分病例仍诊断困难。一组3例小转移淋巴结CT未能检出,原因在于螺旋CT对5 mm以下的淋巴结检出率极低,而薄层增强扫描可有助于提高小淋巴结的检出率及淋巴结密度、形态的显示。

血管周围的淋巴结对比显示明显、检出率较高,而病灶旁淋巴结往往与肿块融合不易分辨,该组3例转移淋巴结与肿块融合,误认为是肿块的一部分而漏诊,因此诊断时一定要注意肿块旁有无可疑淋巴结。该组1例脾动脉旁转移淋巴结CT平卧位扫描未能检出,术后回顾发现右侧卧位淋巴结清晰显示。原因在于消瘦病人腹部脂肪少,淋巴结显示困难,而多体位扫描可有助于提高淋巴结的检出率。该组3例淋巴结直径8~12 mm且强化,术后病理为炎性淋巴结肿大。较大、有强化的炎性淋巴结与转移鉴别困难,有待于进一步研究总结经验。该组另外3例低分化腺癌淋巴结直径<5 mm,术后病理证实为转移淋巴结;4例高/中分化腺癌淋巴结直径5~8 mm且中度/明显强化,术后病理未发现转移。研究显示诊断淋巴结转移还应结合胃癌原发灶的组织学类型,对于低分化腺癌,即使淋巴结直径小于5 mm,特别是簇状生长的小淋巴结,也多发生转移;相反,对于高/中分化癌,淋巴结直径10 mm以上的转移率高,10 mm以下的多不发生转移。

淋巴结直径大于5 mm:一组以淋巴结直径大于5 mm作为诊断标准,主要在于淋巴结标准设定过大会造成小的转移淋巴结的漏诊,而过小则造成非转移淋巴结的高估及淋巴结检出困难。

文献报道直径5 mm以下淋巴结的检出率仅

1.1%，且转移率极低（5.1%）；5 mm 以上淋巴结检出率在 45.1% 以上，且转移率在 69% 以上。该组作者对直径 5 mm 以上的淋巴结重点观察，同时结合淋巴结的强化、形态作为诊断标准。一些学者报告 57 例胃癌的淋巴转移研究，CT 对淋巴结转移的诊断准确性为 78.9%，与病理分期一致性良好（$P<0.05$）。另外，研究显示，转移淋巴结多呈明显、环状、不均匀强化，淋巴结短 / 长径之比多≥ 0.7，多呈蚕蚀状、囊状、花斑状或串珠状，压迫和包绕血管或融合成团块状。

一组对直径大于 5 mm 的淋巴结重点观察，同时结合淋巴结的强化、形态作为诊断标准，可较准确反映胃癌淋巴结转移，该组 CT 对非转移淋巴的诊断准确性为 72.2%，转移淋巴结的准确性为 85.1%，与手术病理一致性良好（$P<0.05$）。一组 65 例胃癌 CT 与病理对照显示：18 例非转移淋巴结，CT 准确诊断 13 例，高估 5 例，这 5 例淋巴结直径均 >5 mm 且有强化，术后病理为非转移淋巴结。47 例淋巴结转移，CT 正确诊断 40 例，低估 7 例，其中 3 例转移淋巴结较小 CT 未能检出；3 例转移淋巴结与肿块融合而误认为是肿块的一部分；1 例淋巴结 CT 已检出但直径 <5 mm，判断非淋巴结转移。分析其原因可能与单排螺旋 CT 扫描层厚较厚有关。

关于 MRI 对胃癌 N 分期的研究：MRI 对胃癌 N 分期的研究报道差异较大，其主要原因是评判胃癌淋巴结转移和 N 分期的标准不尽统一。多数作者借鉴 CT 检查指标，以短轴 >8mm 作为胃癌转移性淋巴结的诊断标准。对于胃癌 N 分期，美国癌症联合会（AJCC）修订的新标准主要以受累淋巴结的数目分类，而以往的胃癌 N 分期则强调受累淋巴结与原发肿瘤间的距离。如前所述，MRI 成像序列对比研究显示，屏息 FSE 序列 T_2WI 诊断胃癌转移性淋巴结的敏感性明显优于 T_1WI SE 序列或动态增强 FMPSPGR 序列，但也有报道，于动态增强早期在明显强化的胃壁和胃周血管衬托下，胃癌转移性淋巴结显示更清晰。

总体上说，MRI 胃癌 N 分期的诊断准确度较低，仅为 52%~65%，有报道其诊断敏感度和特异度也仅为 52% 和 53%，其主要原因是以淋巴结大小为诊断标准来判断胃癌淋巴结转移难以与淋巴结的炎症性或反应性肿大相鉴别，此外，对于 MRI 冠状或矢状影像上腹腔淋巴结的解剖学分布尚需进一步深入研究。

离体标本实验研究：Dux 等（1997）的胃癌离体标本实验研究显示，依据转移性淋巴结与肿瘤病灶有相同的 MRI 信号特征作为胃癌淋巴结浸润的判断标准而不考虑淋巴结大小，胃癌转移性淋巴结的检出率为 94%，敏感度和特异度分别为 87% 和 60%，以 TNM 分期新标准诊断胃癌 N 分期的准确度可达 80%，而根据旧的 TNM 分期标准判断胃癌 N 分期的准确度仅为 40%。

关于胃癌的 N 分期的研究：N 分期，淋巴结的转移是涉及病人预后的重要因素，螺旋 CT 扫描较常规 CT 更具优势。不少作者报道，利用螺旋 CT 探测淋巴结，小于 5mm 者检出率为 1.1%，5~9mm 为 21.7%，10~14mm 为 23%，而直径 >14mm 的淋巴结约 82.6% 受侵。

多数学者仍将直径≥ 15mm 作为判断标准。他们也认为对于直径小于 14mm 的淋巴结有无癌变难以判断。Fukuya 等（1995）认为较大的但强化程度低或短轴 / 长轴的比值小的淋巴结不支持转移。转移淋巴结的特征多为直径 <10mm 但强化程度很高，或直径 >10mm 但强化 CT 值 >100HU，及短轴 / 长轴 >0.7。对 N_1 和 N_2 的鉴别，Davis 等（1997）报道螺旋 CT 检出 N_1 和 N_2 淋巴结敏感度为 24% 与 43%。这与 Sendler 等（1995）报道相似，N_1 的敏感度不及 N_2。

原因可能为 N_1 淋巴结贴近胃癌及胃壁，不及 N_2 易于显示，N_2 淋巴结与周围强化血管极易区别。一些学者报告 57 例胃癌的淋巴转移研究，其中 20 例 N_0 中 CT 准确诊断 15 例，5 例 CT 示胃周孤立淋巴结，直径约 5~8 mm 且有强化，CT 误诊为有淋巴结转移而高估为 N_1，术后病理为非转移淋巴结，其中 4 例胃病变为中分化腺癌，1 例低分化腺癌。

11 例 N_1 中 6 例 CT 诊断正确，2 例 CT 未发现肿大淋巴结而低估为 N_0，但术后病理显示胃周有转移淋巴结；1 例转移淋巴结与肿块融合，CT 误诊为肿块的一部分而低估为 N_0；2 例血管旁淋巴结直径 8~12 mm 且轻度强化，CT 误诊为淋巴结转移而高估为 N_2，但术后病理证实为非淋巴结转移。

26 例 N_2 中 CT 正确诊断 24 例，2 例术后病理证实血管旁多发小淋巴结转移，术前 CT 仅检出 1~2 个淋巴结，且认为其直径 <5 mm 而判断非转移淋巴结，该病例为低分化腺癌。

炎性淋巴结误诊为转移淋巴结：一些伴有长期胃炎的胃癌患者可出现淋巴结炎性肿大，一般炎性肿大淋巴结无强化或轻度强化，但个别病例出现明显强化时，与转移淋巴结鉴别困难，一组 7 例炎性淋巴结误诊为转移淋巴结。一般认为转移淋巴结多肿大明显且有强化，淋巴结短 / 长径之比≥ 0.7，或呈蚕蚀状、囊状、花斑状、串珠状、团状，或侵犯包绕血管；然而早期癌浸润的淋巴结或强化不明显的孤立小淋巴结，CT 鉴别仍很困难。

螺旋 CT 三期增强扫描对 N 分期的准确性为 85.7%，由于门静脉期脏器强化率及血管显示率最高，因此门静脉期对血管旁淋巴结转移的检出率较高。Nishimata 等（2003）的实验也证实了上述的结论，对于术前 N 分期，内镜超声和 MSCT 的总体准确率、敏感性和特异性分别为 79.1%、57% 和 9.5%；75%、57.4% 和 89.3%。

螺旋 CT 三期增强扫描对 N 分期的准确性为 85.7%，由于门静脉期脏器强化率及血管显示率最高，因此门静脉期对血管旁淋巴结转移的检出率较高。Nishimata 等（2003）的实验也证实了上述的结论，对于术前 N 分期，内镜超声和 MSCT 的总体准确率、敏感性和特异性分别为 79.1%、57% 和 9.5%；75%、57.4% 和 89.3%。

第三节　误诊病例简介：以阻塞淋巴管、深静脉为首发症状的右肩转移性胃癌

胃癌的转移途径主要有直接蔓延、淋巴转移、血行转移及腹腔种植等。胃癌的淋巴转移一般按照胃的淋巴引流顺序进行，但也存在着跳跃式淋巴结转移，这主要是因为癌细胞堵塞了某些淋巴管，而另一些淋巴管重新形成，这样癌细胞可沿着不断开放的淋巴管播散，形成远处转移。

有作者报告一例患者为胃角的低分化癌，易发生早期转移，但是右肩部软组织及组织间隙转移甚是少见。主要表现为转移灶引起的右肩背部明显肿胀，持续性疼痛，无胃部明显不适。该病例影像学表现也主要为软组织肿胀，无确切肿块影，因此很容易误诊、漏诊。

该例胃癌转移至右颈肩部软组织及组织间隙，右锁骨下、腋下的深静脉、淋巴管受压或堵塞，从而中断了右上臂的淋巴、血液回流径路，减少了淋巴引流的容量，结果间质液中的蛋白不能清除，导致蛋白溶度增高，胶体渗透压下降，毛细血管的液体量增加导致水肿。

并且富含蛋白质的淋巴液可以刺激间质中的成纤维细胞增殖和释放胶原蛋白，于是皮下组织发生纤维化、硬化，进一步限制淋巴引流。由此恶性循环形成严重广泛的右肩背部及右前臂水肿肿胀，皮肤变硬。

第六章　胃癌部分检查技术

第一节　漏诊病例简介：临床要求与全面观察

一组作者报告一例老年患者因腹痛做MSCT检查，临床要求观察肝、胆、脾与结肠，诊断报告称上述部位未见异常，但未观察胃，临床也未做胃镜。次日该患者在外院纤维胃镜检查胃，并做活检病理，结果是未分化癌。再行回顾性观察和分析CT图像，确实可以看到胃大弯胃壁局限性增厚，但当时却被忽略。

我们认为，一次影像检查，在扫描范围内的器官和组织都属于观察范围，尽管临床要求重点观察一些器官和组织，其他部位器官和组织也应一视同仁地认真观察，如有异常，还应加以报告，这对病人总有益处；切记不能只观察临床要求观察的部位器官和组织。

因为临床医生工作常与其临床经验密切相关，一些经验欠缺的门诊临床医生，常常只关心病人当时的临床症状与体征，对病人全身情况及病史缺乏全面的了解，并且只重视与目前临床症状有关的部位器官和组织，这对影像诊断医生来说，这也许可能就成为一个诊断陷阱。

第二节　MSCT在胃癌诊断中的临床应用

胃癌是我国最常见的恶性肿瘤之一，其发病率居消化道肿瘤第一位。近年来城市胃癌死亡率呈下降趋势，死因顺位由第一位降为第三位，位于肺癌、肝癌之后，农村胃癌死亡率略有上升，居第一位。

胃癌的病因目前尚未清楚，大量研究资料表明与环境、饮食营养失衡，N-亚硝基化合物及一些高危因素如遗传、萎缩性胃炎、肠上皮化生、胃溃疡等有关。近年来，胃幽门螺杆菌与胃癌的关系得到国际广泛重视。

胃气钡双重对比造影检查是诊断胃癌最常用和首选的影像检查方法之一，其对观察胃内病变的形态及对病变的定位、定性等方面均有优越性。胃双重对比造影与内镜及活检、脱落细胞学检查密切配合，对提高早期胃癌的检出率和诊断率已取得显著成绩。同时，随着超声、CT和MRI在临床诊断中的广泛应用，对胃癌的诊断、术前分期和疗后随诊等方面发挥着重要作用。MSCT具有扫描速度快、大容量及后处理速度快的特点，其2DCT的多平面重建技术及3DCT图像在胃癌病例的检查中得到较为广泛的应用。3DCT主要包括仿真内镜、表面遮盖技术和透明技术。

MSCT沿Z轴安装有多排探测器，并与多个数据采集系统相连，CT管球每旋转1周便可获得多层图像，这种将多排探测器与螺旋容积扫描相结合技术大大提高了扫描速度及图像质量，实现了1次屏气获得大范围薄层扫描图像，其多平面重建图像与512×512矩阵横断面图像的空间分辨率相近。

仿真内镜、表面遮盖技术、透明技术三种图像是将螺旋CT扫描获得的容积数据传送至图像工作站，经三种后处理方式重建而成。仿真内镜图像是采用透视法容积再现和飞越法显示技术来显示肿瘤形态，类似胃镜的显示效果。表面遮盖技术是只选择胃腔内气体为成像阈值而对胃壁内表面成像，图像类似于钡餐造影的单对比像。而透明技术图像上的每个像素是由其投影线上所有体素总和，其图像类似于气钡双对比造影像。

早期癌：螺旋 CT（包括 MSCT）2D 图像对早期癌的诊断各家报道不一。文献报道螺旋 CT 的 2D 图像对早期癌诊断准确性为 16.7%~61.5%。一些作者报道正常胃壁在 CT 多表现为 2~3 层结构，分别相当于黏膜层、黏膜下层及肌 - 浆膜层，当黏膜层增厚并明显强化时提示为早期癌。另有作者采用常规 CT 报道，当胃壁呈单层结构时，早期癌可表现为仅见胃壁明显强化而无胃壁增厚，但上述表现仅占该组病例的 23%。

大部分正常胃壁呈单层结构，正常胃壁的黏膜层与其他部位如鼻腔、鼻咽部等黏膜相同，在增强早期均有明显强化，如果没有胃壁局限性增厚，与正常黏膜难以鉴别。

2DCT 对早期癌的诊断主要与其病理类型有关，对隆起病变检出率高，而对平坦型、凹陷型检出率低。此外，也与 CT 机性能、扫描参数及增强技术等因素有关。

既往有关 3DCT 在早期癌的研究报道很少。有学者采用 MSCT 仿真内镜技术对大组早期胃癌病例（94 例，均经手术、病理证实）和正常对照（68 例）进行研究，结果显示对早期胃癌的检出敏感性、特异性为 84% 和 91%。

另有学者报道 CT 仿真内镜对一组胃隆起型病变（38 例）检出的敏感性和特异性分别为 92% 和 100%，检出病变大小为 5mm 到 30mm，与该组胃镜结果相似。

我国的早期胃癌大体类型分布与国外不同。如在日本最多见的是Ⅱ c 型，占 70.7%，而在我国仅占 39.5%。此外Ⅲ型及Ⅱ b 型在我国分别占 22.9% 和 10.5%，而在日本则分别仅占 3.2% 和 1.0%。

关于胃癌的分期：螺旋 CT 对 T_2 和 T_3 期胃癌诊断有较高的准确率，但仍存在分期高估和低估，主要系由于 CT 无法检出肿瘤的微小浸润和鉴别炎症纤维化。

但依据病变处浆膜面是否光滑和胃周脂肪间隙内有无条索影仍有助于鉴别 T_2 和 T_3 期胃癌。MSCT 对 T_4 期胃癌诊断报道不一，准确率为 80%~100%。多数学者采用肿瘤与相邻脏器间脂肪间隙消失为诊断 T_4 期标准，而 Fukuya 等采用与肿瘤相贴邻的脏器内密度发生变化为诊断 T_4 期标准，该组病例中有 11 例表现肿瘤与相邻脏器间脂肪间隙消失，而病理证实仅有 3 例为受侵，其中多平面重建图像改变分期 5 例，但该组仍有低估及高估。

一组研究资料结果表明，MSCT 已基本消除了多平面重建图像中的呼吸伪影，多平面重建连续图像提示部分横断面显示病变周围脂肪间隙内的点状、条状影实为血管影，可排除部分 T_2 期高估为 T_3 期病例，同时通过多方位观察肿瘤与相邻脏器的关系，可排除部分 T_3 期高估为 T_4 期病例，但多平面重建也同样存在假阳性和假阴性，对比横断面及多平面重建分期准确率两者间无显著性差异。

目前，认为多平面重建的优势主要有两个方面：①有助于肿瘤定位，特别是对位于胃角处和胃大弯的病变；②有助于提供 T 分期、N 分期的信心。一组 55 例贲门癌病例分析显示，多平面重建更有助于显示肿瘤侵犯食管下段情况。

胃癌淋巴结转移：螺旋 CT 对于胃癌淋巴结转移的敏感性、特异性报道各家差异较大，采用的诊断标准不一致是原因之一。有的学者以淋巴结大小为标准，也有以淋巴结强化程度为标准，或将两者结合。一些作者报道采用 MSCT 以淋巴结直径超过 5mm 为转移标准，敏感性为 96.3%，特异性为 64.3%。另组 MSCT 研究资料以淋巴结短径≥ 5mm 为标准的敏感性、特异性、准确率分别为 68.9%、80.0%、70.1%。

CT 对 N 分期低的主要原因是 CT 无法准确鉴别增大的淋巴结是炎症或反应性淋巴结增生还是由转移所致，也无法检出小而有转移的淋巴结，而大多数胃癌的转移淋巴结较小，故 N 分期低估者多。

Fukuya 等研究显示，随着淋巴结的增大，转移率上升，<5mm、5~9 mm、10~14 mm 和 >14 mm 的淋巴结中，分别有 5.1%、21.7%、23%、82.6% 的淋巴结出现转移。Fukuya 等报道当增强扫描检出的淋巴结 CT 值≥ 100HU，淋巴结短径与长径比值 >0.7 时多为转移，而这一结果只对淋巴结大于 9mm 的较为准确。

有作者认为淋巴结的强化程度与增强扫描时间、注射对比剂速度及对比剂用量等多因素有关，因此，Fukuya 等研究结果有待于进一步研究。

多平面重建图像更有利于淋巴结定位，特别对于胃左血管周围及胃大弯淋巴结。一组研究结果表明，有 5 例多平面重建图像对淋巴结定位增添信息，纠正横断面 3 例 N_2 期（胃左血管旁）低估为 N_1 期（肿瘤旁），2 例血管断面误诊为 N_1 期，但横断面、多平面重建总的 N 分期敏感性、特异性、准确率无显著性差异。

Filippone 等报道 MSCT 对结、直肠癌研究，结果显示横断面 N 分期准确率为 59%，而多平面重建图像 N 分期准确率为 80%，两者间统计学有显著性差异，认为多平面重建提高 N 分期的原因是淋巴结大小测量更加准确，同时多平面重建图像有利于区别直肠周围的小血管与淋巴结。上述结果可能与结、直肠的解剖特点及周围脂肪较多而易于检出淋巴结及与血管相鉴别有关。

贲门癌：贲门是胃的特殊部位，其黏膜下层、肌层和浆膜下有丰富的淋巴网，并与食管的淋巴管相通。从贲门与食管交通的淋巴管网引流入上纵隔，最后汇入胸导管，向右侧引流经食管贲门支和胃左动脉网到腹腔动脉组淋巴结，左侧从胃后壁经大弯到腹膜后淋巴结。沿这些引流淋巴管，常见的第一站转移淋巴结为贲门旁、食管下段和胃小弯淋巴结，第二站为沿胃左动脉、脾动脉、脾门和网膜的淋巴结。晚期转移至腹腔动脉旁、肝门、腹膜后、纵隔和锁骨上淋巴结。贲门癌沿黏膜下淋巴管网浸润是导致外科手术切缘不净的重要原因。因此，一些作者认为在对贲门癌患者行 CT 检查时，建议采用以左膈上 3cm~5cm 为扫描起点，目的为检出食管下段淋巴结。

肝转移和腹腔转移：螺旋 CT 对肝转移的敏感性较高，主要因为螺旋 CT（特别是 MSCT）明显降低和 / 或消除了呼吸、运动伪影，一次注药可完成多时相扫描，肝脏对比好，不易遗漏小转移灶，有文献报道其对肝转移的敏感性和准确性达到 100% 和 94.4%。但对肝表面的粟粒样转移不易检出。胃癌肝转移多表现为单发或多发低密度结节，可伴有环形强化。腹腔转移表现为腹膜、网膜和肠系膜密度增高、片状增厚、结节状模糊影，网膜饼及腹腔积液等。

文献报道 CT 对腹腔转移的敏感性仅 30%~60.5%。因此，为避免不必要的探查术，Lehnert 等研究显示，对临床分期（采用 CT、MRI、超声等）可疑 T_4 期和肝转移、腹腔转移的病例行腹腔镜检查，可提高手术切除率。有作者建议对于女性病例，临床分期（采用 CT、MRI、超声等）可疑 T_4 期和肝转移、腹腔转移者，还应注意卵巢有无转移。

进展期胃癌：有关 MSCT 的 3D（仿真内镜、表面遮盖技术、透明技术）技术在早期胃癌的研究报道较少，对进展期胃癌的研究较多，主要有以下四个方面：图像质量、伪影情况、病变的诊断可信度及大体分型。

研究结果显示，MSCT 的 3D（仿真内镜、表面遮盖技术、透明技术）图像满意度高，伪影主要为滞留液产生，部分病例可有轻度的环形伪影，考虑与螺旋 CT 数据的插入算法有关。

有作者报道仿真内镜对胃癌诊断的敏感性为 97%，特异性为 75%，准确性为 95%。也有文献报道仿真内镜对进展期胃癌的大体分型准确率为 92.3%，高于双对比造影（86.5%）和电子内镜（84.3%）。表面遮盖技术和透明技术的大体分型能力与双对比造影接近，两者在单独应用时，评价胃癌的价值有限。

一组贲门癌病例研究显示，仿真内镜加 2DCT 的分型符合率（84%），略高于两者单独分型符合率（$P>0.05$），说明仿真内镜有助于鉴别溃疡与肿瘤表面的不规则生长，而 2DCT 的原始横断面图像、多平面重建图像可显示部分表浅溃疡。表面遮盖技术和透明技术的优势在于显示胃的轮廓，而对胃黏膜细节显示不如仿真内镜。特别是贲门肿瘤侵犯食管下端造成食管下段、贲门口狭窄或食管下段生理性收缩，2DCT（横断面、多平面重建图像）在显示病变本身及侵犯食管情况要优于 3D 图像。总之，MSCT 在胃癌的诊断、术前分期和治疗后随诊等方面发挥着重要作用。但 MSCT 对早期癌诊断、T_4 期判断及淋巴结检出、有无转移等方面有局限性，只有将 2DCT 与 3DCT 紧密结合，才能充分发挥 MSCT 的作用。

第七章 胃癌的少见表现

第一节 钙化性胃癌

钙化性胃癌非常少见,其钙化至今报道 3 种类型:黏液湖性钙化、沙粒性钙化、异位性骨化。钙化是钙化性胃癌的显著特征,关于其钙化有 4 种机制:钙化瘢痕组织或者是肿瘤吞噬了肉芽组织;由于肿瘤的快速生长,导致肿瘤营养不良,坏死组织沉积钙化;钙化的产生与肿瘤的特殊分泌有关;由于体内血钙水平过高引起肿瘤的转移性钙化。

碱性环境是钙化性胃癌中钙化的必要因素,其体现在以下几个方面:高黏蛋白组织在黏蛋白物质和相对碱性环境易于发生钙化;营养不良性钙化常发生在胃黏液腺癌的局部缺血坏死组织;变性蛋白束钙化是由于磷酸盐与钙离子在碱性环境下生成磷酸钙。

钙化型胃癌钙化可成点状、粟粒状及胃壁的线性沉积。钙化性胃癌的钙化灶不仅可以见于原发灶,还可以见于转移灶,如淋巴结、肝脏及结肠周围软组织等。

钙化性胃癌的癌细胞常常呈腺样或弥漫浸润分布,肿瘤组织的细胞、腺腔内及间质内富含黏液形成黏液湖,增强 CT 常可见胃壁间低密度带或胃壁呈全层低密度带,黏液湖也是黏液性腺癌的特征之一。钙化性胃癌的侵袭性与预后紧密相关,正常胃壁细胞之间连接比较紧密,钙化性胃癌细胞之间具有分离趋向。细胞间黏附的丧失和细胞外基质的降解是肿瘤侵袭和转移的重要因素。

目前关于胃癌的转移及侵袭机制热点关注,主要包括基质金属蛋白酶 2(MMP-2)、E- 钙黏附素、环氧化酶(COX)和 DNA 含量的研究。

MMP-2 是 MMPs 家族成员,称作明胶酶,其主要依赖降解Ⅳ、Ⅴ型胶原及明胶等以介导炎症细胞迁移和肿瘤细胞突破基底膜屏障,促进肿瘤细胞侵袭性生长和发生转移,MMP-2 的表达有利于胃癌细胞获得侵袭力、发生转移和向恶性方向发展。

E- 钙黏附素是细胞膜上的一种跨膜糖蛋白,其生物学行为主要控制细胞的移动以及促进细胞发生黏附,在胃黏液腺癌、印戒细胞癌及低分化腺癌中呈低表达导致癌细胞侵袭及转移。环氧化酶是花生四烯酸合成前列腺素的限速酶, COX-2 在肺癌、乳腺癌、结肠癌及胃癌中都呈现高表达,与胃癌的生物学行为及淋巴结转移密切相关。DNA 含量也是胃癌细胞生物学特征之一,其含量变化直接影响胃癌的生物学特性及预后。

综上所述,钙化性胃癌是属于特殊性胃癌的罕见病例,钙化性胃癌具有特殊的 CT 表现:①胃壁明显增厚,黏膜粗糙紊乱,呈浸润性生长,与周围组织界限不清;②增厚的胃壁间常有低密度带,也就是所谓病理的黏液湖;③肿瘤组织内常可见弥漫性的斑点状、粟粒状钙化及特殊性钙化。

钙化性胃癌组织学分为黏液腺癌、印戒细胞癌以及低分化腺癌,虽然在浸润深度、远处转移、根治手术与否以及临床分期存在差异性,但是 3 种类型的钙化性胃癌的总体生存率却没有显著差异。

与非钙化性胃癌相比,钙化性胃癌复发、转移概率较高,预后较差。每 1 例钙化性胃癌的生物学行为、CT 表现及病理基础都不尽相同,收集并总结这些病例可以提高对特殊类型胃癌的诊断水平,同时可以帮助人们对于胃肠道肿瘤的生物学行为的更加整体深入的了解。

第二节　胃癌合并胃脂肪瘤

胃脂肪瘤是一种较少见的胃良性肿瘤，约占胃良性肿瘤的2.2%，文献多为个案报道。胃脂肪瘤与胃癌同时发生更少见。胃脂肪瘤起源于胃间叶组织，由成熟的脂肪组织组成，肿瘤位于胃黏膜下，而胃癌起源于胃黏膜上皮，因此病灶主要位于胃黏膜表面，可以向黏膜下发展，两者互不相关。因此，理论上讲同一患者既有胃癌又有胃脂肪瘤是完全可以的，但临床少见，两者可发生于胃的不同部位，也可发生于同一部位。一例两者都位于胃窦部。

胃脂肪瘤属黏膜下肿瘤，胃镜只能提示黏膜下占位，当合并胃癌时，向腔内生长的胃癌组织进一步掩盖了胃脂肪瘤的征象，使胃镜无法显示胃黏膜下占位，而CT能显示胃壁肿块的全貌，特别是脂肪瘤具有特征性的密度和CT值。

因此CT很容易显示胃脂肪瘤，即使有胃癌组织重叠也无妨，关键是不要将胃脂肪瘤的低密度影误为胃溃疡内的气体影，测量其CT值或调整图像的显示窗条件可以避免漏诊。

第三节　胃癌与十二指肠溃疡同存

Bateson(1972)回顾(1962—1972年期间)胃肠X线检查6 080例，发现1 761例患十二指肠球部溃疡，272例胃癌，208例良性胃溃疡，180例食管裂孔疝，172例食管癌。其中，十二指肠溃疡与胃癌同存者仅2例，十分少见，表示十二指肠溃疡患者比正常人群中的胃癌发病率低，分析其原因，大概与胃酸水平较高有关。

第八章 胃淋巴瘤

第一节 胃的孤立性霍奇金病

此病相当少见，1938 年以前文献报告仅 14 例，直到 1970 年还不到 100 例。此病主要依靠胃肠 X 线检查发现，其 X 线表现与胃癌极为相似，难以分辨，一般为手术组织学检查作出诊断。术后可再行淋巴造影等检查，以了解它处有无淋巴瘤的征象。

第二节 进展期胃癌与胃淋巴瘤鉴别

详见本书 本卷 本篇 第三章 第二节 进展期胃癌与胃淋巴瘤鉴别。

第三节 误诊病例简介：胃非霍奇金 B 细胞淋巴瘤与胃溃疡

患者，女，46 岁。中上腹胀痛伴黑便 1 周入院。门诊电子胃镜提示，食管：黏膜光滑柔软，血管纹理清晰，扩张度好。贲门：见一大小约 0.8cm 息肉。胃体小弯侧见巨大溃疡，污苔附着，病变侵及胃底及胃角，活检质脆。胃窦：黏膜见点状充血，未见出血及溃疡，蠕动尚可。幽门：呈圆形，开闭尚可。十二指肠：球部及降部未见异常；内镜诊断：胃溃疡(性质待定)、HP(+)。病理检查：灰白色黏膜组织四枚，最大者大小为 0.2cm×0.1cm×0.1cm，最小者大小为 0.1cm×0.1cm×0.1cm。常规病理诊断：胃体黏膜活检标本：溃疡性病变，溃疡灶旁黏膜固有层及黏膜肌间质可见多量体积较大且具有非典型的淋巴细胞样细胞浸润，需做免疫组化及原位杂交检测进一步协助诊断，另 HP(+)。

免疫组化检测：阳性：CD20，Bcl-6，CD10，MUM1，PAX-5，CD79α，CD3(反应性 T 细胞+)，CD43(反应性 T 细胞+)，CD5(反应性 T 细胞+)，TIA-1(反应性 T 细胞+)，CD45RO(反应性 T 细胞+)，CD7(反应性 T 细胞+)，Ki-67(+，局灶约 90%)；阴性：EBV，EMA，CyclinD1，CD56，CD30，CDX-2，ALK，CD15，TdT，CK18，CK(P)，Mucin-2，Bcl-2，MPO，CD21，CD23，CD35，粒酶 B。免疫组化诊断：胃体黏膜活检标本：结合免疫组化及原位杂交检测结果、消化内镜及影像学检查，诊断为非霍奇金 B 细胞淋巴瘤。(注：因内镜取材局限，倾向于弥漫大 B 细胞淋巴瘤，生发中心源性，GCB 型胃肠道淋巴瘤约占淋巴瘤的 0.9%，以非霍奇金淋巴瘤多见。(图 23-8-1))

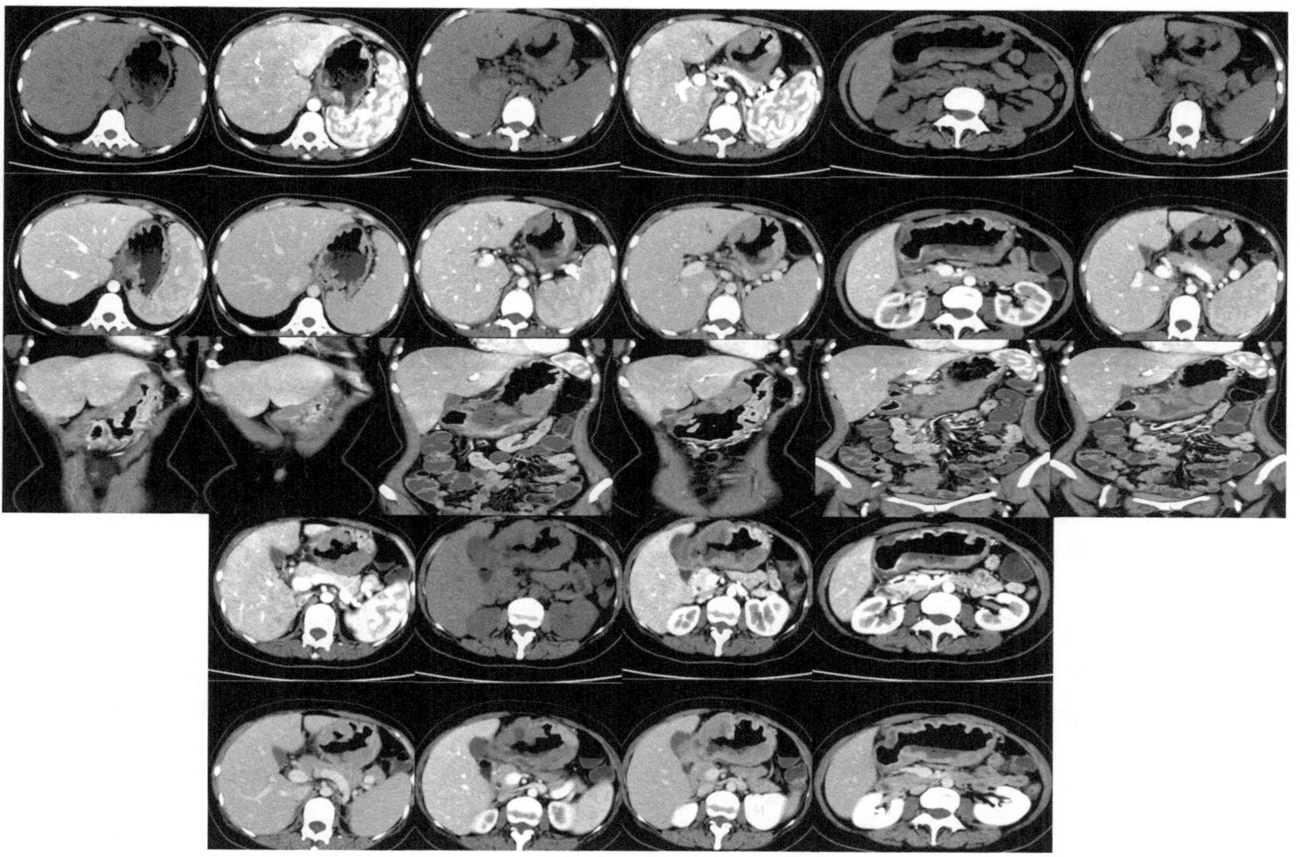

图 23-8-1　胃非霍奇金 B 细胞淋巴瘤与胃溃疡

第九章 胃间质瘤

第一节 胃肠道间质瘤的 CT

胃肠道间质瘤由 Mazur 等(1983)根据肿瘤的分化特征提出。目前,已得到国内外学者的公认,应用于临床和病理诊断。

胃肠道间质瘤是一种少见的肿瘤,占全部胃肠道肿瘤的 0.1%~0.3%,胃是其好发部位(占 50%),其中约 1/2 发生于胃体,发生于胃窦和贲门者各占 1/4。

过去多诊断为平滑肌瘤、平滑肌母细胞瘤或平滑肌肉瘤,但电镜与免疫组织化学表明,肿瘤内并没有平滑肌或施万细胞,而是由不同数量的梭形细胞和上皮样细胞组成。

依据梭形细胞和上皮样细胞的比例可分为梭形细胞型、上皮样细胞型以及梭形细胞和上皮样细胞混合型. 在光学显微镜下与神经鞘瘤、平滑肌瘤不易区分。临床诊断比较困难,免疫组织化学和电子显微镜检查目前已成为确诊胃肠道间质瘤的主要病理手段。

胃肠道间质瘤的免疫组织化学检查表现为 CD117 和 / 或 CD34 阳性。一组病例中 CD117(+)8 例, CD34(+)8 例, Vim(+)5 例,文献报道间质瘤表达 Vim 为 100%,低于文献报道,而平滑肌源性或神经源性肿瘤不表达 CD117 或 CD34,据此可确诊。

胃肠道间质瘤的生物学行为从良性到显著恶性不等,如何准确判断胃肠道间质瘤的良恶性一直是面临的难题之一。

目前,对胃肠道间质瘤生物学行为的认识仍存有分歧,由于较难划分良、恶性,部分研究者提倡依据某些特征将胃肠道间质瘤分为高危组和低危组,如肿瘤直径≥ 5 cm 和 / 或核分裂数≥ 2 个 /10 高倍视野(HPF),复发、转移率大,视为高危组;肿瘤直径 <5 cm 和 / 或核分裂数 <2 个 /10 HPF,则为低危组。

根据瘤体与胃肠道管壁的关系可分为 4 型:黏膜下型,肿瘤从黏膜下向腔内生长突出,与管壁有蒂相连(该组有 2 例);肌壁间型,肿瘤同时向腔内外生长突出(该组有 7 例);浆膜下型,肿瘤从浆膜下向壁外生长突出,与管壁基底有蒂相连(该组有 1 例);胃肠道外型,肿瘤起源于胃肠道管壁以外的腹内其他部位。

肿块大多数呈膨胀性生长,为境界清楚的孤立性圆形或椭圆形,偶见分叶状或多发性。肿块可出血、坏死、囊变等,部分内部可出现点状钙化,由此可以解释 CT 表现密度不均匀。

第二节　胃肠道间质瘤(低危险度)

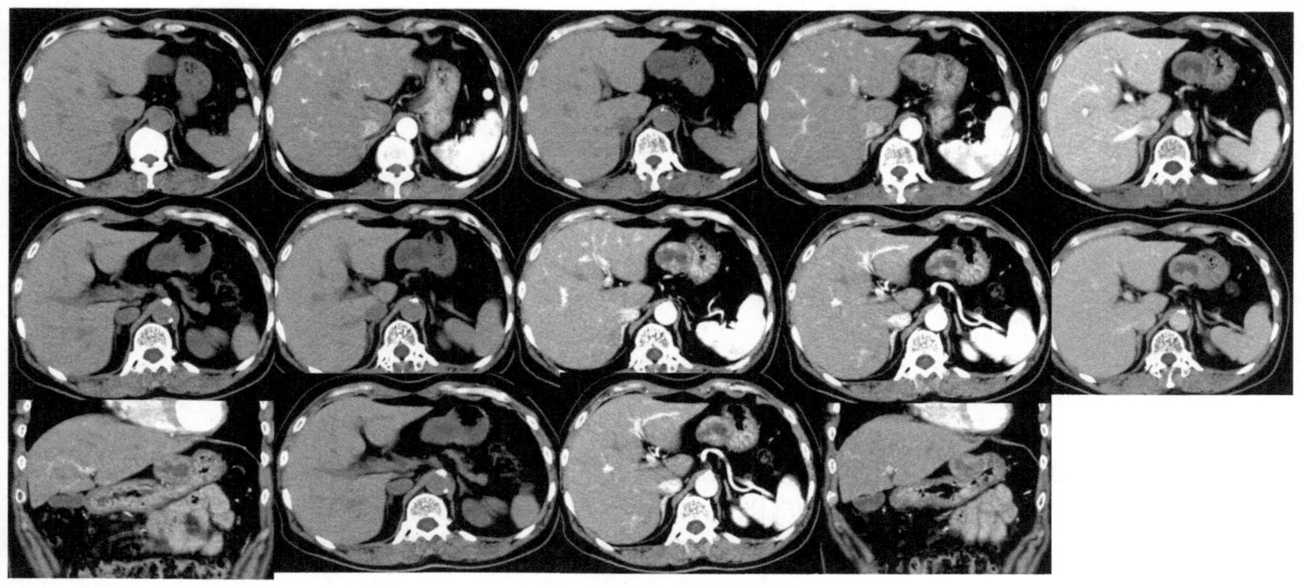

图 23-9-1　胃肠道间质瘤(低危险度)

患者,女,68 岁。体检发现腹部肿块 20 余天入院。

手术所见:探查见肿瘤位于胃窦小弯侧胃壁肌层,侵及浆膜层,大小 3.5cm × 3.5cm × 2.5cm,切面灰白,质中,中央可见出血及坏死,与周围界限欠清。

病理检查:胃大部切除标本:远端胃组织一块,大小 13cm × 7cm × 3cm,小弯侧长 9cm,大弯侧长 16cm,上切缘周径 4.5cm,下切缘周径 10cm,紧靠下切缘可见一椭圆形肿物,肿物位于胃壁肌层,大小 3.5cm × 3.5cm × 2.5cm,切面灰白,质中,中央可见出血及坏死,与周围界限欠清。胃大弯侧附大网膜组织一具,大小 7cm × 7cm × 2cm,网膜及胃周脂肪组织均未触及淋巴结及肿大结节。远端切缘(缝线处)标本:胃组织一块,大小 4.5cm × 2cm × 1.5cm。常规病理诊断:胃大部切除标本:梭形细胞肿瘤,待做免疫组化检测进一步明确肿瘤类型,可见肿瘤组织位于胃壁肌层,局部见坏死,胃上下两处切缘及送检远端切缘均为阴性,大网膜组织未检出淋巴结,亦未见肿瘤组织累及。

免疫组化检测:阳性: CD117, CD34, DOG1, Vimentin, H-caldesmon, Calponin(灶 +), Actin, Ki-67(+, <5%);阴性: Desmin, SMA, S-100, CD57, CK(P)。免疫组化诊断:胃大部切除标本:胃肠道间质瘤(GIST,低危险度),可见瘤组织位于胃壁肌层,局部见坏死,建议做 c-kit 和 PDGFRA 基因检测以应用于肿瘤靶向治疗药物的选择(图 23-9-1)。

第三节　胃底胃肠道间质瘤(低危险度)

患者,男, 51 岁。进食梗阻感 1 年,上腹隐痛 2 个月余,黑便 4 天入院。

病理检查:胃底肿瘤切除标本胃组织一块,大小 8cm × 5cm × 3cm,黏膜下可见一类圆形结节状肿物,大小 4.5cm × 3.5cm × 3cm,切面灰白灰褐,质中偏软,与周围组织界限较清,其余黏膜未见异常。

免疫组化检测:阳性: CD117, DOG1, CD34, H-caldesmon, Ki-67(+, <5%);阴性: CD57, Actin, desmin, SMA, S-100。免疫组化诊断:胃底肿物切除标本:胃肠道间质瘤(GIST,低危险度)(图 23-9-2)。

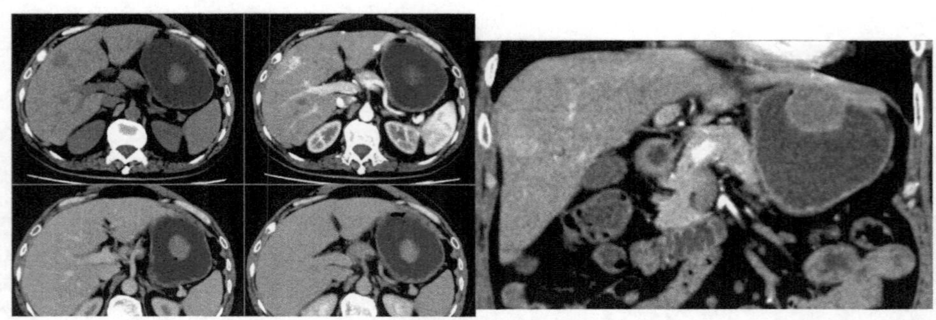

图 23-9-2　胃底胃肠道间质瘤（低危险度）

第四节　胃间质瘤良、恶性区别研究

胃肠道间质瘤是原发于胃肠道、大网膜和肠系膜的 KIT（CD117 干细胞因子受体）染色阳性的梭形细胞或上皮样细胞的间质肿瘤，是消化道最常见的间叶源性肿瘤，主要发生于胃（60%~70%），占胃部肿瘤的 1%~3%。CT 在 GIST 的诊断中发挥着重要作用。

良、恶性判定标准：有关良、恶性的诊断，文献虽报道不少，胃间质瘤生物学行为从良性到显著恶性不等，如何准确判断胃间质瘤的良、恶性一直是病理工作者面临的难题之一。

由于较难划分良、恶性，部分研究者提倡依据某些特征将胃间质瘤分为高危组和低危组，如肿瘤直径≥ 5 cm 和 / 或核分裂数≥ 2 个 /10 HPF，复发、转移率大，视为高危组；肿瘤直径 <5cm 和 / 或核分裂数 <2 个 /10 HPF，则为低危组。也有根据肿瘤大小和核分裂象数目分为极低恶性、低度恶性、中度恶性和高度恶性 4 组。各组间虽有统计学意义，但这种分组仅参考了肿瘤大小和核分裂 2 个指标。该组良、恶性的诊断采纳 Miettinen 和 Lasota（2001）的判断指标作为参考。以往认为胃间质瘤良性多于恶性，但近年来研究发现恶性多于良性，发病部位以胃为多见。该组病例恶性 34 例（34/43），多于良性。并且原病理诊断的良性病例中，有 3 例经随访发现有复发及转移，现被列为恶性组探讨。

病理学诊断往往与生物学行为不一致，文献报告仅 30%~38% 的胃间质瘤有恶性的组织学特征，却有 68% 的肿瘤出现临床转移。所以，不少病理学者认为，胃间质瘤的恶性潜能常难以预测，没有明确的良、恶性界限，一些组织学上判断为良性的胃间质瘤也可发生转移，认为用低危状态来描述比用良性更确切。所以在判断胃间质瘤的良、恶性时，不能单靠病理组织学诊断，这就显得探讨胃间质瘤的 CT 征象越来越重要。因此，胃间质瘤即使诊断为良性，也有可能具有潜在恶性，在治疗前需确诊。

该组资料中，良性（交界性）相当于恶性程度低的间质瘤，恶性相当于中等及高等程度的间质瘤。该研究的目的，亦即探讨胃间质瘤的良性（恶性程度低的）和恶性（中等及高等程度的）与螺旋 CT 征象间相关性。

胃间质瘤的生长方式与其良、恶性及预后关系密切：通过该组胃间质瘤的生长与病理及随访结果的对照研究表明，呈现腔内 / 外生长的胃间质瘤，越倾向于恶性。该组 43 例分析，<5 cm 腔内 / 外型间质瘤只有 2 例，而 >10 cm 的胃间质瘤，只有腔外型和腔内 / 外型，而腔内型未见到。并且 17 例腔内 / 外型者，只有 1 例为良性。说明胃间质瘤的大小与生长方式之间关系也很密切，瘤体越大，越倾向于腔外生长或腔内 / 外生长。

胃间质瘤的生物学特性表明，大多胃间质瘤由小到大，是从良性到恶性直至高度恶性的转变过程，说明胃间质瘤在生长过程中与 C-kit 和血小板源性生长因子受体（PDGFRA）等基因的突变有关，并且不少胃间质瘤患者经伊马替尼治疗后，出现了耐药性，也说明了耐药性与 C-kit 基因的突变有关。因此，胃间质瘤生长过程中，C-kit 和血小板源性生长因子受体等基因的突变是胃间质瘤向高度恶性发展和产生耐药性的根本原因。通过该项研究分析验证了生长方式与预后的关系：腔内 / 外型 > 腔外型 >

腔内型。

综上所述，螺旋CT对分析胃间质瘤的生长方式与病理及预后的关系具有重要价值。

第五节　胃底胃肠道间质瘤(低危险度)

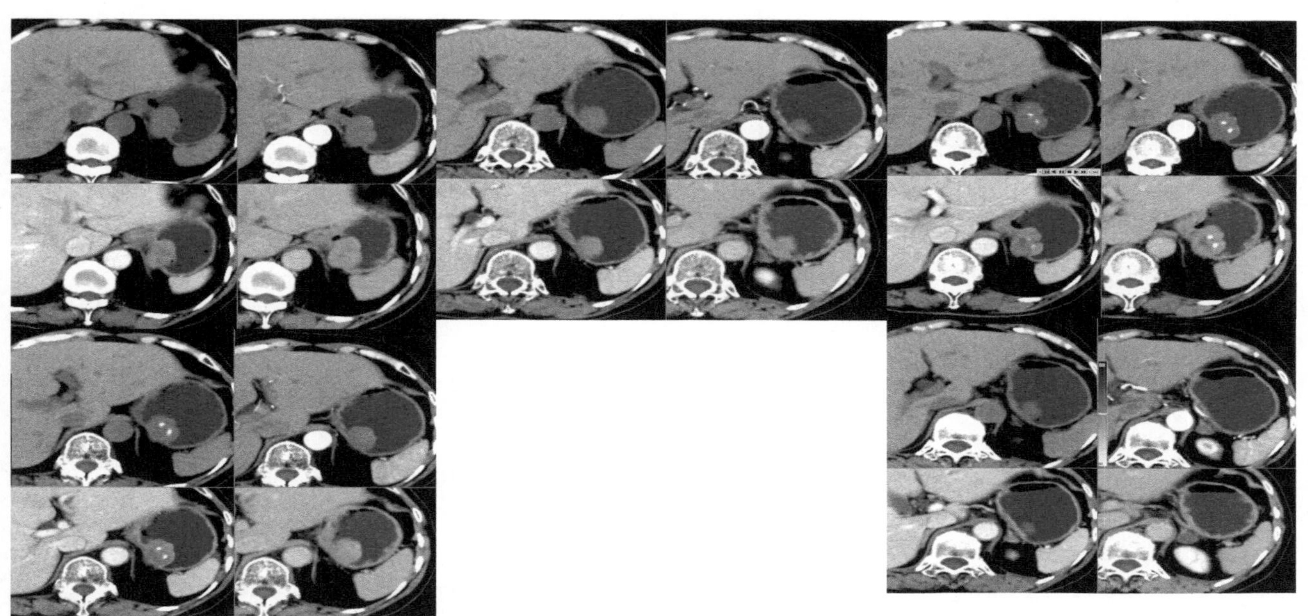

图 23-9-3　胃底胃肠道间质瘤(低危险度)

患者，女，70岁。因反复反酸嗳气半年入院。就诊外院行胃镜检查示：胃底见一大小约3.0cm隆起性赘生物，中央凹陷，界清，表面光滑。

病理检查：胃底黏膜下隆起ESD切除病灶标本：结节状肿物一块，大小3.5cm×3cm×2.5cm，肿物位于黏膜下，切面灰白，质中偏韧。常规病理诊断：胃底黏膜下隆起ESD切除病灶标本：胃底梭形细胞肿瘤，局部胶原化钙化，待做免疫组化检测明确肿瘤类型。

免疫组化检测：阳性：CD117，CD34，DOG1，Nestin，H-caldesmon，Ki-67(+，约1%)；阴性：Actin，Desmin，SMA，S-100。免疫组化诊断：胃底黏膜下隆起ESD切除病灶，胃肠道间质瘤(GIST，低危险度)(图23-9-3)。

第六节　转移性胃间质瘤

胃间质瘤的复发率极高，即使经手术彻底切除，复发率仍高达40%~80%。通常复发的部位在局部或肝脏，但是周围淋巴结转移很少见。一组22例转移性胃间质瘤患者中，血行转移发生率达72.7%(16/22)，而肝脏占血行转移的59.1%(13/22)。

由于恶性胃间质瘤血供极其丰富，而且发现时瘤体常常较大，伴发囊变、坏死以及出血的概率高，手术时难免瘤体破裂，术后种植转移的概率高。该组有6例术后发生种植转移，因此术中应注意完整切除和防止肿瘤破裂，避免术后种植转移。

该组中，5例CT示肿大淋巴结，其中3例术后病理均被证实为慢性反应性增生或慢性炎症改变，未见肿瘤样细胞。因此，本病极少淋巴结转移，小于2 cm的胃间质瘤可以考虑局部切除，而不需做局部淋巴结清扫。对较小的腔外生长的胃间质瘤也可采用腹腔镜下切除术。因此，胃间质瘤只要能做到早期发现，就可以在微创手术下得到很好治疗。

该研究结果表明，胃间质瘤以血行转移为主，以肝脏最多见,其次为种植转移,而淋巴结转移最少见。

目前研究认为,原癌基因 c-Kit 获得性功能突变是发生胃肠道间质瘤的主要分子机制,而没有 c-Kit 突变的胃肠道间质瘤可能与血小板源性生长因子受体(PDGFRA)获得性功能突变有关。手术治疗,包括腹腔镜下切除术仍是胃间质瘤的主要治疗方法。

转移性胃肠道间质瘤患者的中位生存期约为 20 个月,而传统的化疗药对不能手术或转移的胃肠道间质瘤无效。

近年的酪氨酸激酶抑制剂伊马替尼(Imatinb, STI-571)和舒尼替尼(Sutent, SU11248),通过阻断 Kit 和血小板源性生长因子受体膜内的酪氨酸激酶在胃肠道间质瘤的治疗中取得了可观的临床效果,成为分子靶向药物治疗实体瘤成功的典范。由于伊马替尼的费用昂贵,仅有少数患者能够承担。因此,该组资料较少,随访时间最长的 1 例仅 3 年。

该组 11 例胃间质瘤转移患者接受伊马替尼治疗后较未接受治疗组中位生存期明显延长,近期疗效观察,效果满意。有文献报道 1 例转移性胃肠道间质肿瘤患者每天口服伊马替尼 400 mg,达到迅速而持久的完全缓解,并持续 1 年余。因此,伊马替尼对转移性胃间质瘤的疗效肯定,可用于肿瘤广泛粘连、转移无法完整切除或有肿瘤残余者以及术后复发者。

综上所述,螺旋 CT 对分析胃间质瘤转移的特征和疗效的关系具有重要价值,能有效指导临床实践。

第七节　胃底小的胃肠道间质瘤

患者,女, 64 岁。因体检发现胃息肉 21 天入院。21 天前外院电子胃镜示:慢性浅表性胃炎伴痘疣状改变,胃底息肉?门诊拟胃息肉收治住院。

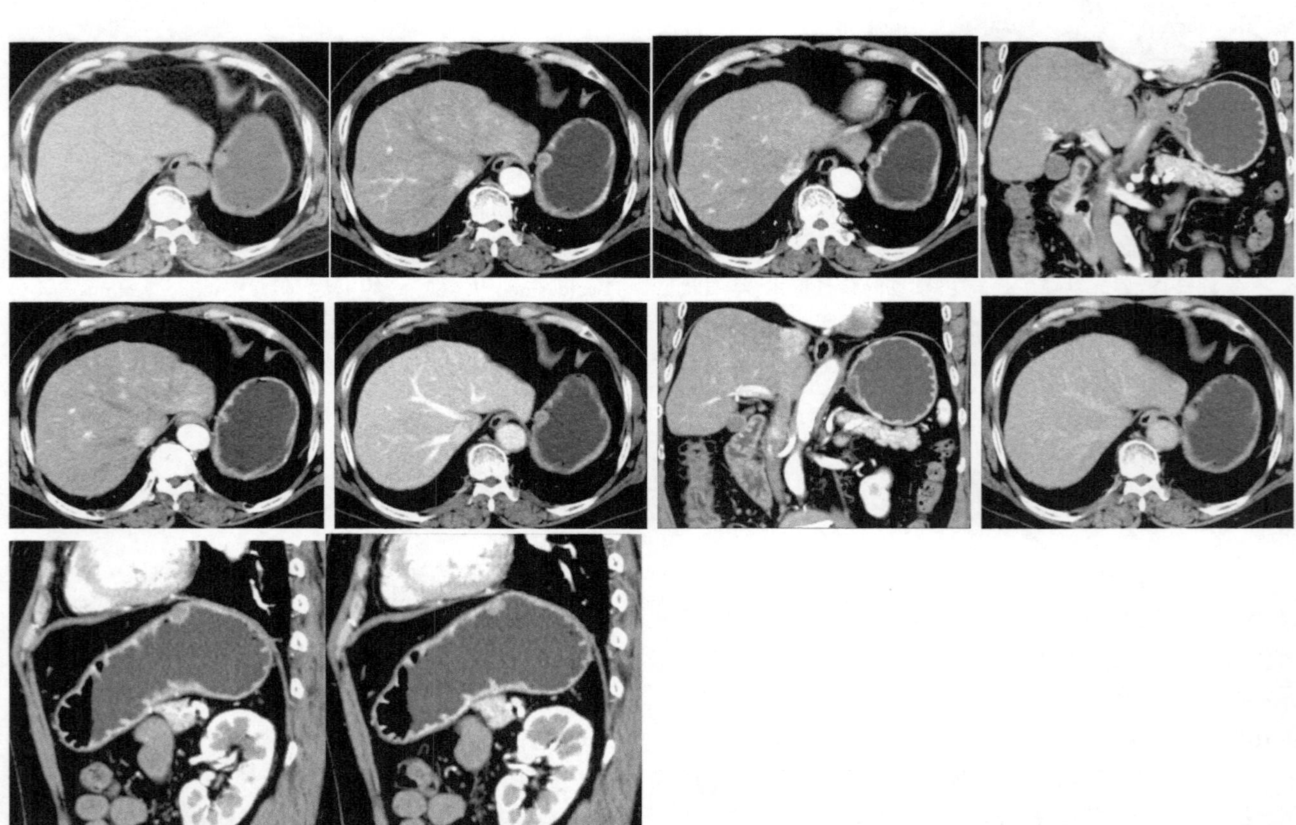

图 23-9-4　胃底小的胃肠道间质瘤

手术：内镜下胃占位病变黏膜下剥离术（ESD 治疗）。

病理检查：胃底病灶切除标本：结节状组织一块，大小 1.5cm × 1.0cm × 0.9cm，切面灰白，质中。

免疫组化检测：阳性：CD34，CD117，DOG-1，Vimentin，Actin（灶+），Calponin（灶+），H-caldesmon（灶+），Ki-67（+，<5%）；阴性：CK（P），S-100，SOX-10。常规病理诊断：胃底病灶切除标本：梭形细胞肿瘤，待做免疫组化检测进一步明确诊断。免疫组化诊断：胃底病灶切除标本：胃肠道间质瘤（GIST，极低危险度）。（图 23-9-4）

第十章　其他胃恶性肿瘤

第一节　胃类癌

病理学：Ⅰ型肠嗜铬样细胞类癌为胃体、底部多发 <1 cm 的黏膜结节。镜下，Ⅰ型与Ⅱ型肠嗜铬样细胞类癌均由圆形或多角形细胞构成，细胞核均一、居中，核仁小，颗粒状染色质。瘤细胞排列成小梁状或菊花团样，其间偶尔可见呈带状或条索状排列的细胞浸润，但通常局限在黏膜或黏膜下。多数Ⅰ型、Ⅱ型肠嗜铬样细胞类癌没有或罕有核分裂相，反映其良性生物学行为。但也有 5% 的Ⅰ型肠嗜铬样细胞类癌出现局限性的淋巴结转移。Ⅱ型肠嗜铬样细胞类癌也是多发，但大小不一，且更倾向于转移，其转移发生率为 10%~30%。Ⅲ型肠嗜铬样细胞类癌常为单发，直径 >2 cm。最常见于胃体、底部，可以侵入胃壁较深，组织学上可见淋巴管与血管受侵。

临床表现：大部分胃类癌为肠嗜铬样细胞类癌，分为 3 个亚型：Ⅰ型与自体免疫性萎缩性胃炎相关；Ⅱ型发生于Ⅰ型多发性内分泌肿瘤综合征（MEN-1）并发 Zollinger-Ellison 综合征（ZES）患者；Ⅲ型不并发于萎缩或肥大性胃炎，为散发病例。

Ⅰ型肠嗜铬样细胞类癌最多见，占胃内分泌肿瘤的 74%，患者常无临床症状，往往因其他原因作胃镜时偶然发现。高胃泌素血症或胃窦部 G 细胞增生常见。Ⅱ型肠嗜铬样细胞类癌占 6%，临床常出现 Zollinger-Ellison 综合征和胃泌素增高导致的肥大性胃炎的表现。Ⅲ型肠嗜铬样细胞类癌占 13%，临床表现无特殊，与其他胃肿瘤类似。

影像学研究：Ⅰ型与Ⅱ型肠嗜铬样细胞类癌在双对比钡餐检查中表现为胃体、底部多发，边缘光滑，1~2 cm 的肿块。CT 增强扫描可见肿块强化。在 Binstock 等（2001）的研究中，小于 1 cm 的肿瘤 CT 检测不到。较大肿瘤黏膜面可出现溃疡。

钡餐显示龛影或 CT 显示局部对比剂聚集、肿块表面有气体都利于溃疡的诊断。对于Ⅰ型多发性内分泌肿瘤综合征与 Zollinger-Ellison 综合征患者，钡餐可显示弥漫性胃黏膜皱襞增厚及黏膜皱襞呈结节状，还可见龛影。

由于胃液分泌过多导致胃壁敷钡不良或钡剂呈片絮状。CT 可见胃壁明显增厚和无数黏膜或壁内结节。增强动脉期可见增厚胃壁强化。

高胃泌素血症患者怀疑胃类癌行 CT 扫描应特别注意扫描技术，胃腔充盈良好、服中性对比剂、在动脉期与门静脉期扫描能最大限度检出胃壁病灶及肝转移灶。

Ⅲ型肠嗜铬样细胞类癌为胃体、底部单发较大肿块，表面可见溃疡。由于此型类癌有明显恶性倾向，CT 扫描应仔细观察有无胃周淋巴结及肝转移。

鉴别诊断：Ⅰ型与Ⅱ型肠嗜铬样细胞类癌的鉴别诊断应包括多发增生性息肉、家族性腺瘤样增生性息肉病、青年性息肉病、Peutz-Jeghers 综合征等多种能产生多发性息肉样肿块的病变。临床病史及检查肠道其余部位有助于鉴别诊断卡波西肉瘤和转移也可表现为多发结节样。Ⅲ型肠嗜铬样细胞类癌还应与腺癌、淋巴瘤、间质瘤鉴别。

第二节　胃低度恶性肌成纤维细胞肉瘤

低度恶性肌成纤维细胞肉瘤非常少见，是 WHO（2002）软组织肿瘤分类中明确列出的一种独立的肿瘤类型，主要由分化程度不同的肌成纤维细胞组成的罕见的梭形细胞肉瘤。

低度恶性肌成纤维细胞肉瘤最常见的发生部位是头颈部，包括面部、口腔、上下颌、耳后、扁桃体等，约占1/3，其次为躯干、四肢等。

低度恶性肌成纤维细胞肉瘤诊断目前主要依据病理。瘤细胞为肌成纤维细胞，它是一种同时具有平滑肌细胞和成纤维细胞特征的间叶细胞，其来源的肿瘤在超微结构和免疫组织化学上均具有成纤维细胞和平滑肌细胞的某些特点，细胞呈梭形或多角形，细胞核至少有局灶性中度非典型性，核大、深染、不规则。

Coffin 等（1998）报道低度恶性肌成纤维细胞肉瘤免疫组织化学常表现为：Vimentin 强阳性，SMA 阳性，肌特异性肌动蛋白（MSA）阳性，Desmin 呈灶性阳性，CK、CD68（KP21）、CD30 偶见灶性阳性。

一些作者报道的1例额部的低度恶性肌成纤维细胞肉瘤 CT 表现为软组织肿块及颅骨的破坏。MRI 表现为 T_1WI 呈中等偏低信号，T_2WI 呈等低混杂信号伴少许小斑片状高信号，增强扫描呈明显强化。另有作者报道1例上颌窦内的低度恶性肌成纤维细胞肉瘤 CT 表现为边界不清的软组织肿块伴窦壁及窦周骨质结构破坏。

胃的低度恶性肌成纤维细胞肉瘤需与胃间质瘤鉴别。一般直径 <5 cm 的胃间质瘤多为良性，CT 平扫密度均匀，边界清晰，边缘光滑，肿块边缘可见斑点状及弧形的钙化影，增强扫描多呈均匀轻中度强化，少数呈明显强化，病灶可见压迫周围组织，但无浸润征象；而直径 >5cm 的多为交界性或恶性胃间质瘤，CT 平扫密度不均匀，其内常可见囊变、坏死区，肿块通常边缘不规则，边界不清楚，多呈结节状浸润性生长，向周围组织浸润，增强扫描多为不均匀轻中度强化，其内常可见斑片状无强化区。

一例低度恶性肌成纤维细胞肉瘤影像表现为边界不清肿块，密度不均匀，中心有坏死区，与交界性或恶性间质瘤颇为相似，但是该病灶体积相对偏小，与交界性或恶性胃间质瘤肿块较大的特点有所不同。

第三节　胃粒状细胞肌胚细胞瘤

此病相当罕见。Naidech 等（1972）报告2例，加上文献报道7例共9例。此肿瘤可分三型：最常见类型为一个小的单个的黏膜下肿瘤；第二型为肿瘤的恶性变种；第三型为一有蒂的龈瘤状新生物附着于新生婴儿的前肠上。此肿瘤起源于肌胚细胞或雪旺细胞，尚存争论。另有作者报告2例，一为较大团块（直径4cm）伴中心性溃疡，一为单个小的黏膜下结节。

第四节 误诊病例简介:胃神经内分泌瘤与间质瘤

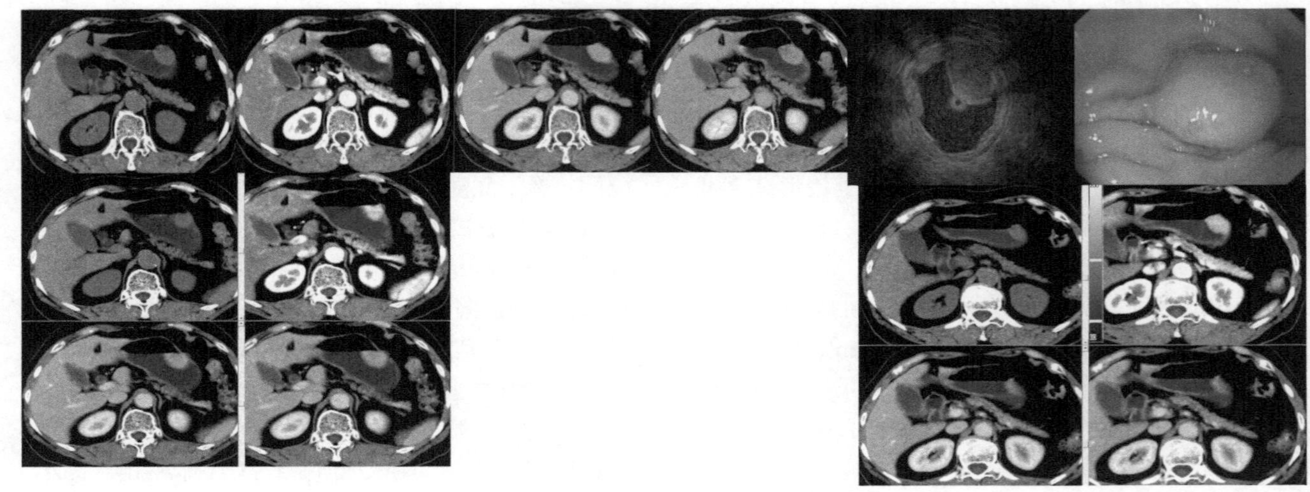

图 23-10-1 胃神经内分泌瘤与间质瘤

病例,女,68 岁。体检发现胃体黏膜下肿物 2 天入院。超声内镜见:胃体大弯侧见一大小约 4.1cm×2.5cm 黏膜呈半球形隆起,表面见一溃疡。超声下见以 12M 细径探头探查,病灶位于胃固有肌层,呈均质低回声团块,切面大小约 22.6 mm×20.3mm,后方浆膜层结构清楚。诊断:胃体黏膜下肿物伴表面溃疡形成(固有肌层间质瘤可能)。

手术所见:内镜下胃黏膜隆起 ESD 术见胃体中部大弯侧见一约 3.0cm 黏膜隆起,顶部凹陷,浅溃疡形成。病理检查:内镜下胃肿物病灶切除标本见结节状肿物一块,大小 3.5cm×2.5cm×1.3cm,切面灰红质中。常规病理诊断见内镜下胃肿物病灶切除标本:腺上皮肿瘤,良、恶性和肿瘤分型待免疫组化明确诊断。

免疫组化检测:阳性:CgA,Syn,Villin,CK-P,CK-L,CK-H(局灶 +),Ki-67(+,<2%);阴性:CDX2,CD34,CD117,CK7,CK20,Mucin-2。免疫组化诊断:内镜下胃肿物病灶切除标本:神经内分泌瘤,G1,低级别。备注(与预后评估相关的指标):肿瘤最大直径约 2.8cm;肿瘤侵犯黏膜固有层及黏膜下层;未见脉管和神经受累;核分裂象数 <2/10HPF;Ki-67 阳性指数 <2%;本例生物学行为属于恶性潜能未定肿瘤。(图 23-10-1)

第五节 原发性胃恶性黑色素瘤

黑色素瘤主要发生于富含黑色素细胞的表皮与真皮交界处,如皮肤、眼球、脑膜等,也可发生于胃肠道等部位,但原发于胃肠道的恶性黑色素瘤罕见。黑色素瘤分泌的黑色素颗粒具有顺磁性作用,能缩短 T_1 和 T_2 弛豫时间,故大部分黑色素瘤 MRI 具有特征性影像表现。

Isiklar 等(1995)将颅内黑色素瘤切除后依据黑色素瘤细胞内不同含量的黑色素在 MRI 的表现将其分为 4 型:黑色素型,T_1WI 为高信号,T_2WI 为低信号,质子密度像呈等或高信号;不含黑色素型,T_1WI 为低或等信号,T_2WI 和质子密度像为高或等信号;混合型,与前两型的任何一型都不相同;血肿型,MRI 只表现血肿特征。一例影像主要表现为:CT 示胃壁呈弥漫不规则增厚,胃腔缩小,部分呈肿块状向胃腔内突出,增厚的胃壁内可见不规则溃疡,增强后呈中度欠均匀强化;MRI 示增厚的胃壁在 T_1WI 上呈欠均匀的等、稍高信号,T_2WI 呈尚均匀的较高信号,其中见有纤维分隔、结节样表现。

恶性黑色素瘤主要应与弥漫性浸润性胃癌、胃淋巴瘤等鉴别。弥漫性浸润性胃癌常见胃黏膜“白线征”，黏膜溃疡多见，胃壁受侵范围常小于胃壁的50%，胃周肿大淋巴结多局限于一个区，MRI 多表现为 T_1WI 呈等低信号、T_2WI 呈等高信号，增强扫描动脉期即开始强化，静脉期仍有大量对比剂滞留在迂曲、变形的肿瘤血管内，该例 T_2WI 上所表现的结节样征象与胃癌不同。胃淋巴瘤黏膜溃疡少见，胃壁受累范围广，常大于胃壁的 75%，但胃腔常不狭窄，大部分胃淋巴瘤密度均匀，多不发生较大片状坏死和液化，增强后呈轻度强化，常有多个分区的胃周淋巴结肿大等影像表现，该例胃腔狭窄与淋巴瘤明显不同。

第六节　误诊病例简介：胃体部神经内分泌肿瘤（类癌）与平滑肌瘤伴大溃疡

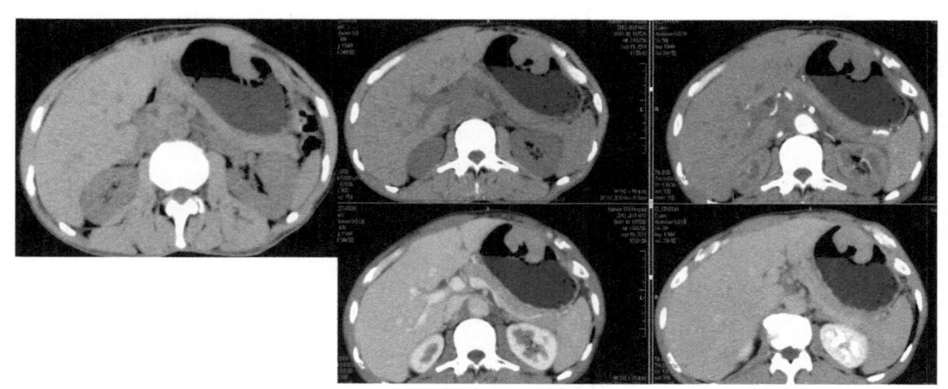

图 23-10-2　胃体部神经内分泌肿瘤（类癌）与平滑肌瘤伴大溃疡

患者，男，64 岁。腹痛伴解黑便 1 个月余入院。门诊胃镜提示胃占位，行 CT 进一步检查。

CT 诊断：胃体部前壁占位，考虑平滑肌瘤伴大溃疡，胃癌待排。门诊病理检查：胃内镜活检标本见灰白、灰褐黏膜组织 6 枚，大者 0.2cm × 0.1cm × 0.1cm，小者 0.1cm × 0.1cm × 0.1cm。病理诊断：胃体部黏膜慢性非萎缩性胃炎，重度，伴局灶性肠上皮化生。局部黏膜坏死，并见少量小细胞呈巢状聚集，性质不明，建议试做免疫组化或再次送检，以便确诊。HP(+)。

病理检查：近端胃及网膜切除标本见大弯长 12.5cm，小弯侧长 5cm，贲门切缘直径 1.2cm，胃切缘长 6cm，在距胃切缘 1cm 处可见一隆起型肿物，体积 5cm × 4cm × 2.5cm，肿物中央溃疡，肿物切面灰白，浸润至深肌层，质中，与周围界限尚清，网膜 9cm × 8cm × 1cm，未触及明显结节。常规病理诊断：胃类癌，溃疡型，体积 5cm × 4cm × 2.5cm，浸润至深肌层，贲门及胃切缘均阴性，网膜阴性，食管残端阴性。

免疫组化检测：阳性：CgA，Syn，CK19（神经内分泌细胞）；阴性：CK20，EMA，NSE。免疫组化诊断：上述结果提示胃体部神经内分泌肿瘤（类癌）（图 23-10-2）。

第七节　胃原发外周原始神经外胚叶肿瘤

外周原始神经外胚叶肿瘤（pPNET）是一种少见的具有多向分化潜能的高度恶性小圆形细胞肿瘤。迄今，原始神经外胚叶肿瘤的病理诊断尚无统一标准，目前一般采用病理 - 免疫组织化学 - 细胞遗传学方法联合诊断。原则上一是要取得诊断原始神经外胚叶肿瘤的直接证据，二是要鉴别属于其他类型的小细胞肿瘤。经典原始神经外胚叶肿瘤细胞有 Homer-Wright 菊形团或非典型菊形团排列。电镜下瘤细胞浆内有神经内分泌颗粒及微丝，致密核心颗粒是确诊原始神经外胚叶肿瘤的重要指标。原始神经外胚叶肿瘤免疫组织化学诊断标准主要为与 EWS 基因重组有关的异染色质基因 M IC2 产物 P30/32m IC2 单克隆抗体阳性并至少有两种以上不同神经标记的表达。

外周原始神经外胚叶肿瘤多发于儿童及青少年,平均发病年龄17岁,男性略多于女性,临床表现为软组织肿块及腹痛等非特异性症状,胃起源原始神经外胚叶肿瘤极为罕见。上述症状外,大多伴有上消化道出血,一例患者以上消化道出血为主要临床表现。肿瘤恶性程度高,易发生远处转移和复发,预后极差,该例患者属晚期,已侵及邻近组织及周围血管,并伴有肺内、纵隔、腹腔及腹膜后多发淋巴结转移。对于外周原始神经外胚叶肿瘤,CT缺乏特异性征象,但发生于青少年、边界不清、密度不均、少钙化的快速增大的疼痛性肿块应想到外周原始神经外胚叶肿瘤的可能。胃的原发原始神经外胚叶肿瘤同样缺乏特异性诊断标准,如发现腹腔巨大占位,与胃关系密切,并有病灶向胃内突入, CT平扫显示病变密度不均,见坏死囊变区。肿瘤实性部分增强后呈轻~中度强化,并可见肿瘤侵及周围组织。应考虑胃原始神经外胚叶肿瘤的可能性。对于外周原始神经外胚叶肿瘤,术前行CT平扫及增强检查,可显示肿瘤的形态、大小、病变对邻近组织的侵犯程度,并可发现扫描范围内是否有远处转移,对手术可切除性评估非常有价值,并可协助临床判断治疗效果。

综上所述,胃原发原始神经外胚叶肿瘤,极为罕见,好发于老人,临床表现无特异性,最终确诊需临床、组织学、免疫组织化学及分子遗传学综合诊断。影像学表现虽缺乏特异性,但可明确肿瘤范围及对周围组织的侵犯及远处转移病灶,为临床治疗提供指导和帮助。

第十一章　胃其他肿瘤和囊肿

第一节　胃脂肪瘤与 CT

胃脂肪瘤属间质性肿瘤，临床少见，多位于黏膜下，可以很大，偶尔有蒂，多为良性。

临床上无症状，并发溃疡时，可有腹痛、呕血、黑便或贫血。当肿瘤生长于贲门部可致吞咽困难，生长于幽门处可致梗阻。胃镜检查时难以与胃平滑肌瘤、纤维瘤等鉴别。胃镜活检因肿瘤常位于黏膜下，难以取到病灶组织，不能获得满意结果，有时需用深活检技术。CT 不仅能准确显示病变所在的部位、形态、密度、大小、数目、边界、毗邻关系，还能对病灶内所含的组织成分进行分析；采用恰当的窗技术，更有利于病变的显示和定性。

鉴别诊断：胃脂肪瘤需与平滑肌瘤、脂肪肉瘤及黏液囊肿等常见病变鉴别。脂肪肉瘤虽亦含脂肪成分，但其密度不均，多呈囊实性，其内可有分隔和钙化，增强时病灶有强化。平滑肌瘤和平滑肌肉瘤通常病变较大，偏心性生长，表现为软组织密度肿块，中心常有低密度坏死灶。黏液囊肿 CT 值为液体样密度，囊壁偶可见“蛋壳”状钙化。

第二节　胃粒状细胞肌胚细胞瘤

详见本书 本卷 本篇 第十章 第三节 胃粒状细胞肌胚细胞瘤。

第三节　误诊病例简介：胃底梭形细胞肿瘤与胃息肉

患者，女，55 岁。因反酸二个月余入院。外院胃镜示：胃底黏膜下肿物，间质瘤？慢性非萎缩性胃炎伴糜烂。CT：胃底结节，三期增强有强化，血供可，邻近可见低密度影为气泡。CT 诊断：胃底壁结节性质待定，息肉？间质瘤？病理检查：胃底黏膜下隆起 ESD 切除标本：灰褐色结节样肿物一块，大小 1.5cm × 1.3cm × 1.0cm，切面灰白，质中。病理诊断：胃底黏膜下隆起 ESD 切除标本：梭形细胞肿瘤，待做免疫组化检测进一步明确肿瘤类型（图 23-11-1）。

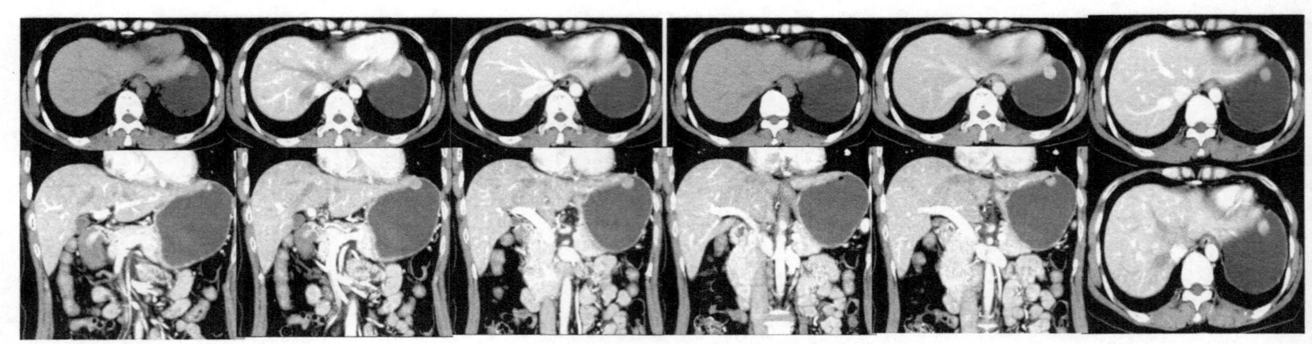

图 23-11-1 胃底梭形细胞肿瘤与胃息肉

第四节 胃癌合并胃脂肪瘤

详见本书 本卷 本篇 第七章 第二节 胃癌合并 胃脂肪瘤。

第五节 胃血管瘤

胃血管瘤是一种位于黏膜下或浆膜下的血管畸形,由 Lammers(1893)首次报道,临床少见,合并肝脏多发血管瘤更罕见。

本病源于中胚层残余组织,其病因及发病机制尚不明确。病理学上血管瘤分为毛细血管型、海绵状型、静脉型(包括蔓状血管瘤)和混合型。

胃血管瘤约占不明原因胃出血的 20%,以胃体及胃窦部多发,呕血和黑便往往是其主要临床表现。由于本病临床症状无特殊性,因而术前确诊困难。

胃镜一般能发现病变、明确部位和诊断,但如出血较多,影响视野,常遗漏病变。胃镜活检时可能会引起出血,要慎行。

CT 不仅可以显示病变的大小、位置和生长方向,还能了解病变与周围脏器的关系,为临床提供可靠信息。CT 平扫表现为低密度影,增强后呈“渐进性强化”为海绵状血管瘤的特征性表现,混合型血管瘤在 CT 上不易与海绵状血管瘤鉴别。

MRI 对血管瘤的诊断准确率高, MRI 信号在一定程度上可以反映血管瘤的组织病理学特征,为定性诊断提供依据。

第六节　误诊病例简介：胃体神经鞘瘤与胃窦黏膜腺癌

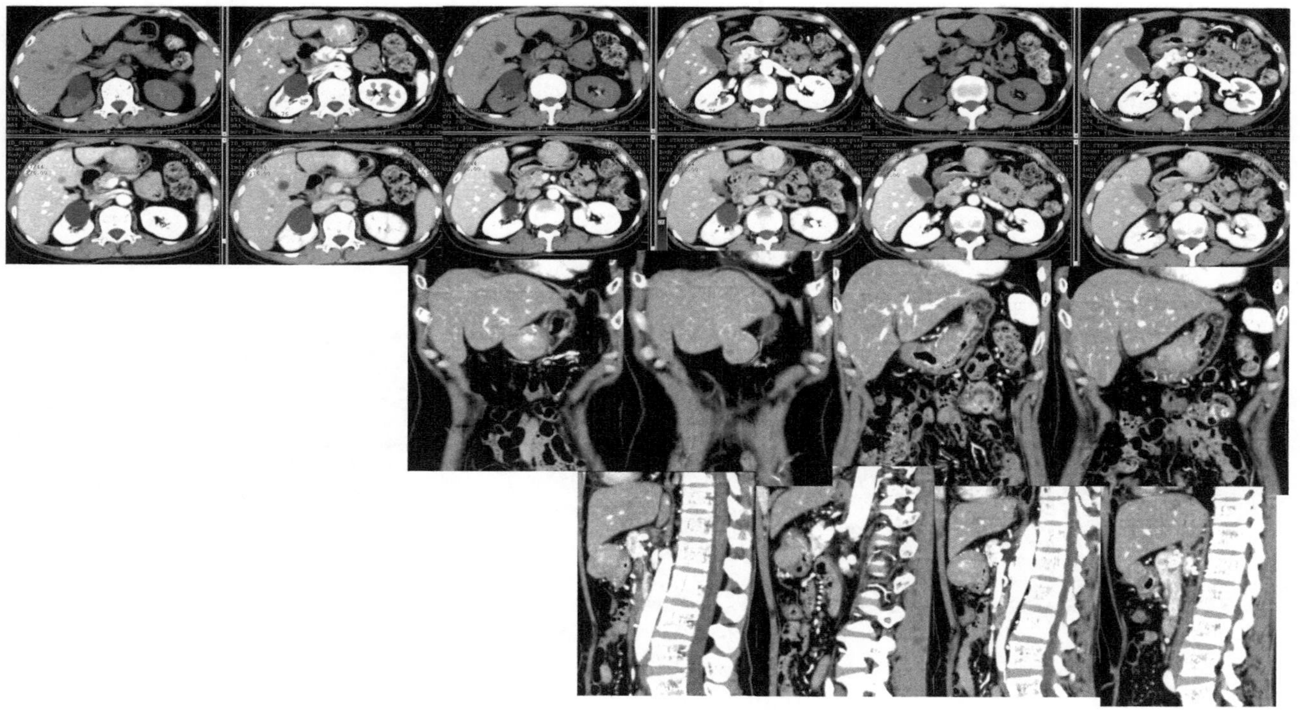

图 23-11-2　胃体神经鞘瘤与胃窦黏膜腺癌

患者，女，52 岁。反复上腹痛 3 个月余入院。

病理检查：胃肿瘤根治切除标本示胃体梭形细胞肿瘤，3.5cm × 3.4cm × 3cm，待免疫组化进一步确诊。胃窦黏膜腺癌，Ⅰ级，直径 1cm，浸润至黏膜下层。两切缘均(-)。胃小弯淋巴结(-)，0/5。胃大弯淋巴结(-)，0/5。大网膜(-)，0/3。

免疫组化检测：阳性：S-100(+++)，Vimentin(+++)，Nestin(++)，Ki-67(局部 10%)；阴性 CD117，DOG1，SMA，Calponin。免疫组化诊断：胃肿瘤根治切除标本示胃体梭形细胞肿瘤，3.5cm × 3.4cm × 3cm，免疫组化支持神经鞘瘤。其他情况参见常规组织学报告。建议临床随访(图 23-11-2)。

第七节　误诊病例简介：胃窦部神经鞘瘤与间质瘤

神经鞘瘤是神经鞘膜细胞发生的良性肿瘤，为最常见的外周神经良性肿瘤之一，又称施万细胞瘤。好发于颅内神经根、脊神经、周围神经干，发生于消化道者极少见，仅占全身神经鞘瘤的 0.2%；而胃神经鞘瘤则占整个消化道神经鞘瘤的 90%，多为良性，恶性者占 6%~7.7%。胃神经鞘瘤好发于胃体部，其次为胃底，胃窦部较少见，多见于 30~50 岁。胃神经鞘瘤临床上缺乏特异性表现和体征。少数患者表现为腹痛、腹胀。发生在胃窦部和胃幽门区的神经鞘瘤可引起幽门梗阻。

上消化道钡餐检查主要表现为向腔内突出的结节状或分叶状充盈缺损，其黏膜面有时可出现浅龛影。MSCT 能够清楚地显示胃神经鞘瘤的部位、范围、大小、界面，也有利于观察病灶内部有无囊变、钙化等，以及显示对邻近脏器的压迫和侵犯情况。同时还可以观察其他部位的转移灶。

一些学者将胃神经鞘瘤 CT 表现归纳为 3 型：巨块型，表现为巨大“哑铃”状软组织肿块，直径达 15 cm，肿块实质部分轻度较均匀强化，中间少许坏死区为低密度不强化；胃壁结节型，多位于胃体小弯侧，表现为胃黏膜下或肌层向腔内生长的圆形或类圆形软组织肿块，直径一般不超过 5 cm，边界清楚，密度较均匀，平扫肿块密度较软组织密度稍低，轻度强化，该类型文献报道常伴有肿块内斑点状钙化；胃壁局限增厚型，此型较少见，应注意与浸润型胃癌鉴别，。浸润型胃癌壁僵硬，管腔狭窄更明显，边界不清，增强扫描明显强化。

上消化道钡餐检查和 CT 检查可对本病定位诊断，而定性诊断有一定难度，需与胃间质瘤及胃癌相鉴别。该例误诊为间质瘤。因本病发病率低，无特异的临床症状和体征，好发部位及影像表现与间质瘤的影像表现有重叠，常被忽略，需依赖术后病理和免疫组织化学方法确诊；胃神经鞘瘤 S-100 蛋白表达阳性，而胃间质瘤 CD117 和 CD34 表达阳性。

第八节　胃底平滑肌瘤

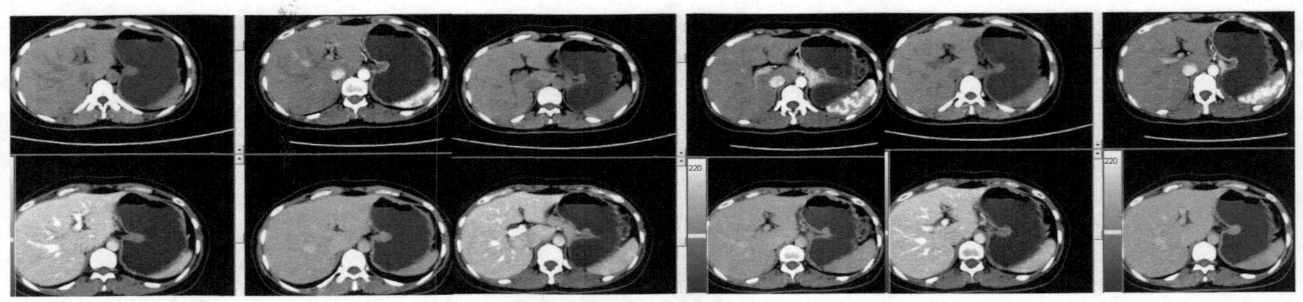

图 23-11-3　胃底平滑肌瘤

患者，女，35 岁。因腹痛 8 天入院。手术所见：胃镜下手术：胃底贲门下方大弯偏后壁见一约 0.8cm × 2.0cm 黏膜隆起，表面光滑，不规则。切开后见病灶位于固有肌层，不规则。

病理检查：胃底病灶切除标本见灰白色不规则组织一块，大小 3cm × 1cm × 1cm，切面灰白，质中。常规病理诊断：胃底病灶切除标本见梭形细胞肿瘤，待做免疫组化检测进一步明确诊断。

免疫组化检测：阳性：Actin，Desmin，SMA，H-caldesmon，Calponin，Ki67（+，1%）；阴性：DOG1，CD117，CD34，P53，S-100，Nestin。免疫组化诊断：胃底病灶切除标本：平滑肌瘤（图 23-11-3）。

第九节　胃少见的原发性肿瘤及误诊分析

MSCT 对胃部病变的显示优势：CT 检查前充分的胃肠道准备、甘露醇或清水充盈胃肠道、检查前肌注诺仕帕 20 mg 抑制肠道蠕动，降低管壁张力，使胃肠道管腔扩张较好，能较好地显示管腔内外及管壁的病变。薄层 CT 轴位图像结合 MPR 图像能清楚显示胃部肿瘤的部位、范围、边界、病灶内有无坏死囊变、钙化等，更能发现腔外生长的肿瘤及肿瘤对邻近脏器、组织累及情况，尤其是三期增强扫描对肿瘤的强化特点更有助于胃部肿瘤的鉴别诊断。因此 MSCT 检查已经成为胃部肿瘤的常规检查，尤其是黏膜下肿瘤的首选检查。

影像学研究：胃部原发性肿瘤分为上皮性肿瘤和非上皮性肿瘤，上皮性肿瘤以类癌及腺瘤少见。非上皮性肿瘤以神经鞘瘤及原发性淋巴瘤较少见，神经纤维瘤、脂肪瘤、脂肪肉瘤及脉管源性肿瘤（如血管瘤、淋巴管瘤、血管球瘤）罕见。该组 17 例已包含胃少见原发性肿瘤的大部分病理类型。

胃息肉伴有上皮异型性改变被称为腺瘤。腺瘤分为三型：肠型、小凹型及幽门腺型，以肠型腺瘤多见（≥ 50%），在西方国家约占胃息肉的 10%，近 40% 病例伴有高级别异型性增生，癌变率约 2.5%~50%。约 10% 的腺瘤患者同时伴有胃其他部位的肿瘤。该组病例中，1 例为管状腺瘤合并胃底部腔内型间质瘤。1 例为绒毛状管状腺瘤，无恶变。

若CT显示病变边界不清、密度不均匀及不均匀强化则要考虑到腺瘤恶变的可能。

类癌起源于胃肠道的黏膜下层的嗜铬细胞，临床非常少见，约占消化道恶性肿瘤的1%~1.5%，发生于胃部更少见；因其常伴类癌综合征，所以肿瘤较小时易发现，肿瘤易侵犯邻近组织，易通过淋巴和血行转移。该组1例类癌因为未出现明显类癌综合征，所以病灶较大，伴较多坏死、囊变及钙化，并累及邻近胰腺。

原发性胃淋巴瘤原发于胃黏膜固有层和黏膜下层的淋巴组织，以非霍奇金淋巴B细胞型多见，可见于任何年龄。其CT表现具有以下特点：①病变累及范围广，常累及两个及以上部位，胃体、胃窦部同时累及，该组5例均累及两个或以上部位；②病变横向生长多见，常侵犯>50%胃周径，胃黏膜完整，增强后动脉期呈细线状强化，因为胃淋巴瘤起自黏膜和黏膜下层的淋巴组织，所以病变往往先在黏膜固有层和黏膜下层蔓延，再向腔内、外侵犯；③梗阻征象少见，原因是淋巴细胞增殖未破坏正常细胞，无纤维组织增生，管壁有一定的扩张度、柔软度。该组病例均无明显梗阻征象；④病变密度均匀并轻中度均匀强化，由于胃淋巴瘤细胞核浆比大，血供相对缺乏，因此胃淋巴瘤密度多均匀，内部很少坏死或坏死灶较小，该组所有病例均呈轻中度均匀强化，无一例出现坏死区；⑤病灶较少侵犯周围脂肪，周围脂肪间隙多清晰，该组5例中有3例周围脂肪间隙内可见多发小淋巴结，其余2例周围未见明显淋巴结。

胃肠道神经鞘瘤是一种极为少见的肿瘤，占整个神经鞘瘤的0.2%，它起源于胃肠道壁肌间Auerbach神经丛神经鞘施万细胞。显微镜下主要由伴有微小梁状结构的梭形细胞构成，肿瘤细胞周围可见淋巴细胞套状浸润；免疫组织化学：梭形细胞胞浆S-100蛋白和NSE呈强阳性反应，而CD117、CD34、肌源性标记物结合蛋白和肌动蛋白阴性。良性多见，恶性少见。CT表现为跨腔外、内生长为主的黏膜下肿块，边界清楚，密度多较均匀，增强后动脉期轻度均匀强化，静脉期均匀渐进性中度强化；肿瘤可坏死囊变，钙化少见。

该组3例神经鞘瘤术前均诊断为间质瘤，其中1例伴病灶内囊变。

胃神经纤维瘤罕见，胃黏膜下、肌层和浆膜下均可发生，起源于交感神经纤维；大部分肿瘤小且无症状，临床表现无明显特异性；术前常误诊为胃间质瘤。胃神经源性肿瘤确诊须依靠组织学及免疫组织化学检查。

胃血管源性肿瘤临床罕见，胃血管瘤约占胃良性肿瘤的1.7%，起源于中胚层残余组织，病因及发病机制尚不明确。Kaijser将胃肠道血管瘤分4型：即多发性静脉扩张型、海绵状血管瘤、毛细血管瘤和血管瘤病。胃海绵状血管瘤最常见于胃窦部黏膜下层，临床表现无特异性。术前内镜、选择性腹腔内动脉造影、CT增强可帮助诊断，确诊需病理证实。CT表现为胃壁不均匀增厚，增强后渐进性强化，病变黏膜层完整、呈细线样强化，可伴钙化。该组1例病变有小点状钙化，典型的渐进性强化特点，术前诊断为血管源性病变。

胃血管球瘤罕见，属于间叶性肿瘤，好发于胃窦部胃黏膜下，临床无特异性症状。CT表现为胃窦部黏膜下软组织肿块，密度均匀、边界清楚，偶见钙化点，增强后动脉期散在不均匀小斑片状强化，门静脉期及延迟期持续不均匀明显强化，并向中心充填，周围包膜轻度强化。

钙化性纤维性假瘤，病因及性质未明，多见于年轻女性，好发于四肢，腹膜及胃肠浆膜层少见。病理镜下可见大量胶原纤维和玻璃样变，在退行性变的基础上出现灶状或遍及瘤体的砂砾样钙化。CT常表现为边界清楚的较高密度肿块，有时可见明显的钙化，轻度强化。该例病变位于胃底部大弯侧黏膜下，平扫密度较高。

胃脂肪瘤是罕见的良性间叶组织来源的肿瘤，约占胃良性肿瘤的3%，多单发，常见于胃体、窦部黏膜下。CT平扫显示病灶内脂肪组织密度，增强后无强化。

鉴别诊断：胃间质瘤：胃部少见的黏膜下肿瘤主要与胃间质瘤相鉴别：间质瘤病灶常较大，易囊变、坏死，为富血供肿瘤，动脉期多为不均匀明显强化、黏膜层常不完整，静脉期呈持续明显强化，强化程度高于动脉期，强化程度比神经鞘瘤明显。

神经鞘瘤：神经鞘瘤多密度均匀、边界清楚，动脉期轻度均匀强化、黏膜层多完整连续且呈细线样强化，静脉期中度强化；部分病灶可有囊变，但钙化少见。

钙化性纤维性假瘤平扫密度常较高，可有斑片状或大片状钙化，轻度不均匀强化。

总之，胃血管源性肿瘤有一定的CT特征性表现，平扫及三期增强扫描诊断不难，但由于其少见或罕见,临床及影像医师较难想到而常常误诊,所以对于有钙化且典型的渐进性充填明显强化的胃部病变,要想到血管源性肿瘤的可能。胃神经源性肿瘤在临床上常常误诊为胃间质瘤,鉴于两者对放化疗不敏感,均首选手术治疗,所以在诊断胃间质瘤时,需想到神经鞘瘤的可能。原发性胃淋巴瘤首先采用保守治疗、化疗和放疗,不同于胃癌首选手术治疗,因此治疗前明确诊断对选择治疗方案具有重要的意义。

第十节　胃窦囊肿

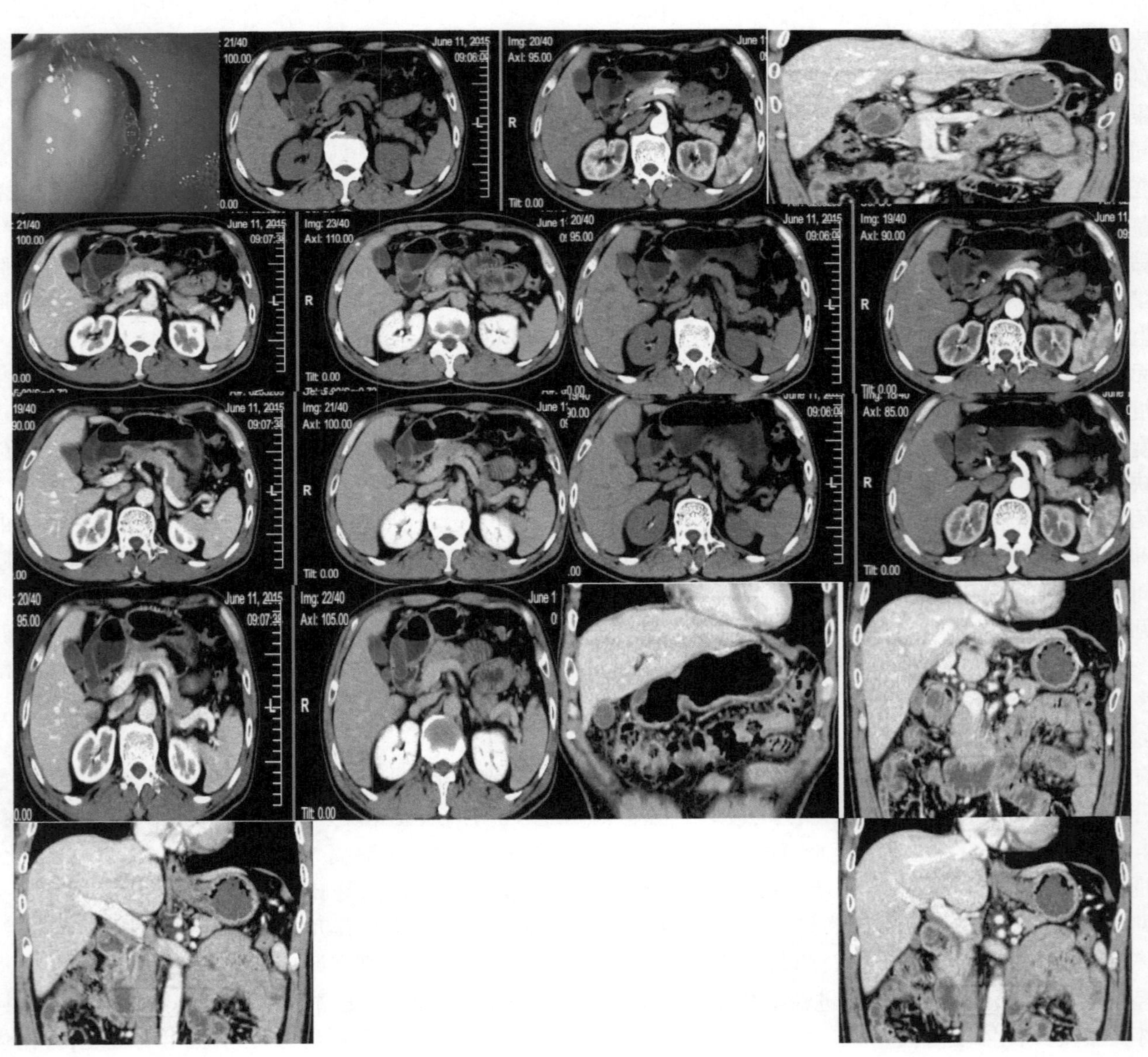

图 23-11-4　胃窦囊肿

患者,男,56 岁。体检发现胃部占位 2 年余。

病理检查:胃窦囊肿 ESD 切除标本:送检胃壁组织一

块,包括黏膜层、黏膜肌层及部分黏膜下层组织。黏膜层呈慢性浅表性胃炎,重度,伴轻度肠化。结合内镜,可符合胃窦囊肿。HP 阴性(图 23-11-4)。

第十一节 胃窦后壁巨大息肉脱垂入空肠

胃息肉是胃黏膜上皮向腔内生长的局限性隆起性病变,关于其发病率,目前尚无确切统计资料。国外早期尸检报告:胃息肉发病率在 0.33%~0.90%,胃镜检出率在 0.4%~1.0%。一些作者的研究显示胃息肉检出率高达 12.6%。

临床表现:有研究显示女性发病率较男性高。发病年龄偏高,60~69 岁为高发年龄。

胃息肉的临床表现缺乏特异性,常因其他疾病在胃镜检查中被发现,被认为是胃癌前病变。主要临床表现为上腹痛及堵胀感。临床上较少见,巨大者更为罕见,未见涉及到影像学的报道。目前国内多将胃息肉分为以下几类:腺瘤性息肉、增生性息肉、混合性息肉、炎性息肉、胃底腺息肉、炎性纤维样息肉及其他。

一些学者研究了 365 例胃息肉的临床特点,发现:胃息肉主要发生于胃体和底部,其次是胃窦和贲门,其中,胃底腺息肉绝大多数分布在胃体和底部;增生性息肉以胃窦部为主,其次为胃体和底部;炎性息肉以贲门和胃体和底部为主;腺瘤性息肉主要分布在胃窦部。

影像学研究:胃息肉的 X 线平片表现为孤立的圆形、卵圆形软组织充盈缺损,可带蒂或广基状与胃壁相连,轮廓清楚,表面光整或呈乳头状改变,也可多发呈簇状或散在分布,其大小差异较大,在低张气钡双对比造影下表现最典型。胃息肉 CT 及 MRI 表现常呈表面光滑,带蒂或广基底,且周围胃壁正常。

鉴别诊断:典型胃息肉超声、X 线钡餐、CT 及 MRI 均可提示诊断;不典型时应与以下几种疾病鉴别:①胃腺瘤 CT 表现与胃息肉相似,需要结合其他检查;②胃癌 CT 表现为胃壁异常增厚及腔内或腔外不规则肿块影,增强扫描明显强化,有时可见淋巴结转移,并侵犯邻近器官;③胃淋巴瘤表现为胃壁广泛性或节段性浸润增厚,较胃癌增厚明显,增强扫描强化不及胃癌明显,较少侵犯邻近组织及器官,并伴有多发淋巴结肿大;④胃平滑肌瘤良性者常 <3 cm,多为等密度,恶性者常 >5 cm,内部密度不均,分叶状,增强扫描不均匀强化。但确诊需依靠病理。

一例患者反复腹痛 18 年,胃内形成巨大息肉,并脱垂入空肠肠腔内,出现梗阻性黄疸。可能由于肿物生长缓慢,脱垂入十二指肠后,十二指肠代偿性扩张、息肉压迫十二指肠乳头部以及推挤胰头等,引起胆、胰管出口阻塞。胃息肉脱垂进入空肠后,其中可见一长条状影贯穿于胃腔与十二指肠球部(一些作者将其称之为"牵引黏膜桥征")。此需与胃黏膜脱垂鉴别,前者充盈缺损位置不恒定,但形态固定,不随触诊改变,回复胃腔后胃内可显示大小、形态完全一致的充盈缺损阴影,胃黏膜纹大多正常;后者胃黏膜脱垂一旦回复胃内时,球部充盈缺损阴影即消失,胃内不再显示与球部充盈缺损大小、形态一致的阴影,而只显示胃黏膜皱襞增粗、紊乱等表现,据此可以鉴别。

第十二节 胃底胃肠道间质瘤

患者,男,61 岁。上腹部胀痛 2 个月余入院。病理检查:胃底肿物切除标本示灰红色不规则组织一块,大小 8cm × 6.5cm × 4cm,切面灰红灰褐,质中。病理诊断:胃底肿物切除标本:胃底梭形细胞肿瘤,倾向胃肠道间质瘤(GIST),体积较大,大小 8cm × 6.5cm × 4cm,提示中等危险度(图 23-11-5)。

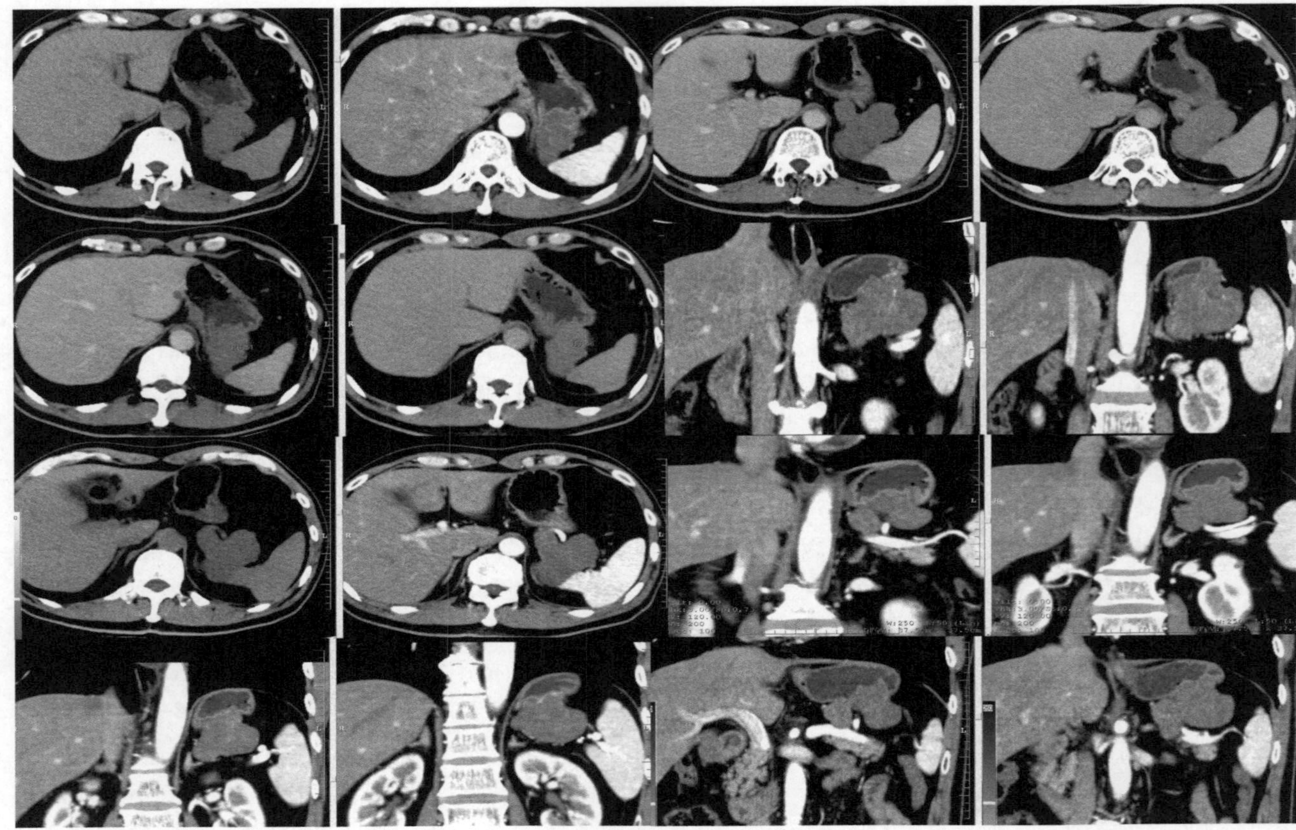

图 23-11-5 胃底胃肠道间质瘤

第十二章　关于胃黏膜

第一节　胃黏膜的乳头样形状变异

胃肠道正常结构的难见的变异常常使内窥镜大夫与放射科大夫解释困难，特别在依靠组织学与分泌物研究诊断不同的胃炎时尤其如此。例如，胃黏膜的乳头样形状变异则常与肥大性胃炎混淆。Magnus 和 Rodgers(1938)首先提出乳头样形状(etat mammelonne)表现，只描述见于胃，黏膜肌收缩使横断面呈沟状，形成正常黏膜呈粗大结节，这些沟明显时，在组织学上黏膜深裂口可深达肌层，而黏膜正常。内镜医师考虑此种改变为正常。

Carey(1940)、Selesrick 和 Kinsella(1953)指出肉眼难以将之与肥大性胃炎区别，只在此征象上诊断肥大性胃炎，应更谨慎。Ylvisaker 等(1955)与 Palmer(1954)指出，大多数病人内镜检查时考虑为肥大性胃炎，但活检正常。

放射科大夫也考虑此种情况充盈钡剂表现为针状影，为正常变异(Wolf，1961)。此情况最大胃酸排出量居正常范围，故可除外肥大性高分泌胃炎。认识此症将减少误诊为肥大性胃炎，甚或黏膜溃疡。Stone 和 keat(1973)专门讨论了这种变异。

第二节　胃底平滑肌瘤病例

详见本书 本卷 本篇 第十一章 第八节　胃底平滑肌瘤。

第三节　胃窦的黏膜隔

远侧胃的闭锁或膜状梗阻十分少见，截至 1972 年，文献报告仅 50 例，多为胚胎发育异常引起，常为婴幼儿。X 线平片可见胃扩张，有的可见气液平。当黏膜隔中央穿孔后，症状与体征可减轻和延迟，甚至到成人才被发现。钡餐检查在胃窦部可见新月形充盈缺损，近侧胃可有扩张；有时大量钡剂可遮蔽此膜，尤其当膜中央穿孔较大，胃排空较接近正常的时候，更是如此。

Haddad 等(1981)专门讨论成人的胃窦黏膜隔，发现黏膜隔仅几毫米厚，由黏膜与黏膜下层构成，其位置距幽门远近不一，隔膜均与胃的长轴保持垂直成角，膜的穿孔可为中心性，也可为偏心性。虽然本病少见，但在任何年龄的胃窦梗阻诊断不明时，都应想到本病的可能。

第四节　误诊病例简介：胃体小弯异位胰腺与间质瘤

详见本书 本卷 第二十篇 第十九章 第六节　误诊病例简介：胃体小弯异位胰腺与间质瘤。

第五节　一些诊断陷阱

胃肠蠕动:胃肠蠕动与胃肠壁内肌束走行方向可造成引起诊断混淆的收缩或凸起。

由于胃角区所有三层肌肉较为纤细,常可导致胃角与幽门之间出现一凸出,伪似溃疡形成。与之相近,幽门由于吊带肌的收缩也可引起一凸起,不在大弯侧就在小弯侧,这就是所谓隆凸性缺陷,它是假性溃疡,不是真溃疡,此凸起表现并不见于每个图像上。如此类凸起持久存在,则应认真搜寻伴存的真正的消化性溃疡。在急性感染时,此种凸起可加重和更恒定更明显,变得特别突出。另外,在幽门肌高张的情况下,可出现成人性增生性幽门狭窄,伪似真性狭窄。

胃的排空时间:利用核素显像可测量胃的排空时间。Griffith 等(1966)测出为 70 分钟,Fridrich 等(1970)为 64 分钟, Harvey 等(1970)为 56 分钟,Van Dam(1974)为 23~77 分钟,平均 47 分钟。不同作者测出数值不同,解释为技术细节的差异和进餐成分的不同所致。Moore 等(1981)用放射性核素技术监测研究固态食物与液态食物在胃的排空情况,发现液态食物排空比固态食物快。在固态餐中,较大体积和较大重量的液体排空慢于较小体积及较小重量的液体。幽门窦区的运动,在固态食物和液态食物标记,都比较恒定。了解上述胃排空的特点,对胃的 X 线观察有一定的益处。

吻壁现象:双对比检查方法本身可产生一些陷阱,吻壁现象即为其一。

在钡剂被覆胃肠道黏膜,气体扩张肠曲时,应努力寻找另外的线形影和新月形影,有时,相对胃肠壁可互相粘贴,尤如接吻,产生假的线影或其他阴影。

此类吻壁现象常常是使用压迫后产生的暂时现象,松压后,此现象即刻消逝。

如还有怀疑,可设法使该段胃肠壁更行扩张,此现象则理应消失,如不消失,则多为真性病变所致。

幽门管与贲门星:幽门管本身即可误为一溃疡,幽门管不是表现为钡剂聚集呈环状,就是为一星状阴影伴向四周放射的皱襞。在胃底,与此类似,胃食道连接区轴位观可貌似玫瑰,又称做贲门星,均勿误为病变。

悬挂小滴或钟乳石现象:此现象常可成为溃疡型息肉错误诊断的一个原因,事实上此现象只是暂时的表现,复查或随访常可澄清是非。

第十三章　胃的炎症

第一节　息肉型胃炎与胃癌

息肉型胃炎是慢性胃炎的一种，其X线表现可与肿瘤混淆，一般将其分为三类，即：单个息肉型、多个息肉型与肿块型。

大多数息肉状隆起皆由粗大的炎症黏膜皱襞卷曲而成，也可由局部黏膜层、黏膜下层甚至肌层的慢性炎症或/和水肿引起。

肿块型多出现于胃窦部，X线表现多为单个肿块状充盈缺损，常呈分叶，其直径一般为3cm以上；常见1~2条短条带状钡影覆盖于充盈缺损上，此带影多纡曲，加压观察可见其形态、长短和走向略有改变；缺损边缘多有1~2条黏膜皱襞向四周伸延；充盈缺损周围一般均有胃窦炎表现；此肿块影甚柔软，胃蠕动保存，偶尔肿块影较硬，蠕动消失，术前及术中尤其容易误诊为胃癌。

第二节　诊断困难的放射治疗后的胃炎

有作者报告2例病人因肾癌行肾切除术及放射治疗，由于放射性胃炎而造成诊断困难。

例1：62岁，男性，钡餐前6个月曾行放射治疗，一直感到上腹不适。例2：63岁，男性，在钡餐检查前9年曾行放射治疗，现亦感胃肠不适，曾于放射治疗后3年因结肠脾曲狭窄而行左半结肠切除术，考虑为放射治疗所致。

此二例皆显现胃窦部狭窄与不规则，但例1之胃镜检查与例2之追踪胃肠检查均未见胃癌征象。此即为继发于放射治疗的伴有良性纤维化的慢性胃炎。

放射治疗后继发结肠癌与严重胃肠出血，也已有报告。

第十四章　消化道出血与胃

第一节　肿块状胃壁静脉曲张

胃壁发生静脉曲张时,钡剂造影的典型表现为多发的黏膜下结节,如同一串位于胃壁的葡萄。然而,偶尔堆积成团的静脉曲张或肿块状静脉曲张会表现为一较大的、息肉样的胃底肿物,影像学上易被误诊为新生物。

许多作者认为依靠钡剂造影区分肿块状静脉曲张与息肉样癌、淋巴瘤或胃肠道基质肿瘤(平滑肌肉瘤)是很难的,甚至是不可能的。

Carucci 等(1999)回顾性地分析了 86 例胃壁静脉曲张患者的影像学资料,12 例(14%)为堆积成团的静脉曲张,即肿块状静脉曲张。12 例中的 5 例经证实为胃壁静脉曲张,5 例在其他检查结果和 / 或临床随访发现的基础上被推测为静脉曲张。分析此 10 例患者的影像学资料,测量病灶大小、部位及形态学表现。

肿块状静脉曲张平均大小为 6.8cm(范围 3~11cm)。8 例病人的病灶累及了胃底的中后部,1 例累及贲门中央区,1 例累及胃底前下部。侧面观,这些肿块状静脉曲张表现为表面光滑的黏膜下波浪形、边界不连续的肿块;正面观表现为团块样聚集的粗大、弯曲的皱襞逐渐移行于周围黏膜中。

认识到肿块状胃壁静脉曲张的临床意义非常重要,因为它比其他类型的胃壁静脉曲张更易出血。此项研究中,50% 有肿块状静脉曲张表现的病人伴有急性上胃肠道出血。因其更容易发生胃肠道出血,所以应密切随访。

Carucci 等(1999)指出,在影像学诊断的胃壁静脉曲张的病人中,14% 为肿块状胃壁静脉曲张,比以往所认为的肿块状静脉曲张更常见。

胃底肿块状静脉曲张在气钡双对比造影上有共同的 X 线表现,侧面观表现为波浪形轮廓、边界不连续的光滑的肿块,正面观呈团块状聚集的粗大、弯曲的皱襞,周边部与邻近黏膜相互移行。

认识肿块状静脉曲张在钡剂双对比造影时的特征性表现是非常重要的,这样就不会误诊为胃的新生物。

第二节　胃间质瘤伴出血

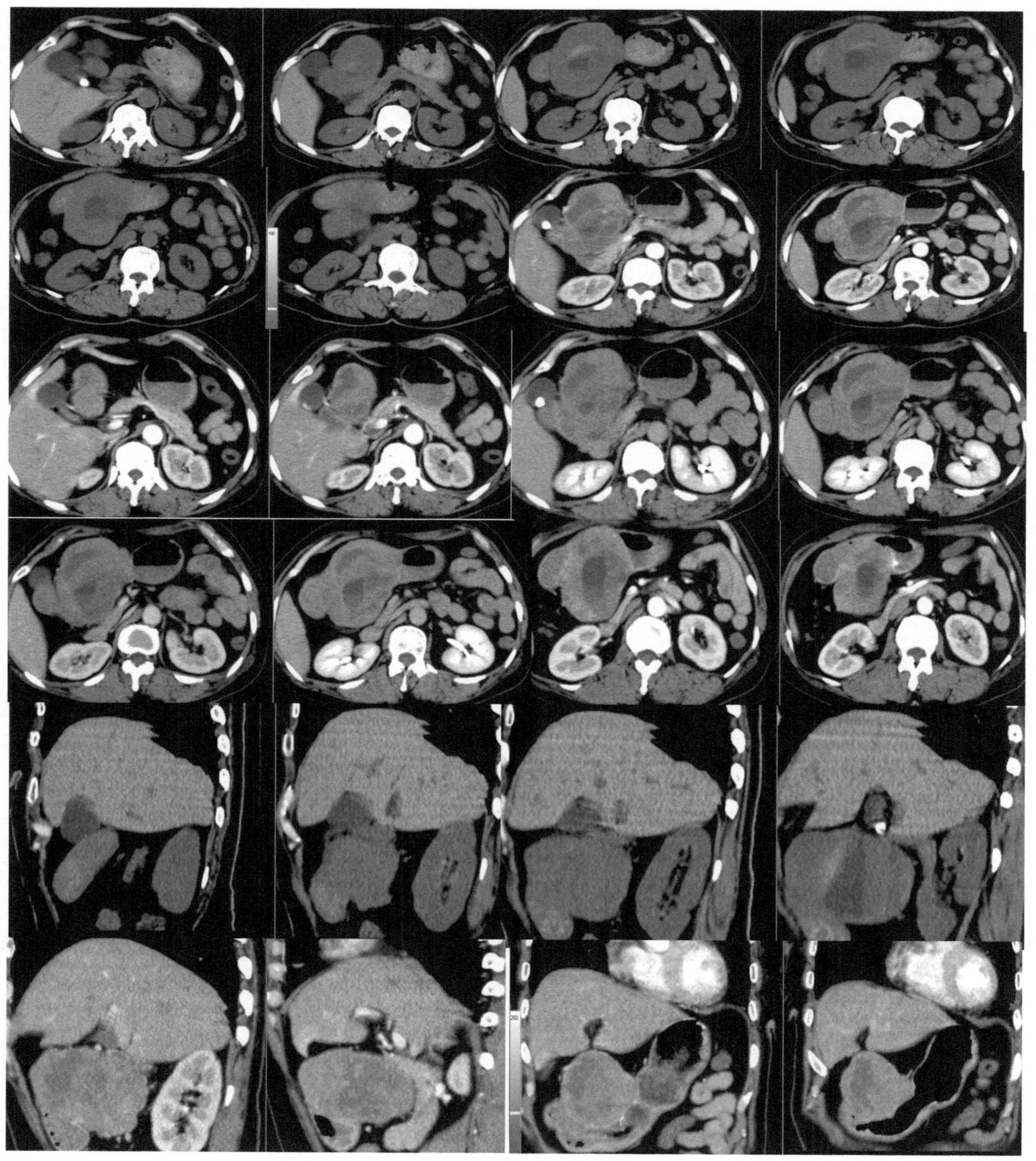

图 23-14-1　胃间质瘤伴出血

患者,女,55 岁。头晕、胸闷、上腹部疼痛三天入院。

胃镜:胃镜标本病理提示慢性轻度萎缩性胃炎(活动期)伴轻度糜烂及中度肠化,局灶区腺体呈轻度不典型增生,HP(+),未见肿瘤组织,建议切除肿瘤送检。

手术所见:胃窦胃角处可见一大小约 8 cm × 7 cm × 6 cm 的肿块,质地硬,未突破浆膜层,表面血管丰富,与胰腺及腹腔干无粘连。脾门、肝十二指肠韧带、贲门旁、胃左动脉旁未见明显淋巴结肿大。肝内无扪及肿块,腹主动脉旁无肿大之淋巴结,肝总动脉旁无肿大之淋巴结,盆腔无扪及种植病灶。

病理诊断:胃间质瘤伴出血(图 23-14-1)。

第三节 Dieulafoy 病

Dieulafoy 病是上消化道严重出血的少见原因之一,其基本病理特征为胃黏膜下增粗并走行异常的畸形小动脉破裂出血,又名胃黏膜下恒径动脉破裂出血,多发生在距贲门 6cm 以内的胃壁,也可发生于消化道的其他部位。黏膜下的异常小动脉直径可达 1~4mm,粗于胃壁内逐渐变细的正常小动脉(直径仅 0.1~0.2mm),具有正常的血管结构,无动静脉畸形和动脉瘤的表现,血管表面的黏膜呈糜烂、浅溃疡改变,多在血压增高、饮酒、药物、粗糙食物及应激等因素的诱发下,黏膜下动脉发生破裂出血,在血栓和凝血块的作用下出血可自行停止。Dieulafoy 病以间歇性反复性呕血或 / 和柏油样便为主要症状,以往诊断主要依靠内镜、选择性腹腔动脉造影、超声内镜和剖腹探查。内镜检查为 Dieulafoy 病的首选检查方法。

随着 CT 技术的发展,MSCTA 对于腹腔血管性病变的诊断价值已得到公认,大部分的血管狭窄、堵塞及其他形态和走行的异常等 MSCTA 均能清晰显示,并采用多种后处理技术,可准确显示病变血管的空间位置和解剖关系,对诊断和指导手术治疗具有一定意义。

第十五章　胃的假性病变

第一节　误诊病例简介：青少年胃反应性结节性纤维性假瘤误诊为胃恶性肿瘤

胃反应性结节性纤维性假瘤，Yantiss（2003）最早报道了5例成年人胃肠道及系膜的反应性结节性纤维性假瘤，他为了区分胃肠道间叶组织来源的肿瘤性病变与胃肠道及其系膜的反应性非肿瘤性病变，将后者命名为“胃肠道及系膜反应性结节性纤维性假瘤”。迄今为止，该病文献报道不足20例。

反应性结节性纤维性假瘤各个年龄段均可发生，一般发病年龄较大，临床表现无特异性，多偶然发现或伴有腹痛、肠梗阻、出血或腹膜炎的症状，或以急腹症就诊。胃肠道反应性结节性纤维性假瘤是一种伴有肌成纤维细胞反应性增生的炎性纤维性病变，是对外伤、炎症的炎性反应性增生，与炎性肌成纤维细胞肿瘤不同。通常认为反应性结节性纤维性假瘤的组织学来源是起自胃肠道浆膜下的多潜能细胞，随着多潜能细胞不断增殖，逐渐发展成为肿瘤样病变。影像学上表现为胃肠道浆膜下的单发或多发类圆形、分叶状或不规则形肿块，病灶多较早累及浆膜层，表现为与周围组织的粘连，而黏膜层较晚累及，多表现为基本正常或炎症表现，这与起源于黏膜或黏膜下层的胃癌具有显著的区别。

该病变可以浸润至固有肌层或黏膜下层，乃至胃肠壁全层，可合并溃疡或穿孔。已报道的大部分病例都有腹部器质性疾患或既往有腹部手术史，推测反应性结节性纤维性假瘤的发生与长期消化道溃疡、阑尾炎、术后粘连、异物等因素有关。

反应性结节性纤维性假瘤的镜下病理显示胶原基质的背景上散在或呈束状分布的星形或梭形成纤维细胞，同时可见淋巴细胞、浆细胞浸润，其中梭形细胞是来源于浆膜下的多潜能细胞。所有已报道的病例免疫组化表现为vimentin阳性，大部分的梭形细胞肌动蛋白（SMA）阳性，S-100阴性，间变性淋巴瘤激酶阴性，CD34阴性。该例有长期消化道溃疡的病史，反复刺激浆膜下多潜能细胞的反应性增生，而逐渐发展成为肿瘤样病变。病灶主要位于胃浆膜层、肌层及黏膜下，病灶邻近的胃黏膜增厚，局部形成溃疡，胃黏膜呈现胃炎、胃溃疡的影像学表现。

Gauchottea（2009）报道反应性结节性纤维性假瘤于CT平扫呈等密度，增强扫描呈渐进性强化（病灶富含纤维成分）；MRI显示病灶于T_1WI呈均匀低信号，T_2WI呈明显低信号。该例CT表现与之类似，这可能和反应性结节性纤维性假瘤内部成纤维细胞的含量有关，若病灶富含成纤维细胞成分，CT上则表现为平扫等密度，增强扫描呈渐进性强化；MR T_2WI呈低信号。由于反应性结节性纤维性假瘤在影像学上多表现为恶性征象（如较早侵犯浆膜层，与周围组织粘连明显等），易被误诊为恶性肿瘤，所以反应性结节性纤维性假瘤一般多行大范围手术切除。实际上，反应性结节性纤维性假瘤预后较好，至今尚未发现复发或转移的病例。结合该例和文献描述，可以认为反应性结节性纤维性假瘤在影像学上的一些表现，如浆膜下的肿块，较早侵及浆膜层，黏膜层基本正常或炎性改变等，再加上胃创伤、手术或炎症等病史，可为反应性结节性纤维性假瘤诊断提供帮助，以避免不必要的大范围组织切除。

第二节　胃的假瘤

贲门和食管胃连接区的轴面CT图像是显示管壁增厚的一个过渡层面,易被误认为软组织肿块。在CT图像上,多达1/3的病人在食管胃连接区存在此现象,它显示于静脉韧带裂平面。轴面CT图像中,此现象与食管胃连接区的不易完全充盈及其斜行汇入胃贲门有关。

当胃充分扩张时,不在食管胃连接区的管壁局限性增厚,除非能证明其为正常结构,否则应考虑为病变。

第三节　CT诊断陷阱之一:胃底和胃憩室及充盈液体的脏器

仰卧位时,胃底是胃的最低部位。CT图像上,它向后延伸到左肾上腺水平和左肾顶部。CT检查时,胃腔内有空气和/或有对比剂时有利于辨认。大多数胃憩室起源于胃底的食管胃连接区的后方。憩室是属先天或后天性的仍存在争议。在胚胎发育期,憩室可陷入并位于腹膜后。因为其位置靠后,憩室通常与左肾上腺相邻或重叠。CT图像上,当憩室内充满液体时,它们可酷似肾上腺肿块。采用薄层CT扫描,通常可辨认出与憩室分开的肾上腺。此外,憩室内如含有气体或对比剂时,则更有利于确定其性质。

充满液体的胃底是腹部最常见的假肿瘤,只有在仰卧时才能看见,不应将之混淆为左肾上腺的肿块。与此相类似,十二指肠球部轴位观察可伪似右上腹一块影,充盈液体的乙状结肠可貌似盆腔包块。

第四节　幽门管与贲门星

详见本书 本卷 本篇 第十二章 第五节　一些诊断陷阱。

第五节　关于瀑布胃的诊断陷阱

在瀑布胃,少量钡剂经贲门入胃后,扩张的胃底部首先充盈,在充盈达一定程度后,钡剂即以细流沿胃体后壁向下流到胃体大弯侧。当胃体充盈后,正位观察见胃呈现中间狭窄,上、下方扩张的哑铃形胃,如不认识可误为胃狭窄。在胃底部小弯侧贲门入口以下,常在服钡后看到龛影状阴影,此即为胃贲门以下小弯侧黏膜内积存钡剂所造成的假性壁龛。

胃窦大弯侧常可见一长期存在的切迹影,切迹的深度及部位多因人而异,它与幽门的距离也各人不同,此即为胃内正常组织结构之一,称中间沟,常被误为器质性病变。

在右侧卧位点片,有时在幽门部见到一类似有中央龛影的十二指肠球部溃疡的阴影,此影实际上是由幽门管内存留少量钡剂重叠于幽门周围放射状黏膜所构成。脾和肝左叶靠近左膈下,与胃底部前后壁黏膜皱襞彼此重叠,可形成胃底部的外形不规则的软组织影。

第六节　胃反应性结节状纤维性假瘤

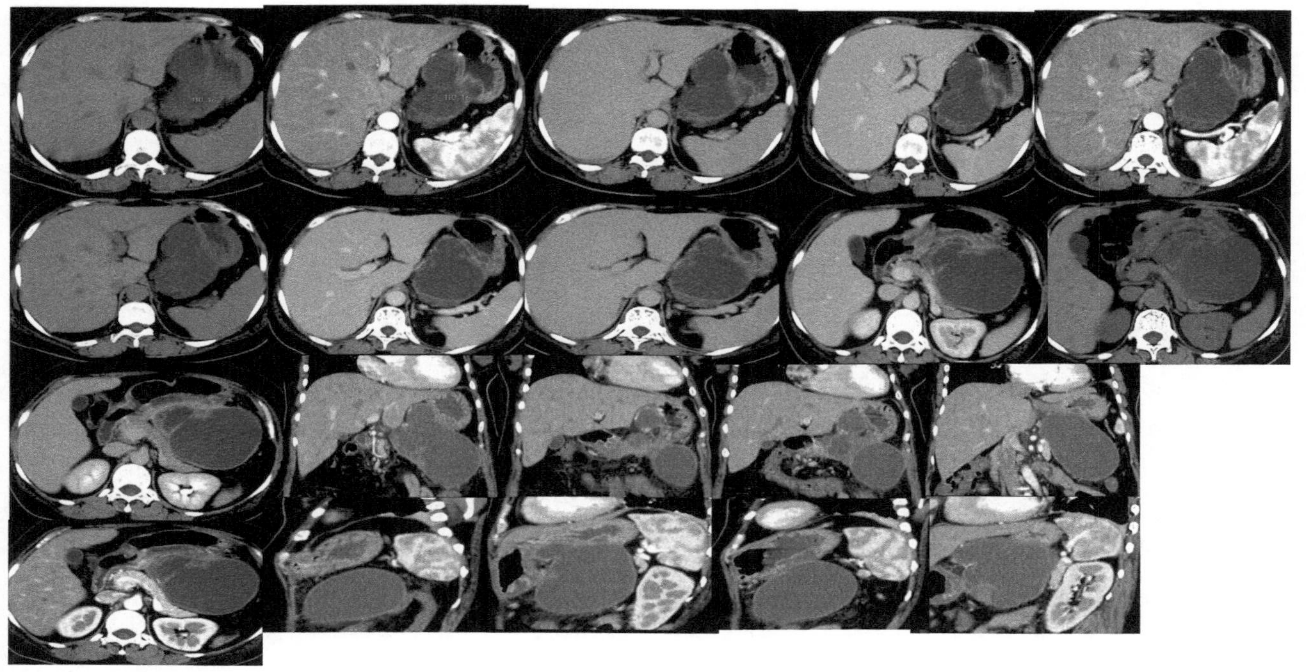

图 23-15-1　胃反应性结节状纤维性假瘤

患者，女，48 岁。因左上腹部外伤后疼痛伴发热约 20 天入院。

手术所见：无腹水，胃体后壁近胃角处可见一大小约 11cm × 9cm 囊实性肿物，内含透明清亮液体，壁较厚，由外向内侵犯胃壁肌层，并与胃体后壁浆膜层、大网膜广泛粘连，后方与胰腺包膜紧密粘连，胃旁未见明显淋巴结肿大。左下腹壁皮下扪及一脂肪瘤约 5 cm × 3cm 大小。

病理检查：腹腔占位切除标本：部分胃组织及囊性肿物一具，总体积 13cm × 12cm × 5cm，其中部分胃组织大小 7cm × 4.3cm × 3.5cm，胃黏膜皱襞存在，胃角后壁见一囊性肿物，肿物大小 10.5cm × 9cm × 1.8cm，表面呈黑褐色，送检前已剖开，囊内壁呈黑褐色，壁厚 0.1~1cm，局部区呈实性，实性区大小约 5cm × 3cm × 2.8cm，切面灰褐，质中偏脆，肿物部分区界限不清，与胃壁相融合。腹壁脂肪瘤切除标本：淡黄色组织一块，大小 4.5cm × 2.2cm × 1cm，切面淡黄质中偏软，大部有包膜。

常规病理诊断：腹腔占位切除标本初步诊断梭形细胞肿瘤，需作免疫组化检测进一步明确类型。肿瘤组织自外向内侵至胃浆膜纤维脂肪组织，贴近胃壁肌层，腹壁脂肪瘤切除标本示脂肪瘤。

免疫组化检测：阳性：Actin，SMA，CD68，CD163，H-caldesmon（灶 +），Catenin-β（点状 +），S-100（散在 +），CD34（血管内皮 +），Ki-67（+，约 8%）；阴性：DOG1，CD117，Desmin，ALKP80，CK（P）。免疫组化诊断：腹腔占位切除标本：结合免疫组化检测结果及组织学图像，符合反应性结节状纤维性假瘤，肿瘤组织自外向内在胃浆膜纤维脂肪组织中延伸，并贴近胃壁肌层，建议治疗后复查及随访。

胃肠道及系膜反应性结节状纤维性假瘤（RNFP）是一种不同于炎性肌成纤维细胞肿瘤的伴有肌成纤维细胞反应性增生的炎性纤维性病变，常发生于腹部手术后。镜检：少量梭性细胞或星形细胞杂乱稀疏的分布于玻璃样变的胶原间质中，部分胶原呈瘢痕样改变，间质内有多少不等的淋巴细胞呈斑片状分布，病灶周边可见残留和内陷的神经束和脂肪组织。免疫组化：Vimentin（+），CD117（+），α-SMA（+），MSA（+），ALK-1（-），CD34（-）。鉴别诊断：炎性肌成纤维细胞肿瘤（组织学）；胃肠道（外）间质肿瘤。（图 23-15-1）

第七节 胃的假性溃疡

胃的膜角:胃的膜角与幽门隆起缺陷是胃小弯处的两个生理性向外的膨凸,在钡餐时可误为溃疡。胃肌分三层,外层或浅层为纵行纤维,它一般与食管及十二指肠纵肌相连,浅层不覆盖全胃而分成二条分离的纵束:一为大弯束,继续延伸进入幽门区成为十二指肠纵肌层;一为小弯束,走行到胃角区时其中心纤维终止,束周围纤维从中心线散开,留下一纵行纤维缺如或减少区。最连续和最复杂的肌层为中层或环肌层,它起于食管环行肌浅层,延伸至全胃,最后汇集为十二指肠环肌层。

在胃窦远端,此层形成二确切的环行束,与中间纤维一块构成幽门括约肌,向小弯汇集成结节或隆起,向大弯分散,而留下一个坚度甚差的中间纤维插进的扇形区,在幽门括约肌近端有一区,Forssell(1913,1934)称为膜角,肌纤维稀疏分散,位于幽门前区小弯缘处。

胃肌纤维最内层为斜行纤维,发自于食管环肌深层,斜纤维变化大,且不完全,最终融合于胃远端及邻近的环肌层。在胃底处,斜纤维厚而明显,抵胃窦区时变薄和稀疏,在小弯区,它平行小弯走行,然后分散或斜行走向大弯远端。沿小弯缘此纤维宽度变化小,在小弯区产生一黏膜的沟畦,此现象常显露于胃镜,已命名为 Magenstrasse 区(Keet,1955)。

膜角或膜角缺陷,为远侧小弯区内纵肌层局限性缺损,相当于幽门前区一个膨凸,常见于蠕动的不同阶段。Torgersen(1942)更扩大膜角的概念,他令人信服地观察到相当于反刍动物的重弁(瓣)胃(omasum)或中胃,他描述此区解剖更为详细。

膜角处胃肌三层纤维在不同程度上缺如或相对减少,则产生一个无运动区或膨凸,常见于幽门前区透视观察时。有时此膨凸表现相当于近侧中央纵行纤维的突然终止,此纤维的终止个体差异较大,导致膨凸与幽门的距离各人不一,在小弯远侧正常膜角出现的程度常不相同,持久存在的时间也不尽一致,它一般随蠕动而变化,通常可完全消逝。

双对比钡餐检查时,此膨凸持续存在与保存钡剂并不少见,在大多数情况下,它的形状和构造常有变化,这在连续照片或透视观察或录像与摄电影时观察得十分清楚。

但在点片上,它也显示为一龛影,与真正的溃疡容易混淆,更甚者,此膜角缺陷可在一定病理情况下变得持久存在,与活动性溃疡龛影极难区别。当活动性溃疡病存在时,此膜角缺陷常变得较明显且持续显示,如真正溃疡位于其邻近区域,此征也更为明显。虽然气钡检查时可以见到其中钡剂残存,但假龛影的黏膜总是完整的。

幽门隆起缺陷:幽门管是胃壁肌层产生第二个假溃疡处,幽门隆起缺陷的名字已应用于幽门管中的假性龛影,见于小弯侧、大弯侧或两侧之幽门管中部。

Bremner(1968)对此现象产生的机制作了解释,他提示为幽门管的黏膜脱垂于幽门括约肌两个肌性圆环之间,在X线检查不同时相时,脱垂的黏膜可以产生一个暂存钡剂的小的菱形影从幽门管突出。在钡剂检查时,此类小的假性龛影可以暂时性地见于不少(约14%)正常人中。此假龛影多只存在片刻,连续细致地观察和照片可见它的一系列变化和消失。

在一定病理情况下,幽门隆起缺陷可以变得凸出和持续存在,使诊断极为困难,例如在幽门溃疡、幽门痉挛以及幽门高张力状态时,就是这样。

第十六章　关于胃的血管

第一节　CTA 显示胃周动脉及其变异

随着外科学的发展，腹腔镜下胃癌 D2 根治术和进展期胃癌多脏器联合切除根治术在技术上的安全性和可行性初步得到证实，但手术复杂且难度相对较大，其难点之一是寻找、辨识胃周血管及其发育变异和重要血管周围相关淋巴结的有效清除。另外，对邻近侵犯的胃癌联合切除扩大根治术的实施，术前也要考虑到胃周主要血管及脏器的结构关系以及对手术的潜在影响，以前有一些胃癌术中肝动脉受损的报道。

一项 67 例研究采用最大密度投影和容积再现技术对腹腔干、胃左动脉、肝动脉的显示率达到 100%，胃右动脉的显示率为 52.24%（35/67），并检出 12 例胃周主要动脉的发育变异以及与肿瘤解剖关系密切血管，对手术方式的选择、判定与实施有重要指导意义。

腹腔干及胃周血管存在多种变异，术前无 CTA 指导时，由于血管变异，在腹腔镜下远端胃切除术中发生了重要血管肝动脉受损的意外事件，从而导致转换为开腹术以修复肝动脉，还有在胃癌手术期间肝动脉受损的报道。该研究中，通过术前 CTA 检出腹腔干及肝动脉相关变异者 12 例（17.9%），有 4 例影响手术方案和进程的变异，分别为 2 例副肝左动脉和 2 例替代肝左动脉起源于胃左动脉，其中 1 例接受腹腔镜手术，因术前充分明了血管变异（迷走肝左动脉发自胃左动脉）而改变了手术入路。全部患者均成功完成腹腔镜下手术，未转开腹手术。即使开腹手术，血管变异和肿瘤侵犯血管也会影响手术方式的制定与实施。

胃左动脉及肝动脉的变异对手术方式的影响较大，术前对胃左动脉、肝动脉及相关血管变异的识别非常重要。术前了解变异血管的存在，避免可能的术中意外损伤及严重出血，进而影响手术进程或导致严重的并发症以致危及患者生命。肝左动脉变异容易导致意外损伤而发生肝左叶坏死。

无论是腹腔镜手术还是开腹胃癌手术，重要血管的侵犯将直接影响到手术的实施。该研究 CTA 发现 4 例胃癌对血管浸润破坏，其中有 2 例为胃左动脉受累。对于胃左动脉受侵病例，提示术中应谨慎处理此动脉及清除相关第 7 组淋巴结。另发现 1 例脾动脉受累及部分脾组织缺血坏死，此发现解释了患者的持续低热并提示尽早实施手术。由于 CT 提示未发现远隔转移灶，该患者选择尽早实施扩大根治术，术后患者恢复良好。

综上所述，术前 CTA 能准确显示胃周动脉及其发育变异和肿瘤对血管侵犯情况，有助于手术方案的选择与制定。由此能减少或避免手术中对血管的误伤，减少术中失血的可能和降低手术风险，有助于腹腔镜手术的顺利实施和真正达到微创的目的，也有助于胃癌开腹手术的安全实施。在胃癌术前 CT 评估中，仅需要增加动脉期扫描即可实施完成，因此具有较高的成本 - 效益比，值得在临床推广。

第二节　胃的动脉性压迹

脾动脉常常产生胃的后内部分轮廓的缺损，特别在老人，当此动脉迂曲或呈动脉瘤状，此压迹尤其明显,而且可伪似新生物引起的充盈缺损。与此相似,主动脉也可产生胃的压迹。熟知这些压迹,将避免误诊和不必要的探查手术。

脾动脉近侧段靠近胃切迹,如挤压该处可产生一缺损。脾动脉更远段常在靠近贲门处推挤胃壁导致缺损。这些缺损各有不同,从一小的局灶性变形到较长的搏动性压迹。此类缺损的范围有时不容易观察,除非在合适的角度和体位摄制点片,发现压迹,不然则常致误诊。

脾动脉对胃的压迹一般总是宽而浅的,具有壁外病变的特点,覆盖此缺损的黏膜皆完整无损。脾动脉的钙化或胃壁的局限性搏动增加(电视透视观察)有时出现,则利于确定血管的位置和压迹的性质。腹主动脉瘤产生胃的块状缺损容易识别,但主动脉迂曲造成胃的挤压,则既不常见,又难认识。

第三节 肿块状胃壁静脉曲张

详见于本书 本卷 本篇 第十四章 第一节 肿块状胃壁静脉曲张。

第四节 胃静脉曲张的诊断陷阱

胃静脉曲张的诊断常有困难,上消化道钡餐检查,甚至内镜都可将胃黏膜皱襞的突起或恶性病变误诊为静脉曲张。

Marshall 等(1978)在胃底发现有黏膜皱襞突起或肿块 3 例,其中 2 例皆为钡餐和胃镜误诊,而通过 X 线血管造影及脾门静脉造影确诊。

食管静脉曲张的存在,提示可疑及胃静脉曲张。

第十七章　胃的其他疾病

第一节　误诊病例简介：胃结核

胃结核是人体各器官结核病中罕见的疾病，在所有常规尸检中，胃结核检出率为 0.03%~0.21%。胃结核可分为原发性和继发性 2 类。原发性指患者体内其他部位没有结核病灶，由体外结核杆菌吞咽入胃致病。继发性大多数继发于空洞型肺结核，由口腔咽下含有大量结核杆菌的痰液，导致胃部发生感染。发病年龄以 20~40 岁最多，占 81.3%。女多于男。胃结核的病理可表现为结核性溃疡龛影、结核球、结核性脓肿，或比较弥漫的浸润。胃结核好发部位是幽门部，可出现幽门梗阻；部分病例出现上腹部包块。

影像学研究：X 线及 CT 表现为：胃溃疡型，有类似于胃溃疡及癌性溃疡的表现；充盈缺损型，圆形或不规则形充盈缺损，软组织肿块或囊性块影；胃窦狭窄型，胃外淋巴结核压迫或浸润胃壁，致胃窦变窄，部分侵及十二指肠。这些往往没有特异性，确诊有赖于病理。

一例发生在胃壁的结核性脓肿，表现为与胃壁相连的不均匀性密度的囊性块影，CT 扫描口服对比剂未见其进入包块内，故考虑上腹部包裹性炎性（结核）脓肿侵犯胃壁和前腹壁，而没有想到是直接来源于胃，这是该例定位错误的主要原因；由于患者没有明显的上腹部症状，也就未行消化道钡透和胃镜检查，若术前胃镜检查钳取深处及多点取材也许会明确诊断。由于胃结核的临床表现没有特异性，常被误诊为其他胃疾病，除非有病理证实，否则诊断实属困难，对身体其他部位有明显结核病变，同时伴有上腹部不适，疼痛等症状应警惕胃结核可能。必须指出的是，对于胃结核病人无论采用何种手术方式，术后均应常规应用抗结核治疗 6~12 个月，才能达到彻底的治愈。

第二节　胃支气管瘘

Gondos 等（1971）报告 1 例女性 63 岁病人，胃底部溃疡穿孔且通过横膈，形成左下叶一个脓腔及胃 - 支气管瘘，上胃肠道钡餐检查，此脓肿与支气管腔皆显示。此穿孔宽约 2.5cm。手术证实 X 线诊断且确定穿孔原因。横膈穿孔，随之而来是胸腹腔交通，常为膈下脓肿的一个并发症，在抗生素应用之前并不少见。此种横膈穿孔可能是胸腔积脓或是与支气管树交通的结果，非常少见，膈下脓肿也可穿入胃，形成胃 - 支气管瘘。一个胃溃疡的穿透及穿孔进入胸腔实属少见，有作者统计 1871—1971 共 100 年间仅 5 例报告。

第三节　胃异位胰腺

详见本书 本卷 第二十篇 第十九章　胰腺先天异常和发育变异。

第四节 胃肠道间质瘤,伴黏液样变性

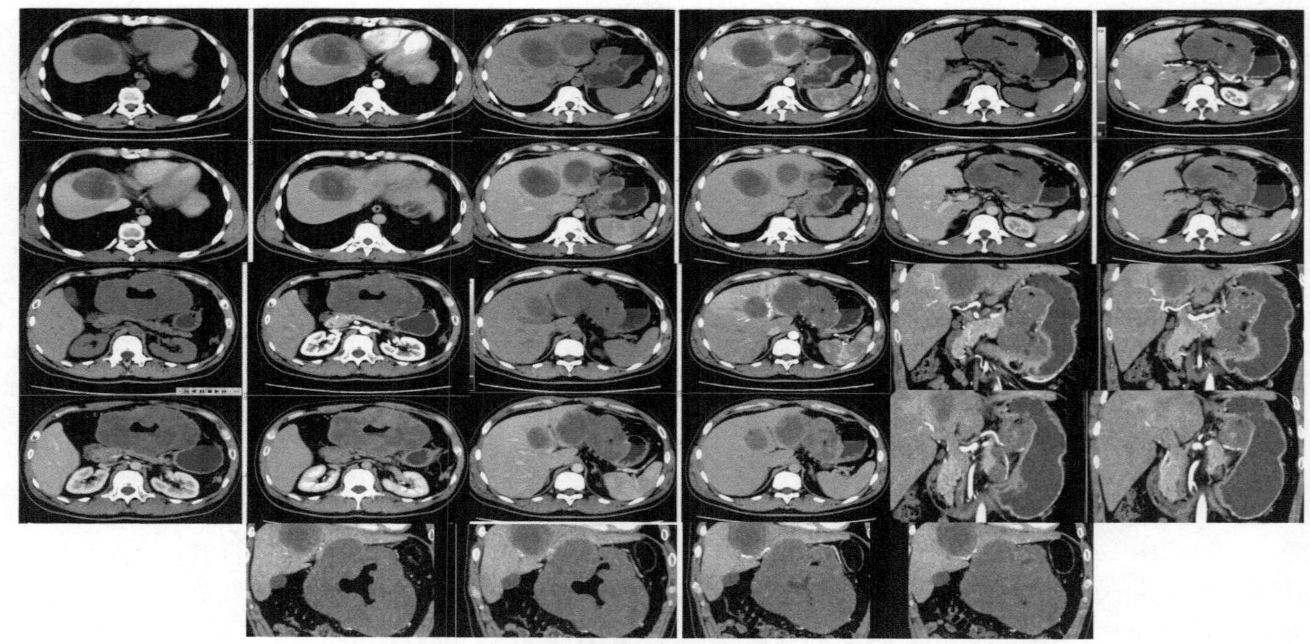

图 23-17-1 胃肠道间质瘤,伴黏液样变性

患者,男, 42 岁。因间歇性酒后黑便 1 年,腹痛、腹胀 1 个月余入院。

查体:上腹可触及一肿块,约 14cm × 15cm,质中,边界不清,表面不整,活动度欠佳,轻触压痛,与周围组织无明显粘连。

胃镜:胃体占位伴穿孔?病理:“胃窦黏膜活检标本”:慢性中度浅表性胃炎(活动性)伴轻度糜烂,另见少量炎性渗出物。HP(-)。肠镜未见明显异常。

病理检查:腹腔占位穿刺活检标本:穿刺组织一堆,长 0.5~1.4cm,直径 0.1cm。常规病理诊断:腹腔占位穿刺活检标本示梭形细胞肿瘤,富于黏液样物质。待做免疫组化检测进一步明确诊断。

免疫组化检测:阳性:CD117,CD34,DOG1(局灶+),Vimentin, Bcl-2, Nestin, CD99(弱+), PAS 染色, AB 染色, Ki-67(+,<5%);阴性:CK(P),CK5/6,CD31,S-100,Actin,Desmin,SMA,H-caldesmon,Calponin,MC,CR。免疫组化诊断:腹腔占位穿刺活检标本结合免疫组化检测结果,符合胃肠道间质瘤,伴黏液样变性。穿刺标本不适于肿瘤分级(图 23-17-1)。

第五节 植物性胃石与肠梗阻

胃石是指进食某些食物、药物或不能消化的物品、食物异物等在胃内聚集形成特殊的凝固物或硬块。根据胃石的成分可分为植物性胃石、动物性胃石、药物性胃石、混合性胃石四类。其中植物性胃石是某些果蔬与胃液作用结成的硬性团块,当植物性胃石通过幽门进入肠道,嵌顿在肠道某一部位即导致肠梗阻。在形成植物性胃石的果蔬中,以柿子、山楂居多。

植物性胃石形成的机制：柿子、山楂等食物中含有大量的鞣酸、果胶及树胶，不成熟的果实中其含量更高，可高达25%。鞣酸、胃酸可与蛋白质结合成不溶于水的鞣酸蛋白而沉淀于胃内，果胶和树胶遇酸即形成凝胶，也可与食物残渣聚积，形成巨大团块。在空腹时游离胃酸增多，更容易与鞣酸、果胶发生凝聚形成结石。食用山楂、柿子后再饮酒更易形成胃石，原因可能是酒中的乙醇能加速蛋白质的凝固，饮酒量愈大，酒精度数愈高，愈易形成胃石，且速度愈快。

空腹生食柿子或山楂等果蔬数小时或数天内，植物性胃石在胃内形成，引起一系列的临床症状，如上腹部饱胀、下坠感、恶心、返酸等，体检上腹部有轻度压痛，有时可扪及光滑可移动的包块。

影像学研究：针对胃内植物性胃石的检查手段多样。X线钡餐可以观察其大小、形态、活动度、胃黏膜的改变及有无伴发溃疡形成，是最常用的检查手段。B超不但可以显示病变的特异性表现，还可显示相应部位胃壁的层次结构，且快捷、方便。胃镜除具有明确诊断的作用，还可以利用特殊的治疗仪器结合某些化学药物治疗较松散的植物性胃石。

当植物性胃石通过幽门进入肠道嵌顿于肠道的某个病理或生理性狭窄区域，即引起肠梗阻，出现相应的临床症状。植物性胃石所致肠梗阻起初一般为单纯的机械性肠梗阻，具有肠梗阻的一般临床表现，但当临床诊治延误时，肠管持续扩张，肠壁变薄，肠腔压力升至一定程度时即可导致肠壁血供障碍，致肠壁缺血甚至坏死。

针对肠道中的植物性胃石上述检查手段尚存不足：肠梗阻是X线钡餐检查的禁忌证；肠梗阻时肠腔内积气较多，极大影响了B超的检查效果；植物性胃石一般嵌顿于小肠内，胃镜及肠镜难以窥及。

而CT检查方便快捷、成像清晰、具有动态性，且禁忌证及影响因素少，已成为临床诊断肠梗阻的首选影像学检查。常规检查结合连续薄层及三维重建可以清楚、直观地显示肠梗阻的位置、范围、肠管扩张的程度，更可以多平面显示梗阻点情况，有助于确定梗阻原因。

CT在植物性胃石所致肠梗阻诊断中的作用：确定有无肠梗阻。所有病例均发现梗阻近端肠管扩张、肠壁变薄、肠腔内气-液平面、远端肠管萎陷等明确的梗阻征象。确定肠梗阻的部位及原因。这是肠梗阻诊断中最具有临床指导意义的一点。两者通常相互依存，互为指示。以往大多数文献通常通过寻找移行带，即扩张和萎陷肠管之间的交界区来判断梗阻部位，进而寻找梗阻原因。但有作者指出，可能会首先发现植物性胃石，其表现为腹部肠管中的类圆形团块，其内软组织密度影与气体密度影相间混杂呈"蜂窝"状结构。其中软组织密度影因成分单一，所以密度较均匀，且略低于同层面的肌肉密度；增强扫描团块无强化。

根据以上较典型的CT征象，可以初步诊断植物性胃石。找到梗阻原因即可确定梗阻部位，但有时在具体区分空肠梗阻和回肠梗阻时有一定难度。通常空肠梗阻扩张肠腔位于上中腹偏左，肠壁的黏膜皱襞呈连续的环状或弹簧状；回肠的中下段梗阻扩张肠管分布于中下腹，扩张的回肠黏膜皱襞较平滑。当梗阻位于空、回肠交界区周围时，则需要根据扩张与萎陷肠管的相对长度及肠黏膜皱襞形态综合判断。

确定肠梗阻的程度。梗阻程度是依据远端肠管的萎陷程度、残留气体及液体的量判断。完全性肠梗阻时梗阻近端肠管显著扩张，远端肠管极度萎陷甚至不能辨认；不完全性肠梗阻时梗阻远端肠管内仍可见一定量的气体和液体。

CT增强扫描能明确肠梗阻部位及其周围肠管血运情况，明确是否有坏死肠管，为手术方案提供客观依据。根据CT增强扫描团块有无强化，可将肠道内植物性胃石与肿瘤鉴别开来。提供除肠道以外其他部位的异常征象。该组有3例扩张肠管周围脂肪间隙内可见渗出，2例可见盆腔积液。综上所述，结合植物性胃石较典型的CT影像学表现及明确的肠梗阻征象，可以初步诊断植物性胃石所致的肠梗阻。

附具体研究资料：有作者报告植物性胃石引起的肠梗阻14例，其中完全性肠梗阻11例，不完全性肠梗阻3例。十二指肠梗阻1例，空肠梗阻5例，回肠梗阻8例。均于梗阻部位发现植物性胃石，其CT表现为：梗阻部位呈类圆形团块，其内软组织密度影与气体密度影相间混杂呈"蜂窝"状，增强扫描团块无强化。其中多发者2例，单发者12例；胃石最大者直径约5.3cm，最小者直径约2.7cm。另外，3例扩张肠管周围脂肪间隙内可见渗出，2例可见盆腔积液。2例行CT增强扫描者，梗阻肠道未见血供异常。

第六节 牙刷穿透胃壁致右髂窝脓肿

胃内异物多为患者有意吞服,当异物较大、较硬时,胃壁的收缩力不足以使之变形经幽门排出,而胃液对绝大多数异物消化作用小,异物可长期滞留胃内,如果异物锐利可穿透胃壁进入腹腔。一例胃内整支牙刷,长度 > 20 cm,异物较长不易通过幽门,穿透胃壁顶于右侧髂骨,长时间挤压致右髂窝脓肿,右侧髂骨化脓性骨髓炎。

胃内异物引起胃穿孔较多见,但引起有髂窝脓肿及右侧髂骨化脓性骨髓炎尚少见报道。该例患者由于病史提供有误,按照异物为牙刷头则主要考虑穿透部位为小肠,然而异物为长约 20 cm 的整支牙刷,穿透胃壁顶在右髂窝内致右髂窝脓肿。

第七节 胃窦局限性血管炎

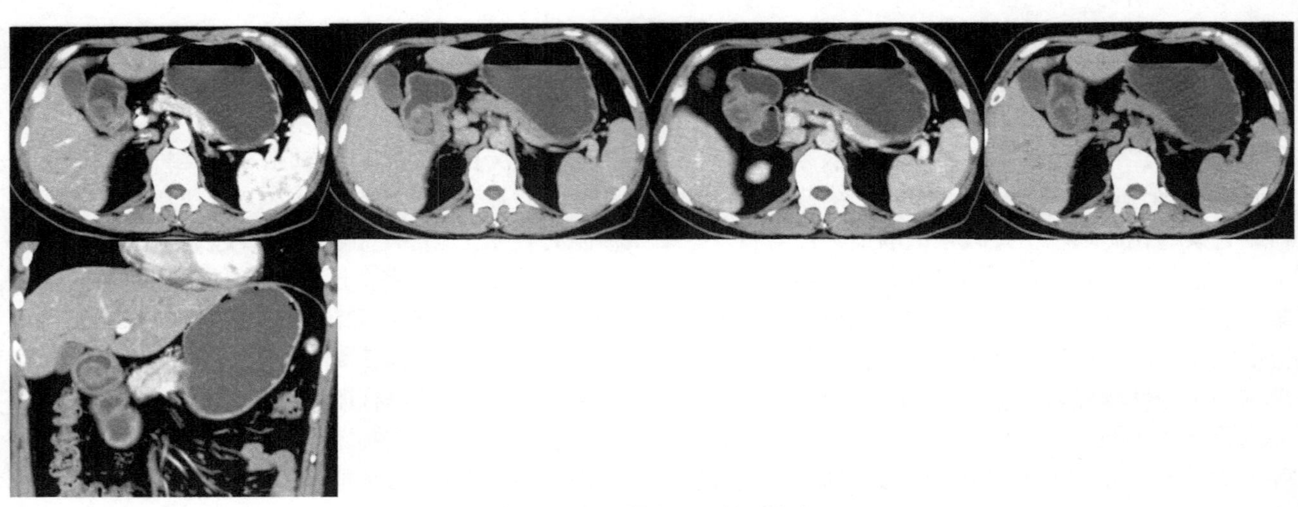

图 23-17-2 胃窦局限性血管炎

患者,女,45 岁。

CT:胃腔充盈良好,胃窦部可见大小约为 3.7cm ×2.8cm 的突向胃腔内的囊实性占位, CT 值 7~46HU,边界清楚,增强扫描时,实性部分中度强化,其 CT 值三期分别为 55HU、63HU、68HU,余胃壁未见明显增厚及异常强化;周围未见明显肿大淋巴结。CT 诊断:胃窦部囊实性占位性质待定,建议进一步胃镜检查病理确诊。

内镜病理检查:胃窦病灶 ESD 切除标本:胃组织一块,大小 4.5cm×3.5cm×0.5cm,黏膜面可见散在不规则隆起,长径 0.2~0.4cm,切面灰白灰褐,质中。病理诊断:胃窦病灶 ESD 切除标本:呈慢性中度非萎缩性胃炎,伴轻度肠化,间质淋巴滤泡形成,黏膜下可见大小不等的血管壁呈玻璃样变及纤维素性变性,伴多量炎细胞浸润,待做免疫组化检测及组织化学特染进一步协助诊断。

免疫组化诊断:胃窦病灶 ESD 切除标本呈慢性中度非萎缩性胃炎,伴轻度肠化,间质淋巴滤泡形成,黏膜下可见大小不等的血管壁呈玻璃样变及纤维素性变性,伴多量炎细胞浸润,结合免疫组化检测及组织化学特染结果,符合血管炎的病理学表现,建议治疗后复查(图 23-17-2)。

第八节　关于胃壁增厚

胃位于上腹部，胃底位于左侧膈下，向下延伸到脊柱右侧。在有高位横行胃的人，其胃底和胃体可于同一平面显示，胃底靠后，胃体靠前。幽门管位于胃窦远端的后方，与三角形的十二指肠球部相连。在CT图像上，当胃被扩张时，胃壁厚度为1~3mm；但当胃萎陷时，则可超过2cm。假如胃未被充分扩张，表现为胃壁增厚，则可酷似炎症和肿瘤病变引起的胃壁增厚。如果胃壁增厚是同心性的、对称的，且主要累及胃的近端，病变通常是良性的。

正常的黏膜皱襞主要见于胃底，然后均匀地沿胃的大弯侧延伸，直达胃窦。在CT图像上这种增厚的皱襞在大弯侧更明显，它们横行贯穿于一个明显增厚的胃轮廓中。此种表现经常被视为一种正常变异，它与黏膜皱襞肥大或胃的不完全扩张有关。

如果对胃壁增厚的原因有疑问，那么用水或发泡剂扩张胃腔或使病人取俯卧位或侧卧位再行CT扫描，可以帮助排除胃部病变。

在胃已充分扩张的情况下，如果增厚的黏膜皱襞呈局限性异常改变，那么与胃炎和肿瘤有关的病变应予排除。此时，需要结合上消化道造影或内镜检查作进一步评估。

胃壁CT观察：正常成人胃大致呈“J”形位于腹部左上象限。活体X线钡餐透视下胃可分为4型：角型胃、钩型胃、瀑布型胃及长胃。其中，钩型胃最多，角型胃次之。然而，与传统X线立位充盈像不同，MSCT采用卧位扫描，由于没有立位胃充盈时向足侧的重力作用，胃壁向足侧方向的牵拉明显减弱，造成胃的位置相对上移，而卧位时脊柱对胃的托垫作用也较立位时明显，因此，一项47例研究中，长胃可能误判为钩型胃，从而使得长胃例数偏少，可能造成结果有所偏差；而瀑布型胃未见显示也可能是由此造成的。

在多平面重建冠状位图像上观察正常成人胃分4区：食管与胃交界区为贲门；贲门平面向上左上方膨出的和贲门延续的为胃底；胃角切迹右侧至十二指肠之前为胃窦；胃底与胃窦之间的部分为胃体。

胃壁厚度与其充盈状态密切相关，有资料表明，在口服温水800~1 000 ml时胃腔充盈最佳，胃壁显示最为清楚。该项研究要求所有患者检查前口服温开水800~1 000 ml，以达到胃部的良好充盈，并且给予654-220mg，降低胃张力，以免胃蠕动影响胃壁厚度的正确测量。

胃腔充盈良好时，胃壁呈柔软、光滑线样，黏膜平坦舒展，胃壁与周围组织分界清楚，厚度均匀，贲门及胃窦处胃壁略厚，胃底及胃体部较薄，多数研究表明，正常胃壁充分展开情况下厚度一般<5 mm。该项研究显示在充分扩张的情况下，虽然贲门部及胃窦部胃壁明显厚于其余区域胃壁，但是各区胃壁厚度以及胃壁总平均厚度均<5 mm。

增强扫描正常胃壁动脉期通常多呈2~3层结构：内层相当于黏膜层，呈明显强化；中层相当于黏膜下层，呈相对低密度；外层通常为轻度强化，呈现中等密度，相当于肌肉-浆膜层。中层强化程度相对低可能与黏膜下层内含粗大的胶原纤维束和大量的弹性纤维，且血供较黏膜层和肌肉浆膜层少有关。

该项研究中，动脉期胃壁有30例呈现3层结构，占63.8%，2层结构有17例，占36.2%。延迟期47例胃壁均呈均一强化的单层结构。

有作者认为，3层结构的破坏是早期胃癌的CT表现。该项研究采用常规单次给药三相增强扫描方法对胃壁形态及结构进行研究。

文献报道MSCT 2次给药3次扫描方法更利于清晰显示胃壁的层状结构；传统CT增强扫描延迟期小动脉、小静脉以及淋巴结呈现等密度，而此2次给药三相增强扫描的延迟期第2次给药使得小动脉、小静脉强化，淋巴结表现为部分边缘强化，从而将小动、静脉以及淋巴结有效的加以区分，更有利于对淋巴结的鉴别及分期。

MSCT分辨率高、扫描速度快、重建层厚薄，1次屏气可完成整个胃部的扫描，加上低张药物及阴性对比剂水的应用，使得MSCT对于胃本身的观察可以基本达到与X线钡餐透视同样的效果，并能够准确判断胃周围组织及其他脏器情况，结合多平面重建技术，可为临床提供更为丰富的信息，并对胃部肿瘤的MSCT研究奠定良好的基础。

第九节 误诊病例简介：胃黏膜下巨大陈旧性血肿与左上腹囊液性肿块性质待定

胃壁由黏膜层、黏膜下层、肌层和浆膜层组成，正常情况下各层之间紧密结合，几乎无法将它们分离。黏膜层和黏膜下层之间有细小血管网分布，在病理过程中黏膜下小血管几乎不可能出血，一般只有在黏膜发生溃疡累及到黏膜下血管时才有可能出血，但出血后不大可能出现黏膜下血肿。而腹部钝器外伤发生黏膜下血肿更是不大可能，因为胃是一个空腔脏器，有相当大的缓冲空间，腹部钝器伤很难伤及胃。

经查阅相关文献，没有有关胃黏膜下血肿的报道，一例是经手术病理证实的胃黏膜下陈旧性血肿，术前诊断是左上腹囊液性肿块性质待定。这实属较为罕见的病例，临床上很少见到，所以在术前诊断上有一定的难度。通过该病例的报道，希望能够为今后在遇到有腹部钝器伤的患者做影像学检查时，如果在胃区出现有囊液性包块时，应该考虑到有胃黏膜下血肿的可能；同时如果在腹腔胃区出现囊液性包块时，应该将胃黏膜下血肿纳入鉴别诊断。

第十节 误诊病例简介：异物导致慢性胃穿孔与胃窦占位

胃破裂常发生于饱餐后胃的钝性创伤。常见于儿童。胃前壁最易破裂，其次是胃大弯、胃小弯，最不易破裂的是胃后壁。许多病人创伤位于左侧，最常见于累及脾的创伤。从鼻胃管中可以引流出浓稠的血液。气腹、口服对比剂和胃内容物的外漏均可在 CT 上显示。

一例患者为尖锐异物导致胃穿孔，临床工作中比较少见，患者术前未提供详细病史，术中发现异物为鱼刺，再次追问病史，有吃鱼后右上腹痛，未予重视，病情自行缓解，术前的 CT 已提示异物可能性，但病变较大，有手术指征，且需排除肿瘤可能。

超声内镜下的 5 层结构，第 1 层为强回声带，第 2 层为低回声带，组织学上共同代表黏膜层；第 3 层为强回声带，组织学上代表黏膜下层；第 4 层为低回声带，组织学上代表固有肌层；第 5 层为强回声带，组织学上代表浆膜层，该例患者超声内镜显示第 1、2 层完整，可能与异物尖锐，导致穿孔部位较小，加之半年病史，局部黏膜已经完全修复有关，也使临床医师无法完全排除肿瘤性病变。

CT 平扫发现病变边缘的条形高密度，形状规则，边界清晰， CT 值达 192 HU，提示可能为骨性组织，鱼刺的 CT 值低于人类骨骼的 CT 值，大约 300~800 HU，也可能与部分容积效应有关，增强扫描动脉期可见与病变相邻的肝左叶外下段（Ⅲ段）、左叶内侧段（Ⅳ段）及肝右叶前下段（Ⅴ段）出现一过性高密度异常灌注，范围较广泛，边界尚清晰，与致炎因子引起的动脉充血和血管通透性的增加有关。CT 诊断：胃窦部占位，炎性病变可能性大，不除外异物所致。

延迟期病变与周围的胃窦壁和肝左叶关系密切，分界不清，但胃窦壁层次清晰，倾向于炎性粘连，而非肿瘤性病变侵犯；病变中央部分液化坏死区密度均匀一致，内壁光整，未见壁结节，也提示炎性病变，对于异物的显示冠状位最大密度投影重建图像清晰，而容积再现图像可以对异物与周围组织器官的空间关系进行准确的评价。

总之，影像医师在诊断的过程中要注意细节和特殊征象的观察，仔细分析，同时充分运用各种后处理图像，尤其注意追问临床医师没有注意到的病史，往往对诊断和鉴别诊断有非常重要的作用，而这也是影像医师容易忽略的。

第十一节　诊断陷阱：胃底憩室与左侧肾上腺区疾病

患者，女，52 岁。

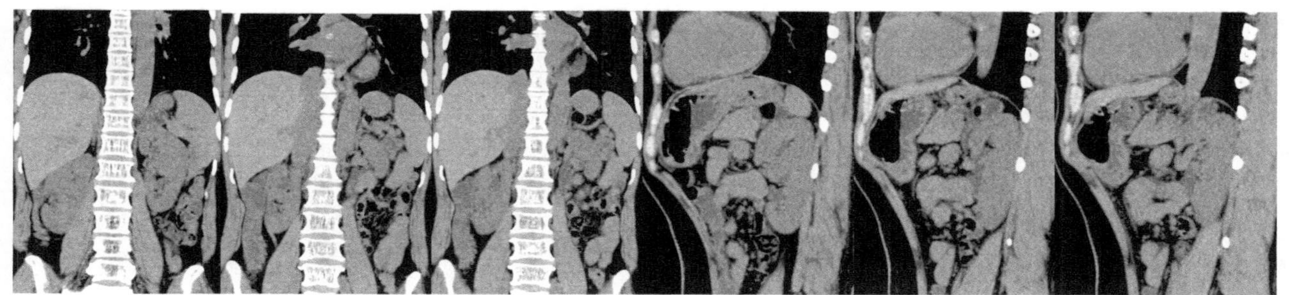

图 23-17-3　胃底憩室与左侧肾上腺区疾病

CT 所见左侧肾上腺区附近囊状影像，胃镜证实为胃底憩室。这是左侧肾上腺区容易引起混淆为恶性占位性病变的疾病之一（图 23-17-3、图 23-17-4）。

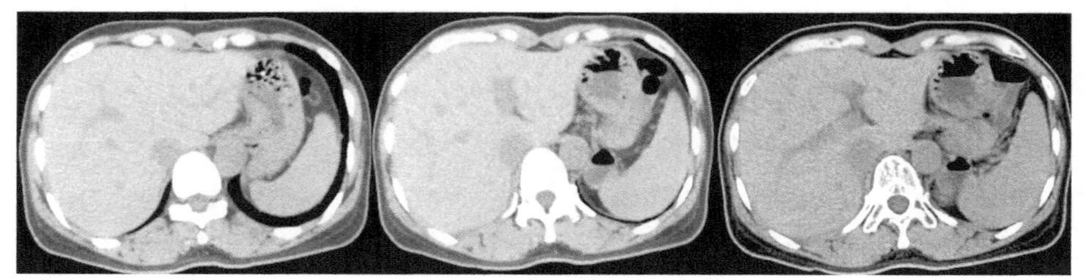

图 23-17-4

第十二节　一些诊断陷阱

肝左叶突入胃底形成压迹：肝左叶突入胃底形成压迹的表现有多种多样，一般为圆弧形，圆弧的程度各不相同，有的很平坦，有的还可呈现成角形凸入胃内，使胃内表现锐角凹陷。

脾对胃的压迹：脾对胃的压迹一般在大弯侧，然而有时脾从上方，即膈顶向下压迫胃底，导致胃底穹隆变形成为平坦状或显现不规则，伪似胃的肿物。

胰腺对胃的压迹：偶尔在胃的后壁可见胰腺对胃的压迹，这常出现于少年。

肋缘对胃的压迹：肋缘也可对胃形成压迹，多出现于胃的外侧和前方，比较局限。

发育性胃憩室：胃憩室的典型位置在胃食管连接区，有作者称之为发育性胃憩室。

胃与假腹水：邻近肝区超声横切扫描发现明显包块影，其前部无回声，后部有回声，疑为腹水；口服饮料后再行横切扫描，见该包块整个均存回声，事实证明该包块为胃。

胃与胰腺假性囊肿：在幽门梗阻者或饮入大量液体为膀胱超声检查作准备的病人，超声扫描见充盈液体而扩张的胃佯似左上腹囊性包块，细心观察此结构的蠕动，从而确认为胃，有时还需请病人饮水一杯，以显示胃中的微小气泡的旋涡，有作者认为这可能是区别胃与胰腺假性囊肿的重要方法。偶尔，大的小网膜囊及胰腺假性囊肿佯似扩张且充盈液体的胃，而真正的胃却萎陷缩小位于假性囊肿前方。

胃溃疡穿孔:胃溃疡穿孔入小网膜囊,造成口服对比剂外渗,充满对比剂的小网膜囊在CT图像上酷似充盈对比剂的肠袢,同时可见腹腔气体液体职聚类似充气扩张的结肠肠袢。

腹部X线正位平片的诊断陷阱:有作者注意到,在腹部的仰卧位片,充满液体的胃底部形似肿瘤,在平片和断层摄影均一样。此假肿瘤在血管造影时亦不透光,因而不易鉴别。在俯卧位腹部平片上,液体充盈的胃窦可伪似右上腹肿块影,也得到钡餐的证实。腹部平片上,气体充盈的胃底部使膈下脾阴影向外侧移位,形似肿瘤。胃气泡内的肝左叶影也可形似肿瘤。充盈液体的胃窦及胃幽门透亮皱褶影可伪似伴存裂隙的胆囊结石。在腹部平片上,胃内容物的影像,有时可伪似左肺下叶基底支气管扩张的改变。

CT:胃位于上腹部,胃底位于左侧膈下,向下延伸到脊柱的右侧。在有高位横行胃的人,其胃底和胃体可于同一横断层面上显示,胃底靠后,胃体靠前。幽门管位于胃窦远端的后方,与三角形的十二指肠球部相连。在CT图像上,当胃被扩张时,胃壁厚度为1~3mm,但当胃萎陷时,则可超过20mm。假如胃未被充分扩张,表现为胃壁增厚,则可酷似炎症和肿瘤病变引起的胃壁增厚。如果胃壁增厚是同心性的、对称的,且主要累及胃的近端,病变通常是良性的。

正常的黏膜皱襞主要见于胃底,然后均匀地沿胃的大弯侧延伸,直达胃窦。在CT图像上,这种增厚的皱襞在大弯侧更明显,它们横贯于一个明显增厚的胃轮廓中。此种表现经常被视为一种正常变异,它与黏膜皱襞肥大或胃的不完全扩张有关。

如果对胃壁增厚的原因有疑问,那么用水或发泡剂扩张胃腔或使病人取俯卧位或侧卧位行CT扫描,可以帮助排除胃部病变。在胃已充分扩张的情况下,如果增厚的黏膜皱襞呈局限性异常改变,那么与胃炎和肿瘤有关的病变应予排除。此时,需要结合上消化道造影或内镜检查并作进一步评估。

第十八章　胃手术后

第一节　Biliroth Ⅰ式术后改变

胃肠钡餐造影表现：胃窦及十二指肠球部切除，胃体部与十二指肠吻合，在胃体小弯侧缝合切口，因此胃体小弯侧为缝合端。吞钡造影时，钡剂通过贲门进入残胃，钡剂可和残胃中存留，残胃为胃底及胃体的一部分。

残胃小弯侧由于缝合，可出现沿小弯至吻合口的隆起样改变，隆起处表面较光整，一般无溃疡性改变，但黏膜不规整，走行较僵直。此种改变，勿误为占位性病变。

Billroth Ⅰ式手术吻合口一般在1~1.5cm左右，可见胃黏膜结构延伸至吻合口处，吻合口以下为十二指肠，呈羽毛状黏膜皱襞。Billroth Ⅰ式术后检查要观察有无吻合口狭窄，钡剂有否顺利进入十二指肠，注意胃肠动力改变。

临床上Billroth Ⅰ式术后经常在术后7天至1个月内出现胃动力减弱现象，表现为进食后不能排空，呕吐胃内容物。这时经常需要影像检查证实，并除外吻合口狭窄，考虑到有吻合口过窄或吻合口漏的可能，此时采用泛影葡胺造影，泛影葡胺造影时，重点是观察胃动力改变，即在透视下观察胃是否有蠕动，如胃蠕动消失，证明为胃动力减弱，如胃蠕动正常，而泛影葡胺不能进入十二指肠，则说明有吻合口狭窄的可能性，应建议在吻合口水肿消失后，再次进行复查。

CT表现：Billroth Ⅰ式多为胃或十二指肠溃疡治疗所采用的术式，但部分胃癌也可采用此种术式。胃十二指肠溃疡术后较少采用CT检查，在有术后并发症的患者，如对包裹性积液、肠梗阻等患者，CT检查是较好的选择；胃癌患者术后应常规行CT扫描，作为以后随诊复查对比的依据。

Billroth Ⅰ式手术后的CT检查时也需饮水或气体以充盈胃腔，平扫时可以吞服产气剂，增强扫描可以饮水，一般在上机前饮水500 ml，上机后再饮水300~500ml，以尽可能充盈胃腔，然后立即行CT扫描，对于无禁忌证的患者可肌肉注射平滑肌松弛剂654-2 10~20mg，既可以减少胃肠蠕动，又可以松弛胃壁，有利于观察胃内及吻合口处的改变。

Billroth Ⅰ式CT可见残胃的胃底及胃体部分，可以显示吻合口的位置，CT可以观察吻合口周围有无肿块，吻合口以远肠管的走行。CT的优势是显示胃周围、腹腔及腹膜后有无淋巴结肿大，还可以观察腹腔内的实质脏器。

第二节　Billroth Ⅱ式术后改变

胃肠钡餐造影表现：胃大部切除，十二指肠球部也同时切除，缝合闭锁十二指肠降段，将空肠上提与残胃做端侧吻合，此种手术胃体小弯侧仍需要缝合，但由于是与空肠侧壁吻合，因此吻合口可以适当增宽。吞钡造影时，钡剂通过贲门进入残胃，钡剂即可由吻合口大部分进入空肠，残胃小弯侧也由于缝合的原因，沿胃小弯至吻合口处也可见隆起样改变，与Billroth Ⅰ式相似，吻合口处有时可见到手术金属夹影。

在Billroth Ⅱ式手术吻合口一般在2~3cm左右，可见大弯侧及前后壁的黏膜自然延伸至吻合口处，吻合口以下为空肠，空肠皱襞呈环形排列，蠕动活跃,肠腔排空钡剂后,空肠黏膜呈羽毛状影像,也可呈雪花样钡剂残留。

Billroth Ⅱ式术后一般不发生吻合口狭窄,钡剂在大多数病例能较快进入空肠。在 Billroth Ⅱ式术后检查时,应注意钡剂可能较快地自胃进入空肠,以致胃内钡剂存留较少,进入空肠较多,影响检查,必要时可以采用半卧位或同时采用右前斜位,尽量使钡剂暂时较多的留存在胃内,转动体位,使钡剂均匀涂抹在胃缝合端及吻合口,注意钡剂是否可以进入输入袢及输出袢,有无输入袢梗阻等改变。

CT 表现:CT 检查的作用与 Billroth Ⅰ式相同,在胃十二指肠术后并发症观察方面有一定的价值,在 Billroth Ⅱ式术后可以观察输入袢有无异常扩张,以证明有无输入袢梗阻。Billroth Ⅱ式手术后 CT 检查前准备与 Billroth Ⅰ式相同。胃空肠吻合术后 CT 可以观察残胃,也可以观察吻合口的位置,CT 可显示与胃吻合的空肠,输入袢肠管一般在吻合口右侧,输出袢空肠在吻合口左侧。由于空肠上提与胃吻合,空肠走行于胆囊与结肠的内侧上方,而输出段以远的空肠也会改变其位置走行,应注意观察鉴别。

第三节 贲门胃底切除术后改变

钡餐造影表现:其表现与食管下端癌术后钡餐造影表现相似,胃提至胸腔内,与食管切除后的下端相吻合,其钡餐造影表现与食管癌术后造影表现相似,参见食管癌的手术后改变。CT 表现:CT 扫描时可见胃位置上移至胸腔内,与食管吻合的为胃底,胃壁厚度均匀,胃腔略变形、拉长,正常情况下吻合口厚度环周较均匀,不应形成软组织肿块。胃周无淋巴结肿大。

第四节 全胃切除术后改变

胃体癌或胃底癌胃体大部侵犯时,多采用全胃切除术,可以避免因保留胃窦而出现残胃溃疡、残胃癌等并发症。全胃切除术后,空肠与食管吻合,一般需加用金属吻合器。

钡餐造影表现:吞钡后,对比剂经食管小肠吻合口,迅速进入空肠内,并向下运行。吻合口以上为食管纵行黏膜结构,而吻合口以下为空肠黏膜,其皱襞呈环形排列,钡剂进入小肠后迅速随蠕动向前输送。全胃切除术后,钡餐造影检查为首先选择的常规检查方法。操作也较方便,一般不需卧位。CT 表现:CT 可在上腹部观察到小肠的位置改变,上腹小肠位置一般发生变化。检查时为利于前后对比,扫描位置条件及摄片窗宽窗位尽可能在多次检查时都保持一致。CT 也可显示吻合口的位置。最主要的是观察上腹部腹腔无有无软组织肿块及腹腔和腹膜后淋巴结有无肿大。

第五节 胃术后缝合处的肉芽肿

一些学者报告 4 例胃术后缝合处的肉芽肿,在术后钡餐检查中常难以诊断而引起误诊。对于此种情况,应该考虑的诊断包括有胃手术后变形、术后肿瘤复发、新生肿瘤、脓肿、恶性溃疡、粘连或几种疾病合并出现。该组 4 例皆无症状,只是术后钡餐时才发现胃内或邻近的十二指肠球部有多个充盈缺损而类似息肉样肿瘤,其中 3 例再手术,活检发现为缝合肉芽肿,第 4 例由内窥镜检发现。

对缝合肉芽肿有用的间接诊断资料是胃的手术史,缝合材料不被吸收,钡餐检查发现手术吻合部位胃壁有轮廓清楚的充盈缺损,内窥镜检见吻合处胃腔内黏膜完整的光滑凸起,胃细胞学检查阴性,并且无其他任何系统性的异常表现。胃大部切除术后残胃有时呈现类似肿瘤的充盈缺损,如出现于晚期胃癌术后的残胃,则更易误为胃癌复发。

第六节　胃大部切除术后假性肿瘤变形

有作者报告 4 例胃大部切除术后假性肿瘤变形，4 例皆作胃镜检查，1 例行手术探查，这 4 例都认为是手术缝合嵴或褶皱造成。另有作者报告 2 例经追踪观察，结合手术缝合情况，考虑可能为手术后缝合嵴加上水肿造成。此种肿瘤变形都在吻合口或胃切除残端缝合处附近，残端病理检查无癌浸润，局部胃壁较柔软，其形态有一定的可变性，均在术后第一次钡餐时发现。

第二十四篇　十二指肠

第一章　十二指肠恶性肿瘤

第一节　十二指肠恶性淋巴瘤

十二指肠恶性淋巴瘤极为少见，仅占胃肠道肿瘤的0.1%，其中1/3为原发性。

病理学：肿瘤质软，表面血管丰富，有的还存在囊性变，可与周围脏器粘连，有的出现邻近淋巴结转移。当肿瘤累及肝外胆管或/和胆胰管十二指肠连接区时，可引起梗阻性黄疸。

临床表现：男女性别差异不大。可有上腹痛、消瘦、贫血、黄疸、黑便等症状。体检时，有的病人可扪及右肋下包块。

影像学研究：CT表现多样，可以是单发肿块、多发肿块或浸润性病变。肿块光滑柔软，易引起肠套叠，但很少引起肠梗阻。在十二指肠降段或/和水平段，可见实性肿块，其下方可有分叶。浸润性病变使肠壁增厚，破坏小肠皱襞，侵及黏膜下层，抑制肠蠕动，受累肠段呈动脉瘤样扩张，见于50%的病例。外生性的肿块易出现溃疡。发生于小肠系膜者，增大后浸润邻近的小肠袢，产生“三明治”征象，其内可见被包绕的肠系膜血管。由于肿块柔软，肠系膜血管很少受到损害。

十二指肠低张双对比造影：十二指肠低张双对比造影是以往诊断十二指肠恶性淋巴瘤的主要手段。一般都行CT、超声、ERCP、PTC、血管造影、内窥镜检等综合影像手段，以期达到早期正确诊断的目的，为手术提供更多信息。在造影时见到的十二指肠恶性淋巴瘤肠管动脉瘤样扩张，脑回样压迹颇具特征性，此种改变是由于淋巴瘤向深部浸润，破坏肠壁固有肌层及神经丛，使肠管失去张力所致。胃窦及十二指肠充盈较慢，球部和/或降段明显扩大。胃窦部偏大弯侧巨大不规则存钡区，并有环绕存钡区的充盈缺损，存钡区与十二指肠不易分开。在降段可有脑回压迹动脉瘤样改变。病变处肠壁僵硬，可伴有龛影形成，黏膜皱襞破坏消失，肠管轮廓不规则。有的病人可触及肿块，呈动脉瘤样囊状息肉样改变。有的病例在PTC检查时，可显示肝外胆管下端梗阻。

鉴别诊断：原发性十二指肠恶性淋巴瘤应与十二指肠腺癌、十二指肠平滑肌肉瘤、局限性炎症及十二指肠结核等进行鉴别诊断。

误诊病例简介：有作者报告一例最初即诊断为十二指肠癌并淋巴结转移，可能与肿瘤侵及肠管较明显且较深（深肌层深部）而其他部位淋巴结肿大不十分明显有关。但十二指肠淋巴瘤肠壁常呈环行增厚，与肿大的淋巴结常融合成较大的团块，而肠腔仍通畅，肠梗阻及近段肠管扩张不明显。

第二节　误诊病例简介：十二指肠空肠低分化癌或肉瘤样癌与肠壁血肿

病例，男，52岁。肺癌6月，放疗后1个月，腹部胀痛7天入院。半年前CT发现左下肺团块影，行左肺下叶基底段活检，病理报告：结合形态学改变及免疫组化结果，符合非小细胞肺癌，倾向腺癌，遂行抗感染和放射治疗。后CT复查见左下肺癌较前进展，且伴阻塞性肺炎，又现空洞，纵隔淋巴结肿大。在放射治疗基础上又加用化疗，病情渐稳定。近日出现腹部胀痛，昨日出现发热，最高体温38.4℃。

胸腹部CT诊断：十二指肠与空肠交界处异常密度影，较三天前增大，考虑血肿（肠壁内血肿？），肿瘤卒中待排；肠梗阻；空肠上段肠壁增厚；腹腔及腹膜后多发肿大淋巴结。

手术所见:十二指肠水平部至空肠起始段见巨大肿瘤,大小约 20cm × 15cm,肿物表面破溃崩裂,腹腔内及腹膜后大量暗红色血凝块及破溃组织,肿物与腹膜后腹主动脉旁周围组织、胰腺、脾脏及后腹膜形成广泛侵蚀性破溃粘连、固定,无法分离。可见肿物侵蚀空肠处已全程穿透肠壁,破溃处近半圈肠壁可见肠液从穿孔处流出。

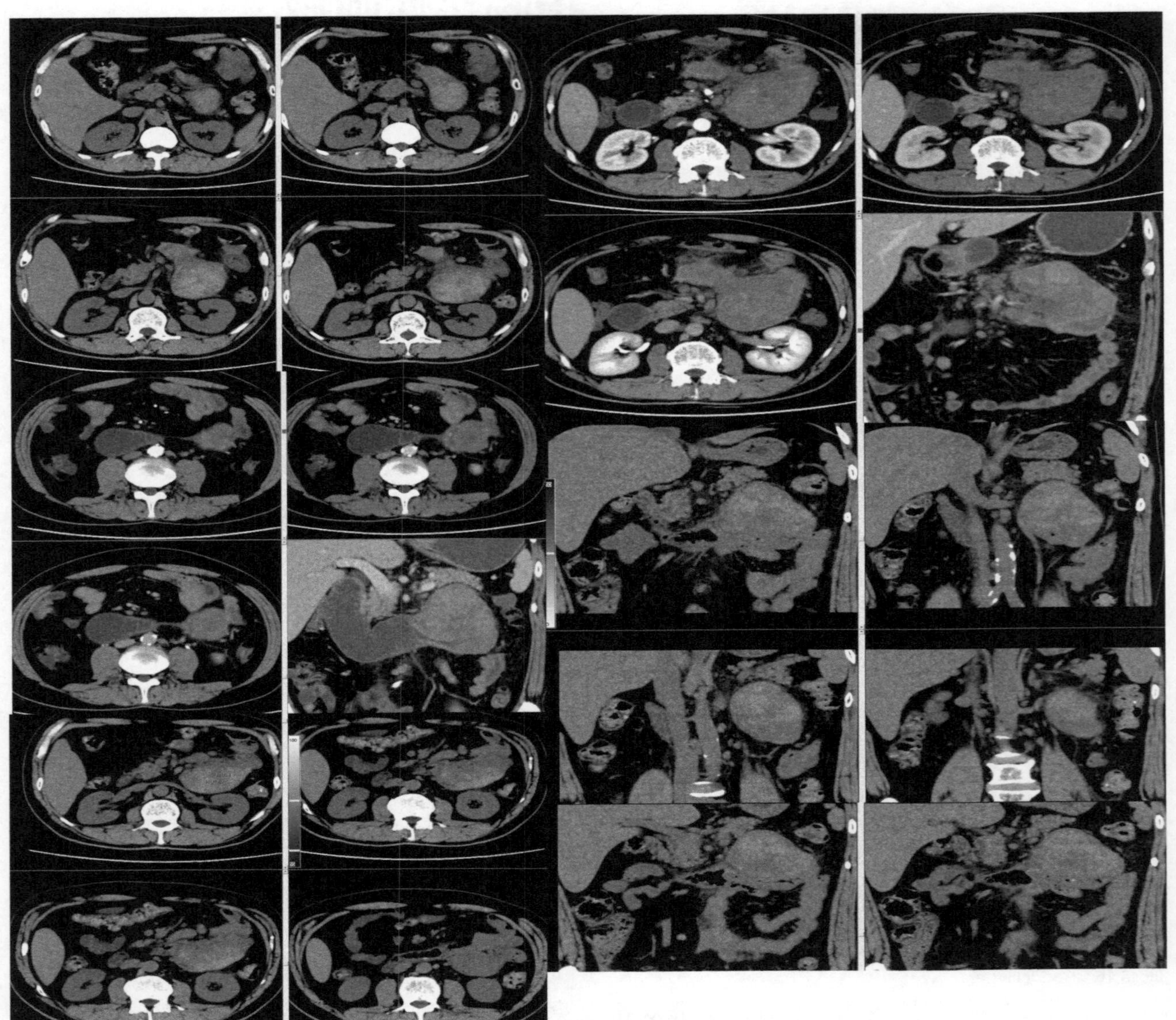

图 24-1-1 十二指肠空肠低分化癌或肉瘤样癌与肠壁血肿

病理检查:十二指肠空肠肿物活检标本:暗褐色组织一堆,总体积 6.5cm × 4.5cm × 1.4cm,切面暗红、质中。常规病理诊断:十二指肠空肠肿物活检标本:大量血凝块中见少量异型细胞聚集,待免疫组化进一步协助诊断。免疫组化检测:阳性:CK(P),CK(L),CK7,CK19,Vimentin,TTF-1,Ki-67(+,约 90%);阴性:CK(H),CK5/6,CK20,NapsinA,Villin,CDX2,CD56,E-cadherin,SyN,CgA,CA199,PSA,P504Sd;阳性:CK7,CK19,Vimentin,TTF-1,Ki-67(+,约 90%);阴性:CK(H),CK(L),CK5/6,CK20,NapsinA,Villin,CDX2,CA199,PSA,P504S。免疫组化诊断:十二指肠空肠肿物活检标本:大量血凝块中见少量异型细胞聚集成片,无巢状结构。结合免疫组化及病史,考虑为低分化癌或肉瘤样癌,可能来源于肺(图 24-1-1)。

第三节　原发性十二指肠癌及误诊分析

原发性十二指肠癌极为少见，其发病率约为0.019%~0.05%，约占胃肠道恶性肿瘤的0.35%。在小肠，原发性癌最常见于十二指肠乳头区周围，该处病变常常表现为套餐巾的小环。它们通常呈中度分化的产生黏液的肿瘤，肿瘤常侵犯固有肌层的整个厚度，常见神经周围性侵犯和淋巴结的转移。原发性十二指肠癌可发生于乳头上部、乳头周围和乳头下部，在乳头周围占40%~60%，在病理上与胆胰管十二指肠连接区癌很难区别。（有关乳头区的肿瘤请详见本书 本卷 第十九篇 胆胰管十二指肠连接区疾病有关章节。）

病理学：小肠腺癌是最常见的小肠恶性肿瘤，多见于十二指肠。十二指肠癌占小肠腺癌的39.8%，大多数为乳头腺癌。在大体病理形态上通常将其分为息肉肿块型和浸润狭窄型，有时两者可同时并存。前者乳突状肿块向肠腔内生长，后者伴有纤维组织增生，引起收缩，导致肠腔狭窄，甚至肠道阻塞。

临床表现：原发性十二指肠癌早期可无明显症状或仅表现为非特异性症状如腹痛，上腹不适。伴随病变进展，癌肿因沿肠壁蔓延、浸润致肠腔狭窄，此时患者常出现上腹饱胀、呕吐、体重下降等症状。癌肿若累及乳头部可出现阻塞性黄疸。

影像学研究：Bosse将X线表现分为环形狭窄型、偏心性非对称性狭窄型、息肉样型、溃疡型、浸润型等五种类型。上垣惠二等（1974）根据低张十二指肠造影所见将十二指肠球部癌分为浸润型和隆起型：浸润型表现为十二指肠球部的变形，可形成溃疡，与十二指肠溃疡有类似表现；隆起型与良性肿瘤有类似表现。又将球部以外的十二指肠癌X线表现分为三种：以多发的充盈缺损为主要所见；以不规则的溃疡为主要所见；以内腔狭窄为主要所见。采用低张十二指肠造影可很好地显示病变形态，易于诊断。但是，有时与胰头癌、连接区癌鉴别困难。当看到多发的充盈缺损和大而不规则的溃疡时，要考虑原发性十二指肠癌的可能。

CT：为了发现异常，准确地做出诊断，首先必须熟悉十二指肠正常结构的CT图像。正常十二指肠降段与胰腺关系密切，附于胰头，在胆囊和肝下缘内侧，右肾和肾上腺的前方，近端结肠和结肠系膜的后方；肝外胆管在十二指肠球部和降段的后方穿过，然后走行于降段的内侧，终止于胆胰共同管；十二指肠水平段和升段沿着胰腺体部和尾部的下缘走行，横过中线在肠系膜上动脉与静脉之后，左肾静脉之下。CT表现多样。典型表现为肠壁局限性增厚引起肠腔变窄，亦可为息肉样肿块或浸润性病变。病变僵硬，含有纤维，早期产生梗阻。冠状位3D CT影像有助于显示十二指肠第3段及其与胰腺的关系。小肠腺癌的肝脏转移灶表现为低密度，增强扫描的门静脉期显示最佳。

有作者列出下述CT表现：①病变区不规则肿块，CT值为40~90HU，肿块内均有不规则含气肠腔；② CT清楚显示肿块与周围脏器的关系：肿块可侵及胰头部、下腔静脉、肠系膜上静脉；十二指肠降段长条状肿块与胰头间多个淋巴结增大；肿块与周围肠管（含对比剂）有粘连；③可观察肝、胰、肾、肾上腺及腹膜后间隙与肿块的关系，发现肝内转移灶；④增强扫描显示肿块有不同程度的非均匀性强化。

在对比剂的衬托下，癌肿表现为突入腔内的不规则或息肉样肿块，可伴有局部肠壁增厚，增强扫描时肿块有较明显强化。癌肿沿肠壁周径方向的浸润引起管腔狭窄是CT较易发现的征象，狭窄段多表现为十二指肠壁的局限性非对称性环周增厚，狭窄前段常表现为较明显的肠腔扩张。癌肿侵及周围脂肪组织，表现为高密度影。胰腺受侵时，出现胰腺体积增大，与十二指肠间的脂肪间隙消失。MSCT在显示溃疡、黏膜改变、肠蠕动等方面有一定的局限，所测肿瘤大小均略小于肿瘤实际范围，气钡双重造影可以显示十二指肠内肿瘤的大小、黏膜改变及溃疡，优于MSCT，且能通过透视动态观察肠壁是否僵硬来判断良、恶性。但是MSCT可明确原发性十二指肠癌的肿瘤位置，向周围器官的浸润及淋巴结转移等情况，这是气钡双重造影所无法代替的，当晚期原发性十二指肠癌癌肿增大导致肠道梗阻趋向完全时，对比剂无法通过，MSCT就成为唯一有效的检查方法。

必须注意的是CT检查和胃肠钡餐检查在十二指肠癌诊断中具有相辅相成的作用。因为，多年来胃肠造影检查对十二指肠癌的诊断已有较为丰富的经验,一般已能检出并做到诊断与鉴别诊断,而CT扫描可提供肿瘤向腔外生长的形态和范围,以及肠管外蔓延和转移的情况,这对制定治疗方案及术前计划极有帮助。由于CT应用于胃肠道病变的诊断经验不多,有的患者却是由于腹部肿块而先行CT扫描,此时,应补作胃肠道钡餐检查,以便两者结合,提高诊断水平。

鉴别诊断:特别要注意的是,许多正常的发育变异和腹部手术后的改变常常被误诊为异常,如:小肠旋转不良,十二指肠环呈不完全的C形。十二指肠空肠曲位置也常变化,近端小肠可位于右上腹。有时,不充盈对比剂的小肠曲很像腹内肿物,但只要口服足够的对比剂或改变体位(俯卧位或侧卧位)扫描,或在不同时间扫描,其形态常有改变,即可避免误诊。

由于十二指肠周围有许多器官,邻近组织的肿瘤亦可直接侵犯十二指肠,最常见的是胰癌,其次是胃癌、胆囊癌、胆管癌、右肾及右肾上腺和结肠的恶性肿瘤也可侵犯十二指肠。

原发性十二指肠癌的特点是,肿块包绕十二指肠,表现为软组织肿块中心或偏心部有不规则充气的肠腔。

十二指肠平滑肌瘤:当原发性十二指肠癌仅表现为肿块时要与十二指肠平滑肌瘤相鉴别,十二指肠平滑肌瘤表现为向腔内或腔外膨胀性生长的软组织肿块,密度均匀一致,体积较小,直径多不超过5 cm,边界清楚,无邻近肠壁增厚,而原发性十二指肠癌表现为浸润性生长,与周围肠管边界不清。

十二指肠淋巴瘤:原发性十二指肠癌既表现肿块又表现肠管狭窄时,要与十二指肠淋巴瘤鉴别,十二指肠淋巴瘤较少见,MSCT可显示十二指肠肠壁的增厚以及周围肿大的淋巴结对肠管的推挤,增厚的肠壁与周围肿大的淋巴结融合在一起,与十二指肠癌的不同是,尽管肿块大,肠管移位、变形明显,但梗阻及肠管扩张并不显著,原发性十二指肠癌表现为肿块与肠管壁的不均匀增厚,当肿块增大时常伴有胃扩张及肠梗阻。

胰头癌:胰头癌侵入十二指肠表现为肿块时,要与原发性十二指肠癌胰头受侵相鉴别,胰头癌常表现为肿块与十二指肠分界不清,十二指肠壁凹凸不平,多有胰体尾部萎缩,增强扫描肿块不强化。原发性十二指肠癌则表现为肿块影及十二指肠管壁不规则增厚,肿块在增强时有强化,胰头与十二指肠间脂肪间隙消失。

胆胰管连接区周围癌:胆胰管连接区癌部分肿块突入十二指肠内要与原发性十二指肠癌相鉴别,胆胰管连接区周围癌的影像表现主要包括胆胰管连接区原发肿瘤和继发于低位胆管梗阻的近端胆管的广泛扩张及胰管的扩张,发生率分别可达75%和67%。MSCT表现:薄层扫描可见肝内外胆管扩张,胆囊扩大且薄壁提示为病理性胆囊扩张胆总管下端的狭窄,截然中断及胆管壁的增厚;增强扫描,可见肿瘤强化,并可见十二指肠壁的偏心性狭窄。十二指肠降部癌表现为:十二指肠管壁增厚、狭窄及管腔内肿块影。少数情况下,MSCT诊断和鉴别诊断困难时还需进行磁共振胆胰管造影检查(MRCP)。

原发于胃、右半结肠转移到十二指肠的转移瘤:胃与右侧结肠的原发性癌在癌组织未穿透肠壁肌层时,较少发生淋巴道转移。一旦穿透肌层,则转移率明显增加,一般转移至癌所在的局部淋巴结,再沿淋巴引流方向到达十二指肠区域淋巴结,从而转移到十二指肠。

继发性十二指肠肿瘤侵犯肠腔,首先是偏于肠腔的一侧而不是包绕肠管,并伴有压迫移位。MSCT除直接显示癌肿所在的原发肠管外还表现为所在的区域淋巴结肿大,发生于胃和右侧结肠的转移癌常伴有癌肿的坏死,表现为肿块内低密度灶,增强扫描后低密度灶不强化,而原发性十二指肠癌肿块内坏死少见。

误诊病例简介:有作者报告5例腺癌在手术中均见肿块,而CT仅1例见明显肿块,其余4例表现为偏侧性或环行肠壁增厚,分析其原因可能为普通CT是横断扫描,而手术为立体的,如果结合三维重建则有助于明确其大体轮廓。十二指肠周围脂肪间隙的显示情况是判断肿瘤有无向周围结构侵犯的重要标志。该组CT均明确显示了肿瘤向周围的侵犯情况、淋巴结肿大及肝脏转移灶,与手术和病理一致。但1例CT发现小肠系膜2枚肿大淋巴结者手术见质地较软、边界清晰,术后病理未见癌转移,可能为反应性增生。CT对发现淋巴结肿大较敏感,但难以判断是否为转移性肿大。以往认为CT对溃疡不易诊断,但仔细分析仍能找到溃疡的征象,表现为底部高低不平或光整的凹陷。

第四节　十二指肠平滑肌肉瘤

十二指肠平滑肌肉瘤少见，占所有十二指肠恶性肿瘤的 10%~33%，其中一半病例肿瘤位于降段，而球部仅占 6%。十二指肠平滑肌肉瘤病理上可分四型：腔内型、腔外型、腔内外型、壁间型。

临床表现：十二指肠平滑肌肉瘤好发年龄为 40~60 岁，性别无明显差异。临床症状有腹痛、便血、贫血、体重减轻、腹部扪及包块。肿瘤较小或腔外型多无症状。

影像学研究：上胃肠道 X 线钡剂造影显示肿瘤的肠腔内部分呈圆形，卵圆形或分叶状充盈缺损，表面黏膜多较光滑，提示黏膜上病变，合并溃疡者可见脐凹征。

超声检查：可显示肿块回声不均匀，内部低回声区为组织液化坏死区。

纤维镜检：可见肿瘤的肠腔内部分表面黏膜光滑，有时可见溃疡。因取材深浅不同，病理学上常表现为炎症或正常。深取材可望能明确诊断。

CT 表现：为不规则分叶状肿块，边界清或不清，密度不均，其内低密度区如水样密度，被认为是组织坏死所致，极少发生钙化，增强扫描通常表现为边缘强化，中心无强化，似囊性病变。CT 图像可清楚显示肿瘤与周围组织器官的关系。

第五节　十二指肠弥漫性大 B 细胞淋巴瘤

患者，女性，33 岁。因反复腹胀 1 个月余入院。胃镜检查示十二指肠球部巨大溃疡。

手术所见：十二指肠球部和肝门部可触及一大小约 7cm × 6cm × 6cm 肿块，质地硬，肿物跟肝门部分界不清，大网膜可触及多枚肿大淋巴结，肝总动脉旁可触及肿大淋巴结，胃小弯侧未触及肿大淋巴结。

免疫组化诊断：胰十二指肠切除标本：十二指肠弥漫性大 B 细胞淋巴瘤，大小 7 cm × 6 cm × 5.2 cm，侵犯浆膜外脂肪组织、胰腺、胆管及神经；肿瘤耐药及预后免疫组化检测结果供临床参考。送检淋巴结有些结节为肿瘤结节，瘤细胞形态类似十二指肠肿瘤，经免疫组化证实为弥漫性大 B 细胞淋巴瘤（图 24-1-2）。

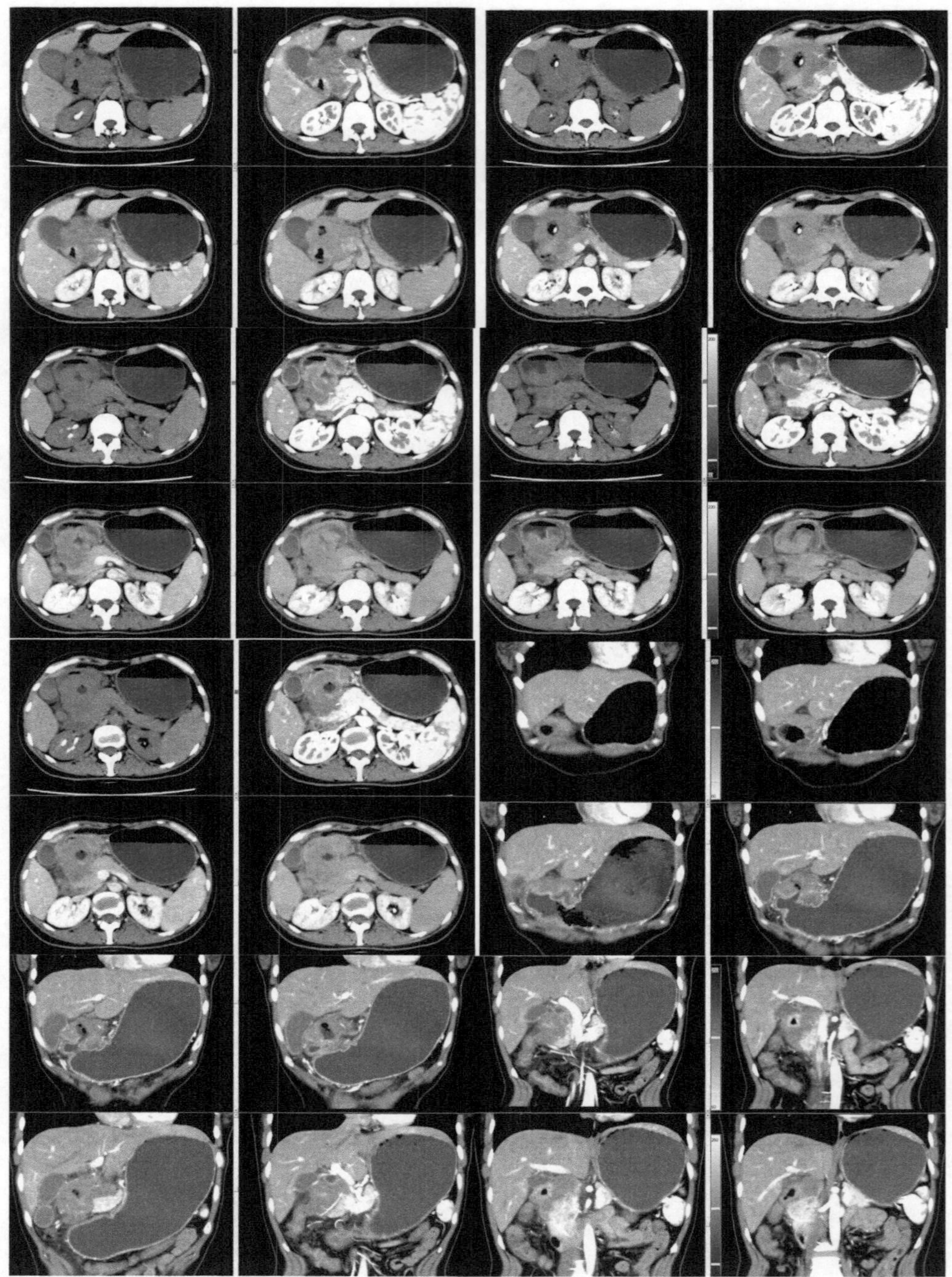

图 24-1-2 十二指肠弥漫性大 B 细胞淋巴瘤

第二章　十二指肠间质瘤

第一节　十二指肠间质瘤 MSCT

CT 显示十二指肠病变的优势与术前准备

目前诊断十二指肠肿瘤的检查方法包括上消化道钡餐和内镜检查，它们主要显示黏膜病变对腔内及腔内外生长的肿瘤检出率高，但对腔外生长的肿瘤难以发现。

与上述传统方法比较，MSCT 具有多通道的快速采集、静脉注射单次扫描覆盖范围大、微体素成像、亚毫米层厚、更高的空间分辨率及强大的图像后处理功能等优点，可清晰显示十二指肠形态，肠壁及腔内外改变，可清楚准确显示肿瘤的具体部位、形态、大小及向腔内外侵犯的范围。

扫描前的准备，有作者采用术前饮水 500ml 及术前 20 min 山莨菪碱 20 mg 肌肉注射。低张药有利减少肠道蠕动而产生的伪影，有文献提倡饮用 1%~3% 阳性对比剂，有作者认为口服高密度对比剂易与 CTA、多平面重建后处理图像的兴趣结构重叠遮盖且增强扫描时强化的肠管与肠腔内阳性对比剂呈等密度均不利于肠壁结构显示，而水作对比剂与强化的病灶有良好的对比，也易于观察肠壁结构、肠壁血运。

常规对比剂剂量多为 80~120 ml，流率为 3~5 ml/s，有作者的经验是对比剂剂量 80 ml，流率 3 ml/s，足以得到高质量图像。注射对比剂后 30 s、60 s 扫描可获取动脉期和静脉期图像，动脉期 MSCTA 可显示富血供的肿瘤及其具体供血动脉，门静脉期则利于显示肿瘤的强化特点及肿瘤与病灶、邻近组织的关系。

MSCT 三维重建技术可同时获得横轴位、冠状面、矢状面影像，能清楚地显示肿瘤与周围结构的关系和有无局部及远处转移等，为临床治疗提供帮助。薄层重建图像虽然信噪比较原始图像低，但薄层重建图像显示微小病变及病变与十二指肠的关系较 10 mm 层厚图像好。

该组有 2 例原始 10 mm 层厚增强图像未显示病变具体部位，而 1.25 mm 薄层重建图像清晰显示病变与十二指肠肠壁的关系，多平面重建多方位图像显示病变与肠道关系较原始轴位像好。有时病变和供血动脉很难在同一 CTA 图像上显示，该作者初步经验是多视角旋转及适当增强多平面重建层厚可显示病变与供血血管。多平面重建应选择以病灶原始图像层面为中心，选择最佳层厚和成像角度。

十二指肠间质瘤的特点及 CT 征象与良、恶性的鉴别：该组病例资料表明，十二指肠间质瘤好发于中老年，年龄为 35~70 岁，男性多见，男女比例为 9∶5。好发于第二段（7/14）且多为腔内型（5/7），球部没发现，第三、四段多为腔外型（5/7）。恶性间质瘤多见（8/14），且倾向于腔外生长，与文献报道相符。根据免疫组化超微结构将间质瘤概括分为平滑肌分化、神经分化、平滑肌和神经双向分化以及未分化 4 型。

CT 表现平扫为等密度或低密度肿块，良性间质瘤直径多≤ 5 cm，多向腔内生长且局限于一侧肠壁，圆形或类圆形、边界清楚，密度均匀，呈轻度均匀性强化，邻近肠壁无增厚，相邻组织未受侵犯，多单支动脉供血。恶性间质瘤形状不规则有分叶征，多向腔外生长，局限于一侧肠壁，直径多 >5 cm，等或低密度、密度不均匀，部分可见囊变坏死及气体影，增强后明显不均匀强化，邻近肠壁不均匀增厚，多侵犯周围组织或远处转移，由多支动脉供血。

良、恶性间质瘤的鉴别不难，有作者认为潜在恶性是病理学分类，影像学并无特征性表现，CT 难以鉴别。

有作者回顾分析误诊的病例发现潜在恶性间质瘤多直径≤ 5 cm,平扫密度均匀,与肠壁等密度,但肿瘤多向腔外生长,邻近肠壁不均匀增厚及强化,肿瘤明显不均匀强化且能重建出单支供血动脉,多不侵犯周围组织及不易坏死囊变,可与恶性鉴别。

鉴别诊断:(1)十二指肠腺癌以乳头周围多见,常表现为局部肠壁增厚及肠腔环形狭窄而产生胃肠道梗阻症状,也可表现为局部肿块,肿块内常坏死、囊变形成溃疡。增强后轻至中度强化,腺癌早期可发生局部或肠系膜淋巴结转移。十二指肠降部多为良性间质瘤,肿瘤多向腔内生长且局限于一侧肠壁,局部黏膜破坏中断,与邻近正常肠壁分界清,轻度均匀强化,不引起消化道梗阻症状,两者容易鉴别。

(2)胰头癌侵犯十二指肠与十二指肠较大的外生间质瘤较难鉴别,但前者多有胆管梗阻及消化道梗阻症状, MSCTA、多平面重建及最大密度投影重建肿瘤供血血管帮助定位以致鉴别,十二指肠外生间质瘤多由胃十二指肠动脉供血, MSCTA、最大密度投影重建可见此血管受压向中线移位且多位于肿瘤的内侧,而胰头癌多见胃十二指肠动脉受压位于肿瘤外侧。

误诊病例简介:该组作者曾将1例十二指肠壁内异位胰腺误诊为间质瘤,回顾性分析发现病变密度、强化方式及程度与胰腺一致;另有1例十二指肠壁内血肿呈等密度,有轻度不均匀强化现象。因此在诊断十二指肠间质瘤时要考虑到以上两种少见病,以免误诊。

第二节　十二指肠球部胃肠道间质瘤

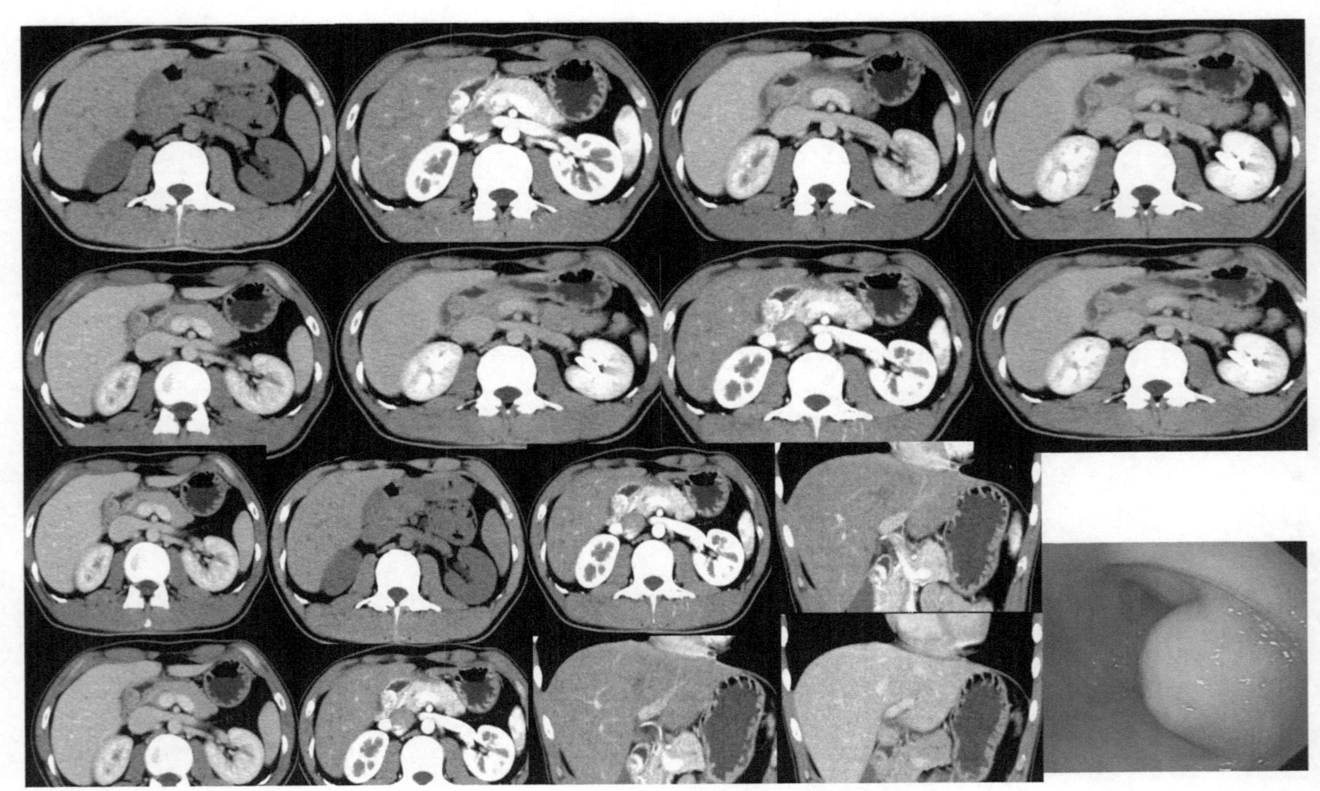

图 24-2-1　十二指肠球部胃肠道间质瘤

患者,男, 29 岁。胃镜检查示:十二指肠球部黏膜下隆起;胆汁反流性胃炎;HP(-)。

手术所见:肿物位于十二指肠前外侧壁,球部近降部水平,约 2cm × 2cm × 2cm,质中,边界清楚,活动度良好,与周围组织无粘连,未突破浆膜层。病理检查:免疫组化检测:阳性:CD117,CD34,DOG1,Nestin,Ki-67(+,约 2%);阴性:Actin, Desmin, Calponin, S-100。免疫组化诊断:十二指肠及远端部分胃切除标本:胃肠道间质瘤(GIST,极低危险度),瘤细胞较丰富，并建议做 c-kit 基因检测以应用于肿瘤靶向治疗药物的选择（图 24-2-1）。

第三节　十二指肠胃肠道间质瘤

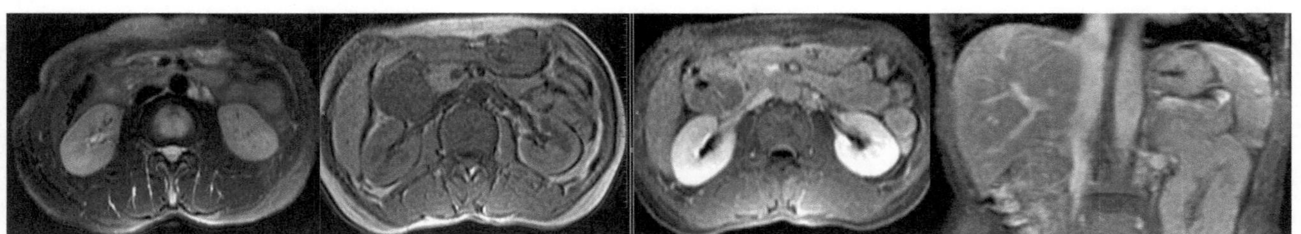

图 24-2-2　十二指肠胃肠道间质瘤

患者，女性，52 岁。间断右腹部疼痛不适 10 年。病理检查：十二指肠肿物切除标本：灰褐色不规则结节一枚，体积 4.5cm × 4cm × 3.5cm，带少许肠壁组织，切面灰白伴有出血，质偏软。常规病理诊断：十二指肠肿物切除标本见十二指肠肠壁梭形细胞肿瘤，体积 4.5cm × 4cm × 3.5cm，伴小灶性出血坏死。待免疫组化进一步确诊。

免疫组化检测：阳性：CD117（+++），DOG1（+++），Nestin（+++），Vim（++），SMA（灶性 +），Ki-67（约 10%）；阴性：S-100。免疫组化诊断：十二指肠肿物切除标本示十二指肠壁胃肠道间质瘤（GIST）。注：根据肿瘤大小（最大径 4.5cm）和核分裂（<5/50HPF）等形态学表现，可归纳为“可能良性（低度危险）”组，建议临床随访（图 24-2-2）。

第三章　十二指肠肿块

第一节　非乳头区十二指肠肿瘤

十二指肠毗邻结构较多且复杂,病变较大时常侵犯周围脏器而给临床治疗带来困难,故早期发现至关重要。十二指肠乳头区肿瘤由于较早引起胆管梗阻症状易于发现;而非乳头区十二指肠肿瘤(即不包括胆胰共同管、胆总管下端以及胰头部的肿瘤)发病率很低,且早期无特异性临床表现,诊断困难,易延误治疗。十二指肠肿瘤临床少见,占整个消化道恶性肿瘤的0.35%,占小肠恶性肿瘤的33%~45%。发生于十二指肠乳头部以外的肿瘤,即不包括胆胰共同管、胆总管下端以及胰头部的肿瘤,则更是少见,且其早期临床表现隐匿而难以诊断,容易造成误诊。

有作者报告11例患者中就有4例合并转移,且有1例因合并十二指肠球部溃疡而长期按消化性溃疡诊治,忽视了降部范围较广的腺癌,以致确诊时已为晚期。

十二指肠降部的肿瘤多呈息肉型,较大者阻塞十二指肠肠腔后,临床多表现为消化道出血(呕血、黑便、贫血)和肠梗阻(恶心、呕吐、腹部胀痛)的症状;降部和水平部移行区及水平部的肿瘤大部分呈缩窄型,临床以肠梗阻为主要表现。故出现上述症状者应想到十二指肠病变的可能。该组降部6例中有5例为息肉型,降部和水平部移行区3例中1例肿块型,2例缩窄型,水平部肿瘤亦为缩窄型。十二指肠肿瘤最常见的为腺癌,占77%,其次为胃肠间质瘤和淋巴瘤,另外还有类癌、未分化癌、鳞癌等。该组因病例数有限,仅见腺癌、恶性胃肠间质瘤和非霍奇金淋巴瘤,另外还见1例腺瘤性息肉和1例十二指肠肠壁血肿。

十二指肠肿瘤或肿瘤样病变的病理及临床:十二指肠降部的肿瘤多呈息肉型,较大者阻塞十二指肠肠腔后,临床多表现为消化道出血(呕血、黑便、贫血)和肠梗阻(恶心、呕吐、腹部胀痛)的症状;降部和水平部移行区及水平部的肿瘤大部分呈缩窄型,临床以肠梗阻为主要表现。故出现上述症状者应想到十二指肠病变的可能。十二指肠肿瘤最常见的为腺癌,占77%,其次为胃肠间质瘤和淋巴瘤,另外还有类癌、未分化癌、鳞癌等。

CT诊断与手术病理的对比及原因分析:该研究发现5例腺癌在手术中均见肿块,而CT仅1例见明显肿块,其余4例表现为偏侧性或环行肠壁增厚,分析其原因可能为常规CT是横断扫描,而手术为立体的,如果结合三维重建则有助于明确其大体轮廓。

十二指肠周围脂肪间隙的显示情况是判断肿瘤有无向周围结构侵犯的重要标志。该组CT均明确显示了肿瘤向周围的侵犯情况、淋巴结肿大及肝脏转移灶,与手术和病理一致。但1例CT发现小肠系膜2枚肿大淋巴结者手术见质地较软、边界清晰,术后病理未见癌转移,可能为反应性增生。CT对发现淋巴结肿大较敏感,但难以判断是否为转移性肿大。以往认为CT对溃疡不易诊断,但仔细分析仍能找到溃疡的征象,表现为底部高低不平或光整的凹陷。

胃肠间质瘤:胃肠间质瘤是一类独立的来源于胃肠道壁间叶组织的非定向分化肿瘤,以往常称之为平滑肌瘤及肉瘤,近年发现其有多种免疫表型和分化,因而得名。恶性胃肠间质瘤常为腔外生长,基本不引起肠腔梗阻,肿块体积较大而边界清晰,中央常见液化坏死,周边为均匀明显强化的软组织密度。该组3例胃肠间质瘤均为腔外生长,2例中央见液化坏死,坏死边缘凹凸不平,术前CT已诊为胃肠间质瘤,术后病理亦得到证实。另1例密度均匀,与十二指肠癌不易鉴别，术后经免疫组织化学确诊，CD117(+)、CD34(-)、SMA(+)、Desmin(-)、S-100(-)、Ki-67 阳性率 <5%。

淋巴瘤：十二指肠淋巴瘤多为非霍奇金淋巴瘤，表现为肠壁增厚及周围淋巴结肿大、肠管受推挤，有时与十二指肠癌并淋巴结转移不易区分。该例最初即诊断为十二指肠癌并淋巴结转移，可能与肿瘤侵及肠管较明显且较深（深肌层深部）而其他部位淋巴结肿大不十分明显有关。但十二指肠淋巴瘤肠壁常呈环行增厚，与肿大的淋巴结常融合成较大的团块，而肠腔仍通畅，肠梗阻及近段肠管扩张不明显。

腺瘤性息肉：十二指肠腺瘤性息肉是源于黏膜上皮的少见的良性肿瘤，症状、体征和影像学检查均无特异性，该例术前诊断为十二指肠癌，术后病理确诊为腺瘤性息肉。如能见到明显的蒂则有助于诊断。该例肝内外胆管和胰管扩张是由于胆囊切除术后胆管代偿和胆总管结石引起梗阻所致。

肠壁血肿：十二指肠肠壁血肿非常少见，仅见个案报道，并且常有外伤史。该组 1 例为 8 岁男性患儿，无明显外伤史但凝血功能较差，腹痛伴呕吐 5 天，左侧脐上扪及包块，临床最初疑为肠套叠，仔细分析 CT 表现诊断应该不难，表现为肠腔内高、低混杂密度囊样病灶，边界清晰，无强化。

第二节　关于十二指肠肿瘤 CT 检查注意事项

尽管肿瘤仅累及十二指肠某一段，但由于远处转移特别是肝脏转移发生率高，因此扫描范围宜从肝脏膈面开始，连续扫描至脐平面。观察肿瘤及肠壁的适宜窗宽为 300~800HU，窗位 50~100HU。十二指肠肿瘤 CT 诊断必须使肠腔内对比剂充盈良好，观察未充盈或充盈不佳肠袢的肠壁细微病变十分困难，甚至形成“假肿瘤”征象混淆诊断。

肠腔充盈良好的标准是内径大于 2cm。目前多采用口服对比剂充盈肠腔，有高密度对比剂、水、脂性对比剂及空气等，以高密度对比剂应用最为广泛。高密度对比剂主要包括 1.5%~2% 的钡混悬液与 2%~3% 的含碘水溶液。服用前病人宜禁食 4 小时。检查前 15~30 分钟口服 400ml 对比剂充盈胃及十二指肠。

常规使用静脉注射对比剂进行增强扫描，以利更好地观察原发与转移病灶，鉴别淋巴结与血管组织。十二指肠的 CT 研究主要包括肠腔，肠壁及肠系膜三部分。充盈良好的十二指肠，肠腔内径正常为 2.0~3.5cm，肠腔内密度均匀，高密度口服对比剂与肠液混合后 CT 值一般在 150HU 左右。肠壁正常厚度在 1~3mm 之间，大于 4mm 即为异常。若肠壁局限性或环形增厚大于 15mm 则强烈提示为肿瘤所致。在测量肠壁厚度时，必需注意被测肠管应充盈良好且与扫描平面平行或垂直，否则测量值将偏大。

正常肠壁密度均一，CT 值为 50~75HU，增强后 CT 值可升至 100HU 左右。

肠系膜在 CT 图像上表现为均一的脂肪密度，CT 值为 -75 到 -125HU，其内可见条索状或点状血管分支，偶尔也可见淋巴结，但正常的血管与淋巴结直径均小于 4mm，大于 5mm 即为异常，大于 15mm 则多提示为肿瘤所致。

第三节　十二指肠上部肿瘤及肿瘤样病变

十二指肠肿瘤及肿瘤样病变较为少见，以往国内外有关十二指肠病变的报道大多为十二指肠第二、三段肿瘤，且以个案报道为多，某些正常或异常的非肿瘤性改变也可在影像上呈现似肿瘤样表现，而对十二指肠上部（球部或球后部）的各种肿瘤及肿瘤样病变研究的报道甚少。

此外，由于十二指肠位于各种重要结构的中间，这些结构的病变也可累及十二指肠，而且，胃窦及幽门部的正常或异常病变也可突入十二指肠上部。因此，正确判定病变存在与否以及病变性质，对制定适当的治疗方案极其重要。

小肠肿瘤占全部消化道肿瘤的 1.7%。一般认为约 20% 小肠肿瘤发生于十二指肠，而且多发生于十二指肠的第二、三段，真正发生于十二指肠球及球后的肿瘤非常少见，由于十二指肠局部解剖较复杂，邻近脏器又较多，而且各种十二指肠球及球后部肿瘤及肿瘤样病变在钡餐造影时均表现为腔内较小的充盈缺损,因此加强对其影像学表现的认识,以区别肿瘤的良、恶性及与肿瘤样改变,对确定适当的治疗方案非常重要。

胃肠钡餐造影:该组 15 例因各种腹部症状或常规体检而做胃肠钡餐造影时发现十二指肠上部有腔内充盈缺损而做进一步检查。最后结果证实 86.7% 病例都有各种良、恶性病变,说明 X 线钡餐造影仍是发现十二指肠及其他胃肠道疾病的最基本的首选检查方法。但也有 2 例最后确定为正常十二指肠黏膜,故钡餐检查仍有一定的假阳性(13.3%),值得注意。

钡餐造影除在发现病变上有很大价值外,在对病变的良、恶性定性上也有作用,它可以根据病变区黏膜皱襞有无破坏及胃肠道形态和动力学变化、观察肠壁是否僵硬来判断良、恶性;尤其对有定性诊断意义的"桥"形皱襞的显示优于 CT,CT 不能充分显示黏膜的细微情况,对病灶表面及周围黏膜聚集显示不如钡餐清楚。

"桥"形皱襞和充盈缺损周围黏膜聚集对良性病变的定性有诊断意义。该组中 2 例有"桥"形皱襞的布氏腺腺瘤和 1 例充盈缺损周围有黏膜聚集的炎性肿块,均在钡餐造影时确诊为良性病变;充盈缺损表面呈菜花状合并幽门管增宽等对胃黏膜脱垂或胃腺瘤十二指肠球脱垂有诊断价值;表面不光滑伴黏膜集中则有利于炎性病变的诊断;卵圆形、圆形者中良性病变较多(7/11 例, 63.64%);不规则形者可见于恶性肿瘤或炎性肿块;出现龛影对平滑肌瘤诊断有利;而肠壁增厚、肠腔狭窄、充盈缺损表面呈鹅卵石状对淋巴瘤(该组中有 2 例)有特征性诊断意义;表面光滑则无助于良、恶性的区别。另外,良性病变多位于球部(8/11 例, 72.7%),而同时累及球部及球后部者则良恶性病变各占半数。总之,该组中多半数(60%)病例可从钡餐检查时判断其良、恶性,其余少半数(40%)病例,包括 2 例为正常十二指肠皱襞的假阳性者,在钡餐造影时均未能做出良、恶性的判断。

CT:CT 是钡餐造影外的可供选择的重要的检查方法,它可以直接显示十二指肠腔内、肠壁和肠腔外病变及有无远处转移等,这都是钡餐造影所不及的。CT 检查有助于确定病灶范围或显示有无淋巴结转移,对肿瘤分期有重要意义。Kazeroon(1992)认为 CT 对检出诊断恶性十二指肠肿瘤的敏感性为 94%,特异性为 50%,准确性为 82%,如结合十二指肠腔外其他改变,则其特异性为 100%,准确性为 86%,可见 CT 诊断的敏感性高,而特异性低。向肠腔内外生长而引起的肠壁不规则增厚是 CT 诊断恶性肿瘤的指征。

该组中 8 例 CT 发现异常者最后都证实有异常(66.7%),肠壁不规则增厚者为恶性肿瘤,肠腔外有淋巴结者则应多考虑淋巴瘤,该组 4 例恶性肿瘤中 2 例显示肠壁不规则增厚合并有腔外淋巴结肿大;仅有腔内肿块而无肠壁增厚者多为良性肿瘤。仅有肠壁规则增厚者可见于恶性肿瘤或炎性肿块。病变的边缘清楚与否则无助于区别良、恶性。

对从胃突入十二指肠的肿瘤样病变,在 CT 上也常能明确病变和胃的关系,而做出正确诊断。1 例 CT 表现为正常肠黏膜,从而纠正了钡餐造影中的假充盈缺损。该组 CT 正确定性为 62.5%。但 CT 可漏检较小的肠腔内病变,该组中 2 例布氏腺腺瘤和 1 例炎性肿块因病灶较小均未能在 CT 上见到,因此 CT 的假阴性达 25%。此外, CT 在区别规则肠壁增厚及腔内肿瘤良恶性中的作用不肯定,该组中类癌和炎性肿块引起的肠壁规则性增厚以及类癌和平滑肌瘤引起的腔内肿瘤,都难以在 CT 上区分其良、恶性。可见 CT 在发现和鉴别十二指肠上部较小病变上还有一定的限度。

内镜检查:内镜检查可较早发现十二指肠肿瘤,同时内镜可直接观察病变的形态、范围和部位,并可取活检,使病变在术前得到明确诊断。但对较小的黏膜下肿块内镜并不一定都能显示,即使发现病灶,也不一定能取得满意病理结果;对因肠腔狭窄内镜不能通过者,也无能为力。该组 2 例布氏腺腺瘤,在内镜检查时,尽管参考钡餐造影所见,但仍未能发现病灶,假阴性为 13.3%;因此内镜检出也有它的限度。

该组的结果显示钡餐造影所见到的十二指肠上部的充盈缺损中的假阳性为 13.3%,因此有条件时应对他们做进一步检查,不能贸然手术。在进一步检查的方法中无创性的 CT,愈来愈受到重视,但 CT 假阴性率达 25%,而且 37.5% 病例在 CT 上不能区别病变的良、恶性,说明常规 CT 也并不是十二指肠病变理想的检查方法。综上所述,对十二指肠上部肿瘤及肿瘤样病变,钡餐造影比 CT 和胃镜检查能发现较多病变,在定性诊断上各有所长和限度。由于十二指肠上部地方狭小,形态走行变化复杂,病灶常较小,检出较困难,而影像表现又常缺少特异性,定性诊断也较困难，并有一定的假阴、阳性率。因此，对钡餐造影时发现的充盈缺损最好结合临床和CT、内镜结果进行综合分析，全面地观察腔内病变的大小范围、黏膜改变、溃疡形态、肠壁是否僵硬以及肠壁或肠外侵犯程度和淋巴转移情况，以确定正确的治疗方案，如仍不能肯定时，应及早做包括手术在内的各种有创性检查。

第四节　十二指肠血管瘤

十二指肠血管瘤极少见，其病因尚不清楚。

一般以为此病源自于中胚层的胚胎残余，血管内皮细胞增大，导致微小动脉，毛细血管和微小静脉之间产生异常交通或扩张。组织学显示厚壁或壁厚薄不匀，扩张并充满血液的动静脉血管组织。有时组织学上很难确定其为血管畸形抑或真性肿瘤。

有作者指出，十二指肠血管瘤系真性肿瘤，不同于血管结构不良。术前诊断较为困难。

一些作者报告一例十二指肠血管瘤，钡餐造影仅见黏膜增粗，三次内镜检查仅发现十二指肠降段黏膜增厚及出血点，不能明确诊断。选择性腹腔动脉造影及肠系膜上动脉造影显示，十二指肠降段有直径6mm的异常血管团，由胰十二指肠上下动脉供血，并可见早期静脉引流及引流静脉增粗。切除标本病理表现为黏膜下血管增多，壁厚薄不均。术后9个月再次复发，在原吻合口上方找到5mm×6mm大小呈紫色血管瘤，病理证实为黏膜下层血管瘤表面破损。

有作者指出，消化道血管瘤诊断困难，疑及上胃肠道或直肠血管瘤时应首选内镜检查，疑及小肠及十二指肠血管瘤者，应首选血管造影。血管造影对出血诊断的敏感率为58%~86%，动物实验发现，出血速率在>0.5ml/min时，可显示对比剂外溢，并可同时显示异常血管。

在活动性出血时施行血管造影可提高阳性率。Thompson等（1984）报告出血后6小时以上再做血管造影可导致28%的病例难以找到出血部位。

也有作者报道，小肠镜为诊断小肠出血的有效方法。钡剂检查对于未突入腔内的黏膜或黏膜下血管瘤无能为力，对于病变范围较大的血管瘤虽可发现，却很难定性，钡餐检查的意义，在于除外其他常见原因所致的消化道出血。

第五节　十二指肠的假性息肉

Nelson等（1975）报告7例十二指肠的假性息肉，追踪随访6个月到15年，均未发现十二指肠异常。这些假息肉位于十二指肠上曲凹陷部，一直持续存在，可能是十二指肠上曲内侧面冗长疏松黏膜的堆积所致。

第六节　十二指肠袢伪似脓肿

在超声检查时，十二指肠袢能位于胆囊与右肾之间而伪似一脓肿，纵切扫描表现为肝下间隙内有混淆的液体积聚，考虑脓肿，实时观察却可见该影可移动，后来证实为十二指肠袢。

第七节　邻近的肠袢

在CT平扫时，邻近的肠袢，如十二指肠，也可造成误诊，它可伪似动脉瘤或腹腔动脉瘤的破裂。充盈不佳或未充盈的肠袢，邻近动脉时可表现为软组织肿块，酷似血栓或邻近的血肿。

第四章　十二指肠乳头

第一节　十二指肠乳头癌

十二指肠乳头癌指来源于十二指肠乳头部黏膜、共同管内黏膜、主胰管和总胆管共同开口处的壁间黏膜上皮的癌瘤,不包括总胆管末端癌或胰头癌等向乳头部的扩散。占全部十二指肠癌的 1/2~3/4,多见于老年患者,无性别差异。组织细胞学以腺癌和乳头状腺癌为主,黏液腺癌占极少数。十二指肠乳头癌手术切除率高于胆总管癌和胰头癌,因此有必要予以鉴别,力争术前准确诊断。

1. 影像学研究　十二指肠乳头癌的 CT 表现为胰腺钩突底部层面,十二指肠降段内侧肠壁向腔内突出软组织肿块充盈缺损影,呈圆形、分叶状和菜花状,以圆形多见。密度多均匀,无钙化及囊变,边缘多清楚。肿块与十二指肠肠腔断面呈"双环征",且内环相切。增强扫描,动脉期病灶多呈轻至中度均匀强化,静脉期、延迟期强化仍较明显。

肝内外胆管呈普遍性一致性扩张,呈蔓状或软藤状,胆总管和胰管明显扩张并于共同管区突然截断,断面平直,该组病例均伴有胆囊增大。正常肝外胆管管径为 3~11mm,平均为 5~6 mm,左、右肝内胆管管径为 2~9mm,平均为 3~4mm。肝内胆管管径达 5 mm 为轻度扩张,6~8 mm 为中度扩张,9 mm 以上为重度扩张。

形态学上分为枯树枝状(CT 像上肝内可见胆管显示,如树枝状由粗到细,管壁规则,与门静脉分支伴行且宽度相当)、蔓状(肝内胆管迂曲增粗,分支增多,超出邻近门静脉的管径及支数但未见囊袋状影)、软藤状(肝内胆管明显迂曲扩张,达肝包膜下,并见多数囊袋状影)。

一些作者报道肝内、外胆管一致性扩张呈软藤样改变提示肿瘤可能性大。还有作者认为肝外胆系(肝外胆管和胆囊)同步一致性重度扩张为肿瘤性胆管扩张,他们认为胆管下端肿瘤梗阻后,胆汁排泄障碍,致肝内外胆管和胆囊内压力均增高,肝内胆管因周围有肝组织的支撑且离梗阻端较远,而肝外胆管及胆囊仅有少量支撑组织且离梗阻端较近,故肝外胆管和胆囊首先发生重度扩张,而肝内胆管重度扩张发生较晚且较轻。

胰管扩张,呈管状或串珠状,与扩张的胆总管构成"双管征",是判断梗阻位于共同管以下的可靠依据。该组中有 1 例胰管不扩张。多数主胰管与胆总管汇合进入共同管,而开口于十二指肠乳头,故乳头部肿瘤多数易堵塞主胰管使之扩张。主胰管也可不与胆总管汇合而单独开口于十二指肠,当此部发生肿瘤时就不会阻塞胰管引发扩张,只有当肿瘤足够大而压迫堵塞主胰管的另一开口时,才会导致胰管扩张。

十二指肠肠腔受压变形、变窄,肿瘤上部肠腔多不梗阻扩张,十二指肠乳头癌是围绕十二指肠乳头生长的肿瘤,此处又是胆胰管连接区的出口,早期极易引起胆系梗阻症状,容易早期发现,并且肠管前、后、外侧壁未被侵犯,扩张良好,不易引发肠梗阻。

2. 鉴别诊断　胆总管远端癌:在胆总管远端管腔内见圆形软组织结节或胆总管增厚,增强扫描肿瘤呈均匀或不均匀明显强化和管壁不规则的环形强化,胆总管在胰头平面呈"截断"改变,肝内外胆管多成比例显著扩张,胆囊增大,多无胰管扩张,这是与十二指肠乳头癌鉴别的重要征象。

胰头癌:平扫示胰头钩突增大、变形,密度不均匀,可有钙化灶及囊变,增强扫描病灶强化不明显,而胰腺正常实质可明显均匀强化,在此衬托下瘤体显示清楚,边缘不规整,易侵犯胰周组织及血管,早期即出现胰管扩张明显,当病灶进展侵犯胆总管胰内段时，亦可引起胆系明显扩张，多平面重建显示梗阻处胆总管呈偏心性不规则狭窄，这与十二指肠乳头癌多平面重建显示胆总管突然中断、梗阻处胆总管断面变直明显不同。

胆胰管十二指肠连接区癌：即壶腹癌。胰头前方隆起，胆管下端软组织肿块，常呈膨胀性向腔内外生长，并向十二指肠肠腔内突出，增强扫描后肿块强化，常伴有出血或坏死并易侵犯胰头和周围淋巴结。肝内外胆管呈普遍性一致性扩张，伴胆囊增大和胰管扩张。鉴别要点是其发生位置较十二指肠乳头癌稍高，往往在肿瘤发生部位的层面可见胰腺钩突，肿瘤在管腔内生长增大到一定程度时，向上可达到胰腺钩突水平，向下可突入肠腔，而十二指肠乳头癌主要表现为突入肠腔内的软组织肿块，二者在CT影像上鉴别较困难。

十二指肠乳头区息肉：息肉密度均匀，边界光滑锐利，增强扫描病灶强化不明显。

十二指肠乳头水肿：乳头水肿表现为十二指肠内的充盈缺损，边缘光滑，无进行性黄疸，治疗后复查可明显好转或消失。

十二指肠乳头区软组织密度结石：软组织密度结石可见“新月征”和“靶征”，增强扫描病灶不强化，胆总管壁均匀环形增厚，肝内胆管多轻度扩张，与肝外胆管扩张不成比例。

第二节　十二指肠乳头异位与胆胰管合流异常的相关性分析

详见本书 本卷 第十九篇 第十章 第六节　十二指肠乳头异位与胆胰管异常连接。

第五章 关于十二指肠溃疡

第一节 胃癌与十二指肠溃疡同存

详见本书本卷第二十三篇第七章第三节 胃癌与十二指肠溃疡同存。

第二节 十二指肠慢性溃疡合并梗阻性黄疸

十二指肠溃疡是一种常见病，90%以上发生在十二指肠球部,前壁较常见,活动性溃疡周围黏膜常有炎性水肿。溃疡浅者仅累及黏膜肌层,深者达肌层甚至浆膜层,穿破浆膜层引起穿孔,溃疡愈合时周围黏膜炎症、水肿消失,边缘上皮细胞增生覆盖溃疡面,其下的肉芽组织纤维化,变为瘢痕,瘢痕收缩使周围的黏膜皱襞向其中纠集。由于十二指肠管壁较薄,水肿及瘢痕组织形成容易导致肠管管腔狭窄。梗阻性十二指肠溃疡患者通常都有长期的十二指肠溃疡病史。溃疡患者中只有约5%~10%合并胃出口的梗阻,其中80%是由于十二指肠溃疡引起。

梗阻性黄疸也常见,引起梗阻性黄疸的原因很多,以胆管病变较多。十二指肠溃疡致梗阻性黄疸却很少见,原因是十二指肠溃疡的好发部位与乳头距离较远,因此十二指肠溃疡成为梗阻性黄疸的病因少有报道。结合一组手术与内镜证实的8例所见,由十二指肠溃疡引起梗阻性黄疸的病理基础是十二指肠慢性溃疡引起的较大范围的瘢痕、肉芽组织增生及炎性水肿并累及乳头部所致。由于十二指肠大部分位于腹腔上部深处,紧贴腹后壁,除其始、末两端被腹膜包裹,成为腹膜内位器官,较为活动之外,其余大部分被腹膜覆盖而固定于腹后壁,是小肠最为固定的部分,其活动度有限,为需较长扫描时间的MRI扫描提供了解剖基础。

SSFSE序列其优点是对磁化率效应不敏感,扫描速度快,屏气时间短,明显减少了运动伪影(包括呼吸、肠蠕动、心血管搏动等产生的伪影),特别适用于不合作患者及屏气困难者。MRI对位置较固定的肠管显示效果较好,并且在肠管充盈良好的状态下显示小肠黏膜皱襞。一些作者在低张下行MRCP,在十二指肠乳头部病变的诊断中取得较好的效果。

该组资料表明,在不需低张的情况下,冠状位T_2WI序列及MRCP可清晰显示十二指肠降部高信号的羽毛状黏膜皱襞结构,可同时显示十二指肠病变、扩张的胆管以及两者之间的关系,因此对十二指肠溃疡导致的梗阻性黄疸有较高的诊断价值。

十二指肠溃疡引起的梗阻性黄疸主要需与十二指肠腺癌鉴别,十二指肠癌好发于乳头部,病变多较局限,呈结节状,较大的十二指肠癌常形成软组织肿块影或较大的充盈缺损,病变少有累及十二指肠球部或球后部,黏膜皱襞消失多为局限性。

十二指肠溃疡所致的梗阻性黄疸具特征性的MRI与MRCP表现,对患者的治疗具有较大的参考价值,部分患者保守治疗效果好,该组有4例经保守治疗黄疸与右上腹痛消失后出院,其中1例1年后再次发作,经保守治疗好转至今。3例因合并幽门梗阻手术治疗,另1例因合并肠穿孔手术治疗。

第六章　十二指肠乳头区憩室

第一节　十二指肠乳头旁憩室

十二指肠是消化道憩室常见部位之一，十二指肠憩室患者常常没有临床症状。但部分十二指肠憩室，尤其是乳头旁憩室除可并发憩室炎外，还易合并胆胰疾病，从而产生一系列消化道症状，临床称之为乳头旁憩室综合征或 Lemmel 综合征。乳头旁憩室是指发生于十二指肠乳头周围 2~3 cm 范围内的憩室，又称胆管口连接区周围憩室。是临床常见的消化系统疾病，由于其特殊的解剖位置，除并发憩室炎以外，还常常合并胆系及胰腺疾病。

乳头旁憩室的检查手段：20 世纪 70 年代以来，随着内镜及逆行胆胰管造影（ERCP）在临床的广泛应用，乳头旁憩室报告日渐增多。由于乳头旁憩室常与胆胰疾病合并存在，其临床表现相似，所以，临床常注意诊断胆胰疾病，而忽视可能造成这些疾病的乳头旁憩室的诊断。

影像学检查在诊断乳头旁憩室方面具有特殊地位。既往主要依赖胆系造影检查和钡餐检查，目前常用的检查方法包括钡餐检查、CT、MRI、MR 胆胰管成像（MRCP）以及 ERCP。但是，消化道造影（钡餐检查）只能局限于胃肠形态及功能改变，不能诊断肝、胆、胰疾病，有其局限性；而 ERCP 是有创性检查，设备要求相对较高，也不适于广泛开展。同时，相当一部分病例系因出现 Lemmel 综合征的表现，临床疑为胆胰病变及肝脏病变而首先做 CT 检查，为偶然发现。因此，提高 CT 诊断乳头旁憩室水平具有重要实际意义。

而且，随着 MSCT 的相关研究不断深入，薄层 CT 影像及多平面重建技术的广泛应用，乳头旁憩室的检出率可以大大提高。在一组 67 例中，MSCT 影像可以清楚地显示乳头旁憩室的位置、大小、形态及密度，以及并发的胆胰病变。经 CT 检查发现乳头旁憩室并发乳头旁憩室综合征高达 70.15%。

乳头旁憩室的 CT 诊断与分型：乳头旁憩室在 CT 上典型表现为突出于十二指肠壁外的囊袋状影，呈圆形、椭圆形或分叶状，憩室的密度依据囊内容的不同、检查前有无口服水剂或阳性对比剂以及有无气体进入而呈不同表现。最常见为胰腺头部右后方半圆形含气体腔影，可见液平面，若口服高密度对比剂后表现为高密度对比剂进入憩室内。该组憩室最多的表现是含气液平面囊袋状影（32/67），与部分学者的报道不完全一致，可能与该组患者检查前严格禁食及口服大量水剂有关。十二指肠憩室炎增强扫描表现为憩室壁轻中度强化。根据憩室与十二指肠乳头或胆管口乳头的关系可以进行分型。

一些作者根据乳头旁憩室开口位置以及与十二指肠乳头的关系将其分型为三：十二指肠乳头开口于乳头旁憩室为中央型；乳头旁憩室开口于十二指肠降段乳头一侧为乳头周围型；乳头旁憩室开口于十二指肠升段近侧上壁为升段毗邻型。有作者根据 MSCT 检查，将其分为四型：乳头上型、乳头缘型、乳头水平外侧缘和乳头下型。这两种分型都是在结合 ERCP 的基础上建立的，不适于完全依赖 CT 横断面影像进行分型。该项研究采用的新型分型方法，根据横断面上憩室与十二指肠乳头的关系将其分为四型，这种分型方法简便、实用，结合多平面重建影像，诊断更加明确。

63 例共 67 个憩室：Ⅰ型 32 个，憩室位于括约肌复合体腹侧，或多或少伸向胰腺；Ⅱ型 17 个，憩室位于括约肌复合体背侧；Ⅲ型 14 个，憩室呈二叶型，伸至复合体腹背两侧；Ⅳ型 4 个，小的憩室位于小乳头腹侧。

憩室与乳头旁憩室综合征的关系：十二指肠憩

室最多见于降部内侧乳头周围,约占60%~70%。好发于降部乳头旁,可能与下述三因素有关:①该处为胚胎发生学和解剖学上的薄弱区;②胆胰管下端括约肌收缩牵拉十二指肠壁对乳头旁憩室的形成有一定作用;③肠腔内压力的增高使该薄弱区的肠壁向外疝出,久之则形成憩室。该理论也说明憩室的发生率随年龄的增长而增高,该组病例平均年龄(66.63±12.62)岁。研究提示,胆胰疾病与乳头旁憩室密切相关,尤其胆总管结石的发生与乳头旁憩室的关系更为密切,而且憩室与乳头距离越近胆结石发生率越高。一般认为乳头旁憩室与胆石症发生有关,与胰腺炎关系密切是由于胆石症的存在,即首先易发生胆总管结石,继之发生胆源性胰腺炎。

一项研究报道93例憩室,发生于十二指肠降部64例,占68.8%。螺旋CT检查组35例降部憩室发现胆囊结石9例(25.7%),胆总管结石3例(8.6%),胰腺炎2例(5.7%)。另有报道降部憩室83例,发现胆囊结石22例(26.5%),胆总管结石7例(8.4%),胰腺炎5例(6.0%)。

该组病例中乳头旁憩室并发乳头旁憩室综合征的发生率高达70.15%,高于上述文献报道。其中,Ⅰ型的发生率尤高,可达87.50%。考虑可能的原因为降部内侧为胆总管通过部位,憩室较大或腔内有潴留液,可直接压迫胆总管下端所致。憩室炎和乳头炎可造成胆汁淤滞和/或伴有细菌感染。提示对于Ⅰ型乳头旁憩室要加以注意及给予必要的处理。当然,该组病例略少,还需加大样本量,进一步总结。

综上所述,128层MSCT对乳头旁憩室的检出率高,可进行分型诊断,并且能够发现与乳头旁憩室关系密切的胆胰病变,有重要的临床意义。

第二节 误诊病例简介:十二指肠腔内憩室

十二指肠憩室绝大多数为腔外憩室,腔内憩室非常罕见,文献报道不足100例。

一般认为,十二指肠腔内憩室的发生与肠壁先天性发育异常有关,肠管局部残留的隔或蹼突向腔内形成腔内憩室,并在肠蠕动的作用下逐渐增大,形成风向袋状结构。

与腔外憩室不同,十二指肠腔内憩室的两面均被覆黏膜层,黏膜层下只有薄的纤维肌层,血供很差,易发生缺血坏死或穿孔。除少数患者憩室与肠壁的全周附着外,大多数情况下其附着点小于肠壁周径的一半,当憩室附着于肠壁全周时,食物只能通过位于憩室中央或周边的小孔进入十二指肠远段。十二指肠腔内憩室可合并其他先天性畸形,如唐氏综合征、肠旋转不良或各种疝、肛门闭锁、胆管畸形、环状胰腺和先天性心脏病等。

诊断十二指肠腔内憩室的主要方法为上消化道造影。典型表现为十二指肠腔内充满钡剂的囊袋状结构及其周围的边界光整的线样透亮线,称为风向袋征,线样透亮线代表憩室壁。并发十二指肠梗阻时,梗阻近段十二指肠及胃腔明显扩张。

CT横断面典型表现为双腔征,十二指肠局部层面见双重管腔,内含液体及肠内容物,有时还能见到内层管壁不连续、局限性断裂,代表憩室的裂孔,同时通过各断面的重建CT图像,可以清楚地看到风向袋征。憩室局部增厚时表现为十二指肠腔内肿块。

鉴别诊断:虽然风向袋征是十二指肠腔内憩室的特异性表现,但有时需与十二指肠息肉、十二指肠肿瘤、胆总管囊肿、肠套叠等鉴别,这时内窥镜检查对鉴别诊断有帮助,在十二指肠内壁上可见盲袋状结构。

CT表现为双腔征时,主要应与肠套叠鉴别。前者2层管壁间间隙较宽,间隙内只能观察到液体密度影即肠液,而后者2层管壁间间隙窄,间隙内能观察到被套入的肠壁外的脂肪密度影。对十二指肠腔内憩室的认识不足是该例术前未能正确诊断的主要原因,因此掌握该病的典型症状及影像表现,提高认识是正确诊断的有效手段。

第三节 诊断陷阱:十二指肠乳头旁憩室与胆胰管下端恶性占位性病变

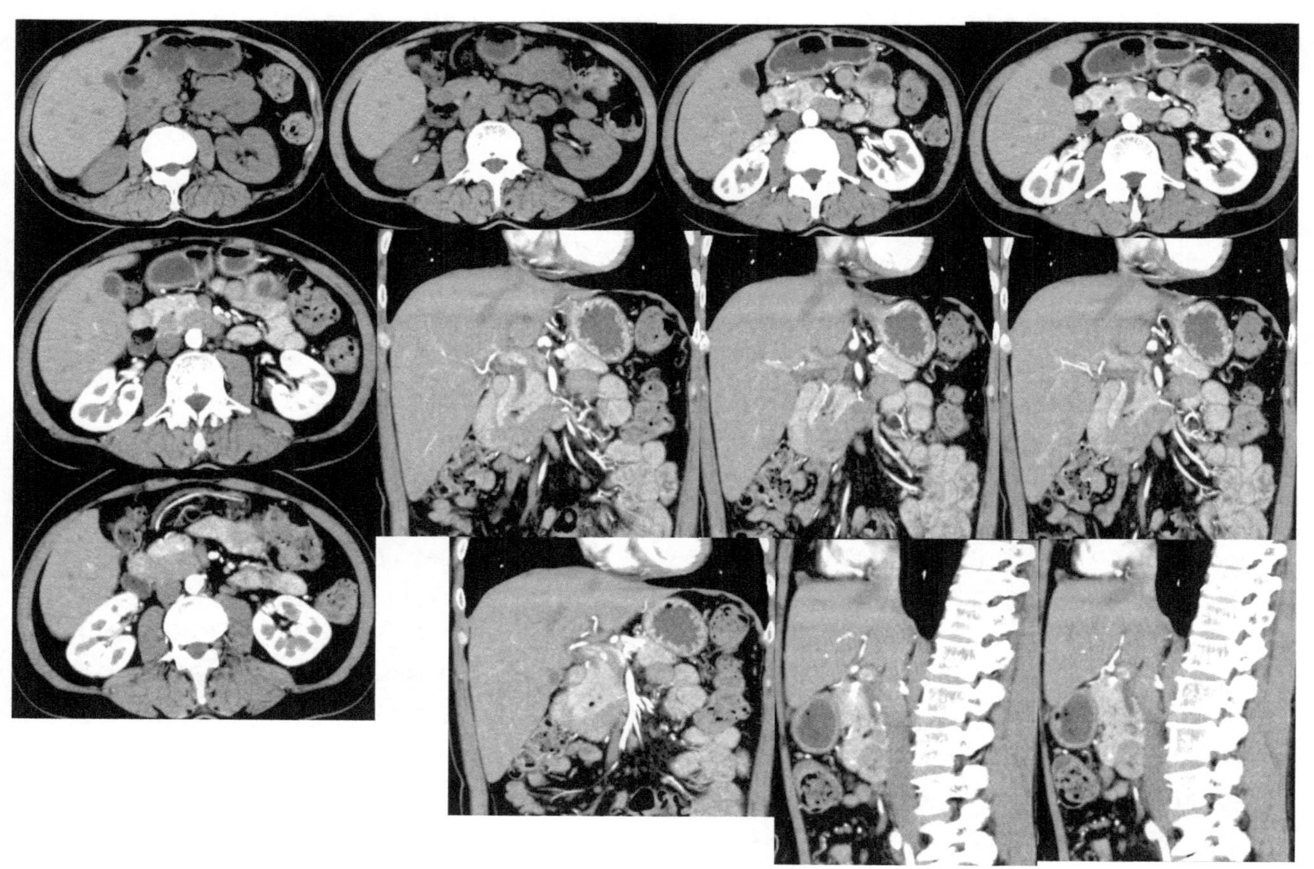

图 24-6-1 十二指肠乳头旁憩室与胆胰管下端恶性占位性病变

患者,女,51岁。

CT:影像表现不典型的十二指肠乳头旁憩室充满食物残渣和少量气体,伪似胆胰管下端的恶性占位性病变,可导致误诊。但该病例胆管与胰管都不扩张,无梗阻表现,临床也无任何症状。冠状位重建图像显示尤其清楚(图 24-6-1)。

第四节 乳头区憩室和憩室内乳头

详见本书 本卷 第十九篇 第四章 第二节 乳头区憩室和憩室内乳头。

第七章　十二指肠梗阻和狭窄

第一节　十二指肠结石性梗阻

十二指肠结石性梗阻可分为二类:胆石性梗阻,一般均可见到胆系 - 十二指肠瘘存在,结石的化学成分也是一个诊断依据;肠石性梗阻,肠石系在肠道内自行聚结而成,一般仅在肠道有淤滞时,且在碱性溶液内形成,因此,常常发生在结肠或小肠下段。国内文献报告胆石、粪石、异物引起肠梗阻仅占肠梗阻病例的 0.48%,而国外报告胆石性肠梗阻约占肠梗阻病例的 1.5%~3.0%。

临床表现:上腹部阵发性疼痛伴恶心、呕吐。

影像学研究:胆石性肠梗阻的梗阻部位, 90% 位于回肠下段,位于十二指肠者较少见。胆石直径在 2.5cm 以上,常不通过十二指肠空肠曲而引起梗阻。钡餐检查显示结石的边缘光整的卵圆形充盈缺损,应与肠息肉及其他肠道良性肿瘤相区别。

肠息肉多见于结肠,发生于十二指肠者罕见,而且息肉质软,有一定的活动度,临床往往有出血史。其他良性肠道肿瘤,自肠壁突向肠腔,往往呈半圆形压迹,局部黏膜受压变平。胆石四周轮廓完全衬托出来,透过胆石影还可见整齐排列的十二指肠皱襞,与它们完全不同。

在肠石性梗阻,胃肠钡剂检查可见胃内有空腹贮留,梗阻近侧十二指肠明显扩张,梗阻处可见充盈缺损,异物(胆系结石、肠石或其他异物)引起的梗阻,充盈缺损常可以移动,表面不规整,可有少量钡剂附着于上,呈不规则条纹状和小斑片状,周围肠壁光滑柔软,黏膜皱襞清晰完整,无肠壁浸润变硬现象。钡剂通过常常受阻,胃排空大大延迟,服钡四小时后复查,可能大量钡剂仍存留于胃与近侧十二指肠内。

一组作者报告一例十二指肠结石性梗阻发生在十二指肠升段,其大小约 7cm × 10cm,分析其原因可能与该病例胃部分切除术后胃酸减少,并且局部肠管与周围发生粘连,导致不易消化吸收的肠内容淤滞于该处有关。

第二节　十二指肠外压性狭窄

十二指肠降段外压性狭窄常导致误诊。我们曾见一例胆囊癌压迫十二指肠降段,黏膜改变不显著;一例慢性胆囊炎急性发作,胆囊肿大压迫十二指肠降段外侧且有内瘘形成,钡餐检查见十二指肠降段有 3cm × 7cm 腔内充盈缺损,表面不光整,局部肠管僵硬,低张检查亦未见缓解;一例右半横结肠癌粘连压迫十二指肠降段外侧而致偏心性狭窄,上下分界清,近端肠管扩张。

这些病例手术病理证实皆为外来的压迫、粘连、浸润,但术前反复检查、会诊却甚难分辨为外来或内在疾病所致,是炎症或是肿瘤亦难辨别,文献上亦有类似报告,说明该区结构毗邻复杂,邻近脏器影响甚大,故在上述情况下,宜多分析,多观察,或进一步进行断面影像学检查,尽可能减少误诊。

第三节　弯曲引起的狭窄

肠管弯曲导致狭窄从而引起误诊，这在小肠气钡双重造影是屡见不鲜的，这实际上不是器质性病变，为一特殊的假病变。由于肠管弯曲、扭折和纠集，有时在十二指肠球部与降段的连接处出现所谓的弯曲性假病变或假肿瘤，这是一个环状充盈缺损，位于十二指肠曲内侧，常伴钡剂的中央性聚集，实质上它是由于十二指肠黏膜冗赘和皱褶所致。在钡剂检查时，施行加压照片可显示此类“病变”，以不同角度的方位进行多角度观察，则显露出它并不是一个真正的病变。在肠曲其他部位也可出现与之类似的表现。

第四节　十二指肠结核

关于感染与发病：结核菌感染十二指肠，可通过摄食，痰液经肠黏膜侵入，或通过血行播散与淋巴通道进入黏膜下，或由邻近感染的器官通过浆膜直接蔓延。Thoeni 等（1979）提出胆系可能也是一个感染途径。Balikian 等（1967）在胃十二指肠结核病例中，观察到一种逆行扩散现象。十二指肠血供比较丰富，且位于淋巴组织近旁，有利于结核菌感染，因此，十二指肠结核的发病率不低，一般都高于胃结核（Tishler 等，1979）。

一些作者报告 7 例十二指肠结核，其中 4 例十二指肠周围有巨大的淋巴结结核包块，1 例有结核性腹膜炎病史，1 例为结核性十二指肠胆囊瘘，另 2 例有十二指肠胃幽门延续病变。7 例均以十二指肠结核感染为主，其中 5 例的结核感染明显与周围淋巴结结核有关。

第五节　十二指肠淤积症

十二指肠淤积症是指各种原因引起的十二指肠远端或十二指肠与空肠交界处的梗阻，致十二指肠近端扩张、肠内容物淤积产生的一种临床综合征。引起本症的原因甚多，传统上认为肠系膜上动脉压迫十二指肠是最常见的原因，又称为肠系膜上动脉综合征。

临床表现：十二指肠淤积症属于少见病，可发生在任何年龄，以消瘦的中青年女性多见，平均发病年龄为 15~50 岁，以 20~30 岁多见，十二指肠淤积症没有特异的临床表现，主要是十二指肠梗阻症状，表现为进食后上腹胀痛，伴轻至重度持续性或痉挛性疼痛，常于餐后数分钟或数小时发生顽固性呕吐，呕吐后不适症状消失，症状呈间歇性反复发作，持续数天后可自行缓解，数天以至数月无症状；症状呈间歇性发作，并可因体位的改变而缓解，部分患者取仰卧位时症状加重，而俯卧位、膝胸位、左侧位时症状缓解。

由于多种原因引起十二指肠阻塞，以致阻塞部位近端扩张，食糜壅积而产生临床综合征，通常认为肠系膜上动脉压迫十二指肠形成十二指肠淤积症者居多。

影像学研究：十二指肠淤积症的诊断需密切结合临床及辅助检查，传统的消化道钡餐检查具有简便易行、价廉经济等特点，对于十二指肠淤积症的影像诊断具有重要价值，特别是动态观察方面更具优势，钡餐检查 X 线主要征象为十二指肠水平或升段出现光滑的压迹，钡剂通过受阻、近端扩张，出现明显的十二指肠逆蠕动，远端肠腔瘪陷，钡剂排空延迟，变换体位时如侧卧或俯卧时钡剂可迅速通过十二指肠水平都进入空肠。

一组资料分析显示十二指肠淤积症患者的 CT 影像所见与钡餐检查是相一致的，在仰卧位 CT 扫描时胃、十二指肠球部、降段及部分水平或升段有不同程度扩张，肠系膜上动脉与十二指肠水平段形成压迹，压迹处肠管变窄、压迹前段的肠管扩张。

消化道钡餐造影存在严重的不足,难以观察肠系膜上动脉与十二指肠的关系、难以显示肠管外部的病理改变,MSCT扫描具有无创性检查的优点,对于十二指肠淤积症具有较高的诊断价值,可以弥补消化道钡餐造影的不足、提高对病变的检出率和诊断的准确率。

腹部彩色多普勒超声及纤维内镜检查也应用于十二指肠淤积症的影像检查,彩色多普勒超声检查可以显示肠系膜上动脉与十二指肠的解剖关系,但难于观察胃、十二指肠的形态变化;胃镜检查可直接观察胃十二指肠管腔内的形态改变,也难以观察胃十二指肠管腔腔外形态。

近些年来, MSCT血管造影已成为临床诊断血管病变的重要检查方法,具有准确定性、定位诊断的优势,为进一步研究肠系膜上动脉与十二指肠淤积症的关系提供了良好的影像研究平台。MSCT除了能清晰显示胃及十二指肠的形态变化外,CT增强后进行血管的三维重建(即CT血管造影)可明确肠系膜上动脉和腹主动脉之间的解剖关系,显示肠系膜上动脉对于十二指肠的压迫状态。

MSCT血管造影可以媲美血管造影,CT血管造影能够精确测量肠系膜上动脉与腹主动脉的夹角以及肠系膜上动脉后壁与腹主动脉前壁之间的距离,非常有利于十二指肠淤积症的诊断。有资料表明肠系膜上动脉与腹主动脉的夹角正常为30º~ 50º,十二指肠淤积症患者这一夹角多半<30º,夹角内肠系膜上动脉压迫处的十二指肠水平段前后管径常常<10 mm,而近端十二指肠腔扩张、前后径>30 mm,而夹角<15º,常常导致肠系膜上动脉压迫十二指肠水平段产生十二指肠淤滞的症状。该组资料分析结果表明虽然多数患者十二指肠水平段前后管径小于10 mm,但正常人群中仰卧位时部分人的十二指肠水平段前后管径也可小于10 mm、肠系膜上动脉与腹主动脉的夹角也可小于30º、甚至夹角小于15º,并未出现十二指肠淤积症的临床表现。

十二指肠的CT形态因人而异、差异较大, CT分析十二指肠形态时应灵活判断,利用CT肠系膜上动脉造影测量肠系膜上动脉与腹主动脉间距及夹角用以判断是否存在十二指肠淤积症应十分慎重,需防止误判,人类肠系膜上动脉与腹主动脉间距及夹角变异较大,况且造成十二指肠水平段梗阻的原因并不能全部归结为肠系膜上动脉的压迫。

导致十二指肠淤积症的原因是多方面的,文献报道以下几方面的原因可以导致十二指肠淤积症:①十二指肠悬韧带过短致使十二指肠位置较高,可引起肠系膜上动脉对十二指肠压迫;②肠系膜上动脉根部病变例如淋巴结增大、纤维化及粘连的纤维组织横跨十二指肠可导致十二指肠淤积症;③脊柱前突可导致肠系膜上动脉和腹主动脉之间的角度过小;④内脏下垂牵拉肠系膜常为本病的重要病因,瘦长体型及各种原因的消瘦可以削弱肠系膜对十二指肠水平部的支撑作用导致十二指肠淤积症;⑤腹腔手术后粘连、牵拉肠系膜可造成肠系膜上动脉对十二指肠水平部的压迫;⑥十二指肠功能异常、肿瘤、肠结核、克罗恩病等诸多病变均可引起十二指肠淤积症。

十二指肠淤积症包含有肠系膜上动脉综合征,就肠系膜上动脉综合征而言,测量肠系膜上动脉和腹主动脉之间的夹角可能有助于诊断,但对于非肠系膜上动脉压迫十二指肠而出现的十二指肠淤积症病例,就不能机械性地套用测量值来作为诊断标准。

有关肠系膜上动脉和腹主动脉的形态改变与十二指肠淤积症发病之间的关系,有待进一步研究方可做出定论。CT诊断十二指肠淤积症有其局限性,CT难以观察到胃十二指肠的蠕动、难以动态显示十二指肠的功能变化,消化道钡餐检查可以弥补CT在这方面的不足,两种检查方法相互取长补短。值得注意的是十二指肠淤积症虽然不是消化系统常见疾病,但往往容易误诊、漏诊,临床上十二指肠淤积症需与胃十二指肠溃疡、慢性胃炎、胃神经官能症、幽门梗阻等常见的上消化道疾病鉴别。CT结合消化道钡餐、纤维内镜等多种影像手段,利用不同影像检查手段的相互补充,对本病的诊断和鉴别诊断是非常必要的。

第六节　十二指肠的占位性病变

这是十二指肠梗阻和狭窄的常见病因,请详见本书 本卷 本篇 各有关章节。

第八章　十二指肠先天异常与发育变异

第一节　先天性巨十二指肠

病因学与病理学：先天性巨十二指肠，又称为先天性巨大型十二指肠扩张。先天性巨十二指肠可见于下述三种情况：

（1）十二指肠膜式狭窄：系先天性十二指肠隔膜或蹼，是由于胚胎期肠管腔化过程异常而形成。先天性十二指肠隔膜症分为完全闭锁和膜式狭窄两种。十二指肠隔膜，多发生于十二指肠乳头附近，隔膜孔直径从 2mm 至 10mm 不等，并且大多数呈偏心性，隔膜通常为 1 个，也可以是 2 个，Anderson（1984）报告一例甚至多达 4 个隔膜。在成人，十二指肠膜式狭窄不少见，有作者统计约占整个膜式狭窄的 30%~35%。膜式狭窄可位于十二指肠各处，位于十二指肠空肠交界处者，是引起婴幼儿和儿童先天性巨十二指肠的重要原因。

（2）肠壁肌间神经因素：是由于肠壁肌层内神经丛的神经节细胞减少或完全缺如，使病变肠段失去正常蠕动，经常处于收缩状态，而造成痉挛性梗阻，使肠内容物通过发生障碍，导致痉挛近端肠管出现明显扩张。

（3）特发性：此型先天性巨十二指肠是十二指肠既无器质性狭窄，又无肌间神经丛的神经节细胞发育障碍，病因不明。有作者认为，先天性巨十二指肠有家族性倾向。

临床表现：自出生以来，经常出现呕吐，呕吐物为胃内容物或水。可出现腹胀，腹胀明显时，食欲减退或拒食。面部或双下肢有时可见水肿。查体可见营养不良的表现，诸如面色苍白、眼睑及面部水肿、下肢凹陷性水肿。腹部膨隆，胀气明显，可出现移动性浊音。临床印象多为营养不良性水肿。

影像学研究：插管进行钡餐检查前，务必观察胃贮留情况，设法尽量抽吸贮留的胃肠道内容物，然后注入稀钡混悬液。可见十二指肠环形肠黏膜皱襞显示，十二指肠明显扩张，其直径可达 10 厘米以上，同时可发现扩张肠曲远端有狭窄，可为环形偏心性狭窄（膜状或短节段状），狭窄远端肠曲无异常。如遇婴幼儿上消化道不全梗阻的病例，宜采用导管法进行造影检查，这样做的优点是：可将胃肠道内容物抽吸得较为干净，以保证检查的顺利进行；可在注入钡混悬液同时进行观察，对明确诊断大有帮助；检查完毕后，可将钡混悬液尽量抽出，以免造成完全性肠梗阻。

成人十二指肠球部扩张，可为先天性或后天获得性，后者的起因以肠系膜上动脉压迫升段起始处为最常见。十二指肠亦可因肠壁肌层无神经节，或神经节细胞中毒性，或退行性改变而扩张。巨大十二指肠球部与溃疡的关系，学者们意见不一。有作者认为球部内容物潴留是产生溃疡或炎症的原因，另一些作者则认为溃疡导致球部的局部淤张和潴留，我们认为，孰因孰果应视具体病人而论，不宜笼统地概括。

第二节　巨大十二指肠重复畸形

在消化道重复畸形中，以小肠多见，约占总数的 57%，而小肠重复畸形绝大多数位于回肠末段，其次位于十二指肠的第二段。但巨大十二指肠重复畸形罕见。

肠重复畸形病理分为4型：①肠外囊肿型；②肠内囊肿型；③管型或双肠腔型；④胸内消化道重复畸形。十二指肠重复畸形多发生在十二指肠圈内侧，常不与肠道相通，呈囊性，所以临床上又称为肠源性囊肿。囊肿大小及形态表现多样，小的仅蚕豆大小，大的可占据大部分腹腔。如病变较小，消化道造影表现为十二指肠降部或水平部的充盈缺损，不具有特征性表现；肠外囊肿型，且囊肿较大，并有入口和出口则囊肿显影，消化道造影有特征性表现。

鉴别诊断：先天性小肠狭窄、内脏转位、胃扭转、巨大十二指肠憩室等，根据消化道造影及临床表现各有其自身特点，易于鉴别。

第三节　成人完全性环状胰腺并急性胰腺炎

详见本书 本卷 第二十篇 第十九章 第二节　成人完全性环状胰腺并急性胰腺炎。

第四节　十二指肠一些发育变异

十二指肠空肠曲韧带只是腹膜组织，无肌纤维，而十二指肠悬肌却含有大量肌肉组织。十二指肠空肠曲韧带是十二指肠空肠曲左前上部与横结肠系膜根部之间的斜行（由左上斜向右下）腹膜部分，曾被称作十二指肠空肠腹膜皱褶。而十二指肠悬肌上部起于右膈脚，下部附着于十二指肠空肠曲的右后部（由右上斜向左下），因此，此韧带与悬肌不仅表现方向不同，而且两下端附着部位也不相同，两者下端在左右位置关系上还稍有距离。此韧带下端右侧的肠管是固定于腹膜后位的十二指肠末端，而其左侧则为可移动的空肠起始部。因此，韧带下端连于肠管处的位置，实为十二指肠与空肠的确切界限。

而悬肌是在腹膜后位，手术时不宜用它作为标志，并且，其下端附于肠管处的位置变异也较大，它对十二指肠起着悬吊和支持的作用。

绝大多数人的十二指肠走行为逆时钟性，但也有一定变异，即少数人的球部，却先向右后方或左后方走行，然后顺时钟下降，直接与空肠相连接。

有作者报告十二指肠先天异常，不存在十二指肠环，空肠上段完全在右上腹，在超声检查时疑为腹膜后肿块，在CT扫描图像上清楚可见腹膜后间隙右肾上前方出现10cm×10cm×5cm大小团块影，其内可见小的气泡，后手术证实为异常走行的十二指肠及空肠上段附近粘连，引起其上方肠袢出现梗阻所致。

十二指肠球后面沿降部内侧下降到胆胰共同管。在进行CT诊断时应注意，一些发育变异或先天性异常可能与主要病变相混淆，十二指肠憩室充盈气体可能被误认为是肠穿孔，十二指肠旋转不良加上未完全充盈对比剂可能难以和肿瘤区别。

第九章　十二指肠创伤

第一节　十二指肠肠壁内血肿

十二指肠肠壁内血肿少见，自 Mc Langhlan（1938）首先报道十二指肠肠壁内血肿以来，Janson 和 Stockinger（1975）总结文献报告共有 182 例，至 1986 年共报道儿童病例 130 余例。

1. 病因学　（1）腹部外伤：是最常见的原因，复习文献，70% 以上的病例皆有腹部外伤史。十二指肠易受损伤，是因为它固定在后腹膜，当腹部受暴力损害时，十二指肠挤压于椎体上而受到损伤。骤然举重，或搬运重物，使腹肌猛力收缩，腹压急剧升高也同样可引起小肠或肠系膜的损伤。Winthrop（1986）报道腹部钝性外伤是引起十二指肠肠壁内血肿的最常见原因，其中儿童病例占 90%。十二指肠肠壁内血肿好发于儿童且多见于十二指肠及空肠上段，其原因为：①儿童身体两侧前肋弓缘位置较高，且较成人分开，加之腹肌尚未发育完全，对上腹保护甚差；②十二指肠及近段空肠由屈氏韧带固定于后腹膜，对外伤的应变能力较其他部分小肠弱；③十二指肠有双重血供，肠壁黏膜及浆膜下有丰富的血管丛，钝性外伤的剪力易引起血管丛的撕裂出血，使肠壁及其系膜形成血肿。

（2）抗凝血药物的应用：经过抗凝血药物治疗的患者，大约 3%~4% 有胃肠道出血。

（3）出血性疾病：如白血病、血友病、Henoch 紫癜、多发性骨髓瘤、淋巴肉瘤及肿瘤的浸润等。

（4）医源性：如幽门成形术、腹腔血管造影、小肠黏膜活检等。

（5）原因不明。

2. 临床表现　十二指肠肠壁内血肿的主要症状为腹痛，血肿较大时可向肠腔内凸出，引起肠腔狭窄梗阻，出现胆汁性呕吐。腹部有不同程度的触压痛，有时可扪及包块，如出血量多则可出现贫血及低灌注状态。腹部钝性外伤史是诊断十二指肠肠壁内血肿的关键病史。

3. 影像学研究　十二指肠肠壁内血肿的影像学表现变化较大，这与肠壁内血肿的大小、范围、黏膜的肿胀程度，肠腔内分泌物，及有无合并肠系膜血肿等，有着密切的关系。外伤患者的血肿比较局限，其他原因所致的血肿常常比较广泛，甚至蔓延至空肠，肠管表现僵直。

X 线腹部平片：腹部平片很重要，有的病例依此即可作出诊断。平片可显示：①不同程度的十二指肠梗阻，若肠管狭窄较严重，则表现胃十二指肠明显扩张；②血肿较大时，腹部可见密度增高的软组织块影，并压迫周围脏器移位；③若肠腔内有气体，则可能显示肠腔狭窄，肠壁增厚及肠腔内血肿或软组织阴影；④若血肿破入后腹膜，则呈现右侧腰大肌影消失。

上消化道钡餐：这是显示十二指肠及空肠肠壁内血肿传统的方法，也是较好的方法。典型表现为：①十二指肠黏膜呈弹簧圈样；②向十二指肠肠腔内凸出的边缘光整的肿块影，可造成十二指肠肠腔变形，不同程度的狭窄（狭窄处黏膜可呈纵行排列，形似毛笔尖等），甚至钡流受阻，近端十二指肠及胃扩张；③空肠肠壁内血肿一般不出现肿块，累及的黏膜因出血水肿增厚，形如堆砌的硬币。

超声：一般血肿位于腹主动脉及下腔静脉前方，多呈长条状左右方向延伸，其长轴常与身体纵轴垂直，呈混合性回声，有液性暗区及回声增强的血块，并可见条索状分隔。随时间的延长及血肿成分的改变，肿块的回声随之减低呈囊性。

胰腺假性囊肿一般位于脾静脉的前方，其位置多偏前偏高，且回声及形态皆与肠壁血肿不同，B 型超声易于鉴别。

CT:十二指肠肠壁内血肿的CT图像决定于损伤的时间及周围组织的密度。在急性期,肿块密度为50~80HU,一周后血肿密度降低至20~50HU,到慢性期其密度更低。同时,CT可显示血肿部位肠壁增厚,肠腔狭窄及黏膜异常。

MRI:MRI对于出血时间超过48~72小时的血肿有诊断价值。T_1WI上,血肿表现为很高的信号,与脂肪信号相同,但其分布与脂肪不同,可资区别;T_2WI上也可表现为高信号。三周后的血肿在MRI表现具特征性,呈同心圆表现,外层有一薄层暗的边缘,T_1WI显示高信号,内缘较清楚。

第二节 十二指肠壁内血肿

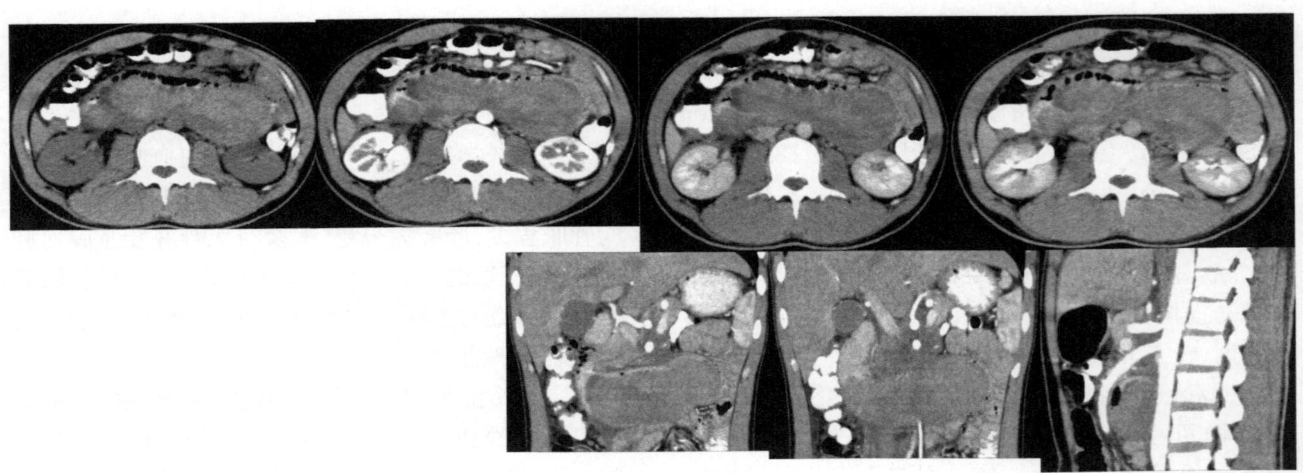

图 24-9-1 十二指肠壁内血肿

患者,男,25岁。外伤致上腹部疼痛不适3天入院。患者缘于3日前在建筑工地作业时,不慎被重物砸伤腰背部及头部,当时急诊就诊外院,行CT头颅未见明显异常,头皮外伤予以清创缝合后出院,后于昨日下午出现腹部疼痛不适,并伴有呕吐,呕吐物为胃内容物,无畏寒、发热、腹胀、腹泻等不适,急诊就诊我院,门诊以"腹痛"收住入院,患者自发病以来,精神睡眠一般,食欲差,大小便正常,体重无明显减轻,体力明显下降。CT:腹膜后见巨大混杂密度影,大小约14.1 cm × 5.4 cm × 4.5cm,CT值35~ 64HU,增强后未见明显强化,周围组织受推压,与十二指肠降段及水平段后壁关系密切,局部肠腔变窄,腹腔干及肠系膜上动脉起始段显示清楚。CT诊断:十二指肠壁内血肿可能性大。该例经临床保守治疗痊愈出院(图24-9-1)。

第十章　十二指肠瘘

肝外胆管十二指肠乳头旁瘘

由慢性穿透性十二指肠溃疡所致的肝外胆管十二指肠瘘，是指在肝外胆管十二指肠后段的胆肠内瘘，Kourias 报告 3 000 例胃切除术中有 9 例（占 0.3%），Michowitz（1984）报告因十二指肠溃疡而手术的 550 例中有 3 例（占 0.54%）。

由于纤维十二指肠镜检查及 ERCP 的广泛开展，发现了更多的肝外胆管十二指肠瘘，发生在十二指肠壁内段及胰腺段，大多由于胆管下段结石嵌顿、梗阻、感染，导致胆管壁溃烂向十二指肠穿孔，自行引流减压而形成瘘道，这常常是机体自行排石的一种特殊过程，也可看作肝外胆管结石的一类并发症。肝外胆管十二指肠乳头旁瘘是胆肠内瘘的一种较特殊类型，它可引起腹痛、发热等胆系感染症状。如果在施行胆系手术前和术中未能发现及处理此症，术后仍常常有胆管炎症状残存。

临床表现：性别差异不大。年龄 25~58 岁，平均 50.3 岁。病程最长 30 年，平均 11 年 5 个月。病史在 10 年以上者 18 例（约占 70%）。

影像学研究：超声检查可发现胆系结石，个别病例为肝门胆管癌合并胆管结石。CT 扫描可见肝内外胆管结石伴胆管扩张，少数病例仅见肝内外胆管扩张。ERCP 与 PTC 可见肝内外胆管结石伴胆管扩张，部分病例可见胆管积气，部分病例胆管僵硬，普遍呈枯树支状，胆管扩张一般较明显，肝外胆管直径大于 2cm 者约占总例数的 70%，肝外胆管最粗者达 4.5cm。胃肠钡剂检查有的病例伴存乳头区憩室，瘘口也可开口于憩室内。为证实是否为憩室可于胆系检查后行胃肠钡剂检查，可见典型的囊袋状憩室影。

纤维十二指肠镜检查所见：内镜入十二指肠后，可见突于十二指肠降部内侧纵行隆起皱襞远端表面的乳头，上缘有皱襞复盖，下呈人字小带，一般瘘口位于乳头尖附近，其直径约 0.5~1.0cm。瘘口多呈不规则的星状，无正常乳头形态及开口特征，有时瘘口可被黏膜覆盖，从乳头开口插入导管可从瘘口折回至肠腔，改从乳头附近瘘口插管则极易使胆系显影。

当发现瘘口后，应注意观察有无胆汁流出，并可用生理盐水冲洗，偶见碎石渣从瘘口流出。瘘口多位于乳头开口正上方或右上方，与胆管走行的解剖关系一致。

个别乳头及瘘口均位于大的乳头区憩室内。在镜下应注意鉴别憩室与瘘口，憩室边缘较整齐有唇，开口多呈圆形，也可在十二指肠乳头附近开口，但上无横行皱襞，下无人字小带，其内常可见到食物残渣，拨开残渣后可能见到憩室底部，导管向内插入即折回肠腔，向内注入对比剂可见其全部溢出，同时肠道可见对比剂，但胆管不显影。按 Ikeda 等（1975）分类，瘘口位于乳头开口近侧纵行皱襞的十二指肠内壁为 1 型，瘘口位于纵行皱襞上方横行皱襞内为 2 型。

诊断依据有：①有长期胆系疾病史，如上腹痛、发热、黄疸，说明有胆管梗阻及胆系感染；②内镜直视下经瘘口插管注入对比剂，可获得肝外胆管显影；③ X 线静脉法胆系造影，胆系不显影时，应想到有无胆肠内瘘的存在；④腹部 X 线平片、CT 及 MRI 检查时显示胆系积气，说明存在胆肠内瘘，而且瘘孔较大；⑤钡餐检查可见钡剂返流入胆管，患者有典型的返流性胆管炎症状；⑥手术切开胆管后，见有十二指肠液逆流入胆管，应想到胆肠内瘘的可能性，但需与胆胰管下端括约肌松弛症鉴别。

第十一章　十二指肠其他疾病

第一节　右侧十二指肠旁疝

十二指肠旁疝是腹内疝(发病率 0.2%~0.9%)中最常见的一种,约占全部内疝的 53%,男女发病率约 3∶1;十二指肠旁疝分为左、右侧 2 种亚型,以左侧常见,右侧约占 25%。

腹内疝为小肠梗阻的少见病因(约占 0.5%~4.1%),腹内疝易并发肠绞窄或缺血。十二指肠旁疝常表现为饱食、剧烈运动或突然改变体位后出现恶心、呕吐并上腹剧烈疼痛,症状可追溯至儿时。也有报道出现不寻常的左腰部疼痛、呕吐等症状。

腹部平片是首选的影像检查方法,部分患者可见肠梗阻征象,一例患者没有肠梗阻表现。胃肠道造影显示位于十二指肠降段后下方的由小肠肠管聚集而成的较大且固定的卵圆形团块。CT 表现为右中腹部一簇小肠肠袢被膜性结构包绕所形成的团块,可见肠梗阻,表现为肠管扩张,管腔内气液平面,该例患者为囊袋状团块,梗阻致近端肠管扩张,无明确气液平面。可以并发肠扭转及急性肠缺血,导致部分小肠绞窄、坏死,表现为小肠走行僵直、肠壁增厚,肠系膜血管扭曲成旋涡状。少见肠套叠。还可见血管的改变,包括:肠系膜血管充血,肠系膜上动脉、肠系膜上静脉的空肠支环绕至主干的右后方,以供应疝入的空肠。还可发现其他发育异常,如肠系膜上静脉位于腹侧或左侧,或无十二指肠水平段。有时还能见胰头受压下移,胃潴留。对十二指肠旁疝的解剖位置、影像及临床表现的熟知是诊断十二指肠旁疝的关键。检查手段主要选 MSCT 平扫加增强扫描,多进行图像后处理,处理技术主要选择多平面重建和最大密度投影。

第二节　十二指肠结石

肠内结石可分为三类:粪石,多见于结肠;混合性肠结石,或植物团块;药物性结石,多见于小肠中。一般认为,胃内异物如能通过幽门,基本上就可通过全消化道,但少数异物也可能在乙状结肠直肠交界处或回盲部停顿,在十二指肠球部嵌顿者却甚为少见。

有作者报道,原有十二指肠球部溃疡史十几年,后来食入柿,导致出现腹痛、恶心、呕吐。钡餐检查见胃蠕动弱、张力低、有少量潴留液、幽门开放延迟、十二指肠球部内可见一边缘光滑整齐,表面有细条索状钡纹的充盈缺损,直径约 3cm,不活动,球外形及远侧肠管未见异常。手术见球部有直径 2cm 左右的溃疡瘢痕,球内可摸到直径约 3cm 的质硬光滑包块,切开肠壁发现为一黄褐色植物团块。

由于十二指肠球部容积有限,加上球部有溃疡瘢痕,导致植物团块嵌顿于球部,引起不全性上消化道梗阻。结石嵌顿于球部,不能活动,边缘又光滑,可伪似良性肿瘤。但是,如密切结合病史,注意充盈缺损表面有斑纹的表现,即可作出正确诊断。

第三节　十二指肠邻近病变

在低张十二指肠造影时，十二指肠邻近脏器的占位性病变基本 X 线征象有：十二指肠管壁边缘呈结节状受压或充盈缺损，侵蚀破坏或出现双重轮廓；十二指肠曲圆钝扩大，呈三角形或倒 3 字形，管腔弥漫性或局限性狭窄，狭窄段以上扩张；管壁僵硬，扩张受限，失去正常的光滑度；黏膜皱襞粗大，迂曲，扁平，变直，呈不规则的锯齿状，棘状突出或破坏中断；十二指肠乳头光滑或不规则增大，失去正常形态；发现溃疡或憩室。

第四节　十二指肠弯曲部假性病变

在十二指肠第一段与降段连接处常可见钡剂积聚，形似溃疡；或出现充盈缺损而形似肿块，前已述及可形似息肉。这些假性病变的出现可能与下述三因素有关：解剖生理的弯曲引起变形、紊乱和失真；括约肌的作用（Albot 等曾报告十二指肠有三个分离的括约肌）；外在的压迫。假性溃疡的特殊 X 线表现是弯曲的黏膜皱襞中央有圆形的钡剂积聚，多位于十二指肠内面，在不同角度和体位的投照中，其形态有显著的变化，而与真性病变有所区别。

真正十二指肠肿瘤十分少见，通常为息肉状，其范围可大可小，小者如腺瘤，大者为广泛转移性肿瘤，此类肿瘤如正好位于十二指肠球部尖端，则与该处黏膜皱襞所形成的假性病变难以区别，透视观察及连续点片摄影可见后者形态变化明显，有助于鉴别。Burrell 和 Toffler（1976）报告十二指肠曲的假性病变 64 例，不少均经内镜检和 / 或手术证实，该作者对此进行详细讨论。在十二指肠球部，钡剂双对比结肠检查时，不仅能见到淋巴滤泡增生，而且有时还能见到增生的布氏腺。

第五节　胆囊病变引起胃流出道梗阻

Furtado（1974）报告 2 例胆囊病变引起胃流出道梗阻。1 例为 63 岁老妇，呕吐清水 5 天，X 线检查见胃扩张，十二指肠球部明显畸形。手术示胆囊底粘连于十二指肠球部，胆囊内含多数透光结石，一些结石在球部内发现，胆囊与球部粘连处附近已穿孔。另例为 40 岁男性，腹痛，上胃肠道检查示十二指肠曲完全性梗阻，伴一大的钙化性包块，手术见为胆石挤压肠袢导致梗阻。2 例腹部平片均未见梗阻征象。

第六节　一些诊断陷阱

在仰卧位及俯卧位时钡餐照片，正常胆囊或扩大的胆囊可压挤十二指肠球部，不留心则会误为球部变形。肝外胆管有时压迫十二指肠球部可产生一斜行的条状透光带。在双对比胃造影时，十二指肠曲扩大，偶尔是由于高位横结肠使胃上移而导致十二指肠曲较正常明显扩大。在仰卧位及俯卧位时钡餐照片，正常胆囊或扩大的胆囊可压挤十二指肠球部，不留心则会误为球部变形。除十二指肠球部和一短段球后部分外，十二指肠位于腹膜后。十二指肠水平部位于肠系膜上动脉和肠系膜上静脉的后方以及主动脉和下腔静脉的前方。倘若无既往手术史，而十二指肠的这部分缺失，则强烈提示为小肠旋转不良。小肠的其余部分（空肠与回肠）位于腹膜腔内。

第十二章　十二指肠疾病的影像学检查

第一节　CT 显示十二指肠病变

目前诊断十二指肠肿瘤的检查方法包括上消化道钡餐和内镜检查,它们主要显示黏膜病变对腔内及腔内外生长的肿瘤检出率高,但对腔外生长的肿瘤难以发现。与上述传统方法比较, MSCT 具有多通道的快速采集、静脉注射单次扫描覆盖范围大、微体素成像、亚毫米层厚、更高的空间分辨率及强大的图像后处理功能等优点,可清晰显示十二指肠形态,肠壁及腔内外改变,可清楚准确显示肿瘤的具体部位、形态、大小及向腔内外侵犯的范围。

扫描前的准备,有作者采用术前饮水 500ml 及术前 20 min 山莨菪碱 20 mg 肌肉注射。低张药有利减少肠道蠕动而产生的伪影,有文献提倡饮用 1%~3% 阳性对比剂,有作者认为口服高密度对比剂易与 CTA、多平面重建后处理图像的兴趣结构重叠遮盖且增强扫描时强化的肠管与肠腔内阳性对比剂呈等密度均不利于肠壁结构显示,而水作对比剂与强化的病灶有良好的对比,也易于观察肠壁结构、肠壁血运。

常规对比剂剂量多为 80~120 ml,流率为 3~5 ml/s,有作者的经验是对比剂剂量 80 ml,流率 3 ml/s,足以得到高质量图像。注射对比剂后 30 s、60 s 扫描可获取动脉期和静脉期图像,动脉期 MSCTA 可显示富血供的肿瘤及其具体供血动脉,门静脉期则利于显示肿瘤的强化特点及肿瘤与病灶、邻近组织的关系。

MSCT 三维重建技术可同时获得横轴位、冠状面、矢状面影像,能清楚的显示肿瘤与周围结构的关系和有无局部及远处转移等,为临床治疗提供帮助。薄层重建图像虽然信噪比较原始图像低,但薄层重建图像显示微小病变及病变与十二指肠的关系较 10 mm 层厚图像好。

十二指肠镜和钡餐检查一直是十二指肠病变的首选检查方法。但对十二指肠水平段及升段的病变,十二指肠镜难以到达病变部位,而钡餐检查仅能发现肠腔内的病变,对肠壁和周围结构无法显示。随着技术的更新, CT 对胃肠道的显示越来越清晰,且 CT 检查除可发现十二指肠腔内的病变外尚可显示肿瘤向腔内外的生长情况及对周围血管、脏器的侵犯,并了解淋巴结及腹腔有无转移。如果结合二维和三维图像重建,对十二指肠病变的诊断及肿瘤的分期将更加准确,也会为临床治疗提供更多更可靠的信息,从而避免不必要的剖腹探查,减轻患者的痛苦。总之, MSCT 可以很好地显示非乳头区十二指肠肿瘤和肿瘤样病变及其与周围解剖结构的关系,在病变的定性方面也有一定的价值,能为临床治疗方案的选择提供可靠的信息。

第二节　十二指肠在 X 线腹部正位片上的诊断陷阱

在腹部正位片上,充盈气液或充盈液体的十二指肠球部重叠于肾上腺区,偶尔可伪似肾上腺肿瘤。在腹部平片上,液体充盈的十二指肠球部可伪似右上腹肿块影,在仰卧位,肿块影较难辨认,钡餐检查证实该软组织包块实为十二指肠球部所致。

第二十五篇　空、回肠疾病

第一章　淋巴瘤

第一节　小肠动脉瘤性淋巴瘤

Norfray 等 (1973) 报告 2 例小肠动脉瘤性淋巴瘤，观察此病早、晚期 X 线表现的变化。淋巴瘤不引起纤维性反应，它沿小肠长轴浸润，肠曲变得无力与扩张。

半卧位 X 线平片示腹部包块伴气液平；排泄性泌尿系造影或钡灌肠可见泌尿系或结肠被挤压移位；小肠检查可见急性肠腔扩张，早期伴存“粗糙”黏膜表现，晚期即见黏膜完全性破坏；邻近肠袢为肿瘤侵犯的肠壁所推移；因为动脉瘤段肠袢蠕动缺如，远端肠袢常见延迟充盈；残余食物与分泌物混合造成扩张肠段钡剂呈现斑驳状。

鉴别诊断包括：局限性肠炎，任何原因的纤维化继发肠袢扩张、硬皮病、皮肌炎、重复囊肿和美克尔憩室。黏膜与肠壁的表现有助于鉴别诊断。

第二节　误诊病例简介：回肠 T 细胞相关性（巨大）淋巴瘤伴破裂与肠壁型间质瘤

患者，女，50 岁。于 2 个月前无明显诱因出现腹泻，呈水样便，每天约 3~8 次，无里急后重，无黏液脓血便，反复多次于外院就诊，给予输液治疗，症状无明显缓解，进而出现下腹隐痛、腹胀，进食后明显，于上周就诊我院行胃镜检查提示“浅表性溃疡”，行腹腔 CT 检查，近期体重减轻约 6 kg。

CT：腹腔下部内可见一巨大囊性异常混杂密度影，大小约 17.7 cm × 8.4 cm × 11cm，囊腔两侧可见与回肠相通，病灶内可见多量含脂肪和钙斑的内容物，管壁不规则增厚，最厚处 2.4cm。局部边界欠清楚，周围肠管、子宫、膀胱受压移位。CT 诊断：下腹部囊性占位，肠壁型间质瘤？建议 CT 增强扫描、小肠镜检查。次日 CT 增强扫描：增强三期扫描管壁实性部分呈中度强化，CT 值 73~78HU，局部边界欠清楚，周围肠管、子宫、膀胱受压移位。CT 诊断：下腹部囊性占位，考虑来源于回肠肠壁型间质瘤。

手术所见：距回肠末端 50cm 见 18cm × 10cm × 8cm 肿物，已破溃，并被大网膜与周围组织粘连包裹，破溃肠管内有肠内容溢出，无明显外溢，肿瘤占据下腹部及盆腔，侵犯膀胱、子宫陷凹，系膜根部及腹主动脉旁见肿大淋巴结。

病理检查：回肠肿瘤切除标本：肠管一段，长 40cm，直径 2cm，在距一端 15cm，另一端 20cm 的肠壁及肠系膜处可见一结节样肿物，肿物大小 7cm × 5cm × 2.5cm，切面灰白质软，呈鱼肉状，与周围界限不清。肠系膜淋巴结：灰白色组织一块，大小 0.6cm × 0.4cm × 0.4cm。常规病理诊断：回肠肿瘤切除标本：初步诊断非霍奇金淋巴瘤，瘤组织浸润肠壁全层及肠系膜，待做免疫组化及原位杂交检测进一步分型。肠管一侧切缘为阴性，另一侧切缘及另送肠系膜淋巴结可见瘤组织累及。

免疫组化诊断：回肠肿瘤切除标本：回肠 T 细胞相关性淋巴瘤伴破裂（图 25-1-1）。

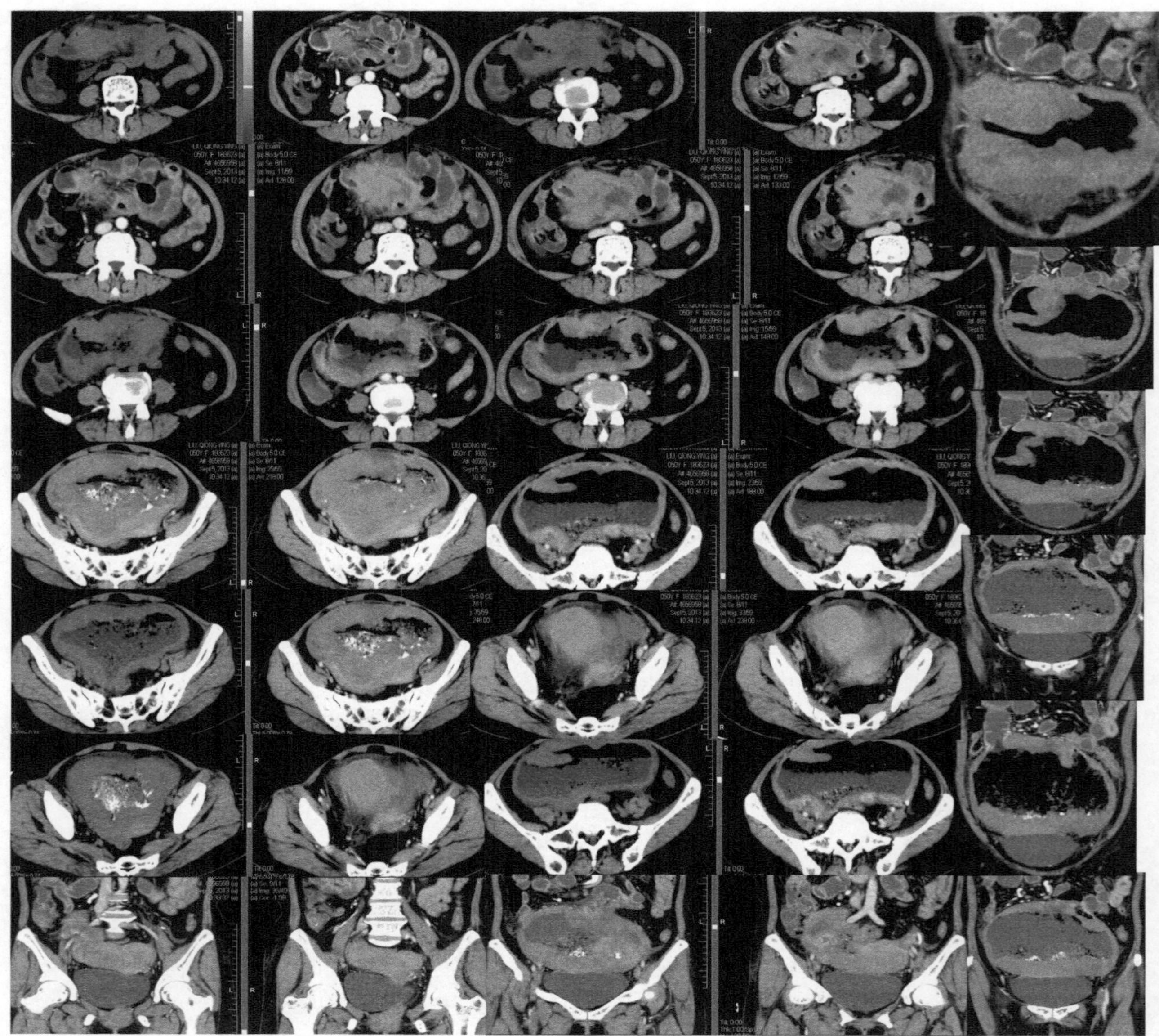

图 25-1-1　回肠 T 细胞相关性(巨大)淋巴瘤伴破裂与肠壁型间质瘤

第三节　小肠与阑尾弥漫性大 B 细胞淋巴瘤

患者,女,47 岁。右下腹闷痛 5 个月余入院。

手术所见:肝、脾、胰、胃、十二指肠、空肠、回肠、结肠均未见异常,盆腔及腹膜未见种植转移,末段回肠距回盲部约 15cm 处,可见一肿物生长侵犯出浆膜外,肿瘤直径约 7cm 大小,与阑尾粘连,质硬,肠系膜见数个肿大淋巴结。

病理检查,阑尾及小肠肿瘤切除标本见:①恶性肿瘤伴坏死,倾向淋巴瘤,待做免疫组化及原位杂交检测进一步分类,肿物位于浆膜下,侵犯内外肌层;肠管近、远切端均为阴性,肠周及肠系膜检出淋巴结 4 枚,均未见肿瘤组织累及;②阑尾呈慢性炎,未见肿瘤组织累及。免疫组化诊断:阑尾及小肠肿瘤切除标本:免疫组化及原位杂交检测支持弥漫大 B 细胞淋巴瘤(生发中心 B 细胞样型)(图 25-1-2)。

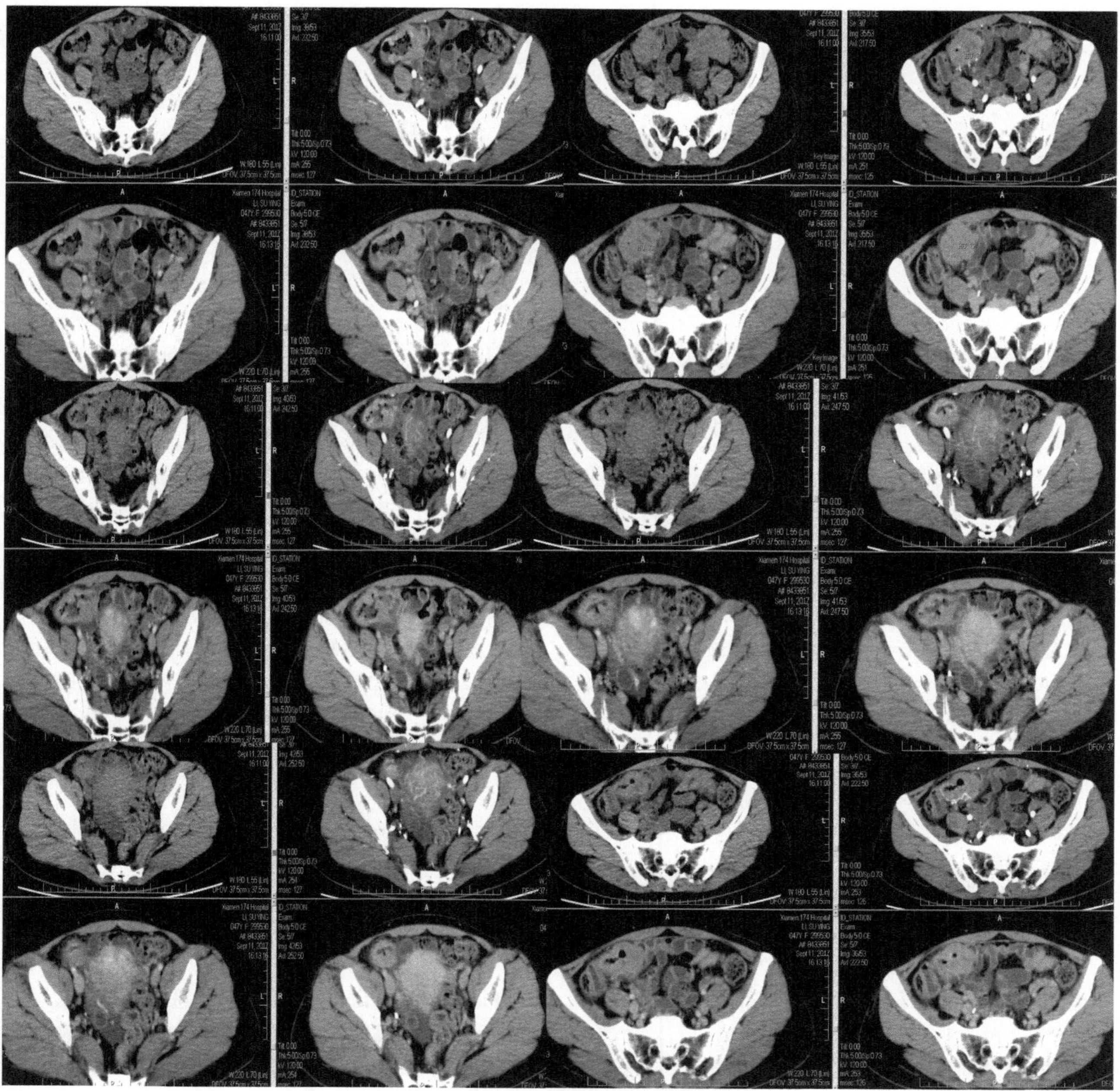

图 25-1-2　小肠与阑尾弥漫性大 B 细胞淋巴瘤

第二章 小肠间质瘤

第一节 不典型小肠恶性间质瘤的 MSCT 表现(误诊讨论)

胃肠道间质瘤 (GIST) 是消化道最常见的原发性间叶组织源性肿瘤，最常见于胃，小肠次之。以前病理学上多将其诊断为平滑肌源性或神经源性肿瘤，随着免疫组织化学、电子显微镜等的发展应用，目前国内外学者多认为它是具有非定向分化特征的间质肿瘤。

典型的小肠间质瘤 CT 表现为不规则实性或囊实性肿块，肿块多富血供，可有囊变、坏死，钙化少见，囊变、坏死可明显或较轻，钙化多呈斑点状。当小肠间质瘤完全囊变或伴有粗大、包环样钙化时，则诊断困难；为加深此类肿瘤的认识，一些作者回顾性分析经手术病理证实的 7 例不典型小肠恶性间质瘤 (6 例完全囊变，5 例有粗大或包环样钙化) 的 CT 表现及其病理基础，以期能对有此征象的小肠间质瘤的诊断及认识有所帮助。

胃肠道间质瘤是一类通常表达 C-kit(CD117) 的以富于梭形和上皮样细胞为特征的间叶组织源性肿瘤，涵盖了过去长期将其诊断为消化道平滑肌(肉)瘤或神经源性肿瘤。胃肠道间质瘤可发生于任何年龄，临床中以 50 岁以上的中老年人多见，男女发病率各家报道不一，一组 7 例，男 3 例，女 4 例，发病年龄 45~75 岁，平均 (58.3 ± 9.3) 岁，与文献报道相符。

临床表现以腹部包块、腹部不适及消化道出血多见。

根据瘤体内各自成分的比例优势，小肠恶性间质瘤可分为实性、囊实性或完全囊性。囊性肿瘤瘤体内囊性成分≥ 90% 以上，实性肿瘤瘤体内实性成分≥ 90% 以上，囊实性肿瘤瘤体囊性及实性成分介于 10%~90%。

该组 7 例不典型小肠恶性间质瘤，6 例为囊性肿瘤，1 例为实性肿瘤。

肿瘤的强化形式分为均质或不均质强化，强化程度分为轻度强化、中度强化、明显强化。以动脉期为参照标准，轻度强化为瘤体动脉期强化较平扫期增加 10~20 HU；中度强化为瘤体动脉期强化较平扫期增加 20~40 HU；明显强化为瘤体动脉期强化较平扫期增加 40 HU 以上。

该组 7 例不典型小肠恶性间质瘤，1 例囊实性肿瘤实性成分呈轻度强化，6 例囊性肿瘤的囊壁及囊内分隔呈轻度强化，随时间的延迟其强化程度略增加，并可出现壁结节样强化。

实性肿瘤以梭形细胞为主，大多呈交叉串状和栅栏状排列，瘤体内可出现明显的出血、胶原化、黏液样变，致瘤体密度不均；囊性肿瘤多为瘤体内陈旧性出血或液化、坏死所致，肿瘤细胞呈束状分布，胞界不清，核呈长卵圆形。

关于小肠肿瘤良、恶性的鉴别，CT 并无优势，参照 Fletcher 及 Miettinen 等的良、恶性标准，恶性指标有：①肿瘤浸润性，可侵犯局部黏膜、肌层和邻近器官；②瘤体浸润脉管或瘤体血管瘤栓形成；③肿瘤性坏死；④邻近或远处器官的转移；⑤核分裂象 >10/50 HPF；⑥肿瘤直径 >4.0cm。

该组 7 例不典型小肠间质瘤均表现为恶性，6 例出现了肿瘤性坏死，7 例核分裂象均 >10/50 HPF，6 例瘤体直径 >5 cm，仅 1 例瘤体短径 <4 cm (3.5 cm)，但长径 >4 cm(4.8 cm)，肺转移 1 例，肝脏转移 2 例。与文献报道相符。

小肠间质瘤钙化少见，且常见于恶性间质瘤。Hasegawa 等 (1998) 报道的 9 例中仅 1 例在手术标本中见到了钙化，CT 未见显示。

该组 7 例瘤体，5 例 CT 及手术标本均见到了钙化，且钙化均为粗大或包环样，与文献报道有一定差异，提示粗大或包环样钙化亦可是恶性间质瘤的一个征象。

该组 7 例不典型小肠恶性间质瘤，首次诊断正确者仅 1 例，误诊为小肠腺癌 2 例，误诊为复杂性肠源性囊肿 1 例，误诊为畸胎瘤 3 例。

根据该组 CT 表现并结合相关文献报道，不典型小肠恶性间质瘤有以下特征：①小肠边界清晰的椭圆形肿块，可完全囊变，实性肿瘤平扫呈等或稍高密度，囊性肿瘤呈低密度；②肿瘤有完整的包膜，瘤体周边可见粗大或包环样钙化影；③完全囊变的肿瘤可有厚壁，厚度不均匀，可引起肠穿孔改变；④增强扫描动脉期，实性肿瘤呈轻度强化，静脉期及延迟期强化可进一步持续，此特点与瘤体内血窦丰富，无动静脉瘘形成，窦内血流缓慢有关；⑤肿瘤囊性成分不强化，囊壁及囊内分隔轻度强化，且随时间延长，囊内分隔强化程度略增加，可有壁结节样的强化；⑥瘤体多呈外生性生长，较少引起肠梗阻，此表现与小肠腺癌及小肠克罗恩病有一定的差异；⑦瘤体直径多 >4 cm。

尽管 CT 在评估小肠间质瘤的良、恶性中并无明确诊断价值，但 CT 在发现早期病变、显示瘤体与系膜及肠管的解剖关系、评价肿瘤的直供及与周围血管的关系上具有明显的优势。

通过该组病例研究表明，粗大或包环样钙化可见于小肠恶性间质瘤，同时小肠恶性间质瘤亦可完全囊变，此 2 种征象在不典型小肠恶性间质瘤的诊断中具有一定的参考价值。

有关不典型小肠恶性间质瘤的 CT 表现还有待进一步积累、总结。但通过该项研究表明，不典型小肠恶性间质瘤可完全囊变，并可伴有粗大或包环样钙化，增强扫描，瘤体实性成分呈轻度强化；肿瘤囊性成分无强化，但囊壁及囊内分隔可有轻度强化，随增强时相的延长强化略增加，并可有壁结节样强化。

因此，充分认识上述不典型小肠恶性间质瘤的 CT 表现，可拓展临床及影像医师对此类肿瘤的诊断认识，对于提高该肿瘤的诊断认识及指导临床治疗有一定的作用。

第二节 胃肠道间质瘤

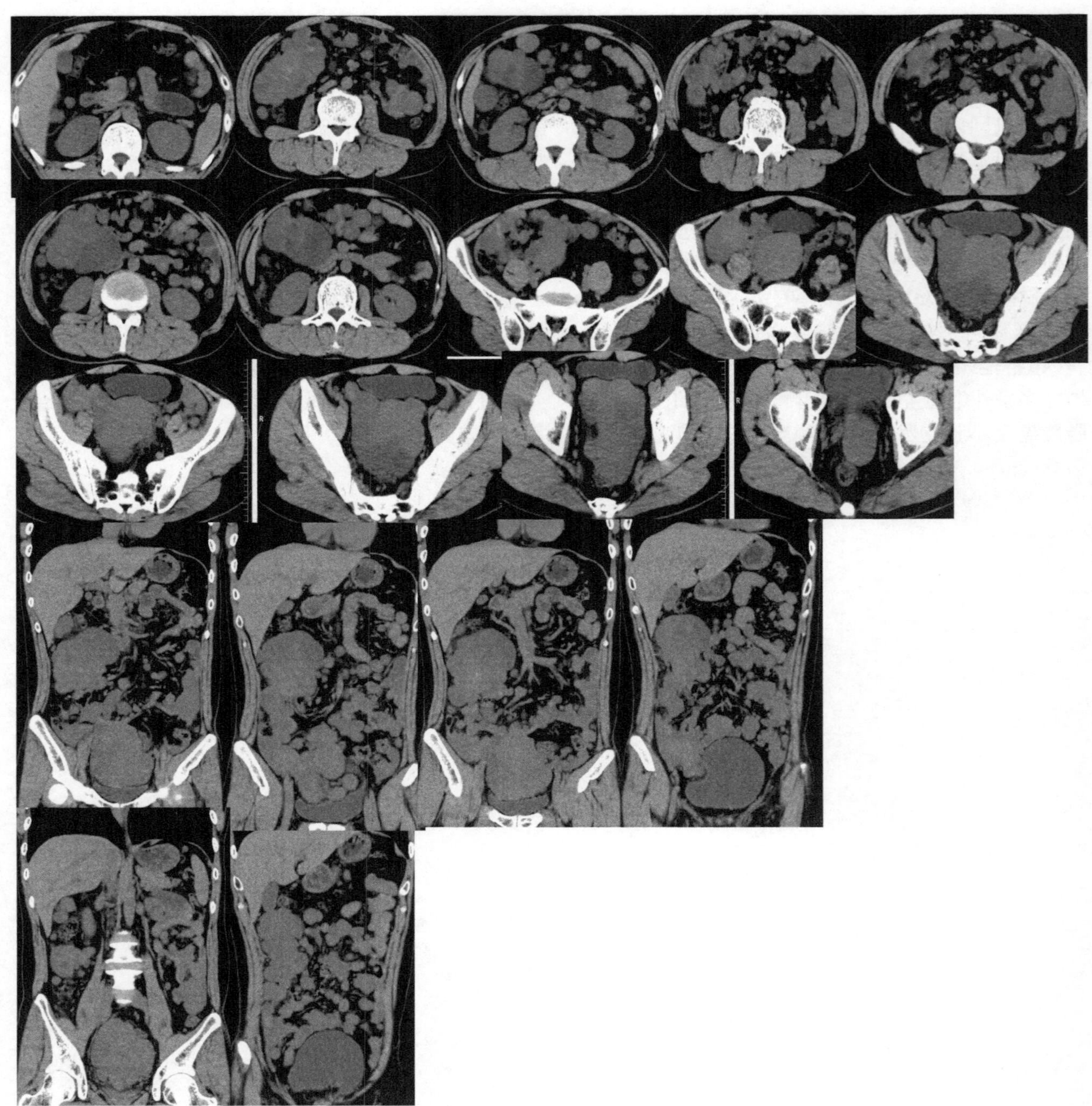

图 25-2-1 胃肠道间质瘤

患者,男, 44 岁。腹痛 3 天入院。患者自诉 3 天前出现腹部闷痛,症状逐渐加重,起床活动、走路时明显,伴有大便习惯改变,稀便,色黑、每天约 2~3 次,伴反酸、闷痛。

病理检查:灰褐色穿刺组织一堆,总体积 0.2cm × 0.2cm × 0.1cm。常规病理诊断:腹腔肿物穿刺活检标本:梭形细胞肿瘤,待免疫组化检测进一步明确肿瘤类型。免疫组化诊断:腹腔肿物穿刺活检标本:免疫组化检测结果支持胃肠道间质瘤。注:请注意肿瘤位置是否在胃肠道,偶尔胃肠道间质瘤可发生在胃肠道外的组织(图 25-2-1)。

第三节　不同侵袭危险度的小肠间质瘤

胃肠道间质瘤 (GIST) 是消化道最常见的间叶组织来源的具有潜在恶性的肿瘤，60%~70% 发生在胃部，20%~30% 发生在小肠，而胃肠道其他部位(如大肠、网膜、肠系膜及食管)的发生率不足 10%。有报道起源于小肠壁的间质瘤较起源于胃壁的肿瘤具有更高的侵袭性。

Fletcher 等 (2002) 报道的美国国立卫生研究院 (NIH) 会议的分类原则作为危险级别的判断标准：极低危险，肿瘤直径≤ 2cm，核分裂象 <5/50 高倍镜视野 (HPF)；低危险，肿瘤直径 2~5cm，核分裂象 <5/50HPF；中危险，肿瘤直径 <5cm，核分裂象 6~10/50HPF，或直径 5~10cm，核分裂象 <5/50HPF；高危险，肿瘤直径 >5cm，核分裂象 >5/50HPF，或肿瘤直径 >10cm，无论任何程度的核分裂象，或任意大小肿瘤，但核分裂象 >10/50HPF。

病理及临床生物学特性：胃肠间质瘤的概念是由 Mazur 等 (1983) 提出，是发生在胃肠道最常见的间质来源的肿瘤，组织学上富含梭形细胞、上皮样细胞或多形性细胞，呈束状、弥漫状排列，免疫表型上表达 CD117，遗传学上存在频发性 ckit 基因以及血小板源生长因子受体 α 基因。好发部位以胃最多见，小肠其次，然后是胃肠道其他部位。患者多为 40 岁以上，临床症状主要取决于肿瘤的大小、部位，但大多数患者没有临床症状。

目前普遍认为胃肠间质瘤为恶性或潜在恶性肿瘤，而发生于小肠的间质瘤较其他部位相同大小的间质瘤更具侵袭性，临床上多采用恶性程度分级来评估，因此病变的危险度就成了目前临床上最关心的问题。恶性程度越高，死亡率越高，复发和转移也就越常见。

间质瘤最主要的两大转移途径是血源播散和腹膜种植，肝脏和腹膜是最常见的转移部位，且原发灶大部分为来源于小肠的间质瘤。骨、肺和脑转移非常罕见，仅有个案报道。对于淋巴转移仍有争议，以前的报道认为淋巴转移很少见，如发现腹腔内广泛淋巴结转移应考虑其他疾病。最近的研究表明淋巴途径也是间质瘤的转移途径，特别是 <40 岁的年轻人，转移率高达 25 %。

MSCT 征象以及与侵袭危险度相关性：有资料表明间质瘤恶性程度与 CT 表现之间存在一定相关性。一组 32 例不同危险度组胃肠间质瘤间肿块形态是否规则、密度是否均匀、脂肪间隙是否清晰、有无血管样强化的差异均有统计学意义，并且肿块的形态是否规则在低危与中危、高危间有统计学意义，肿瘤的密度是否均匀在低危和高危间有统计学意义，说明肿瘤的危险性越高，形态越不规则，密度也就越不均匀。这些与 Wong 等 (2011) 认为肿瘤直径 >5 cm、不均匀强化、中间囊变及中央坏死提示恶性程度较高基本相符。

根据美国国立卫生研究院规定的危险级别判断标准，可以看出肿瘤危险程度主要是根据肿块直径的大小来划分的。该组研究中的肿块经病理证实后发现随着恶性度的增高，平均直径也逐渐增大，因此该研究未将肿块的大小做统计学分析。另外有文献认为钙化为恶性间质瘤的指标，但该组病例钙化少见，仅有 2 例，1 例为低度恶性，1 例为高度恶性。

由于肿瘤的生长依赖于新生血管的生成，MSCT 的增强扫描及重建图像可清晰的显示肿瘤血供的基础病理特征。该组结果表明 32 例胃肠间质瘤中动态增强中静脉期强化程度均高于动脉期，其中 29 例呈中高度明显强化，18 例可见血管样强化及大部分可见间隔样强化。这与一些学者报道的小肠相对较常见的其他肿瘤如淋巴瘤不强化或轻度强化、腺癌不均匀明显强化但静脉期强化程度低于动脉期等相比有明显的不同。

此外，该组病例中强化峰值在低危、中危及高危 3 组肿块间差异无统计学意义。因此肿瘤实质部分呈中高度明显强化、静脉期强化程度高于动脉期可作为胃肠道间质瘤表现特征之一，而强化峰值不能成为胃肠间质瘤侵袭危险度的评估指标。

该组胃肠间质瘤发生的部位以空肠最多，最少为十二指肠，这与一些文献报道相仿。但是各发生部位侵袭危险度未见明显差异。由于 5 例病灶呈向腔外生长型(即浆膜下型)被误诊为混合生长型(即肌壁间型)，因此未对肿瘤的病理学类型进行统计学分析，但是该组病理结果显示以腔外型生长比例较高。腔内生长者可以产生中心溃疡,严重者出现肿块内气液平或穿孔。32 例肿瘤中 14 例侵犯周围组织,其中高危 9 例,中危 4 例,低危 1 例,提示侵袭危险度越高,出现周围侵犯的可能性越大,但侵袭危险度较低的病例也可出现周围侵犯。该组 1 例低危、3 例中危及 5 例高危病例出现肠系膜侵犯,4 例高危和 1 例中危病例发生肝转移。

术前见淋巴结肿大者 3 例,术后病理均显示为淋巴结反应性增生,这与文献报道 >40 岁的患者淋巴转移少见相符。据报道间质瘤导致肠梗阻少见,可能与肿瘤生长于黏膜下层的平滑肌层及外生性生长有关,该组仅 1 例发生肠梗阻。

小肠属于空腔脏器,由于胃肠道钡餐造影检查重点显示肠腔内病变,对腔外侵犯情况难以定性及判断,因此对胃肠间质瘤危险性评估作用有限;MRI 具有良好的软组织分辨力和多种功能成像,并且有文献报道 DWI 对间质瘤危险度的评估,但是 DWI 图像本身易受呼吸运动、胃肠道蠕动及气体等很多因素影响。ROI 取值部位和范围也会影响结果,诊断及评估时仍需结合其他多项指标,并且 MRI 对钙化的显示不够直观,加上检查价格相对较贵。因此一些作者认为 MSCT 由于具有良好的空间分辨力及强大的后处理功能,成为了胃肠间质瘤危险性评价的首选方法,从而为临床制定合理的治疗方案提供参考。

第四节 小肠胃肠道间质瘤(中等危险度或潜在恶性)

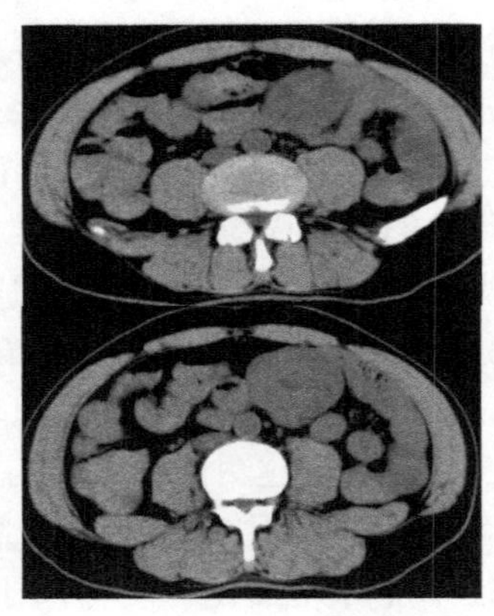

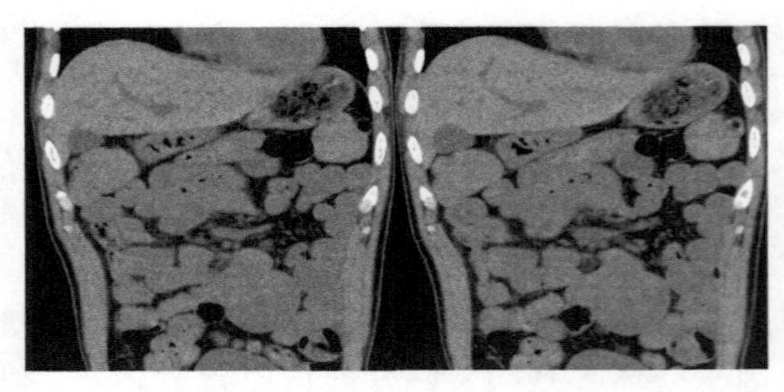

图 25-2-2 小肠胃肠道间质瘤(中等危险度或潜在恶性)

患者,男,45 岁。无明显诱因出现恶心、呕吐,呕吐进餐食物,无呕吐咖啡色胃内容物及鲜红色血迹,随后排大量柏油样黑便 2 次,每次量约 250ml,呈糊状,伴头晕、心慌、盗汗、四肢抽搐及肢端发凉,家属诉患者伴有意识不清,持续数秒钟后意识恢复正常,无腹痛、发热,无摔倒、偏瘫、失语等。

病理检查:小肠肿瘤切除标本:肠管一段,长 7cm,直径 2.5cm,距一切缘 4.5cm,距另一切缘 4cm 的肠表面见一结节状肿物,大小 6.5cm × 5cm × 4.5cm,肿物切面灰红灰黄,质中,肠系膜处未检出淋巴结样物。常规病理诊断:小肠浆膜梭形细胞肿瘤,大小,伴多灶性出血坏死,与肠壁粘连并浸润肌层,倾向胃肠道间质瘤 (GIST),待免疫组化协助确诊。小肠黏膜慢性炎,两切缘均阴性。

免疫组化检测:阳性:CD117(+++),DOG1 (+++),CD34(+),Vimentin(+++),Nestin(+++),Ki-67(+,<5%);阴性:S-100,SMA,CK(P),Calponin。免疫组化诊断:小肠肿瘤切除标本:胃肠道间质瘤 (GIST,中等危险度或潜在恶性)(图 25-2-2)。

第五节 小肠系膜恶性间质瘤

胃肠道间质瘤是一种较少见的肿瘤,表现为一种不成熟的梭形细胞或上皮细胞增殖。由 Mazur

和 Clark(1983) 首次报道。绝大多数胃肠道间质瘤存在 c-kit 前癌基因变异，表达 CD117 和 CD34。该病多见于 55~65 岁，中位年龄 60 岁。好发部位依次为胃 60% ~70%、小肠 20% ~30%、结直肠 5%、网膜、肠系膜 3% ~4%。腹部 CT 表现为低密度肿块，中心可有坏死液化。临床上早期多无症状，随着肿瘤的生长才出现相应的症状，主要表现为消化道出血、腹部肿块、腹痛和消化道梗阻等。触诊可触及肿块。

第六节　小肠胃肠道间质瘤

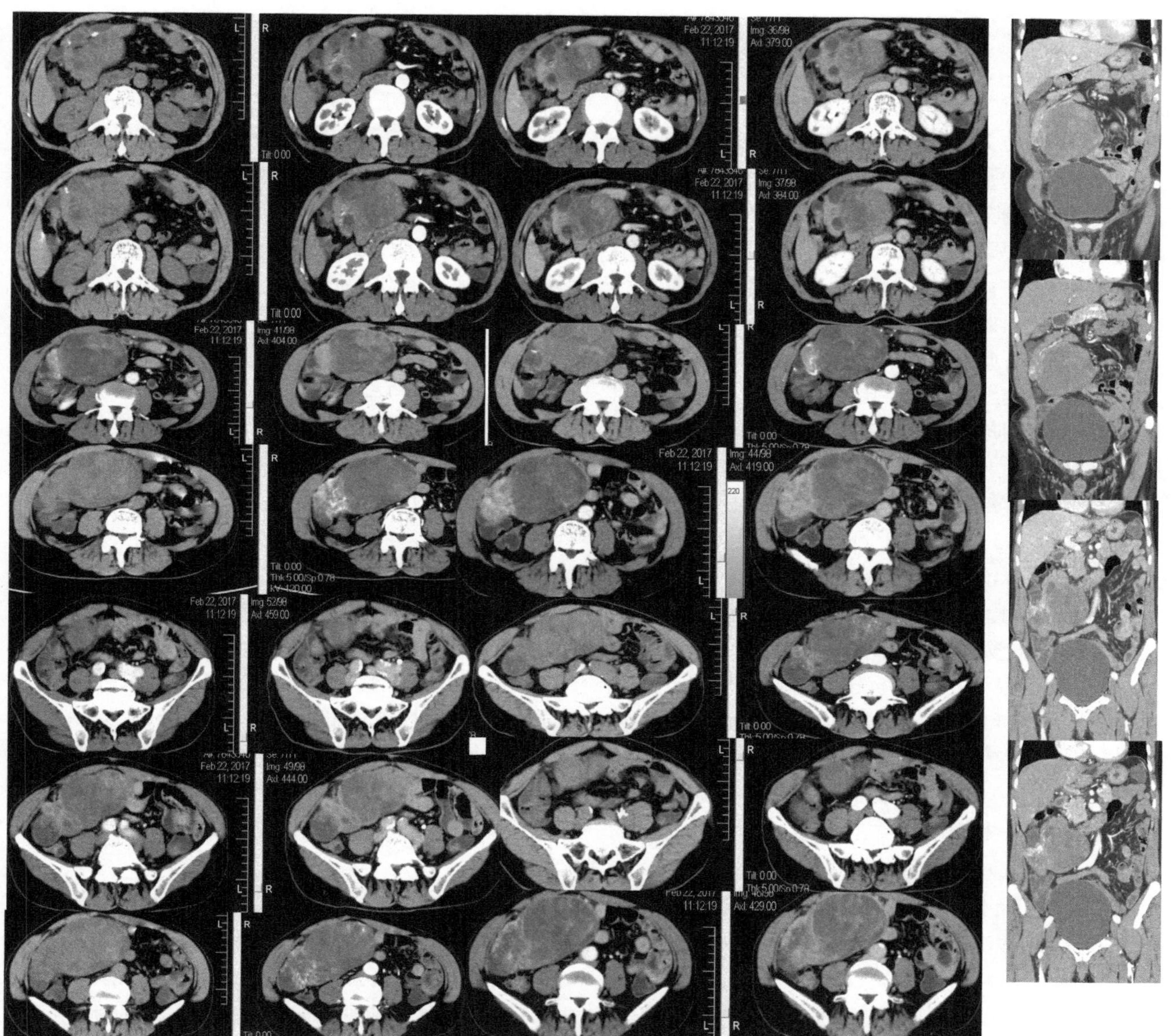

图 25-2-3　小肠胃肠道间质瘤

患者，男，68 岁。发现腹部肿物 20 余天入院。患者缘于 20 天前无意间发现下腹部一肿物，就诊外院行彩超提示：左侧腹腔混合回声肿块可能。

手术所见：距离屈氏韧带约 10cm 处空肠上段可见肿瘤，约 15cm × 10cm × 8cm 大小，质中偏软，包膜完整，肿物似未侵出浆膜层，但有丝絮状附着物与周围肠管及大网膜粘连，肠管轻度水肿扩张。

病理检查:“小肠肿瘤切除标本”:灰褐色结节状肿物一块,大小 14.5cm×9cm×6.5cm,切面灰白暗褐,伴出血及大片坏死,质中偏软,肿物周围大部区域有包膜,局部附着肠管一段,长 9cm,管腔直径 1.5cm,肿物与肠壁局灶粘连,肠黏膜皱襞存在,未见明显异常。常规病理诊断:“小肠肿瘤切除标本”:梭形细胞肿瘤伴坏死,可见瘤组织疑似起源于小肠固有肌层。

免疫组化检测:阳性:CD117, DOG-1, Vimentin, Catenin-β(浆+), Ki-67(+, 约 10%), Bcl-2, NSE(灶+), P53(+, 约 30%);阴性:CD34, H-caldesmon, SMA, Desmin, Actin, CD99, S-100, Sox-10, CK(P), MyoD1, Myogenin, Calponin, CD57。免疫组化诊断:胃肠道间质瘤(GIST,高危险度),瘤细胞较丰富(图 25-2-3)。

第七节 关于小肠间质瘤及小肠肿物的影像诊断思维

小肠间质瘤是起源于小肠干细胞的间叶起源的肿瘤,好发部位为十二指肠和空肠。小肠间质瘤在胃肠道肿瘤中所占比例不足 1%,然而随着对小肠间质瘤认识的提高,以往所诊断的部分胃肠道平滑肌瘤和神经鞘瘤应归属胃肠道间质瘤范畴,因而小肠间质瘤发病率逐年上升趋势。小肠钡餐检查和纤维肠镜检查难以观察腔外情况,对小肠间质瘤的检查效果不理想;此外,小肠间质瘤的恶性程度相对于其他部位胃肠道间质瘤要更高,在所有的胃肠道间质瘤中小肠间质瘤预后最差,因而认识小肠这一特殊部位胃肠道间质瘤的影像表现和生物学特性更具意义。小肠间质瘤的生物学行为为潜在恶性,其发病年龄在 55~65 岁,临床上可无明显症状,也可表现为腹痛、黑便等消化道症状。

小肠间质瘤影像表现有三大特点:①肿块大小形态特点。小肠肿瘤多为不规则形态肿块,肿块较大,肿块长径最大可达 30 cm。②肿块位置。好发生在十二指肠和空肠,回肠较少,腔外生长,形成腔外肿块,较少发生梗阻。③生长方式特点。生长特点表观为膨胀生长方式,即表现为即使小肠间质瘤肿块很大,肿块对周围器官及结构仅仅挤压、推移的膨胀性生长的改变,少见包埋、浸润周围结构。

综上所述,小肠 GIST 的 CT 表现为边界清晰的肿块,肿块通常比较大,强化明显,伴出血和坏死,腔外生长,少有肠梗阻。

MRI 表现为实性部分 T_1WI 呈低信号,T_2WI 呈高信号,增强后明显强化,瘤内出血可因时间不同而在 T_1WI 及 T_2WI 上呈现多样的 MRI 信号。高风险小肠间质瘤可出现腹腔淋巴结肿大及远处器官转移。

影像医生需读懂“病理学家的二个共识”。第一个共识:胃肠道间质瘤的病理诊断共识。组织学上小肠间质瘤与平滑肌肿瘤、神经鞘瘤光镜下均表现为间叶源性梭型细胞,部分亚型无法在组织学上做出明确诊断。针对这一问题,病理学家通过组织学结合免疫组化对胃肠道间质瘤病理诊断达成的共识是:①组织学形态符合典型胃肠道间质瘤、CD117 和 DOG1 阳性;②组织学形态符合典型胃肠道间质瘤、CD117 和 DOG1 阴性的病例,病理学进一步的检测存在 c-kit 或 PDGFRA 基因的突变,才能诊断;③组织学符合典型胃肠道间质瘤、CD117 和 DOG1 阴性的病例,病理学进一步检测无 c-kit 或 PDGFRA 基因的突变,排除其他类型的肿瘤,如平滑肌肿瘤、神经鞘瘤和神经纤维瘤等,可做出野生型胃肠道间质瘤的诊断。

第二个共识:胃肠道间质瘤的良恶性判定的共识。小肠间质瘤作为潜在恶性肿瘤,病理学家根据肿瘤的部位、大小及核分裂比例、是否发生破裂等来评估胃肠道间质瘤的恶性风险达成共识,胃肠道间质瘤分为良性、恶性潜能未定和恶性三大类,风险度分为极低风险、低风险、中等风险和高风险。

小肠肿物主要包括上皮性肿瘤、非上皮样肿瘤、内分泌肿瘤和肿瘤样变,小肠间质瘤属于非上皮样肿瘤。

小肠肿物的影像诊断思维分为四步,第一步为定位,应结合 CT 薄层及三维重建多角度观察明确病变来源及位置,准确的定位直接影响后续的定性;第二步为定性,即观察肿块影像特点进而做出明确的诊断,定性的细节包括以下方面:①分析病变影像表现,即病变的直接征象,包括病变的大小、形态、密度及瘤内情况,小肠肠壁、管腔及周围间接征象。②鉴别小肠肿瘤与非肿瘤病变,根据病变影像表现鉴别小肠肿瘤与非肿瘤病变,因为小肠肿瘤需要手术,而炎性肠病可以保守治疗。③对小肠肿瘤做出影像定性诊断。需要强调的是应认识到影像方法对定性诊断的局限性，尽可能的多收集临床信息可获得更准确的影像定性诊断；第三步为病灶手术可切除性的评估，包括肿块邻近肠管系膜累及情况，手术切除范围，周围淋巴结情况；第四步为病理结果判读，病理结果将决定生物学行为预测及术后随访。

小肠占位的四步影像诊断思维：第一步，结合CT薄层及MPR多角度观察明确病变定位于十二指肠水平段。第二步，定性为小肠间质瘤，即观察肿块影像特点进而做出明确的诊断，理论依据包括：①肿块的特点为肿块大，强化明显，肿块腔外生长，管腔狭窄程度轻，因而不易发生肠梗阻。②鉴别小肠肠壁无明显水肿，周围无渗出，累及范围局限，明显形成肿块，因而为小肠肿瘤，而非小肠非肿瘤病变。③小肠GIST的诊断和鉴别诊断。小肠间质瘤最需要鉴别的是小肠淋巴瘤和小肠腺癌，小肠淋巴瘤肿块较柔软，这主要是由于肌层和自主神经丛的弥漫破坏而不引起促结缔组织反应. 导致病变小肠壁张力减弱和顺应性下降，肠管扩张形成空腔样的肿块，强化程度低而均匀。小肠腺癌黏膜破坏形成腔内肿块，管腔狭窄，这点亦不同于小肠间质瘤的腔外生长特点。第三步，该病灶局限，累及肠管范围小，腹腔无淋巴结肿大，手术可完全病灶局限切除达到根治。第四步，该病例镜下病理结合免疫组化CD117阳性，病理确诊为小肠间质瘤。肿瘤大小为3.5 cm，核分裂比例≤ 5个/50 HPF为低风险，转移和肿瘤相关病死率小于2%，随访时间为6个月，持续5年。

总之，小肠间质瘤具有肿块大、强化明显、腔内外生长、肠腔狭窄与梗阻少见等影像学特点. 认识小肠间质瘤影像特征和病理复杂性的特点，有助于理解小肠占位的影像诊断思维在小肠间质瘤临床实践中的重要意义。

第三章　空回肠其他恶性肿瘤

第一节　空回肠类癌

病理学:空回肠类癌常较小,极少超过 3.5 cm。相反,其转移灶却可长得很大而使原发灶被忽视。30% 的病例为多发肿瘤。肠嗜铬细胞类癌可表现为肠壁内多发坚硬小结节,也可像息肉样向管腔内突出并可导致肠套叠。更典型的表现是,肿块透过肠壁累及浆膜下和邻近肠系膜,若累及范围广,则局部组织受刺激而出现大量成纤维反应并导致肠腔狭窄、成角等。

镜下,可见位于肌层纤维之间的明显瘤细胞巢。这些瘤细胞索带浸润肌层,在浆膜下形成局灶性瘤结节。瘤细胞浸润生长并分泌 5- 羟色胺使局部组织出现致密纤维化,这种改变尤以黏膜下和邻近肠系膜明显。肿瘤分泌物可使邻近或远隔肠系膜血管壁增厚、管腔变窄或阻塞,这种表现被称为“弹力血管硬化”,从而导致肠缺血。

临床表现:大部分空回肠类癌是含 P 物质、产生 5- 羟色胺、嗜银阳性的肠嗜铬细胞肿瘤。一般来讲,绝大部分小肠肠嗜铬细胞类癌表现为恶性生物学行为,产生肝脏及淋巴结转移。患者常无症状,若有症状则往往由于肿块局部占位效应或转移至它处引起。肿块可导致小肠梗阻,缺血或出血。某些患者有长期间断性的腹部绞痛及体重减轻、虚弱、腹胀、腹泻、恶心或呕吐。当出现肝脏及腹膜后淋巴结转移时常产生类癌综合征。

影像学研究:空回肠类癌依据其肿块的大小、肠系膜累及范围、有无转移灶等出现不同的表现。肠壁黏膜和黏膜下多发息肉或结节样小病灶适合用小肠钡剂造影来检查。典型病灶常位于回肠末端,为孤立或多发圆形光整的结节或仅见黏膜隆起,通常表现为边界光滑的充盈缺损,而肠腔显示不对称性狭窄较少见,在病变的早期阶段出现肠梗阻或肠套叠的情况十分少见。随着病变向黏膜下浸润,逐渐出现肠壁增厚,有时可见环形或向心性肠腔狭窄。

当病变进一步发展,肠系膜纤维化形成时,常常可见肠壁较广泛的甚至是弥漫性的狭窄、僵硬、成角以及黏膜皱襞僵硬、毛糙等改变。时间更长的病灶会使相应肠道血管受压、阻塞导致小肠出现慢性缺血的改变。病灶表面黏膜可因溃疡而出现龛影。多发小病灶 CT 扫描常无法检出,但大的息肉样病灶可以检出。

MRI T_1 增强压脂可显示中度强化的多发结节或局部肠壁增厚。CT 也可显示肠壁对称或不对称增厚,这多是肿瘤浸润致黏膜下纤维化的结果,偶尔也可由肠壁缺血所致。

而肿瘤浸润及黏膜下纤维化还可导致肠壁僵硬成角或弯曲(也称“发夹样弯曲”),钡餐透视可直观显示受累肠道的僵硬固定及弯曲成角,CT 则可发现肠壁增厚、扭曲。通常断面影像即足以确定肠道僵硬成角的改变,但有时仍需 CT 冠状重建来观察。

肠嗜铬细胞类癌还可直接侵犯血管,引起血管堵塞导致局部或广泛肠缺血。肠缺血的表现包括肠壁增厚呈环形低密度,靶征,晕环征等。肿瘤浸润透过肠壁伴随邻近组织纤维化或出现肝转移时 CT、MRI 显示较好。可见肠壁向心性狭窄及狭窄处软组织肿块。局部纤维化导致的肠道弯曲纠结、成角可引起完全或不完全性肠梗阻。58%~64% 的小肠类癌在得到诊断时已出现肝脏或淋巴结转移。肠系膜转移时可见肠系膜内多发肿大淋巴结、边缘清楚或有毛刺边缘不规则的肿块。肿瘤分泌的激素还可作用于肠系膜淋巴结,使得肠系膜挛缩以及肠系膜上出现 CT 可显示的软组织密度线状影。一般讲,这些线状影多继发于局部纤维化而非肿瘤浸润。

CT 所示肠系膜肿块边缘毛刺化程度表现为肿块周围辐射状软组织密度线状影，与组织学上纤维化程度相关。这种纤维化可沿肠系膜血管排列呈“日光辐射”或“车轮”样表现。偶尔，肠系膜和腹膜腔病灶较广泛，形成粟粒样腹膜种植、多发较大肿块或网膜饼。

70% 肠系膜淋巴结转移可见钙化。钙化可以呈浅淡点状，也可粗大致密或弥漫。肠系膜肿块可出现强化，偶尔肿块内可见低密度区，代表肿瘤退变或坏死。空回肠类癌肝转移瘤通常是富血供病灶，在增强动脉期显示较好。病灶中央坏死或退变可无强化，因此在 CT、MRI 增强扫描时可表现为环形强化。鉴别诊断包括转移瘤、小肠腺癌、淋巴瘤、间质瘤。肠道特征性的固定成角、肠系膜肿块边缘毛刺强烈提示类癌。此外，克罗恩病和局限性缺血性肠炎也可出现类似类癌的改变。

第二节　麦克尔憩室类癌

麦克尔（Meckel）憩室内的类癌常单发、较小、没有症状，多是意外查出。

若产生症状则多是腹痛、出血、体重减轻、恶心、呕吐、腹泻等。生物学行为类似回肠类癌。由于病灶非常小，影像手段常难检出，但有时可见肝脏及淋巴结转移灶。

第三节　回肠原发性黑色素瘤

恶性黑色素瘤是一类起源于神经脊黑色素细胞的恶性肿瘤，恶性程度很高，其发病率约占全身恶性肿瘤的 1%~3%，近年来发病率呈上升趋势。本病好发于中老年人，90% 以上起源于皮肤，人体含有黑色素细胞的组织（如胃肠道、呼吸道、眼脉络膜等）也可发病；发生于小肠的黑色素瘤多为转移性（约占小肠转移性肿瘤的 50% 以上）。小肠原发性黑色素瘤罕见，临床及影像学表现缺乏特征性，术前诊断困难，误诊率高达 78%，预后差。

Sachs 等（1999）提出以下诊断标准：单发，无小肠外原发病灶，且无引流区域外淋巴结肿大，诊断后存活 1 年以上。腹痛（60%）、梗阻（47%）、呕吐（41%）、消化道出血（30%）和肿块（10%）等常为其主要的临床症状。

小肠气钡双重造影诊断本病的敏感性约为 58%，常规腹部 CT 的敏感性为 66%，多表现为肠腔内孤立性、偏心性肿块，浸润性生长，单发病灶常累及较大范围的肠管，肿块较大时可引起梗阻症状，常伴区域淋巴结转移；CT 增强扫描肿块呈明显均匀强化，病变区肠道黏膜破坏，肠壁水肿等，但均缺乏特异性。MSCT 增强扫描旨在明确肿瘤浸润程度，有无区域淋巴结转移，寻找肿瘤血管，评估可切除性及切除范围。

一例采用小肠 MSCT 检查技术，显示病灶、小肠肠腔、肠壁、肠系膜及其血管、淋巴结等，并进行肿瘤评估。发现肿瘤与周围组织局部分界欠清，未见明显区域淋巴结转移；最大密度投影、容积再现示肿瘤供血动脉为回结肠动脉，病变较局限，可行手术切除，切除范围包括肿瘤本身及其侵犯部分，与术中所见基本一致。

DSA 检查示肿瘤供血动脉增粗，局部可见狭窄、僵直现象，实质期见局限性团块状染色，肿瘤血管结构紊乱，静脉早显；该例因消化道出血行 DSA 检查，检查过程中未见新鲜出血。胃肠道内镜检查对本病的诊断价值有限。某些黑色素瘤，即使病理切片常规镜检也较难与其他分化较差的肿瘤相区别，联合应用 HMB45、Malen-A、S-100、Vimentin 等免疫组织化学指标，其特异性可达 90% 以上，且敏感性高。

小肠黑色素瘤恶性程度极高，预后差，5 年生存率低，早期行局部广泛性切除及区域淋巴结清扫术似可延长生存期但该种手术往往难以彻底，患者术后多死于转移或复发。

第四章 小肠包块

第一节 病理误诊病例简介:小肠炎性肌纤维母细胞瘤与间质瘤

小肠炎性肌纤维母细胞瘤是一种极少见的独特的间叶性肿瘤,虽然来源为间叶组织,但它有别于小肠间质瘤及平滑肌瘤。小肠炎性肌纤维母细胞瘤发生于成人小肠,并向小肠内生长,产生持续套叠的较为少见。

小肠炎性肌纤维母细胞瘤是一种少见而独特的由肿瘤性肌纤维母细胞、淋巴细胞、浆细胞等炎症细胞组成的肿瘤,表现为低度恶性或交界性肿瘤的特点。小肠炎性肌纤维母细胞瘤已被WHO列入软组织类肿瘤,多发生于儿童及青年患者。小肠炎性肌纤维母细胞瘤可发生于任何部位,好发于肺、腹部,肿块形态随发生部位不同而不同,形态及组织学变化多样,影像学表现为侵袭性占位性肿块,极易误诊。小肠炎性肌纤维母细胞瘤的发病原因与机制尚不清楚。小肠炎性肌纤维母细胞瘤可发生于消化系统任何部位,甚至可发生于麦克尔憩室内以及胆系内。大多发生于小肠系膜上或环小肠壁生长,发生于小肠腔内的小肠炎性肌成纤维细胞瘤与其他发生于小肠肠腔内的实质性占位肿瘤相比,气钡双对比造影检查时影像学表现无特异性,均表现为腔内肿块和不规则的充盈缺损,易误诊为恶性肿瘤。

小肠炎性肌纤维母细胞瘤患者症状与发生部位有关,发生于回肠的小肠炎性肌纤维母细胞瘤可引起回结肠的套叠,引发一系列消化道症状,发生于近段空肠的小肠炎性肌纤维母细胞瘤有肠穿孔的危险。一例发生于空回肠交界处,并造成了小肠与小肠的持续性套叠,引起消化道出血及不完全梗阻。

小肠炎性肌纤维母细胞瘤肉眼观多呈局限性或多灶性实质性肿块,也可呈息肉状,大小不等,直径1.0~20.0 cm,有时可有完整的包膜。镜下肿瘤主要由梭形细胞、数量不等的胶原细胞、淋巴细胞及浆细胞组成。

一些作者认为当组织含有丰富的梭形细胞,梭形细胞夹杂炎性细胞而形成类似纤维组织细胞瘤时,如发生在胃肠道则常被误诊为平滑肌瘤或间质瘤,所以要根据免疫组化来鉴别间质瘤与小肠炎性肌纤维母细胞瘤,仅凭HE染色见到肿瘤主要由丰富的梭形细胞组成就诊断为间质瘤是不可靠的。

Khoo等(2005)报道间质瘤的免疫组化结果为CD117(+)100%,CD34(+) 76.9%,Vimentin(+)61%,S-100(+)46. 1%,SMA(+)11.5%,Desmin(+)0%。有文献报道肌纤维母细胞间变型淋巴瘤激酶(ALK)阳性表达,小肠炎性肌纤维母细胞瘤的ALK阳性率可达60%(44/73),免疫组化抗ALK抗体有益于鉴别小肠炎性肌纤维母细胞瘤、平滑肌瘤和小肠间质瘤。该例ALK呈阳性表达,与文献报道一致。

附:具体病例资料:病例,男,64岁,20天前无明显诱因自觉中上腹不适,进食后感中上腹饱胀。每1~2天排质软、成形黑便一次,量中等,双下肢乏力,病程中无黏液脓血便。14天前在外院住院给予制酸、止血、输血等处理,自觉近3天大便颜色有所好转,但隐血仍呈阳性。患者病程中体重下降1.5~2 kg,既往有高血压、前期收缩及心脏肥大病史,有慢性便秘及高血糖病史。胃镜:慢性浅表性胃炎。腹腔超声:腹腔未探及游离液性暗区,腹膜后未见明显肿块,肝、胆、胰、脾未见异常。小肠气钡双对比造影:空、回肠交界处见一段肠管狭窄,对比剂通过缓慢,远端见一腔内“充盈缺损”,大小约5.0cm×3.5 cm,边缘光滑,狭窄段肠管外层可见“弹簧”状小肠黏膜,黏膜增宽,狭窄段肠管近端扩张不明显,气钡对比造影诊断:成人小肠内占位伴小肠套叠。手术:肿瘤位于距回盲部约150 cm的空回肠交界部位,局部肠管套叠长约20.0 cm,外套小肠肠管血流障碍,肿瘤直径约5.0 cm,向肠腔内突起,质韧,未穿出浆膜,周围未见肿大淋巴结。病理检查：病变小肠肠管一段长约 18.0cm，距一切缘 6.0cm 处见 3 cm × 3 cm × 2 cm 蒂息肉样物，切面灰白。镜下见肿瘤由梭形细胞组成，两切缘未见异常。病理诊断为间质瘤。

1 年后复习病例时，再将手术标本蜡块行免疫组化处理，镜下：HE 染色，见肿瘤由梭形细胞夹杂有大量炎性细胞及淋巴细胞组成，ALK(+)、CD117(-)、CD34：灶性 (+)、CD3(-)、CD15(-)、CD20(-)、CD30(-)、SMA：灶性 (+)、肿瘤细胞 S-100(-)。免疫组化诊断：小肠炎性纤维母细胞瘤。3 年后回访，患者术后未行任何化疗及后续治疗，生存、生活状态良好。

第二节　误诊病例简介：大部分钙化的空肠炎性肌纤维母细胞瘤与畸胎类肿瘤

炎性肌纤维母细胞瘤是一种少见的间叶组织肿瘤，其病因及发病机制尚不明确。以往曾被称为炎性假瘤、炎症性肌纤维母细胞增生等。大体病理和组织形态学上可被误诊为恶性肿瘤。基本病理改变为大量细长梭形的肌纤维母细胞及纤维母细胞增生伴不同程度的浆细胞、淋巴细胞等慢性炎性细胞浸润。文献报道瘤体内可有玻璃样变性、钙化及黏液样变性。全身各部位均可发生，最常见于肺部。可以发生于任何年龄，儿童和青少年较常见。

临床表现多为局部包块，因发生部位不同而伴随症状各异，部分病例无明显临床症状。据文献报道其影像学表现多样，缺乏特异性征象，较常见的 CT 及 MRI 表现是平扫多为单发软组织肿块，其边界清楚或不清，增强扫描呈均匀或不均匀轻、中度甚至显著强化。

一例为 41 岁中年男性，常规 B 超检查时意外发现，临床无特殊症状和体征。肿瘤发生于空肠上段，肿瘤下移至盆腔且几乎完全钙化，增强后仅边缘强化。CT 检查拟诊为畸胎类肿瘤，来源未确定。MRI 检查表现为以长 T_1 信号、稍长 T_2 信号为主的不均质肿块。如果没有 CT 检查还会误诊为平滑肌肿瘤、纤维瘤或间质瘤等，三者钙化少见，结合 CT 所见容易和上述肿瘤区别。

由于慢性炎性细胞的浸润，肿瘤与周围组织粘连并牵拉，术前定位、定性均与手术病理结果相差甚远，再加上瘤体如此多量的钙化使其具有了所谓的鲜明的“特征性”，这也是术前误诊的主要原因。文献报道本病钙化少见，钙化发生率在 5.0%~17.5%，且多为发生于肺内的肿瘤。一些学者报道的 18 例中 3 例有不同程度的钙化灶，均发生与肺内，钙化发生率为 17. 6%。另有作者报道的 1 例瘤体中心有大面积骨化。该例瘤体几乎完全钙化且来源于空肠上段，实属少见。手术切除是治疗炎性肌纤维母细胞瘤的首选方法。由于炎性肌纤维母细胞瘤有染色体 2p23 重排，使其具有克隆能力，同时瘤体具有侵袭、较少量的转移行为及局部复发倾向。所以术后定期复查很有必要。该例手术切除已 3 年，复查至今未见复发及远处转移。

第三节 小肠梭形细胞肿瘤

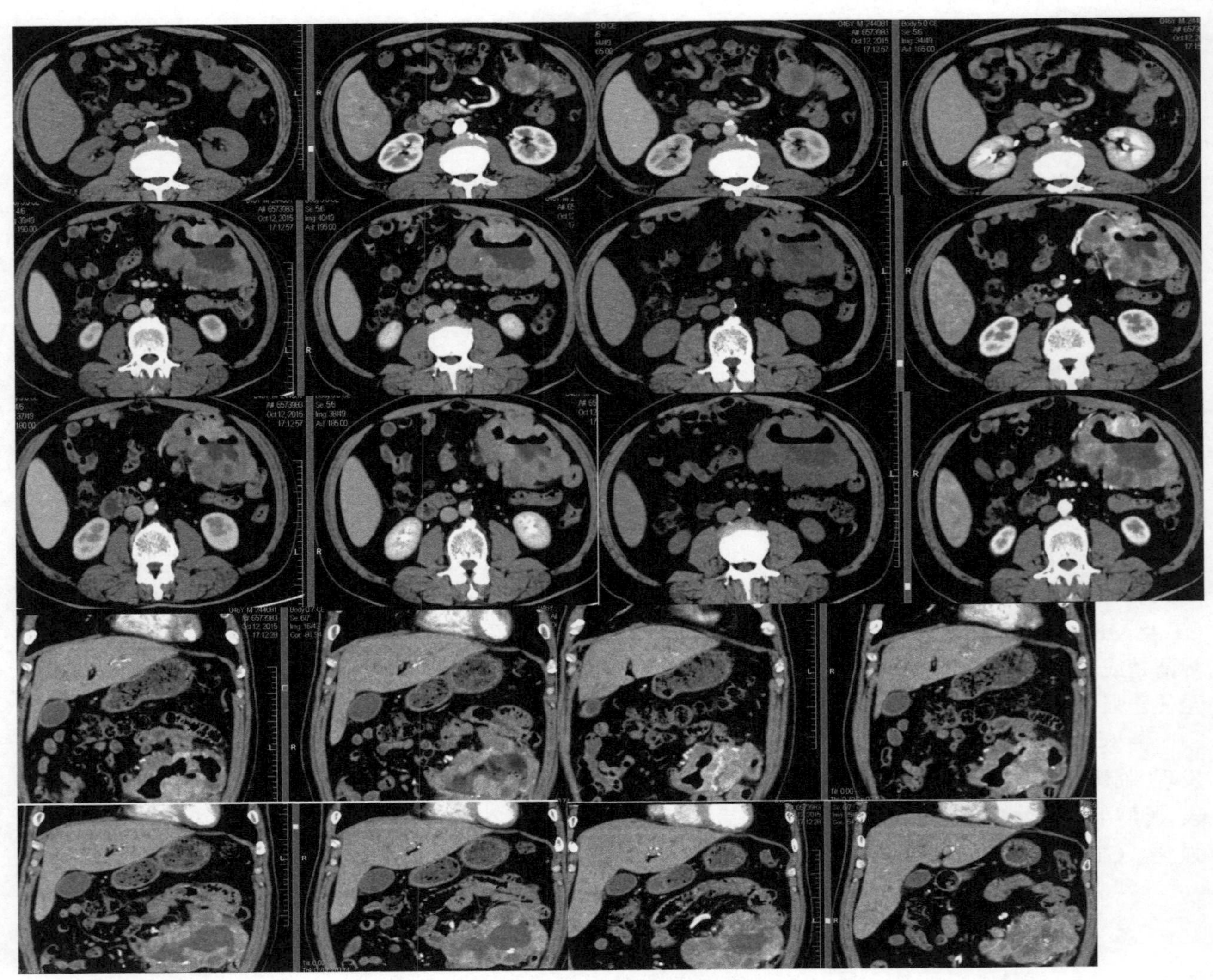

图 25-4-1 小肠梭形细胞肿瘤

患者,男, 47 岁。患者缘于 2 个月前无意间扪及中腹部一肿物,约“拳头”大小,随体位变化而改变位置,无明显疼痛及腹部不适,两月来肿物无明显增大,来医院进一步诊治。

手术所见:中腹部空肠距屈氏韧带 80cm 处可扪及空肠肿瘤 13cm × 8cm × 6cm 大小,质硬,肿物有浸出浆肌层,浸润系膜,肠系膜根部、腹主动脉旁未见肿大淋巴结。

病理检查:小肠肿物切除标本:肠管一段,长 33cm,一切缘周径 5.5 ㎝,另一切缘周径 2 ㎝,距一切缘 2.5cm、另一切缘 23cm 肠壁处见一隆起型肿物,肿物大小 13.5cm × 8cm × 6cm,其肠腔黏膜面呈溃疡形成,切面呈囊性,内含暗红色样物,囊内壁粗糙,壁厚 0.4~2.2 cm,其余肠腔黏膜皱襞存在。于肠外膜及肠周检出淋巴结样物数枚,直径 0.8~2.5cm,切面均灰白灰褐,质中。病理诊断:小肠肿物切除标本:梭形细胞肿瘤,待做免疫组化检测进一步明确肿瘤类型,肠管两切缘均未受肿瘤组织累及。肠外膜及肠周检出淋巴结 5 枚,均未见肿瘤组织转移(图 25-4-1)。

第四节　误诊病例简介：回肠系膜淋巴管肌瘤病并累及肠系膜淋巴结 50/55 枚

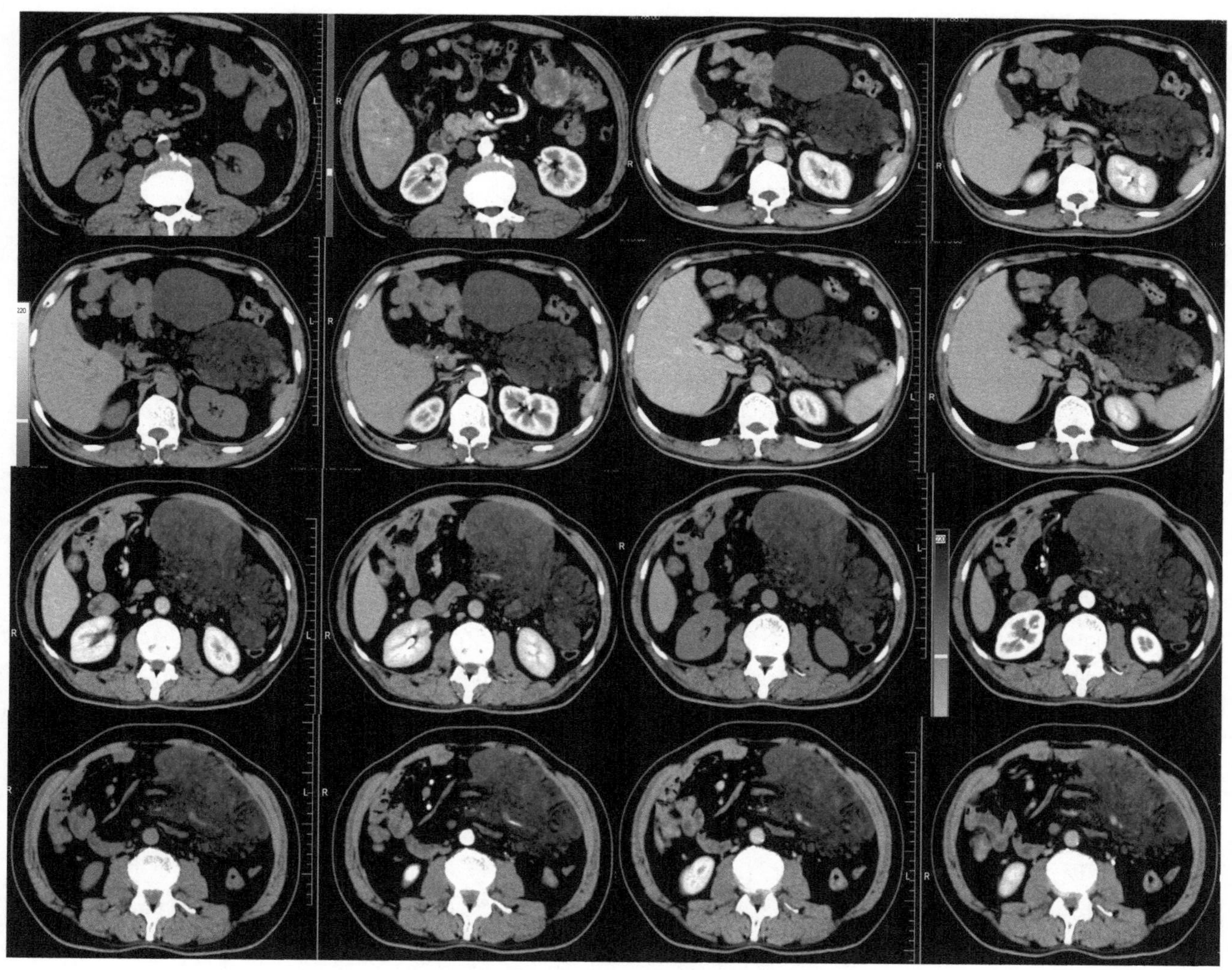

图 25-4-2　回肠系膜淋巴管肌瘤病并累及肠系膜淋巴结 50/55 枚

患者，男，56 岁。因发现左上腹包块 10 年余入院。

CT：左中腹部一不规则混杂密度肿块，大小约 11 cm × 8 cm × 13cm，CT 值 -43~21HU，增强扫描强化不明显，肿块边界欠清楚，邻近肠系膜增厚呈饼状，其内见多发肿大淋巴结，周围肠道受推压。CT 诊断：脂肪肉瘤可能，转移性肿瘤？

病理检查：回肠系膜肿物切除标本：肠系膜上见一巨大肿物，大小 17cm × 13cm × 12cm，切面灰褐淡黄，海绵状，有乳糜样和血性液体流出，质中偏软。部分与回肠壁粘连。其余稍正常，肠系膜增厚，肿物与周边肠系膜界线不清，肠系膜检出淋巴结 55 枚。

病理诊断：回肠系膜肿物切除标本：回肠系膜淋巴管肌瘤病并累及肠系膜淋巴结 50/55 枚。上下切缘均阴性。（说明）该病按 WHO 定义是由组织学和免疫组化特征的血管周上皮样细胞 (PEC) 构成的间叶性肿瘤，即 PEComa。它代表一组肿瘤家族，其中有血管周上皮样细胞 (PEC) 是经常出现在 PEComa 肿瘤中。在这家族中包括肺、肝、肾的血管平滑肌脂肪瘤、肺和肺外透明细胞“糖”瘤，以及淋巴管肌瘤病。PEComa 可发生在腹内和躯体软组织及多种器官。多数病例似乎具有良性过程。但也有少数亚型可发生转移（图 25-4-2）。

第五章　炎症性肠病

第一节　炎症性肠病

炎症性肠病是一组原因尚不明确的慢性非特异性肠道炎症，主要包括溃疡性结肠炎和克罗恩病，有10%~20%的炎症性肠病病人不能确定是克罗恩病还是溃疡性结肠炎，只能定义为“不确定性大肠炎”或“不确定性结肠炎”。目前认为炎症性肠病是多种因素相互作用的结果，主要包括环境、遗传、感染、免疫及精神心理等，其诊断和鉴别诊断主要依靠内镜病理。在炎症性肠病的诊断和治疗过程中，由于其临床表现无特异性，诊断有一定的难度，并且诊断一旦成立，即要求临床医生对该病做出全面的评估，即定度、定期、定型、定范围及判断有无并发症。当治疗一段时间后，其临床疗效如何以及下一步的治疗方案如何制定等一系列问题单靠临床医生来解决是相当困难的，因此需要临床、内镜、病理和影像等多学科的合作。

临床表现：炎症性肠病主要发生于青壮年，男女发病率无明显差异，溃疡性结肠炎和克罗恩病的临床表现有较多重叠，不易鉴别。溃疡性结肠炎临床主要表现为腹痛、腹胀、腹泻、黏液脓血便等消化系统症状，同时可伴有消瘦、贫血、低蛋白血症及水电解质紊乱等全身表现和多种肠外表现。克罗恩病临床主要表现为腹痛、腹泻、腹部包块、肠梗阻及肛门直肠周围病变等消化系统症状、体征，可伴有发热、营养障碍等全身性表现和肠外多个系统损害等。

病理学：虽然溃疡性结肠炎和克罗恩病临床表现类似，但病理变化不同，且各有一定的特征性。溃疡性结肠炎主要见于大肠，尤其是直肠和乙状结肠，病变呈连续性分布，局限于黏膜和黏膜下层。肉眼下溃疡性结肠炎几乎都累及直肠，其病理表现依发展的不同阶段而异，急性期黏膜弥漫性充血并可见大小不等的浅溃疡；较晚期病变呈现为广泛“潜掘状”溃疡及黏膜桥形成；随病变进一步发展，损伤与修复交替进行则可见炎性息肉形成；炎症消散期或非活动期，黏膜恢复正常或皱襞消失，溃疡减少，可有少量息肉持续存在，严重病例也可表现为肠管纤维化导致肠腔瘢痕性缩窄。内镜活检示溃疡性结肠炎的病变主要位于黏膜和黏膜下层，急性期于黏膜固有层炎症细胞增加，出现隐窝脓肿(即隐窝内中性粒细胞聚集)；静止期或消退期则只表现轻微的异常，表现为腺体分支且不规则，腺体基底与黏膜肌层之间存在缝隙，出现潘氏细胞(内分泌细胞)增生以及黏膜固有层内出现脂肪细胞岛。

而克罗恩病属系统性肉芽肿性炎症，可累及从口腔至肛门的全部胃肠道，尤以回肠末端和邻近结肠为高发，可累及肠壁各层。肉眼下最明显的两个特征是好发于小肠末端及病变常呈节段性分布，病灶轮廓清楚，被正常的肠管分隔开来(即跳跃性分布)。内镜活检最具有诊断意义的表现是累及肠壁全层的裂隙状溃疡和肉芽肿(卵石征)形成，肉芽肿主要由上皮样细胞和多核巨细胞组成，通常没有坏死，或仅有局限于中心区域的小坏死灶。

尽管炎症性肠病病理变化有一定的特异性，但并非获得病变标本就可以获得病理诊断。由于内镜活检标本组织量较小，且多只取材到黏膜层，因此对溃疡性结肠炎及克罗恩病的诊断较手术标本更困难。同样，仅部分结肠有病变的克罗恩病类似于溃疡性结肠炎，其镜下炎症仅累及黏膜表层，而不累及黏膜固有层，大体病变呈弥漫性、连续性，甚至表现为全结肠炎。因此，结合临床病史、内镜及影像学表现有利于做出正确的诊断。

内镜检查：目前，电子肠镜为炎症性肠病诊断和鉴别诊断的主要筛查工具，并可起到初步诊断的作用。溃疡性结肠炎肠镜所见主要包括:①黏膜弥漫性充血、水肿,粗糙呈细颗粒状,血管纹理模糊,质脆易出血,可附有脓性分泌物;②病变明显处可见黏膜糜烂或多发性溃疡;③慢性病变可见假息肉及黏膜桥,结肠袋变钝或消失。结肠镜黏膜活检组织学可见弥漫性炎症细胞浸润,活动期表现为表面糜烂、溃疡、隐窝炎及隐窝脓肿:慢性期表现为隐窝结构紊乱,杯状细胞减少。溃疡性结肠炎内镜分级为:0级,黏膜正常;Ⅰ级,黏膜血管充血、水肿和颗粒状改变,血管网模糊;Ⅱ级,在Ⅰ级基础上,黏膜更加糜烂;Ⅲ级,在Ⅱ级基础上,黏膜溃疡形成;Ⅳ级,在Ⅲ级基础上,黏膜明显增厚、肠腔狭窄;Ⅴ级,发生中~重度不典型增生或癌变。

克罗恩病内镜所见的重要改变为:病变呈节段性分布,见纵行溃疡,溃疡周围黏膜正常或增生呈鹅卵石样,肠腔狭窄,炎性息肉,病变肠段之间黏膜外观正常。

克罗恩病的内镜分级为:0级,黏膜正常;Ⅰ级,炎症改变;Ⅱ级,溃疡形成;Ⅲ级,黏膜明显增厚、肠腔狭窄;Ⅳ级,瘢痕期;Ⅴ级,发生中~重度不典型增生或癌变。

肠镜的主要缺点是不能观察整个肠壁和肠壁外的病变,部分病人不能耐受检查,甚至检查中出现肠出血、肠穿孔等并发症。

超声检查:近年由于各种超声设备及技术的进步,其作为一种实时、无创、便捷、廉价的检查方法已越来越受到临床的关注,经腹超声在炎症性肠病诊察中已显示出较好的应用价值。目前超声对炎症性肠病的诊断方法主要有:传统肠道超声、静脉注射对比剂超声成像、口服对比剂的肠道超声、能量多普勒超声及门静脉、肠系膜动脉的彩色多普勒超声检测。

克罗恩病最常见的超声表现包括:①肠壁增厚(≥4mm),病变肠段结构模糊或消失(正常肠壁超声下分5层,从内到外依次为强回声黏膜层,低回声黏膜肌层,强回声黏膜下层,低回声肌层,强回声浆膜层);②肠壁僵硬,结肠袋消失;③深溃疡形成,黏膜下层的强回声界限中断;④肠腔狭窄、肠壁微血管增多、脓肿及瘘管形成等。溃疡性结肠炎最常见的超声表现也是肠壁增厚,但因为病变主要局限于黏膜层和黏膜下层,肠壁层次基本保持正常,其肠壁血流信号及肠系膜淋巴结肿大情况不如克罗恩病。超声诊断的主要限度是敏感性和特异性不高,对设备和操作者的依赖度高。

X线检查:怀疑小肠病变者可做胃肠钡餐检查,结肠病变则需做钡剂灌肠检查。

溃疡性结肠炎的X线征象主要有:①黏膜粗乱和/或颗粒样改变;②多发性浅表溃疡,表现为肠壁边缘毛糙呈锯齿状改变以及小龛影,也可有炎症性息肉而表现为多个小的圆形或卵圆形充盈缺损;③病变严重时,结肠袋消失,肠管缩短、变细、僵直,可呈“铅管”状。

克罗恩病的X线表现为:黏膜皱襞粗乱、纵行性溃疡或裂沟、卵石征、假息肉、多发性肠狭窄、瘘管形成等,病变呈节段性分布。虽然X线小肠钡餐或结肠钡剂灌肠检查对起自肠壁且向腔外生长的病变的检出不理想,且操作者的检查方法和个人经验对结果有明显影响,但是其容易显示肠壁黏膜的特征性改变,对于炎症性肠病的初步诊断具有重要价值。

MSCT检查:由于上述各种检查方法的局限性,寻找一种敏感性、特异性和性价比均高且能全面观察肠壁和肠道外病变的技术成为炎症性肠病诊断急需解决的问题。MSCT可具备上述优势。自Vining等(1994)首次报道螺旋CT结肠成像技术(SCTC)以来,通过研究人员的不断努力,CTC的实验和临床应用取得了很大进展。近年来,随着MSCT技术的不断进步和工作站图像重建软件的发展,MSCT为炎症性肠病的诊断提供了更多、更有价值的信息,而且对诊断炎症性肠病肠道外病变具有独特的优势。

CT小肠成像是结合了MSCT和小肠钡剂造影优点的小肠检查方法,该检查方法简便、易行、廉价。MSCT为无创伤性检查,通过调节窗宽、窗位和各种重建技术有助于观察整个胃肠道情况,也能够很好地显示肠壁和肠外的异常改变。口服等渗水溶液具有无毒、廉价、较少引起呕吐、肠道不吸收及病人易接受等优点,还可以刺激肠蠕动,有利于对比剂快速通过小肠,较短时间内达到充盈肠管的目的。扩张良好的小肠壁厚度应小于3 mm,充盈欠佳时小肠壁较厚,但此时小肠黏膜皱襞变得明显,尤其分层强化的特点可与病变区别。同样情况下,结肠壁的厚度应小于5 mm。

溃疡性结肠炎的CT表现:①肠壁增厚。肠壁厚度平均为7.8 mm,增厚的肠壁为连续性改变,病变段肠壁的厚度大致均匀,表现为对称性的改变,或有分层现象,表现为“靶征”或“双晕征”:②黏膜面的改变,黏膜面多发小溃疡和灸性息肉,运用合理的窗宽、窗位,可清楚显示出结肠腔内黏膜面锯齿状凹凸不平的改变,而非病变区的黏膜面则是光滑的;③肠管形态的改变,可见病变区肠腔变细等表现;④肠系膜改变,病变区肠系膜密度升高、模糊,同时伴有系膜血管束的边缘不清。一些作者除发现溃疡性结肠炎病人病变区结肠系膜密度增高、模糊及系膜血管束边缘不清外,还发现肠系膜淋巴结肿大,直径多在 5~10 mm,且无融合倾向,推测可能是溃疡性结肠炎活动期的一个征象。

克罗恩病的 CT 表现:①肠壁增厚,口服对比剂后肠壁平均厚度 >4 mm 即为增厚,通常为 11~13 mm;②肠壁强化程度增加,克罗恩病活动期增强 CT 动脉期和静脉期肠壁均较邻近正常肠壁强化程度增加,以静脉期更明显;③并发症表现,可见肠管周围蜂窝织炎、炎性肿块、脓肿、瘘管和肠梗阻等,CT 诊断这些并发症较 X 线钡剂造影具有更多优势。

一些学者将克罗恩病病人肠壁增厚和强化模式分为 4 种类型,并发现不同肠壁增厚类型与炎症活动度有关, A 型和 B 型提示克罗恩病处于活动期,而 C 型和 D 型提示克罗恩病处于静止期。炎症波及小肠黏膜下, CT 可见全肠壁增厚,但此表现并非为炎性病变特有,在肿瘤及缺血性病变亦较常见。疑有炎性病变时,须仔细观察邻近小肠系膜,小肠系膜脂肪受累时通常表现为条状模糊密度影。此外,炎症可发生蜂窝织炎或脓肿。CT 可很好显示克罗恩病肠外并发症,如小肠系膜脂肪沉积、蜂窝织炎、脓肿和瘘。

肠系膜血管增粗、增多、密集时称为"梳征",此表现是活动性克罗恩病的特征之一,其机制为病变引起肠系膜静脉狭窄、阻塞,静脉回流障碍,供血小动脉扩张、充血,导致肠系膜小血管增粗、增多。所以"梳征"和肠壁厚度及肠壁增厚模式均可作为判断克罗恩病是否活动的重要指标。

另外,研究表明,克罗恩病时肠黏膜强化程度和肠壁厚度与病变的活动度高度相关。急性期增强 CT 可见肠壁增厚并呈分层表现:最内层为黏膜层,其强化程度与病变活动度有关,居中的环状低密度为水肿的黏膜下层,外层高密度为肌层。随着病变迁延,增厚肠壁的层次消失,呈均匀高密度,提示肠壁纤维化,为慢性期表现。有作者研究指出, CT 小肠成像对克罗恩病活动期的敏感度、特异度、阳性预测值及阴性预测值分别为 94%、40%、96% 及 38%。另据报道 CT 肠道成像在术前诊断炎症性肠病肠道瘘管的准确度高达 86%,并且可为临床医生提供肠道外病变的信息,从而有助于及时调整治疗方案。

肠道 MSCT 和其他检查方法相比具有影像清晰,提供的信息量大,禁忌证少,病人耐受性好,结果相对稳定且不受操作者经验影响等优点,但它属于辐射性检查,应注意大范围和多期扫描中的辐射剂量问题。

MRI 检查:早期 MRI 因为呼吸运动或肠道蠕动产生的严重伪影使肠道成像质量下降, MR 肠道成像一度被认为价值不大。随着 MRI 设备软、硬件发展和肠道对比剂的应用,肠道影像质量有了很大提高,有研究报道该检查技术对炎症性肠病诊断的敏感性和特异性不亚于 CT。溃疡性结肠炎的 MRI 表现主要有:肠壁增厚、肠壁的异常强化、病灶周围多发淋巴结和结肠皱襞减少。溃疡性结肠炎急性期由于黏膜和黏膜下层肿胀,使 MR T_1 和 T_2WI 成像均呈高信号;慢性期结肠壁在 T_1 和 T_2WI 成像上均呈低信号。

克罗恩病的 MRI 表现包括:①病变肠壁因炎性充血致肠壁强化幅度增加,据此可准确反映病变范围,且炎性肠壁的增强程度与炎性程度密切相关,中~重度炎症肠壁的血管通透性大,因此其较正常和轻度炎症的肠壁强化更明显;②肠壁厚度 >4 mm,可与周围蜂窝织炎粘连、融合而边界不清,开始时常表现为偏心性肠壁增厚,随着病变的进展也可表现为肠壁环形增厚;③多节段性病变或跳跃性病变,表现为多个肠段的肠壁增厚和强化幅度增加,其间隔为正常厚度和正常强化的肠段。

MRI 无电离辐射的优点使其更适于年轻病人的长期观察随访,在临床上具有很好的应用前景。但目前 MRI 对炎症性肠病活动性的定量评估尚无统一标准,而制定一个统一的量化标准还需多中心大样本研究。此外, MRI 的局限性如检查费用昂贵、耗时较长且有较多禁忌证如体内金属植入物、幽闭恐惧症等也限制其广泛应用。

核医学检查:核医学检查具有较高的敏感性,有助于确定受累肠段和了解并发症,并可区别炎症性肠病是处于活动期抑或静止期。^{99m}Tc-HMPAO 标记的白细胞单光子发射计算机体层摄像术 (SPECT) 对临床已有炎症性肠病症状但其他检查尚未发现病变的病人有一定的诊断价值。正电子发射体层摄像术 (PET) 与常规 CT 结合的 PET/CT 是目前最佳的成像技术，具有高敏感性和定量探测机体各种代谢过程的优点对判断疾病的活动性有一定的价值。

综上所述，炎症性肠病的各种影像学诊断方法各有优缺点，普通X线对炎症性肠病及并发症不敏感，MRI和放射性核素检查性价比不高，经腹超声检查受操作者自身操作经验等因素影响较多。尽管确诊炎症性肠病依赖于内镜病理，但该检查技术费时且病人顺应性差，相对而言，MSCT虽然具有电离辐射的缺点，但同时具备适用面广、性价比高、诊断特异性高等优势，对于急诊病人，MSCT是唯一最适合的检查方法，能为准确诊断和并发症的处理能提供重要的信息。

有研究报道通过调节扫描参数能降低约30%的辐射剂量，且炎症性肠病病人一年平均用于诊断的辐射剂量与人们自然状态下所接受的电离辐射剂量基本相同。所以，具备以下情况者应行低张MSCT检查：①临床上高度怀疑炎症性肠病者；②X线检查拟诊为炎症性肠病者；③内镜病理确诊为炎症性肠病、经临床治疗判断疗效者；④炎症性肠病治疗后复发及再治疗后的随访等。

第二节　炎症性肠病

患者，男，20岁。

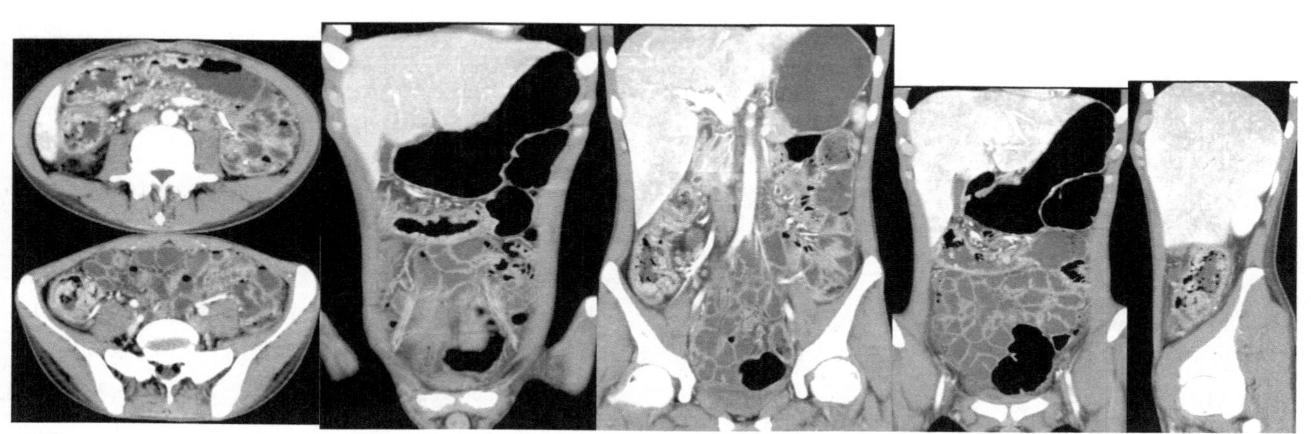

图 25-5-1　炎症性肠病

手术后病理诊断：右半结肠溃疡性结肠炎，炎症性肠病（图25-5-1）。

第六章　空、回肠克罗恩病

第一节　空回肠克罗恩病与MRI

小肠克罗恩病的影像学检查：小肠灌肠气钡双对比造影一直是小肠克罗恩病的主要影像学检查方法，它可显示炎症早期增生的淋巴滤泡、颗粒状隆起及其中心的口疮样溃疡，进展期的溃疡结节、“卵石征”、肠管变形、狭窄、僵硬、瘘管、窦道、病变的不对称性和跳跃性分布。近几年，CT应用于胃肠道疾病的诊断逐渐增多，它可显示小肠克罗恩病增厚的肠壁和肠系膜、纤维脂肪增生、蜂窝织炎、脓肿、窦道和瘘管，可发现传统小肠灌肠不能发现的肠管周围病变。

MRI具有软组织对比度好，对对比剂增强敏感，既无射线辐射，又能显示肠管外组织结构的特点。多组对照研究表明，显示正常和病变肠壁，增强后的MRI比CT更优越。并且，诊断炎症性肠病的敏感度和特异度以及对肠壁增厚、瘘管和脓肿的显示，MRI也明显优于小肠灌肠。因此，Umschaden等(2000)认为MRI可代替传统小肠灌肠诊断肠道慢性炎症和大多数克罗恩病结肠镜检查的随访。

肠壁强化增加：Low等(1997)及Knollmann等(2002)认为，炎性肠壁的异常增强可准确反映病变的范围，注射Gd-DTPA增强后，由于病变肠壁炎性充血，强化较邻近正常肠壁增加。有作者报告一组13例即是以肠壁的异常增强作为克罗恩病的病变肠管，共36个肠段增强后强化增加，增强后病变肠壁与邻近正常肠壁的信号强度比在注气灌肠组≥1.9，在水成像组≥1.3。Koh等(2001)认为增强后病变肠壁与正常肠壁信号强度的比值>1.3即为克罗恩病的活动期。水成像组病变肠壁增强百分比≥96%，最高达223%，而正常肠壁增强百分比则≤78%。Knollmann等(2002)在实验研究中发现，炎性肠壁的增强程度与炎症程度密切相关，中度炎症肠壁比正常和重度炎症的肠壁强化更明显，因为中度炎症的血管通透性比正常和重度炎症的血管通透性更大。该组病例中3个病变节段的肠壁厚度仅2~3mm，但增强百分比已达150%，增强后病变肠壁与正常肠壁的信号强度比达1.8~2.1，而邻近正常肠壁只增强了76%。这是因为炎症早期的肠壁无明显增厚时，由于炎性充血，肠壁增强已很明显，这与Low等(2000)的研究结果一致。

Low等(2000)发现，经内镜和病理证实的轻微炎症，只有轻度或无肠壁增厚，但已有异常强化。这表明，肠壁的异常增强较肠壁增厚能更敏感地发现早期的炎性病变。病变肠壁部分呈均匀一致强化，部分呈分层强化，表现为内层与外层呈显著高信号，为炎性充血的黏膜层和浆膜层，中层呈相对低信号，为水肿的黏膜下层和肌层，此征象为活动性炎症的特异性表现。

肠壁增厚：克罗恩病为侵犯肠壁全层的肉芽肿性炎症，尤以黏膜下层为重，由纵横交错的刀切样溃疡与周围水肿、增生的黏膜形成颗粒状或岛屿状隆起，称之为“卵石征”。刀切样溃疡以肠系膜侧为重，以纵形溃疡为特征。

由于水肿、淋巴管扩张、胶原纤维增生和黏膜下层增宽导致肠壁增厚，急性期以水肿和痉挛为主，慢性期主要为纤维组织增生，导致肠腔狭窄，甚至肠梗阻。该组病例表明，肠壁厚度≥10mm的重度增厚肠壁主要为环形对称性增厚，肠壁厚度<10mm的增厚肠壁中多以肠系膜侧增厚为重(非对称性)，部分系膜侧肠壁已明显增厚，但对侧的肠壁厚度仍正常。这是由于克罗恩病早期的溃疡和炎症以系膜侧肠壁为重，随着病变的发展，系膜对侧的肠壁也明显增厚，而使整个肠壁增厚呈均匀的环形。这种肠壁

偏心性增厚与病理上肠系膜侧病变严重的特点一致。因此，以系膜侧肠壁增厚为主是克罗恩病的MRI特点。

多个节段性病变：克罗恩病可侵犯整个消化道，但以小肠发病率最高，其中以末段回肠最多见，并且常常呈节段性侵犯多处消化道，表现为多个肠段肠壁增厚和强化增加，其间隔以正常厚度和强化的肠段，称之为跳跃性病变。该组13例中，回肠全部受侵，并以回肠远段受侵最多（10例），其次为第4、5、3组和回盲部，未见第2组小肠和十二指肠受累。并且常常为多节段受累，同时累及2个及2个以上节段者占85%，每例同时累及2~5个节段，每个节段长约4~32 cm。仅少数（5%）累及1个节段。这种多节段性、跳跃性病变亦为克罗恩病的MRI特点。

肠管外病变表现：克罗恩病的溃疡为刀切样深溃疡，可穿透肠壁引起肠管周围的蜂窝织炎和脂肪纤维增生，MRI表现为带脂肪抑制的T_2WI上肠管周围脂肪信号增高，边缘模糊，增强后明显强化。蜂窝织炎局限并伴纤维组织增生，可形成炎性肿块，T_2WI呈局限性高信号，增强后明显强化，边界较清楚，周围肠管分离移位。

该组病例中3例以肠管外炎性肿块为突出表现，肠腔狭窄，而病变肠壁仅1个或2个节段呈轻、中度增厚，强化增加。这表明，部分克罗恩病的MRI主要表现为炎性肿块和肠管狭窄，而无多节段肠壁炎症。

若炎性肿块进一步液化坏死，可形成脓肿，呈长T_1、长T_2信号，增强后边缘强化，坏死区无强化。炎症穿透邻近肠管、膀胱、腹壁，形成瘘管，同时可伴肠系膜和后腹膜淋巴结肿大。该组病例2例瘘管形成，1例回肠末段与腹壁形成外瘘，1例为第5组小肠与升结肠形成内瘘，瘘管周围均已形成明显强化的蜂窝织炎和炎性肿块，这时常有发热、血象增高和腹部可触及的包块等临床表现。

肠外并发症的诊断非常重要，因为其临床治疗方案不同。在显示肠管外并发症时，MRI较传统小肠灌肠和CT具有更多的优越性。

Rieber等（2000）对2组克罗恩病进行MRI研究，结果为诊断脓肿的敏感性分别是77.8%和100.0%，诊断瘘管的敏感度分别是70.6%和83.3%；而传统小肠灌肠诊断脓肿的敏感度均为0%，诊断瘘管的敏感度分别是17.7%和17.0%。两组病例中，MRI诊断脓肿和瘘管的敏感度均高于传统小肠灌肠，是因为传统小肠灌肠只能显示脓肿引起的肠腔变形、狭窄和移位的间接征象，并且肠管重叠多，因此，传统小肠灌肠很难发现肠外较小的脓肿和瘘管，而MRI应用脂肪抑制技术、多序列、多轴面和钆对比剂增强逐层扫描，无肠管重叠，很易发现肠管外的脓肿。

MRI两种检查方法的各自特点：为了标记和扩张肠道，清楚显示肠壁和病变，须使用足量的对比剂充分扩张肠管。在一组研究中，有作者应用了小肠插管注入气体和口服等渗甘露醇溶液两种肠道对比剂。通过对两种方法的初步研究，该作者认为，注气灌肠的优点为：注入的气体在肠腔内弥散快，与肠壁的信号对比度高，肠管可充分扩张，轻微的肠壁增厚即可显示，该组6例小肠直径均扩张到20 mm以上；缺点为：气体在FSPGR序列屏气扫描时磁敏感伪影明显，在SE序列存在一定呼吸运动伪影，但图像质量仍以SE序列的为好，并且小肠插管可使患者感到不适。

水成像的优点为：行SSFSE和FSPGR序列屏气快速扫描均无呼吸运动伪影和磁敏感伪影，图像质量明显优于注气灌肠组，而且扫描时间短，口服液体简便易行；缺点为：口服的对比剂对小肠的扩张程度不及注气灌肠显著。

总之，MRI是诊断小肠克罗恩病的一种敏感的检查方法，小肠克罗恩病的MRI主要表现为常常累及回肠尤其是回肠远段的节段性肠壁增厚，轻、中度肠壁增厚以系膜侧为主，重度增厚呈均匀的环形，增强后肠壁强化显著增加，炎症易穿透肠壁在肠管周围形成蜂窝织炎和炎性肿块。

第二节　MSCT小肠造影与克罗恩病

详见本书 本卷 第二十二篇 第九章　克罗恩病　MSCT小肠造影。

第三节　有关鉴别诊断

一、感染性肠病

溃疡性结肠炎：溃疡性结肠炎是一种病因不明的直肠和结肠的慢性非特异性肠病，以直肠、乙状结肠多见，CT 发现肠外病变的敏感性和特异性较高。典型的溃疡性结肠炎 CT 表现为：①结肠壁连续、均匀性增厚。②肠黏膜改变：CT 可发现龛影、充盈缺损及肠壁边缘“锯齿”样改变等征象。③肠管病变：肠管变细、缩短、僵直，呈“铅管”样改变，结肠袋变浅消失。④肠系膜增粗，密度增高，系膜淋巴结肿大，系膜血管增多。⑤肠壁分层现象：重症患者可见肠壁分层呈“双晕征”。⑥肠外病变：CT 可发现肠瘘、腹腔脓肿、蜂窝织炎、腹腔内少量游离气体、瘘管形成等并发症，CT 结肠造影检查时可见腹腔内、肠管间渗出的对比剂影，腹腔脓肿呈多囊、薄壁、分隔样改变。

肠结核：肠结核是由结核分枝杆菌侵犯肠道引起的慢性特异性肠道感染性疾病，好发于中青年女性，回盲部多见。临床主要表现为腹痛、腹泻、便秘、右下腹包块等征象。X 线钡餐检查可见肠壁不均匀增厚，黏膜增粗紊乱，龛影形成，息肉样充盈缺损及“激惹征”。CT 可见肠壁增厚，腹膜后及系膜区肿大淋巴结，系膜区血管束增多、扩张、扭曲。内镜检查可见回盲瓣肿胀变形，瘢痕或假性息肉形成，不规则穿透性溃疡（多为环形溃疡）、系膜区淋巴结肿大，干酪样坏死形成。

伪膜性肠炎：伪膜性肠炎是一种好发于结肠和小肠的急性纤维素渗出性炎症，多见于老年人、重症患者及免疫功能低下的患者。临床上患者以腹泻、腹痛、黏液样脓血便为主要表现。内镜检查见病变肠黏膜充血、水肿、糜烂，表面覆盖有白苔样伪膜，病灶间肠黏膜正常。

二、缺血性肠病

缺血性结肠炎：缺血性结肠炎是由于结肠供血不足引起肠壁缺氧损伤导致的肠道炎性病变，好发于脾区结肠，临床以腹痛、腹泻、血便为主要症状，老年人多见，可突然起病，病情变化快。X 线钡餐检查结肠多有指压样痕迹。内镜检查可见肠壁增厚，肠腔狭窄，肠壁增厚处多有蓝黑色斑点分布。CT 造影检查结肠血供减少，侧支循环形成。

肠系膜动脉 / 静脉栓塞：肠系膜动脉 / 静脉栓塞是肠系膜缺血的常见诱因，患者常有心脏疾病、动脉瘤或动脉粥样硬化的病史。临床上患者常表现为剧烈腹痛、恶心、呕吐等征象，X 线钡餐检查可见肠壁增厚，黏膜下“指压征”。内镜检查可见黏膜出血、糜烂、坏死及纵行溃疡形成，CT 血管成像可见血管内血栓形成。

三、结缔组织病性肠病

系统性红斑狼疮（SLE）性肠病：系统性红斑狼疮性肠病的病理基础是由系统性红斑狼疮引起肠壁和肠系膜血管炎及血管内血栓形成，引起肠缺血，临床以腹痛、腹泻、柏油样病变为主要表现，CT 可见肠壁水肿、增厚，受累肠段呈“靶征”或“双环征”，肠系膜水肿，系膜区血管增多、增粗、排列紊乱呈“梳”状或“栅栏征”。

白塞病：白塞病是一种以细小血管炎为病理基础的慢性多系统性疾病，属于结缔组织性疾病，可累及口、眼、生殖器、循环、消化等多个系统，以回肠及回盲部溃疡为主要症状，患者以腹痛、腹泻、腹部肿块为主要征象。X 线钡餐检查可见肠壁弥漫性增厚，肠腔狭窄，病理学检查可见肠壁血管玻璃样变性，纤维蛋白及血栓沉积。

四、肿瘤性、息肉性肠病

小肠恶性淋巴瘤：淋巴瘤是原发于淋巴组织的恶性肿瘤，约有 20% 发生于淋巴组织以外的器官，以消化道最常见，好发于回盲部，临床以腹部包块、腹痛、腹泻、便秘为主要表现。CT 主要表现为肠壁增厚、肠腔变形、肠管扩张或狭窄、肠腔内或外的软组织肿块。该肿瘤为低血供，通过三维重组可发现被肿瘤包绕的血管，增强扫描肿瘤轻度强化，并发溃疡时，可见典型“牛眼征”。X 线钡餐检查可分为肿瘤型、溃疡型及浸润型。肿瘤型可见肠腔内多发结节状充盈缺损，溃疡型可见不规则龛影形成，并可见“半月征”及“指压迹征”，浸润型可见肠腔狭窄变形。

多发性肠息肉病:多发性肠息肉病多有家族史,患者以便血、腹痛、大便次数增多为主要表现。内镜检查可见结肠弥漫分布大小不等的息肉,数目多>100个,以直肠、乙状结肠居多。X线钡餐检查表现为肠腔内多发边界光滑锐利的类圆形充盈缺损,也可为分叶状或绒毛状充盈缺损。

小肠间质瘤:小肠间质瘤病灶大,富血供,易囊变或坏死,增强扫描动脉期及静脉期明显不均匀强化,通过三维CT血管造影可以找到肿瘤的供血血管。

第七章 小肠梗阻

第一节 误诊病例简介:小肠脂肪瘤伴异位胰腺致小肠套叠

成人肠套叠较少见,多由于肿瘤及术后粘连和肠动力性病变等引起。脂肪瘤是小肠少见的良性肿瘤,异位胰腺是先天性畸形,可发生在消化道的任何部位,异位胰腺组织散存于脂肪瘤样组织中引起成人肠套叠少见。

CT扫描肠套叠可表现为靶征、彗星尾征或肾形征等征象。靶征表现为鞘部、套入部最内壁和返折壁3层结构,它反映了套叠的各层肠壁、肠腔及肠系膜间的解剖关系,是肠套叠最常见的特征性CT征象。

因肠道迂曲及排列位置、方向不规则,CT扫描与肠套叠长轴呈平行关系时,可表现为彗星尾征或肾形征,即肠系膜脂肪及血管卷入所致。彗星尾征是套叠近端肠系膜血管牵拉聚拢的征象,其组成尚包括套入近端肠管。肾形征或肾形肿块为套鞘部游离缘与套入部近端肠管及肠系膜的CT斜切面影像,其中游离的套鞘呈弧形围绕套入部状如肾轮廓外形,而套入部近端肠管、肠系膜状若肾蒂。彗星尾征均与肾形征相伴出现,是肠套叠除靶征外的又一较常见的特征性CT征象。靶征见于各型肠套叠,而彗星尾征及肾形征多见于小肠型肠套叠。

肠套叠的CT表现有一定特征性,诊断相对较容易,但病因有时难以确定,应重点观察套叠头部,寻找隐匿的原发病灶。

小肠脂肪瘤所致肠套叠表现为套头部圆形或椭圆形均一脂肪密度肿块,不同于肠套叠靶征内弧形的肠系膜脂肪而易于鉴别确诊。一例CT检查示类圆形分层状靶形肿块,盆腔内示不规则肾形肿块,套头部肠腔内见椭圆形脂肪密度肿块,CT值为-97 HU,即考虑到脂肪瘤并肠套叠的诊断,但对脂肪密度中央部斑点状软组织肿块(异位胰腺组织)认识不足,术前未能给予明确诊断。

第二节 腺瘤、息肉和脂肪瘤同时并存引起成人肠套叠

成人肠套叠多为继发性肠套叠,由息肉或肿瘤等病变引起。有作者报告一例,也为继发性肠套叠,且套叠主要由腺瘤、息肉和脂肪瘤同时并存引起;息肉数量多,约30枚,类型比较特殊,病理上呈管状绒毛状,部分有蒂或无蒂,此类型息肉易引起肠套叠;小肠脂肪瘤较少见,该例的脂肪瘤在胃肠钡餐检查时不能诊断,而在CT上由于脂肪瘤密度较低,CT值特殊,故能得以诊断。空肠脂肪瘤、多发炎性息肉及腺瘤同时存在致肠套叠者少见,该例钡餐检查有典型表现:肠管明显扩张,内可见一细长条充钡肠管及多个菜花状充盈缺损,对确定病变的大小、位置及范围有价值,“贝壳”状改变可能是套入肠管的头部;CT可见典型的同心圆表现,多层密度不均肿块,以及套入的肠管。

第三节　柿石性小肠梗阻

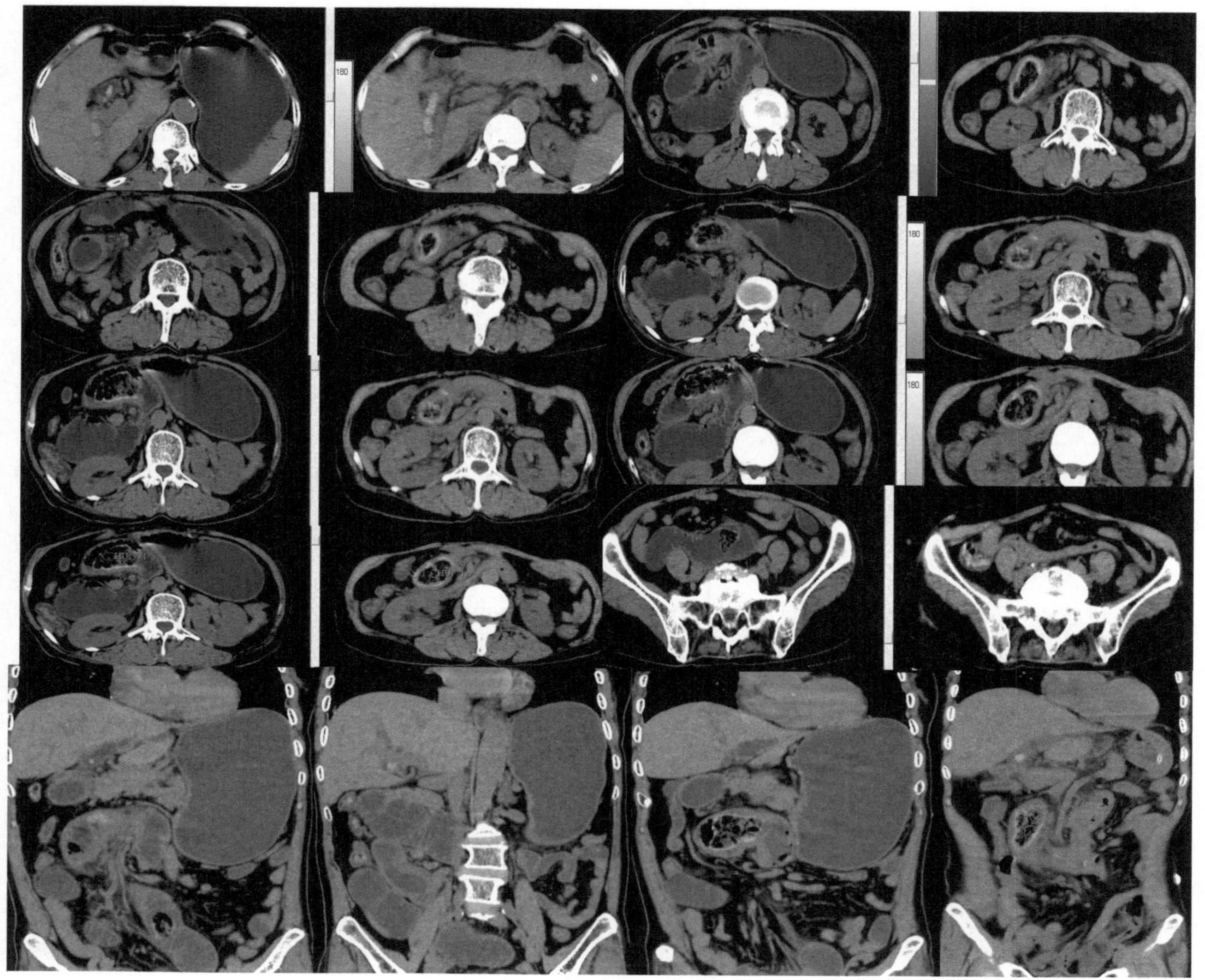

图 25-7-1　柿石性小肠梗阻

患者，女，64 岁。反复上腹部疼痛 1 年余，加重 10 天入院。

外院胃镜检查提示：胃多发息肉，胃结石，慢性非萎缩性胃炎。电子肠镜：慢性直肠、乙状结肠炎，结肠结石。建议内镜取石术。

CT 示肝总管、左肝管近端段、右肝管及肝分支内见铸形结石，肝管及肝内积气。胆囊无明确显示，胰尾部部分缺如，请结合临床。十二指肠水平部至空肠段肠腔内多个类圆形高密度影，内部密度不均，十二指肠上段及胃扩张。左肾上腺区数个结节灶。盆腔积液。

此例在 X 线检查立位平片有肠胀气及液平面，结合实验室、B 超检查，可以确诊肠梗阻。外院胃镜和肠镜均见到胃结石和肠结石。通过 CT 可见到梗阻点，肠腔内气体与液平面的比例或肠腔扩张的程度及对其梗阻原因的诊断，但确诊还需通过详细询问病史、发病季节、发病人群及发病前是否空腹进食大量柿史，尽量在术前明确，从而制定相应的治疗计划，避免绞窄性肠梗阻、肠坏死的发生（**图 25-7-1**）。

第四节 MSCT诊断肿瘤性肠梗阻

肿瘤性肠梗阻占机械性肠梗阻的27.3%~32.4%。中老年机械性肠梗阻绝大多数为肿瘤引起。一般存在以下3种情况:

腔内型:隆起性病灶。起源于肠管壁一侧,呈广基或带蒂生长,形成肿块突入肠腔,部分或全部阻塞肠腔时,临床出现肠梗阻症状。常见有脂肪(肉)瘤、腺瘤(癌)和较大息肉恶变,常常需与肠腔内粪块和异物引起梗阻鉴别,普通CT平扫时极易误诊。

管壁型:浸润性病灶。起源于管壁,呈环形浸润生长,使管壁僵硬,管腔狭窄,如结肠癌在钡剂灌肠时所见的"苹果核"征;病灶也可偏心性生长,肿块部分突入腔内引起梗阻,与腔内型广基生长病灶鉴别在于后者同时向腔外生长侵犯腔外结构。

肠外型:病灶起源于肠外组织形成肿块,对肠管形成外压性狭窄;也见于肠道周围恶性肿瘤侵犯肠壁和肠外。

对肿瘤病灶的显示:肠梗阻是否存在、梗阻程度、部位及病因的判断,近10年来国内外有较多文献报道。普通CT和单层螺旋CT检查虽然很大程度上弥补了单凭临床经验或仅借助普通X线和/或内镜检查的局限性和盲区,提高了术前诊断准确性,但由于肠道解剖、肿瘤性肠梗阻的病理特点等和单层螺旋CT性能的局限性,时间分辨率和容积数据Z轴分辨率低,不能短时间内进行大范围扫描,重建图像粗糙,不能全面立体显示病灶,也不能对病灶及周围情况等做出更加精细的显示,为手术方案制定提供的信息非常有限。

MSCT时间分辨率和Z轴分辨率高,多平面重建图像质量好,重建出来的冠状位、矢状位及斜位图像能观察到较长的肠袢和梗阻点的病灶,克服了由于肠道迂曲走行使轴位像难以见到整段肠管的缺点,直观清楚地影像使诊断更加容易和准确。

而且,重建图像特别是冠状位图像与临床医师手术时所见病灶及腹部的周围结构相同,更符合其观察和判断习惯,使外科医师术前心中有数。一组选用的口服和结肠灌注对比剂浓度不同,更能清楚地显示梗阻部位及程度。该组9例腔内型病灶。在多平面重建像上大多能显示病灶某处与肠壁相连,其密度与肠壁密度相同,增强扫描时有相同的强化表现,如血管重建时有血管进入则可肯定为肿瘤。

对肿瘤血管的显示:Matsuki等(2004)利用4排SCT三维血管成像显示腹腔镜胃切除术前患者胃周血管,获得良好的临床效果。近年来,肿瘤血管已成为肿瘤学研究的热点,在临床实践中,临床医师非常需要以最简单和无创的方法明确肿瘤血供情况,确定手术方案或先进行介入治疗、增加病灶可切除性,减少手术中出血问题。

该组利用最大密度投影后处理技术显示肿瘤供血血管27例,占69.2%,其中17例因肿瘤对周围结构侵犯明显,临床外科医师评价肿瘤可切除性低,先采用DSA肿瘤血管选择性介入化疗和栓塞治疗。介入治疗后13例病灶被成功切除,4例因有远处转移仅作姑息性介入治疗和梗阻近端肠管造瘘术解除梗阻症状;其余10例因梗阻明显而对周围侵犯较轻或考虑为良性肿块者而直接手术,肿瘤血管结构在手术时得到证实。

该组仍有12例未能明确显示肿瘤的供血血管,推测可能与部分肿瘤为低血供(如该组1例空肠脂肪瘤,增强扫描各期强化均不明显)和部分肿瘤由于供血血管较细,以及4排MSCT的分辨率低有关。

肿瘤的TNM分期:肿瘤的TNM分期对临床治疗和患者预后均十分重要。该组27例肠道原发性恶性肿瘤性肠梗阻病例MSCT的TNM分期对原发病灶、淋巴结转移和远处转移总的诊断准确性分别为92.6%、85.2%和100%,与文献报道相似,但对直径<0.5 cm的淋巴结检出率不及文献报道。能引起肠梗阻的肿瘤常常相当大并已为晚期,故该组病例中未见T_1、T_2期病例。该组误将1例T_1划分为T_4,是因为肿块外脂肪间隙很薄,无法分辨。1例N_0、1例N_1期假阳性,病理报告为炎性淋巴结增大,2例N_2期假阴性,其淋巴结直径<0.5 cm,MSCT未发现,可能与4排MSCT分辨率不够高和扫描层厚不够薄有关。但总体上讲,MSCT能很好地对病灶进行TNM分期。

总之,MSCT扫描及多平面重建、最大密度投影等后处理技术是诊断肿瘤性肠梗阻的重要方法,对引起梗阻的肿瘤的定位、定性及恶性肿瘤的TNM

分期判断准确性很高，对肿瘤血管能较好显示，对评估肿瘤可切除性、制定治疗方案具有重要的意义。

第五节　“假肾征”在诊断肠套叠中的价值

“假肾征”是指超声波检查时见到的中心呈高回声周围被低回声区包绕的肾形肿块回声。肠套叠时出现的“假肾征”是由两部分组成，即套入部的肠管、套鞘。据扫描断面的不同，肠套叠的影像也大不一样。纵切面表现为肾形的肿块，形成“假肾征”或“夹心面包征”。横切面时呈“靶环样”，为新月样低回声带组成的同心圆。即“牛眼征”或“同心圆征”。

当肠管形成肠套叠时，静脉回流受阻，从而导致该套入部发生水肿，水肿的套入部在超声波上为低回声。脂肪呈高回声，而淋巴结节和血管为低回声。肠套叠的这种结构形成了声像图的特殊表现，在长轴切面形成“假肾征”。在横切扫描时，在套入部分的末端表现为较低的同心圆状回声，主要代表套入并发生水肿的肠管。在肠套叠中央的部分，较高回声为肠系膜部分，低回声区为淋巴结和血管，形成“同心圆征”（靶环征）。

虽然“假肾征”和“靶环征”对诊断肠套叠具有高度的敏感性和特异性，但其他原因的肠壁水肿，如坏死性小肠结肠炎、肠扭转和乙状结肠扭转，也可有类似的征象。但在横切面上，新月状高回声是肠系膜的脂肪，低回声是为淋巴腺结节或者血管，这是肠套叠所特有的，借此可排除假阳性。肠套叠的影像学诊断方法通常采用常规 X 线平片、钡剂或空气灌肠以及超声。有报道，肠套叠出现的“假肾征”可使超声诊断本病的敏感度及特异度达到 100%。因此“假肾征”及与其相关的征象，对诊断该病是非常有帮助的。

第六节　肠梗阻的少见病因

Medden 等（1982）在慢性腹膜透析病人中发现 2 例经透析导管腹膜开口形成小肠疝而引起的急性小肠梗阻，这是腹膜透析极少见的并发症。巨大的美克尔憩室引起肠梗阻常常多于出血，在新生儿，这多由于扭转所致；而在成人，则通常由粘连和占位效应引起。钡剂检查和腹部侧位片常有助于诊断。

在肠梗阻的病因中应包括此类病因，在不全性、间断型和慢性肠梗阻的病因区别诊断中更应想到本征，Miller 等（1981）特别强调此点。

第七节　小肠假性梗阻

小肠假性梗阻常为一种慢性疾患，患者有梗阻的症状和体征，但却寻找不到确切的阻塞部位。急性小肠假性梗阻常有病因可寻，而慢性者则多为特发性，无明确病因。Golladay 和 Byrne（1981）对本症进行细致探讨，研究胃肠道自律性的生理特征，将本症与机械性梗阻对比分析，并详细讨论了本症的鉴别诊断。

Schuffler 和 Deitch（1980）与 Bryne（1981）分别对慢性特发性小肠假性梗阻及其综合征进行讨论，本症 X 线平片均可见肠梗阻征象，胃肠道节段性运动紊乱、降低、甚或缺如，但皆未发现确切阻塞的地方。如临床上疑及本症，宜行小肠灌钡造影和测压法进行诊断，不可轻率地进行有害的剖腹探查术。

第八节 腹内疝

腹内疝为肠梗阻的少见原因,其发病率低,尸检率仅为 0.2%~0.9%,在肠梗阻病例中的发生率不超过 6%。但是,腹内疝容易形成闭袢,发生肠管绞窄、缺血、坏死,死亡率超过 75%,病情危急,因此早期诊断和手术治疗十分必要。MSCT 具有扫描速度快、薄层扫描、多维后处理重建技术及 CTA,在明确肠梗阻诊断、判断内疝的部位及分型、评价有无肠管绞窄坏死等严重并发症方面有着明显优势,已成为诊断腹内疝的首选检查方法。

腹内疝的定义及基本分型:腹内疝是指腹腔脏器或组织离开原来的位置,通过腹腔内的正常或异常的孔道、裂隙进入腹腔内某一解剖间隙。这些正常或异常的疝口及间隙便是腹内疝发生的特定解剖学基础。

Meyers 根据解剖部位提出腹内疝的传统分型,经 Sala 等(2013)统计,腹内疝及其发病率包括十二指肠旁疝(53%)、盲肠周围疝(13%)、小网膜孔疝(8%)、经肠系膜疝(4%~8%)、乙状结肠周围疝(6%)、吻合口后方疝(5%)、经网膜疝(1%~4%),以及发生在盆腔的内疝(6%)如膀胱上疝、子宫阔韧带疝、道格拉斯疝等。一些学者按照致病原因,将腹内疝分为原发性和继发性 2 类。前者是指在胚胎发育过程中肠管旋转或腹膜附着异常等先天性因素所致腹膜隐窝大而深,腹膜、网膜或肠系膜存在缺损,肠管等内容物经此疝入,如十二指肠旁疝、小网膜孔疝、肠系膜裂孔疝等;后者多为后天因素如手术、外伤、炎症等所致腹膜或肠系膜的异常孔隙,多表现为经系膜疝、吻合口后疝等。近年来,由于手术引起腹腔粘连型内疝有明显增加的趋势,且发生率较高,因此一些学者将该类内疝纳入分型。一组 15 例中,粘连束带疝 4 例,占 26.7%,在发病前均有腹部手术史。

临床表现:腹内疝的临床症状差异很大,轻者可无症状,或出现间歇性轻度消化不良,如恶心,进食后呕吐,不特异的腹部不适等;重者出现急性肠梗阻症状,表现腹痛、腹胀、恶心、呕吐,停止排气排便等。症状严重程度与内疝的持续时间、是否可复性、有无绞窄性等有关。

影像学研究:闭袢性肠梗阻:因疝口较小,小肠等内容物不断疝入其中,梗阻近段扩张和积液进行性加重,疝口附近肠壁水肿,在疝口极易形成闭袢并发肠梗阻。该组共有 13 例 MSCT 表现闭袢性肠梗阻,其特征性征象包括:①根据疝入肠管的长度和分布不同,扩张、积液、聚集的小肠可呈“C”、“U”或“W”形状,其中,“C”字征最具代表性。在不同的扫描层,也可表现为“咖啡豆征”或“假肿瘤征”;②疝颈处肠管因疝口的收缩、邻近肠管和肠系膜的挤压,输入袢和输出袢逐渐变细形成鸟嘴状突起,称“鸟嘴征”。当 2 个以上“鸟嘴征”“对吻”时,多提示闭袢。

肠系膜及血管的改变:因肠管的位置及形态发生改变,伴随着肠系膜及血管移位、扭转,腹内疝的肠袢或多或少存在血运异常:①肠系膜因淤血水肿,系膜及网膜脂肪密度增高,呈“云雾状”;②疝口附近可见肠系膜血管聚集、增粗充血、拉伸、移位和扭曲,称之为“血管纠集征”“缆绳征”“旋涡征”;③肠袢因绞窄缺血缺氧,肠壁向内渗出导致肠腔积液、明显扩张,肠壁因缺血水肿、增厚,密度异常,增强扫描可见缺血肠壁强化减低、强化延迟或不强化,CT 上通常表现为由管壁、肠系膜脂肪以及肠腔内气体等不同组织密度交错分布的影像,呈“靶环征”或“同心圆征”;④间接征象,肠壁间积气征、肠系膜静脉和/或门静脉气栓征、肠系膜积气、腹水、气腹等,往往提示肠袢存在绞窄坏死。

占位效应:闭袢导致疝口内的小肠扩张、积液,相互挤压成团,邻近组织受压推移,出现占位效应,但大多局限在上、中、下腹某个固定区域,根据疝的位置及与相邻组织脏器的关系,有助于腹内疝诊断并大致分型:

左侧十二指肠旁疝:一般位于屈氏韧带左侧、胃和胰腺之间,也可见于胰尾后方或横结肠与左肾上腺之间,并见供应该段的肠系膜血管向疝口移位、纠集、增粗,肠系膜下静脉及左升结肠动脉位于疝口前界并向左侧移位;

右侧十二指肠旁疝:通常位于右中上腹,十二指肠降段后方,CT 表现为一簇异常聚集扩张的小肠肠袢,被肠系膜上动脉、静脉的空肠支环形包绕,肠系膜上动脉、右结肠静脉位于疝口前界,受压向前推移。如在 CT 上未发现十二指肠水平段，有利于此型的诊断。与左侧十二指肠旁疝相比，右侧型疝囊一般较大，且比较固定，难自行复位。

盲肠周围疝：在 CT 上表现为盲肠及升结肠后外方的聚集扩张的小肠肠袢，可占据右结肠旁沟，盲肠受压向前、内侧移位。

肠系膜裂孔疝：患者多有胃肠手术史，尤其是 Roux-en-Y 吻合术，CT 表现因疝口位置及疝入肠管的长度而异，疝入的肠管因无疝囊包绕限制而差异巨大，可表现为紧贴腹壁的扩张积液的异位肠袢，无网膜脂肪被覆，多位于结肠外侧，致邻近结肠向中心移位。

乙状结肠系膜周围疝：可见疝入降结肠左后方的扩张小肠肠袢，疝口多位于降结肠和左侧腰大肌之间。

黏连索带疝：患者一般有腹部手术史，CT 表现为闭袢性肠梗阻，大多伴有肠管绞窄，出现缺血、坏死，CT 可以较好地显示闭袢梗阻的部位，在多平面重建冠、矢状位图像上追踪肠管走向，有时可以发现黏连束带状结构。

盆腔内疝：如道格拉斯窝疝，CT 显示盆腔扩张积液的肠管，压迫直肠、乙状结肠向背外侧移位，压迫子宫向腹侧移位。

鉴别诊断：主要与黏连或扭转所致的肠梗阻相鉴别。

黏连性肠梗阻：在黏连性肠梗阻，一般梗阻部位移行带光滑，无肠袢移位、聚集成团等征象，肠系膜血管走行大致正常。

肠扭转：与肠扭转鉴别，两者有相似之处，均有肠袢及肠系膜移位征象，但肠扭转无疝口，可以相鉴别。

综上所述，根据腹内疝发病原理，发生部位及 MSCT 典型表现如闭襻性肠梗阻，肠系膜改变，不同类型腹内疝的占位效应，对多数病例能做出正确诊断并大致分型。MSCT 对腹内疝肠梗阻分级的探讨有助于评估病情，指导手术方案的选择。

第九节　腹膜腔内疝及其误诊与漏诊的分析

详见本书 腹盆下卷 第一篇 第三章 第三节　腹膜腔内疝及其误诊与漏诊的分析。

第八章 小肠淋巴管扩张症

小肠淋巴管扩张症影像学检查

小肠淋巴管扩张症,由 Waldmann 等(1961)首次报道,是一种蛋白丢失性肠病,因各种原因导致小肠淋巴回流障碍,肠淋巴管扩张破裂,淋巴液漏出,从而导致蛋白质、脂肪及淋巴细胞的大量丢失。

1. 发病机制 小肠淋巴管扩张症分为原发性和继发性。正常小肠淋巴管主要分布于小肠黏膜固有层、黏膜下层及浆膜层,汇入肠干后经乳糜池、胸导管回流入左静脉角,进入血液循环。当淋巴回流受阻后,可造成淋巴液反流,继而导致小肠淋巴管扩张、瓣膜功能受损、破裂,淋巴液从扩张的淋巴管漏入肠腔或腹腔,造成乳糜泻、乳糜性腹腔积液,蛋白质、脂肪及淋巴细胞三种营养成分从胃肠道大量丢失。病理镜下可见病变肠段黏膜或黏膜下淋巴管扩张。继发性多为自身免疫性疾病、肿瘤、感染、肝硬化门静脉高压、缩窄性心包炎、慢性右心功能不全、腹部外伤、手术损伤等原因造成淋巴管及周围组织炎症、粘连、狭窄,使淋巴回流不畅。

2. 临床表现 一组 21 例直接淋巴管造影和造影后 CT 检查均显示淋巴管系统有不同程度的梗阻征象,其中 3 例可见对比剂直接进入肠腔内。该组病例中,1 例合并肝硬化门静脉高压,1 例既往有缩窄性心包炎,3 例有胸腹部手术史,影像学检查显示梗阻部位与手术部位一致,考虑此 5 例为继发性小肠淋巴管扩张症可能性大,但即便继发性小肠淋巴管扩张症,也可能存在先天性淋巴管发育缺陷因素。其余 16 例未发现继发因素,同时有肢体原发性淋巴水肿和淋巴管造影等影像学检查所见的先天性淋巴管发育缺陷的佐证,符合原发性小肠淋巴管扩张症特征。

3. 影像学研究 直接淋巴管造影:正常直接淋巴管造影可依次显示同侧下肢淋巴管、腹股沟和髂淋巴管、同侧腰淋巴干、乳糜池、胸导管和胸导管末端以至对比剂入血的影像。正常时淋巴液沿管道向心性流动,对侧腰干、肠淋巴干所属的淋巴管不会显影。

只有当淋巴系发育缺陷(淋巴管闭塞、瓣膜损害)或后天因素导致淋巴管病变,造成管腔内压力增高,使对比剂反流。如胸导管回流不畅或末端梗阻,对比剂可沿肠干反流到肠系膜所属淋巴管,轻则表现为肠系膜上动脉周围淋巴管扩张显影,重则在荧光屏动态监视下观察到对比剂直接进入肠腔现象。

该组病例中侧位摄片可见腹膜后显影的淋巴管位于脊柱前方,对比剂反流显影的肠干所属淋巴管位于腹腔内。有 3 例在透视下可见随肠管蠕动,对比剂明显进入小肠的直接征象,具有特征性诊断价值,但所占的比例较低,与淋巴管梗阻的程度和肠壁淋巴管有无破口有关。

直接淋巴管造影可直接显示胸导管出口以下的全程淋巴管系统,在评估淋巴管异常的累及范围、选择临床治疗方案等方面具有重要意义。

MSCT:MSCT 以其快速的扫描速度、更高的空间分辨力和强大的图像后处理技术,能无创地获得优质的多方位图像,显示清晰的解剖细节。直接淋巴管造影后行 CT 平扫,既能保留造影征象,又能弥补其不足。该组 21 例均为自然状态下行 CT 检查,检查前未行胃肠道饮水充盈,平扫可见病变处小肠肠管扩张积液,肠腔内漏出的淋巴液含有脂性成分,导致其 CT 值略低于正常小肠液体密度。增强扫描增厚的肠壁呈三层靶环样改变,内环为软组织密度影,由充血、肿胀及炎性变的肠黏膜组成,静脉期及延迟期强化明显;中间环为低密度,为黏膜下层的水肿及脂肪堆积、扩张的含乳糜的淋巴管组成,强化不明显;外环为增厚的肌层和浆膜层组成,中度强化。

该组在增强扫描的 8 例中,7 例肠壁增厚,其中 5 例可见此征象,另 2 例病变肠段肠壁均匀性强化,病理显示小肠黏膜下散在扩张淋巴管、多灶性血管扩张并淤血,考虑固有层内淋巴管扩张程度不及增生扩张的小血管,从而使管壁均匀强化,未能形成低密度的中间环。

淋巴回流障碍，淋巴液聚集，淋巴管扩张，腹腔或腹膜后也可以形成囊性淋巴管瘤，表现为沿血管淋巴管走行的囊性低密度影，增强扫描囊内成分未见强化，该组中有 3 例合并淋巴管瘤。Mazzie 等(2003)认为儿童中失蛋白性肠病患者，如未找到其他病因，CT 扫描见弥漫性小肠管壁增厚肿胀，合并腹腔积液及肠系膜水肿可提示原发性小肠淋巴管扩张症的可能。

直接淋巴管造影与造影后 CT 对小肠淋巴管扩张症检查的优缺点：直接淋巴管造影可直观显示淋巴管走行及发育，查找梗阻部位，了解侧支循环及淋巴反流通路，并可动态观察胸导管末端的入血情况，具有独特的优势。如能显示对比剂进入肠腔是诊断小肠淋巴管扩张症的金标准。

但 DSA 透视下观察，图像空间分辨率较低，无法全面了解胸腹部的细微解剖结构，难以显示淋巴管系统以外胸腹腔的异常情况，如不能对本病所致的肠壁和肠腔状态、腹腔积液和胸腔积液及肠系膜水肿的程度及其他伴随征象等进行观察。

而直接淋巴管造影后 CT 扫描可以弥补上述不足，不仅具有直接淋巴管造影的部分诊断价值，而且在显示异常淋巴管结构累及的部位、范围和程度上更为准确和细致，但 MSCT 在显示淋巴管的连续性和胸导管末端入血情况不及直接淋巴管造影，且无法捕捉造影时的瞬间动态影像，故二者对病变观察角度不同，无法互相替代，联合检查可以相互弥补，提高诊断的阳性率。根据该组经验，在二者检查的时间顺序上应有所要求，对疑似本病者应先进行胸、腹部 MSCT 增强检查，再择期进行直接淋巴管造影和造影后 CT 平扫，如此可以获得较全面、准确的检查信息，不会因致密的对比剂伪影干扰而影响观察周围的细微结构。

不提倡淋巴管造影后行 CT 增强检查，反流显影的淋巴管与强化的小血管有时不易区分。另外，对疑似本病者进行 CT 检查前，应禁食和禁水，以利在自然状态下观察消化道内存留液体，对判断肠壁和肠腔病变程度和范围有一定的帮助。

4. 鉴别诊断　本病需要与以下疾病进行鉴别。

局限性淋巴管扩张症：局限性淋巴管扩张症的发病机制不明，有作者推测本病的发生是由于黏膜下淋巴管的炎症致使淋巴管闭塞，形成局部淋巴管扩张。其病理表现与小肠淋巴管扩张症完全一致。但局限性淋巴管扩张症的病变局限，不会造成淋巴液的大量丢失，影像学在病变程度和范围上与小肠淋巴管扩张症都会有较大的不同。

小肠黏膜下淋巴管瘤：腹腔及腹膜后淋巴管瘤诊断不难，但小肠黏膜下淋巴管瘤较少见，小肠镜及肉眼所见为多囊性肿物，病检见有较多扩张淋巴管，形成多个淋巴囊肿并伴内皮细胞增生。一般不伴有低蛋白血症。影像学检查意义不大。

综上所述，直接淋巴管造影与造影后 CT 联合检查对小肠淋巴管扩张症的诊断具有重要意义。

第九章　小肠创伤

第一节　延迟性小肠破裂

延迟性小肠破裂作为小肠破裂的一种特殊类型，多指小肠在损伤后24小时至数天内发生破裂。延迟性小肠破裂在早期腹膜刺激征不明显，腹腔诊断性穿刺受超声、X线检查多为阴性结果，容易造成临床漏诊、误诊，小肠破裂的延迟诊断是影响手术预后的主要因素，严重者可危及患者生命。

1. 发病机制　延迟性小肠破裂作为小肠破裂的一种特殊类型，分析原因可能有以下几个方面：腹部受到钝击伤后使肠管及系膜推移，受脊柱挤压产生挤压伤，肠壁破裂是不完全性的，早期仅有肠壁浆膜层的破裂，黏膜层受到碾挫伤肿胀，但黏膜层尚完整，局部肠壁的完全性得到保持，肠壁充血、水肿、渗出，MSCT表现为肠壁弥漫性增厚，肠系膜间隙脂肪密度增高（50~70 HU之间）。小肠间系膜脂肪间隙模糊、密度增高，肠壁弥漫性增厚、周围积液及点状积气。此时没有肠道内容物的外溢，所以没有明显的腹膜刺激征出现；临床表现只有受伤部位局部隐痛，全身状况尚可，少数患者还可出现症状隐匿期，即腹痛逐渐减轻的表现。

随着病情的发展，当损伤的黏膜受到肠道内容物的作用，受伤部位的肠黏膜发生缺血、坏死，局部继发化脓性炎症，加上进食、活动等因素，使肠道内压力增大，导致受伤后24 h或数天后肠管才出现完全破裂，局部出现渗液，肠道气体溢出，临床腹痛再度加重，并出现发热、腹胀、血液中性粒细胞升高等感染征象。

一组阳性病例中有3例受伤后24 h出现肠壁肿胀，周围少量液体外渗（3/15），有10例受伤3天内出现肠管周围积液、局限性小泡状游离性气体等征象（10/15），有2例患者受伤后1周内才出现肠管周围积液、渗出等腹膜炎征象（2/15）。

小肠受到损伤后，由于肠壁的破裂口较小，空、回肠腔内气体较少，肠腔压力低，局部的肠道渗出物较少，局部血凝块阻塞伤口或裂口炎性渗出、黏膜外翻导致肠内容物暂时不外溢，再加上受伤后应激反应肠袢相互靠拢或大网膜的覆盖，使早期腹膜炎征象不明显，临床症状轻微，肠管前方可见小泡状游离气体。当受伤数小时或数天后由于进食或运动导致肠蠕动恢复，肠气增多，肠腔内压力升高，导致堵塞物脱落，肠道内容物逐渐外渗，气体溢出，临床才逐渐出现腹痛加剧，腹膜炎及腹膜刺激征征象。

小肠受到减速撞击后产生剪切伤，肠腔相对完整，但肠壁出现挫伤，肠系膜水肿或斑片状出血，血肿形成，导致肠管局部缺血、肿胀，或者较大的肠系膜血管血栓形成导致继发性肠管坏死，当数小时或数天后局部肠管坏死加重或肠腔内压力增大时，病变处肠管出现破溃而导致肠道内容物外漏，临床出现腹膜炎症状，手术中可发现缺血性肠狭窄及较深的溃疡形成，镜下可见看到嗜铁细胞、血肿及异物反应性改变，这也可能是导致小肠迟发性破裂的原因之一。部分患者由于腹部多脏器损伤后合并腹腔实质脏器破裂出血、腹腔积血或腹膜后血肿，肠壁挫伤早期缺血、肿胀或肠壁破裂口较小，肠麻痹导致临床腹膜炎征象被掩盖，数天后肠管出现感染坏死，肠腔内容物外渗才出现明显腹膜炎征象。

2. 影像学研究　临床常见的小肠破裂通过诊断性腹腔穿刺及超声探查腹腔积液、X线透视膈下游离性气体等常规检查手段较易作出诊断。但延迟性小肠破裂早期腹腔积液较少，且多局限在肠管周围间隙内，诊断性腹腔穿刺结果往往为阴性，腹部超声检查对少量肠间积液由于受到肠气、肠液的干扰，诊断敏感度及特异性不高；由于早期腹腔游离气体较少，且局限于肠周间隙，膈下往往看不到游离性气体影，使早期的小肠破裂得不到充分的影像学证据；而临床医师仅靠临床经验及体征进行诊断，容易造成误诊、漏诊，延误治疗。

MSCT 较高的空间及密度分辨率为早期诊断延迟性小肠破裂提供了充分的影像学基础，使用 MSCT 薄层扫描及重建技术可以早期发现小肠破裂局部肿胀、增厚的肠壁及肠系膜脂肪间隙少量的渗出、漏出液和游离性小气泡影；发现肠管外游离气体是诊断肠破裂的重要征象，MSCT 可发现腹腔内 5 ml 以上的游离气体，X 线平片则需 50 ml 以上才可出现膈下游离性气体征象，所以 MSCT 对早期诊断小肠破裂具有较高的敏感性及特异性。

有报道认为，对于胃肠道损伤的患者 CT 检查的敏感性为 64%，特异性为 97%，另有报道阳性率达 83.3%。一组 16 例病例中 MSCT 术前诊断阳性 15 例，敏感性达 94%，高于一些报道，可能为例数较少之故。一般认为，在 CT 检查扫描过程中患者应尽量屏气，避免腹式呼吸，减少呼吸伪影造成的图像模糊，扫描时速度要快，使用无间距螺旋扫描，尽量减少肠管蠕动造成的运动伪影；如病人条件允许，应行 MSCT 平扫 + 增强扫描，这样可以增加肠管周围对比度，更加清楚地显示增厚的肠管及肠间积液、积气，增强扫描可提高肠系膜血管损伤的检出率，同时了解肠系膜动、静脉是否存在血栓等情况。

扫描完成后进行图像薄层重建，在工作站进行图像冠状位及矢状位重建，结合横轴位图像可准确判断小肠病变的位置及肠管走行形态，有助于甄别正常小肠内少量气体和积液造成的误判；要把有无局限性游离小气泡作为重点观察和判断。

另外，由于腹部损伤患者多为急诊患者，病情特殊，行腹部 MSCT 检查前不能进行有效的肠道准备（如口服对比剂、清洁肠道等），或由于患者合并胸腹部其他脏器损伤，不能有效配合检查，部分 MSCT 检查阴性者也不能除外小肠破裂的可能性。

该组病例中就有 1 例在住院观察期间，腹痛缓解后又持续性加重，临床出现持续性低热及腹部局限性压痛，临床科室高度怀疑延迟性小肠破裂，后经剖腹探查证实。

对于腹部外伤患者应提高警惕，虽然腹痛暂时缓解也应留院观察，早期行腹部 MSCT 检查，如结果阴性也应结合病情随时复查，争取早期诊断延迟性小肠破裂，早期手术治疗，减少术后并发症。该组病例中有 2 例患者是在住院观察期间 1 周内再次行 MSCT 检查诊断小肠破裂。延迟性小肠破裂早期征象不典型，延迟诊断往往增加术后并发症及死亡率，给患者造成不必要的痛苦。MSCT 以其特有的高密度分辨率及高空间分辨率可以清晰观察到受伤局部肠管肿胀、增厚情况及肠系膜脂肪间隙内少量渗出积液和 / 或少量游离积气，相对于诊断性腹腔穿刺及超声、X 线检查在延迟性小肠破裂的早期诊断中具有显著优势，随着 MSCT 的逐渐普及，值得临床推广应用。

第二节　腹腔游离气体与胸腔积气

腹部创伤病人的腹腔肠外积气征象常由于小肠破裂引起，X 线片上显示游离气体是紧急剖腹术的指征之一。然而在许多钝性创伤病人，CT 虽显示有腔外游离气体但并没有小肠破裂。有研究报道 18 例钝性创伤的 CT 扫描结果，只有 4 例（约占 22%）被证明有小肠破裂。

另有研究报道 118 例钝性创伤的腹部 CT 扫描，7 例见到游离的腔外积气，但均无小肠穿透伤。在这两项研究中所有气腹的病人几乎都有胸部创伤，有气胸或机械通气。这意味着空气可能由胸腔进入了腹腔。

第十章 肠壁积气和成人小肠中气体

第一节 肠壁积气

肠壁积气是空腹脏器壁内(浆膜下、黏膜下或二者)积气,肠道任何部分均可受累。在原发性或特异性积气,主要发生在结肠,而无另外胃肠道受累, X 线表现一般为多发性小气泡聚集。继发性积气伴存于各种胃肠病变, X 线表现通常呈线状分布透光影。另外的分类是:①囊状积气,存在于空腹脏器壁内(通常在结肠);②间质气肿,气体出现于空腔脏器壁内,为非囊状积气,不伴产气微生物的感染;③产气感染。气腹可为肠积气的并发症,依赖其病因而出现症状或不出现症状。

Bryk(1973)报告 2 例小肠肠壁积气伴气腹:一例为穿孔性十二指肠溃疡伴广泛空肠积气,表现为肠梗阻;一例穿孔性空肠憩室出现空肠积气与大量气腹,但腹部症状轻微。此二例肠积气可能是因为气体从穿孔处分离浆膜下而生,这是小肠积气的少见原因。

至此,文献上已报告的肠壁积气的原因有 19 种:慢性肠炎,特异性或非特异性;慢性肺病;继发于化学性(碱)狭窄的食管梗阻;肠梗死;肠梗阻;肠寄生虫;坏死性大、小肠炎;腹膜炎;胃蜂窝织炎;胃镜检后;乙状结肠镜检后;肠吻合术后;幽门狭窄与溃疡伴胃流出道梗阻;硬皮病;乙状结肠扭转;溃疡性结肠炎伴有毒的巨结肠;肠脂质营养不良(Whipple 病);十二指肠溃疡穿孔;空肠憩室穿孔。

第二节 成人小肠内的气体

传统观念一直认为小肠内出现空气均属病理情况,事实证明远非如此,此传统观念是错误的,应予摒弃。Zahnd 等(1981)研究 827 例成人腹部常规平片,均为仰卧位,照片前皆未准备肠道。其中 553 例为住院者, 274 例为一般门诊病人,男性 429 例,女性 398 例,均无急腹症、腹痛、小肠和大肠疾病。

所有照片取自胃肠造影及尿系、生殖系、胆系造影之前的腹部平片,腰椎及骨盆照片。该作者发现,住院病人中大约一半,门诊病人中大约 1/3 在小肠内均出现气体,小肠内空气又以空肠为多,空肠腔平均横径 25mm(20~30mm),回肠为 20mm(15~25mm),这些测量值符合于钡餐检查所见,小肠壁平均厚度为 1.5mm。

第三节 “透光”伪影

应用双对比技术检查时,一肋骨或骶髂关节斜位重叠于胃肠充气钡的影像上,可伪似一息肉的茎。如误将脊柱椎弓根影像诊断为一息肉,则使人非常困窘。灌肠管尖端有一圆孔,切勿将此孔影像误认为息肉。灌肠管尖端的气囊投影有时也可铸成假病变,故有作者专门强调对直肠的反复照片总应在气囊放气以后再做。

第四节　分成小腔的气腹酷似肠壁内气体

在 X 线腹部平片上发现弯曲的透光影，多表示肠壁内有气体，为肠壁血管梗死的 X 线征象。Kressel 等（1977）报告一例表现与此类似者，手术发现气体不在肠壁内，而是紧靠存活肠袢的乱成一团的肠袢的浆膜外腹膜腔积气所致。

对于肠袢外气体有许多解释，在腹部手术后持续长达 38 天腹腔内可见气体存在（Felson，1968），而该病例已达 70 天仍见气体；腹膜腔脓肿常有肠壁外气体可见，但该例在气体存在处并未发现脓肿；肠壁内气体外出穿过浆膜层也可引起壁外积气，但该例照片后几小时手术，壁内并未发现气体。Koss（1952）和 Nelson（1972）报告肠梗阻是引起肠壁内积气的原因之一，Koss 描述 1 例急性肠梗阻伴肠气囊病，在肠袢之间和粘连带中，如同在肠壁内均有气囊存在。该例术时未见肠腔内气体，梗阻在此也不是原因。

第十一章 肠道缺血

第一节 肠缺血

肠缺血是肠血流(动脉或静脉)减少引起的一种复杂的疾病状态。随年龄增长发病率增加。据估计在急性腹痛病例中约1%为缺血性肠病。在过去的30年中,尽管对本病的认识和诊断的敏感性都有提高,但其发病率和死亡率仍然很高,其中急性肠系膜缺血的死亡率超过60%。血管造影被认为是肠缺血的标准检查方法,但由于系有创性检查,可能引起并发症,因此使用较少。随着CT的广泛应用,对肠缺血的诊断取得了一定的成功。

肠系膜缺血病因主要包括3方面:①动脉血流减少或闭塞;②静脉血流减少或闭塞;③低血流量状态。根据肠系膜缺血的发生时间及临床表现分为急性和慢性。

血栓栓塞所致的动脉闭塞是急性肠系膜缺血的最常见原因,栓子常来自左房、左室或心脏瓣膜。肠系膜上动脉栓塞占全部病例的50%。发生在动脉粥样硬化斑块基础上的血栓形成占25%,且常发生于有慢性肠系膜缺血的病例。

动脉狭窄超过管腔横断面积的50%~80%才出现临床症状。非闭塞性肠系膜缺血占急性肠系膜缺血病例的30%,发生于低血流量状态(如低血压、脓毒血症、心衰、洋地黄治疗),原因可能是血管收缩或痉挛。

急性肠系膜缺血少见的原因是静脉血栓形成,可发生于门静脉高压、高凝状态或外伤的病例。有腹部疾病(如胰腺炎、胰腺癌、憩室炎)的病人也是高危人群。

慢性肠系膜缺血典型发病年龄在50岁以上。大多数病人是吸烟者,1/3以上有高血压、冠状动脉疾病或脑血管疾病。典型表现为反复的餐后腹痛,常位于上腹部或中腹部,1~2小时后缓解。多数病人还可出现体质下降。慢性肠系膜缺血大多来自肠系膜动脉粥样硬化,后者可引起管腔狭窄和血流灌注减少。肠系膜动脉粥样硬化是否会引起肠系膜缺血症状取决于管腔狭窄程度和侧支循环建立的程度。

影像学研究:临床疑为肠系膜缺血的病例行CT检查主要有两方面原因:第一,有助于发现受累肠袢和肠系膜的缺血性改变;第二,通过评价肠系膜血管的动脉粥样硬化、血栓、闭塞、肿瘤压迫或侵犯及外伤,有时可以发现病因。

但第一代和第二代CT诊断肠系膜缺血准确性的报道并不令人满意。由于螺旋CT可提供更窄的准直、更快的扫描速度以及经静脉团注定时增强,因此对肠系膜血管和肠壁的显示能力大大提高。MSCT对于肠系膜血管和小肠的观察优于单排探测器螺旋CT。

CT检查技术:目前一般采用口服低密度对比剂(主要应用水500~1 000ml)。与高密度对比剂相比主要有两方面优势:第一,低密度对比剂不干扰三维(3D)重建效果,因此不用大量的数据编辑即可很好地显示肠系膜血管及其分支;第二,肠腔内低密度对比剂使肠壁的强化显示更佳,因而可以采集到功能方面的信息。MSCT在显示肠系膜血管方面明显优于单排探测器螺旋CT。MSCT扫描速度更快,大大消除了呼吸和运动伪影,而且可更准确地控制团注对比剂的时机,获得动、静脉期图像;MSCT允许准直更窄,可达0.5~1mm层厚,从而降低小血管分支的部分容积效应。

使用3D重建技术观察肠系膜血管小分支的走行及管腔明显优于横断层面影像。3D重建技术主要有3种:遮蔽表面显示、最大密度投影和容积再现。遮蔽表面显示由于仅使用了一定密度阈值内的数据，因此对显示肠壁信息不充足，而且由于仅表面得以显示，故有较多的伪影、噪声和肠壁细节信息的丢失。

最大密度投影仅显示由计算机产生的特定方向线束上的最亮体素，对显示远端血管有一定价值，但丢失了空间关系信息。

容积再现是最为先进的重建方法，与遮蔽表面显示不同，它获得最终图像需要编辑所有数据，同时可以调节参数使强化肠壁得到最佳显示，此外，可调节容积数据，模拟出类似传统的小肠造影影像。与最大密度投影不同，容积再现既可以准确显示血管，又可以显示邻近结构，保留了空间关系信息。

CT 表现：急性肠系膜缺血：最常见的 CT 表现为肠壁环周增厚，因黏膜下水肿或炎症所致，一般壁厚不超过 1.5cm。肠壁可表现为密度减低，反映水肿和炎症，有时可因黏膜下出血表现为高密度。增厚的肠壁可密度均一或表现出“晕征”，还可出现肠系膜水肿或积液。

增强后由于受累肠袢血流减少表现为强化程度减低，在某些病例由于充血可表现为强化程度增加，延迟强化或持续强化也有报道。

肠壁增厚虽然是最常见的 CT 表现，但并非特异，还可见于其他炎性、感染性或肿瘤性疾病。肠管扩张也是常见表现，可能是由于正常蠕动功能破坏所致，扩张的肠腔内常充满液体，也不具特异性。

肠壁积气相对少见，但特异性高，肠道内气体进入受损肠壁，提示已发生不可逆损害，受累肠壁全层梗死，是急症手术的指征。肠壁积气还可见于其他病变，如胶原血管性疾病、激素应用和肺疾病，依靠病史不难鉴别。肠壁内气体还可进入肠系膜静脉或肝内门静脉分支，甚至形成腹腔内游离气体，均是预后不良的征象。

急性肠系膜缺血受累肠袢的范围决定于缺血原因和侧支循环建立的程度。如果是大的血管病变（如肠系膜上动脉、肠系膜上静脉），则整个小肠及右半结肠和横结肠均可受累。房颤病人的栓子可仅累及一段小肠。低血流量状态可引起肠管的广泛缺血，由此导致的非闭塞性肠系膜缺血可在 CTA 图像上表现为动脉分支变细，与传统的血管造影表现一致。

慢性肠系膜缺血：多为肠系膜动脉粥样硬化斑块引起管腔狭窄，导致血流减少。由于病程可达数年，典型病例多建立起侧支循环保证了肠管血供。MSCT 横断层面影像和 3D 影像可显示这些解剖通道。肠系膜动脉起始部的粥样硬化斑块钙化在老年人相对常见，大部分病人并无缺血的症状。与急性肠系膜缺血不同，慢性肠系膜缺血病人除非并发急性血栓栓塞，小肠形态通常正常。

其他原因所致的肠缺血：各种原因所致的机械性和绞窄性梗阻包括肿瘤、肠套叠、腹疝、肠扭转等均可引起受累肠袢血供的减少。CT 表现为肠管扩张、肠壁增厚、肠系膜水肿或积液等。梗阻段肠袢延迟增强提示绞窄，是急症手术指征。

肠外伤：“休克肠”是外伤后低血容量休克引起的长时间低灌注所致。典型 CT 表现为肠管扩张、充满液体，静脉注入对比剂后明显持续强化等。休克肠可在血容量恢复后好转。

第二节　关于小肠“狭窄”

近年有作者报道，在小肠偶尔也出现类似的“狭窄”，十分像局部缺血的 X 线表现。

气钡充盈不良的肠曲也可伪似疾病，当该肠曲完全扩张时，此“病变”也即刻消逝。

需要注意，不要在排空后照片上诊断苹果心病变，只有在肠曲膨胀时才能去评估它的内径大小。

第三节　小肠梗死肠壁内积气的难见表现

肠壁内积气众所周知为小肠坏死的 X 线征象，常显示为细薄的线状透光影，与肠轴平行走行，Wiot 和 Felson（1961）首次报告 2 例。另有作者报告 2 例类似征象，壁内积气显示为细而连续的、固定的新月形线状与肠轴平行走行的透光影。一些作者称壁内积气为肠坏死常见征象，而气体聚积偶尔呈环状，部分或完全围绕肠曲。

有作者认为肠坏死壁内积气不变地呈现线状，而另外学者发现气体积聚可呈现少见的曲线状或环形，走行垂直于肠轴，彼此间分离 2~6mm，稍类似于瓣状逐渐集中，在横卧、直立照片所见相同，24 小时后照片仍未见变化。

唯一与此情况可能混淆的是肠气囊病，其气体呈囊状积聚，沿着肠的边缘走行，且气体积聚一般较大，与此不同。壁内积气与肠腔内气体的区别是：前者立卧位保持一样的表现；24 小时后照片也变化不大；为曲线状集聚，而肠腔内积气无一定形状。

第十二章　空肠和回肠的其他疾病

第一节　导致肠壁增厚的良性疾病

许多良性疾病可引起环状或对称性肠壁增厚，厚度通常小于 1cm。肠壁既可表现为均匀软组织密度，又可表现为高低密度混杂的环状影，即所谓“双晕征”或靶征。此征象由肠黏膜下水肿和 / 或脂肪沉积等引起，于螺旋 CT 增强血管期观察最佳。

可见于一些生理性或疾病状态，如克罗恩病、缺血性肠炎、感染性肠炎、放射性肠炎、嗜酸性胃肠炎、Henoch-Schonlein 紫癜及门静脉高压引起的肠水肿。

肠壁出血表现为肠壁增厚，平扫呈高密度。

小肠良性疾病，通常为节段性，病处小肠系膜脂肪多增厚，密度升高，呈条状。

第二节　回盲瓣逆行脱垂

当回盲瓣黏膜皱襞过多而形成一唇状突起时，可造成回盲瓣的逆行性脱垂。此突起的瓣在盲肠内产生一充盈缺损。用手扪压或 / 和依靠钡柱的静水压力，凸出的回盲瓣逆行脱垂，造成回肠末端逐渐变尖。瓣装置的这些变化能伴装为病理情况，然而细心地观察可辨别此类变异。回盲瓣逆行脱垂首先由 Rigler 和 Lasser（1951）报告，钡灌肠检查时，在盲肠内可见一光滑的圆形充盈缺损，此缺损颇为柔软，扪压能改变其形状，用手扪压或 / 和钡柱的静水压，减轻盲肠内的充盈缺损，造成末端回肠的环状缺损。这些征象容易复制，空气造影时更为明显。结肠镜检查有助诊断，手术证实诊断。此症为良性，唇状突起处可见溃疡，为胃肠出血的一个原因。

鉴别诊断有淋巴瘤可产生套迭进入盲肠；回盲瓣的原发性腺癌甚少见，但也可出现类似套叠；回盲瓣类癌慢性套叠也有个案介绍。

瓣的逆行脱垂性质柔软，容易脱垂于末端回肠内或外，瓣连接处无肠梗阻。回盲瓣脂肪过多在盲肠内产生一个巨大的压迫，然而真性脂肪过多很少出现逆行脱垂，脂肪过多者瓣的脂肪沉着远远多于本症。

第三节　回盲瓣的脂肪瘤样肥大抑或是肿瘤

在腹部 CT 图像上，经常可以见到回盲瓣，它位于盲肠的内侧壁，距盲肠盲端大约 3~4cm 处，CT 扫描时，偶可见到轻微增厚的回盲瓣达 2~3cm。

在增厚的回盲瓣内含脂肪密度影提示为良性脂肪瘤样浸润，没有临床意义。低密度脂肪影可以排除炎症或肿瘤性病变，它是一个偶然的发现，不需要进一步检查。

第四节 小肠出血性梗死

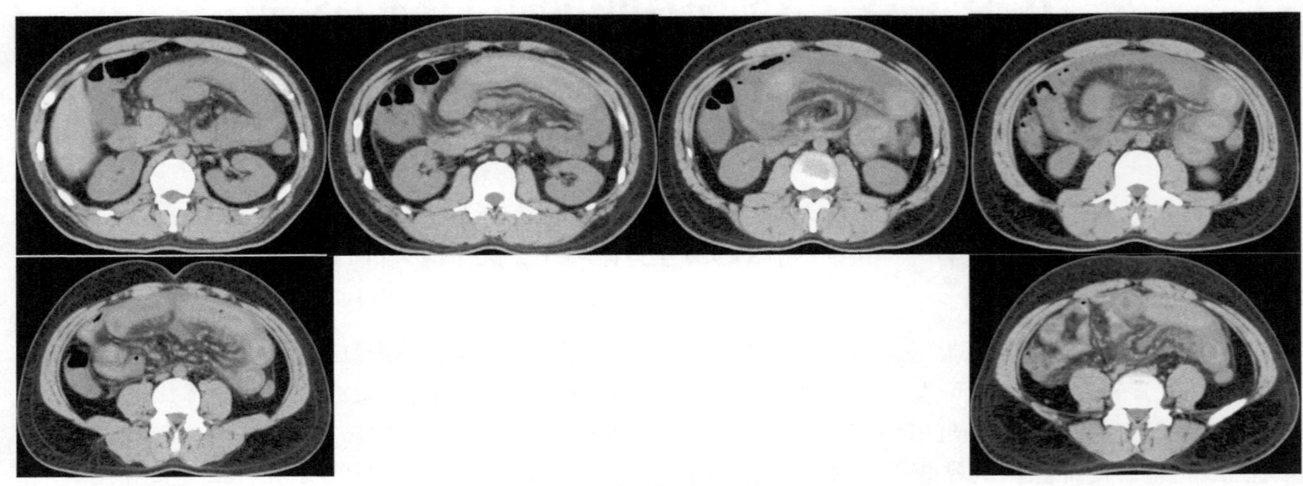

图 25-12-1 小肠出血性梗死

患者,男,37 岁。因腹痛 4 天入院。

手术所见:小肠约 1.5 米坏死发黑出血,周围组织水肿,肠系膜增厚,内见黑色血凝团块,腹腔内积血性液体 200ml。逐层进腹,护皮,距曲氏韧带 50cm,超声刀离断坏死小肠肠系膜,在系膜根部,予以止血,发现血管断端处血栓形成,尽量取出血栓,将坏死小肠予以切除。

病理检查:部分空回肠切除标本:肠管一段,长 40cm,一切缘周径 3cm,另一切缘周径 6cm,肠管内充满血性液体,肠壁呈暗褐色,壁厚 0.5~0.7cm,皱襞明显,未见明显坏死及其他明显异常。病理诊断:部分空回肠切除标本:镜下示肠管黏膜表面糜烂、脱落及坏死,黏膜下层水肿,血管扩张及充血,并肌层断裂,浆膜层显著充血水肿伴出血;结合临床及大体所见,符合肠出血性梗死的病理学改变(图 25-12-1)。

第五节 小肠发育变异和诊断陷阱

除十二指肠球部和一短段球后部分外,十二指肠位于腹膜后。十二指肠水平部位于肠系膜上动脉和肠系膜上静脉的后方以及主动脉和下腔静脉的前方。倘若无既往手术史,而十二指肠的这部位缺失,则强烈提示小肠旋转不良。小肠的其余部分(空肠与回肠)位于腹膜腔内。

壁厚:当小肠腔内被水充盈时,其正常的环行皱襞即清晰可见。CT 扫描时,若肠腔内充满阳性对比剂,其壁就很难辨认。它的壁厚不超过 1~2mm。扩张的小肠袢的壁厚如大于 3mm 时,应可疑病变。然而,当未充分扩张时,正常的肠壁呈环行增厚,且酷似小肠本身病变。在充分扩张的情况下,如果小肠壁厚在其最宽处超过 3mm,应怀疑肿瘤性或炎性病变。一些继发的征象也能把正常萎陷的小肠袢和病变区分开来,这包括肠周围脂肪线的显影,肠系膜淋巴结肿大,肠腔外气体或液体的聚集以及小肠壁的靶征或晕征。

靶征:多层靶征(2~3 层同心环状的不同密度影)不是一个特异的征象,但当它出现时,可暗示异常小肠壁的存在,且通常可除外恶性病变。静脉团注对比剂后,黏膜层和肌层被强化,靶征可解释为夹在环行影中间的低密度区,它代表水肿的黏膜下层。在对比增强 CT 图像上,靶征在以下情况下会出现:克罗恩病、溃疡性结肠炎、感染性肠炎、缺血性肠炎、放射性肠炎、肠水肿和与烧伤后炎性病变有关的脂肪沉积。

评估腹腔与盆腔的 CT 图像时，常遇到的问题是如何把部分充盈和萎陷的小肠袢与腹腔内病理性增厚的肠袢和软组织块影区分开。

如果阳性对比剂未能使小肠腔充分充盈，则这些小肠袢可被误认为病变，例如肠系膜和腹膜的转移瘤。此时，可从一系列相邻 CT 层面上继续追踪它的走行，就可望将萎陷的肠袢与腹膜腔的肿瘤区分开来。只要可能，都应预先策划 CT 扫描程序。

此外，口服对比剂后延迟扫描可将小肠和肿瘤鉴别开。被液体充分充盈并含气体的小肠袢可酷似脓肿，二者的区别在于肠系膜脂肪线和占位效应，这在前者出现，而后者则无。偶尔对两者的鉴别发生困难时，还可应用口服对比剂后的延迟 CT 扫描，将被气体、液体充盈的小肠与肿瘤、脓肿等区分开。

小肠的长度：关于小肠的长度，报告颇不一致，一方面由于测量时条件不同，所得结果各异，另一方面个体变异也相当大。一般说来，活体情况下，用吞入细管至胃肠道的方法测量得的小肠长度数字过于偏小；而尸解时，肠管失去紧张度，牵拉时会变长，在这样情况下进行测量，其结果则偏大。

常见型与变异型：小肠肠袢的分支数目，可分为常见型与变异型，分别占统计数的 80% 和 20% 左右，一般认为，它们与先天发育有关，与个体的体型关系不大，至于与性别有无关系，尚待研究。肠袢的走行方向与途径也可分为常见型与变异型，它除与先天发育有关外，与体型及高矮胖瘦还有一定关系。决定腹腔脏器的毗邻关系的因素是先天发育，但是，个体的体型、体位、姿势、空腔脏器的空虚与充盈对它还有一定的影响。作为发育变异，肠管可介入肝与膈之间（Chilaiditi 综合征）。

第六节　一些诊断陷阱

肠袢类似肿块：有作者报告，偶尔 CT 扫描在结肠肝曲上部充有不规则对比剂，并紧贴肝穹隆外上方，被误为钙化的肝肿块。肠袢类似肿块，肠袢类似肿瘤复发，无对比剂的肠袢形成假肿瘤等在文献上均有不少报告，常用口服对比剂后再重复扫描，一般可澄清问题。

邻近的肠袢：邻近的肠袢如十二指肠也可造成误诊，它可伪似动脉瘤或腹腔动脉瘤的破裂。充盈不佳或未充盈的肠袢邻近动脉时，可表现为软组织肿块，酷似血栓或邻近的血肿。

胃内含有大量黏液：有作者注意到，当胃内含有大量黏液时，可引起十二指肠和近端小肠钡剂造影时出现异常，表现为雪花状充盈不良，似乎肠袢内含有大量的分泌物。

大量肠系膜脂肪：大量肠系膜脂肪可导致全腹小肠表现异常，可见小肠袢均变细小，且分布疏散。

淋巴样组织：有作者报告 3 岁男孩回肠末端出现“卵石影”。此正常变异是由于这段小肠有大量的淋巴样组织引起，不应误认为炎症性小肠疾病的证据。另有作者报告一例 16 岁男孩和 62 岁健康老人回肠末端也出现类似淋巴样增生引起的卵石样表现。

扩张的膀胱：有作者报告一例 3 岁儿童扩张的膀胱使小肠和结肠向上移位显著，导出 300ml 尿液后上述移位完全消失。

假蛔虫：偶尔回肠末端的黏膜皱襞在钡餐检查时表现伪似蛔虫病。

第七节　空肠与回肠的少见病

小肠团块性淀粉样变性病：Pandarinath 等（1978）报告 1 例小肠团块性淀粉样变性病，其钡餐检查类似多发性小肠肿瘤，其临床表现为消化道出血。尽管胃肠道淀粉样浸润常见，但小肠团块性淀粉样变性却难见到。此病例从十二指肠到回肠均可见散在的结节，该作者称文献上仅见 1 例相似的情况。

硬化性纤维性腹膜炎：Gold 和 Redman（1972）报告 1 例硬化性纤维性腹膜炎的血管造影表现十分类似于回肠类癌。类癌常侵犯小肠系膜，引起显著的纤维性反应、缩短与增厚，系膜的扭曲反映在系膜血管的变形，为风琴状或星状排列。应当注意到，凡是能引起系膜纤维化反应的疾病，皆可造成类似的血管造影表现。

肠性脂质营养不良：肠性脂质营养不良（即

Whipple 病)的淋巴造影表现与犯及淋巴系统的恶性肿瘤淋巴造影表现极难区别。该病与淋巴瘤只靠临床进行鉴别是不容易的。虽然此病的许多症状与体征也见于淋巴瘤,但其常见的腹泻在淋巴瘤却极少见到。

第十三章　小肠疾病影像检查技术

第一节　小肠磁共振水成像

小肠比较影像学：目前小肠影像检查方法主要有口服法小肠钡餐造影、插管法小肠气钡造影、MSCT、肠系膜血管造影等。口服法小肠钡餐造影操作简单，患者无痛苦，诊断准确性较低；插管法小肠气钡造影诊断准确性较高，操作复杂，患者有一定痛苦。上述检查经常因肠袢重叠误诊，难以直接观察肠壁和肠腔外组织。MSCT显示肠壁增厚和肠腔外病变有明显优势，对肠壁及肠腔总体结构显示欠佳，不能提供小肠功能状态信息，检查过程有X线辐射。肠系膜血管造影为有创性检查，不能直接显示肠管病变。

小肠磁共振水成像：小肠磁共振水成像为无创性检查，适应证广，结合常规腹部MRI，小肠的整体性显示较好，软组织分辨率高，能显示肠腔内外组织结构，可进行多平面成像，无X线辐射。一组小肠磁共振水成像检查效果良好。可以认为小肠磁共振水成像是一种新型有效的小肠影像学检查方法。小肠磁共振水成像检查需要良好的肠道清洁准备，肠道内容物易形成伪影，甚至误诊。小肠肠管需充盈足量对比剂，以充分扩张肠管，瘪陷状态的小肠易掩盖病灶，有时会误诊为肠壁增厚。

目前国内外小肠影像学检查方法的研究集中在肠腔的充盈和扩张，肠道对比剂主张用等渗液体，并且不被人体过快吸收，否则达不到扩张肠管的目的。扩张肠管的方法主要有口服或经小肠导管注入大量的水、钡剂、钆剂、超顺磁性氧化铁溶液等。该组小肠磁共振水成像选择等渗的生理盐水或葡萄糖盐水作为肠道对比剂，对人体无害，患者耐受性好，无副作用；生理盐水或葡萄糖盐水易被小肠少量吸收，该组选择检查前30 min口服肠道对比剂，小肠肠管得到良好充盈，肠壁显示清楚。使用低张药物以抑制肠蠕动，消除蠕动伪影，提高了图像质量。该组检查前10 min静脉注射山莨菪碱20 mg，肠蠕动抑制效果良好。

克罗恩病主要表现为小肠多发节段性肠壁增厚，小肠肿瘤主要表现为肠壁增厚和肿块，两者增强扫描均有中等程度以上强化，十二指肠肿瘤除上述征象以外常合并胆总管和胰管扩张，一组18例小肠磁共振水成像和腹部MRI序列很好地显示上述征象，敏感性达100%，特异性77.8%(14/18)。该作者认为：小肠磁共振水成像对小肠肠壁增厚和小肠肿块的诊断价值较高。腹部平片是诊断小肠梗阻的常用方法，大多数情况无法明确梗阻原因。利用肠梗阻潴留液体行小肠磁共振水成像，可提高诊断小肠梗阻的准确性，对明确梗阻原因有帮助。一组3例梗阻近段小肠获得满意显示，对梗阻原因的判断基本准确。

小肠磁共振水成像较其他小肠影像学检查方法具有适应证广，操作简单，诊断敏感性、特异性高，无痛苦和无X线辐射等优点，是一种新型有效的影像学检查方法。能比较清晰地显示小肠正常解剖结构和病变组织，对克罗恩病和小肠肿瘤等肠管增厚或肿块性病变具有较高的诊断价值，显示小肠梗阻部位比较准确，对判断小肠梗阻原因具有一定的价值。

第二节　腹腔多发占位性病变 - 胃肠道间质瘤病例

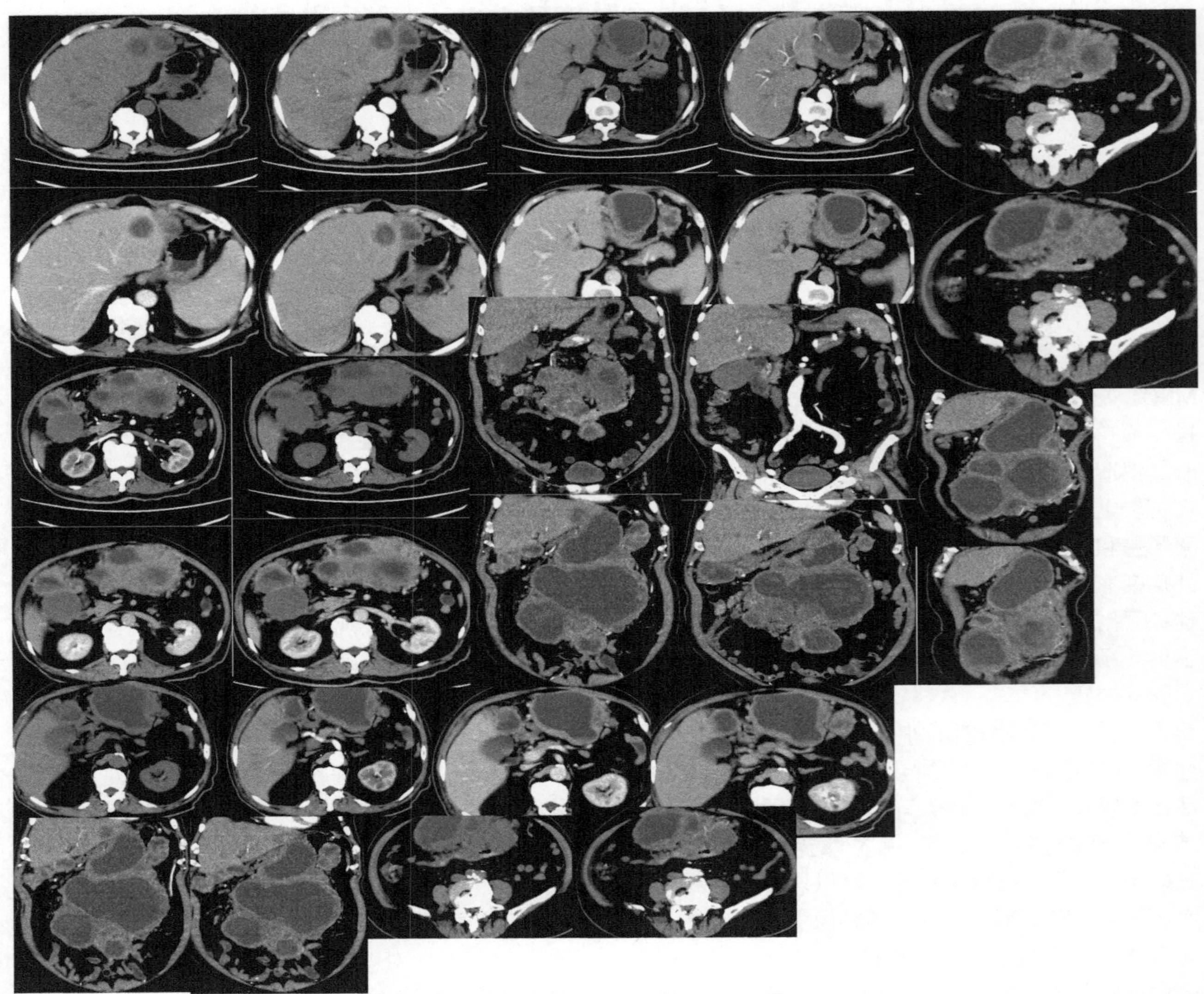

图 25-13-1　腹腔多发占位性病变 - 胃肠道间质瘤

患者，男，79 岁。腹胀 1 个月余入院。

病理检查：腹腔包块穿刺组织：灰白色条索状组织两条，分别长为 1.2cm 和 1cm，直径均为 0.1cm，另见灰白色组织一枚，大小 0.1cm × 0.1cm × 0.1cm。常规病理诊断：腹腔包块穿刺组织：梭形细胞肿瘤，需做免疫组化进一步确诊。免疫组化检测：阳性：CD34，CD117，DOG1，Vimentin，Bcl-2，NSE（局灶 +），Ki-67（+，约 20%）；阴性：CK（P），CK（H），CK（L），Calponin，EMA，Actin，Calretinin，MC，CA199，S-100，PSA。免疫组化诊断：腹腔包块穿刺组织：胃肠道间质瘤（图 25-13-1）。

第三节　肠壁CT增强后的密度改变

分析肠壁的异常形态主要是通过两个方面：①静脉增强后肠壁的密度改变；②钡剂灌肠后肠管的形态特点。一组作者提出，可将肠壁CT增强后的密度改变分类为五种模式：白密度、灰密度、水晕征、脂肪晕征及黑密度。

（1）白密度：白密度代表肠壁的大部分均匀强化。这仅仅应用于静脉增强之后，有时候，没有口服对比剂可更好地评价肠管，因为腔内对比剂会填满腔内空隙而造成混淆。结肠周围的供血血管可以出现扩张。这种白密度可能有两种病理生理学基础：血管扩张和/或血管内壁的损伤及伴随的增宽的裂隙的漏出。休克肠管（受钝器外伤后的低血压患者，小肠弥漫性缺血）是后者的典型例子。低灌注引起血管对大分子和白蛋白的通透性增加，这导致弥漫性的肠壁增厚和肠壁强化，后者是因为缓慢灌注和对比剂分子的漏出造成的。对低血容量的成功纠正可逆转休克肠管，这暗示了白密度部分代表着可逆的缺血性改变，有重要的临床意义。

白密度至少和同层面的静脉血管密度相近，或者更高，但它依赖于静脉注射对比剂的量和速度以及扫描时机。无强化或低强化对肠缺血更有特异性，但缺血部分也可能出现增强，这是因为血管通透性和灌注改变造成的。肠壁的增强和肠管的炎性病变有关，反应充血和血管增生改变，这在急性炎症中有典型表现。血管增生表现为肠系膜的血管扩张和迂曲。回肠系膜缘直管动脉的增粗和间距增加被称为梳征。

鉴别诊断：白密度一般发生在肠管炎性病变和血管疾患中。在恶性病变中少见。

注意事项：当前的方法是利用静脉强化的自身的标准。假如肠壁强化程度相当于或高于同层面的静脉，它应该被分类为白密度。因此，建立肉眼上的密度对比很实际有效。

（2）灰密度：灰密度定义为增厚的肠壁，轮廓欠清，强化后密度相当于强化的肌肉密度。‘灰密度’的分类，介于白密度和水样密度之间。灰密度是五种密度中最少特异性的，它一般用于良性和恶性疾病的鉴别。Macari和Balthazar注意到肠壁增厚小于2cm多为良性病变，增厚大于3cm通常发生在肿瘤中。但在这两组病变中存在相当多的重叠，最后解释这种情况应当结合形态学观察。如钡剂造影，因为它能动态观察、触诊和透视，这是传统CT所不能做到的。

鉴别诊断：灰密度和伴随的形态学特征用于区分良性和恶性疾病。

注意事项：一般造成小肠或结肠的假阳性的原因是未完全的肠腔扩张。假如怀疑结肠不完全扩张，要采用灌肠后CT扫描。这也可应用于怀疑假阴性的情况。例如，怀疑小肠不完全的肠腔扩张，就要加服对比剂后立刻重复该层面扫描。小肠壁增厚的假阳性经常发生，特别是空肠。由于口服对比剂的不均匀的分层和肠腔内容物的影响，也可造成假阳性。

（3）水晕征：水晕征表示增厚的肠壁中的一层，这种肠壁是由两个或三个连续的、对称性的增厚层组成：内层和外层为高密度，中间层为灰密度。水晕征的灰密度层被认为代表水肿，位于黏膜下层。靶征的内层和外层被认为分别是黏膜和黏膜肌层，高密度是明显强化的结果。水晕征作为肠壁损伤的观察是很有价值的，表示为急性反应。而且，小肠或大肠的许多病理情况可以产生这些征象，恶性病变很少出现这种‘水晕征’。

鉴别诊断：出现‘水晕征’的一般诊断包括肠道炎性疾病、血管疾患、感染性疾病和放射性损害。它罕见于恶性病变中。

注意事项：CT值测量和组织学的相互关系推断水晕征的病理生理基础很有可能是水肿。要合理利用形态学特征，除非有可以肯定的其他恶性征象，否则都应该诊断为良性。静脉增强后环形结构更明显，不增强可能不被发现。当肠腔内有水样密度的对比剂时，可更好地评价靶征中的黏膜层密度。

（4）脂肪晕征：脂肪晕部分指增厚肠壁的三层靶征中的中间层，也称黏膜下层，呈现脂肪密度。假如测量黑环的CT值，将大大地低于-10HU。无论如何，它很少与单纯的肠系膜或腹膜后的脂肪密度相等，这可能因为部分容积效应，或者同时存在的水肿。黏膜肌层的外缘可能清楚也可能模糊。在小肠观察到脂肪晕，可诊断克罗恩病，它可独立作为慢性期的征象。可是,在克罗恩病病人的肠管中,除了可以观察到脂肪晕征外,还可能发现其他肠管异常,没有脂肪晕而含其他密度部分,这种更多表明是急性期或亚急性期。在一个无症状的30年前曾经作过放射治疗的病人上观察到小肠脂肪晕征。小肠脂肪晕也可由细胞减数疗法引起。在结肠,这征象是相同的,但鉴别诊断上包括溃疡性结肠炎。有研究显示溃疡性结肠炎比克罗恩病更常见到脂肪晕征。细胞减数疗法也是结肠脂肪晕征的原因。

鉴别诊断:脂肪晕征的一般见于小肠克罗恩病,结肠溃疡性结肠炎或克罗恩病。少见的诊断包括细胞减数疗法和慢性放射性肠炎。

注意事项:壁内的脂肪可能为正常的发育变异,存在于没有胃肠道症状或胃肠道病史的病人的末段回肠和结肠。黏膜肌层是薄而均一的,厚度上很少超过1mm。围绕的肠系膜很少有异常。正常的脂肪晕征更常常出现在不扩大的或稍扩大的肠袢中。正常的变异不伴随其他肠壁的异常和局部肠系膜的改变(包括淋巴结增大)。最后诊断应该重视病史。

(5)黑密度:黑密度部分相当于气肿。除了少见的,大的囊性积气,所有的气肿都应该认为是急性肠管损伤的一部分。尽管气肿通常被认为是危及生命的损伤的征象,偶然也可见于肠腔吻合术后。任何伴随有黏膜损伤的情况都可能产生壁内积气。

鉴别诊断:一般诊断包括缺血、感染和外伤。在医源性的损伤中少见。

难点主要在于:①区别壁内少量的积气和邻近黏膜的肠腔内气体;②区别气体是位于黏膜内或是黏膜外血管;③区别盲肠、升结肠壁上的气泡和位于食物残渣与黏膜间的气体。采取不同体位重新定位和重新扫描,有时可以消除这种疑惑。

另外还应该检查肠系膜上静脉及下静脉和肝脏是否有静脉内的气体来支持气肿的诊断。

联合密度模式:一种疾病可能在不同肠管表现出不同的密度模式。这种现象可能是代表了几种同时存在的不同的病理生理学改变。肠道炎性疾病是这种现象的典型例子。要按照其所属不同的种类来分析肠管的每一部分。

结论:这里介绍的是一种肠壁异常形态的分类方法,它是以肠壁密度、分层结构的变化为基础的,并辅与形态学特点作补充。它可能有助于模棱两可的病例的诊断。尽管这种分类方法更有助于区别良、恶性疾病,但是它也可应用来区别一般的非肿瘤的肠道疾病。它的优点是以五种普通CT密度为基础,缺点是不易很好识别。也许这种方法能启迪放射学学者深入研究肠壁病变。

第二十六篇　大肠疾病

第一章　大肠癌

第一节　大肠癌的少见表现

一组作者指出转移性结肠癌可以类似感染性结肠炎。有作者综合文献提出大肠癌的数种不寻常的表现。一组学者对大肠癌的少见表现作了介绍，包括癌肿的多发性、大肠癌腹腔内转移、大肠癌穿孔、大肠癌侵犯胃及十二指肠、大肠癌侵犯回肠、大肠癌钙化等。

第二节　异物所致炎性肉芽肿误诊为肿瘤

52 年前，作者曾见 1 例中年女性患者，因左下腹不适且扪及包块，临床考虑卵巢囊肿及腹部恶性肿瘤而行钡剂胃肠检查。钡剂灌肠时，钡剂抵达乙状结肠远端即受阻，检查被迫中止。再做钡餐发现，从降结肠下段开始肠管逐渐变细，乙状结肠中远段明显狭窄，呈“C”形固定于包块后方，肠黏膜尚可。X 线诊断左下腹炎性包块，淋巴肉瘤不能除外。手术病理证实为乙状结肠周围鱼刺引起慢性肉芽肿，伴脓肿形成。

对该病例术后仔细追问，患者方想起 6 年前曾在吃鱼后不久突感剧烈腹痛，后对症治疗缓解。较大的异物经过胃肠道，常常难以通过幽门及回盲部，乙状结肠直肠连接处为结肠最窄处，鱼刺通过前二狭窄处后，被阻于大肠最窄处，并穿出肠壁，这是十分少见的情况。

第三节　升结肠黏液腺癌病例

患者，男，36 岁。因腹痛 19 个月，右下肢肿胀 1 个半月入院。11 个月前在外院就诊诊断为回盲部黏液腺癌（外生型）伴肺部多发转移，行化疗 6 周期，右侧胁腹部肿块破溃 8 个月。入院诊断为“腹部巨大肿块伴双肺转移”。

病理检查：升结肠黏膜活检标本：灰白色组织二枚，大小 0.5cm × 0.4 cm × 0.2 cm。病理诊断：升结肠黏膜活检标本示溃疡病灶及大小不等的黏液湖形成，其中有少数细胞核异型，周围腺体呈低级别上皮内瘤变，但结合临床，恶性肿瘤不能排除。

腹部肿瘤窦道组织新生物活检标本：破碎灰红色组织一堆，大小 1.5 cm × 1.5 cm × 0.7 cm。病理诊断：腹部肿瘤窦道组织新生物活检标本结合病史为转移性黏液腺癌。（图 26-1-1）

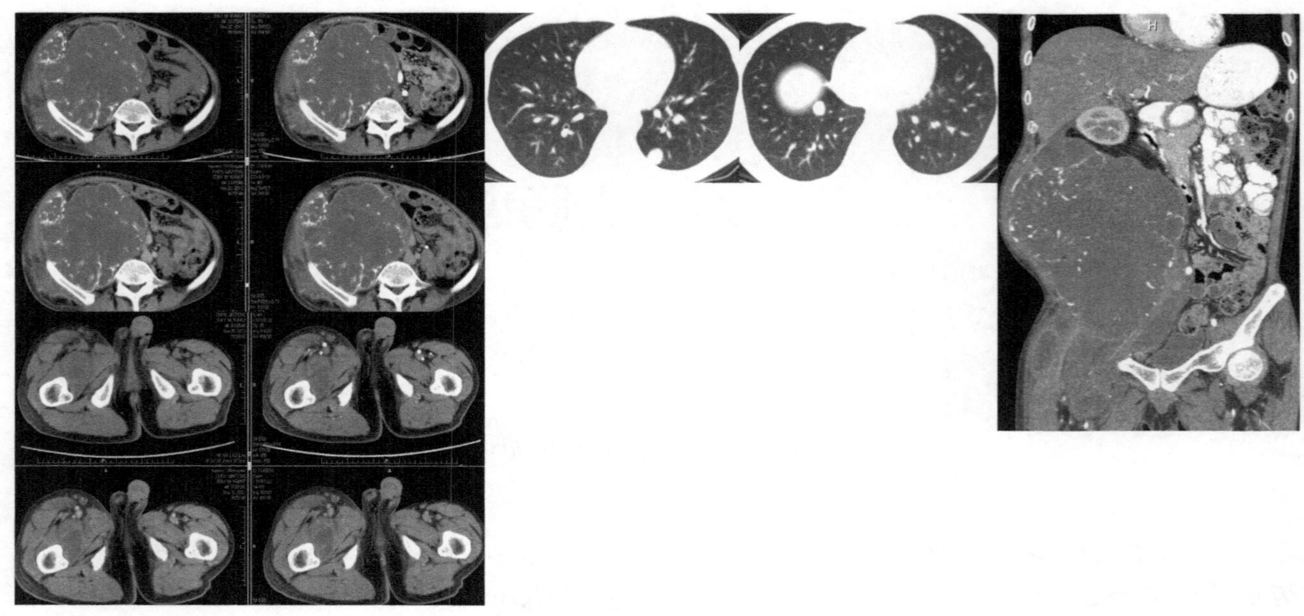

图 26-1-1 升结肠黏液腺癌病例

第四节 多个误诊病例简介:非大肠病变与大肠癌

骨肿瘤与直肠癌:40 多年前,我们曾检查一例老年患者,主诉排便困难半年,逐渐加重,指肛检查扪及硬块,直肠明显偏心性狭窄,几家医院门诊外科临床均诊断为直肠癌。钡剂灌肠照片见直肠近端完全性梗阻,直肠为一巨大蜂窝状骨瘤挤压移位。手术病理证实该骨瘤为遗传性多发性骨软骨瘤病,起自左侧坐骨棘,几乎占据整个小骨盆腔。该患者左股骨下端及左肱骨上端亦有类似骨软骨瘤,其子亦有三个部位的骨软骨瘤。

纤维索带与大肠癌:一组作者报告 4 例钡剂检查显示大肠腔内与壁内包块,诊断为大肠肿瘤,但手术证实为粘连带与纤维索带所致。可以提示粘连的特征性表现为:覆盖包块的黏膜完整;肠曲或邻近内脏受侵的征象;以前曾手术或有腹部盆部感染性疾病历史;横结肠和 / 或乙状结肠之肠脂垂局部病变。

例 1 为远端横结肠壁上 3cm 大小充盈缺损,乃由胃结肠韧带下部分到横结肠前表面一宽的纤维束所致;例 2 为横结肠近侧有 5cm 大小无柄息肉状充盈缺损,乃由粘连固定的回肠肠曲附着于该处所致;例 3 为乙状结肠有 2.5cm 大小无柄息肉状充盈缺损,手术见该处壁外一脓肿,一条 2cm 宽 0.5cm 厚的纤维条带从脓肿壁发出,粘连到乙状结肠,造成肠壁局限性凹入;例 4 为中段横结肠内广基息肉状充盈缺损,为纤维结缔组织粘连到横结肠所造成。

35 年前作者钡餐检查曾见一例胃小弯处约 1cm 宽, 0.5cm 深的充盈缺损,黏膜不规则,局部蠕动差,患者年迈,术前诊断为胃癌,手术发现却是一粘连带跨越附着小弯所致。

腹部手术后常见粘连与纤维索带,除非肠袢出现局限性固定(即"粘连中心")或发生肠梗阻,X 线检查时是难以察觉这些索带的。有作者报告,粘连引起结肠的缩窄性病变可类似于癌的餐巾环变形。

发生粘连的机制尚不完全清楚,并非凡是腹部手术均要产生,有作者指出,肠壁的纤维索带可出现于不同的病变时,可能是肠脂垂炎症的结果。这包括血管闭塞及随后的梗死、急性或慢性炎症、坏疽性或 / 和扭转性病变等。在上述任何一种病理过程之后,肠壁皆可能以纤维结缔组织粘连到附近肠袢或器官。由粘连造成的上述假性肿瘤出现于钡剂灌肠时难与淋巴囊肿、局限血肿、子宫内膜异位、脂肪瘤、转移癌、息肉及癌区别,其临床表现常为腹痛、恶心、呕吐、体重下降或黑便,皆为非特异性的。

粪结类似大肠新生物:50 年前,作者所在医院曾有一次会诊,讨论一老年患者盲肠有不规则充盈缺损，较大，两次钡剂灌肠均见该影变化不大，扪诊“包块”相当硬，透视下推压形状及位置几无变化，检查者认为系盲肠癌，手术却发现实为盲肠的粪结粘连肠壁。

另有学者报告 2 例，1 例粪结在乙状结肠，1 例粪结在结肠肝曲扩大部分，后者手术时发现沿着末段小肠与右侧结肠的肠系膜根部有一 30cm 长的缺损，且有肠扭转，并造成间歇性机械性肠梗阻。此 2 例术前皆诊断为癌。在结肠内，大的散在的粪便团块，尤其是粪块粘连肠壁固定不动时，很容易同结肠内新生物混淆，此种粪块即称粪结，它常见于直肠、乙状结肠、盲肠及其他部位。

近年来，钡餐检查常常使用胃复安之类促进胃肠排空的药物，钡剂得以迅速进入大肠。如用此法检查结肠，检查前务必清洁洗肠，否则难以观察，或者造成误诊。

第五节　炎性病变类似于大肠癌

非特异性结肠溃疡：非特异性结肠溃疡是一种临床和 X 线诊断都颇感困难的少见病，迄今只有 100 多例报道，Gardiner 和 Bird(1980)报告 4 例非特异性结肠溃疡钡灌肠检查表现类似环状结肠癌。因本病少见，术前诊断较难，它可表现如同急腹症，病变常发生在盲肠，且易穿孔。临床表现取决于溃疡的部位及有无合并症存在。盲肠和升结肠溃疡的症状酷似急性阑尾炎，而横结肠与左半结肠之病变临床发病突然，类似于癌肿、梗阻或憩室炎。钡灌肠检查约 75% 病例有异常发现，但溃疡本身却难见到。

此病 X 线表现为：环状狭窄伴锥形边缘，偶现充盈缺损；受累节段肠管痉挛伴不完全充盈；黏膜不规则。有作者指出，气钡双重造影对诊断本病是必要的，其 X 线征象为：溃疡龛影；环形水肿带；局限性激惹；局限性肠动力亢进；局部痉挛及触痛；瘢痕性改变引起狭窄以及穿孔造成气腹。

盲肠远侧的孤立性结核：盲肠远侧的孤立性结核病变十分少见。MacDonald 和 Middleton(1976)报告 1 例大肠远端结核酷似癌肿，经乙状结肠镜检、穿刺活检及细菌培养、治疗随访证实。Chawla(1971)收集英文文献中远段大肠的节段性肠结核 77 例，他本人报告的 750 例肠结核中，盲肠以外的孤立性病灶只有 10 例。大肠远侧段结核而不累及回盲部者诊断十分困难，老年患者的孤立性肠结核，只用 X 线检查确实难与恶性病变鉴别。病变为多发性，病人年轻则更可能是结核。不少作者指出，鉴别增生性肠结核与癌肿极为困难，甚至手术时也是如此。大多数恶性狭窄是孤立的，长 2~6cm，轮廓不整齐，有腔内充盈缺损，僵硬及轮廓逐渐变尖。而且，恶性狭窄较良性病变淤积更明显。结肠原发性硬化性癌如发生于年轻人，显示良性狭窄表现者，诊断尤其困难。

结肠感染性纤维性息肉：Ferin 和 Skucas(1983)报告 1 例结肠感染性纤维性息肉在气钡灌肠时误为肿瘤，且为组织学证实。此病又名嗜酸性肉芽肿性息肉。极少见于大肠，在 X 线检查与手术时，其表现酷似新生物而诊断困难。此病与肠道及骨的嗜酸性肉芽肿关系不大。Morson 和 Dawson(1979)称之为感染性纤维性息肉。

自 Vanek(1949)报告 6 例侵犯胃以来，只有几例犯及胃、小肠的报告。犯及大肠者仅 2 例报告(Matsuzaki 等，1979；Zimmerman，1979)，一位于升结肠，一位于横结肠，X 线上皆类似于新生物。它可出现于盲肠，但实际上它是发生于末端回肠或回盲瓣，脱垂进入盲肠。小时无蒂，长大则可见蒂，它可发生溃疡与出血。目前，其正确诊断只有仰赖于组织学。

急性阑尾炎伴存脓肿：急性阑尾炎伴存脓肿常常产生一确切的盲肠的外压性变形，如脓肿较大或出现播散，胃肠道其他部分也可受累。脓肿通常产生外压变形和良性特点，但偶尔可极其类似于恶性病变。Halls 和 Meyers(1977)报告 3 例非典型性急性阑尾炎，其临床与 X 线表现皆提示为恶性病变。急性阑尾炎的诊断一般临床即可作出，但症状不典型者则需 X 线检查帮助，当外在压迫出现于距盲肠有一定距离的大肠时，X 线解释则感困难。

盲肠后阑尾炎：Meyers 和 Oliphant(1974)报告 3 例上升的盲肠后阑尾炎，其炎症显示于盲肠与升结肠的非通常的部位，一误为升结肠的浸润，一误为结肠原发性癌，一误为腹膜外淋巴瘤。Joffee(1974)讨论了急性穿孔性阑尾炎的不寻常的 X 线表现,其中1例乙状结肠出现凹陷和缺损,类似结肠原发性黏膜下肿瘤。

乙状结肠狭窄:Phillips(1974)报告数例2~12cm长的乙状结肠的狭窄出现于输卵管卵巢脓肿,狭窄大多长于5cm,黏膜尚完整,其中1例狭窄区有一陡峭的近侧边缘提示为肿瘤所致。Halls和Meyers(1977)之3例均在内窥镜检查见到直肠乙状结肠黏膜连结处近端的环形病变,钡灌肠见不同长度狭窄,其中1例逆行灌注为完全性梗阻,次日顺行检查方获成功,曾按直肠癌治疗。所有3例乙状结肠狭窄皆不像继发于盆腔脓肿通常所见的光滑变尖,其狭窄变形及异常黏膜常提示为恶性病变,术前诊断均为癌肿,手术病理方确诊。此3例阑尾均不充盈,盲肠有不同程度的变形。

第六节 结肠恶性肿瘤少见CT表现

结肠恶性肿瘤一般表现为肠腔内外软组织密度肿块,肠壁增厚和/或伴肠腔狭窄,多数可正确诊断,但有些肿瘤影像表现不典型,极易误诊。

关于结肠黏液腺癌:结肠黏液腺癌青年人多见,恶性程度高,黏液腺癌含有大量细胞外液为特点,在癌实质中黏液成分占半量以上,肿瘤高黏液成分CT表现为肿块内均质或不均质的囊性密度,病理学显微镜下观察细胞外黏液形成大片“黏液湖”,分隔成岛状或小巢状腺癌上皮细胞漂浮于“黏液湖”中,肿瘤间质血管稀少并受到“黏液湖”推挤、压迫,使得对比剂进出肿瘤间质不但量少且缓慢。一组1例黏液腺癌增强后CT值由30~37 HU缓慢升至50~55 HU,强化微弱以致肉眼不易查别,延迟期囊性病灶内出现强化肠壁,一些作者认为结肠黏液腺癌能延迟强化,某些学者报道的囊性黏液腺癌无强化可能是延迟时间不够,但相关文献强化时间未作详述,有待进一步探讨。黏液腺癌腹膜播种概率高是其特征之一,这与肿瘤腹膜播种因子有关,如CT见腹膜强化结节强烈提示肠癌诊断。

此类肠癌另一特征表现是肿瘤内邻近肠腔、系膜甚至腹膜上出现不规则沙砾样或斑片状钙化,形成机制相对复杂。有作者认为肠壁内外出现钙化斑可能系肿瘤细胞直接浸润或种植所致,另有报道认为黏液腺癌钙化与软骨钙化成分上有类似,并认为钙化性结肠癌预后较差,一些作者认为钙化可能系肿瘤细胞坏死出现的一种反应。

由于忽略钙化邻近肠壁显著不规则增厚,该组1例黏液腺癌误诊为肠结核,肠结核病变虽以回盲部为中心,但肠壁多为轻度增厚,局部钙盐沉积反而少见,当肠壁增厚大于15 mm是癌性肠壁增厚的特征。肠结核轮廓多为锯齿状且肠壁变形较为对称,而该例肠腔变形明显不对称,且病变肠袢僵直、挛缩。

肿瘤坏死与腹腔脓肿:由于肿瘤中心血供不足引发瘤内坏死囊变,可表现为含气的假囊肿,CT容易误诊为腹腔脓肿,对照手术病理来看,肠癌浸润浆膜外形成巨大肠外肿块容易继发坏死。黏液腺癌肿瘤内的黏液成分、肿瘤囊变坏死物与脓肿脓液密度应有所不同,一组前者密度相对较高,平扫CT值高于30 HU,肿瘤囊变坏死物CT值仅10~20 HU,坏死肿瘤内残存癌肿组织会使瘤壁毛糙不整并有强化,据此可与腹腔脓肿鉴别。

绒毛状腺瘤:绒毛状腺瘤系结肠良性肿瘤,瘤体分泌细胞多,表面有大量黏液随粪便排出,临床表现为慢性腹泻、黏液血便,常误诊为黏液性结肠炎或肠道感染而延误治疗,以至发生恶变。绒毛状腺瘤瘤体较大,一般发现时已达3 cm以上,一组个别可达14 cm,癌变与腺瘤大小有关,腺瘤越大,癌变的概率越大,但是,腺瘤增大后才发生癌变,还是腺瘤恶变后才迅速增大尚无定论。癌变腺瘤最多见于乙状结肠、直肠,这可能因为这些部位大便稠厚、停留时间长,粪便内致癌物多并长期刺激肠道黏膜所致,对发生在直肠、乙状结肠腺瘤应高度警惕癌变可能。一组部分腺瘤病变肠段较长,肠黏膜表面呈丝绒或粗颗粒状,甚至有乳头状突起凹凸如天鹅绒地毯,病变区肠壁及肠壁新生物血供丰富,增强CT值达到115~120 HU,一些作者认为系腺瘤增生及伴发肠道炎症刺激了病变肠段血管增生,但肠轮廓光滑及肠周间隙清晰也是此类病变特征之一。

淋巴瘤:全身淋巴瘤尸检约44%在镜下见累及结肠,肿块型CT表现为结肠壁结节样隆起,浸润型通常累及较长一段肠壁,表现为环形浸润向心性狭窄,当肿瘤侵及固有肌层内自主神经丛则肠壁肌张力下降而肠腔扩张,由于病变沿黏膜下层向深层浸润，故肠黏膜表面仍光整。部分肠浸润型淋巴瘤表现为巨块状病灶，在 MR T_2WI 为等或略高信号，不同于其他肿瘤和炎症，因此 T_2WI 对淋巴瘤诊断有重要价值。此外，MR 软组织分辨力明显高于 CT，一组 1 例直肠淋巴瘤就观察到肠壁内外肿块的直肠浆膜分界面，证明淋巴瘤是跨越或沿脏器解剖结构生长，通常肿瘤内原有组织解剖结构存留而无明显破坏。

弥漫型淋巴瘤几乎均伴病灶广泛播散，可累及整个结肠，结肠表面布满多发结节样隆起，一般无蒂、表面较光整，大小 2~5 cm，数目可上百个，病变范围广泛是因其有多中心生长特性，像葡萄串一样，称为葡萄串征。

直肠套叠：直肠套叠临床少见，主要继发于直肠恶性肿瘤，以直肠癌最多见，病变钻入邻近柔软肠管引发套叠，病变头端易被误漏诊。直肠位置特殊，直肠套叠在 CT 扫描及多平面重建上会出现不典型征象如“猪鼻孔征”“山字征”，一般认为这些都是“靶征”的变形，但不论形态如何，肠管都存在肠系膜脂肪组织及肠系膜血管，采用薄层扫描及多方位重建即可明确肠套叠诊断。

多发性胃肠癌：多发性原发性大肠癌是指大肠同时性发生多于 2 个互不相连的原发癌灶，据对手术切除的 324 例进行期大肠癌的统计，同时性多发大肠癌有 23 例，占 7.1%，也就意味着每 14 例进行期大肠癌就有 1 例可能是多发癌，其中包括进行期癌合并大肠其他部位早期癌。一组 1 例降结肠、乙结肠多发低分化腺癌，同时伴有胃低分化腺癌，术前漏诊胃癌，故该组作者认为有必要对大肠多发癌给予高度的重视，在大肠 CT 检查时，不同肠段甚至不同胃肠组织不能仅满足于发现 1 个癌灶，应整个大肠、甚至整个消化道全程检查，尤其是有肠腔狭窄或出现梗阻的病例更应引起警惕，认真观察出现狭窄或梗阻的近侧段肠管壁，并作多平面重建观察以免遗漏病变。

第七节　回盲部隆起型中分化腺癌伴套迭病例

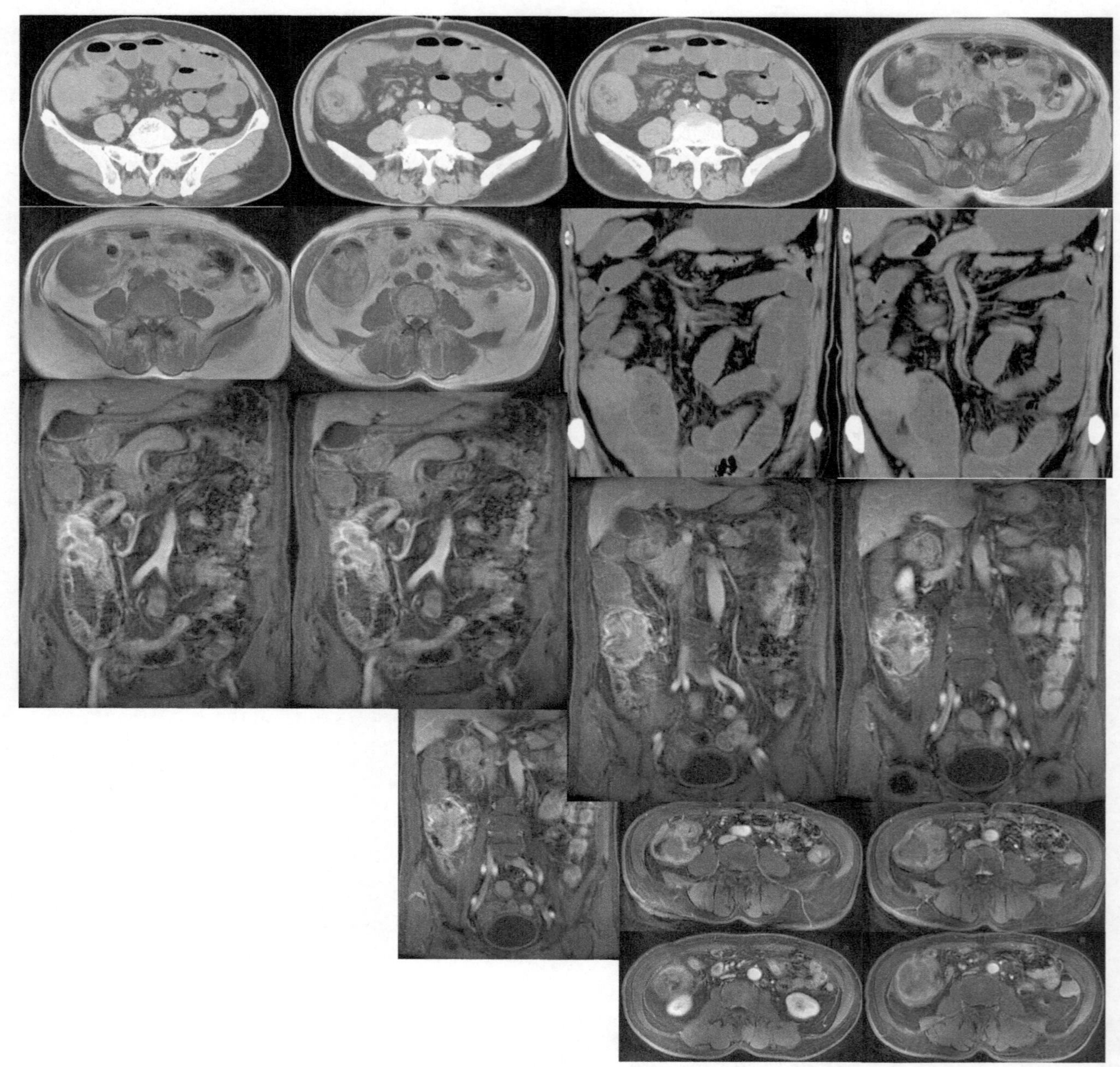

图 26-1-2　回盲部隆起型中分化腺癌伴套迭

患者,男,75 岁。

术后病理证实:回盲部隆起型中分化腺癌,浸润至肠外膜外纤维脂肪组织,5.5cm × 5cm × 2.7cm。十二指肠绒毛状 - 管状腺瘤伴低级别上皮内瘤变,呈菜花样，5cm × 4cm × 2cm(图 26-1-2)。

第八节　人工智能及影像组学在结直肠肿瘤中的应用简介

随着信息技术的迅速发展和计算机算法的不断革新，人工智能（AI）已广泛涉及临床诊疗的诸多环节。其中，人工智能与影像学的结合具有巨大的发展潜力，并已初步应用于临床。

影像组学是人工智能在肿瘤影像方面的应用热点，它通过高通量地提取影像特征，结合机器学习等人工智能算法，为结直肠肿瘤的精确诊断、个体化治疗提供更多信息。

人工智能技术：评估新辅助放化疗的疗效对结直肠癌的临床决策至关重要，能否利用人工智能早期预测疗效是许多研究者关注的问题。Liu 等（2017）基于直肠癌患者新辅助治疗前后的 T_2WI 和扩散加权成像（DWI）图像，利用线性支持向量机构建组学分数以预测新辅助治疗后的病理学完全缓解，独立验证的受试者操作特征（ROC）曲线下面积（AUC）为 0.979 9。

Horvat 等（2018）采用随机森林预测直肠癌新辅助治疗的病理学完全缓解，并对随机森林和传统阅片的预测效能进行对比，发现随机森林的诊断特异性更高，而敏感性与传统阅片无显著差异。Bibault 等（2018）开展了一项多中心的回顾性研究，在放疗计划 CT 图像的基础上应用深度学习预测直肠癌新辅助治疗的病理学完全缓解，并与支持向量机和 TNM 分期比较，五折交叉验证的结果表明深度神经网络的准确性最佳。

Shi 等（2019）的研究也取得了类似的结果，他们基于多序列 MRI 构建卷积神经网络，十折交叉验证发现联合治疗前和治疗中 MRI 图像构建的模型可用于预测病理学完全缓解，AUC 为 0.83。另 1 项关于预测直肠癌新辅助治疗疗效的研究基于 T_2WI 分别构建支持向量机、贝叶斯网络、神经网络和 K 最近邻分类，并对 4 种方法进行集成学习，结果表明集成学习分类器的预测效能最优，独立验证的 AUC 为 0.95，准确性为 90%。

影像组学：肿瘤在生长演变过程中，内部异质性不断变化，不同分期的肿瘤可能存在影像特征上的差异，这为影像组学评估肿瘤分期提供了理论基础。

Liang 等（2016）在门静脉期 CT 上构建组学标签，发现组学标签可作为独立预测因素对Ⅰ～Ⅱ期和Ⅲ～Ⅳ期结直肠癌进行分类。

Huang 等（2016）针对结直肠癌淋巴结转移的术前预测展开研究，共筛选 24 个特征构建组学标签，多因素回归结果表明组学标签是淋巴结转移的独立预测因素，整合组学标签和临床数据的预测模型一致性指数（concordance index, C-index）为 0.778。

Chen 等（2018）联合 3 种影像方法（超声内镜、超声弹性成像、CT）分别计算组学分数，并在感兴趣区（ROI）的放置上同时关注肿瘤周围组织和淋巴结，结果表明，相比于单一影像方法模型，多模态模型在直肠癌淋巴结转移的区分度、临床净获益上均有所提升。

结直肠癌患者出现肝转移提示预后不良，早期预测肝转移将对结直肠癌的治疗决策提供指导。有研究者提出对肝脏进行 CT 纹理分析有望预测同时性结直肠癌肝转移，但该研究样本量相对较少。一些作者发现，基于 T_2WI 构建的影像组学列线图可预测直肠癌同时性肝转移，准确性为 0.844。

挑战与展望：尽管人工智能及影像组学等相关研究方兴未艾，但应该认识到，人工智能与影像的融合仍处于起步阶段。首先，目前应用于临床的商业化人工智能影像产品多集中于单纯的图像识别、病变检出和良恶性判断等，人工智能仅作为影像医师的辅助工具以减少重复性工作，避免漏诊，提高阅片效率。而对于肿瘤影像而言，人工智能及影像组学在预测肿瘤的表型、预后、疗效评估等方面的探索尚未成功转化应用于临床。

其次，腹部肿瘤种类多、腹部器官在影像上组织对比度低、胃肠道形态及位置常不固定等因素导致肿瘤在自动分割上具有挑战性，目前大多数研究仍依赖人工分割，这个过程需要耗费大量的时间和精力，难以友好地融入影像医师的日常诊断流程中。

此外，在临床上应用人工智能技术同样带来一些伦理、社会层面的问题，诸如医疗责任的划分、数据处理流程中患者隐私的保护等，未来有待更深入的讨论及立法规范。

综上所述，当下医学影像已经步入大数据时代，作为人工智能和影像大数据共同促进的时代产物,人工智能影像的发展具有巨大的价值和广阔的前景。相信在不远的将来,人工智能及影像组学会克服现有不足,进一步帮助影像医师实现更高效、准确的诊断,并对临床实践产生深远的影响。

第二章　大肠淋巴瘤

第一节　大肠淋巴瘤

胃肠道是原发性结外非霍奇金淋巴瘤（NHL）最常见部位。胃是最常见的发病部位，约占原发性胃肠道淋巴瘤的50%，其次是小肠，而结肠和食管较少见。原发性大肠淋巴瘤罕见，占所有大肠肿瘤的0.05%~1%，在胃肠道淋巴瘤中约占10%，占直肠原发肿瘤的0.1%。

1. 病理学　在大肠原发性淋巴瘤中以盲肠和直肠最常见，两者占60%，但也可有多段肠管受侵。大肠淋巴瘤主要为非霍奇金淋巴瘤，以低分化最常见。大肠原发性淋巴瘤起源于大肠黏膜固有层或黏膜下层的淋巴组织，常在黏膜固有层或黏膜下层沿器官长轴生长。大体病理主要分4型：①浸润型；②肿块型；③溃疡型；④混合型。

2. 临床表现　临床表现非特异性，与消化道疾病的临床表现相似。发病年龄多见于50岁以上，男性多于女性。

3. 影像学研究　原发性大肠淋巴瘤：原发性大肠淋巴瘤CT主要表现为肠壁的明显增厚，通常不伴有结缔组织的增生，有时肠壁增厚形成巨大软组织团块。肿块向肠系膜侵犯时，可以形成巨大的空洞性病灶。肿块向肠壁外生长时，可有溃疡甚至穿孔而形成瘘道。瘘道可发生在结肠与脾或结肠与空肠等脏器之间。在大肠淋巴瘤中，有时广泛受累的大肠表现为无数小的、固定的息肉。此时，极易与家族性多发性息肉病及淋巴样增生相混淆。然而，后两者病变息肉的大小较为均匀一致，而前者息肉大小不一。同时，淋巴瘤的发病年龄通常在50岁以上，有助于鉴别。

有作者将本病概分为三型：①局部肿块型，表现为肠腔内息肉样肿块，呈软组织样均匀等密度；②弥漫型，表现为肠壁的弥漫性增厚，肿块周围的脂肪间隙多清晰；③当肿瘤侵及固有肌层的自主神经丛时，导致肠壁肌张力下降，也可表现为特殊的征象“动脉瘤样扩张”。

以下几点有助于大肠淋巴瘤的诊断与鉴别：①淋巴瘤表现为单发或多发结节或肿块，边缘清楚，大小不一，可互相融合成分叶状肿块；②淋巴瘤累及肠段较长，肠壁较厚，但由于病变区缺乏纤维结缔组织反应增生，使其肠腔变窄不明显，一般没有肠梗阻的表现；③大肠淋巴瘤较少见溃疡病变，即使出现溃疡，其周围环堤也较光整；④淋巴瘤常有全周性肠壁增厚，轮廓较光整，少向周围脂肪浸润，也较少直接侵犯邻近器官；⑤淋巴瘤可表现为多发弥漫性浸润，而大肠癌则相对较少；⑥淋巴瘤可伴有腹腔、盆腔或腹膜后淋巴结明显肿大，可融合成团，大肠癌的转移淋巴结较小，很少融合成团，多发生在区域性淋巴结。

一些作者报道在免疫缺陷的病人中发生淋巴瘤的机会明显高于普通人群，尤其是罕见部位（如直肠），应加以警惕。另外，尚有直肠淋巴瘤未经治疗而自行消失的个案报道。

大肠淋巴瘤沿肠系膜浸润和侵犯后腹膜时，CT表现与小肠淋巴瘤表现相似。

结肠外周T细胞淋巴瘤：结肠外周T细胞淋巴瘤（PTCL）罕见。根据病变累及范围分为局限型和广泛型两种，前者指病变仅局限在1个结肠节段；后者指病变累及2个或2个以上结肠节段。将钡灌肠表现与结肠镜下所见、切下的大体标本对照。根据临床病史、钡灌肠表现，每例均作临床拟诊。有作者报告4例广泛型结肠外周T细胞淋巴瘤，几乎累及结肠各段。双对比灌肠表现为结肠黏膜多个大小不等的地图样或鹅口疮样溃疡，直径2~30mm，3例在溃疡之间见正常的黏膜岛或假性息肉，2例伴管腔多处环状狭窄，4例伴回盲部变形，其中3例见开放的回盲瓣。影像学诊断结肠炎性病变，考虑为结肠结核或克罗恩病。

结肠镜检查，该组4例均见多个大小不等呈地图样或鹅口疮样溃疡，与双对比钡灌肠表现相似，也考虑结核性肠炎或克罗恩病。

作手术的2例广泛型结肠外周T细胞淋巴瘤中，1例作了全结肠切除，见全结肠黏膜多个地图样溃疡或溃疡之间未受损的正常黏膜和假性息肉；另1例因结肠穿孔作了横结肠切除，见黏膜多个地图样溃疡，且伴有6cm长管腔狭窄，而穿孔处未见有溃疡。上述大体标本所见与钡灌肠表现及结肠镜检查结果一致。

2例局限型结肠外周T细胞淋巴瘤，1例位于横结肠，另1例位于降结肠，钡灌肠均表现为地图样溃疡且有管腔环状狭窄。1例见假性息肉，1例见管腔内一偏心生长的肿块。1例影像学诊断考虑结肠癌，另1例考虑结肠淋巴瘤。结肠镜下所见与钡灌肠检查结果类似，1例诊断结肠淋巴瘤，另1例诊断结核性肠炎。

Lee等(2001)指出，结肠外周T细胞淋巴瘤有广泛型和局限型两种，双对比钡灌肠主要表现为广泛的黏膜溃疡，类似炎性肠病，与较为常见的结肠B细胞淋巴瘤明显不同，后者则以息肉样肿块、局部浸润或形成巨大腔样病变为主。

4.鉴别诊断　大肠淋巴瘤需与结肠癌鉴别。前者肿块边缘多较清晰光滑，后者多不规则，且淋巴瘤病变范围虽广泛，但较少向周围组织浸润。结肠癌常可伴病变周围淋巴结增大，多 <2 cm，而淋巴瘤往往不仅是局部的淋巴结肿大，而是腹腔或盆腔多发的淋巴结受累，并且较大，有时可融合成团。单纯根据影像表现有时无法鉴别结肠淋巴瘤与结肠癌，需结肠镜活检及免疫组织化学染色确诊。

5.误诊病例简介　有作者报告一例老年女性，患者有30年的系统性红斑狼疮病史，并服用过免疫抑制剂，可能与其发生淋巴瘤有重要关系。发生淋巴瘤后结肠壁正常组织结构受到肿瘤组织破坏，尤其是当肿瘤侵及固有肌层的自主神经丛时，导致肠壁肌张力下降，引起管腔的扩张并表现为特殊的“动脉瘤样扩张”，在此基础上极其容易发生坏死、破裂穿孔。

该例患者行急诊全腹CT扫描，当时仅发现胃肠道内大量内容物影，结肠明显扩张，尤以降结肠“动脉瘤样扩张”显著，降结肠见肠壁坏死水肿征象，肠周及腹膜密度增高(提示穿孔)，诊断消化道梗阻、穿孔并不困难，但连续上下层面未能发现明显软组织肿块征象，影像科和临床上都未能考虑到是结肠淋巴瘤导致穿孔的诊断。

而老年人发生穿孔在临床上原因更是多方面的，可以是长期便秘粪石对肠壁的直接损伤，或肠道梗阻导致压力增高，也可能是肠壁缺血坏死溃疡穿孔等，但多数是由结肠癌所致，所以易被误诊为结肠癌。在以穿孔为首发症状就诊时，掩盖了肿瘤性病变，更容易导致漏诊及误诊，因此在日常工作中应重视从临床上详细了解基础病(便秘、糖尿病高血压及服用激素等)，以利于分析、鉴别诊断。

第二节　弥漫性大B细胞淋巴瘤病例

患者，男，65岁。发现左下腹肿块伴疼痛一月余入院。手术内容：剖腹探查+腹膜后肿瘤切除+左肾上腺切除+左半结肠切除+横结肠-降结肠端端吻合+脾切除+左侧输尿管支架置入术。

免疫组化病理诊断：腹腔巨大肿瘤根治标本(无法明确原发部位)：弥漫性大B细胞淋巴瘤，生发中心型，肿瘤累及肠壁、肾上腺、腹膜及腹膜后(图26-2-1)。

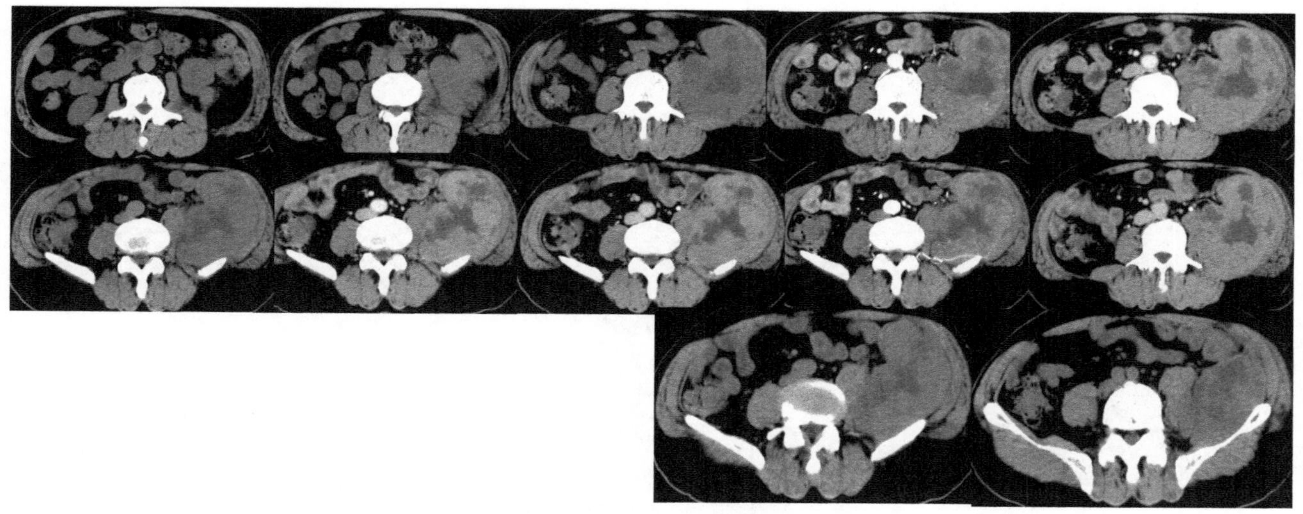

图 26-2-1 弥漫性大 B 细胞淋巴瘤

第三节 结肠外周 T 细胞淋巴瘤与结肠炎性病变

结肠外周 T 细胞淋巴瘤少见。为了评价其双对比钡灌肠表现，Lee 等（2001）收集病变局限在结肠及邻近淋巴结的结肠外周 T 细胞淋巴瘤 6 例，男 3 例，女 3 例，年龄 30~44 岁。6 例均作了经结肠镜活检，3 例施行了手术治疗（全结肠切除、右半结肠切除及部分结肠切除各 1 例）。2 例还作了小肠钡剂检查。免疫组化检查显示，2 例来源于 T 细胞；4 例来源于 NK 细胞。3 例与 EB 病毒有关，3 例呈血管中心性侵犯。临床症状为腹痛 4 例，便血 4 例，腹泻 3 例，发热 3 例，消瘦 2 例，便秘 1 例。2 例继发结肠穿孔。根据 Ann Arbor 分期，2 例病变局限在结肠（Ⅰ B 期），4 例累及邻近淋巴结（Ⅱ B 期）。对双对比钡灌肠作回顾性阅片时，观察病变部位、范围，溃疡形态和大小，有无息肉、肿块，管腔有无环状狭窄以及回盲部有无变形。根据病变累及范围分为局限型和广泛型两种，前者指病变仅局限在 1 个结肠节段；后者指病变累及 2 个或 2 个以上结肠节段。将钡灌肠表现与结肠镜下所见、切下的大体标本对照。根据临床病史、钡灌肠表现，每例均为临床拟诊。研究结果表明，4 例广泛型结肠外周 T 细胞淋巴瘤，几乎累及结肠各段。双对比灌肠表现为结肠黏膜多个大小不等的地图样或鹅口疮样溃疡，直径 2~30mm，3 例在溃疡之间见正常的黏膜岛或假性息肉，2 例伴管腔多处环状狭窄，4 例伴回盲部变形，其中 3 例见开放的回盲瓣。影像学诊断结肠炎性病变，考虑为结肠结核或克罗恩病。

结肠镜检查，4 例均见多个大小不等呈地图样或鹅口疮样溃疡，与双对比钡灌肠表现相似，也考虑结核性肠炎或克罗恩病。作手术的 2 例广泛型结肠外周 T 细胞淋巴瘤中，1 例作了全结肠切除，见全结肠黏膜多个地图样溃疡或溃疡之间未受损的正常黏膜和假性息肉；另 1 例因结肠穿孔作了横结肠切除，见黏膜多个地图样溃疡，且伴有 6cm 长管腔狭窄，而穿孔处未见有溃疡。2 例局限型结肠外周 T 细胞淋巴瘤，1 例位于横结肠，另 1 例位于降结肠，钡灌肠均表现为地图样溃疡且有管腔环状狭窄。1 例见假性息肉，1 例见管腔内一偏心生长的肿块。1 例影像学诊断考虑结肠癌，另 1 例考虑结肠淋巴瘤。结肠镜下所见与钡灌肠检查结果类似，1 例诊断结肠淋巴瘤，另 1 例诊断结核性肠炎。结肠外周 T 细胞淋巴瘤有广泛型和局限型两种，双对比钡灌肠主要表现为广泛的黏膜溃疡，类似炎性肠病，与较为常见的结肠 B 细胞淋巴瘤明显不同，后者则以息肉样肿块、局部浸润或形成巨大空腔样病变为主。

第四节 降结肠T细胞淋巴瘤病例

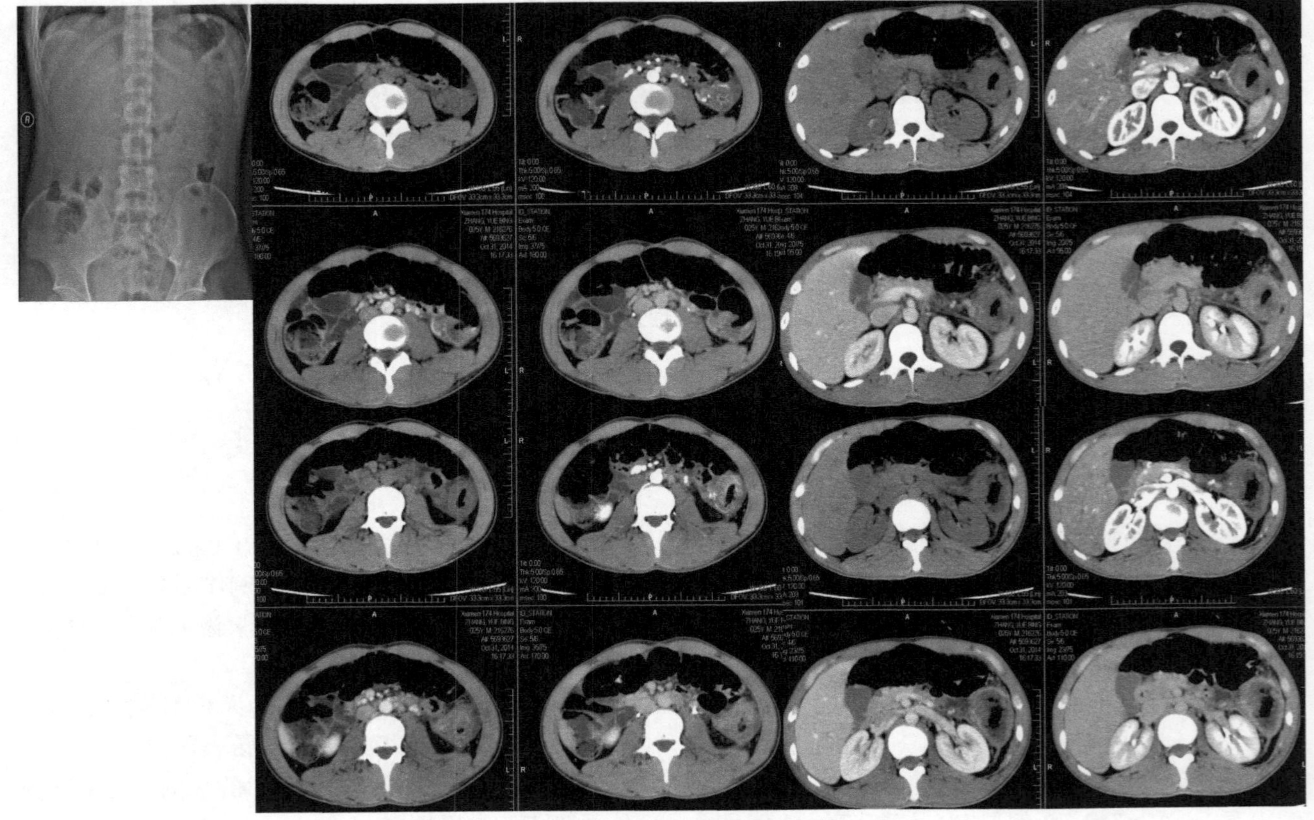

图 26-2-2 降结肠 T 细胞淋巴瘤

患者,男,25岁。缘于20天前无明显诱因出现左腹部闷痛,呈持续性,平卧时较好转,立位时明显,门诊行腹部立位片示:低位不全性肠梗阻。

腹部立位片:右下腹小肠见多发小气-液平面。

CT:左半结肠肠壁不均匀增厚,最厚处2.3cm,平扫CT值50HU,增强三期中度强化,CT值72~77HU,周围脂肪间隙模糊,周围多发肿大淋巴结,肠外侧脂肪间隙模糊。左侧结肠旁沟及盆腔积液。

手术所见:降结肠脾区肿瘤约11cm×5cm×5cm大小,质硬,肿物侵犯浆肌层,与脾脏下极粘连,向后侵及后腹膜、胰尾部被膜、左肾包膜的纤维脂肪组织。肿瘤以上肠管扩张明显,肠壁轻度水肿,结肠系膜血管根部及腹主动脉旁未见明显肿大淋巴结。

病理检查:结肠黏膜活检标本见灰白色黏膜组织六枚,最大者大小为0.3cm×0.2cm×0.1cm,最小者大小为0.1cm×0.1cm×0.1cm。常规病理诊断见结肠黏膜活检标本:镜下可见大量的坏死及上皮样细胞,初步考虑低分化癌肿,待免疫组化进一步明确。

免疫组化检测:阳性:LCA,CD3,CD43,CD45RO,MUM1(局灶),Ki-67(+,约80%);阴性:CK(P),CK(L),CK(H),CD34,CD10,CD68,CD163,Bcl-2,Syn,CgA,TDT,Bcl-6,EMA,CD1a,CyclinD1,CD20,CD79a,S-100,Lambda链,Kappa链。免疫组化诊断:结肠黏膜活检标本:肠黏膜坏死,间质中的少量上皮样细胞经免疫组化证实为T细胞来源,结合常规病理形态特点考虑肠病型T细胞淋巴瘤,但肿瘤成分少,诊断依据欠充分,建议避开坏死组织重新活检,或外院会诊,请与病理科联系。

病理检查:降结肠肿瘤:肠管一段,长27cm,直径3~5.5,距一切端5 cm,另一切端8 cm处见一隆起型肿物,肿物大小10.5 cm×4 cm×4 cm,切面灰白,质脆,侵及全层,肿物周围黏膜皱襞暗红色,网膜大小8 cm×6 cm×2 cm,网膜未触及淋巴结,肠周找到淋巴结14枚,直径0.7 cm~1 cm,切面灰白质中。胰腺表面粘连组织:灰白色碎组织一堆,总体积 2.5 cm × 2 cm × 2 cm,切面灰白质中。常规病理诊断:降结肠恶性肿瘤切除标本见降结肠恶性淋巴瘤,隆起型,大小 10.5 cm × 4 cm × 4 cm,伴显著坏死,侵及浆膜层,待免疫组化进一步分型。两切缘均为阴性。肠周淋巴结恶性淋巴瘤,类似肠道病变，10/13。胰腺表面粘连组织:纤维组织中见散在片状异型细胞浸润,倾向淋巴瘤,待免疫组化进一步确认与肠道病变是否相同类型。免疫组化诊断:“降结肠恶性肿瘤根治标本”:降结肠 T 细胞淋巴瘤,符合肠病型 T 细胞淋巴瘤,大小 10.5 cm × 4 cm × 4 cm,伴显著坏死,侵及浆膜层。详见常规组织学报告。肠周淋巴结与“胰腺表面粘连组织”均为 T 细胞淋巴瘤,考虑来源于降结肠。出院诊断:降结肠恶性淋巴瘤 Ⅳ期;不全性肠梗阻(图 26-2-2)。

第三章 大肠其他肿块

第一节 肠管恶性黑色素瘤

恶性黑色素瘤是一种常见于皮肤的高度恶性肿瘤,起源于黏膜者少见,而胃肠道恶性黑色素瘤以转移性病变居多,原发性者罕见,且临床表现缺乏特异性。

1. 病理学 恶性黑色素瘤是一种少见的来源于黑色素细胞的肿瘤,预后极差。常见于皮肤,其次是皮肤以外的部位,如眼、脉络膜、柔脑膜、口腔、鼻黏膜、咽部、食管、气管以及阴道和肛管直肠黏膜。原发于黏膜尤其是消化道的黑色素瘤均为少数。

免疫组织化学学指标 HBM45 及 Melan A(MART-1)具有很高特异性(90%~100%),S-100 蛋白可出现在神经鞘瘤、胶质瘤、神经内分泌癌细胞、色素细胞及组织细胞增殖,朗格汉斯细胞,偶见于未分化癌,其他免疫及指标阴性(如 CK、LCK),可作为排他性诊断。

2. 临床表现 临床表现主要有便血,其他症状有腹泻、肛门坠胀和肿块,类似痔和直肠癌等常见病。一组 4 例肠道病例均为中老年人,多数年龄>70 岁。1 例小肠病例以肠梗阻发病,此前无特征表现。

3. 影像学研究 肛管直肠病变表现为大小不等软组织密度肿块。该组 2 例位于齿线 1.5 mm 以上,可视为“原发的直肠黑色素瘤”。不同病例密度不等,但多均匀。肿块巨大者密度较低。术前 3 个月未提示巨大肿块,无明显肠梗阻症状;增强后强化不明显,可能与对比剂剂量相对不足有关。另 1 例病变显著强化且伴有腔内出血,与临床表现一致。3 例直肠周围间隙清晰,盆腔未见肿大淋巴结。肛管-直肠的黑色素瘤少见,而直肠原发性病变更为罕见,其 CT 表现多为蕈伞形肿块,也可形成充填肠腔的肿块而无梗阻征象。也有少数病例报道有肠壁增厚,类似原发癌。1 例小肠病变为多发肠壁增厚或肿块伴有多节段肠梗阻。空肠近段病变以肠管对称性增厚为主;远端病变也可见管壁增厚,且可见环形及中心脂肪密度,而相应近侧空肠囊状扩张,提示有肠套叠并肠梗阻。

一般认为,胃和小肠是皮肤黑色素瘤远处转移的好发部位。为区分转移和复发,有作者提出临床标准,包括:是否为孤立病灶;就诊时除区域淋巴结外,有无其他转移性病变;确诊后无病生存期不少于 12 月。此外,在组织病理学上,正常组织与肿瘤细胞间存在移行带提示原发。该组 1 例虽经全面检查未发现皮肤和黏膜的原发灶,但按上述标准仍不能除外转移性病变。因为有些转移性黑色素瘤根本找不到原发灶,属于原发部位不明的黑色素瘤。

4. 鉴别诊断 本病因其少见、无特征性形态表现以及预后极差,其误诊率及死亡率均高。临床上常误为原发上皮肿瘤(直肠癌),应予以鉴别,其他包括胃肠间质癌(或称基质癌)、淋巴瘤。

直肠癌:直肠癌为常见病。临床上有便血时视其混有黏液的程度(直肠指诊)可以大致区分于癌-黑色素瘤-痔。前者多混有较多黏液,后者以便(鲜)血为主,而黑色素瘤多无或少有黏液,与“痔”类似。CT 图像上肛管直肠癌多表现为管壁增厚或环形狭窄,息肉和肿块较少,巨块者罕见。强化多较均匀,伴有淋巴结肿大。

胃肠间质瘤:为最常见的胃肠道间叶性肿瘤,起源于胃肠固有肌层,具有腔外生长和坏死囊变倾向,无肠壁环状受累,罕有肠梗阻。发生于直肠者多为恶性,可呈腔内息肉或壁内肿块。体积较大,伴脏器转移,少有淋巴结肿大。发生于肛门-直肠也可呈巨大肿块,致肠壁局限性膨隆,有出血、囊变及边缘显著化。腔外生长及不均强化可资鉴别。

淋巴瘤:该组小肠多发病变表现为肠壁增厚及肿块,均质密度伴肠梗阻,与淋巴肠壁浸润类似。但淋巴瘤常为继发,多伴有淋巴结广泛而显著肿大及多脏器受累,强化较轻及均匀。鉴别诊断有赖于全身检查及手术病理。

由于此病为少见疾病,该组收集病例有限,且时间跨度长,检查手段略有差异。如早期病例仅有病理组织学资料;另外,不同免疫组织化学指标也存在相对敏感性和特异性问题;虽然 MRI 对此病有特殊征象提示诊断,但由于其腹部相对适用性不及 CT,仅行 1 例 MRI 检查,且病变淋巴结并未见特征性信号,有待于更多的资料积累。

总之,肠管恶性黑色素瘤为少见疾病,原发于肛门直肠者病例罕见,可表现为息肉或蕈伞形肿块及巨大肿块,可不伴有肠梗阻;小肠病变表现多样,可有管壁增厚、肿块及肠梗阻。CT 在确定病变部位、范围、继发改变及术后随访有一定作用,诊断有赖于手术及病理。

第二节 大肠类癌

病理学:肉眼观盲肠嗜铬细胞类癌类似盲肠腺癌,因为两者都较大、呈息肉样、表面可见溃疡;而镜下观则类似空回肠肠嗜铬细胞类癌。直肠 L 细胞类癌常常表现为孤立、<1 cm 的黏膜下结节或局部肠壁呈斑块状增厚。镜下 L 细胞类癌常为嗜银性肿瘤,瘤细胞排列成小梁状,或较少见的情况下呈腺泡、腺体及管状结构。

临床表现:多数大肠类癌发生在直肠及盲肠。盲肠类癌多为肠嗜铬细胞类癌,而多数直肠类癌显示 L 细胞分化。结肠类癌的典型临床表现为腹痛及体重减轻;而超过一半的直肠类癌患者没有症状,常在行常规指检或内镜筛查时发现。若直肠类癌出现症状,则多为出血、疼痛、便秘。结肠类癌转移病灶可产生类癌综合征,但直肠类癌则否。

影像学研究:近端结肠类癌为息肉样腔内肿块,钡剂造影多表现为充盈缺损,肠腔局部狭窄,可并发肠套叠,与息肉样腺瘤及腺癌无法鉴别。CT、MRI 平扫见肿块内低密度或长 T1、长 T2 退变坏死区,增强扫描肿块有轻至中度强化。直肠类癌常是壁内较小肿块,较少见情况下,恶性程度较高的病灶可侵犯邻近盆腔结构。

第三节 升结肠胃肠道型神经鞘瘤病例

患者,男, 52 岁。因发现腹部渐大肿物 40 年,间断便血 1 年余入院。 查体:右腹脐水平略上方可扪及一直径约 8cm 肿物,质地硬,边界欠清,无压痛,活动度差。5 天前肠镜检查:升结肠近肝曲一 4cm × 5cm 广基黏膜下隆起,间质瘤?病理诊断:升结肠黏膜活检标本:呈黏膜慢性炎及息肉状增生,黏膜间质所见的肌样纤维经免疫组化检测证实为平滑肌,未见间质瘤成分。手术所见:肿瘤大小 18 cm× 10 cm × 10 cm,质地硬,表面光滑,基底位于升结肠靠近肝曲处,周围可见大网膜包裹,肠系膜淋巴结无明显肿大。

病理检查:升结肠肿物切除标本:肠管一段,长 15cm,一切缘周径 3cm,另一切缘周径 4cm,距一切缘 6cm、距另一切缘 4 ㎝处肠腔内见一隆起型肿物,肿物根部向肠腔外突出,形成一巨大肿物,大小 18cm × 9.5cm × 9cm,肿物切面灰黄,质韧,其余肠黏膜皱襞明显。肠周检出淋巴结样物五枚,直径 0.4~1cm。横结肠上切缘标本:灰白色组织一块,大小 2cm × 1.5cm × 0.5cm,切面灰白,质中。升结肠下切缘标本:管状组织一块,大小 2.5cm × 2cm × 1.2cm,切面灰白,质中。病理诊断:升结肠梭形细胞肿瘤,大小 18cm × 9.5cm × 9cm,位于黏膜下层,大部分向浆膜外隆起。倾向胃肠道间质瘤,待免疫组化进一步协助诊断。免疫组化诊断:升结肠肿物切除标本示升结肠梭形细胞肿瘤,CD117、Ki-67 阴性,CD34 阳性,考虑为胃肠道型神经鞘瘤,大小 18cm × 9.5cm × 9cm,位于黏膜下层,大部分向浆膜外隆起(注:胃肠道间质瘤少数可为 CD117 阴性,故不能完全排除,建议进一步检测有无 c-Kit 和 PEGFRA 基因突变进一步确诊)(图 26-3-1)。

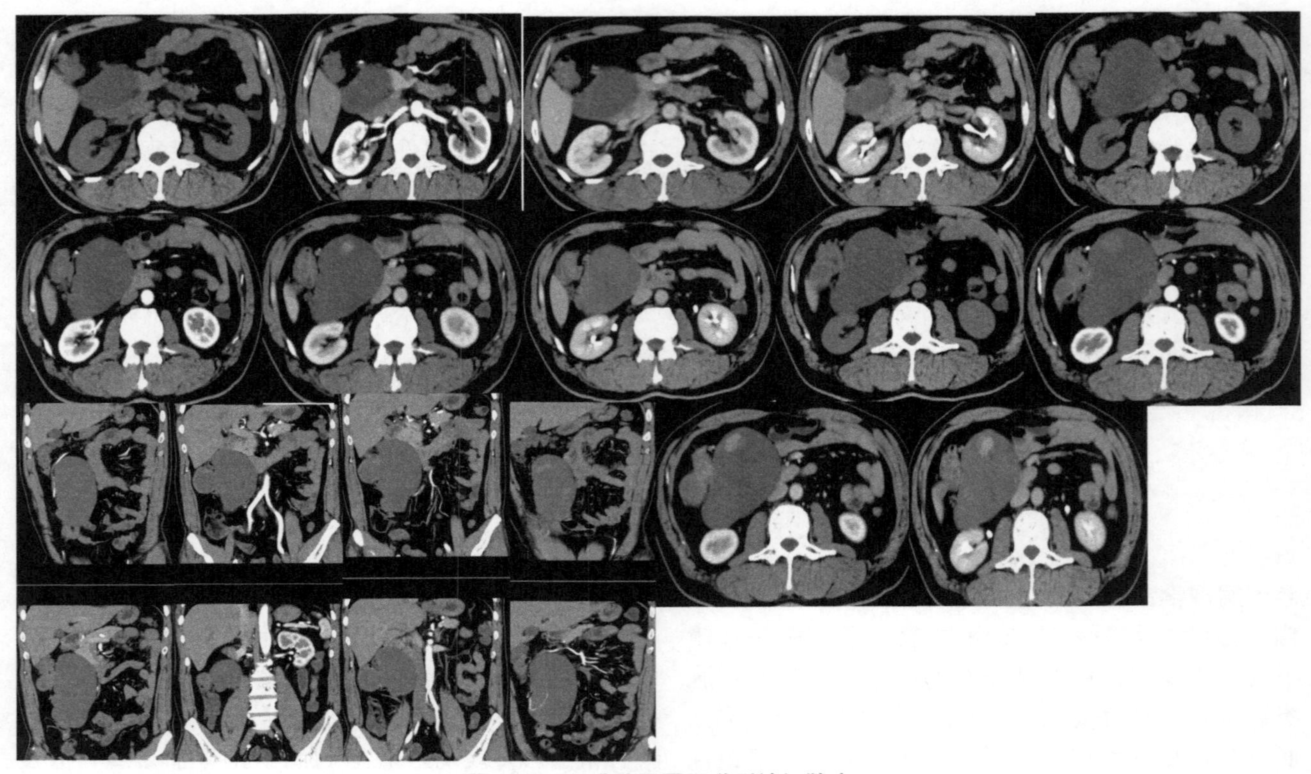

图 26-3-1 升结肠胃肠道型神经鞘瘤

第四节 结肠绒毛状肿瘤

结肠腺瘤被认为是结肠癌的前期病变,可分为管状腺瘤、绒毛状腺瘤及绒毛管状腺瘤,所占比例分别为 75%、10% 和 15%。

1. 病理学 绒毛状腺瘤是结肠中较少见的腺瘤,典型的绒毛状腺瘤无蒂,表面呈绒毛和乳头状突起,常伴有黏液覆盖。显微镜下可见叶状突起,表面被覆异型增生的腺上皮,绒毛结构超过腺腔结构的 80%。绒毛管状腺瘤由管状和绒毛状结构混合而成,两者比例在 4∶1 和 1∶4 之间。常出现程度不同的异型增生,生物学特性与绒毛状腺瘤相同。一般来说,肿瘤中绒毛成分越多,癌变的危险性越大,相同大小的绒毛状肿瘤,其癌变率是管状腺瘤的 10 倍。

2. 临床表现 绒毛状腺瘤是一种具有恶变倾向的良性病变,可发生在消化道的任何部位。结肠绒毛状腺瘤好发于直肠和乙状结肠,好发年龄在 50~80 岁,一组中病变发生在直肠和乙状结肠 7/8 例,年龄均在 50 岁以上。大部分直肠腺瘤不引起症状,偶尔会引起直肠出血、排便习惯的改变,该组病人黏液便或血便 5 例,排便习惯改变 2 例。

绒毛状腺瘤可能会引起蛋白质中富含类黏蛋白和钾的丢失,引起低蛋白血症、低钾、低钠血症等,肿瘤生长到一定程度,可能会阻塞肠腔,该组 8 例均无电解质紊乱及肠梗阻症状。1 例为胃癌术后复查腹部 CT 发现,无明显腹部症状。

3. 影像学研究 结肠绒毛状肿瘤是一种血供丰富的病变,该组 8 例均明显强化,强化幅度达 40 HU。其 CT 表现多样,典型者增强后实性部分明显强化,周边可见无强化水样密度影,这对应于绒毛间的黏液。

这种水样密度可以出现在肿瘤内部坏死区,但如果是坏死的话,密度通常不会这么均匀,而且更易出现在肿块的中心部分,而不是周边。再者,如果是表面的坏死或肠腔内液体,它会随着肠管的蠕动而排出。直肠气体密度影并没有和相接触的液体形成气 - 液平面,两者的交界面不规则,这更说明了液体是肿瘤的一部分，肿瘤对肠腔是一种推挤的改变。

因此，该组认为如果 CT 出现以下征象，可以考虑绒毛状肿瘤。黏膜来源的混杂密度肿块，其内有不规则水样密度。增强后肿块内实性部分明显强化，在水样密度对比下显示更清晰，呈脑回状、树叶状改变。如果水样密度影周边见到不规则气体影，两者交界面并不形成气 - 液平面。但是对于一些较小病变，由于表现不典型，这些诊断分析不太适用。绒毛状肿瘤可表现为腔内息肉样病变，也可表现为局部肠壁的增厚。

有文献报道，在行 CT 增强扫描的时候，对比剂可能会渗入到肿块内部的黏液中去，引起其密度增高，看起来像是有强化，影响其特征性的表现，造成对病变的误诊。黏液密度甚至可以高到被误认为肠腔内的对比剂，以至于掩盖病变，无法在 CT 上发现病变。

因此，如果临床上怀疑绒毛状肿瘤，应该在口服对比剂到达结肠前行 CT 扫描（例如口服造影剂后 45~60 min），这样不会掩盖绒毛状肿瘤特征性 CT 表现。扫描前行结肠充气有助于显示病变形态及特征。如果扫描结果可疑时，在口服对比剂到达盆腔后延迟扫描有助于腔内粪便和黏膜肿块鉴别开来。该组术前对比较典型的 3 例病变诊断正确，余 5 例由于表现不典型，所以没有进行延迟扫描及结肠充气。

《2006 年结直肠腺瘤切除术后肠镜监视指南》认为绒毛状腺瘤，或腺瘤直径≥ 1 cm 均为高危性腺瘤。由于其恶变常在基底部，因此对于直径 >1 cm 的任何腺瘤，即使活检未见癌变，均主张切除。Hendricks 等（1989）报道 13 例绒毛状肿瘤，其中 8 例恶性，7 例均 >2 cm。在良恶性鉴别中，恶性病变通常更大，该组 8 例平均长径 3.3 cm，其中 1 例局部癌变，4 例合并不同程度不典型增生。

4. 鉴别诊断　鉴别诊断包括炎性息肉及管状腺瘤、结肠癌、淋巴瘤、炎症性肠病等。

非腺瘤样息肉和管状腺瘤：通常体积较小，其 CT 及临床表现与不典型绒毛状肿瘤难以区分，确诊需依赖病理结果。

结肠癌：结肠绒毛状肿瘤是结肠癌的癌前病变，肿块型结肠癌常引起便血、消瘦及腹部肿块等症状，累及直肠时可有里急后重，肛门指诊可扪及质硬肿块，CT 可表现为分叶状偏心肿块，但其主要向黏膜下浸润生长，密度常不均匀，常可见坏死区，强化不均匀，而绒毛状肿瘤是向肠腔内生长，可相鉴别。

结肠淋巴瘤：临床症状主要有腹痛、乏力及消瘦等，CT 可表现为黏膜下肿块，密度均匀，增强后轻度强化，坏死少见，与绒毛状肿瘤鉴别不难。

炎症性肠病：如溃疡性结肠炎、克罗恩病等常发生于青壮年，临床表现多与绒毛状肿瘤相似，但其有发作期与缓解期相互交替的特征，CT 可表现为肠壁增厚，增厚多较广泛或多发节段性分布，壁厚较均匀，与绒毛状肿瘤肠壁局限性增厚或局部肿块可相鉴别。

综上所述，结肠绒毛状肿瘤表现形式多样，对于典型的结肠绒毛状肿瘤，CT 可以做出正确诊断；但对于一些较小的及表现不典型的绒毛状肿瘤，往往难以做出正确的诊断。

第五节　右半结肠黏膜下脂肪瘤，肠外膜局部区呈化脓性炎伴脓肿形成

患者，男，37 岁。反复腹痛 1 个月，无疼痛，无发热畏寒、寒战等不适。

病理检查：冰冻病理：右半结肠肿物切除标本：结肠及周围脂肪组织一堆，总体积 17cm × 12 cm × 3.8 cm，距一侧切缘 5 cm，距另一切缘 10 cm 处肠黏膜下见一脂肪瘤样结节，大小 5.5 cm × 4 cm × 1 cm，切面淡黄质软，包膜完整；于肠外膜处见一结节样肿物，直径 2.5 cm，质硬，似钙化组织。冰冻病理诊断：右半结肠肿物切除标本：初步考虑结肠黏膜下脂肪瘤；阑尾组织呈急性炎伴周围脓肿，且与结肠外膜周围脂肪组织粘连及被包裹；肠外膜处见一钙化样质硬结节，无法冰冻取材，可能需常规脱钙；以上需常规石蜡切片后进一步证实。

病理诊断：右半结肠肿物切除标本：肠黏膜下脂肪瘤，肠外膜局部区呈化脓性炎伴脓肿形成，并检出 2 枚淋巴结呈反应性增生，且肠壁局灶见一枚纤维钙化结节形成，建议切除后复查（图 26-3-2）。

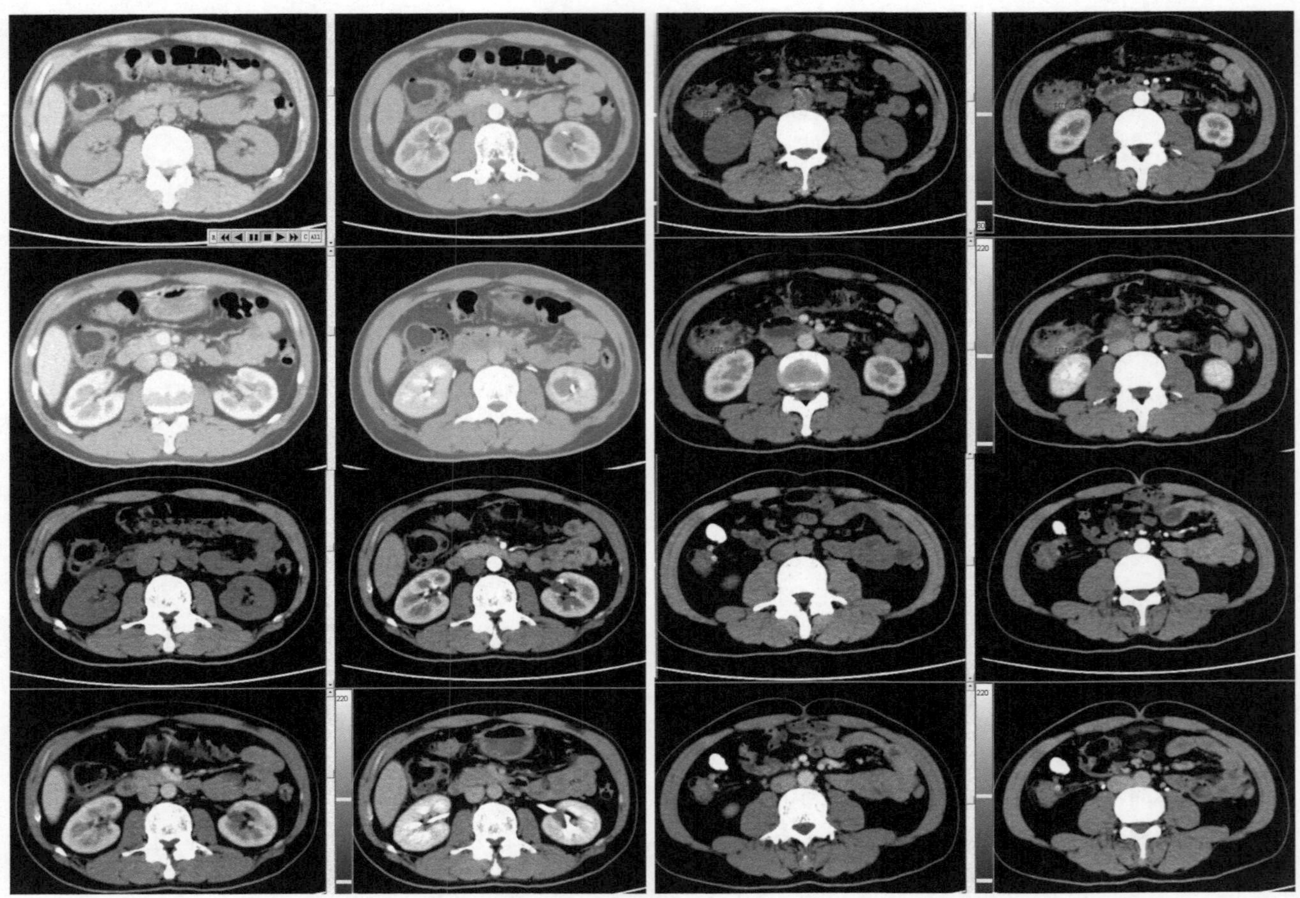

图 26-3-2 右半结肠黏膜下脂肪瘤，肠外膜局部区呈化脓性炎伴脓肿形成

第六节 Gardner 综合征

Gardner 综合征的临床表现具有多样性，典型的 Gardner 综合征表现为三联征，即结肠多发息肉性病变、多发性骨瘤或骨疣、形态各异的结肠外软组织肿物。

当临床中发现上述病变以二联或三联征出现时，一定要引起对该疾病的重视，结合必要的影像检查如 X 线钡餐、CT、MRI 以及病理学，可做到对该疾病的早期诊断与治疗。

Gardner 综合征多发生于 30~40 岁，男女均可发病，此病和遗传因素有关，一般有明显的家族史，癌变倾向明显，其临床表现不一，可表现为肠内及肠外多种临床征象。肠内主要表现为腹部不适、黏液样脓血便、腹泻等症状，肠外表现复杂多样，可表现为骨瘤、多发性硬化性纤维瘤、结肠外恶性肿瘤等。

本病需与色素沉着息肉综合征(Peutz-Jeshers 综合征)、家族性腺瘤性息肉病(肠镜检查可见全结肠弥漫分布大小不等的息肉，数目可多于 100 个，以直肠、乙状结肠居多)、Turco 综合征、神经纤维瘤病和胃肠道来源的间质瘤或间质肉瘤相鉴别。

胃肠道来源的间质瘤或间质肉瘤是消化道最常见的间叶组织源性肿瘤，境界清晰，肿块多为单发，富血供，多有液化坏死，CT 增强扫描可有较明显均匀或不均匀强化。

第七节　胃肠道间质瘤(高危险度)

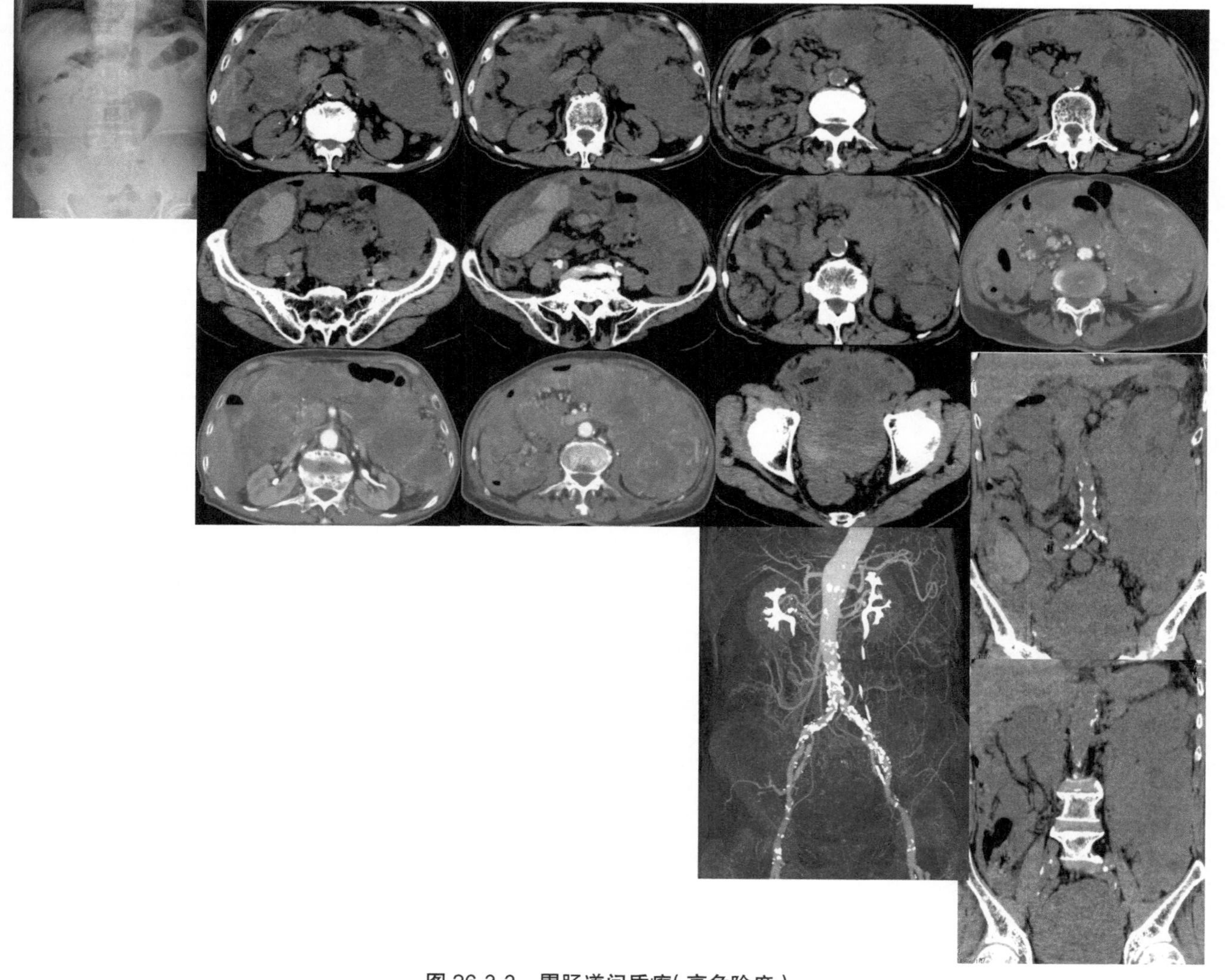

图 26-3-3　胃肠道间质瘤(高危险度)

患者,男, 72 岁。无明显诱因出现腹胀,以下腹部明显,无明显腹痛,伴排便费力,大便量少,无恶心呕吐,无畏寒发热,就诊我院,化验尿常规提示蛋白 +、血常规:血红蛋白94g/L、腹部立位片示低位不全梗阻。门诊以“不全性肠梗阻”收住入院。

CT:平扫示肠管弥漫性病变,考虑肿瘤可能性大,建议 CT 增强扫描;右侧肠管内高密度影,考虑出血可能;腹腔少量积液。CT 增强扫描:腹腔病变,考虑肿瘤可能性大,建议进一步检查确诊。

手术所见:腹腔内数百个大小不等肿瘤结节遍布壁腹膜、肠系膜、网膜、肠管等处,最大肿瘤与部分小肠、肠系膜粘连,形成包裹,大小约 6 cm × 5cm,位于右侧腹部,腹腔肠管广泛粘连,腹腔内肿瘤破裂出血,腹腔积血约 300ml,肝脾、胃、盆腔等脏器无法显露,考虑患者为晚期肿瘤并肿瘤腹腔广泛侵犯转移,无法行肿瘤切除手术,告知患者家属病情,请患者儿子进入手术室观看后,患者家属决定放弃进一步手术,取壁腹膜、肠系膜、网膜、肠管等处肿瘤结节送病理检查,吸尽腹腔内渗出血液,确认无明显活动性出血,予关闭腹腔,术毕麻醉苏醒后带气管插管返回病房。

病理检查:腹腔肿瘤切除标本:不规则肿物一堆,总体积

9cm × 5.5cm × 1cm,切面均灰白质中,偏软。常规病理诊断:腹腔肿瘤切除标本示恶性间叶性肿瘤,待做免疫组化检测进一步明确肿瘤类型(图 26-3-3)。

免疫组化检测:阳性: CD117, DOG1, Vim, SMA(散在+);阴性: CD34, Actin, Desmin, CK(P), EMA, CK(L), Ki-67(约 5%)。免疫组化诊断:腹腔肿瘤切除标本:胃肠道间质瘤(高危险度),并建议作 c-kit 基因检测以应用于肿瘤靶向治疗药物的选择。

第四章　大肠炎症

第一节　原发性肠脂垂炎：急腹症的鉴别诊断

肠脂垂为沿结肠带两侧分布的许多小突起，长度 0.5~5.0cm，由浆膜及其所包含的脂肪组织形成，肠脂垂内有各自独立的动静脉供血。整个结肠约有 100~150 个肠脂垂，主要分布在横结肠及乙状结肠。

1. 病理学：原发性肠脂垂炎是由于肠脂垂发生扭转，造成肠脂垂内的血管闭塞、脂肪坏死。原发性肠脂垂炎是一种少见的原因不明性疾病，该病早期酷似外科急腹症，在临床表现上难以与阑尾炎、憩室炎、胆囊炎或妇科急症等疾病鉴别。早期诊断困难，容易误诊。

继发性肠脂垂炎，则是因为附近的组织先有一些如憩室炎、阑尾炎及胆囊炎等炎症反应，再侵犯到肠脂垂而导致后者发炎。比较少见的原因则是肠套叠和出血。

2. 临床症状：临床症状根据受累结肠的节段不同而异，最常见的症状是局限性的短期腹痛。此外，30% 患者伴有反跳痛，20% 患者伴恶心和呕吐，极少数患者伴发肠梗阻症状。只有大约 7% 的患者伴有血液内白细胞增多。最常见的临床诊断是急性憩室炎、急性阑尾炎、胆囊炎。在大多数情况下本病是一种良性自限性疾病，通常不需要手术治疗，因此正确的识别本病的影像学表现对于本病的治疗意义较大。临床上本病需要与阑尾炎相鉴别。由于本病是一种自限性疾病，可能有很多病例未见报道，因此发病率不详。现有临床数据显示，本病发病率约为 0.88×10^{-5}/ 年。

3. 影像学研究：超声和 CT 在急腹症的诊断中起着至关重要的作用，MRI 在肠脂垂炎的诊断报告甚少。本病的超声表现为腹部压痛最为明显部位的椭圆形强回声团块，此团块不可压缩，紧贴于结肠壁。团块中央可表现为低回声或者环状低回声。在大多数情况下此病灶位置较为固定，不随呼吸上下移动。与憩室炎鉴别的关键在于彩色多普勒显示病灶中央无血流信号。CT 增强扫描显示肠脂垂炎通常表现为肠壁旁的椭圆形或类圆形的脂肪密度病灶，周围肠管结构正常，病灶周边常可见环状强化。病变常与四周的脂肪混合在一起。邻近的结肠在少数情况下也可能发生炎症反应。乙状结肠、降结肠和横结肠较易受累，升结肠和盲肠受累少见。常见病因是中央动脉的血栓形成，可表现为病变中央的条状或圆形高密度影，有时 CT 扫描难以显示。本病较为罕见的表现为整个大网膜坏死。病变常在几周内经临床证实，6 个月内无任何残留表现。MSCT 能准确地显示结肠及结肠旁沟的解剖结构，并且能发现病变，确定病变的部位、大小、范围及与周围组织的关系，是目前诊断原发性肠脂垂炎有效的手段。结合冠状位和矢状位重组图像，能更全面、直观地反映病变形态及范围。Gomez 等（2008）认为原发性肠脂垂炎的典型 CT 表现为结肠旁沟内椭圆形或火焰状脂肪密度肿块，增强后呈环形强化，且邻近肠壁无增厚及肠管周围无积液征象。

一组 5 例原发性肠脂垂炎均发生于结肠旁沟，其中位于乙状结肠周围 3 例，盲肠周围 1 例，升结肠周围 1 例。其中乙状结肠发生率最高，其结果与 Sánchez-Pérez 等（2010）和 Gurses 等（2007）报道的一致。5 例 CT 平扫均表现为结肠旁沟内椭圆形的含脂肪密度的肿块影，3 例 CT 增强后呈均匀的环形强化，其结果与 Gomez 等（2008）的报道一致。

正常的肠脂垂在腹部或盆腔 CT 上显示不清，仅仅在腹腔或盆腔积液的衬托下才可显示；肠脂垂发生病理变化时，覆盖其表面的脏层腹膜亦增厚，同时伴有其他炎性改变，在 CT 上则表现为肿块呈环形强化,并与四周的脂肪混合在一起,肠脂垂中心密度可以增高,代表可能有血栓形成。从该组病例手术病理结果来看,5 例组织病理显示致病的肠脂垂外脏层腹膜覆盖纤维白细胞渗出物,其对应的 CT 平扫均表现为位于结肠旁沟的椭圆形的含脂肪密度肿块影,CT 增强后椭圆形的肿块呈环形强化,对照病理结果,环形强化影为增厚的脏层腹膜。因此一般认为高密度的环形强化影是原发性肠脂垂炎的特征性表现。

实际工作中,腹部 CT 平扫与增强往往是分开进行的,如只有 CT 平扫,对该病的诊断有一定的困难,但是结合患者有急腹症的临床症状(固定的腹部疼痛),除了要想到引起急腹症的常见原因外,还应该想到原发性肠脂垂炎,如果 CT 平扫发现结肠旁沟内的含脂肪密度的肿块影,应高度怀疑原发性肠脂垂炎,CT 增强后的环形强化表现将进一步明确诊断。

4. 鉴别诊断　原发性肠脂垂炎主要需与继发性肠脂垂炎相鉴别。

继发性肠脂垂炎:阑尾炎、憩室炎、胆囊炎等都是引起继发性肠脂垂炎的常见原因。周围肠壁增厚、肠管外游离气体影以及局部脓肿等也是继发性肠脂垂炎的影像学征象,依此可对两者进行鉴别。

阑尾炎:原发性肠脂垂炎与阑尾炎的鉴别诊断关键是显示阑尾,阑尾正常可排除阑尾炎;阑尾肿大和阑尾周围炎性改变,是急性阑尾炎最重要的 CT 征象。

结肠憩室炎:肠周的类圆形脂肪密度病灶及含脂肪成分的病变常要与结肠憩室炎相鉴别,憩室炎好发于老年患者,常可见肠壁受累。

外伤、肠系膜脂膜炎及大网膜肿瘤:少数病例需要与外伤、肠系膜脂膜炎及大网膜肿瘤相鉴别,前者多需要结合病史进行诊断,而后两者通常不会急性发作,且有其特定好发部位。

原发性肠脂垂炎属于外科急腹症的一种不太常见的原因,由于解剖位置的特殊性,肠脂垂炎在临床上表现为部位固定的腹痛,CT 和超声对其诊断有至关重要的作用。MSCT 及三维重建能较好地显示其影像学特征,排除其他继发性炎症,本病常不需要手术干预。

第二节　炎症性肠病

详见本书 本卷 第二十五篇 第五章 第一节　炎症性肠病。

第三节　慢性溃疡性结肠炎的不常见的并发症

慢性溃疡性结肠炎恶变早已为人熟知,其中腺癌为最常见的恶变表现。一些学者报告 2 例病人为此病的少见的恶性并发症表现,一为结肠淋巴瘤,一为结肠多发性类癌,二例皆有慢性溃疡性结肠炎 10 年以上的病史。

第四节　克罗恩病病例之一

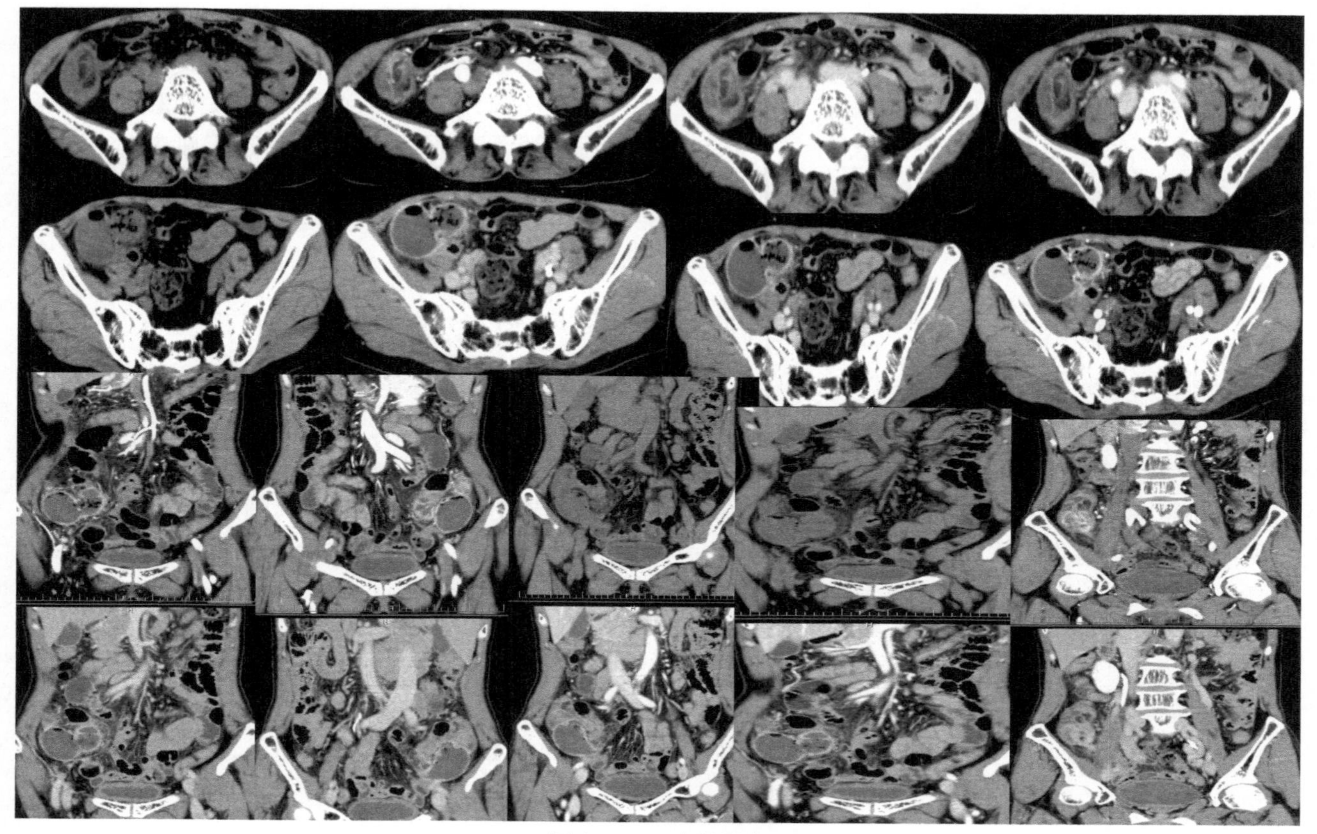

图 26-4-1　克罗恩病

患者，女，54 岁。腹痛 2 周入院。

内镜检查：插镜至回肠末段，回盲瓣呈唇型，阑尾窝存在，阑尾周边黏膜呈半球型隆起（约 3 cm ×3cm），表面充血呈分叶状，局部糜烂，予活检 7 块，质软易出血，其余所见肠黏膜未见明显异常，无充血糜烂，无溃疡、息肉、肿瘤及异常隆起，血管纹理清晰，肠腔内无血迹。内镜术后病理诊断：回盲部黏膜活检标本：黏膜组织呈急慢性炎伴糜烂，未见肿瘤组织，建议再取或深取活检。手术所见：回盲部可见肿物生长穿出浆膜外，约 5cm×5cm 大小，质硬，与大网膜等粘连成团，腹腔内少量黄色脓液，结肠系膜根部见数个肿大淋巴结。术中送快速病理示（回盲部肿物）："肿块与腹壁粘连组织"良性病变。

病理检查：冰冻病理：肿块与腹壁粘连组织示灰红色组织一块，大小 0.7cm×0.5cm×0.2cm。肠道肿物：灰白灰红色肿物一块，大小 1.7cm×1.3cm× 1.0cm，切面灰白质中偏脆。冰冻病理诊断：第一次送检肿块与腹壁粘连组织：见纤维组织增生伴出血与慢性炎细胞浸润，可能与下述肠壁病变相关。第二次送检肠壁组织：见炎细胞浸润及炎性肉芽组织，局部深达浆膜层，考虑为肠壁慢性溃疡性病变。

常规病理：回盲部肿物及周围组织：升结肠一段，长 13cm，肠管直径 1.5cm，小肠一段，长 4.5cm，直径 1cm，在回盲部见一质硬区，大小 5cm×4cm× 2cm，切面灰白质中，肠管层次不清，其余黏膜灰白，皱襞明显，肠周检出淋巴结 22 枚，直径 0.5~1.5cm。常规病理诊断：回盲部肿物及周围组织示肠壁慢性溃疡，深达浆膜层，伴贯壁性炎细胞浸润，大致符合克罗恩病（Crohn disease）表现，但未见典型肉芽肿形成。小肠及结肠黏膜慢性炎。肠系膜淋巴结 22 枚，直径 0.2~1.5cm，部分淋巴结反应性增生（图 26-4-1）。

第五节　转移性癌误诊为结肠炎

Meyers 等(1975)报告起初临床和 X 线检查诊断为溃疡性或肉芽肿性结肠炎,最后确诊为转移性癌的 12 个病例。

其临床症状为腹泻且偶有血性黏液、里急后重及胀气,特征性 X 线表现为:黏膜增厚、结节状包块、多发偏心性狭窄、病变不对称、假性小囊形成及边缘刺状突起,且常常犯及回肠。这些表现与结肠炎症性病变,尤其是克罗恩病有不少相同之处,从而造成误诊。

结肠转移性癌可由血行播散、直接蔓延、腹腔内种植等引起,最常见的血源性播散来源是乳腺癌。原发病灶可沿肠系膜反折或直接毗邻处蔓延至结肠。

第六节　肉芽肿性结肠炎之少见的结肠中毒性扩张

结肠的中毒性扩张出现于肉芽肿性结肠炎是难见的,大多为人不认识的并发症,而它出现于溃疡性结肠炎却很易识别。一些作者报告 2 例肉芽肿性结肠炎伴存结肠中毒性扩张,其中 1 例在患病几年后又有两次中毒性扩张。结肠之中毒性扩张通常出现于溃疡性结肠炎,且横结肠最易受犯,然而现已报告中毒性扩张也出现于阿米巴结肠炎。

在溃疡性结肠炎,炎症常局限于黏膜;而在肉芽肿性结肠炎,炎症则常在壁内,肉芽肿且具特征性组织学表现。在肉芽肿性结肠炎,壁内炎症及纤维化,可能是中毒性扩张的原因。在此 2 例,中毒性扩张不为抗副交感神经传导药物、鸦片类药物及低血钾症引起,也未发现任何机械性梗阻因素引起,其横结肠直径在 6~7cm。

当胃肠病人出现结肠中毒性扩张时,考虑诊断不能只限于溃疡性结肠炎,阿米巴及肉芽肿性结肠炎亦应考虑。这即是一征多病,宜结合各方面综合分析,才能减少误诊。

第七节　克罗恩病

详见本书 本卷 第二十二篇 第九章　克罗恩病。

第八节　慢性缓泻性结肠炎

慢性缓泻性结肠炎的 X 线研究十分重要,因为临床诊断可能延误。

当服用缓泻剂史未被医师诱出,或为病人有意否定时;当病人慢性体重下降、便秘或腹泻或电解质紊乱时,应怀疑本症。

X 线钡剂灌肠所见异常多出现于右半结肠,表现为结肠短缩、结肠袋消失,偶尔结肠扩张。盲肠、回盲瓣与末端回肠常受累及。结肠黏膜象可见黏膜侵蚀而呈现不规则,横结肠可见纵行黏膜纹。当停服缓泻剂后一段时间,这些异常表现可以减少,甚至消失。

本症鉴别诊断一般不难,因为溃疡性结肠炎和肉芽肿性结肠炎发作时常有发热,出血,分泌物增加,X 线观察其病变肠段的运动是特征性的。并且本症最不犯及直肠与乙状结肠。

第九节　炎性病变类似于大肠癌

详见本书 本卷 本篇 第一章 第五节 炎性病变　类似于大肠癌。

第十节　异物所致炎性肉芽肿误诊为肿瘤

详见本书 本卷 本篇 第一章 第二节 异物所致　炎性肉芽肿误诊为肿瘤。

第十一节　克罗恩病病例之二

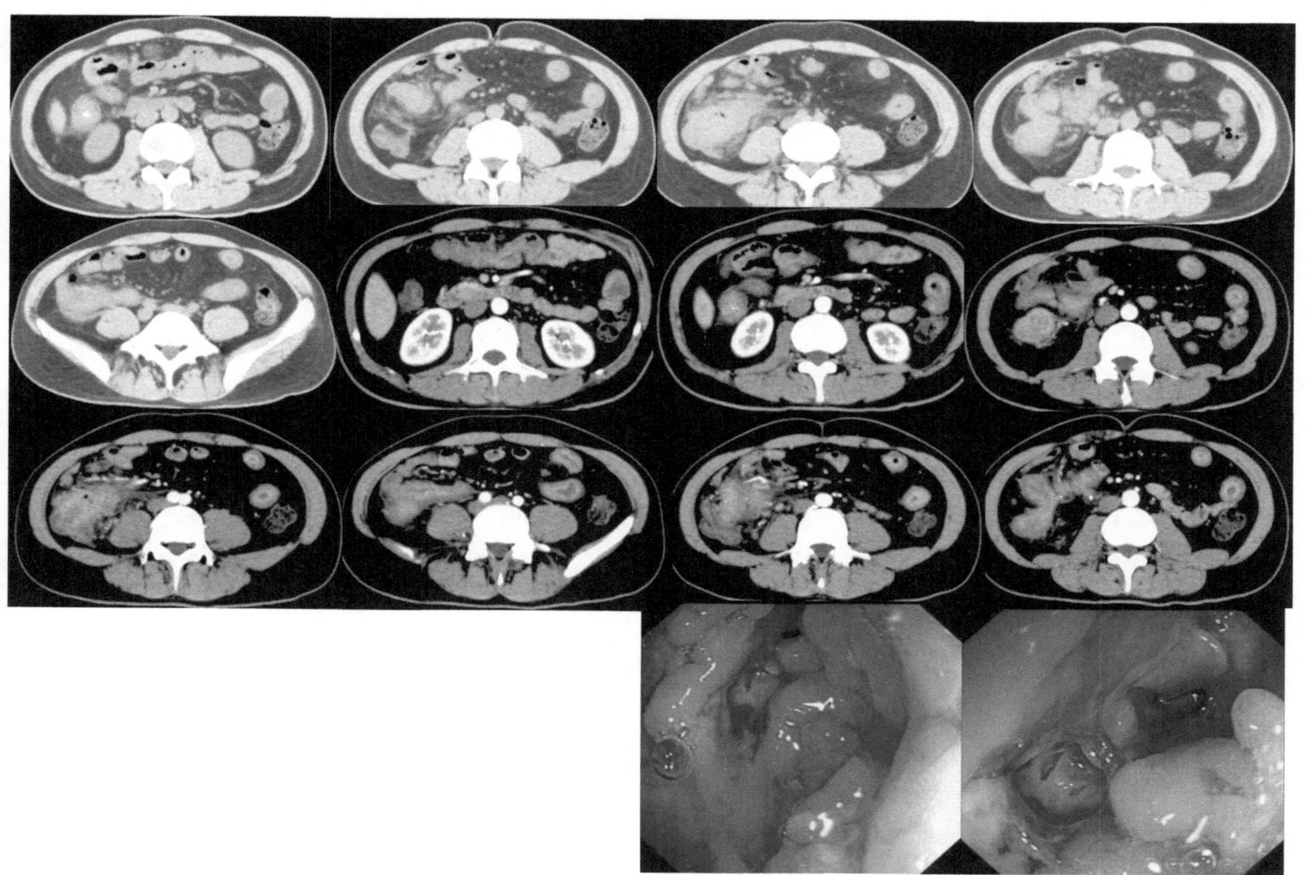

图 26-4-2　克罗恩病

患者，男，31 岁。内镜除考虑克罗恩病外，还怀疑小肠结肠瘘、结肠多发溃疡。可见卵石征，肠壁明显增厚，侵犯周围淋巴结。病理诊断：慢性黏膜炎症及炎性肉芽组织，为溃疡性病变（图 26-4-2）。

第五章 回盲部疾病

第一节 回盲瓣逆行脱垂,回盲瓣的脂肪瘤样肥大抑或是肿瘤

详见本书 本卷 第二十五篇 第十二章 第二节 回盲瓣逆行脱垂;第三节 回盲瓣的脂肪瘤样肥大抑或是肿瘤。

第二节 回盲部少见病

一些作者提出回盲部少见病有六种:类癌、套叠的美克尔(Meckel)憩室、神经纤维瘤、阑尾腺癌、末端回肠的转移性腺癌以及肿瘤样的肠结核。了解这些病变的情况,对术前诊断确诊颇有帮助。

第三节 诊断的混淆

有作者报告幼儿出现腹痛和包块,拟诊为肠套叠(回盲套叠),本应首先做钡剂灌肠进行诊断,但却先做普通CT扫描,结果普通CT提示为一孤立的腹腔内或腹膜后包块,反而造成诊断的混淆。CT图像上,鼻胃管可伪装成几种不同的结构,在广泛腹水病人鼻管可在胃中扭折,向颅侧或足侧再扫描可见鼻胃管的含水银的尖端,水银可引起条纹伪影。

第四节 误诊病例简介:回盲部腺癌与类癌、恶性间质瘤

患者,男,80岁。因血压、血糖高20余年,血透9月,乏力3天入院。住院期间突发大量鲜红色血便伴血凝块,CT发现:回盲部见一混杂密度肿块,大小约5.0cm×5.0cm,其内密度欠均匀,见多发钙化灶,边界模糊,与右半结肠分界欠清,腹腔肠道扩张积气,右上腹部肠道纠集,肠壁未见明显增厚,肠腔内容物呈高密度,肠外侧脂肪间隙模糊。CT诊断:回盲部占位,考虑恶性肿瘤,类癌?恶性间质瘤?建议MRI检查。

手术所见:肝、脾、胰、胃、十二指肠、空肠、回肠均未见异常,盆腔及腹膜未见种植转移,回盲部可见肿物生长侵犯出浆膜外,肿瘤约5 cm大小,与外侧及后侧腹膜粘连,质硬,内有液化坏死,结肠系膜根部及腹主动脉旁数个肿大淋巴结。

病理检查:回盲部肿物切除标本:升结肠一段,长8cm,直径5cm,升结肠切端周径4cm,紧靠小肠切端,见一溃疡型肿物,大小4.0cm×2.5cm,环绕管壁,肿物切面灰白质脆,侵及肌层。另附小肠一段,长3cm,直径1.5cm,于肠周检出淋巴结样物6枚。病理诊断:回盲部腺癌,Ⅰ级,溃疡型,大小4.0cm×2.5cm,浸润至浆膜层,伴多个小脓肿形成。升结肠及小肠切缘均阴性。肠周围淋巴结(-),0/6。

第六章　盲肠疾病

第一节　误诊病例简介:盲肠炎与肿瘤

盲肠炎,又称中性粒细胞减少性结肠炎,主要见于非白血性白血病、其他免疫抑制情况(如获得性免疫缺陷综合征)或恶性肿瘤化疗后。黏膜改变常局限于盲肠和升结肠,特征性表现是弥漫性水肿和浅表溃疡形成,CT 表现为盲肠及升结肠壁明显水肿增厚,肠腔变窄,也可伴有结肠周围脂肪内条索影或积液。

该组病例特点是盲肠及升结肠呈环状明显水肿,与阑尾炎有明显区别,阑尾炎盲肠往往呈局限或偏侧水肿。严重病例可引起脓毒症、脓肿形成、肠穿孔、肠坏死、出血等,但从 CT 表现很难与引起盲肠、升结肠及末段回肠壁增厚的克罗恩病、感染性或缺血性肠炎鉴别,但结合临床病史, CT 上病变的特定部位可做出正确诊断。

由于当初缺乏经验,有 1 例误诊为肿瘤,但结肠镜活检为炎症,经广谱抗生素和营养治疗病情好转,1 周后复查 CT 盲肠完全恢复正常。

第二节　盲肠腺癌需与慢性炎症性病变鉴别

盲肠腺癌占所有结肠癌的 1/4,共同的 MSCT 特点是:明显不对称的肠壁增厚,病变范围较局限,增强后呈中等度强化,没有肠穿孔的情况下也会有局部浆膜面轻微浸润的征象。盲肠癌与小肠癌不一样,很少引起肠梗阻,病变很长时间都没有临床症状,常向腔外生长,往往长得比较大才被现,肿瘤与邻近正常结肠分界明显。

盲肠癌主要需与慢性炎症性病变鉴别,该组部分病例 64 层 MSCT 动脉期薄层高分辨图像肿瘤内见斑点状无强化低密度区,多系含黏蛋白成分,认为这种征象诊断回盲部腺癌较有特征性,慢性炎症及淋巴瘤密度较均匀。

一些作者认为 MSCT 肠系膜浑浊征有助于回盲部恶性肿瘤与炎性病变的鉴别,肠系膜脂肪受炎性细胞、液体(水肿、淋巴液和血液)、肿瘤浸润及纤维化时,形成不规则条、片状高密度影称为肠系膜浑浊征,恶性肿瘤的肠系膜浑浊征较局限,而炎症性病变的肠系膜浑浊征较明显和弥散。

第三节　误诊病例简介:盲肠腺瘤

国内报道大肠腺瘤好发于左半结肠和直肠,病理上分为管状腺瘤、管状绒毛状腺瘤和绒毛状腺瘤,大肠腺瘤的癌变与腺瘤的大小、解剖部位、外形和病理类型有关,腺瘤直径 >2 cm 者易癌变,乙状结肠及直肠腺瘤易癌变,广基底腺瘤较带蒂腺瘤癌变率高,绒毛状腺瘤癌变率最高,管状腺瘤癌变率低。由于缺乏经验,该组 2 例腺瘤术前均误诊,但回顾性分析 CT 表现仍具有特征性,腺瘤 CT 上表现为突向肠腔内带蒂的或广基底的与肠壁相连的软组织密度肿块,用不同方位的多平面重建图像观察发现腺瘤蒂更有助诊断。

第四节 盲肠发育变异

位置变异:盲肠的位置变异很大,随肠道胚胎发育过程进展,盲肠的旋转和下降的程度可有不同,盲肠可位于肝脏下缘、脐周部或深入盆腔内,但大多数盲肠的位置在右髂窝内。

形状变异:盲肠形状变异, Treves(1885)早已典型地分为四型。在早期胎儿,它是短的、圆锥形和宽的基底,伴同它的尖转向上内,趋于回盲连接处。随胚胎生长,盲肠的长度增加较宽度为著,所以它形成一长管状,失去其宽的基底,但一直仍有尖指向回盲连接处的倾向。继续发育,管的下部分停止生长,而上部分变得增大,所以在出生时,狭长的阑尾从一锥形盲肠的尖伸出。这是婴儿型,它可保持于整个一生,约占人群的2%,为 Treves 的四型中的第一型。三条结肠带开始于阑尾,且互相等距。

在第二型,锥形盲肠变成方形,以一个囊在前结肠带的两边过度地生长,这些囊两侧等大,阑尾从它们之间凸出,而不是从锥形的尖伸出,此型约占人群的3%。

第三型为常见型,也称为正常型,该处有两囊,在第二型它们发育基本一致,而在第三型它们的生长速度则不相等,右边的比左边的生长迅速,显而易见的结果是形成新的尖,以右囊生长的下移,而原始的尖,伴阑尾附着处,则被推向左上,指向回盲连接处。此三条结肠带一直从阑尾基底开始,但它们的长度彼此不等,因右边囊生长在前带和后外带之间,推它们向左。此型大约占人群中的90%。

第四型只是一个第三型的过度,右囊更大,同时左囊变得萎缩,所以盲肠最初的尖伴同阑尾,紧靠回盲连接处,而前结肠带走行向内到同一位置,此型约占4%。

Pavlov 和 Petrov(1968)指出,第三型显示为壶腹状者占78%;所谓漏斗型,即为锥形,约占13%;余下9%为中间型。在同一资料中,活动盲肠约占20%,且常见于女性。

第五节 盲肠悬吊

盲肠扭转通常表现为扩张的盲肠移向左上,但扩张的盲肠也可见于腹部任何部位。盲肠横轴旋转可造成盲肠悬吊,扭转的盲肠位于盆腔内。因有回盲瓣存在,可形成闭袢型肠梗阻,盲肠明显扩张呈球形。对此情况缺乏了解与认识,可导致临床和X线诊断的混淆。

第七章　横结肠与升结肠疾病

第一节　横结肠系膜病变的CT研究

横结肠系膜是腹腔内的重要解剖结构，随着CT、MRI的临床应用，得以直观显示其正常走行、分布及其病变。横结肠系膜不但自身可发生病变，而且全身性病变、邻近脏器的病变和远距离转移的病变均可累及横结肠系膜。因此，发现和明确横结肠系膜病变，对病变的性质和肿瘤分级有重要意义。

1. 横结肠系膜正常CT表现　中结肠血管是CT图像上观察横结肠系膜的标志，96.7%的正常人中结肠血管可在CT图像上辨别出来，而肠系膜上动脉、上静脉的显示率为100%。横结肠系膜内的脂肪CT上表现为均匀一致的低密度，其内的淋巴结一般难以显示。在CT图像上，沿横结肠系膜边缘血管可追至横结肠系膜根部。

2. 横结肠系膜病变的CT表现　横结肠系膜水肿是血管渗透压增加，血管内液体渗出所致。非肝源性门静脉高压，如胰头癌压迫包绕肠系膜上血管，致短时间内肠系膜上血管内血流不畅，可致系膜水肿，CT表现为系膜内斑片影，血管边缘模糊，血管增粗，扭曲不明显。肝硬化门静脉高压时，可使门静脉属支静水压升高及血管内白蛋白含量下降，胶体渗透压下降，致肠系膜水肿，CT图像表现为系膜内水雾状、小束状的密度增高影及系膜血管增粗、扭曲、边缘模糊。CT图像上，单纯肠系膜水肿，到肠系膜水肿合并网膜水肿，再到肠系膜、网膜和腹膜后组织水肿，是反映失代偿期肝硬化病情进展的一个影像学指标。

3. 横结肠及邻近脏器炎症累及横结肠系膜的CT表现　急性胰腺炎：急性胰腺炎时，炎性物质或多种化学酶可沿横结肠系膜扩散，造成横结肠系膜血管渗透压增加而出现水肿，CT上表现为系膜内斑片影，血管边缘模糊。

溃疡性结肠炎：溃疡性结肠炎累及横结肠系膜时，CT显示系膜密度增高、模糊，系膜血管边缘不清，为系膜血管充血、水肿、增厚所致。

憩室炎：憩室炎是由憩室颈部闭塞所致的炎性改变，主要发生于降结肠和乙状结肠，可在系膜形成脓肿，并可突破系膜在盆腔内形成脓肿，导致脓毒血症。CT图像上表现为病变肠壁增厚水肿，肠系膜密度增高，可见脓腔。

放射性肠炎：放射性肠炎是由大剂量射线照射引起的，病理改变是由于慢性进行性内膜炎及淋巴管炎所致，可出现肠系膜缩短等改变，多见于远端回肠、乙状结肠和直肠。在某些情况下，横结肠亦可受累。

结核性肠系膜炎：肠系膜结核，CT上表现为系膜增厚成团，系膜内结节状、片状密度增高影。增强扫描呈不均一强化，系膜血管显示不清，见系膜淋巴结增大，并可有环状强化。

结肠囊性纤维化：在结肠囊性纤维化，横结肠受累达50%。CT上表现为肠壁增厚，可达6.4 cm，系膜内密度增高，横结肠及其系膜可有类似改变，但非病变的中心。

4. 横结肠系膜继发癌性病变　邻近脏器癌性病变侵及横结肠系膜：胰腺癌可直接侵及横结肠系膜根部，并可经横结肠系膜蔓延至横结肠。胆管癌亦可侵及横结肠系膜根部，进而累及横结肠系膜。横结肠癌可直接侵及横结肠系膜，结肠癌时可见到沿边缘血管、横结肠系膜根部和胰周增大淋巴结，增大淋巴结可侵及胰腺，从而造成与胰腺癌鉴别困难。

横结肠系膜转移性病变：CT上表现为结节状、饼状、污垢状、囊状，且有不均匀强化或呈条状、粟粒状强化。螺旋CT增强扫描对横结肠系膜转移瘤显示率可达83.3%。

横结肠系膜原发肿瘤的CT表现:肠系膜原发肿瘤少见,其组织来源广泛。其中,良性肿瘤多为纤维瘤、淋巴管瘤、脂肪类肿瘤、神经纤维瘤等;常见恶性肿瘤为肉瘤。淋巴管瘤CT上表现为巨大囊性分叶状肿块,其内有分隔,并推移邻近肠管。横结肠系膜神经纤维瘤CT上表现为横结肠系膜上一界限清楚,活动性差的囊实性肿块,大小约20 cm。

5. 横结肠系膜其他病变 经结肠系膜疝:肠道经横结肠系膜的缺损可形成内疝。CT征象包括:系膜血管增粗扭曲,主要系膜血管移向旁侧,降结肠内移,疝入的小肠扩张,扩张小肠与不扩张的小肠之间可见移行段。疝入的小肠袢前方一般无大网膜,且无疝囊,疝入的小肠与前腹壁相贴,可以见到肠扭转和肠绞窄的征象。

网膜孔疝:网膜孔疝内容物可为全部的小肠、末段回肠和盲肠、横结肠或胆囊。CT表现为:胃后方见疝入的肠管及其系膜和腹腔内的脂肪组织等,疝入肠管的解剖部位见不到原有的肠管;胃向前、外侧移位;小网膜孔扩大,小网膜孔处疝入的肠管的输入和输出袢呈鸟嘴样狭窄,门静脉、肝固有动脉和胆总管受压前移,肝内胆管有扩张。小网膜孔处见因牵拉移位而聚集的受累肠管的系膜血管。

由于横结肠系膜两层腹膜间的间隙与腹膜后间隙相通联,其附着处的解剖及其与胰腺的关系必将影响腹膜后病变和横结肠病变的扩散途径和影像学表现的认识。

第二节 横结肠脂肪瘤并肠套叠

结肠脂肪瘤并发肠套叠临床少见。结肠脂肪瘤发病率低,文献报道约为0.26%,年龄多在40岁以上,好发于女性,病因未明。约半数肿瘤发生于盲肠或升结肠,临床表现无特征性,可有腹痛、腹胀、腹泻及便血,腹痛原因是脂肪瘤引起肠梗阻或肠套叠所致。

影像学研究:成人肠套叠多有器质性病变,在小肠套叠中良性肿瘤占40%,脂肪瘤最为常见;而结肠套叠常由恶性肿瘤所致。对脂肪瘤结肠镜检查可发现肿块,但其是黏膜下病变,活检常为慢性炎症组织,易误诊和漏诊。

对脂肪瘤并发的肠套叠,由于脂肪瘤位于套叠的头端,结肠镜检查常不能发现。有作者报告一例以肠梗阻就诊,经CT检查而发现结肠套叠,表现为分层状靶形肿块及"彗星尾征",还发现套叠前端脂肪密度肿块。CT检查不仅可以发现肠套叠,还可找到引起肠套叠的原因;可以清楚显示肠套叠及其所在部位,套入肠管的长度及头端的肿物,根据肿物的密度、边缘、强化情况,周围结构有无侵及,腹膜后有无淋巴结增大,可大致区分良、恶性。

鉴别诊断:结肠脂肪瘤应与肠套叠前端的肠系膜脂肪鉴别。因肠套叠是指一段肠管及与其相连的肠系膜被套入与其相邻的一段肠管内,因此肠套叠前端的肠系膜脂肪CT表现为不与肠气和肠液相连的脂肪块,而脂肪瘤因位于套叠头部前端可与肠气、肠液相连。脂肪瘤因其CT表现具有特征性,可做出正确诊断。但对大多数肿瘤的定性,仍需结合其他影像学检查。

第三节　横结肠韧带样型纤维瘤病

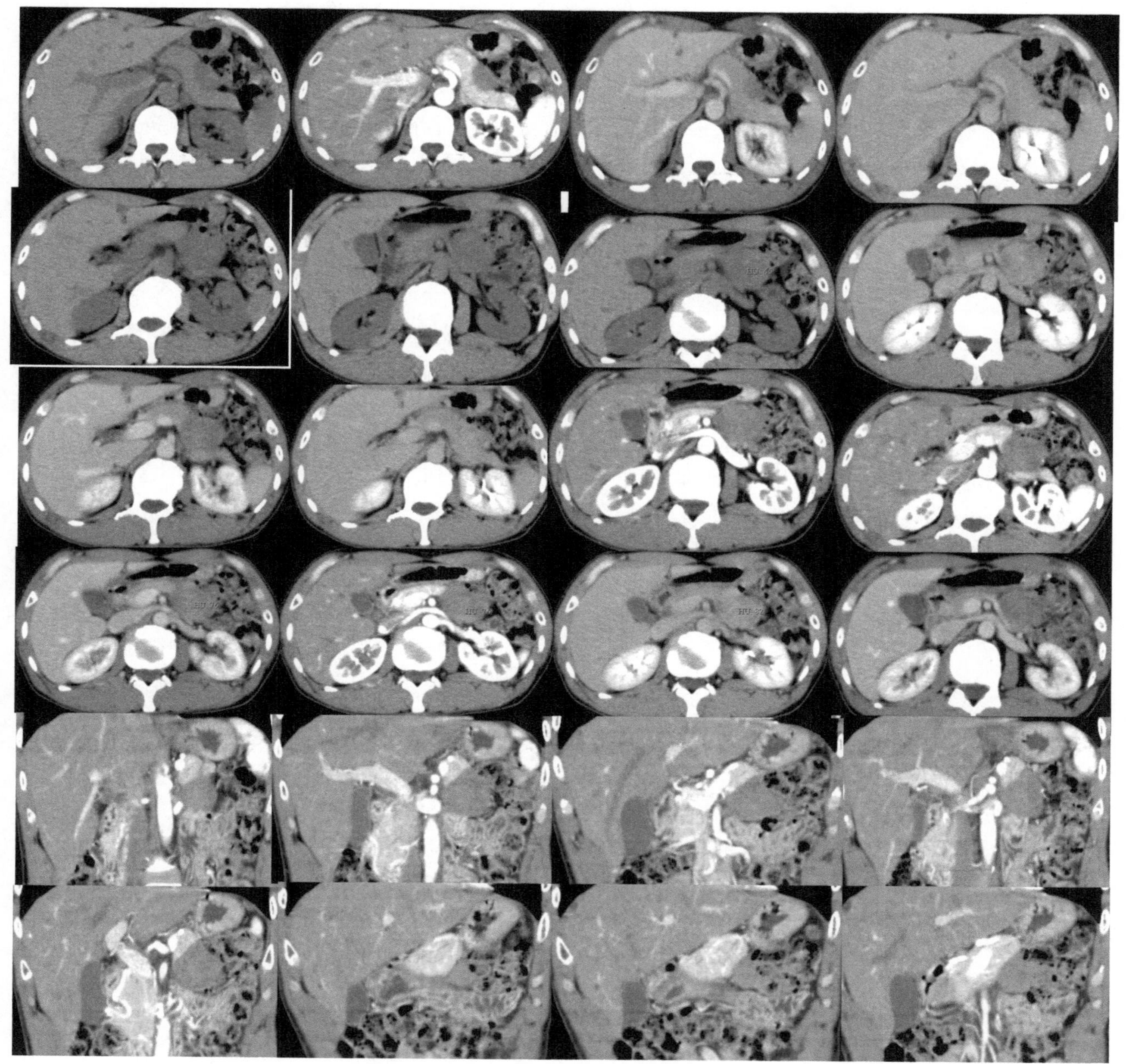

图 26-7-1　横结肠韧带样型纤维瘤病

患者，男，48 岁。因间隙性上腹痛 10 余天入院。

病理检查：胰体尾肿瘤、脾及部分横结肠切除标本：灰褐色不规则组织一块，体积 8.5cm × 5cm × 4.5cm，在中央区有一缺损区，大小 5cm × 3cm × 1.5cm，肿物带有一段肠管，长 6cm，直径 1.5~2.2cm，肿物肠管紧密相连，肿物切面灰白质中；另带脾脏，大小 7.5cm × 7.5cm × 3.5cm，切面紫红，未触及质硬区。常规病理诊断：胰体尾肿瘤、脾及部分横结肠切除标本示横结肠梭形细胞肿瘤，8.5cm × 5cm × 4.5cm，类型待免疫组化确定，肿瘤累及胰腺边缘，结肠两端切缘皆阴性。“结肠吻合口”阴性。“胃壁”阴性。脾脏 7.5cm × 7.5cm × 3.5cm，脾窦轻度充血。胰腺内部未见特异性改变，“胰上缘”淋巴结阴性，0/1。

免疫组化检测:阳性:梭形细胞 VIM(+),CD99(+,弱);阴性:CD117,DOG1,SMA,S-100,CD34,CK,Bcl-2,Nestin。免疫组化诊断:腹腔内纤维瘤病。注:病变累及结肠肠壁肌层及胰腺边缘组织。本病属于韧带样型纤维瘤病中的一个类型,可发生肠系膜、胃结肠韧带、大网膜或后腹膜,为中间型(局部侵袭性)肿瘤,有复发倾向(图 26-7-1)。

第四节 升结肠黏膜下黏液纤维肉瘤

黏液纤维肉瘤是一种少见的软组织类肿瘤,约占所有恶性肿瘤的 1%,临床发病率低,根据发病部位不同而临床表现各异,但均无明显的特异性,多表现为间接受压症状,容易误诊为其他病变。

本病多发生于四肢和躯干,也可发生于腹膜后、结肠、网膜等部位,中老年男性相对多见,临床上一般肿瘤体积多较大,界限可清晰或不清晰,有时可有假包膜,容易浸润邻近的组织器官。

影像学研究:CT 上表现不具特征性,常常表现为较大的软组织肿块,形态不一,多为分叶状,多数肿块边界与周围组织分界不清,侵犯邻近器官,呈现侵袭性生长趋势,肿块中心可发生坏死性低密度区,增强后肿块多以边缘强化为主,随着时间的延迟,强化范围进一步增大,中央坏死区强化较弱,由于肿瘤血供丰富,生长迅速,常常可以发现多支供血动脉,MSCT 重建技术可以术前帮助寻找供血动脉,为手术提供帮助。

MRI 上 T_1WI 和 T_2WI 多以不均匀中等信号为主,黏液区表现为长 T_1、长 T_2 信号,很少伴有出血,增强后实性部分不均匀强化,由于本病少见,文献相关报道较少,该病的影像表现特别是 MRI 表现还需进一步总结。

一例为来源于升结肠浆膜面肿块,向腔外生长为主,因此尽管邻近结肠受压变扁,但是病史较长,梗阻症状不明显,CT 重建可以发现邻近脏器侵袭性生长趋势,邻近腹膜、肾脏下极、肝脏下缘均受累及。由于本病临床表现和影像特征均无特异性,术前诊断困难,最终确诊需要依赖病理和免疫组织化学指标,黏液纤维肉瘤在病理学上相对较具特征性,主要表现为短束状、旋涡状结构,伴有丰富的黏液样结构,免疫组织化学一般只表达 Vimetin 和 CK,而几乎不表达 Desmin、EMA、S-100、CD34。

由于黏液纤维肉瘤容易侵犯邻近组织脏器,一般多采取扩大手术切除为主,辅以放疗和化疗等综合治疗,肿瘤容易复发和转移,若肿瘤恶性程度高,可伴有肺部和骨转移,极少数病例伴有淋巴结转移。

第五节 病理误诊漏诊病例简介:横结肠癌、胃神经鞘瘤与胃间质瘤、胃窦黏膜腺癌

患者,女,52 岁。反复上腹痛 3 个月余入院。CT:左肝外侧叶与胃窦间见大小约 3.8cm×3.9cm 软组织密度肿块影,CT 值 37HU,与左肝外侧叶及胃壁粘连,分界不清,周围见多发淋巴结影,胃窦壁增厚。CT 诊断:左肝外侧叶与胃窦间软组织肿块,来源及性质不明,周围多发淋巴结,建议 CT 增强扫描;胃窦壁增厚,建议进一步检查。

6 天后 CT 增强扫描:左肝外侧叶与胃窦间见大小约 3.8cm×3.9cm 软组织密度肿块影,平扫 CT 值 46~57HU,增强后明显不均匀强化,三期 CT 值分别为:75~101HU、119~130HU 及 136~142HU,与左肝外侧叶及胃壁粘连,分界不清,周围见多发淋巴结影。胃窦壁增厚。CT 诊断:左肝外侧叶与胃窦间软组织肿块,考虑胃浆膜层外生性间质瘤,周围多发淋巴结,建议进一步检查。

手术所见:探查肝脏、小肠肠管、盆腔未见肿瘤转移灶,胃角可见一直径约 4cm 大小肿块突出胃壁,周围游离,与周围组织无粘连,胃壁可见散在结节,其中较大的一个位于胃前壁,直径约 0.5cm,位于浆膜层,胃旁肝固有动脉旁可见数枚肿大淋巴结;横结肠中段可扪及一大小约 2cm×2cm 不规则肿物,质硬,突破浆膜外,与周围组织无粘连,结肠系膜可见数枚肿大淋巴结。

冰冻病理与常规病理:胃壁结节活检标本为不规则软组织一块,大小 1.1 cm×1.0 cm×0.3 cm;横结肠肿物切除标本为肠管一段,长 16cm,一侧切缘直径 15cm,另一侧切缘直径 1.8cm,距一侧切缘 8cm,距另侧切缘 6cm,可见一隆起型肿物,大小 2.0

cm × 2.0 cm × 1.5 cm，切面灰白质中。冰冻病理诊断：横结肠肿物切除标本示腺癌，侵犯浆膜；胃壁结节活检标本为平滑肌和纤维脂肪组织。常规病理诊断：横结肠肿物切除标本示隆起型中分化腺癌（部分为黏液腺癌），侵犯浆膜，未见脉管内癌栓，两侧切缘均阴性，肠管周围检出淋巴结 8 枚，均阴性。胃壁结节活检标本为平滑肌和纤维脂肪组织。免疫组化诊断：横结肠肿物切除标本示隆起型中分化腺癌（部分为黏液腺癌），侵犯浆膜，未见脉管内癌栓。

病理检查：胃肿瘤根治切除标本为部分胃组织，大小 9.5cm × 4.0cm × 4.0cm，胃大弯长 13cm，胃小弯长 8cm，一切缘直径 1.3cm，另一切缘直径 3.5cm，距一切缘 5cm，距另一切缘 3cm，胃体浆膜面见一结节状肿物，大小 3.5 cm × 3.4 cm × 3.0 cm，肿物切面灰白质韧，边界清楚，未侵及黏膜。胃窦部局部黏膜面粗糙，直径 1.0cm。胃小弯周围和胃大弯周围各找到淋巴样物 5 枚。另见大网膜组织一堆，大小共 12 cm × 12 cm × 3cm，找到淋巴样物 4 枚。常规病理诊断：胃肿瘤根治切除标本示胃体梭形细胞肿瘤，大小 3.5 cm × 3.4 cm × 3.0 cm，待免疫组化进一步确诊。胃窦黏膜腺癌，Ⅰ级，浸润至黏膜下层。两切缘均（-）；胃小弯淋巴结（-），0/5。胃大弯淋巴结（-），0/5。大网膜（-），0/3。

免疫组化检测：阳性：S-100（+++），Vimentin（+++），Nestin（++），Ki-67（10%）；阴性：CD117，DOG1，SMA，Calponin。免疫组化诊断：胃肿瘤根治切除标本：胃体梭形细胞肿瘤，3.5 cm × 3.4 cm × 3.0 cm，免疫组化结果支持神经鞘瘤。

第八章 乙状结肠疾病

第一节 巨大的乙状结肠憩室

巨大的结肠憩室通常发生于老年人,几乎总是发生在乙状结肠。病人可能没有临床症状,如有,则与肿块或突发腹痛有关。此种情况的发生可能与活瓣性机制有关。即:只允许气体进入憩室,但不能排出来。假性憩室不同于乙状结肠憩室之处,在于前者没有平滑肌层。在腹部平片上,乙状结肠憩室通常表现为存在于盆腔左侧中的一个巨大光滑的含气体密度影。CT 图像上则可看到一个位置固定的含气囊性薄壁结构毗邻于乙状结肠。憩室内可有液气平面,不应与脓肿混淆。巨大乙状结肠憩室一经证实即应视为手术适应证。

第二节 误诊病例简介:乙状结肠副神经节瘤与腺癌

副神经节瘤是起源于神经节细胞肿瘤,嗜铬细胞瘤用于描述发生在肾上腺髓质的副神经节瘤,其他部位的副神经节瘤按解剖部位及功能命名,一例发生在乙状结肠,按照解剖部位取名乙状结肠副神经节瘤。副神经节瘤的组织学及免疫组织化学特点与发生在身体部位相关,组织学成分主要是主细胞(Ⅰ型)和支持细胞(Ⅱ型),前者量较多,细胞呈圆形、核居中、胞浆内见神经内分泌颗粒,细胞间无桥粒连接。NSE 是副神经节瘤主细胞最敏感的标记,CgA 次之,二者联合应用敏感性可达 100%。免疫组织化学技术不仅有助于最终确诊副神经节瘤,而且能反映其生化和内分泌功能,有助于生物学行为的判断。

肾上腺外副神经节瘤的影像特点:大多数副神经节瘤直径 >3 cm,形态较规则,圆形或类圆形,边界清楚;副神经节瘤由于血供不均,容易出现变性、坏死、囊变,出血或钙化等较常见;由于副神经节瘤血供丰富,所以增强后病灶强化显著,部分区域强化程度与血管强化相近。有学者认为交感副神经节瘤多有粗大供血动脉,所以在部分病例中能见到供血血管,病灶呈早期、进行性延迟强化。据报道发生于罕见部位的副神经节瘤根据肿瘤发生部位不同,影像表现也不同。增强扫描有助于微小肿瘤的发现。大多数副神经节瘤均呈明显强化,这与病灶内含有丰富的毛细血管的病理基础相吻合。

一例发生在乙状结肠,实属少见,病灶密度均匀,增强后强化明显,边界清楚,血供丰富,动脉期病灶内见供血血管,并且呈均匀延迟强化。符合文献报道中肾上腺外副神经节瘤的 CT 表现,病理免疫组织化学也支持副神经节瘤诊断。

该例患者需要与乙状结肠肿瘤,特别是乙状结肠腺癌(Borrmann Ⅰ型)鉴别诊断,腺癌病灶增强后边界清晰,强化明显,与副神经节瘤相似,但延迟期强化明显减退,这一点与副神经节瘤差别很大。所以在乙状结肠肿瘤扫描中,延迟扫描有时是必要的,可以为诊断提供更多丰富信息。

第三节　乙状结肠暂时性腔外的充盈缺损

有作者报告一例乙状结肠暂时性腔外的充盈缺损，乃为人工全髋置换术所使用的结合剂造成的。此缺损在手术后即刻出现，当手术野水肿与出血时，缺损则更为明显。如有不透X线的物质附加于结合剂上，病因诊断则更加明确。

第四节　卵巢癌复发浸润乙状结肠误为粪石

病例，女，36岁。2007-11-07病理诊断（右卵巢）为浆液性乳头状囊腺瘤。2009-6-01病理诊断（右卵巢）为浆液性囊腺癌，伴部分透明细胞癌；（双）输卵管、宫角、左卵巢、网膜及阑尾未见癌。子宫、双侧附件、阑尾及大网膜切除。

MRI初看怀疑为粪石，后看为盆腔肿块。多次超声及MRI一直看成阴道上端肿物，由于子宫及附件均已切除，盆腔空虚，肠袢下降占据原子宫附件的位置，使观察者看到该组组织结构而一直未与乙状结肠联系起来，CT盆腔增强扫描方见乙状结肠肿块。手术病理及免疫组化检测证实卵巢癌复发浸润乙状结肠。

第五节　乙状结肠粪结误为肿瘤

病例，女，65岁。混合痔10年，便秘月余入院。骶前触及包块，直径约6cm。

3月15日CT左侧盆腔附件区见大小为37.1mm×59mm的软组织密度影，平扫CT值33~54HU，增强CT值为60~78HU，强化欠均匀，周围见较多迂曲增粗的盆腔血管环绕；肿块与周围肠管分界欠清。乙状结肠区见较大含气及脂肪密度肿块影，其内呈多层结构，近段结肠扩张积气。膀胱充盈较好，壁光整，腔内密度均匀。直肠壁较均匀增厚，管腔变窄，增强呈点灶状明显强化。子宫形态结构未见改变，周围界清。肝脏体积不大，包膜光整，实质密度均匀，肝门结构清晰，实质强化均匀。胆囊形态饱满，壁光整，腔内密度均匀。胰腺形态及结构未见异常，实质密度均匀。脾脏体积不大，约为5个肋单元，实质强化均匀。双肾轮廓光整、体积不大，肾实质未见异常征象。CT诊断意见：左侧附件区实性肿块病变，乙状结肠区肿块影，怀疑左侧盆腔附件区恶性病变，伴存乙状结肠肠套叠？请结合内镜检查进一步诊断。直肠壁增厚并明显强化，结合临床病史符合痔改变。

3月17日MRI：盆腔内未见异常信号灶。乙状结肠局部积气、可见数个较大球形低信号（T_1/T_2）灶，边缘清楚，乙状结肠局部腊肠样扩张。对比近期CT图像，该信号位置有所变化。子宫前倾前屈位，信号较均匀。双侧附件区未见明显肿块灶。子宫与直肠和膀胱间隙存在。膀胱充盈好，壁无增厚，内未见异常灶。双侧腹股沟区见淋巴结。左侧股骨头和股骨颈骨质呈片状长T_2信号。左侧股骨头尚无变形。MRI诊断意见：①盆腔内未见明显肿块灶；②乙状结肠内球形信号，考虑为干燥的粪便，建议排便后复查；③左侧股骨颈部骨折后所见，股骨头坏死？

第六节　诊断陷阱：尿滞留引起乙状结肠-直肠的假性狭窄

乙状结肠-直肠段是各种原因容易引起狭窄的区域之一，因其位于盆腔内易于受压。膨胀的膀胱外压引起此段狭窄者文献述及甚少。

Bryk（1967）在讨论钡灌肠对盆部包块鉴别诊

断时,较详细地论及了膨胀膀胱对此段的影响。Simpkins 和 Young(1971)在讨论大肠狭窄时,提及膨胀膀胱可成其原因。膨胀膀胱致乙状结肠 - 直肠狭窄的 X 线表现颇具特征性。腹部平片见盆腔内均匀一致软组织块影,伴或不伴结肠积气。钡灌肠见此段在侧位片上呈双凹狭窄,骶岬平面尤甚,乃由膀胱与对应之骶岬突起夹击所致。狭窄段边缘光滑,黏膜正常,狭窄可以很明显和恒定,也可在检查期间肠腔口径轻度变化。

正位观察狭窄段可呈不规则外缘,乃因外源性挤压使此肠段不完全充盈的缘故。狭窄上方的乙状结肠下缘可有平滑的凹陷,为膨胀膀胱挤压所致。更甚者,可将乙状结肠向上方举出盆腔。此类病人泌尿系统症状少或无,而与大肠病变有关的临床症状和体征却可非常显著,当钡灌肠有所发现时,狭窄与症状体征符合,使放射科大夫上当,如能记住膨胀膀胱可为狭窄的病因,诊断也就轻而易举了。然而,Kleinhaus 和 Kaftori(1978)介绍 4 个病例中,就有 3 例最初并未如此考虑,其中 1 例甚至因误诊而进行了手术。膀胱膨胀伴尿贮留尽管主要发生在男性,但要记住,女性也可同样发生。鉴别诊断应包括任何大到足以将乙状结肠 - 直肠段压向骶岬的盆腔包块。

第七节　异物所致炎性肉芽肿误诊为肿瘤

详见本书 本卷 本篇 第一章 第二节　异物所致炎性肉芽肿误诊为肿瘤。

第九章　直肠癌

第一节　前列腺癌及直肠癌对盆腔筋膜侵犯

盆腔内有许多重要的筋膜结构，其中最重要的有三组：尿生殖膈、直肠膀胱隔和直肠系膜或直肠系膜筋膜，肿瘤对上述三组筋膜结构的侵犯可以改变术前分期的判断和手术术式的决定。

前列腺癌局部浸润的MRI表现：前列腺癌是老年男性常见的恶性肿瘤，在欧美等地其占男性恶性肿瘤发病率的第一位。文献报道北京和上海地区321例尸检前列腺标本的结果，发现前列腺潜伏癌发病情况：41~50岁为2.2%，51~60岁为9.3%，61~70岁为5.9%，71岁以上为25%。随着年龄的增长，其发病率呈上升趋势。

对于前列腺癌的术前诊断，最重要的是确定其术前分期，而确定周围结构是否有侵犯是确定前列腺癌术前分期的重要指标。尿生殖膈紧邻前列腺尖部，其由三层结构组成，分别为尿生殖膈上筋膜、尿生殖膈下筋膜和会阴深横肌。

位于尖部的前列腺肿瘤极易侵犯尿生殖膈。如果肿瘤没有侵犯，则临床上可以行前列腺全切术；相反，则目前较好的治疗方法是先行局部放疗，待病变范围缩小后再行全切术。确定尿生殖膈受累的范围对放疗计划的制定有重要意义，因为对尿生殖膈部位的照射必然会造成尿道不同程度的损伤，可导致排尿困难。MRI对了解尿生殖膈的受累情况有重要意义。

一组病例中，肿瘤靠近前列腺尖部，前列腺尖部与尿生殖膈分界不清，部分层面显示尿生殖膈上筋膜不连续，其中1例病变累及了会阴深横肌。

盆腔中另一重要筋膜结构为直肠膀胱隔，它是位于直肠与膀胱之间的筋膜结构。该组有2例前列腺癌病灶较大，向后侵犯直肠膀胱隔。对于侵犯尿生殖膈的患者，该组作者进行了术后随访，其中1例患者术后效果良好，另1例由于侵犯范围较大，术后出现了尿漏。

直肠癌浸润周围筋膜的MRI表现：术前准确地评估肿瘤浸润肠壁的程度对于外科手术或术前放疗至关重要。但临床对T_1、T_2期直肠癌均能够局部切除，对治疗的影响不大，且对术后是否给予辅助治疗，主要依赖于组织病理学结果，术前对其进行分期的价值不大。另一方面，MRI不能区分直肠壁的黏膜及黏膜下层与固有肌层，因此不能鉴别T_1、T_2期直肠癌。

MRI对直肠癌浸润程度的准确性受检查技术和设备的影响，其总的准确性为58%~84%。

直肠内线圈能分辨直肠的各层结构，提高了对直肠癌浸润深度（T分期）的准确性，直肠内线圈MRI对T分期的准确性达71%~85%，但在远离线圈的部位信号突然衰减消失，故不能显示直肠及其周围毗邻组织结构以及受肿瘤位置或肠腔狭窄的限制而不能正确放置线圈或放置困难等缺点而制约其在临床中的广泛应用。

相控阵线圈在拥有较大检查野的同时，具有较高的信噪比和较高的空间分辨率。对肿瘤浸润程度的准确性为65%~86%之间，在不同的观察者之间的变化范围很大。Brown等（1999）研究发现其准确性为100%。Wallengren等（2000）采用MRI双对比检查可鉴别直肠高信号的黏膜及黏膜下层和低信号的固有肌层，提高分期的准确性，T_2期的准确性为82%。

Brown等（1999）强调直肠周围脂肪组织内出现广基底的软组织影，且与腔内肿瘤具有相同的信号变化特征，是诊断T_3期肿瘤的可靠依据。Beet-Tan等（2001）的研究表明在直肠周围的脂肪内出现较明显的粗刺状或条带状应归为 T_3 期。

毗邻组织器官受侵 MRI 表现为与毗邻组织器官之间的脂肪间隙消失，是诊断 T_4 期的一个特征。但需注意的是脂肪间隙的变薄模糊并不是可靠的依据，尤其是对位于直肠前壁的癌肿。直肠前缘脂肪层明显变薄甚至缺如，此时由于肿瘤的炎性浸润，常导致脂肪间隙模糊，造成过度分期，进行连续观察有助于提高诊断准确性。

有研究认为 MRI 能准确诊断壁外浸润扩散的情况。采用术后新鲜直肠癌标本进行 MRI 检查，与术前 MRI 和组织病理学比较评估肿瘤壁外浸润扩散的深度，结果表明术后 MRI、术前 MRI 能提供准确的肿瘤壁外扩散的信息且与组织病理学之间有较好的一致性。

直肠周围最重要的筋膜结构是直肠系膜和直肠系膜筋膜。在该项研究中，可见直肠壁浸润、直肠系膜内肿大的淋巴结以及血管聚拢的征象，这些征象对于确定术前分期很有帮助，但其只能作为参考。综上所述，MRI 可以清晰地显示前列腺癌及直肠癌对盆腔筋膜的侵犯，通过其直接及间接征象，可对肿瘤进行正确的术前分期指导临床工作。

第二节　直肠癌浸润周围筋膜的 MRI 表现

术前准确地评估肿瘤浸润肠壁的程度对于外科手术或术前放疗至关重要。但临床对 T_1、T_2 期直肠癌均能够局部切除，对治疗的影响不大，且对术后是否给予辅助治疗，主要依赖于组织病理学结果，术前对其进行分期的价值不大。另一方面，MRI 不能区分直肠壁的黏膜及黏膜下层与固有肌层，因此不能鉴别 T_1、T_2 期直肠癌。

MRI 对直肠癌浸润程度的准确性受检查技术和设备的影响，其总的准确性为 58%~84%。

直肠内线圈能分辨直肠的各层结构，提高了对直肠癌浸润深度（T 分期）的准确性，直肠内线圈 MRI 对 T 分期的准确性达 71%~85%，但在远离线圈的部位信号突然衰减消失，故不能显示直肠及其周围毗邻组织结构以及受肿瘤位置或肠腔狭窄的限制而不能正确放置线圈或放置困难等缺点而制约其在临床中的广泛应用。

相控阵线圈在拥有较大检查野的同时，具有较高的信噪比和较高的空间分辨率。对肿瘤浸润程度的准确性为 65%~86% 之间，在不同的观察者之间的变化范围很大。Brown 等（1999）研究发现其准确性为 100%。Wallengren 等（2000）采用 MRI 双对比检查可鉴别直肠高信号的黏膜及黏膜下层和低信号的固有肌层，提高分期的准确性，T_2 期的准确性为 82%。

Brown 等（1999）强调直肠周围脂肪组织内出现广基底的软组织影，且与腔内肿瘤具有相同的信号变化特征，是诊断 T_3 期肿瘤的可靠依据。Beet-Tan 等（2001）的研究表明在直肠周围的脂肪内出现较明显的粗刺状或条带状应归为 T_3 期。

毗邻组织器官受侵 MRI 表现为与毗邻组织器官之间的脂肪间隙消失，是诊断 T_4 期的一个特征。但需注意的是脂肪间隙的变薄模糊并不是可靠的依据，尤其是对位于直肠前壁的癌肿。直肠前缘脂肪层明显变薄甚至缺如，此时由于肿瘤的炎性浸润，常导致脂肪间隙模糊，造成过度分期，进行连续观察有助于提高诊断准确性。

有研究认为 MRI 能准确诊断壁外浸润扩散的情况。采用术后新鲜直肠癌标本进行 MRI 检查，与术前 MRI 和组织病理学比较评估肿瘤壁外浸润扩散的深度，结果表明术后 MRI、术前 MRI 能提供准确的肿瘤壁外扩散的信息且与组织病理学之间有较好的一致性。

直肠周围最重要的筋膜结构是直肠系膜和直肠系膜筋膜。在该项研究中，可见直肠壁浸润、直肠系膜内肿大的淋巴结以及血管聚拢的征象，这些征象对于确定术前分期很有帮助，但其只能作为参考。

第十章　结直肠癌

第一节　直肠结肠癌诊断与 MSCT

直肠、结肠癌的发病率男性高于女性，发病部位多位于升结肠及乙状结肠。右半结肠癌多以不明原因的腹部包块、腹痛、腹胀、贫血、消瘦等症状为主，左半结肠癌多为腹部包块、大便习惯改变及黏液性血便等，纤维结肠镜和结肠气钡双重造影对直肠、结肠癌的诊断具有重要价值，但纤维结肠镜和结肠气钡双重造影均不能观察肠壁的深层改变和肠壁外情况及其周围脏器的浸润。

1. 影像学研究　CT 作为纤维结肠镜和结肠气钡双重造影的重要补充手段，能清晰显示肿瘤的部位、大小和形态，直接显示肿瘤所形成的软组织肿块及继发征象（肠梗阻、淋巴结转移、局部肠系膜增厚、肝转移等），从而确定肿瘤的侵犯范围及转移情况，对肿瘤进行术前分期，为临床确定治疗及判断预后提供依据。

三期扫描：MSCT 扫描根据静脉注入对比剂后延迟时间可分为门脉期（55~65 s 后）、双期（动脉期 25 s、门脉期 55~65 s）及三期扫描（动脉期 25 s、门脉期 55~65 s、平衡期 3~4 min）。

采用三期扫描能清晰显示肠壁的多层结构，动脉期肠道周边动脉及其肿瘤区强化最为显著，肠周有丰富的脂肪组织，对浆膜层是否侵及突破、淋巴结是否转移容易作出判断；门脉期肝脏显著强化，肠系膜及其脂肪密度增高、模糊，有助于鉴别淋巴结与肿瘤周围小血管，可确定有无肝、腹部转移以及是否门静脉癌栓形成；平衡期可显著提高直肠、结肠癌分期的准确性。

CT 表现：直肠、结肠癌 CT 表现为局部肠壁不规则增厚，呈分叶状软组织肿块或环状、半环状肠壁增厚，边界锐利，肠腔狭窄、不规则，增强后肿块明显强化，肿瘤外侵时肠壁外缘不规则，与周围脏器间脂肪层存在密度改变，提示肿瘤可能已浸润邻近器官。一组 21 例 CT 图像上均能清楚显示肠壁增厚和肿块形态以及较准确测量肿瘤的大小。

MSCT 在诊断腹膜转移有明显优势，腹膜转移一般出现腹水、腹膜增厚、肠系膜与大网膜转移灶。肠系膜转移表现为软组织肿块影，系膜内脂肪密度增高；网膜转移早期为网膜脂肪内不规则软组织密度影，继而出现分散结节，晚期融合后形成“网膜饼”；腹膜增厚为线状或结节型，增强后均有强化。该组 1 例病例出现腹水、腹膜转移。

淋巴结的显示：早期文献认为 CT 对淋巴结的显示较低，为 33%~62%，MSCT 容积扫描及后处理可以有效地提高淋巴结的检出率，淋巴结的大小是诊断转移的重要标志，直肠、结肠癌的淋巴结转移多为小淋巴结，难与炎性及反应性肿大鉴别。

有作者以直径大于 10 mm 来评估淋巴结转移，淋巴结的形态、密度亦是诊断淋巴结转移的重要指标。一些作者指出转移性淋巴结密度高于非转移淋巴结，MSCT 对 B 期、C 期、D 期的直肠、结肠癌诊断符合率很高，但 CT 对直肠、结肠癌有无淋巴结转移的确定有一定的局限性，由于解剖关系，结肠淋巴系统与结肠动脉伴行，小的淋巴结转移不易与血管影区分。

另外，CT 仅能显示淋巴结大小，而不能确定其性质，当淋巴结已有转移而增大不明显（直径小于 10 mm）、增强强化不明显时 CT 难以判断，该组 C 期就出现 2 例术前误判为 B 期情况。

MSCT 检查的局限性：MSCT 不能显示肠道黏膜表面细微病变，对早期直肠、结肠癌仅黏膜破坏而无肠壁增厚的病变容易漏渗，该组术后 1 例仅为 A 期，而术前 CT 判断为 B 期。这是由于黏膜及黏膜下水肿显示肠壁增厚,而目前一般 CT 尚难清楚分辨肠壁各层,误认为病灶已侵及黏膜下肌层。

另外,肠道解剖部位特殊、肠管扩张不好而容易漏诊,为提高 MSCT 检查的准确性,提倡扫描前应做好肠道准备,可行低张结肠水或 3% 泛影葡胺灌注造影 MSCT 检查。

2. 鉴别诊断　良性肿瘤:主要为腺瘤,常表现为腔内或肠壁结节状肿块,邻近肠壁无增厚。恶性肿瘤可有局限、分叶状肿块,常伴边缘毛糙,肠壁不规则增厚,局部或远处转移。

炎性病变:如溃疡性结肠炎、克罗恩病,病变肠壁可增厚,但增厚肠壁多较广泛或多发节段分布,肠周病灶内有气体提示炎性病变。

第二节　双对比检查中结肠直肠癌的误诊和漏诊

Kelvin 等(1981)汇集 6 个医院 5 年多(1976—1980)期间双对比钡剂灌肠检查 31 例原发结肠直肠癌的误诊,并回顾误诊的原因,误诊原因可分三类:

(1)纯认识错误:占 52%。最常见的认识错误是缺乏对钡池与充盈缺损的认识, Kressel 和 Laufer(1979)指出,钡池能显露或覆盖沉降面上的隆起病变,遮蔽非沉降面的隆起病变,该组却未重视钡池的意义,只对边缘凸外的钡池感兴趣,而对边缘凹入(即有一充盈缺损)却有忽略,实际上,这也应高度怀疑包块,源自于新生物或大便块。

对癌肿黏膜表面轴位象表现缺乏认识是第二个认识错误,该组 26 个癌肿仅只 3 个显示轮廓的缺损见于切线位片上。在双对比造影照片上,癌表面的轴位表现十分微妙,当病变仅稍现突起,或肿瘤黏膜表面逐渐倾斜时,癌表面可能只现一线状影。

(2)认识错误与技术不完善合并所致:占 32%。在直肠,缺乏足够地将钡剂引流以显示病变是个大问题。抬高足侧床头使头低足高,或令病人俯卧,即可使足够的空气进入直肠,同时将多余的钡剂引流离开,以显露病变。有 3 例癌肿漏诊是因为照片曝光过度,细心地用一强光源进行观察,即能避免此类漏诊。此 3 例病变皆位于升结肠,左侧卧位观察尤其重要,只有这样才能观察右半结肠的双对比象。肠腔扩张欠佳和黏膜层被覆不良也造成漏诊。此组中仅只 3 例,反复回顾照片都不能观察到病变,考虑为纯技术的漏诊。

(3)解释错误:占 6%。一例表现为慢性溃疡性结肠炎的征象,双对比显示一长而光滑的狭窄区,解释为良性狭窄。关于浸润型癌误诊为溃疡性结肠炎的良性狭窄的报告,James 和 Carl son(1978)曾有介绍。另一例为分叶状直肠包块,错误解释为大的内痔。我们 40 多年前曾见一例中年女性排便困难,却被一位颇有经验的放射科医师误诊,与上述病例恰恰相反,将正常肛门括约肌收缩的不典型表现误为早期直肠癌,最后由外科医师指诊及直肠镜检否认。憩室的存在可构成邻近癌的漏诊,该组有 4 例。2 例憩室及附近节段结肠腔扩张不完全,如给予平滑肌松弛剂,可能有诊断价值;2 例憩室紧贴癌肿,使检查大夫观察时分心,而漏掉了更重要的癌肿。

Seaman(1976)指出,结肠近侧和远端同存癌肿者,近侧癌肿可被漏诊,因为 X 线大夫不愿意再充盈远端癌肿近侧的结肠。应该规范结肠的全程检查,不应因为已发现病变而不再观察病变近侧的结肠,减少漏诊近侧的第二个病变。结肠直肠癌造成的高度梗阻不常见,在绝大多数病例都能安全地检查整个大肠。Abrams 等(1979)报告大肠内同时多发癌的发生率为 5.5%。手术前的发现甚为重要,因为手术者可能在剖腹时扪不到第二个肿瘤。

按该组资料,最常漏诊癌的区域是乙状结肠(9 例)和升结肠(8 例),然而,Hunt(1978)认为癌可在整个大肠被漏诊。在双对比检查中,息肉被漏诊的分布情况与此不同,大多数在乙状结肠。目前发现结肠癌位于升结肠和盲肠的发病率有所上升,因此右半结肠的细心搜寻特别重要,结肠镜并不是常规地足以抵达如此远的地方。该组漏诊的癌,息肉状者多于环状病变。众所周知,大肠癌早期通常为息肉状。该组最终确诊都是反复地双对比钡剂灌肠,其使用频率多为二倍于结肠镜,在双对比钡剂造影怀疑隐藏结肠癌时,结肠镜一般只扮做证实的角色。

然而,在二十一世纪,临床上应用纤维结肠镜检远远超过钡剂灌肠,结肠镜检后如有怀疑,一般都是再做 CT 观察肠壁及周围脏器的问题。

第十一章　直肠与肛的其他疾病

第一节　盆底直肠周围恶性血管外皮瘤

恶性血管外皮瘤是一种发生在间叶组织血管源性肿瘤，可发生于任何年龄、任何部位，男女发病无差异，多成年发病。肿瘤的发生与毛细血管之后的微静脉有关，故全身均可发病，以发生于四肢、腹膜后软组织常见，发生于盆底直肠周围罕见。直肠周围静脉丛丰富，可能是发生该肿瘤的基础。

一例发生部位较为特殊，位于尾骨与直肠之间，肿块与直肠毗邻，并与直肠外壁粘连，造成肿块对直肠肠管的直接压迫，使肠管逐步变窄，患者出现排便不畅，大便变形等类似直肠肿瘤的症状。由于肿块逐渐增大，长期压迫直肠壁，使之局部肠管缺血而形成溃疡，患者便血，肛诊触及肠内肿块，超声探及直肠区域肿块，肠镜检查同样见肠管内肿块，并局部糜烂触之出血，进一步提供了直肠肿瘤的信息。

为了慎重手术，术前做了钡灌肠检查，见局部肠管呈偏心性狭窄，边缘光滑但局部欠规整，考虑直肠外压性病变。由于患者拒绝CT增强扫描，平扫显示的信息缺乏特异性，肿块与直肠界限不清，但直肠内残留钡剂显示明显推移，盆底脂肪间隙清晰，提示盆底直肠周围占位，手术选择了保留肛门。

联想我们曾见到的坐骨棘遗传性骨软骨瘤病引起排便困难的病例，认真深入分析，它们都是中老年人结直肠梗阻应该考虑的少见原因，建议读者博览群书，扩大知识面，敞开思路，考虑内容广泛，多想几个原因总有益处。

第二节　直肠后间隙的动态表现

一些作者按以往描述方法，在钡灌肠充盈直肠后侧位照片测量直肠后间隙99例，均见此间隙前后径增大，超过正常值。经分析证实38.4%病例无病变，为正常发育变异；其余为感染性病变、肿瘤和其他疾病。

因此，该组作者得出结论，骶前直肠后间隙前后径增加不一定就表示为疾病，此间隙的病理性增宽通常皆伴有直肠轮廓的变化、骶骨骨质异常或骶前软组织的其他病变。

几十年的临床经验告诉我们，对待影像诊断中的某项测量值的正常与异常，或某个影像学征象的诊断价值的评价，皆须辨证地看，灵活地使用，千万不可生搬硬套，机械地不折不扣地去比较，去实施。因为，人毕竟是人，不是机械，不是非生命物体，人不仅有生命，是活体，而且有思想，随时都要想到正常范围内至少有15%~20%还存在着发育变异，更何况性别、年龄、体型、体重、体位、呼吸、循环等诸因素对影像学表现都有影响，务须动态观察和分析。这也是我们研究活体形态学的宗旨。

第三节 MSCT 与肛缘定位

术前测量肿瘤下缘与肛缘距离的常用方法有直肠指诊、结肠镜等,但均为间接测量,准确度不高。CT 因其无法直接显示肛缘,所以在这方面应用较少,有文献报道直肠癌影像分期时,常将肛门括约肌作为肛缘。

有作者尝试在 MSCT 矢状面重建图像上进行肛缘的间接定位,筛选出变异度最小,误差在临床测量允许范围内的确定肛缘的解剖标志,使 CT 测量肿瘤下缘与肛缘的距离变得可行,在一定程度上弥补了指诊与结肠镜的不足,从而提高了测量的准确性。

Williams 等(1983)报道,肿瘤在直肠壁内的下行扩散一般都在 2 cm 以内,所以,对直肠癌远端切除不少于 2 cm 就足够了,这为低位直肠癌实行保肛手术提供了理论依据。Heald 等(1982)提出的直肠全系膜切除术也仅要求肿瘤远端切除不少于 2cm 即可,这也进一步提高了低位直肠癌的保肛率。目前普遍的观点是肿瘤与肛缘距离≥ 3 cm,就有可能进行保肛手术。

测量肿瘤下缘与肛缘距离的常用方法有直肠指诊和结肠镜。直肠指诊是一种简单而有效的测量方法,但是有其缺陷,直肠肛缘至其会阴曲之间一段 3.5~4.0cm 的肠管走行较直,当指诊距离 <4 cm,可较准确反映实际距离;而当指诊距离 >4 cm 时,往往略小于实际距离。

有作者对指诊距离大于 4cm 的患者资料进行了线性回归之后提出,实际距离 = 指诊距离 × 1.3-1。

肠镜因其不仅可以观察肿瘤形态、大小等,而且可以取活检,明确诊断,所以在结肠癌的术前检查中必不可少,又因为它可以直视肿瘤,所以也经常应用于测量直肠癌与肛缘的距离,但是肠镜测量的结果并不十分准确,其原因可能为:由于肠镜只能看到腔内情况,所以对于肿瘤下缘判断容易产生偏差;结肠肠腔较宽,肠镜在肠腔内可能弯曲,或与肠腔长轴不平行,这些原因都可导致肠镜得到的数值较实际的数值大。

与指诊及肠镜相比,直肠癌患者行 CT 检查时直肠腔内没有任何器械,处于生理状态。尽管在增强 CT 图像上,直肠癌边缘的确定要明显好于肠镜和直肠指诊,但是由于肛缘在 CT 上无法显示,所以 CT 无法用来准确测量直肠癌下缘与肛缘的距离。

该组作者认为,尽管 CT 不能显示肛缘,但是如能找到与肛缘位置关系较固定的解剖结构,则可以间接确定肛缘位置。解剖标志应在 CT 上能够比较清楚地辨认;位置固定,变异度小;与肛缘的距离较近,这样误差较小;测量方法简单易行;使用该参照物与肛缘之间的对应关系能够方便而准确的找出肛缘的位置。

该组选择了耻骨联合下缘、骶 5 椎体下缘、小骨盆下口正中矢状线(为避免尾骨不同角度对测量的影响,选择第 5 骶椎为正中矢状线的后端)和肛门外括约肌基底袢作为确定肛缘的解剖标志。

研究结果表明,耻骨联合下缘、骶 5 椎体下缘及小骨盆下口到肛缘的距离变异过大,不适于作为肛缘定位的解剖标志。而肛门外括约肌基底袢的下缘与肛缘的距离最为恒定,测量值变异范围在 5 mm 之内,而且受年龄与性别影响较小。

肛门外括约肌可以分为 3 个部分,尖顶袢、中间袢和基底袢,基底袢所在平面与肛管垂直,其后下方即为皮下脂肪。在 CT 图像上虽然无法区分尖顶袢、中间袢和基底袢,但是其最下部即基底袢的下缘。由于与低密度的脂肪相邻,所以可以明确的辨认。因为这个标记满足上述几个条件,可以作为间接测量肛缘的解剖标记。选择正中矢状面的时候,部分患者有痔疮,导致肛门外括约肌基底袢下缘不好辨认,此时可以稍稍改变一点角度,避开病变即可较好显示约肌基底袢下缘(图 26-11-1)。

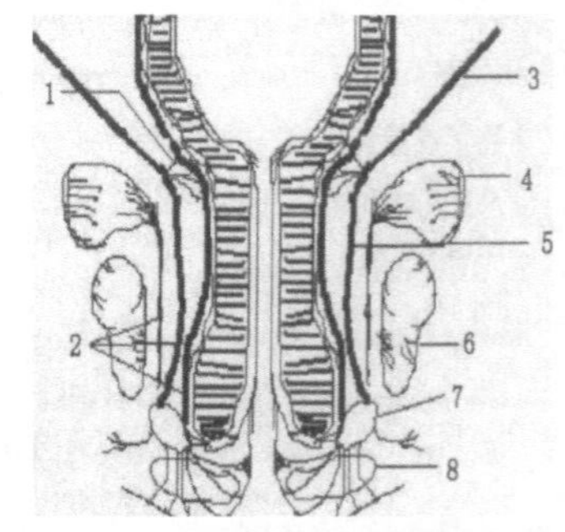

图 26-11-1 直肠下端冠状面结构示意图

1. 裂隙韧带;2. 联合纵肌;3. 提肌板;4. 外括约肌尖顶袢;5. 肛门悬带;6. 外括约肌中间袢;7. 中央腱;8. 外括约肌基底袢

明确肛缘位置之后，在患者的矢状面重建 CT 图像上，可以很方便地沿直肠走行测出直肠癌下缘至肛缘的距离，这种方法有很多优点：可以避免直肠指诊时直肠曲度的影响；避免肠镜弯曲、与肠管长轴不平行的影响；直肠指诊、结肠镜的测量受操作者主观因素影响较大，而 CT 测量受阅片者影响较小；直肠癌患者行 CT 检查时，会常规进行空气灌肠，这样肠管被撑开，可减少肠管松弛、蜷缩的影响等。

但是这种方法也有一些不足之处，首先，对肛缘的估计本身就有一定的误差；其次，CT 图像上所判断出来的肿瘤的下缘与手术医师在手术过程中所判断的下缘未必一致，当肿瘤浸润肠壁造成肠壁僵硬，但是并未明显隆起或增强扫描明显强化时，可造成 CT 上估计不足；再者，直接决定保肛手术是否可行的是直肠经过充分游离之后肿瘤下缘距肛缘的距离，保肛手术要求这个距离大于 6 cm，并不是术前生理状态下肿瘤下缘距肛缘的距离。

测量直肠癌下缘与肛缘的距离并不是决定能否保肛的唯一条件，必须综合考虑肿瘤的分期、病理类型及患者自身情况等才能正确的选择治疗方法。

该研究的不足之处是样本量较小。另外，虽然找到了一种可用于定位肛缘的方法，但是并未实际用来测量直肠癌，该组将会在适当增加样本量的基础上试用此方法来测量真正直肠癌肿瘤下缘与肛缘的距离，并与手术切除新鲜标本作对比，以评价该方法的准确性。

第十二章 关于排粪

动态 MR 排粪成像与 X 线排粪造影

动态 MR 排粪成像与 X 线排粪造影的比较：动态 MR 排粪成像与 X 线排粪造影在测量静息、提肛及排便时肛直角的大小及排便时肛直交界的位置上有一定差异，原因可能与 2 种检查采取的体位不同有关，前者采用卧位，后者采用坐位。有作者研究发现，两种检查测量从静息到排便时肛直角的改变差别不大，这与 Jorge 等(1994)的发现一致，Kelvin 等(2000)发现采用卧位的 MR 成像与采用坐位的透视下膀胱阴道直肠成像在发现器官下垂方面与临床结果差别不大。

将 7 例直肠前膨者前膨程度比较后发现，坐位的 X 线排粪造影比卧位的动态 MR 排粪成像直肠前膨程度更明显，可能与器官重力作用有关，与 Jorge 等(1994)的发现相似。

Shoryon 等(1989)发现正常志愿者也会存在直肠前膨，尤其是 <20 mm 的直肠前膨，其临床意义不明，与便秘等症状无明确相关性，无需特殊治疗。

X 线排粪造影分辨率低，组织标记、肛直交界及耻骨直肠肌后缘难以辨认，而动态 MR 排粪成像分辨率高，软组织对比好，肛直交界位置及参考线(耻尾线)容易辨认。X 线排粪造影在结果评估时重复性较差，在评估肛门直肠结构方面的价值有限，而动态 MR 排粪成像在测量肛直角大小及肛直交界位置时不同观察者之间有较好的一致性。

动态 MR 排粪成像的优势：动态 MR 排粪成像能发现肛门直肠结构及功能方面的异常，虽然由于肛直角及肛直交界的下降与临床症状之间没有较好的一致性使其临床诊断价值受到影响，但由于其分辨率高、安全性好，临床上仍有较好的应用价值。

许多研究发现，较好地了解肛门直肠部的结构和功能可以帮助了解便秘及大便失禁等的发病机制。该研究发现便秘患者有复合性盆底异常，可能与整个盆底结构松弛有关。动态 MR 排粪成像能显示盆底泌尿系统、生殖系统及腹腔脏器情况，可以提供充分的盆底结构信息，有利于治疗方案的制定。

第十三章　下胃肠道出血和大肠憩室

第一节　大肠的憩室病

结肠憩室可任意地出现于结肠的各处，但也有一定的趋势，常出现在系膜结肠带的旁边，及网膜结肠带和独立结肠带的系膜缘。在X线检查时，可清楚地在系独袋和系网袋确定这些憩室。在侧位照片上，可见憩室常出现于后壁（系网袋）。

结肠憩室的发病率随着成人寿命的增长而增加，有作者报告，在60岁以上的人竟高达35%~65%。结肠憩室是构成下消化道出血的一个常见病因，既隐蔽而又大量，在右半结肠则更是那样。结肠憩室病是严重直肠出血最常见的原因，这种出血是典型地急性、大量，常有生命危险，相比之下继发于结肠憩室炎的出血则是轻微的和间断的。

出血明显的原因是有炎症的结肠憩室内衬里高度血管分布的肉芽组织。

结肠憩室出现处与结肠的直血管纵行排列密切相关。研究发现，明显的长的直血管走行于一充血的浆膜下部位，覆盖于每个憩室的顶部，不论是单支或是多数性分支的黏膜下血管，沿着憩室开口的系膜缘分布。血管穿过肠壁处，直接导致肠壁软弱，倾向于形成憩室。直血管从浆膜层到黏膜下层，持续穿通结肠壁，而憩室的形成则是从黏膜层向肠壁外突出。

结肠的节段性肌肉收缩，导致肠腔内压局限性升高，造成黏膜与黏膜下层通过肠壁这自然的软弱处凸出于肠壁外，形成疝样突起，即为憩室。

结肠憩室与血管构造的这种不变的解剖关系值得注意，相当大小的一支动脉（直血管）密切走行于浆膜中，覆盖于憩室，在该处，此血管只以黏膜和少许减弱的肌纤维与憩室腔分开。

在憩室的大量出血的诊断和处理中，首要问题是正确定位出血点，选择性动脉造影可以较容易地完成此事，并可进行介入处理。

对比剂外渗显示于急性憩室出血的所有病例，对比剂进入憩室的范围内显示为环形（或圆形）的积聚，该处即为最活跃的出血处，它可以泛滥到一个或几个结肠袋内并使之显影，有时，还能发现供血的直血管实际的破裂处。

第二节　肠道血管畸形伴血管瘤形成

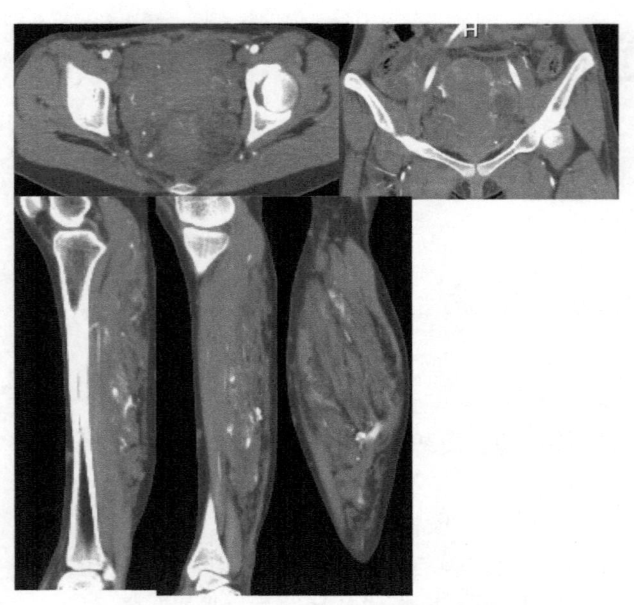

图 16-13-1　肠道血管畸形伴血管瘤形成

患者,女，19 岁。因右下肢肿胀并反复便血 10 余年,右小腿疼痛 25 天入院。曾行盆腔、右侧大腿及小腿 MRI 平扫示:卵巢多发囊性改变,请结合临床;左侧卵巢上方囊性信号;盆腔少量积液;盆腔、右侧臀部、大腿、小腿群血管瘤。肠镜示:直乙状结肠血管畸形,内痔。

手术所见:肝脏各叶完整,未见结节样新生物,胆系、胃、脾门、胰腺、升结肠、横结肠、空肠、回肠均未触及异常,腹主动脉旁、髂动脉旁、骶前未见肿大之淋巴结。左侧隆结肠、乙状结肠及距肛门口约 6cm 直肠可见弥漫性充血,局部血管瘤形成。左侧输卵管系膜可见一大小约 4cm × 3cm 囊肿样肿物,边界清楚,活动度可。

病理检查:结肠、乙状结肠、部分直肠肠管一段,临床已剖开,长 15.5cm,一切缘周径 6.5cm,另一切缘直径 1.6cm,肠黏膜未见异常,在距一切端 1.5cm 处可见肠壁外侧有血管堆积、扭曲,其余未见特殊。

病理诊断:降结肠、乙状结肠及部分直肠病变处肠壁全层可见许多大小不一、扩张不等的动静脉血管,符合肠道血管畸形伴血管瘤形成。左输卵管:系膜囊肿(图 26-13-1)。

第十四章　大肠的影像学检查技术

第一节　大肠双对比技术检查中的诊断陷阱

“透光”伪影：应用双对比技术检查时，一肋骨或骶髂关节斜位重叠于胃肠充气钡的影像上，可伪似一息肉的茎。如误将脊柱椎弓根影像诊断为一息肉，则使人非常困窘。灌肠管尖端有一圆孔，切勿将此孔影像误认为息肉。灌肠管尖端的气囊投影有时也可铸成假病变，故有作者专门强调对直肠的反复照片总应在气囊放气以后再做。

气钡灌肠时钡剂反流入末端回肠：这也是常常引起误诊的原因之一。在气钡灌肠检查时，如尚未出现反流入回肠时，宜令患者俯卧，这样则常常只有空气反流回肠而无钡剂反流。俯卧位观察、照片完成后再行仰卧观察与摄片。

结肠内钡剂过多：大肠双对比检查时，结肠内钡剂过多，则严重影响气钡对比观察，导致错诊和漏诊。此时斜位照片常有帮助，也可令病人排便。但如果再重新插管注气，尽管动作迅速完成，也难免结肠内钡剂凝絮或成为块状，难以观察。

第二节　对大肠影像认识与解释不当导致误诊

气钡双对比灌肠中的认识错误：在气钡双重结肠检查时，结肠直肠新生物可被漏看，其原因不是技术性问题就是认识影像的错误。在气钡灌肠，假阳性率较高，主要是在粪便与息肉之间鉴别困难，特别是直径小于 1cm 者。此种情况又不得不追踪随访，既增加医师的工作量又添增病人的不适。

不少研究指出，直径小于 1cm 的息肉病变中癌的发生率是 1%~2%。假阴性出现的原因可能是认识和 / 或技术性错误。有作者统计 12 个直径大于 1cm 的新生物中就有 3~6 个被不同的 X 线大夫漏看，乙状结肠的息肉样癌竟被 4 位 X 线医师全漏诊，这些主要是对影像的认识、识别能力的问题。

对于 0.5~1.0cm 直径的结肠直肠新生物，在回顾性研究时，约有一半难以确定，几个作者都发现这个情况。目前认为，气钡双对比结肠检查对此类病变敏感性较差，这是方法本身的问题。对于直径大于 1cm 的小癌和息肉，几位 X 线大夫进行讨论性回顾性分析时，发现率较以前常规检查读片时有所增加，但仍有不少遗漏。这是值得认真对待的问题。如何解决呢？ 读片时展开讨论，多找 1~2 个医师读片商量是个好办法，可增加发现率；在作气钡双重结肠检查后，再补以乙状结肠镜检可减少大部分漏诊，因为漏诊的此类新生物绝大多数都位于乙状结肠和直肠。

钡剂的人工伪影：在识别和解释气钡双对比检查的图像时，务须注意不应将钡剂的人工伪影与真正的疾病混淆，在大肠检查时尤其如此。在大肠，黏液、粪渣常引起钡剂凝絮，特别在检查时间延长时，而钡剂凝絮所产生的影像与溃疡性结肠炎的表现极为类似，难以分辨。气钡双对比检查时，即使检查技术十分理想，有时一些钡剂偶然呈现为致密的白点，可出现于胃和大肠，此刻，切勿将此类白点误为糜烂或鹅口疮溃疡。

线影与新月形影：在气钡双重造影检查胃、十二指肠、小肠及大肠时，对任何线状影与新月形影都应特别小心。当某肠袢不能展开时，务须认真观察其对侧壁的轮廓,任何轮廓外的线状影都不属于该肠袢而可能为某处病变的边缘。有作者着重指出,一个大的病变可以表现为只是几条线状影,甚或在正面观时只显示为一条线影;十分大的病变,例如息肉或癌,却可呈现为相当小的线影。

对于气柱中任何另加的线影或新月形影皆宜特别注意,对此类另加的线影未予留心,可能把气钡双重检查名声搞坏,因为某些非常大的病变除非极为注意这些细节,不然就会被漏诊。同样,新月形影亦为有用的征象,应仔细寻找,因为它不是部分被覆钡剂的息肉状病变,就是部分充盈钡剂的溃疡龛影。最后,应牢牢记住,在气钡双重造影时,除了胃小沟、无名沟以外,不应有任何阴影出现于气柱中。

第三节 胆石性肠梗阻的不常见的诊断手段

胆石性肠梗阻是一严重的急症情况,死亡率较高,如早期能正确诊断,常可救治病人性命。X线检查在确立正确诊断方面作用巨大,当其能够对已穿孔漏出的胆石定位时尤其如此。X线征象包括:①肠梗阻;②胆管内存在气体或进入对比剂以示内瘘存在;③胆系外可见胆石;④以前所见之胆囊结石现已完全消失或部分消失。

有作者报告2例借助于结肠钡剂灌肠确诊此病的少见情况。例1为结肠钡灌肠排空后照片观察到一完整的胆石在末端回肠为残钡所覆盖;例2为一个以前所见的大的胆石从胆囊区消失,但胆管内可见气体存留,钡剂灌肠显示乙状结肠一卵圆形充盈缺损,且见横结肠与胆管之间形成瘘道交通。由此看来,钡灌肠对胆石定位有时可起到不小作用。

第十五章　大肠的发育变异和诊断陷阱

第一节　大肠一般情况的改变与误诊

大肠长度、走向及宽度：肠袢的长度、位置和活动程度，及系膜的长度都有很大的变异。通常盆部结肠部分位于盆腔，部分位于腹部。当它有长的结肠系膜时，它可以横过中线。但是，在相当的情况下，盆腔结肠较短，无袢，系膜也较短，肠曲直接从髂段结肠进入盆腔。一个腹膜陷窝，按其性别分别为直肠 - 膀胱陷窝或直肠 - 阴道陷窝，位于直肠中段之上。

正常结肠有许多发育的变异。中间类型的变异，出现于极短的结肠伴少许肠袢，与异常伸长的结肠伴许多肠袢（长结肠）之间。病人直立时，下垂的结肠可进入小骨盆。腔径在个体之间也可有相当的变化。

大肠长度的变化小于小肠，Treves（1885）报告，在胎儿和幼年，大肠的长度较为恒定，全长 33cm 最大的变化只有 12.7cm；成人大肠的平均长度，男性为 142cm，女性为 137cm，其变化的范围为 99~198cm。该作者发现，在大肠与小肠的长度之间无恒定的比率。当整个大肠的长度变长时，通常都是由于或是横结肠，或是乙状结肠，出现难得的变长。一般说来，升结肠平均长度为 20.32cm，降结肠平均长度为 21.59cm，降结肠的长度变化小。

大肠的长度变化可很大，短的不到 1 米，长的可达 2 米以上，长度变化最大处在横结肠和乙状结肠。大肠的直径在盲肠最粗，约 7.5cm，至乙状结肠末端仅约 2.5cm，宽约 4~7cm。大肠的宽度也有差异，一般右半结肠的直径都较左半结肠为宽，但直肠壶腹也较大。

结肠长度、走向及宽度有显著的个体差异，其宽度从盲肠逐渐减小至直肠。升、降结肠固定于腹腔两侧和后方，乙状结肠系膜长、活动度大，可伸展至右中上腹部，然后向下至左下腹与降结肠相连。盲肠和横结肠分别位于髂嵴上方和上腹部，随着年龄增长而下降。结肠袋不显著，黏膜和肌层在直肠有增厚。

结肠节段的位置随体位不同而常有变化，这特别表现在伴有长的结肠系膜（正常腹膜腔内）的盲肠。当系膜长时，盲肠可位于右肋弓下，甚或进入小骨盆；前或后移位也属可能的，这称作活动盲肠。偶尔，盲肠还可位于腹膜后，因其关系固定，不随体位改变其位置，而被称为固定盲肠。

结肠与腹部的比例：有作者注意到 3 岁儿童与成人结肠和腹部比例的差异甚大，婴儿结肠和儿童结肠占腹部的比例远较成人为大，不应误诊为巨结肠。正常青少年结肠有较大的扩张性，可扩张到相当大，这是应该注意的正常情况。大肠的腔径和长度：最常见的变异是结肠的腔径和长度。节段性变异，诸如长乙状结肠或巨大结肠都可出现。在巨大结肠，结肠特别长，而且有许多肠袢。此类巨大结肠、获得性巨大结肠（即中毒性或轻泻诱发者）与先天性者可清楚区别。先天性巨结肠为无神经节所致。

假的“巨结肠”：一些作者注意到 3 岁儿童与成人大肠和腹部比例的差异甚大，在做各种腹部的影像检查时，在图像上常常显示出婴儿结肠和儿童结肠占腹部的比例远较成人为大，这是应该重视的问题，我们不可用一般成人腹部影像学表现的标准去衡量幼儿的大肠，更不应误诊为巨结肠。有作者报告，在临床上做影像学检查时，发现正常青少年大肠肠壁有较大的扩张性，肠腔可以扩张到相当大，远超过以往 X 线诊断“急腹症”规定的标准：大肠肠腔直径不能超过 6cm，这是应该注意的正常情况。

大肠的移动性:有作者报告结肠“过度旋转”伴降结肠冗长,此时盲肠位于中腹部。并非异常。移动性盲肠,排便后盲肠位置发生明显变化,尽管其本身无临床意义,但这样显著的移动容易发生扭转。

弯曲度和位置变异:横结肠和乙状结肠的弯曲度和位置变异较大,横结肠可以横在上腹,也可下垂到盆腔,但多数位置偏前,靠近前腹壁,胃结肠韧带及横结肠系膜连接横结肠的上缘,正常情况下不显影,在胃或胰腺肿瘤或炎症时,可作为病变扩散通道,CT 图像上表现为增厚的致密带。事实上,正常无名沟的宽度、深度和间距的变异范围是较大的,而且同一个体抽样测量误差也相对较大。

左半结肠的结肠袋:左半结肠的结肠袋明显缺乏,在正常人体中并非少见,此现象常常是由于长时间滥用泻药引起的。此类影像可能会被误认为慢性溃疡性结肠炎。了解病人的临床病史和服药情况有助于正确诊断。

第二节 关于结肠息肉

类似结肠息肉的正常解剖重叠及变异:有作者提出类似结肠息肉的正常解剖重叠及变异有:

(1)回盲瓣:脂肪蓄积或脂肪过多可造成回盲瓣增大。有作者认为轻度增大而对称的回盲瓣是一发育变异。有时回盲瓣开口于侧后方,正位投照时可见凸出的回盲瓣类似息肉样隆起,但根据特定的部位,及转至一定的体位是容易区别的。

肠壁皱褶的重叠:肠壁皱褶、结肠瓣及多处肠壁相互重叠时,在双对比相上常可产生类似息肉样的隆起和环影。如能根据解剖结构仔细观察,投照时注意肠曲的展开及各个角度摄片的比较,鉴别往往不难。

骶骨孔:有其特定的解剖部位,两侧一般对称,故骶骨孔投影在肠曲内的透亮影一般容易区别。

阑尾残端或基部凸向肠腔:有时阑尾残端或正常阑尾基部凸入肠腔内可形成一息肉样隆起影,但根据特定的部位,特别是部分充钡时,易于区别。

假的结肠息肉:在气钡双重结肠造影时,健康小儿的淋巴样滤泡可显示群聚的小泡状影,这些影像无临床意义,但易与结肠息肉病混淆。在气钡双重结肠造影时,有作者报告 2 例成人结肠淋巴样滤泡,分别为 43 岁和 63 岁,无临床意义,它表现为局限性数粒小的环状影云集在一起。有作者注意到,在气钡双重结肠造影时,服用蓖麻油产生的结肠内脂肪小滴,形似息肉样病变。在气钡双重造影时,偶尔可见由并列皱褶形成的横结肠“吻状”伪影,与肠轴垂直,形似息肉,转换体位后该影立即消失。

第三节 消化道钡剂检查中的一些诊断陷阱

消化道钡剂检查中出现的假像,有时可以假乱真。诊断时应注意以下几点:应熟悉正常的生理解剖及发育变异;要多深入临床,了解病史;在分析图像时应全面考虑,既要注意管壁是否僵硬,黏膜有无破坏,短期内形态有无改变以及与手术后的基础片对比等等,还要观察邻近脏器的一些变化;对可疑病变应在短期随访复查。有作者指出,在气钡双重结肠造影时,有的结肠看似小肠,可能是由于钡剂充盈无名沟所致。

生理性结肠括约肌:不少作者报告,在钡剂结肠造影和气钡双重结肠造影中,充盈像时生理性结肠括约肌形似环状狭窄的结肠癌肿,形成不规则的环状充盈缺损,但排空后该影像完全消失。了解此类情况有助于避免误诊。

黏膜假溃疡:在钡剂结肠造影时,偶尔可见钡剂充盈肝曲的无名皱褶,形似黏膜溃疡,一般情况下,排便前充盈像未见该皱褶,部分排便后则清楚可见皱褶内的钡剂。

有作者报告,在气钡双重造影时,由于黏液呈线状而引起长条细线透亮影,它与肠轴平行,可以相当长,经历 3~6 个结肠袋,不应与线状溃疡混淆。

影像重叠与陷阱:在气钡双重造影时,斜位照片上偶尔可见结肠后方的骶骨孔投影于结肠上,伪似充盈缺损。一些作者指出,在气钡双重造影时,盆腔静脉石重迭于结肠影像上可伪似结肠憩室。

淋巴滤泡增生：钡剂双对比结肠检查时，常可见到小的直径 1~2mm 的结节状、颗粒状充盈缺损，不应与真正疾病混淆，它们实质上是淋巴滤泡增生，将它与真正病理性小结节或小息肉鉴别开来在临床上是十分重要的。

淋巴样滤泡：在气钡双重结肠造影时，健康小儿的淋巴样滤泡可显示群聚的小泡状影，这些影像无临床意义，但易与结肠息肉病混淆。在气钡双重结肠造影时，有作者报告 2 例成人结肠淋巴样滤泡，分别为 43 岁和 63 岁，无临床意义，它表现为局限性数粒小的环状影云集在一起。

肠外结构挤压：在气钡双重结肠造影时，偶尔可见邻近腰椎棘突挤压结肠，引起降结肠内缘出现假性肿块。在气钡双重结肠造影时，有作者注意到排便前、后显示髂腰肌挤压，引起的乙状结肠移位，表现为乙状结肠被抬向上方，接近肌肉侧呈现浅的充盈缺损，在一些病人中也可以见到升结肠和回肠末端类似的缺损。

腹盆腔的脂肪蓄积：在气钡双重结肠造影时，继发于盆腔脂肪堆积的结肠冗长、上移、狭窄，正侧位图像上均可见及，此类影像不能与盆腔肿瘤引起的变化相混淆。膀胱也可有类似的变化。随着人民的生活水平的不断提高，此类情况出现的概率越来越高。

另有作者指出，在气钡双重结肠造影时，盆腔及回盲部脂肪过多症患者可见直肠和乙状结肠变窄、变直，回盲瓣脂肪浸润显示盲肠内低密度的三角形的充盈缺损由内侧伸入盲肠。CT 扫描清楚显示上述部位周围的大量脂肪。

黏液：有作者报告，在气钡双重造影时，由于黏液呈线状而引起长条细线透亮影，它与肠轴平行，可以相当长，经历 3~6 个结肠袋，不应与线状溃疡混淆。

邻近结构与影像形成的认真分析：有的升结肠引起右肾侧方移位，右肾的肾轴近似于横位，静脉肾盂造影和 CT 扫描清楚可见右肾肾轴由内向外横行的情况。在气钡双重结肠造影时，偶尔可见邻近腰椎横突挤压结肠，引起降结肠内缘出现假性肿块。在气钡双重造影时，斜位照片上偶尔可见结肠后方的骶骨孔投影于结肠上，伪似充盈缺损。此时，认真分析影像的形成常常有益。有学者报告，在钡剂灌肠时，偶尔出现钡剂漏入阴道的情况，其影像可伪似直肠破裂引起的钡剂外渗。在气钡双重造影时，盆腔静脉石重叠于结肠影像上可伪似结肠憩室。

第四节　关于回盲部

盲肠：有作者报告，当结肠“过度旋转”伴降结肠冗长时，盲肠可位于中腹部，不可误认为异常表现。在移动性盲肠，排粪后盲肠位置发生明显变化，尽管其本身无临床意义，但这样显著的移动容易发生扭转。 在肝下盲肠，阑尾正位于右上腹肝缘下，这是值得注意的正常的发育变异。临床上，阑尾的高位常常可引起影像诊断的误诊。

回盲瓣：在气钡双重结肠造影时，大的回盲瓣突入盲肠内缘可出现各式各样的表现，酷似息肉样肿块，且有分叶，此类诊断陷阱不得不认真提防。回盲瓣可逆行脱垂，酷似回肠末端肿瘤，有时出现于气钡双重结肠造影时，偶尔同一次检查甚至可见到脱垂前与脱垂后的情况。

在移动性盲肠，回盲瓣则可从右侧进入盲肠。在气钡双重结肠造影时，盆腔及回盲部脂肪过多症患者可见直肠和乙状结肠变窄、变直，回盲瓣脂肪浸润显示盲肠内低密度的三角形的充盈缺损由内侧伸入盲肠。CT 扫描清楚显示上述部位周围的大量脂肪。

关于阑尾：在肝下盲肠，阑尾正位于右上腹肝缘下，这是值得注意的正常变异。

有作者报告，在低压钡灌肠时，可见正常阑尾基底部套叠入盲肠；中等压力钡灌肠时可见部分还纳及阑尾钡剂充盈；高压灌肠时则见阑尾完全还纳，显示清楚。

第五节 乙状结肠、直肠与肛

乙状结肠:乙状结肠上端的位置一般认为在髂嵴平面,但有作者将其系膜出现处作为起点;下端的位置变异较大,可在第 3 骶椎平面或其上缘,可在左骶髂关节或骶岬平面,这种差别可能与对其下端的标准认识不统一有关,因为有的以乙状结肠系膜消失处为其下界,而临床上又常以第 3 骶椎上缘为其下界。乙状结肠系膜越过左髂血管、精索血管和左输尿管。

乙状结肠的位置和形状变化较大,仰赖于:乙状结肠的长度;乙状结肠系膜的长度及其自由游离的情况;乙状结肠伸张的情况,当伸张时它向上升出小骨盆而入腹腔,当排空时它下沉再进入盆腔;直肠和膀胱的充盈状态(女性还有子宫的状态),当这些脏器膨胀时,乙状结肠即上升。人种的不同,有作者报告人种的不同影响乙状结肠的大小,在埃塞俄比亚,盆腔上肠袢占比例较大,肠袢位置较高,导致乙状结肠扭转的发病率上升。

在钡剂灌肠时,充盈的膀胱可对乙状结肠挤压,导致乙状结肠变形,变窄、移位,在膀胱排空后,上述表现完全消失。

乙状结肠系膜:乙状结肠系膜一般附着于左髂嵴至骶骨岬间区,但上端与下端的位置常有差异,其附着线类似一颠倒的 V 字母,它开始于腰大肌内缘,走行向上内,然后向下,典型终止于第 3 骶椎的前面。有称之为升支和降支,乃表示肠管的系膜的排列。

乙状结肠系膜越过左髂血管、精索血管和左输尿管。肠袢的长度、位置和活动程度,及系膜的长度都有很大的变异。通常盆部结肠部分位于盆腔,部分位于腹部。当它有长的结肠系膜时,它可以横过中线。但是,在相当的情况下,盆腔结肠较短,无袢,系膜也较短,肠曲直接从髂段结肠进入盆腔。一个腹膜陷窝,按其性别分别为直肠 - 膀胱陷窝或直肠 - 阴道陷窝,位于直肠中段之上。

直肠:在 CT 扫描时,有的病人直肠明显扩张,其最大直径可达 10cm 以上,尤其是一些年老病人及便秘病人,这并不一定是异常现象,而可能是一些亚健康的表现。然而,在临床上,我们也见到少数年青人因腹部以外疾病进行 CT 检查时,发现直肠明显扩张,但并无直肠疾病症状,只是想排便而已,排便后再看,一切恢复正常。

"直肠耳":有作者报告 1 例婴儿"直肠耳",在水溶性碘剂灌肠正位盆腔照片上,它表现为直肠两侧局限性如耳状的外突,轮廓光滑,形态圆钝。该影像是由于直肠暂时性突入腹股沟环所致。钡剂灌肠时,偶尔钡剂漏入阴道,其影像可伪似直肠破裂引起的钡剂外渗。

直肠 - 骶骨间隙:一种正常的变异是直肠前壁有一小的轻度囊状隆起,可以认为是直肠膨出。这种变异可发生在男性病人,而不伴任何特殊症状。直肠 - 骶骨间隙(在气钡双重造影时称做直肠后间隙)的变更有着病理学意义。在溃疡性结肠炎、直肠癌导致的直肠的狭窄、直肠壁的放射治疗后纤维化等均影响此间隙的宽度。也可出现正常的发育变异,在肥胖的人,此间隙一般都有增宽。任何直肠 - 骶骨间隙增宽都应当准确评价,特别应该考虑直肠的内部情况。检查者还应当估价直肠的轮廓和直肠壁的弹性的变化。直肠的直径不应低于 5 cm,直肠口径的变化,明显地与直肠的充盈情况、排便、空气的灌入等密切相关。直肠不应比骶骨长。

Teplick 等(1978)按以往描述方法,在钡灌肠充盈直肠后侧位照片测量直肠后间隙 99 例,均见此间隙前后径增大,超过正常值。经分析证实 38.4% 病例无病变,为发育变异;其余为感染性病变、肿瘤和其他疾病。因此得出结论,骶前直肠后间隙前后径增加,不一定就表示为疾病;此间隙的病理性增宽通常皆伴有直肠轮廓的变化、骶骨骨质异常或骶前软组织的其他病变。在气钡双重结肠造影时,侧位片显示排便前、后由于肥胖导致的直肠后空隙增大,而非病理性改变,此类征象在库欣综合征中也可见到。

临床经验告诉我们,对待影像诊断中的某项测量值的正常与异常,或某个 X 线征像的诊断价值的评价,皆须辩证地看,灵活地使用,千万不可生搬硬套,机械地不折不扣地去比较,去实施,因为人毕竟是人,不是机械,不是非生命物体,人不仅有生命,是活体,而且有思想。我们随时随地都要想到正常范围内至少有 15%~20% 还存在着变异,更何况性别、年龄、体型、体重、体位、呼吸、循环等诸因素对影像学表现都可能有影响，务须动态观察和分析。

直肠周围结缔组织：Grabbe(1983)、Sugimura(1990)等都观察到直肠周围结构可在CT、MRI的图像上清晰显示，Grabbe根据盆部CT影像观察，为直肠周围筋膜与间隙进行重新划分。

该作者认为，直肠周围结缔组织从内到外可分为：直肠脂肪性囊，紧贴直肠肌壁，向上与乙状结肠的浆膜下组织相连，这层脂肪性组织可清楚地衬托出直肠肌壁和刚刚侵出直肠肌壁的肿瘤边界；直肠周围筋膜，结构与腹膜类似，极薄，包裹脂肪，它对限制肿瘤的扩散有一定的作用，正常人这层筋膜不能在CT影像上显示出来，当直肠有病理改变时，或病人接受放疗之后，CT影像上出现明显增厚的直肠周围筋膜，Dixon(1981)曾提出，一旦直肠周围筋膜出现，表明直肠肿瘤已不可手术治疗；直肠旁结缔组织，位于最外层，含成成纤维细胞、胶原纤维较多，并在直肠两侧富有血管神经。Grabbe对直肠周围筋膜和筋膜间隙的划分与解剖学者的观点出入较大，还有待于进一步证实。

肛管：有作者指出，在肛门口的稍上方，上皮由单层柱状上皮突然变为复层鳞状上皮，就在这条移行线上，可见许多巨大变异的汗腺，称作肛门腺。白线以下0.8cm，肛管被里为真正的皮肤，它可以为暗白色或褐色，含有汗腺和皮脂腺，上皮带的描述有相当的变异，常见是不同类型的上皮的互相贯通，所以此带彼此可以不硬性分离。

提肛肌压迹：切记注意，小儿直肠的提肛肌压迹可以又深又大，不应误为异常。

气钡双重结肠造影与排便前后：在气钡双重结肠造影时，有作者注意到排便前后显示髂腰肌引起的乙状结肠移位，表现为乙状结肠被抬向上方，接近肌肉侧呈现浅的充盈缺损，在一些病人中也可以见到升结肠和回肠末端类似的缺损。在钡剂结肠造影时，偶尔可见钡剂充盈肝曲的无名皱褶，形似黏膜溃疡，一般在排便前充盈像未见该皱褶，部分排便后则清楚可见皱褶内的钡剂。在钡剂灌肠时，充盈的膀胱可对乙状结肠挤压，导致乙状结肠变形，变窄、移位，在膀胱排空后，上述表现完全消失。

第六节　大肠的位置异常

轴面CT图像上看到的是升、降结肠腹膜后段的横切面像，而对于横结肠和乙状结肠而言，则是其纵剖面像。由于结肠的固有位置，较为粗大，有肠袋结构以及含粪便等特征使得它相对容易被CT所辨认和评估。升、降结肠位于腹膜后，而横结肠、乙状结肠位于腹膜腔内，其肠系膜且可能相当冗长。结肠位置异常是由于某种原因胚胎期肠旋转和固定异常所致。最常见的位置异常是盲肠和升结肠游动。在这种情况下，盲肠和升结肠有一长的系膜，将结肠的这些部分连接到腹膜后，尽管这些病人多无临床症状，但却使病人易于发生盲肠扭转。

结肠位于肝和膈之间(间位结肠)者，少部分病人会出现腹部症状。这是一个潜在的误诊因素。在胸腹部平片上，它可被误认为是膈下脓肿或游离气体。当病人取仰卧位时(2.4%)比直立位(0.3%)更易见到间位结肠。值得注意的是给病人实施经皮肝脏介入治疗时，多数是仰卧位进行的。CT扫描时，依据所见到的结肠袋及其与右半结肠和横结肠的连续性就不难作出间位结肠的诊断。其他较少见的位置异常包括胃后和脾后结肠、肾和腰大肌之间位结肠、胰腺后结肠等。最罕见的是胚胎期肠未旋转，此时整个结肠位于左腹，小肠位于右腹。

第七节　肠道的肝膈间位

肠道的肝膈间位在世界上某些地区(如伊朗为0.22%，在美国为0.02%)的正常人群中是一常见的X线表现，这种情况发生率较高者为慢性肺疾患病人(2.7%)与接近足月的孕妇(2.0%)，而惊人的高发生率见于坏死后肝硬化(有作者报告高达22%)。

推测可能的致病因素甚多：肠道变异、冗长，活动度增加；胸腔下口增大(如妊娠、肺气肿及肝硬化、腹水等)；坏死后肝硬化等疾病引起肝体积缩小，为突入的肠段留下空间，此时多无症状，常为摄胸片时偶然发现；提悬肝脏的韧带无力，加之腹壁松弛使肝下垂;镰状韧带缺如;肝与胃窦或十二指肠粘连;膈神经疾病导致膈肌轻度麻痹而易被充气扩张的肠管向上推举。有作者将肠道肝膈间位又分为完全型和部分型(按其间位肠道多少划分);恒久型和暂时型,后者其现象可时现时消,常随体位改变而变化。

肠道肝膈间位以结肠居多,其X线表现可伪似游离气腹及膈下脓肿,必须妥为鉴别。

肠道肝膈间位特点是右膈顶与肝脏之间透亮区内可见肠纹或结肠袋影;右膈顶位置稍高或正常;右膈运动自如,且其运动与对侧对称。而由气腹所形成的肝膈间透光区内无其他阴影可见,此为重要鉴别点;气腹量如果较多,常见于左右两膈下,可资鉴别。

由膈下脓肿所造成的透光区常有液平可见;且无肠纹或结肠袋影;其膈肌多显著升高,动度减弱甚或消失。参考病史及临床所见,也对鉴别有所帮助。

第八节 结肠壁的厚度

在CT图像上,正常结肠壁的厚度不超过2~3mm。结肠壁的厚度至少应在其呈部分扩张状态的横断面上测量。在任一段扩张的结肠断面上,如其壁厚超过4mm,均应视为异常。

评估结肠时,应当细致观察结肠的扩张程度,因为非扩张结肠段落在不同平面将呈现出厚壁征象而酷似病变。在作出相关的临床推断之前,正确解释结肠壁的真实厚度需要结合结肠的扩张程度。此外,当液体和口服对比剂混合存在于结肠腔内,也会遇到酷似结肠壁增厚的CT表现。在这些结肠节段中,少量气体的存在有助于准确地解释这些现象。

另外,其他一些征象的出现,也有助于澄清可疑结肠壁的异常。结肠袋消失,结肠水肿、冗长、“靶征”以及结肠周围感染等征象的存在都有助于确认结肠壁的病变。

第九节 结肠与肾脏关系

关于结肠与肾脏关系的一项研究结果显示,降结肠大多位于下方肾盏水平(3.6%和10.4%),较少位于肾盂水平(0.8%和6.4%),而很少位于上盏水平(0.4%和1.2%)。这种发育变异在右侧升结肠发生率较低,下盏水平为1%和2.8%,很少见于肾盂水平(0.2%和0.6%),而几乎不发生在上盏水平。

肾后结肠(确实位于肾后缘之后的结肠)在下盏水平有17例(1%),肾门水平5例(0.3%),而肾后降结肠在下盏水平为13例(0.8%)。女性变异较男性更常见,有统计学意义($P<0.001$),而各年龄组之间无显著性差异。该作者指出,腹膜后结肠的位置取决于肾前、后筋膜与结肠侧筋膜汇合点的前后。肾旁间隙内结肠正常解剖位置变异应由CT和排泄性尿系造影评估。在行经皮肾切除或活检前,应先行CT或超声检查,以免术中损伤结肠。

有的升结肠引起右肾侧方移位,右肾的竖轴近似于横位,排泄性尿系造影和CT扫描清楚可见右肾肾轴由内向外横行的情况。

第十六章 大肠的其他疾病

第一节 结肠袋被侵

三排结肠袋，分别可为不同的疾病或病理情况所侵犯，通过对于结肠袋的观察和分析，常常有助于早期发现异常情况，同时对某些疾病作出诊断。

病变进入胃结肠韧带：当胃癌沿着胃结肠韧带扩散时，它首先必定侵犯横结肠上缘的系网袋，而不是侵犯横结肠下缘的网独袋。通过电视透视观察，可以研究该排结肠袋的蠕动收缩、形态、大小以及轴的改变。但要注意，不是所有的系网袋的外在性侵犯情况，都是反映病变进入了胃结肠韧带。因为，正常的胆囊也可局限性造成结肠肝曲及附近此排结肠袋的压迹，当此类压迹成为明显的压痕时，常常表示胆囊有所肿大，这见于胆囊积水、胆囊气肿，有时，肝外胆管囊肿也可出现此征。

病变进入横结肠系膜：研究证明，当病变沿着横结肠系膜扩散时，在系膜平面常常优先地选择向下，在横结肠下缘，沿着系独袋，走向网独袋。胰腺病变，沿着横结肠系膜扩展，它们可以特征性地影响横结肠下排结肠袋。在严重的胰腺炎，外渗的胰酶典型地使网独袋轮廓变平，此酶可以沿着横结肠系膜的范围向左侧播散，对结肠的影响可以特征性地终止于膈结肠韧带平面。此时，横结肠的上轮廓的未受侵犯的系网袋常常表现为假囊性改变。

此类似的方式，胰癌也可直接扩展到横结肠，沿着结肠系膜特征性地，首先或主要地侵犯网独袋。

腹膜内和腹膜外病变的分布：在升结肠和降结肠，两排结肠袋面向腹膜内结构，网独袋关系到外侧结肠旁沟，系独袋关系到内结肠旁沟和小肠肠袢。在这些区域，腹膜内的病变可主要累及此两排结肠袋。与之相反，后面的系网袋是唯一与腹膜外结构病变有关的结肠袋，当腹膜外病变的临床表现隐伏时，它常与腹膜内病变混淆。如病变只累及系网袋这一排，则可清楚地决定异常所在是腹膜外。

上升的盲肠后阑尾炎：上升的盲肠后阑尾炎发生率的范围，从手术病例 26%，到尸解病例的 65%。在这位置上，阑尾可在腹膜内，也可在腹膜外。阑尾炎的许多并发症都与阑尾位置上的发育变异有关，这反映在临床上是区别诊断急性阑尾炎与肝、右肾、胆囊和右肺基底及胸膜的病变。伴发于腹膜腔内上升的盲肠后阑尾的炎症，出现于右结肠旁沟，侵犯升结肠外侧的网独袋；相反，伴发腹膜腔外的上升的盲肠后阑尾炎，主要影响后面的系网袋。阑尾本身还可显示明确的异常，诸如：显著移位、窦道形成以及脓肿腔的显影等。熟悉影像学表现，再联系到上述特征性表现，对于疾病的正确定位和诊断常常有益。

腹部外伤：有的腹部外伤可伴存升结肠和 / 或降结肠的移位，此时，确定受影响的结肠袋是哪一排则非常重要，因为它可用来区别腹膜内出血和腹膜外出血。腹膜内的液体积聚在外侧结肠旁沟，可压迫网独袋；相反，腹膜外出血则关系着结肠袋变平，特别是系网袋。

恶性肿瘤的种植：恶性肿瘤的腹膜内种植及腹腔积液的流动，趋向于局限在升结肠的网独袋。肿瘤栓子的转移，按照壁内动脉的分布，也趋向于犯及结肠袋的反系膜侧。

结肠重复：结肠重复常有一很好发育的平滑肌层，以结肠黏膜画出轮廓，而且粘连，常常交通于结肠。它们典型地沿着系膜缘推移结肠，这就关系着升结肠或 / 和降结肠的系独袋，以及横结肠的系网袋。因为这两段结肠共享一共同的血液供应，而且在大多数病例，只有一简单的系膜。

第二节 大肠破裂

结肠损伤往往由上腹部挤压伤所致。最常见的损伤位置是横结肠、乙状结肠和盲肠。

横结肠的损伤可以引起肌间血肿和没有肠内容物外渗的浆膜撕裂。结肠撕裂伤可发生结肠肠系膜和血管损伤,这些会影响该部分结肠的血液运输。发生于侧方或是背侧的损伤要进行腹部 CT 三维成像,以显示直肠至大肠。病情稳定的腹膜后刺伤病人如果没有结肠穿透伤,可保守治疗。一旦显示结肠穿孔,则需手术治疗。

第三节 关于结肠“狭窄”

关于此类“狭窄”,可出现于结肠许多特殊部位(请参见巫北海总主编:《活体形态学》腹盆上卷,北京,科学出版社,2006 年版),它们有些是由于纵肌或/和环肌纤维的局限性增厚,有些却尚未发现器质性的改变。一些作者认为这些“狭窄”区带也许是由于过度的神经刺激活动所致。区别此类“狭窄”区与器质性病变十分重要,一种方法是重复检查,反复动态观察,了解其变化情况;一种方法就是用药物使肠壁松弛。

有学者指出,既然它们又叫结肠的括约肌,如有怀疑,难辨真伪时,可注射高血糖糖原质分解因子(glucagon),使此种苹果心状“狭窄”松弛,显示正常结肠袋状扩张。

第四节 结肠黏膜下脂肪沉积

在 CT 增强图像上,结肠的“靶征”或“晕征”通常提示该段肠管的炎症或缺血性病变。这是由于夹在增强了的黏膜下层与肌层之间的呈低密度的黏膜下水肿所致。偶尔在结肠硬性癌的病人中可见到“靶征”。靶征也可见于黏膜下脂肪沉积。

它有时出现在长期患慢性肠炎的病人中,并不提示急性炎症。其病因还不完全清楚,但部分可能与病人经常使用激素有关;也有报道黏膜下脂肪沉积出现在没有肠炎病史的病人,可能与接受过大剂量的化疗有关。

第五节 结肠缺血

结肠缺血是老年人最常见的肠血管性疾病。与肠系膜缺血相比,结肠缺血的病人临床表现较轻,常诉轻微腹痛或血性腹泻。大多数病例找不到确切的病因,也没有血管闭塞的证据。多数病人年龄在 70 岁以上,且常伴广泛的动脉粥样硬化,因此一般认为是由于结肠血流减少所致。

结肠受累范围取决于病因,非闭塞性缺血常常较粥样硬化栓子所致的缺血累及范围大。非闭塞性结肠缺血一般累及结肠的交界区,即脾曲和直肠乙状结肠交界处,但任何一段结肠均可受累。CT 表现与肠系膜缺血相似,最常见表现为肠壁增厚,多数为节段性受累,平均受累总的长度为 19cm。肠壁积气、肠系膜血管或门静脉内气体都是预后不良的征象,提示肠壁全层缺血或梗死,但某些良性病变、获得性免疫缺陷综合征晚期也可出现类似征象。

第六节　结肠水肿

在不同病因所致的严重结肠炎和肠缺血性损害的病人中，通常可见到结肠水肿。另外，在肝硬化病人中，经常发生肠水肿，且可通过钡餐检查和胃肠道CT检查诊断。水肿经常发生在小肠，而较少见于胃和结肠。

导致这些病人胃肠道发生水肿的主要因素包括渗透压的降低（低蛋白血症）和门静脉压力的增高（流体静水压增高）。而后者可能起了决定性作用，因为它与肝硬化病人的异常水肿分布范围具有更好的相关性。在结肠中，一些混淆的影像学变化可被误认为急性结肠炎。

肝硬化病人的结肠水肿可类似于任何其他原因引起的结肠水肿。由于黏膜下有低密度水肿区，因此结肠壁增厚，结肠袋也有所改变，也可能存在靶征。而内镜检查时，黏膜却可表现正常。肝硬化引起的结肠水肿，尽管整个结肠都有可能受累，但往往有累及右半结肠的趋势。鉴别诊断则须依据其他CT征象（肝硬化的表现、静脉曲张等）以及相应临床症状。

第七节　结肠孤立性良性溃疡

孤立性或非特异性良性结肠溃疡首先由Cruveilhier（1835）报告，迄今有100多例报告。

溃疡多在盲肠，也可在结肠其他各段，钡剂灌肠时几乎总是误诊为癌，正确诊断往往直到手术病理才能作出。病因学目前尚不甚清楚，估计与此有关的因素是局部血管或神经性障碍、异物损伤、肠内容物淤滞、药物刺激、结肠酸碱度改变等。

Magilner（1972）报告1例小儿，主诉为便血与腹痛，钡灌肠见降结肠有一孤立性溃疡龛影，追踪4个月复查已完全痊愈。一年后因阑尾炎入院手术，见原溃疡处有弥漫纤维性腹膜炎，考虑为结核性。

第八节　关于大肠的内容物

在腹部X线正位片上的诊断陷阱中，需要注意几点：横结肠内的瓜子影，可伪似胰腺钙化。有作者报告盆腔右侧致密影为摄入的骨粉，可被误认为卵巢恶性肿瘤的沙样瘤钙化。盲肠内的杏核可伪似结石。

第九节　大肠的淋巴滤泡

胃肠道淋巴滤泡广泛分布于黏膜下层。特别是儿童的末端回肠淋巴滤泡常聚集成斑片状，突出于黏膜面，称Peyer淋巴丛。Dukes和Bussey（1926）统计成人结肠内的淋巴滤泡分布，平均每平方厘米3~5个，儿童则较成人更多。

Frederick等资料表明成人结肠淋巴滤泡呈节段性分布。最多见的部位是结肠肝曲（62%），其次为降结肠、横结肠，直肠与乙状结肠仅占19%。有81%的病例滤泡分布少于结肠全长的一半。并认为在气钡双重造影检查中，成人淋巴滤泡的检出率为13%。

然而Cole的22例结肠标本的X线与解剖学对照研究，提出结肠黏膜下的淋巴滤泡呈线形分布，并与无名沟走行一致。有作者在25例结肠标本组织学研究中，发现58%的无名沟下有淋巴组织聚集。根据以上资料我们认为，只有提高结肠无名沟的显示率,才有可能提高结肠淋巴滤泡的检出率。Burbige和Sobky又指出成人结肠内的淋巴滤泡,在内窥镜下观察不到。由此可见,正常结肠气钡双重造影淋巴滤泡难以显示,一旦造影显示弥漫分布的小结节状充盈缺损,即可考虑为消化道的淋巴滤泡增生症。

第十节 卡拉兹综合征(Chilaiditi's syndrome)

肝、膈结肠间位(卡拉兹综合征)为结肠位于肝脏和右侧膈肌之间的一种异常。尽管常为意外发现,无重要临床意义,但偶尔可以伴有非特异性的胃肠道症状。偶尔因肠扭转需要手术治疗。肠袢也可以插入肝脏与腹壁之间,类似于腹膜腔内的游离气体。

第二十七篇　阑尾疾病

第一章　炎症

第一节　阑尾周围脓肿误诊为右侧髂窝恶性肿瘤

患者，女，71岁。因发现胃息肉12天入院。门诊胃镜见胃多发性息肉，反流性食管炎。病理检查示胃底腺息肉。拟择日行胃息肉切除术。入院10天后仍有右下腹间歇性疼痛不适。

CT检查示：右髂窝巨大肿块影，约8.4cm×7.5cm×12cm，CT值25~36HU，肿物侵犯右髂窝脂肪、右盆壁软组织、右腰肌下部。右侧髂窝巨大肿块，性质？恶性肿瘤？脓肿并炎性肉芽肿？请结合临床进一步检查；临床查体未触及肿块，认为可能与患者腹壁脂肪较厚，包块位置较深，所以难以触及，但结合其发病过程，考虑急性阑尾炎并发脓肿可能，但恶性肿瘤尚不能排除，拟完善肠镜了解回盲部及阑尾窝情况，请普外科会诊。2日后查房，患者仍然发热，体温最高达38.7℃，仍右下腹痛，结肠镜检查未见明显异常，请普外科会诊，建议转科进一步剖腹探查及治疗。

一周后普通外科病房申请再做CT平扫，CT所见与前次相近，其诊断意见与前次相同，建议CT增强扫描或MR检查。

2日后手术所见：回盲部、右侧卵巢、输卵管、子宫等结构及周围组织相互粘连、包裹，形成脓肿壁，脓肿穿透后腹膜，形成腹膜后巨大脓肿，未见明显肿瘤迹象。用大盐水纱布垫保护于脓肿周围，打开脓肿前壁，有大量黄白色伴恶臭脓液自脓腔流出，脓液量约400ml。脓腔前壁各组织结构溃烂，相互粘连、融合，无法分离，无法辨别阑尾，未见肠瘘。脓腔后壁腹膜后组织未见输尿管、髂血管等结构受累。

误诊病例分析：回顾两次CT检查均可见病变周围网膜都受侵犯，但被忽略；第二次CT检查所见较一周前病变明显有所进展，但却未认识到急性炎症的表现才有如此表现，仍维持原来诊断意见，导致误诊。

第二节　急性化脓性阑尾炎病例

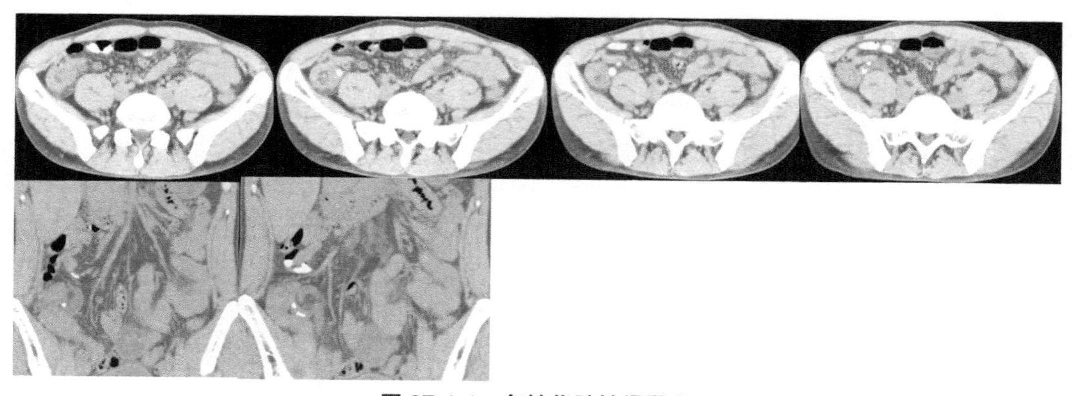

图27-1-1　急性化脓性阑尾炎

患者,男,43 岁。右下腹痛 12 小时入院。

手术所见:阑尾位于回盲部盆位,约长 7cm,肿胀化脓,与周围粘连,腹腔少许脓性渗液,回盲部周围肠管未见异常。病理检查:阑尾切除标本:阑尾一条,长 6cm,表面呈灰褐色,被覆脓苔,切面管腔直径 0.5-0~6cm,腔内含黄褐色样物,壁厚 0.3cm。病理诊断:阑尾切除标本:急性化脓性阑尾炎(图 27-1-1)。

第三节 急性阑尾炎 CT 检查的限度与诊断的问题

由于盲肠的移动度很大,阑尾的位置也各不相同。有位于肝脏下方的高位阑尾;降至小骨盆内的低位阑尾;盲肠后腹膜外阑尾(腰部阑尾);位于左髂窝内或腹腔中部的阑尾。由于判断这些位置的阑尾相当困难,故能导致假阴性的出现。阑尾位置多变给诊断带来一定困难,但阑尾与盲肠的位置关系相对固定,因此 CT 诊断中正确判断回盲瓣与盲肠的位置是寻找阑尾的关键。

应仔细观察整个盲肠,努力寻找回盲瓣等解剖结构标志。由于回肠末端的环形肌层在回盲瓣口处增厚,在 CT 影像上可表现为突向盲升结肠腔内的隆起,形态对称,并以回盲瓣口为中心等特征,有别于病理性肿块,有助于发现起源于盲肠后中部的阑尾。

腹腔内脂肪是 CT 扫描中体内的天然对比物质,阑尾周围常因有肠系膜脂肪包绕而能较清楚地显示其形状。因此对腹腔内脂肪量较少的小孩、体型较瘦的妇女和老人,阑尾常无法清晰显示,阑尾周围炎性改变的判断也存在困难。Lane 等(1999)分析了 5 例阑尾炎假阴性病人的 CT 影像,结果其中 4 例年轻女性病人均因几乎没有肠系膜脂肪存在,影响了阑尾及其周围炎性改变的观察而漏诊。

因此对儿童、妊娠期妇女和体型较瘦的病人疑为阑尾炎时,超声应是较理想的影像学检查方法。但超声常不易显示正常阑尾,且易将末端回肠误认为阑尾,将正常阑尾误认为急性阑尾炎。鉴别诊断中末端回肠与阑尾相反,不附着于盲肠底,也不呈盲端,常能见到蠕动,而且末端回肠常在横断面上显示为卵圆形,而阑尾则为圆形。

阑尾炎的初期,由于仅为黏膜层和黏膜下层的炎症,而阑尾并无明显的增粗,阑尾周围脂肪内未见条索影,此时应充分运用 MSCT 后处理技术,并密切随访观察。

此外,由于阑尾位于腹部位置较低,与生殖腺相邻,故 CT 检查时,应注意采用低剂量扫描方式,尤其在儿童及育龄妇女中应予以重视。

第四节 急性阑尾炎 CT 诊断中的几个问题

扫描层厚与阑尾的显示率有十分密切的关系。有作者报道使用 5 mm 层厚扫描,对于临床怀疑阑尾炎患者诊断敏感性可达到 100%。Wehman 等(2000)的研究中采用 5 mm 层厚扫描,94% 可确定异常阑尾,10 mm 层厚则为 69%。一组病例均以 10 mm 层厚扫描,阑尾总显示率 77.97%(46/59),扫描后重建薄层(1.25 mm)阑尾显示率 89.29%(25/28),扫描后未重建薄层阑尾显示率 67.74%(21/31)。

该组中有 13 例阑尾显示不清,分析有以下原因:①扫描层厚较厚,对阑尾的观察缺乏连续性,容易遗漏;②患者为小儿或成人体型消瘦者,右下腹脂肪组织少,缺乏对比,较难显示阑尾;③坏疽型阑尾炎穿孔阑尾区形成脓肿而导致阑尾无法显示。

阑尾炎但阑尾表现正常:一些作者报告 1 例单纯性阑尾炎和 1 例慢性阑尾炎发病轻,早期 MSCT 表现正常(阑尾直径 <7 mm,阑尾壁厚 <3 mm,无阑尾周围炎),导致漏诊。

远端阑尾炎:有作者报告 2 例蜂窝织炎性阑尾炎,由于炎症发生在阑尾的远端(即远端阑尾炎),而阑尾根部和近端以及盲肠下端缺乏阑尾炎 MSCT 阳性征象,造成假阴性诊断。因此,结合临床资料,及时复查,静脉增强检查观察阑尾壁强化征象,经过减薄多平面重建、曲面重建后观察阑尾全长,可以提高对其的诊断准确率。

阑尾炎但阑尾显示不清:年轻患者和瘦小患者

腹部脂肪少，肠管排列紧凑，偶尔阑尾位置异常，都可以造成阑尾显示不清。该组 1 例单纯性阑尾炎，因阑尾显示不清而漏诊。检查前口服 2.5% 的甘露醇溶液 1 000 ml 左右，静脉增强检查，扩大扫描范围，减薄重建等技术可以提高阑尾显示率，避免漏诊。

残端阑尾炎：阑尾切除术后，阑尾残端保留过长超过 1 cm，或者阑尾石残留等因素，都可以引起炎症复发，即残端阑尾炎。一些学者报告一组 4 例患者阑尾炎术后复查，由于术后阑尾的不显示，1 例腹痛患者简单认为化脓性包块。因此，结合阑尾切除病史，观察阑尾周围炎改变、邻近肠道改变和阑尾炎术后遗留金属夹高密度影等 MSCT 征象，可提示残端阑尾炎的可能。

类似阑尾炎的疾病：有作者报告 1 例阑尾黏液囊肿的 MSCT 征象类似阑尾炎影像学表现，造成误诊。由于临床手术方式不同，黏液囊肿需要防止囊肿破裂、黏液溢出，避免并发腹膜假黏液瘤的危险，因此术前明确诊断有重要临床价值。

无明显阑尾炎临床症状，MSCT 检查发现阑尾囊性扩张（直径 >13 mm），黏膜钙化的影像学征象，提示阑尾黏液囊肿。如果伴有慢性阑尾炎，鉴别诊断比较困难。

此外，克罗恩病、Meckel 憩室炎、右侧附件输卵管病变、盲肠炎和肠脂垂炎的 MSCT 影像学表现都与阑尾炎相似，需要结合临床病史进行鉴别诊断。

一些学者报告 2 例盲肠炎，1 例右侧卵巢来源的盆腔脓肿被误诊为阑尾炎伴周围脓肿。

类似阑尾的组织：右侧扩张的输尿管，回盲区增粗、扭曲的血管，回盲部未充盈而塌陷的肠管等组织结构与阑尾极其相似，容易误认为正常阑尾或炎性阑尾，而忽略真正阑尾的 MSCT 影像学改变，造成误诊。

有学者报告 1 例扩张的输尿管（右侧输尿管末端结石所致）被误认为积液的阑尾，另 1 例回盲部塌陷的回肠被误认为增粗的阑尾，造成假阳性阑尾炎诊断。扩大扫描范围，口服阳性对比剂，减薄重建等技术可以鉴别阑尾，同时排除其他右下腹痛的病因，可避免误诊。

薄层扫描或者扫描后薄层重建：另外，薄层扫描或者扫描后薄层重建对阑尾内部及周围的征象的显示有明显提高。对照该组以层厚、层距 10 mm 扫描，再以 1.25 mm 层厚、层距重建的 28 例，发现薄层重建前后对阑尾粪石的发现率由未重建的 14.3%（4/28）提高到 35.7%（10/28），阑尾积液从 7.1%（2/28）提高到 25%（7/28），阑尾周围炎从 35.7%（10/28）提高到 67.9%（19/28）。因此，薄层扫描或者扫描后薄层重建对阑尾的显示和分型诊断会有很大帮助。

第五节　急性阑尾炎诊断假阴性的分析

有文献报道，容易把一些正常的结构如回肠末端、回盲部的血管误认为阑尾，一组 60 例中，没有发生上述情况。但有 2 例假阴性，后进行回顾性分析，手术均为单纯性阑尾炎，分析原因，为患者体形较瘦小，腹部缺少脂肪衬托，未显示正常的阑尾，盲肠周围也无炎性渗出。所以对早期的急性阑尾炎，临床体症明显，但是阑尾未显示，或未见阑尾周围炎，也不能排除急性阑尾炎，需要随访观察，再根据临床表现是否进展，复查 CT 后再明确诊断。

第六节　有液体充盈的远端回肠酷似急性阑尾炎

一些作者报告，有液体充盈的远端回肠酷似急性阑尾炎，导致误诊。为避免此类情况再现，需要注意检查技术与规范。当怀疑病人有急性阑尾炎时，用口服阳性对比剂充盈末端回肠和小肠是十分必要的，它有助于辨认异常的阑尾，并与有液体充盈的小肠相鉴别。

如怀疑阑尾炎，则病人应于口服阳性对比剂 1~2h 后再行 CT 扫描。可常规在髂嵴水平先获得一幅 CT 图像来证实盲肠内已有口服阳性对比剂的存在。而后，就可静脉注射对比剂行 CT 扫描，开始对可疑的阑尾炎进行评估。

第七节 急性化脓性阑尾炎病例

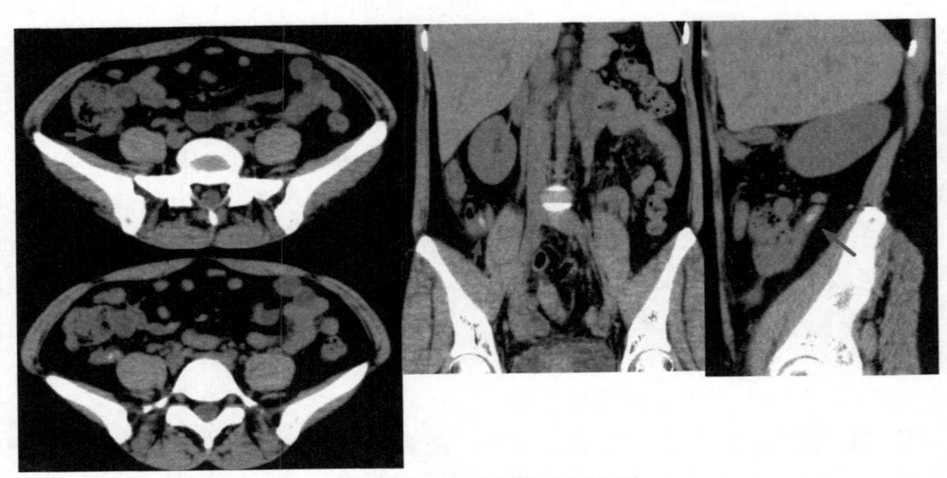

图 27-1-2 急性化脓性阑尾炎

患者，女，35 岁。反复右下腹痛 10 余天，再发 1 天入院。查体：腹肌紧张，右下腹压痛、反跳痛明显，未及包块。实验室检查：白细胞计数 $13.53 \times 10^9/L$，超敏 C 反应蛋白 61mg/L ↑，中性粒细胞 $6.74 \times 10^9/L$ ↑。

手术所见：阑尾位于回盲部后位，约 8 cm × 0.6cm，充血水肿化脓明显，与周围无粘连，腹腔少许脓性混浊渗液，回盲部周围肠管未见异常。病理检查：阑尾一条，长 8cm，表面充血，切面管腔直径 0.1cm~0.2cm，壁厚 0.1cm。病理诊断：急性化脓性阑尾炎（图 27-1-2）。

第八节 老人非急性阑尾炎

急性阑尾炎是外科的常见疾病，其典型临床表现是转移性右下腹痛、麦氏点压痛及反跳痛。实验室检查白细胞比例及中性白细胞计数增高，其预后的关键在于及时的诊断及治疗。

但在实际工作中，并非所有的阑尾炎表现都是典型和容易诊断的，不典型急性阑尾炎大约为 20%，而临床上被误诊为急性阑尾炎而行手术切除者约占 30%，尤其是年龄 >60 岁的老年人，由于其器官和功能退化，加之免疫功能低下，对疼痛的反应迟钝以及多种慢性疾病并存，所以，很多急性阑尾炎临床表现往往不典型。老年人就诊时，经常会病史叙述不清，如果经验不足，很难正确诊断，甚至误诊。

在急性阑尾炎的影像学检查中，以往 X 线平片和 B 超是常用的方法，但是平片只能提示右下腹局限性肠郁张，在诊断上无特异性；B 超易受阑尾解剖位置多变、肠道气体以及腹壁脂肪等干扰导致成像困难而漏诊。

近年来，随着 MSCT 的出现，其强大的三维重建后处理技术的应用，为急性阑尾炎的诊断提供了一种新的影像学检查手段，具有很大的优越性。

阑尾的位置：阑尾的位置变化较多，走行极不规则，常见有内位、内下位、内后位、下位、后位、外位及外后位。该组作者认为诊断的要点，阑尾的显示是关键。

由于阑尾的位置变化较多，走行也不很规律，CT 平扫有时难以发现阑尾的位置，有时容易将回肠末端或血管误认为阑尾，所以必须对原始扫描数据重建后进行三维重建，清楚、直观地显示阑尾的全貌、具体位置、周围是否有渗出以及脓肿形成等征象。该组中有 28 例清晰显示了阑尾位置，为外科手术方案的制定及手术入路的选择提供了较为可靠的依据。

阑尾粪石：在阑尾炎的诊断中，有学者认为阑尾粪石是诊断阑尾炎较为直接和可靠的征象，对诊断有重要意义。该组中，19 例阑尾腔内粪石，结合增粗、肿胀的阑尾及周围渗出，诊断十分明确。1 例临床表现为恶心、呕吐伴下腹疼痛，三维重建也未显示阑尾的形态，但是盲肠周围渗出明显，周围局部肠系膜增厚、粘连，内见结石影，提示阑尾坏疽穿孔伴局限性腹膜炎形成可能大。即刻手术，证实腹腔内黄色渗液 250 ml，阑尾全程坏疽化脓，体部穿孔。

憩室与增粗的阑尾：另有 1 例以右上腹痛就诊，上腹部 CT 诊断为升结肠憩室炎，由于抗炎治疗后未见明显好转，症状加重，后行下腹部 CT 检查，发现所谓的“憩室”实为增粗阑尾，粪石位于腔外，周围见大片低密度模糊渗出影，局部肠系膜粘连，提示阑尾坏疽穿孔伴腹膜炎形成，得到手术及病理证实。分析上腹部 CT 误诊原因为：忽略了回盲瓣及阑尾位置较高，阑尾根部腔内粪石嵌顿，而结肠憩室一般为囊袋样结构，与阑尾“长条”样形状有区别。普遍认为，在不能确诊的情况下，必须行上腹部联合扫描，多平面重建后显示病变的位置和特征。

阑尾脓肿：在实际工作中发现，有部分老年人由于延误了就诊时间，在 CT 检查时阑尾已经形成包块（该组有 2 例），CT 平扫后，发现回盲部软组织密度影，周围境界模糊，立即行 CT 增强扫描，肿块明显“环”状强化，提示阑尾脓肿，经抗炎治疗后，包块缩小，后经手术切除，病理证实。有 2 例为升结肠癌伴阑尾炎，临床表现为右下腹压痛，MSCT 扫描后见盲肠壁不规则增厚，浆膜面模糊，增强扫描不均匀强化，三维重建提示升结肠环状狭窄，考虑升结肠恶性肿瘤可能大，术后病理证实为中低分化腺癌。所以一般认为，CT 平扫及三维重建，显示技术是诊断的关键。

诊断思路：该组作者认为，在老年性不典型阑尾炎的诊断中，可以遵循以下思路：

首先，找到阑尾，如果阑尾增粗 >6 mm，管壁明显增厚、水肿，可以诊断为急性阑尾炎；如果伴腔内粪石及阑尾周围炎，基本可以确诊。单显示阑尾粪石，阑尾形态本身没有变化，不可诊断为急性阑尾炎，因为它也可出现在正常人群中。

其次，如果仅显示阑尾周围炎的征象而未发现异常阑尾，不可盲目诊断为急性阑尾炎，必须通过多平面重建多角度旋转，寻找水肿增粗的阑尾。

阑尾周围炎不具有诊断急性阑尾炎的特异性，它仅是诊断的一个重要标准，因为如盲肠憩室炎、末端回肠炎、盲肠炎、盆腔附件炎等也可出现阑尾周围炎，正确认识这些疾患的影像学表现，并结合临床相关资料，可以提高诊断的正确性，避免阑尾的误切除。

值得注意的是，盲肠憩室炎与阑尾炎因临床表现相似而鉴别诊断困难，但 CT 三维重建，可以清晰显示盲肠囊袋样腔外突起，腔内常见粪石，浆膜面模糊，周围见低密度渗出影。

再次，三维重建未找到阑尾，而显示阑尾周围蜂窝织炎、腔外气体及腔外粪石，应该高度提示阑尾穿孔的可能。由于老年人急性阑尾炎穿孔较多，这些征象有助于诊断。

最后，如果 CT 平扫发现有回盲部包块，必须进行增强扫描。

鉴别诊断：在相当一都分老年患者中，在就诊时已经形成了阑尾脓肿，但急性炎症的表现又不很明显，容易与回盲部肿瘤相混淆。

阑尾脓肿为软组织密度灶，内部密度不均匀，常夹杂液性低密度影，边缘见低密度渗出影，境界模糊，增强扫描中央脓腔无强化，脓壁明显环状强化。而回盲部肿瘤表现为局部肠壁不规则增厚，增强扫描肿块不均匀强化，常有浆膜面、邻近组织受侵及周围肠系膜根部淋巴结肿大，甚至出现肠梗阻征象。

老年人患结肠肿瘤的较多，在阑尾炎性包块与肿瘤之间进行鉴别，十分重要。

综上所述，老年人急性阑尾炎的临床表现和体征常不典型，诊断较难，易发生误诊或漏诊。MSCT 及其三维重建技术的应用，能够准确显示阑尾的位置、形态及周围的病理变化，为快捷、准确诊断提供了有力的技术支持，对老人不典型阑尾炎的诊断及鉴别诊断，具有较高的临床应用价值。

第九节　急性化脓性阑尾炎，局部坏疽，周围脓肿

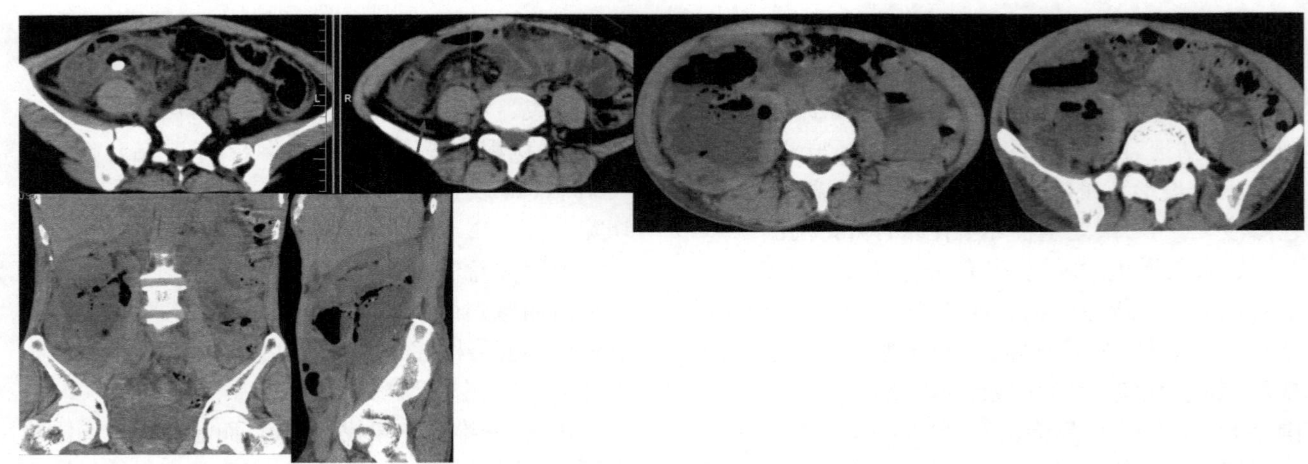

图 27-1-3　急性化脓性阑尾炎，局部坏疽，周围脓肿

患者，男，27 岁。反复右下腹闷痛 9 天入院。查体：右下腹部稍隆起，右下腹腹肌紧张伴压痛、反跳痛，未触及包块。实验室检查：血常规：WBC19.8 × 10^9/L，中性粒细胞 88.4%。

手术所见：阑尾位于回盲部后位，已坏疽穿孔形成巨大腹膜后脓肿，约 300ml，回盲部周围肠管未见异常。病理诊断：急性化脓性阑尾炎，局部坏疽，周围脓肿（图 27-1-3）。

第十节　急性阑尾炎与阑尾的位置

急性阑尾炎影像学分型与解剖学间隙关系：解剖学上阑尾为一蚓状突起，其根部大多位于盲肠后内侧壁，远端变异较大，急性阑尾炎根据其阑尾远端位置可分为回肠前型、回肠后型、回肠下型、盲肠前型、盲肠后型、盲肠下型以及盲肠外型，这种分型方法是根据其阑尾发生与盲肠及末端回肠的关系所分类的，是临床分类常用的方法。随着 MSCT 各向同性技术的完善，通过 3D 工作站可完全对此进行解剖学分型，但有作者通过 CT 图像的分析，认为根据其位置是腹膜腔还是腹膜后以及其指向性，分为腹膜腔型、腹膜后型及盆腔型更有实用意义。

腹膜腔型阑尾炎：腹膜腔型阑尾炎根据其走向可分内前位、上位及外位，由于阑尾完全走行于腹膜腔内，其炎症渗出之液体顺自然腔隙积于相应低点或窦腔位置，由于小肠系膜根部从左上斜向右下，所以右结肠下间隙形成一个相对封闭的三角形，其最低点刚好位于右肠系膜窦的位置，腹腔内前位型阑尾炎渗液可在右下邻近肠系膜窦聚集。

当阑尾炎渗液较少时，可仅表现为右肠系膜窦积液；但当渗液较多时，液体则通过右结肠下间隙越过肠系膜窦流入盆腔间隙。

腹膜腔外位型阑尾炎渗液一组 4 例，3 例可见右结肠旁沟积液，右结肠旁沟是升结肠与右侧腹壁腹膜间形成的腹膜反折沟，向上连接右肝上、下间隙，向下连接右髂窝，是一个相对比较宽大的间隙，腹膜腔外型阑尾炎渗液根据液体力学原理最容易沉积于此，该组病例也得到了证实。由于腹腔和盆腔的连通关系，腹腔型阑尾炎渗液较多时可沿腹腔间隙向盆腔渗漏，这也是该组资料统计显示腹腔型阑尾炎伴有盆腔渗液较多的原因。

腹膜后型阑尾炎：本型定义为腹膜内位阑尾走行在腹膜后或变异的腹膜外位阑尾，由于升结肠是腹膜间位器官，其后部肠壁位于腹膜后肾旁前间隙内，该间隙其实是相对比较疏松的脂肪组织，肾旁后间隙是指肾后筋膜和圆锥侧筋膜后方与腹横筋膜之间的区域，内无脏器，主要含较多脂肪组织。

由于腹膜后间隙空间较小，相对固定，且由于壁层腹膜与脏层腹膜的双重阻隔作用，腹膜后型阑尾炎症渗液多聚集于肾旁前间隙，但是炎症较明显，渗液较多时，仍可通过肾旁后间隙与盆腔侧间隙相通，特别是穿孔性阑尾炎。

穿孔性阑尾炎多由急性单纯性阑尾炎恶化或坏疽性阑尾炎发展而来，阑尾管壁坏死或部分坏死，阑尾腔内积脓，压力升高，阑尾血液循环障碍。穿孔部位多在阑尾根部和近端。阑尾穿孔后，阑尾内容物及气体可进入腹腔或腹膜后间隙引起广泛性腹膜炎或脓肿，正常的解剖间隙及筋膜结构破坏，炎症渗液或脓液的引流聚集更不规则。

该组病例未将穿孔性阑尾炎纳入统计范围，因为一旦阑尾穿孔，其特定的渗液范围或者聚集间隙便没有任何意义。而升结肠旁的右结肠旁沟后方与腹膜后间隙紧邻，炎症的渗液可通过后腹膜在结肠旁沟聚集，该组统计显示结肠旁沟积液在腹膜后阑尾与腹腔阑尾间无统计学意义的主要原因可能在此。

盆腔型阑尾炎：盆腔型阑尾通常阑尾位置相对较低且指向性向下，由于液体的重力关系通常流向盆腔间隙，且由于小肠系膜根部从左上斜向右下，一定程度上阻碍了盆腔间隙的液体向上流入右侧肠系膜窦间隙。

急性阑尾炎积液男性患者通常滞留在直肠膀胱间隙或右直肠旁间隙，女性则为子宫直肠陷凹，相对而言，女性的盆腔积液考虑相关疾病较多，特别是阑尾周围脓肿形成时需与妇科疾病及部分肠道肿瘤性病变鉴别。

由于该组资料未将阑尾脓肿纳入研究范围，仅统计阑尾渗液与盆腹腔间隙的关系，有些盆腔型阑尾炎本身阑尾增粗并不明显，此时就会面临着盆腔积液来源的鉴别的问题，相对而言，盆腔炎会有妇科相关疾病的病史，且 CT 能确定大部分盆腔病变，再结合临床相关病史及超声检查不难鉴别。

通过以上分析可以看出，急性非穿孔性阑尾炎伴渗出患者，根据阑尾炎解剖位置其渗液有一定的规律，MSCT 能对其渗液部位做出准确的判断，可给术前提供有价值的指导。

第二章　阑尾结石

阑尾石与阑尾炎

阑尾区出现粪石、钙化高密度影为阑尾石征象阳性。阑尾石短径≥ 5 mm，位于阑尾近端为梗阻性阑尾石征象，阑尾石位于阑尾腔外附近为腔外阑尾石征象。

病理学统计显示 70% 的阑尾炎因梗阻引起，而阑尾石是最常见的梗阻原因，发生率高达 43 %。阑尾石一旦在阑尾腔内形成，虽然不一定会引起梗阻并诱发阑尾炎，但是当阑尾石偶然嵌顿在阑尾腔的狭窄部分，或阑尾有一时性的痉挛时，梗阻即可发生，容易诱发炎症。

一组 MSCT 影像学资料显示：阑尾石征象诊断阑尾炎的准确性和敏感性不高，分别为 54.9%、37.9%，但特异性较高，为 81.8%，在阑尾炎和非阑尾炎患者中出现的概率无显著差异性，不能鉴别阑尾炎病理分型（ $P>0.05$ ）。因此，不能仅凭阑尾石征象诊断阑尾炎，需结合临床病史和其他阑尾炎征象综合考虑。

梗阻性阑尾石征象多见于炎性阑尾（ $P<0.05$ ），若伴有阑尾壁增厚（ ≥ 3 mm ），壁明显增强，阑尾周围炎等征象，可以明确诊断阑尾炎。由于患者从发病到 CT 检查相距时间不等，因此梗阻性阑尾石征象可以出现在阑尾炎不同病理过程中，无鉴别价值（ $P>0.05$ ）坏疽性阑尾炎患者因阑尾壁坏死穿孔，阑尾石可游离到阑尾腔外附近，即腔外阑尾石征象，提示穿孔性阑尾炎。若同时观察到阑尾壁缺损、阑尾周围蜂窝织炎、腔外气体、脓肿包块等阑尾炎征象，诊断坏疽性阑尾炎特异性高达 100%（ $P<0.05$ ）。因此，梗阻性阑尾石征象有助于阑尾炎的诊断，腔外阑尾石征象诊断坏疽性阑尾炎存在较高的特异性价值。

有学者报道腔外阑尾石也见于蜂窝织炎性阑尾炎和非阑尾炎患者。该组作者认为可能与病例收集，病理观察经验以及将阑尾附近钙化淋巴结影像误认为腔外阑尾石等因素有关。而且，蜂窝织炎性阑尾炎与坏疽性阑尾炎为连续的病理过程，缺乏明确的分界，有时病理分型存在困难，因此腔外阑尾石征象诊断穿孔性阑尾炎更具有临床意义。

该组回顾分析的腹部影像采集层厚为 7.0mm，仅 44 例减薄至 2 mm 重建观察，对阑尾石直径测量存在一定的影响。此外，MSCT 诊断阑尾炎必须排除引起右下腹痛其他疾病（阑尾囊肿、盲肠炎、盲肠憩室炎、肠结核、克罗恩病等）的可能，多平面重建和曲面重建技术对鉴别诊断具有一定的价值。

第三章　阑尾囊性病变

第一节　阑尾黏液囊肿

阑尾黏液囊肿是阑尾呈囊状扩张并腔内有黏液积聚的一类少见病，在阑尾切除术中的发现率为0.07%~0.3%，文献报道术前误诊率达94.6%。

现大多数学者认为其病理基础为先天异常或后天炎症致阑尾根部阻塞，远端黏膜不断分泌黏液，分泌的黏液受阻潴留。随着潴留液的增多，阑尾腔内压力增高，致阑尾壁黏膜细胞变扁，分泌功能减弱，且最终丧失分泌功能，形成阑尾黏液囊肿。引起梗阻最常见的原因是阑尾炎症。也有认为本病是阑尾的新生肿物。个别病例患者癌胚抗原轻度升高，是否具有潜在的恶变可能，需进一步扩大样本来观察。

临床表现：阑尾黏液囊肿以女性多见，主要症状和体征有右下腹痛和腹部肿块。表现为慢性非转移性右下腹疼痛或急性腹痛以及右下腹肿块。其并发症主要有阑尾黏液囊肿破溃，脱落的上皮细胞种植于腹腔内形成腹膜假性黏液瘤；梗阻导致肠套叠；肠扭转导致肠梗阻等。偶尔有病例以泌尿系感染症状而就诊并形成膀胱瘘。

X线检查：X线腹部平片可见局部囊壁弧形、曲线状或点状钙化，由于阑尾壁黏液慢性炎症刺激引起营养不良所致。钡灌肠造影典型征象为阑尾不显影，盲肠内侧壁和/或回肠末端外侧壁见弧形压迹，回肠末端与盲肠形态固定、夹角增大。

超声：超声表现为成分复杂但以囊性成分为主的肿块。回声的强弱依赖于囊内的黏液，但通常透声良好。阑尾黏液囊肿具有长管状外形，易误诊为输卵管积水，追踪肿块起源于盲肠有助于两者鉴别。

CT：阑尾增大，为右侧髂窝区多囊性或索条状病变，或右下腹盲肠周围出现圆形、椭圆形或管状囊性低密度或软组织密度肿块，密度均匀，边缘光滑，偶尔肿块直径最大可达26 cm，为巨大囊肿；一般囊壁薄规则，且均匀光滑，厚度1~3 mm不等，边界清楚，周围无炎症，低密度且密度接近于水；囊壁可有弧线状钙化；有的囊壁较厚且不规则，可伴有壁结节。增强后囊壁可轻度强化或无强化。肿块周围肠系膜脂肪清晰，密度无增高；增强扫描大部分肿块无强化，少部分囊壁有轻度环状强化，肿块越大强化越不明显；盲肠腔可受压、变形，但盲肠壁无水肿增厚。对比剂充分充盈肠管有助于将黏液囊肿与未充盈的肠管区分开来。阑尾黏液囊肿可并发肠套叠、肠扭转等。

误诊病例简介：有作者回顾性分析个别患者钡灌肠及CT表现，主要是因为病变较大（标本上其大小为17cm×5cm×4.5cm），且表现为外压改变，故考虑回盲部占位性病变，间质瘤来源可能性大，导致误诊。

鉴别诊断：诊断阑尾黏液囊肿需与下述疾病鉴别。阑尾周围脓肿：阑尾周围脓肿一般临床症状典型，脓肿壁较厚，边缘轮廓欠清晰，与周围组织粘连明显，周围肠系膜脂肪呈炎性浸润改变，密度增高或消失。阑尾黏液性囊腺癌：阑尾黏液性囊腺癌常常密度不均匀，内有大小不等囊性低密度区，边缘不规则，增强扫描有不均匀强化，有时可见壁结节，周围脂肪层模糊，可推压或侵犯盲肠，使肠壁增厚、僵硬。阑尾淋巴瘤：阑尾淋巴瘤为密度均匀的软组织密度肿块，无低密度区或钙化。增强扫描呈轻度强化，伴肠系膜及腹膜后淋巴结肿大。肠系膜囊肿及卵巢囊肿：根据病变位置，阑尾黏液囊肿位于盲肠与回肠末端之间，盲肠被推向外上方，回肠被推向内下方；而肠系膜囊肿及卵巢囊肿则无盲肠受压移位现象。

第二节 阑尾黏液囊肿与回盲部黏膜下黏液囊肿病例

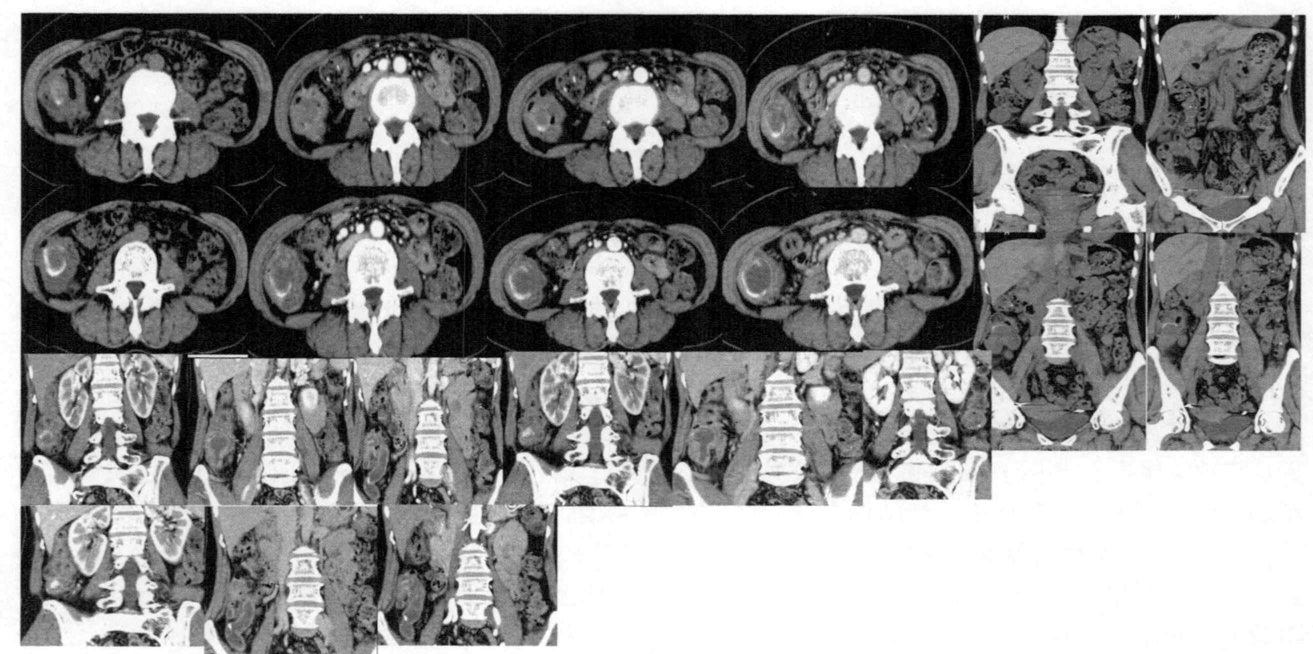

图 27-3-1 阑尾黏液囊肿与回盲部黏膜下黏液囊肿

患者,女, 57 岁。腹痛 2 个月余入院。1 个月前在外院住院期间行肠镜检查示回盲部肿物。病理检查:回盲部切除标本:回盲部切除标本一具,结肠长 21.5cm,结肠切缘直径 2.5cm;回肠长 10cm,回肠切缘直径 2cm;近回盲部见一结节,大小约 4cm × 3.5cm × 2cm,切面见一囊腔,内含胶冻样物;其余肠黏膜皱襞明显,未见明显异常,于肠周脂肪组织检出淋巴结样物二十余枚,直径 0.3~1cm。阑尾长 3cm,直径 1cm,内含胶冻样黏液,与肠壁囊肿相通。病理诊断:回盲部黏膜下黏液囊肿,大小约 4cm × 3.5cm × 2cm,由纤维组织包裹,未见内衬上皮,与阑尾黏液囊肿相通。自检肠系膜淋巴结 21 枚,均呈反应性增生,局部钙化。注:阑尾黏液囊肿与相邻肠壁黏膜下黏液囊肿相通,考虑阑尾黏液囊肿为原发性病变,其内容物侵入相邻肠壁致回盲部黏膜下黏液囊肿形成(图 27-3-1)。

第三节 阑尾黏液性囊腺瘤病例

患者,男,68 岁。发现回盲部黏膜下隆起 1 个月余入院。患者缘于 1 个月前于我院门诊体检行肠镜检查示距回盲部近阑尾窝见一 2.0cm 球形黏膜下隆起,质硬。回盲部黏膜活检标本示送检浅表黏膜,呈黏膜慢性炎伴间质水肿。今门诊拟“结肠肿物”收住入院。手术所见:肿瘤位于回盲部阑尾根部,似阑尾来源,局限于肌层,约 2cm × 3cm × 2cm,质中,边界尚清,活动度良好,与周围组织无粘连,距回盲瓣约 3cm。肠周及系膜根部未及明显肿大淋巴结。

病理检查:回盲部肿瘤切除标本:回盲部及附着的阑尾一段,回盲部大小 4.5cm × 3.5cm × 2cm,阑尾长 6.5cm,阑尾与回盲部交界处膨大,直径 3cm,切开阑尾,可见腔内灰白色胶冻样物,黏膜消失,壁厚 0.1cm。回盲部肿瘤切除标本病理诊断为阑尾黏液性囊腺瘤(图 27-3-2)。

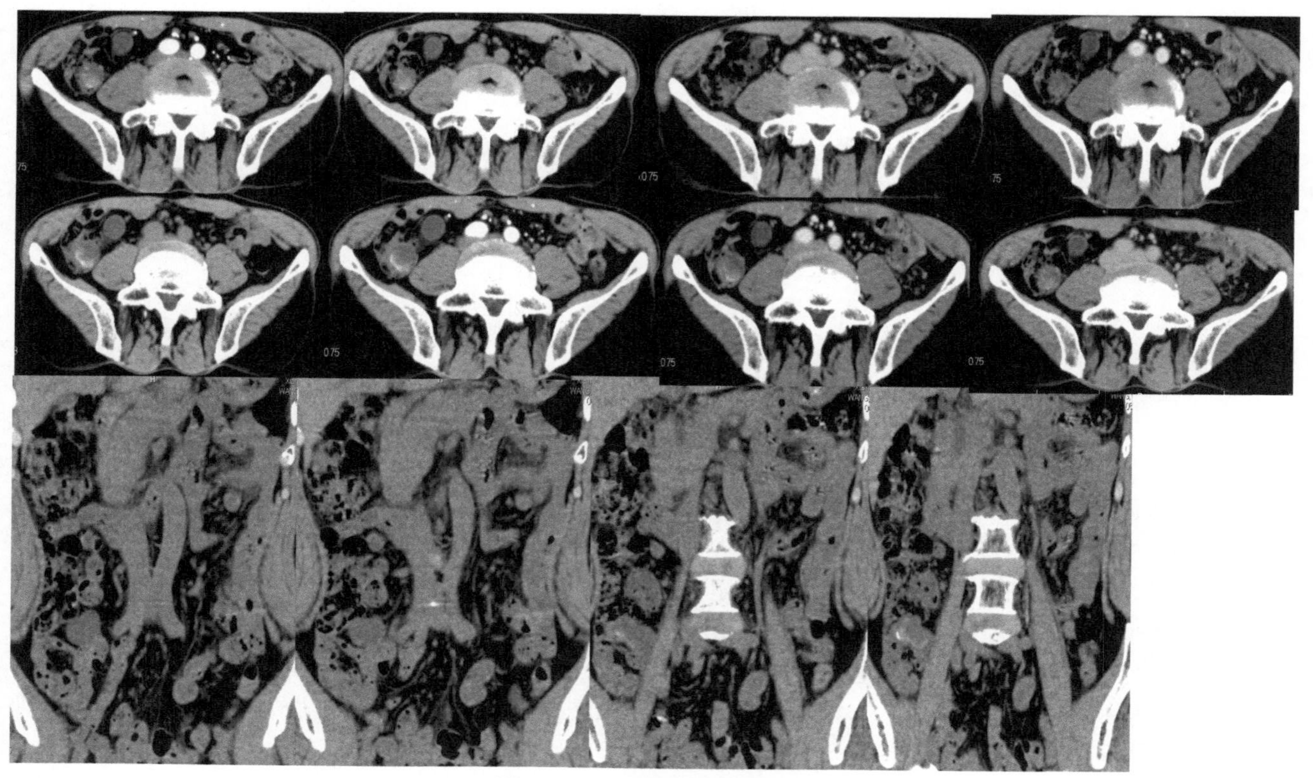

图 27-3-2　阑尾黏液性囊腺瘤

第四章 阑尾肿瘤

第一节 原发性阑尾肿瘤

原发性阑尾肿瘤罕见，仅占胃肠道肿瘤的0.4%。30%~50%的患者与急、慢性阑尾炎临床表现相似，术前诊断困难，误诊率高。不少病例以阑尾炎作手术或病理检查才诊断为阑尾肿瘤，此类患者大多需进行二次手术，因此原发性阑尾肿瘤的术前诊断具有重要的临床意义。

1. 影像学研究　原发性阑尾肿瘤多为上皮性起源，类癌最为常见，其次为囊性黏液肿瘤，而后者是影像检查中最常见到的肿瘤类型。CT检查是术前诊断原发性阑尾肿瘤的有效方法之一，一组术前CT诊断准确率为82.6%，低于文献报道(90%以上)，主要原因为该组病例中包含了3例类癌，仅表现为阑尾增粗而无肿块。阑尾发生炎症时阑尾肿大，但其最大径很少超过15 mm，使用15 mm作为阈值对可能发生的肿瘤进行评价，具有较高的敏感性，该组病例中7例肿大阑尾最大径>15 mm，其中4例伴右下腹部囊性或实性肿块，3例无明显肿块；其余病例中阑尾因肿瘤较大或侵犯而显示不清。

囊性肿瘤：该组病例中16例为囊性肿瘤，包括黏液囊腺瘤9例及黏液囊腺癌7例，两者在组织学上均表现为阑尾腔近端闭塞，黏膜上皮分泌黏液，使扩张的阑尾内充满黏蛋白；黏液囊腺瘤可恶变为阑尾囊腺癌；黏液囊腺癌为高分化肿瘤，有时易诊断为良性肿瘤。

该组中有2例术中诊断为阑尾黏液腺瘤，免疫组织化学等确诊为高分化黏液囊腺癌。

阑尾黏液腺瘤CT表现为右下腹囊性肿块影，壁厚，可有曲线状或斑片状壁钙化，增强后瘤体壁环形强化，内为水样低密度，有线样间隔，间隔可强化。

黏液性腺癌表现为囊性肿块，外形不规则，呈分叶状，囊壁不规则增厚，部分可见乳头状明显强化结节，周边组织浸润等改变，部分患者临床上有癌胚抗原等肿瘤指标不同程度升高；黏液性肿瘤因黏膜上皮分泌旺盛易穿破浆膜形成腹膜假性黏液瘤，该组病例中有5例发生腹腔假性黏液瘤，其中4例为黏液性腺癌，1例为黏液性腺瘤，CT表现为大量腹腔积液，肝脾边缘扇贝样或结节状压迹和腹腔不规则囊实性肿块，其CT值较实质性肿块低。

对阑尾良性黏液肿瘤手术治疗原则是完整切除包括肿瘤在内的阑尾及其系膜，恶性者及时行右半结肠切除术，术中防止黏液外溢致腹腔种植。如果囊肿破裂，必须反复冲洗腹腔和脏器表面黏附的胶冻样物，防止形成腹腔假性黏液瘤。该组病例中4例行单纯阑尾切除3~6个月后二次手术行右半结肠切除术。

实性肿瘤：该组病例中实性肿瘤为结肠型腺癌(3例)、阑尾平滑肌瘤(1例)。3例结肠型腺癌发生于阑尾根部，呈浸润性增长，向回盲部及结肠浸润而形成肿块，临床上出现类似右半结肠癌的表现。CT增强扫描表现为紧邻回盲部不规则软组织肿块，多为不均匀性轻度强化，回盲部可见不同程度受压改变，阑尾闭塞，阑尾腔扩张，但未见囊肿形成；2例钡剂灌肠后行CT扫描，阑尾闭塞口可见“箭头征”。因阑尾腺癌具有右半结肠癌的特点，其生物学行为与结肠癌相近，呈浸润性生长，易淋巴转移，故临床治疗以右半结肠切除术最适合，若有肠系膜淋巴结肿大，必须行淋巴结清扫，术后辅以化疗提高生存率。该组病例中仅1例术前诊断恶性肿瘤行右半结肠切除术。

平滑肌瘤发生在阑尾者罕有报道。肿瘤发生于肌层，肿瘤界清、无包膜，表面光滑，切面灰白、质韧，呈编织状或旋涡状，偶可见钙化、透明变性等，且预后良好。该组仅发现 1 例平滑肌瘤，CT 主要表现为类圆形均质软组织肿块，增强后轻度均质强化，邻近组织无明显改变；该患者行单纯阑尾切除术，预后良好。有文献报道，平滑肌瘤如瘤体过大，向周围浸润，肿块呈分叶形，不均匀性强化多考虑为平滑肌肉瘤。

阑尾肿大：正常阑尾最大管径约为 8~10 mm，当阑尾发生炎症或肿瘤时，阑尾管壁充血水肿致管壁增厚，肿瘤阻塞可致阑尾扩张、管径增粗。该组病例中表现为阑尾肿大者 7 例，其中 4 例伴有右下腹肿块，其余 3 例患者仅表现为阑尾肿大而无右下腹肿块，术后病理证实为类癌。

类癌源于表皮下的神经内分泌细胞，具有恶变倾向，较少转移，多发生在消化道，约 19% 发生于阑尾，阑尾类癌约占所有阑尾肿瘤的 50%~60%，因其缺乏典型临床表现，多在阑尾炎手术发现，术前难以诊断，误诊率极高。其发病率女性高于男性，一般单发，有研究表明肿瘤直径多 <1 cm，>2 cm 者罕见，因肿瘤体积小，CT 发现率极低，尽管类癌是阑尾发病最多的肿瘤，但依靠影像学检查可以证实的不足 10%。有文献报道，薄层螺旋 CT 扫描可以提高类癌检出率；阑尾类癌直径 <1 cm 则近乎良性表现，可行单纯阑尾切除术，预后良好；直径 >2 cm 或肿瘤位于阑尾基部，则预后欠佳，需行回盲部切除甚至右半结肠切除；对肿瘤直径在 1~2 cm 之间患者的处理争议较大，原则上应行根治性切除，尤其肿瘤位于近端或累及系膜者。

2. 鉴别诊断　黏液囊肿：黏液囊肿、黏液囊腺瘤与黏液囊腺癌病理学上相近，CT 上均表现为囊性肿块，均可在腹腔内形成腹腔假性黏液瘤；黏液囊肿，其大小一般较小，阑尾壁较薄，光滑，内无分隔；黏液囊腺瘤内部多不均匀，有分隔，囊壁增厚钙化，黏液囊腺癌囊壁不规则，可见明显强化壁结节。

阑尾脓肿：黏液囊腺癌应与阑尾脓肿区分开，后者临床表现为高热、白细胞明显增高等症状，CT 上表现为阑尾区混杂密度肿块，增强扫描多呈明显环形强化，阑尾周围渗出明显。该组病例中 1 例术前误诊为阑尾脓肿，术后病理证实为黏液囊腺癌。阑尾黏液腺癌癌胚抗原等肿瘤指标增高有助于鉴别。

回盲部结肠癌：回盲部结肠癌临床触诊右下腹可扪及肿块，活动度差，多有便血或脓血便症状，CT 上多表现为结肠内外的肿块，管壁局限性不规则增厚，与阑尾结肠型腺癌鉴别困难；病变范围较广、管壁僵硬多考虑结肠癌，如出现“箭头征”则有助于阑尾结肠型腺癌的诊断。

右侧卵巢囊性肿瘤：此外，女性患者阑尾囊性肿瘤需与右侧卵巢囊性肿瘤鉴别，后者位置偏下，多无回盲部压迫症状，而子宫受压向左移位明显。

综上，CT 对发现阑尾肿瘤较为敏感，当发现阑尾囊状扩张，最大管径超过 15 mm 以及右下腹肿块则可做出肿瘤判断，术前 CT 检查可以提供较多有价值的诊断信息，为临床制定手术方案提供重要依据。

第二节　阑尾黏液性囊腺瘤病例

详见 本书 本卷 本篇 第三章 第三节　阑尾黏液性囊腺瘤病例。

第三节　误诊病例简介：阑尾周围脓肿与盆腔高代谢肿块

患者，男，18 岁。缘于 10 天前无明显诱因出现间断发热，最高达 37.5℃，无规律性，伴腹痛、颈部皮疹，就诊当地卫生院，查血常规示：“白细胞 14.4×10^9/L，中性粒细胞 11.1×10^9/L，余正常”，给予抗炎等处理（具体措施不详）后症状好转，入院 2 天前复查血常规示：“白细胞 20.95×10^9/L，中性粒细胞 16.59×10^9/L，余正常”；无畏冷、发热，无腹胀、腹痛、腹泻，无咳嗽、咳痰、咯血等不适，今为进一步诊治，门诊以“白细胞升高原因待查”收入我院肿瘤科，拟诊：盆腔肿物性质待查；白细胞增多症。入院后检查：血沉 29.0mm/h。电解质肾功能、大便常规、尿常规、血常规、肿瘤标记物：大致正常。骨髓涂片示：正常骨髓象。结肠镜及病理诊断：乙状结肠黏膜活检标本：黏膜慢性炎。外院 PET/CT 检查：右下腹高代谢肿块，肿瘤待排。

手术所见：建立人工气腹，探查见回盲部粘连形成约

6cm×4cm不规则阑尾周围脓肿,并与乙状结肠粘连,余肠管及大网膜未见异常。盆腔少量积液,吸引器吸尽送检以查找肿瘤细胞。明确无明显出血,再次仔细探查明确腹腔内无其他异常后,关闭取出穿刺套管,切口予丝线缝合。出院后,定期复查腹部包块,3个月后入院行阑尾切除术(图27-4-1)。

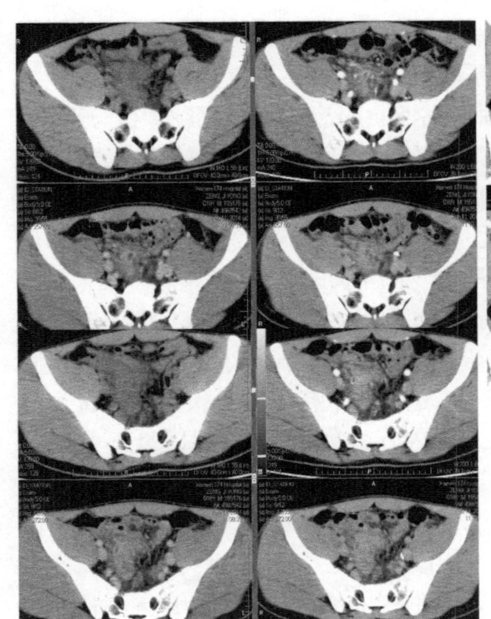

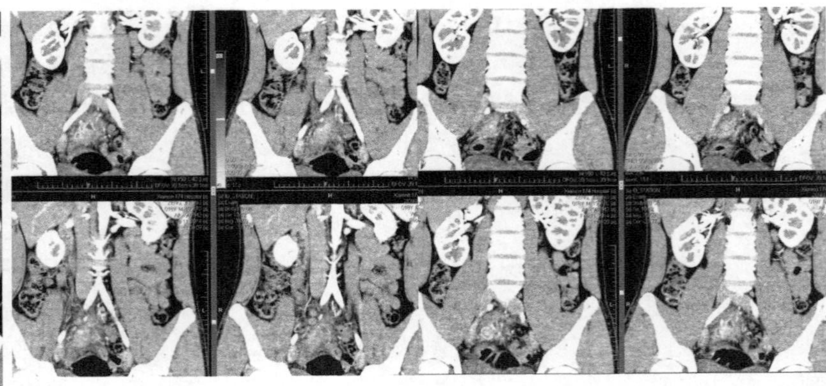

图27-4-1 阑尾周围脓肿与盆腔高代谢肿块

第四节 阑尾类癌

病理学:70%阑尾类癌位于阑尾末端。病灶直径多<1cm,常常是在阑尾切除后作病检时意外发现;直径>2 cm的病灶罕见。镜下,其表现类似空回肠类癌,但通常不穿透阑尾壁、不浸润阑尾系膜。

临床表现:多数阑尾类癌是肠嗜铬细胞类癌;也有少数为肠内分泌细胞类癌。多数阑尾类癌表现为良性临床病程,不发生转移。阑尾类癌临床表现无特殊。

影像学研究:由于阑尾类癌常较小、局限在阑尾内且临床病程多为良性,所以其影像特征报道很少。最初的表现多是肿瘤阻塞阑尾腔所致的阑尾炎性改变,此时常用影像学检查手段如CT、MRI、超声常难发现肿瘤。肠道钡剂造影也仅显示阑尾不显影而无特异性。

在阑尾类癌,通常位于阑尾末梢且体积较小,有时横断面扫描见管壁弥漫性增厚,位于阑尾根部引起梗阻症状的阑尾类癌在CT或超声检查时呈阑尾炎表现,当其钙化或体积较大时似阑尾结石,黏液囊肿较少见。肿瘤长大后可表现为阑尾内的局灶性软组织肿块或弥漫性环周型肠壁增厚,前者在钡剂造影及CT上均可查见,而后者在断面影像上更易发现。罕见情况下,阑尾类癌也可像空回肠类癌那样侵袭性生长并出现淋巴结和肝脏转移。同样,若发生转移则CT、MRI是很好的检查办法。

另外,阑尾类癌有一变异类型——杯状细胞类癌,其表现更类似于腺癌,有着侵袭性生长的潜能,此种情况与腺癌在影像上极难鉴别。

第五章　阑尾的活体形态学

关于阑尾的发育变异

胚胎学发育：有作者将阑尾的胚胎学发育分为四个阶段：①妊娠 3~4 月，是一个锥形下部盲肠节段末端狭窄；②新生儿的阑尾，末端盲肠更为狭窄，从第 3 个月到足月期，由盲肠进入一个相当粗大的阑尾；③在盲肠与阑尾连接处，出现一个突然的过渡区域，阑尾与盲肠的最关连的部位，呈现一致性狭窄，可见于幼儿；④成人阑尾，位于左后盲肠壁，在三条结肠带的连接处，该处它并于阑尾的纵肌层，通常位于回盲瓣以下 2.5~3.5cm。

在人体的发育过程中，盲肠的位置随年龄增长而不断下降，一般小儿盲肠的位置高于成人。少数人，由于胚胎发育过程中肠旋转异常，盲肠和阑尾可有不同的位置，如盲肠下降不全，阑尾可位于肝下或胆囊下方，称高位阑尾；如盲肠下端位于或低于骨盆缘，阑尾可位于盆腔内，称低位阑尾。患有移动性盲肠者，其阑尾可位于中腹及左下腹部。

在中年以后，阑尾的腔可以部分或完全闭塞。阑尾最常见的发育变异，出现在发育的第一阶段和第三阶段，其他阶段也可见发育变异。也有作者认为，阑尾发育成为成人型，不依赖于中肠的旋转和固定。

阑尾动脉：主要的阑尾动脉走行向阑尾尖，首先靠近其后，位于阑尾系膜的游离缘。动脉的末梢实际上位于阑尾壁内，在阑尾炎时可出现栓塞，导致阑尾末端部分坏疽或坏死。阑尾动脉一般起于回结肠动脉，有的起于回结肠动脉的盲肠动脉的前支或后支。阑尾动脉为一终末动脉，它与盲肠血管供应没有交通，因此，阑尾一旦血液供应发生障碍，阑尾即出现坏死。阑尾动脉起于回结肠动脉回肠支者约占 46%，起于回结肠动脉盲肠后支者约占 24%，起于回结肠动脉干者约占 18%，起于回结肠动脉盲肠干者约占 12%。

阑尾动脉为一支者约占 92%，二支者占 8%。当阑尾动脉为双支时，分布于阑尾近侧的一支多数仅供养邻近的盲肠和阑尾根部，最大范围不超过阑尾近侧的 1/3 段。远侧支是供应阑尾的主要动脉。阑尾动脉起点至阑尾尖部，平均长约 56mm，伴行静脉长约 52mm。阑尾动脉外径为 1.5mm，阑尾静脉外径约为 1.7mm。阑尾动脉通常为终末血管。有作者报告 100 例标本阑尾动脉，发现单阑尾动脉有 79 例，其余 21 例为双阑尾动脉，双支起源于不同动脉支者有 16 例，起于同一动脉支者有 5 例。121 支阑尾动脉的起点可分为 6 型：回结肠动脉回肠支，占 33%；回结肠动脉干，18%；回结肠动脉盲肠后支，21%；回结肠动脉盲肠干，12%；回结肠动脉盲肠前支，11%；回结肠动脉结肠支，5%。

有作者报告 1 例阑尾动脉有 5 支，其中 1 支起源于回结肠动脉的结肠支，其余 4 支起源于回结肠动脉干与阑尾支形成的动脉弓上。阑尾动脉若为两支，自近侧起始的一支分布至阑尾尖端，而发出部位较低的一支则分布至阑尾根部或其近侧段。然而供应阑尾的动脉的变异可以很大，常见许多副动脉，80% 的人可有 2 支或更多支动脉供应。

阑尾在腹腔内的位置：阑尾基底与盲肠的相对关系虽固定不变，但因盲肠本身在体内的位置可有变异，阑尾系膜的宽窄又有较大的差别，且阑尾之长短又不甚一致，故阑尾在腹腔内的实际位置和活动范围也就有很大的变异。阑尾在腹腔内的位置，主要取决于盲肠的位置。盲肠一般位于右侧髂窝内，故阑尾的基底部通常在麦（McBurney）氏点上，即髂前上棘与脐部连线的外 1/3 处，但实际上阑尾基底的位置也可略有高低，或稍偏左右。

如盲肠本身位置不正常，则阑尾的位置可随之而有如下四类变异：

盲肠未降：盲肠在腹腔右侧较高的位置，有时甚至在肝的下部，此时阑尾亦居于高位，导致阑尾炎之症状颇似于胆囊炎。

活动盲肠：盲肠系膜过长，能在腹腔内自由活动，阑尾亦可随之移动而远离右下腹。

内脏反位：因胚胎转位的障碍，全身内脏均在相反的位置,盲肠和阑尾亦在左下腹。

盲肠左旋:此与内脏反位不同,乃胚胎发育时中肠未能回转,致盲肠和升结肠仍在腹腔左侧,降结肠也在左侧,此时阑尾也可远离右下腹。

阑尾位于盲肠的内下侧,短的仅数厘米长,个别长者可达20cm左右,其位置也可有较多的变异。

有作者报告,阑尾为盲肠后位者约占28%,盆位约占26%,盲肠下位占22%,回肠后位占22%,回肠前位占2%。盲肠的位置变化,影响着阑尾异位,成人盲肠变异较小,而小儿常有接近于肝下方的高位盲肠,甚至多达21%。

真正的阑尾缺如,非常罕见,但当阑尾为腹膜外位时,阑尾在盲肠后完全为腹膜壁层所掩盖时,要切开腹膜才能找到阑尾,此时应仔细检查,不要误为阑尾缺如。

阑尾的位置随盲肠在腹腔中的位置变动而改变,一般均在右侧髂窝内。在结肠旋转不良时,阑尾可位于肝下或中腹部。有作者统计5万人阑尾的位置,发现阑尾位于右下腹占95.45%,右上腹占3.94%,左上腹占0.58%,左下腹占0.03%。

阑尾可出现的位置有:①可位于盲肠和升结肠下部的后方(盲肠后位或结肠后位);②可下降超过小骨盆缘(盆位或下降位),与右输尿管和女性卵巢关系密切;③可位于盲肠下(盲肠下位);④可位于回肠末端前方,可接触于前腹壁;⑤可位于回肠末段后方。Wakeley(1933)10 000例统计:①占65.3%;② 31.0%;③ 2.3%;④ 1.0%;⑤ 0.4%。虽然上述分类基于大量病例,但其后的文献,不论是解剖学还是外科学,都显示出不少的矛盾。

Buschard和Kjaeldgaard(1973)报告一组(234例尸解)比较若干研究的结果(1885年至1973年),远比Wakeley收集的病例数量多得多,他们将所有位置分类为二组,前组(包括骨盆的和回盲部的)与后组(盲肠后和盲肠下),结论是前组更为常见。Wakeley在其自己的丹麦组内以后组更常见,而在德国组中,此意见正好颠倒。Collins(1932)在第二大组(4 680例)研究中,发现各组比例与Wakeley组恰恰相反:前组与后组分别为78.5%与21.5%(Wakeley组为32.4%与67.6%)。从上述统计数字看,各作者报告的差别相当大,这除了与不同的观察者的观察标准有关外,可能还与人种、民族不同有关。

有作者报告高位阑尾,位于右肾前方。该病例右腰区仅见升结肠,其后方(需将其右后方腹膜剖开)藏着褶贴于腹后壁的部分升结肠、盲肠和阑尾。盲肠及褶向后的升结肠总长达6cm,回肠末段有9cm长的小肠系膜,而紧贴于腹后壁。阑尾自倒置的盲肠末端伸向上方,长7cm,口径0.1cm,位于升结肠上段的后方,而以疏松的结缔组织相连。阑尾的后面紧贴于右肾下部的前面。阑尾的左侧又以结缔组织与十二指肠降部右缘相连。阑尾右侧面被以腹膜,与右肾外前面腹膜相延续,因而阑尾愈着而不能活动,它位于麦氏点上方7cm。

为了提高急性阑尾炎的CT诊断的精确性及效率,还可采用局部阑尾扫描技术。但因盲肠解剖位置的变异,常常带来扫描、诊断、治疗方面的困难,因此应先拍腹部平片或在CT定位像以确定盲肠的位置,采用这种方法,可以在很大限度上缩短扫描时间,减少曝光量、降低CT检查的费用等。

婴儿阑尾位于盲肠尖端,在发育中盲肠呈偏心性生长,成人的阑尾基部则位于盲肠内后侧,回盲瓣下方2.5cm处,外形上从漏斗状(婴儿期)变成丘蚓状盲管。其长短、粗细不一。最长可达20cm,直径约6mm,方向不定。约2/3的人位于盲肠后,其余则位于内下部。因盲肠解剖位置变异,阑尾的解剖位置也并不都在麦氏点。

第二十八篇　门静脉疾病

第一章　肝硬化门静脉高压

第一节　肝硬化合并不同病变对门静脉成像延迟时间的影响

MSCT 门静脉血管成像具有无创、快速、简便、无并发症等优点，对于肝硬化患者术前了解病变程度、门静脉血管情况具有重要意义。在诸多因素固定的情况下，门静脉成像的关键取决于合理的延迟时间，但是根据国内外文献报道门静脉成像的延迟时间各有差异，无统一的标准。一项研究考虑到国人体重较轻、体表面积较小的缘故，采用对比剂剂量为 1.8ml/kg，流率 3.5ml/s，注射流率过高会导致对比剂外渗。

该组采用智能扫描技术测定肝硬化患者门静脉时间 - 密度曲线多获得了较好的结果。早在 20 世纪已有使用智能扫描技术测定门静脉达峰阈值触发扫描的研究报道，近年来在国内也有采用此技术对肝硬化门静脉延迟时间的报道，与 Test bolus 小剂量预注射实验技术和经验扫描延迟技术相比，智能扫描技术能更直接反应门静脉强化峰值和达峰时间。

肝硬化主要改变为肝细胞弥漫性变性坏死、结缔组织增生、肝细胞结节状再生，这种改变反复交错进行，肝小叶结构和血液循环途径逐渐被改建。

正常人全肝血流量为 1 500ml/min，其中门静脉血占 70%~80%，肝动脉血占 20%~30%。以往有报道肝硬化时肝动脉血流星增加，而全肝血流量明显减少，表明肝硬化时门静脉血流减少对全肝血流减少有很大影响，这是由于肝硬化引起门静脉高压、脾大、静脉曲张等一系列并发症导致血液被分流所致。

以往对于肝硬化门静脉成像延迟时间的研究报道比较笼统，时间范围在 40~70s，跨度较大。由于肝硬化病程错综复杂，所以造成不同时期门静脉的延迟时间也不同。正常人脾脏一般不能触及，而肝硬化患者病程达到后期往往伴有脾脏不同程度肿大。脾脏肿大会把大量血液阻留在脾内而使循环血量减少，为了维持有效循环血容量，细胞外液进入血液循环从而稀释血液。当对比剂进入脾脏时，根据血流动力学改变，使得对比剂达峰时间延迟。

根据该组研究结果，脾肿大组门静脉达峰时间较脾正常组延迟 5s 左右，肝实质的达峰时间也较脾正常组延迟 10s 左右，差异均有统计学意义（$P<0.05$）。当肝硬化合并脾肿大患者肝脏还未进入失代偿期时，肝内血管变形和侧支循环不明显，所以脾肿大组的门静脉、肝实质的 CT 值差较脾正常组差异无统计学意义（$P>0.05$）。

该组实验门静脉曲张引起对比剂的门静脉、肝实质的 CT 值差值下降，对比剂的门静脉达峰时间较无静脉曲张组延迟 20s 左右，与多数文献报道的门静脉侧支循环所采用的延迟时间相似，这是由于肝硬化的病理改变造成肝内血液循环的紊乱，血管床缩小、闭塞或扭曲，血管受到再生结节挤压，肝内门静脉、肝静脉和肝动脉小分支之间失去正常关系并相通出现吻合支，围绕门静脉系统形成静脉团，血流形成阻力和侧支分流，血管显示有不同程度的扩张或迂曲。

肝硬化腹水产生的原因有以下几方面：低蛋白血症、肝淋巴液失衡、内分泌因素、肾脏因素。该组实验中肝硬化合并腹水组与无腹水组门静脉和肝实质的延迟时间基本一致，这可能是由于此组病例腹水量仅累及小部分肝脾，肝脏还未进入失代偿期。

国内外对于腹水量的多少对门静脉延迟时间的影响尚无相关文献报道。该组作者估计当腹水量达到一定程度，腹壁张力升高挤压肠壁血管使静脉回流受阻，门静脉在单位时间内的血流量减少，门静脉的增强时间也必定延迟，但这一观点需要在以后的研究中加以证实。

第二节　门脉高压时的钡餐检查

门脉高压引起的食管静脉曲张的特征性表现，是食管造影时食管下端皱襞增厚。吞食钡剂或空气使管腔扩张可能部分地或完全地遮蔽曲张的静脉。对于发现小的静脉曲张，电视透视观察是必要的。有用的技术包括：左前斜位仰卧照片、录像、Valsalva试验、用钡剂被覆黏膜以及抗副交感神经药物的应用等。

门脉高压时的胃静脉曲张通常主要是在胃底。只有胃静脉曲张，而没有食管静脉曲张，提示脾静脉梗阻。它们是多数性的光滑的分叶状充盈缺损(增厚、分叶的皱襞)。气钡双对比造影观察它们为最好，过度膨胀可部分地遮蔽它们。由于胃静脉曲张常常是浆膜下，在面临内镜检查结果为阴性或模棱两可时，放射学检查则可能有阳性发现。

十二指肠静脉曲张时，可产生弥漫性的匐行性的黏膜增厚，而且几乎总是伴存食管静脉曲张。当只有十二指肠静脉曲张时，其原因通常为肠系膜上静脉梗阻。

空肠或回肠静脉曲张通常极为少见，这与结肠静脉曲张一样。

直肠静脉曲张在放射学的表现与食管静脉曲张类似，其范围表现在，从突出的痔，到爬行性的黏膜下包块，一直伸展向上，进入乙状结肠远端。

第三节　肝脏门静脉成像延迟时间选择

详见本书 本卷 本篇 第十三章 第一节　关于门静脉的影像检查技术：肝脏门静脉成像延迟时间选择。

第二章 非肝硬化性门静脉高压

肝硬化以外的门脉高压的原因

门脉高压的大多数病例是相当明确地有滥用酒精导致肝硬化，或病毒性肝炎导致坏死后肝硬化的病史。这些病人有窦性或窦后性梗阻和升高的楔形压。偶尔，此类情况不明确，而且必需进行复杂的肝血管造影和静脉造影，以便确定梗阻的部位是窦后还是窦前，同时还要找出病因。正常的校正的肝的楔形压见于门脉高压病人时，则证明为窦前性门脉高压。窦后性门脉高压的肝外原因，诸如缩窄性心包炎和充血性心力衰竭通常被其他手段诊断，但是，在肝静脉造影时得到的系统静脉压力升高，则可用于确证临床的诊断。在诊断下腔静脉和/或肝静脉的梗阻或/和狭窄时，血管造影的技术是极重要的。

窦前性门脉高压：在美国，窦前性门脉高压的主要原因是门静脉栓塞。通常的病因有：新生儿脐炎、胰腺炎的并发症、新生物侵犯以及肝硬化的血流淤滞。少见的病因有：腹内炎症（诸如：阑尾炎、憩室炎或炎症性肠病）、创伤、凝血性疾病以及特发性。门脉栓塞可以是肝内性、肝外性、部分性或完全性。

门静脉栓塞的影像学表现：非常罕见，在门静脉内的血凝块中或是门静脉壁上出现钙化。门静脉壁上的钙化表现为平行性致密的线状影，它沿着门静脉的走行分布。它们常常不连续和稍不规则。钙化性门静脉血凝块，是整个钙化，没有边缘性密度增浓。任一类型钙化的存在，都意指有门静脉梗阻，常常都是这样，但不一定完全都是这样。

超声能十分可靠地观察门静脉主干及其较大的分支的栓塞，表现为血管腔内的有回声的物质。偶尔，当梗阻是完全性时，和管腔整个被栓子充满时，则可能难以确诊，而且，一个菱形的回声带代替原来见于肝门内的管样透声区。在慢性门静脉栓塞，栓子可能变为机化而且最终再形成管道，可能出现多数的侧支引流血管。

在超声检查时，当见到下述三个一组的表现时，可提示诊断：①肝外门静脉不能看见；②在门静脉区，出现一条光亮的回声索带，表示不是栓子就是门静脉周围纤维化；③在门静脉区内，门静脉周围的侧支引流血管表现为多数性弯曲的管状结构。

对侧支引流血管的多普勒超声检查，可发现门静脉的特征性血流表现。门静脉系统可观察到连续的流动，比较于系统循环，前者受心跳或呼吸运动的影响较少或不受影响。

CT增强扫描可显示门静脉栓塞为一个周围强化的低密度的中心影像。关于周围性强化存在某些争论，是否是围绕血凝块的血流，还是由于静脉的壁所产生的强化。可以想象，两种情况都可能存在。当静脉是闭塞或扩张时，不论是用超声，还是用CT，有肿瘤栓子存在时，改变都是明显的。

肝细胞癌、胆管癌、胰癌以及胃癌是常见的原因。在超声检查时，与肿瘤栓子相关的血管造影的线状和条纹征表现为在有回声的血凝块内的众多小的透声区。相应的CT征象则是血凝块的条纹状强化。

门静脉梗阻的一个间接CT征象是分叶的低密度区，或是出现于CT平扫，或是出现于对比剂滴注肠系膜上动脉后的CT扫描（CTAP）。前者大概是由于局部缺血脂肪浸润，而后者则是类似于肺核素显像时的灌注缺损。

门静脉闭塞的另一个间接CT征象是动态CT扫描时出现动脉-门脉瘘，受侵犯的门静脉分支过早显影出现于动脉期（与主动脉显影同时）。

窦前门静脉梗阻：窦前门静脉梗阻的病人对于肝静脉血的输出不增加阻力。某些门静脉侧支引流出现，但是供应肝的血液的大多数还是来自于肝动脉。肝脏趋向于缩小，门静脉-系统静脉的侧支引流出现。腹腔动脉造影显示肝动脉及其分支扩张与一个较小的肝脏。如果有脾肿大，则可出现脾动脉的扩张。如果栓塞是由于多血管性肿瘤（如肝细胞癌）引起，可能见到肿瘤栓子的条纹状强化，即线状和条纹征。胃冠状静脉和肠系膜下静脉的侧支引流血管出现于静脉期。肠系膜上动脉造影的静脉期，最好观察门静脉-门静脉侧支引流血管,它们通过胰头、胆囊以及肝外胆管,到肝内门静脉支(海绵样变性)。对于门静脉闭塞的真实的描写,还必须做经肝门静脉造影或脾门静脉造影。

窦前性门脉高压的肝内原因包括:血吸虫病、肝内门脉纤维化、肝的部分性结节性变性、类肉瘤病、由于接触氯化乙烯所致的纤维化、钍对比剂、病毒性肝炎、先天性肝纤维化以及胆汁性肝硬化的前期。

肝内门脉纤维化或硬化:肝内门脉纤维化或硬化,属于非肝硬化或其他已知特殊原因的门静脉梗阻的肝内门静脉梗阻。在文献上名称甚为混淆,诸如:特发性门脉高压、原发性门脉高压、非肝硬化性肝内门脉高压、非肝硬化性门脉纤维化、肝内门脉高压以及闭塞性门静脉病。门脉纤维化的范围是变化的,尽管通常范围都较小。肝内门静脉的静脉炎和硬化的病因学,考虑是以往的腹内炎症。动脉性门静脉造影,或直接法门静脉造影通常显示肝内门静脉的突然性梗阻。闭塞处常常比较小,位于肝内门静脉分支远端。门脉纤维化可以出现,但其表现不同于也不提示先天性肝纤维化。肝外门静脉开放,门静脉压升高,在门静脉压与楔形肝静脉压之间有一梯度。在这些病人,自由肝静脉造影显示在大的静脉与其分支之间存在狭窄的夹角,即垂柳征。这是与肝硬化时出现的较宽的夹角相对而言。

肝的部分性结节性变性:肝的部分性结节性变性是一种成人的疾病,可出现门脉高压、脾肿大以及静脉曲张出血。肝活检显示肝实质的结节性变性伴同少量纤维化,无肝硬化或炎症。血管造影征象包括:门静脉压升高伴开放,但由于肝的结节造成的血管紊乱和伸直,而呈现肉眼观为异常的肝内门静脉构筑。整个肝的大小一般在正常范围内。

动-静脉瘘所引起的血流增加:最后,一种少见的,但是属于手术可以矫正的,窦前性门脉高压的原因是由于动-静脉瘘所引起的血流增加,这种瘘出现于肠系膜动脉或肝动脉,与门静脉主干或其主要分支之间。基本的病因包含:肝或腹部的外伤、手术(诸如胃切除术、肠切除术)、经皮肝穿活检、内脏动脉瘤破入门静脉系统、由于系膜内的多血管性肿瘤产生的动-静脉瘘。病人就诊,或是因为静脉曲张出血,或是因为一般的非特异性的不适,诸如体重减轻和不舒服。可以出现上腹部或脐周的杂音。断面影像检查可以提示正确的诊断,但是,内脏血管造影更可以确诊,而且,如果瘘能被栓塞,还可行介入性治疗。

窦后性门脉高压:肝外性窦后性门脉高压可由下述情况引起:长期的三尖瓣闭锁不全、慢性充血性心力衰竭、缩窄性心包炎以及下腔静脉肝后段和/或肝静脉的栓塞(布-加综合征)。

第三章　门静脉高压时的侧支循环

第一节　门脉-系统侧支引流血管与超声检查

一个小的皱缩的肝，只见于肝硬化的进展性病例。在早期，肝的大小或是肿大或是正常。肝硬化超声诊断的标准包括：肝实质回声增强，穿透肝的超声束的减弱，肝内血管（尤其是小分支）显示差。使用上述标准，超声诊断肝硬化特异性约在65%~80%。而其余20%的假阳性病例，一般都是难以区别肝脂肪浸润与肝硬化。

在肝硬化观察到的上述超声表现在慢性肝炎病例也同样可见到。穿透的超声束减少与肝实质回声的增加，能由胶原和/或脂肪沉积来解释。无能力看见门静脉壁可能是由于周围肝实质回声增强轮廓画出这些正常回声的结构。

肝硬化的附带征象包括脾肿大和腹腔积液。在肝硬化的进展性病例，裂隙、轮廓的切迹和结节，偶尔还有大的再生结节都是应该强调观察的。大的再生结节大约与肝实质有着相同的回声性质，但与肝细胞癌比较，它通常则不是相同回声。左叶与尾叶是相对保持不变，比较于皱缩的肝右叶，它们则较大。

实时超声和多普勒超声可以无损伤地评估门-腔侧支引流血管的情况。一般认为，在适当的临床状态下，门静脉的直径大于13mm是门脉高压的特点。正常门静脉直径范围是6.4~12.1mm，而在肝硬化时，门静脉直径平均为12mm。

在X线血管造影，肝硬化组与对照组之间，门静脉直径无明显差异，而且门静脉直径保持恒定，甚或缩小伴存门-肝的梯度增加（因为血流的逆流到侧支）。有作者指出，门静脉（和脾静脉）的大小显示，对肝硬化和门脉高压说来，门静脉扩张是不敏感的，但是，当其存在时，它则可相当准确地提示为门脉高压。

在正常人，在深吸气时，由于横膈下降与肝静脉流出的受压，门静脉系统扩张。在门脉高压时门静脉不再出现扩张，这是因为门静脉已经最大限度扩张的缘故。肠系膜上静脉与冠状静脉的评估是有价值的。在正常情况下，肠系膜上静脉直径从无大于门静脉者，在内径测量上，冠状静脉大于4mm是门脉高压有用的征象。如冠状静脉大于7mm，通常提示门-肝压力梯度大于10mmHg，此时曲张的静脉则容易发生出血。

在门脉高压时，可能出现的门脉-系统侧支引流血管如下：①经肝的静脉，门静脉到胃冠状静脉、脊柱静脉丛、下腔静脉、半奇静脉；②胃食管静脉的侧支引流血管，静脉曲张；③食管旁静脉，胃冠状静脉到奇静脉、半奇静脉、脊柱静脉丛；④胃-肾静脉：胃静脉曲张到左肾静脉；⑤门-冠状到肺静脉，胃食管静脉曲张到左肺静脉；⑥脾-肾静脉，脾静脉到左肾静脉；⑦脾静脉-腔静脉；⑧脾-奇静脉，到半奇静脉、腹后壁静脉；⑨肠系膜下静脉到痔静脉（下部和中部）；⑩胰十二指肠静脉到半奇静脉（在十二指肠空肠曲处）；⑪丛状的腹膜后静脉，腹后壁静脉、结肠和肠系膜静脉到下腔静脉；⑫胸膜心脏周围静脉/腹膜的静脉；⑬脐旁静脉；⑭肠系膜上静脉到右肾静脉；⑮肝内静脉，门静脉到肝静脉。

超声检查最容易识别的静脉侧支引流血管，是胃冠状静脉以及与之伴存的胃食管静脉曲张。在纵切面扫描，确定胃冠状静脉来自于脾静脉或门静脉之后，在胃食管连接区和胃小弯处，以成角的纵切面扫描可见到环状或管状透声的静脉曲张。偶尔在肋下以向颅成角的横切面扫描，通过肝的左叶也可发现食管静脉曲张。脐静脉连接左门静脉到系统循环，是起源于脐，途经表浅腹壁静脉分支而形成（称为蛇女头，Cruveilhier-Baumgarten 综合征）。

在横切面扫描，再通的脐静脉表现为一圆形透声影，位于左段间裂中，周围有镰状韧带内脂肪的回声。在纵切面扫描，追踪它足侧走向脐部，为一管状透声影。当今病理学研究指出，它不是脐静脉本身再通，而是镰状韧带内的脐旁静脉开放。此征象对于门脉高压是有特异性的，由此还可排除窦前性原因。

沿着脾静脉的下缘到中线的左侧进行扫描，有时可发现扩张的肠系膜下静脉。胃 - 肾和脾 - 肾侧支引流血管的静脉在通过脾和左肾的冠状切面扫描时可能见到。来自于脾的脾静脉近端及其分支能在脾门处看见，胃短静脉侧支引流血管位于脾的内侧和脾门的上方。

沿着胃大弯及其邻近的肠系膜可能见到胃网膜静脉曲张。超声检查发现的其他的静脉曲张包括十二指肠旁静脉、门静脉周围静脉以及盆腔内的侧支引流血管的静脉。扩张的胆囊静脉和胆囊周围静脉已有报告见于肝硬化和门脉高压、胆囊癌和门静脉栓塞的病例。

在意欲进行分流手术之前，对侧支引流血管的具体表现的了解是十分重要的。外科医生一般都希望结扎胃冠状静脉的侧支引流血管，和任何其他较大的侧支引流血管静脉，脾能保持向肝的门脉血流和避免出现脑病。如果拟行脾 - 肾分流，脾静脉和左肾静脉的观察，排除主动脉后左肾静脉的存在，对于手术医生说来都是有用的资料。观察不到门静脉是门静脉闭塞的有力证据：空的肝门是一高水平回声的宽的菱形带状影。

可能形成门静脉的血管瘤，或是在肠系膜上静脉与脾静脉汇合处近侧，或是在更远侧。考虑它们不是先天性者，就是门脉高压时形成的。有时伴存肝实质的异常，但是它们的发生发展情况尚不清楚。多数病人皆出现胃肠道出血，分流手术对治疗常有帮助。血管破裂可出现进入腹腔、胆管树或腹膜后腔，常常病危。

附：Cruveilhier-Baumgarten 综合征：为门脉高压性肝硬化伴有脐或脐旁静脉曲张。此征特点为呕血、腹腔积液、脾肿大、脾功能亢进、食管静脉曲张、脐周静脉扩张弯曲呈放射状，酷似水母头或蛇女头，腹壁可见大量弯曲的静脉。通常在剑突区可闻及静脉性杂音，且常伴存震颤。

第二节　自发性肝内型门静脉 - 下腔静脉分流

门静脉 - 下腔静脉分流，属门 - 体分流的一种类型，发生率较低。按病因分为先天性和自发性；按解剖位置分为肝内型和肝外型。

自发性门静脉 - 下腔静脉分流多因肝硬化门静脉高压引起。肝外型是指门静脉肝外段直接发出分支与后方的下腔静脉相连；肝内型是指门静脉右后支经过右叶在右肾上腺区与下腔静脉相连。无论肝内或肝外型，其 CT 表现特点均为门静脉期 CT 增强扫描可见门静脉血管强化，并分别表现为门静脉分支末端与下腔静脉相连。门静脉 CT 成像或多层曲面重建有助于诊断。有作者报告一例，该例在 7 年前曾做肝脏 CT 检查，未发现异常分流，表明不是先天性发育异常所致，而是由于门静脉高压或肝癌进展引起，但其门静脉出肝的机制（先天存在或后天再通）尚待探讨。

明确门静脉分流有重要的临床意义：①有助于门静脉瘤、右肾上腺病变的鉴别诊断；②有助于门静脉畸形的诊断；③门静脉分流患者多伴有血氨升高，易患肝性脑病，发现此分流存在，有助于指导临床治疗；④对于需要手术或介入、腹腔穿刺等操作的患者，发现分流有助于术者提前制定方案；⑤有助于影像科医师在肝脏检查时，要想到门静脉分流的存在及类型；⑥有助于Ⅰc 型分流畸形引起的便血原因的诊断。

第四章　门静脉海绵样变与门静脉胆病

第一节　门静脉海绵样变性

门静脉海绵样变性，是指门静脉主干和/或它的分支完全或部分阻塞后，其周围形成大量侧支静脉或阻塞后再沟通。此时，如无肝窦或窦后阻塞引起的门脉系统血液逆流或继发性门脉高压，侧支静脉内的血液是流向肝内的。过去，曾认为门静脉变性为罕见病例，然而近几年随着影像技术（特别是多普勒超声技术）的发展，对此变性的认识已逐步加深，确诊率也逐步提高。

1. 病因　大多数学者认为，门静脉变性是由于门静脉阻塞（血栓、瘤栓）引起的，其中包括栓塞后侧支引流血管形成和栓塞后再沟通。在成人中，最常见的栓塞病因有肝硬化（尤其是伴有肝细胞癌）、胰腺疾病、肾盂静脉发炎，其他病因有凝血机制障碍、出血性疾病、消化系统感染（如急性胆囊炎、坏死性肠炎，等）、邻近组织肿块和癌症（如胃癌）、手术并发症（如脾切除术后、门静脉吻合术）及布-加综合征。门静脉栓塞的患者大约有50%出现门静脉海绵样变性，出现时间为栓塞后1~12个月；另一些学者认为，这种病变是由于脐肠系膜和肝静脉之间的静脉丛异常增生而来。Leger等（1962）认为出生后脐静脉和静脉导管闭塞的过程可以累及门静脉干和它的属支，在闭塞的门静脉区域便有海绵样静脉形成。

2. 病理学　因门静脉闭塞，许多潜在的门静脉周围小静脉分支扩张开放即形成门静脉海绵状变性。最快可于门静脉阻塞后6~20天内发生。门静脉海绵样变性的侧支血管来源于与淋巴管、胆管、血管伴行的小静脉和新生的静脉管道，这些血管跨过阻塞的门静脉引流远侧的血液进入肝内门静脉分支，在肝门部（胆囊床旁）和肝十二指肠韧带内形成侧支血管网。

3. 影像学研究　核素扫描：Ros等（1986）运用核素扫描检查了1例因红细胞增多症并发的本症患者，其特点为肝门轮廓明显缺损。Mahlstedt（1984）在门静脉海绵样变性患者的静脉内注射^{99m}Tc之后，进行动态观察，在动脉相之后不久，核素于门静脉属支的异常结构内迅速浓聚；在肝实质相，由于核素被网状内皮系统清除，上述变化则迅速消失。该作者认为，比较静态与动态图像可以诊断门静脉海绵样变性。

超声检查：Kauzlaric等（1984）报道2例超声检查发现的本症，分别经血管造影和手术证实。超声表现的特点有：肝外门静脉的正常结构消失；肝门部区域内呈现强回声；在肝门部或管腔内可见到形成不一的管状结构。Weltin等（1985）认为，单纯的超声检查有一定的局限性，应用双功能多普勒检查，通过对脉冲多普勒频谱的分析有助于进一步诊断本症，其特点是在门静脉周围的异常结构内引出门静脉血流。

门静脉血流的多普勒表现的特点是：连续血流频谱，很少或不受心脏及呼吸的影响；与体循环静脉比较，门静脉血流平均值与峰值均较低；多普勒频谱的包络不平或通过扬声器听见低音调的隆隆声。近年，一些学者通过应用双功能多普勒超声检查本症，均获满意结果，由于彩色多普勒超声能够直接观察到门静脉海绵样结构内的血流，为其诊断开辟了新的途径。综上所述，超声诊断本症的主要特点有：超声显示门静脉正常结构消失，其周围或管腔内有形态不一的管状结构；脉冲多普勒超声在异常管状结构内引出门静脉样血流频谱；彩色多普勒超声显示管状结构内有血流。

CT：Mathieu等（1985）应用CT动态扫描检查

本症患者16例,其中肝硬化3例(1例肝细胞癌),3例血小板增多症,2例慢性胰腺炎,2例急性胰腺炎,2例胆管炎,4例其他疾病。CT动态扫描图像的特征是:①门静脉系统的正常结构在肠系膜上静脉与脾静脉汇合处,肝门部及肝内门静脉分支等断面上消失;②在门静脉相,门静脉的位置出现迂曲的血管;③肝血流灌注异常,即注射对比剂15~30秒后,远离肝门的正常肝组织被增强为高密度,到45秒后,整个肝组织均被增强,变为等密度。该作者认为,这一变化是由于周围肝组织通过门静脉海绵样结构供应的血流太少以致肝动脉供血增加,而肝门周围的肝组织通过门静脉海绵样结构供血就足够了。这一观察证明,门静脉阻塞后肝动脉的供血可以增加。

在CT平扫图像上,海绵状变性可与肝门或胰头部的淋巴结肿大或肿块相仿。在慢性门静脉血栓形成的病人中,门静脉本身不能看到,看到的仅仅是侧支血管。在CT增强扫描,门静脉海绵状变性表现为肝门处小静脉血管团,而取代闭合的正常门静脉。

MRI:Ros等(1986)通过0.35T MR,应用自旋回波技术。MRI发现肝门部有大量与门静脉平行的血管结构。MRI不仅能发现门静脉的异常结构,而且还能了解开放的侧支引流血管的血流动力学情况。

血管造影:Kauzlaric等(1984)应用血管造影检查本症2例。1例行腹腔动脉造影,发现肠系膜下静脉扩张,其血流经异常静脉流向肝脏,从而代替了门静脉主干;另1例行术中肠系膜上静脉造影,发现门静脉被栓塞,其周围有大量异常静脉形成的侧支引流血管。早在1979年,Adler用血管造影也证实了1例门静脉海绵样变性。

一些作者对180例肝癌病人做了腹腔动脉和肠系膜上动脉造影,其中98例造影后做了肿瘤切除术和病理检查,对这些病例分析,发现门脉阻塞和门脉内无向肝性或离肝性血流,是肝内门脉海绵变性形成的重要因素。同时该作者还对门脉海绵变性的形态结构及其形成机制进行了探讨。

4. 临床意义　当门静脉阻塞范围较局限时(如仅为主干阻塞),门静脉海绵样变性的侧支静脉可以跨过阻塞部位与叶内开放的门静脉分支相通,使肝脏的门静脉血流灌注保持正常;相反,在门静脉阻塞范围较广泛时,尽管门静脉海绵样变性的侧支静脉参与了门静脉循环,但是,它仍不足以减轻门脉高压,可以引起食管静脉曲张和其他静脉曲张。因此,正确诊断有助于临床采取正确的治疗措施。

第二节　门静脉性胆病

门静脉性胆病,是指由于肝外门静脉梗阻导致胆囊和胆管出现形态学异常和功能障碍的一种疾病。它可累及整个胆系,包括肝内外胆管、胆囊管和胆囊。

肝外门静脉梗阻是导致门静脉高压的常见病因之一,长期肝外门静脉梗阻可导致门静脉侧支循环出现,并形成门静脉海绵样变性。研究发现,肝外门静脉梗阻还可引起胆系的改变。

Fraser和Broun(1944)描述了门静脉高压患者合并胆系异常的改变。Dilawari和Chawla(1992)报道了20例肝外门静脉梗阻患者出现类似硬化性胆管炎的胆系异常改变,在内镜逆行性胆系造影法(ERCP)上表现为胆管局部狭窄、扩张、管壁不规则等。现在又有关于肝外门静脉梗阻合并胆系改变并导致黄疸、腹痛等症状出现的一些相关报道。肝外门静脉梗阻患者合并门静脉性胆系病的发生率为81%~100%。

门静脉性胆系病主要表现为胆管的狭窄和扩张,导致胆汁淤积、梗阻性黄疸、胆管炎和胆结石,严重者可出现继发性胆汁性肝硬化,甚至肝衰竭。但大多数门静脉性胆系病患者仅有影像学表现,而无临床症状出现。

1. 发病机制　本病的发病机制目前尚未完全明确,可能与以下因素有关。

机械性压迫学说:Williams等(1982)描述了肝外胆管静脉曲张压迫胆管的影像学表现,此后研究发现,胆系静脉可能在本病发病中了起到了重要作用。

肝外胆管有两个静脉,一个是Saint静脉丛,位于肝外胆管外周,紧邻肝外胆管外膜,形成致密的网状结构,静脉体积不一,但其直径一般不超过1 mm。Saint静脉丛扩张可以导致肝外胆管内壁不规则狭窄。

另外一个静脉丛是Petren静脉丛，与肝外胆管走行平行，与胃静脉、胰十二指肠静脉和门静脉相通。Petren静脉丛扩张将导致肝外胆管受压，甚至穿透肝外胆管形成胆管内静脉曲张或者上皮下静脉曲张。

门静脉海绵样变性的病理生理过程除了包括门静脉周围侧支循环扩张以外，还包括新生血管和结缔组织的生成，形成类似肿瘤的实体组织，导致肝外胆管受压和成角。

缺血和纤维化学说：Dhiman等（1999）发现5例肝外门静脉梗阻合并胆系病变的患者进行门体分流术后，胆系病变并未完全改善，仅有部分病变消失。这提示机械性压迫并不是导致门静脉性胆系病发生的唯一原因。

长期肝外门静脉梗阻和门静脉海绵样变性可影响小动脉和毛细血管的血供，导致胆系缺血和纤维化形成，引起胆管狭窄和扩张。而且，胆管缺血和纤维化降低胆囊收缩功能，导致慢性胆汁淤积。

感染学说：曾有一些学者在早期研究中提出感染和胆管炎参与了门静脉性胆系病的形成。然而，后期研究发现，绝大多数门静脉性胆系病患者没有感染的症状和表现，并且，胆管炎常常发病于疾病的后期，因此这一学说并没有得到广泛认可。但是胆管炎可以加重门体分流术后胆管狭窄的发生。

2. 临床表现　大多数患者没有临床症状。少数患者出现黄疸、瘙痒、发热、腹痛等表现，发生率为5%~30%。Condat等（2003）报道25例患者中有7例（28%）出现临床症状。易出现临床症状的高危因素包括：高龄、病程长、胆结石和肝功能异常改变。临床表现主要与胆管的完全或不完全性梗阻及合并的感染有关。主要有以下两个方面：

（1）黄疸和瘙痒：与肝外胆管狭窄或肝外胆管结石导致的胆汁淤积有关。如果病情持续进展，可能会发展为继发性胆汁性肝硬化，但少见。

（2）胆管炎：少部分患者可能出现发热、黄疸、腹痛等胆管炎的表现。Macaluso等（2013）报道了1例表现为急性胆管炎的门静脉性胆系病患者。

此外，上述症状常发生于疾病的后期，常常晚于食管胃底静脉曲张导致的上消化道出血。Mangla等（2012）报道1例门静脉性胆系病患者于腹痛、黄疸发病之前的5年内多次出现呕血。

3. 实验室检查　血清胆红素、碱性磷酸酶、γ-谷氨酰转移酶、丙氨酸转氨酶和天冬氨转氨酶轻度至中度升高，提示胆汁淤积和胆管炎。出现继发性胆汁性肝硬化时，可出现白蛋白、胆碱酯酶降低，凝血酶原时间延长。

4. 影像学研究　影像学检查是诊断本病的主要依据，尤其是磁共振胆胰管成像（MRCP）和ERCP。

MRCP：MRCP可以很好显示胆系和门静脉系统，是诊断门静脉性胆系病、肝外门静脉阻塞和门静脉海绵样变性的主要非侵入性检查手段。研究发现，MRCP诊断本病的敏感性与ERCP相同。影像学检查常见的表现为：胆管狭窄，狭窄部位以上的胆管节段性或弥漫性扩张，胆管的串珠样改变，肝外胆管成角，胆结石。门静脉性胆系病最常见的影像学改变为肝内胆管扩张（42%），其次分别为胆囊结石、肝外胆管结石、多发狭窄、肝外胆管扩张。狭窄部位可仅累及肝外胆管或肝内外胆管均受累。肝外胆管的胰上段为最常见的狭窄部位。门静脉性胆系病患者胰头上段肝外胆管成角平均为110°。

ERCP：ERCP对于诊断门静脉性胆系病具有很高的价值，但是由于具有创伤性，因此只有在需要内镜下治疗时推荐应用。

超声：彩色多普勒超声应用广泛，可以检测到肝门区迂曲血管结构，但是由于门静脉海绵样变性可能干扰胆系的检查，因此彩色多普勒超声检查对本病的诊断价值有限。超声内镜检查有助于鉴别胆管静脉血张和胆结石。

CT平扫＋增强扫描：可以很好地显示门静脉海绵样变性和胆系的异常改变。

我们体会到，肝胆系统MRI诊断中出现的误诊不只局限于技术因素所产生的伪影，也可能来自于发育变异或医源性解剖结构的改变，它们的表现可能类似于肝胆病变。认识这些发育变异，可消除误诊，也可减少其他不必要的影像检查或介入处理。

第五章　关于门静脉血流

第一节　门脉血流量的研究

生理因素影响:门脉血流受多种生理因素影响。进餐对门脉血流量的影响显著,进餐后门脉血流量增加,与空腹比较有显著性差异;流速变化不大。这些生理性因素的影响最早在采用廓清法测量肝血流量时就已被注意到了,体位、进餐和药物都可以改变肝脏的血流量。这些因素对正常人和肝硬化病人的影响是不同的,对正常人影响大,对肝硬化病人影响较小。有作者指出,正常人进餐后门脉血流量可增加 80%,肝硬化病人增加 26%,并认为这一指标可以反映肝功能的储备。

单位时间内门脉血流量与体重有关,并显示男、女间有显著性差异,但经体重标化后差异消失,可见性别差异是由体重差异造成的。

肝硬化患者门脉血流量:肝硬化门脉血流量的分布:肝硬化患者门脉血流量可以正常,低于正常,高于正常,这种分布对选择治疗方案有参考价值。

此类情况可以用阻力和动力两种原因加以解释:导致低流量的原因可能是肝硬化时门脉血流阻力增加,导致血流不畅;高流量的原因可能是门脉压力升高,激素代谢失常,体循环血量增多,加之肝内侧支循环的开放,于是大量血液涌入门静脉,致使门脉呈现高动力循环。

这两种机制的共同作用,决定了肝硬化患者的门脉血流量。但是高流量不能代表肝脏的有效循环血量,随着门静脉对肝脏的有效灌注量的减少,肝动脉供血将增加,可由原来的 25% 增加到 50%。

肝硬化门脉血流量与肝功能分级的关系及返流的意义:一般认为,肝硬化门脉血流量与肝功能分级不存在显著性差异。个别病例出现返流,返流是侧支自发性分流减压的结果,是门静脉血流遇到高阻力后的代偿机制。发现返流对选择治疗方案十分有意义。

MRI 门脉血流的检测是一项非创伤性技术,可以用于定量测量门脉血流,并预测食管静脉曲张出血,但肝硬化门脉血流变化十分复杂,尚有待于进一步研究。

第二节　门静脉循环与体循环

虽然门静脉循环是体循环的一部分,但二者却有显著不同之处,值得特别注意。

引流消化系统的各条血管,并不进入从身体下部来的下腔静脉,而是经门静脉到肝窦状隙或血窦。如此,肝脏则可以首先选取从消化道吸收来的营养。在肝脏内,来自门静脉的血与肝动脉来的含氧血相混合,以后肝脏所有的血都注入肝静脉,再经下腔静脉而到达右心房。

第六章　肝动脉－门静脉分流

第一节　肝内肉眼可见的肝－门静脉分流的 MR

门静脉系统与全身静脉系统分流分为三个基本类型：①肝外离肝型分流，放射学检查能很好地显示；②肝内微小或功能性分流，超出一般影像学的分辨能力；③肝内肉眼可见的肝－门静脉分流，在 CT 和超声检查应用之前影像学很少能诊断。

肝－门静脉间的直接交通（肉眼可见的肝内肝－门静脉分流（IPHVS）罕见。

肝内肉眼可见的肝－门静脉分流的病因可能包括：先天性因素、门静脉瘤破裂、肝硬化后静脉导管未闭或重新开放、肝炎实质萎缩等获得性血管功能失调。

CT 和超声能检查出大多数肝内肉眼可见的肝－门静脉分流，但 MR 图像中肝实质及肝内血管的对比更高。MRI 可清楚地显示肝－门静脉分流所表现的“流空现象”。此类肝－门静脉分流分为单发和多发两型病变，前者更多见。

Araki 等（1991）报道 5 例：1 例表现为多发弥漫性分流；4 例为单发性分流；后者呈管状，局灶性扩张或葡萄状改变。在多发分流中，小的分流呈弥漫分布，X 线肝动脉造影常显示不甚清楚。

第二节　诊断陷阱：肝硬化中非肿瘤性肝动脉门静脉分流之 MSCT

近来由于 MSCT 广泛应用于临床，可使肝脏在动脉期一次完成成像，双期扫描的常规使用，提高了对小肝细胞性肝癌的检测能力并且可反映血流动力学的改变，在肝硬化患者 MSCT 扫描的动脉期，对早期小肝癌检测力较强，但常有许多假阳性存在。

硬化肝脏在动脉期可看到高密度灶，在门静脉期呈等密度，经 DSA 造影后发现它们不是恶性病灶，因为肝硬化改变了正常肝脏的结构和肝血流动力学，导致动脉血增加，门静脉血减少。肝动脉与门静脉分支间可形成许多新的交通支，所以在肝硬化中，肝动脉门静脉分流的表现很可能诊断为小肝癌。在肝硬化患者中，确定与小肝癌相似的良性病灶对于肝硬化并发肝癌的治疗前准确诊断是很重要的，肝动脉门静脉分流的诊断标准为：①在硬化肝脏中或远离肝内肝细胞性肝癌的肝实质内，MSCT 扫描的动脉期发现点状、结节样或楔形、不规则的肝脏局部高密度灶，门静脉期呈等密度，多平面重建后形态有所改变；② DSA 造影显示病灶区早期模糊的门静脉小分支；③无碘油沉积。

肝动脉门静脉分流形成机制分析：在双血供的肝脏中出现短暂的肝脏实质强化，反映了肝硬化肝脏结构和肝血流动力学的改变，由于动脉血增加，门静脉血减少，受影响的部位表现为在动脉期呈高密度灶，在门静脉期呈等密度，在动脉期中表现为短暂的强化影，即重分配的动脉血再分布到门静脉血流入的局部区域，门静脉或静脉血流减少而导致肝动脉门静脉分流，是肝脏影像学中相对常见的假病灶原因，但是从小肝癌中区分出这种假病灶并不容易，这被认为是一种肝血管的表现或周边短暂的楔性肝实质的强化，代表灌注紊乱。

在肝硬化及慢性肝炎患者中，肝动脉期检测的高密度灶，在门静脉期呈低密度灶常代表肝细胞性肝癌的存在，而肝动脉门静脉分流常位于肝周边的肝包膜下、胆囊窝及肝门前方，表现为短暂的高密度区，是肝实质在门静脉系统强化前肝局部区域的强化表现。

有作者认为在结构改变的肝硬化中循环改变起了一个重要的作用，肝硬化中小的肝动脉门静脉分流使门静脉血流逆向充填是肝动脉门静脉分流的一个原因。

小的肝静脉受压闭塞也是一个原因，闭塞的肝静脉致肝窦内压力增高，在窦腔与门静脉间有反向压力梯度，在这种情况下肝动脉是唯一的供血动脉；在动脉期扫描时对比剂从高压的动脉血流入低压的门静脉小分支支配区；也有可能高流速的对比剂进入较小的毛细血管间隙内，更有可能造成潜在沟通的肝动脉门静脉之间产生分流。

另外，胆囊周围血管丛的增生和肝周边区直接吻合的动脉门静脉也是肝动脉门静脉分流的主要途径，所以在MSCT双期典型的位于周边楔形或不规则形均匀高密度灶，在动脉期发现这种短暂高密度区，在门静脉期呈等高密度，被认为是肝动脉门静脉分流，因此要从肝细胞性肝癌中鉴别肝动脉门静脉分流，门静脉期的研究是必需的。

MSCT对肝动脉门静脉分流的诊断及鉴别分析：在硬化的肝脏中，非肿瘤的肝动脉门静脉分流在CT图像上表现有时很像小肝癌，在动脉期检测为高密度灶，当肝动脉门静脉分流形态几乎为圆形时，很难与小肝癌区分，这些小病灶没有小肝癌的典型表现，而是表现为动脉期病灶立即全部充填，在其他扫描期内与肝实质的密度一致，包括平扫CT图像。

而密实的小肝癌在三期是不一致的，与门静脉期肝实质的密度比较有下降即可诊断。有作者建议在有肝动脉门静脉分流表现的情况下要行MSCT的多平面重建，一项研究中9个结节样灶经多平面重建后形态均有改变，所以采用这种多向同性的重建方法对于鉴别肝动脉门静脉分流有非常重要的作用。

Oliver和Baron（1998）与Kim等（2001）的研究提出，在肝动脉期对比剂注入开始时，肝实质基本上无强化，因为对比剂未到达门静脉血流及血管周围的间隙，肝动脉期是显示富血供病灶的最佳成像时间。当血管间的沟通发生时，双血供系统引起各血管的血流量发生改变，甚至血流方向也受影响。

在研究肝硬化中的小肝癌时，要考虑肝硬化时血流动力学发生改变，肝动脉门静脉之间有许多的联系，而不是独立系统，这一点是非常重要的，因为临床肝动脉门静脉分流也可是良性表现，并不一定是与肝细胞性肝癌有关的恶性特征之一。

非肿瘤性肝动脉门静脉分流起源于肝硬化的改变是由于高灌注异常，导致假肿瘤形成，有作者的研究中出现非肿瘤性肝动脉门静脉分流表现的高密度灶或由于较小及不典型的轮廓常疑诊为小肝癌，在CT轴位显示结节样病灶，进行多平面重建后显示楔形或不规则形病灶，经DSA造影显示为非恶性肿瘤病灶；Yu等（2000）研究认为，肝动脉门静脉分流的发生与非典型增生结节（DN）或早期分化好的小肝癌有关，但没有被明确报道。

有作者的研究中有2个病灶，均≥1 cm，门静脉期呈等密度，经DSA造影显示为肝细胞性肝癌并有碘油沉积，有作者认为在肝硬化患者的研究中发现的肝动脉门静脉分流与肝细胞性肝癌的发生发展是否有关系尚不清楚，还待进一步研究，所以追踪随访这些患者是非常有必要的。该研究由于病例数较少，未能进行统计学分析，有待进一步收集研究。

虽然大多数的小肝动脉门静脉分流通过DSA证实是非肿瘤性的，但仍然有可能是生长慢的小肝癌潜在病灶的存在，只是未被影像学技术检出。

除了对高危患者进一步细致地追踪检查，没有方法可证实隐藏的肿瘤，CT与DSA不一致原因是否与DSA设备的分辨率以及导管的位置、注射压力的大小及流率等因素影响肝动脉门静脉分流的血流量和范围有关，还待进一步追踪研究。

总之，小的肝动脉门静脉分流是误诊为肿瘤的原因之一，大多数发生在肝脏周边包膜下，表现为动脉期边缘性小的楔形、结节样或不规则形高密度灶，边界较平直，常有正常血管通过，门静脉期呈等密度改变。

由于断层方面和空间关系的原因，非肿瘤性肝动脉门静脉分流可能表现为圆形、结节样，经多平面重建后呈楔形改变可提示肝动脉门静脉分流。如果MSCT得不到可靠的结果，DSA检查对了解血流情况有帮助，DSA易看到门静脉逆流及门静脉小分支早显。MSCT追踪检查有助于确定病灶的性质，或显示小肝癌的发生发展。

第三节 少见的肝动脉 - 门静脉瘘

肝动脉 - 门静脉瘘少见，它们可出现在肝动脉与入肝处门静脉主干之间，也可见于肝动脉分支和肝实质内门静脉分支之间。

Foley 等（1971）报告 5 例肝内的肝动脉 - 门静脉瘘，其中 4 例临床未曾怀疑为此症，只是血管造影才揭露本症的存在。2 例为腹部钝伤所致，2 例为针刺活检引起，1 例为肝硬化自发形成瘘。与系统性的动 - 静脉瘘相比较，本症不引起心排出量的增加，这考虑是由于肝血管窦内阻力改变的缘故。

Trinez 等（1973）介绍一例 30 岁男性患者，有胃肠出血和进食后疼痛，且以进食食物较多而加重，血管造影发现从左肝动脉分支到门静脉系统有一较大的动 - 静脉瘘，从而存在腹腔内血液的偷窃现象，瘘的血液来自肠系膜上动脉，故造成该动脉供应区域的小肠局部贫血；同时，门静脉压的动脉化伴存门脉高压，出现静脉曲张。该作者认为此类系膜动脉的局部贫血是这种难见的动 - 静脉瘘的少见并发症。

第七章　门静脉系血栓形成

第一节　门静脉血栓形成

许多原因可导致门静脉血栓形成,这些可能原因包括:肝硬化和门静脉高压、恶性肿瘤、外伤、血液病、败血症、胰腺炎、阑尾炎、憩室炎和肠炎性疾病。门静脉血栓也是肝移植的一种并发症,发生率达肝移植病例的 10% 之多。

在平扫 CT 图像上,为血凝块的急性血栓呈高密度改变(CT 值 60~80HU)。对比增强 CT 图像上低密度的壁内血栓在门静脉主干或分支内呈充盈缺损样改变。门静脉可因血栓而扩大。CT 的优势在于不仅能检出门静脉血栓形成,而且在许多情况下可确定血栓形成的原因。

在动脉早期 CT 扫描中,增强与不增强的血液在门静脉内混合不均匀时,不要与门静脉内血栓混淆。另外,在早期 CT 增强扫描时,肝动脉强化而门静脉不强化,也不应误为门静脉血栓。如果考虑到上述情况,应进行适当的重复延迟扫描。因为门静脉被周围低密度的脂肪包围,门静脉内血凝块的表现也可能因部分容积效应所造成。在这种情况中,重叠扫描和重建可减小部分容积效应。偶尔,因为门静脉血栓存在而导致肝动脉扩张,不要误认为是开通的门静脉。

第二节　急性门静脉和肠系膜上静脉血栓形成

病因:急性门静脉和肠系膜上静脉血栓形成约占肠缺血疾病的 5%~15%,临床相对少见,可发生于任何年龄。该病病因较多,血液滞缓、静脉壁内膜损伤和血液成分变化是三大主要因素。

临床表现:临床上可分为原发性和继发性,其中原发性多为先天性因素;继发性病因最多见的是获得性血液高凝状态,如肿瘤、腹内感染、腹部手术后、肝硬化、门静脉高压等。一组 19 例中, 9 例为术后并发症, 7 例伴有肝硬化、门静脉高压。由于本病相对少见,症状不典型,容易误诊为其他急腹症。早期临床主要表现为间断性或持续性腹痛、恶心、呕吐等非特异性症状,当病变进展时,症状随之加重,出现肠缺血症状,如不同程度腹胀、肠鸣音消失、肛门停止排气、排便、腹膜刺激症状、腹腔积液、血压下降、黑便等症状,严重者危及生命。

影像学研究:急性门静脉和肠系膜上静脉血栓形成的直接征象主要表现为血管腔不同程度增粗,平扫显示血栓形成部位管腔内高密度, CT 值约 50~70 HU,这与早期血栓中血红蛋白成分有关,随着时间的延长表现为管腔内低密度充盈缺损,增强扫描显示管腔内完全或不完全性充盈缺损,是其明确诊断的最可靠征象。CT 平扫有时未出现典型的静脉管腔内高密度,而仅发现肠系膜周围脂肪密度增高、混浊,静脉血管增粗、密度不均,肠管壁增厚及分层等征象。此时应考虑到本病可能,结合增强扫描,可明确诊断。

间接征象主要表现为:①肝脏灌注异常,由于门静脉或肠系膜上静脉血管栓塞,使得肝脏血供减少,肝脏强化时间延迟,表现为门静脉期肝脏不均匀强化,门静脉期延迟,出现肝脏一过性灌注异常;②肠壁增厚,正常情况下肠壁 >5 mm 为异常, 26%~96% 可出现肠壁增厚,主要与缺血段肠壁水肿、出血、感染有关；③肠管扩张积液，56%~96% 可出现此征象，由于缺血肠管蠕动消失，肠壁渗出液体和血液所致；④肠壁密度异常，平扫显示缺血段肠壁呈低密度或高密度，肠壁相对低密度是由于肠壁水肿明显，增强扫描显示肠壁黏膜与浆膜面强化明显，而黏膜下肠壁水肿积液，呈现“靶征”，肠壁高密度是由于黏膜下层坏死出血所致，增强扫描高密度的肠壁无强化，该征象是判断肠管坏死最敏感的指标；⑤肠系膜周边脂肪密度增高，边缘毛糙，肠系膜血管充血水肿，呈现“缆绳”样改变；⑥肠黏膜水肿，黏膜呈“弹簧”样增厚；⑦腹腔积液渐进性增多，主要与肠管缺血后渗出有关；⑧门静脉海绵样变性，由于门静脉阻塞后形成门体静脉侧支循环所致；⑨肠壁、肠系膜以及门静脉和肠系膜上静脉积气，提示肠管坏死，预后差。

MSCT 对急性门静脉和肠系膜上静脉血栓的诊断：MSCT 平扫和增强扫描是诊断急性门静脉和肠系膜上静脉血栓形成的最快捷、准确的无创检查方法，可以正确判定门静脉和肠系膜上静脉血栓以及侧支静脉异常，其诊断准确率达 90% 以上，特别是对急性者敏感性可达到 100%。MSCT 具有更快速、更大范围、各向同性容积数据采集的能力，同时图像后处理具有更方便、快捷、安全等特点，能够通过强大的三维后处理技术获得高质量的门静脉系统血管全面清晰的图像，不仅可以从任意平面观察栓子的分布范围和管腔内情况，还可以清晰显示门静脉系统走行、门 - 体间侧支循环、测量管腔内径，以及了解腹腔内脏器情况。

第八章　门脉癌栓

第一节　原发性肝癌门脉癌栓

门静脉内栓塞(血栓、癌栓)最常见于伴有肝细胞癌或不伴肝细胞癌的肝硬化门脉高压病人,其次见于胰腺癌、胰腺炎、胆管炎及凝血功能障碍等。此外,还可见于腹部手术后,如脾切除术后可见到脾静脉栓塞向门脉延伸形成门脉主干栓塞。门脉癌栓在肝癌中的发生率为33.8%~90.2%,被认为是肝癌在肝内广泛转移的根源,是晚期肝癌的重要合并症。因此,早期确诊癌栓及其位置,对病变分期,治疗方案的选择和预后评估都具有重要意义

1. 病理病因学　门静脉癌栓的形成多为肝细胞癌侵犯门静脉的小分支,在其内形成微小癌栓,继而生长,伸延,扩展到段,叶,以及门静脉主干。门静脉主干的癌栓进一步生长蔓延,形成肠系膜上静脉或/和脾静脉的癌栓。肝细胞癌合并门脉主干癌栓,其腹腔积液出现率很高,可达80%以上。一方面是由于肝硬化及门脉高压的结果,另一方面肝细胞癌导致肝功能和全身情况恶化,门脉主干癌栓的形成又加剧了门脉高压,这样,腹腔积液很快出现或急剧增加,个别病例还出现肠道水肿。门脉主干癌栓的出现与肝细胞癌的类型有一定关系,一般认为,弥漫型最高,巨块结节型次之,再次为巨块型,结节型出现概率最低。通常是,病灶越大(直径大于10cm),病灶数目越多,主干内癌栓形成的概率亦越高,弥漫型癌栓形成的机会尤其多。

2. 影像学研究　门脉癌栓在CT、DSA和B型超声检查时呈现多种表现,部分征象具有一定的特征性。在CT增强扫描时,门静脉内出现低密度影或充盈缺损,经手术病理证实,为门脉癌栓的可靠而具特征性的征象。

CT:在CT平扫,门静脉主干内癌栓的密度与门静脉本身的密度并无明显差异,仅显示门脉直径增粗。增强扫描时,主要的CT表现为门脉主干内低密度影,与增强前影像比较无明显变化,少数可轻度强化,而形成管腔内低密度充盈缺损。这一类低密度影常延伸至门脉左支和右支或其中一个分支内。很难见到单纯门脉主干内癌栓而分支不受累的病例。

门脉主干旁多出现代偿性增粗的侧支静脉,向肝门伸延分布,部分病例可见胆囊周围静脉增粗呈网格状。侧支血管形成的多少与门脉癌栓形成的速度和门脉高压的程度有关。一般门脉癌栓的形成较为缓慢,且有不同程度的肝硬化和门脉高压,因此,绝大多数病例都有此类表现。门脉主干癌栓形成后,对门静脉壁增强的表现的认识,各学者意见不同。有的发现癌栓形成后,管壁增强的程度较其他静脉壁明显,认为是供应管壁的滋养血管代偿性扩张的结果。由于管腔内癌栓无强化,管壁相对呈较明显的强化,称之为管壁的环形强化表现。在主干尚未完全形成癌栓时,或癌栓的末端可见到癌栓表现为新月状的低密度影。

增强扫描的少见表现是门脉主干的癌栓延续到肠系膜上静脉和脾静脉,此外,偶尔还可见到肠道水肿。在CT平扫时,有的门脉癌栓可偶尔表现为密度不均或高密度影,增强后,门脉内呈充盈缺损,这可能是由于癌栓由肿瘤细胞和血栓混合形成所致。Mori等(1987)认为,CT平扫所示门脉内高密度影,若B型超声诊断门脉癌栓,则可确诊,不必再做CT增强扫描和X线血管造影。

X线血管造影:在X线血管造影时,大多数门脉癌栓表现为门脉内结节状充盈缺损,经手术病理证实,这是一个常见而可靠的特异性征象。

门脉内癌栓依其生长方式不同而有相应的X

线表现：

（1）索状型，肝动脉造影时，在动脉期 3~5 秒就可见门脉内显示数条线状影，提示门脉主干内癌栓形成，称作“线样征”。Okuda 等（1975）认为，“线样征”是由于对比剂进入癌栓的供血动脉，或对比剂逆流到癌栓和门脉壁间的腔隙所致。有作者认为，这些线条状透光影是癌栓内有多数与管径平行生长的新生血管所致。Marks 等（1979）报道，在 67 例肝癌病人中，17 例出现“线样征”的患者，经组织病理学检查，门静脉和肝静脉内均有癌栓形成。

（2）假腺管型：癌栓呈密度不均匀的充盈缺损。

（3）坚实型和硬化型：癌栓呈局限性生长，为圆形或椭圆形边缘清晰的充盈缺损。

当门静脉存在癌栓时，门静脉常有明显增粗，最粗的直径可达 3~4cm。在团块状充盈缺损出现时，缺损边缘有的可形成明显的弧形影，常出现于动脉造影早期，是诊断门脉主干癌栓的可靠征象，有作者称之为杯口征。

门静脉不显影，并不表示一定有门脉癌栓形成，这是值得注意的。

肝静脉内的癌栓：肝静脉内的癌栓与门脉内癌栓表现相似，其部位多在横膈与脊柱连接处的肝静脉内。

影响门脉癌栓影像诊断的因素：CT、DSA、B 型超声作为门脉癌栓的常规检查方法各有优缺点。CT 诊断门脉癌栓，若以增强扫描所见门脉内显示低密度影作为诊断标准，则其诊断特异性高。但是，在下列因素存在时，CT 的诊断敏感性则较低：①增强扫描图像质量差，如患者耐受性差，推注对比剂量少，或推注速度慢，增强扫描效果不良，则可造成癌栓显示不清；② CT 扫描未扫到癌栓所在层面，如病人呼吸配合不佳，或扫描层距较大，或有癌栓的门脉走向与扫描层面平行，导致未能显示有癌栓的平面，造成误诊或漏诊；③癌栓位于门脉三级分支。有作者指出，CT 扫描主要用于诊断门脉主干或一级分支内的癌栓。训练病人良好屏气，采用薄层扫描或重叠扫描，可减少误诊和漏诊。

X 线血管造影在门脉癌栓诊断敏感性方面，较 CT 为高，但是，血管造影也受呼吸、减影质量等因素的影响。血管造影在特异性方面较 CT 为差，主要因为将“门脉不显影”作为诊断门脉癌栓的征象特异性低。因为，除门脉癌栓外，还有多种因素可引起门脉不显影，而在血管造影上却难以鉴别。

B 型超声可多层面灵活探查，且癌栓与血液界面间声阻抗差大，故对门脉癌栓诊断的敏感性高于 CT 和 DSA。B 型超声可根据门脉内血流信号和血液内异常强回声光团来判断门脉内癌栓和门脉高压是否存在。因此，对 DSA 不能鉴别是癌栓阻塞门静脉，还是门脉高压引起的门脉不显影的病例，B 型超声可协助诊断。然而，B 型超声也存在诊断的局限性，由于受腹腔积液，影像重叠等因素的影响，其特异性远不如 CT。

Okuda（1987）认为 B 型超声对门脉内癌栓的检出率最高，其次是血管造影，CT 最次，它们对三级门脉内癌栓的发现率分别是 71.4%、28.6% 和 14.5%

在门脉癌栓的三种常规检查方法中，CT 和 B 型超声为非损伤性的，若以 B 型超声作为筛选手段，以 CT 作为辅助确诊，则可望提高门脉癌栓影像诊断的准确性。

第二节　门脉癌栓与血栓的超声检查

Furuse（1992）报道 21 例肝细胞癌合并门静脉癌栓，并与 14 例门静脉血栓进行比较，发现：①采用连续闪烁阈值（FFT）检查和彩色血流图均证实癌栓比血栓更常见到血流；②脉冲波和逆向连续波是癌栓的特征性表现；③癌栓的血流信号类型可能与 X 线血管造影术显示的线性和条纹征及门动脉侧支形成征象有关。

第九章　门脉先天异常和发育变异

第一节　门静脉先天畸形

Fraser-Hill 等(1990)应用双功能彩色多普勒超声研究了不同类型的门静脉畸形,包括门静脉左支畸形和门静脉右支畸形两大类。

门静脉右支畸形:门静脉右支畸形包括四种右支主干完全缺失的不同类型,具体如下:①门静脉主干分为右后支、右前支及门静脉左支等三支;②门静脉主干分为右前支和门静脉左支,右后支起源于门静脉主干;③门静脉主干分为右后支和左支,右前支起自于门静脉左支,2 型和 3 型是借右后支分出后门静脉的延续方向来区别的,向右为 2 型,向左为 3 型;④门静脉右支及其分支完全缺失,这种畸形与肝右叶缺失相关。其他相关表现有尾叶和左叶内段的代偿性肥大以及门静脉左支水平段更长。另外,可能伴有膈下胆囊。如果肝右叶发育不良,可能其内有源自门静脉主干的细小分支。

门静脉左支畸形:门静脉左支畸形常是由左支水平段缺失引起。此时,门静脉左支存在着长度不同的垂直部。门静脉左支畸形中,门静脉左支的血液多来自肝实质内门静脉右前支和门静脉左支垂直部之间的一条连接血管。

肝内门静脉畸形:在 Atri 等(1992)报道的一项前瞻性研究中,肝内门静脉畸形主要有如下几个方面:①三支门静脉,占 10.8%;②门静脉右后支起始于门静脉主干,占 4.7%;③右前支起始于左支,占 4.3%;④门静脉左支水平段缺失,占 0.2%。这组无右支缺如病例。

门静脉闭锁和门静脉主干先天性狭窄:门静脉闭锁和门静脉主干先天性狭窄非常罕见。这些变异在下面两种情况下显得十分重要:一是拟行肝脏手术时,二是与慢性门静脉栓塞进行鉴别时。在大多数门静脉栓塞的病例中,栓塞的门静脉依然可见;相反,在上述畸形中相关的门静脉常常缺如。

第二节　先天性门 - 腔静脉分流畸形

先天性门 - 腔静脉分流畸形是由于门静脉系统发育异常所致的一种十分少见的肝外门静脉系统血液分流入体静脉系统的畸形,Abernethy(1793)首次报道。有作者统计,国外文献共报道 50 例,其中 I 型 42 例,Ⅱ型 8 例。

一般认为,先天性门 - 腔静脉分流畸形是由于门静脉在胚胎过程中发育异常所致的一种罕见先天性肝外门体静脉分流畸形。在妊娠第 4~10 周时,卵黄静脉系统的肠周卵黄静脉丛有选择性的退化和保留形成门静脉。在此过程中,如果退化和保留发生异常,就可能产生各种畸形,如过度退化会导致先天性门静脉缺如。

先天性门 - 腔静脉分流畸形的共同特点是门静脉系统的血液不流经或少量流入肝脏,而大量分流入体静脉系统。一般临床症状轻微,常在儿童患者中偶然发现,肝功能正常或轻度异常,无肝硬化和门脉高压体征。

Morgan 和 Superina(1994)对先天性门 - 腔静脉分流畸形进行了分型:Ⅰ型,完全型门体静脉分流,肝脏不接受门静脉灌注,即 Abernethy 畸形;Ⅱ型,部分型门体静脉分流,肝脏接受部分门静脉血的灌注(如门肝静脉吻合)。Ⅰ型又被分为 2 个亚型:

Ⅰa型，肠系膜上静脉和脾静脉不汇合，分别汇入体静脉系统；Ⅰb型，肠系膜上静脉和脾静脉汇合形成门静脉干后汇入体静脉系统。Ⅰ型绝大多数为儿童，多见于女性，常伴有其他先天畸形，如胆系闭锁、多脾、心脏缺陷及肝肿瘤等，其门静脉系血液可分流至上腔静脉、下腔静脉、左肝静脉、右心房、髂静脉、左肾静脉等。Ⅱ型更为罕见，以男性为主，极少伴发其他先天畸形，肝肿瘤少见。已报道8例Ⅱ型病例中，男6例，女2例，均为门静脉主干与下腔静脉形成侧-侧吻合，伴肝内增生结节2例。

有作者报告一例为一成年女性，临床症状无特殊，肝功能轻度异常，B超检查仅见肝右叶丰富动脉血流信号之低回声团块及格林森鞘增厚。CT平扫见肝内稍低密度肿块，强化明显，提示为富血供肿瘤。其内星芒状低密度区显示清楚，且见脾门附近扭曲增多的血管及门脉主干较细。

MRI检查T1WI肿块周边呈厚环状稍高信号，中心为星芒状低信号，T2WI肿块中心为星芒状明显高信号。延迟增强扫描见肿块周边及中心均显强化。综合此肿瘤的影像表现为多血供、较均质及有中心星状瘢痕，提示为局灶性结节增生，后经穿刺活检病理学证实。

3D-CE MRA见门静脉系的血液通过迂曲扩张的肠系膜上静脉分支及胃冠状静脉分别引流向肾动脉下方的下腔静脉及上腔静脉，肠系膜上静脉、脾静脉、门静脉主干及肝内分支均显细小，肝脏仍接受少量门静脉血流的灌注，符合Ⅱ型先天性门-腔静脉分流畸形。但该病例有许多独特之处：①年龄与性别：该病例为19岁成年女性，而Ⅱ型以男性儿童多见，成人仅1例报道。②门静脉系血液与体静脉汇合的方式：该病例发育不良的门静脉主干并不直接与腔静脉发生侧-侧吻合，大量门静脉系血液从肠系膜上静脉、脾静脉经迂曲扩张的异常血管分别引流至体静脉，与Ⅰa型的门体静脉联系方式相似。③并发肝肿瘤：该病例并发肝内局灶性结节增生。

Ⅱ型病例中，仅有2例报道并发肝脏增生结节，并发局灶性结节增生者未见报道。而在Ⅰ型病例常并发肝肿瘤，并发局灶性结节增生者10例。所以该病例虽属先天性门-腔静脉分流畸形Ⅱ型，但具备许多Ⅰ型的特点，介于Ⅰ型与Ⅱ型之间，提示先天性门-腔静脉分流畸形的分型值得进一步研究。

并且不同的检查方法也可能对其分型产生影响。Kalifa等（1978）报道1例3岁男孩的Ⅱ型病例，经下腔静脉将导管插入肠系膜上静脉造影，显示出了发育不良的门静脉，而经肠系膜上动脉行门静脉造影，却不能显示出门静脉。这就提示，有些本属于Ⅱ型的病例可能由于检查方法不全面而错误地归于Ⅰ型。

至于先天性门-腔静脉分流畸形并发局灶性结节增生的机制还不十分清楚，一般认为是由于门静脉系的血液分流入体静脉，导致肝脏缺乏门脉血的灌注，对肝脏发育、功能及再生能力产生影响，从而发展为结节性增生、肝癌、其他良恶性肿瘤及肿瘤样病变。总之，先天性门-腔静脉分流畸形是一种十分罕见的先天畸形，随着检查设备和技术的进步，必将会有更多的病例得以诊断，对先天性门-腔静脉分流畸形认识也必将更加深刻而全面。

第三节　先天性肝内门静脉-肝静脉瘘

门静脉-肝静脉瘘属肝内门体静脉分流的一种类型，比较罕见，Golli等（2000）统计2000年以前肝内门体静脉分流的病例报道少于50例，其中约1/2病例继发于肝硬化门静脉高压。

近年来随着医学影像技术的飞速发展，特别是MSCT广泛应用于临床，病例报道数逐年增加。

Tanoue等（2003）将肝内门体静脉分流分为2种类型。第1种为肝内门静脉肝静脉通路型，该类型中常出现（69%）动脉瘤样的分流道，其中又分为单支分流道和多支分流道2个亚型，前者较多见，常不伴有肝硬化。第2种为肝内门静脉-肝周静脉通路型，其中亦分为肝内门静脉-肝周静脉-下腔静脉通路型和肝内门静脉-下腔静脉通路型2种亚型，后者常见，继发于肝硬化门静脉高压基础上。

一例属第1种类型的第一亚型，表现为动脉瘤样的分流道，无肝硬化病史。另外，该例病变部位符合Mayayo Sinués等（2004）报道的多位于肝脏周边部或肝包膜下。

肝内门体静脉分流的出现常继发于肝硬化、门静脉高压（约占40%以上），其他原因还包括外伤性、医源性及先天性等。

该例患者相关实验室检查结果证实无肝硬化,无外伤史及医源性损伤史,考虑为先天因素所致。其形成机制为胚胎期门静脉和肝静脉系统发育过程中两者间出现未闭合的交通支,出生后也未闭合,成年后偶然被发现。

肝内门体静脉分流的临床表现取决于其病因和分流量的大小,由肝硬化门静脉高压因素造成的肝内门体静脉分流,患者常出现低血糖症或血氨明显升高,并可继发肝性脑病;先天性肝内门体静脉分流患者多无临床症状,但部分分流量大者可出现精神障碍,少数发生低血糖。该例患者最终诊断盆腔炎治疗后很快康复,临床上无低血糖及肝性脑病。该病如分流量较小,无相关的脑病则不必治疗,但仍需监测血氨水平,饮食尽量减少蛋白质的摄入量。如分流量较大,出现脑病或肝功能损害则需要介入性血管栓塞治疗。

该病的诊断主要依靠影像学检查,其中彩色多普勒血流显像(CDFI)的优势在于可以显示病灶局部的血流方向及血液流率,有利于该病的诊断、鉴别诊断以及治疗方法的选择,并可作为随诊观察的重要检查方法。MRI 也可以很好地显示分流道及瘘口情况,但与 MSCT 相比,空间分辨率较低,检查时间相对较长是其不足之处。DSA 是目前诊断该病的金标准,但属有创性检查。MSCT 检查方便、快捷,具有多种图像后处理功能,可以准确、直观、多角度地显示病变全貌及分流道的走行和范围,是诊断该病的重要手段。

第四节 先天性门静脉缺如

门静脉血对维持肝细胞的功能,结构和再生具有重要作用,先天性门静脉缺如伴内脏的静脉回流到下腔静脉是一种极罕见的先天性异常。截至 1992 年,文献报道 9 例先天性门静脉缺如中 6 例有先天性心脏病(1 例右位心, 1 例永存动脉干和卵圆孔未闭,房间隔及室间隔缺损各 2 例), 3 例的下腔静脉异常,表现为奇静脉或半奇静脉与下腔静脉连续和左侧下腔静脉。经动脉门静脉造影对这种极罕见的异常病例的诊断是必要的。

Matsuoka(1992)报道 1 例 22 岁女性病人,因易疲劳而入院,肝脏肿大,盆腔扪及肿块,脊柱侧凸畸形,转氨酶升高,血氨降低。腹部 X 线照片示肝肿大,盆腔肿块和半侧椎体脊柱侧凸; CT 和超声图像示右肝叶内有一肿块,子宫纤维化,另有一非常短的门静脉引流到下腔静脉的肾上段。门静脉肝内分支也缺如;肝动脉造影示肝右叶肿瘤血供丰富;经肠系膜上动脉的门静脉造影证实肠系膜上静脉直接引流到肾上段下腔静脉,肠系膜上静脉肠系膜下静脉及脾静脉汇合如常,导管能通过下腔静脉插到内脏静脉;从肝右叶活组织检查表明在正常肝组织内无门静脉分支,病理检查肝内肿块为局灶性结节增生;盆腔肿块切除证实为子宫平滑肌瘤。

第五节 门静脉 - 系统静脉的腹膜后侧支通路

几个作者已报告从门静脉到系统静脉的侧支通道,称之为腹膜后管道。

Ishikawa 等(1980)介绍 6 例此类病案,均行 CT 增强扫描进行观察。这些潜在的侧支通道一般考虑大慨与胚胎心下静脉的发育有关。

Creed 等(1982)指出,此类无回声结构和囊性表现常见于淋巴瘤类病变,由于它们的均质性而与扩张的异常血管结构难以区别。如果出现搏动,实时超声可有助于区别。多普勒超声对观察流动甚有益处。

由于此侧支通道结构较大,常规不增强的 CT 平扫未能见到它与正常血管结构相关, CT 也难诊断。对于怀疑淋巴瘤者,如需摒除血管异常结构,增强扫描是必须的。

当发现门静脉高压伴存腹膜后包块时,应疑及有静脉曲张存在,此刻血管造影对于完全除外静脉曲张是十分必要的。

第六节　门静脉-腔静脉之间可能出现的侧支循环

门静脉重要的头向侧支循环有:胃左、胃短静脉→食管静脉丛→食管静脉→奇静脉;胃左、胃短静脉→膈静脉→纵隔静脉→头臂静脉;脾静脉→膈静脉→肋间静脉→奇静脉;脾静脉→腹膜后 Retzius 静脉→腰升静脉→奇静脉。

门静脉重要的尾向侧支循环有:肠系膜下静脉→直肠静脉丛→髂静脉→下腔静脉;脾静脉→腹膜后 Retzius 静脉→肾静脉;脾静脉→左肾静脉,脾静脉与左肾静脉短路发生率高达 15.7%;胃左静脉→左肾静脉,胃左静脉与左肾静脉短路发生率约占 5.6%。

腹膜后吻合:腹膜后吻合为肠系膜静脉与脊柱旁静脉网的连接,侧支循环走向上腔静脉与下腔静脉。

Sappey 静脉:在肝裸区,肝静脉有无数小支与体循环中的膈静脉吻合,被称为 Sappey 静脉。

Retzius 静脉:在腹膜后,肠系膜静脉分支及门静脉干和下腔静脉分支相吻合,称 Retzius 静脉,进入下腔静脉。Retzius 静脉是众多的,但典型的是很小的静脉,从器官无腹膜覆盖的表面,走行到体壁。诸如:升结肠、降结肠、十二指肠与胰腺、肝、以及来自于腹膜后的门静脉的支流(如脾静脉和肠系膜上静脉的一部分),这些小静脉使门静脉内血液进入腰静脉、下肋间静脉和腔静脉系统的膈支。Retzius 静脉连接门静脉系的脾支、系膜干与下腔静脉的分支。这些属于整个腹膜后的静脉侧支,位于腹部脏器周围,在膈与腹壁之间。

胃后静脉:胃后静脉出现率约为 62%,分布于胃后壁的上部,穿出胃壁处绝大多数都在距贲门 5cm 范围内,主干经膈胃韧带到膈下,然后经网膜囊后壁腹膜后向下注入脾静脉,此静脉位置隐蔽,常被忽略。大约 71% 的胃后静脉与胃后动脉伴行。

食管胃底处小静脉:食管胃底处小静脉汇合成一细小静脉支,离胃壁后,经小网膜囊壁层腹膜后汇入门静脉,其走行虽是胃左静脉的位置,但仅引流食管下段及贲门胃底部的血液,而胃壁绝大部分是由粗大的胃右静脉引流。

交通支:门脉系与腔静脉系之间有若干交通支,当门静脉内压力升高时,因血液的返流将引起交通支扩张。这包括胃底及食管下端;直肠下段及肛管;腹壁;腹膜后交通支。在腹膜后,许多肠系膜上静脉与肠系膜下静脉属支与下腔静脉属支相互吻合,亦称作 Retzius 丛。

腹膜后-椎旁静脉曲张:肠壁静脉(Retzius 静脉)及 Sappy 静脉与腹膜后-椎旁静脉相连,门静脉高压时呈丛状或蔓状扩张,平扫时可拟似腹膜后淋巴结肿大。

第七节　门静脉发育变异

门静脉分支的位点多变。有作者报告 32 例尸检,门静脉肝内分支者占 25.8%,在肝被膜处分支者占 25.8%,在肝外分支者占 48.4%。门静脉分支位点对肝内门体分流支架的放置非常重要,因为门静脉分支点是施行门静脉穿刺的最佳位点。

三分支型门静脉是尸检中最常见的门静脉变异,此类变异在进入肝门之后,门静脉主干立即分成左支、右前支和右后支。

在超声和经动脉门静脉血管造影 CT(CTAP)的研究中曾报道一种门静脉变异,即门静脉左支缺乏水平段。在此类变异中,流向肝左叶的血液来自于门静脉右前支发出的迷走血管。这些血管先形成门静脉左支的垂直段,然后形成正常分支。

在超声和 MRI 上描述过的其他门静脉变异,包括门静脉右前支或右后支起源于门静脉左支和整个门静脉右支缺如,导致肝右叶较小,并接受起源于门静脉左支的多支迷走血管供血。总之,门静脉的发育变异并非少见,识别这些变异有助于更好地进行病变定位和制订肿瘤切除的手术计划。

第八节 少见的副门脉形成

门脉发育变异,特别是少见的副门脉形成,文献上报道较少,一些作者报告在门脉 X 线造影中发现 6 例副门脉,它们均位于门脉主干的右侧,表现为与之并行的但管腔较细的另一条门脉,约为门脉主干管径的 1/5~1/3;2 例走行较直,4 例呈迂曲蛇行状,其长度与门脉主干相似或稍长;6 例均来自肠系膜静脉区,其中 4 例源于肠系膜上静脉,1 例源于肠系膜下静脉,1 例来源难以确定;其引流部位均为肝脏右叶。5 例门脉造影中胃冠状静脉同时显示,3 例引流入脾静脉,1 例引流入副门静脉,另 1 例有 2 支冠状静脉分别汇入脾静脉与副门静脉。成人门脉由胚胎卵黄静脉和脐静脉演变而成。胚胎期卵黄静脉与脐静脉之间存在多处吻合而呈丛状。由于血流动力学因素,血液有探索最直接通路的趋势。

在某些因素作用下,门脉系统可以发生发育变异。门脉肝外段少见的先天发育变异包括:重复门脉、十二指肠前门脉、小的静脉血管直接从邻近区域引流入肝以及副门脉形成等。

副门脉形成的临床意义主要表现于下述 12 个方面:

(1)外科分流术:适当的分流道大小的设计对于保障手术成功,且在达到满意分流效果的同时,降低发生肝性脑病的危险有着决定性意义。副门脉存在的情况下,设计分流道大小应将副门脉引流部分血液入肝这一点考虑在内。

(2)经颈静脉门 - 体静脉分流:术中从肝静脉穿刺门脉主支,有可能穿中副门脉。在这种情况下,若不了解存在此种发育变异,而将副门脉误为门静脉继续操作,即使在肝静脉至副门脉之间建立了分流道,由于副门脉管径细小,血流量少,亦将因分流量不足而不能起到充分降低门脉压力的作用。

(3)胃冠状静脉栓塞:胃冠状静脉汇入副门脉或部分汇入副门脉,将给栓塞带来很大困难,使栓塞无法进行或栓塞不完全。门脉高压时,胃冠状静脉形成离肝性血流,成为胃底食管静脉曲张的主要供血血管。经颈静脉门 - 体静脉分流中,同时行胃冠状静脉栓塞,对于胃底静脉曲张破裂引起急症大出血患者的抢救,以及经颈静脉门 - 体静脉分流后再出血的预防均有重要意义。

动脉性门脉造影 CT 中肝实质染色不均的可能原因:副门脉的存在有可能解释动脉性门脉造影 CT(CTAP)中局灶性肝实质染色不均匀现象。副门脉与门脉在对比剂浓度上和时相上的差异,可能是造成其各自供血区在动脉性门脉造影 CT 中表现染色浓度不均的原因之一。

第九节 门静脉先天性异常

门静脉系统的先天性异常可以直到成人都未被发现。当由于其他原因进行影像学检查时,意外发现门静脉系统的先天性异常可引起诊断的混淆,熟悉正常解剖情况与它们的先天异常,有助于我们正确解释门静脉系统的影像表现。

正常解剖:脾静脉、肠系膜上静脉与肠系膜下静脉在胰颈后方汇合形成门静脉,门静脉收集胃肠道腹段、胆囊、胰腺以及脾脏的血液,汇集进入肝脏。门静脉通过肝十二指肠韧带上升到达肝门,而分为左、右侧门静脉。在横断面影像上,右侧门静脉及前、后侧分支通常在同一平面。在该层面或向头侧上一层面可见到左侧门静脉,左侧门静脉水平走行一短段后转向头侧,然后水平分支到肝左叶的外段和内段。

十二指肠前门静脉:此类异常是由肠旋转异常和胰腺、脾、或心脏的先天异常造成。十二指肠前门静脉通过十二指肠或胰头的前面,因此,在 CT 和 MRI 图像上在胰头前可清晰地看到一圆形结构。

双门静脉:为少见的发育异常,系两个分离的门静脉上升到达肝门。在影像学上表现为肝门结节或团块状病变,不要与其他实质性疾病如淋巴结肿大相混淆,CT 增强扫描对于区别血管结构与其他病理性情况常有帮助。

门静脉瘤:可为先天性病变,是少见的实质性疾病。CT 增强扫描时，门静脉分支示踪可以区别门静脉瘤与高血供肿瘤。门静脉瘤亦可由动脉 - 门静脉瘘和门静脉高压引起。

肝外的门静脉瘤潜在的并发症包括：栓塞、破裂以及局部的压迫。

肠系膜上静脉转位：在横断面图像上，肠系膜上静脉通常位于肠系膜上动脉的右前方。相反，在中肠转位不良的患者，肠系膜上静脉常位于肠系膜上动脉的左前方。当肠系膜上静脉和肠系膜上动脉移位出现时，多提示肠转位不良。然而，肠系膜上静脉和肠系膜上动脉移位，也可由腹腔包块引起。

门静脉属支的变异：门静脉系统及其属支，包括胆囊和胃冠状静脉之间的交通支变异，必须充分认识，因为这些畸形静脉引流，在 CT 增强扫描时，可导致肝内假性病变。这些畸形静脉能直接交通肝左叶内段的外周门静脉血管，或左侧门静脉，而不是直接引流到右侧门静脉，或门静脉主干。在此区域内，动态 MR 扫描的动脉相或螺旋 CT 扫描，偶尔可见到这些门静脉属支变异所产生的早期强化的假性病变，乃因从这些迷走的静脉引流通过门 - 腔静脉分流，而比之于通过门静脉系统，更迅速进入肝脏。这些高灌注异常不能误认为疾病。

肝内门 - 腔静脉分流：在横断面图像上，可以看见肝内门 - 腔静脉分流，但较肝外门 - 腔静脉分流少见。这些分流可引起脑病。在 Mori 等（1987）报道一组 16 例病人中，有 11 例出现脑病，足见影像诊断的重要性。

肠系膜血管畸形：少见，其原因尚不清楚。尽管少见，但是当患者发生胃肠道出血而无门静脉高压时，应考虑到此畸形的存在。

第十章　关于门腔静脉间隙

第一节　门腔静脉间隙

门腔静脉间隙是上腹部的一个重要解剖结构，其影像学价值自 Kenneth 等(1985)首次应用 CT、MR 进行研究以来，逐渐为人们所熟悉。

门腔静脉间隙的解剖结构：门腔静脉间隙是门静脉和腔静脉之间的一个狭窄间隙，理论上讲，门腔静脉间隙是一个不规则立方体结构，有相对明确的边界，在不同体位的 CT 像上，其范围相对固定。

在 CT 轴位像：前缘为门静脉后壁，后缘为腔静脉前壁，左缘为门腔静脉左缘连线，右缘为门腔静脉右缘连线。冠状位：上缘为门静脉分叉的水平线，下缘为脾静脉与肠系膜上静脉汇合处水平线。矢状位：上缘为门静脉断面上缘水平线，下缘为胰腺断面下缘水平线。

解剖学上门腔静脉间隙由三部分组成，分别是：①门静脉后间隙：为门静脉后壁与网膜囊前壁腹膜之间的间隙，内含淋巴结、胆总管、副右肝动脉和胰十二指肠上后动静脉血管等。门静脉后间隙淋巴结主要有两组：网膜孔淋巴结和胰十二指肠上淋巴结，引流肝内外胆管的淋巴液。②腹膜内间隙：实质上就是网膜孔所在的位置，是小网膜囊与腹膜腔之间的通道。③腔静脉前间隙：为网膜囊后壁腹膜与腔静脉前壁之间的间隙，其内主要有肝尾状叶的乳状突和尾突，副神经节及脂肪组织等。

正常门腔静脉间隙的影像表现：

(1)血管：最常见的是源于肠系膜上动脉的副肝右动脉，显示率为 15%~23%，其次是肝右动脉的尾叶支、胰十二指肠上后动静脉，肝固有动脉一般行走在门静脉的腹面，部分变异的肝右动脉有时也会行走在门腔静脉间隙内。肝右动脉和副肝右动脉均可在通过追踪其起源而辨认出来，其余血管基本不易分辨，只能根据解剖部位和走行方向进行推测。

(2)胆管：肝外胆管在门静脉的侧后方下行，进入胰头，汇合主胰管，正常管径的胆管在轴位上显示率约 3%，需要从多层面或多平面重建进行观察，扩张的胆管则非常容易观察。

(3)尾状叶：门腔静脉间隙不同水平的层面，内容不尽相同，在较高层面上，主要是尾状叶。尾状叶是门腔静脉间隙内最大的结构，一般它位于肝右叶后上边缘，密度等同于肝脏密度，形态变化很大，从长条形到圆形或不规则形均可见到。由于形态变化，有时尾状叶在轴位像上与肝右叶呈分离状态，此时应进行多层面观察分析，或者结合冠状位和矢状位图像观察，以免将尾状叶误认为淋巴结。

(4)网膜孔：正常情况下网膜孔在 CT 上并不能显示，但可以根据解剖结构分析其位置，它位于肝后间隙与左侧的小网膜囊之间，在轴位上为一横行的狭长间隙，但当患者出现腹水或气腹时，CT 通常可以清晰显示，表现为局部液体或气体密度影，形态为横行条状。

上腹部病变对门腔静脉间隙的影响：尾状叶增大：尾状叶增大常见于肝硬化、肝静脉阻塞和占位性病变，肝硬化患者尾状叶增大多由于肝细胞再生引起的肝叶比例失调所致；由于尾叶引流静脉直接汇入下腔静脉，肝静脉阻塞一般不直接引起尾叶变化，但是长期病变常导致右叶萎缩，尾状叶代偿增大。由于解剖上尾状叶紧邻胃窦、门静脉、肝总动脉和胰头，因此尾状叶增大常推压邻近器官组织，引起变形和移位，除此之外，尾状叶增大有时伴有本身密度的改变。

尾状叶增大的评价方式及诊断标准文献报道较少，近年来有学者认为 MSCT 的容积扫描，自动或手工测量肝脏体积，精确度较高。然而不同个体尾状叶的体积和形态差异很大，国内外报道正常人群肝脏体积的绝对值差异也较大，可能与被检者的身高、年龄、体重和体表面积有关。显然用体积的绝对值来衡量尾状叶的变化，可信度较低。有作者采用尾状叶与肝右叶体积之比来衡量尾状叶的大小，排除了身高和体重等影响因素，有一定的科学价值，可信度较高。以超过 0.1 作为尾状叶增大的诊断标准，是因为国内外对正常人群的观察结果均不超过 0.1，更客观的评价方法和标准有待于进一步的研究和探讨。尾状叶与肝右叶分离时，应注意与门腔静脉间隙淋巴结及邻近病变的直接侵犯进行区别，除进行多层面及多平面图像观察分析外，尚可结合组织密度及增强时 CT 值的变化进行鉴别。

血管迂曲增多：走行于门腔静脉间隙内的血管较少，CT 检查时偶尔见到，一般不超过 2 支。上腹部病变患者出现门腔静脉间隙血管增多，主要是由于门静脉主干栓塞或发育异常，引起门静脉海绵样变或侧支引流静脉增多所致，恶性肿瘤引起侧支供血动脉增加亦可导致门腔静脉间隙内血管影增多。

综上所述，门腔静脉间隙内含有一些重要的组织结构，上腹部良恶性疾病在一定时期会引起门腔静脉间隙内的组织结构发生改变，正确认识门腔静脉间隙内组织结构的正常表现及病变征象，有助于上腹部多种疾病的影像诊断。

第二节　门腔静脉间隙淋巴结

无明显上腹部病变的患者中 70% 左右在 CT 像上可见门腔静脉间隙淋巴结。

网膜孔淋巴结可通过走行在肝十二指肠韧带内的肝固有动脉和门静脉来辨认，它一般位于门静脉的侧后方，而肝固有动脉在此平面越过门静脉向前走行。

正常门腔静脉间隙淋巴结在轴位上呈卵圆形或矩形，边缘规则，前后径明显小于横径，其前后径最大不超过 1.3 cm，密度近似邻近的胰腺、胆管或尾叶的乳状突。80% 的正常淋巴结不强化，显示为低密度。

门腔静脉间隙内的淋巴结主要是网膜孔淋巴结和胰十二指肠淋巴结，其增大的诊断标准有多种，有些学者采用 1.0 cm 作为正常上限，也有作者认为短径超过 1.5 cm 才能认定淋巴结增大，因而报道门腔静脉间隙淋巴结增大的发生率也不相同，最高可达 89%。

有学者通过影像和病理对照研究，其结果表明用 1.3 cm 作为标准，假阳性率最低。

采用前后径 >1.3 cm 这一诊断标准，同时结合淋巴结的形态轮廓和密度改变，综合评价门腔静脉间隙淋巴结的改变，阳性率为 66.7%。

在实际分析过程中，除前后径超过 1.3 cm 外，淋巴结呈不规则外形或分叶，出现低密度中心，也是诊断淋巴结病变的依据，尤其当淋巴结中心出现低密度时，无论其形态和大小如何，均可被认为是淋巴结病变。不同病变引起淋巴结改变的形式及影像表现基本相同，组织病理学研究表明，除淋巴瘤外，无论良、恶性病变，其淋巴结改变的病理变化均为反应性增生，极少数为病变的恶性浸润和转移。

第三节　门腔间隙

门静脉与下腔静脉之间的较小的间隙称为门腔间隙。门静脉是在第二腰椎平面由脾静脉与肠系膜上静脉汇合而成，然后经肝十二指肠韧带走向肝门进入肝内。下腔静脉是在第 4、5 腰椎水平由左、右髂总静脉汇合形成，沿着腹主动脉右侧上行，穿过十二指肠第一段与胰头后方，再经肝右叶与尾叶之间的腔静脉窝、横膈，到达胸腔。

门腔间隙内的结构：在门腔间隙内有许多解剖结构：肝尾叶的尾突与乳状突、门腔淋巴结、副右肝静脉或替代右肝静脉、胰十二指肠上后血管、胆囊管和网膜孔。

肝尾突与乳状突：尾叶位于肝脏的后上方，左侧被横裂（静脉韧带裂），下方被肝门，右后侧被腔静脉沟所限制。在肝门平面，尾叶经尾突与肝右叶相连续。尾突为一尾状突起，它构成网膜孔的上缘，位于门静脉与腔静脉之间，是门腔间隙内的最大的解剖结构。尾叶左下方有一圆形突起——乳状突，它向前下伸入门腔间隙的内侧缘，并可以位于腹腔动脉的起始处的前方尾叶属于左半肝，但尾突的血液供应来自于门静脉右支。

Auh 等（1984）对 50 例正常肝脏的 CT 图像与 5 具尸体进行研究，得出肝尾叶的解剖与 Gray's 解剖学陈述的基本相同，但他提到乳头突可伸向左前方并折入小网膜囊上隐窝。他还提到尾突与乳头突之间可有一条小沟，在横断面解剖尸体上与 CT、MRI 图像上出现尾突与乳头突不相连，乳头突表现为一孤立的卵圆形软组织影，而可能被误认为胰头或门腔淋巴结病变或肝外病变。Dodds（1990）曾对肝尾叶的解剖，胚胎演变及病理学进行讨论，文中也提到肝尾叶尾突与乳头突在 CT 图像上的特殊表现的解剖基础。

门腔淋巴结：Zirinsky 等（1985）通过研究 5 具尸体与 123 例 CT 图像，认为 CT 图像上门腔淋巴结的显示率为 102/123，并指出正常的门腔淋巴结在横断图像上为卵圆形或长形结节影，类似于邻近的胰腺组织、胆系组织或肝尾叶尾突或乳状突。

异常的门腔淋巴结也呈卵圆形或长形结构，但趋向于分叶或呈现外形不规则。正常门腔淋巴结的最大前后径的上限为 13mm。在 CT 图像上，绝大多数门腔淋巴结的 CT 密度值低于门静脉和腔静脉。MRI 显示门腔淋巴结的信号强度介于门静脉、腔静脉与胰腺组织之间。

Engel（1989）认为网膜孔淋巴结也即门腔淋巴结。Dorfman（1991）在 CT 图像上测量上腹部淋巴结后提出，正常门腔淋巴结的最短径的上限为 10mm。

门腔血管：门腔血管包括副右肝静脉或替代右肝静脉，胰十二指肠血管弓的分支。副右肝动脉在大多数情况下来源于肠系膜上动脉，并且常常走行于小网膜内，位于门静脉与胆管的后方进入肝内。副左肝动脉或右肝动脉也可起源于胃十二指肠动脉或主动脉，可与肝动脉的正常分支一起成为肝脏的供血动脉，也可替代肝动脉成为一部分肝脏的唯一供血动脉而被称为异常替代动脉。右肝动脉可起源于肠系膜上动脉并走行于肝十二指肠韧带内，位于门静脉的后方。胰十二指肠血管是胃十二指肠血管发出的胰十二指肠上后血管，与肠系膜血管发出的胰十二指肠下后血管，在胰头后方形成胰十二指肠后血管弓，以及胰头前方的胰十二指肠前血管弓构成。尸体解剖或 CT 扫描门腔血管的显示率均不高。

胆囊管：左、右肝管在肝门末端发出，在肝动脉的前方向下走行后汇合成肝总管，右肝管垂直下行，左肝管斜向左上方行走，两者呈 V 字型于肝门处联合。肝总管在小网膜的右侧游离缘下行约 25mm 后，胆囊管呈锐角加入形成胆总管。有时胆囊管也可在肝十二指肠韧带内下行一段距离后再汇入胆总管。在这种情况下，胆囊管可伸向门静脉的后外方或门静脉后方、腔静脉前方，也即在门腔间隙内。

网膜孔：小网膜是由肝门移行至胃小弯和十二指肠上部的双层腹膜构成。它由左和右两部分组成，连接肝与十二指肠上部的部分称为肝十二指肠韧带，它构成小网膜的游离缘，其中含有三个重要结构，即位于最右侧并紧靠小网膜右缘的肝外胆总管，其左侧的肝固有动脉以及位于两者之后的门静脉。肝十二指肠韧带为网膜孔的前缘，下腔静脉与覆盖在其前面的腹膜构成网膜孔的后界，在此，网膜孔位于门静脉与腔静脉之间。

在异常情况下，可出现三类情况：（1）门腔间隙内某些解剖结构的病变可引起门腔间隙内的结构改变，诸如肝尾突肿瘤，脓肿，网膜孔积液或积脓、门腔淋巴结肿大等。

（2）邻近脏器如肝、胆、胰、十二指肠、胃的病变也可侵犯到门腔间隙。

Baker（1987）报道胆系癌、肝细胞癌、胆囊癌均可出现肝门或肝十二指肠韧带包块。

Tsutomu Araki 与 Engel（1988）分别报告了肝细胞癌最常出现的腹腔淋巴结肿大为门静脉淋巴结（即门静脉行径中的淋巴结）；胆系癌最易侵犯网膜孔与胰十二指肠上后淋巴结。

Mori（1989）认为，当肝的脓肿、血肿、胆汁瘤邻近肝门或 / 和肝十二指肠韧带时可扩散到肝十二指肠韧带，他还指出邻近肝门处的胆系病变也可扩散到肝十二指肠韧带。

（3）远处器官和全身性疾病也可侵犯门腔间隙。Meyers（1987）指出，胃癌、食管癌、肺癌以及淋巴瘤均可出现肝十二指肠韧带淋巴结肿大。同年 Baker 也指出，转移性疾病与淋巴瘤 / 白血病均可出现肝门与肝十二指肠韧带包块。

第四节　门腔间隙病变

详见本书 腹盆下卷 第一篇 第八章 第七节　门　　腔间隙病变。

第十一章 门静脉瘤

第一节 门静脉瘤

静脉瘤常发生在腘静脉、颈静脉、隐静脉,门静脉瘤(PVA)临床罕见,约占全身静脉瘤的3%。Barzilai等(1956)首次以个案报道该病。病理改变为门静脉瘤壁的内、中膜变薄以及结构的破坏。发病原因尚不十分清楚,可分为先天性与后天性。

病因:一般认为先天发育异常是其主要原因,Yang等(2003)报道的18例门静脉左支门静脉瘤中40%都合并有门静脉变异,与正常组门静脉变异发生率间的差异存在统计学意义;Gallagher等(1993)及Gomez等(2004)报道的2例宫腔内胎儿门静脉瘤病例更加支持此观点。

而后天性的患者往往有胰腺炎、门脉高压、外伤、肿瘤等病史,Ozbek等(1999)与一些作者的报道表明门静脉高压与门静脉瘤的发病有关但并非其发生的根本因素。

部位及分型:门静脉瘤多发生于肠系膜上静脉与脾静脉汇合处、门脉主干与肝内门脉分支的分叉处,这种分布可能与血管分叉处所受血流冲击力较大所致。

根据其发生部位分为肝内型、肝外型,临床上以肝外型多见。患者常无临床症状,多为体检发现或表现为轻微腹痛症状,若门静脉瘤伴随并发症,则会出现相应的临床症状与体征,如瘤体破裂、胆管受压则可出现梗阻性黄疸、胆汁淤积以及胆石症、血栓性门脉高压等。

一组所报道病例,为老年女性,临床表现无特殊,为常规检查偶然发现,增强MSCT未发现门脉变异,无门脉高压、外伤、胰腺炎等病史,亦无并发症的出现。

诊断标准:关于门静脉瘤的诊断标准,国内外文献报道不尽一致,门静脉的局限性增宽是诊断的主要依据。一些作者认为门静脉肝内或肝外段的局限性扩张,肝内段直径 >1.5 cm,肝外段直径 >2.0 cm,则可诊断门静脉瘤。但是门静脉在正常或者门脉高压时变化比较大,所以也有学者认为如果门静脉局部宽度明显大于相邻段的门静脉,尤其是异常增宽的门静脉呈梭形或囊状时可诊断为门静脉瘤。一般认为后者观点更具合理性。

影像学研究:CT平扫对门静脉瘤的确诊有困难,常需要结合增强CT,其强化表现是诊断门静脉瘤的主要依据,最大密度投影及容积再现重建能清楚、直观、全面地显示瘤体的来源、部位、形态、大小、与邻近结构关系、有无合并血管畸形及血栓形成等。

CT平扫门静脉瘤常表现为低密度,边界清楚,密度多较均匀,动态CT增强扫描后清楚显示门静脉管腔局部呈囊状或梭形扩张,强化时相同门静脉,且以门脉期显示最佳。

鉴别诊断:由于CT扫描技术及后处理技术的进步,门静脉瘤的诊断不难,主要与门脉高压所致的门静脉增宽相鉴别,前者主要为门静脉局限性的扩张,门静脉主干及其分支、属支一般无增宽,而门脉高压所致的门静脉增宽为弥漫性改变。

第二节 肝外型门静脉瘤

门静脉瘤临床较为少见。Barzilai 和 Kleckner(1956)首次报道。随着新的检查设备应用于临床,对该病的诊断数量逐年上升。关于发病原因有三种学说:主要是先天性血管缺陷,其他原因所致的门静脉高压、胰腺炎对胰腺周围血管壁的消化作用。

患者多无症状,体检时偶然发现,少数患者可出现腹痛症状。

门静脉瘤分为肝内型和肝外型两类,肝外型居多。肝外型的门静脉瘤多发生于脾静脉与肠系膜上静脉汇合处。该例属肝外型,发生于常见部位。门静脉大多表现为梭形和囊状扩张。

Doust 等(1976)研究发现在健康人群中,门脉最大径不超过 1.5cm,在肝硬化患者中不超过 1.9 cm。有学者提出门静脉瘤的诊断标准为肝外门静脉扩张超过 2.0cm,肝内门静脉横径超过 1.5 cm。

彩色超声、螺旋 CT、MRI、血管造影检查对该病均有很好的诊断价值。彩色超声可直接显示局部扩张的瘤体及瘤体内异常血流,同时还可以显示瘤体内有无血栓。

螺旋 CT 及 MRI 可直观显示瘤体的部位、形态、大小以及瘤体与周围组织结构的关系,同时还可评价肝脏、胰腺、脾脏实质脏器有无病变及其他血管发育异常,三维重建技术更能清晰显示瘤体的形态、大小、空间位置关系。两种方法可取代有创性血管造影检查。

第十二章　关于门静脉周围

第一节　门静脉周围的晕圈

肝三联(肝动脉、门静脉和胆管的统称)疏松结缔组织内积液或淋巴管扩张可导致门静脉周围晕圈的出现。这种晕圈表现为门静脉分支周围的低密度,可被误认为胆管扩张。两者不同的是,门静脉周围的水肿通常在门静脉分支的两侧,而扩张的胆管仅在门静脉的一侧,这是两者很重要的鉴别特征。尽管门静脉周围水肿的CT表现不具有特征性,但在充血性心力衰竭、肝炎、肝移植受体或肝外伤后的病人中,门静脉周围水肿是常见的异常征象。

门静脉周围淋巴结肿大或肿瘤,可因中心性淋巴管阻塞而出现门静脉周围晕圈。一旦门静脉周围晕圈在CT上被确认,应仔细寻找其可能的病因及相应的肝脏疾病。

第二节　门静脉周围脂肪

CT上门静脉周围脂肪也呈低密度,毗邻于门静脉分支,不要误认为扩张的中央胆管。门静脉周围脂肪除门静脉近端外不伸入肝实质。

第三节　门静脉周围窦性扩张和肝紫癜

门静脉周围窦性扩张和肝紫癜是由类固醇引起的肝内的血管性紊乱。前者多相关于口服避孕类固醇,后者则主要与男性激素、促合成代谢的类固醇有关。虽然有的学者相信这些疾病是单独的病理生理情况的一部分,但是介于两者之间的差别大概是专有的。

1. 病理学　在门静脉周围窦性扩张,肝的外表面为棕色,或浅蓝色,或为正常。镜下观,有扩张的血管窦,内衬以内皮细胞和枯否细胞,主要分布在门静脉周围地带。

在肝紫癜,肝的外表面显露大小不等的多发性蓝黑色的凸起。镜下观,在肝细胞被覆的陷窝间隙内充满血液。这些含血液的小池可与邻近的血管窦或肝静脉分支互相交通。

2. 临床表现　在门静脉周围窦性扩张的病人,除了肝肿大与血沉升高是恒定以外,表现的症状和体征是变化的。1/5的病人有腹痛,多半源于肝包膜膨胀。肝功能试验正常或轻度升高。在口服避孕剂停止之后,临床表现与生化指标有所改善。

肝紫癜传统地出现于有令人衰弱的疾病的病人,诸如:癌转移、结核病、糖尿病、以及慢性肾病。目前,本症还伴存于促合成代谢的男性激素和避孕类固醇的使用后。

然而,当其作为口服避孕剂的并发症出现时,它总是局限于邻近腺瘤处。常见肝肿大,而且黄疸和严重的肝功损害可以见到。肝功异常是肝紫癜的结果,还是基本疾病的表现,目前尚不清楚。由于紫癜的破裂进入腹腔,可能出现严重的腹痛。死亡可以是休克或肝功衰竭的结局。如果上述基本疾病能获得成功的治疗或未继续再用类固醇，肝紫癜可以逆转。

3. 影像学研究　核医学：在两类疾病，肝的硫胶显像均可显示肝肿大，局灶性缺损提示门静脉周围窦性扩张的肝内包块。虽然可能产生肝内血肿，但是为什么出现局灶性缺损，目前还不明白。

血管造影：肝静脉造影通常正常。肝动脉造影显示多发性小的造影剂聚集，其大小变化于仅仅肉眼可见到直径1厘米。此征象出现在动脉相晚期，而在实质相和静脉相时更为突出。有的病例在镜下显示门静脉周围窦性扩张，而在影像诊断却表现为肝紫癜。

在肝紫癜，血管造影显示征象类似于门静脉周围窦性扩张。个别病例，在肝血管造影片上，大多数紫癜间隙未显影而显示小的透光区。在脾门静脉造影片上，有作者报告少数小儿病例显示小的阴影，相当于紫癜池。

在肝动脉造影片，门静脉周围窦性扩张与肝紫癜的鉴别诊断，应当包括：主要是多发性的小的血管瘤，和遗传性出血性毛细血管扩张症的多发性毛细血管扩张。有的继发于使用促合成代谢类固醇的肝紫癜病人，在楔形肝静脉造影观察到，在血窦染色之前出现周围性间隙的6mm大小的丛团显影。在药物4个月后再重复检查，显示周围性间隙的消退，残余的0.5mm肝-门静脉管道考虑相当于持久存在的扩张的血管窦。

有的肝紫癜病人超声检查是有帮助的。如果口服避孕药是病因学因素，真正的诊断大概是门静脉周围窦性扩张。由于肝硫胶显像为多发性充盈缺损，肝功能又是正常，超声检查更有必要。超声可显示肝肿大伴一非特异性异质的实质性回声组织（有回声的和无回声的两者都有），在右叶表现最为突出。血管造影与活检对于肝紫癜的诊断是不矛盾的。

第四节　门静脉周围晕：肝病的一个CT征象

门静脉周围晕，是指增强CT影像中门静脉或亚段门静脉周围的环形低密度区。

Lawson（1993）复习3 777例腹部增强CT图像，并对照临床与实验室检查，经皮或手术活检结果等资料后指出，门静脉周围晕可能是肝门三管道（门静脉、肝动脉、胆管）周围疏松结缔组织内增多的液体或扩张的淋巴管。由于约80%的肝内淋巴经肝段淋巴管引流至肝门区，肝门肿物可能阻塞肝脏淋巴引流，造成远侧门静脉周围淋巴水肿，最常见于恶性淋巴结肿大，也可见于炎症与良性肿瘤。肝外伤患者可见出血引起的门静脉周围晕征。

充血性心力衰竭所致肝淤血，重度肝炎或小静脉阻塞性病变可造成肝脏淋巴生成过多，超过淋巴引流能力，继发门静脉周围水肿，形成门静脉晕征。肝移植后的门静脉晕征可能与术后淋巴管紊乱，淋巴向心性引流障碍有关。该作者认为，门静脉周围晕虽然无特异性，但确为一病理征象，应提示临床对肝脏全面检查，以找到可能存在的病因。

第五节　肝的门静脉周围的透光区或水肿

1. 病因　肝源性：急性肝炎、肝硬化、肝脓肿、肿瘤导致的继发性淋巴管阻塞、肝移植术后、肝外伤；非肝源性：中心静脉压力增高、低蛋白血症、菌血症、门静脉周围淋巴肿大、急性胆囊炎、急性胰腺炎、炎性肠病。

常见于：胆管扩张（假性）、全身血容量增多、肝淤血、急性肝炎、上行性胆管炎、肝移植术后、肝外伤；不常见于：肝门淋巴结病、肝硬化、肝门静脉栓塞、原发性硬化性胆管炎、脂肪肝、获得性免疫缺陷综合征（AIDS）胆管病、肝细胞癌、胆管癌、肝转移瘤及淋巴瘤。

2. 发生机制　任何增加肝细胞外液产生，或阻碍淋巴循环的因素，都能引起肝的门静脉周围水肿。发生机制为：门静脉周围疏松蜂窝组织易被水分充分膨胀。常见的水通路包括：淋巴管的淋巴液、胆管内的胆汁、血管内的血液。

3. 常见的诊断陷阱　将门静脉周围的水分误认为扩张的胆管;将栓塞的门静脉分支误认为胆管;鉴别诊断的主要手段是 MRCP 和 ERCP。

4. 有助于常用诊断的线索　胆管扩张:仅存在于门静脉的一侧;表现为肝的门静脉周围透亮区,又称为晕圈征(从晕圈征定义看,应围绕门静脉一圈,事实上不是一圈,而是一侧)。胆管梗阻也可引起肝的门静脉周围水肿;肝内胆管直径小于邻近肝的门静脉分支的一半。

全身血容量增多:血容量增多,例如创伤患者复苏后血流过快;肝产生的淋巴液多于淋巴管的引流量;还有一条线索是膨胀的下腔静脉。

肝的被动充血:充血性心力衰竭、缩窄性心包炎、三尖瓣关闭不全;导致肝的门静脉周围淋巴水肿;肝静脉与下腔静脉同时膨胀是一条线索。

急性肝炎:任何原因(包括酒精性、病毒性、毒物性);常导致明显肝的门静脉周围水肿和/或胆囊壁水肿。

上升性胆管炎:任何形式(包括上升性胆管炎、原发硬化性胆管炎、化脓性胆管炎),获得性免疫缺陷综合征胆管炎、化疗后胆管炎。其机制是胆管壁增厚,胆管周围水肿,胆管可能阻塞;任何一个因素都能引起或导致类似肝的门静脉周围水肿。

肝移植术后:移植过程中淋巴系统被分离;淋巴系统功能的重新启动需要一段时间;肝的门静脉周围水肿常见,且可持续数周。胆管坏死可作为肝移植的并发症出现;胆管仅有动脉供血,肝动脉狭窄或栓塞在梗死前引起胆管坏死;这些液体常填满肝内水分聚集的并行胆管。肝外伤:血流沿着肝门血管胆管束进入分支;可被误认为扩张的胆管或肝实质深部裂口;肝的门静脉周围血流并非肝外伤唯一表现,常局限于一个肝叶内的血肿或裂口。

5. 有助于不常用诊断的线索　肝硬化:可引起肝的门静脉周围水肿和/或类似的表现;可引起胆管周围囊肿(膨大的胆管周围腺体)。

门静脉栓塞:未强化的肝的门静脉分支可被误诊为扩张的胆管或肝的门静脉周围水肿;肝硬化(门脉高压)、高凝状态、门静脉血栓静脉炎等引起。

原发性硬化性胆管炎:引起胆管不规则狭窄及上游胆管扩张;胆管扩张可致类似肝的门静脉周围水肿征象;超声常见胆管壁变厚及门静脉周围水肿。

脂肪肝:血管周围区域表现类似水肿;在 CT 图像上常可导致误诊;脂肪变性在 MRI 和超声不会被误诊为水肿;在肝短轴断面常呈现为球形。

肝细胞性肝癌:常引起非特异的淋巴水肿和浸润或阻塞胆管或肝的门静脉;肝细胞性肝癌易侵犯肝的门静脉,可以寻找强化的瘤栓。

胆管癌:外围的或门静脉处的胆管;分枝状无强化结构的可能的病因(包括扩张的胆管、肝的门静脉周围水肿、增厚的胆管壁)。

肝转移肿瘤及淋巴瘤:任何肝脏恶性肿瘤都可引起淋巴过量渗出,导致肝的门静脉周围水肿;肿瘤阻塞胆管,有时难与部分病例的肝的门静脉周围水肿相鉴别。

第十三章　关于门静脉的影像检查技术

第一节　肝脏门静脉成像延迟时间选择

肝脏门静脉成像技术已在临床上得到广泛的应用,其成像技术的优化尤其是对正常人门静脉成像技术的优化已在多篇文献得到报道并取得良好的效果。

但对于肝硬化患者由于其一系列病理生理改变,使得门静脉成像质量较差。这一系列病理生理改变包括门静脉高压导致门静脉血流明显减慢,对比剂很难在门静脉内形成较高的峰值;肝内门静脉的分支明显变细,分支减少;大量侧支循环的开放使得对比剂从侧枝分流,而主干峰值降低;肝实质动脉血供增加,导致门脉期肝实质与门静脉密度差减小。

延迟时间选择的方法:延迟时间是门静脉成像技术的核心,是门静脉成像质量的关键。扫描时间过早,则门静脉强化不明显。扫描时间过晚则错过门静脉强化峰值,且肝实质与肝静脉均强化而影响门静脉图像的分辨率,造成诊断困难。

目前国内外对延迟时间的确定一般采用 3 种方式。

第一种技术是固定延迟时间,国内较多研究采用此种方式,其延迟时间从 40~70 s 不等,且均未区分正常人与肝硬化患者。此种方法虽然操作简单,但其并未考虑个体因素及生理及病理因素的影响,缺乏个体化设计。而一组研究发现当对比剂注射速度为 5 ml/s,延迟 60 s 扫描时,不仅错过门静脉强化峰值,而且肝静脉内对比剂浓聚,严重影响门静脉三维观察。

第 2 种技术是注射对比剂后监测门静脉内的 CT 值,当达到预先设定的阈值时即开始扫描。这一技术以 GE 公司的 Smart Prep 技术和飞利浦公司的 Bolus Tracking 技术为代表。它在一定程度上体现了门脉成像延迟时间的个体化,但也存在一定的缺点:阈值的设定,这一阈值就是门脉强化峰值而它本身受个体生理和病理因素的影响;对于门静脉内 CT 值的监测易受到呼吸运动、血管搏动等因素的影响,尤其是门静脉主干直径较小者更甚;一次注射对比剂无法完成对肝脏动脉期的扫描,将影响常规检查。

第 3 种技术即先注入小剂量(12~20m1)对比剂,采用同层动态扫描技术测定门静脉内的时间-密度曲线,找到门静脉密度的峰值时间后,再注入大剂量对比剂并在该峰值时间行门脉成像,这一技术以西门子公司的 Test Bolus 技术为代表。此项技术能在门静脉峰值时间进行扫描,不影响肝脏动脉期扫描,受呼吸及搏动影响相对较小。有作者曾采用此种方法(小剂量 20m1)未获得成功。

一组研究采用此项技术并加大对比剂剂量,采用对比剂 40 ml 注射,对 135 例纳入对象进行同层动态扫描均取得良好的效果。对于同层动态扫描层面的选择,根据以往研究结果及该组研究预试验,门静脉胰头部虽然受呼吸运动影响最小,但由于其接近门静脉起始部,而来自脾静脉与肠系膜静脉的血流常常混合不均,这会直接影响门静脉内的时间密度曲线的准确性。而肝门平面及其稍下方处门静脉主干直径大,受呼吸运动影响较小且门静脉内血液混合较均匀。故该组研究采用肝门平面作为同层动态扫描的标准层面。

对于患者所受辐射剂量问题,该组研究经计算后得出完成上述一次检查患者所受到辐射剂量远低于安全标准。故该组研究认为 Test Bolus 技术在肝内门静脉成像技术中是一项安全、易行,且能较好体现个体化设计的方法。

肝硬化患者门静脉扫描延迟时间的优化:门静脉延迟时间受多个生理因素的影响,包括每个个体的体型、体重、心输出量、基础代谢率、肝肾功能及对比剂注射速率等;该组研究在设计时也充分考虑了上述因素,故所纳入研究的肝硬化患者与正常人在身高、体重及年龄方面均无统计学差异。

同时该组65例肝炎后肝硬化患者与70例正常人主动脉强化峰值时间及峰值均无统计学差异,故大大减少了体型、体重、心输出量等因素对该研究的影响。该组研究采用Test Bolus技术对65例肝炎后肝硬化患者与70例正常成人组研究发现,在总剂量为40 ml,注射速度相同(5 ml/s)的情况下肝硬化患者门静脉强化时间(42.3 s)明显长于正常人(34.4 s),二者存在统计学差异。且肝硬化患者门静脉强化峰值明显低于正常人。

这一结果与其他作者的研究结果不同,但其他作者的研究中肝硬化患者仅12例,包括3种不同的肝硬化(肝炎后、血吸虫和酒精性),且并未对患者做出Child分级。而不同病因造成的肝硬化对肝内门静脉血流动力学的影响是不同的,故该组纳入的肝硬化患者均为肝炎后肝硬化。在该组研究中30例Child A级肝硬化患者门静脉平均延迟时间为40.5 s,而35例Child B、C级患者门静脉强化平均延迟时间为43.9 s。虽然该组中二者之间无统计学差异,但可以看出Child A级肝硬化患者门静脉平均延迟时间稍短于Child B、C级患者。

无论是肝硬化还是正常人其肝实质强化的峰值时间均落后门静脉15~20 s,这与以往研究结果相仿。而16层螺旋CT完成整个肝脏的扫描仅仅需要7~10 s,这就非常有利于门静脉成像延迟时间的设定。

肝硬化患者门静脉成像峰值与正常人有差异,在注射速度相同(5 ml/s)的情况下肝硬化患者门静脉强化时间(42.3 s)明显长于正常人(34.4 s),Child B、C级肝硬化患者门静脉强化峰值时间(43.9 s)稍长于Child A级肝硬化患者(40.5 s),但二者之间并无统计学差异。对于肝硬化患者肝内门静脉成像该研究推荐其延迟时间可采用Test bolus技术确定,或为43 s左右。

第二节 肝硬化合并不同病变对门静脉成像延迟时间的影响

详见本书 本卷 本篇 第一章 第一节 肝硬化合并不同病变对门静脉成像延迟时间的影响。

第十四章　门静脉其他疾病及活体形态学

第一节　门静脉积气

肝内门静脉积气，最常伴存于肠道的梗死。其他原因包括：溃疡性结肠炎、坏死性肠结肠炎、小肠梗阻、脓腔内脓肿、胃溃疡以及肺炎。门静脉积气的预后是不一定像以往想象得那么可怕。

X线检查：门静脉积气的放射学典型征象是肝内的树支状线条气体密度影，且多为较小的周围性分支的阴影。而在胆系积气，则倾向于汇集在中央区的较大的胆管内。这个差异的解释是，门静脉血流是离心性的，相反，胆汁流动则呈向心性。

门静脉积气在平片上的其他伴存征象包括，系膜血管内积气和/或肠壁积气。

超声检查：当腹部X线平片尚属正常时，超声能发现婴儿坏死性肠结肠炎的门静脉积气。门静脉积气的超声表现类似于身体它处的积气征象。光亮的线状或汇集的回声，伴存或不伴存声影，存在于门静脉主干及其分支，或在肠系膜上静脉内。

超声图像与X线平片一样，门静脉积气也是以周围性分支较为显著，而胆系积气则以中央区较为明显。不久以前，气体可能在实时检查时发现只是在门静脉内断断续续流动，高的回声，不恒定的细小气泡影。可能观察到肠蠕动与气泡的胀裂同时发生。这些细小气泡也能见于从周围血管优先地进入肝实质的非下垂部分。迅速流动的回声常常见于大血管内，这对于区别门静脉积气与正常情况说来是重要的。正常的回声一般振幅较低，而且为连续流动，它们源于红血球的集合。

CT扫描：对于门静脉积气的特别的搜寻，少有用CT扫描。通过CT图像，能鉴别门静脉积气与胆系积气，当在X线平片上两种积气均出现时。当然，在观察气体存在于门静脉和其他伴随的部位（系膜血管和/或肠壁）时，CT扫描比X线平片敏感得多。

第二节　门静脉受侵

门静脉受侵的X线血管造影表现有四：

（1）线样征或条纹征，这是门脉瘤栓的直接征象，具有可靠的瘤栓诊断价值。此征象的成因有二：①门脉瘤栓的血供源于肝动脉，因而出现于腹腔动脉-肝动脉造影的动脉期，在3.0~3.5秒时最为清晰；②在瘤栓内部，以及瘤栓与门脉壁之间，存在纵向走行的衬以单层内皮细胞的血液间隙，因而表现为沿门脉或其分支行走的一束纤细血管影。

（2）肝动脉-门静脉瘘。

（3）门静脉或其分支不显影，或出现充盈缺损。

（4）门静脉海绵样变性。

第三节　门静脉异常

Koc等（2007）分析研究了1212例患者的常规腹部CT图像，发现门静脉异常很常见，发生率为

27.4%，最常见的为门静脉呈三分叉状，共有 139 例（12.4%）。门脉分支缺如或血供异常很少见。下腔静脉异常的发生率为 23%，高于以前的研究结果。

第四节　门静脉造影的一些问题

Viamonte 等（1977）专门著文讨论经肝门静脉造影中的陷阱。

在此种造影时，肠系膜上静脉或门静脉内的充盈缺损，栓塞与肿瘤是常见的原因，但绝非唯一原因，某支动脉挤压上述静脉也可被误认为血管内病变所致的充盈缺损。

对于门静脉的某一肝内分支的隐蔽性闭塞，如果门静脉直接法造影在正位照片上未使所有肝实质充分显影，必须用侧位照片补充检查，否则，极易导致误诊。

门静脉造影时，肝的充盈缺损原因甚多，诸如：肝内血肿、恶性肿瘤（原发或继发）、错构瘤、囊肿、脓肿或血管畸形。动脉造影、核素显像、超声、CT 和针刺活检对这些充盈缺损病因的确定皆具重要价值。Fulenwider 等（1979）在外科杂志上评价门静脉血流的血流动力学问题，对门静脉造影时的门静脉假性灌注提出讨论，且认为它是一种血管造影的错觉。

第二十九篇　急腹症与腹盆创伤

第一章　急腹症

第一节　小肠梗阻

详见本书 本卷 第二十五篇 第七章　小肠　梗阻。

第二节　腹部空腔脏器穿孔MSCT

CT检查对腹部空腔脏器穿孔的定性诊断：腹腔游离气体是诊断腹部空腔脏器穿孔的可靠依据，X线检查有助于确定穿孔的存在，但不能确定其部位和原因。CT可迅速准确地判断腹腔游离气体，但常规腹部软组织窗（窗宽200 HU，窗位40~60HU）气体与脂肪均成低密度的黑色，难以区分腹内气体抑或脂肪，造成漏诊。此时，适当调节窗宽、窗位，特别是采用大窗宽、低窗位（窗宽500~800 HU，窗位-30~30 HU）则可容易区分腹腔内脂肪和气体。较大的窗宽，还能同时清晰地显示腹腔内的脂肪、积液、空腔器管壁及实质性脏器的边界。

可以认为，对急腹症疑有空腔脏器穿孔患者，全腹CT扫描图像同时采用常规腹部窗和大窗宽、低窗位两种窗技术进行观察非常必要，可以有效地避免仅有少量游离气体的腹部空腔脏器穿孔病例的漏诊。

一组15例中，1例乙状结肠粪块性肠梗阻，术前CT仅诊断为乙状结肠粪块性肠梗阻，遗漏了肠穿孔的诊断。回顾分析其原因就是因为仅采用常规腹部软组织窗观察，未能有效识别出腹腔和腹膜后游离气体。

CT对腹腔空腔脏器穿孔的定位诊断：一些作者所认定的剑突下隐窝（左、右肝上间隙及肝脏前方与腹壁下之间间隙的总称）是该组病例中游离气体征出现最多的部位，15例中有13例；其次是肝下肝圆韧带间隙，15例中有9例，此部位出现的游离气体量较少，呈小泡状沿肝圆韧带间隙排列。

该组病例肝下肝圆韧带间隙积气同时都伴有剑突下隐窝积气。以上两个部位的积气手术证实的穿孔部位从胃至乙状结肠、子宫均有发生。可见两者确是腹膜空腔脏器穿孔后气体容易积聚的部位，且容易辨认，但作为孤立的征象，其对穿孔部位的诊断价值有限。

该组病例中有4例出现小网膜囊区积气征，穿孔部位2例发生在十二指肠球部，2例发生在胃。因此网膜囊区积气征可作为是胃十二指肠穿孔定位的征象。

穿孔脏器周围局限性积气11例（含网膜囊区积气4例），根据气体所在部位，及伴随的肠壁增厚、肠腔周围脂肪间隙密度增高、积液、直观地显示脏器穿孔破裂口、异物等征象可以明确提示穿孔部位。其中直接显示脏器穿孔破裂口3例、异物（硬鱼骨）刺穿肠壁1例诊断价值最大。

值得注意的是，胃十二指肠溃疡穿孔由于疾病及周围解剖结构关系，除网膜囊区积气外，脏器周围局限性积气、邻近脂肪间隙密度增高或少量积液的征象不容易确定，但患者常有典型的溃疡病病史，结合临床资料，术前可以确诊。该组病例中有1例乙状结肠直肠交界处粪块性梗阻穿孔，出现了腹膜后间隙的大量游离气体。由于直肠上段是腹膜间位器官，其穿孔后气体逸出后可进入腹膜后间隙。因此CT出现腹膜后间隙的游离气体征应考虑十二指肠、升结肠或降结肠等腹膜间位或外位段肠管的穿孔。

CT 对腹腔空腔脏器穿孔的病因诊断及合并症的显示:腹部 X 线平片是急性腹部空腔脏器穿孔首选的检查方法,但通常不能直接显示引起胃肠道穿孔的疾病,而 CT 检查则可根据引起穿孔的原发病的 CT 表现及穿孔后引发的相应 CT 征象做出较为准确的病因学诊断。该组肠结核穿孔 1 例,异物(硬鱼骨)致乙状结肠穿孔 1 例,粪块性乙状结肠穿孔 1 例,子宫积脓自发穿孔 1 例均可在术前得以明确诊断。胃十二指肠溃疡穿孔 7 例,腹部外伤致空回肠穿孔 4 例,根据病史亦可以明确诊断。另外, CT 还可以了解周围脏器及合并症情况,为临床提供更全面、更准确的诊断。该组 15 例中,CT 发现腹腔少量积液 6 例、腹腔大量积液 5 例、胆系积气 1 例、两侧胸腔积液 2 例以及肠梗阻 4 例等有重要参考价值的影像学征象。

鉴别诊断及注意事项:腹腔内游离气体大多为胃肠穿孔或损伤所致,但胃肠道外器官子宫穿孔亦能导致腹腔游离气体,该组即有 1 例由子宫积脓自发穿孔引起。因子宫积脓其感染细菌多为厌氧菌,可产生气体,子宫穿孔时,气体随脓液进入腹腔,引起腹腔游离气体。

自发性子宫穿孔导致气腹临床上少见,多发生在老年女性,一些作者报道病例均误诊为消化道穿孔。因此,临床上如遇到老年女性急腹症患者有游离气腹时,应考虑到本病的可能,避免误诊。

此外尚需与下列情况鉴别:女性生殖道与腹腔沟通,在一定条件下如阴道冲洗,产前胸膝位锻炼,腹内压改变等可使外界气体由女性生殖道进入腹腔;腹膜腔产气杆菌的感染,如产气荚膜杆菌感染;先天性胃肠道结构异常,如肠憩室破裂、肠道气囊肿破裂;医源性因素,因诊断或治疗所需而进行人工气腹、剖腹产术后、输卵管扩张术、尿潴留膀胱造瘘误伤腹腔、腹腔穿刺术等,结合临床病史可区别。CT 能准确地判断腹腔游离气体的有无、部位和多少,并能为穿孔部位、病因、合并症的诊断提供有价值的信息,及时做出诊断,减轻患者的痛苦,可作为腹部空腔脏器穿孔的有效检查方法。

第三节　原发性肠脂垂炎:急腹症的鉴别诊断

详见本书 本卷 第二十六篇 第四章 第一节　原发性肠脂垂炎:急腹症的鉴别诊断。

第四节　坏死性小肠结肠炎

详见本书 本卷 第三十篇 第三章 第三节　坏死性小肠结肠炎。

第五节　儿童急性阑尾炎

详见本书 本卷 第三十篇 第三章 第四节　儿童急性阑尾炎。

第六节　胆石性肠梗阻

详见本书 本卷 第十七篇 第七章 第九节　胆石性肠梗阻。

第七节　成人肠套叠的CT表现

成人肠套叠的CT表现及病理基础：成人肠套叠多为继发性肠套叠，由息肉或肿瘤等病变引起。其大体病理为套头部病变、套鞘部肠管、折返部肠管、套入部肠管及卷入的肠系膜脂肪、血管等。根据肠套叠大体病理可将其分为头、体、尾部，套入部前端即为头部，尾部以套鞘部肠管尾端折返部为界，之后为尾部，头部与尾部之间为体部，体部的长短取决于套入的深度。肠套叠CT表现即为肠套叠病变各部位在CT不同扫描层面、不同角度上显示。

头部：多为原发病变所在，显示为规则或不规则肿块，呈偏心性者其边缘可见肠系膜脂肪影。口服对比剂后，在套入部头部周围常可见薄层高密度对比剂呈弧形或环状分布。脂肪瘤的CT表现具有特征性，但需与卷入的肠系膜脂肪鉴别。部分肠套叠病例体部很短，头部表现复杂不规则，尾部无典型征象时易误诊为肠道原发肿瘤。口服对比剂可显示肠管的特征，例如清晰显示套入部肠管的结肠袋形，密度逐渐减低。对比剂进入不规则的套叠靶块内有助于与非肠套叠的肠道原发肿瘤鉴别。因此检查前口服对比剂是非常必要的。

体部：靶征是肠套叠体部最多见的特征性CT征象之一，一组20例均可见，它反映肠套叠头、体部的各层肠壁、肠腔及肠系膜间的解剖关系。

最内层为套入部肠管，其外为陷入的肠系膜，因含有脂肪而呈低密度。最外层为套鞘部肠管及折返部肠管，二者间有间隙存在，但常无法显示。靶块多呈圆形或类圆形，或呈同心圆状，为轴位或接近轴位时的表现。由于套叠长轴与CT扫描层面角度的不同，也可呈肾形、香蕉形或不规则状肿块。体部靶块内，常可见套入的肠系膜脂肪及血管影，由于肠系膜偏于肠管一侧，因此靶块内脂肪常呈偏心性分布。肠系膜脂肪及血管影卷入肠腔，也为肠套叠的重要征象之一。体部短或不规则的病例内可无肠系膜脂肪及血管影显示。

尾部：（1）彗星尾征：为套叠尾部多见的CT表现，即套叠近端肠系膜血管牵拉聚拢的征象，该组见8例。彗星尾征均与肾形肿块相伴出现。该肾形肿块，为套鞘部游离缘与套入部近端肠管及肠系膜的CT斜切面图像，其中游离的套鞘呈弧形围绕套入部，状若肾轮廓外形，而套入部近端肠管、肠系膜状若肾蒂；此时，所谓彗星尾的组成还应包括套入近端肠管。

（2）双肠管征：该组6例尾部可见套入部肠管套入至体部逐渐变细，肠系膜脂肪及血管随同套入，CT像上同时直观地可见套入部及套鞘部肠管，为肠套叠特征性征象，称之为双肠管征，为扫描线与肠管长轴一致或接近一致时套叠体尾部的CT表现，多见于套入较深、体部较长的病例。肠腔内有对比剂时更易显示，其体部轴位则表现为靶征，中央为套入部肠管，对比剂呈高密度，周围为脂肪，外层为套鞘肠管。部分病例可在适当斜切面的多平面重建图像上显示。双肠管征对肠套叠诊断的特异性高，说明其为肠套叠体尾部常见的特征性征象。双肠管征可见于各型肠套叠，但其在各型肠套叠中的发生率，由于该组样本量较小，尚需进一步搜集病例研究。

（3）部分病例尾部仅表现为肠管轻度扩张，少量积液积气，该组3例，无明显特征性。尾部无梗阻表现也无其他特征3例。成人肠腔相对较大，一般不容易发生完全性梗阻，表现为梗阻近端肠腔扩张积液积气，远端肠腔不完全萎陷，梗阻点多为肠套叠的体部末端，即套入部肠管入口处附近。

其他征象：肠壁增厚多见于肠道原发肿瘤，结肠癌、淋巴瘤等恶性肿瘤及肠管缺血水肿坏死增厚。如果肠壁节段性环形增厚超过2~3 mm，肠系膜结构模糊、腹腔积液，螺旋CT增强扫描肠壁强化减弱或不强化，延迟扫描强化正常，说明肠缺血水肿；肠壁密度增加、肠壁积气、肠系膜出血说明肠管严重缺血或梗死。腹膜后及肠系膜淋巴结肿大及远处转移提示套叠病因为恶性。

CT分型：根据肠套叠的肠管类型将肠套叠分为小肠-小肠型，小肠-结肠型（包含回-结肠型，回-回-结肠型，回-结-结肠型），结-结肠型。

肠套叠CT分型依据主要在于观察套叠头部及尾部的位置及CT表现。小肠-结肠型及结-结肠型头部在结肠，可根据结肠的门框型分布特点及结肠袋形定位，尾部观察有无结肠袋形、肠黏膜情况及肠系膜情况定位，如彗星尾征。

头部无结肠特征者考虑小肠-小肠型。头部有结肠特征、尾部有小肠特征考虑小肠 - 结肠型。小肠 - 结肠型多为回 - 结肠型,尾部位于回盲部。尾部有小肠特征且不位于右侧髂窝正常回盲部,头部又有结肠特征者考虑回 - 结 - 结肠型。尾部有小肠特征且位于右侧髂窝正常回盲部,头部有结肠特征,体部发现双重套叠考虑回 - 回 - 结肠型。尾部有结肠特征者考虑结 - 结肠型。靶征、双肠管征见于各型肠套叠,肾形肿块伴彗星尾征主要见于尾部为小肠的肠套叠,可能和小肠系膜的特点有关。横结肠、乙状结肠套叠系闭袢性梗阻,更易引起肠坏死,对这类患者应尽早明确诊断,减少并发症和病死率,因此明确肠套叠 CT 分型有重要意义。

病因诊断:由于成人型肠套叠多为继发性病变,应尽量寻找原发病灶,注意鉴别良、恶病变。根据肠套叠形成原理,多由于头部病变运动受阻而近端肠管蠕动加强及近端肠管压力增高致套入,因此 CT 诊断时首先应重点观察套叠头部,该组 20 例肠套叠于套叠头部发现原发病灶 16 处。

肠套叠小的原发病变易被掩盖而不易发现,套叠肠管的复杂表现也掩盖原发病变的许多特征,因此原发病变定性诊断困难,但良恶性病变仍有其一定特征性,解套后 CT 检查对原发病变的检出及定性很有利。

增强扫描对进一步显示病因肿块的特点有帮助;恶性肿瘤导致的肠套叠 CT 检查可显示其他脏器及淋巴结转移等。目前螺旋 CT 对原发病变的诊断仍有较大限制,值得进一步研究。

随着螺旋 CT 的普及和诊断水平的提高,成人肠套叠的发现率近年来明显增高,说明成人肠套叠并非很少见。在肠套叠头体尾部发现任一特征性 CT 征象,均可诊断肠套叠,各征象不需同时具备。因此对肠套叠特有征象的认识有助于提高诊断水平。

由于螺旋 CT 对肠套叠诊断的诸多优势,如定位准确,部分可了解病因情况,对肠腔内外及腹腔情况了解全面,对病变血供及有无肠管坏死可及时作出评判,应将其作为成人肠套叠的首选检查方法。

第二章　腹盆创伤

闭合性腹部创伤的CT诊断

肝、脾、肾的损伤如下。

单纯实质裂伤：CT表现为脏器内局限性呈纵形、横行或斜形裂伤，形态为条状、梭状或楔形的低密度阴影，CT值多为9~30 HU，发生于肝、脾者CT值偏高，发生于肾者CT值偏低。

实质脏器的粉碎伤：CT表现为局限性与广泛性2种，局限性为脏器一侧损伤为主，表现为节段性与小片状，甚至呈大片状低密度影，其内密度均匀，界线较清，CT值一般在10 HU左右；广泛性损伤表现为脏器体积多增大，呈膨胀性改变（以脾脏最为明显），其内密度不均，有条状及斑片状低密度影，可见小块与大块状稍高密度影，常伴有包膜下、腹腔内及腹膜后不同程度积血。

实质内血肿：可见脏器内圆形或卵圆形稍高密度影或低密度影，低密度影多见于肝脏，若为高密度血肿周围可见环状低密度影与正常的实质分开呈“环堤”状改变伴不同程度包膜下积液。

包膜下出血：即所谓的哨兵小块征，表现为脏器周围双边状、新月状及梭形略低密度影或高密度影或混杂密度影。

肾脏损伤的其他表现：肾脏属腹膜后脏器，肾脏外伤还可见肾周血肿，血液贮于前后肾周间隙之间，常偏于肾周脂肪囊一侧，常表现为较大范围的弧形宽带状高密度灶。

肋骨骨折刺伤肝、脾或腰椎骨折刺伤肾：可见受伤脏器内块状或斑片状低密度影，其附近可见到骨折的病灶，同时出现包膜下与腹腔内积血，部分病例可见腹膜后血肿。

胰腺损伤：CT表现与肝、脾、肾的损伤有所不同，常见胰腺增大，胰周脂肪层增厚模糊、胰周大量渗出等，可以是局部，也可以是弥漫性的，有时可见到肠系膜上动脉起始部周围水肿、横结肠系膜增厚以及胸腔渗出灶，其附近可见椎体骨折与腹膜后血肿表现。

腹盆部空腔脏器的损伤：腹腔内可见少量或较多量游离气体与腹腔内少量积血，少数病例可见肠系膜或腹膜后血肿。肠管破裂可见肠系膜向损伤处纠集、包绕，并形成局部血肿，在手术中可见大网膜游离到病灶处将其进行包绕，打开包裹其内可见血液与肠腔内容物如粪便等。膀胱损伤表现为膀胱充盈极差，盆腔内可见少量或较多的积液（这与损伤时间的长短及损伤时膀胱内尿潴留量有关），少数病例可见膀胱轻度充盈，但其正常形态改变，两侧不对称，呈斜形状改变，多数病人常无尿，并有骨盆骨折。

闭合性腹部创伤CT扫描的必要性：早期诊断与及时治疗对闭合性腹部创伤患者的愈后是密切相关的，CT扫描不但能准确地做出闭合性腹部创伤的程度与哪一脏器损伤的诊断，还可估量腹腔内与包膜下积血的量，给临床治疗提供很有价值的资料，对制订手术方案起较大作用，为手术顺利进行赢得了宝贵的时间。

当然，诊断性腹腔穿刺术和腹腔灌洗术以及B超检查是很有必要的，但CT检查更是不可缺少的，尤其是诊断性腹腔穿刺术与诊断性腹腔灌洗术检查阴性者而临床上又不能排除腹腔内脏器损伤的情况下，更应行CT扫描，以明确诊断。该组8例肝脏损伤、11例脾脏损伤、1例胰腺损伤及2例肠管损伤的患者，术前B超、诊断性腹腔穿刺术与诊断性腹腔灌洗术检查均未能提供其损伤的证据，通过CT检查得以发现并经手术进一步证实。

CT扫描对闭合性腹部创伤处理的价值：CT扫描对闭合性腹部创伤的诊断与提供手术方案均有很大的意义，对其行手术或保守治疗也有一定的帮助，近年来手术保脾与非手术保脾的成功率明显提高，通过非手术治疗获得痊愈达46.6%。该组作者认为CT表现为单纯性包膜下积血量较少者，局限性肝、脾、肾损伤，单纯肝脾脏器血肿或并有包膜下积血量少者以及腹腔内未见阳性出血征象者，肾脏非碎裂者在临床密切观察下均能行非手术治疗。

闭合性腹部创伤CT检查的适应证及应注意的问题:患者就诊时一般病情较重,相当部分病人诊断性腹腔穿刺术与诊断性腹腔灌洗术检查不能得到明确诊断,所以该组作者认为如有下列情况尤其需要做CT检查:腹痛与腹部压痛明显并有腹膜刺激征者;腹痛与腹部压痛明显而诊断性腹腔穿刺术与诊断性腹腔灌洗术检查阴性者;伴有任何高危因素而临床又无法明确腹腔内脏器损伤情况者;仅有低危因素、意识清楚但腹痛始终不减者;临床症状体征与患者的伤情不一致者。虽然加行增强扫描的诊断准确率比平扫高,但该组作者认为在实际工作中,主要由于需做CT检查的闭合性腹部创伤患者就诊时一般病情较重较急,甚至处于休克昏迷状态,行增强扫描危险性很大,这在其他作者已有提及,故除非非常必需,增强扫描不做为好,该组病例中只有病情较轻、诊断不明确且多有责任纠纷的6例行增强扫描。

未能明确诊断的患者多可通过密切观察、复查随防得以明确诊断,这在可疑脾破裂患者中尤为重要,与迟发性脾破裂相比,迟发性肝破裂是很罕见的。

CT扫描的局限性:虽然CT扫描对腹腔脏器的损伤的诊断与治疗有很大的帮助,但有时腹腔闭合性损伤的CT征象并不明显,特别是胰腺与肠管损伤后,即刻做CT检查容易使其漏诊,若怀疑胰腺损伤可做薄层CT扫描或在12~24 h内复查。肠管损伤时CT虽能发现腹腔内游离气体,但对其损伤的部位难以确定,对其损伤程度及几处损伤更难确定,甚至不少病人漏诊而在手术时才发现病灶,对腹膜后与肠系膜损伤产生血肿者CT扫描有时也不敏感,甚至出现漏诊。总之,要注意观察伤员临床症状的变化与CT征象的改变,并要及时地随防复查,以免延误失去治疗的良好时机。

第三章　消化道出血

第一节　消化道出血的常见病因及其DSA诊断

消化道出血的发病率为(17~144)/10万人，消化道疾病及全身性疾病均可引起。大量出血者，除有呕血、血便外，同时伴有因血容量减少而导致的周围循环衰竭而危及生命。临床常见的病因有消化性溃疡、食管贲门黏膜撕裂综合征、Dieulafoy病、血管畸形、憩室、息肉、肿瘤、弥漫性溃疡性结肠炎、外伤、重症急性胰腺炎以及医源性损伤等。

胃肠钡餐、内镜、放射性核素扫描及胶囊内镜在不同时期、不同方面对动脉性消化道出血的诊断均起到了重要作用。消化道钡餐检查能较好显示腔内占位性或明显外压性病变，但不能显示黏膜下的血管病变，并要求在出血静止期检查，限制了其在处理急症患者时的应用。纤维内镜检查最直观，其阳性检查结果对引导选择性血管造影检查及介入治疗有积极的意义，但当出血量比较大时，肠腔内充满血液，内镜的使用就受到限制。

ECT核素扫描在定性诊断方面最敏感，出血量在0.05~0.12 ml/min时即可测出，并且由于^{99m}Tc在血液循环中滞留的时间长，检查时间跨度长，故适用于一些间隙性或少量消化道出血的患者，其最大缺点是不能精确定位，对下一步治疗的指导意义有限。

血管造影检查通过显示对比剂外溢及肠腔内的对比剂异常集聚等消化道出血的直接征象，或通过判断导致出血的基础病变的供血动脉来源进行定位诊断，是对消化道出血进行定位的最直观的检查方法。

Nussbaum等(1963)经动物实验表明，当出血量达到0.5 ml/min以上，选择性血管造影即能显示对比剂外溢征象而明确出血部位。同时，血管造影还能显示基础病变异常血管的形态、分布、大小、范围及其与周围血管及器官的关系等间接征象，借此推测病变的性质，进行定性诊断。

更重要的是，在血管造影检查发现了出血灶之后，在无相关禁忌证的情况下能够立即实行介入治疗止血，迅速改善失血症状。

与常规血管造影方法相比较，DSA对显示血管结构具有独到的优势。它利用同一部位造影前后2次成像相减原理，避免了非血管组织的重叠，单独显示血管结构，也可清晰显示一些常规造影不易发现的小病灶，更有利于介入栓塞治疗时的定位。

同时，每秒时间内多幅采集技术使对比剂在血管内呈一个动态显影过程，充分地显示动脉、毛细血管及回流静脉，对血管内对比剂外溢、静脉早显等异常征象的实时观察特别有利。连续的血管造影图像，可清晰显示肿瘤的供血动脉及引流静脉、肿瘤血管、肿瘤染色、肿块与邻近血管及脏器的关系，从而进行可能的定性诊断。

由于肿瘤性病变最终需要外科手术根治，在介入处理过程中，还可以在靶血管放置弹簧圈或其他标志物，为外科医师手术提供可靠的导向信息。

对于血管畸形，DSA能够清晰显示出异常血管团的形态特征和病变范围，明确有无静脉早显。动脉瘤血管造影表现一般比较典型，可使荷瘤血管呈卵圆形扩张，或者囊袋状偏于动脉壁一侧。更重要的是，多角度的DSA检查能够全面了解动脉瘤与荷瘤动脉的关系，清晰显示瘤蒂，以指导治疗方案的制订。

DSA对肿瘤性疾病和血管性疾病等异常血管的检出率较高，而对消化道炎性病变、憩室及息肉等检出率相对偏低，导致定性诊断困难。为提高动脉性消化道出血的血管造影检出率，应综合分析临床症状和在血管造影检查前进行的其他检查，针对最有可能出血的血管进行超选择插管造影。通过导管对靶血管灌注扩血管药物，行药物性血管造影也有助于异常血管的发现。另外，在出血活动期进行血管造影检查，尽量避免临床止血药物的干预，亦能提高出血的检出率。

第二节　胃肠出血的少见原因

主动脉 - 肠瘘极为少见，主要出现于腹主动脉的动脉瘤，多继发于腹主动脉手术后。在大量胃肠出血的区别诊断中，此瘘应考虑为原因之一。此瘘的病因学讨论，包括动脉硬化、霉菌性动脉瘤、梅毒性动脉瘤和创伤后动脉瘤、腹腔内或腹膜后新生物、偶尔为非特异性感染或直接创伤所致。

手术后出现的瘘已报告见于主动脉手术后或腹部血管手术后感染。大多数瘘都出现于动脉瘤与十二指肠之间，Ammann 等（1973）报告 4 例，其中 1 例曾行胃切除术，1 例瘘位于动脉瘤与乙状结肠之间，此症预后不良。

新生儿上消化道出血较少见，大约有一半病儿无器质性改变或凝血障碍。一般说来，食管炎、胃炎、食管溃疡或应激性溃疡、及出血性素质已知为上消化道出血的常见原因。

Cairo 等（1981）首例报告了胃畸胎瘤引起的反复上消化道出血。随后又出现胃排空障碍。腹部 X 线平片示一大钙化性包块使充气胃轮廓外移，触诊为硬而固定无触痛包块。钙化块中有一下颌骨伴存牙结构。超声见平段波混杂密集波，手术切除证实为 10cm × 15cm × 10cm^3 大的良性畸胎瘤。畸胎瘤常见出现在骨盆、纵隔、腹膜后和颈部，约有 1/3~1/2 具有钙化。胃的畸胎瘤占小儿畸胎瘤不到 1%，几乎总是良性，它常位于大弯，且男孩多于女孩。一例颇为少见，因其引起上消化道出血，且部位又在小弯，而又是新生女婴。

胃静脉曲张的诊断常有困难，上消化道钡餐检查，甚至内镜都可将胃黏膜皱襞的突起或恶性病变误诊为静脉曲张。

Marshall 等（1978）在胃底发现有黏膜皱襞突起或肿块 3 例，其中 2 例皆为钡餐和胃镜误诊，而通过 X 线血管造影及脾门静脉造影确诊。食管静脉曲张的存在，提示可疑及胃静脉曲张。

第三节　消化道出血与胃

详见本书 本卷 第二十三篇 第十四章　消化道出血与胃。

第三十篇　小儿腹盆部疾病（上）

第一章　胃十二指肠疾病

第一节　十二指肠壁内血肿及误诊病例简介

单纯十二指肠壁内血肿是临床少见疾病，大多数由外伤造成，也有报道发生于抗凝治疗、血友病、特发性血小板减少性紫癜、骨髓瘤等出血性疾病，还可由急性胰腺炎、医源性操作不当引起。Desai 等(2003)报道该病多发生于儿童。一组 5 例中 3 例为 12 岁以下的儿童。

1. 临床表现　十二指肠壁内血肿临床多因腹痛就诊，表现为无放射性的脐周疼痛，中上腹压痛、反跳痛，轻度腹肌紧张，移动性浊音阴性，可呕吐含胆汁的胃内容物，有轻度或中度发热，若继发破裂或者穿孔则可造成陈旧血液和 / 或小肠液渗入腹膜后间隙或腹膜腔，导致严重感染。多数学者认为十二指肠壁内血肿形成与其解剖位置相关。由于屈氏韧带的固定使十二指肠及上段空肠活动度减小，又紧贴腹后壁，其降段、水平段属腹膜后位器官。靠近腰椎，而十二指肠的供血动脉前后、上下吻合成弓，钝性外伤的剪切力易造成血管丛撕裂，使肠壁及系膜形成血肿。多数病例血淀粉酶正常，但尿淀粉酶可较正常升高 2~3 倍。有作者考虑可能由于胰头与十二指肠降段有共同的血供，当胰十二指肠下动脉损伤时，十二指肠表现为壁内血肿，胰头部分则可有少量坏死，释放出胰蛋白酶原，表现为患者血淀粉酶轻度升高，而患者就诊时多为发病 3 天以后，因此也只能检出尿淀粉酶有轻度升高。

2. 影像学研究　B 超可显示腹部包裹局限的液性暗区，但由于十二指肠位置深在，加之肠气的干扰，对十二指肠壁内血肿常不能明确显示，且对血凝块定性不准确。上消化道造影可发现十二指肠的梗阻，但对鉴别导致梗阻的原因价值不大。

十二指肠壁内血肿 CT 平扫表现为十二指肠走行一致或相邻的高或等密度的软组织肿块影，边界多较清晰、光滑，形态多不规则，密度不均匀，边缘呈环形高密度和中心有融冰样高密度为其特征，这与血肿吸收的进程相吻合；但对于病程时间较长的血肿可呈液性均匀低密度影，此时则需与肠壁、系膜的囊性病变鉴别。

口服碘水对比剂则有部分病例可见受压移位的肠管和变窄的管腔，而由于肠管的蠕动收缩，此征象并不是所有病例都能见到。血肿段及血肿近段肠壁肿胀、增厚，多与局部血肿压迫和缺血有关，有作者利用 GE CT 扫描仪的体积计算软件可初步估算血肿的体积，与术中所见血肿量误差不超过 10%。

增强扫描肿块无强化是其特点，可以与十二指肠或网膜来源的肿瘤性病变鉴别，间接征象为近端的小肠及胃有不同程度地梗阻、扩张。

腹部钝伤所致的十二指肠断裂或穿孔需手术修补，未并发穿孔的血肿则可采用非手术治疗。有作者分析 7 例腹部钝伤病人的 CT 图像对鉴别十二指肠穿孔与血肿的价值。其中 3 例为十二指肠穿孔或断裂，4 例血肿，所有穿孔的病例及 1 例血肿经手术证实。

分析图像发现：4 例十二指肠肠壁血肿病人中有 3 例显示肠壁增厚(厚于 3mm)，2 例有腹腔内积液，1 例气腹，2 例见右肾周间隙及肾前间隙内积液，1 例伴存实质脏器损伤。3 例十二指肠穿孔病人，均见有十二指肠肠壁增厚，2 例腹腔内积液，2 例气腹，3 例都有右侧肾前间隙积液及实质脏器的损伤，2 例有右肾前间隙积气，2 例右肾前间隙口服对比剂外渗。3 例穿孔者均见肠腔外积气或 / 和对比剂外渗，此征象未见于不伴发穿孔的血肿病人。

该作者认为，CT 对鉴别腹部钝伤所致的十二指肠穿孔与无穿孔的血肿可提供较大的帮助，右肾前间隙积气及口服对比剂外渗仅见于穿孔者,而其他征象特异性较差。

3. 鉴别诊断　CT 诊断时需与十二指肠的肿瘤性病变进行鉴别。十二指肠良性肿瘤主要包括腺瘤和间质来源肿瘤。腺瘤多发生于十二指肠第一、二段,表面光滑,呈球形,向腔内生长,易与十二指肠壁内血肿鉴别;间质来源的肿瘤中脂肪瘤及错构瘤有其特征的 CT 值易鉴别,平滑肌瘤与血管瘤因有不同程度的强化,与十二指肠壁内血肿无强化的特征也可鉴别。而十二指肠恶性肿瘤多有浸润性生长的特征,且腹膜后有淋巴结转移可以资鉴别。

本病由于临床少见,常以脐周渐进性加重的腹痛就诊,且以儿童多见,容易误诊为阑尾炎或急性胰腺炎,但白细胞计数常正常或偏高,血淀粉酶多数正常,尿淀粉酶轻度升高,临床不易确诊。CT 对明确诊断有显著意义,同时还可以帮助判断血肿出血量的多少、梗阻的严重程度,对合并肠壁坏死、穿孔者更具提示意义。

4. 误诊病例简介　有作者报告一例 8 岁男性患儿,无明显外伤史但凝血功能较差,腹痛伴呕吐 5 天,左侧脐上扪及包块,临床最初疑为肠套叠,仔细分析 CT 表现诊断应该不难,表现为肠腔内高、低混杂密度囊样病灶,边界清晰,无强化。

第二节　一些诊断陷阱

在婴儿和成人,胃与全腹部的比例不同,婴儿胃比例相对较大,需注意避免与婴儿胃胀气混淆。哭闹时正常婴儿胃可明显充气扩张,扩张的大小有时可达到惊人的程度。

在双对比胃造影时,胃窦部的功能性和瞬间蠕动不应与黏膜隔膜混淆,这在婴幼儿尤其常见。

第二章　胃肠道疾病

第一节　新生儿胃肠穿孔 X 线征

新生儿腹腔内游离气体为诊断胃肠穿孔的可靠依据,但仅依赖气腹征象来诊断胃肠道穿孔,易造成漏诊和误诊,有作者报告一组 56 例新生儿胃肠穿孔中有 17 例无膈下游离气体。所以熟悉胃肠道穿孔的特殊 X 线征象,才能提高新生儿胃肠道穿孔的早期诊断率。

X 线直接征象: X 线表现为两侧膈下大量异常透亮的游离气体影,两膈面抬高,腹腔脏器下移、聚拢,易于诊断。特殊 X 线征:胃泡征消失提示胃穿孔可能;马鞍征,膈下马鞍状积气影;足球征,穿孔大量积气卧位时的表现,大量气腹构成显著腹胀,两侧腹壁内缘光滑,形如"足球"易漏诊,多由于先天性胃壁肌层缺损,结肠穿孔引起(该组 12 例)。

中等量膈下游离气体: X 线表现为两侧膈下中等量异常透亮的游离气体影,腹腔脏器略下移、聚拢,易于诊断。特殊 X 线征:胃泡征消失、马鞍征、足球征、镰状韧带征(卧位时可以观察到气腹衬托显示镰状韧带)、腹腔积液征(该组 16 例)。

少量膈下游离气体: X 线表现为两侧膈下少量异常透亮的游离气体影,仔细观察不难诊断。特殊 X 线征:新月征、线样征存在于左侧膈下有时要与胃泡积气鉴别,极易漏诊;镰状韧带征、木梳征、肠间隔增宽征(该组 9 例)。

极少量膈下游离气体: X 线表现为两侧膈下线状、点状异常透亮的游离气体影,极易漏诊,必须细心观察。特殊 X 线征:线样征、点状积气征、三角形积气征(水平侧位时的 X 线表现,该组 2 例)。

间接征象:X 线表现为无膈下游离气体,或由于游离气体被包裹且游离气体量的多少和投照体位不同而表现各异。

假囊肿征:胃、结肠、阑尾穿孔漏出气体于大网膜后方被包裹形成,于中腹部示囊状透亮影,与肠管和胃不能延续。

网膜囊积气和积液征:穿孔发生在胃后壁或十二指肠后壁上方者,游离气体或液体进入小网膜囊内,此时在腹腔内不再出现气腹征象,而在仰卧位片于上腹部相当于脊柱或脊柱旁区显示局限性透亮影,有的可位于脊柱与胃小弯之间呈新月状透亮影,在直立位片有时呈现液平面;侧位:小网膜内气影位于胃的后方。

镰状韧带征:在腰椎右旁可见纵行或弯曲线状致密影。铅笔征:部分充气肠管内外缘均可见且很光滑,像铅笔所画。肠壁积气征:沿增宽的肠壁可见线样或点状串珠状积气。木梳征:围绕肠系膜分布的肠管在肠管间游离气体的衬托下形似木梳。腹膜后充气征:游离气体位于腹膜后方。腹腔包裹性积气征:腹腔游离气体被组织粘连包裹,表现形式多样,应多体位摄片观察。腹腔积液征:穿孔并发腹膜炎的表现。肝缘投影征:有时少许气体逸至肝肾陷窝,衬出肝下缘的轮廓,在其下方呈现新月状透亮影。气粪混合征:腹腔外围肠管出现气粪混合影像。此外,纵隔积气及皮下气肿征,胸部改变等也有一定的参考意义。

新生儿胃肠道穿孔病情危急,不同部位、不同原因的胃肠道穿孔表现各异,熟知和掌握其特殊 X 线征,对新生儿胃肠道穿孔的早期诊断和防止漏诊,降低患儿死亡率有重要作用。

第二节　新生儿上消化道出血

新生儿上消化道出血较少见，大约有一半病儿无器质性改变或凝血障碍。一般说来，食管炎、胃炎、食管溃疡或应激性溃疡及出血性素质已知为上消化道出血的常见原因。

第三节　小儿胃肠道特点

小儿胃肠道发育成熟从出生持续到3~4岁，发育过程中的胃肠道在解剖生理方面均不同于年长儿和成人。了解和熟悉这些特点有利于从影像学角度显示病变和判断病因。

（1）生后随着呼吸和啼哭，空气迅速积聚在胃肠道内且通过迅速，出生后3~8小时内气体已抵达结肠。

（2）胃肠道内充满了气体，形成气量丰富的因素有：①啼哭和喂奶过程中吞咽的空气约占70%；②腹肌发育差，菲薄的腹肌致腹壁松弛，造成肠壁血液循环相对缓慢而影响肠腔内气体的吸收；③食管下括约肌、贲门和幽门功能不全，使吞咽气体易进入胃肠道内，胃内气体也易返流入食管；④回盲瓣功能不全，气体易从结肠返流至小肠；⑤肠道发育不成熟以致肠腔内气体不易排空；⑥仰卧生理体位使气体易积聚在胃肠道内。

（3）小肠和结肠的解剖标志不明显。空肠黏膜纹浅细，结肠无袋形。随着年龄增长解剖结构逐渐显示。

上述的婴幼儿胃肠道解剖生理反映在X线腹部平片上，具有以下5个特征：①除右上腹肝区致密影外，全腹腔为分布均匀的充气胃肠道占有，以致腹腔向两侧及前方膨隆。②胃底充气位于左上腹，胃体横行伸展至上腹部中央。胃囊充气容量受啼哭和喂奶影响而有较大的变化，甚至可占据整个左侧中上腹腔。由于贲门松弛，食管下端可有气体充盈。③充气肠腔形态特殊，呈多角形或类圆形，相互交错呈网格状。肠肌菲薄，肠腔张力低，气量中多但腔内压力不高，以致充气肠腔相互挤压，在腹部平片上形成多角形或类圆形。偶尔小肠腔内可见到少许短浅液平。④依靠解剖位置区分大小肠。小肠位于腹腔中央和前方，结肠位于腹腔两侧和后方，乙状结肠和直肠位于小骨盆腔内。侧位片示升、降结肠呈纵行管状充气位于脊柱前方，直肠则位于骶尾椎前方。乙状结肠冗长，位于小骨盆腔上方，可伸展致右侧中下腹部前方。⑤网格状致密影系肠壁软组织所构成，边缘光整锐利，厚度约1~2mm，容易受肠腔气量的影响而改变其厚度。

第三章　肠道疾病

第一节　儿童一过性小肠套叠

若胃肠道的一部分(套叠的套入部)陷入一个相邻的部分(套叠的鞘部),就会发生肠套叠。尽管它在儿童中十分常见,却少见于成人,后者的发生率只有5%。

在CT图像上,肠-肠套叠表现为一个复合性肿块,且CT表现具有多样性,但通常是一段带有肠系膜和血管的萎陷肠管(套入部)位于一段相邻扩张的肠管内(鞘部)。其横断面的表现是由一个外周的肠圈(鞘部)包裹着一个萎陷的肠袢(套入部)及其邻近的肠系膜脂肪成分。

在成人,超过90%的肠套叠是由肿瘤引起的。但肠套叠的确切原因在CT上却不易被分辨出来,从而难以靠它来确立诊断。不伴肠梗阻的管腔内肠系膜脂肪的轻度一过性肠套叠有时可被CT发现,但却无临床意义。这种肠套叠,可见于有肠炎、胰腺炎、腹泻、肠水肿的病人,或为特发性。对这些病人的CT表现应予谨慎解释,在拟行手术前,须有足够的临床证据和充分的小肠检查。找到一个诱发此病的因素是重要的,因为大多数非肿瘤性病变引起的一过性肠套叠并不需要外科手术。

第二节　儿童慢性特发性小肠假性梗阻综合征

Byrne等(1977)报告本症11例,4例无症状,全由X线检查作出诊断,且皆做食管动力学研究。所有病例都有腹部平片、钡餐检查和钡灌肠检查。

有症状者平片示小肠曲扩张,常伴气液平,造影示运动障碍,食管下1/3收缩差为运动异常的特征,胃排空延迟伴十二指肠扩张。全部病例小肠中钡剂皆清楚可见特征性的顺行——逆行往返的蠕动。3例可见钡剂通过小肠缓慢,到达盲肠时间在7小时以上;6例可见钡灌肠时排粪异常,表示结肠运动的障碍。形态学变化包括不同程度的小肠袢的节段性扩张、膨胀、结肠袋消失、结肠冗长等。10例运动性研究均见吞咽时食管下1/3段原发性蠕动收缩幅度降低。活检对本症无诊断意义。

第三节　儿童急性阑尾炎

急性阑尾炎是小儿最常见的外科急腹症之一,小儿阑尾壁很薄,病变发展很快,极易引起暴发性腹膜炎而死亡,故临床早期诊断早期治疗十分重要。

儿童阑尾炎的临床病理特点:儿童阑尾的解剖不同于成人,其壁薄,阑尾系膜动脉细小,故易发生栓塞,早期即可发生穿孔、坏疽,穿孔率较成人高,且年龄越小,穿孔越多。同时,儿童盲肠活动度大,急性阑尾炎时炎性渗出快,大网膜较短且薄,即使阑尾穿孔,也难以限制炎症的扩散。

儿童阑尾炎的诱因及发病机制与成人也有差异。在儿童常见的诱发因素有上呼吸道感染、扁桃体炎、秋季腹泻、暴饮暴食、急性胃肠炎等,该组患儿均有类似诱因。

其发病机制主要有三:①阑尾管腔的阻塞。常见的因素有阑尾黏膜下层淋巴滤泡增生、肿胀,在青少年儿童急性阑尾炎中占 60%;粪石、异物或寄生虫虫体及虫卵阻塞,约占 35% 左右,其中粪石是引起大龄儿童急性阑尾炎的重要原因;阑尾本身病变或畸形;盲肠和阑尾周围病变,如炎症、憩室、息肉、肠套叠、肿瘤等,导致阑尾腔的阻塞。②细菌感染。主要为大肠杆菌、肠球菌及脆弱类杆菌等。一般有直接侵入、血源性感染和邻近感染的蔓延 3 种途径。③神经反射因素。

各种原因的胃肠道功能紊乱反射性引起阑尾环形肌和阑尾动脉的痉挛性收缩。前者可加重阑尾腔的阻塞使引流更为不畅,后者可导致阑尾的缺血、坏死,加速急性阑尾炎的发生和发展,如儿童秋季腹泻等。

儿童阑尾炎的临床表现与成人相比也不典型。儿童神经系统发育尚不健全,机体调节和应激能力较差,加上语言表述不清,使得儿童阑尾炎的临床症状和体征表现不典型,疼痛定位不准,如经典的转移性右下腹疼痛的病史常常不能表达或确定,从而导致临床诊断困难,有学者报告,约有一半的患儿均没有此典型表现。

值得一提的是,右下腹压痛、肌紧张和反跳痛仍然是儿童最重要的临床体征,并为手术证实。此外,肛指检查、腹腔穿刺等方法,对于非典型阑尾炎仍然有非常重要的诊断价值。儿童阑尾炎病理上也有特点,且与年龄段有关,常分为 4 型:①卡他型阑尾炎,主要发生在大龄儿童的早期,及时治疗可自愈,但也易转为化脓、坏疽型阑尾炎;②化脓型阑尾炎,多见于婴幼儿,从黏膜下层开始,各层均有化脓性细胞浸润,表现为阑尾肿大、猩红,有脓苔,临床上表现腹痛及高热,局部压痛明显,很快扩散为腹膜炎,特别是 3 岁以下婴儿,就诊时多有腹膜炎或脓肿形成;③坏疽型阑尾炎,多见于学龄儿童,因阑尾系膜血管栓塞,阑尾迅速坏死、穿孔,但纤维蛋白脓苔性粘连较早,故容易形成局限脓肿,有学者报告约 1/3 病例可形成阑尾脓肿;④梗阻型阑尾炎,多为学龄儿童,以蛔虫或蛲虫性阑尾炎最多见,阑尾外表无明显变化,临床上腹痛、压痛、发热均不严重,病情发展缓慢,有慢性中毒症状,可发生以蛔虫为中心的多发性腹内脓肿,诊断困难。

影像学研究:一般正常生理状况下,儿童阑尾的大小、形态和位置因人而异,阑尾基底部与盲肠的关系比较固定,但尖端方向很不一致,常见有 5 种方位,即盆腔位、盲肠后位、盲肠下位、回肠前位和回肠后位。

值得注意的是,正常儿童阑尾呈蚯蚓状,其管径不超过 6 mm,在 CT 上不易显示。一些作者在手术视野下对正常儿童阑尾进行测量发现:0~3 岁阑尾外径为(4.9 ± 0.8)mm,3~6 岁阑尾腔外径为(5.1 ± 0.9)mm。Leite 等(2005)也认为正常阑尾直径 <6 mm,故该组病例以此可作为判断阑尾是否增粗、增大的参考标准。

儿童急性阑尾炎的 CT 征象主要表现为阑尾外径增粗、管壁增厚,管径 >6 mm,严重者可超过 10 mm 以上,这是诊断儿童阑尾炎最直接、最重要和可靠的征象。增粗的阑尾在 CT 上表现为环形均匀增厚,阑尾腔内因含液体多呈低密度,极少数可含气体,呈"同心圆"样改变。可伴有单发或多发的阑尾粪石;阑尾腔内粪石,也是协助诊断儿童阑尾炎最重要而可靠的征象之一,出现率占儿童阑尾炎的 50% 左右,在阑尾炎脓肿中占 20%~30%。CT 表现为圆形或不规则形高密度影,同时伴阑尾腔扩大。

阑尾穿孔并阑尾脓肿形成,是诊断阑尾炎及其并发症的可靠征象。脓肿常位于盲肠周围或结肠后方,由于阑尾位置、长度不同,盲肠的活动性以及渗液的可流动性,脓肿可远离盲肠,位于盆腔、肠曲间甚至膈下。CT 平扫阑尾穿孔及其周围形成的脓肿表现为中心液体密度、或含气体(气 - 液面)的团块影,其壁厚薄不均。增强扫描,脓肿壁明显强化,腔内容物不强化。

阑尾盲肠周围炎,主要表现为阑尾周围脂肪层内出现片絮状或条纹状稍高密度的炎性渗出影,邻近筋膜、肠系膜水肿、增厚,局部渗液(如右侧结肠旁沟积液);盲肠、升结肠肠壁增厚,系盲肠、升结肠受累时改变,CT 不仅显示盲肠壁增厚,末端可呈尖角样改变,且盲肠腔扩张、积液。

肝脓肿、粘连性小肠低位梗阻等是急性阑尾炎常见的并发症。

值得重视的是,在上述 CT 表现中阑尾增粗及阑尾腔粪石两大征象,是儿童急性阑尾炎早期最常见和最可靠的诊断依据,也是临床早期诊断和及时手术的可靠指征。

儿童急性阑尾炎的诊断主要靠病史、查体及一些实验室检查。近几年来由于螺旋 CT 尤其是

MSCT 的应用，越来越受到小儿外科医生的欢迎，因为 CT 具有扫描时间短、容积扫描、可进行多平面重建、三维重建，多层面、多角度显示腹部及盆腔的解剖结构，可精确显示阑尾炎及其周围组织的病变，为临床提供可靠的客观依据。

CT 诊断急性阑尾炎的主要依据是显示异常的阑尾和阑尾周围的炎性改变。因此，高质量地显示阑尾及其周围结构是 CT 检查是否成功的关键。然而，阑尾的显示与 CT 扫描的参数及质量有重大的关系。

Weltman 等(2000)采用 5 mm 层厚进行扫描，94% 可确定异常阑尾，而 10mm 层厚则为 69%。由此看来，层厚对于阑尾的显示十分重要，因此，该组病例在局部感兴趣区常规采用 3mm 或 5mm 薄层扫描。同时，除常规轴面图像外，应常规行图像后处理，尤其使用 MSCT 薄层扫描后的多平面重建图像，可较完整地显示阑尾的全貌和走向，对于判断阑尾的增粗、粪石、脓肿、盲肠及其周围结构的改变等细节都明显优于一般 CT 轴面图像。

静脉注射对比剂行增强扫描，对阑尾炎及其并发症的诊断也十分有价值，可以显示阑尾壁、阑尾脓肿壁及周围组织的蜂窝织炎的强化及其程度，有利于准确诊断。

有学者建议，在阑尾炎 CT 扫描前 30min 给予口服对比剂，或者经肛门灌注对比剂，可帮助提高阑尾、结肠和盲肠的显影效果，对确定病变性质有所帮助，尤其是对右下腹混杂密度包块价值更大。在实际工作中，对于大龄儿童或青少年可以采用，对于婴幼儿不宜采用，因为往往不能配合，或者易于惊醒而影响 CT 扫描的镇静和制动；其次，高密度阳性对比剂可充盈阑尾腔，掩盖阑尾腔内粪石，对于阑尾粪石发生率高的儿童来说更不适宜。

关于 CT 对于儿童阑尾炎的诊断价值，Jonathan 等(2000)报告 CT 诊断儿童阑尾炎的敏感度、特异度和准确度分别是 95%~97%、91%~99% 和 96%；See 等(2008)认为 CT 对于阑尾炎诊断的精确度达 93%~99%，且对表现模棱两可、怀疑急性阑尾炎的病例，比超声的敏感度和特异度更高。

对于儿童阑尾炎的 CT 征象需要综合分析和评价，且有 4 点值得注意：①如果没有发现阑尾增粗、增大或阑尾腔粪石等直接征象，而仅有盲肠周围的炎性改变，应慎重诊断。因为这种征象不具有特异性，盲肠憩室炎、肠结核病、盆腔炎等均可有类似改变。②仅有阑尾粪石，没有阑尾增粗、阑尾周围组织的炎性改变，也不能盲目诊断为急性阑尾炎，因为在正常情况下阑尾腔有可能存留粪石。③关于阑尾穿孔的评估，当发现阑尾周围蜂窝织炎、腹腔脓肿、阑尾壁强化伴缺损和阑尾周围积气等征象时，应高度考虑为穿孔性阑尾炎的直接表现。④穿孔性阑尾炎的阑尾直径往往显著大于非穿孔性阑尾炎的直径，显著肿大的阑尾可肯定阑尾炎的诊断，但不能作为阑尾穿孔依据。

第四章　肝脏疾病

第一节　儿童肝占位性病变

详见本书 本卷 第八篇　儿童肝占位性病变。

第二节　小儿肝钝伤

肝是腹腔内最大的实质性脏器,也是损伤发生率最高的脏器。小儿肝钝伤占儿童腹部损伤的10%~30%。

小儿肝脏的解剖生理特征:成人肝大部分位于右上腹部,小部分位于左上腹部,上方有横膈,后方有脊柱,前方有肋弓遮护,一般成人轻微的腹部钝伤不至于引起肝损伤,但在小儿的腹部钝伤中这种肝损伤的机会就明显上升。这主要是与小儿的解剖生理特征有关:

与成人相比,小儿肝右叶的前区被肋弓遮护不完全,容易受到外伤;小儿肝不仅占腹腔较大容积,而且比较脆弱,缺乏弹性,即使轻微外伤也很容易引起损伤,如剧烈振动可致韧带附着周围肝损伤。小儿的肋骨尚未发育成熟,腹部肌肉及腹膜均比较薄弱,缺乏对肝的保护和对外来致伤力的缓冲作用,这是比较重要的因素;小儿不能对突发致伤的危险环境作出应变的保护性反应,容易受伤;小儿喜动好奇,爬高越险,发生钝性损伤的机会较多。

1. 肝钝伤的原因和机制　肝损伤可分两大类:一是直接损伤,如刀伤、枪伤等;另一种是交通事故、高处坠落等钝性损伤。临床上以后者更为常见,在小儿更是如此。

肝钝伤的发生机制,可以是当下肢着地坠落或在未系安全带发生交通事故的状态下,由于突然减速使腹腔内脏器产生剧烈振动,以致引起肝镰状韧带和三角韧带附着处周围的肝损伤,严重者,甚至可累及到肝后面的下腔静脉和肝静脉;也可以是在强烈的致伤力的作用下,肝动幅过大,以至发生从肝门部和下腔静脉为固定点的肝辐射状损伤。

2. 影像学研究　检查技术:肝损伤常伴脾或其他脏器损伤,病人伤情往往较重,应先行急救,待生命体征基本稳定后,再做CT检查。肝钝伤的CT检查包括平扫和增强扫描,有些损伤(如血肿)在平扫时即可显示,而增强后反而可变为等密度导致漏诊,平扫加增强扫描可发现更多的损伤。一般行全腹部扫描,但不少病人常伴有胸部甚至盆腔的损伤,故应根据实际情况,在检查腹部的同时加做上述部位的CT扫描。增强扫描多采用非离子型对比剂,以240或300 mg/(ml·kg)2~3 ml/s快速团注有利于观察正在出血的损伤。有作者指出,对小儿腹部钝伤采用超高速动态CT扫描可大大减少伪影和检查时间,明显提高CT图像的质量,且有助于外伤性假性动脉瘤及动-静脉瘘的显示。

CT表现:肝右叶钝伤多于左叶,其中绝大多数位于后段。Stalker等(1986)报道48例肝钝伤,其中肝右叶损伤占40例,而且后段占31例。这可能因右叶体积较大,后面为脊柱和肋骨,钝伤时易使肝撞击于骨架上致伤有关。通常右叶损伤程度轻而浅表,左叶损伤程度重而复杂。依照肝钝伤的程度和类型不同,CT扫描中可有下述各种表现:

肝挫伤:最轻微的肝损伤仅为局部组织充血水肿及微血管血液外渗。CT平扫为边界不清的较低密度区,增强扫描能强化,但比周围肝组织密度略低,局部结构可轻度扭曲。

肝撕裂:指肝实质内的线状或星状缺损,未侵及肝表面,CT平扫为低密度,增强时不强化。

肝破裂:为肝实质损伤的严重类型,还可侵及肝表面包膜破裂。CT平扫为较宽不规则低密度带,增强扫描表现为明显的低密度区,周围有强化,边界十分清楚。如果断裂的肝失去血液供应,或见门静脉截断征,增强时该肝组织不强化。肝破裂时,肝实质内的出血灶可呈圆形或卵圆形的均匀高密度区,增强时不强化,呈相对低密度。肝包膜下的血肿可呈月牙形或凸透镜状高密度区,并可压迫其下的肝组织变扁。

门脉周围轨迹征(或门脉周围晕征):为肝三联结构中的小血管破裂出血,血液沿门静脉周围阻力较小的结缔组织鞘蔓延所致。增强扫描见门静脉及其分支周围有管状低密度影。长轴断面上呈树枝状轨迹征,横断面上呈环形影,此征象在小儿腹部钝伤中并不罕见,且提示损伤的严重性。

但是,此征并非肝外伤所特有,充血性心力衰竭所致肝淤血,重度肝炎或小静脉阻塞性病变等,可造成肝淋巴液生成过多,超过淋巴引流能力,继发门静脉周围水肿,形成门静脉周围晕征。因此,对此征象的评价要同肝损伤的其他征象结合起来考虑。

腹腔内及腹膜后积血:发生率大约为67%,积血多发生于肝脏周围、Morison隐窝、左结肠旁沟、右结肠旁沟或盆腔内隐窝处。积血也可发生于腹膜后间隙,表现为肾上腺周围积血使肾上腺移位,下腔静脉周围积血表现为下腔静脉周围的低密度晕轮影。

合并症:肝钝伤的患儿常可合并胆汁肿、胰腺炎、胆汁性腹膜炎、延迟出血或感染。胆汁肿是由于胆管破裂,胆汁漏至肝实质内或肝外积聚形成,可表现为低密度囊状影,并压迫、推移周围组织。当肝组织损伤坏死软化或感染,于伤后CT随访可见肝区内有气体影。

肝钝伤的动态变化:轻微肝损伤经2~3周保守治疗后,CT平扫和增强扫描可恢复正常表现或低密度改变范围缩小,程度减轻。而血肿经一至数周后,由于血液被完全溶解吸收,CT表现为范围缩小,密度逐渐降低接近液体。在恢复良好的病例中,门脉周围晕征短期内就可消失。病变发展和并发症的出现均可在短期复查CT扫描中得到观察,长时间CT随访则可了解损伤痊愈状况。

CT检查对小儿肝钝伤治疗和随访的作用:CT除了提供肝损伤及其程度的诊断外,更重要的是CT诊断分型有利于协助临床治疗。CT分型主要包括肝损伤部位、程度、范围以及出血情况。一般认为,肝钝伤的诊断分类越细致,越有利于临床治疗,当然预后也越好,故有作者提出对于肝钝伤患者进行CT、超声、X线血管造影等综合影像学检查,以便尽可能做出详细的肝钝伤分类诊断,但这在实际工作中有时较难做到,一般肝钝伤病人病情多较严重,难以完成各种影像学检查。因此,不少学者认为肝钝伤的患儿只需要尽可能及早做CT检查,并主张将CT扫描中的肝钝伤分为A.挫伤,B.撕裂伤,C.破裂三种类型。这样,不仅分型简单实用,而且完全能够反映肝损伤的实际程度,便于临床及时制定恰当的治疗措施,为治疗赢得时间。A型损伤以接受内科保守治疗为主,同时要注意密切观察,短期内行CT检查,了解血肿大小的变化和损伤愈合情况;B型表浅性裂伤,多主张先保守治疗,对症处理和临床观察,部分因病情发展出血不止或血肿逐渐增大等需要采用手术治疗;C型肝破裂,一经诊断应立即手术治疗,因其容易合并反复出血、胆汁瘘、肝脓肿等并发症。CT扫描中发现有对比剂外渗,提示急性出血,尚可行肝动脉栓塞止血,但在小儿很少应用。

一些作者将一组经保守治疗的肝钝伤按损伤范围分级进行CT随访,发现轻度(损伤范围小于一叶的25%)、中度(范围小于一叶的50%)、重度(范围大于一叶的50%)损伤痊愈时间分别为3个月、3~6个月和9个月,并认为肝钝伤的CT分级有助于预后的判断和随访。

第五章 小儿黄疸

婴儿梗阻性黄疸的鉴别诊断

近年来,高胆红素血症发生率有上升趋势,以高胆红素血症为主诉入院的婴儿占婴儿住院例数的首位,可高达30%~50%。婴儿梗阻性黄疸的鉴别诊断一直是个难题,比较常见的两种病因是婴儿肝炎综合征和胆系闭锁,两者治疗方式、预后不同。

婴儿肝炎综合征多采用非手术疗法;胆系闭锁则必须手术,研究显示,先天性胆管闭锁术后10年生存与手术时年龄密切相关,60天前74%,90天后19%,120天后为0,因此,早期诊断早期治疗先天性胆管闭锁,有利于改善预后、提高患儿生存率。一般强调40~60 d内完成Kasai手术,或择期行肝移植术,否则会因肝硬化、肝功能衰竭死亡。故必须早期诊断胆系闭锁,才能提高治愈率。

影像学研究:先天性胆管闭锁的诊断有多种影像学方法,如B超可根据肝门纤维块来鉴别肝炎和先天性胆管闭锁,但是由于患儿年龄较小合并肝发育障碍,以及超声仪固有分辨率的限制,使小于0.5cm×0.5cm的纤维块很难被B超发现。彩色多普勒超声可以显示门静脉周围的纤维块,但也对肝内外胆管显示差。核素扫描在婴儿梗阻性黄疸的鉴别诊断中起重要作用,其敏感性虽高达100%,但特异性仅60%,且难以直接观察解剖关系。

据报道磁共振胆管成像在鉴别诊断婴儿黄疸的符合率可达100%,MRI可多序列、多平面扫描,又无电离辐射,还可以显示肝门周围的纤维块,MRCP可以显示胆系的全貌。但是婴儿不能行呼吸安静配合,因而不适合呼吸控制法下检查,也给这项检查带来了诸多不便,不易广泛应用。

核素显像:放射性核素肝胆显像是一种安全、简单、无创伤性和准确的鉴别诊断婴幼儿黄疸的方法,^{99m}Tc-亚氨二醋酸类(^{99m}Tc-IDAs)肝胆显像是目前临床用于早期鉴别诊断婴儿黄疸最常用的方法之一,对先天性胆系闭锁诊断的敏感度可达97%,特异度82%,准确度91%,但是当血中胆红素浓度过高(>102μmol/L)或肝内胆管胆汁淤滞,由于显像剂与胆红素结构类似,均经阴离子传输进入肝细胞,二者存在竞争抑制作用,从而影响胆系显像,不易与胆管闭锁鉴别。

在日常诊疗过程中,^{99m}Tc-MIBI显像剂多应用于心肌显影,其体内代谢特点之一就是经肝胆系统排泄。MIBI与EHIDA显像剂不一样,分子结构与胆红素不同,故胆红素和^{99m}Tc-MIBI显像剂的肝胆摄取排泄过程无明显竞争抑制作用,^{99m}Tc-MIBI的肝胆排泄不受血胆红素水平的影响,而是由多药耐药相关蛋白(MRP)和P糖蛋白(P-gp)调控。所以该组探讨了利用MIBI的特性来鉴别诊断高胆红素病因可能性,报道的两例高胆红素患儿血胆红素均>212μmol/l。

从显像图像上可以看出二乙基乙酰苯胺亚氨二醋酸(^{99m}Tc-EHIDA)显像胆系未见胆汁排泄征象,而^{99m}Tc-MIBI影像则能很好地显示胆汁排泄通畅。通过分析对比以上两种显像剂影像学表现,并经随访证实^{99m}Tc-MIBI可用于婴儿黄疸的鉴别诊断,尤其在胆红素水平很高的情况下较^{99m}Tc-EHIDA更具有优势。

一例报道为黄疸鉴别诊断提供了值得进一步探索的新方法,由于病例数少,且未在胆系闭锁病例中观察,其临床应用价值有待进一步研究。

MRI与MRCP:MRI可显示肝胆管及肝门周围的情况,并且可多层面成像及对病变的综合诊断做出全面的评价,以指导临床合理治疗。

第六章 小儿胆系疾病

第一节 先天性胆总管囊肿自发穿孔

胆胰管连接异常所致的胰液反流是先天性胆总管囊肿穿孔的主要病因之一。胆胰管连接异常在囊性扩张型胆总管囊肿为胆管→胰管连接型(C-P型),连接部近端胆管发生狭窄,胰液逆流入胆管少;梭形扩张型胆总管囊肿则为胰管→胆管连接型(P-C型),连接管相对狭窄,胰液易逆流入胆管。

自发性胆管穿孔与胆总管囊肿是同源于胆胰管连接异常的不同临床阶段的胆系疾病,胰液反流引起反复发作的胆管炎、黏膜破坏、胆管壁弹性纤维变性,胆管逐渐扩张,胆汁聚集,囊肿内压升高,胆管缺血坏死,引起胆总管囊肿自发性穿孔,继发胆汁性腹膜炎。一组25例中22例术中胆系造影发现胆胰管连接异常,腹水及胆管内胆汁淀粉酶不同程度升高。

胆系血供60%来自胰十二指肠后上动脉,38%来自肝动脉,这些血管沿胆总管侧边走行,胆总管与胆囊管交界部处于血供的末梢,血供最差,这是胆管穿孔好发于此处的主要原因。一组胆总管囊肿穿孔部位在胆囊管与胆总管交界部占72%(18/25),与文献报道一致。

文献报道胆总管囊肿自发穿孔与胆总管远端有蛋白栓子造成的梗阻有关,该组术中于胆胰管连接段多次发现牙膏样黏稠蛋白栓子。由此可见,胆胰管连接异常使胰液进入胆管造成局部组织损伤,胆管梗阻使胆总管囊肿内压升高,在胆管血供先天性发育缺陷的基础上加重了局部缺血,以上因素共同作用造成胆管穿孔。

小儿胆总管囊肿自发性穿孔少见,其临床特点与成人胆管穿孔有着明显的不同,有腹膜炎表现者腹部压痛以右上腹为著,但部分病例早期并不表现出典型的急性腹膜炎症状,晚期常以腹胀、腹水为其主要临床表现,常规腹腔穿刺可明确腹水为胆汁性渗液。

但是非胆总管囊肿性肝外胆管穿孔(包括胆囊穿孔)和十二指肠溃疡穿孔也可出现胆汁性腹水,因此本病的诊断需借助影像学检查以明确胆总管囊肿及其穿孔的存在。

胆总管是否扩张的判定标准:正常2~6岁胆总管直径2~4 mm,6~10岁为2~6 mm,10~12岁为3~6 mm。当其直径>6 mm时即为胆总管扩张。如果胆总管囊肿的直径小于胆总管囊肿长度的1/3即为梭型胆总管囊肿,否则为囊型胆总管囊肿。

如前所述,梭型胆总管囊肿与囊型胆总管囊肿不仅是形态上的不同,在病因、临床等方面也存在较大差异。胆总管囊肿自发性穿孔易发生于梭型病例,该组胆总管囊肿穿孔病例中梭型占18例,囊型仅占7例。

胆总管囊肿穿孔主要表现为由于胆汁漏出胆总管囊肿和/或胆囊张力明显减低,胆总管囊肿局部囊壁皱缩,胆囊萎缩,伴腹腔积液。该组23例显示胆总管囊肿和/或胆囊张力减低、囊壁皱缩并腹腔积液。胆总管囊肿囊壁的缺损是胆总管囊肿自发性穿孔的直接征象。但由于穿孔一般较小,常规CT检查较难发现。该组病例胆总管囊肿囊壁多显示模糊,仅3例显示比较明确的囊壁缺损,与穿孔口较小,断层层面较厚有关。

有学者采用螺旋CT薄层增强扫描多平面重建诊断胆管穿孔的报道。但该组作者认为,在已经出现胆总管囊肿囊壁皱缩、胆囊缩小、胆管周围及腹腔积液等典型征象时,为了显示缺损口而施以薄层或增强扫描,难免有增大辐射剂量之虞。

解剖学上胆总管走行于肝十二指肠韧带中,因此胆总管囊肿自发性穿孔时首先在胆管周围出现胆汁漏出、蜂窝织炎或假性囊肿形成,继而胆汁性腹水向小网膜囊及大腹腔内积聚,也可沿肝十二指肠韧带向肾旁及肾周间隙等腹膜后间隙处引流积聚。该组 1 例可见胆总管囊肿旁局限性包裹积液,假性囊肿形成。

超声可清晰显示胆总管囊肿及其穿孔后合并的腹水,但由于婴幼儿胃肠道内积气较多,超声易受肠气干扰而误诊。

磁共振胆胰管成像(MRCP)能精确地显示胆胰管系统结构,但当有大量腹水或小网膜囊积液时,肝外胆管和胰管可被掩盖。一般认为作为急诊处置,CT 检查可以对胆总管囊肿自发性穿孔及其合并的胆汁性腹膜炎做出明确诊断,为手术方案的制订提供足够的术前参考信息。并且,CT 有助于胆总管囊肿自发性穿孔与消化道穿孔、肠梗阻、胰腺炎等儿童常见急腹症的鉴别诊断。总之,自发性穿孔是胆总管囊肿的一种少见并发症,并且常常是儿童胆总管囊肿明确诊断前的首发表现,临床表现不典型,易被误漏诊。CT 检查可根据胆总管囊肿外形缩小、张力减低、囊壁皱缩或缺损、胆囊缩小、腹腔积液等典型征象做出明确诊断。

第二节　先天性气管胆管瘘

先天性气管胆管瘘是气管与胆管的异常通道,若瘘道起自支气管,又称先天性支气管胆管瘘。本病非常罕见,自 Neuhauser 等(1952)首次报道截止至 2011 年(英文文献)共报道 27 例,其中新生儿 15 例。仅有较少报道发生于成人。国内万方数据库共报道 3 例,均为成年患者。先天性(支)气管胆管瘘的发病机制尚有争议。一种观点认为其属于上消化道的重复畸形,是气管与肝内胆管憩室的异常连通;另有一些人认为它是异常支气管芽与异常胆系的联通。Tommasoni 等(2000)报道瘘管常起源于气管隆突,约占 55%,右主支气管占 30%,左主支气管占 10%。瘘管穿过后纵隔,经过食道裂孔进入腹腔。所有瘘管的胆管端无一例外地开口在左半肝。Kumagai 等(2011)认为瘘管是在胚胎发育过程中肝芽与肺芽最接近的部分残留形成的,所以所有的异常通道均发生于左半肝。

先天性(支)气管胆管瘘伴左侧引流胆管或总胆管的发育不良或缺如的发生率可高达 36.5%。一例患儿即合并肝外胆管闭锁,产生的胆汁只能通过瘘管引流至气管,持续的胆汁刺激使支气管、肺组织发生慢性炎症,进而导致肺实变和不张,临床表现为反复发作、持续难治性肺炎。该例先天性气管胆管瘘在新生儿期即表现为反复发作的咳嗽、气促、呕吐;胸部 X 线示肺炎、肺不张。该组作者认为,对于持续的胆汁性呕吐伴反复发作、持续的难治性肺炎的患儿,应怀疑此病,早期明确诊断,尽早手术处理。

先天性(支)气管胆管瘘的其他合并畸形包括膈疝、食管闭锁伴气管食管瘘等。在不合并胆管闭锁或其他畸形的患者,临床症状可不显著,可能导致瘘管直到成年才被发现。

在一些国家纤维支气管镜常为先天性(支)气管胆管瘘主要检查手段。但纤维支气管镜只能显示瘘管开口,而无法了解瘘管远端情况,同时给患儿带来一定痛苦。也有部分采用 CT 重建技术和磁共振胰胆管造影显示瘘管的报道。该例新生儿采用低剂量 64 层螺旋 CT 检查和重建可显示支气管胆管瘘的起点、行径及终点;可清楚显示肝内胆管气体,术前即可确诊,并为术前准备提供充足信息;而术中造影则可以进一步明确肝外胆管闭锁。

第三节　误诊病例简介:小儿胆总管管状乳头状腺瘤与胆总管囊肿

有作者报告小儿胆总管管状乳头状腺瘤误诊一例。肝外胆管的良性肿瘤性病变是指左右肝管至胆胰管十二指肠连接区的胆管良性肿瘤。肝外胆管良性肿瘤病变少见。常见的良性肿瘤起源于胆管的腺上皮,2/3 为息肉、腺瘤,男:女 =1.3:1,平均发病年龄 58 岁,好发部位依次为乳头部(47%)、胆总管(27%)、肝总管(15%)。

肝外胆管腺瘤为息肉样外观,大小不等,大体呈结节状,绝大多数为单发,可有蒂或无蒂。显微镜下腺瘤分3型:管状腺瘤、乳头状腺瘤、管状乳头状腺瘤,其中以管状腺瘤最为常见。肝外胆管腺瘤常常引起梗阻性黄疸,同时伴有不同程度的右上腹疼痛。

分析该例误诊原因:①本病发生率低。胆总管腺瘤较胆总管囊肿的发生率低,尤其是小儿患者。文献记载小儿胆管腺瘤极为罕见。②临床病史无特征性。患儿以"脐周及右上腹痛伴恶心、呕吐"为主诉,无梗阻性黄疸、腹部肿块等症状;同时患儿3年前在外院曾诊断为先天性胆总管囊肿,此病史对诊断有误导作用。③MRCP征象无特征性。胆总管腺瘤当瘤体较小时, MRCP多不能显示胆总管内结节状的软组织信号影,但可显示瘤体梗阻引起的胆总管扩张、胆囊增大、胆囊管增粗。一般表现为扩张的胆总管形态欠规则,下部呈鸟嘴样狭窄,常因反复合并的胆管炎、胆管结石而表现出胆汁淤积、分层现象、信号不均、壁欠光整等,但这些征象可见于多种疾病,对于小儿患者,先天性胆总管囊肿合并胆管炎、胆管结石引起梗阻时,亦可表现出胆汁淤积、分层现象、信号不均、肝内外胆管扩张、胆囊增大等。④因术中观察扩张的胆总管壁增厚,内壁较毛糙、内有4枚结石样物质,未见明显的软组织肿块,考虑系"胆总管囊肿"并反复发生胆管炎和胆管结石导致胆管壁增厚并与周围结构粘连.所以术后仍诊断为"先天性胆总管囊肿"。

胆总管腺瘤缺乏特有的症状和体征, B超是最基本的检查手段,口服/静脉胆系造影和ERCP可显示扩张的胆管腔内单个(偶为多个)的充盈缺损及胆管狭窄、阻塞等征象,CT、MRCP有时可显示出扩张的胆管腔内的肿瘤呈软组织结节影。

以上影像学检查均可能显示出肿瘤结节,但不能鉴别腺瘤、息肉、未钙化结石等。胆总管腺瘤术前确诊困难,最后定性诊断需要病理切片检查证实。

第四节　新生儿胆胰管下端括约肌闭锁不全

本症十分少见。Frates(1965)报告2例,均伴存十二指肠闭锁和环状胰腺。Kirks 和 Baden(1973)报告一例唐氏综合征患者,出现完全性远段十二指肠梗阻伴存本症。Rosenblatt(1967)报告2例空气返流入胆系伴十二指肠梗阻。Caffey(1972)也曾举例介绍十二指肠狭窄婴儿钡剂返流入胆系。在X线照片上,肝影内可见线状空气条纹影,在新生儿期,此类表现通常表示空气位于门静脉系统内,在胆管树内者极少。一般说来,在常规腹部X线检查中,对于门静脉系统积气与胆系积气难以区别,在新生儿尤甚,但是,如从影像上能够确定胆外胆管蒂或胆囊的所在,则可排除门静脉积气的可能性。

Atkinson等(1977)在讨论本症时指出,十二指肠远端梗阻的病例出现本症,可能源于十二指肠内压高于胆管树处腔内压的升高。有的病例手术发现无确切的胆胰下端共同管,此类解剖结构的变异也为本症的一个原因。

第七章 小儿胰腺疾病

第一节 MR诊断小儿环状胰腺

环状胰腺是胰头的胰腺组织于十二指肠乳头以上呈环状或钳状压迫十二指肠降部的先天性畸形，分为完全型和不完全型。完全型者胰腺组织环绕十二指肠降部，无间隙；不完全型者胰腺组织环绕肠管周径的2/3~4/5，有1.0~1.5cm的间隔区，间隔区位于前壁或外侧壁。

环状胰腺是胰腺胚胎时期发育异常所致。同时临床上常见合并多种畸形，提示本病与基因表达异常相关。临床上大多数环状胰腺为不完全型，压迫程度多不严重，约有近半数患者至成年后才出现症状。主要症状为十二指肠部分或完全梗阻，呕吐是最常见症状，少数伴有黄疸，重症发病较早。

腹部平片可见高位梗阻征象。胃肠钡餐造影示十二指肠降部一局限外压性狭窄，长度为1.0~4.5 cm，边缘光滑，黏膜皱襞存在并完整；狭窄近端的十二指肠扩张，严重时胃也扩张且胃内有潴留。但胃肠钡餐造影不能直接显示胰腺和胆胰管。

超声显示十二指肠降部肿块，并有压迫梗阻。但由于解剖关系的复杂性及超声显像的特性，很少病例显示十二指肠降部通过胰头中心这种典型的特征。CT和MRI均可见十二指肠腔狭窄和围绕十二指肠降段的软组织块影，与胰头在同一水平，类似肿大的胰头。平扫与增强扫描其密度、信号均与正常胰头一致。

磁共振胆胰管造影(MRCP)示主胰管在胰头部向右侧呈环状包绕十二指肠降部并向左侧横向走行，体尾主胰管变短，胰管和胆管汇合的共同管很短。MRCP与MRI相结合可获得胰腺和胆胰管的整体影像表现。

第二节 胰母细胞瘤

胰母细胞瘤发生于幼儿，Horie(1977)认为此瘤出现在器官发育阶段，即胚胎第八周胰腺发育见与腺泡相似的错构状态，故称为胰母细胞瘤，由于它属于胰腺上皮性肿瘤，也被称为幼儿癌。有作者报告3例胰母细胞瘤，他回顾1932—1976年共有11例报告。再检索1977—1995年有13篇论文涉及胰母细胞瘤的描述，病例数计23例。本病影像诊断的病理基础为具有包膜，肿块巨大，坏死囊变发生率高等。

另有作者报告1例8岁男孩。因左上腹包块就诊，包块约拳头大小，质硬固定。患儿近2个月来有食欲减退，消瘦和上腹痛等症状。CT扫描示胰尾巨大占位，卵圆形，大小约8.0cm×13.0cm，囊壁厚薄不均，最厚处达2.8cm，可见密度不均的条状囊壁钙化，囊内液性密度区之CT值为4.2HU，其间混有散在和聚集成团的钙斑。肿块内因液化坏死而形成所谓假-假性囊肿。CT增强扫描，示囊壁瘤块有明显强化，肝内有多个大小不等的低密度区。手术见胰尾巨大肿块，与脾门粘连，肝左右叶均有质地坚硬的肿块。遂作胰尾及脾切除术。瘤细胞主要有两种形态：一种为扁平(鳞状)细胞，组成扁平小体；另一种为低柱状细胞，围成腺样结构；在上述两种细胞间为过渡细胞。病理诊断为胰母细胞瘤。该例甲胎蛋白试验阴性。

由于胰母细胞瘤的手术切除预后优于成人胰腺癌，提高对本病的认识，在术前做出正确诊断，将有助于患者得到有效的治疗。

第三节　胰腺胚胎细胞瘤

胰腺胚胎细胞瘤是儿童罕见的胰腺原发肿瘤，为描述该病在MR、CT及超声的特点，Montemarano等(2000)分析了病理确诊的10例病人，男性6例，女性4例，年龄2~20岁，平均年龄6.8岁，中位年龄11.2岁。9例有手术结果，无病例随访。10例均行CT检查，超声检查7例，3例行MRI。

影像学描述内容：肿瘤大小，起源器官，肿瘤边界及形态，肿瘤均匀程度，钙化，增强程度，腹水，胆管和/或胰管扩张，局部侵犯，淋巴结肿大，血管包埋，血管侵犯，转移部位及MRI的信号强度。

研究结果表明，肿瘤最大直径5~14cm(平均8.6cm)，5例起源于胰腺，局限于胰头、胰体和胰尾各1例，位于体尾部2例。其余5例中的4例超声和CT很难确定肿瘤起源胰腺或肝脏，其中1例MRI考虑来源于肝脏，但不能排除肝脏外生性肿瘤，第10例肿瘤巨大，影像学难以确定其起源。

CT显示6例肿瘤边界清晰，3例部分清晰，1例边界不清，有浸润存在。超声描述肿瘤边界与CT相一致，但1例CT示边界清晰而超声示不清晰。行MRI 3例中2例MR表现肿瘤边界与CT相同，第3例MRI示肿瘤边界清晰但CT示部分清晰。7例肿瘤呈圆形而光滑，2例分叶状，1例不规则且有浸润。2例于静脉给对比剂前后均行CT，显示肿瘤强化，其余8例通过与邻近血管比较提示肿瘤强化。1例在MRI上肿瘤呈明显强化。CT和超声示7例肿瘤高度不均匀，2例中度不均匀，1例均匀。在超声和MRI上，肿瘤的不均匀性一般不如CT增强后明显。

肿瘤在T_1WI上为低或中等信号强度，与脾一致，在T_2WI上呈高信号强度，稍低于脾。1例肿瘤在钆剂增强后稍高于脾强度。2例肿瘤有钙化。影像学上无法确认血管受侵，1例胰体肿块7.5cm，而手术发现门静脉主干已受侵；另1例胰头有巨大肿物，CT和超声均示胆管及胰管扩张，手术证实肿物在胰头水平压迫和侵犯总胆管。2例CT和超声证明有盆腔转移，但均未发现肠系膜、门静脉及网膜淋巴结肿大。影像学及手术均证实有2例肝转移。1例网膜、腹膜及盆腔转移的患儿在镰状韧带区还有多发肝脏肿块，因肿块邻近原发灶，影像学无法确定为局部侵犯、转移或为淋巴结肿大。2例出现腹水，其中1例门静脉受侵，另1例有盆腔转移。10例均未发现淋巴结肿大。

Montemarano等(2000)认为，胰腺胚胎细胞瘤质地不均匀，边界清晰，多数可能起源于胰腺及肝脏，肿瘤浸润性强，易发生局部血管、肠管侵犯及远处转移。当儿童出现上腹部包块尤其是源于胰腺及肝脏时，应考虑此病的可能性。

第四节　胰腺损伤

胰腺损伤在儿童腹部闭合性损伤中并不常见，与成人多数为贯通伤的损伤机制不同，儿童胰腺损伤绝大多数为腹部钝挫伤。由于儿童膈肌活动度大，腹壁相对较薄，肋缘相对较高，作用于上腹部的各种外力容易将胰腺向较坚硬的脊柱挤压，产生损伤。同时随着交通事故发生率不断提高，外伤性胰腺炎所占比例逐渐增大，一组18例中，共有8例，约占总数的44.5%。

由于胰腺位于腹膜后，解剖位置较深，损伤后症状较轻微及隐匿，常无腹膜刺激症状。上腹部外伤病史及中上腹疼痛有压痛是小儿诊断可疑胰腺损伤的主要依据，多数患儿可有呕吐，而典型腰背部放射痛在儿童中较少见。

尤其单纯胰腺钝挫伤，临床表现不明显，因而往往延误诊断，直至形成假性胰腺囊肿时才被发现(如该组3例腹部钝挫伤后，早期仅出现腹痛及发热等非特异性症状)。

若胰腺损伤较重，液体可积聚于网膜囊内，则表现为上腹明显压痛和腹肌紧张,也可因腹肌受刺激而出现局部疼痛,该组 9 例(Ⅱ级 6 例,Ⅲ级及Ⅳ级各 1 例)。

若胰液外渗,即胰瘘,则易经网膜孔或破裂的网膜进入腹腔后,可很快出现局限性或弥漫性腹膜炎,临床特征明显,该组 2 例(Ⅲ级及Ⅳ级各 1 例)。

可见,在小儿胰腺损伤中,较轻型损伤(Ⅰ级、Ⅱ级)较多见,重型损伤(Ⅲ级、Ⅳ级及Ⅴ级)较少见,该组Ⅰ级 + Ⅱ级共 13 例(72.2%),Ⅲ级 + Ⅳ级共 5 例(27.8%),无Ⅴ级病例,这与既往同类报道相似,也是小儿胰腺损伤的一大特点。

在胰腺损伤中,多数学者认为胰淀粉酶及脂肪酶升高的诊断意义不大,在非常严重的胰腺损伤中,淀粉酶及脂肪酶可表现正常。该组所有病例入院时均进行了血常规及血清淀粉酶水平检查,但均未行脂肪酶检查,其中白细胞升高 12 例,血清淀粉酶升高仅 9 例,另有 9 例患儿 24 h 后复查血及尿淀粉酶均明显升高,因此,当患儿入院时单独血清淀粉酶水平低并不能排除胰腺损伤的可能性。

当影像学检查不能确定诊断,临床表现无立即剖腹探查根据,但患儿有持续难以解释的腹痛时,重复检查血清淀粉酶水平对诊断胰腺损伤尤为重要。同时也应当明确,仅血清淀粉酶升高既无诊断特异性,又无法判断胰腺损伤的范围,但假性胰腺囊肿形成后,囊液淀粉酶的测定及囊壁标本的病理检查则是确诊的金标准。该组 18 例中单发 4 例,结合临床病史考虑为胰腺损伤后遗改变,合并急性胰腺损伤同时存在 6 例。

胰腺损伤包括实质损伤及胰管损伤,CT 能直接显示实质部分的损伤,而并发症的发生与主胰管的损伤密切相关。对于怀疑胰腺损伤患儿,在病情条件许可情况下, MSCT 增强扫描应作为首选检查方法。在增强条件下,相对平扫更容易发现胰周血肿、积液、胰实质损伤及断裂。该组除 4 例通过术中探查确诊外,10 例均经 CT 平扫加增强扫描,4 例仅行 CT 平扫。胰腺损伤 CT 的直接征象包括胰腺肿大、胰腺裂伤、胰管断裂,胰腺内出血、积液。间接征象包括胰周被膜和肾周筋膜增厚、小网膜囊、胰周及肾旁间隙积液、胰周及腹膜后出现炎性反应和胰周假性囊肿的形成。虽然 CT 在直接显示胰管损伤存在困难,但可以根据胰腺实质损伤程度间接判断胰管是否可能破裂,少数病例也可在多排螺旋薄层 CT 显示实质破裂处与胰管相通。

结合该组病例资料,该组作者认为有下列情况之一者,应想到有胰管或主胰管损伤可能:①胰腺完全断裂;②胰腺断裂大于胰腺直径的 1/2(特别是胰颈、胰体中上部的断裂);③胰腺实质内较大血肿;④胰腺实质严重挫伤或碎裂;该组病例手术记录 3 例有胰管损伤,CT 提示 2 例。有条件者可进一步行磁共振胰胆管造影(MRCP)或内镜逆行胰胆管造影(ERCP)。

尽管急性、慢性胰腺炎引起胰腺假性囊肿相对多见,且与损伤性胰腺假囊肿的病理改变及 CT 表现相同,但两者假囊肿形成时间有所不同,损伤性胰腺假囊肿形成约为 2 周,而前者为 4 周左右,结合临床病史不难区分。

该组 4 例 CT 仅表现为单纯性胰腺假囊肿,结合临床考虑为损伤后遗改变,而另 6 例则是同时合并急性胰腺损伤。由于胰腺损伤的病理变化为进行性,在损伤早期,CT 可呈假阴性,该组 1 例门诊首次 CT 平扫呈阴性表现,血清淀粉酶亦无异常,入院后复查 CT 见胰颈处裂伤伴胰周积液 / 血。因此,结合临床实验室检查,及时进行必要的 CT 复查,对漏诊及误诊尤为重要。综上所述,小儿胰腺损伤临床相对少见,但死亡率及并发症较高,临床需高度警惕胰腺损伤的可能性。MSCT 结合外伤病史,外伤部位及临床症状和体征可以对本病做出准确诊断;同时除了可以确定病变性质外,还可以明确病变范围,以及全面了解腹部复合损伤的情况。因此, MSCT 是目前诊断本病首选的检查方法。

第八章　小儿脾脏疾病

第一节　脾硬化性血管瘤样结节性转化

详见本书本卷第二十一篇第八章　脾硬化性　　血管瘤样结节性转化。

第二节　多脾综合征伴腹腔脏器转位

多脾综合征，指多脾伴有先天性心血管异常和内脏位置异位，是一种十分少见的先天性多系统发育畸形组成的综合征。由 Baillie(1788)首先报道，之后逐渐为人们所认识。脾脏起源于中胚层，是人体唯一见于左侧的器官。在胚胎发育第 5~6 周，自脐管回纳到腹腔内进行自身旋转，当这一阶段发生障碍，即可形成多脾综合征。多脾综合征的特征为脾的数目可为 2~6 个，合并有下腔静脉肝内段中断并奇静脉连续，房、室间隔缺损或其他心血管畸形，腹部内脏异位，胃肠道异常等，临床症状多与心血管畸形有关，肠道旋转不良可引起肠梗阻、腹部不适。虽然多脾综合征少见，但不应误认为肿瘤性病变，尤其是进行 B 超检查时，应建议进行 CT 或者 MRI 检查。其结节可多个和大小不一，但增强表现符合脾脏的强化规律，即动脉期呈花斑样强化，静脉期及延迟期强化均匀，多可明确诊断。同时还应检查心脏、肝脏、胰腺及胃肠等，除外是否有相伴随的病变。同时在发现有心脏先天性畸形及胃肠道位置异常时，要进一步检查脾脏有无异常。

第三节　脾尖部的重叠引起 CT 误诊

有作者在小儿腹部 CT 检查时报告 1 例左侧肾胚胎瘤病儿，该肿瘤呈现明显低密度包块，且向左侧伸延累及左肾前上缘。但是，超声检查与手术均发现左肾健存，该肾受侵犯的阴影实际上为脾的尖部重叠所致。

第四节　婴儿急性脾扭转

脾脏由各韧带和腹壁肌肉的张力维持其解剖位置，当各韧带先天性发育异常，发生韧带松弛，脾蒂过长，形成游走脾。早期游走脾在腹腔内活动范围很大，可由横膈疝入胸腔或下移到盆腔内，甚至进入巨大的腹股沟管内。晚期游走脾与周围组织发生粘连时可使之固定。Abell 统计 95 例游走脾，其中 88 例为女性，年龄为 6~80 岁，最常见的症状是腹部包块。脾蒂发生扭转大多为顺时针方向，最多可达 12 圈。急性脾扭转表现为突然发生腹痛，扭转将造成血液循环障碍，充血及坏死。慢性脾扭转可无自觉症状,如脾动脉完全闭塞可使脾组织发生纤维化,逐渐萎缩。游走脾主要靠影像学检查确诊。CT 不仅可以显示游走的脾脏,CT 增强扫描还可能了解扭转后脾脏的血运情况,是术前诊断较理想的方法。

第九章　小儿门静脉疾病

儿童门静脉海绵样变性

门静脉海绵样变性是门静脉主干和/或分支完全或部分阻塞后，门静脉压力增高，其周围逐渐形成大量侧支血管和/或阻塞后再通，因此这些侧支血管在大体标本切面上呈海绵状血管瘤样改变，故有此名称。本病并发上消化道出血高达 80%，因此，及时诊断和早期治疗意义重大。

原发性和继发性：门静脉海绵样变性病因尚不完全清楚，分为原发性和继发性。

原发性病因常见于儿童患者，主要是门静脉或其主要分支先天畸形，如缺失、狭窄或闭塞，患儿易合并其他先天畸形，可累及心血管、气管、肾脏及胃肠道等，一组 22 例中 18 例(82%)为先天发育异常所致门静脉海绵样变性，其中 5 例患儿合并心血管、胆管或气管、支气管畸形。继发性病因是指原有正常的门静脉系统的管腔结构，由于肿瘤侵犯、门静脉炎、血栓形成等导致门静脉血流受阻(成人多见)，该组仅 4 例(18%)由于瘤栓或血栓所致。

主要包括两种情况：①继发于新生儿脐炎等门静脉系统炎症的门静脉及其主要分支的血栓栓塞症。该组所有患儿均无新生儿脐炎病史，3 例患儿形成门静脉系统血栓。②门静脉外压性狭窄或闭塞，血液系统疾病(如凝血机制异常、真性红细胞增多症等)等继发门静脉血栓形成，该组仅 1 例，为肝右叶内胚窦瘤压迫门静脉主干狭窄。

临床表现：目前普遍认为有侧支循环建立、脾肿大、腹腔积液等门静脉高压表现以及影像学上有门-门、门-体侧支循环形成和门静脉海绵样变性征象，便可以确诊。但门静脉海绵样变性缺乏特异性临床表现，早期临床诊断困难，常在出现消化道出血后才就诊。该组 22 例中 16 例出现呕血、便血后，进一步检查发现门静脉海绵样变性合并门静脉高压、食管胃底静脉曲张。无症状或症状轻的门脉海绵样变性患者可保守治疗，症状重者需要手术治疗。

分型：一般临床分为Ⅳ型：Ⅰ型，海绵样变性限于门静脉，无临床症状，无脾脏增大；Ⅱ型，海绵样变性限于门静脉，同时有脾大，肝硬化；Ⅲ型，海绵样变性累及门静脉和肠系膜上静脉，脾静脉；Ⅳ型，海绵样变性累及整个门静脉系统。临床根据病变分型不同，采用不同的治疗和手术方式。因此，确定病变范围及严重程度对于治疗具有指导价值。

影像学研究：临床诊断主要依靠影像学检查。既往，传统的数字减影血管造影(DSA)是评价血管病变的金标准，但其为有创检查，并发症多，不利于临床上的广泛应用。近年来，随着螺旋 CT 技术的发展，特别是 64 排 MSCT，其微创、快捷和强大的重组功能等优点，特别是 CT 血管成像(CTA)，不但能够清晰显示细小的血管和门静脉的病变，还能立体显示迂曲侧支血管的起止、行径、扩张程度和累及范围。

门静脉系统阻塞后导致门静脉远端高压，门静脉属支及侧支循环开放，形成两种分流，即：门-门分流和门-体分流，门-门分流指向肝性侧支循环——胆支(胆囊静脉丛和胆管周围静脉丛)开放，主要是向肝脏提供营养性物质；门-体分流指将门静脉的部分血流引向压力较低的体循环，即离肝性侧支循环——胃支、胰十二指肠后上静脉、脐旁静脉开放，可降低门静脉高压程度。

正常情况下门静脉周围仅见肝固有动脉伴行，胆管及胆囊壁及其周边无小血管断面，在门静脉海绵样变性中，胆丛和胆总管周围侧支血管开放具特征性，为门静脉栓塞后特有的一组侧支循环路径。CT 表现为胆囊、胆管壁增厚和/或管腔不规则狭窄，病理基础是胆囊、胆管壁及其附近的侧支静脉丛，致胆囊、胆管壁增厚，甚至胆管受压狭窄，形成所谓“假性胆管癌征”，严重时可引起梗阻性黄疸。该组 22 例出现胆管周围静脉丛曲张，16 例出现胆囊静脉丛曲张。另外，该组 22 例中，门-体侧支血管有胃静脉和食管胃底静脉曲张者最多，共 21 例(95%)，胰十二指肠后上静脉曲张 5 例，脐静脉曲张 1 例，腹膜后静脉曲张 8 例，还出现了脾-肾静脉

或胃 - 脾静脉分流,肠系膜下静脉直肠静脉丛曲张,肠系膜上静脉汇入左髂内静脉,肠系膜静脉汇入下腔静脉。

该组研究发现儿童门静脉海绵样变性的门 - 体分流可以是多种多样的,除了成人病例所描述的常见门 - 门分流和门 - 体分流外,还出现了腹膜后静脉,脾 - 胃 - 肾静脉分流,肠系膜静脉直接汇入腔静脉系统,可能在胚胎发育中形成或生后代偿能力强,侧支循环可广泛形成。

门静脉系统特殊的解剖结构及复杂的血流成分、血流速度缓慢,致栓塞易发生于门静脉系统。儿童发生门静脉栓塞较少,该组仅 4 例,其中 1 例是瘤栓,3 例为血栓。

肝动脉期异常灌注,表现为动脉晚期肝脏周边区的异常明显强化灶,呈斑片状高密度影。有学者认为,肝脏由肝动脉及门静脉双重血供,门静脉主干及叶分支完全或部分阻塞后,门静脉供血诱发肝动脉供血随即代偿增加,这种代偿一般发生在肝脏的周边区,因为肝门区周围的血供通常由海绵样变的侧支循环来提供。该研究仅 3 例患儿表现出肝动脉期灌注异常,可能是由于儿童代偿机制较强,易形成侧支循环,肝脏血供较好。

Valerie 等(2006)发现门静脉海绵样变性能够引起肝脏尾状叶及第Ⅳ段增生,左外叶的萎缩,称为萎缩 - 增生复合体。尾状叶及第Ⅳ段的增生主要原因是其与海绵样变性的肝门静脉较近使门静脉血流能够得以维持。该研究中 11 例(50%)出现肝叶比例失调,表现为左外叶萎缩及尾状叶饱满、增生,此征象较成人少见,原因可能是患儿年龄偏小,肝脏形态异常未完全形成。

儿童与成人门静脉海绵样变性的差异:该组认为儿童与成人门静脉海绵样变性不同点有:①病因不同,儿童先天性为主,成人继发性为主;②儿童侧支循环形成较成人更广泛、多样;③肝左叶萎缩,尾叶肥大等肝形态异常征象较成人少见;④肝脏异常灌注征象更少见。

综上所述,MSCT 不仅能显示门静脉海绵样变性后形成的侧支循环,提供直观的诊断,还能显示肝脾大小、形态、肝脏的灌注情况、各段血流改变以及侧支循环走行情况等,可为临床治疗提供较明确的资料以方便正确选择治疗方案。

虽然该研究采用了低剂量 CT 扫描技术,但 MSCT 仍存在辐射、需使用碘剂,不能测定流向、流速和流量等缺陷。对于儿童门静脉海绵样变性,应首选彩超筛选,然后有针对性的进行 CT 检查,以降低辐射损伤。

第十章　小儿其他疾病

小儿常见腹部肿瘤

小儿腹部肿瘤并不少见，X线平片可显示肿瘤的钙化和肿瘤对其他脏器的推移;超声检查是发现小儿腹部肿瘤最主要的影像学方法;CT扫描用于进一步确诊小儿腹部肿瘤,定性,制定手术或化疗方案以及治疗后随访;磁共振扫描用于进一步定性,观察肿瘤对椎管或大血管的侵犯等。儿科病儿由于不配合、易运动且解剖部位较小,造成CT和磁共振检查与成人患者相比较为困难,而且图像质量较成人稍差。小儿CT和磁共振检查时,对于年龄较小不能合作者需给予镇静或麻醉,镇静剂一般用10%的水合氯醛,口服或肛门注射,剂量为每公斤体重0.4~0.5毫升。对于要做增强扫描者,应先开放静脉,然后给予镇静剂。

由于CT检查时间较短,与磁共振相比,噪声也很低,绝大多数病儿使用镇静剂即可完成检查,少数磁共振检查镇静不成功者,可采用氯胺酮麻醉,此时需用经皮血氧饱和度仪监护。小儿CT检查必须考虑射线剂量问题,在检查中,特别是在复查随访时,应尽量采用低剂量扫描技术或直接增强扫描等,并注意放射线防护。

肝母细胞瘤:肝母细胞瘤是小儿最常见的肝脏恶性肿瘤,男孩多见,婴幼儿无痛性腹部肿块是最常见的症状,90%病例在3岁以下,60%在1岁以下,为婴幼儿肝脏内巨大的、边界清楚的肿块,血清甲胎蛋白阳性。肝母细胞瘤CT表现为婴幼儿肝内边界清晰的肿块,通常单发,肿块较大,周围的肝脏结构受压移位,CT平扫低密度居多,也可等密度,可有钙化及坏死,约有半数的病人可出现钙化。增强扫描可见肿块血供丰富,动脉期高密度,门脉期强化程度低于正常的肝脏组织。肝母细胞瘤磁共振表现为T_1WI低信号，T_2WI高信号,也可因出血、坏死而表现为多种信号。DSA血管造影可见肿瘤血管和肿瘤染色,肝动脉化疗也是肝母细胞瘤的治疗方法之一。

肝血管内皮瘤:肝血管内皮瘤最多见于婴幼儿,女孩的发病率是男孩的2倍,是新生儿期最常见的能引起症状的血管性病变之一，85%的病例在6个月之前出现症状,腹部肿块伴有杂音和充血性心力衰竭,可导致消耗性凝血病(血小板减少症)。经过几个月或者几年有无需治疗自然消退的可能,约有一半的婴幼儿伴有皮肤血管瘤。肝血管内皮瘤CT平扫为低密度,可有钙化。增强扫描早期外围强化,随着时间推移,对比剂逐渐进入中心部分,肿瘤呈不均匀的高度强化,病灶内可见粗大的血管。CT随访可见肿块明显减小并可发生钙化。

磁共振表现为T_2WI高信号，T_1WI低信号,肿块的内部及外围可见粗大的滋养/引流血管流空表现。肝血管内皮瘤血管造影表现为肝动脉扩张、扭曲,早期肝静脉显影,病灶部位对比剂异常聚积,降主动脉在腹腔干水平以上粗大,腹腔干水平以下相对细小。

肾母细胞瘤:肾母细胞瘤,也称Wilms瘤,相当常见，80%患病小儿小于5岁,平均年龄为3.6岁,但新生儿和小婴儿中少见，5%~10%的病例是双侧的。临床表现常为无症状腰部肿块。通过外科手术切除,术后化疗等治疗,治愈率超过90%。肾母细胞瘤CT平扫表现为在肾脏位置有一较大的实质性肿块,密度不均匀,偏低,肿块边界清楚,在CT中约15%有钙化。CT增强扫描表现为强化不等,密度不均匀,有低密度坏死区的边界清晰或有假包膜的实质性肿块,明显强化的残留肾脏位于肿瘤外侧。肾母细胞瘤可局部侵犯肾周脂肪和淋巴结。在诊断时约有20%的病人CT可见已发生肺部转移。瘤栓可侵犯肾静脉和下腔静脉。肾母细胞瘤如过中线,往往推移大血管而不是包绕大血管。肾母细胞瘤MR表现与CT表现相似,为T_1低信号和T_2高信号,信号不均匀。MRA有助于在术前确定受影响的血管的情况。

排泄性尿系造影是以前的常用方法,现在较少用。外科手术前肾动脉栓塞和化疗术有助于手术切除肿瘤,但由于影响术后病理观察故开展并不广泛。

神经母细胞瘤:神经母细胞瘤为原发于神经嵴细胞的恶性肿瘤,相当常见,通常表现为无痛性腹部肿块。多见于2岁以前小儿。大约95%的神经母细胞瘤病人尿中儿茶酚胺水平(VMA)升高。根据Evans解剖分期(预后-存活率%),一期肿瘤限于原发器官(存活率90%);二期肿瘤扩散在原发器官附近,但不超越中线(75%);三期肿瘤超越中线(30%);四期肿瘤远处转移(10%)。

但另有4S期,患儿在1岁以内,肿瘤远处转移至皮肤,肝脏和骨髓,但患儿大多预后好,肿瘤不需治疗能自行消失,存活率接近100%。

神经母细胞瘤CT平扫为较大的不规则肾外肿块,可由于坏死,出血表现为肿块密度不均匀,85%以上CT上可看到钙化。CT增强扫描表现为轻度不均匀强化,肿块浸润性生长,可包绕大血管如腹腔干、肠系膜动脉和主动脉,肿块可沿神经孔蔓延侵入椎管,常常转移至肝和骨。神经母细胞瘤MR表现为T_1低信号和T_2高信号的肾外肿块,冠状位扫描可清晰显示肿块与肾脏的关系,MR最有利于发现肿瘤侵入椎管内情况,对肿块包绕血管也可很好显示。DSA血管造影可见血管被推移,很难找到较大的供血动脉。

盆腔横纹肌肉瘤:小儿盆腔横纹肌肉瘤并不罕见,肿瘤可原发于膀胱、阴道、宫颈、子宫、盆腔壁、前列腺和睾丸周围组织。发病高峰在2~6岁。临床上可表现为盆腔巨大肿瘤,伴有继发性尿路症状如排尿困难等。小儿盆腔横纹肌肉瘤CT表现为盆腔不均匀的中度强化的肿块,肿瘤往往很大,可为葡萄簇状,也可为团块状或表现为膀胱壁增厚。肿瘤发展快,播散可通过局部扩散、淋巴结转移和血源性转移至肺、肝和骨。小儿盆腔横纹肌肉瘤MR表现可见肿块表现为T_1稍低信号和T_2高信号,可为混杂信号,肿块有强化。MR矢状位扫描对盆腔横纹肌肉瘤与周围结构的关系显示较好。

骶尾部畸胎瘤:骶尾部畸胎瘤大多数肿瘤在出生数天内就被诊断,如为外生性肿块很容易诊断,如为完全内生性肿瘤有时会延误诊断,可表现为尿路症状、尿潴留或便秘。骶尾部畸胎瘤内含有头发、牙齿、软骨和脂肪等,仅17%的畸胎瘤属恶性。男女比例为1∶3或1∶4。骶尾部畸胎瘤CT表现为可看到脂肪成分和钙化的囊实性肿块,有时可见脂肪液面和骨骼影。MR表现与CT表现类似,信号混杂,MR对钙化显示差,但MR对肿块与椎管的关系显示很好。CT或MR可以明确肿块的范围和有助于外科制定手术方案。

第三十一篇　腹盆部
影像学检查技术

第一章　腹盆部影像学检查

磁共振胃肠道成像

长期以来，不断蠕动的胃肠道不仅被认为是磁共振成像（MRI）的盲区，而且为了避免在邻近组织器官成像时形成运动伪影，常常采用预饱和带抑制其信号。近年来，随着高性能梯度系统的广泛采用，快速成像序列的影像质量大大改善，磁共振成像的应用范围也越来越广。磁共振应用研究人员开始把胃肠道——这一通常意义上的磁共振检查盲区，作为磁共振成像的兴趣区，使得胃肠道疾病诊断及其相关方面的研究充满乐观前景。

磁共振胃肠道成像的研究主要有以下3个方向：①通过扫描序列优化、扫描前准备及对比剂应用等方法，改善胃肠道影像的质量；②利用胃肠道MRI进行生理、药理等基础研究；③观察胃肠道，研究MRI对胃肠疾病的诊断价值。

成像方法优化：胃肠道处于不停的蠕动中，而且该蠕动是一种顺序性的紧张活动，也就是说，同一时点胃肠道各部分活动状态具有不一致性，所以胃肠蠕动形成的伪影无法采用生理信号触发来抑制。目前普通采用扫描前使用解痉剂（口服山莨菪碱或静脉注射 buscopan or glucagon）来减弱肠蠕动，同时采用快速的扫描序列来抑制肠道蠕动对影像质量的影响。

增加肠壁与胃肠道内容物及邻近组织的对比度。

T_1 对比度：胃肠道周围的肠系膜、大小网膜，都是富含脂肪的组织，为了减少这些脂肪高信号对胃肠显示的影响，几乎所有MR胃肠扫描的研究均选择脂肪抑制的 T_1WI序列。同时，采用胃肠道内的负性对比剂，来减低胃肠内容物的信号。有报道使用肠导管，向肠腔内注入一定量的气体，一方面使小肠扩张便于肠壁病变的显示，同时在肠腔形成低信号，在低信号的气体和被抑制的肠周脂肪组织衬托下，正常肠管壁呈高信号。Thomas等（2002）采取连续3天口服加钡餐作为负性对比剂，使肠内容物呈低信号，而免除了检查前清洁灌肠，结果显示，这种方法简便经济，病人容易接受而且检查结果可靠（与结肠镜检结果相比）。

多数胃肠道成像通过静脉注射Gd-DTPA，提高胃肠壁的信号强度，增加其与肠内容物和周围组织的对比而且有利于胃肠肿块性质的鉴别。但使用细胞外对比剂，病变的定性很大程度上取决于兴趣区的首过动力学信息，而快速动态成像，受对比剂在兴趣区停留时间的限制，影像的空间分辨力有限，从而难以检出一些小的病变。Zuo等（2002）进行了锰对比剂用于胃肠道MR扫描的动物实验，结果显示锰对比剂可被消化道黏膜上皮选择性摄取，且在胃肠道黏膜停滞的时间明显长于Gd-DTPA，从而有充分的数据采集时间，可提高影像的空间分辨力。

T_2 对比度：主要通过给肠腔注水，这样既可降低肠道的紧张性又可作为正性对比剂，形成肠腔高信号，与肠壁的低信号形成明显的对比。Thomas等（2002）利用饮水降低小肠紧张性，他们在水中加入甘露醇或甲基纤维素等物质，减少水的重吸收，从而更好地降低小肠紧张性。

扫描序列及技术：为了消除呼吸运动和肠蠕动造成的伪影，MR腹部成像应选用屏气扫描的快速序列，而且空间分辨力要足够高，以便显示小肠常见的溃疡、息肉等小病变。同时要尽量提高信噪比以获得满意的影像质量。只有在配有高性能梯度系统的高场系统上，选用相控阵表面线圈才能满足以上要求。

T_1WI一般选用2D或3D梯度回波序列，与2D序列相比，3D序列可提供更高的空间分辨力和信噪比。在西门子MR系统上，VIBE是普遍采用的序列，它在保证影像分辨力和信噪比足够高的前提下，缩短了扫描时间，使覆盖整个肠道系统仅需22~25秒。

T_2WI一般选用单次激发的TSE或HASTE序列，HASTE序列可产生重 T_2WI 每个层面影像采集时间 <1秒，从而使呼吸运动伪影最小，此外该序列

还有一个优点，即对化学位移伪影不敏感，故其影像可用来进行肠壁厚度的定量测量。

该序列的缺点，除了长回波链引起的模糊伪影外，它对磁敏感性伪影比较敏感，故肠腔气体的存在可产生信号缺失伪影。此外，HASTE 序列显示肠系膜和短 T_2 组织，如淋巴结和纤维组织不理想。

梯度回波序列家族的新宠真实稳态进动快速梯度回波（true FISP）序列，用于胃肠道成像，可提供更高的信噪比和空间分辨力，对磁敏感性伪影也不敏感，故可免用解痉药。该序列特别适合显示肠系膜，在高信号的脂肪和低信号的血管和淋巴结间，形成良好的对比分辨力。要检测克罗恩病活动与否，可采用脂肪抑制的 TSE。

总之，充分的肠腔扩张、匀质的肠腔填充、屏气采集的快速扫描序列、兼有 T_1WI 和 T_2WI 以及对比度增强是理想的肠道 MR 检查的基础。一个完整的 MR 检查程序应包括：SSTSE、HASTE、true FISP 和脂肪抑制的 T_1WI FLASH 序列。SSTSE 用于监测肠腔对比剂等的注入进程或进行透视扫描；HASTE、ture FISP 用于显示解剖结构和发现病变；用对比剂后的 3D FLASH 有助于病变性质的判定。

第二章　CT 与腹盆部疾病

第一节　CT 检查意外发现胃肠疾病

一般说来，食管胃肠疾病主要依靠双对比钡剂造影和内窥镜检查，CT 扫描对此类疾病不是首选的检查法。有时用 CT 检查其他器官疾病时，可同时发现食管胃肠的异常。

一些作者报告一组 1 000 例腹部 CT 扫描中有 4 例意外发现胃肠病变，分别是重复胃、特发性胃幽门肥厚、分房性腹膜炎以及穿孔性结肠癌。由于胃内含液体和空气，胃壁外面有脂肪层以及邻近结肠的充气，CT 图像有时不仅能确定胃壁的情况，而且可观察胃的皱襞。

有作者指出，CT 对于评价消化道原发性恶性肿瘤的范围，以及了解腹部可扪及包块与胃肠道的关系颇有价值。偶尔，CT 扫描可清楚显示含有脂肪的回盲瓣及回盲部，少见情况下 CT 还可观察到胆胰管十二指肠连接区的十二指肠乳头。

第二节　CT 灌注有利于肿瘤的分期

目前在影像学检查中，还一直沿用通过测量淋巴结的大小来判断是否发生了转移。

研究表明，即使很小的淋巴结，其内亦可见异型性细胞；相反，部分较大的淋巴结内可能仅为炎性反应，所以单纯测量大小的方法易致假阳性和假阴性，对指导临床正确分期有一定的局限性。初步的研究结果表明，CT 灌注可通过定量分析淋巴结强化判断转移情况而有助于临床分期。而且，CT 灌注亦能显示隐匿性肝转移，可显示大小仅为 500μm 的小转移灶，进一步提高了对胰腺癌分期的能力。

第三章 其他影像学检查技术

第一节 胃肠疾病的核素检查

怀疑下消化道出血的病人行 Tc 标记红血球扫描,可见示踪剂集中于盆腔中部,与较早的扫描图像进行细致对比,显示为膀胱内示踪剂聚集。

标记效率研究指出注射人体内的 Tc 只有 80% 是结合于红血球,而游离的 Tc 是经尿系分泌排泄。有作者报告根据上述图像却误诊为乙状结肠出血,内镜观察否认乙状结肠出血,无乙状结肠疾病的征象。

有多种不同的原因引起美克尔憩室 ^{99m}Tc 显像的假阳性。有作者报告一例 3 岁女孩大便隐血试验阳性,近有急性胃肠出血史, ^{99m}Tc 显像示右中腹示踪剂聚集,提示为美克尔憩室。手术见肠系膜有一 10cm 大小囊性包块,紧密粘连于近段回肠,这是一个大的回肠重复囊肿,其中有胃黏膜。出血的原因是附近回肠的一个溃疡。

利用核素显像可测量胃的排空时间。各个作者报告测量结果不同:有的作者测出为 70 分钟,有的为 64 分钟,有的作者为 56 分钟,另有作者测量为 23~77 分钟,平均 47 分钟。不同作者测出数值都不相同,解释为技术细节的差异和进餐成分的不同所致。

第二节 胃肠疾患与超声检查

有时在右髂窝发现“肾样”包块,实际上却是盲肠内嵌塞的粪块。超声扫描见膀胱后方有包块挤压膀胱,CT 图像证实该包块实为肠袢。间或见到明显的子宫包块延伸到骶骨,在纵切和横切均见如此,但清洁洗肠后此包块完全消逝,说明也是粪块。

有作者报告,在子宫切除术后,超声检查怀疑有脓肿位于直肠子宫陷凹内,清洁洗肠后此脓肿影仍无变化,但 4 天以后再复查却见该影完全消失,后证实为盲肠积液。

邻近肝区横切扫描发现明显包块影,其前部无回声,后部有回声,疑为腹水;口服饮料后再行横切扫描,见该包块整个均存回声,事实证明该包块为胃。

十二指肠袢能位于胆囊与右肾之间而伪似一脓肿,纵切扫描表现为肝下间隙内有混淆的液体积聚,考虑脓肿,实时观察却可见该影可移动,后来证实为十二指肠袢。

超声检查时偶尔在左侧见到两个肾影,事实上靠前方者为结肠脾曲,结肠壁较厚,靠后方者才是真正肾脏。Engel 和 Deitch(1980)在超声横切扫描时发现网膜充盈盆腔可伪似盆腔内囊性包块。在幽门梗阻者或饮入大量液体为膀胱超声检查作准备的病人,超声扫描见充盈液体而扩张的胃佯似左上腹囊性包块,细心观察此结构的蠕动,从而确认为胃,有时还需请病人饮水一杯,以显示胃中的微小气泡的旋涡,有作者认为这可能是区别胃与胰腺假性囊肿的重要方法。

第三节　肝脏术中超声

详见本书本卷第三篇第十五章　肝癌与超声。

第四章 关于伪影

第一节 腹部和盆腔血管多普勒超声伪影

根据多普勒原理,超声显像不仅可用于解剖结构的探测,且还能用于血流显像。然而,令人遗憾的是,伴随着超声与组织相互作用的多普勒信号的处理过程可产生伪影。如果不能清楚地理解和正确辨别伪影,则可导致误诊。此处就多普勒显像伪影产生的原因给予解释,并讨论如何识别在常规多普勒、彩色多普勒显像及能量多普勒显像的过程中出现的伪影。重点放在腹部和盆腔血管,偶尔以颈动脉为例解释一些多普勒伪影产生的原理。

基本原理:根据下面的公式,从背离超声探头运动的反射体反射回来的声波将会成倍地伸展。$(1+v/c)/(1-v/c)\approx 1+2v/c$(当 v/c 小于 1 时)

式中 v 是反射体的运动速度,c 是声波传播速度,在人体组织内约为 1 540m/s。而对于朝向探头运动的反射体,则 v 为反向,回声将成倍的被压缩。

发射的声波信号频率 f_0 为正弦波,f_0 可以为连续波,或者为脉冲波。只有与超声束共线的速度成分对多普勒频移的产生有作用。频移大小的表达式可写为 $2f_0 \cdot v/c \cdot \cos\theta$,θ 为声速与血流方向间的夹角。虽然多普勒频移微不足道(如对于流速为 75cm/s 的血流来讲,频率的变值约 0.1%),但却可以通过将回声信号与原始信号的 f_0 参照对比,从而获得很精确的测量。事实上,由一组运动速度稍有差异的反射体反射回来的声波速度谱可通过 Fourier(傅里叶)分析或相关分析方法进行测定和分析。

聚焦带移行过渡区:位于探头聚焦带内的组织可反射较强的回声信号。现在新的探头往往提供多重聚焦带,操作者应注意仔细调节,使不同聚焦带之间有一均匀的过渡,从而获得一无缝隙的均匀图像。但常见的情况是,因聚焦带间过渡调节不好,可能会出现一条回声增强的区带,既可出现于灰阶图像上,也可见于彩色多普勒显像图上。在灰阶图像上其边缘笔直;在彩色多普勒显像中此带显示为彩色编码伪影,提示存在血流,但此区域的所谓血流显像色彩混乱,且不存在可见的血管。

折返:脉冲多普勒每接收一次相应区域的回声反射信号所对应的时间,为声波在探头与兴趣区间的来回距离所需时间。对于静止的反射体,每一取样区域的回声信号转化为的电压相同,这样相对于时间来说,它的表现是平坦的(有时偶然带有噪音导致的波动)。但如果是运动的反射体,取样容积区域内的回声信号转化的电压是不同的,随时间延续将是脉冲式的。

只要作为结果而发生的回声到回声位置产生的频移小于声波的半个周期,样本的时间依赖性将在多普勒频移范围内振荡。如果反射体移动很快,或者脉冲重复频率很慢以至于脉冲间隔大于半个声波周期,那么这就违背了尼奎斯特标准,多普勒频移将按脉冲重复频率的整数倍折返到基线的下方或成为负向频移,而误认为有反向血流。

伴有折返的频谱图显示顶端被截去,波峰显示在基线下方,同时彩色多普勒上折返显示为五彩多色区,代表着彩色图谱信号边缘上的包裹。且在彩色图谱上可见经过一明亮的色带后,颜色会突然改变,这种亮带色彩提示血流折返前的极限速度。

在真正有血流反向的情况下,彩色血流图上显示为一连续色彩变化,即在血流显色改变前与原色彩之间有一黑色色带,这一黑色色带表示零速度血流。

折返的校正:折返可通过下列方法来校正:①降低探头的频率;②移动基线;③提高脉冲重复频率以扩展可探测频率范围;④增大多普勒声束与血流方

向的夹角(这样可减少多普勒频移);⑤应用连续多普勒超声取样。增加脉冲重复频率减少了折返的可能,但增加了距离错判的可能性。令人满意的折中方案是依临床情况而定。从连续多普勒原理上来讲,其重复频率是无限的,因而可明确地测定血流速度,但对血流异常的起源处却无法确定。

振铃伪影/彗尾伪影:在高反射体如钙化、手术剪、鼻胃管及中空结构等的远方可发现有类似彗星尾形状的回声。由于这些物质前、后面的声学不匹配,结果产生了以上类似彗星尾巴的混响回声。它们空间排列紧凑,密度渐减,且呈线状构型。从物体反射回来的二次回声,因时间延迟作用看起来好像其在运动,这样在彩色多普勒或能量多普勒显像中可有色彩编码显示。在胆囊腺肌症及前列腺淀粉样变时,可观察到这种彗星尾状彩色编码伪影,这些彩色编码区可误为血流信号。因此,首要的任务是正确识别它们。

无回声区域的彩色伪影:彩色或灰阶预置的变化可能会使无回声的区域填入色彩。当彩色预先设置到低敏感状态时,可能会产生因噪声而致的无回声区的彩色编码。有作者曾在阴囊水性囊肿、囊性肿块和1例有悬浮碎屑的脓肿中遇见过这种伪影。令人困惑的是这种情况可见于肝囊肿,这好像是相邻的心脏搏动传导的结果。有趣的是,无回声区域内如有色彩显示,就提示有液体流动。囊肿中液体运动亦可通过能量多普勒显示。注意彩色显示局限于囊肿本身,其周边组织无任何闪烁的伪影。

在与心脏邻近的囊肿中,搏动传入囊肿,从而在频谱多普勒上显示它有一个动脉血流信号。有作者报道彩色多普勒在区分胸腔积液与胸膜增厚中的价值(液-彩征)。

重复/镜像伪影:重复和镜像伪影不仅出现于灰阶显像,亦可发生于彩色多普勒和能量多普勒图像中。如果一支血管位于一个能改变超声束方向的强反射体附近,那么就可出现它的镜像。超声仪会认定在真正的血管旁有另一与其相似的结构,其内有血流,且可呈现血流显色。令人奇怪的是,在彩色血流多普勒中,这种镜像可显示与真实血管同向或反向的血流,这种情况尤其值得注意。出现重复和镜像伪影的物理学原理源于真实血管与超声束间有一α夹角,而作为镜面反射体与声束又成β夹角,正如光学原理中所述,血管映像和镜像间的夹角和真正血管与镜像间的夹角是相同的。这样,血管映像与血流方向成γ角,$\gamma=2\beta-\alpha$,临界角$\gamma=90^{o}$。

若$\gamma<90^{o}$,映像血管的血流方向与真实血管血流方向一致;但若$\gamma>90^{o}$,则两者的血流方向相反,且色彩颜色也随之改变。有两种有趣的特殊情况:①血管与镜面平行(如下面讨论的颈动脉伪影),则$\gamma=\alpha=\beta$,两者血流方向完全相同。②镜面与声束垂直,则$\beta=90^{o}$,血管和其映像内的血流方向(和颜色)总是相反的。在这种情况下,若α也接近90^{o},则血管及其映像就易被误作真实血管的伴行血管。并且当α和β都接近90^{o}时,探头角度的微小波动就可使镜像的血流方向向前或向后,与真实血流方向间产生同向或反向翻转,色彩也随之改变。

不论是纵切面还是横切面,这种伪影出现最多的部位是阴囊和下腔静脉。由于肺尖的高反射影像,锁骨下动脉和/或锁骨下静脉及股血管和颈血管也是镜像伪影经常出现的部位。

颈血管的镜像伪影曾被称为颈动脉鬼影,反射体是血管壁本身。当超声声束轴线与显像的血管成90^{o}角时,会发生镜像伪影,伪影具有与真实血管相似的频谱表现。由于探头发出的声束向两侧分散,声束的一侧可见血流方向轻度朝向探头。而另一侧血流方向却背离探头。在频谱分析中,两种方向同时显示,频谱看起来像在基线两侧的镜像。在彩色多普勒中,可通过自相关技术来选定优势方向。这项技术来源于每一取样处的平均多普勒频移,即指定给每一像素——正向或负向频移。

颈动脉伪影(鬼影):Middleton和Melson(1990)细致地描述了这种伪影。指的是颈血管镜像伪影,最常见的部位为颈总动脉。这种伪影的产生是由于颈动脉显像时,较深一侧动脉管壁强反射的结果。这种反射导致了颈动脉壁、管腔和腔内血流镜像的产生,因而伪影内也可显示血流。颈血管镜像伪影还有下列特征:信号强度低于真实血管的信号强度;随能量输出增加,伪影显示更清楚;无论矢状面还是横切面,颈动脉伪影都将显示在紧贴颈动脉的深侧;图中有相应于此种伪影的灰阶图像;真正的颈动脉和颈动脉伪影在频谱波形中显示为相似的血流类型;但伪影的频谱波形偏弱,这可能与其位置深在声束能量衰减有关。在列举的颈动脉伪影的病例中,相应的灰阶图像也有显示。有作者报告此类伪影,几天后再进行扫描,仍可显示颈动脉伪影,但颈动脉和伪影之间的距离有所增加。

组织震动:在狭窄、动静脉瘘或搏动增强区域的周围，可能观察到血管周围区域有彩色编码显示。这代表着高速血流的血流动力学能量向其毗邻组织的传播，即组织震动。

色彩编码表现为不连贯的深红或深蓝色。血管周围组织震动使潜在的细节模糊不清，结果难以明确识别组织震动的原因。事实上，可通过改变灰阶显像来显示潜在的血管，但灰阶显像不能显示组织的震动。活检后病人的动静脉瘘附近可有组织震动。过去这种情况常发生在用 14G 针活检后。如继发于股血管导管术后的动静脉瘘可显示组织震动，且常见相关的动脉血流喷射到邻近的静脉内。此外，新近接受肾移植的病人也可能仅仅因为继发于移植的肾动脉痉挛而在脐水平出现组织震动。这种现象可在移植后 24~48h 被观察到，不要误认为动静脉瘘。尤其要考虑到大多数尸体移植应用的是 Carrel 补片，而活体移植则是通过端 - 端吻合进行。

杂乱伪影：静止结构（血管壁、血管周围组织等）的搏动可产生强烈的低频多普勒频移，这在频移的波形中显示于基线的上下区域，它可被误认为是频谱的增宽和 / 或血流反向。

管壁滤过设置可消除这种杂乱反射。动脉取样时需要高通过滤器，而低通过滤器允许记录发生在循环中静脉侧的低多普勒频移。要正确调节仪器的这些过滤器装置，以免消除正常血流信号。据 Burns 等（1990）报道，谐波显像可大大减少杂乱反射的发生，优于单纯多普勒显像。

线性频率干扰：来自输人电源的 60Hz（欧洲为 50Hz）频率干扰，可在频谱图上显示为与基线相邻和 / 或平行的一条直线。当这些线状回声远离基线时，与血流频谱不同，易于识别。但当显示在紧邻基线上方或下方时，可被误认为血流频谱。通常因其振幅很低，所以酷似静脉血流或舒张期动脉血流。然而，频率干扰的图形单调，没有舒张期血流中可见的频谱声音逐渐降低等特点，也不像静脉血流那样，随着呼吸频谱会发生变化。所以，识别这种伪影的途径之一是注意其缺乏生理改变。

彩色取样框边缘：对彩色信号的处理需要强大的计算机功能。为了获取高帧频图像，可应用彩色取样框来进行适当大小的取样，它将允许只对某一特定区域的彩色血流信号进行处理，以加快计算机对信号的处理。彩色取样框给出了将获取的血流信号范围的边界。

双功能扫描中图像的更换：在获取频谱信息时，当扫描图像更换时信息会缺失。必须对频谱中的这种缺失间隙正确认识，不要误认为是一个心动周期的结束。因此，应当注意避免混淆不完整的波形。

与超声对比剂相关的伪影与误诊：近年来，随着新型超声诊断仪的出现，其临床应用也发生了变化。对设备制造商的一大挑战是生产出来的仪器设备能够获取对比剂的信号，而不是记录对比剂产生的伪影或引起的血流速度估测错误。超声对比剂可能给图像分析带来伪影和误诊。

超声对比剂应用的基本原理：传统的超声显像源于声阻抗不同的组织间界面反射产生的回声信号，多普勒显像则是通过发射和接收的声波频率不同而形成图像。能量多普勒则是利用以上两种图像形成的方式，在探测血流方面优于彩色多普勒，但无法探测血流方向，这种多普勒成像技术使频谱多普勒技术比双功能多普勒功能更强大。不尽如人意的是，和其他任何显像方法一样，超声显像中一直存在着真实信号和噪声并存的现象。近来发展起来的谐波成像技术，能大大提高信噪比。这就允许主要记录特殊的对比剂发生的谐波，而大大减少无用的组织信号。

彩色外溢：超声对比剂可影响声束的轴向和侧向分辨力，尤其当应用彩色多普勒显像时，对比剂的增强信号作用使得血管边界外会出现血流或实际上无血流的区域有血流显示，可误认为有血管存在。这样就丧失了空间分辨力，各个独立的血管会混为一大片的色彩溢出区。消除此伪影的最好方法就是减小彩色探测范围，这样可以在更短的时间内获得更多的扫描线，从而提高分辨力。

频谱多普勒假性流速增加：实际上，应用超声对比剂并没有增加血流速度，但这些对比剂引起的后散射，使先前低于阈值频移的信号获得了增强并记录下来。这在新的超声仪中，通过增加动态范围可得以校正。现在市场上有售的可以应用的新型超声设备的动态范围为 90~100dB，而陈旧的仪器动态范围仅为 60dB。

第二节　MRI运动伪影的形成与处理

运动导致的MRI伪影最常见，可分为生理性运动伪影与自主性运动伪影。

MRI时，运动和流动伪影主要来自胸、腹部、盆腔及椎管等部位，尤其是在皮下脂肪和血管流经处，常常产生垂直于相位编码方向的条纹状或重叠伪影，严重降低图像的质量。

运动伪影主要见于相位编码方向，是由于周期性运动频率与相位编码频率不一致（相位编码时间长于频率编码时间）导致的磁化组织相位移动。以呼吸运动为例，原始数据在吸气和呼气中交替获取，使胸腔部位的显示发生偏移，皮下脂肪有高强度信号的组织会出现伪影。

MRI图像上运动伪影产生的机制非常复杂，影响运动伪影的因素包括：运动的方式和运动方向，还取决于不同的成像参数，磁场强度、表面线圈、运动结构的亮度以及不同的成像参数。有多种技术可用于减少或消除MRI时的运动伪影，运动伪影的前处理抑制技术包括变换相位和频率编码方向、使用空间预饱和脉冲、流动补偿序列、PROPELLER技术、脂肪抑制序列、物理抑制技术及口服药物镇静或抗胆碱药物减少胃肠蠕动，以及包括呼吸门控、呼吸补偿、导航回波和呼吸触发技术在内的呼吸运动伪影抑制技术。

运动伪影的后处理矫正技术可在不需要额外硬件或MRI序列的条件下抑制运动伪影，但由于其难度大，国内外学术界研究较少。运动导致的MRI伪影最常见，可分为生理性运动伪影与自主性运动伪影，前者是由心脏大血管搏动、呼吸运动、胃肠蠕动、血流及脑脊液流动等所致；后者是由咳嗽、吞咽运动、眼球转动及病人的躁动不配合所致。

MRI成像时，运动伪影主要来自胸、腹部、盆腔及椎管等部位，尤其是在皮下脂肪和血管流经处，它们常常产生垂直于相位编码方向的条纹状或重叠伪影，严重降低图像的质量。

运动伪影的前处理抑制技术：有多种技术可用于减少或消除MRI成像时的运动伪影，恰当的抑制技术取决于特殊硬件和软件、患者的临床状况以及特定的成像部位等。运动伪影的前处理抑制技术包括变换相位和频率编码方向、使用空间预饱和脉冲、PROPELLER技术、脂肪抑制序列、药物及物理抑制技术，以及包括呼吸门控、呼吸补偿、导航回波和呼吸触发技术在内的呼吸运动伪影抑制技术。

改变相位和频率编码方向：MRI时，相位编码的时间要大大超过频率编码的时间，在具体扫描过程中，通常是将成像层面的最小径线方向作为相位编码的方向，以降低相位编码步的数量。正确选择相位编码方向，可以消除或减弱一些运动伪影。例如，腹部的轴面成像可显示由呼吸引起的高信号脂肪周期性运动伪影；与此同时，腹主动脉内搏动的血流也会产生在相同方向上的伪影，这些伪影可能会使胰腺图像模糊。通过交换梯度方向，这些伪影将自左至右出现，因此图像质量得到提高。

空间预饱和脉冲：由于伪影的强度与产生伪影的运动解剖结构的强度成正比，如果该解剖结构不需要成像，那么降低它的信号强度可以降低伪影的强度。预饱和技术的理论基础就是在成像脉冲激发前使用90ºRF脉冲将容易产生运动伪影而又不是感兴趣区的部位饱和掉，即在成像扫描时让这一部分的组织不再产生共振信号。这样，在成像过程中，即便这部分组织产生了运动，也不会产生运动伪影。一个典型的例子即是在颈椎及脊髓MRI检查时，可在扫描定位像上的椎体前缘加上与颈椎相平行的饱和带，可有效抑制轻微的吞咽运动以及颈内动脉搏动所致的运动伪影。

呼吸运动伪影抑制技术：一种方法是减少图像采集时间，从而在患者有限的屏气时间内完成图像采集，即所谓的屏气快速扫描；第二种方法是使用呼吸运动周期控制MRI图像采集，即呼吸门控或呼吸触发技术。

屏气快速成像：极快的成像速度由于图像采集时间非常短，因而可部分减少呼吸运动伪影。短TR时间（40~250 ms）的FSE序列和GRE序列可在约5~30秒的单次屏气时间内采集图像，快速SE成像序列可有效抑制肺部MRI时的呼吸运动伪影。现今，已有多种快速成像序列已应用于抑制运动伪影，如FSE、GRE、HASTE和RASE序列成像。

呼吸门控技术：门控技术是利用额外的设备来监控人体某些器官的运动情况，以此控制激发以及数据采集时刻。胸部 MRI 检查时,呼吸门控技术可通过传感器监视呼吸情况,以调整相位编码与运动刷期同步,通常是和呼气末采集数据。呼吸门控技术通常延长成像时间 2~3 倍以上,因而限制了其在长 TR 时间 MRI 序列的应用。

呼吸补偿技术:呼吸补偿机制可使脏器各位点处统一呼吸相位时进行信号采集,亦在一定程度上减少运动伪影。最常见的呼吸补偿方式是中心排列相位编码(COPE)和呼吸排列相位编码(ROPE)。这些技术的基本原理是在扫描过程中检查呼吸运动,以呼吸时相决定 K- 空间线填充顺序的方法,重排相位编码步阶或采集视野,在吸气顶峰时采集 K- 空间的高频部分,呼气末期采集 K- 空间的低频部分,使得受运动严重影响的分量分布在傅利叶数据矩阵的边缘,从 K- 空间数据中去除了呼吸周期的影响。这些技术极大地减少了扫描时间。

导航回波技术:呼吸导航回波触发采样使用射频脉冲激发一个垂直于肝 - 肺界面的条带状区域,利用空气和组织的信号差别确定右侧膈肌的空间位置,将此空间位置信息用于前瞻性触发采样或者回顾性图像编码,从而达到控制呼吸的影响和提高成像精度的目的。呼吸导航回波触发采样可以使患者在自由呼吸状态下完成检查,不受屏气时间的限制,有利于提高图像的空间分辨力,缩短数据采样时间。

呼吸触发技术:触发是指数据采集在某个重复运动的指定相位被触发而开始,呼吸触发技术是在当 TR 时间与平均呼吸时相相等时采集 MRI 图像,与呼吸门控技术不同的是,其可在呼吸时相的每一点采集 MRI 层面图像数据,抑制呼吸运动伪影。呼吸触发 FSE 序列的成像时间明显短于常规 T_2WI 成像,且前者可明显提高图像质量,因而呼吸触发 FSE 序列已被大多数影像中心所采用。

脉冲序列参数:短 TE 成像技术可在不需添加特殊硬件设备的条件下抑制多种运动相关伪影,如心脏搏动、血液流动、呼吸运动和肠蠕动所致的伪影。且短 TE 成像技术不需监测患者运动,也不延长成像采集时间。其可在单次屏气时间内采集图像,并可联合应用信号平均技术提高图像质量。

信号平均技术:信号平均技术是指用多组数据来减少随机噪声和伪影,重复数也叫信号平均数或采集次数。信号平均技术的原理是基于随机噪声或伪影为随机相位,而 MRI 信号则为规律相位这一事实,多次重复数据的平均后,使伪影或噪声在一定程度上互相抵消,而规律性的 MRI 信号得到进一步增强。从而抑制运动结构的信号,并增强静止组织信号。信号平均技术可明显抑制包括心脏搏动、血液流动、呼吸运动和肠蠕动在内的多种运动伪影。

PROPELLER 技术:GE 公司研发的 PROPELLER 技术即“周期性旋转重叠平行线采集和增强后处理重建方法”,也称为螺旋桨扫描技术,专门解决和消除运动伪影。

西门子公司也推出类似 PROPELLER 的技术——Syngo BLADE“刀锋”防躁动成像技术。PROPELLER 技术的原理是基于 K- 空间中心部分是决定图像的对比度和信噪比的主要因素,由于 PROPELLER 技术采用一种独特的 K- 空间采集填充方式,应用辐射状的“叶片”以“螺旋桨扫描技术”重叠式充填 K- 空间中心部分,K- 空间中心部分的数据量明显多于边缘部分,因而主要用于克服运动和磁敏感性伪影。

脂肪抑制序列:伪影的亮度取决于运动结构的亮度,即运动结构越亮,伪影越明显,这尤其见于 T_1WI 上运动的脂肪组织,因而脂肪抑制序列图像可有效地减小此类伪影的显示。目前,脂肪抑制 MR 成像法主要有四种,即脂肪饱和序列、反转恢复序列、反相位成像及基本原理与反相位成像相似的 Dixon 法。其中 STIR 序列和 ChemSat 序列是 MRI 脂肪抑制技术最常用的方法。

物理抑制技术:腹部 MRI 检查时,腹带加压包扎是既往常用的方法。腹部加压包扎通过限制腹式呼吸,减少腹部脏器的上下移动,降低运动伪影。乳腺 MRI 成像时,让患者穿着紧身 T 恤、使用乳腺夹或气囊装置,或填充线圈底部,均可用于减少运动伪影。

药物:其他可用于抑制腹部 MRI 成像时的运动伪影技术为联合应用阴性肠管对比剂及低张药物以消除胃肠道蠕动造成的伪影和图像模糊。对不配合的儿童及婴儿进行 MRI 检查时,采用口服水合氯醛(0.5ml/kg)的方法使其在睡眠状态下进行 MRI 扫描;昏迷烦躁的患者可给予肌肉注射安定。

运动伪影的后处理矫正技术:在目前的磁共振成像领域,绝大多数临床应用都是采用二维傅里叶变换的成像技术。由于线性平移运动会在 K 空间内产生相位偏移,因而发生弥散现象,污染整个图像。关于相位偏移的修正算法,有前处理和后处理两种方式。前处理主要有快速扫描、门控扫描或可校正的重建模式等方法。过去多数研究工作是关于前处理的；至于伪影消除的后处理研究，由于难度大，国内外学术界研究较少。

自 Wood 等（1985）提出周期性运动的理论模型后，多位学者进行了运动伪影的后处理矫正技术研究，包括线性平移运动的相位修正、基于相位恢复的图像平面内线性平移运动伪影的消除、在成像域内用自动聚焦的方法消除图像平面内线性平移运动伪影、熵中心标准的自动后处理技术、自动校正技术、类似最小化熵中心标准的“自动聚焦”算法、基于频谱移动消除频率编码方向的伪影及一些学者提出的逆向迭代修正法用于消除由于刚性平移运动造成的 MRI 伪影。

第四节　流动相关伪影

螺旋 CT 是 CT 扫描技术的一个重大进展，由于螺旋 CT 扫描快捷并可重建，又有很好的组织对比，使病变的显示更加清楚，同时也使 CT 扫描较少受到呼吸运动的影响，消除呼吸运动所致的病变遗漏。但是，螺旋 CT 尚有一些不足，这主要包括静脉团注时机的选择和为了更好地显示不同器官需要不同的扫描参数，还有一些可能导致误诊的血液流动伪影。

混合不匀：血管的强化程度取决于血池的大小和与选择扫描时机有关的心输出量。例如，如果静脉血管在对比剂注射后扫描得过早，强化和未强化的血液混合不匀可以导致静脉内血栓的假象，这在邻近肾静脉连接处的下腔静脉中最常见。

在此水平，自肾脏的强化高密度血液（循环时间相对较短），与从下肢回流的未强化低密度血液（具有较长的循环时间）相遇，结果形成了下腔静脉中心低密度“充盈缺损”的表现，继续向头侧流动，这两种类型静脉血相互混合，从而密度变得较为均一。这种现象也可以在髂总静脉汇合处见到。当经足静脉注射对比剂增强时，强化和未强化的血液在下腔静脉的远端混合，这时出现一种异常流动现象，使问题变得更为复杂。在静脉增强前后进行延时扫描或重复扫描有助于鉴别这种伪影，受累静脉扩张（内有血栓）和侧支循环存在也有助于这种血流伪影和血管内血栓的鉴别。

分层强化：当血液流动特别缓慢时，静脉血管可以出现分层强化。运用螺旋 CT 扫描常要求 Valsalva 动作进行长时间屏气，这种现象更易发生，此时，对比增强的较高密度血液将会沿静脉的后壁分布。在腔静脉瓣功能不全时，腔静脉内血液将出现返流。当右心房因三尖瓣功能不全而增大时，对比剂实际上绕过了体循环。因为存在来自右心房的返流，所以可以看到下腔静脉内强化的出现早于主动脉，这种表现不要与从足部注射对比剂相混淆。

静脉的“中断”：流动相关伪影的另一个原因是下腔静脉的“中断”，特别是在运用螺旋技术扫描时更易出现。在深吸气时，由于邻近膈肌的下腔静脉局部塌陷和回心静脉血流减少或停止，大多数仰卧位病人出现这种现象。这将导致下腔静脉内强化的和未强化的血液混合延迟，使任何以前存在的流动伪影更明显，造成血栓形成的假象。但在正常平静呼吸状态下行 CT 增强扫描，一般不会出现下腔静脉的中断。

虽然流动伪影较常见于大口径的血管，但它也可以出现在像门静脉和肠系膜上静脉这样的小血管中。这些血管中的流动伪影在普通 CT 增强扫描时比较少见，但在螺旋 CT 增强扫描时，由于血管增强明显和快速扫描技术的使用，这些伪影较为常见。这些伪影可类似于静脉内血栓，为了解决这一问题，可以在有疑问的血管段进行延迟扫描。

假血栓：可见到与部分容积效应有关的假血栓现象，这种现象见于在被低密度脂肪包绕的门静脉或下腔静脉。此时螺旋扫描有助于明确诊断，因为容积扫描获得的原始数据可用各种层厚和间隔进行图像重建。右侧卵巢静脉的假血栓现象也可以看到，它常见于多产妇女，继发于瓣膜功能不全和左侧卵巢静脉逆流。在螺旋 CT 增强扫描早期，可以见到两侧卵巢静脉增强的不对称性。

伪似肿大的淋巴结：有作者报告扩大的左侧卵巢静脉在 CT 平扫和增强扫描中可伪似肿大的淋巴结、左肾盂积水及双下腔静脉，它位于腹主动脉的左侧和左输尿管的前方，仔细观察邻近的上下层面进行分析，一般都能避免此类误诊。与此类似的情况有腹主动脉周围迂曲的侧支静脉，在横断图像上，也可伪似肿大的淋巴结,但在增强扫描时,此类情况即可澄清。

左和右性腺静脉:在早期扫描中,下腔静脉和右侧性腺(睾丸或卵巢)静脉只有少量或没有静脉给予的对比剂,但是肾静脉强化较早,如有左侧卵巢静脉头侧部分的瓣膜功能不全或缺如,可出现强化血液返流入左卵巢静脉的情况。这是因为两侧卵巢静脉的正常回流不同:右侧卵巢静脉直接回流入下腔静脉,而左侧卵巢静脉汇入左肾静脉。其结果是,左侧卵巢静脉强化而右侧卵巢静脉尚未强化,这好像右侧卵巢静脉内有“血栓”存在。此时观察下腔静脉,如未出现强化,可以避免这种误诊;如下腔静脉强化时,行延迟 CT 扫描才可以完全排除假血栓的诊断。虽然许多问题同静脉注射对比剂的时机和流动伪影有关,但静脉注射对比剂优点很多,能够把正常血管结构、血管正常发育变异同病变区别开来。

第五节 MRI 与伪影

MRA 的缺陷和伪影:平面内饱和:在顺序采样的二维和三维 TOF MRA 中,采集平面的定向对流入增强效应十分关键。如果血管走向平行于采集平面,在 RF 脉冲之间,自旋质子磁距不能有效恢复。虽然采用大的翻转角在一定程度上有帮助,但由于对周围组织的饱和也同时降低,图像的对比度下降。由于血管走向的复杂性,总会遇到一段血管与激发平面平行的情况,比如在腹部血管和髂血管成像时,当 T_1 大于 TR 时,就会发生平面内饱和。当血液沿扫描平面流动时,就相当于流经的距离拉长,故在反复施加 RF 脉冲的情况下,磁矩就来不及恢复至磁场的方向。对比剂增强三维 MRA 就不存在这个问题。正如前面讨论过的,这种技术的对比度是基于钆对比剂的 T_1 缩短作用而不是流入增强效应。

二维 TOF 存在的另一个常见伪影是所采集图像之间由于屏气的呼吸时相不同所引起的体素迁移。有时,轴面二维 TOF GRE 序列显示了肝动脉,腹侧还有一个较大的血管,这很容易被错认为是意外发现的门静脉;而该例病人实际上是门静脉闭塞和腔静脉改建术后病人,在同一病人冠状位三维对比剂增强 MRA 像中,大血管事实上是肠系膜侧支血管。由于门静脉高压,可见食管静脉曲张和脾肿大。冠状位三维对比剂增强 MRA 清楚地显示了这些解剖结构。二维 TOF 原始数据的最大信号强度投影重建,由于不同屏气呼吸时相数据之间的体素迁移,显示解剖结构的准确性稍差,分析诊断时要结合整个成像体素数据来考虑。

狭窄过高估计伪影:对狭窄的过高估计是一直存在于二维、三维 TOF MRA 技术中的问题,多由最大信号强度投影采用的方式所导致。最大信号强度投影算法通过调整录入数据的阈值来降低噪声。这样,低强度的背景信号以及血管的低信号部分便从形成的平面投影中取消。要获得好的最大信号强度投影像,血管信号至少要高于背景信号 2 个标准差。

在血管狭窄时,血流模式突然改变,结果出现两种重要改变影响成像结果:第一是不同流速成分导致严重的体素内失相位,引起信号缺失;第二是由于背景的投影信号强于血管的信号,致使最大信号强度投影不能投影出来自相散体素的低强度血管信号。这一效应在使用对比剂团注后进行的二维 TOF 成像中有所减弱。相应的 X 线血管造影像也显示在感兴趣区对比剂充盈缺损。即使采取足够小的体素,体素内相散也在所难免。

有作者报告,双侧肾脏对称灌注,可见右肾动脉闭塞,这被灌注检查的时间 - 强度曲线所证实。该病人左肾动脉起始处亦见明显狭窄,但同侧肾脏血液灌注正常,提示为假性狭窄。

增大成像矩阵提高空间分辨力可减小体素内相散,但这也不能彻底解决血管连接处的体素内相散的问题,比如肾动脉起始部。这时,仔细查看每一幅原始图像再来判断最大信号强度投影的图像就显得十分重要。

饱和带与最大强度投影伪影:在二维 TOF 中,特别是当对正常情况下呈三相搏动式流动的外周血管成像时,一些序列参数(如切层和移动饱和带)的定位十分重要。Masui 等(1995)等首先注意到这些参数对腘动脉成像的作用。在下肢动脉行程上观察到多个水平带状伪影,而且它们的表现形式随 RF 脉冲和饱和脉冲之间的距离而变化。如果 RF 脉冲足够大,在舒张早期,它们在进入成像层面之前先进入饱和带。这时,旨在饱和反方向血流的饱和脉冲也同时饱和了正常血流。三维 TOF 多层块部分重叠成像时也会出现相似的伪影，如果重叠容积选择不恰当，边缘就会出现信号强度不等，引起一种称作“威尼斯盲”或“百叶窗帘”的伪影，在颅内 MRA 像中经常见到。

最大信号强度投影后处理伪影：以斜视角观察，最大信号强度投影会显示不同信号强度的图像，当斜面投影的信号强度低于原始图像背景信号 2 个标准差时就会发生这种情况。要获得理想的最大信号强度投影像，保证背景信号强度的均匀性很重要。这在对细小血管或血流缓慢的血管成像时几乎是不可能的。这种情况下，可依靠原始图像或图像数据的多平面重建做出诊断。此外，也可对一小的靶区域使用最大信号强度投影以改善血管的对比度。例如，通过在图像 FOV 内划定一个小的兴趣区，便可从 FOV 中剔除重叠的和不需要显现的血管。总之，靶区最大信号强度投影可改善对比度，也可明显缩短后处理时间，并减弱整个最大信号强度投影时出现的血管缺失伪影。在弯曲的血管，如移植肾动脉或脾动脉，最大信号强度投影像中可见多个重叠圈。有时通过变化角度也很难找到合适的多平面重建定向而准确显示狭窄病变。偶尔，外部物体（如过滤器）的存在可能会使最大信号强度投影图像模糊。故有必要再次强调：对于带有过滤器的病人，原始图像是诊断的重要依据。

对比剂增强三维 MRA 中团注对比剂到达时间的选择不当：在对比剂增强三维 MRA 中，血管和周围组织的最佳对比度噪声比，需要根据不同病人的血流特征和循环时间准确选择对比剂到达兴趣区的时间。在采集填充 K- 空间中心的图像数据时，应恰好是感兴趣血管的对比剂浓度峰值。根据对比剂推注的情况，首过浓度峰值应呈钟形，数据采集窗应确定得与浓度 - 时间曲线相吻合。这样，数据采集窗的中心部分正好对应峰值，否则，在血管的边缘会出现明显的环状伪影。如果对比剂到达较迟，所得图像将很难显示出血管病变。

反之，如果对比剂过早地到达，外周静脉将叠加于动脉血管上。所以，要获得最佳图像，对每个病人都应该在采集信号之前先测得流经时间，或者在一次屏气间不间断扫描以使体素迁移伪影最小化。数据采集时血液的实际 T_1 取决于注射后血液的首过浓度，首过浓度和对比剂到达的时间取决于病人的循环时间和心输出量。不适当的时间选择可导致动脉显影不佳，也可导致静脉信号重叠于图像中。在运行对比剂增强扫描序列时，有必要采集几组数据，以便在对比剂到达静脉时也获得静脉图像。如果对比剂推注速度得当，对比剂到达时间选择准确，便可同时获得对比度良好的动、静脉时相的 MRA 图像。

不适当三维层块定位而引起的伪影：在腹部对比剂增强三维 MRA 中，腹部的冠状平面将包括大部分胸主动脉和整个腹主动脉。由于不依赖血管的几何结构，血管走向与成像平面相平行的冠状面最适合于对比剂增强三维 MRA 扫描，因为这样采集单元最少，采用数据实时保存来提高空间分辨力。但是，在主动脉延长、主动脉瘤和髂动脉拉长扭曲的病人，正确定位三维扫描层块常较为困难。如果血管的一部分未包括进扫描层块，那么，在冠状面或斜面的最大信号强度投影像中，就会出现假性狭窄。如果采用矢状面投影，常常可证实为假性狭窄。髂动脉未被包括进成像层块是这种现象的常见例子。

察看矢状面最大信号强度投影像或原始图像以确定血管或动脉瘤是否完全包括在冠状层块内十分重要。当可疑阻塞的远端血管信号强度与阻塞近端血管相同，而且也无侧支循环建立时，应想到这种伪影的可能。可通过增加层块的厚度使最大信号强度投影中的血管各部分全部包括在其内，以避免这一弊端。

如果保持空间分辨力不变，增加层块厚度无疑会延长扫描时间，这样，缩短 TR（要求高性能的梯度）有助于在不损失空间分辨力的前提下，缩短扫描时间获得大的层块厚度。增加层块厚度而不增加层块内单元，可在相同的扫描时间内获得较大的覆盖范围和良好的信噪比（SNR），但是空间分辨力下降。有时，尤其是对大的胸主动脉瘤成像时，有必要将扫描层块由冠状面变为矢状面。

屏气呼吸时相不同所导致的伪影：在对比剂增强的三维 MRA 中，常用相减运算进一步降低背景信号以改善最大信号强度投影效果。这就要求两次扫描的层块间无体素位移。但是如两次屏气膈肌位置不同，在多个二维 TOF 数据组和不同体素间的信号相减，就不能完全消除背景信号。使用三维对比剂增强 MRA 技术时，应保证扫描时间很短，以在一次屏气间完成多次扫描。使用片层插入技术，可使一次扫描的时间缩短至 6~8s，从而可在病人深吸气后的屏气期间完成 3~4 次扫描。这样便可很好地减去背景信号。

折叠伪影（包绕伪影）：当 FOV 未将整个扫描

区的人体结构包括在内时便会产生折叠伪影,位于FOV之外而被RF脉冲激发的解剖结构会投影到图像的另一边。在MRA扫描中,病人取仰卧位,双臂放在身体两侧,当有静脉血管的手臂未被包进操作者设定的矩形FOV内时,它就会叠加到图像的对侧。

大多数情况下,这并不会影响图像质量,因为兴趣区位于图像的中心,而折叠伪影出现在图像的边缘。但折叠伪影有时会被误诊为异常血管,比如肾下极的副肾动脉。如果高信号的结构(如胸壁的皮下脂肪)叠加在感兴趣血管的同一平面上,可能遮掉血管信号,导致狭窄或闭塞的误诊。这种伪影可通过增大FOV来消减。但是,增大FOV会损失空间分辨力而引发其他问题,比如小血管显示不出来。有时可借助于改变病人的姿势(如将注射对比剂的一侧上肢置于头上)来消除伪影。

金属支架伪影:交织钛丝做成的支架在MRI图像上常常可显影,这些支架只在其放置的部位产生很弱的MRI伪影。由于GRE脉冲序列没有180º重聚脉冲,在这样的支架部位会产生磁敏感性伪影。但是,MRA可很好地显示支架远端的血流。大多数MRA技术采用对比剂增强法来准确地识别支架的位置。

原始图像上在支架部位显示局灶性的信号缺失。在对血管(如肾动脉)内放置支架的病人进行诊断时,由于磁敏感性效应,TOF图像中的信号缺失会比较显著,通常会引起类似狭窄的伪影,所以同时依靠原始图像结合最大信号强度投影图像进行诊断甚为重要。

脉冲序列相关性伪影:进行MRA扫描要求根据组织和血液的固有特性确定最佳的脉冲序列参数。选择合适的序列对在合理的时间内获得满意的对比度十分重要。比如,有时采用黑血技术把流体从其他亮信号的结构中区分开来。在腹主动脉水平行轴面扫描时,应注意管腔内的信号改变。腔内的信号不均匀是因为血流速度变化而导致血管未呈完全的流空信号。在这种情况下,使匀速的血液信号归零毫无意义。

现在,通过采用片间采样和插值技术使整个片层厚度减小,可大大提高三维序列的空间分辨力。这对减小体素内相散是必要的。此外,通过提高时间分辨力,可使三维序列的多次重复扫描在一次屏气完成。这样,同一体素和不同三维数据组间同一采集单元的位置吻合,便于在三维数据组间进行减影(即从注射对比剂后的图像中减去注射对比剂前的图像),获得理想的结果。

参考文献

[1] 中华医学会. 病毒性肝炎防治方案 [J]. 中华肝脏病杂志，2000，8：324.

[2] 中华肝脏病学会脂肪肝和酒精性肝病学组. 非酒精性肝病诊断标准 [J]. 中华肝脏病杂志，2003，11：71.

[3] 中华医学会肝脏病学分会脂肪肝和酒精性肝病学组. 酒精性肝病诊断标准 [J]. 中华肝脏病杂志，2003，11：72.

[4] 中华肝脏病学分会脂肪肝和酒精性肝病学组. 非酒精性脂肪性肝病诊疗指南 [J]. 中华肝脏病杂志，2006，14：161.

[5] 中华医学会肝病学分会脂肪肝和酒精性肝病学组. 非酒精性脂肪性肝病诊疗指南（2010 年修订版）[J]. 中华肝脏病杂志，2010，18：163.

[6] 中华人民共和国卫生部. 原发性肝癌诊疗规范（2011 年版）[J]. 临床肿瘤学杂志，2011，16（10）：929.

[7] 中国抗癌协会肝癌专业委员会，中国抗癌协会临床肿瘤学协作专业委员会，中华医学会肝病学分会肝癌学组，等. 原发性肝癌规范化病理诊断方案专家共识 [J]. 中华肝脏病杂志，2011，19：254.

[8] 中华医学会血液学分会 / 中国医师协会血液科医师分会. 铁过载诊断与治疗的中国专家共识 [J]. 中华血液学杂志，2011，32：572.

[9] 中国胃肠胰神经内分泌肿瘤病理专家组. 中国胃肠胰神经内分泌肿瘤病理学诊断共识 [J]. 中华病理学杂志，2011，40（4）：257.

[10] 溶酶体贮积病医疗协作组《中国戈谢病诊治专家共识》编委会. 中国戈谢病诊治专家共识 [J]. 中华医学杂志，2011，91（10）：665.

[11] 中华医学会肝病学分会脂肪肝和酒精性肝病学组. 中国非酒精性脂肪性肝病诊疗指南（2010 年修订版）[J]. 中国医学前沿杂志（电子版），2012，4（7）：4.

[12] 中华医学会放射学分会腹部学组. 肝胆特异性 MRI 对比剂钆塞酸二钠临床应用专家共识 [J]. 中华放射学杂志，2016，50：641.

[13] 中华医学会肝病学分会，中华医学会消化病学分会，中华医学会内镜学分会. 肝硬化门静脉高压食管胃静脉曲张出血的防治指南 [J]. 中华内科杂志，2016，55（1）：57.

[14] 中华医学会影像技术分会，中华医学会放射学分会.MRI 检查技术专家共识 [J]. 中华放射学杂志，2016，50（10）：724.

[15] 中华医学会影像技术分会，中华医学会放射学分会.CT 检查技术专家共识 [J]. 中华放射学杂志，2016，50（12）：916.

[16] 中华医学会放射学分会腹部学组. 肝胆特异性 MRI 对比剂钆塞酸二钠临床应用专家共识 [J]. 中华放射学杂志，2016，50（9）：641.

[17] 中华人民共相国卫生和计划生育委员会医政医管局. 原发性肝癌诊疗规范（2017 年版）[J]. 中华消化外科杂志，2017，16（7）：635.

[18] 中华医学会放射学分会腹部学组. 磁共振成像对比剂钆贝葡胺肝脏应用专家共识 [J]. 中华肝胆外科杂志，2017，23（9）：577.

[19] 巫北海. 静脉法胆道造影的体会 [J]. 重庆医药，1976，X 线诊断专辑：56.

[20] 巫北海. 关于静脉法胆系造影中显影的生理和病理的浮浅认识 [J].《中西医结合治疗急腹症》放射诊断交流会，放射学讲座，山东昌潍，1977：41.

[21] 巫北海. 肝外胆管结石 X 线诊断（上）[J]. 人民军医，1978，（3）：53.

[22] 巫北海. 肝外胆管结石 X 线诊断（下）[J]. 人民军医，1978，（4）：59.

[23] 巫北海.X 线检查中不常见的意外死亡 [J]. 重庆医药，1983，（2）：30.

[24] 巫北海，何庆奎. 鱼刺致左下腹炎性肉芽肿 1 例报告 [J]. 人民军医，1985，（5）：80.

[25] 巫北海，胡清锡. 胆囊憩室内结石一例报告

[J]. 临床放射学杂志,1985,4(4):178.

[26] 巫北海主编.X线解剖图谱 正常·变异 [M]. 重庆:科学技术文献出版社重庆分社,1985.

[27] 巫北海.X线检查时的意外死亡与休克 [J]. 中华放射学杂志,1985,19(5):307.

[28] 巫北海. 胃肠癌瘤X线诊断的误诊 [J]. 全国消化系早期癌瘤放射学诊断新进展讲座, 1987:143.

[29] 巫北海. 大肠癌瘤X线误诊病例的分析 [J]. 实用放射学杂志,1988,4:104.

[30] 马奎,巫北海. 药物性结肠炎 [J]. 国外医学临床放射学分册,1988,11(3):151.

[31] 巫北海,冉隆中,宁德辰,等.ERCP中肝外胆管内径的观察分析 [J]. 中华放射学杂志,1988,22(增刊):38.

[32] 巫北海主编. 实用影像诊断手册 [M]. 重庆:科学技术文献出版社重庆分社,1988.

[33] 巫北海. 努力减少X线诊断的误诊与漏诊 [J]. 中级医刊,1988,23(12):41.

[34] 巫北海主编. 医学影像正常解剖——《X线解剖图谱 正常·变异》续编 [M]. 重庆:科学技术文献出版社重庆分社,1989.

[35] 巫北海. 胰头段胰管的动态观察 [J]. 实用放射学杂志,1989,5:220.

[36] 巫北海,陈友全,宁德辰.ERCP胰头段胰管的动态解剖观察 [J]. 实用放射学杂志, 1989, 4(5):173.

[37] 巫北海. 胆囊管低位汇入及其有关问题 [J]. 全国肝胆胰脾影像学专题座谈会资料汇编. 1990:108.

[38] 张万强,巫北海. 胰腺结石 [J]. 国外医学临床放射学分册,1990,13(1):8.

[39] 巫北海,王其源. 胆囊管低位汇合的解剖形态学观察——附ERCP检查63例报告 [J]. 重庆医药,1990,19(6):1.

[40] 周永碧,巫北海,李智华. 逆行胰胆管造影发现胆囊管变异的临床意义 [J]. 中华外科杂志,1990,28(6):328.

[41] 罗小明,巫北海."早期胰癌"影像诊断的几个问题 [J]. 国外医学临床放射学分册,1999,13(3):18.

[42] 黎海涛,巫北海. 非扩张型胆管阻塞性胆汁淤积的影像诊断. 国外医学临床放射学分册, 1990,13(2):88.

[43] 罗小明,巫北海. 胰、胆管癌的内镜诊断进展 [J]. 内镜,1990,7(1):45.

[44] 游箭,巫北海. 胆管结石的CT诊断 [J]. 第三军医大学学报,1990,12(2):125.

[45] 巫北海.X线动态观察. 胆总管括约肌段 [J]. 第三军医大学学报,1990,12(4):309.

[46] 巫北海,戴帜主编. 矮身材的防治 [M]. 成都:成都科技大学出版社,1991.

[47] 张爱梅,巫北海. 胆石性胰腺炎 [J]. 国外医学临床放射学分册,1991,14(2):75.

[48] 张爱梅,巫北海. 胆石性胰腺炎的影像学检查评价(附21例分析)[J]. 第三军医大学学报, 1991,13(2):130.

[49] 宁德辰,巫北海. 原发性胆囊癌的影像学诊断 [J]. 中华放射学杂志,1991,25(增):44.

[50] 张万强,巫北海. 胰腺结石并发胰腺癌的X线诊断(附三例报告)[J]. 中华放射学杂志,1991,25(6):365.

[51] 巫北海. 胆胰管十二指肠连接区的动态解剖学观察 [J]. 临床医学影像杂志,1991,2(3):197.

[52] 丁仕义,巫北海,初铭忠. 胆胰管十二指肠连接区癌的影像诊断特点 [J]. 中华医学杂志, 1991, 71(3):170.

[53] 王绍岩,巫北海. 手术损伤性胆管狭窄的影像学诊断(附54例分析)[J]. 中华放射学杂志, 1991,25(4):260.

[54] 吕维富,巫北海. 胰腺分裂的影像诊断及其与特发性胰腺炎的关系 [J]. 国外医学临床放射学分册,1992,15(2):67.

[55] 吕维富,巫北海. 胰腺微囊腺瘤的病理和影像学表现 [J]. 国外医学临床放射学分册, 1992, 15(2):70.

[56] 丁仕义,巫北海. 胆胰管十二指肠连接区癌的影像诊断 [J]. 国外医学临床放射学分册,1992,15(2):73.

[57] 郑大伟,巫北海. 胆管囊肿的影像诊断 [J]. 国外医学临床放射学分册,1992,15(2):77.

[58] 巫北海,王其源. 胆囊管与肝外胆管低位汇合的ERCP观察 [J]. 中华外科杂志, 1992, 30(5):336.

[59] 向武昌,巫北海. 慢性胰腺炎影像学诊断进展 [J]. 实用放射学杂志,1992,8(2):113.

[60] 向武昌,巫北海. 慢性弥漫性胰腺炎的影像学诊断(附 84 例分析)[J]. 中华放射学杂志, 1992, 26(5):333.

[61] 张万强,巫北海. 胰腺结石的影像学诊断 [J]. 临床放射学杂志,1992,11(1):15.

[62] 丁仕义,巫北海. 关于胆管结石 X 线解剖分型的探讨 [J]. 第三军医大学学报, 1992, 14(2):191.

[63] 巫北海,吕维富. 异常胰胆管连接与胰胆系病变(一)胆囊炎、胆石症、胆管炎和胰腺炎 [J]. 中华放射学杂志,1993,27(12):840.

[64] 丁仕义,巫北海. 胆胰管十二指肠连接区癌影像诊断 [J]. 癌症,1993,12:365.

[65] 向武昌, 巫北海. 假肿瘤性胰腺炎 11 例报告 [J]. 中华消化杂志,1993,13:181.

[66] 张万强,巫北海. 胰腺疾病的介入放射学 [J]. 国外医学临床放射学分册,1993,16(1):4.

[67] 李小玲,巫北海. 胰腺 CT 扫描中口服造影剂的分析 [J]. 第三军医大学学报,1993,15(3):261.

[68] 巫北海.54 例胆囊管与肝外胆管低位汇合的 ERCP 观察 [J]. 内镜,1993,10(2):82.

[69] 汪庆华,巫北海. 胆囊的介入放射学 [J]. 国外医学临床放射学分册,1993,16(1):8.

[70] 郑大伟,巫北海. 胆管囊肿的影像诊断 [J]. 实用放射学杂志,1993,9(2):129.

[71] 黎孝勇,巫北海. 慢性胰腺炎并发肝外胆管局限性狭窄 [J]. 国外医学临床放射学分册, 1993, 16(2):77.

[72] 董陆平,巫北海.Caroli 氏病的影像诊断 [J]. 国外医学临床放射学分册,1993,16(2):80.

[73] 吕维富,巫北海. 异常胰胆管连接与胰胆系病变 [J]. 国外医学临床放射学分册, 1993, 16(2):83.

[74] 向武昌,巫北海. 假肿瘤性胰腺炎 11 例报告 [J]. 中华消化杂志,1993,13(3):181.

[75] 张爱梅,张登武,巫北海.ERCP 在儿童胰腺炎中的应用 [J]. 国外医学临床放射学分册, 1993, 16(3):144.

[76] 姚茹国,巫北海.Mirizz's 综合征的 CT 表现 [J]. 实用放射学杂志,1993,9:531.

[77] 周代全,巫北海. 动脉性门静脉造影 CT[J]. 国外医学临床放射学分册,1993,16(3):202.

[78] 孙金城,吕维富,巫北海. 原发性硬化性胆管炎:临床及影像学诊断 [J]. 国外医学临床放射学分册,1993,16(3):206.

[79] 巫北海. 专家评述:学习实事求是,力争实事求是 [J]. 中华放射学杂志,1993,27(12):815.

[80] 张宗蓉,巫北海. 小肝癌的影像诊断 [J]. 国外医学临床放射学分册,1994,17(2):75.

[81] 巫北海,黎孝勇. 慢性胰腺炎并发胆总管狭窄(附 28 例报告)[J]. 中华放射学杂志, 1994, 28(1):54.

[82] 董陆平,姚茹国,巫北海.Caroli 氏病的 CT 诊断(附 2 例报告)[J]. 实用放射学杂志, 1994, 10(1):52.

[83] 巫北海,刘启芬. 胆囊管残留过长的 X 线诊断(附 33 例报告)[J]. 实用放射学杂志, 1994, 10(9):386.

[84] 巫北海主编. 影像诊断中的误诊 [M]. 成都:四川科学技术出版社,1995.

[85] 黄学全,巫北海. 脾肿瘤的影像学诊断进展 [J]. 国外医学临床放射学分册,1995,18(2):75.

[86] 巫北海,廖军. 肝门胆管梗阻影像诊断 [J]. 实用放射学杂志,1995,11(增):120.

[87] 张伟国,巫北海. 动态增强 MRI 在原发性肝癌诊断中的应用 [J]. 国外医学临床放射学分册, 1995,18(2):84.

[88] 巫北海,张平. 应当重视十二指肠乳头区憩室——乳头周围憩室和憩室内乳头的影像学分析 [J]. 医学临床与研究,1995,4(4):43.

[89] 秦伟,巫北海. 肝肿瘤成像的一些新概念 [J]. 国外医学临床放射学分册,1995,18(2):90.

[90] 黄学全,巫北海. 脾灶性非肿瘤病变的影像学诊断进展 [J]. 国外医学临床放射学分册, 1995, 18(4):215.

[91] 周代全,巫北海. 胆囊结石化学成分与体外 CT 扫描表现的相关研究 [J]. 第三军医大学学报, 1995,17(4):470.

[92] 巫北海. 对"Oddi 括约肌闭锁不全一例"一文的浅见 [J]. 中华放射学杂志,1996,27:152.

[93] 颜红兵,巫北海.Budd-Chiari 综合征及其影像学诊断 [J]. 国外医学临床放射学分册, 1996, 19(2):66.

[94] 周代全,巫北海. 胆囊结石化学类型的体外预测:影像学研究进展 [J]. 国外医学临床放射学分册,1996,19(2):74.

[95] 周代全，巫北海，许汝福. 胆囊结石化学类型的计算机辅助诊断 [J]. 放射学实践（中文版），1996，11（3）：93.

[96] 秦伟，巫北海. 异常胰胆管连接与胆系肿瘤 [J]. 国外医学临床放射学分册，1996，19（2）：76.

[97] 巫北海. 肝外胆管括约肌段透光线条影 X 线研究 [J]. 解剖学杂志，1996，19（3）：189.

[98] 巫北海，秦伟，周代全. 原发性肝细胞癌侵犯胆管的影像学观察 [J]. 中华放射学杂志，1996，30（6）：444.

[99] 巫北海，马翔宇. 胆胰管下端占位性梗阻的影像学表现 [J]. 第三军医大学学报，1996，18（3）：246.

[100] 周代全，巫北海. 胆囊结石 X 线特征与化学类型的相关性研究 [J]. 中国医学影像学杂志，1996，4（3）：146.

[101] 巫北海，周永碧，李智华，等. 肝门胆管癌的影像学诊断 [J]. 实用放射学杂志，1996，12（4）：197.

[102] 黎海涛，巫北海. 肝外胆管梗阻性病变影像诊断学进展 [J]. 国外医学外科学分册，1996，23（6）：325.

[103] 巫北海. 专家论坛：质量保证和质量控制与诊断医师密切相关 [J]. 中华放射学杂志，1996，30（5）：367.

[104] 巫北海. 述评：我国肝胆胰脾医学影像学的发展前景. 中华放射学杂志，1996，30（6）：437.

[105] 巫北海，牟玮. 专家经验谈：学习，学习，再学习——浅谈调整知识结构以促进介入医学的发展 [J]. 介入医学杂志，1997，2（4）：153.

[106] 巫北海. 述评：欲穷千里目，更上一层楼——国人胆系影像诊断学研究的回顾和展望 [J]. 中华放射学杂志，1997，31（增）：5.

[107] 黎海涛，巫北海. 肝外胆管梗阻病变 CT 诊断的评价 [J]. 中华放射学杂志，1997，31（1）：25.

[108] 巫北海，何泽清. 胆胰管下端括约肌段良性狭窄的影像学表现 [J]. 中华放射学杂志，1997，31（增）：59.

[109] 黎海涛，巫北海. 肝外胆管梗阻性病变 CT 诊断的计算机辅助系统 [J]. 第三军医大学学报，1997，19（2）：217.

[110] 秦伟，巫北海. P 型和 B 型异常胰胆管连接犬模型的建立及其 X 线表现分析 [J]. 第三军医大学学报，1998，20（2）：142.

[111] 陆明，巫北海. 复发性肝类癌 1 例 [J]. 中国医学影像技术，2001，17：507.

[112] 巫北海总主编. 活体形态学·腹盆上卷 [M]. 北京：科学出版社，2006.

[113] 程红岩，贾雨辰，王培军，等. 肝胆疾病影像学 [M]. 上海：上海科学技术出版社，2005.

[114] 周康荣，严福华，曾蒙苏. 腹部 CT 诊断学 [M]. 上海复旦大学出版社，2011.

[115] 陈凡. 放射诊断学征象 [M]. 武汉：同济大学出版社，1995.

[116] 全冠民，陈敏，袁涛. CT 和 MRI 诊断 - 重点、热点问题精讲第 1 辑（修订版）[M]. 北京：人民军医出版社，2012.

[117] 全冠民，袁涛，耿左军. CT 和 MRI 诊断 - 重点、热点问题精讲. 第 2 辑 [M]. 北京：人民军医出版社，2013.

[118] 全冠民，陈为军，袁涛. 磁共振基本病例诊断·鉴别诊断·CT 对照 [M]. 北京：人民军医出版社，2012.

[119] 陈克敏. 能谱 CT 的基本原理与临床应用 [M]. 北京：科学出版社，2012.

[120] 杨天和. 少见病影像诊断分析 [M]. 福州：福建科学技术出版社，2016.

[121] 钱斌，胡晓华，陈宏伟，等. 肝脏上皮样血管内皮瘤 CT 与 MRI 特征及病理对照 [J]. 中华放射学杂志，2012，46（2）：172.

[122] 李丽英，吴秀蓉. 混合型肝癌的 CT 和 MRI 表现 [J]. 中华放射学杂志，2012，46：701.

[123] 赵晶，赵心明，欧阳汉，等. 肝细胞腺瘤的影像表现及与病理结果的对照分析 [J]. 中华放射学杂志，2012，46（12）：1096.

[124] 严福华. 重视腹部 CT 和 MR 新技术的量化研究和临床应用 [J]. 中华放射学杂志，2013，47：101.

[125] 郁义星，林晓珠，陈克敏，等. CT 能谱成像在鉴别肝癌和局灶性结节增生中的价值 [J]. 中华放射学杂志，2013，47：121.

[126] 梁亮，曾蒙苏，纪元，等. 自身免疫性胰腺炎合并腹部其他组织器官受累的影像表现 [J]. 中华放射学杂志，2013，47：220.

[127] 宋凤祥，周建军，施裕新，等. 胆管内乳头状肿瘤的动态增强 CT 表现 [J]. 中华放射学杂志，

2013,47:430.

[128] 刘海龙,刘敏,刘艳,等.脾脏窦岸细胞血管瘤的影像表现 [J]. 中华放射学杂志,2013,47:440.

[129] 李雪丹,刘屹,任克,等.胆汁流动伪影的MR 胆胰管成像表现 [J]. 中华放射学杂志, 2013, 47:850.

[130] 石喻,郭启勇,张兰,等.3.0 T MR 弹性成像评价健康者及慢性肝病患者肝弹性值的初步研究 [J]. 中华放射学杂志,2013, 47(11):1005.

[131] 李若坤,曾蒙苏,强金伟,等.肝硬化结节癌变的磁敏感加权成像表现与病理的对照研究 [J]. 中华放射学杂志,2013,47(11):1014.

[132] 陈枫,赵大伟,冯骥良,等.硬化型肝癌的影像表现 [J]. 中华放射学杂志,2014,48(1):43.

[133] 刘于宝,李萌,钟小梅,等.胆管导管内乳头状肿瘤的影像表现 [J]. 中华放射学杂志,2014,48(2):128.

[134] 盛若凡,曾蒙苏,饶圣祥,等.小肝细胞肝癌和肿块型肝内小胆管细胞癌的 MRI 表现特征 [J]. 中华放射学杂志,2014,48:288.

[135] 应明亮,肖文波,许顺良,等.脾脏硬化性血管瘤样结节性转化的 CT 及 MRI 表现 [J]. 中华放射学杂志,2014,48:777.

[136] 梁亮,曾蒙苏,纪元,等.IgG4 相关性疾病腹部病变的少见及不典型影像表现 [J]. 中华放射学杂志,2014, 48(11):887.

[137] 应世红,赵艺蕾,滕晓东,等.胆管导管内乳头状黏液性肿瘤的影像表现和形态分型 [J]. 中华放射学杂志,2015,49(1):42.

[138] 鲁果果,高雪梅,程敬亮,等.单、双指数模型扩散加权成像鉴别诊断肝脏良、恶性肿瘤的价值 [J]. 中华放射学杂志,2015, 49(1):47.

[139] 刘广宇,孙浩然,白人驹.胆系结石金属成分与 MRI 信号的相关性研究 [J]. 中华放射学杂志, 2015,49(2): 107.

[140] 丁怀银,孙晓东,朱西琪,等.无胆管扩张的肝内胆管细胞癌的 MRI 特征及其病理基础 [J]. 中华放射学杂志,2015,49(2):113.

[141] 李若坤,曾蒙苏,强金伟,等.MR 磁敏感加权成像对肝硬化背景下小肝癌的诊断价值 [J]. 中华放射学杂志,2015,49(7):520.

[142] 陈枫,赵大伟,文硕,等.肝内肿块型胆管癌的 CT、MRI 动态增强表现以及与病理分化程度的关系 [J]. 中华放射学杂志,2015,49(11): 843.

[143] 施莺燕,胡克非,胡俊,等.儿童朗汉斯细胞组织细胞增生症累及肝脏的影像表现 [J]. 中华放射学杂志,2016,50(4):243.

[144] 黄志强.肝外伤治疗观念上的转变 [J]. 中华创伤杂志,2000,16(4):255.

[145] 陆才德,卢长江,吴胜东,等.肝内胆管乳头状瘤病的临床病理特征和诊治分析:附九例报告 [J]. 中华肝胆外科杂志,2010,16:328.

[146] 廖冠群,郃升.黏胆症的研究进展 [J]. 中华消化外科杂志,2011,10:155.

[147] 严茂林,王耀东,魏少明,等.肝内胆管黏液性肿瘤的诊断与治疗 [J]. 中华普通外科杂志, 2013,28:669.

[148] 陈敏华,严昆,戴莹,等.肝超声造影应用指南(中国)(2012 年修改版)[J]. 中华超声影像学杂志,2013, 22:696.

[149] 丁庆国,成翠娥,蒯新平,等.磁共振扩散加权成像在胰腺囊性病变中的鉴别诊断价值 [J]. 中华胰腺病杂志,2013,13:382.

[150] 张溢,李锐,张晓航,等.肝血管平滑肌脂肪瘤超声造影、增强 CT 特点及其与病理分型的关系 [J]. 中华医学超声杂志:电子版, 2013, 10(11): 929.

[151] 何敏,王坚,陈涛,等.黄色肉芽肿性胆囊炎的诊治分析 [J]. 中华肝胆外科杂志,2013,19:232.

[152] 严茂林,王耀东,魏少明,等.肝内胆管黏液性肿瘤的诊断与治疗 [J]. 中华普通外科杂志, 2013,28:669.

[153] 陈枫,赵大伟,冯骥良,等.硬化型肝癌的影像表现 [J]. 中华放射学杂志,2014,48(1):43.

[154] 郝春鹍,王旭.胃神经鞘瘤的影像学表现二例并文献复习 [J]. 中华临床医师杂志(电子版), 2014,8:1588.

[155] 王影,余深平,李子平.肝细胞癌影像诊断及肝脏影像报告和数据管理系统 [J]. 中华临床医师杂志(电子版),2014, 8:2548.

[156] 亓昌珍,章士正,刘义涛,等.多层螺旋 CT 小肠造影对克罗恩病活动度的评估价值 [J]. 中华医学杂志,2015,95:2006.

[157] 曹广文."癌症进化发育学"理论框架及其在乙肝致癌预防中的作用 [J]. 中国科学基金, 2015, 29(5):323.

[158] 高回青,胡春洪,郁义星,等. 能谱 CT 定量分析在鉴别肝癌和肝脓肿中的价值 [J]. 中华肝脏病杂志,2016, 24(9):676.

[159] 王铮,苏丹柯,赖少侣,等. 肝内肿块型胆管细胞癌不典型 CT 表现与病理对照分析 [J]. 中华肿瘤防治杂志,2016,23:30.

[160] 李爽,张德发,陆伟,等. 超声内镜对食管静脉曲张套扎术后复发的预测作用 [J]. 中华消化内镜杂志,2016, 33(4): 223.

[161] 唐磊,李子禹,付佳,等. 胃癌侵犯胰腺的 CT 影像学特征及在原发灶可切除性判断中的意义 [J]. 中华消化外科,2017, 16(3): 304.

[162] 唐磊. 胃癌术前影像学精准分期存在的争议与困惑 [J]. 中华胃肠外科杂志,2016,19(2):165.

[163] 陕飞,李子禹,张连海,等. 国际抗癌联盟及美国肿瘤联合会胃癌 TNM 分期系统(第 8 版)简介及解读 [J]. 中国实用外科杂志,2017,37(1): 15.

[164] Amin MB, Edge SB, Greene FL, et al[J]. AJCC Cancer Staging Manual. 8th ed. New York: Springer,2017.

[165] Amin MB, Greene FL, Edge SB, et al.The Eighth Edition AJCC Cancer Staging Manual: continuing to build a bridge from a population-based to a more "personalized" approach to cancer staging[J]. CA Cancer J Clin, 2017, 67(2): 93.

[166] An H, Shi Y, Guo Q, et al.Test-retest reliability of 3D EPI MR elastography of the pancreas. Clin Radiol,2016,71(10): 1068.e7.

[167] Bai DS, Wu C, Yang LX, et al. UBAP2 negatively regulates the invasion of hepatocellular carcinoma cell by ubiquitinating and degradating Annexin A2[J]. Oncotarget, 2016,7(22): 32946.

[168] Bang CS, Song IH. Impact of antiviral therapy on hepatocellular carcinoma and mortality in patients with chronic hepatitis C: systematic review and meta-analysis[J]. BMC Gastroenterol, 2017, 17(1): 46.

[169] Behbahani S, Hoffmann JC, Stonebridge R, et al.Clinical case report: Sclerosing hemangioma of the liver, a rare but great mimicker[J]. Radiol Case Rep, 2016, 11(2):58.

[170] Bellentani S. The epidemiology of non-alcoholic fatty liver disease[J]. Liver Int, 2017, 37 Suppl 1: 81.

[171] Bruix J, Reig M, Sherman M. Evidence-based diagnosis, staging, and treatment of patients with hepatocellular carcinoma[J]. Gastroenterology, 2016, 150(4): 835.

[172] Bucsics T, Krones E. Renal dysfunction in cirrhosis: acute kidney injury and the hepatorenal syndrome[J]. Gastroenterol Rep (Oxf), 2017, 5(2): 127.

[173] Buettner S, van Vugt JL, IJzermans JN, et al. Intrahepatic cholangiocarcinoma: current perspectives[J]. Onco Targets Ther,2017,10:1131.

[174] Buechter M, Penndorf V, Canbay A, et al. Multimodal therapy of recurrent and refractory bleeding from esophageal varices – case report and review of the literature[J]. Z Gastroenterol, 2016, 54(12): 1320.

[175] Carneiro FO, Retes FA, Matuguma SE, et al. Role of EUS evaluation after endoscopic eradication of esophageal varices with band ligation[J]. Gastrointest Endosc, 2016, 84(3): 400.

[176] Chalasani N, Younossi Z, Lavine JE, et al. The diagnosis and management of nonalcoholic fatty liver disease: practice guidance from the American Association for the Study of Liver Diseases[J]. Hepatology, 2018, 67(1): 328.

[177] Chan KL, Lade S, Prince HM, et al. Update and new approaches in the treatment of Castleman disease[J]. J Blood Med, 2016,7:145.

[178] Chen BB, Tien YW, Chang MC, et al. PET/MRI in pancreatic and periampullary cancer: correlating diffusion-weighted imaging, MR spectroscopy and glucose metabolic activity with clinical stage and prognosis[J]. EurJ Nucl Med Mol Imaging, 2016, 43: 1753.

[179] Chiang AL, Lee LS. Clinical approach to incidental pancreatic cysts[J]. World J Gastroenterol, 2016,22:1236.

[180] Correa-Gallego C, Maddalo D, Doussot A, et al. Circulating plasma levels of microRNA-21 and microRNA-221 are potential diagnostic markers for primary intrahepatic cholangiocarcinoma[J]. PLoS One,2016,11(9):e0163699.

[181] Cui HY, Wang SJ, Miao JY, et al. CD147 regulates cancer migration via direct interaction with Annexin A2 and DOCK3-β-catenin-WAVE2 signaling[J]. Oncotarget, 2016, 7(5): 5613.

[182] Diehl AM, Day C. Cause, pathogenesis, and treatment of nonalcoholic steatohepatitis[J]. N Engl J Med, 2017, 377(21): 2063.

[183] Di Tommaso L, Roncalli M. Tissue biomarkers in hepatocellular tumors: which, when, and how[J]. Front Med(Lausanne), 2017, 4:10.

[184] Duchartre Y, Kim YM, Kahn M. The Wnt signaling pathway in cancer[J]. Crit Rev Oncol Hematol, 2016, 99: 141.

[185] Esnaola NF, Meyer JE, Karachristos A, et al. Evaluation and management of intrahepatic and extrahepatic cholangiocarcinoma[J]. Cancer, 2016, 122(9):1349.

[186] European Association for the Study of the Liver, European Association for the Study of Diabetes, European Association for the Study of Obesity. Clinical Practice Guidelines for the management of non alcoholic fatty liver disease[J]. J Hepatol, 2016, 64(6): 1388.

[187] Fan JG, Kim SU, Wong VW. New trends on obesity and NAFLD in Asia[J]. J Hepatol, 2017, 67(4): 862.

[188] Gani F, Nagarajan N, Kim Y, et al. Program death 1 immune checkpoint and tumor microenvironment: implications for patients with intrahepatic cholangiocarcinoma[J]. Ann Surg Oncol, 2016, 23(8): 2610.

[189] Gong X, Wei W, Chen L, et al. Comprehensive analysis of long non-coding RNA expression profiles in hepatitis B virus-related hepatocellular carcinoma[J]. Oncotarget, 2016, 7(27): 42422.

[190] Guo Z, Cao M, Zhang D, et al.Simultaneous SPECT imaging of multi-targets to assist in identifying hepatic lesions[J]. Sci Rep,2016,6:28812.

[191] Han TT, Du M, Zhang X, et al. Quantitative assessment of early liver fibrosis in rats using ^{13}N-NH_3-H_2O PET/CT[J]. Nucl Med Commun, 2016, 37:92.

[192] Hartl J, Denzer U, Ehlken H, et al. Transient elastography in autoimmune hepatitis: timing determines the impact of inflammation and fibrosis[J]. J Hepatol, 2016, 65(4):769.

[193] Healey R, Corless L, Gordins P, et al. Do anti-smooth muscle antibodies predict development of autoimmune hepatitis in patients with normal liver function? A retrospective cohort review[J]. Autoimmun Rev, 2016, 15(7): 668.

[194] Heimbach JK, Kulik LM, Finn RS, et al. AASLD guidelines for the treatment of hepatocellular carcinoma[J]. Hepatology,2018,67(1):358.

[195] Hong CS, Byun JH, Kim JH, et al.Thread sign in biliary intraductal papillary mucinous neoplasm:a novel specific finding for MRI[J]. Eur Radiol, 2016,26(9):3112.

[196] Ismail MM, Morsi HK, Abdulateef NA, et al. Evaluation of prothrombin induced by vitamin K absence, macrophage migration inhibitory factor and Golgi protein-73 versus alpha fetoprotein for hepatocellular carcinoma diagnosis and surveillance[J]. Scand J Clin Lab Invest,2017,77(3):175.

[197] Joo I, Lee JM, Lee DH, et al.Preoperative assessment of pancreatic cancer with FDG PET/MR imaging versus FDG PET/CT plus contrast-enhanced multidetector CT: a prospective preliminary study[J]. Radiology, 2017, 282:149.

[198] Kanno A, Masamune A.Okazaki K.et al.Nationwide epidemiological survey of autoimmune pancreatitis in Japan in 2011[J]. Pancreas,2015,44:535.

[199] Kaur M, Dalal V, Bhatnagar A, et al. Pancreatic tuberculosis with markedly elevated CA 19-9 levels: a diagnostic pitfall[J]. Oman Med J, 2016, 31: 446.

[200] Kim WJ, Hwang S, Lee YJ, et al.Clinicopathological features and long-term outcomes of intraductal papillary neoplasms of the intrahepatic bile duct[J]. J Gastrointest Surg, 2016, 20(7): 1368.

[201] Kopec AK, Luyendyk JP.Role of Fibrin(ogen)in progression of liver disease: guilt by association[J]. Semin Thromb Hemost,2016,42:397.

[202] Kumar PA, Singh G, Joseph JB, et al. Pancreatic tuberculosis: a puzzle for physicians. A rare case and review of literature[J]. J Clin Diagn Res,

2016,10:PD29.

[203] Lahooti A, Sarkar S, Laurent S, et al.Dual nano-sized contrast agents in PET/MRI: a systematic review[J]. Contrast Media Mol Imaging, 2016, 11: 428.

[204] Lammert F, Gurusamy K, Ko CW, et al. Gallstones[J]. Nat Rev Dis Primers, 2016,2:16024.

[205] Lamontagne RJ, Bagga S, Bouchard MJ. Hepatitis B virus molecular biology and pathogenesis[J]. Hepatoma Res, 2016, 2:163.

[206] Lee SJ, Kim SY, Kim KW, et al.Hepatic angiomyolipoma versus hepatocellular carcinoma in the noncirrhotic liver on Gadoxetic Acid-Enhanced MRI: A diagnostic challenge[J]. AJR,2016, 207:562.

[207] Lee SL, Ku YM, Jeon HM, et al.Impact of the cross-sectional location of multidetector computed tomography scans on prediction of serosal exposure in patients with advanced gastric cancer[J]. Ann Surg Oncol, 2017, 24(4): 1003.

[208] Lens S, Alvarado E, Marino Z, et al. Effects of all-oral anti-viral therapy on HVPG and systemic hemodynanucs in patients with hepatitis C virus-associated cirrhosis[J]. Gastroenterology, 2017, pii:S0016-5085(17)35922-X.

[209] Li F, Yan H, Wang J, et al.Non-invasively differentiating extent of liver fibrosis by visualizing hepatic integrin alphavbeta3 expression with an MRI modality in mice[J]. Biomaterials,2016, 102:162.

[210] Li P, Liu J.Diagnostic value of MRI and computed tomography in anorectal malignant melanoma[J]. Melanoma Res, 2016, 26:46.

[211] Lim JK, Flamm SL, Singh S, et al. American gastroenterological association institute guideline on the role of elastography in the evaluation of liver fibrosism[J]. Gastroenterology, 2017, 152(6): 1536.

[212] Liu WB, Wu JF, Du Y, et al. Cancer evolution-development: experience of hepatitis B virus-induced hepatocarcinogenesis[J]. Curr Oncol, 2016, 23(1):e49.

[213] Liu WB, Cao GW. Cancer evolution-development: novel theory based on studies of inflammation-cancer transformation[J]. Chin J Cancer Biother, 2017, 24(2): 103.

[214] Luetkens JA, Klein S, Traeber F, et al. Quantitative liver MRI including extracellular volume fraction for non-invasive quantification of liver fibrosis: a prospective proof-of-concept study[J]. Gut, 2017,pii: gutjnl-2017-314561.

[215] Luli S, Di PD, Pem P, et al. A new fluorescence -based optical imaging method to non-invasively monitor hepatic myofibroblasts in vivo[J]. J Hepatol,2016,65:75.

[216] Montalbano M, Georgiadis J, Masterson AL, et al. Biology and function of glypican-3 as a candidate for early cancerous transformation of hepatocytes in hepatocellular carcinoma (Review)[J]. Oncol Rep, 2017, 37(3): 1291.

[217] Muller P, Messmer M, Bayer M, et al. Non-alcoholic fatty liver disease (NAFLD) potentiates autoimmune hepatitis in the CYP2D6 mouse modeI[J]. J Autoimmun, 2016, 69:51.

[218] Nieberler M, Reuning U, Reichart F, et al. Exploring the role of RGD-recognizing integrins in cancer[J]. Cancers (Basel),2017,9:116.

[219] Omata M, Cheng AL, Kokudo N, et al. Asia-Pacific clinical practice guidelines on the management of hepatocellular carcinoma:a 2017 update[J]. Hepatol Int, 2017,11(4): 317.

[220] Pan LH, Yao M, Cai Y, et al. Oncogenic Wnt3a expression as an estimable prognostic marker for hepatocellular carcinoma[J]. World J Gastroenterol, 2016, 22(14): 3829.

[221] Pan L, Yao M, Zheng W, et al. Abnormality of Wnt3a expression as novel specific biomarker for diagnosis and differentiation of hepatocellular carcinoma[J]. Tumour Biol, 2016,37(4):5561.

[222] Park CC, Nguyen P, Hernandez C, et al. Magnetic resonance elastography vs transient elastography in detection of fibrosis and noninvasive measurement of steatosis in patients with biopsy-proven nonalcoholic fatty liver disease[J]. Gastroenterology, 2017, 152(3):598.

[223] Peleg N, Issachar A, Sneh-Arbib O, et al. AST to Platelet Ratio Index and fibrosis 4 calculator scores for non-invasive assessment of hepatic fibrosis in patients with non-alcoholic fatty liver disease[J].

Dig Liver Dis, 2017, pii: S1590-8658(17)30879-4.

[224] Petta S, Wong VW, Camma C, et al. Improved noninvasive prediction of liver fibrosis by liver stiffness measurement in patients with nonalcoholic fatty liver disease accounting for controlled attenuation parameter values[J]. Hepatology, 2017, 65(4):1145.

[225] Pozzi-Mucelli RM, Rinta-Kiikka I, Wunsche K, et al. Pancreatic MRI for the surveillance of cystic neoplasms: comparison of a short with a comprehensive imaging protocol[J]. Eur Radiol, 2017, 27: 41.

[226] Rockey DC, Elliott A, Lyles T. Prediction of esophageal varices and variceal hemorrhage in patients with acute upper gastrointestinal bleeding[J]. J Investig Med, 2016, 64(3): 745.

[227] Saad K, Theis S, Otto A, et al. Detailed expression profile of the six glypicans and their modifying enzyme, notum during chick limb and feather development[J]. Gene, 2017, 610: 71.

[228] Saha SK, Zhu AX, Fuchs CS, et al. Forty-year trends in cholangiocarcinoma incidence in the U.S.: intrahepatic disease on the rise[J]. Oncologist, 2016,21(5):594.

[229] Schnabl B, Farshchi-Heydari S, Loomba R, et al. Staging of fibrosis in experimental non-alcoholic steatohepatitis by quantitative molecular imaging in rat models[J]. Nucl Med Biol, 2016, 43:179.

[230] Shaker O, Alhelf M, Morcos G, et al. miRNA-101-1 and miRNA-221 expressions and their polymorphisms as biomarkers for early diagnosis of hepatocellular carcinoma[J]. Infect Genet Evol, 2017, 51:173.

[231] Shaker MK, Abdel Fattah HI, Sabbour GS, et al. Annexin A2 as a biomarker for hepatocellular carcinoma in Egyptian patients[J]. World J Hepatol, 2017, 9(9): 469.

[232] Shen S, Lin Y, Yuan X, et al. Biomarker nucroRNAs for diagnosis, prognosis and treatment of hepatocellular carcinoma: a functional survey and comparison[J]. Sci Rep, 2016, 6:38311.

[233] Shi Y, Xia F, Li QJ, et al. Magnetic resonance elastography for the evaluation of liver fibrosis in chronic hepatitis B and C by using both gradient-recalled echo and spin-echo echo planar imaging: a prospective study[J]. Am J Gastroenterol, 2016, 111(6): 823.

[234] Shiha G, Ibrahim A, Helmy A, et al. Asian-Pacific Association for the Study of the Liver (APASL) consensus guidelines on invasive and non-invasive assessment of hepatic fibrosis: a 2016 update[J]. Hepatol Int, 2017, 11(1):1.

[235] Singh VP, Rajesh S, Bihari C, et al.Xanthogranulomatous cholecystitis: what every radiologist should know[J]. World J Radlol, 2016, 28, 8:183.

[236] Sun Y, Zhou J, Wang L, et al. New classification of liver biopsy assessment for fibrosis in chronic hepatitis B patients before and after treatment[J]. Hepatology, 2017, 65(5):1438.

[237] Sureka B, Singh VP, Rajesh SR, et al. Computed tomography and magnetic resonance findings in xanthogranulomatous cholecystitis: retrospective analysis of pathologically proven 30 cases-tertiary care experience[J]. Pol J Radiol, 2017, 82:327.

[238] Vasconcelos RN, Dolan SC, Barlow JM, et al. Impact of CT enterography on the diagnosis of small bowel gastrointestinal stromal tumors[J]. Abdom Radiol, 2017, 42:1365.

[239] Viggiani V, Palombi S, Gennarini G, et al. Protein induced by vitamin K absence or antagonist- Ⅱ (PIVKA- Ⅱ) specifically increased in Italian hepatocellular carcinoma patients[J]. Scand J Gastroenterol, 2016, 51(10): 1257.

[240] Wang L, Pan L, Yao M, et al. Expression of oncofetal antigen glypican-3 associates significantly with poor prognosis in HBV-related hepatocellular carcinoma[J]. Oncotarget, 2016, 7(27): 42150.

[241] Wei M, Lu L, Lin P, et al. Multiple cellular origins and molecular evolution of intrahepatic cholangiocarcinoma[J]. Cancer Lett, 2016, 379(2):253.

[242] Wong VW, Chan WK, Chitturi S, et al. Asia-Pacific Working Party on Non-alcoholic Fatty Liver Disease Guidelines 2017-Part 1: Definition, risk factors and assessment[J]. J Gastroenterol Hepatol, 2018, 33(1): 70.

[243] Wu Y, Liu H, Ding H. GPC-3 in hepatocellular carcinoma: current paspectives[J]. J Hepato-

cell Carcinoma, 2016,3: 63.

[244] Xiao SM, Xu R Tang XL, et al.Splenosis with lower gastrointestinal bleeding mimicking colonical gastrointestinal stromal tumour[J]. World J Surg Oncol, 2017,15(1):78.

[245] Xu J, Li J, Zheng TH, et al. MicroRNAs in the occurrence and development of primary hepatocellular carcinoma[J]. Adv Clin Exp Med, 2016, 25(5): 971.

[246] Yao M, Wang L, Fang M, et al. Advances in the study of oncofetal antigen glypican-3 expression in HBV-related hepatocellular carcinoma[J]. Biosci Trends, 2016, 10(5): 337.

[247] Younossi ZM, Koenig AB, Abdelatif D, et al. Global epidemiology of nonalcoholic fatty liver disease-Meta-analytic assessment of prevalence, incidence, and outcomes[J]. Hepatology, 2016, 64(1): 73.

[248] Yu X, Wu Y, Liu H, et al.Small-Animal SPECT/CT of the Progression and Recovery of Rat Liver Fibrosis by Using an Integrin αvβ-targeting Radiotracer[J]. Radiology,2016,279:502.

[249] Yuan BH, Li RH, Yuan WP, et al. Harms and benefits of adoptive immunotherapy for postoperative hepatocellular carcinoma: an updated review[J]. Oncotarget, 2017, 8(11): 18537.

[250] Zhang C, Liu H, Cui Y, et al.Molecular magnetic resonance imaging of activated hepatic stellate cells with ultrasmall superparamagnetic iron oxide targeting integrin alphavbeta(3) for staging liver fibrosis in rat modeI[J]. Int J Nanomedicine, 2016, 11: 1097.

[251] Zhang CY, Yuan WC, He P, et al.Liver fibrosis and hepatic stellate cells: etiology, pathological hallmarks and therapeutic targets[J]. World J Gastroenterol,2016,22:10512.

[252] Zhang D, Guo Z, Zhang P, et al. Simplified quantification method for in vivo SPECT/CT imaging of asialoglycoprotein receptor with ^{99m}Tc-p(VLA-co-VNI) to assess and stage hepatic fibrosis in mice[J]. Sci Rep,2016,6:25377.

[253] Zhang X, Cuo Q, Shi Y, et al.(99m)Tc-3PRGD2 scintigraphy to stage liver fibrosis and evaluate reversal after fibrotic stimulus withdrawn[J]. Nucl Med Biol, 2017, 49:44.

[254] Zhang Y, Li T, Qiu Y, et al. Serum microRNA panel for early diagnosis of the onset of hepatocellular carcinoma[J]. Medicine(Baltimore), 2017, 96(2): e5642.

[255] Zheng W, Yao M, Sai W, et al. Diagnostic and prognostic significance of secretory clusterin expression in patients with hepatocellular carcinoma[J]. Tumour Biol, 2016, 37(1): 999.

[256] Zhu B, Wei L, Rotile N, et al.Combined magnetic resonance elastography and collagen molecular magnetic resonance imaging accurately stage liver fibrosis in a rat model[J]. Hepatology, 2017,65:1015.

本卷有关医学影像词汇

在研究误诊时，我们发现不少误诊都源自于对中文的英译原文理解和翻译错误，而同一外文词条下的中译又五花八门，一些翻译者相当随意，其中在缩略语上的随意性更是达到登峰造极，导致不少读者理解的混淆和概念的混乱。因此，我们将专业的医学影像词汇收集起来，介绍给读者，使其在临床上随时可查阅，以减少诸如此类的混淆和错误。

本书各卷书末所附的医学影像词汇，为便于读者查阅和使用，均按英文字母次序排列：有缩写词者按缩写词英文字母次序排列；无缩写词者按首位单词首位字母排列。缩写词相同者，酌情同排于一个词条或多个词条。同一英语词条，不同中译文者均排于同一词条；同一中文词条，不同英语译文者亦排于同一词条。

A

acute appendicitis，AA（急性阑尾炎）

AA（花生四烯酸）

aplastic anemia，AA（再生障碍性贫血）

acute aortic dissection，AAD（急性主动脉夹层）

atypical adenomatous hyperplasia，AAH；atypical adenomatous hyperplasis，AAH（不典型腺瘤样增生），AAH（非典型腺瘤样增生）

aggressive angiomyxoma，AAM（侵袭性血管黏液瘤，即血管黏液瘤），又称为 deep angiomyxoma（深部血管黏液瘤）

acute aortic syndrome，AAS（急性主动脉综合征），又称为急性胸痛综合征，包括一组有相似临床症状的异质性疾病：典型的 acute aortic dissection，AAD（急性主动脉夹层）、intramural hematoma，IMH（主动脉壁内血肿）和 penetrating atherosclerotic ulcer，PAU（穿透性粥样硬化性溃疡）

American Association for the Study of Liver Diseases，AASLD（美国肝病学会，美国肝病研究学会，美国肝脏病学会，美国肝病研究协会，美国肝脏病研究协会）

AAT（胰蛋白酶）

automated border detection，ABD（自动边缘识别技术）

ABI（踝 - 臂血压指数）

arterial blood pressure，ABP（动脉血压）

allergic bronchopulmonary aspergillosis，ABPA（变应性支气管肺部曲菌病，即过敏性支气管肺曲霉病）

absolute molar concentration of adenosine triphosphase（三磷酸腺苷的绝对摩尔浓度）

anabolic charge，AC（合成代谢负荷）[AC=PME/（PME+PDE）]

abdominal cocoon，AC（腹茧症）

anticarbonic anhydrase，ACA（抗碳酸苷脱水酶），ACA Ⅱ、Ⅳ（抗碳酸苷脱水酶Ⅱ、Ⅳ）

ACA（抗心磷脂抗体），AECA（抗内皮细胞抗体），ASMA（抗平滑肌抗体）

acinar cell carcinoma，ACC（腺泡细胞癌）

accessory fissures（肝脏的副裂隙），pseudoaccessory fissures（假副裂），inferior accessory fissure（下副裂）

accessory liver（附加肝叶，副肝）

accordion sign（手风琴征）

acinar cell carcinoma of pancreas，ACCP（胰腺腺泡细胞癌）

angiotensin converting enzyme inhibitors，ACEI（血管紧张素转换酶抑制剂）

acute collection of fluid，ACF（急性液体积聚）

auto-correlation function，ACF（自相关函数）

ACG（美国胃肠病学院）

acetylcholine，Ach（乙酰胆碱）

air cast imaging，ACI（空气投影成像，也称大肠三维表面覆盖成像）

airway centered interstitial fibrosis，ACIF（气道中心性间质纤维化）

acoustic radiation force impulse(声辐射力脉冲成像技术)
American College of Radiology, ACR(美国放射学院,美国放射学会)
acute coronary syndrome, ACS(急性冠状动脉综合征)
a-1-ACT(抗胰糜蛋白酶,免疫组织化学检查内容之一),a-1-AT(a抗胰蛋白酶)
actin(肌动蛋白,免疫组织化学指标之一)
active alcoholic cirrhosis(急性酒精性肝硬化)
Acetazolamide,ACZ(乙酰唑胺)(商品名 diamox)
aortic dissection,AD(主动脉夹层)
Alzheimer's disease, AD(老年性痴呆,即阿尔茨海默病)
American Diabetes Association, ADA(美国糖尿病协会)
apparent diffusion coefficient, ADC(表观扩散系数,ADC值)
Apparent Diffusion Coefficient Map(表观扩散系数图)
lesion-liver ADCratio(病灶与周围肝实质的ADC值比)
ADC-time curve(表观扩散系数-时间曲线)
adenoacantuoma(胰腺腺鳞癌,又称腺棘癌)、muco-epidermoid carcinoma(黏膜表皮样癌)
adenomatous heperplasia(腺瘤样增生), adenomatosis(腺瘤病), adenomatous hyperplastic nodules(腺瘤性增生结节)
adenomyosis(腺肌症)
ADM(阿霉素)
ADP(二磷酸腺苷)
autosomal dominant polycystic kidney disease, ADPKD(显性遗传性多囊肾病), autosomal dominant polycystic liver disease, ADPLD(显性遗传性多囊肝病,常染色体显性多囊肝)
adverse drug reaction,ADR(化疗的不良反应)
automatic exposure control,AEC(自动曝光控制)
AES(肛门内超声)
atrial fibrillation,AF(心房颤动,即房颤)
autofluorescence bronchoscopy, AFB(自发荧光支气管镜)
alpha fetoprotein, AFP(甲胎蛋白,甲胎蛋白测定,或胎甲球试验),AFP-L3(甲胎蛋白异质体3)
alcoholic fatty liver, AFL(酒精性脂肪性肝病), alcoholic fatty liver disease,AFLD(酒精性脂肪性肝病,酒精性肝病)
American Gastroenterological Assoaation,AGA(美国胃肠病学院和美国胃肠病学会)
AG(阿拉伯半乳聚糖),ASG(去唾液酸糖蛋白)
advanced gastric cancer,AGC(进展期胃癌)
agenesis(发育不全), hypoplasia(发育不良)
adverse grug reaction, AGR(药物不良反应,化疗的不良反应)
alcoholic hepatitis, AH(急性酒精性肝炎), alcoholic cirrhosis, AC(酒精性肝硬化), ALD(酒精性肝病)
adenomatous hyperplasia, AH(腺瘤样增生),即 macroregenerative nodules(巨再生结节); atypical adenomatous hyperplasia, AAH(不典型性腺瘤样增生)
apnea hypopnea index, AHI(呼气暂停低通气指数,呼吸紊乱指数)
adenomatoid hyperplasia of the liver, AHL(肝脏腺瘤样增生)
accessory hepatic vein, AHV(副肝静脉)或肝短静脉, inferior right hepatic veins, IRHV(肝右后下静脉)
anisotropy index,AI(各向异性指数)
acquired immunodeficiency syndrome, AIDS(获得性免疫缺陷综合征,艾滋病)
autoimmune hepatitis, AIH(自身免疫性肝炎),AIH-PBC-PSC重叠综合征(自身免疫性肝炎、原发性胆汁性肝硬化、原发性硬化性胆管炎重叠综合征)
autoimmune pancreatitis, AIP(自身免疫性胰腺炎), AIP有两个类型:即Ⅰ-AIP型和Ⅱ-AIP型;Ⅰ-AIP型为 lymphoplasmacytic sclerosing pancreatitis, LPSP(淋巴浆细胞硬化性胰腺炎),Ⅱ-AIP型为 idiopathic duct-centric pancreatitis, IDCP(非酒精性导管破坏性胰腺炎、特发性导管中心性胰腺炎)或 granulocyte epithelial lesion, GEL(粒细胞上皮内浸润性胰腺炎)。focal AIP, f-AIP(局限性AIP)
acute interstitial pneumonia,AIP(急性间质性肺炎)
average intensity projection,AIP(平均密度重建)
American joint committee on cancer, AJCC(美国癌症联合委员会,美国癌症联合会,美国癌肿联合委

员会）

American joint committee on cancer，AJCC（美国癌症联合委员会）/ international union against cancer，UICC（国际抗癌联盟），AJCC/UICC（美国癌症联合会 / 国际抗癌联盟）

anomalous junction of pancreaticobiliary duct，AJPBD（胰胆管异常合流），

anomalous pancreaticobiliary ductal union，APBDU（异常胰胆管连接）

acute kidney injury，AKI（急性肾损伤）

AKP（血清碱性磷酸酶，血清磷酸酶），GTP（γ- 谷氨酰转氨酶），GGT（g- 谷氨酰转移酶）

as low as reasonably achievable，ALARA（合理可行尽量低的原则）

Albumin，Alb（白蛋白）

alcoholic cirrhosis（酒精性肝硬化）

alcoholic liver disease，ALD（酒精性肝病），ALD/NAFLD Index，ANI（酒精性肝病 / 非酒精性脂肪肝病指数）

ALEH（拉丁美洲肝病学会）

acute liver failure，ALF（急性肝衰竭）

antilactoferrin，ALF（抗乳铁蛋白），ALF（抗乳铁蛋白抗体）

algorithm（计算机辅助探测算法）

aliasing（折叠伪影）

abnormal localization of immature precursor，ALIP（幼稚前体细胞异常定位）

anaplastic lymphoma kinase，ALK（渐变性淋巴瘤激酶）

activin receptor-like kinase-1，ALK-1（活化受体激酶基因）

alkaline phosphatase，ALP（碱性磷酸酶）

arterial liver perfusion，ALP（肝动脉灌注）

alpha-1-antitrypsin（a-1- 抗胰蛋白酶）

amyotrophic lateral sclerosis，ALS（肌萎缩性侧索硬化）

alanine aminotransferase，ALT（谷丙转氨酶，丙氨酸转氨酶，丙氨酸氨基转移酶）；GGT（g- 谷氨酰转肽酶）；aspartate aminotrans-ferase，AST（天冬氨转氨酶，天门冬氨酸氨基转移酶）

actual liver volume，ALV（实际肝体积）

anti-mitochondrial antibody，AMA（抗线粒体抗体），AMA-M2（抗线粒体抗体 M2 型）

appendical mucous cyst，AMC（阑尾黏液囊肿）

amehcabscess（阿米巴肝脓肿），entamoeba histo1ytica（溶组织内阿米巴），amebic trophozoites（滋养体，阿米巴营养子）

American Pancreatic Association（美国胰腺学会）

aminopr-opyl bond elut cartridge（氨基丙基键洗脱药桶）

amiodarone（胺碘酮）

angiomyolipoma，AML（血管平滑肌脂肪瘤），AML（血管平滑肌脂肪瘤）分为 classical AML，CAML（经典型血管平滑肌脂肪瘤）和 epithelioid AML，EAML（上皮样血管平滑肌脂肪瘤）；hepatic epithelioid angiomyolipoma，HEA（肝脏上皮样血管平滑肌脂肪瘤），hepatic epithelioid angiomyolipoma，HEAML（肝上皮样血管平滑肌脂肪瘤）

acute myeloid leukemia，AML（急性骨髓粒细胞性白血病，急性髓细胞白血病）

anorectal malignant melanoma，AMM（肛管直肠恶性黑色素瘤）

AMNP（阴离子磁赤铁矿）

acute mountain sickness，AMS（急性高山病）

amyloidosis（肝淀粉样变）

antinuclear antibody，ANA（抗核抗体），antinuclear antibodies，ANAS（抗核抗体）

anabolic steroids（蛋白同化甾类，代谢性甾体激素）

ANCA（抗中性白细胞胞浆抗体），p-ANCA（核旁型抗中性粒细胞胞浆抗体）

anaplastic lymphoma kinase（间变性淋巴瘤激酶）

avascular necrosis of femoral head，ANFH（股骨头缺血坏死）

angiogenesis（肿瘤血管生成，血管生成）

angiography-assisted CT（血管造影 CT）

angiosarcoma（血管肉瘤）

angiostatin（血管抑素）

aggressive non-Hodgkin’s lymphoma，ANHL（进展性非何杰金淋巴瘤）

annular array ultrasonography（环形矩阵超声）

array processor，AP（阵列处理器）

acute physiology and chronic health evaluation，APACHE（急性生理和慢性健康评估）

Asian Pacific Association for the Study of Liver Disease，APASLD，APASL（亚太肝病研究学会，亚太肝病学会）

anomalous pancreaticobiliary junction，APBJ(胰胆管合流异常)

adenomatous polyposis coli，APC(腺瘤性结肠息肉病)

aperture(视角)

accessory pancreatic duct，APD(副胰管)

abdomino-perineal excision，APE(腹-会阴联合切除术)

arterioportal fistula，APF(肝动脉-门静脉瘘)

apoptosis(细胞凋亡)，又称 programmed cell death，PCD(程序性细胞死亡)

APP-PS1(β 前体蛋白-早老素 1 联合转基因)，APP-PS2(β 前体蛋白-早老素 2 联合转基因)

apparent portal perfusion(表观门脉灌注)

aspartate aminotransferase-to-platelet ratio index，APRI(丙氨酸氨基转移酶血小板指数)

ALT-to-platelet ratio index，APRI(天冬氨酸转氨酶/血小板指数)

arterioportal shunt，APS(肝动脉-门静脉分流，肝动脉门脉瘘，肝动脉-门静脉瘘)

anterior pararenal space，APS(肾旁前间隙)，posterior pararenal space，PPS(肾旁后间隙)

amine precursor uptake and decarboxylation，APUD(脱羧基化，胺前体摄取脱羧化)

amine precursor uptake and decarboxylation，APUD(胺前体摄取脱羧细胞神经内分泌肿瘤罕见，归类于弥散的神经内分泌细胞肿瘤)

amine precursor uptake and decarboxylation，APUD(摄取胺前体和脱羟基，胺前体摄取脱羧细胞弥散的神经内分泌细胞)，Szijj 还把这类肿瘤描述为“apudoma”

acoustic quantification，AQ(声学定量检查)

Aquaporin-4，AQP-4(水通道蛋白 4)

anorectal angle，ARA(肛直角)

acoustic radiation force impulse，ARFI(声辐射力脉冲成像，超声声辐射力脉冲成像技术)

anorectal malignant melanoma，ARMM(肛管直肠恶性黑色素瘤)

ARPKD(常染色体隐性多囊性肾脏疾病)，ADPKD(常染色体显性多囊性肾脏疾病)

arsenic poisoning(慢性砷中毒)

arteriohepatic dysplasia(动脉肝性发育不良或 Alagille 综合征)

arrhythmogenic right ventricular cardiomyopathy，ARVC(致心律不齐性右心室心肌病)

arterial sequestration，AS(动脉性肺隔离症)，也称 anomalous systemic arterial supply to relatively normal segments of the lung，ASANL(正常肺异常体循环供血)

anomalous systemic artery，ASA(异常体循环动脉)

achalasia sphincter ani internus，ASAI(肛门内括约肌失弛缓综合征)

apical sodium-dependent bile acid transporter，ASBT(胆汁酸转运体)

adenosquamous cell carcmoma，ASC(腺鳞癌)

ASI(轴面源像)

Primitive neuroectodermal tumor，PNET(发生于胸肺部的原始神经外胚层瘤)，或称 Askin 瘤

arterial spin labeling，ASL(动脉血流自旋标记法，动脉血质子自旋标记法)，arterial spin labeling technigue，ASL(动脉自旋标记技术)，分为 continuous arterial spin labeling，CASL(连续式)和 pulsed arterial spin labeling，PASL(脉冲式)。FAIR 是 PASL 的一种，分别采用选层与非选层的反转恢复脉冲对成像层面进行射频激发，将所得图像减影得到灌注图像。

AsMA(抗平滑肌抗体)

arteriosclerotic occlusive disease，ASO(动脉硬化闭塞)

anterior superior pancreatico-duodenal vein，ASPDV(胰十二指肠上前静脉)，posterior superior pancreatic-duodenal vein，PSPDV(胰十二指肠上后静脉)，anterior and posterior inferior pancreatico-duodenal vein，AIPDV and PIPDV(胰十二指肠下前和下后静脉)

array spatial sensitivity encoding technique，ASSET(并行采集空间敏感性编码技术)

aspartic aminotransferase，AST(天冬氨酸转氨酶，天冬氨酸氨基转移酶)

selective arterial calcium stimulation and hepatic venous sampling，ASVS(选择性动脉钙刺激静脉采血测定胰岛素)

adipose tissue，AT(脂肪组织)

a-AT，a-1-AT(a 抗胰蛋白酶，抗胰蛋白酶，免疫组织化学检查内容之一)

Aneuploid tumor，AT(非整倍体肿瘤)

AT Ⅱ（血管紧张素Ⅱ）
adenosine triphosphate, ATP（三磷酸腺苷）
area under the curve，AUC（曲线下面积），Az 值，area under the ROC curve，AUC（ROC 曲线下面积）
area under the receiver operating characteristic curves，AUROC（受试者操作特征曲线下面积）
Auerbach's 神经丛（奥氏神经丛）
autoimmune disease（自身免疫性疾病）
autosomal dominant polycystic kidney disease（常染色体显性遗传多囊肾疾病）
aortic valve area, AVA（主动脉瓣口面积）
advanced vessel analysis, AVA（高级血管分析）
AVP（精氨酸血管加压素）
AVS（动静脉短路），APVS（肝动脉 - 门静脉短路），AHVS（肝动脉 - 肝静脉短路）
axial field of view（纵向视野）

B

diffusion gradient factor（扩散梯度因子，即 b 因子，又称 b 值）
biliary ascariasis, BA（胆系蛔虫病）
β- actin（β 肌动蛋白）
biliary atresia, BA（胆管闭锁）
bronchiolo-alveolar carcinoma，BAC（细支气管肺泡癌）
back projection（反投影法）
back-propagation（反向传播）
bronchoalveolar lavage, BAL（支气管肺泡灌洗）
balance-FFE（平衡快速梯度回波），balance fast field echo，B-FFE（小角度激发平衡式快速场回波，平衡快速场回波），Balance-FFE（平衡式稳态自由进动梯度回波序列）是 Philip 公司序列，Siemens 公司又称 true fast imaging with steady state procession, True FISP（真稳态进动快速成像）
Bankart 病变（前下关节盂前缘病变）
blood-brain barrier, BBB（血脑屏障）
black brown spots, BBS（黑棕色斑）
B-catenin（b- 链蛋白），β-catenin（β- 连环蛋白）
bcl-2 是 B-cell lymphoma/lenkmia-2（B 细胞淋巴瘤 / 白血病 -2）的缩写
Binsvanger disease，BD（Binsvanger 病），又称为 subcortical arteriosclerotic encephalopathy，SAE（皮层下动脉硬化性脑病）
base density, BD（片基灰雾）
beam averaging（声束平均）
blood flow, BF（血流量）[ml/100ml/min]
basic fibroblast growth factor，bFGF（碱性成纤维生长因子，碱性成纤维细胞生长因子）
benign fibrous histiocytoma，BFH（良性纤维组织细胞瘤）
benign gallbladder lesions, BGL（胆囊良性病变）
breath-hold DWI with MPG pulses in X，Y，Z Direction，BH600ALL（X、Y、Z 轴扩散梯度憋气 DWI）、
breath-hold DWI with MPG pulses in Z direction，BH-600SI（Z 轴扩散梯度憋气 DWI）
biliary cystadenoma and cystadenocarcinoma（胆系囊腺瘤与囊腺癌，胆管囊腺类肿瘤）
biliary hamartoma（胆管错构瘤，胆管性错构瘤），也称胆管微小错构瘤或 Von Meyenburg complex（von Meyenburg 综合征）
Biliary stenting（胆管内支架）
bilioma（肝内胆汁瘤，胆汁漏），intrahepatic biloma（肝脏胆汁瘤）
breast imaging reporting and data system，BI-RADS（乳腺影像报告和数据管理系统）
bizarre（补丁样）
Blue berry juiee, BJ（兰浆果液）
BLADE（刀锋伪影校正）
basal-like breast carcinoma，BLBC（基底细胞样乳腺癌）
benign metastasizing leiomyoma，BLM（良性转移性平滑肌瘤）
blooming effect（模糊效应）
$β_2$microglobulin，$β_2$M（$β_2$ 微球蛋白），$β_2$ microglobulin amyloidosis，A$β_2$M（$β_2$ 微球蛋白淀粉样变性病）
bone mineral content, BMC（骨矿含量）
bone mineral density，BMD（骨密度），bone mineral density, BMD（骨矿物质密度，即骨矿含量与骨密度之比）。BMD 定量测量的方法从最初的 RA（X 线吸收法）、SPA（单光子吸收法）、DPA（双光子吸收法）发展到 DXA（双能 X 线吸收测定法）
body mass index, BMI（体重指数，体质量指数）

biomedical microimaging，BMMI（生物医学显微图像学）

bronchiolitis obliterans，BO（闭塞性细支气管炎）

bronchiolitis Obliterans interstitial pneumonia，BOIP（闭塞性细支气管炎性间质性肺炎）

bronchiolitis obliterans organizing pneumonia，BOOP（闭塞性细支气管炎性机化性肺炎）

blood oxygenation level-dependent，BOLD（血氧水平依赖，血氧合水平依赖，血氧水平依赖成像），blood oxygenation level-dependent functional magnetic resonance imaging，BOLD-fMRI（血氧水平依赖功能磁共振成像）

Bolus Tracing（对比剂示踪技术）

Back Propagation，BP（误差反向传播模型）

base pair，bp（碱基对）

biliary papillomatosis，BP（胆管内乳头状瘤病）

benign prostate hyperplasia，BPH（良性前列腺增生）

blue rubber bleb nevus syndrome，BRBNS（蓝色橡皮大疱痣样综合征）

Breath-hold imaging（屏气成像）

idiopathic bronchiolocentric interstitial pneumonia，BrIP（特发性细支气管中心性间质性肺炎）

Brucellosis（布鲁士菌病）

Behcet's syndrome，BS（白塞综合征）

body surface area，BSA（体表面积）

balance steady state free precession，B-SSFP（平衡稳态自由进动）

balance turbo field echo，Balance-TFE，B-TFE（平衡式稳态自由进动梯度回波序列）

British Transplant Society，BTS（英国移植学会）

broadband ultrasound attenuation，BUA（振幅衰减）

blood urea nitrogen，BUN（血液尿素氮）

bursting heart syndrome（心脏爆裂综合征）

blood volume，BV（血容积，血容量）[ml/100ml]

bone volume fraction，BVF，BV/TV（骨体积分数），bone surface/bone volume ratio，BS/BV（骨表面积体积比），trabecular thickness，TbTh（骨小梁厚度），trabecular number，TbN（骨小梁数目），trabecular spacing，TbSp（骨小梁间隙）

C

^{11}C-HED（^{11}C-对羟麻黄碱）

C-Ⅲ，type Ⅲ collagen（Ⅲ型胶原蛋白）

C-Ⅳ，type Ⅳ collagen（Ⅳ型胶原蛋白，Ⅳ型胶原）

CA199、CA125、CA153（癌相关抗原）

cancer antigen 153，CA153（癌抗原153）

carbohydrate antigen，CA199（糖链抗原，癌抗原199，消化道癌抗原）

cerebral amyloid angiopathy，CAA（脑淀粉样血管病）

computer aided diagnosis，CAD（计算机辅助诊断），computer-aided detection，CAD（计算机辅助监测系统），computer aided detection/diagnosis，CAD（计算机辅助检测和诊断）

coronary atherosclerotic heart disease，CAD（冠状动脉硬化性心脏病）

coronary angiography，CAG（冠状动脉造影），coronary artery angiography，CAG（冠状动脉血管造影）

Chronic active hepatitis，CAH（慢性活动性肝炎）

Cajal（卡哈尔）细胞，ICC（间质细胞），interstitial cell of Cajal，ICC（胃肠道Cajal细胞），interstitial cell of Cajal，ICC（胃肠道Cajal间质细胞）

calcium iodate（碘酸钙）

calibration drift（偏斜校准）

Calot三角（胆囊三角）

chronic necrotizing aspergillosis，CAN（慢性坏死型曲菌病），又称为semiinvasive aspergillosis（半侵袭性曲霉病）

cancellation（相消伪影）

candida albicans（白色念珠菌）

controlled attenuation parameter，CAP（受控衰减参数）

computer-assisted polyp detection，CAPD（计算机辅助息肉检出）

congenital absence of portal vein，CAPV（先天性门静脉缺如）

Carney三联征（肺软骨瘤、胃平滑肌肉瘤和肾上腺外副神经节瘤）

Caroli病（先天性肝内胆管扩张症，也称胆管交通性海绵状扩张，一般将Caroli病合并先天性肝纤维化时称Caroli综合征），Caroli disease/Caroli syndrome（卡罗利病/卡罗利综合征）

classification and regression tree，CART（分类与回归决策树）

CAS（计算机辅助外科）

continuous arterial spin labeling，CASL（持续性动脉自旋标记）

cavernous hemangioma（海绵状血管瘤）

cavernous transformation of portal vein（门静脉的海绵样改变）

congenital bronchial atresia，CBA（先天性支气管闭锁）

congenita biliary dilatation，CBD（先天性胆管扩张症），common bile duct dilatation，CBD（总胆管扩张症）

cerebral blood flow，CBF（脑血流量）

cerebral blood volume，CBV（脑血容量）

conventional colonoscopy，CC（传统结肠镜，常规结肠镜）

cranio-caudal view，CC（头足轴位）

choledochal cyst，CC（胆总管囊肿）

choline+creatine/citrate，CC/C 比值（[Cho（胆碱）+Cre（肌酸）/ Cit（枸橼酸盐）] 比值）

cholangiocarcinoma，CCA（胆管癌）

cholangiocellular carcinoma，CCC（胆管细胞癌，胆管细胞型肝癌），intrahepatic mass-forming cholangiocarcinoma，IMCC（肿块型胆管细胞癌），intrahepatic cholangiocarcinoma，ICC（肝内胆管细胞癌）

CCD panel sensor（CCD 平面传感器）

charge coupled device，CCD（电子耦合原件）

criss-cross heart，CCH（十字交叉心脏）

cholecystokinin，CCK（胆囊收缩素）

anti-cyclic citrullinated peptide，CCP（抗环瓜氨酸肽抗体）

chromophobe cell renal carcmoma，CCRC（嫌色细胞肾癌）

Crohn disease，CD（克罗恩病，Crohn 病）

celiac disease，CD（谷蛋白敏感性肠病：即腹病、乳糜病），也称 nontropical sprue（非热带性口炎性腹泻）

CD31（血小板内皮细胞粘连分子）

CD34（血管源性物，人造血祖抗原），（CD34）为原始造血组织分化抗原，已有的研究表明 CD34 在 GIST 有较高的表达率

CD-68（巨噬细胞，免疫组织化学指标之一）

CD117（c-kit 原癌基因的蛋白产物，为Ⅲ型酪氨酸激酶生长因子受体，属免疫球蛋白超家族成员）

color doppler flow imaging，CDFI（彩色多普勒血流显像技术，彩色多普勒血流成像，彩色多普勒血流显像法），color Doppler energy，CDE（彩色多普勒能量），color Doppler ultrasound，CDUS（彩色多普勒超声技术）

congenital dislocation of the hip，CDH（先天性髋脱位）

CDH（先天性膈疝）

cDNA microarray analysis（cDNA 微点阵分析法）

conventional digital radiography，CDR（常规数字 X 线摄影）

capsule endoscopy，CE（胶囊内镜）

carcino-embryonic antigen，CEA（癌胚抗原）

CEA（颈动脉内膜切除术）

contrast-enhanced color Doppler sonography，CECD（造影多普勒血流显像法）

contrast-enhanced MR angiography，CE-MRA（对比增强 MR 血管成像），three-dimensional dynamic contrast-enhanced MR angiography，3D CE MRA（三维动态增强磁共振血管成像），three-dimensional contrast-enhanced MRA，3D CE MRA（三维增强 MRA）

central obesity（中心型肥胖）

central volume principle（中心容积定律）

central-peripheral phenomenon（中心 - 边缘现象）

c-erbB-2（癌基因）

maximum contrast enhancement ratio，CER_{max}（最大强化率）

ceruloplasmin（蓝胞浆素）

contrast-enhanced ultrasonography，CEUS（对比增强超声），contrast-enhanced ultrasound，CEUS（实时超声造影）

cerebral fat embolism syndrome，CFE（脑脂肪栓塞综合征）

calcifying fibrous pseudotumor，CFPT（钙化性纤维性假瘤）

congestive gastropathy，CG（充血性胃病），或 portal hypertensive gastropathy，PHG（门脉高压性胃病）

chromogranin A，CgA（嗜铬蛋白 A，嗜铬素 A）

Camna-Gandy bodies，CGB（Camna-Gandy 小体，亦称铁质沉着结节）

chronic granulomatous disease，CGD（慢性肉芽肿病）

congestive hepatopathy，CH（淤血性肝病）

common hepatic artery, CHA(肝总动脉), accessory left hepatic artery, aLHA(副肝左动脉), accessory right hepatic artery, aRHA(副肝右动脉)

chronic hepatitis B, CHB(慢性乙型肝炎), chronic hepatitis C, CHC(慢性丙型肝炎)

combined hepatocellular carcinoma and cholangiocarcinoma, cHCC-CC(混合型肝细胞癌 - 胆管细胞癌,混合型肝癌), Combined HCC–Cholangiocarcinoma(结合型肝癌)

chemical shift imaging(化学位移成像)

confluent hepatic fibrosis(融合性肝纤维化)

congenital hepatic fibrosis, CHF(先天性肝纤维化)

ciliated hepatic foregut cyst, CHFC(纤毛前肠性肝囊肿,纤毛性肝前肠囊肿)

Chiba 针(千叶针)

Chilaiditi's syndrome(肝、膈结肠间位,卡拉兹综合征)

childhood fibrous tumor with psammoma bodies(伴有砂粒体结构的儿童纤维性肿瘤)

cavernous hemangiomas of the liver, CHL(肝海绵状血管瘤)

chloromas(局灶性肝的白血病浸润,绿色瘤)

choline, Cho(胆碱)

cholangiocarcinoma(肝内胆管癌), cholangiocellular carcinoma, Intrahepaticcholangiocarcinoma(胆管细胞型肝癌)

choledochal cyst(胆总管囊肿),又称 congenetal biliary dilatation(先天性胆总管扩张症)

choledochocele(胆总管囊状膨出), choledochal deverticulum(胆总管单发憩室)

choledochocele, type 3 choledochal cyst(总胆管壁内囊肿,又称Ⅲ型肝外胆管囊肿)

cholestatic type of HCC(淤胆型肝细胞性肝癌)

Cholesterinosis(胆囊胆甾醇沉积病),又称 strawberry gallblad-der(草莓胆囊), fishscale gallbladder(鱼鳞胆囊)

Chol+Unsat peak, 5.4ppm~5.6ppm(胆固醇和不饱和脂肪酸的混合峰)

Choline peak, 3.2ppm(胆碱峰)

chrondrocalcinosis(软骨钙化症)

cardiac index, CI(心指数)

cine(电影)

Cine PC MRI(电影相位对比磁共振成像)

congenital intrahepatic porto-systemic venous shunts, CIPSVS(先天性肝内门 - 体静脉分流,先天性肝内门静脉 - 体静脉分流)

cirrhotic nodule(硬变结节)

Cisapride Tablets(西沙必利)

clinically isolated syndrome, CIS(临床孤立综合征)

cisplatin(顺铂)

color kinesis, CK(彩色室壁动力分析)

CK(角蛋白, 细胞角蛋白,免疫组织化学检查内容之一), cytokeratin, CK(细胞角蛋白 18), CK19(细胞角蛋白 19), CKPan(细胞角蛋白)

CK19(胆管上皮)

claypipestem(粘土烟管状)

chronic liver disease, CLD(慢性肝脏疾病)

Clear Cell Type HCC(透明细胞型肝癌), Combined HCC–Cholangiocarcinoma(混合型肝癌), Sarcomatoid HCC(肉瘤样肝癌), Fibrolamellar HCC(纤维板层型肝癌), Sclerosing HCC(硬化性肝癌)

centrilobular fibrosis, CLF(小叶中心性纤维化)

cross-linked iron oxide, CLIO(交联氧化铁微粒,交联化氧化铁)

^{11}C-MET(^{11}C- 蛋氨酸)

circumferential margin involvement, CMI(环周切缘癌浸润)

curved multiplanar reformation, CMPR(曲面多层面重建)

cytomegalovirus, CMV(巨细胞病毒)

cirrhotic nodular, CN(肝硬化结节)

cryptococcus neoformans, CN(新型隐球菌)

complicated normal appendix, CNA(复杂病变正常阑尾), noncomplicated normal appendix,

NCNA(非复杂病变正常阑尾)

central neurocytoma, CNC(中枢神经细胞瘤)

calcineurin inhibitor, CNI(钙调磷酸酶抑制剂)

chronic necrotizing pulmonary aspergillosis, CNPA(慢性坏死性肺曲霉病)

contrast to noise ratio, CNR(对比噪声比)

category name retrieval test, CNRT(种类名称提取测试)

cardiac output, CO(心肌每分输出量)

Codman 瘤(成软骨细胞瘤,又称软骨母细胞瘤)

colloid carcinoma(黏液腺癌,又称胶样癌)

CO_2 -DUS（二氧化碳微泡超声血管造影，二氧化碳微泡超声动态检查）
cometlike echo（彗星样回声）
condition associated with a hyperdense liver（伴同高密度肝脏的疾病）
confluent hepatic fibrosis（融合性肝纤维化）
congenital microcolon（先天性细小结肠症，又称胎儿型结肠）
connectivity algorithm（连接算法）
cryptogenic organizing pneumonia，COP（隐源性机化性肺炎），原称 BOOP
chronic obstructive pulmonary disease，COPD（慢性阻塞性肺疾病）
cyclooxygenase，COX（环氧合酶），cyclooxygenase2，COX-2（环氧化酶 2）
chronic periaortitis，CP（慢性主动脉周围炎）
CP（铜蓝蛋白）
cerebral peduncle，CP（大脑脚）
collagen proportionate area，CPA（胶原蛋白面积比率）
choroid plexus cysts，CPC（脉络丛囊肿）
congenital portacaval shunt，CPCS（先天性门腔静脉分流异常，先天性门 - 腔静脉分流畸形）
centraI pontine myelinolysis，CPM（脑桥中央髓鞘溶解症），CPM 与 extrapontine myelinolysis，EPM（脑桥外髓鞘溶解症）合称渗透性髓鞘溶解症。
CPMG（Carr-purcell-meiboom-gill）
cerebral perfusion pressure，CPP（脑灌注压）
curved planar reconstruction，CPR；curred multiplanar reformation，CPR（曲面重建，曲面重组）
creatine，Cr（肌酸），Creatine peak，3.0ppm（肌酸峰）
computed radiography，CR（计算机 X 线摄影术）
colorectal cancer，CRC（结 / 直肠癌）
cerebral radiation injuries，CRI（放射性脑损伤）
circumferential resection margin，CRM（环周切缘）
cross-sectional moments of inertia（横截面的惯性力矩）
cross-sectional MPR（横断面多平面重组）
crow-foot（喜鹊足征）
CRP（C- 反应蛋白）
clinic-radiologic-pathologic diagnosis，CRP diagnosis（临床 - 影像 - 病理诊断）
cherry-red spots，CRS（樱桃红样斑点）
cathode ray tube，CRT（阴极射线管），CRT（Cathode Ray Tube 显示器）
3-demensional conformal radiotherapy，3DCRT（三维适形放射治疗），chemotherapy-radiation therapy，CRT（放化疗）
carcinosarcoma，CS（癌肉瘤）
chemical shift imaging，CSI [（多体素的）化学位移成像，即 MR 波谱分解成像技术]，即 in phase imaging/opposed phase imaging，IPI/OPI（同相位 / 反相位成像）
cholesterol polyps，CSP（胆固醇息肉）
cystic and sotid pseudo-papillary tumor，CSPT（胰腺囊实性假性乳头状瘤）
adrenal-spleen chemical shift ratio，CSR（肾上腺肿块 - 脾化学位移成像信号比）
cortical spinal tract，CST（皮质脊髓束）
cystic-solid tumor of pancreas，CSTP（胰腺实质性囊性肿瘤）
CT（计算机断层检查），HRCT（高分辨力 CT），micro-CT（显微 CT），peripheral QCT，pQCT（周围骨定量 CT），QCT（定量 CT），volumetric QCT，vQCT（容积 QCT），electric beam CT，EBCT（电子束 CT），dual-source CT，DSCT（双源 CT）
computed tomography angiography，CTA（CT 血管成像），CT 血管造影，或 CT 动脉造影，CT arteriography，CTA（动脉造影 CT）
computed tomography during arterial portography，CTAP（动脉法门静脉造影 CT 扫描，动脉期 CT 门脉造影，动脉性门静脉造影 CT，动脉性门脉 CT 成像检查，经动脉门静脉造影性 CT，经肠系膜上动脉 - 门脉增强肝脏 CT 扫描，经动脉门静脉 CT 成像）；spiral CT during arterial portography，SCTAP（螺旋 CT 动脉门脉造影），three-dimensional CTAP，3D-CTAP（动脉性门静脉造影 CT 三维重建像）
3D CT cholangiography，3D CTC（三维 CT 胆系造影）
CT colonography，CTC（结肠 CT，CT 结肠成像技术）
connective tissue disease，CTD（结缔组织病）
CT enterography，CTE（CT 小肠成像，小肠 CT 成像）
CT-enteroclysis，CT-E（插管法 CT 扫描）

spiral CT during gastric arteriography，CTGA（动脉造影期行双期螺旋 CT 扫描）

CT during hepatic arteriography，CTHA（经肝动脉注入对比剂 CT 增强扫描，动脉造影 CT，肝动脉造影 CT）

cytotoxic T lymphocyte，CTL（细胞毒性 T 淋巴细胞），CTLA-4（细胞毒性 T 淋巴细胞相关抗原 4）

$CT_{L/S}$（肝脾密度之比），CT_{LP}（无血肝实质密度，CT_{LP} =[L-0.3（0.75P+0.25A）]/0.7）

spiral CT portography，CTP（螺旋 CT 门静脉造影，CT 门静脉血管成像）

CT perfusion，CTP（多层螺旋 CT 灌注成像），CT perfusion，CTP（CT 灌注成像），CTPI（CT 灌注成像）

cavernous transformation of the portal vein，CTPV（门静脉海绵样变）

computed tomography portal venography，CTPV（CT 门静脉成像）

cardiothoracic ratio，CTR（心胸比率）

carpal tunnel syndrome，CTS（腕管综合征）

CT severity index，CTSI（CT 严重性指数，CT 严重指数评分，急性胰腺炎时用）

computed tomography virtual colonoscopy，CTVC（CT 虚拟结肠镜，CT 仿真肠镜，CT 仿真结肠镜成像）

CT virtual choledochoscopy，CTVC（胆系 CT 仿真内镜）

combined CT venography and pulmonary angiography，CTVPA（CT 肺动脉造影联合间接法下肢静脉造影）

coefficient of variation，CV（变异系数，可重复性的变异系数），CV= 标准差 / 平均值

cardiovascular disease，CVD（心血管疾病）

cerebral venous malformation，CVM（脑静脉性血管畸形），又名 cerebral venous angioma，CVA（脑静脉性血管瘤），或 developmental venons anomaly，DVA（脑发育性静脉异常）

cerebrovascular reactivity，CVR（脑血管反应性）

cerebral venous sinus thrombosis，CVST（脑静脉窦血栓形成）

cerebral venous thrombosis，CVT（脑静脉血栓形成）

CYP450S（人类细胞色素 P450）

cystic metastases-hypervascular metastases with necrosis，or cystic metastases（mucinous CA）[囊性转移——富血管性转移伴坏死和囊性变或囊性转移（如黏液腺癌）]

cystohepatic duct（囊肝管）

cytokeratin（细胞角蛋白）

D

two dimension，2D（二维），three dimension，3D（三维），four dimension，4D（四维）

double end gel electrophoresis，2-DE（双向凝胶电泳）

2D TOF MRA（心电门控二维时间飞跃 MR 血管成像），3D TOF-MRA（三维时间飞跃法 MR 血管成像）

3D constructive inference in steady state，3D-CISS（三维稳态构成干扰序列）

3D FSPGR（无间隔三位扰相梯度回波，三维快速扰相梯度回波）

three-dimensional proton MR spectroscopic imaging，3D MRSI（3D 氢质子磁共振波谱成像）

3D-volumetric interpolated breath-hold examination，3D-VIBE（三维容积式内插法屏气检查）

dielectric artifact，DA（电解质伪影）

degree of anisoropy，DA（各向异性程度）

3，3'-diaminobenzidine，DAB（二氨基联苯胺）

pancreatic ductal adenocarcinoma，DAC（胰腺导管腺癌），ductal adenocarcinoma of pancreas，DACP（胰腺导管上皮癌）

diffuse alviolar damage，DAD（弥漫性肺泡损害）

diffuse alveolar hemorrhage，DAH（弥漫性肺泡出血）

death-associated protein kinase-1，DAPK1（死亡相关蛋白激酶）

data acquisition system，DAS（数据采集系统）

dendritic cell，DC（树突状细胞）

DC（扩散系数）

average fiffusion coefficient，DCavg（平均扩散系数图）

double-contrast barium enema，DCBE（双对比钡灌肠，结肠双重对比造影）

double-contrasted MRI，DC-MRI（双对比增强 MR 成像，双增强 MR 成像）

decompensation cirrhosis，DCC（失代偿期肝硬化）

dynamic contrast-enhanced，DCE（动态增强成像），dynamic contrast enhanced MRI，DCE-MRI（动态

对比增强 MRI）

Doppler Color Flow Imaging，DCFI（多普勒彩色血流成象）

ductal carcinoma in situ，DCIS（导管原位癌）

dilated cardiomyopathy，DCM（扩张型心肌病）

double contrast radiography of small intestine，DCR（小肠气钡双对比造影）

decompression sickness，DCS（潜水减压病）

death domain，DD（死亡域）

duodenal diverticulum，DD（十二指肠憩室），periampullary diverticula，PAD（十二指肠乳头旁憩室），juxta-papillary duodenal diverticulum，JPD；juxta-papillary diverticulum of duodenum，

JDD）（十二指肠乳头旁憩室）

developmental dysplasia of the hip，DDH（发育性髋关节发育不良）

DDP（顺铂）

double end gel electrophoresis，2-DE（双向凝胶电泳）

dead-endevolution（末路进化）

iterative decomposition of water and fat with echo asymmetry and least squares estimation，DEAL（多回波迭代水脂不对称回波分解与最小二乘估计）

deconvolution method（去卷积法，对去卷积法）

decoupling（去耦联）

delirium tremens（震颤性谵妄）

Denonvilliers 筋膜（直肠膀胱隔）

diethylnitrosarmne，DEN（致癌剂）

de novo carcinogenesis（重新癌发生）

dual energy subtraction，DES（双能减影）

desmin（结蛋白，免疫组织化学检查内容之一）

desoplastic strom（促结缔组织增生的基质）

display field of view，DFOV（重建范围）

distal gastric cancer，DGC（远侧胃癌），proximal gastric cancer，PGC（近侧胃癌）

dual gradient echo MRI，DGE-MRI（双梯度回波 MR 成像）

diabetes insipidus，DI（尿崩症）

desquamative interstitial pneumonia，DIP（脱屑性间质性肺炎）

diaphragmatic slips（膈带）

DIC（弥散性血管内凝血）

diamagnetic agents（逆磁性）

Dynamic incremental bolus CT，DIB-CT（进床式团注增强动态 CT）

dripinfususion cholangiography，DIC（静脉胆系造影术，静脉滴注胆系造影），helical CT during drip infusion cholangiography，DIC-CT（滴注胆管造影螺旋 CT）

digital imaging and communication in medicine，DICOM［医学数字成像和传输，医学数字影像和通信（标准），医学数字成像与通信标准］

diffuse nodular hyperplasia without fibrous septa（无纤维间隔的弥漫性结节增生），又名 NRH（结节性再生性增生），也称为 noncirrhotic regenerative nodules，NRN（不伴有肝硬化的大再生结节），或巨再生结节

diffusion gradient factor（扩散梯度因子）

diffuse steatosis（弥漫性脂肪变性，脂肪浸润），diffuse hepatic steatosis（弥漫性肝脂肪变性），focal steatosis（局灶性脂肪变性）

diffuse malignancy（弥漫性恶性病变）

drug-induced liver injury，DILI（药物性肝损伤）

disarray（弥漫性紊乱）

disease-free survival rate（无病生存率）

Disse’s space（窦周间隙）

Dixon’s 技术（自旋回波）

diffuse large B-cell lymphoma，DLBCL（弥漫大 B 细胞淋巴瘤）

direct lymphography，DLG（直接淋巴管造影，直接淋巴管造影术）

Data Mining，DM（数据挖掘）

DL-MRGIH（黑腔 MR 胃肠水成像）

dynamic MRI，D-MRI（动态 MRI）

dimethyl sulfoxide，DMSO（二甲亚砜）

dysplastic nodule，DN（退变结节、不典型增生结节），曾称为腺瘤样增生、发育不良结节、异型增生结节等。根据其细胞异型性程度，DN 又分为 low grade DN，LGDN（低级别）和 high grade DN，HGDN（高级别）两类

DN with subfocus of HCC（非典型性结节伴微灶性肝细胞癌）

diffuse nodular hyperplasia，DNH（弥漫性结节增生）

difference of Gaussian，DOG（高斯差分）

discovered on GIST21，DOG1（功能未知蛋白）

Doppler（多普勒），Doppler effect（多普勒效应），Doppler shift（多普勒频移），Doppler tissue velocity, DTV(多普勒组织速度图), Doppler tissue acceleration, DTA(多普勒组织加速度图), Doppler tissue energy, DTE(多普勒组织能量图), Doppler tissue pulse wave, DTPW(多普勒组织频谱图), Doppler tissue M-mode, DTM-mode(多普勒组织M型)

dysplastic nodules in cirrhosis(肝硬化发育不良结节)

dysplastic focus(非典型增生或异型增生灶)

dome(上凸,圆屋顶状)

dominant negative(显性阴性)

diabetic osteoporosis,DOP(糖尿病性骨质疏松症)

dihydroxyphenylalanine,DOPA(二羟苯丙氨酸)

DOTATOC(DOTA-Tyr^3-octreotide,DOTATOC)

dual-photon absorptiometry,DPA(双能光子测量仪)

dorsal pancreatic artery, DPA(胰背动脉), transverse pancreatic artery, TPA(胰横动脉), magnificent pancreatic artery, MPA(胰大动脉)

disconnected pancreatic duct syndrome, DPDS(胰管中断综合征)

duodenal papilla ectope, DPE(十二指肠乳头开口异位)

delay phase image,DPI(延迟成像)

diagnostic peritoneal lavage, DPL(诊断性腹腔灌洗术)

disseminated peritoneal adenomucinosis, DPAM(弥散性腹膜黏液腺瘤病)

DPP(诊断性腹腔穿刺术)

descending perineum syndromes, DPS(会阴下降综合征)

digital radiography, DR(数字X线照片检测法,数字化X线摄影术)

dialysis-related amyloidosis, DRA(透析相关性淀粉样变性)

digital rectal examination,DRE(直肠指检)

droplets(脂肪微滴)

destruction spondyloarthropathy,DSA(破坏性脊柱关节病)

digital subtraction angiography, DSA(数字减影血管造影)

dynamic susceptibility contrast-enhanced, DSC(动态磁敏感对比剂增强)

dynamic susceptibility contrast-enhanced perfusion MR imaging,DSCE-MR(动态磁敏感性对比增强MR灌注成像)

dual-source CT,DSCT(双源CT)

dual source CT coronary angiography, DSCTCA(双源CT冠状动脉血管成像)

duodenal stasis disease,DSD(十二指肠郁积症)

diffusion-sensitizing gradient pulse, DSGP(扩散敏感梯度脉冲)

doubling time,DT(倍增时间)

diffusion tensor imaging, DTI(扩散张量成像)

dual TE sequence(双重回波时间序列)

ductal plate(胆管板)

duct-penetrating sign(胰管穿过征)

duplex Doppler US(双功能多普勒超声), doppler ultrasonography,DUS(多普勒超声)

Dual Energy Monoenergetic(双能单能谱分析软件)

diastolicv velocity,DV(舒张期末流速)

distribution volume,DV(分布容积)

deep venous thrombosis,DVT(深静脉血栓)

dual-energy x-ray absorptiometry, DXA, DEXA(双能X线吸收仪,双能X线吸收测量法)

double-resonance(双共振)

diffusion weighted imaging,DWI(扩散加权成像)

dynamic first-pass bolus tracking of susceptibility contrast agent magnetic resonance imaging(磁敏感性对比剂动态首过示踪磁共振成像)

dynamic first-pass bolus rtacking of susceptibility contrast agent magnetic resonance imaging(对比剂团注示踪法)

dynamic illustration of defecography(排粪造影解剖学划线或动态插图)

diffusion weighted imaging with back-ground body signal suppression, DWIBS(背景信号抑制扩散加权成像序列)

dysplastic(非典型增生), dysplastic focus(异型增生灶)

dysplastic nodules in cirrhosis(肝硬化发育不良结节)

E

electroanatomic mapping,EAM(电解剖标测系统)

epithelial angiomyolipoma, EAML(上皮样血管平滑肌脂肪瘤)

European Association for the Study of the Liver, EASL (欧洲肝病学会,欧洲肝病协会), European Association for the Study of Liver Disease, EASLD(欧洲肝病学会)

enteropathy-associated T-cell lymphoma, EATL(肠病相关 T 细胞淋巴瘤)

EB 病毒(人类疱疹病毒)

electric beam computed tomography, EBCT(电子束 CT)

endobronchial ultrasound, EBUS(支气管内超声探查)

endocardial cushion defect, ECD(心内膜垫缺损), complete endocardial cushion defect, CECD(完全型心内膜垫缺损), partial endocardial cushion defect, PECD(部分型心内膜垫缺损)

esophageal capsule endoscopy, ECE(胶囊内镜)

electrocardiography, ECG(心电图), ECG/VCC(心电 / 心向量)

echinococcus granulosus(细粒棘球蚴), unilocular (单室性)棘球蚴病, echinococcus multilocularis (多房棘球蚴), alveolar(泡状)棘球蚴病, hydatid matrix [棘球囊基质,亦称 cystic sand(囊沙)]

Kulchitsky 细胞(肠黏膜的嗜银细胞)或 enterochromaffin cells, EC(肠嗜铬细胞), entero-

chromaffin-like, ECL(肠嗜铬样)细胞

eclamptic(子痫)

extracellular matrix, ECM(细胞外基质)

emission computed tomography, ECT(发射型计算机体层扫描术)

enhancement degree, ED(强化程度)

ED(有效剂量)

edoscopic laser doppler velocimetry(内镜激光多普勒血流仪)

exposure data recognizer, EDR(曝光数据识别)

ethylenediamine tetraacetic acid, EDTA(乙二胺四乙酸钠)

extraductal ultrasonography, EDUS(管外超声检查)

end-diastolic volume, EDV(舒张末期容量,或舒张末期容积)

electroencephalography, EEG(脑电图)

extra-vascular extra-cellular space, EES(间质)

ejection fraction, EF(左室射血分数)[EF=(EDV-ESV)/EDV)=(舒张末期容积 - 收缩末期容积)/舒张末期容积]

Effective-Z(有效原子序数)

eosinophilic gastroenteritis, EG(嗜酸细胞性胃肠炎,又被译作嗜酸性粒细胞性胃肠炎)

early gastric cancer, EGC(早期胃癌), advanced gastric cancer, AGC(进展期胃癌)

epidermal growth factor, EGF(表皮生长因子), EGFR(表皮生长因子受体)

extrahepatic growing hepatocellular carcinoma, EG-HCC(外生型肝细胞癌)

esophagogastric varices, EGV(食管胃静脉曲张)

epithelioid hemangioendothelioma, EH(上皮样血管内皮细胞瘤,曾被称为组织细胞样血管内皮细胞瘤、硬化性内皮样肉瘤)

early hepatocellular carclnoma, eHCC(早期肝细胞癌)

extrahepatic cholangiocarcinoma, EHCC(肝外胆管癌)

epithelioid hemangioendothelioma, EHE(上皮样血管内皮瘤,上皮样血管内皮细胞瘤病), hepatic epithelioid hemangioendothelioma, HEHE(肝上皮样血管内皮瘤), Neoplasms of the perivascular epithelioid cell, PEComas, PEC(血管周围上皮样细胞瘤), pulmlonary epithelioid hemangioendothelioma, PEH(肺上皮样血管内皮瘤),又称 IVBAT(血管内支气管肺泡肿瘤)

eosinophilic hepatic infiltration, EHI(肝脏嗜酸性粒细胞浸润,又称为局灶性嗜酸性粒细胞性坏死、嗜酸性粒细胞性脓肿、局部嗜酸性浸润)

extrahepatlc portal venous obstruction, EHPVO(肝外门静脉梗阻)

echointensity, EI(回声强度)

enzymeimmunoassay, EIA(酶免疫分析法)

early lung cancer action project, ELCAP(国际早期肺癌行动计划)

electro magnetic radiation(电磁辐射), electro magnetic spectrum(电磁波谱)

electron-hole pair(电子空穴对), electronic cassette (电子暗盒), electronic linear scanner(电子线形扫描器), electronic pair effect(电子对效应), electronic phased array scanner(电子相控阵扫描器)

enzyme-linked immunosorbent assay, ELISA(酶联免

疫吸附法），enzyme linked immunosorbent assay，ELISA（固相夹心法酶联免疫吸附实验）
endobronchial metastasis，EM（支气管内转移瘤）
epithelial membrane antigen，EMA（上皮膜抗原，上皮细胞膜抗原，免疫组织化学检查内容之一）
embryo（胚芽）
extent of mesorectal invasion，EMI（直肠系膜受侵的程度）
extramedullary plasmacytoma，EMP（髓外浆细胞瘤）
epithelial-to-mesenchymal transition，EMT（上皮 - 间质转化）
emphysematous cholecystitis（气肿性胆囊炎，又称气性胆囊炎）
ENBD（鼻胆管引流），EPT（内窥镜乳头切开术），EST（括约肌切开术）
European Neuroendocrine Tumor Society，ENETS（欧洲神经内分泌肿瘤学会）
endothelial nitric oxide synthase，eNOS（内皮型一氧化氮）
enuclcation sign（摘除征）
EO%（嗜酸性粒细胞百分比）
ethoxybenzyl，EOB（乙氧基苯甲基），ethoxybenzyl diethylenetriaminepentaacetic acid，EOB-DTPA（乙氧基苯甲基）
Ethiodol-Oil-Emulsion-13，EOE-13 （乙碘油乳剂 -13）
eosinophilic inclusions（嗜伊红包涵体）
excretory phase，EP（分泌期）
single shot spin echo，EPI（单次激发自旋回波）
echo planar imaging，EPI（回波平面成像，或平面回波成像），spin echo-echo planar imaging，SE-EPI（T_2 加权），gradient echo-echo planar imaing，GE-EPI（重 T_2 加权），inversion recovery echo planar imaging，IR-EPI（T_1 加权），echo planar imaging diffusion-weighted magnetic resonance imaging，EPI-DWI（扩散加权平面回波成像）
EPIC（胰腺外炎症评分系统）
extrapontine myelinolysis，EPM（脑桥外髓鞘溶解症）
early postoperative inflammatort small bowel obstruction，EPISBO（术后早期炎症性小肠梗阻），early postoperative small bowel obstruction，EPSBO（术后早期小肠梗阻）
effector cell protease receptor-1，EPR-1（效应细胞蛋白酶受体 -1）
estrogen receptor，ER（雌激素受体）
endoscopic retrograde cholangiography，ERC（内镜逆行性胆系造影）
endo-rectal coil，ERC（直肠内线圈）
endoscopic retrograde cholangio-pancreatography，ERCP（经内镜逆行胆胰管造影术，X 线内镜逆行胆胰管造影）
extracellular signal-regulated kinase，ERK（细胞外信号调节激酶）
ERS（欧洲呼吸病学会）
endolymphatic sac，ES（内淋巴囊）
ectopic splenic autotransplantation，ESAT（自体异位脾种植）
extended-spectrum beta-lactamase，ESBL（超广谱 b 内酰胺酶）
extracapsular spread，ESC（包膜外受侵）
extracellular fluid space，ESC（细胞外间隙）
extrapleura solitary fibrous tumor，E-SFT（胸膜外孤立性纤维瘤）
electrospray ionization tandem mass spectrometry，ESI-MS/MS（电喷雾电离质谱分析）
EST（括约肌切开术）
end-systo1ic volume，ESV（收缩末期容量，或收缩末期容积）
endothelin-1，ET-1（内皮素 -1），ET（内皮素）
ejection time，ET（射血时间）
enhancement-time curves，ETCs（增强 - 时间曲线）
echo train length，ETL [回波序列（链）长度]
EUS（增强超声），EUS（声学造影超声），endoscopic ultrasonography，EUS（内镜超声，超声内镜），endosonography guided fine needle aspiration，EUS-FNA（内镜超声引导下行细针穿刺活检）
esophageal vein，EV（食管静脉），coronary gastric vein，CGV（胃冠状静脉），short gastric vein，SGV（胃短静脉），gastroepiploic vein，GEV（胃网膜静脉），gastrocolic trunk，GCT（胃结肠干）
esophagogastric variceal bleeding，EVB（食管胃静脉曲张破裂出血）
evidence-based radiology（循证放射学）
extramedullary hematopoiesis（髓外造血）

F

fractional anisotropy，FA（部分各向异性，部分各向异性图，各向异性分数，各向异性分量，各向异性指数，各向异性比值）

flip angle，FA（反转角度）

ferric ammonium citrate，FAC（枸橼酸铁铵）

flow-sensitive alternating inversiong recovery，FAIR（流入敏感性交替反转恢复技术，血流敏感性的交替反转恢复）

flow sensitive alternating inversion recovery with an extra radiofrequency pulse，FAIRER（外在射频脉冲的的血流敏感性交替反转恢复）

flow-sensitive alternating inversion recovery exempting separate T_1 measurement，FAIREST（流速敏感交替反转恢复免除独立 T_1 测量）

fast acquisition with multiple excitation，FAME（多次激发快速采集技术）

the fast gradient echo-echo train，fast GRE ET（快速梯度回波链）

FAT（肝内脂肪含量），fatty liver disease（脂肪性肝病），liver steatosis and fatty liver（脂肪肝）

fat globules（脂肪液滴），droplets，fat droplets（脂肪小滴）

fatty metamorphosis（脂肪变态）

fatty replacement of pancreas（胰腺脂肪替代），又称为 lipomatosis（脂肪过多症）、fat infiltration（脂肪浸润）、adipose atrophy（多脂肪性萎缩）

fast low-angle-shot-GRE（二维快速小角度激发成像梯度回波序列）

free-breathing DWI with MPG pulses in X，Y，Z direction and inversion recovery for fat saturation，FB600ALL+FS（自由呼吸反转恢复脂肪抑制DWI）

fat saturation，FATSAT，又称 CHEMSAT/CHESS（脂肪饱和序列）

fetal bovine serum，FBS（胎牛血清）

FC（血流补偿）

FC（纤维结肠镜）

FCD（纤维性骨皮质缺损）

F-18 fluorocholine，FCH（^{18} 氟胆碱）

Food and Drug Administration，FDA[（美国）食品及药物管理局，美国食品药品监督局]

fluorodeoxyglucose，FDG（脱氧葡萄糖，氟脱氧葡萄糖），F-18 fluorodeoxy-D-glucose，FDG（^{18} 氟脱氧葡萄糖），^{18}F-fluorodeoxyglucose，^{18}F-FDG（^{18}F- 氟脱氧葡萄糖），fluorodeoxyglucose，

FDG（脱氧葡萄糖）

field echo，FE（场回波）

γ-Fe_2O_3（磁赤铁矿），Fe_3O_4（磁铁矿）

finite element，FE（有限元），finite element analysis，FEA（有限元分析）

feathered contour（羽毛样）

Feridex（菲立磁）

ferucarbotran（超顺磁性氧化铁）以及 mangafodipir trisodium（磁性物质）

Ferucarbotran，Resovist（铁羧葡胺，拜耳先灵医药，德国）

ferumoxides（超顺磁性氧化铁），Ferumoxides 或 SPIO（超顺磁性三氧化二铁制剂），

Ferumoxtran-10 或 US-PIOs（超小超顺磁性三氧化二铁制剂）

fat embolism syndrome，FES（脂肪栓塞综合征）

^{18}F-FET（氟代乙基酪氨酸）

fat fraction，FF（脂肪分数），FFA（游离脂肪酸）

full field digital mammography，FFDM（全视野数字化乳腺摄影，全数字化乳腺摄影）

^{18}F-fluorodopamine（^{18}F- 氟多番）

^{18}F-FMISO（^{18}F- 氟硝基咪唑）

fast Fourier transform，FFT（快速傅里叶变换）

fibroblast growth factor-2，FGF-2（成纤维细胞生长因子），fibroblast growth factor 21，FGF21（成纤维细胞生长因子）

focal ground glass opacity，fGGO（局灶性磨玻璃密度影）

fast gradient echo，FGRE（快速梯度回波）

fat index，FI（肝脂肪变性指数），liver fat content，LFC（肝脏脂肪含量），fatty liver disease，FLD（脂肪性肝病），alcoholic fatty liver disease，AFLD（酒精性脂肪性肝病），alcoholic liver disease，ALD（酒精性肝病），relative lipid content，RLC（肝细胞相对脂肪含量）

fibrosis 4 score，FIB-4（纤维指数评分）

Fibrolamellar HCC（纤维板层型肝癌），fibrolamellar hepatocellular carcinoma，FL-HCC（纤维板层型肝细胞癌）

fibrosarcoma(纤维肉瘤)

fibroscan(瞬时弹性成像),FibroScan(瞬时弹性超声,肝脏瞬时弹性超声),是利用脉冲回波超声采集数据测量肝脏硬度,从而评价肝纤维化程度的一种超声技术

fibrous protein amyloid(淀粉样纤维蛋白沉积)

free induction decay,FID(自由感应衰减),free indication decay signal,FID(自由感应衰减信号)

balance steady state free precession, B-SSFP(平衡稳态自由进动),不同厂家分别称为快速平衡稳态成像,稳态采集快速成像,快速 T_2WI 序列即快速稳态进动采集序列,快速成像稳态采集,三维稳态进动快速成像,快速稳态自由进动序列,fast imaging employing steady-state acquisition, FIESTA(快速稳态进动成像)、fast imaging with steady-state precession,FISP(稳态进动快速成像)和真实稳态自由进动,真稳态进动快速序列, true fast imaging with steady-state precession, true FISP(真实稳态自由进动序列)和(three-dimensional Fourier transformation, 3DFT)

international federation of gynecology and obstetrics, FIGO(国际妇产科协会)

fast inversion recovery motion, FIRM(快速反转恢复运动抑制序列), fast inversion recovery motion insensitive sequence,FIRM(快速 T_1WI,即反转恢复运动抑制序列)

fluorescein isothiocyanate, FITC(异硫氰酸荧光素)

Fitz-Hugh-Curtis syndrome(菲-科综合征)

fluid attenuated inversion recovery, FLAIR [液体衰减反转恢复成像,液体抑制的(流动衰减)反转恢复,液体衰减反转恢复序列]

fast low-angle shot, FLASH(快速小角度激发),gradient-echo fast low-angle shot, FLASH(梯度回波快速小角度激发)

flash-filling(闪现充填)

fibrolamellar carcinoma, FLC(纤维板层肝细胞癌),纤维板层型肝细胞癌, fibrolamellar hepatocellular carcinoma,FL-HCC(肝纤维板层样肝癌)

fatty liver disease,FLD(脂肪性肝病)

focal liver lesion,FLL(肝脏局灶性病变)

fatty liver index,FLI(脂肪肝指数)

flip-flop(翻转征)

floating gallbladder(游离胆囊,漂浮胆囊)

flythrough(漫游,漫游技术)

fast multiplanar spoiled gradient-echo, FMPSPGR(快速多层面扰相梯度回波)

functional MR imaging,fMRI(功能 MR 成像)

fine needle aspiration, FNA(细针穿刺活检), FNAB(经皮穿刺细针抽吸活检)

false negative, FN(假阴性), false negative fraction, FNF(假阴性概率)

focal nodular hyperplasia, FNH(肝局灶性结节性增生)

fine needle percutaneous transhepatic cholangiography,FNPTC,FPTC(细针经皮肝穿胆系造影)

FOBT(大便潜血试验)

Focal fatty changes and focal sparing(局灶性脂肪变和局灶性肝岛)

focal nodular hyperplasia(局灶性结节状增生)

field of view,FOV(视野)

flat panel detector,FPD(平板探测器)

false positive, FP(假阳性), false positive fraction, FPF(假阳性概率)

fast recovery fast spin echo,FRFSE(快速恢复快速回波脉冲系列,快速恢复快速自旋回波,快速恢复自旋回波序列)

free receiver operating characteristic, FROC(无条件限制性 ROC)

framingham risk score, FRS(Framingham 危险积分)(有关冠心病)

fat saturation,FS(脂肪抑制)

fibroscan,FS(单维瞬变弹性图)

flow-sensitive dephasing, FSD(血流敏感散相,血流敏感梯度)

FSD-bSSFP(平衡稳态自由进动序列非增强 MRA), balance steady-state free precession, bSSFP(平衡稳态自由进动)

fast spin echo, FSE; fast turbo spin echo, FSE)(快速自旋回波,快速自旋回波序列,快速自旋回波系列)

FSIR(MR 脂肪抑制序列)

FSPGR(二维快速损毁梯度重聚序列),three dimension fast spoiled gradient recalled echo, 3D-FSPGR(三维快速扰相梯度回波)

fast spoiled gradient echo, FSPGR(快速干扰梯度回波,快速扰相稳态梯度回复采集)

fast spin echo, FSE（2D 快速自旋回波序列）

FT 图（扩散张量的示踪图），fiber tractography，FT（纤维束示踪技术图）

fecal tagging, FT（标记粪便法）

5-Fu（5- 氟尿嘧啶），5-FUDR（5- 氟尿嘧啶脱氧核苷）

full width at half maximum, FWHM（全宽半高值）

G

γ-GABA（γ- 氨基丁酸）

gallbladder adenomyomatosis, GAM（胆囊腺肌瘤病）

gap（缺损区）

glyceraldehyde-3-phosphate dehydrogenase，GAPDH（三磷酸甘油醛脱氢酶）

gastric antral vascular ectasia，GAVE（胃窦血管扩张症）

gastrinoma triangle（胃泌素瘤三角区）

gastric bare area, GBA（胃裸区）

adenomyomatosis of gallbladder，GBA（胆囊腺肌增生症，又称胆囊腺肌瘤病、腺体增生性胆囊炎，胆囊壁憩室症）

wall-thickening type gallbladder cancer, GBC（厚壁型胆囊癌）

gallbladder ejection fraction, GBEF（胆囊排胆分数）

giant cell interstitial pneumonia, GCIP（巨细胞间质性肺炎）

gastriccoronary vein, GCV（胃冠状静脉），left gastric vein, LGV（胃左静脉）

gadolinium, Gd（钆）

Gd-BOPTA，gadobcnatc（钆贝葡胺），gadobenate dimeglumine, Gd-BOPTA（钆贝葡胺，贝酸二甲葡胺钆），商品名 Multihance（莫迪斯，博莱科公司，意大利）

Gd-DOTA（钆特酸葡甲胺）

Gadolinium diethylenetriamine pentaacetic acid，Gd-DTPA（二乙三胺五醋酸钆），gadolinium diethylenetriamine pentaacetic acid，Gd-DTPA（钆二乙烯五胺乙酸，钆喷酸葡胺）

gadolinium ethoxybenzyl pentaacetic acid，Gd-EOB-DTPA，gadoxctic acid（钆塞酸二钠注射液），商品名普美显，gadolinium ethoxybenzyl diethylene-triamine pentaacetic acid，Gd-EOB-DTPA（钆塞酸二钠），商品名 Primovist（普美显，美国；拜耳先灵医药，德国）

gadolinium ethoxybenzyl diethylenetriamine pentaacetic acid，Gd-EOB-DTPA，gadoxetate disodium，Gd-EOB-DTPA（钆塞酸二钠），Gd^{+}-EOB-DTPA 是一种 gadolinium，Gd （钆）与 EOB-DTPA（ethoxybenzyl diethylenetriamine pentaacetic acid）螯合物的二钠盐，在 Gd^{+} -DTPA（钆 - 喷替酸葡甲胺）分子结构上添加了脂溶性的 ethoxybenzyl，EOB（乙氧基苯甲基）而形成，通用名为 gadoxetic acid（钆塞酸）二钠，商品名为普美显

Gd-PBCA-NP（Gd-DTPA 聚氰基丙烯酸正丁酯纳米微粒）

gradient echo, GE（梯度回波）

granulocytic epithelial lesions，GEL（上皮粒细胞病变），granulocytic epithelial lesion, GEL（粒细胞上皮损害）

general considerations（总体设计）

gastroenteropancreatic neuroendocrine tumors，GEP NET（胃肠胰神经内分泌肿瘤）

gastroenteropancreatic neuroendocrine neoplasm，GEP-NEN（胃肠胰神经内分泌肿瘤）

gastroesophageal varices，GEV（胃食管静脉曲张），esophageal varices，EV（食管静脉曲张），isolated gastricvarices, IGV（孤立的胃静脉曲张）

GFAP（血管周围瘤细胞胶质纤维酸性蛋白，胶质纤维酸性蛋白，免疫组织化学检查内容之一）

GFR（肾小球滤过率）

Gamna-Gandy bodies，GGB（铁质沉着结节，亦称 Gamna-Gandy 小体）

ground-glass opacity，GGO（磨玻璃密度影），simple GGO or pure GGO（单纯磨玻璃影）或者 nonsolid nodule（非实性结节）；pure GGO, pGGO（纯磨玻璃影）；complex GGO（混杂磨玻璃影）或 sub-solid nodule（亚实性结节）；mixed GGO（混合性磨玻璃影）

gamma glutamyl tranzpehtidaze，GGT（谷氨酰转酞酶，γ- 谷氨酰胺转肽酶，γ- 谷胺酰转移酶），gamma-glutamyl transferase, GGT（g- 谷氨酰转移酶）

GILT（胃肠道雪旺细胞肿瘤），GIGT（胃肠道神经节细胞肿瘤），GIFT（胃肠道纤维性肿瘤）

gastrointestinal mesenchymal tumor，GIMT（胃肠道间叶源性肿瘤）；extragastrointestinal stromal tumors，EGIST（胃肠道外间质瘤），消化道以外的

腹腔软组织,如网膜、肠系膜、腹膜后等处亦可发生与 GIST 形态、免疫表型及分子遗传特征类似的肿瘤,称为 EGIST; gastrointestinal stromal tumors, GIST(胃肠道间质瘤)

Glu/Gln(谷氨酸和谷氨酰胺,代表神经递质), glutamate, Gln(谷氨酸盐), Glutarate, Glu(谷氨酸), glutamic acid, Glu(谷氨酸), Glx(谷氨酸盐), Glx(谷氨酰胺和谷氨酸复合物)

glucagonoma(胰高血糖素瘤)

glutathione-S-transferase(谷胱甘肽 -S- 转移酶)

glycogen storage disease, glycogenosis(糖原贮积病,糖原沉积症); von Girke's disease(Ⅰ型糖原沉积症)

gastric mucosal blood flow, GMBF(胃黏膜血流)

ganglioneuroma, GN(节细胞神经瘤,又称神经节细胞瘤、节细胞神经纤维瘤)

ganglioneuroblastoma, GNB(节细胞神经母细胞瘤,节细胞成神经细胞瘤)

gastroesophageal varices, GOV(胃食管静脉曲张)

gangliocytic paraganglioma, GP(节细胞性副神经节瘤)

glypican-3, GPC-3(磷脂酰肌醇蛋白多糖 -3)

gradient-dual-echo MRI(梯度双回波磁共振成像),又称化学位移成像(同 / 反相位成像)

generalized autocalibrating partialy parallel acquisitions, GRAPPA(全面自动校准部分并行采集)

grading of recommendations assessment development and evaluation, GRADE(推荐分级的评估,制定与评价)

the Grading of Recommendations Assessment, Develonnent and Evaluation, GRADE(分级系统)

Granulomatous diseases of the liver(肝脏肉芽肿性疾病)

generalized autocalibrating partialy parallel acquisitions, GRAPPA(全面自动校准部分并行采集)

gradient-recalled acquisition spin-echo, GRASE(梯度恢复采集自旋回波)

GRASS(稳态梯度回波重聚)

gradient recalled echo, GRE, gradient echo, GRE, gradient echo, GE(梯度回波,梯度回波序列), 3D GRE(三维梯度回波序列采集)

gradient echo T_1-weighted, GRE T_1W(梯度回波 T_1WI)

gradient-recalled echo echoplanar imaging, GRE-EPI(单脉冲梯度回波 - 回波平面成像), gradient-echo plannar imaging, GRE-EPI(梯度回复回波 - 回波平面成像)

GRE(扰相梯度回波)T_1WI 序列,该序列在不同的产家采用不同的名称,如 fast low angle shot, FLASH,西门子公司(快速小角度激发)、spoiled gradient recalled acquisition in steady state, GE 公司(SPGR)、fast field echo, FFE,飞利浦公司(快速场回波)

gradient and spin echo, GRASE; gradient spin-echo, GSE(梯度自旋回波)

gradient inversal pulse(梯度翻转脉冲)

gradient magnetic field(梯度磁场)

gradient phase dispersion(梯度相位发散), gradient phase effect(梯度相位效应)

GRF(释放生长激素释放因子)

GRGCS(日本胃癌规约)

groove pancreatitis(沟部胰腺炎)

high-resolution peripheral quantitative computed tomography, HRpQCT(高分辨力周围骨定量 CT)

Grynfelt-Lesshaft 三角(上腰三角), Petit 三角(下腰三角)

Gs(明胶海绵)

granulocytic sarcoma, GS(粒细胞肉瘤)

gastric schwannoma, GS(胃神经鞘瘤)

glycogen storage disease, GSD(糖原贮积病)

Grayscale standard Display Function, GSDF(灰阶标准显示函数)

gemstone spectral imaging, GSI(宝石能谱成像,能谱成像,能谱扫描模式)

graft-versus-host disease, GVHD(移植物抗宿主病)

genome-wide association studies, GWAS(全基因组关联研究)

H

hepatic adenoma, HA(肝腺瘤), hepatocelluar adenoma, HA(肝细胞腺瘤), hepatocelluar adenoma, HCA(肝腺瘤)

hyaluronic acid, HA(透明质酸), serum hyaluronic acid, HA [血清透明质酸(肝纤维化的一种标志物)]

Hepatic Arterial Chemoembolization, HAE; Hepatic

Arterial Chemoinfusion，HAI（肝动脉内化疗栓塞术），Preventive HAI/HAE，P-HAI，P-HAE（预防性肝动脉内化疗栓塞）

hepatic alveolar echinococosis，HAE（肝泡状棘球蚴包虫病，肝泡状棘球蚴病，肝泡型包虫病，肝泡球蚴病，恶性包虫病）为泡状棘球绦虫的幼虫引起

hepatic arterial fraction，HAF（肝动脉分数），hepatic arterial fracture，HAF（肝动脉灌注分数）

hepatic artery index，HAI（肝动脉指数）

hepatic artery perfusion index，HAI；HAI=HAP/（HAP+PVP（肝动脉灌注指数）；hepatic arterial perfusion，HAP（肝动脉灌注量），portal venous perfusion，PVP（门静脉灌注量），total liver perfusion，TLP（全肝总灌注量），hepatic arterial perfusion index，HPI（肝动脉灌注指数），hepatic arterial perfusion index，HAPI（肝动脉灌注指数），portal venous perfusion index，PPI（门静脉灌注指数）

hepatic angiomyolipoma，HAML（肝血管平滑肌脂肪瘤）

half-Fourier FSE（半傅里叶快速自旋回波）

high-resolution magic angle spinning MRS，HR-MAS MRS（高分辨魔角自旋 MRS）

half scan（半扫描技术）

hepatic artery pseudoaneurysm，HAP（肝动脉假性动脉瘤）

hepatic arterial perfusion，HAP；HAP = BF × HAF（肝动脉灌注量）

hepatic artery stenosis，HAS（肝动脉狭窄）

hepatic angiosarcoma，HAS（肝脏血管肉瘤）

half-Fourier acquired single-shot turbo spin echo，HASTE（半傅里叶单次激发快速自旋回波），half fourier acquisition single shot turbo spin echo，HASTE（半傅里叶采集单次激发快速自旋回波），half-Fourier acquisition single-shot-turbo-spin-echo，HASTE（半傅里叶采集单次激发快速自旋回波序列）

hepatic artery thrombosis，HAT（肝动脉栓塞）

hepatitis A virus，HAV（甲型肝炎病毒）

hepatic arteriovenous shunting，HAVS（肝动静脉分流），hepatic arterio-hepatic venous shunting，HAH-VS（肝动脉 - 肝静脉分流），hepatic arterioportal-venous shunting，HAPVS（肝动脉 - 门静脉分流）

hepatic biliary cystadenoma，HBC；hypatobiliary cystadenoma，HBC（肝内胆管囊腺瘤），hepatobiliary cystadenocarcinoma，HBCC（肝内胆管囊腺癌）

hepatitis B core antigen，HbcAg（乙型肝炎核心抗原），hepatitis B e antigen，HBeAg（乙型肝炎 e 抗原），hepatitis B surface antigen，HbsAg（乙型肝炎表面抗原）

HBeAb（乙型肝炎 e 抗体），HbcAb（乙型肝炎核心抗体，核心抗体）

抗 -HBs（乙型肝炎表面抗体），抗 -HBc（乙型肝炎核心抗体），抗 -Hbe（乙型肝炎 e 抗体）

hepatic blood flow，HBF（肝血流量），global hepatic blood inflow，HBF（全肝血流量）

HBS（肝区闪烁扫描）

hepatitis B surface antigen，HBsAg（乙型肝炎表面抗原），HBeAg（乙型肝炎 e 抗原）

hepatitis B virus，HBV（乙型肝炎病毒），hepatitis C virus，HCV（丙型肝炎病毒），hepatitis D virus，HDV（丁型肝炎病毒），hepatitis E virus，HEV（戊型肝炎病毒），hepatitis G virus，HGV（庚型肝炎病毒）

hepatic blood volume，HBV（肝血容量）

hepatoblastoma（肝母细胞瘤或肝胚细胞瘤，肝胚胎瘤）

histoplasma capsularum，HC（荚膜组织胞浆菌）

hepatocellular adenoma，HCA（肝细胞腺瘤），hepatocellular adenomatosis，HCAs（肝腺瘤病）

HCV-associated dysmetabolic syndrome，HCADS（丙型肝炎病毒相关代谢异常综合征）

Hepatocellular Carcinoma，HCC（肝细胞性肝癌，肝细胞癌），Small Hepatocellular Carcinoma，SHCC（小肝细胞性肝癌，小肝细胞癌）

welldifferentiated HCC（高分化肝癌）、classical HCC（古典肝癌）[早期肝癌]，Early hepatocellular carcinoma，eHCC（早期肝癌，早期肝细胞癌）

hilar cholangiocarcinoma，HCC（肝门胆管癌），hilar cholangiocarcinoma，HC（肝门胆管癌），hilar cholangiocarcinoma，HCCA（肝门部胆管癌）

human chorionic gonadotropin，HCG（绒毛膜促性腺激素）

hepatic cavernous hemangioma，HCH（肝海绵状血管瘤）

hepatic computed tomographic perfusion，HCTP（肝脏

CT 灌注成像)
hepatitis C virus, HCV(丙型肝炎病毒), hepatitis D virus, HDV(丁型肝炎病毒), hepatitis E virus, HEV(戊型肝炎病毒), hepatitis G virus, HGV(庚型肝炎病毒)
hypotonic duodenography, HD(低张十二指肠造影)
Hirschsprung disease, HD(先天性巨结肠,先天性巨结肠病,又称肠管无神经节细胞症,或称 Hirschsprung 病), Hirschsprung alied disease, HAD(先天性巨结肠类缘病)
high-grade dysplastic nodule, HDN(高度不典型增生结节或发育不良结节)
HDL(高密度脂蛋白)
HDRBC(热变性红细胞)
hematoxylin eosin, HE 染色(苏木素 - 伊红染色)
hepatic epithelioid hemangioendothelioma, HEH, HEHE(肝脏上皮样血管内皮瘤)
hemolysis, elevated serum level of liver enzymes, and low platelets syndrome, HELLP(溶血、肝酶升高和低血小板综合征, HELLP 综合征)是以溶血、肝酶升高、血小板减少为主要临床表现的综合征
hemangiomas(血管瘤), hemangiomatosis(血管瘤病), Large, heterogeneous hemangioma(大的不均质的血管瘤), rapidly filling hemangioma(对比剂快速填充的血管瘤), hyalinized hemangioma(玻璃样变的血管瘤), pedunculated hemangioma(外生性的血管瘤), hemangioma with capsular retraction(伴有包膜皱缩的血管瘤), hemangioma enlarging over time(血管瘤的进行性增大)
hemangioendothelioma(血管内皮细胞瘤), hemangioendothelioma [(上皮样)血管内皮细胞瘤]
hemochromatosis(血色素沉着病,血色素沉着症)
hemosiderosis(含铁血黄素沉着症)
hepatic adenoma(肝腺瘤)
hepatic artery aneurvsm(肝动脉动脉瘤:创伤性或炎症性)
Hepatic Arterial Lipiodol Angiography(肝动脉乙碘油造影)
hepaticangiosarcoma(肝血管肉瘤)
hepatic congestion(肝充血)
hepatic hydatid disease(肝包虫病), hydatid cysts(包虫囊肿), ectocyst(外囊), endocyst(内囊,亦称内生发层), daughter cyst(子囊)
hepatic peliosis(肝紫斑病,肝紫癜症), peliosis hepatis(肝紫癜症)
hepatic peribiliary systs(肝内胆管周围囊肿)
hepatofugal(离肝性), hepatofugal flow(离肝血流)
hepatolenticular degeneration(肝豆状核变性)
Hep Par1(肝细胞抗原)
heterotopic liver(异位肝),又可称 mobile liver(迷走肝)
heterotopic pancreas(异位胰腺),又称为 aberrant pancreas(迷走胰腺)
hepatic fat fraction, HFF(肝脏脂肪含量)
high grade dysplasitic nodule, HGDN(高级别异形增生结节)
hepatocyte growth factor, HGF(肝细胞生长因子)
hereditary hemorrhagic telangiectasia, HHT(遗传性出血性毛细血管扩张症),也称 Rendu-
Osler-Weber 病。hepatic hereditary hemorrhagic telangiectasia, HHHT(肝脏 HHT)
hypoxic-ischemic encephalopathy, HIE(新生儿缺氧缺血性脑病)
high intensity focused ultrasound, HIFU(高强度聚焦超声)
hypoxia inducible factor1, HIF-1a(乏氧诱导因子)
hypoxic-ischemic injury, HII(缺氧缺血损伤)
high-resolution three dimensional constructive inference in steady state, high-resolution 3D-CISS MRI(高分辨三维稳态重建 MR 成像)
Hill-sachs 病变(肱骨后外侧骨质病变),反 Hill-sachs 病变(肱骨头前内侧骨质病变)
hospital information system, HIS(医院信息系统)
HISORt 诊断标准,分别取 histology(组织学)、imaging(影像)、serology(血清学)、other organ involvement(其他器官累及)和 response to immunosuppressive therapy(免疫抑制剂治疗应答)的首字母,至少两项以上符合可诊断 IgG4-SC
Histoplasmosis(组织胞浆菌病)
human immunodeficiecy virus, HIV(人类免疫缺陷病毒,人类免疫缺损病毒)
hodgkin lymphoma, HL(何杰金淋巴瘤)
human leucocyte antigen, HLA(人类白细胞抗原)
hepatolenticular degeneration, HLD(肝豆状核变性)
hemophagocytic lymphohistiocytosis, HLH(嗜血细胞综合征)

HMB-45（蛋氨酸羟基类似物）

hyaline membrane disease，HMD（肺透明膜病），又称 neonatal respiratory distress syndrome，NRDS（新生儿特发性呼吸窘迫综合征）

hepatic multifocal nodular fatty infiltration，HMNFI（肝脏多灶性结节状脂肪浸润）

proton magnetic resonance spectroscopy，^{1}H-MRS（氢质子磁共振波谱，质子磁共振波谱）

HMT（肝转移癌）

hepatocyte nuclear factor 1a，HNF1a（肝细胞核因子1a）

HNF-1a-inactivated hepatocellular adenoma，HNF-1a-inactivated HCA（肝细胞核因子 1a 突变型肝细胞腺瘤）

hepatic osteodystrophy，HOD，HO（肝性骨营养不良），也称 hepatic bone disease，HBD（肝性骨病）

homoeostasis model assessment insulin resistance，HOMA-IR（胰岛素稳态评估模型胰岛素抵抗指数）

holo sign（晕征）

Homer-Wringt（H-W）菊形团

Helicobacter pylori，HP（幽门螺旋杆菌，幽门螺杆菌）

histoplasmosis，HP（组织胞浆菌病）

peliosis hepatis，HP（肝紫癜症）

HPC（血管外皮瘤）

hepatic perfusion disorders，HPD（肝脏灌注异常，肝的异常灌注）

HPF（高倍镜视野）

hepatic perfusion index，HPI（肝实质肝灌注系数，肝脏灌注指数）；hepatic arterial perfusion index，HPI（肝动脉灌注指数）

hepatic portal perfusion，HPP（门静脉灌注量，门静脉肝灌注值，肝的门静脉灌注量）

hepatopulmonary syndrome，HPS（肝肺综合征）

hyperparathyroidism，HPT（甲状旁腺功能亢进）

human papilloma virus，HPV（人乳头瘤病毒）

high resolution CT，HRCT（高分辨率 CT）

hemodynamic response function，HRF（血流动力反应功能）

high-resolution magic angle spinning MR spectroscopy，HRMAS MRS（高分辨魔角旋转磁共振波谱）

horse-radish peroxidase，HRP（辣根过氧化物酶）

hepatorenal syndrome，HRS（肝肾综合征）

hepatic stellate cell，HSC（肝星形细胞），hepatic stellate cells，HSCs（肝星状细胞）

HSC（造血干细胞），hematopoietic stem cell transplantation，HSCT（造血干细胞移植）

hysterosalpingography，HSG（X 线子宫输卵管造影）

hepatic sclerosing haemangioma，HSH（硬化性血管瘤）

hepatic sinusoidal obstructive syndrome，HSOS（肝窦阻塞综合征），又称为 hepatic veno-occlusive disease，HVOD；veno-occlusive disease of the liver，VOD（肝小静脉闭塞症）

heat shock protein，HSP72（72 ku 热休克蛋白）

human herpes simplex virus，HSV（单纯疱疹病毒）

HT_2 FSE（二维重 T_2 快速自旋回波序列）

5-hydroxytryptamine，5-HT（5- 羟色胺），5-hydroxytryptophan，5-HTP（5- 羟色胺酸）

5-hydroxyindoleacetic acid，5-HIAA（5- 羟吲哚乙酸）

hounsfield unit，HU（X 线衰减系数，CT 值单位）

human adapted（人工调节）

HVJ-Es（hemagglutinating virus of Japan envelopes）

half value layer，HVL（半价层）

hepatic venous pressure gradient，HVPG（肝静脉压力梯度）

hyperintense vessel sign，HVS（高信号血管征）

hydatid disease（echinococcus granulosus）[包虫病（细粒棘球蚴）]

hydrops of gallbladder（胆囊积水，又称为胆囊积液，阻塞性胆囊炎）

hypervascular metastases（富血管性肝转移）

hypoplastic（发育不全的），rudimentary（发展不健全的）

I

inflammatory abdominal aortic aneurysms，IAAAs（炎性腹主动脉瘤）

immunoglobulin G4-associated cholangitis，IAC（IgG4 相关胆管炎）

The International Association for the Study of Lung Cancer，IASLC（国际肺癌研究会，国际肺癌研究协会，国际肺癌研究联合会）

inflammatory bowel disease，IBD（炎症性肠病，结肠炎性病变，炎性肠病）

indeterminate colitis, IC(不确定性大肠炎或不确定性结肠炎)

International-Club of Asates,ICA(国际腹水俱乐部)

iodine concentration in portal venous phase, Ica/Icp(肝动脉/门静脉期碘含量比值)

intrahepatic cholangiocarcinoma, ICAC(肝内胆管(腺)癌,肝内胆管细胞癌)

intercellular adhesion molecule, ICAM(细胞间黏附分子)

ICC(间质细胞)

intrahepatic cholangiocellular carcinoma, ICC(肝内胆管细胞癌)

intrahepatic cholangiocarcinoma, ICC(肝内胆管癌,又称胆管细胞癌或周围型肝内胆管癌)

intestinal bypass for obesity(因为肥胖而作肠道旁路)

interstitial cell of Cajal,ICC(胃肠道 Cajal 细胞)

intraclass correlation coefficient, ICC(组内相关系数,组间相关系数)

iodine concentration difference, ICD(碘浓度的差异)

indocyanine green,ICG(吲哚氰绿,靛氰绿)

IDA(亚氨基二乙酸,乙酰苯胺亚氨二醋酸), ^{99m}Tc-HIDA(^{99m}锝-二甲基乙酰苯胺亚氨二醋酸), ^{99m}Tc-EHIDA(^{99m}锝-二乙基乙酰苯胺亚氨二醋酸), ^{99m}Tc-p-BIDA(^{99m}锝-对丁基乙酰苯胺亚氨二醋酸)

icteric type hepatoma(黄疸型肝细胞性肝癌), cholestatic type of HCC(淤胆型肝细胞性肝癌)

idiopathicduct centric pancreatitis, IDCP(特发性导管中心性胰腺炎), idiopathic duct-centric chronic pancreatitis, IDCP(特发性导管中心性慢性胰腺炎)

IDCS(指突状树突细胞肉瘤)起源于淋巴组织中的IDC(指突状树突细胞),又称为 IRCS(指突状网状细胞肉瘤)、ICS(指突状细胞肉瘤)

IDF(国际糖尿病联盟)

idiopathic demyrlinating optic neuritis, IDON(特发性脱髓鞘性视神经炎)

intradiverticular papicla, IDP(憩室内乳头)

intraductal secretin test, IDST(导管内的胰泌素实验)

intraductal ultrasonography, IDUS(导管内超声), intraluminal ultrasonography(腔内超声)

interictal epileptiform discharges, IEDs(发作间期痫样放电)

intraepithelial neoplasia, IEN(上皮内瘤样病变)

IEPI(隔行扫描 EPI)

interferon, IFN(干扰素)

immunoglobulin, Ig(免疫球蛋白)

IG(导管内生长型)

IGF(胰岛素样生长因子)

IgG4-related disease, IgG4-RD(IgG4 相关疾病), immunoglobulin G4-related disease, IgG4-RD(IgG4 相关性疾病)

immunoglobulin G4-associated autoimmune hepatitis, IgG4-AIH(IgG4 相关自身免疫性肝炎)

immunoglobulin G4-related sclerosing cholangitis, IgG4-SC(IgG4 相关硬化性胆管炎)

^{123}I-GLP-1(胰高糖素样肽)

isolated gastric varices, IGV(孤立性胃静脉曲张)

infusion hepatic angiography, IHA(灌注性肝动脉造影)

intrahepatic cholangiocarcinoma, IHCC(肝内胆管细胞癌)

intrahepatic peripheral cholangiocarcinoma, IHPCC(周围型肝内胆管细胞癌)

intrahepatic content of lipid, IHCL(肝内脂肪含量,肝内脂质相对含量,肝脏脂质相对含量)

infantile hemangioendothelioma(婴儿血管内皮瘤)

Infantile hepatic hemangioendothelioma, IHH(婴儿型肝血管内皮瘤)

infantile hepatic hemangio-endothelioma, IHHE(婴儿型肝脏血管内皮细胞瘤)

infantile hepatitis syndrome, IHS(婴儿肝炎综合征)

idiopathic interstitial pneumonia, IIP(特发性间质性肺炎)

intestinal lymphangiectasia, IL(小肠淋巴管扩张症), primary intestinal lymphangiectasia, PIL(原发性小肠淋巴管扩张症), secondary intestinal lymphangiectasia, SIL(继发性小肠淋巴管扩张症), finite lymphangiectasia, FL(局限性淋巴管扩张症)

interleukin, IL(白细胞介素), interleukin 6, IL-6(白细胞介素 6)

interleukin 6 signal transducer, IL6ST(白细胞介素信号传导因子)

intestinal malrotation, IM(肠旋转不良)
intrahepatic mass-forming cholangiocarcinoma, IMCC(肝内肿块型胆管细胞癌)
intramural hematoma, IMH(主动脉壁内血肿)
inflammatory myofibroblastic tumor, IMT(炎性肌纤维母细胞瘤),曾称为炎性假瘤、肌纤维母细胞瘤、肺外炎性假瘤、浆细胞假瘤、组织细胞瘤、假性淋巴瘤、纤维黄色瘤、炎性纤维肉瘤、浆细胞肉芽肿、炎症性肌纤维母细胞瘤、炎性成肌纤维细胞瘤和黄瘤性炎性假瘤
intestine inflamematory myofibroblastic tumor, IMT(小肠炎性肌纤维母细胞瘤)
IMT [(颈动脉内)中膜厚度]
inducible nitric oxide synthase, iNOS(诱导型一氧化氮合酶)
in-phase(同相位)
INR(国际标准化比值)
insufficiency fracture(微细骨折或应力性骨折)
interhepatic duct(肝间管)
intraductal papillary mucinous tumor(导管内乳头状黏液瘤),又称 ductectatic cystadenoma(导管扩张囊腺瘤)、cystadenocarcinoma(囊腺癌)、ductectatic mucinous tumor(导管扩张黏液瘤)
International Working Party on Hepatology(国际肝病工作组)
intrahepatic arterioportal shunts(肝内动脉-门静脉分流)
index of NASH, ION(脂肪性肝炎指数)
Iotroxate(碘曲克)
iopanoic acid(碘番酸)
intraoperative ultrasonic, IOUS(术中超声)
inflammatory pseudotumor, IP(炎性假瘤)
in-phase, IP(同相位), in-phase, IP(同相), in-phase/opposed-phase, IP/OP(梯度回波同/反相位)
invasive pulmonary aspergillosis, IPA(侵袭性肺曲霉菌病)
inferior phrenic arteries, IPA(膈下动脉,下膈动脉)
ileal pouch-anal anastomosis, IPAA(回肠储袋肛管吻合术)
intrapancreatic accessor spleen, IPAS(胰腺内副脾,胰腺内异位副脾)
intrahepatic peripheral cholangiocelluar carcinoma, IPCC(肝内周围型胆管细胞癌)
idiopathic pulmonary fibrosis, IPF(特发性肺纤维化),亦即 UIP(usual interstitial Pneumonia, UIP)
inflammatory pseudotumor of the liver, IPL(肝脏炎性假瘤,肝脏的炎性假瘤)
IPM(炎性胰腺肿块,炎症性的胰腺肿块,又称假肿瘤性胰腺炎、炎症性的假性胰腺肿瘤)
intraductal papillary mucinous adenoma, IPMA(导管内乳头状黏液性腺瘤), intraductal papillary mucinous borderline tumor, IPMBT(导管内乳头状黏液性交界性肿瘤), intraductal papillary mucinous carcinoma, IPMC(胰腺导管内乳头状黏液性腺癌)
intraductal papillary mucinous tumor, IPMT, IPMTs[(胰腺内)导管内乳头状黏液性肿瘤,胰管内乳头状黏液瘤]
intraductal papillary mucinous neoplasm, IPMN(导管内乳头状黏液性肿瘤), intraductal papillary mucinous neoplasm of the bile duct, IPMN-B(胆管导管内乳头状黏液性肿瘤,胆管内黏液性乳头状肿瘤), intraductal papillary mucinous neoplasm of the pancreas, IPMN-P(胰腺导管内乳头状黏液性肿瘤)
intraductal papillary neoplasm of the bile duct, IPNB(肝内胆管乳头状肿瘤,胆管导管内乳头状肿瘤), intraductal papillary neoplasm of the bile duct, IPN-B(胆管的导管内乳头状肿瘤,胆管内乳头状肿瘤)
idiopathic pneumonia syndrome, IPS(特发性肺炎综合征)
intrahepatic portosystemic venous shunt, IPSVS(肝内门体静脉分流)
inflammatory pseudotumor, IPT(炎性假瘤)
indirect portal-venography, IPVG(间接门静脉造影)
insulin resistance, IR(胰岛素抵抗)
IR-β(β胰岛素受体)
inversion recover, IR(反转恢复,反转恢复序列)
impulse redsidue function, IRF(推动剩余函数)
idiopathic retroperitoneal fibrosis, IRF(特发性腹膜后纤维化)
time of arrival, IRF To(对比剂到达时间,到达时间)
iron overload(肝脏铁过载):如多次输血
internal rectal prolapse, IRP(直肠内脱垂), rectal mucosal prolapsed, RMP(直肠黏膜脱垂),

internal rectal intussusceptions,IRI(直肠内套叠)
isotropic MR imaging(各相同性图像)
ischemic-type biliary lesions,ITBL(缺血胆系损害)
intrahepatic biloma(肝脏胆汁瘤)
intravenous cholangiography,IVC(静脉法胆系造影)
iliac vein compression syndrome, IVCS(髂静脉受压综合征),也称 Cockett 综合征或 May-
Thurner 综合征
intravoxel incoherent motion, IVIM(体素内不均一运动)
intravenous leiomyomatosis, IVL(静脉内平滑肌瘤病)
intravenous pyelography, IVP(静脉肾盂造影), intravenous urography, IVU(静脉尿路造影)
ivy sign(常春藤征)
International Working Party,IWP(国际肝病工作组)

J

JAMA(美国医学会杂志)
juxtapapillary diverticulum of duodenum, JDD(十二指肠乳头旁憩室)
JGCA(日本胃癌学会)
judgment of line orientation test, JLOT(直线方向判断测试)
JSH(日本肝病学会)
jigsaw pattern(拼图样)
junctional zone,JZ [联合带,结合带(子宫)]

K

Kaposi(卡波西肉瘤)
Katayama' s syndrome(急性血吸虫病)
kilobase,kb(千碱基对)
Kawasaki disease, KD(川崎病,又称皮肤黏膜淋巴结综合征)
rate constant of backflux,K_{ep}(血液回流常数)
Keratin(角蛋白,免疫组织化学检查内容之一)
kilo electron voltage,keV(千电子伏)
Ki-67(细胞增殖标记), Kiel 67 antigen, Ki-67(Ki-67 抗原), Ki-67 labeling index, Ki-67LI(Ki-67 抗原标记指数)
kidney injury molecule,KIM(肾损伤因子)
Kimura 病(嗜酸性淋巴肉芽肿,又称木村病)
KIT(CD117 干细胞因子受体)
Klatskin 瘤(肝门部胆管细胞癌)
Klippel-Trenaunay-Weber syndrome(克 - 特 - 韦综合征,是系统性血管瘤的一部分)
kPa(千帕)
KPS(通透性参数图)
klebsiella rhinoscleromatis,KR(克雷伯鼻硬结杆菌)
transfer constant,K^{trans}(血管通透性常数)
Kulchitsky 细胞(肝内毛细胆管的神经内分泌细胞)
Kulchisky 细胞(消化道和支气管黏膜腺体的嗜银细胞)

L

liver adenomatosis,LA(肝腺瘤病)
lactate,Lac(乳酸),Lacticacid,Lac(乳酸)
left anterior descending, LAD(左前降支), left circumflex, LCX(左回旋支), left main artery, LMA(左主干)
Laennec type(雷奈克肝硬化,微结节型肝硬化)
liver attenuation index, LAI(肝密度指数,肝衰减指数,为平均肝密度减去平均脾密度,即肝、脾的 CT 值之差)
lymphangioleiomyomatosis,LAM(淋巴管肌瘤病)
liver acquisition with volume acceleration, LAVA(肝脏容积加速采集,肝脏加速容积采集,肝脏快速容积扫描,肝容积采集加速序列,肝脏快速容积成像序列,肝脏三维容积超快速多期动态增强成像技术,肝脏三维容积超快速采集成像)
Liver acquisition with volume acceleration, LAVA CE-MRA(肝脏三维容积超快速多期动态增强成像技术)
linear blending, LB(线性融合), nonlinear blending, NLB(非线性融合)
large bowel obstruction, LBO(大肠梗阻), SBO(小肠梗阻)
liver cirrhosis, LC(肝硬化)
laparoscopic cholecystectomy, LC(腹腔镜胆囊切除术)
LC-1(抗 1 型肝细胞溶质抗原抗体)
littoral cell angioma,LCA(脾窦岸细胞血管瘤)
Liquid Crystal Display, LCD(平面显示器)
Langerhans cell histiocytosis, LCH(朗格汉斯细胞组织细胞增生症),即 Langerhans 细胞组织细胞病,以前曾称为 HX(组织细胞增多症 X)。可分为

Letterer-Siwe disease, LSD,即勒-雪综合征(勒-雪病)、Hand-Schuller-Christian disease,韩-薛-柯病, HSCD,即韩-薛-柯综合征(黄脂瘤病)和eosinophilic granuloma, EG,即嗜伊红细胞肉芽肿(嗜酸细胞性肉芽肿)3 型

laser capture microdissection, LCM(激光捕获显微切割技术)

large cell neuroendocrine carcinoma, LCNEC(大细胞神经内分泌癌)

low-dose CT, LDCT(低剂量 CT), low dose computed tomography, LDCT(低剂量 CT)

lumbar disc herniation, LDH(腰椎间盘突出)

laetate dehydrogenase, LDH, lactic dehydrogenase, LDH(乳酸脱氢酶)

low density lipoprotein, LDL(低密度脂蛋白)

living donor liver transplantation, LDLT(活体肝移植)

low-grade dysplastic nodule, L-DN(低级别异型增生结节), high-grade dysplastic, H-DN(高级别异型增生结节)

low-dose digital radiogrophic device, LDRD(低剂量数字 X 线机)

lea body mass(去脂肪体质量)

leakage current(漏电流)

Lemmel's syndrome(乳头旁憩室综合征)

leptin(瘦素)

Leptospirosis(钩端螺旋体病)

lesion detection(早期检测), lesion characterization(定性诊断)

lesion loads(病灶负荷)

liver fatty acid binding protein, LFABP(肝脏脂肪酸结合蛋白)

left gastric artery, LGA(胃左动脉)

low-grade endometrial stromal sarcoma, LGESS(低级别的子宫内膜间质肉瘤)

low-grade myofibroblastic sarcoma, LGMS(低度恶性肌纤维母细胞肉瘤)

liver hemochromatosis, LHC(肝血色素沉着症)

lumbar intervertebral foramen, LIF(腰椎间孔)

laser imaging fluorescence endoscopemeter, LIFE(荧光支气管镜)

light emission life(光发射寿命)

lymphocytic interstitial pneumonia, LIP(淋巴细胞型间质性肺炎)

Lipid peak, 1.3ppm; 1ppm=10^{-6}(脂峰)

lipid(类脂质), microscopic fat, intracellular lipid(镜下脂质), intracellular microscopic lipid(肝细胞内含镜下脂质)

lipiodol-CT, Lip-CT(碘油 CT 扫描)

lipoatrophic diabetes(脂肪萎缩性糖尿病)

lipomatous pseudohypertrophy(脂肪瘤样假性肥大)

lipomatous tumor(脂肪瘤性肿瘤), lipomatous nodules(脂瘤性结节), lipopeliosis(脂肪性肝紫癜症)

liver imaging reporting and data system, LI-RADS(肝脏影像报告和数据管理系统)

Liver Cancer Study Group of Japan(日本肝癌研究会)

liver steatosis and fatty liver(脂肪肝), fatty liver disease(脂肪性肝病)

LKM-1(抗 1 型肝肾微粒体抗体)

lupus mesenteric vasculitis, LMV(狼疮性肠系膜血管炎)

laminin, LN(层粘连蛋白,层黏蛋白)

lymph node micrometastase, LNMM(淋巴结微转移)

lymphotropic nanoparticle enhanced MR imaging, LN-MRI(磁共振纳米颗粒淋巴结增强成像)

lesion-to-normal hepatic tissue ratio, LNR(病灶与周围正常肝组织碘浓度比值)

Lp(碘化油), Lp-TACE(含药碘油栓塞)

levator plate angle, LPA(提肌板角)

labile plasma iron, LPI(不稳定的血浆铁)

lipopolysaccharide, LPS(脂多糖)

lymphoplasmacytic sclerosing pancreatitis, LPSP(淋巴浆细胞硬化性胰腺炎)

liver stiffness measurement, LSM(肝脏硬度,肝脏硬度值)

liver spleen ratio, LSR(肝/脾 CT 比值)

LT(肝移植)

long time low rate angiography, LTLRA(长时间低流率造影)

lipiodal ultra fluid, LUF(碘油超悬液)

LUS(腹腔镜超声)

large vestibular aqueduct syndrome, LVAS(大前庭水管综合征)

lymphatic vessel density, LVD(淋巴管密度)

left ventricular end diastolic volume, LVEDV(左室舒张末期容积), left ventricular end systolic volume, LVESV(左室收缩末期容积), left ventricular ejection fraction, LVEF(左室射血分数), left ventricular myocardial mass, LVMM(左室心肌质量), left ventricular single-shot volume, LVSV(左室每搏输出量)

lipid water ratio, LWR(脂水比)

lymphoid hyperplasia(淋巴样增生)

lymphatic vessel endothelial hyaluronan receptor 1, LYVE-1(淋巴管内皮透明质酸受体1)

lympho-myeloproliferative disorders(淋巴-骨髓增生性疾病)

M

mycobacterium avium intracellulare, MAC(分枝杆菌复合体,鸟型胞内分支杆菌复合体)

macroregenerative nodules(肝硬化的巨再生结节)

macroscopic fat(肉眼可见脂肪)

mean apparent diffusion coefficient, mADC(平均表观扩散系数值)

magnetic dipole moment(磁偶极距)

magnetic susceptometry(磁化率测量法)

malignant fibrous xanrhoma(恶性纤维组织细胞瘤,又称为恶性纤维黄色瘤)、fibrous xanrhosarcoma(纤维黄色肉瘤)

mucosa-associated lymphoid tissue, MALT(黏膜相关性淋巴样组织或淋巴样增生)

mucosa associated lymphoid tissue, MALT(黏膜相关淋巴组织淋巴瘤), mucosa-associated lymphoidtissue lymphoma, MALT, MALToma(黏膜相关结外边缘带B细胞淋巴瘤), mucosa associated lymphoid tissue lymphoma, MALT-ML(黏膜相关淋巴组织型淋巴瘤)

mixed adenoneuroendocrine carcmoma, MANEC(混合腺神经内分泌癌)

mangafadipir(锰福地吡), Mangafodipir trisodium(锰福地吡三钠),为胰腺特异性对比剂

mean arterial pressure, MAP(平均动脉压)

mild acute pancreatitis, MAP(轻症急性胰腺炎), severe acute pancreatitis, SAP(重症急性胰腺炎)

major aortopulmonary collateral arteries, MAPCAs(主肺动脉侧枝动脉)

macrovesicular steatosis, MaS(大泡性脂肪变性)

myocardial bridging, MB(心肌桥), myocardial bridge, MB(心肌桥)

mural coronary artery, MCA(壁冠状动脉)

MCAO(阻塞一侧大脑中动脉), tMCAO(短暂性大脑中动脉阻塞); pMCAO(永久性大脑中动脉阻塞)

mild cognitive impairment, MCI(轻度认知损害,轻度认知功能障碍)

mucinous cystic neoplasms, MCN(黏液性囊性肿瘤), pancreatic mucinous cystic neoplasm, MCN(胰黏液性囊腺肿瘤,胰黏液性囊腺性肿瘤)为黏液性囊腺瘤或癌的统称, pancreatic mucinous cystic cystadenoma, MCA(胰黏液性囊腺瘤), pancreatic mucinous cystic cystadenocacinoma, MCC(胰黏液性囊腺癌)

pancreatic mucinous cystic neoplasm, MCN(胰腺黏液性囊腺肿瘤),包括 pancreatic mucinous cystic cystadenoma, MCA(黏液性囊腺瘤)、pancreatic mucinous cystic cystadenocacinoma,

MCC(黏液性囊腺癌)和介于二者间的 pancreatic mucinous cystic borderline cystadenoma,

MCB(交界性黏液性囊腺瘤)

mucinous cystic tumour, MCT(黏液性囊性肿瘤,囊性黏液肿瘤)

microcomputed tomography, μCT(显微CT)

mean diffusivity, MD(平均扩散系数,平均扩散度,平均扩散率)值

multi-slice helical CT(多层螺旋CT), multirow detector CT, MDCT(多列探测器CT), multidetector CT, MDCT(多探测器螺旋CT), multidetector-row spiral CT, MDCT(多层螺旋CT), multidetector row computed tomography, MDCT(单源多层CT)

maximum depth of the intraluminal appendiceal fluid, MDIAF(阑尾腔内液体最大直径)

multi-drug resistance, MDR(多重耐药)

myelodysplastic syndrome, MDS(骨髓异常增生综合征,骨髓增生异常综合征)

maximum enhancement percentage, ME%(最大强化百分比)

Medusa's head(海蛇头征)

melanotic melanoma(黑色素性黑色素瘤)

mesenchymal hamartoma（间充质（间叶）错构瘤——以囊性为主）

model of end stage liver disease，MELD（终末期肝病模型）

Multiple endocrine neoplasia，MEN（多发性内分泌肿瘤），multiple endocrine neoplasm syndrome，MENS（多发性内分泌肿瘤综合征），multiple endocrine neoplasia type 1，MEN1（多发内分泌肿瘤 1 型，又称 Wermer 综合征）；multiple endocrine neoplasia type 2，MEN2（多发内分泌肿瘤 2 型）

Menetrier 病（肥厚性胃炎）

Mercedes-Benz（麦尔舍德什 - 本茨征）

Mesenchymal hamartoma（间叶性错构瘤），hepatic mesenchymal hamartoma，HMH（肝脏间叶性错构瘤），mesenchymal hamartoma of the liver，MHL（肝脏间叶错构瘤，肝脏间叶性错构瘤）

mixed epithelial and stromal tumor of the kidney，MEST（肾混合性上皮间质瘤）

methionine，MET（甲基蛋氨酸）

Metoclopromide（胃复安，甲氧氯普胺，灭吐灵）

metabolic syndrome，MetS（代谢综合征）

metaphseal fibrous defect，MFD（干骺端纤维缺损）

malignant fibrous histiocytoma，MFH（恶性纤维组织细胞瘤）

mixed function oxidase system，MFOS（微粒体功能氧化酶系统，功能氧化酶系统）

mass-forming type，MF type（肿块型），periductal-infiltrating type，PI type（胆管周围浸润型），intraductal growth type，IG type（管内生长型）

major histocompatibility complex，MHC（主要组织复合体，主要组织相容性复合物）

micro-HCC，MHCC（微小肝癌）

minimal hepatic encephalopathy，MHE（轻微肝性脑病）

myo-inositol，MI（肌醇）

Michaelis-Gutman 小体（软化斑小体）

microcystic adenoma（微囊腺瘤），又称 cystadenoma（囊腺瘤）、serous adenoma（浆液腺瘤）、glycogen-rich adenoma（富糖原腺瘤）

microscopic fat，intracellular lipid（镜下脂质）

minimum intensity projection，MinIP（最小强度投影）

maximum intensity projection，MIP[最大密度投影，最大密度投影法，最大（信号）强度投影]

MION（单晶氧化铁）

the maximal long-axis diameter，MLAD（长轴最大径，最大长轴直径），the maximal shortaxis diameter，MSAD（最大短轴直径），MSAD/MLAD=（淋巴结直径比 = 淋巴结最大短轴直径 / 淋巴结最大长轴直径）

mycobacterium kansasii，MK（堪萨斯分支杆菌）

metastatic liver carcinoma，MLC（转移性肝癌）

metastatic liver leimyosarcoma，MLL（肝脏转移性平滑肌肉瘤）

medio-lateral oblique，MLO（内外侧斜位）

multiple myeloma，MM（多发性骨髓瘤）

MM（心肌质量 = 心肌的体积 × 心肌的密度）

methylmalonic acidemia，MMA（甲基丙二酸血症），即 methylmalonic aciduria（甲基丙二酸尿症）

MMc（丝裂霉素）

macromolecular contrast media，MMCM（大分子对比剂）

malignant myoepithelioma，MME（恶性肌上皮瘤）也称 myoepithelial carcinoma，MC（肌上皮癌）

modern medical imaging，MMI（现代医学影像学）

multifocal micronodular pneumocyte hyperplasia，MMPH（多灶性微结节性肺细胞增生）

matrix metallopotienases，MMP，MMPs（基质金属蛋白酶，金属蛋白酶）

monomicrobial nonneutrocytic bacterascites ，MNB（中性粒细胞不增高单株细菌性腹水）

mangafodipir trisodium，MnDPDP（锰福地吡三钠，锰 -DPDP，Mn-DPDP）

molecular imaging（分子成像）

mosaic pattern（镶嵌征，镶嵌征象，马赛克征）

membranous obstruction of the inferior vena cava，MOVC（下腔静脉膜性阻塞）

autoimmune pancreatitis，MP（自身免疫性胰腺炎）

meconium peritonitis，MP（胎粪性腹膜炎）

main pancreatic duct，MPD（主胰管）

myocardial performance index，MPI（心肌运动指数）

malignant peripheral nerve sheath tumor，MPNST（恶性周围神经鞘瘤，恶性外周神经鞘瘤）

multiplanar reformat，MPR（多平面重建），multiplanar reformation，MPR（多平面重组），multi-plane reconstruction，MPR（多平面重建），multiplanar reconstruction，MPR（多层面重建）

main portal vein, MPV(门静脉主干), left portal vein, LPV(门脉左支), right anterior portal vein, RAPV(右前支), right posterior portal vein, RPPV(右后支)
multiplanar volume reconstruction, MPVR(多平面容积重建,多平面容积再现), multiple position volume reconstruction, MPVR(多方位容积重建)
magnetic resonance angiopraphy, MRA(磁共振血管成像)
MR cholangiography, MRC(磁共振胆系成像, MR胆系成像), CE-MRC(钆贝葡胺增强胆管成像)
MR colonography, MRC(结肠 MRI), magnetic resonance colonography, MRC(磁共振结肠成像)
MR CISS(constructive interference in the steady state 序列)
magnetic resonance cholangiopancreatography, MRCP [磁共振胆胰管成像(造影)]
MR dacryocystography, MRD(MR 泪道成像)
magnetic resonance defecography, MRD(磁共振排粪造影)
magnetic resonance elastography, MRE(磁共振弹性成像, MR 弹性成像)
MR enterography, MRE, MR enteroclysis, MRE(MR 小肠成像)
mesorectal fascia, MRF(直肠系膜筋膜)
MR gastro-intestinal hydrography, MRGIH(MR 胃肠水成像)
magnetic resonance hydrometry, MRH(磁共振液体比重测定法)
MRI enteroclysis images(MRI 灌肠影像学)
MRI oximetry(MRI 血氧定量)
MR myocardial perfusion imaging, MRMPI(MR 心肌灌注成像)
macroregenerative nodules, MRN(大再生结节)
MR pancreatography, MRP(MR 胰管成像)
magnetic resonance portography, MRP(磁共振门静脉成像)
multi-drug resistance protein, MRP(多药耐药相关蛋白,多耐药蛋白载体), multidrug resistance protein 2, MRP2(多药耐药蛋白 2,多药抵抗蛋白 2)
MR pulmonary perfusion, MRPP(磁共振肺灌注)
magnetic resonance renoglam, MRR(磁共振肾图)
magnetic resonance spectroscopy, MRS(磁共振波谱)
maximal relative signal increase, MRSI(最大相对信号增加率)
MR severity index, MRSI(MR 严重指数)
mean residence time, MRT(平均滞留时间)
MR Venography, MRV(MR 静脉成像法)
magnetic resonance virtual cholangioscopy, MRVC(MR 胆系仿真内镜)
MR water imaging(磁共振水成像)
metabolic syndrome, MS(代谢综合征)
maximal slope, MS(最大的倾斜度)
musclespecifieactibody, MSA(特异性肌源性抗体)
maximum short axis diameter, MSAD(短轴最大径)
MSC(间叶干细胞)
multiple-slice spiral CT, MSCT(多层螺旋 CT)
multislice spiral CT cholangiography-multiplanar reconstructtion, MSCTC-MPR(MSCT 胆系多平面重建成像技术)
multislice spiral computed tomography enterography, MSCTE(多层螺旋 CT 小肠造影)
multi-slice CT enterography, MSCTE(MSCT 小肠造影)
muli-slice row CT portography, MSCTP(MSCT 门静脉成像)
maple syrup urine disease, MSUD(枫糖尿病)
MT(磁化传递), magnetization transfer imaging, MTI(磁化传递成像), MTR(磁化传递率)
MTBE(甲基叔丁醚)
4,5-simethylthiazaoly, MTT)(四甲基偶氮唑盐
malignant triton tumor, MTT(恶性蝾螈瘤)
mean transit time, MTT, MTT=BV/BF(平均通过时间)
methotrexate, MTX(甲胺喋呤)
mucinous cystic tumor(黏液囊性瘤), 又称 cystadenoma(囊腺瘤)、cystadencarcinoma(囊腺癌)、macrocystic adenoma(巨囊腺瘤)
MUC-1(黏糖蛋白 -1)
mucobilia(黏胆症)
multiacinar regenerative nodule(多小叶性再生性结节)
multiple transverse folds(多发胃窦横纹)
mutlislice cone-beam tomography, MUSCOT(多层面锥形线束体层摄影)

mean velocity, MV(平均流速)

microvessel count, MVC(微血管数)

microvascular density, microvessel density, MVD(微血管密度)

micro-vascular decompression, MVD(神经微血管减压术)

myocardial velocity gradient, MVG(心肌运动速度阶差)

mesenteric venous thrombosis, MVT(肠系膜上静脉血栓形成)

myelolipomas(髓质脂肪瘤)

myoglobin(肌红蛋白)

N

N-acetylaspartate, NAA(N-乙酰天门冬氨酸,氮-乙酰天门冬氨酸)

normal-appearing brain tissue, NABT(看似正常脑组织),实际上通过进一步检查却发现与真正的正常脑组织有很多差异,说明可能是早期病理改变的表现

neoadjuvant chemotherapy, NACT(新辅助化疗方法)

nicotinamide adenine dinucleoride dhosphate, NADPH(烔酰胺腺嘌呤二核苷磷酸)

nonalcohoLic fatty liver, NAFL(单纯性脂肪肝), nonalcoholic fatty liver disease, NAFLD(非酒精性脂肪性肝病,非酒精性脂肪肝)

normal appearing gray matter, NAGM(正常表现灰质,表现正常脑灰质)

NAFLD activity score, NAS(非酒精性脂肪性肝病活动度积分)

non-alcoholic steatohepatitis, NASH(非酒精性脂肪性肝炎,脂肪性肝炎)

Navigator(导航者), navigation(导航技术), navigator(模拟导航技术)

normal-appearing white matter, NAWM(看似正常白质,正常表现白质,表现正常脑白质),实际上通过进一步检查,却发现与真正的正常白质有很多差异,说明可能是早期病理改变的表现

nonbronchial systemic arteries, NBSA(非支气管性体动脉)

National Comprehensive Cancer Network, NCCN(美国国立综合癌症网络,美国国家综合癌症网)

necrotic cystic degeneration, NCD(坏死液化囊性变)

the National Council on Radiation Protection and Measurements, NCRP(国际辐射保护与测量委员会)

N-CTC(阴性法CT胆管造影), P-CTC(阳性法CT胆管造影)

negative CT cholangiopancreatography, N-CTCP(阴性法CT胆胰管成像)

neuroendocrine carcinoma, NEC(神经内分泌癌), mixed adenoendocrine carcinoma, MANEC(混合性腺神经内分泌癌)

neuroendocrine neoplasm, NEN(神经内分泌肿瘤),包括类癌; low grade, G1(低度恶性); intermediate grade, G2(神经内分泌肿瘤,中度恶性); neuroendocrine carcinoma, small or large cell carcinoma, high grade, G3(小细胞或大细胞神经内分泌癌,高度恶性)

neuroendocrine tumor, NET(神经内分泌肿瘤,神经内分泌瘤)

neuroendocrine tumors of the pancreas, NETP(胰腺神经内分泌肿瘤)

pancreatic neuroendocrine tumor, PNET(胰腺神经内分泌肿瘤)

neuroendocrine neoplasms of pancreas, pNENs(胰腺神经内分泌肿瘤)

neurendocrine tumorlets(神经内分泌性微小瘤)或 tumorlets of carcinoid(类癌型微小瘤)或肺微小瘤

neurofibromatosis(神经纤维瘤病)

neurolipoidosis(神经类脂质病)

number of excitation, NEX(激励次数)

nonalcoholic hepatic steatosis(非酒精性肝脂肪变性)

non-functioning neuroendocyine tumors of the pancreas, NFNTP(无功能性胰腺神经内分泌肿瘤), non-functioning pancreatic endocrine tumors, NF-PETs(非功能性胰内分泌肿瘤)

NAFLD fibrosis score, NFS(非酒精性脂肪性肝病纤维化积分)

nodular goiters, NG(结节性甲状腺肿)

neutrophil gelatinase-associated lipocalin, NGAL(中性粒细胞明胶酶相关脂质运载蛋白)

neonate hepatitis, NH(新生儿肝炎)

normalized iodine concentration, NIC(标准化碘浓度)

neonatal intrahepatic cholestasis caused by citrin Deficiency，NICCD(Citrin 缺陷导致的婴儿肝内胆汁淤积症)

NIEC(the new italian endoscopic club)

National Instituition of Health，NIH 美国国家健康学会,美国卫生部,美国国立卫生研究院()

NIM(肠神经分布异常)

NNPCs(无功能性胰岛细胞癌)

nodular type(结节型)，massive type(巨块型)，diffuse type(弥漫型)，trabecular type(梁状型)，pseudoglandular type(假腺管型)，compact type(实体型),scirrhous type(纤维硬化型)

nodule-in-nodule(结节中结节)

non-ossifying fibroma,NOF(非骨化性纤维瘤)

nonalcoholic hepatic steatosis(非酒精性肝脂肪变性)

non-slice selective GRE(非层面选择梯度回波序列采集)

nosocomial,SBP(院内感染自发性细菌性腹膜炎)

nontumorous perfusion defect，NPD(非肿瘤性灌注缺损,又称为假阳性病变)

necrosis of peripancreatic tissue，NPT(胰周组织坏死)，hemorrhage of peripancreatic tissue，HPT(胰周组织出血)

negative predictive value,NPV(阴性预测值)

NPV(可切除肿瘤的预测值)，PPV(不可切除肿瘤的预测值)

neonatal respiratory distress syndrome，NRDS(新生儿特发性呼吸窘迫综合征),又称 hyaline membrane disease,HMD(肺透明膜病)

diffuse nodular hyperplasia without fibrous septa(无纤维间隔的弥漫性结节增生),又名 nodular regenerative hyperplasia，NRH(结节性再生性增生或肝弥漫性纤维再生结节),也称为 noncirrhotic regenerative nodules，NRN(不伴有肝硬化的大再生结节或巨再生结节)

Nodular regenerative hyperplasia，NRH(肝脏再生结节性增生,结节性再生性增生,再生性结节增生,纤维再生结节,肝腺瘤病,肝脏非硬化性结节,腺瘤样增生)

neurofilaments,NS(神经丝)

nonsteroidal anti-inflammatory drugs，NSAIDs(非甾体类消炎药物)

non-small cell lung cancer,NSCLC(非小细胞肺癌)

neuron-specific enolase,NSE(神经特异性烯醇化酶,神经元烯醇化酶,免疫组织化学检查内容之一)

nonspecific interstitial pneumonia,NSIP(非特异性间质性肺炎)

NTBI(非转铁蛋白结合铁)

Na/taurocholate cotransporting polypeptide，NTCP(钠-牛胆酸盐协同转运多肽)

nontuberculous mycobacteria，NTM(非结核分枝杆菌)

nuclear crowding(核簇集)

nutritional ischemia(营养性缺血)

O

organic anion transporter，OATP(OATP8)，organic anionic transporting polypeptides,OATP(有机阴离子转运系统,有机阴离子转运多肽),organic anion transporting polypeptide 1B3，

OATP1B3(有机阴离子载体多肽 1B3),转运多肽中的 OATP 8,也称为 OATP1B1/3)

obstructtive jaundice(梗阻性黄疸)

osteocalcin，OC(骨钙素),也称 bone gamma- carboxyglutamic- acid-containing proteins，BGP(骨 g-羧谷氨酸包含蛋白)

oral cholecystography,OC，OCG(口服胆囊造影)

obeticholic acid,OCA(6-乙基鹅去氧胆酸)

occlusive colorectal carcinoma，OCC(闭塞性结肠直肠癌,阻塞性结肠癌)

osteochondritis disease,OCD(剥脱性骨软骨炎)

oriental cholangiohepatitis，OCH(东方人胆管性肝炎)

oral contrast-enhanced helical CT cholangiography，OCHCTC(口服对比剂螺旋 CT 胆管造影)

octreotide(奥曲肽)

obstructed defecation syndrome，ODS(出口梗阻型便秘)

obstructive jaundice,OJ(梗阻性黄疸)

oligovascularity(嗜血管性肿瘤)

orthotopic liver transplantation,OLT(原位肝移植)

osteochondral lesions of the talus，OLT(距骨骨软骨损伤)

outer medullary blood flow,OMBF(肾外髓血流量)，inner medullary blood flow,IMBF(内髓血流量)

osteonectin,ON(骨连接蛋白)

outlet obstruction constipation, OOC（出口梗阻型便秘）
osteopontin,OPN（骨桥蛋白）
Organ Procurement and Transplantation Network, OPTN（器官获取和移植网络）
osteoporosis,OP（骨质疏松）
opposed-phase,OP（反相位,反相）
osteoprotegerin, OPG（护骨素）, receptor activator of nuclear factor kB, RANK（NK-kB受体活化因子）, receptor activator of nuclear factor kB ligand, RANKL（NK-kB受体活化因子配体）
RANKL/OPG（NK-kB受体活化因子配体/护骨素系统）
RANKL/OPG（核因子κB受体活化因子配体和骨保护素系统）
ovarian dermoid（卵巢皮样囊肿）
ovarian-type stroma,OS（卵巢样间质）
obstructive sleep apnea hypopnea syndrome, OSAHS（阻塞性睡眠呼吸暂停低通气综合征）
obstructive sleep apnea syndrome, OSAS（阻塞性睡眠呼吸暂停综合征）
hereditary hemorrhagic telangiectasia, HHT（遗传性出血性毛细血管扩张症）,
又名 osler-weber-rendu disease（Osler-Rendu-Weber综合征）
osteopenia（骨量减少）
out-of-phase（异相位）
overlapping reconstruction（重叠重建技术）
overtreatment（过度治疗）

P

"4P"医疗,即 prediction（预测）、personalization（个性化）、prevention（预防）和 participation（参与）医疗
"5 P"征：pain（疼痛）、paresthesia（感觉异常）、paralysis（麻痹）、pulselessness（无脉）和 pallor（苍白）
pancreatic cancer,PAC（胰腺癌）
pancreatic acinar cell carcinoma, PACC（胰腺腺泡细胞癌）
PACE(prospective acquisition and correction 技术）
picture archiving and communication system, PACS（图像存储与通讯系统,图像存储与传输系统）
Pancreatic arthritis syndrome（胰性关节炎综合征）
periampullary diverticula, PAD（十二指肠乳头旁憩室）
pulmonary artery hypertension,PAH（肺动脉高压）
plasminogen activator inhibitor-1, PAI-1（纤溶酶原激活剂抑制剂）
pancreatic fat deposition（胰腺脂肪沉积）
PAN（结节性多动脉炎）
pANCA（抗中性粒细胞抗体）
pancreatic intraepithelial neoplasia, PanIN（胰腺上皮内瘤变）
papillary cystic-tumor of pancreas（胰腺乳头状囊实性肿瘤,又称实性乳头状瘤、乳头状囊性瘤、实性假乳头状上皮瘤）
paracolonic streakiness（结肠旁条纹征）
paragangliomas[副神经节瘤(嗜铬细胞瘤)]
parallel factor（并行采集因子）, parallel imaging-DWI（平行采集序列）
parasiticblood supply（寄生性供血）
perianeurysmal retroperitoneal fibrosis, PARF（动脉瘤周围腹膜后纤维化）
pyrrolozidine alkaloids,PAs（吡咯里西啶类生物碱）
PAS（过碘酸-雪夫反应）
pulmonary artertial systolic pressure,PASP（肺动脉收缩压）
Pulmonary acceleration time, PAT（三尖瓣返流至返流血流速度达峰值时间）
patchy（补丁）,patchy mosaic（片状镶嵌）
penetrating aortic ulcers,PAU（穿透性主动脉溃疡）
penetrating atherosclerotic ulcer,PAU（穿透性粥样硬化性溃疡）
Prussian blue,PB（普鲁士兰）
portal biliopathy, PB（门静脉性胆病,门静脉性胆系病）
perineal body,PB（会阴中心腱）
primary biliary cirrhosis, PBC（原发性胆汁性肝硬化）
PBC（原发性胆汁性胆管炎）
polybutylcyanoacrylate, PBCA（聚氰基丙烯酸正丁酯）
PBD（经皮肝穿胆管引流）
pulmonary blood flow,PBF（肺血流量）
portal blood inflow,PBF（门脉血流量）

pancreaticobiliary maljunction, PBM(胆胰管合流异常,胰胆管合流异常)

peripheral blood monocyte, PBMC(外周血单个核细胞)

peribronchiolar metaplasia-interstitial lung disease, PBMILD(细支气管周围化生性间质性肺疾病)

phosphate buffered saline, PBS(磷酸盐缓冲液)

mulmonary cryptococcosis,PC(肺隐球菌病)

PC(磷酸胆碱)

phase contrast, PC(相位对比,相位对比法), PC MRA(相位对比 MRA)

pure cystic,PC(纯囊性),cystic-solid,CS(囊实性), cystic subtype, Cs(囊性亚型), cystic subtype of metastases(转移的囊性亚型)

type- Ⅲ -procollagen, PC Ⅲ (Ⅲ型前胶原), type- Ⅳ -collagen,C Ⅳ(Ⅳ型胶原)

primary clear cell carcinoma of the liver, PCCCL(原发性透明细胞型肝癌)

pCEA(多克隆性癌胚抗原)

peak contrast enhancement ratio, pCER(最大对比强化率)

pubococcygeal line, PCL(耻尾线,耻骨联合下缘到最后一个尾骨关节的连线)

phase-contrast magnetic resonance imaging, PC-MR (相位对比法磁共振成像), real time interactive duplex PC-MR(实时交互式相位对比法磁共振成像法)

cystic pancreatic neoplasm,PCN(胰腺囊性肿瘤)

proliferating cell nuclear antigen, PCNA(增殖细胞核抗原)

Pneumocystis carinii pneumonia,PCP(卡氏肺囊虫肺炎,卡氏肺孢子虫肺炎)

polymerase chain reaction, PCR(聚合酶链反应)

PCR-SSCP(聚合酶式反应 - 单链构象多态性)

phosphocreatine, Pcr(磷酸肌酸), inorganic phosphate, Pi(无机磷), phosphomonoester, PME(磷酸单酯),phosphodiester,PDE(磷酸双酯)

procalcitonin,PCT(降钙素原)

positive-contrast CT cholangiography, P-CTC(阳性法 CT 胆管造影)

Penicillium marneffei(马尔尼菲青霉菌)

primary colonic malignant lymphoma,PCML(原发性大肠淋巴瘤,结肠原发性淋巴瘤), PTCL(结肠外周 T 细胞淋巴瘤)

proliferating cell nuclear antigen, PCNA(增殖细胞核抗原)是 DNA 合成酶的辅助蛋白,亦称周期素, PCNA labeling index, PCNALI(增殖细胞核抗原标记指数)

percutaneous hepatography(经皮肝造影)

Pulsed Doppler, PD(脉冲多普勒,脉冲多普勒超声), power Doppler flow imaging, PDI(能量多普勒血流显像法)

portal ductopathy,PD(门静脉性胆系病)

perineum descending,PD(会阴下降)

pancreatico-duodenectomy,PD(胰十二指肠切除术)

pancreas divisum, PD(胰腺分裂), incomplete pancreas divisum,IPD(不全性胰分裂)

pancreatic ductal adenocarcinoma, PDA(胰腺导管腺癌)

PDGFRA(血小板源性生长因子受体)

pulmonary embolism, PE(肺栓塞), pulmonary embolism, PE(肺动脉栓塞),即 pulmonary thromboembolism,PTE(肺血栓栓塞症)

portal fraction,PE(门脉血流分数)

periportal sinusoidal dilatation and peliosis hepatis(门静脉周围窦性扩张和肝紫癜)

primary epiploic appendagitis, PEA(原发性肠脂垂炎), second epiploic appendagitis, SEA(继发性肠脂垂炎)

pearl necklace sign(珍珠项圈征)

perivascular epithelioid cell, PEC(血管周上皮样细胞), perivascular epithelioid cell(PEC,一类血管周围上皮样细胞瘤,共同表达黑色素细胞标志物, HMB-45)家族,统称为 perivascular epithelioid cell tumors,PEComas(血管周上皮样细胞肿瘤)

PEI(经皮酒精注射)

peliotic(紫癜型), peliosis hepatis(肝紫癜), peliosis-like lesion(紫癜样病变)

Penicillium marneffei(马尔尼菲青霉菌)

peribiliary plexus(胆管周围血管丛途径), peribiliary plexus routes(胆管周围血管丛途径)

perivascular lymphedema(血管周围淋巴水肿)

permeability imaging(通透性成像)

positron emission tomography, PET(正电子发射计算机体层成像)

pancreatic endocrine tumor, PET(胰腺内分泌肿瘤),

functioning PETs（功能性内分泌肿瘤）
Peutz-Jeshers 综合征（色素沉着息肉综合征）
proportion of fatty degenerative cells，PFDC（脂肪变性细胞所占百分比）
pelvic floor dysfunction disease，PFDD（盆底功能障碍性疾病）
pelvic floor spasm，PFS（盆底痉挛）
portal flow velocity，PFV（门静脉流速）
PGs（前列腺素），prostaglandin F_2，PGF_2（前列腺素 F_2）
prostacyclin，PGI（前列环素），prostacyclin，PGI_2（前列环素）
primary gastric lymphoma，PGL（原发性胃淋巴瘤），primary gastrointestinal lymphoma，PGIL（原发性胃肠道恶性淋巴瘤，原发性胃肠道淋巴瘤）
polypoid gallbladder lesions，PGL（胆囊息肉样病变）
P-gp（P 糖蛋白）
peliosis hepatis，PH（肝紫癜）
Pulmonary hypertension，PH（肺循环高压）
primary hepatic angiosarcoma，PHA（原发性肝血管肉瘤）
phakomatoses（斑痔性错构瘤病）
phased-array coils（相控阵线圈），phased-array coil（阵列线圈）
phase cancellation artifact（相位消除伪影）
phase cycling（相位循环）
pleomorphic hyanilizing angiectaic tumor of soft parts，PHAT（软组织多形性透明变性血管扩张性肿瘤）
pedunculated or exophytic hepatocellular carcinoma，P-HCC or E-HCC（外生型肝癌）
extrahepatic hepatocellular carcinoma，EHCC（外生型肝癌）
extrahepatic growing hepatocellular carcinoma，EG-HCC（外生型肝癌）
primary hepatocellular carcinoma，PHC（原发性肝细胞癌）
pheochromocytoma，PHEO（嗜铬细胞瘤）
portal hypertensive gastropathy，PHG（门静脉高压性胃病）
primary hepatic lymphoma，PHL（原发性肝脏淋巴瘤）
primary hepatic neuroendocrine carcinoma，PHNEC（原发性肝脏神经内分泌癌），primary hepatic neuroendocrine tumor，PHNET（原发性肝脏神经内分泌肿瘤）
phrygian cap deformity（自由帽畸形，僧帽畸形或变异）
phsiological overstreching（生理性过度拉长）
inorganic phosphate，Pi（无机磷酸），inorganic phosphate，Pi（无机磷酸盐）
proliferative index，PI（增殖指数）
pulsation index，PI（搏动指数），pulsatility index，PI（搏动指数），pulsatility index，PI（脉动系数）
post-paracentesis circulatory dysfunctiori，PICD（大量放腹水后循环障碍）
periductal infiltrating intrahepatic cholangiocarcinoma，PIICC（胆管周围浸润型肝内胆管癌）
primary intestinal lymphangiectasia，PIL（原发性小肠淋巴管扩张症），secondary intestinal lymphangiectasia，SIL（继发性小肠淋巴管扩张症）
P-IPMN（胰腺导管内乳头状黏液性肿瘤）
pitch 值（螺距）
pyruvate kinase de-ficiency，PKD（丙酮酸激酶缺乏）
pulmonary lymphangiomyomatosis，PLAM（肺淋巴管肌瘤病）
PLB（经皮肝组织活检）
primary carcinoma of liver，PLC（原发性肝癌）
polycystic liver disease（PLD）[多囊性（成人型）肝脏疾病]
plexiform fibrohistiocytic tumor（丛状纤维组织细胞瘤）
polypoid lesions of the gallbladder，PLG（胆囊息肉样病变，又称胆囊隆起样病变）
peritumoral lymphatic vessel density，PLVD（癌周淋巴管密度）
pseudo-membranous colitis，PMC（假膜性结肠炎，伪膜性结肠炎）
pancreatic microcystic adenoma，PMCA（胰腺微囊腺瘤）
peritoneal mucinous carcinomatosis，PMCA（恶性腹膜黏液腺瘤病）
pancreatic mucinous cystic borderline cystadenoma，PMCB（胰交界性黏液性囊腺瘤）
pancreatic mucinous cystic neoplasm，PMCN（胰腺黏液性囊腺肿瘤），包括 pancreatic mucinous cystic

cystadenoma，PMCA（黏液性囊腺瘤）、pancreatic mucinous cystic cystadenocacinoma，PMCC（黏液性囊腺癌）和介于二者间的 pancreatic mucinous cystic borderline cystadenoma，PMCB（交界性黏液性囊腺瘤）

polymorph nuclear，PMN（中性粒细胞）

pseudomyxoma peritonei，PMP（腹膜假性黏液瘤）

pancreatic necrosis，PN（胰腺坏死）

pancreatic neuroendocrine neoplasms，PNEN（胰腺神经内分泌肿瘤）

peripheral neurocetodermal tumor，PNET（外周神经外胚层瘤）

primitive neuroectodermal tumors，PNET（原始神经外胚层瘤），peripheral primitive neuroectodermal tumors，pPNETs（外周性原始神经外胚层瘤），peripheral primitive neuroectodermal tumors，pPNET（外周原始神经外胚叶肿瘤）

paroxysmal nocturnal hemoglobinuria，PNH（阵发性夜间血红蛋白尿）

pulmonary nodule of mass，PNM（肺结节或肿块）

Podoplanin（肾小球足突细胞膜蛋白）

polarization transfer（极化传递）

pelvic organ prolapse，POP（盆腔器官脱垂）

portal cavernoma（肝门海绵状血管瘤）

portal fraction（门脉分数）

portosystemic encephalopathy（门体循环性脑病）

posterior hepatic notch sign（肝脏右后缘切迹征）

postnecrotic necrosis（坏死后的坏死）

pancreatic phlegmon，PP（胰腺蜂窝组织炎）

pancreatic pseudocyst，PP（胰腺假性囊肿）

PPD（结核菌素纯蛋白衍化物试验）

PPD（乳头区憩室）

primary pulmonary Hodgkin disease，PPHD（原发性肺何杰金病）

portopulmonary hypertension，PPHTN（门脉性肺动脉高压）

portal perfusion index，PPI，portal venous perfusion index，PPI（门静脉灌注指数）

ppm（parts per miilion），ppm 表示 10^{-6}

peripheral primitive neuro-ectodermal tumor，pPNET（外周原始神经外胚层肿瘤，外周原始神经外胚叶肿瘤，外周神经上皮瘤）

primary pulmonary Non-Hodgkin lymphoma，PPNHL（原发性肺非何杰金淋巴瘤）

positive predictive value，PPV（阳性预测值）

progesterone receptor，PR（孕激素受体）

point resolved spectroscopy，PRESS（点分辨技术，点解析波谱），point resolved selective spectroscopy，PRESS（点分辨波谱，点分辨选择波谱，单体素点分辨波谱）

percutaneous radiofrequency ablation，PRFA（经皮射频消融术）

puborectalis rectocele muscle hypertrophy，PRMH（耻骨直肠肌肥厚）

primary heptatic angiosarcoma（肝脏原发性血管肉瘤）

procollagen type Ⅲ peptide，P Ⅲ P（血清前胶原肽）

periodically rotated overlapping parallel lines with enhanced reconstruction，PROPELLER（螺旋桨扫描技术）

periodically rotated overlapping parallel lines enhanced reconstruction，PROPELLER（周期性旋转重叠平行线采集和增强后重建技术）

principle of selectiwe excitation technique，ProSET（频率选择激励技术）

protein plug（蛋白栓）

prototypic automated polyp detector software（自动息肉检出软件）

puborectalis syndrome，PRS（盆底失弛缓征，又称耻骨直肠肌综合征），spastic pelvic floor syndrome，SPFS（盆底痉挛综合征）

permeability of capillary vessel surface，PS；permeability surface area product，PS；permeability surface，PS（表面通透性，渗透表面积乘积，又称为毛细血管表面通透性）

prostate-specific antigen，PSA（前列腺特异抗原），prostate specific antigen，PSA（前列腺特异抗原），PSA（前列腺血清特异性抗原）

pseudoaneurysm，PsAn（假性动脉瘤）

primary sclerosing cholangitis，PSC（原发性硬化性胆管炎）

primary squamous cell carcinoma of liver，PSCCL（肝脏原发性鳞状细胞癌）

pancreatic size index，PSI（胰腺大小指数）

PSPDA（胰十二指肠上后动脉），ASPDA（胰十二指肠上前动脉），GDA（胃十二指肠动脉），AIPDA

（胰十二指肠下前动脉），PIPDA（胰十二指肠下后动脉）

pancreatogenic segmental portal hypertension，PSPH（胰源性区域性门静脉高压症）

primary sjgren's syndrome，PSS（原发性干燥综合征）

pancreatic secretory trypsin inhibito，PSTI（胰蛋白酶抑制剂）

prothrombin time，PT（凝血酶原时间），prothrombin activity，PTA（凝血酶原活动度）

pancreatic tuberculoses，PT（胰腺结核）

percutaneous transhepatic cholangiography，PTC（X线经皮穿肝胆系造影，经皮肝穿刺胆系造影，经皮肝穿胆管造影）

percutaneous transluminal coronary angioplasty，PTCA（经皮经腔冠状动脉血管成形术）

percutaneous transhepatic cholangiographic drainage，PTCD（经皮肝穿胆系引流术，经皮肝穿胆管引流），PTCD或PTBD（经皮穿肝内胆管减压术，或经皮穿肝内胆管引流术）

peripheral T-cell lymphomas，PTCLs（外周T细胞淋巴瘤）

PTCS（经皮经肝脏胆管镜检查）

Posttransplant Lymphoproliferative Disorder，PTLD（实性器官移植后淋巴增殖性疾病）

percutaneous needle biopsy，PTNB（经皮针吸活检）

percutaneous transhepatic portal catheterization，PTPC（经皮经肝门静脉置管分段取血测定胰岛素）

PTPC（经皮穿刺门静脉采血）

PTRA（经皮肾动脉成形）

portal vein aneurysm，PVA（门静脉瘤）；portal venous blood flow，PVBF（门静脉血流）；CT angiography of portal vein，PVCTA（门静脉CT血管成像）；portal vein perfusion，PVP（门静脉灌注量），PVP = BF × (1-HAF)；portal venous perfusion index，PPI（门静脉灌注指数）；portal vein thrombosis，PVT（门静脉系统血栓，门静脉血栓形成）；mean portal vein velocity，PVVmean（门静脉平均血流速度）；portal vein stenosis，PVS（门静脉狭窄）；portopulmonary hypertension，PPHTN（门脉性肺动脉高压）

p53-up-regulated modulator of apoptosis，PUMA（p53正向细胞凋亡调控因子）

peak velocity，PV（峰值流速）

portal venous blood flow，PVBF（门静脉血流）

peripancreatic vascular invasion，PVI（胰周血管侵犯）

perivascular lucencies，PVLs（血管周围低密度影）

portal venous perfusion，PVP（门静脉灌注量）；PVP = BF × (1-HAF)

PVR（肺循环血管阻力）；PVR=(mPAP-PCWP)/CO（mPAP:肺动脉平均压；PCWP:肺毛细血管楔压；CO:心输出量）

perspective volume rending，PVR（容积再现）

portal vein stenosis，PVS（门静脉狭窄）

perfusion weighted imaging，PWI（灌注加权成像）

PWSEA（瘤周楔形强化区）

peripheral zone，PZ（外周带）

Q

quantitative computed tomography，QCT（定量CT），peripheral QCT，pQCT（周围骨定量CT），volumetric QCT，vQCT（容积定量CT）

QHA（肝动脉血流量）

quantitative-magnetization transfer imaging，qMTI（定量磁化传递成像）

QPv（门静脉血流量）

quantitative ultrasound，QUS（定量超声）

quantization（量化）

quantum mottle（量子斑点）

R

routine angiography，RA（肝总动脉常规造影）

Relative Anisotropy，RA（相对各向异性，相对各向异性值）

renin angiotensin aldosterone system，RAAS（肾素-血管紧张素-醛固酮系统）

relative apparent diffusion coefficient，rADC（相对表观扩散系数）

Ranson 分数，急性胰腺炎分级时用

rapid acquired of relaxation enhancement，RARE（半傅里叶快速采集弛豫增强序列，快速采集弛豫增强序列），hybrid RARE（合成的RARE）

Rokitansky-Aschoff sinuses，RAS（罗-阿窦）

Rathke cleft cysts（Rathke囊肿，拉克囊肿）

Ray sum（透明重建，表面透明法，透明法）

^{82}Rb(Rubidium-82)-PET

renal blood flow,RBF(肾血流量)

respiratory bronchiolitis interstitial lung disease, RB-ILD(呼吸性细支气管炎性间质性肺疾病)

rectocele,RC(直肠前膨出,直肠前突)

repeatable coefficient,RC(可重复性系数)

rotate clip,RC(转动剪辑)

RCA(右冠状动脉)

rCBF(相对脑血流速度)

relative cerebral blood volume, rCBV(相对脑血容量)

RCD(残留胆囊管)

right colic vein, RCV(右结肠静脉), right superior colic vein, RSCV(右结肠上静脉), superior right colic vein, SRCV(上右结肠静脉), middle colic vein,MCV(中结肠静脉)

relative enhancement,RE(相对强化程度)

response evaluation criteria in solid tumors, RECIST(实体瘤的疗效评价标准)

region growing image segmentation process(区域增长图像分段处理功能)

reticuloendothelial system,RES(网状内皮系统)

retention(对比剂留存)

reticulated mosaic pattern(网状镶嵌征)

retraction of the liver capsule(肝包膜回缩)

radiofrequency,RF(射频脉冲)

rheumatoid factor,RF(类风湿因子)

restriction fragment length polymorphism, RFLP(限制性片段长度多态性分析)

Arg-Gly-Asp,RGD(精氨酸 - 甘氨酸 - 天门冬氨酸)

right gastro-epiploic vein,RGEV(胃网膜右静脉)

RF(类风湿因子)

RFI(肾血流指数,RFI= 肾血流量 / 肾体积)

rhabdoid tumour(横纹肌样瘤)

regional hepatic blood flow, rHBF(局部肝组织血流量)

regional hepatic blood volume, rHBV(局部肝血容量,局部肝组织血容量)

recurrent HCC,RHCC(复发性肝癌)

right hepatic vein, RHV(肝右静脉), left hepatic vein,LHV(肝左静脉),middle hepatic vein,MHV(肝中静脉), inferior right hepatic vein, IRHV(右后下肝静脉)

resistive index, RI(阻力指数), resistance index, RI(阻力指数),resistance index,RI(阻力系数)

RIs[肾脏(多点的)阻力指数]

radioimmunoassay,RIA(放射免疫法)

radiology information system,RIS(放射科信息系统,放射信息系统)

RITA(射频热消融)

replaced left hepatic artery, rLHA(替代肝左动脉), replaced right hepatic artery, rRHA(替代肝右动脉)

root mean square, RMS(均方根值), root-mean-square variation(变异均方根)

relative mean transit time, rMTT(相对平均通过时间)

regenerative nodule, RN[再生性病变(结节),再生结节], regenerative hepatic nodules(退行性肝结节), cirrhosis regeneration nodules, RN, regenerating nodules in cirrhosis(肝硬化再生结节), mono-acinar RN(单腺泡再生结节), multiacinar RN(多腺泡再生结节), macroregenerative nodule, MRN(巨再生结节,大再生结节), multiacinar regenerative nodule(多小叶性再生性结节),LRN(低度再生结节), regenerative nodules in Budd-Chiari syndrome(and other vascular disorders)[布 - 加综合征中再生结节(和其他血管性疾病中的再生结节)]

reactive nodular fibrous pseudotumor, RNFP(反应性结节性纤维性假瘤)

renal oncocytoma,RO(肾嗜酸细胞腺瘤)

receiver operating characteristic curve, ROC(受试者操作特性解析,受试者操作特性曲线,受试者工作特性曲线)

region of interest ,ROI(兴趣区), regions of interest, ROIs(感兴趣区)

ratio of main pulmonary artery to aortic diameter, rPA(主肺动脉与升主动脉横径比值)

relative pulmonary blood flow,rPBF(相对肺血流量)

recurrent pyognic cholangitis, RPC(复发性化脓性胆管炎),或 oriental cholangiohepatitis, OCH(东方人胆管性肝炎)

retroperitoneal fibrosis, RPF(腹膜后纤维化, Ormond's 病)

regional portal hypertension, RPH(区域性门脉高

压症）

red point lesions，RPL（黏膜表面细小红点灶）或 scarlatina rash（猩红热样疹）

RR（相对危险度）

relative speed，RS（相对感度）

Ray sam（透明法重建技术），ray sum，RS（透明技术）

right superior colic vein，RSCV（右结肠上静脉，结肠右上静脉）

relative signal intensity，RSI（相对信号强度）

Radiological Society of North America，RSNA（北美放射学会）

road map mode（路标方式），road map test，RST（道路地图检测）

relative tissue blood flow，rTBF（相对组织血流量）

relative tissue blood volume，rTBV（相对组织血容量）

RTP（放射治疗计划）

reversal transcription-polymerase chain reaction，RT PCR（逆转录聚合酶链反应）

rise value，RV（增幅）

RVSP（右室收缩压），RVSP=SBP·[1-（RC/1.03）]（SBP 代表系统收缩压，RC 表示曲率即 CIVS/CFW，其中 CIVS 表示室间隔曲度，CFW 代表左室游离室壁曲度）

S

sensitivity，S（感光度，敏感性，灵敏度），sensitivity，SEN（敏感性）

S100-protein，S100-P（S-100 蛋白）

serum-ascites albumin gradient，SAAG（血清 - 腹水白蛋白梯度）

sampling（抽样）；sample volume（取样容积）

sclerosing angiomatoid nodular transformation，SANT（硬化性血管瘤样结节性转化，脾脏硬化性血管瘤样结节性转化）

Sappey 上静脉位于镰状韧带上部，接受来自胸内和膈下血管的供血；Sappey 下静脉位于镰状韧带下部，接受腹部和脐旁静脉的供血

specific absorption rate，SAR（特异吸收率）

sarcoidosis（心脏结节病）

Sarcoidosis（类肉瘤病）

sarcomatoid hepatocellular carcinoma；Sarcomatoid HCC（肉瘤样肝细胞癌）

severe acute respiratory syndrome，SARS（严重急性呼吸综合征）

sleep apnea syndrome，SAS（睡眠呼吸暂停综合征）

subcutaneous abdominal adipose tissue，SAT（皮下脂肪）

saturation（饱和），saturation artifact（饱和性伪影）

Shwachman-Bodian-Diamond syndrome，SBDS（Shwachman-Bodian-Diamond 综合征）

barium small-bowel follow through，SBFT（X 线小肠钡餐造影，口服钡剂小肠造影）

spontaneous bacterial peritonitis，SBP（自发性细菌性腹膜炎）

small bowel volvulus，SBV（小肠扭转）

sarcomatoid carcinoma，SC（肉瘤样癌）

SC（硬化性胆管炎）

shift clip，SC（移动剪辑）

small cell carcinoma，SCC（小细胞癌），small cell/oat cell carcinoma（小细胞 / 燕麦细胞癌）

sclerosing cholangitis with autoimmune pancreatitis，SC- AIP（自身免疫性胰腺炎相关硬化性胆管炎）

schistosomiasis（血吸虫病），schistosoma（血吸虫也称裂体吸虫），S.japonicum（日本血吸虫），S. mansoni（曼氏血吸虫），S.haematobium（埃及血吸虫）

small cell 1ung cancer，SCLC（肺小细胞癌）

serous cystic neoplasm，SCN；serous cystadenoma，SCN（浆液性囊腺瘤）

solid-cystic papillary tumors of the pancreas，SCPTs（胰腺囊实性乳头状瘤）

serum creatinine，SCr（血肌酐）

spiral CT angiography，SCTA（螺旋 CT 血管成像）

spiral CT during arterial portography，SCTAP（螺旋 CT 动脉门脉造影）

spiral CT colonography，SCTC（螺旋 CT 结肠成像技术）

SD（信号衰减）

sodium dodecyl sulfate polyacrylamide gel electrophoresis，SDS-PAGE（十二烷基硫酸钠—聚丙烯酰胺凝胶电泳）

secretin-stimulated diffusion-weighted magnetic resonance imaging（胰泌素刺激的 MR 扩散加权成像）

spin echo，SE（自旋回波）
soluble egg antigen，SEA（可溶性卵抗原）
spin-echo plannar imaging，SE-EPI（自旋回波 - 回波平面成像）
sensitivity encoding，SENSE（敏感性编码，敏感（度）编码，敏感梯度编码）
sclerosing encapsulating peritonitis，SEP（硬化包裹性腹膜炎）
serum hyaluronic acid，HA [血清透明质酸（肝纤维化的一种标志物）]
serum ferritin，SF（血清铁蛋白）
screen-film mammography，SFM（乳腺屏片系统）
solitary fibrous tumor，SFT（孤立性纤维瘤）
sarcomatoid hepatocellular carcinoma，SHC（肝肉瘤样癌）
sclerhous hepatocellular carclnoma，SHCC；Sclerosing HCC（硬化型肝癌）
small hepatocellular carclnoma，SHCC（小肝癌），small hepatocellular carcinoma，sHCC（小肝细胞癌）
subclinical hepatic encephalopathy，SHE（亚临床期肝性脑病）
shear elasticity（剪切弹性模量），shear viscosity（剪切黏性）
sclerosing hemangioma of lung，SHL（肺硬化性血管瘤）
sinus histocytosis with massive lymphadenopathy，SHML（窦组织细胞增生症伴巨大淋巴结病），又称 Rosai-Dorfman 病
small hepatic metastatic tumor，SHMT（小的肝内转移瘤）
siderotic regenerative nodule（铁沉着再生结节）
shouldered margins（垫肩征）
signal intensity，SI（信号强度），signal intensity-time curve，SI-T 曲线（信号强度 - 时间曲线）
splenic index，SI（脾的大小指数，脾长径乘以脾厚度）计算出的 SPI（脾门指数，脾指数除以门静脉平均血流速度）
small intrahepatic mass-forming cholangiocarcmoma，SIMCC（肿块型肝内小胆管细胞癌）
similar Hexheimer reaction（类赫反应），与驱梅治疗时 Hexheimer reaction（赫克斯海默反应）相似，也称作 paradoxical reaction，PR（矛盾反应）
sinusoidal growth pattern（窦性生长），replacing growth pattern（置换性生长），pseudocapsular growth pattern（假包膜性生长方式）
Sip（正相位信号强度），Sop（反相位信号强度）
siphoning effect（虹吸效应）
singnal intensity ratio，SIR（信号强度比）
systemic inflammatory response syndrome，SIRS（全身炎症反应综合征）
SLA/LP（抗可溶性肝抗原抗体 / 抗肝胰抗体）
systemic lupus erythematosus，SLE（系统性红斑狼疮）
slice thickness artifacts（薄片厚度伪影）
slope method（斜率法）
snakeskin-like pattem，SLP（类似蛇皮样）或 mosaic-like pattern，MLP（马赛克样改变）
sludge（胆泥），sludge ball（胆泥球）
superior mesenteric artery，SMA（肠系膜上动脉）
smooth muscle actin（平滑肌肌动蛋白）
anti-smooth muscle antibody，SMA（平滑肌源性抗体，抗平滑肌抗体）
superior mesenteric artery compressing syndrome，SMACS（肠系膜上动脉综合征）
styrene- maleic acid neocarzinostatin（抗肿瘤药物 SMANCS）
smart heart（冬眠心肌）
Smart Prep（智能扫描技术）
simultaneous acquisition of spatinal barmonics，SMASH（空间谐波同步采集）
structure model index，SMI（结构模型指数）
Slab MIP，SMIP（薄层最大密度投影）
secretin-enhanced magnetic resonance cholangiopancreatography，s-MRCP（激发促胰液素分泌 MRCP，胰泌素磁共振胆胰管成像，激发促胰液素分泌 MRCP，胰泌素刺激后 MRCP，促胰液分泌物质（如胰泌素）刺激下的动态 MRCP）
sliding multislice MRI，SMS MRI（动床多层 MRI）
submucosal vein，SMV（食管深层固有静脉，位于黏膜下层，又称黏膜下静脉）
superior mesenteric venous thrombosis，SMVT（肠系膜上静脉血栓形成）
siderotic nodule，SN（铁沉积结节）
sinus node artery，SNA（窦房结动脉）
solitary necrotic nodule，SNN（孤立坏死结节，孤立

性坏死结节）

single nucleotide polymorphisms，SNP（单核苷酸多态性）

signal noise ratio，SNR（信噪比）

SNS（交感神经系统）

Society of Abdominal Radiology（美国腹部放射学会）

serous oligocystic adenoma，SOA（寡囊型浆液性囊腺瘤），也称巨囊性浆液性囊腺瘤，或 serous macrocystic adenoma（大囊性浆液性囊腺瘤）

sphincter of Oddi dysfunction，SOD（胆胰管下端括约肌功能障碍，Oddi 括约肌功能障碍）

solid papillary epithelial neoplasm（实性乳头状上皮性肿瘤），又称 solid pseudopapillary tumor（实性假乳头状瘤）、papillary cystic tumor（乳头状囊性瘤）

Somatostain（生长抑素），somatostatinoma（生长激素释放抑制激素瘤）

secondary osteonecrosis of the knee，SON（膝关节继发性骨坏死）

spontaneous osteonecrosis of the knee，SONK（膝关节自发性骨坏死），又命名为膝关节 idiopathic osteonecrosis（特发性骨坏死），或 primary osteonecrosis（原发性骨坏死）

speed of sound，SOS（超声声速）

solitary plasmacytoma，SP（孤立性浆细胞瘤），solitary plasmacytoma of bone，SPB（孤立性骨浆细胞瘤）

single photon absorptiometry，SPA（单光子骨矿分析仪）

sampling perfection with application optimized contrasts using different flip angle evolutions，

SPACE（可变反转角优化对比成像序列，三维质子加权快速自旋回波序列）

Spectrally selective Attenuated Inversion Recovery，SPAIR（脂肪抑制序列），Philips 公司的（Spectral Inversion Recovery，SPIR）序列，GE Healthcare 的 SPECIAL（SPECtral Inversion At Lipids）序列，spectral saturation inverision recovery，SPIR（频谱饱和反转恢复法脂肪抑制术）

spectral attenuated inversion recovery，SPAIR（频率选择反转脉冲）

small peripheral cholangiocarcinoma，sPCCC（周围型小胆管细胞癌）

single photon emission computed tomography，SPECT（单光子发射计算机断层成像）（简称 ECT）

spastic puborectal muscle，SPFS（耻骨直肠肌肉痉挛），spastic pelvic floor syndrome，SPFS（盆底痉挛综合征）

spoiled gradient-recalled imaging，SPGR（扰相梯度回波成像，扰相梯度回波），T_1WI 序列

SPI（脾门指数，为脾指数除以门静脉平均血流速度）

superparamagnetic iron oxide particles，SPIO（超顺磁性氧化铁微粒，超顺磁性氧化铁颗粒，超顺磁性氧化铁纳米颗粒，超顺磁性氧化铁）

spoiled gradient echo（毁损梯度回波，扰相梯度回波）

splenocele（脾疝）

splenopneumopexy（脾肺固定术）

split-echo acquisition of FSE signals，SPLICE（分裂回波快速自旋回波采集技术）

solitary pulmonary nudole，SPN（孤立性肺结节），SPN-to-aorta ratio（SPN 与主动脉增强峰值比）

spoke wheel（轮辐征）

solid pseudopapillary tumor，SPPT（实性假乳头状瘤）

subperitoneal space，SpS（腹膜下间隙）

solid-pseudopapillary tumors of pancreas，SPTP（胰腺实性假乳头状瘤），或称 solid pseudo-

papillary neoplasm，SPN（胰腺实性假乳头状肿瘤），solid pseudo-papillary carcinoma，SPC（实性假乳头状癌），solid pseudopapillary tumors，SPT（实性假乳头状瘤）

superconducting quantum interference device，SQUID（超导量子干涉仪）

somatostatin receptor scintigraphy，SRS（生长抑素受体闪烁成像），somatostatin，SS（生长抑素），somatostatin analogues，SSA（生长抑素类似物），SSTR（生长抑素受体）

synovial sarcoma，SS（滑膜肉瘤）

steepest slop，SS（最大斜率）

single slice spiral CT，SSCT；single-slice CT，SSCT（单层螺旋 CT）

shaded surface display，SSD（遮蔽表面显示，表面遮蔽显示法，表面遮盖法）

single-shot echo-planar DWI, SS-EPI-DWI（单次激发平面回波磁共振扩散加权成像）

steady state free precession sequence, SSFP（稳定自由进动成像序列）

SSh-FSE（单次激发快速 SE）

single-shot fast spin echo, SSFSE（单次激发快速自旋回波，屏气单次激发快速自旋回波，单次发射快速自旋回波，单次激发快速自旋回波序列），SSFSE-MRCP（单次激发厚层投射磁共振胆胰管成像）

slice sensitivity profile, SSP（螺旋层面灵敏度），slice selection（选层），slice thickness（层厚）

single shot rapid acquisition relaxation enhancement（半傅里叶 SS-RARE）

single-shot turbo spin echo, SSTSE（单次激发厚层快速自旋回波）

spasmodic torticollis, ST（痉挛性斜颈）

slab thickness, ST（投影块厚度），thin-slab（薄块），thick-slab（厚块）

steal phenomenon（盗血现象）

stimulated-echo acquisition mode, STEAM（激励回波采集方法，激励回波采集序列，激发回波序列，激励回波脉冲序列）

steatotic（脂肪变型）

stedy-state methods（梯度回波稳态法）

Short T_1 inversion recovery, STIR（短 T_1 反转恢复）

short time inversion recovery, STIR（短时反转恢复）

short inversion time inversion recovery, STIR（短反转时间反转恢复技术）

stool labeling（标记粪便）

storage disease（贮积病）

straight border sign（平直边缘征）

straining-levator reflex（排便肛提肌反射，排粪肛提肌反射）

stress fracture（应力性骨折），俗称 march fracture（行军骨折），亦称 fatigue fracture（疲劳骨折）

soluble tumor necrosis factor receptor, sTNFR（可溶性肿瘤坏死因子受体）

stress urinary incontinence, SUI（压力性尿失禁）

stump appendicitis（残端阑尾炎）

subvesical ducts（囊下胆管）

sump effect（血池效应）

superparamagnetic agents（超顺磁性）

surface rendering（遮蔽表面显示，又称为表面再现）

susceptometer（超导磁强计）

standardized uptake volume, SUV（标准摄取值，标准化摄取值）；SUVratio（标准摄取率）

super vena cava syndrome, SVCS（上腔静脉阻塞综合征，上腔静脉综合征）

surface/volume ratio, SVR（面积 / 体积的比），surface/mass ratio, SMR（面积 / 质量的比）

susceptibility weighted MR imaging, SWI（磁敏感成像技术）

single energy x-ray absorptiometry, SXA（单能 X 线吸收测量仪）

Syn（乳头间瘤细胞突触素，突触素，免疫组织化学检查内容之一）

T

Tesla, T（特斯拉）

T_1-map（T_1 值图）

T_2 shine-through; T_2 shine-through effect（T_2 穿透效应）

time attenuation curve, TAC（时间 - 密度曲线）

transcatheter arterial chemoembolization, TACE（经导管动脉化疗栓塞，介入性动脉栓塞治疗，复合性栓塞治疗，经肝动脉栓塞化疗，经导管动脉栓塞治疗），或 Transcatheter Hepatic Artery Chemoembolization, TACE（经导管肝动脉化疗栓塞治疗），Lp（碘化油），Lp-TACE（含药碘油栓塞）

transarterial embolization, TAE（经导管动脉栓塞术，经动脉栓塞）；TAI（动脉内灌注）

Tagging-MRI（MRI 标记技术）

Takayasu's 动脉炎（大动脉炎）

thrombosis angiitis obliterance, TAO（血栓闭塞性脉管炎，也称 Buerger 病）

transabdominal sonography, TAS; transabdominal US, TAUS（经腹部超声）

percentage of total body fat, TBF%（总体脂率，总体脂占体重的百分比）

total bilirubin, TBIL; total bilirubin, TBil（血清总胆红素，总胆红素），DBIL（直接胆红素），IBIL（间接胆红素）

tracheobronchomegaly, TBM（气管支气管巨大症，又称 Mounier-Kuhn 综合征）

transient bone marrow edema, TBME（一过性骨髓水

肿）

typical carcinoid，TC（典型类癌），atypical carcinoid，AC（非典型类癌）

total cholesterin，TC（总胆固醇）

TCC（胆囊穿刺胆管造影）

transcranial Doppler ultrasound，TCD（经颅多普勒超声）

^{99m}Tc-diethy iminodiacetic acid，^{99m}Tc-EHIDA（二乙基乙酰苯胺亚氨二醋酸），^{99m}Tc-IDAs（^{99m}Tc-亚氨二醋酸类），^{99m}Tc-iminodiacetic acid（^{99m}Tc-亚胺酮醋酸）

TCD（经颅多普勒超声）

transcription factor 1，TCF1（转录因子 1）

time-density curve，TDC（时间-密度曲线）

tissue doppler imaging，TDI（组织多普勒成像）

tumefactive demyelinating lesion，TDL（肿胀性脱髓鞘病变）

transient elastography，TE（超声瞬时弹性成像技术，瞬时弹性成像，超声弹性成像）

echo time or last echo time，TE 或 TE last（回波时间）

transesophageal echocardiography，TEE（经食管超声心动图）

temporary window（时间窗或范围）

temporal parenchymal enhancement（一过性肝实质强化）

triangular fibrocartilage complex，TFCC（三角纤维软骨复合体）

transferrin，Tf（转铁蛋白），transferrin receptor，TfR（转铁蛋白受体）

thin film transistor，TFT（薄膜晶体管）

triglyceride，TG（甘油三酯），triglyceride，TG（血脂）

transforming growth factor，TGF（转化生长因子）

transforming growth factor-a，TGF-a（胃黏膜转化生长因子）

transforming growth factor beta，TGF b（转化生长因子 b）

tGLVP（特利加压素，三甘氨酸-赖氨酸-加压素）

transient hepatic attenuation difference，THAD[一过性肝实质强化差异，一过性肝密度差异，一过性强化差异，一过性（短暂性）肝密度差异，一过性肝脏密度（衰减）差异，一过性衰减差]

transient hepatic echogenicity difference，THED（一过性回波差异）

third inflow（第三血供）

transient hepatic intensity difference，THID（一过性肝脏信号强度差异）

transient hepatic perfusion disorders，THPD（肝实质一过性灌注异常，肝脏一过性灌注异常）

transient hepatic parenchymal enhancement，THPE（一过性肝实质强化，一过性（暂时性）肝实质强化）

tissue harmonic imaging，THI（组织谐波显像）

THK_{max}（最大厚度）

transient hepatic parenchymal enhancement，THPE（一过性肝实质强化）

Three-point Dixon（3 点自旋回波法）

three-segment sign（三节征）

threshold value（有效阈值）

T_1 high resolution isotropic volume excitation，THRIVE（T_1 高分辨力各向同性容积激发）

inversion time，TI；time of inversion，TI（反转时间）

Transient Ischemic Attacks，TIA（一过性脑缺血，短暂性脑缺血发作）

time signal –intensity curve，TIC（时间-信号强度曲线，时间-信号曲线）

time-to-inflow deceleration，TID（达到最大信号强度的时间）

total imaging matrix，TIM（全身成像矩阵技术）

tissue inhibitor of metalloproteinase，TIMP（金属蛋白酶组织抑制因子）

trans jugular intrahepatic porto-systemic shunt，TIPSS 或 TIPS（经颈静脉肝内门-体分流术，经颈静脉门-腔静脉分流，或经颈静脉门-体静脉分流）

T/L（肿瘤与肝信号强度比值）

total liver perfusion，TLP（全肝总灌注量，肝总灌注量），TLP=HAP+PVP

toll-like receptor4，TLR4（Toll 样受体 4）

thalassanemia，TM（地中海贫血）

total mesorectal excision，TME（全直肠系膜切除术）

triple negative breast cancer，TNBC（三阴性乳腺癌）

tumor necrosis factor，TNF（肿瘤坏死因子）

transient osteoporosis，TO（一过性骨质疏松）

time of flight，TOF（时间飞跃法）

TORSOPA（体部相控阵列线圈）

time resolved echoshared angiographic techniqueMRA，TREAT MRA（时间分辨回波分享 MRA virtual non-enhanced, VNE(虚拟平扫), true non-enhanced, TNE(真实平扫)

veno-occlusive disease, VOD(静脉 - 阻塞性疾病,肝静脉 - 阻塞性疾病,肝静脉闭塞症)

volume of interest, VOI(兴趣容积,兴趣向量)

Type Ⅰ a glycogen storage disease(Ⅰ a 型糖原贮积病)或 Von Gierke 病

Von Meyenburg 综合征(胆管性错构瘤,即胆管微小错构瘤)

vancomycin resistant enterococci, VRE(万古霉素耐药肠球菌)

VP(血管加压素)

vessel probe, VP(血管探针)

volumetric quantitative computed tomography, vQCT(容积定量 CT)

volume rendering, VR(容积再现,容积再现法,容积重建), volume ratio, VR(容积比率), Volume Ratio, VR(容积比), 1-VR(1- 容积比), 3DVR(三维容积重建), volume rendering technique, VRT(容积再现技术)

variance of residence time, VRT(驻留时间方差)

vascular-vaculor organelle, VVO(血管内皮细胞内囊泡)

varicella zoster virus, VZV(水痘带状疱疹病毒)

W

Waldeyer 韧带(直肠骶骨韧带), Waldeyer 筋膜(骶前筋膜)

wash-in rate(信号增高率)

water or fat subtraction techniques(水或脂肪减影技术)

water peak, 4.7ppm(水峰)

whole body diffusion weighted imaging, WB-DWI(MR 全身扩散加权成像)

WC(腰围)

Hepatolenticular degeneration, WD(肝豆状核变性); Wilson's disease(威尔逊病,肝豆状核变性)

Water diarrhea hypokalemia and achlorhydria syndrome(WDHA 综合征)

WECT(水灌肠 CT)

Wegener's granulomatosis, WG(韦格纳肉芽肿)

World Gastroenterology Organization, WGO(世界胃肠病学组织)

WGVC(Working Group on Virtual Colonoscopy)研究组

WHCC(分化良好的典型肝细胞肝癌)

Whipple 病(肠脂质营养不良,肠源性脂肪代谢障碍)

white in black(黑底白影)

World Health Organization, WHO(世界卫生组织)

waist to hip ratio, WHR(腰臀围比值)

wedged hepatic venous pressure, WHVP(肝静脉楔入压,肝静脉楔压)

wireless capsule endoscopy(胶囊内镜)

Wirsung 管(主胰管,腹胰管); common channel(共同管); Santorini 管(副胰管,背胰管)

window level, WL [窗位(窗水平)], window technology(窗口技术), window width, WW(窗宽)

white light bronchoscopy, WLB(普通纤维支气管镜)

walled-off necrosis, WON(胰腺包裹性坏死)

wraparound liver(包围肝)

Wiener spectrum, WS(威纳频谱)

wall-thickening type of gallbladder cancer, WTGC(厚壁型胆囊癌)

X

X-ray absorption(X 线吸收)

X-ray maximum linear dose(X 线最大的线性剂量)

X-ray spectrum(X 线谱), extensively drug-resistant, XDR(泛耐药)

xanthogranulomatous cholecystitis, XGC(黄色肉芽肿性胆囊炎)

X-ray defecography, XRD(X 线排粪造影)

Y

^{99}Y-minigastrin(小胃泌素)

Z

Zeeman effect(塞曼效应)

Gastrinomas(胃泌素瘤),也名 Zollinger-Ellison syndrome, ZES(卓 - 艾综合征)

ZOOM-EPI(区域放大倾斜多层 EPI)

常用文献类型及对应的标志代码: M(普通图书), C(会议录), G(汇编), N(报纸), J(期刊); 常用电子文献载体及对应的标志代码: CD(光盘), OL(联机网络)